THIRD EDITION

HEART FAILURE

A Companion to Braunwald's Heart Disease

Douglas L. Mann, MD

Lewin Chair and Professor of Medicine, Cell Biology, and Physiology
Chief, Cardiovascular Division
Washington University School of Medicine
Cardiologist-in-Chief
Barnes-Jewish Hospital
St. Louis, Missouri

G. Michael Felker, MD, MHS

Professor of Medicine
Chief, Heart Failure Section
Division of Cardiology
Duke University School of Medicine
Durham, North Carolina

ELSEVIER

ELSEVIER

1600 John F. Kennedy Blvd.
Ste 1800
Philadelphia, PA 19103-2899

HEART FAILURE: A COMPANION TO BRAUNWALD'S HEART DISEASE, THIRD EDITION ISBN: 978-1-4557-7237-7

Notices

Knowledge and best practice in this field are constantly changing. As new research and experience broaden our understanding, changes in research methods, professional practices, or medical treatment may become necessary.

Practitioners and researchers must always rely on their own experience and knowledge in evaluating and using any information, methods, compounds, or experiments described herein. In using such information or methods they should be mindful of their own safety and the safety of others, including parties for whom they have a professional responsibility.

With respect to any drug or pharmaceutical products identified, readers are advised to check the most current information provided (i) on procedures featured or (ii) by the manufacturer of each product to be administered, to verify the recommended dose or formula, the method and duration of administration, and contraindications. It is the responsibility of practitioners, relying on their own experience and knowledge of their patients, to make diagnoses, to determine dosages and the best treatment for each individual patient, and to take all appropriate safety precautions.

To the fullest extent of the law, neither the Publisher nor the authors, contributors, or editors assume any liability for any injury and/or damage to persons or property as a matter of products liability, negligence or otherwise, or from any use or operation of any methods, products, instructions, or ideas contained in the material herein.

Library of Congress Cataloging-in-Publication Data

Heart failure (Mann)
Heart failure : a companion to Braunwald's heart disease / [edited by] Douglas L. Mann, G. Michael Felker.—Third edition.
p. ; cm.
Complemented by: Braunwald's heart disease / edited by Douglas L. Mann, Douglas P. Zipes, Peter Libby, Robert O. Bonow, Eugene Braunwald. 10th edition. [2015].
Includes bibliographical references and index.
ISBN 978-1-4557-7237-7 (hardcover : alk. paper)
I. Mann, Douglas L., editor. II. Felker, G. Michael, editor. III. Braunwald's heart disease. 10th ed. Complemented by (expression): IV. Title.
[DNLM: 1. Heart Failure. WG 370]
RC681
616.1′2—dc23

2014039592

Executive Content Strategist: Dolores Meloni
Senior Content Development Specialist: Anne Snyder
Publishing Services Manager: Catherine Jackson
Project Manager: Rhoda Bontrager
Design Direction: XiaoPei Chen

Printed in China

Last digit is the print number: 9 8 7 6 5 4 3 2 1

To

Laura, Erica, Jonathan, and Stephanie
Claire, William, and Caroline

Contributors

Kariann Abbate, MD
Postdoctoral Clinical Fellow
Columbia University Medical Center
New York, New York
Disease Management in Heart Failure

Luigi Adamo, MD, PhD
Division of Cardiology
Department of Medicine
Washington University School of Medicine
St. Louis, Missouri
Alterations in Ventricular Structure: Role of Left Ventricular Remodeling and Reverse Remodeling in Heart Failure

Larry A. Allen, MD, MHS
Assistant Professor of Medicine
Division of Cardiology
University of Colorado School of Medicine
Aurora, Colorado
Decision Making and Palliative Care in Advanced Heart Failure

Efstathia Andrikopoulou, MD
Department of Internal Medicine
Thomas Jefferson University Hospital
Philadelphia, Pennsylvania
Disease Management in Heart Failure

Piero Anversa, MD
Professor of Anesthesia and Professor of Medicine
Departments of Anesthesia and Medicine
Division of Cardiovascular Medicine
Brigham and Women's Hospital
Harvard Medical School
Boston, Massachusetts
Cellular Basis for Myocardial Regeneration and Repair

Pavan Atluri, MD
Assistant Professor of Surgery
Division of Cardiovascular Surgery
Department of Surgery
University of Pennsylvania School of Medicine
Philadelphia, Pennsylvania
Cardiac Transplantation

Kenneth M. Baker, MD, FAHA, FIACS
Professor and Vice Chair, Department of Medicine
Director, Division of Molecular Cardiology
Director, Cardiovascular Research Institute
Mayborn Chair in Cardiovascular Research
Texas A&M Health Science Center
College of Medicine
Baylor Scott & White Health
Temple, Texas
Molecular Signaling Mechanisms of the Renin-Angiotensin System in Heart Failure

George L. Bakris, MD
Professor of Medicine
Director, ASH Comprehensive Hypertension Center
The University of Chicago Medicine
Chicago, Illinois
Alterations in Kidney Function Associated with Heart Failure

Sukhdeep S. Basra, MD, MPH
Section of Cardiology
Baylor College of Medicine
Houston, Texas
Treatment of Heart Failure with Preserved Ejection Fraction

Robert O. Bonow, MD, MS
Max and Lilly Goldberg Distinguished Professor of Cardiology
Vice Chairman, Department of Medicine
Director, Center for Cardiac Innovation
Northwestern University Feinberg School of Medicine
Chicago, Illinois
Heart Failure as a Consequence of Ischemic Heart Disease

Biykem Bozkurt, MD, PhD
The Mary and Gordon Cain Chair
W.A. "Tex" and Deborah Moncrief, Jr., Chair
Professor of Medicine
Medicine Chief and Cardiology Chief, DeBakey Veterans Affairs Medical Center
Director, Winters Center for Heart Failure Research
Associate Director, Cardiovascular Research Institute
Baylor College of Medicine
Houston, Texas
Heart Failure as a Consequence of Dilated Cardiomyopathy

Michael R. Bristow, MD, PhD
Professor of Medicine
Division of Cardiology
University of Colorado Health Sciences Center
Aurora, Colorado
Adrenergic Receptor Signaling in Heart Failure

Angela L. Brown, MD
Associate Professor of Medicine
Department of Medicine
Division of Cardiology
Washington University School of Medicine
St. Louis, Missouri
Management of Heart Failure in Special Populations: Older Patients, Women, and Racial/Ethnic Minority Groups

Javed Butler, MD, MPH
Professor of Medicine
Chief of Cardiology
Co-Director, Heart and Vascular Center
Stony Brook University
Stony Brook, New York
Epidemiology of Heart Failure

Blase A. Carabello, MD
Professor and Chair, Department of Cardiology
Medical Director of the Heart Valve Center
Mount Sinai Beth Israel Hospital
New York City, New York
Heart Failure as a Consequence of Valvular Heart Disease

Jay N. Cohn, MD
Professor of Medicine
Rasmussen Center for Cardiovascular Disease Prevention
Cardiovascular Division
University of Minnesota Medical School
Minneapolis, Minnesota
Disease Prevention in Heart Failure

Wilson S. Colucci, MD
Professor of Medicine and Physiology
Boston University School of Medicine
Chief, Section of Cardiovascular Medicine
Boston Medical Center
Boston, Massachusetts
Oxidative Stress in Heart Failure

Anita Deswal, MD, MPH
Professor of Medicine
Section of Cardiology
Michael E. DeBakey Veterans Affairs Medical Center
Winters Center for Heart Failure Research
Baylor College of Medicine
Houston, Texas
Treatment of Heart Failure with Preserved Ejection Fraction

Adam D. DeVore, MD
Division of Cardiology
Duke University School of Medicine
Duke Clinical Research Institute
Durham, North Carolina
Quality and Outcomes in Heart Failure

John P. DiMarco, MD, PhD
Professor of Medicine
Department of Medicine
Division of Cardiac Electrophysiology
University of Virginia
Charlottesville, Virginia
Management of Arrhythmias and Device Therapy in Heart Failure

Abhinav Diwan, MD
Assistant Professor of Internal Medicine
Center for Cardiovascular Research
Cardiovascular Division
Department of Medicine
Washington University School of Medicine and John Cochran Veterans Affairs Medical Center
St. Louis, Missouri
Molecular Basis for Heart Failure

Shannon M. Dunlay, MD, MS
Assistant Professor of Medicine
Cardiovascular Diseases and Health Care Policy and Research
Mayo Clinic
Rochester, Minnesota
Pulmonary Hypertension

Gregory A. Ewald, MD
Associate Professor of Medicine
Medical Director, Cardiac Transplant and Mechanical Circulatory Support Program
Washington University
St. Louis, Missouri
Circulatory Assist Devices in Heart Failure

Justin A. Ezekowitz, MBBCh, MSc
Associate Professor of Medicine
Division of Cardiology
University of Alberta
Director, Heart Function Clinic
Mazankowski Alberta Heart Institute
Edmonton, Alberta, Canada
Management of Comorbidities in Heart Failure

James C. Fang, MD
Professor of Medicine
Chief, Division of Cardiovascular Medicine
University of Utah Health Sciences Center
Salt Lake City, Utah
Hemodynamics in Heart Failure

G. Michael Felker, MD, MHS
Professor of Medicine
Chief, Heart Failure Section
Division of Cardiology
Duke University School of Medicine
Durham, North Carolina
Contemporary Medical Therapy for Heart Failure Patients with Reduced Ejection Fraction

Victor A. Ferrari, MD
Professor of Medicine and Radiology
Director, Cardiovascular Magnetic Resonance
Penn Cardiovascular Institute
Interim Director, Echocardiography Laboratory
Division of Cardiovascular Medicine
Perelman School of Medicine
University of Pennsylvania Medical Center
Philadelphia, Pennsylvania
Cardiac Imaging in Heart Failure

James D. Flaherty, MD, MS
Associate Professor of Medicine
Division of Cardiology
Northwestern University Feinberg School of Medicine
Chicago, Illinois
Heart Failure as a Consequence of Ischemic Heart Disease

John S. Floras, MD, DPhil, FRCPC, FACC, FAHA, FESC
Canada Research Chair in Integrative Cardiovascular Biology
Director, Research, University Health Network and Mount Sinai Hospital Division of Cardiology
Professor, Faculty of Medicine, University of Toronto
Toronto, Ontario, Canada
Alterations in the Sympathetic and Parasympathetic Nervous Systems in Heart Failure

Viorel G. Florea, MD, PhD, DSc
Associate Professor of Medicine
University of Minnesota Medical School
Minneapolis Veterans Affairs Health Care System
Minneapolis, Minnesota
Disease Prevention in Heart Failure

Thomas L. Force, MD
Professor of Medicine
Division of Cardiology
Vanderbilt University School of Medicine
Nashville, Tennessee
Molecular Basis for Heart Failure

Gary S. Francis, MD
Professor of Medicine
Cardiovascular Division
University of Minnesota
Minneapolis, Minnesota
Clinical Evaluation of Heart Failure

Hanna K. Gaggin, MD, MPH
Instructor in Medicine
Harvard Medical School
Cardiology Division
Department of Medicine
Massachusetts General Hospital
Boston, Massachusetts
The Use of Biomarkers in the Evaluation of Patients with Heart Failure

Vasiliki V. Georgiopoulou, MD
Assistant Professor of Medicine
Division of Cardiology
Emory University
Atlanta, Georgia
Epidemiology of Heart Failure

Mihai Gheorghiade, MD
Professor of Medicine and Surgery
Division of Cardiology
Northwestern University Feinberg School of Medicine
Chicago, Illinois
Heart Failure as a Consequence of Ischemic Heart Disease

Joshua M. Hare, MD
Louis Lemberg Professor of Medicine
Cardiovascular Division
Founding Director, Interdisciplinary Stem Cell Institute
Chief Science Officer
Leonard M. Miller School of Medicine
Miami, Florida
The Restrictive and Infiltrative Cardiomyopathies and Arrhythmogenic Right Ventricular Dysplasia/Cardiomyopathy

Adrian F. Hernandez, MD, MHS
Associate Professor of Medicine
Division of Cardiology
Duke University School of Medicine
Director, Outcomes Research
Duke Clinical Research Institute
Durham, North Carolina
Quality and Outcomes in Heart Failure

Joseph A. Hill, MD, PhD
Professor of Medicine and Molecular Biology
Chief of Cardiology
Departments of Internal Medicine (Cardiology) and Molecular Biology
University of Texas Southwestern Medical Center
Dallas, Texas
Molecular Basis for Heart Failure

Toru Hosoda, MD, PhD
Assistant Professor
Departments of Anesthesia and Medicine
Division of Cardiovascular Medicine
Brigham and Women's Hospital
Harvard Medical School
Boston, Massachusetts
Cellular Basis for Myocardial Regeneration and Repair

James L. Januzzi, Jr., MD
Hutter Family Professor of Medicine
Harvard Medical School
Roman W. DeSanctis Endowed Distinguished Clinical Scholar in Medicine
Cardiology Division
Department of Medicine
Massachusetts General Hospital
Boston, Massachusetts
The Use of Biomarkers in the Evaluation of Patients with Heart Failure

Mariell Jessup, MD
Professor of Medicine
Department of Medicine
Cardiovascular Division
University of Pennsylvania School of Medicine
Philadelphia, Pennsylvania
Cardiac Transplantation

Susan M. Joseph, MD
Assistant Professor of Medicine
Department of Medicine
Division of Cardiology
Washington University School of Medicine
St. Louis, Missouri
Management of Heart Failure in Special Populations: Older Patients, Women, and Racial/Ethnic Minority Groups

Daniel P. Judge, MD
Associate Professor of Medicine
Director, JHU Center for Inherited Heart Disease
Division of Cardiology
Section of Heart Failure/Cardiac Transplantation
Johns Hopkins University
Baltimore, Maryland
Heart Failure as a Consequence of Genetic Cardiomyopathy

Andreas P. Kalogeropoulos, MD, PhD, MPH
Assistant Professor of Medicine
Division of Cardiology
Emory University
Atlanta, Georgia
Epidemiology of Heart Failure

Garvan C. Kane, MD, PhD
Assistant Professor of Medicine
Division of Cardiovascular Diseases
Mayo Clinic
Rochester, Minnesota
Pulmonary Hypertension

David A. Kass, MD
Abraham and Virginia Weiss Professor of Cardiology
Professor of Medicine
Professor of Biomedical Engineering
The Johns Hopkins Medical Institutions
Baltimore, Maryland
Alterations in Ventricular Function in Systolic Heart Failure

Eric V. Krieger, MD
Adult Congenital Heart Service
University of Washington Medical Center and Seattle Children's Hospital
Department of Medicine
Division of Cardiology
University of Washington School of Medicine
Seattle, Washington
Heart Failure as a Consequence of Congenital Heart Disease

Rajesh Kumar, PhD
Associate Professor
Division of Molecular Cardiology
Department of Medicine
Texas A&M Health Science Center
College of Medicine
Baylor Scott & White Health
Central Texas Veterans Health Care System
Temple, Texas
Molecular Signaling Mechanisms of the Renin-Angiotensin System in Heart Failure

Daniel Lenihan, MD
Professor of Medicine
Division of Cardiovascular Medicine
Vanderbilt University
Nashville, Tennessee
Managing Heart Failure in Cancer Patients

Annarosa Leri, MD
Associate Professor of Anesthesia and Medicine
Departments of Anesthesia and Medicine
Division of Cardiovascular Medicine
Brigham and Women's Hospital
Harvard Medical School
Boston, Massachusetts
Cellular Basis for Myocardial Regeneration and Repair

Gregory Y. H. Lip, MD, FRCP, FACC, FESC
Professor of Cardiovascular Medicine
University of Birmingham Centre for Cardiovascular Sciences
City Hospital
Birmingham, United Kingdom
Alterations in the Peripheral Circulation in Heart Failure

W. Robb MacLellan, MD
Professor of Medicine
Head, Division of Cardiology
University of Washington
Seattle, Washington
Stem Cell–Based and Gene Therapies in Heart Failure

Douglas L. Mann, MD
Lewin Chair and Professor of Medicine, Cell Biology, and Physiology
Chief, Cardiovascular Division
Washington University School of Medicine
Cardiologist-in-Chief
Barnes-Jewish Hospital
St. Louis, Missouri
Role of Innate Immunity in Heart Failure
Alterations in Ventricular Structure: Role of Left Ventricular Remodeling and Reverse Remodeling in Heart Failure
Contemporary Medical Therapy for Heart Failure Patients with Reduced Ejection Fraction

Ali J. Marian, MD
Professor of Molecular Medicine (Genetics) and Internal Medicine (Cardiology)
Center for Cardiovascular Genetics
Institute of Molecular Medicine
University of Texas Health Sciences Center at Houston and Texas Heart Institute
Houston, Texas
Heart Failure as a Consequence of Hypertrophic Cardiomyopathy

Daniel D. Matlock, MD, MPH
Assistant Professor of Medicine
Department of General Internal Medicine
University of Colorado School of Medicine
Aurora, Colorado
Decision Making and Palliative Care in Advanced Heart Failure

Mathew S. Maurer, MD
Professor of Medicine
Department of Medicine
Division of Cardiology
Columbia University Medical Center
New York, New York
Management of Heart Failure in Special Populations: Older Patients, Women, and Racial/Ethnic Minority Groups

Dennis M. McNamara, MD, MS
Director, Center for Heart Failure Research
Professor of Medicine
University of Pittsburgh Medical Center
Pittsburgh, Pennsylvania
Heart Failure as a Consequence of Viral and Nonviral Myocarditis

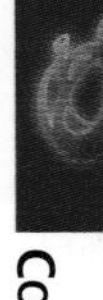

Robert J. Mentz, MD
Assistant Professor of Medicine
Division of Cardiology
Duke University School of Medicine
Durham, North Carolina
Contemporary Medical Therapy for Heart Failure Patients with Reduced Ejection Fraction

John Mignone, MD, PhD
Division of Cardiology
University of Washington
Seattle, Washington
Stem Cell–Based and Gene Therapies in Heart Failure

Carmelo A. Milano, MD
Professor of Surgery
Surgical Director, Cardiac Transplant and Mechanical Circulatory Support Program
Duke University
Durham, North Carolina
Circulatory Assist Devices in Heart Failure

Alan R. Morrison, MD, PhD
Section of Cardiovascular Medicine
Yale University School of Medicine
New Haven, Connecticut
Cardiac Imaging in Heart Failure

Wilfried Mullens, MD, PhD
Department of Cardiology
Ziekenhuis Oost–Limburg, Genk Belgium
Faculty of Medicine and Life Sciences
Hasselt University
Belgium
Surgical Treatment of Chronic Congestive Heart Failure

Adam Nabeebaccus, MRCP
King's College London British Heart Foundation Centre of Excellence
London, United Kingdom
Cellular Basis for Heart Failure

Jose Nativi Nicolau, MD
Assistant Professor of Medicine
Division of Cardiovascular Medicine
University of Utah Health Sciences Center
Salt Lake City, Utah
Hemodynamics in Heart Failure

Jing Pan, MD, PhD
Associate Professor
College of Medicine
Texas A&M Health Science Center
Temple, Texas
Molecular Signaling Mechanisms of the Renin-Angiotensin System in Heart Failure

Walter J. Paulus, MD, PhD
Cardiologist and Professor in Cardiovascular Physiology
Department of Physiology
Institute for Cardiovascular Research VU (ICaR-VU)
VU University Medical Center
Amsterdam, The Netherlands
Alterations in Ventricular Function: Diastolic Heart Failure

Linda R. Peterson, MD
Associate Professor, Medicine
Division of Cardiology
Washington University School of Medicine
St. Louis, Missouri
Alterations in Cardiac Metabolism

Tamar S. Polonsky, MD, MSCI
Assistant Professor of Medicine
The University of Chicago Medicine
Chicago, Illinois
Alterations in Kidney Function Associated with Heart Failure

J. David Port, PhD
Professor of Medicine and Pharmacology
Division of Cardiology
University of Colorado Health Sciences Center
Aurora, Colorado
Adrenergic Receptor Signaling in Heart Failure

Christopher P. Porterfield, MD, MPH
Department of Medicine
Division of Cardiac Electrophysiology
University of Virginia
Charlottesville, Virginia
Management of Arrhythmias and Device Therapy in Heart Failure

Florian Rader, MD, MSc
Staff Physician
Heart Institute
Hypertension Center of Excellence
Cedars-Sinai Medical Center
Assistant Professor of Medicine
David Geffen School of Medicine at UCLA
Los Angeles, California
Heart Failure as a Consequence of Hypertension

Margaret M. Redfield, MD
Professor of Medicine
Division of Cardiovascular Diseases
Mayo Clinic
Rochester, Minnesota
Pulmonary Hypertension

Michael W. Rich, MD
Professor of Medicine
Department of Medicine
Division of Cardiology
Washington University School of Medicine
St. Louis, Missouri
Management of Heart Failure in Special Populations: Older Patients, Women, and Racial/Ethnic Minority Groups

Joseph G. Rogers, MD
Professor of Medicine
Medical Director, Mechanical Circulatory Support Program
Duke University
Durham, North Carolina
Circulatory Assist Devices in Heart Failure

Marcello Rota, PhD
Assistant Professor
Departments of Anesthesia and Medicine
Division of Cardiovascular Medicine
Brigham and Women's Hospital
Harvard Medical School
Boston, Massachusetts
Cellular Basis for Myocardial Regeneration and Repair

John J. Ryan, MD
Assistant Professor of Medicine
Division of Cardiovascular Medicine
University of Utah Health Sciences Center
Salt Lake City, Utah
Hemodynamics in Heart Failure

Can Martin Sag, MD
King's College London British Heart Foundation Centre of Excellence
London, United Kingdom
Cellular Basis for Heart Failure

Douglas B. Sawyer, MD, PhD
Chief of Cardiac Services and Leader of Cardiovascular Service Line
Maine Medical Center
Portland, Maine
Oxidative Stress in Heart Failure
Managing Heart Failure in Cancer Patients

Joel Schilling, MD, PhD
Assistant Professor of Medicine, Pathology, and Immunology
Section of Advanced Heart Failure and Cardiac Transplantation
Division of Cardiology
Washington University School of Medicine
St. Louis, Missouri
Alterations in Cardiac Metabolism

P. Christian Schulze, MD, PhD
Associate Professor of Medicine
Department of Medicine
Division of Cardiology
Columbia University Medical Center
New York, New York
Alterations in Skeletal Muscle in Heart Failure

Ajay M. Shah, MD, FMedSci
BHF Chair of Cardiology
James Black Professor of Medicine
King's College Hospital
Director
King's College London British Heart Foundation Centre of Excellence
London, United Kingdom
Cellular Basis for Heart Failure

Eduard Shantsila, PhD
University of Birmingham Centre for Cardiovascular Sciences
City Hospital
Birmingham, United Kingdom
Alterations in the Peripheral Circulation in Heart Failure

Albert J. Sinusas, MD, PhD
Section of Cardiovascular Medicine
Yale University School of Medicine
New Haven, Connecticut
Cardiac Imaging in Heart Failure

Karen Sliwa, MD, PhD
Professor
Hatter Institute for Cardiovascular Research in Africa
Department of Medicine and IDM
University of Cape Town
Soweto Cardiovascular Research Unit
University of Witwatersrand
South Africa
Heart Failure in the Developing World

Francis G. Spinale, MD, PhD
Professor
Cardiovascular Translational Research Center
Departments of Surgery, Cell Biology, and Anatomy
University of South Carolina School of Medicine
WJB Dorn Veteran Affairs Medical Center
Columbia, South Carolina
Myocardial Basis for Heart Failure: Role of Cardiac Interstitium

Martin St. John Sutton, MBBS
John Bryfogle Professor of Medicine
Division of Cardiovascular Medicine
Perelman School of Medicine
University of Pennsylvania Medical Center
Philadelphia, Pennsylvania
Cardiac Imaging in Heart Failure

Randall C. Starling, MD, MPH
Professor of Medicine
Department of Cardiovascular Medicine
Section of Heart Failure and Cardiac Transplant Medicine
Cleveland Clinic—Kaufman Center for Heart Failure
Cleveland, Ohio
Surgical Treatment of Chronic Congestive Heart Failure

Lynne Warner Stevenson, MD
Professor of Medicine
Harvard Medical School
Director of Cardiomyopathy and Heart Failure
Heart and Vascular Institute
Brigham and Women's Hospital
Boston, Massachusetts
Management of Acute Decompensated Heart Failure

Simon Stewart, PhD, NFESC, FAHA, FCSANZ
NHMRC Principal Research Fellow
Director, NHMRC Centre of Research Excellence to Reduce Inequality in Heart Disease
Baker IDI Heart and Diabetes Institute
Melbourne, Victoria, Australia
Heart Failure in the Developing World

Carmen Sucharov, PhD
Assistant Professor of Medicine
Division of Cardiology
University of Colorado Health Sciences Center
Aurora, Colorado
Adrenergic Receptor Signaling in Heart Failure

Aaron L. Sverdlov, MBBS, PhD, FRACP
NHMRC CJ Martin Fellow
Section of Cardiovascular Medicine
Boston University School of Medicine
Boston, Massachusetts;
Department of Medicine
The Queen Elizabeth Hospital
University of Adelaide
Australia
Oxidative Stress in Heart Failure

Heinrich Taegtmeyer, MD
Professor of Medicine
Department of Internal Medicine
Division of Cardiology
The University of Texas–Houston Medical School
Houston, Texas
Alterations in Cardiac Metabolism

W. H. Wilson Tang, MD
Professor of Medicine
Department of Cardiovascular Medicine
Heart and Vascular Institute
Cleveland Clinic
Cleveland, Ohio
Clinical Evaluation of Heart Failure

Michael J. Toth, PhD
Associate Professor of Medicine
Departments of Medicine and Molecular Physiology and Biophysics
University of Vermont College of Medicine
Burlington, Vermont
Alterations in Skeletal Muscle in Heart Failure

Anne Marie Valente, MD
Boston Adult Congenital Heart Disease and Pulmonary Hypertension Program
Brigham & Women's Hospital, Boston Children's Hospital
Departments of Medicine and Pediatrics
Harvard Medical School
Boston, Massachusetts
Heart Failure as a Consequence of Congenital Heart Disease

Loek van Heerebeek, MD, PhD
Cardiologist
Department of Physiology
Institute for Cardiovascular Research VU (ICaR-VU)
VU University Medical Center
Amsterdam, The Netherlands
Alterations in Ventricular Function: Diastolic Heart Failure

Frederik H. Verbrugge, MD
Department of Cardiology
Ziekenhuis Oost–Limburg, Genk Belgium
Faculty of Medicine and Life Sciences
Hasselt University
Belgium
Surgical Treatment of Chronic Congestive Heart Failure

Ronald G. Victor, MD
Burns and Allen Chair in Cardiology Research
Director, Hypertension Center of Excellence
Associate Director, Cedars-Sinai Heart Institute
Professor of Medicine, David Geffen School of Medicine at UCLA
Los Angeles, California
Heart Failure as a Consequence of Hypertension

Ian Webb, MRCP, PhD
Consultant Cardiologist
King's College Hospital
King's College London British Heart Foundation Centre of Excellence
London, United Kingdom
Cellular Basis for Heart Failure

David Whellan, MD, MHS, FACC, FAHA
Professor of Medicine
Jefferson Medical College
Philadelphia, Pennsylvania
Disease Management in Heart Failure

Foreword

Heart failure presents a major global health challenge, affecting an estimated 38 million patients worldwide. Despite striking advances in the diagnosis and treatment of a variety of cardiovascular disorders during the past three decades, the prevalence of heart failure is increasing. Indeed, heart failure may be considered to be the price of successful management of congenital, valvular and coronary disease, hypertension, and arrhythmias. While both the morbidity and mortality in patients with these disorders have improved markedly, they often associate with myocardial damage, which, if prolonged, can commonly cause heart failure.

With the progressive aging of the population, the incidence and prevalence of this condition continue to rise. In high-income countries, heart failure is now the most common diagnosis in patients over the age of 65 admitted to hospitals. In medium- and low-income countries, the case fatality rates of heart failure are two to three times greater than in high-income countries. The costs of caring for these patients are immense, in large part because of their hospitalizations, which, paradoxically, increase as their lives are prolonged.

On a more positive note, there has been enormous progress in this field, with important new information obtained about the disordered pathobiology, diagnosis, and treatment of heart failure. Indeed, heart failure has now become a well-recognized subspecialty of cardiovascular medicine and surgery.

This third edition of *Heart Failure* is a magnificent text that covers every important aspect of the field. It represents the efforts of 100 authors, who are experienced and recognized experts. Douglas L. Mann, the founding editor, has been joined as co-editor of this edition by G. Michael Felker, who brings enormous clinical expertise, clinical investigative experience, and energy to this effort.

Heart Failure will be of enormous interest and value to clinicians, investigators, and trainees who are concerned with enriching their understanding of and caring for the ever growing number of patients with this condition. We are proud of this important companion to *Heart Disease: A Textbook of Cardiovascular Medicine.*

Eugene Braunwald

Douglas P. Zipes

Peter Libby

Robert O. Bonow

Preface

The editors are pleased to present the third edition of *Heart Failure: A Companion to Braunwald's Heart Disease* as the latest update of a unique learning platform that is intended to provide practitioners, nurses, physicians-in-training, and students at all levels with the critical tools they need to remain current with the rapidly changing scientific foundations and clinical advances in the field of heart failure. The print version of the third edition, which has been revised extensively, is complemented by a new online version that is updated frequently with the results of late-breaking clinical trials, reviews of important new research publications, and updates on clinical practice authored by leaders in the field. These online supplements are selected and edited superbly by Dr. Eugene Braunwald.

As with the first and second editions, the goal in organizing this textbook was to summarize the current understanding of the field of heart failure in a comprehensive bench-to-bedside textbook. The third edition is not merely an update of prior editions of the Heart Failure Companion, it is an attempt to envision what a "modern" textbook on heart failure should provide, recognizing that many readers of this book may pursue board certification in heart failure. The extensive revisions for the third edition would not have been possible without the addition of Dr. G. Michael Felker as a co-editor. His expertise in biomarkers, clinical trials, and advanced heart failure, combined with his consummate editorial skills, has strengthened the content and quality of the entire book enormously. The overarching vision for the third edition was to develop a leaner, more readable, textbook that also provided expanded coverage of those areas of clinical heart failure that have evolved as distinct clinical niches. Twenty-seven of the 47 chapters in this edition are new, including 4 chapters covering topics that were not addressed in prior editions. We have added 67 new authors, who are highly accomplished and recognized in their respective disciplines. All chapters carried over from the second edition have been thoroughly updated and extensively revised. Finally, beginning with the third edition, we have included updated summaries of practice guidelines for acute heart failure, heart failure with reduced ejection fraction, heart failure with preserved ejection fraction, and the use of cardiac devices.

A detailed rendering of all of the changes in the new edition is not feasible within the confines of this preface. However, the editors would like to highlight several of the exciting changes in the third edition, beginning with Section II on mechanisms of disease progression in heart failure, which contains entirely new chapters on mechanisms of diastolic heart failure, left ventricular remodeling, alterations in the peripheral circulation, and alterations in renal function and skeletal muscle function. Section III on the etiological basis for heart failure features entirely new chapters on the epidemiology of heart failure, the genetics of heart failure, heart failure in developing countries, as well as heart failure as a consequence of viral heart disease and congenital heart disease. There is also a new chapter on restrictive cardiomyopathy that was not present in the second edition. The section on the clinical assessment of heart failure (Section IV) has been strengthened with new chapters on cardiac imaging and the use of biomarkers, and the addition of a chapter on the hemodynamic assessment of heart failure that was not covered in the second edition. Section V on the treatment of heart failure has been revised extensively. Twelve of the 16 chapters in this section are new, including chapters on pulmonary hypertension and co-morbidities that were not present in the second edition. As noted above, we have also included summaries of the latest practice guidelines in heart failure in Section V.

The extent to which the third edition of *Heart Failure: A Companion to Braunwald's Heart Disease* proves useful to those who seek to broaden their knowledge base in an effort to improve clinical outcomes for patients with heart failure reflects the expertise and scholarship of the many talented and dedicated individuals who contributed to the preparation of this edition. It has been a great pleasure to work with them, and it has been our great fortune to learn from them throughout this process. In closing, the editors recognize that a single text cannot adequately cover every aspect of a subject as dynamic or as expansive as heart failure. Accordingly, we apologize in advance for any omissions and shortcomings in the third edition.

Douglas L. Mann, MD

G. Michael Felker, MD, MHS

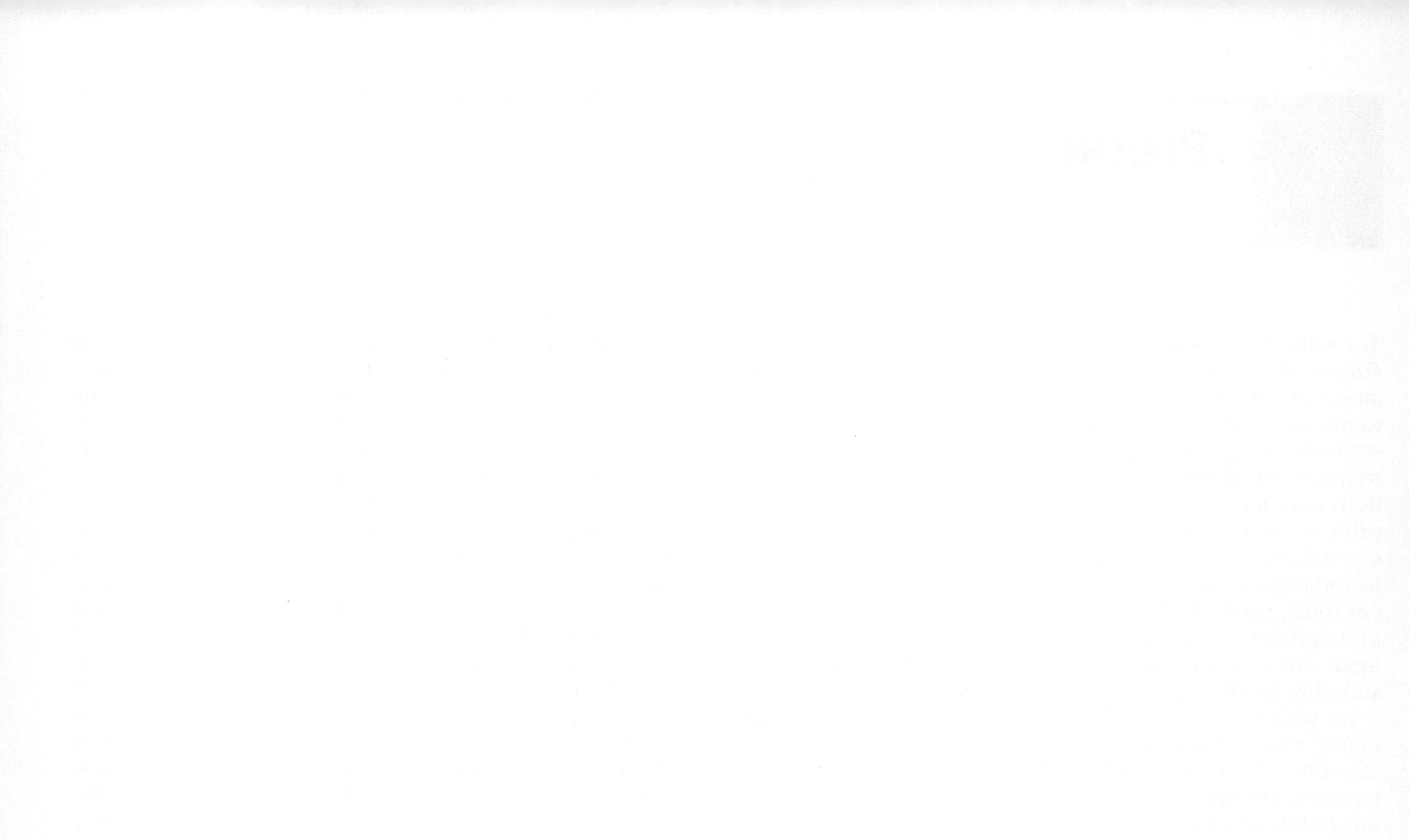

Acknowledgments

No textbook of the size and complexity of *Heart Failure: A Companion to Braunwald's Heart Disease* can come about without support from a great many individuals. We would like to begin, first and foremost, by thanking Dr. Eugene Braunwald for providing us with the inspiration, as well as the opportunity, to edit the third edition of the Heart Failure Companion. We would also like to extend our thanks to Drs. Bonow, Libby, and Zipes, whose continued guidance is sincerely appreciated. The editors would be entirely remiss if they did not acknowledge the unswerving support of Elsevier, who approved of the concept of publishing a comprehensive heart failure textbook in 2001 and who has continued to provide the requisite support to allow the editors to refine the original vision with each subsequent edition of the Heart Failure Companion. We would like to formally acknowledge and thank the following members of the Elsevier staff without whom the third edition would not have happened: Dolores Meloni, Executive Content Strategist, for always believing in and championing the Heart Failure Companion; Anne Snyder, Senior Content Development Specialist, for quietly holding everything (mainly the editors) together and keeping everything on time; and Rhoda Bontrager, Project Manager, whose attention to detail on the copyediting was remarkable. Dr. Mann would also like to thank his administrative assistant, the indefatigable Ms. Mary Wingate, for making all aspects of his professional life possible.

Contents

Look for these other titles in the Braunwald's Heart Disease Family

Douglas L. Mann, Douglas P. Zipes, Peter Libby, and Robert O. Bonow
Braunwald's Heart Disease: A Textbook of Cardiovascular Medicine

Braunwald's Heart Disease Companions

Pierre Théroux
Acute Coronary Syndromes

Deepak L. Bhatt
Cardiovascular Intervention

Elliott M. Antman and Marc S. Sabatine
Cardiovascular Therapeutics

Ziad F. Issa, John M. Miller, and Douglas P. Zipes
Clinical Arrhythmology and Electrophysiology

Christie M. Ballantyne
Clinical Lipidology

Darren K. McGuire and Nikolaus Marx
Diabetes in Cardiovascular Disease

Henry R. Black and William J. Elliott
Hypertension

Robert L. Kormos and Leslie W. Miller
Mechanical Circulatory Support

Roger S. Blumenthal, JoAnne M. Foody, and Nathan D. Wong
Preventive Cardiology

Catherine M. Otto and Robert O. Bonow
Valvular Heart Disease

Mark A. Creager, Joshua A. Beckman, and Joseph Loscalzo
Vascular Medicine

Braunwald's Heart Disease Review and Assessment

Leonard S. Lilly
Braunwald's Heart Disease Review and Assessment

Braunwald's Heart Disease Imaging Companions

Allen J. Taylor
Atlas of Cardiovascular Computed Tomography

Christopher M. Kramer and W. Gregory Hundley
Atlas of Cardiovascular Magnetic Resonance Imaging

Ami E. Iskandrian and Ernest V. Garcia
Atlas of Nuclear Cardiology

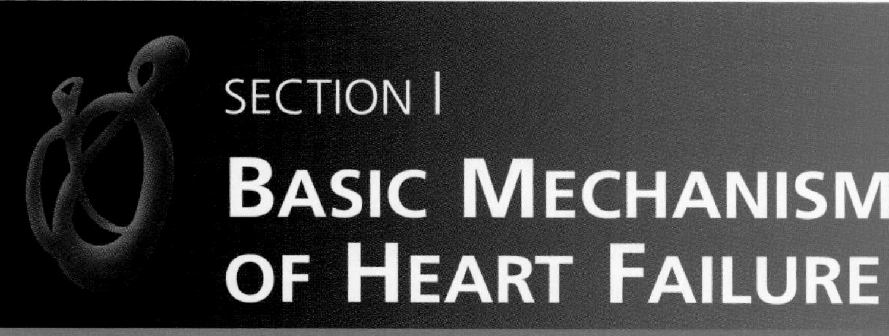

SECTION I
BASIC MECHANISMS OF HEART FAILURE

1 Molecular Basis for Heart Failure

Abhinav Diwan, Joseph A. Hill, and Thomas L. Force

Heart failure is a multisystem disorder characterized by profound disturbances in circulatory physiology and a plethora of myocardial structural and functional changes that adversely affect the systolic pumping capacity and diastolic filling characteristics of the heart. A discrete inciting event, such as myocardial infarction or administration of a chemotherapeutic agent, may be identifiable as a proximate trigger in some cases. However, in the vast majority, contributory risk factors (hypertension, ischemic heart disease, valvular disease, or diabetes) or genetic and environmental causes are uncovered during the diagnostic workup. These adverse processes affect myocardial biology and trigger cardiomyocyte hypertrophy, dysfunction, and cell death. They also provoke alterations in the extracellular matrix and vasculature, and promote neurohormonal signaling as an adaptive response that paradoxically worsens the pathophysiology. At the cellular level, loss of cardiac myocytes occurs focally with an acute myocardial infarction, or diffusely with some chemotherapeutic agents and with viral myocarditis. This leads to sustained hemodynamic stress, which results in increased hemodynamic load on the surviving myocardium. Simultaneously, molecular changes are triggered in various cardiac cell types, either in response to the inciting stress, or as a secondary consequence of increased hemodynamic load, culminating in contractile dysfunction, altered relaxation and stiffness, fibrosis, and vascular rarefaction.

Evolution of the disease process involves inexorable progression of these cellular and molecular changes in the face of ongoing stress, often despite state-of-the-art antiremodeling therapies. When the process reaches the end stage, mechanical support or heart transplantation is required. Elucidation of the molecular and cellular bases of these changes during the course of heart failure pathogenesis is therefore paramount in developing the next generation of therapeutic approaches to address the growing epidemic of heart failure. For the convenience of the reader, a glossary of abbreviations used is presented at the end of Chapter 1.

INVESTIGATIVE TECHNIQUES AND MOLECULAR MODELING

Contemporary molecular investigation into the pathogenesis of heart disease has been driven by parallel advances in preclinical modeling, genetic manipulation, and imaging technologies, coupled with rapid refinements in high-throughput sequencing technology. Together, this has permitted integration of unbiased approaches with candidate gene-based reductionist strategies to interrogate cellular pathways in animal models of heart failure and in specimens from patients with heart failure. Simultaneously, the framework for understanding normal cardiac growth and development, as well as physiological myocardial function, has been refined. With these advances, insights gained from genomewide analyses of human disease and small animal preclinical studies can be tested in large animal models. As a consequence, a pipeline-based approach has emerged for development and evaluation of therapeutic strategies.

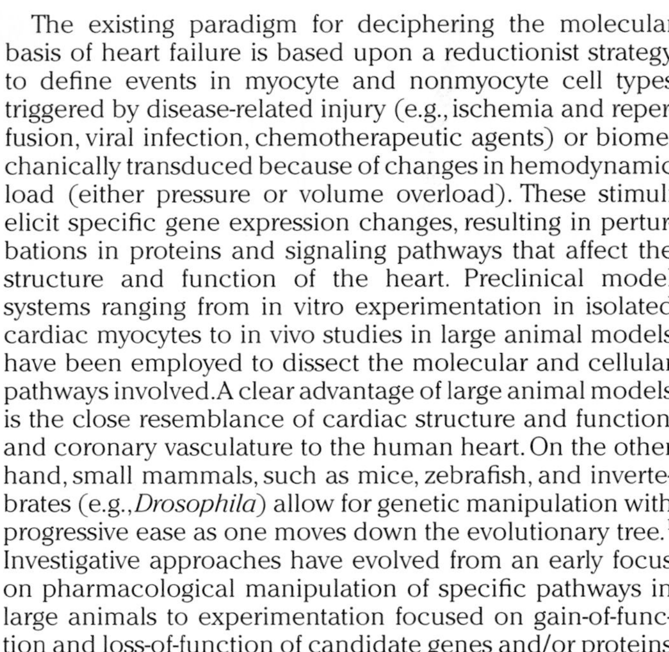

The existing paradigm for deciphering the molecular basis of heart failure is based upon a reductionist strategy to define events in myocyte and nonmyocyte cell types triggered by disease-related injury (e.g., ischemia and reperfusion, viral infection, chemotherapeutic agents) or biomechanically transduced because of changes in hemodynamic load (either pressure or volume overload). These stimuli elicit specific gene expression changes, resulting in perturbations in proteins and signaling pathways that affect the structure and function of the heart. Preclinical model systems ranging from in vitro experimentation in isolated cardiac myocytes to in vivo studies in large animal models have been employed to dissect the molecular and cellular pathways involved. A clear advantage of large animal models is the close resemblance of cardiac structure and function, and coronary vasculature to the human heart. On the other hand, small mammals, such as mice, zebrafish, and invertebrates (e.g., *Drosophila*) allow for genetic manipulation with progressive ease as one moves down the evolutionary tree.[1] Investigative approaches have evolved from an early focus on pharmacological manipulation of specific pathways in large animals to experimentation focused on gain-of-function and loss-of-function of candidate genes and/or proteins in small animals to recapitulate human pathology.

In vitro techniques in isolated cardiac myocytes have evolved from the development of the isolated neonatal rat cardiac myocytes by Paul Simpson, to studies in isolated adult cardiac myocytes,[2] and the recent emergence of reprogrammed induced pluripotent stem (iPS) cell technology.[3] Neonatal rat and mouse cardiac myocytes continue to be widely used, because these cells are easily isolated and cultured. Also, they respond to hypertrophic stimuli with an increase in cell size associated with increased protein synthesis and changes in gene expression, mimicking the cardiomyocyte hypertrophic response in vivo. This model system allows the study of cellular changes occurring in hemodynamic overload-induced hypertrophy. A major shortcoming of neonatal cardiomyocytes, however, is the incompletely developed sarcomere architecture and sarcoplasmic reticulum network. To overcome these limitations, techniques to isolate calcium-tolerant adult cardiac myocytes have been developed to allow for measurement of contraction, relaxation, and calcium transients. These cells are also amenable to gene transfer with viral vectors. Given that the mouse is the predominant mammalian model for genetic manipulations, isolated field-paced cultured adult myocytes are an attractive model system to assess the effect of genetic manipulations on cardiac myocyte function.

A major breakthrough in defining patient-specific and disease-specific alterations in cardiac myocytes was achieved with the observation that isolated somatic cells, such as fibroblasts obtained from a skin biopsy, can be reprogrammed with a cocktail of transcription factors to acquire characteristics of stem cells.[4] These so-called induced pluripotent stem cells (iPS cells) can be subsequently transdifferentiated to beating cardiac myocytes in vitro, with the structural and functional characteristics of adult cardiac myocytes. While rapid refinements in the technology are being made to minimize the impact of reprogramming manipulations and ensure suitability of this model as being representative of human cardiomyocytes, more work is needed. That said, studies with iPS cells have already begun to reveal insights into the cellular mechanisms of genetic cardiomyopathies and arrythmogenic ion channel mutations.[3] The ability to conduct genome editing with zinc-finger nucleases and TALENs (transcription-activator like effector nucleases)[5] offers tremendous promise to manipulate the molecular pathways in patient-specific iPS cells.

While in vitro systems are well suited to the study of myocyte cell biology, in vivo modeling is required to determine the effect of disease processes on organ structure and function. The prerequisites for an ideal model system are (1) a high degree of similarity to human cardiac structure and function; (2) ease of surgical manipulation with development of structural and functional changes mimicking human pathology; (3) superior fidelity to implement targeted genetic interventions to perturb molecular pathways and mimic human genetic alterations; and (4) suitability for application of analytical assays in the live organism to permit serial evaluation in a high-throughput fashion. None of the currently available model systems offers all these advantages, necessitating use of combinations to interrogate the wide range of pathophysiological, molecular, and cellular changes observed in cardiac disease.

Large animal models are well suited to studies involving disease-related stresses, such as valvular stenosis or regurgitant, ischemia/reperfusion, pressure overload, and cardiomyopathy (e.g., pacing-induced heart failure or coronary microembolization).[1] These allow for evaluation of hemodynamic and neurohormonal events on disease progression; however, these animal models do not allow for genetic manipulations. Small mammals, particularly mice, have served as a close-to-ideal workhorse system for experimental in vivo studies. Techniques for genetic perturbations, surgical intervention, and assessment of cardiac structure and function with noninvasive and invasive approaches have been developed over the last three decades. Despite persistent concerns regarding translation of findings from the mouse to humans, many observations regarding disease pathophysiology mimic those observed in human disease. Indeed, data obtained in murine models are the backbone of contemporary understanding of the molecular basis for heart failure. At the other extreme, model systems such as zebrafish and the fruit fly are ideally suited for rapid and high-throughput modeling to unveil the effects of genetic perturbations; these models, however, can be less informative with respect to alterations in myocardial structure and function or circulatory pathophysiology.

A transgenic gain-of-function approach is typically employed to evaluate whether a particular gene or its product, by virtue of its structure or its functional involvement in a particular signaling pathway, is *sufficient* to stimulate myocardial pathophysiology. Forced cardiac expression of proteins is conventionally achieved by driving their expression with cardiomyocyte-specific promoters, such as Mlc2v and α-MHC.[6] This strategy achieves a high level of gene expression in the early embryonic heart or starting at birth, respectively. For proteins that may have lethal effects following forced expression, or when temporal evaluation of the effects of forced expression are to be studied, conditional bitransgenic systems are employed where the expression of the protein of interest can be switched on or off with drug administration (typically tetracycline derivatives or mifepristone).[6]

A loss-of-function approach is designed to determine whether a certain gene (or its product) is *necessary* for a specific phenotype. One approach is to forcibly overexpress a modified protein that has dominant-negative effects by virtue of its structure or function. The potential limitations of this methodology are the unpredictable effects of a modified protein, which may be difficult to discern experimentally, and the possibility of noncanonical effects of high-level protein expression, whereby even inert proteins may induce pathology.[6] A more scientifically robust strategy is gene ablation, which has been achieved using homologous recombination in embryonic stem cells. This strategy has permitted the evaluation of nonredundant functional roles of mammalian proteins in normal development and homeostasis, and in pathophysiological processes relevant to human disease states.[6]

To overcome limitations pertaining to systemic effects of germline gene ablation, tissue-specific ablation has been achieved in the heart using Cre-Lox (or flp-FRT: flippase, flippase recognition target) technology.[6] Cardiomyocyte-specific gene deletion may be achieved in the embryo with Cre expression driven by the Nkx2.5 promoter (knocked into the Nkx locus), or conditionally, at any age, with Cre expression induced by tamoxifen treatment in Cre-ER (mutant estrogen receptor)-expressing (α-MHC promoter–driven) Mer-Cre-Mer transgenic mice.[6] Simultaneously, a "toolbox" has been developed to target diverse cell types at various developmental stages, driving an explosion of knowledge in cardiac development.[7] Another exciting advance has been the successful targeting of genes in cardiac fibroblasts with an inducible fibroblast-specific promoter (Periostin-Cre).[8] Coordinated international efforts have created repositories of targeted genes, with an ever-expanding list of available targets. This is likely to facilitate further expansion of experimentation with these technologies in the near future.

With its development, genetic manipulation offered a powerful experimental system to understand the role of specific genes and proteins in cardiac homeostasis. Interactions among genetic changes and various stressors could be examined with the advent of microsurgical techniques to mimic human heart disease. Examples of such approaches include induction of pressure overload or myocardial infarction. Pressure overload can be induced by thoracic aortic constriction or pulmonary artery banding.[1] Induction of myocardial infarction can be performed either by reversible ligation or permanent occlusion of murine coronary arteries to simulate ischemia-reperfusion injury or permanent infarction, respectively.[1] This can also be performed in a closed-chest model to minimize inflammatory changes related to the surgery, thereby more closely mimicking human disease.[9] Miniaturization of invasive hemodynamic monitoring has been achieved with development of micromanometer-tipped catheters for pressure measurement, and conductance catheters for pressure-volume loop assessment of load-independent indices. Noninvasive cardiac assessment by echocardiography and magnetic resonance imaging has also advanced significantly. Finally, telemetry-based cardiac rhythm monitoring has permitted rapid throughput evaluation of arrhythmic phenotypes in mutant mouse models.

The isolated perfused working heart preparation and the ejecting heart model offer experimental approaches well suited to investigating cardiac function and metabolism in the setting of disease (e.g., ischemia-reperfusion injury) coupled with pharmacological perturbations in genetically manipulated mice.[1] Together, these techniques comprise a comprehensive "toolkit" that allows for detailed evaluation of molecular pathways in the context of pathological stresses.

MOLECULAR DETERMINANTS OF PHYSIOLOGICAL CARDIAC GROWTH, HYPERTROPHY, AND ATROPHY

Based on early studies in rodents, cardiomyocytes have traditionally been regarded as terminally differentiated cells that rapidly exit the cell cycle early in the postnatal period. Cardiomyocytes manifest increases in cell size and nuclear division leading to binucleated and even multinucleated mature cells, but true cell division appears to occur at a low frequency. As a consequence, cardiomyocyte hypertrophy has been understood as the dominant response of adult cardiac myocytes to injury, as opposed to the hyperplasia observed in tissues with robust regenerative capabilities. Indeed, cardiomyocyte loss due to cell death has been considered largely irreplaceable. Recent work has challenged these notions, and rapidly accumulating evidence indicates that adult cardiac myocytes may be renewed from a pool of resident stem cells in the myocardium throughout life, albeit at a rate much lower than that observed prior to the early postnatal period.[10] Simultaneously, studies have revealed that the mammalian heart retains regenerative capacity in response to injury in the immediate postnatal period with generation of new cardiomyocytes from existing ones to restore normal myocardial architecture after surgical apical resection,[11] and prevent cardiac dysfunction after ischemia-reperfusion injury in 1-day-old mouse pups.[12] Importantly, this regenerative potential is lost in 7-day-old mice,[11,12] associated with transcriptional downregulation of positive cell cycle regulators and induction of cell cycle inhibitors.[13] This has triggered an explosion of interest in understanding the determinants of homeostatic regenerative capacity and the mechanisms underlying the lack of robust regenerative capacity in the face of injury after the early postnatal period. Intense efforts are also being directed toward developing strategies to enhance the regenerative potential of resident cardiac stem cells and reprogramming mature cardiomyocytes to allow them to divide. Alternatively, exogenously administered cells and/or their products are being explored to enhance cardiac regeneration.[14]

Cardiac hypertrophy has been conceptualized as "physiological" to indicate normal postnatal growth and the cardiac enlargement observed with the increased workload demands of pregnancy or exercise conditioning; conversely, "pathological" hypertrophy is observed in response to disease-related stress, such as hemodynamic overload or myocardial injury.[15] Hypertrophy serves to normalize wall stress occurring with increased hemodynamic load, thereby diminishing oxygen consumption, and is largely viewed as an adaptive response. In pathological states, however, hypertrophy may be considered maladaptive, because it often progresses to a decompensated state with development of cardiomyopathy and heart failure. While these descriptive terms reflect the nature of the inciting stimulus and the probable outcome, it is the specific intracellular signaling events that are closely correlated with the outcome. Indeed, the hypertrophic response may match the stimulus but not track its pathological characteristics. In a study where intermittent pressure overload was induced with reversible transverse aortic constriction, quantitatively less severe hypertrophy

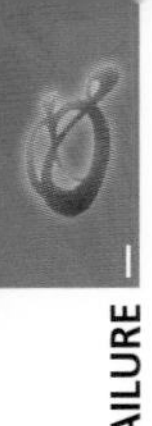

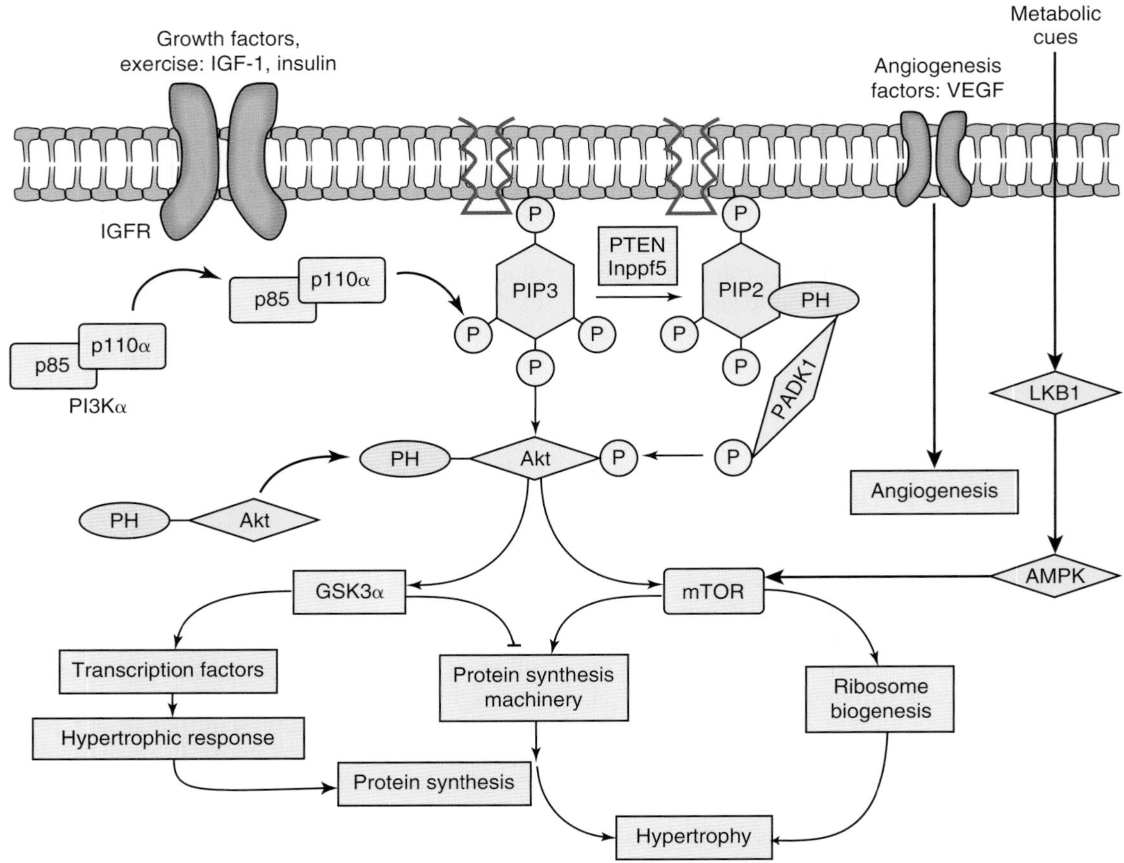

FIGURE 1-1 Molecular signaling in physiological hypertrophy. Normal growth and exercise induce cardiac hypertrophic signaling via IGF-1 release. IGF-1 binds the membrane-bound IGF receptor (IGFR), leading to autophosphorylation and recruitment of PI3K isoform p110α to the cell membrane. PI3Kα phosphorylates phosphatidylinositols in the membrane at the 3′ position in the inositol ring, generating phosphatidylinositol triphosphate (PIP3). Protein kinase B (Akt) and its activator PDK1 associate with PIP3, resulting in Akt activation, which also requires phosphorylation by PDK2 (mTORC2) for full activity (not shown). Activated Akt phosphorylates and activates mTOR, resulting in ribosome biogenesis and stimulation of protein synthesis. Akt also phosphorylates GSK3 (both α- and β-isoforms), resulting in repression of its antihypertrophic signaling (see later discussion). The phosphatases, PTEN and Inppf5, dephosphorylate PIP3 to generate PIP2 and shut off the signaling pathway. Physiological hypertrophy may be triggered by metabolic cues (circulating fatty acids) and requires coordinated induction of angiogenesis.

was observed as compared with persistent pressure overload.[16] However, the key pathological characteristics of maladaptive pressure-overload hypertrophy were comparable and resulted in functional decompensation with both intermittent and persistent pressure overload, suggesting that it is the nature of the inciting stress, not its frequency or intermittency that is most relevant.

Normal embryonic and postnatal cardiac growth, termed *cardiac eutrophy,* and physiological hypertrophy of the adult heart share important traits that distinguish physiological from pathological hypertrophy. Physiological hypertrophy is associated with normal contractile function and normal relaxation. Myocardial collagen deposition is not observed, and capillary density is increased in proportion to the increase in myocardial mass. Additionally, favorable bioenergetic alterations are observed with enhanced fatty acid metabolism and mitochondrial biogenesis. Also, the characteristic expression of the "fetal gene program" seen in pathological hypertrophy is not observed with physiological hypertrophy.[15]

Physiological hypertrophy is typically mild (≈10% to 20% increase over baseline) and regresses without permanent sequelae upon termination of increased hemodynamic demand.[17] Indeed, induction of physiological hypertrophy by exercise, and molecular manipulation of cardiac growth signaling pathways induced primarily in physiological hypertrophy (vide infra), have been reported to prevent or ameliorate the effects of pathological hypertrophy and heart failure.[18]

Eutrophy occurs via activation of signaling pathways similar to those observed in exercise-induced hypertrophy (**Figure 1-1**). At birth, a dramatic increase in circulating thyroid hormone levels transcriptionally upregulates the synthesis of contractile and calcium handling proteins in the heart, and induces a myosin heavy chain isoform shift.[15] Concomitantly, the peptide growth factor, insulin-like growth factor (IGF)-1, is secreted primarily from the liver in response to growth hormone released from the pituitary gland, stimulating physiological growth. An essential role for IGF-1 in normal growth is evidenced by growth retardation and perinatal lethality in IGF-1 and IGF receptor (IGFR-1) null mice.[15]

Development of physiological cardiac hypertrophy in response to exercise is also triggered by IGF-1, levels of which are increased in trained athletes and in cardiomyocytes in response to hemodynamic stress.[19] Indeed, IGF-1 signaling is required for exercise-induced hypertrophy; the hypertrophic response to swimming was completely suppressed in mice with cardiomyocyte-targeted ablation of the IGF-1 receptor.[20] Interestingly, induction of IGF-1 production and secretion by cardiac fibroblasts is observed in pressure-overload hypertrophy, mediated via activation of Kruppel-like transcription factor, KLF-5.[8] This has been implicated in provoking cardiomyocyte hypertrophy by paracrine signaling to preserve cardiac function in the short term, possibly by maintaining an adequate adaptive hypertrophy response.[8] Thus, the primary effect of IGF-1 on cardiac myocytes appears to be stimulation of eutrophic and physiological growth.

Insulin signaling also transduces physiological cardiac growth, in addition to governing metabolism, as mice with ablation of the insulin receptor manifest reduced cardiomyocyte size with depressed myocardial contractile function. Insulin receptor ablation also attenuates development of exercise-induced hypertrophy.[20] Additionally, ablation of the insulin receptor exacerbates pathological hypertrophy, suggesting an increased propensity for decompensation in the absence of protective physiological hypertrophy signaling.[21]

IGF-1 and insulin signaling converge on heterodimeric lipid kinases, termed *PI3Ks* (see Figure 1-1), which catalyze the formation of phosphatidylinositol-3,4,5-trisphosphate. PI3P recruits downstream effectors such as Akt via a PH-3 domain. Phosphoinositide phosphatases, namely PTEN and Inpp5f , extinguish PI3P signaling. Type I PI3 kinases (PI3Kα, β, and γ) mediate signaling downstream of the IGFR, the insulin receptor, and integrins (vide infra). Class I PI3Ks are heterodimers composed of a regulatory subunit (p85α or p85β, or their truncated splice variants p50α or p55α) and a catalytic subunit (p110α, p110β, or p110δ). Whereas genomic ablation of PI3K (p110α) is embryonic lethal at day 9.5 of gestation, expression of a dominant-negative mutant of p110α in the postnatal heart reduces adult heart size and blunts development of swimming-induced hypertrophy.[15] Additionally, a gain-of-function approach with forced cardiac expression of p110α results in cardiac growth with characteristics of physiological hypertrophy; ablation of PTEN kinase promotes cardiac growth,[22] confirming a role for this pathway in physiological cardiac hypertrophy. PI3K (p110α) is also essential for maintaining ventricular function via membrane recruitment of protein kinase B/Akt (see Figure 1-1). Ablation of Akt1 and/or Akt2 downstream of PI3K activation—as well as its activator, PDK1—reduces cardiac mass, further demonstrating the essential role for this signaling pathway in normal cardiac growth.[15]

C/EBPβ, a transcription factor repressed by Akt activation, was discovered in a genetic screen for transcriptional determinants of swimming-induced hypertrophy.[23] Furthermore, its conditional ablation resulted in increased cardiomyocyte proliferation and mild hypertrophy, which retained features of physiological hypertrophy.[23] This study suggested an exciting possibility that exercise may promote cardiomyocyte proliferation, potentially via activation of the transcription factor CITED4 and repression of SRF. C/EBPβ inhibition also ameliorated pressure overload-induced hypertrophy, bolstering the paradigm that stimulation of physiological hypertrophy pathways may offer benefits by hitherto undiscovered mechanisms.

Metabolic reprogramming and angiogenesis are other essential components of the physiological hypertrophy response. Indeed, targeted ablation of LKB1 (an activator of AMP kinase, which is activated in response to energy deficit)[24] and of vascular endothelial growth factor (VEGF), a proangiogenic signaling protein (in *vegfb* null mice), provokes reduced postnatal cardiac size and vascular rarefaction.[15] Conversely, transgenic expression of VEGF stimulates cardiomyocyte growth with elongated cardiomyocytes and preserved cardiac function, phenocopying physiological hypertrophy.[25]

Despite these observations, it is critical to proceed cautiously with strategies to stimulate physiological hypertrophy in hopes of ameliorating pathological hypertrophy. This is underscored by the observations that forced cardiac expression of IGF-1 initially produces functionally compensated ventricular hypertrophy that evolves over time into pathological hypertrophy with fibrosis and systolic dysfunction.[26] Also, forced cardiac expression of its pivotal downstream signaling effector, Akt, results in compensated hypertrophy, which transitions to cardiac failure because of inadequate angiogenesis.[27] Mechanistically, it is plausible that exuberant cardiomyocyte hypertrophy, whether initially physiological or pathological, may outstrip concordant angiogenesis and exceed the capacity for oxygen and nutrient delivery needed to meet the demands of the hypertrophied myocyte. This may explain the rare clinical observations of irreversible ventricular hypertrophy and dilation observed in athletes after long-term participation in endurance sports with a strength component, such as rowing and cycling.[28]

Cardiomyocyte size is remarkably plastic[29]; the heart undergoes atrophy with a reduction in hemodynamic load or metabolic demand as may occur in conditions of weightlessness and bed rest, such as with a spinal cord injury. This may involve inhibition of growth pathways, as suggested by rapid declines in cardiac mass observed with experimental deactivation of overexpressed Akt or induction of antihypertrophic signaling pathways (vide infra). A parallel induction of proteolytic and catabolic pathways, such as activation of the ubiquitin-proteasome system, facilitates the atrophic response. Indeed, activation of muscle ring finger 1 (MuRF 1) ligase has been demonstrated to be essential for regression of pressure-overload hypertrophy and steroid treatment-induced atrophic signaling.[30]

Cardiac growth and atrophy are also observed as physiological responses to metabolic demand, as demonstrated in fascinating studies in Burmese pythons, wherein a large meal induces a 40% increase in cardiac mass rapidly over 48 hours, and a 50% increase in stroke volume.[31] These dramatic changes revert to baseline values as the meal is digested over a period of days. The increased cardiac mass is due to cardiomyocyte hypertrophy (and not hyperplasia), is associated with transcriptional induction of synthesis of contractile elements with activation of PI3K-Akt and mTOR pathways, and is mechanistically driven by increased circulating free fatty acids and stimulation of fatty acid uptake and oxidation in the myocardium.[31]

MOLECULAR DETERMINANTS OF PATHOLOGICAL HYPERTROPHY

Cardiac hypertrophy, occurring in response to injury, hemodynamic overload, or myocardial insufficiency, has been conceptualized as a compensatory response to normalize wall stress as defined by Laplace's relationship ($S = PR/2H$, where S is wall stress [force per unit area], P is the intraventricular pressure, R is the radius of the ventricular chamber, and H is the wall thickness).[32] Hypertrophy is measured at the organ level using electrocardiographic, echocardiographic, and/or magnetic resonance imaging (MRI) indices of myocardial mass and cardiac size. In pressure overload, cardiomyocytes enlarge in the short axis by adding sarcomeres in parallel. In volume overload, sarcomeres are added

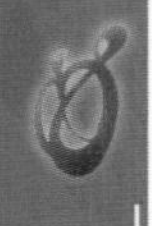

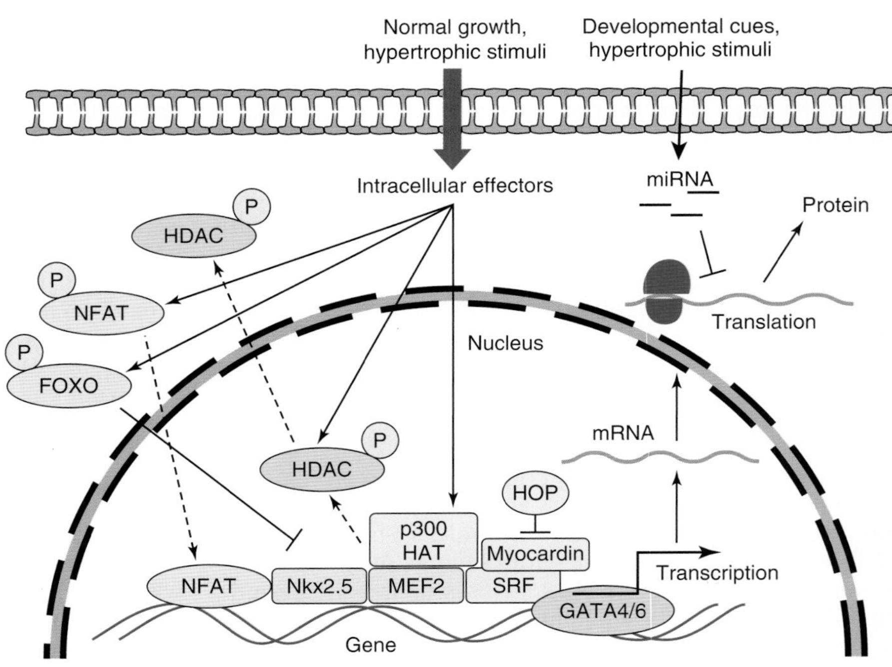

FIGURE 1-2 Regulation of gene expression in normal growth and pathological hypertrophy. A common set of transcription factors determine normal cardiac growth and pathological hypertrophy, such as GATA4, Nkx2.5, SRF, MEF2, and NFATs. Hypertrophic signaling pathways result in phosphorylation of histone deacetylases (HDACs) with export out of the nucleus, permitting histone acetylation by histone acetyltransferases (HATs), with activation of gene transcription to generate messenger RNA (mRNA). mRNA is spliced to yield a mature form, which recruits the protein synthesis machinery leading to protein translation. MicroRNAs (miRNAs) inhibit mRNA translation and/or enhance mRNA degradation to negatively regulate translation. FoxO3 family and Wnt transcription factors (not shown) negatively regulate hypertrophic growth.

in series, lengthening the cell.[33] Hypertrophic remodeling is then characterized as "concentric" (increased wall thickness without dilation) or "eccentric" (chamber dilation with a mild increase in wall thickness). A purely physical perspective to the mechanics of hypertrophy conceptualizes the primary change in ventricular geometry (i.e., wall thickening) as helpful in normalizing wall stress[32] and postponing the inevitable functional decompensation and adverse remodeling (wall thinning and chamber dilation). Although this may be the mechanical basis for the "compensated" state of hypertrophy, the near-inevitable development of heart failure and cardiomyopathic decompensation indicates that the quality of the myocardium rather than its quantity may be a more important determinant of development of heart failure.[34] Indeed, in pathological hypertrophy, the characteristic gene expression changes, cardiomyocyte dysfunction and altered neurohormonal responsiveness (reviewed in Harvey and associates[33]), are in striking contrast to those observed during normal cardiac growth and physiological hypertrophy, and portend adverse outcomes. Interestingly, studies in animal models have suggested that reactive hypertrophy after hemodynamic overloading may be entirely dispensable to functional compensation, and even undesirable.[35] Therefore, interrupting pathological hypertrophic signaling may be a desirable therapeutic endpoint in heart failure.

Transcriptional Regulation of Pathological Cardiac Hypertrophy

A hallmark of pathological hypertrophy in the adult heart is reexpression of embryonic cardiac genes, a process often referred to as the *fetal gene program*, because this aspect of the cardiac response to stress or injury recapitulates aspects of cardiac development.[33] The earliest detectable change (within hours of increasing afterload or stimulating cultured cardiomyocytes to hypertrophy with norepinephrine) is induction of regulatory transcription factors c-fos, c-jun, jun-B, c-myc, and Egr-1/nur77, and heat shock protein (HSP) 70, thereby mimicking changes observed with cell cycle entry. Induction of these "early response genes" drives expression of other genes in the fetal program. The prototypical gene, atrial natriuretic factor (ANF), is expressed early during heart development through the coordinated interactions of Nkx2.5, GATA4, and PTX transcription factors, but only in the atria of normal adult hearts.[33] A robust induction of ventricular ANF expression (and related BNP [B-type natriuretic peptide]) is observed in pathological hypertrophy and heart failure. In fact, increased BNP secretion from the stressed heart is used widely as a biomarker of heart failure.[36] Other elements of the fetal gene program induced in pathological hypertrophy and heart failure encode sarcomeric genes, such as β-MHC, MLC2v, α-skeletal actin, and β-tropomysin, proteins that are prominent in the embryonic, but not adult, ventricle.

Cardiac gene expression in pathological hypertrophy is driven by the reactivation of many developmentally regulated transcription factors (**Figure 1-2**). GATA4 and GATA6 are two such zinc-finger DNA binding transcription factors that are individually essential for heart tube development and myocyte proliferation during embryogenesis.[37,38] Both of these transcription factors are also essential for homeostatic expression of various cardiomyocyte genes in the adult heart, including ANF, BNP, ET-1, α-skeletal actin, α-MHC, β-MHC, cardiac troponin c, and AT1Ra; their individual or combinatorial ablation results in progressive cardiomyopathy.[37,38] In pressure-overload hypertrophy, upregulated GATA4 and GATA6 protein levels play key roles in mediating pathological hypertrophy, such that their individual transgenic expression is sufficient to induce hypertrophy.[38] Furthermore, cardiomyocyte-specific deletion of either markedly attenuates development of pressure-overload hypertrophy, resulting in accelerated decompensation. Importantly, pathological hypertrophic stimuli result in GATA4 activation and nuclear translocation with induction of VEGF expression. This may be essential for sustaining angiogenic responses in pressure-overload hypertrophy,[37] underscoring its critical role in this setting.

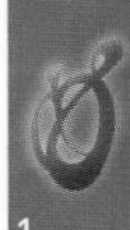

Prohypertrophic signaling pathways, such as activation of MAP kinase cascades downstream of Gαq-coupled α_1-adrenergic (α_1A) receptors, trigger activation of GATA4.[37] Antihypertrophic signaling such as that mediated by GSK3β, a kinase downstream of PI3K-Akt, regulates normal cardiac growth in some scenarios but also converges upon the NFAT and GATA transcription factors to regulate pathological hypertrophic signaling. GATA4 also complexes with other transcription factors such as Nkx2.5, MEF2, a coactivator, p300, SRF, and NFAT to affect cardiac gene expression (see Figure 1-2).[37] SRF (serum response factor) is another cardiac-enriched transcription factor that coordinately induces sarcomerogenesis with other transcription factors, including SMAD1/3, Nkx2–5, and GATA4.[37] Cardiomyocyte-specific ablation of SRF in the adult heart results in progressive development of cardiomyopathy with disorganization of the sarcomeres and heart failure.[37] SRF also interacts with myocardin and HOP transcription factors.[37] HOP antagonizes SRF signaling, and conditional ablation of HOP results in aberrant cardiac growth with evidence for both lack of myocyte formation and excess cardiomyocyte proliferation.[37] Myocardin acts as a cardiac and smooth muscle-specific co-activator of SRF, and is essential for embryonic cardiomyocyte proliferation[39] and maintenance of normal sarcomere organization in the adult heart. Signaling by the G13 subunit of heterotrimeric G proteins downstream of prohypertrophic agonists (e.g., angiotensin II and endothelin-1) transduces activation of pathological hypertrophy genes through RhoA-GTPase-mediated activation of myocardin.[40]

There has been much speculation about the functional impact of reexpression of the fetal gene program in pathological hypertrophy.[33] It has been postulated that an increased ratio of β-MHC/α-MHC isoforms impairs myocardial contractility because of the relative inefficiency of the β-isoform, culminating in reduced sarcomere shortening, prolonged relaxation, and adverse remodeling. While this may have a major impact in the adult mouse ventricle, which predominantly expresses the faster α-isoform, its relevance in the adult human heart, wherein 90% of the myosin heavy chain is the β-isoform, is less clear. In contrast, downregulation of the gene encoding the sarcoplasmic reticulum Ca^{2+} ATPase (SERCA) affects the activity of this important Ca^{2+} pump, which is responsible for the rapid diastolic reuptake of calcium into the sarcoplasmic reticulum.[33] This has been established as an important mechanism for the contractile dysfunction observed in human heart failure and forms the basis for experimental gene therapies currently under evaluation.[41]

Multiple studies focusing on transcriptome profiling of cardiac pathology have identified a panoply of gene expression changes in both human heart failure and animal models of pathological hypertrophy (www.cardiogenomics.org). These myocardial mRNA signatures and the different patterns of gene expression in normal, early failing, late failing, and recovering hearts might be useful as prognostic biomarkers and help guide therapeutics.[42] Also, in the past decade, there have been dramatic advances in sequencing technologies. A rapidly accumulating list of individual variations in genetic sequence (termed *single nucleotide polymorphisms*) and their combinations, through genome-wide association studies, holds the promise to uncover novel targets for further mechanistic exploration in heart failure.[43]

Another layer of complexity in gene regulation has been revealed by studies of microRNAs (miRNAs). These are short, noncoding, naturally occurring single-stranded RNAs that negatively regulate gene expression by promoting degradation of mRNAs and/or inhibiting mRNA translation, thereby suppressing protein synthesis (see Figure 1-2). MicroRNAs are abundantly expressed in the myocardium and differentially regulated in animal models and human heart failure.[44] MicroRNAs are essential for homeostatic gene regulation, as targeted cardiomyocyte-specific ablation of Dicer, an enzyme essential for miRNA processing, causes heart failure with profound transcriptional dysregulation of cardiac contractile proteins.[44] Upstream signaling pathways alter miRNA expression in response to developmental cues and hypertrophic stimuli, such as the regulation of miR-1 and miR-133 from a common precursor by SRF and MEF2. These transcription factors control cardiomyocyte proliferation during development and downregulate miR-1 and miR-133, facilitating prohypertrophic pathways in swimming-induced and pressure-overload hypertrophy.[44] Another group of miRNAs is localized to the myosin heavy chain genes, miR-208a, miR-208b, and miR-499 (termed *MyomiRs*). These have been shown to regulate transcriptional repressors and thyroid hormone signaling to transduce myosin heavy chain gene expression changes observed in pathological hypertrophy.[44] Importantly, targeted deletion of miR-208a prevented reexpression of the fetal gene program and attenuated pathological remodeling with pressure overload.[44]

Recent exciting discoveries point to a critical role for upregulation of the miR-15 family at birth by suppressing cardiomyocyte proliferation in the immediate postnatal period.[45] Indeed, miR-15 inhibition with locked nucleic acids stimulates continued cardiomyocyte proliferation after birth and induces regeneration of myocardium when administered after myocardial infarction in adult mice. This restores the regenerative capacity otherwise observed only in 1-day-old pups.[12] Therefore, targeting the regulation of gene expression with miRNA-targeted strategies holds promise in developing novel therapeutics to treat heart failure.

Cellular Mechanisms of Impaired Cardiomyocyte Viability (see also Chapter 2)

Hypertrophy of the ventricular myocardium is an independent risk factor for cardiac death,[46] and is observed with near-universal prevalence in patients with heart failure. Left ventricular hypertrophy may in part underlie the diastolic dysfunction observed in HFpEF.[47] In addition, in patients with HFrEF, pathological left ventricular hypertrophy manifests inexorable progression from a compensated or nonfailing state, to dilated cardiomyopathy and overt failure.[32,34] It is important to recognize that while the essential feature of cardiac hypertrophy is increased cardiomyocyte size/volume, other myocardial alterations, such as fibroblast hyperplasia, deposition of extracellular matrix proteins, and a relative decrease in vascular smooth muscle and capillary density[33] also contribute to the progression from functionally compensated pathological hypertrophy to overt heart failure.

Activation of Cell Death Pathways

Evidence for cardiomyocyte "drop-out" due to death or degeneration is observed in failing hearts and in pathological hypertrophy before the development of cardiomyopathy.[33] The extant literature indicates that hypertrophied cardiac myocytes are likely to die from a number of different processes, and cardiomyocyte death can be a causal factor in cardiomyopathic decompensation, although the relative contribution of specific pathways appears to vary with pathological context.[48] Cardiomyocyte death may be programmed (i.e., cell suicide) by apoptosis, necrosis, or autophagy[48] or accidental (as in conventional necrosis due to interruption of vascular supply). Histological evidence for all forms of death is seen in end-stage human cardiomyopathy.[49]

Apoptosis, derived from the Greek expression for "the deciduous autumnal falling of leaves" (apo, means away from and ptosis, means falling), is an orderly and highly regulated energy-requiring process that mediates targeted removal of individual cells during development without provoking an immune response. The rates of apoptosis, measured as apoptotic indices (e.g., number of TUNEL-positive nuclei/total nuclei), parallel the rates of cell division and are highest in the outflow tract (≈50%); intermediate in the endocardial cushions, which are sites of valve formation, and in left ventricular myocardium (10% to 20%); and lowest in the right ventricular myocardium (≈0.1% at birth).[48] In rats, both cardiomyocyte apoptosis and mitosis in the left ventricular myocardium virtually cease soon after birth, and within the first 2 weeks of life in the right ventricle. Abnormal persistence of apoptosis in right ventricular myocardium contributes to the pathogenesis of arrhythmogenic right ventricular dysplasia, a disorder caused by mutations provoking abnormal localization of desmosomal proteins leading to suppression of Wnt signaling.[50] This stimulates de novo adipogenesis from resident cardiac stem cells to cause right ventricle-specific cardiomyocyte apoptosis and fibro-fatty replacement associated with arrhythmias and sudden death.[51] Apoptotic cardiomyocytes are extremely rare in normal adult myocardium (1 apoptotic cell per 10,000 to 100,000 cardiomyocytes).[48] Together with reactivation of the fetal gene program in hypertrophied and failing hearts, the prevalence of cardiomyocyte apoptosis is markedly increased in chronic cardiomyopathies.[52] Apoptotic cardiomyocyte death may also play a role in the transition of pressure-overload hypertrophy to dilated cardiomyopathy.[48] Emerging evidence suggests that necrosis, a form of cell death associated with rupture of the plasma membrane and inflammatory infiltration, may also be programmed and controlled by the cell.[48] The death machinery that orchestrates these processes exhibits crosstalk at multiple levels, whereby features of either or both forms may be dominant in a specific pathophysiological setting.

Cell death may be initiated by ligand-dependent signaling from the cell exterior through the extrinsic or receptor-mediated pathways; conversely, it may occur by induction of the death machinery within the cell, through mitochondrial pathways (**Figure 1-3**).[48] Sustained experimental pressure overload is sufficient to induce expression of the prototypical death-promoting cytokine, TNF-α,[53] and TNF signals via the type 1 TNF receptor (TNFR1) to stimulate cardiomyocyte hypertrophy and apoptosis, and provoke contractile dysfunction.[54] A potentially causal role for

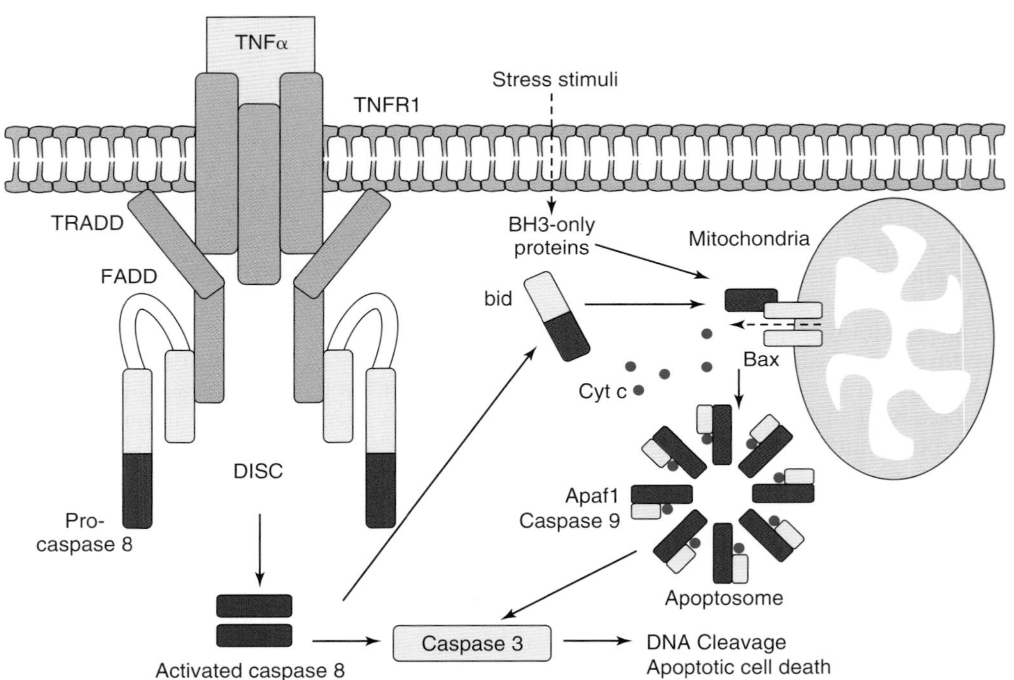

FIGURE 1-3 Cell death signaling in heart failure. Cell death machinery is activated via an "extrinsic pathway," when death-inducing ligands such as TNF/Fas engage cognate receptors, or an "intrinsic pathway" triggered by stress-mediated transcriptional induction or activation of prodeath BH3 domain-only proteins. TNF-α binds the TNF receptor 1 (TNFR1) homotrimer, resulting in recruitment of proteins via death domains, namely TRADD and FADD; and procaspase 8 and assembly of DISC (death inducing signaling complex). This causes cleavage activation of caspase 8, which cleaves and activates the effector caspase, caspase 3. Activated caspase 3 proteolyzes cellular substrates and causes cell death. BH3 domain-only Bcl2 family proteins get activated in response to stress stimuli (as with transcriptional induction of BNIP3L/Nix with pathological hypertrophic signaling; see text for details) to permeabilize mitochondria. The extrinsic pathway is also amplified by caspase 8-induced cleavage of bid, the truncated form of which, t-bid, interacts with multidomain proapoptotic Bcl2 proteins Bax and Bak (not shown) to engage the intrinsic pathway. This results in mitochondrial outer membrane permeabilization and release of cytochrome c (cyt c), which associates with the adaptor protein Apaf-1, ATP, and procaspase 9, forming the apoptosome, with activation of caspase 9. Activated caspase 9, in turn, activates caspase 3. This process is opposed by Bcl2 and Bcl-xl (not shown), and inhibitor protein XIAP. Smac/DIABLO and Omi/HtrA2 are released during mitochondrial permeabilization (not shown) and bind to XIAP, relieving its inhibitory effect. Also released are DNAses: AIF (apoptosis inducing factor) and EndoG, which cause internucleosomal DNA cleavage.

elevated levels of this cytokine is suggested by elevated TNF-α plasma levels that are correlated with the degree of cardiac cachexia in end-stage heart failure.[55] Death receptor signaling downstream of TNFR1 is triggered by TNF binding to a receptor homodimer, resulting in formation of the DISC (death inducing signaling complex) with recruitment of adaptor protein FADD and caspase 8 (an upstream member of a family of executioner cysteine proteases). Activated caspase 8 then cleaves caspase 3 and Bid, a proapoptotic Bcl2 family member. Activated caspase 3, the effector caspase, activates a nuclear DNAase (CAD-caspase-activated DNAse) that results in internucleosomal cleavage of DNA and chromatin condensation. Generation of truncated tBid links the extrinsic pathway to activation of the intrinsic pathway. This leads to their simultaneous activation in TNF-induced cardiomyocyte apoptosis in the setting of TNF-induced depletion of anti-apoptotic signaling proteins in the mitochondria.[54] While elevated TNF levels signal to provoke myocardial hypertrophy with increased cardiomyocyte apoptosis, adverse ventricular remodeling, and systolic dysfunction in rodent models, endogenous TNF signaling is cytoprotective in ischemia-reperfusion injury.[56] This indicates that precise context-dependent modulation of TNF signaling may be required to attenuate cell death in pathological hypertrophy.

The intrinsic mitochondrial pathway of programmed cell death is triggered by stress-induced upregulation or activation of BH3-domain only prodeath proteins (see Figure 1-3),[48] such as with Gαq/PKC/SP-1-mediated transcriptional induction of BNIP3L/Nix in pathological hypertrophy. Nix targets and permeabilizes mitochondria to induce release of prodeath mediators such as cytochrome c. Nix-induced mitochondrial permeabilization may be direct via outer membrane permeabilization (MOMP), or may occur via Nix-targeting to the ER, triggering ER-mitochondrial crosstalk to provoke calcium overload and mitochondrial permeability transition pore (MPTP) opening.[57] In the cytosol, cytochrome c binds to the adaptor protein Apaf-1 (apoptotic protease activating factor-1), resulting in sequential recruitment and cleavage-mediated activation of caspase 9 and caspase 3. Together with release of AIF (apoptosis inducing factor) and endoG from the mitochondrial intermembranous space, this results in activation of PARP and DNA cleavage in the nucleus (see Figure 1-3) and cell death. Stress-induced cardiomyocyte death is an important determinant of pathological hypertrophy and decompensation, because cardiomyocyte-specific ablation of Nix attenuates pressure overload-induced ventricular remodeling and programmed cell death.[48]

Calcium overload-induced opening of the mitochondrial permeability transition pore is also implicated in programmed necrosis. Inhibition of MPTP formation with ablation of ppif (the gene encoding cyclophylin D), a critical mitochondrial matrix component of the permeability pore, reduces cell death provoked by ischemia-reperfusion injury.[48] However, a subsequent study reported a critical physiological role for cyclophylin D-mediated mitochondrial Ca^{2+} efflux in maintaining adequate mitochondrial function to match metabolic demand. In this study, mice with cyclophylin D deficiency developed exaggerated hypertrophy and heart failure with exercise or pressure overload, which was corrected by transgenic restoration of cyclophylin D levels.[58] This indicates a paradigm similar to that observed with TNF signaling, whereby a precise modulation of the mitochondrial permeability pore will be required to therapeutically address programmed necrosis in heart failure.

In pathological hypertrophy, cardiomyocyte necrosis may also be triggered by ischemia due to mismatch between the degree of hypertrophy and vascular supply. An adequate blood supply for growing myocardium is critical to normal cardiac function, and capillary density is closely coupled to myocardial growth during development.[15] As discussed earlier, pathological hypertrophy is associated with relative vascular rarefaction (as compared with normal capillary density observed with physiological hypertrophy) with decreased capillary density, decreased coronary flow reserve, and increased diffusion distance to myocytes. There is a temporal correlation between decreased capillary density and cardiomyocyte "dropout" during decompensation in both human disease and experimental animal models.[27] Indeed, in pressure overload-induced hypertrophy, impairment of angiogenesis with cardiomyocyte-specific GATA4 ablation (and resultant deficiency of angiopoietin and Vegf)[37] and sustained increases in p53 (with suppression of HIF1α signaling) accelerate progression to decompensated heart failure.[59] Conversely, restoration of angiogenesis with p53 inhibition or exogenous administration of proangiogenic agents markedly attenuates cardiomyocyte death in this setting, confirming a central role for this paradigm in decompensation.

Also relevant to this discussion is the observation that both myocyte and nonmyocyte cell types produce placental growth factor (PGF) in response to hypertrophic stress in the myocardium, which stimulates angiogenesis and paracrine stimulation of cardiomyocyte hypertrophy via IL-6 generation.[60] Studies suggest that this angiogenic response could be stimulated further to prevent decompensation of pressure-overload hypertrophy.[60] Additionally during physiological hypertrophy of pregnancy, proangiogenic signaling via PGC1α (peroxisome proliferator activating factor γ coactivator α) counters the antiangiogenic effects of a VEGF inhibitor secreted by the placenta, termed *sFLT-1*.[61] Deficiency of the angiogenic response provokes peripartum cardiomyopathy, pointing to a critical need for coordinated increases in angiogenesis and myocyte size to maintain physiological hypertrophy.

Cell Survival Pathways

Countervailing pathways promoting cell survival play critical roles in regulating cell death during pathological cardiac remodeling. One such pathway is elicited by the IL-6 family of cytokines, comprising IL-6, cardiotrophin, and LIF, and signaling via a shared membrane receptor, viz., the gp130 glycoprotein that has intrinsic tyrosine kinase activity (**Figure 1-4**). Binding of ligand induces gp130 homodimerization or oligomerization with β-subunits of other cytokine receptors, stimulating autophosphorylation on receptor cytoplasmic tails and activating intrinsic tyrosine kinase activity. This permits binding of adaptor proteins Grb2 and Shc to SH2 binding domains to activate Janus kinases (JAKs) that phosphorylate STAT transcription factors. Activated STAT dimers then migrate to the nucleus to (1) regulate gene expression; (2) activate SH2 domain-containing cytoplasmic protein tyrosine phosphatase (SHP2), which subsequently activates the MEK/ERK pathway; and (3) activate the Ras/mitogen-activated protein kinase leading to MAPK activation and extracellular signal-regulated kinase (ERK) signaling (see Figure 1-4). A simultaneous transcriptional

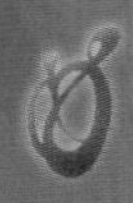

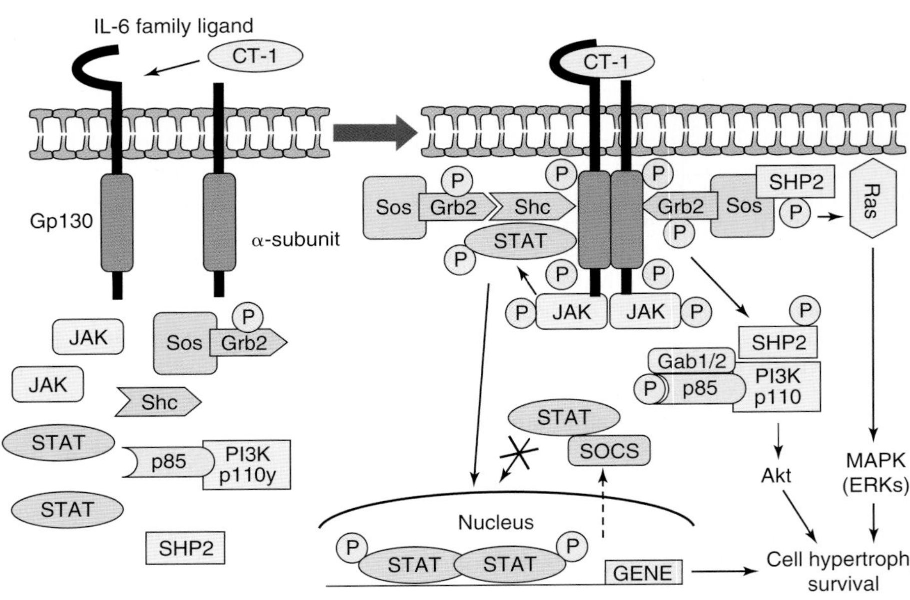

FIGURE 1-4 Gp130-mediated survival signaling in heart failure. Ligand-induced homodimerization of Gp130, a transmembrane receptor protein, or heterodimerization with α-receptor subunits for IL-6 cytokine family members, such as CT-1, LIF, or oncostatin M, causes tyrosine autophosphorylation and recruitment and activation of JAK1/2. Subsequently, two major intracellular signaling cascades are triggered: (1) Signal transducer and activator of transcription (STAT)-1/3 pathway with STAT dimerization and translocation to the nucleus with activation of gene transcription. This pathway is opposed by induction of SOCS proteins, which bind to and prevent STAT translocation. (2) SH2-domain-containing cytoplasmic protein phosphatase (SHP2)/MEK/Extracellular signal-regulated kinase (ERK) pathway. Additionally, Grb2 binding with Gab1/2 causes PI3K-mediated Akt activation. These pathways signal to promote cardiomyocyte hypertrophy and survival.

upregulation of SOCS family proteins via STAT signaling provides for feedback inhibition of these pathways (see Figure 1-4). Gp130 activation is transiently observed early after the onset of pressure overload, and this survival pathway is deactivated during the transition to failure, possibly related to interruption of gp130-JAK-STAT signaling by stress-induced SOCS3, and the resulting suppression of STAT3 signaling. Importantly, ablation of gp130 provokes exaggerated cardiac myocyte apoptosis with fulminant heart failure with pressure-overload hypertrophy.[62]

Signaling through gp130 also protects against viral myocarditis by accelerating viral clearance, whereas cardiomyocyte-specific gp130 gene ablation, or expression of the gp130 inhibitor, SOCS3, accelerates the myocarditis.[63] Sustained activation of the gp130 pathways can, however, be counterproductive, as observed in a study with a constitutively active mutant with sustained STAT3 activation, which caused prolonged inflammation, adverse postinfarction remodeling, and ventricular rupture in the subacute period after a myocardial infarction.[64] Additionally, SOCS3 signaling is critical for appropriate feedback inhibition of the pathway, as cardiomyocyte-specific ablation of SOCS3 results in altered myofilament Ca^{2+} sensitivity, resulting in contractile dysfunction and heart failure, which can be rescued by concomitant gp130 ablation.[65]

Autophagy (i.e., to eat self [Greek]) is a lysosomal degradative pathway essential for breaking down intracellular constituents to recycle defective proteins and mitochondria and to replenish nutrients during periods of deprivation. Autophagy of intracellular constituents is critical for cardiomyocyte survival during the early perinatal period of starvation, as mice deficient of key autophagy proteins, such as ATG5 and ATG7 (both essential for the initial step of autophagosome formation), develop fatal myocardial deterioration.[66,67] Autophagy is also essential for cardiomyocyte homeostasis in adult mice, because adult-onset cardiomyocyte-specific ablation of ATG5 results in fulminant heart failure, and postnatal onset of ATG7 deficiency leads to insidious development of cardiomyopathy with aging.[68] Stimulation of autophagy enhances cardiomyocyte survival during myocardial ischemia, as mice expressing a dominant-negative mutant of AMPK are unable to mount an effective autophagic response to ischemia and manifest larger infarct sizes as compared with control. Interestingly, perinatal onset of ATG5 deficiency is well tolerated and yet induces rapid decompensation in the setting of pressure overload,[68] suggesting an essential role for basal autophagy. Foci of degenerated cardiomyocytes with autophagic vacuoles are observed in human dilated cardiomyopathy and aortic stenosis,[49] indicating that this pathway likely plays an important role in human pathophysiology.

Interestingly, other studies have suggested that induction of autophagy may be potentially deleterious in certain forms of cardiac injury. In particular, mice with haploinsufficiency of Beclin-1 demonstrate decreased infarct size with ischemia-reperfusion injury and attenuation of pressure overload-induced adverse ventricular remodeling.[68] Whether these effects are due to a role for Beclin-1 in autophagy, or involve Beclin-1-induced signaling via other mechanisms,[68] remains to be fully delineated. Therefore, although the evidence suggests a predominantly prosurvival role for autophagy, further studies are needed to clarify whether autophagy in dying cells is causal, compensatory and adaptive, or an associated but unrelated response.

Mitochondria and Metabolic Remodeling in Pathological Hypertrophy

The heart is a mitochondria-rich organ that depends upon oxidative phosphorylation via the Krebs cycle to satiate its massive demands for energy required for continuous contraction (see also Chapter 16). At birth, a metabolic shift in substrate preference occurs, moving from reliance on glucose to fatty acids, and accompanied by a surge in mitochondrial biogenesis. This surge in postnatal mitochondrial biogenesis is required to permit normal cardiac growth and function, because mice deficient in both PGC1α and β-isoforms (that play redundant roles in induction of the mitochondrial biogenesis program) manifest rapid development of cardiomyopathy in the early neonatal period.[69] Activation of PGC1α and stimulation of mitochondrial biogenesis occur with exercise-induced physiological hypertrophy via PI3K (but not Akt) activation. PGC1α and β are transcriptional coactivators that drive activation of the transcription factors NRF1, NRF2, and ERRα. These proteins, in turn, stimulate biogenesis of nuclear DNA-encoded mitochondrial proteins and TFAM, which drives transcription in the mitochondrial genome. They also function in concert with PPAR transcription factors to regulate metabolic gene expression in the heart. Cardiomyocyte-specific ablation of TFAM mimics the phenotype observed with combinatorial PGC1α and β ablation, with development of insidious cardiomyopathy observed in heterozygous null mice and fulminant cardiomyopathy leading to embryonic lethality in the context of homozygous ablation.[70] These findings lend further support to the premise that maintenance of a "normal" mass of normally functioning mitochondria is critical for cardiac homeostasis.

Pathological cardiac hypertrophy is associated with a shift in cardiac metabolism back to glucose, with transcriptional downregulation of the fatty acid metabolism machinery associated with repression of both PGCα and β (see also Chapter 16).[71] Importantly, in these studies, genetic ablation of the PGC1α/PPAR/ERR signaling axis accelerated decompensation in pressure-overload hypertrophy. Multiple mitochondrial abnormalities were observed with transition from a compensated to decompensated state, and magnetic resonance spectroscopy demonstrated reduced "high-energy" phosphate stores (phosphocreatine or PCr) in pressure overload-induced ventricular hypertrophy that progressively decline during the transition to heart failure.[71] It is suspected, based primarily on correlative evidence, that inadequate mitochondrial biogenesis and/or impaired quality control result in an inability to maintain a normal complement of mitochondria, provoking decompensation and heart failure. Accordingly, stimulation of mitochondrial biogenesis to induce a favorable metabolic shift is currently being evaluated as a strategy to treat heart failure.

Neurohormonal Signaling and Cardiomyocyte Dysfunction

Activation of the sympathetic nervous system in heart failure commences early as an adaptive response to maintain cardiac function and adequate cardiac output. Persistent sympathetic activation, however, becomes progressively maladaptive over time, because catecholamines are toxic to cardiomyocytes (see also Chapter 6).[72] In vivo, persistent activation of catecholamine signaling pathways, such as by chronic infusion of isoproterenol, causes cardiomyopathy associated with cardiomyocyte loss.[73] These effects are largely blocked by pharmacological inhibition of the β_1-receptor and the L-type calcium channel.

There are nine subtypes of adrenergic receptors (three each of α1, α2, and β), and β_1-receptors are the most abundant subtype in the myocardium, present in a 10:1 ratio as compared with α-receptors. Catecholamine signaling via cardiomyocyte β-adrenoceptors regulates increases in myocardial contractility by modulating inotropy and chronotropy. The β_1-adrenoreceptor signals via the stimulatory G protein (Gαs) to activate adenyl cyclase, resulting in cyclic AMP production, which acts as a second messenger to activate protein kinase A (**Figure 1-5**). In comparison, signaling downstream of the β_2-adrenoreceptor couples to both Gαs and the inhibitory G protein, Gαi, but results primarily in inhibition of adenyl cyclase and downregulation of cAMP levels. In normal myocardium, β_1-receptors constitute approximately 80% of all β-adrenoreceptors.[73] However,

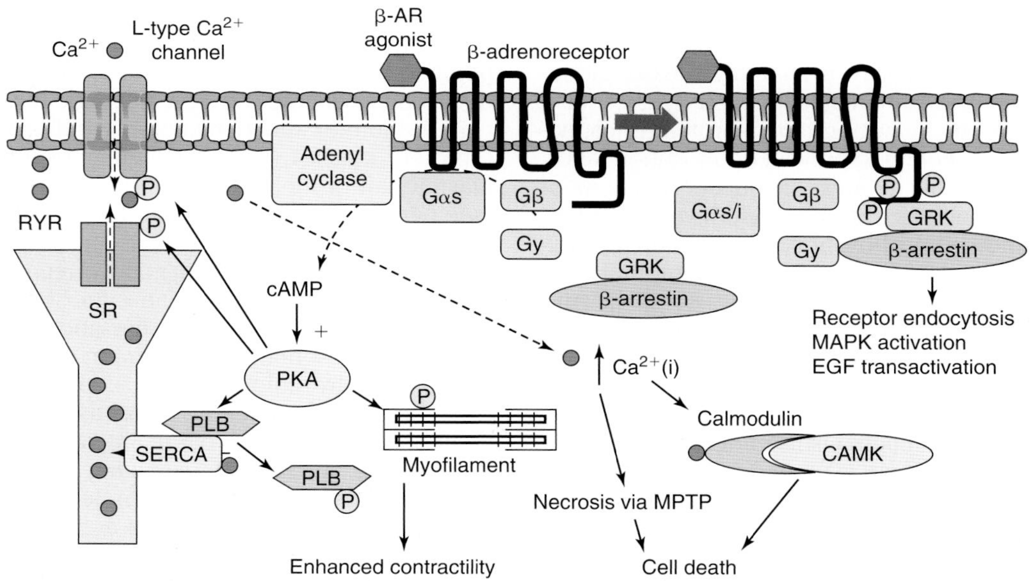

FIGURE 1-5 β-adrenoreceptor signaling in heart failure. Catecholamine binding to the seven transmembrane myocardial β_1-adrenoreceptors activates Gsα signaling, with displacement of bound GDP by GTP, and association with Gβ and Gγ forming the heterotrimer at the receptor. This causes cyclic AMP generation via stimulation of adenyl cyclase, which activates PKA. PKA phosphorylates the L-type calcium channel, enhancing Ca^{2+} entry, and RYR enhancing calcium release from the SR, increasing intracellular calcium (Ca^{2+}(i)) available for excitation contraction coupling. PKA phosphorylates phospholamban, derepressing SERCA activity with enhanced SR Ca^{2+} reuptake, and phosphorylates troponin on the myofilaments, with the net effect of enhancing contractility. Termination of G-protein signaling occurs with GTPase activity of Gsα causing GDP formation and cAMP being degraded by phosphodiesterases (not shown). Additionally, activated β-adrenoreceptors are phosphorylated at their cytoplasmic tails by G-protein receptor kinases, causing receptor endocytosis. Increased Ca^{2+}(i) with chronic adrenoreceptor signaling causes necrotic cell death via calmodulin-mediated CaMkinase activation and mitochondrial permeability transition pore formation (MPTP) (see text). β_2-adrenoreceptor activation stimulates Giα with inhibition of adenyl cyclase (not shown). A delayed phase of signaling downstream of β_1-adrenoreceptor may also be activated by GRK-mediated recruitment of β-arrestin with transactivation of EGF with enhanced survival signaling (see text).

heart failure is associated with desensitization of β_1 adrenoreceptor signaling, preferential internalization and degradation of β_1-receptors, and a proportionate increase in β_2-adrenoceptor-mediated inhibitory G(i) signaling.[73] The latter occurs via redistribution of β_2-adrenergic receptors from T-tubules to the cell surface,[74] an event that shifts the localized compartmentalization of G(i)-mediated cAMP responses to diffuse intracellular effects. Gα subunit signaling is suppressed via GTPase activation, which is enhanced by RGS (regulators of G-protein signaling) proteins. In an exciting discovery, the beneficial effects of cardiac resynchronization therapy in the failing myocardium were found to be transduced by an increase in RGS2/RGS3 protein levels and a shift from G(i) to G(s) signaling.[75] Interestingly, a burst of β_2-receptor-mediated inhibitory G(i) signaling may also transduce the reversible myocardial dysfunction of the mid and apical segments of the left ventricular myocardium (which harbor a proportionately greater abundance of β_2-receptors as compared with basal segments) observed in catecholamine-mediated stress cardiomyopathy (also referred to as *Takotsubo cardiomyopathy*).[76] Together, these studies underscore the potential for therapeutically targeting G(i) signaling in various forms of heart failure.

In cardiomyocytes, membrane depolarization-induced calcium entry into the cytoplasm is rapidly induced through L-type Ca^{2+} channels, triggering Ca^{2+}-induced Ca^{2+} release from the sarcoplasmic reticulum through the ryanodine receptor and culminating in mechanical contraction.[77] During diastole, membrane repolarization is associated with rapid reuptake of Ca^{2+} through SR uptake mediated by the sarcoplasmic reticulum ATPase (SERCA). The β_1-adrenoceptor/Gsα/PKA signaling axis increases contractility via PKA-mediated phosphorylation of phospholamban to relieve inhibition on SERCA and promote diastolic calcium uptake into the SR. This results in increased SR Ca^{2+} loading and larger systolic Ca^{2+} transients that augment contractility. PKA also phosphorylates both L-type Ca^{2+} channels to enhance Ca^{2+} entry and ryanodine receptors, acting at multiple levels to increase Ca^{2+} availability for excitation-contraction coupling. PKA-mediated phosphorylation also enhances relaxation by activating type-1 protein phosphatase (PP1) inhibitor-1 protein to prevent dephosphorylation of phospholamban at Ser16, and via phosphorylation of contractile proteins, such as troponin I and myosin binding protein C. In addition, PKA phosphorylates phosphodiesterases (PDEs), which are located in the same membrane subcompartment as the β-receptor signaling complex and mediate hydrolysis of cAMP. This, in turn, potentiates cAMP-mediated signaling events by preventing its feedback inhibition (see Figure 1-5).

Genetic manipulation of adrenergic receptors and their effectors have uncovered mechanisms underlying catecholamine toxicity.[73] While forced expression of low levels of β_2-receptors enhances cardiac function, expression at much higher levels provokes dilated and fibrotic cardiomyopathy. In contrast, forced expression of the β_1-receptors provokes hypertrophy progressing to failure. Signaling via β-receptors does not appear to transduce pressure-overload hypertrophy, because it progresses similarly in combined β_1- and β_2-receptor knockout mice relative to wild-type controls.[78] Importantly, targeted ablation of β_1-receptors results in absence of contractile response to adrenergic agonists, underscoring an essential role for β_1-receptors in transducing the effects of catecholamines to govern contractility.[73] In contrast, disruption of β_2-receptors has minimal consequences, such as impaired isoproterenol-mediated vasodilation and differences in energy metabolism.

β_1- and β_2-receptors have distinct effects on cardiomyocyte apoptotic cell death, related to the specifics of each G-protein coupling pathway. Signaling via the Gαs-coupled β_1-receptors (but not β_2-receptors) stimulates cell death via reactive oxygen species and activation of the JNK family of MAP kinases, leading to mitochondrial cytochrome c release and mitochondrial permeability transition pore opening.[73] Sustained β_1 signaling also increases intracellular free Ca^{2+} via the L-type Ca^{2+} channel, resulting in activation of CaMKIIδ and cardiomyocyte apoptosis.[79] Indeed, CaMK inhibition with forced expression of a dominant-negative CaMKIIδ mutant attenuates cardiomyocyte apoptosis, prevents hypertrophy and left ventricular remodeling, and protects against isoproterenol-induced cardiomyopathy. At physiological levels, activation of β_2 adrenoceptor signaling switches from the stimulatory Gsα pathway to the inhibitory Giα signaling pathway by means of receptor phosphorylation by PKA activated downstream of the Gsα subunit. This, in turn, triggers dissociation of the Gβγ subunit from Giα, resulting in activation of the PI3K-Akt survival pathway (see Figure 1-5).

Cyclic AMP generation also activates transcription. Indeed, a counterbalance among cAMP response element binding ATF/CREB family transcription factors, namely CREB2 and CREM, appears to regulate transcription downstream of β_1-adrenergic receptors. CREB2 antagonism with forced cardiac expression of a dominant-negative isoform results in dilated cardiomyopathy with progressive left ventricular (LV) remodeling, cardiac dysfunction, and heart failure, whereas CREM inactivation rescues cardiomyocyte hypertrophy, fibrosis, and left ventricular dysfunction in β_1-adrenoceptor-overexpressing mice.[80] Also, enhanced β_1-adrenergic signaling results in activation of NGF1a-binding protein (Nab1), a transcriptional repressor of early growth response (Egr) transcription factors, which attenuates pressure-overload hypertrophy and prevents its decompensation.[81] These studies point to a fine balance in transcriptional activation that determines cell fate with β_1-adrenergic receptor signaling.

Activation of the β_1-receptors leads to recruitment of G-protein kinases (GRKs), which phosphorylate the cytoplasmic tail of the receptor and inhibit receptor signaling (see Figure 1-5).[82] GRK-mediated recruitment of β-arrestins 1 and 2 also mediates internalization of the receptors in clathrin-coated pits, resulting in downregulation of signaling. The internalized receptors can either be recycled back to the plasma membrane upon cessation of stimulus, or targeted for lysosomal and ubiquitin–proteasome-mediated degradation by ubiquitination of β-arrestin. However, the GRK-β-arrestin complex also acts as a scaffold for recruitment of tyrosine kinases of the Src family, resulting in activation of the MEK-1-ERK signaling cascade to mediate prohypertrophic effects. The complex nature of the temporal and spatial consequences of activation of this pathway is highlighted by divergent pathways that are activated downstream (discussed later).

GRK2, 5, and 6 are predominantly expressed in the myocardium.[83] Activation of GRK2 and GRK5 modulates cardiac function, because forced cardiac expression of either is sufficient to attenuate isoproterenol-mediated increases in contractility. Conversely, their cardiac ablation or dominant-negative inhibition results in enhancement of the contractile response.[83]

GRK2 plays a critical role in cardiac development, and its activation has differential effects depending upon the chronicity of the inciting stimulus. Indeed, loss of GRK2 prevents adverse ventricular remodeling in the setting of chronic isoproterenol infusion by downregulating β_1-receptor signaling, but its inhibition prevents heart failure after myocardial infarction likely by preventing receptor downregulation in the acute setting.[83] In pressure-overload hypertrophy, GRK2 expression increases with stimulation of β_2-receptor phosphorylation to enhance inhibitory G(i) signaling. In this setting, inhibition of G(i) with pertussis toxin rescues contractile dysfunction and prevents cardiac decompensation.[84] The protective effects of nitric oxide stimulation in this setting may also be transduced by preventing GRK2-mediated downregulation of β_1-adrenergic receptors.[83] Interestingly, enhanced GRK2 signaling in the adrenal gland has been implicated as the culprit in provoking sympathetic hyperactivation in heart failure by downregulating adrenal α_2-adrenoreceptors and preventing the feedback inhibition of catecholamine release. These studies suggest that GRK2 inhibition may be a therapeutic strategy, targeting multiple elements of heart failure pathophysiology.[83] Activation and nuclear localization of GRK5 is observed downstream of Gαq signaling in pressure-overload hypertrophy, where it functions as a histone deacetylase to activate the transcription factor MEF2 and provoke pathological hypertrophic signaling.[85]

A novel survival pathway is triggered by GRK-mediated recruitment of β-arrestin to the receptor, which leads to cleavage of heparin-binding EGF ligand by a membrane-bound matrix metalloprotease.[82] EGF receptor transactivation in this fashion protects against catecholamine-induced cardiomyopathy by enhancing survival signaling. Indeed, β-adrenergic blockers may vary in their clinical efficacy in patients with heart failure because of their ability to provoke signaling through this novel pathway.[86]

CASCADES THAT TRANSDUCE HYPERTROPHIC SIGNALING

As discussed previously, pathological cardiomyocyte hypertrophy is a central event in the pathogenesis of cardiac failure, such that persistent and progressive activation of hypertrophic signaling cascades in hypertrophied myocytes can lead to failure. Reactive hypertrophy with cardiac injury results in decreased intrinsic contractility of hypertrophied myocytes because of changes in contractile protein isoforms, the calcium cycling apparatus, and metabolic efficiency.[87] This further impairs global cardiac function, stimulating more hypertrophy and ultimately cardiomyocyte death, accelerating decompensation and the transition to dilated cardiomyopathy. This section examines the current state of knowledge regarding biochemical and molecular events that promote, transduce, and ultimately produce heart failure.

Biomechanical Sensors of Hypertrophic Stimuli

It is widely accepted that the major stimulus for hypertrophy is increased wall stress that results from elevated hemodynamic load, globally or regionally in response to injury, as sensed by individual myocytes and perhaps by other resident cell types in the heart. Mechanical deformation or stretching cultured cardiomyocytes on deformable substrates provokes reactive hypertrophy with upregulation of early response and fetal genes and increased protein synthesis in the absence of DNA synthesis.[33] In vivo, cardiomyocytes are intricately connected to the extracellular matrix (ECM), such that stretch is transduced via the intercellular and ECM connections via proteins located on the cell surface and subcellular adhesion complexes, termed *costameres*, and via stretch-sensing proteins within the cardiomyocyte Z-line (**Figure 1-6**).[15]

Transient receptor potential (TRP) channels are present within the plasma membrane at the cell surface and transduce stretch-activated Ca^{2+} current in cardiac myocytes (see Figure 1-6).[15] A subset of these channels is also activated by diacylglycerol (DAG), a key signaling molecule downstream of prohypertrophic Gαq signaling. Studies have confirmed an important role for two family members, TRPC1 and TRP6, in transducing pressure-overload hypertrophy in mouse models.[88] A recent study has ascribed an important role for the TRP vanilloid 4 (TRPV4) channel in transducing pulmonary edema in heart failure.[89] In this study, TRPV4 expression was found to be increased in lungs from patients with heart failure-induced pulmonary edema, and blockade of these channels by an orally administered chemical inhibitor prevented increases in vascular permeability and pulmonary edema.

Integrins, a diverse family of cell surface receptors, comprise α- and β-subunits in various combinations, each with an extracellular domain that interacts with extracellular matrix proteins and a short cytoplasmic tail that interacts with the cytoskeleton at the focal adhesion complex (see Figure 1-6).[90] Accordingly, studies have established that stretch and neurohormonal signaling activate hypertrophic pathways downstream of integrin signaling through multiple pathways, including (1) recruitment and activation of focal adhesion kinase (FAK), a tyrosine kinase; (2) activation of Src family members, which are membrane-bound SH2 domain-containing tyrosine kinases; (3) tyrosine phosphorylation of Grb2-associated binder (Gab) family proteins, with docking and activation of PI3K/Akt and ERK1/2 signaling; (4) activation of the serine/threonine kinase integrin-linked-kinase (ILK); and (5) recruitment of adaptor proteins, such as melusin and vinculin.

Shp2 (Src homology region 2, phosphatase 2), a phosphatase that tonically inhibits prohypertrophic FAK signaling, is inactivated by stretch to stimulate hypertrophy. The following lines of evidence[90] suggest that the integrin-costamere signaling axis plays an essential role in cardiac homeostasis and transduction of hypertrophic stress: (1) Cardiomyocyte-specific ablation of FAK prevents pressure overload-induced hypertrophy and induction of ANF, and in vivo siRNA-mediated FAK antagonism prevented and even reversed established pressure-overload hypertrophy with transverse aortic constriction. (2) Cardiomyocyte-specific gene targeting of ILK or the β_1-subunit results in spontaneous cardiomyopathy. (3) Ablation of melusin, a striated muscle-specific protein that interacts with the cytoplasmic tail of β_1-integrin, prevented the myocardial hypertrophic response to pressure overload. (4) Talin, a protein located in costameres, is observed to be upregulated with pressure overload, and cardiomyocyte-specific Talin-2 ablation attenuates pressure-overload hypertrophy and contractile dysfunction.[91]

Another sensing apparatus for mechanical stretch is postulated to exist within structural proteins in the Z-disc, where

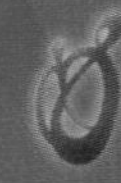

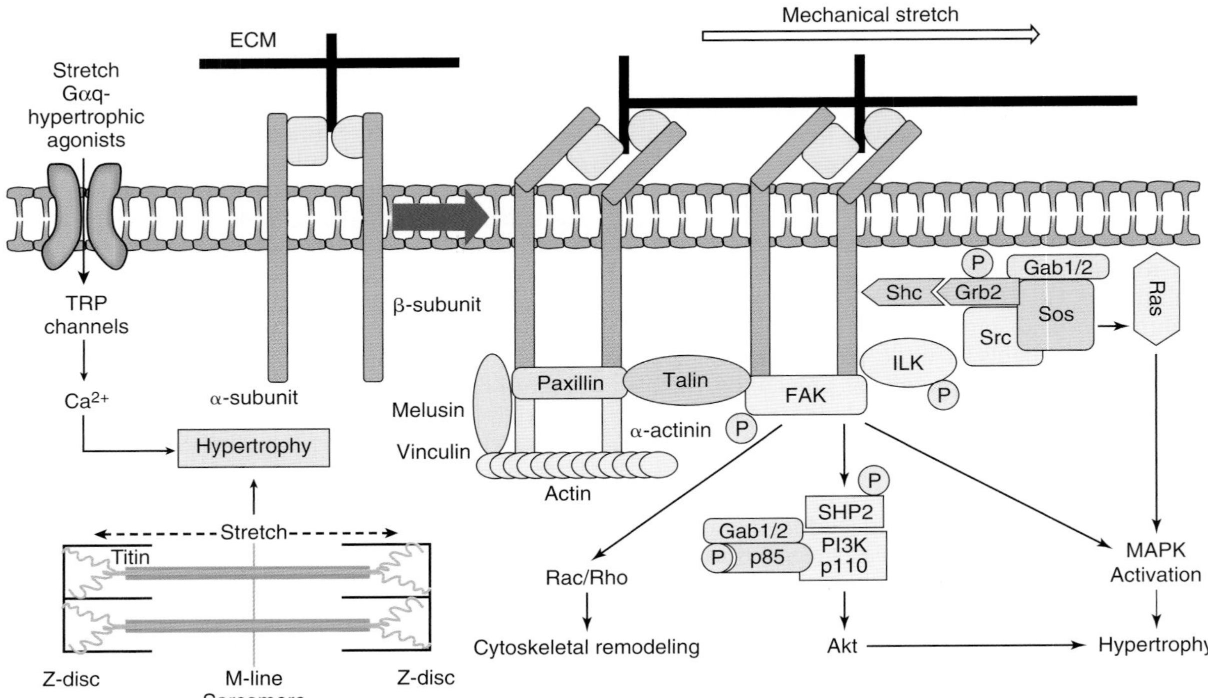

FIGURE 1-6 Cellular transduction of biomechanical stress. Integrins are heterodimeric proteins formed by the association of various combinations of single-transmembrane α- and β-subunits, which are attached to extracellular matrix proteins, such as laminin and fibronectin. Biomechanical stress induces changes in conformation and integrin clustering, resulting in assembly of the focal adhesion complex comprising the kinases FAK, Src, and ILK, along with adaptor proteins vinculin, paxillin, talin, α-actinin, and melusin that connect the integrins to the cytoskeletal elements (actin). Stretch-mediated phosphorylation and activation of FAK and ILK causes MAPK (ERK) activation and Akt activation via the SHP2/PI3K pathway resulting in hypertrophic signaling. Additionally FAK activates small G proteins Rac and Rho (see below), which transduce cytoskeletal reorganization in hypertrophy. Integrin signaling also activates Ras via Shc/Grb2/Gab1/2-mediated Src kinase activation, which transduces hypertrophic signaling via MAPK (ERK) activation. Stretch and hypertrophic agonists also cause activation of transient receptor potential (TRP) channels, resulting in Ca^{2+} entry that stimulates progrowth signaling. Titin (blue) is a giant sarcomeric protein that acts as a molecular spring to connect the Z-disc to the M line, and senses stretch to activate signaling via its C-terminal kinase domain.

the small LIM-domain protein MLP (muscle LIM protein) is anchored and transduces stress stimuli.[92] Titin, a large sarcomeric protein component of the thin filament anchors the Z-disk at one end and extends to the M line at the other; it is postulated to function as a molecular spring providing passive stiffness to the cell and acting as a biomechanical sensor with stretch-induced activation of its C-terminal kinase domain at the M-line (see Figure 1-6).[93] A recent exciting discovery has implicated mutations in the gene coding for Titin as the most common cause of familial dilated cardiomyopathy (observed in 25% of all cases).[94] Titin is also a major determinant of resting cardiomyocyte elasticity, and hypophosphorylation of its more compliant isoform N2B (which is transcriptionally induced as an adaptive response in pathological hypertrophy) has been implicated as a cause of diastolic stiffness in patients with heart failure with preserved ejection fraction (HFpEF).[93] Of note, telethonin, a titin-associated protein localized to the Z-disc in normal cardiomyocytes, can be mislocalized within the nucleus in human heart failure, and its ablation in cardiomyocytes prevents hypertrophy and induces massive apoptosis in response to pressure overload.[95]

Neurohormonal and Growth Factor Signaling (see also Chapters 5 and 6)

Pathological hypertrophy is also transduced via autocrine and paracrine release of neurohormones and growth factors that signal through highly specialized cognate receptors.[33] Mechanical stretch induces autocrine secretion of angiotensin II, endothelin-1, and peptide growth factors, such as FGF. Also, conditioned medium from stretched myocytes provokes hypertrophy in unstretched cardiomyocytes, attesting to the presence of a paracrine and/or autocrine signaling pathway for hypertrophy. In vitro studies suggest that integrins may also upregulate angiotensin II generation to transduce hypertrophic stimuli.[90] Interestingly, pressure-overload hypertrophy may be transduced by stretch-triggered signaling via activation of the AT1 receptor without the need for angiotensin,[96] suggesting redundancy at the cell membrane level in transduction of mechanical load to the cardiomyocyte. Additionally, mechanical stretch provokes production of neurohormones, growth factors, and cytokines by nonmyocytes in the heart, leading to cardiac fibroblast proliferation, and acting as an amplification loop to increase neurohormonal effects on cardiomyocytes.

Neurohormones, such as epinephrine, angiotensin II, and endothelin, signal via heptahelical transmembrane receptors coupled to heterotrimeric G proteins. G proteins comprise three polypeptide chains: α, β, and γ (**Figure 1-7**). The α-subunits are organized into four primary groups, Gαs, Gαi, Gαq, and Gα12/13, and are largely responsible for determining activation of downstream signaling effectors. Signaling through Gαq-coupled receptors by Ang II and other neurohormones activates phospholipase C, which catalyzes hydrolysis of phosphatidyl inositol 4,5 bis-phosphate (PIP2) to inositol 1,4,5 triphosphate (IP3) and diacylglycerol (DAG). DAG and IP3 activate protein kinase C (PKC), a family of powerful growth-stimulating serine/threonine kinases. IP3 also interacts with IP3 receptors (IP3Rs) to trigger

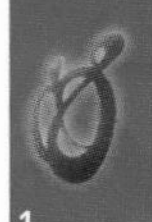

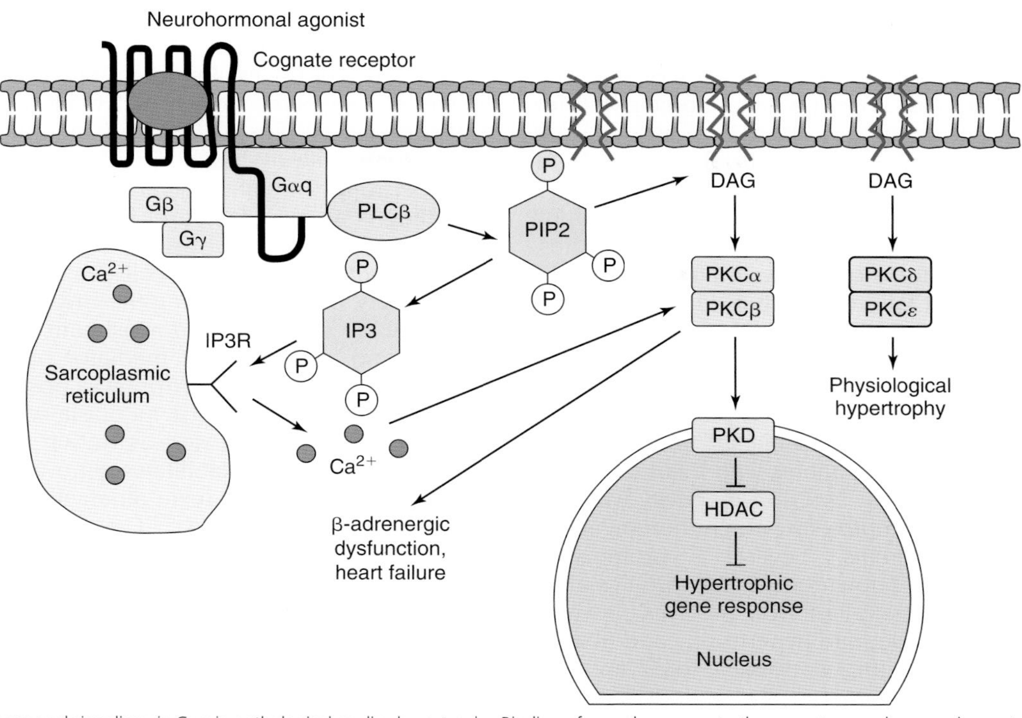

FIGURE 1-7 Neurohormonal signaling via Gαq in pathological cardiac hypertrophy. Binding of neurohormones to the cognate neurohormonal receptor causes GTP exchange and activation of the Gα subunit, with dissociation from the Gβγ subunit and recruitment of PLCβ to the cell membrane. PLCβ causes hydrolysis of PIP2 with generation of IP3 and DAG. IP3 binds to IP3 receptors (IP3Rs) on the sarcoplasmic reticulum, triggering Ca^{2+} release, which elicits PKC activation along with DAG for classical PKCs (α and β). Novel PKCs (δ and ε) are activated by DAG alone. See text for details of PKC signaling in heart failure. Classical PKCs activate PKD, which phosphorylates class II HDACs (5 and 9), resulting in export from the nucleus and derepression of hypertrophic gene transcription.

intracellular Ca^{2+} release, which can activate signaling through Ca^{2+}-dependent PKCs, Ca^{2+}-calmodulin-dependent kinases (CaMKs), and calcineurin. Cytosolic Ca^{2+} also interacts with DAG to activate PKC (see Figure 1-7). PTEN is a phosphatase that dephosphorylates the 3' position on IP3 and shuts down this signaling pathway. Another arm of signaling is triggered by the dissociated (free) Gβγ subunits, leading to recruitment and activation of PI3Kγ to the sarcolemma to facilitate interaction with phosphoinositides (see Figure 1-7).

α-Adrenergic Receptors

As discussed earlier, heart failure is associated with sympathetic activation and increased circulating levels of catecholamines that activate α_1-adrenergic receptors leading to Gαq activation. There are three subtypes: α_1A/C, α_1B, and α_1D, of which the first two are present in the human and mouse myocardium, but are not observed to be differentially regulated in heart failure.[97] In vitro, norepinephrine and phenylephrine stimulate cardiomyocyte hypertrophy, which is marked by increases in protein synthesis, induction of early response genes, reactivation of the fetal gene program, and increases in cell size. Studies investigating the in vivo role of these receptors in hypertrophy point to redundancy in signaling via the two cardiac-expressed α_1-adrenergic receptor subtypes, as individual genetic ablation of the α_1A/C or α_1B receptors alone reveals a role in blood pressure modulation without an effect on cardiac hypertrophy. In contrast, combinatorial ablation of both subtypes together points to an essential role for α_1-receptor signaling in normal postnatal cardiac growth and hypertrophy. Indeed, the double knockout hearts were 40% smaller than wild type, with reduced cardiomyocyte cross-sectional area and mRNA content, decreased ERK (but not Akt) activation, and a lack of reduction in blood pressure (i.e., at similar afterload). Interestingly, mice with combinatorial α_1A and α_1B ablation manifest an equivalent hypertrophic response with pressure overload as compared with controls, along with markedly decreased survival, decreased upregulation of fetal genes, and increased cell death and fibrosis. These findings may stem from lack of prosurvival signaling via the ERK pathway. Together, these studies indicate that α-adrenergic receptors play a crucial role in normal cardiac growth, but are redundant for pathological hypertrophic signaling, primarily regulating cell survival in this setting.

Angiotensin Signaling

Angiotensin II (Ang II), a powerful vasoconstrictor, derives from sequential cleavage of circulating angiotensinogen by renin and angiotensin-converting enzyme (ACE). Reducing Ang II levels via pharmacological inhibition of ACE is a cornerstone of therapy for cardiomyopathy and heart failure in humans (**see also Chapters 5 and 34**).

Endothelin

Endothelin-1 (ET-1) is a 21-amino acid polypeptide cleaved from a larger precursor by endothelin converting enzyme primarily by endothelial cells, and to a smaller extent in cardiomyocytes and fibroblasts. ET-1 signals via the ET1A and ET1B receptors, which are both coupled to Gαq, such that ET1 is sufficient to induce cardiomyocyte hypertrophy in vitro. Although ET1 appears to be a part of the autoregulatory loop with Ang II, as ET1 receptor blockade antagonizes AngII-mediated hypertrophy, it does not play a nonredundant role in transducing pathological hypertrophy.[33]

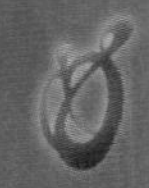

Gαq/PLC/PKC Signaling Axis

Redundancy in signal transduction at the receptor level in pathological hypertrophy prompted evaluation of heterotrimeric G proteins, Gαq and G11, as potential nodal points for targeting pathological signaling. Indeed, Gαq and G11 are critical mediators of pathological hypertrophic signaling, as combined cardiomyocyte-specific ablation of Gαq and G11 prevents development of pressure-overload hypertrophy and attenuates fetal gene expression and fibrosis with preservation of myocardial function.[98] The importance of this pathway to human heart failure is further demonstrated by the observation that polymorphisms in the gnaq (Gαq) gene with a single base pair change from GC to TT at position -694/-695 in the promoter results in increased Gαq promoter activity. This is associated with increased prevalence of left ventricular hypertrophy in normal subjects[99] and increased mortality in African American patients with heart failure.[100]

Gαq signaling is terminated by GTPase activity, which is markedly enhanced by RGS proteins, which thereby act as negative regulators of G proteins.[101] Several RGS proteins are expressed in the heart. RGS2 downregulates Gαq/G11 signaling, and transgenic expression of RGS proteins prevents development of pressure-overload hypertrophy and fibrosis via inhibition of Gαq signaling. Conversely, RGS2 ablation worsens pressure-overload hypertrophy without affecting the physiological hypertrophic response to swimming exercise. Importantly, activation of protein kinase G via inhibition of phosphodiesterase 5 (PDE5) caused sustained localization of RGS2 to the Gαq receptors and prevented development of pressure-overload hypertrophy.

Phospholipase Cβ (PLCβ) is a prototypical downstream effector of Gαq and Gβγ signaling (see Figure 1-7). Activation of PLCβ via Gαq receptors has been observed in pathological hypertrophy in vivo.[102] Of the four isoforms, $PLC\beta_1$ and β_3 are expressed in the heart. While in vitro studies suggest an essential role for PLCβ isoforms in transducing Gαq-mediated hypertrophic signals, in vivo confirmation of this will require tissue-specific targeting. This is due to the observation that germline $PLC\beta_1$ knockout mice develop seizure activity, and $PLC\beta_3$ knockout mice harbor abnormalities in neutrophil chemotaxis and skin ulcers, but no apparent abnormalities in normal cardiac development. Levels of PLCε, another cardiac-expressed phospholipase (which is downstream of nonreceptor tyrosine kinase signaling such as with Ras), are observed to be elevated in human dilated cardiomyopathy, and in response to isoproterenol treatment and pressure overload. Germline ablation of PLCε results in contractile dysfunction with reduced β-adrenergic responsiveness, and exaggerated catecholamine-induced cardiomyopathy and decompensation, indicating an essential role in modulating β-adrenoceptor signaling in heart failure.

Activation of PKCs downstream of Gαq/PLCβ has emerged as a key mediator of altered myocardial contractility and cardiomyocyte survival in pathological hypertrophic signaling (see Figure 1-7).[102] In the heart, the functionally important PKC isoforms are PKCα and β ("conventional" PKCs, which are activated by DAG with a requirement for Ca^{2+}); PKC δ and ε ("novel" PKCs, activated by DAG without a requirement for Ca^{2+}); and PKC ζ and ι/λ ("atypical" PKCs, that bind PIP3 and ceramide, but not DAG or PMA). Upon activation, PKCs translocate to specific subcellular locations, such as PKCα to the membrane, $PKC\beta_1$ to the nucleus, and PKCε to the myofibrils; PKCδ redistributes in a perinuclear location.

In the rodent heart, Gαq signaling in pressure-overload hypertrophy and heart failure upregulates PKCα and translocates PKCε to the membrane.[103] PKCα activation negatively regulates myocardial contractility but not the hypertrophic response.[104] Indeed, inhibition of PKCα prevents contractile dysfunction without affecting the degree of hypertrophy in pathological hypertrophic states.[104] PKCβ signaling is also not required for transducing hypertrophy with pressure overload or phenylephrine.[103] PKCδ appears to be a critical modifier of cell death in response to ischemic injury, without affecting the myocardial hypertrophic response. PKCε is activated downstream of pressure-overload stimuli, and is a potential mediator of postnatal cardiac growth and adaptive hypertrophy, as postnatal PKCε inhibition results in myocardial hypoplasia with heart failure.[103] Additionally, PKCε-mediated activation of aldehyde dehydrogenase in ischemia facilitates removal of reactive oxygen species (ROS)-induced toxic aldehydes and offers cardioprotection in this setting.[105] Ca^{2+}-dependent, nonconventional PKCs also activate protein kinase D (PKD) (**Figure 1-8**). Protein kinase D directly phosphorylates class II HDACs (histone deacetylases), resulting in their export from the nucleus and derepression of transcription. PKD1 activation is involved in transducing hypertrophy, as siRNA-mediated knockdown of PKD1 prevents hypertrophic cardiomyocyte growth by agonists that signal via Gαq and Rho GTPase. Also, cardiomyocyte-specific deletion of PKD1 prevents pressure-overload hypertrophy with preserved cardiac function and prevention of remodeling.[106] In myocardial ischemia, calpain-mediated cleavage of PKCα releases a constitutively active fragment PKMα, which activates PKD with nuclear to cytoplasmic transport of the transcriptional repressor HDAC5 and activation of pathological gene transcription.[107] These studies with modulation of PKC pathways highlight the qualitative nature of hypertrophic signaling, wherein differential activation of divergent pathways downstream of common nodal points determines its adaptive or pathological nature.

Mitogen Activated/Stress Activated Protein Kinase (MAPKs/SAPKs) Signaling Cascades

Activation of G protein–coupled receptors generates dissociated Gβγ subunits, which crosstalk with small GTPase proteins (see later discussion) or directly activate mitogen activated protein kinases (MAPKs).[104] Multiple other signaling pathways, such as receptor tyrosine kinases, serine/threonine kinases (e.g., downstream of transforming growth factor-β [TGF-β] signaling), Janus-activated kinases (JAK-STAT activation via the gp130 receptor), and stress stimuli such as stretch, activate MAPK pathways. MAPKs are three tiered cascades consisting of a MAPKKK (MAP3K or MEKK), a MAPKK (MEK), and a MAPK, the transducer of the signal downstream from the cascade. There are three major groups of MAPKs: extracellular signal regulated kinases (ERK), c-Jun N-terminal kinases JNKs (also known as stress-activated protein kinase and/or SAPKs and p38s. Specific MAPKKs activate specific MAPKs: MAPKK1/2 for ERK1/2, MAPKK3/6 for p38s, and MAPKK4/7 for JNKs. At the next tier, each MAPKKK can activate different MAPKK-MAPK pathways, suggesting a mechanism for integration of upstream signaling. MAPKs phosphorylate multiple substrates, including enzymes and transcription factors with overlapping specificity that regulate cardiac gene expression ("immediate early response" factors), cell survival, mRNA translation

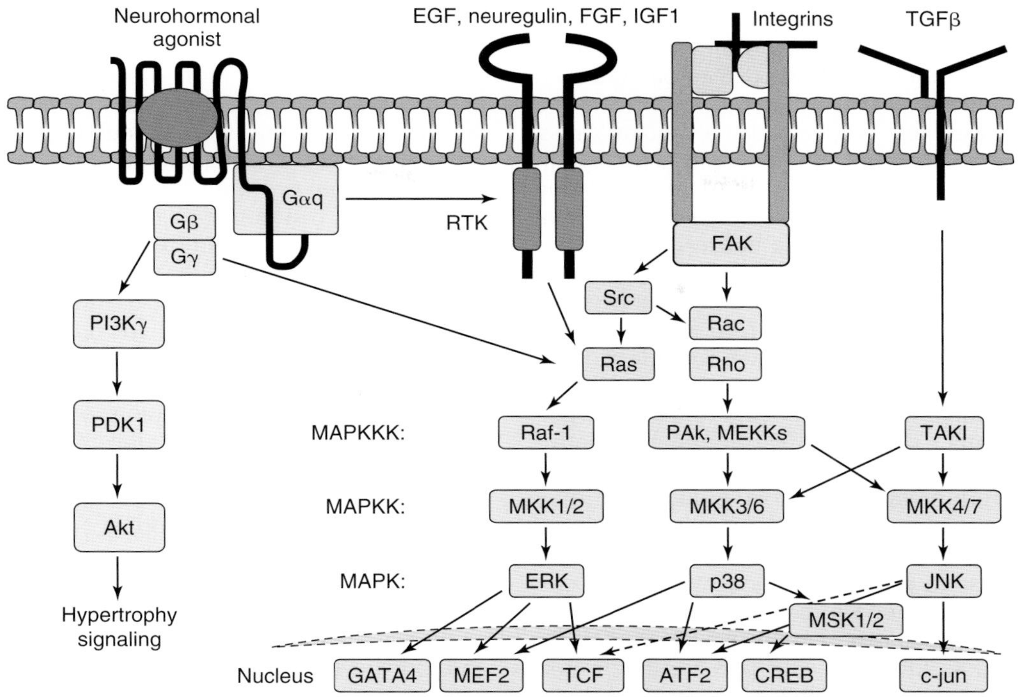

FIGURE 1-8 Neurohormonal activation of MAPK signaling in pathological hypertrophy. Activated Gαq protein causes activation of small G proteins such as Ras either directly via the released Gβγ subunits or via crosstalk with receptor tyrosine kinases (RTKs), which are activated by growth factors such as EGF, neuregulin, FGF, and IGF-1 (see later in text). This leads to stimulation of the mitogen-activated protein kinase (MAPK) signaling cascades. MAPKs are also activated by integrin signaling and TGF receptor-mediated activation of TAK1. MAPK cascades are organized into three tiers: MAPKinase kinase kinases (MAPKKKs) that activate MAPKinase kinases (MAPKKs), which subsequently activate MAPKinases. MAPKs signal redundantly via multiple transcription factors (see details in text). Gβγ subunits of the Gαq signaling complex also activate PI3Kγ, resulting in Akt activation and hypertrophy signaling.

(eIF4E), and mRNA stability. Specificity for downstream substrates is primarily determined via docking interactions to integrate downstream signaling. For example, while p90RSKs are phosphorylated primarily by ERK1/2, MAPKAPK2 is phosphorylated by p38-MAPK, and Msk1/2 may be phosphorylated by either ERK1/2 or p38-MAPK.

At the top tier of kinases are the MAPKKKs (see Figure 1-8) such as mammalian sterile 20-like kinase 1 (Mst1), which is a mammalian homolog of Hippo, a master regulator of cell death, proliferation, and organ size in *Drosophila*.[108] Forced expression of Mst1 elicits an apoptotic cardiomyopathy. Rassf1A (Ras-association domain family 1 isoform A), a Ras-GTP binding protein, acts as an activator of Mst1 and appears to play divergent roles in cardiomyocytes and fibroblasts.[109] Whereas cardiomyocyte-specific ablation of Rassf1A protects against pressure overload-induced hypertrophy and decompensation, germline ablation of Raasf1A results in markedly enhanced myocardial fibrosis with cardiac-pressure overload.[109] These discrepant findings were resolved by the observation that loss of Rassf1A in cardiac fibroblasts results in enhanced TNF-α generation, with increased cell death and fibrosis in the heart. Another upstream serine threonine kinase, Lats2, activates Mst1, and its transgenic expression results in reduced heart size. Conversely, expression of a dominant-negative Lats2 mutant results in hypertrophy, indicating that the Lats2-Mst1 pathway is also a negative regulator of cardiomyocyte size.[110] In aggregate, these studies illustrate how the same pathway may promote cardiomyocyte apoptosis but suppresses fibroblast activation, highlighting the need for targeting specific cell types for desirable effects.

Subsequent stepwise activation of kinases culminates in the activation of the effector kinases (see Figure 1-8).[108] ERK1/2 is activated via Gαq signaling in response to hypertrophic agonists (e.g., Ang II, PE, ET1, and stretch) in vitro and by pressure overload in vivo.[104] Accumulated evidence suggests a predominant role for the ERK signaling axis in promoting hypertrophy, and the p38 and JNK axes in regulating cell death and fibrosis. Forced expression of MEK-1-ERK1 causes concentric hypertrophy, via activation of the calcineurin-NFAT pathway without adverse ventricular remodeling.[104]

A role for the ERK pathway in hypertrophic signaling was interrogated with combinatorial gene ablation studies, wherein ERK2 was silenced in a cardiomyocyte-specific manner,[111] or inferred from studies with transgenic expression of MEK-1. Interestingly, while MEK-1 activation provoked concentric hypertrophy, ablation of both ERK1/2 did not affect normal cardiac growth or development of pressure-overload hypertrophy. Rather, it resulted in dilated, eccentrically hypertrophied chamber morphology with lengthening of myocytes and contractile dysfunction mimicking observations with volume overload-induced hypertrophy. ERK1/2-mediated phosphorylation of GATA4 at serine 105 is critical for its ability to transduce pathological cardiac growth, as knock-in mice homozygous for a nonphosphorylatable mutant at this locus did not manifest hypertrophy in response to pressure overload or angiotensin II infusion.[112] Rather, these stimuli led to rapid development of cardiac failure, indicating that ERK1/2-GATA4-mediated cardiac growth is predominantly consistent with physiologically hypertrophied myocardium.

ERK5 is related to ERK1/2 with a similar activation motif, and is activated in the heart in response to gp130 signaling (by LIF or cardiotrophin 1). Similar to ERK1/2, forced cardiac expression of MEK-5 (activator of ERK5, also called *big ERK*) triggers eccentric cardiac hypertrophy associated with the addition of sarcomeres in series, and cardiomyocyte-specific ablation of ERK5 attenuated pressure overload-induced hypertrophy and fibrosis.[113]

p38 and JNK kinases were originally discovered as "stress-responsive kinases" on account of their rapid activation in response to stressful stimuli.[108] Of the four genes encoding p38's, p38α is the most abundant in the heart, with minimal p38β detected. p38 and JNK signal via transcription factors c-jun, ATF2, ATF6, Elk-1, p53, and NFAT4. Loss-of-function modeling with transgenic expression of dominant-negative mutants of p38α or p38β, as well as p38α gene ablation, revealed an antihypertrophic effect in exercise-induced and pathological hypertrophy. Similarly, stress-induced JNK signaling (c-Jun N-terminal kinases) appears to be antihypertrophic, because mice with either dominant-negative repression or combined ablation of JNK1 and 2, exhibit increased basal and pressure overload-induced cardiac mass with depressed calcineurin-NFAT signaling. Combinatorial ablation of JNK1, 2, and 3 increases cardiomyocyte apoptosis in response to pressure overload with rapid cardiomyopathic decompensation, indicating a prominent role for these stress-induced kinases in cell survival signaling.[108]

The terminal MAPKs ERK, JNK, and p38 are inactivated by dephosphorylation at serine/threonine residues by a family of dual specificity phosphatases. This feedback inhibition is critical for maintaining basal cardiac function, because combinatorial ablation of DUSP1 and DUSP4 provokes cardiomyopathy with unrestrained activation of p38. This progressive cardiomyopathy and cardiac dysfunction was prevented with pharmacological p38 inhibition, indicating a redundant role for these two phosphatases (as individual knockout was of no consequence) in cardiac homeostasis.[114]

Ask-1 is a MAPKKK that is upregulated in the myocardium by angiotensin stimulation via AT1R-induced oxidative stress and NFkB activation.[108] Activation of Ste20/oxidant stress response kinase 1 (SOK-1), an Mst family member known to be activated by oxidant stress, mediates Ask-1 activation in this setting. Ask-1 ablation significantly attenuates cardiomyocyte apoptosis and cardiomyopathic decompensation induced by angiotensin infusion in response to pressure overload or coronary artery ligation, yet without an effect on hypertrophic signaling. Conversely, overexpression of Ask1 induces cardiomyocyte apoptosis and accelerates development of heart failure via activation of the calcineurin axis.[115] Indeed, Ask1 physically interacts with subunit B of calcineurin (PP2B), resulting in enhancement of Ask1 activity by calcineurin-induced dephosphorylation. Ask1-p38α signaling is a negative regulator of adaptive hypertrophy, as mice with Ask1 ablation display increased cardiomyocyte hypertrophy when subjected to swimming exercise, as is also observed in p38α-deficient mice subjected to the same stimulus.[116] This was associated with reduced PP2A activity, with resultant increases in phosphorylation and activation of Akt.

One of the central kinases upstream of ERKs is Raf-1 (and the related B-Raf).[108] Deletion of Raf-1 led to increased cardiomyocyte death with LV dysfunction and dilation in mice. However, this did not appear to be due to ERK inhibition. Rather, the apoptosis signal regulating kinase (ASK1) was activated (as were Jnks and p38), and deleting ASK1 rescued the LV dilatation and dysfunction. Thus, Raf-1 is a critical regulator of cell death in the heart, acting through ASK1.

IP3-Induced Ca^{2+}-Mediated Signaling

Gαq signaling results in generation of IP3, which interacts with intracellular receptors to generate Ca^{2+} fluxes, which are localized to microdomains and lead to compartmentalization of Ca^{2+}-induced signaling (**Figure 1-9**).[102] This segregates the signaling effects of local Ca^{2+} alterations from the global Ca^{2+} transients that determine contraction. For example, β_2-adrenergic receptors are associated with caveolin-3 protein within caveolar microdomains in cardiomyocytes, and this allows for the regulation of L-type Ca^{2+} channel activity with β_2-dependent activation, which is prevented by disruption of the caveolar architecture.[117] Other examples of spatially localized IP3-induced Ca^{2+} release that affect signaling are calsarcin-mediated regulation of Ca^{2+}-induced activation of the prohypertrophic phosphatase calcineurin at the Z-disk and perinuclear CaMK signaling to influence gene transcription via export of HDACs[118]. IP3R-mediated Ca^{2+} release is sufficient to transduce a mild hypertrophic phenotype in mouse myocardium, and regulates the hypertrophic response to various Gαq agonists. However, this axis is not required for pressure overload-induced hypertrophy, as indicated by studies with transgenic expression of an IP3 "sponge" in cardiomyocytes.[119]

Calcineurin/NFAT Axis and CaMK Signaling

IP3-mediated release of intracellular Ca^{2+} downstream of hypertrophic Gαq signaling activates the calcineurin and CaMK pathways (see Figure 1-9).[102] Calcineurin (Cn), a serine/threonine phosphatase (also known as protein phosphatase 2B, PP2B), is stimulated by Ca^{2+} binding to calmodulin and dephosphorylates the transcription factor NFAT at an N-terminal serine residue.[120] This allows for NFAT translocation to the nucleus. The functional protein is a dimer comprising two subunits, A and B. Cn is encoded by three genes (CnA α, β, and γ) and CnB by two genes (CnB1 and B2), of which the mammalian heart only expresses CnAα, CnAβ, and CnB1. In vitro stimulation of cardiomyocytes with hypertrophic stimuli (PE, AngII, ET-1) activates calcineurin, and forced expression of activated calcineurin results in pronounced cardiac hypertrophy progressing to heart failure.[121] Calcineurin activity is increased in human compensated LV hypertrophy, in the myocardium of patients with heart failure, and in animal models of both pressure overload-induced and exercise-induced cardiac hypertrophy.[120] Studies employing pharmacological inhibition of calcineurin activity with FK506 and cyclosporine have demonstrated that calcineurin transduces pathological hypertrophic signaling both in vitro, in response to PE, Ang II, and ET1, and in response to pressure overload in vivo.[121] Confirmatory evidence for calcineurin signaling in pathological hypertrophy has emerged from studies in mice harboring ablation of the CnAβ gene. This results in an 80% reduction in calcineurin activity and results in attenuated cardiomyocyte hypertrophy in response to pressure overload or infusion of neurohormones. Calcineurin is localized at the Z-disc in a complex with calsarcins, providing access to NFAT proteins.[120] Ablation of calsarcin-1 increases pressure overload-induced calcineurin signaling, resulting in rapid progression to heart failure. Signaling via FGF23 with activation of the calcineurin-NFAT pathway has also been implicated in development of LV hypertrophy in patients with chronic kidney disease, who often develop heart failure with preserved ejection fraction (HFpEF).[122] This could be

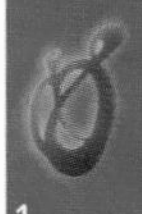

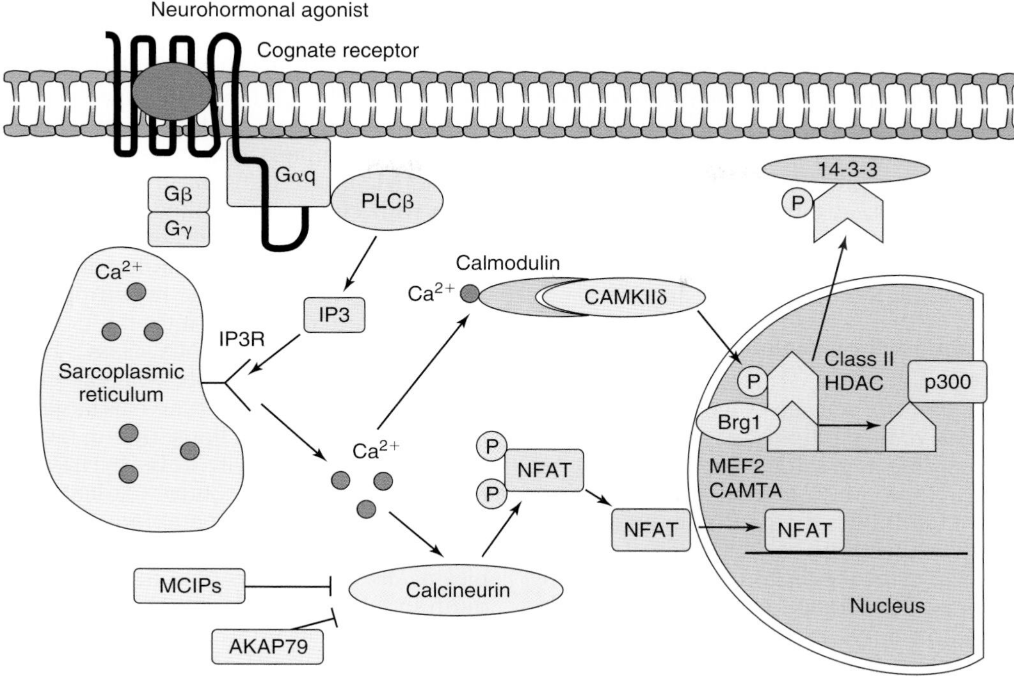

FIGURE 1-9 Neurohormonal activation of calcineurin and CAMK signaling. Gαq/Gα11-mediated production of IP3 via PLCβ causes release of intracellular Ca^{2+} from the SR via the IP3Rs, leading to activation of the protein phosphatase, calcineurin. Calcineurin dephosphorylates NFAT transcription factor, resulting in its nuclear translocation and activation of hypertrophy gene transcription. AKAP79 and MCIPs are endogenous inhibitors of calcineurin activity. The increased cytoplasmic calcium concentration (Ca^{2+} (i)) also causes activation of CAMKs via interaction with calmodulin. CAMKs phosphorylate class II HDACs, resulting in HDAC translocation out of the nucleus and binding to 14-3-3 protein in the cytoplasm. This allows histone acetylation by HAT p300, derepressing hypertrophic gene transcription mediated by transcription factors such as MEF2 and CAMTA. Brg1 is a transcriptional modulator that associates with HDACs on the MHC gene promoters to enhance β-MHC *(MYH7)* and suppress α-MHC *(MYH6)* transcription. Brg1 gets turned off at birth during normal growth and is reactivated in pathological hypertrophy signaling to affect the shift in myosin heavy chain gene expression.

a significant step forward in our understanding of the mechanisms in this population.[47]

Activation of calcineurin (and the NFAT axis) is triggered by elevated cytosolic Ca^{2+}, and the source of the elevated Ca^{2+} levels has been the subject of extensive investigation. Potential candidates include the L-type Ca^{2+} channel (LTCC),[123] the T-type Ca^{2+} channel,[124] and transient receptor potential channels (TRPCs). The LTCC mediates Ca^{2+}-induced Ca^{2+} release during each depolarization, which drives excitation-contraction coupling. Mice with heterozygous germline deletion or cardiomyocyte-specific ablation of the α_1c subunit of the LTCC manifest mild reductions in LTCC current in adulthood, with mild impairment in cardiac function and development of cardiac hypertrophy with aging.[125] When these mice were subjected to swimming (physiological exercise) or pathological stress (pressure overload or isoproterenol infusion) in young adulthood, exaggerated hypertrophy and rapid development of heart failure was observed. This was driven by activation of the calcineurin-NFAT axis because of elevated cytosolic Ca^{2+}. A subsequent study, which selectively targeted LTCCs located only in caveolin-3 microdomains, ablated Ca^{2+} influx-mediated NFAT activation with minimal reduction in basal Ca^{2+} current, indicating that focal LTCC-mediated Ca^{2+} release in microdomains may trigger pathological signaling via calcineurin-NFAT pathway.[126]

In the heart, all four NFAT isoforms are present, and NFAT transcription factors are essential for normal cardiac development.[120] Ablation of NFATc2 and NFATc3, but not NFATc4, protects against pressure overload and angiotensin-induced hypertrophy with attenuated expression of fetal genes, without affecting development of exercise-induced adaptive hypertrophy.[120] The upstream regulators of NFAT signaling reflect the extensive crosstalk between various signaling pathways and include GSK3β (which is discussed further below), p38, and JNK MAP kinases.[108] These factors generally phosphorylate and inactivate NFAT by facilitating nuclear export, accounting for some of the observed antihypertrophic actions.

Calcineurin signaling is restrained by modulatory calcineurin inhibitory proteins, or MCIPs, which bind to calcineurin to inhibit its activity.[120] MCIP1 gene transcription is activated in the heart by calcineurin-mediated NFAT signaling, providing a negative feedback loop for repression of calcineurin signaling, whereas MCIP2 expression is induced by thyroid hormone signaling. Forced expression of MCIP1 is antihypertrophic and results in a reduction in unstressed adult heart weight (by 5% to 10%), and attenuates both physiological hypertrophy induced by swimming and pathological hypertrophy induced by calcineurin activation or pressure overload.[120] MCIP1 overexpression also attenuates development of pathological hypertrophy after myocardial infarction with preservation of systolic function. This suggests a beneficial effect of preventing pathological hypertrophy signaling in the surviving myocardium. Also, suppression of calcineurin signaling via induction of MCIP1 confers antihypertrophic signaling downstream of the vitamin D receptor.

While these studies indicate that enhanced MCIP1 signaling is primarily antihypertrophic, loss of function by MCIP1 gene ablation did not lead to overt phenotypic abnormalities, indicating that basal MCIP1 levels do not regulate eutrophic cardiac growth.[120] Rather, MCIP1 ablation paradoxically attenuated the hypertrophic response to pressure overload, and combinatorial ablation of both MCIP1 and MCIP2 attenuated both swimming-induced and pressure overload-induced hypertrophy. This indicates that regulation of hypertrophy via MCIP1 may be bimodal, wherein endogenous levels are required for hypertrophic signaling, and elevated levels can inhibit other prohypertrophic pathways. A small EF hand domain-containing protein and integrin-binding protein-1 (CIB1) was recently discovered in a screen for mediators of calcineurin-induced pathology and identified as another critical mediator of calcineurin-mediated pathology in pressure-overload hypertrophy and dysfunction.[127]

Signaling via Ca^{2+}/Calmodulin-Dependent Protein Kinase (CaMK)

Increased cytosolic Ca^{2+} also activates CaMKs, a family of enzymes that phosphorylate multiple Ca^{2+} handling proteins to regulate myocardial contractility (see Figure 1-9). All four CaMKs, I-IV, can activate MEF2-mediated transcription of fetal genes in vivo.[79] CaMKIIδ is the predominant cardiac isoform, and forced expression of CaMKIIδb (nuclear isoform) or CaMKIIδC (cytosolic isoform) in cardiomyocytes is sufficient to cause pathological hypertrophy. CaMKIIδ isoforms bind to and phosphorylate HDAC4, a class II histone deacetylase, resulting in its export from the nucleus. This leads to derepression of cardiac gene expression. Ablation of CaMKIIδ attenuates pressure overload-induced hypertrophy via inhibition of HDAC4.[128] Aldosterone-mediated ROS generation causes oxidation and activation of CaMKII, which may explain its deleterious cellular effects in cardiac myocytes,[129] because myocardial CaMKII inhibition, or NADPH oxidase deficiency, prevented aldosterone-induced activation of MMPs and cardiac rupture after myocardial infarction. Additionally, mitochondria-localized CaMKII modulates mitochondrial calcium uniporter activity and regulates susceptibility to mitochondrial permeability transition under stress. Accordingly, inhibition of mitochondrial CaMKII prevents MPTP-driven mitochondrial calcium overload and cell death in ischemia-reperfusion injury.[130]

Epigenetic Regulation of Transcription in Cardiac Hypertrophy

Reversible acetylation of histone proteins governs steric access of transcription factors, such as MEF2 and CAMTA, to the chromatin machinery. Histones are nuclear proteins within the nucleosome, a compact structure consisting of chromatin genomic DNA tightly coiled around histone octamers. This structure prevents access of transcription factors to DNA and represses gene expression. Histone acetyltransferases (HATs) acetylate conserved lysine residues in histone tails, neutralizing their positive charge, resulting in destabilization of histone-histone and histone-DNA interactions. This limits access of DNA binding proteins, such as transcription factors, to DNA (see Figure 1-9). Thus, HATs generally stimulate gene expression. In contrast, histone deacetylases (HDACs) counter this effect, promoting chromatin condensation and repressing transcription (see Figure 1-9).

HATs belong to five families, and p300 and CREB binding protein (CBP) are the most abundant HAT family members in cardiac muscle. P300 binds to and acts as a transcriptional coactivator for GATA4, MEF2, and SRF, and dominant-negative p300 prevents the acetylation and coactivation of GATA4 downstream of G signaling, resulting in a cardiomyopathy.[120] Evidence supporting therapeutic targeting of p300 in prevention and treatment of pathological hypertrophy has emerged from studies of p300 HAT inhibition by curcumin (a polyphenol abundant in the spice turmeric). Pretreatment with curcumin prevented development of hypertrophy and cardiac decompensation in response to pressure overload or phenylephrine infusion in vivo in mice.[131] Treatment of mice with curcumin resulted in compensated myocardial hypertrophy after induction of pressure overload or phenylephrine infusion and was sufficient to cause regression of cardiomyocyte and cardiac hypertrophy.[131]

HDACs are classified into three categories based on homology with yeast HDACs. Class I HDACs comprise primarily a catalytic domain, whereas class II HDACs have phosphorylation sites that serve as targets for signaling pathways and interact with transcription factors. Class III HDACs require NAD for activity. Class II HDACs (HDAC4, HDAC5, HDAC7, and HDAC9) control cardiac growth by translocation across the nuclear membrane to the cytoplasm. HDACs are commonly associated with MEF2 proteins in the nucleoplasm. MEF2 activity is held in check in the adult myocardium by binding to class II HDACs (HDAC4, 5, and 7). This repression is relieved by phosphorylation of HDACs by Ca^{2+}/calmodulin kinases (CaMK), which causes HDAC export out of the nucleus, and enhances association of p300 with MEF2, promoting gene transcription.[120] By this mechanism, multiple hypertrophic signaling pathways, including MAPKs, calcineurin, CaMKII, and protein kinase D, converge on MEF2 activation by class II HDAC export, relieving transcriptional repression. Indeed, MEF2D-mediated transcriptional activation plays an essential role in stress-induced fetal gene regulation with cardiomyocyte-specific MEF2D deletion preventing development of hypertrophic ventricular remodeling in response to pressure-overload stress.[132]

Forced expression of class II HDACs, HDAC5, and HDAC9 prevents hypertrophy in response to agonists such as phenylephrine or serum in vitro.[120] In contrast, HDAC5- and HDAC9-null hearts develop spontaneous cardiac hypertrophy with derepression of MEF2 activity, as well as profoundly exaggerated hypertrophy in response to pressure overload.[120] Their response to swimming-induced hypertrophy is not altered, suggesting these HDACs predominantly regulate pathological hypertrophy. Spatial regulation of this signaling occurs through local inositol 1,4,5-trisphosphate receptors (InsP3Rs) situated in the nuclear envelope, where IP3 produced in response to Gαq-coupled endothelin (ET-1) receptor activation causes local Ca^{2+} release, CaMKII activation, and HDAC5 export.[118] This provides a mechanism to separate Ca^{2+}-mediated transcriptional changes from the beat-to-beat cycling that determines contractility.

In contrast to class II HDACs, class I HDACs (HDACs 1, 2, 3, and 8) stimulate cardiac growth. HDAC2-null mice are resistant to myocardial hypertrophic stimuli, and HDAC2 transgenic mice manifest an exaggerated hypertrophic response involving HDAC2-mediated suppression of the gene encoding inositol polyphosphate-5-phosphatase f (Inpp5f), resulting in activation of Akt-PDK1 signaling with constitutive activation of GSK-3β.[133] Additionally, chemical inhibition of GSK3β (see later discussion) results in resensitization to the hypertrophic response in vivo in HDAC2-deficient hearts, implicating increased GSK3β-mediated antihypertrophic signaling in the absence of HDAC2 as the mechanism for suppression of hypertrophy. Pharmacological inhibition of histone deacetylases by Trichostatin A and

Scriptaid, two broad-spectrum HDAC inhibitors, or SK7041, an HDAC class I-specific inhibitor, suppresses hypertrophy by a dominant effect on class I HDACs.[133]

Deacetylation mediated by class III HDACs (Sirt2 family of kinases) requires NAD+ and produces 2'-O-acetyl-ADP-ribose (O-AADPR) and nicotinamide. Both Sirt1 and Sirt2 are induced by ischemia/reperfusion injury in the heart, but while ablation of Sirt1 protects against cardiac myocyte death,[134] Sirt2 signaling triggers cardiomyocyte death. This appears to be due to acetylation of RIP1 kinase by Sirt2, which mediates activation of programmed necrosis via TNF-α-mediated activation of the RIP1-RIP3 complex. Mice with Sirt2 ablation are relatively protected against programmed necrosis in ischemia/reperfusion injury.[135] Sirt3 activation in the myocardium confers antihypertrophic signaling via FoxO3-mediated induction of ROS scavenging enzymes. Mice with Sirt3 ablation developed spontaneous hypertrophy with dysfunction and fibrosis at 10 weeks of age.[136]

Recently, epigenetic regulation by a chromatin remodeling protein, Brg1, has been assigned an important role in maintaining fetal gene expression in the myocardium before birth.[137] Brg1 associates with HDAC2 and HDAC9 on the α-MHC promoter and with PARP on the β-MHC promoter to suppress or activate transcription, respectively, in the fetal state. Expression of Brg1 is extinguished soon after birth to depress transcription in the postnatal period but is rapidly reactivated with pressure overload and other hypertrophic stresses to provoke reexpression of the fetal gene program.

Crosstalk Between Gαq and PI3K/Akt Hypertrophic Signaling Pathways

Gαq/phospholipase C pathways also crosstalk with the PI3K/Akt signaling axis in transducing pathological hypertrophy signals (**Figure 1-10**).[102] Gαq-coupled receptors activate PI3Kγ, an isoform that is different from the α-isoform, which is activated in physiological hypertrophy mediated by the IGF-1 pathway. The mechanism of activation also differs. PI3Kα is activated by receptor tyrosine kinase-mediated phosphorylation. PI3Kγ binds to Gβγ dissociated from Gαq after ligand interaction, providing access to membrane phosphoinositides (see Figures 1-8 and 1-10). PI3Kγ (p110γ) signals through Akt and is required for pressure overload-induced hypertrophy.[102,120] Also, in contrast to brief activation of p110α by exercise in stimulating physiological hypertrophy, activation of p110γ is sustained downstream of Gαq signaling and recruits additional signaling pathways, namely the phospholipase Cβ and calcineurin/NFAT axis to determine the pathological nature of hypertrophy.[102,120] PI3Kγ null mice develop rapid cardiac dilation despite maintaining preserved ventricular contractility in response to pressure-overload stress. This is due to increased β-adrenoreceptor-CREB-mediated transcriptional activation of MMPs and extracellular matrix breakdown.[138]

Signaling downstream of Akt is divergent (see Figure 1-10), which may also help determine whether the hypertrophy is adaptive or maladaptive. One axis involves activation of mTOR (mammalian target of rapamycin) kinase and induction of protein synthesis. mTOR exists in

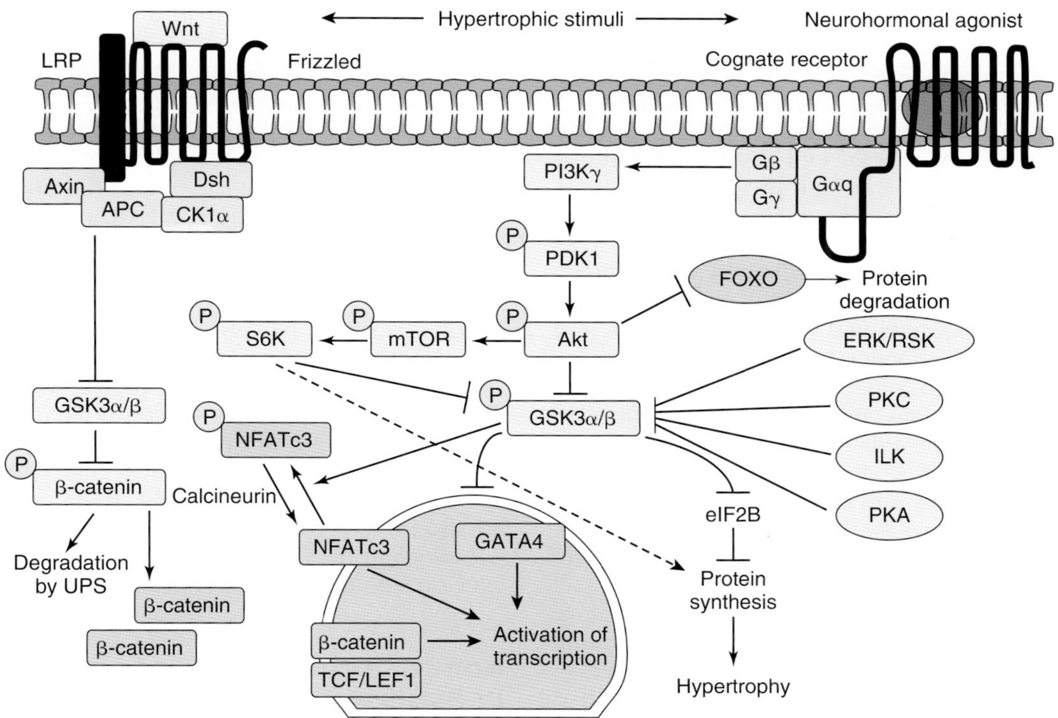

FIGURE 1-10 Regulation of hypertrophy via Wnt/β-Catenin and Akt/mTOR/GSK3β signaling. Wnt signaling is activated by hypertrophic stimuli to assemble the LRP-Frizzled-Dishevelled receptor signaling complex together with other proteins, Axin, APC, and CK1α, which induces dephosphorylation of GSK3α/β to relieve the tonic inhibition and prevent degradation of β-catenin by the ubiquitin-proteasome system. This causes accumulation of β-catenin, which translocates to the nucleus to associate with transcription factor TCF/LEF1, and initiate hypertrophic gene transcription. In response to neurohormonal receptor activation, Gαq and Gβγ subunits dissociate. Subsequently, Gβγ-mediated PI3Kγ activation leads to Akt activation and stimulation of protein synthesis via mTOR and suppresses antihypertrophic signaling via GSK3β. Akt also phosphorylates and causes export of FoxO transcription factors from the nucleus, suppressing protein degradation via the ubiquitin-proteasome pathway. GSK3α/β exerts tonic inhibition on multiple prohypertrophic transcription factors and its phosphorylation relieves this inhibition resulting in hypertrophic signaling. Inhibition of GSK3α/β is a nodal point for convergence of hypertrophic signaling pathways and also occurs via phosphorylation by PKA (downstream of Gsα), PKCs (downstream of Gαq), ERK/ribosomal S6 kinases (downstream of small G protein signaling), and ILK (downstream of integrin signaling).

two complexes: mTORC1 or mTORC2. Raptor is rapamycin sensitive and is the predominant mass-regulating complex downstream of Akt. mTORC2, with Rictor and Sin, controls the actin cytoskeleton and determines cell shape. Signaling downstream of mTor plays a central role in mediating pathological hypertrophic signaling, because conditional ablation of mTOR in the adult myocardium provokes rapid onset of cardiomyopathy with widespread apoptosis, altered mitochondrial ultrastructure, and accumulation of eukaryotic translation initiation factor 4E-binding protein 1.[139] Also, cardiomyocyte-specific ablation of Raptor results in inhibition of mTORC1 and spontaneous development of cardiomyopathy with lack of hypertrophy in response to pressure overload.[140] These findings suggest a primary role for mTOR in facilitating cardiomyocyte hypertrophy and survival in response to stress.

A second Akt pathway leads to phosphorylation and suppression of glycogen synthase kinase (GSK3β) with disinhibition of hypertrophic signaling (see Figure 1-10). GSK3β is tonically active in the myocardium and its phosphorylation by Akt relieves downstream antihypertrophic signaling.[141] GSK3β is also phosphorylated and activated by protein kinase A (PKA) and in response to activation of the Gαq/PKC/ERK/p90 ribosomal S6kinase axis, thereby derepressing downstream hypertrophic signaling. In vivo, pressure overload causes rapid phosphorylation of GSK3β within 10 minutes after transverse aortic constriction is applied, pointing to early recruitment of the kinase in the hypertrophic response.[141] Germline ablation of GSK3β results in embryonic lethality with lack of cardiac differentiation of embryoid bodies, congenital defects, and markedly hypertrophied ventricular chamber resulting from increased cardiac myocyte proliferation.[141] This indicates a prominent developmental role for GSK3β.

In myocardial ischemia, GSK3β activation, via a constitutively active knock-in, reduced infarct size, whereas dominant-negative GSK-3β expression or heterozygous ablation worsened ischemia-induced cell death with parallel modulation of ischemia-induced autophagy.[141] In contrast, virtually opposite observations were made with reperfusion injury, the reasons for which are not clear. GSK3β may play a prominent role in suppressing cardiomyocyte proliferation in response to stress, because adult-onset inducible GSK-3β null mice demonstrate less ventricular dilation and postinfarct remodeling associated with increased cardiomyocyte proliferation, with ischemia/reperfusion injury.

Just as GSK-3β, GSK3α signaling is antihypertrophic. In contrast to GSK3β, germline ablation of GSK3α did not elicit developmental abnormalities, but resulted in progressive cardiomyocyte hypertrophy and dysfunction. Pressure overload was associated with a markedly enhanced hypertrophic response that rapidly transitioned to dilation, along with markedly impaired β-adrenergic responsiveness.[141] GSK3α mice subjected to ischemia/reperfusion injury before spontaneous development of hypertrophy also manifest exaggerated hypertrophy and worse postinfarction remodeling as compared with wild-type mice.[142] Taken together, these data suggest a prominent role for GSK3β in suppressing cardiomyocyte proliferative capacity, whereas GSK3α signaling may be predominantly antihypertrophic in the adult myocardium.

A novel mechanism for the antihypertrophic effects of GSK3β signaling may be through the canonical Wnt signaling axis, which is under tonic repression by GSK3β-mediated signaling (see Figure 1-10).[50] Wnts are extracellular proteins that signal either from cell to cell as membrane-bound proteins or as secreted proteins via heptahelical Frizzled receptors and single transmembrane-pass coreceptors known as *low-density lipoprotein receptor-related proteins* (LRPs). Tonic activity of GSK3β phosphorylates β-catenin, a transcription factor, at three sites, targeting it for degradation by the ubiquitin-proteasome system. With activation of Wnt signaling via Frizzled-LRP receptors, the entire complex is recruited to the receptor with scaffolding proteins, resulting in phosphorylation of LRP and Dishevelled, which inhibits GSK3β and prevents GSK3β-mediated phosphorylation of β-catenin. In this form, β-catenin accumulates in the nucleus and forms a complex with a transcription factor TCF/LEF1 (T-cell-specific transcription factor/lymphoid enhancer factor 1) by displacing a binding protein Groucho, thereby activating gene transcription.

Wnt signaling plays an important role in the cardiac response to hypertrophic stimuli, as mice with adult-onset cardiomyocyte-specific β-catenin ablation displayed marked attenuation of hypertrophy in response to pressure overload with reduced expression of c-fos and c-jun, without any adverse consequence on myocardial function. Furthermore, mice with cardiomyocyte-specific overexpression of a dominant inhibitory mutant of Lef-1 manifest profound cardiomyocyte growth impairment with reduced heart weight, contractile dysfunction, and early death.[50] In contrast, β-catenin stabilization leads to decreased cardiomyocyte size, with upregulation of the atrophy-related protein IGFBP5. The signaling pathways connecting hypertrophic stimuli to β-catenin signaling appear complex. This is because, in contrast to the insights gained from β-catenin ablation in pressure overload, it was the gain-of-function of β-catenin with stabilization and increased expression, and not cardiomyocyte-specific ablation, that attenuated angiotensin II-mediated hypertrophy.[50]

In addition to stimulating protein synthesis, Akt suppresses protein degradation via phosphorylation of FoxO (O family of forkhead/winged-helix) transcription factors.[143] Akt-mediated phosphorylation of FoxOs suppresses their transcriptional activity by facilitating interaction with 14-3-3 proteins, leading to export from the nucleus and targeting for ubiquitin-proteasomal degradation (see Figure 1-10). This prevents expression of proapoptotic genes and upregulation of the E3-ligase atrogin-1/MAFbx. Atrogin-1 is a cardiac and skeletal muscle-specific F-box protein that binds to Skp1, Cul1, and Roc1 (the common components of SCF ubiquitin ligase complexes), and regulates muscle atrophy. Atrogin-1 also ubiquitinates and activates FOXO to suppress Akt-mediated hypertrophy signaling. Therefore, suppression of atrogin-1 may provide another explanation for Akt-mediated pathological hypertrophic signaling when Akt is activated via Gαq signaling (see later discussion).

Non-IGF Growth Factor Signaling in Hypertrophy

Cardiac myocytes elaborate peptide growth factors in response to stress, including the prototypical growth factors neuregulin, EGF, and TGF-β (**Figure 1-11**). Neuregulin, a member of the epidermal growth factor (EGF) signaling pathway, activates tyrosine kinase receptors (ErbB2, ErbB3, and ErbB4), leading to dimerization, tyrosine autophosphorylation, and recruitment of downstream signaling

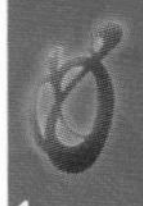

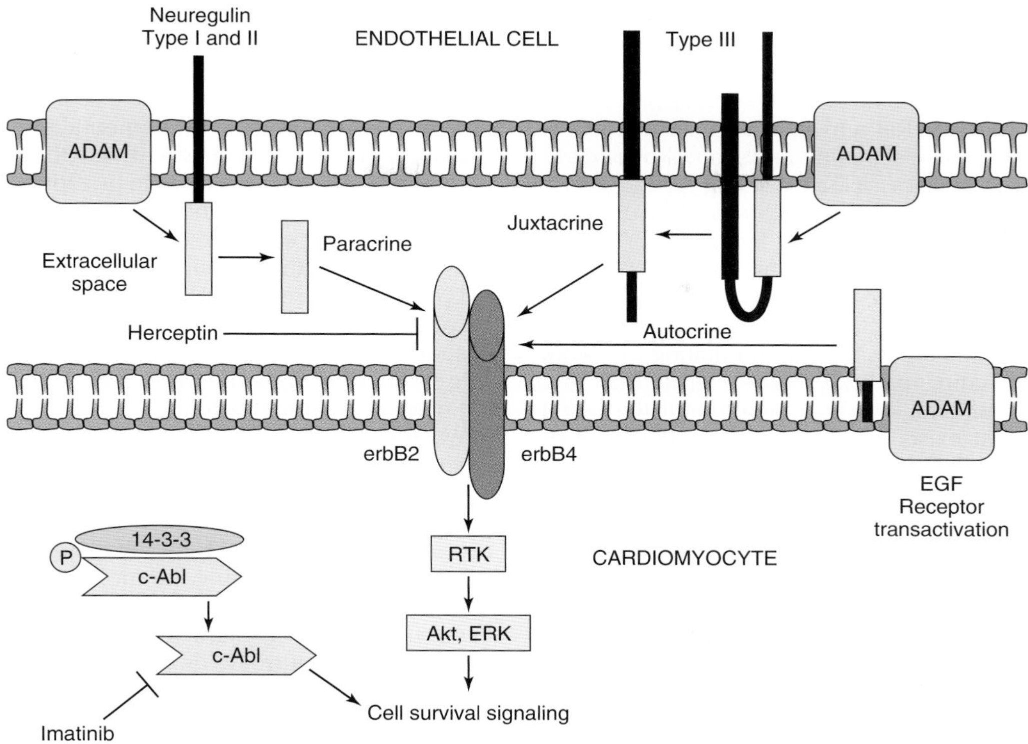

FIGURE 1-11 Neuregulin/EGF/c-Abl signaling in hypertrophy. Neuregulins are transmembrane proteins of the EGF family, present mainly on endothelial cells as three different types (I, II, and III). Proteolytic cleavage by ADAM (A disintegrin and metalloproteinase) family enzyme provokes exposure of an EGF-like signaling domain, which interacts with erbB2 and erbB4 receptors, resulting in receptor tyrosine kinase activation. EGF signaling is also activated by GRK-β-arrestin-mediated EGF cleavage by ligand-occupied seven transmembrane neurohormonal receptors. Neuregulins and EGF activate Akt and ERK signaling pathways to promote cell survival in the heart. Chromosomal translocation with formation of Bcr-cAbl fusion protein is implicated in the pathogenesis of chronic myeloid leukemia. Inhibition of endogenous c-Abl protein by imatinib (an antibody directed against the c-Abl protein [Imatinib]) and antagonism of the ErbB2/4 receptor by herceptin (an antibody-based chemotherapeutic agent used to treat breast cancer) antagonize c-Abl and neuregulin-mediated survival signaling, respectively, and this results in cardiomyocyte death and heart failure.

effectors.[144] All three isoforms of neuregulin are cleaved by membrane-bound metalloproteinases, producing an activated fragment that is released or associates with EGF receptor to provoke paracrine and juxtacrine signaling, respectively. Neuregulin is induced by pressure overload in the endothelium during development of concentric hypertrophy, and its levels decline along with those of cardiomyocyte ErbB2 and ErbB4 with transition to cardiomyopathic decompensation.[144] Neuregulin signaling primarily regulates cardiomyocyte survival, as endothelial cell-derived neuregulin protects cardiomyocytes against ischemic injury, but not hypertrophy.[144] Importantly, cardiomyocyte-specific ablation of ErbB2 or ErbB4 receptors results in spontaneous development of cardiomyopathy, accompanied by increased cardiomyocyte apoptosis.[144] These findings implicate the loss of neuregulin-mediated survival signaling as a major mechanism for the cardiotoxicity observed with use of trastuzumab, an antibody directed against the ErbB2 receptor, as a chemotherapeutic agent.

The transforming growth factor family is a large group of polypeptide growth factors. They are divided into two groups: the TGF/activin subfamily and the bone morphogenic proteins (BMP). TGF-β_1 is secreted in a latent form and is tethered to the extracellular matrix. Its stimulus-induced proteolytic cleavage allows interactions with its cognate cell-surface receptors, TGFβRI and TGFβRII, which are serine-threonine kinases that phosphorylate and activate downstream signaling proteins called *Smads*. Upon activation, Smad transcription factors translocate to the nucleus and activate gene transcription. TGF-β signaling also activates MAPKs (see later discussion) such as the TAK1 (TGF-activated kinase)-MEK-4-JNK1 and TAK1-MEK-3/6-p38 axes, and tyrosine kinase pathways, such as Ras/ and RhoA/p160 Rho-associated kinase (ROCK). TGF-β_1 signaling mediates angiotensin-induced hypertrophy as TGF-β_1-null mice manifest a markedly attenuated hypertrophic response with minimal fibrosis and ANF gene induction with preservation of myocardial function.[108] TAK1 is a MAP-KKKinase activated downstream of TGF-β and transduces p38 activation. An unexpected role for TAK1 signaling in regulating AMPK activation, and thereby regulating cellular energy stores, was discovered when forced expression of TAK1 in the heart elicited Wolf-Parkinson-White-like physiology with preexcitation,[145] recapitulating the phenotype with expression of an activated AMPK mutant. Smad 4 is the canonical transcription factor downstream of TGF-β signaling, and given the prohypertrophic effects of TGF-β_1 and its downstream MAPK kinase TAK1, it was unexpected that cardiomyocyte-specific gene ablation of Smad 4 would result in spontaneous cardiac hypertrophy with reexpression of fetal genes and activation of the MEK-1-ERK1/2 pathway.[108] This suggests that Smad4 signaling acts in an antihypertrophic manner in opposition to TGF-β-induced MAPK activation. Growth differentiation factor 15 (gdf15), another TGF-β family member induced by pressure overload, provokes antihypertrophic signaling. Indeed, forced cardiac expression of GDF15 attenuates pressure-overload hypertrophy and fibrosis, without affecting basal cardiac structure and function or expression of the fetal gene expression program.[108]

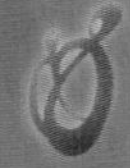

Role of Small G Proteins

Peptide growth factors and G protein–coupled receptors also transduce neurohormonal and stretch-induced hypertrophy via nonreceptor tyrosine kinases such as Src, serine-threonine kinases such as Raf, and small G proteins such as Ras. Ras is the prototypical signaling molecule downstream of receptor tyrosine kinases (RTKs) causing MAPK activation by recruitment of adaptor proteins Shc and Grb2, which bind the guanine nucleotide exchange factor (GEF) named *Sos* (Son of Sevenless) and activate Ras. The phosphotyrosine residues on the RTKs also interact with other proteins that have intrinsic catalytic activity, such as Src family tyrosine kinases, PI3Kγ and PLCγ, thereby mediating crosstalk between these signaling pathways (see Figure 1-8). Ras, along with Rac, Rho, and Rab, is a member of the small G-protein family that exists bound to GDP in the inactive state. Upon stimulation, GDP is exchanged for GTP and followed by a conformational change resulting in stimulation of mitogen activated protein kinase (MAPK) cascades. Intrinsic GTPase activity then extinguishes the signal, returning the G protein to its basal state. GEFs are proteins that facilitate GTP exchange, and GAPs promote inactivation by activating the GTPase activity. Ras and Rac1 are activated by Gαq agonists (PE, Ang II, endothelin-1, and mechanical stretch) and are sufficient to induce hypertrophy.[146] In contrast, mice with forced cardiomyocyte expression of Rho A do not develop hypertrophy and instead develop fatal cardiomyopathy.[146] RhoA activates Rho kinases, namely ROCK1 and ROCK2. Interestingly, ROCK1 deletion markedly reduces fibrosis in mice subjected to pressure overload, suggesting activation of maladaptive signaling pathways downstream of Rho in pressure-overload hypertrophy.[146] Rac1 also transduces hypertrophic signaling via increased generation of reactive oxygen species by NADPH oxidase signaling. Indeed, cardiomyocyte-specific gene ablation of Rac1 attenuates myocardial oxidative stress and hypertrophy in response to Ang II infusion.[146] Interestingly, Rad, another small G protein, is significantly downregulated in human heart failure and has an antihypertrophic role, as Rad knockout mice developed increased cardiac hypertrophy in response to pressure overload.[147]

A recent study has identified an essential role for a nonreceptor tyrosine kinase, c-Abl, in cardiomyocyte homeostasis (see Figure 1-11). This was based on the observations that some patients with chronic myelogenous leukemia, who were treated with imatinib (Gleevec), a small molecular inhibitor of the fusion protein Bcr-Abl, developed LV dysfunction.[148] Modeling of this process in mice revealed imatinib-induced cardiomyocyte death due to both apoptotic and necrotic pathways leading to myocardial dysfunction. Activation of ER stress and JNK activation were implicated in this process.

FUTURE DIRECTIONS

We have witnessed a breathtaking pace of discovery in the elucidation of the molecular basis of heart failure. Although the information presented above is inadequate to fully chronicle all the developments, we have tried to present a framework for understanding the complex and intricate signaling processes that govern cardiac growth, development, and pathology. Investigators and clinicians alike are acutely aware of the current limitations of heart failure therapeutics, with persistent high morbidity and mortality, and the nature of investigation has been increasingly refocused toward evaluating and developing therapeutic targets. Simultaneously, ground-breaking basic discoveries continue to be made, which often challenge the existing dogma, and stimulate innovation to tackle fundamental questions. One such discovery in recent years has been the appreciation that cardiomyocytes may continue to be replenished in the adult myocardium, which harbors a complement of resident cardiac cells that could be expanded and recruited to assist with cardiac repair. Another exciting possibility is the potential to predict disease risk and response to therapy based on an individual's genetic makeup. Given recent advances in sequencing technology and systems biology approaches, "big science," with its unbiased approaches to understanding disease, is rapidly taking center stage.

We are poised to enter an era of increased risk for cardiovascular diseases, driven by the current epidemic of obesity and westernization of cultures all over the world. The next generation of cardiac investigators will likely redirect their research efforts to tackle these challenges, while continuing to invest in understanding the molecular underpinnings of cardiac development and homeostasis. With rapid advances in our understanding of the molecular basis for heart failure continuing, the future holds exciting prospects that some of the therapeutic strategies highlighted in this chapter will be translated into clinical use in a safe and cost-effective manner.

References

1. Houser SR, Margulies KB, Murphy AM, et al: Animal models of heart failure: a scientific statement from the American Heart Association. *Circ Res* 111:131–150, 2012.
2. Louch WE, Sheehan KA, Wolska BM: Methods in cardiomyocyte isolation, culture, and gene transfer. *J Mol Cell Cardiol* 51:288–298, 2011.
3. Bellin M, Marchetto MC, Gage FH, et al: Induced pluripotent stem cells: the new patient? *Nat Rev Mol Cell Biol* 13:713–726, 2012.
4. Takahashi K, Tanabe K, Ohnuki M, et al: Induction of pluripotent stem cells from adult human fibroblasts by defined factors. *Cell* 131:861–872, 2007.
5. Gaj T, Gersbach CA, Barbas CF, III: ZFN, TALEN, and CRISPR/Cas-based methods for genome engineering. *Trends Biotechnol* 31:397–405, 2013.
6. Davis J, Maillet M, Miano JM, et al: Lost in transgenesis: a user's guide for genetically manipulating the mouse in cardiac research. *Circ Res* 111:761–777, 2012.
7. Degenhardt K, Singh MK, Epstein JA: New approaches under development: cardiovascular embryology applied to heart disease. *J Clin Invest* 123:71–74, 2013.
8. Takeda N, Manabe I, Uchino Y, et al: Cardiac fibroblasts are essential for the adaptive response of the murine heart to pressure overload. *J Clin Invest* 120:254–265, 2010.
9. Dewald O, Frangogiannis NG, Zoerlein MP, et al: A murine model of ischemic cardiomyopathy induced by repetitive ischemia and reperfusion. *Thorac Cardiovasc Surg* 52:305–311, 2004.
10. Bergmann O, Bhardwaj RD, Bernard S, et al: Evidence for cardiomyocyte renewal in humans. *Science* 324:98–102, 2009.
11. Porrello ER, Mahmoud AI, Simpson E, et al: Transient regenerative potential of the neonatal mouse heart. *Science* 331:1078–1080, 2011.
12. Porrello ER, Mahmoud AI, Simpson E, et al: Regulation of neonatal and adult mammalian heart regeneration by the miR-15 family. *Proc Natl Acad Sci U S A* 110:187–192, 2013.
13. Mahmoud AI, Kocabas F, Muralidhar SA, et al: Meis1 regulates postnatal cardiomyocyte cell cycle arrest. *Nature* 497:249–253, 2013.
14. Anversa P, Kajstura J, Rota M, et al: Regenerating new heart with stem cells. *J Clin Invest* 123:62–70, 2013.
15. Maillet M, van Berlo JH, Molkentin JD: Molecular basis of physiological heart growth: fundamental concepts and new players. *Nat Rev Mol Cell Biol* 14:38–48, 2013.
16. Perrino C, Prasad SV, Mao L, et al: Intermittent pressure overload triggers hypertrophy-independent cardiac dysfunction and vascular rarefaction. *J Clin Invest* 116:1547–1560, 2006.
17. Fagard R, Aubert A, Lysens R, et al: Noninvasive assessment of seasonal variations in cardiac structure and function in cyclists. *Circulation* 67:896–901, 1983.
18. Scheuer J, Malhotra A, Hirsch C, et al: Physiologic cardiac hypertrophy corrects contractile protein abnormalities associated with pathologic hypertrophy in rats. *J Clin Invest* 70:1300–1305, 1982.
19. Neri Serneri GG, Boddi M, Modesti PA, et al: Increased cardiac sympathetic activity and insulin-like growth factor-I formation are associated with physiological hypertrophy in athletes. *Circ Res* 89:977–982, 2001.
20. Kim J, Wende AR, Sena S, et al: Insulin-like growth factor I receptor signaling is required for exercise-induced cardiac hypertrophy. *Mol Endocrinol* 22:2531–2543, 2008.
21. Boudina S, Bugger H, Sena S, et al: Contribution of impaired myocardial insulin signaling to mitochondrial dysfunction and oxidative stress in the heart. *Circulation* 119:1272–1283, 2009.
22. Zhu W, Trivedi CM, Zhou D, et al: Inpp5f is a polyphosphoinositide phosphatase that regulates cardiac hypertrophic responsiveness. *Circ Res* 105:1240–1247, 2009.
23. Bostrom P, Mann N, Wu J, et al: C/EBPbeta controls exercise-induced cardiac growth and protects against pathological cardiac remodeling. *Cell* 143:1072–1083, 2010.
24. Ikeda Y, Sato K, Pimentel DR, et al: Cardiac-specific deletion of LKB1 leads to hypertrophy and dysfunction. *J Biol Chem* 284:35839–35849, 2009.
25. Bry M, Kivela R, Holopainen T, et al: Vascular endothelial growth factor-B acts as a coronary growth factor in transgenic rats without inducing angiogenesis, vascular leak, or inflammation. *Circulation* 122:1725–1733, 2010.
26. Delaughter MC, Taffet GE, Fiorotto ML, et al: Local insulin-like growth factor I expression induces physiologic, then pathologic, cardiac hypertrophy in transgenic mice. *FASEB J* 13:1923–1929, 1999.

27. Shiojima I, Sato K, Izumiya Y, et al: Disruption of coordinated cardiac hypertrophy and angiogenesis contributes to the transition to heart failure. *J Clin Invest* 115:2108–2118, 2005.
28. Pelliccia A, Maron BJ, De Luca R, et al: Remodeling of left ventricular hypertrophy in elite athletes after long-term deconditioning. *Circulation* 105:944–949, 2002.
29. Hill JA, Olson EN: Cardiac plasticity. *N Engl J Med* 358:1370–1380, 2008.
30. Willis MS, Rojas M, Li L, et al: Muscle ring finger 1 mediates cardiac atrophy in vivo. *Am J Physiol Heart Circ Physiol* 296:H997–H1006, 2009.
31. Riquelme CA, Magida JA, Harrison BC, et al: Fatty acids identified in the Burmese python promote beneficial cardiac growth. *Science* 334:528–531, 2011.
32. Grossman W, Jones D, McLaurin LP: Wall stress and patterns of hypertrophy in the human left ventricle. *J Clin Invest* 56:56–64, 1975.
33. Harvey PA, Leinwand LA: The cell biology of disease: cellular mechanisms of cardiomyopathy. *J Cell Biol* 194:355–365, 2011.
34. Katz AM: The cardiomyopathy of overload: a hypothesis. *J Cardiovasc Pharmacol* 18(Suppl 2):S68–S71, 1991.
35. Sano M, Schneider MD: Still stressed out but doing fine: normalization of wall stress is superfluous to maintaining cardiac function in chronic pressure overload. *Circulation* 105:8–10, 2002.
36. Braunwald E: Biomarkers in heart failure. *N Engl J Med* 358:2148–2159, 2008.
37. Oka T, Xu J, Molkentin JD: Re-employment of developmental transcription factors in adult heart disease. *Semin Cell Dev Biol* 18:117–131, 2007.
38. van Berlo JH, Elrod JW, van den Hoogenhof MM, et al: The transcription factor GATA-6 regulates pathological cardiac hypertrophy. *Circ Res* 107:1032–1040, 2010.
39. Huang J, Elicker J, Bowens N, et al: Myocardin regulates BMP10 expression and is required for heart development. *J Clin Invest* 122:3678–3691, 2012.
40. Takefuji M, Wirth A, Lukasova M, et al: G(13)-mediated signaling pathway is required for pressure overload-induced cardiac remodeling and heart failure. *Circulation* 126:1972–1982, 2012.
41. Jessup M, Greenberg B, Mancini D, et al: Calcium Upregulation by Percutaneous Administration of Gene Therapy in Cardiac Disease (CUPID): a phase 2 trial of intracoronary gene therapy of sarcoplasmic reticulum Ca2+-ATPase in patients with advanced heart failure. *Circulation* 124:304–313, 2011.
42. Margulies KB, Bednarik DP, Dries DL: Genomics, transcriptional profiling, and heart failure. *J Am Coll Cardiol* 53:1752–1759, 2009.
43. Kathiresan S, Srivastava D: Genetics of human cardiovascular disease. *Cell* 148:1242–1257, 2012.
44. Quiat D, Olson EN: MicroRNAs in cardiovascular disease: from pathogenesis to prevention and treatment. *J Clin Invest* 123:11–18, 2013.
45. Porrello ER, Johnson BA, Aurora AB, et al: MiR-15 family regulates postnatal mitotic arrest of cardiomyocytes. *Circ Res* 109:670–679, 2011.
46. Levy D, Garrison RJ, Savage DD, et al: Prognostic implications of echocardiographically determined left ventricular mass in the Framingham Heart Study. *N Engl J Med* 322:1561–1566, 1990.
47. van HL, Franssen CP, Hamdani N, et al: Molecular and cellular basis for diastolic dysfunction. *Curr Heart Fail Rep* 9:293–302, 2012.
48. Konstantinidis K, Whelan RS, Kitsis RN: Mechanisms of cell death in heart disease. *Arterioscler Thromb Vasc Biol* 32:1552–1562, 2012.
49. Hein S, Arnon E, Kostin S, et al: Progression from compensated hypertrophy to failure in the pressure-overloaded human heart: structural deterioration and compensatory mechanisms. *Circulation* 107:984–991, 2003.
50. Rao TP, Kuhl M: An updated overview on Wnt signaling pathways: a prelude for more. *Circ Res* 106:1798–1806, 2010.
51. Lombardi R, da GC-H, Bell A, et al: Nuclear plakoglobin is essential for differentiation of cardiac progenitor cells to adipocytes in arrhythmogenic right ventricular cardiomyopathy. *Circ Res* 109:1342–1353, 2011.
52. Olivetti G, Abbi R, Quaini F, et al: Apoptosis in the failing human heart. *N Engl J Med* 336:1131–1141, 1997.
53. Baumgarten G, Knuefermann P, Kalra D, et al: Load-dependent and -independent regulation of proinflammatory cytokine and cytokine receptor gene expression in the adult mammalian heart. *Circulation* 105:2192–2197, 2002.
54. Haudek SB, Taffet GE, Schneider MD, et al: TNF provokes cardiomyocyte apoptosis and cardiac remodeling through activation of multiple cell death pathways. *J Clin Invest* 117:2692–2701, 2007.
55. Levine B, Kalman J, Mayer L, et al: Elevated circulating levels of tumor necrosis factor in severe chronic heart failure. *N Engl J Med* 323:236–241, 1990.
56. Kurrelmeyer KM, Michael LH, Baumgarten G, et al: Endogenous tumor necrosis factor protects the adult cardiac myocyte against ischemic-induced apoptosis in a murine model of acute myocardial infarction. *Proc Natl Acad Sci U S A* 97:5456–5461, 2000.
57. Diwan A, Matkovich SJ, Yuan Q, et al: Endoplasmic reticulum-mitochondria crosstalk in NIX-mediated murine cell death. *J Clin Invest* 119:203–212, 2009.
58. Elrod JW, Wong R, Mishra S, et al: Cyclophilin D controls mitochondrial pore-dependent Ca(2+) exchange, metabolic flexibility, and propensity for heart failure in mice. *J Clin Invest* 120:3680–3687, 2010.
59. Sano M, Minamino T, Toko H, et al: p53-induced inhibition of Hif-1 causes cardiac dysfunction during pressure overload. *Nature* 446:444–448, 2007.
60. Accornero F, van Berlo JH, Benard MJ, et al: Placental growth factor regulates cardiac adaptation and hypertrophy through a paracrine mechanism. *Circ Res* 109:272–280, 2011.
61. Patten IS, Rana S, Shahul S, et al: Cardiac angiogenic imbalance leads to peripartum cardiomyopathy. *Nature* 485:333–338, 2012.
62. Hirota H, Chen J, Betz UA, et al: Loss of a gp130 cardiac muscle cell survival pathway is a critical event in the onset of heart failure during biomechanical stress. *Cell* 97:189–198, 1999.
63. Yajima T, Yasukawa H, Jeon ES, et al: Innate defense mechanism against virus infection within the cardiac myocyte requiring gp130-STAT3 signaling. *Circulation* 114:2364–2373, 2006.
64. Hilfiker-Kleiner D, Shukla P, Klein G, et al: Continuous glycoprotein-130-mediated signal transducer and activator of transcription-3 activation promotes inflammation, left ventricular rupture, and adverse outcome in subacute myocardial infarction. *Circulation* 122:145–155, 2010.
65. Yajima T, Murofushi Y, Zhou H, et al: Absence of SOCS3 in the cardiomyocyte increases mortality in a gp130-dependent manner accompanied by contractile dysfunction and ventricular arrhythmias. *Circulation* 124:2690–2701, 2011.
66. Komatsu M, Waguri S, Ueno T, et al: Impairment of starvation-induced and constitutive autophagy in Atg7-deficient mice. *J Cell Biol* 169:425–434, 2005.
67. Kuma A, Hatano M, Matsui M, et al: The role of autophagy during the early neonatal starvation period. *Nature* 432:1032–1036, 2004.
68. Lavandero S, Troncoso R, Rothermel BA, et al: Cardiovascular autophagy: concepts, controversies and perspectives. *Autophagy* 9, 2013.
69. Lai L, Leone TC, Zechner C, et al: Transcriptional coactivators PGC-1alpha and PGC-lbeta control overlapping programs required for perinatal maturation of the heart. *Genes Dev* 22:1948–1961, 2008.
70. Larsson NG, Wang J, Wilhelmsson H, et al: Mitochondrial transcription factor A is necessary for mtDNA maintenance and embryogenesis in mice. *Nat Genet* 18:231–236, 1998.
71. Abel ED, Doenst T: Mitochondrial adaptations to physiological vs. pathological cardiac hypertrophy. *Cardiovasc Res* 90:234–242, 2011.
72. Mann DL, Kent RL, Parsons B, et al: Adrenergic effects on the biology of the adult mammalian cardiocyte. *Circulation* 85:790–804, 1992.
73. Lohse MJ, Engelhardt S, Eschenhagen T: What is the role of beta-adrenergic signaling in heart failure? *Circ Res* 93:896–906, 2003.
74. Nikolaev VO, Moshkov A, Lyon AR, et al: Beta2-adrenergic receptor redistribution in heart failure changes cAMP compartmentation. *Science* 327:1653–1657, 2010.
75. Chakir K, Depry C, Dimaano VL, et al: Galphas-biased beta2-adrenergic receptor signaling from restoring synchronous contraction in the failing heart. *Sci Transl Med* 3:100ra88, 2011.
76. Paur H, Wright PT, Sikkel MB, et al: High levels of circulating epinephrine trigger apical cardiodepression in a beta2-adrenergic receptor/Gi-dependent manner: a new model of Takotsubo cardiomyopathy. *Circulation* 126:697–706, 2012.
77. Bers DM: Calcium cycling and signaling in cardiac myocytes. *Annu Rev Physiol* 70:23–49, 2008.
78. Palazzesi S, Musumeci M, Catalano L, et al: Pressure overload causes cardiac hypertrophy in beta1-adrenergic and beta2-adrenergic receptor double knockout mice. *J Hypertens* 24:563–571, 2006.
79. Swaminathan PD, Purohit A, Hund TJ, et al: Calmodulin-dependent protein kinase II: linking heart failure and arrhythmias. *Circ Res* 110:1661–1677, 2012.
80. Lewin G, Matus M, Basu A, et al: Critical role of transcription factor cyclic AMP response element modulator in beta1-adrenoceptor-mediated cardiac dysfunction. *Circulation* 119:79–88, 2009.
81. Buitrago M, Lorenz K, Maass AH, et al: The transcriptional repressor Nab1 is a specific regulator of pathological cardiac hypertrophy. *Nat Med* 11:837–844, 2005.
82. Shenoy SK, Lefkowitz RJ: Beta-arrestin-mediated receptor trafficking and signal transduction. *Trends Pharmacol Sci* 32:521–533, 2011.
83. Belmonte SL, Blaxall BC: G protein coupled receptor kinases as therapeutic targets in cardiovascular disease. *Circ Res* 109:309–319, 2011.
84. Zhu W, Petrashevskaya N, Ren S, et al: Gi-biased beta2AR signaling links GRK2 upregulation to heart failure. *Circ Res* 110:265–274, 2012.
85. Martini JS, Raake P, Vinge LE, et al: Uncovering G protein-coupled receptor kinase-5 as a histone deacetylase kinase in the nucleus of cardiomyocytes. *Proc Natl Acad Sci U S A* 105:12457–12462, 2008.
86. Wisler JW, DeWire SM, Whalen EJ, et al: A unique mechanism of beta-blocker action: carvedilol stimulates beta-arrestin signaling. *Proc Natl Acad Sci U S A* 104:16657–16662, 2007.
87. Mudd JO, Kass DA: Tackling heart failure in the twenty-first century. *Nature* 451:919–928, 2008.
88. Wu X, Eder P, Chang B, et al: TRPC channels are necessary mediators of pathologic cardiac hypertrophy. *Proc Natl Acad Sci U S A* 107:7000–7005, 2010.
89. Thorneloe KS, Cheung M, Bao W, et al: An orally active TRPV4 channel blocker prevents and resolves pulmonary edema induced by heart failure. *Sci Transl Med* 4:159ra148, 2012.
90. Sheikh F, Ross RS, Chen J: Cell-cell connection to cardiac disease. *Trends Cardiovasc Med* 19:182–190, 2009.
91. Manso AM, Li R, Monkley SJ, et al: Talin1 has unique expression versus talin 2 in the heart and modifies the hypertrophic response to pressure overload. *J Biol Chem* 288:4252–4264, 2013.
92. Knoll R, Hoshijima M, Hoffman HM, et al: The cardiac mechanical stretch sensor machinery involves a Z disc complex that is defective in a subset of human dilated cardiomyopathy. *Cell* 111:943–955, 2002.
93. LeWinter MM, Granzier HL: Titin is a major human disease gene. *Circulation* 127:938–944, 2013.
94. Herman DS, Lam L, Taylor MR, et al: Truncations of titin causing dilated cardiomyopathy. *N Engl J Med* 366:619–628, 2012.
95. Knoll R, Linke WA, Zou P, et al: Telethonin deficiency is associated with maladaptation to biomechanical stress in the mammalian heart. *Circ Res* 109:758–769, 2011.
96. Zou Y, Akazawa H, Qin Y, et al: Mechanical stress activates angiotensin II type 1 receptor without the involvement of angiotensin II. *Nat Cell Biol* 6:499–506, 2004.
97. Jensen BC, O'Connell TD, Simpson PC: Alpha-1-adrenergic receptors: targets for agonist drugs to treat heart failure. *J Mol Cell Cardiol* 51:518–528, 2011.
98. Wettschureck N, Rutten H, Zywietz A, et al: Absence of pressure overload induced myocardial hypertrophy after conditional inactivation of Galphaq/Galpha11 in cardiomyocytes. *Nat Med* 7:1236–1240, 2001.
99. Frey UH, Lieb W, Erdmann J, et al: Characterization of the GNAQ promoter and association of increased Gq expression with cardiac hypertrophy in humans. *Eur Heart J* 29:888–897, 2008.
100. Liggett SB, Kelly RJ, Parekh RR, et al: A functional polymorphism of the Galphaq (GNAQ) gene is associated with accelerated mortality in African-American heart failure. *Hum Mol Genet* 16:2740–2750, 2007.
101. Zhang P, Mende U: Regulators of G-protein signaling in the heart and their potential as therapeutic targets. *Circ Res* 109:320–333, 2011.
102. Dorn GW, Force T: Protein kinase cascades in the regulation of cardiac hypertrophy. *J Clin Invest* 115:527–537, 2005.
103. Palaniyandi SS, Sun L, Ferreira JC, et al: Protein kinase C in heart failure: a therapeutic target? *Cardiovasc Res* 82:229–239, 2009.
104. van Berlo JH, Maillet M, Molkentin JD: Signaling effectors underlying pathologic growth and remodeling of the heart. *J Clin Invest* 123:37–45, 2013.
105. Chen CH, Budas GR, Churchill EN, et al: Activation of aldehyde dehydrogenase-2 reduces ischemic damage to the heart. *Science* 321:1493–1495, 2008.
106. Fielitz J, Kim MS, Shelton JM, et al: Requirement of protein kinase D1 for pathological cardiac remodeling. *Proc Natl Acad Sci U S A* 105:3059–3063, 2008.
107. Zhang Y, Matkovich SJ, Duan X, et al: Receptor-independent protein kinase C alpha (PKCalpha) signaling by calpain-generated free catalytic domains induces HDAC5 nuclear export and regulates cardiac transcription. *J Biol Chem* 286:26943–26951, 2011.
108. Rose BA, Force T, Wang Y: Mitogen-activated protein kinase signaling in the heart: angels versus demons in a heart-breaking tale. *Physiol Rev* 90:1507–1546, 2010.
109. Del Re DP, Matsuda T, Zhai P, et al: Proapoptotic Rassf1A/Mst1 signaling in cardiac fibroblasts is protective against pressure overload in mice. *J Clin Invest* 120:3555–3567, 2010.
110. Matsui Y, Nakano N, Shao D, et al: Lats2 is a negative regulator of myocyte size in the heart. *Circ Res* 103:1309–1318, 2008.
111. Kehat I, Davis J, Tiburcy M, et al: Extracellular signal-regulated kinases 1 and 2 regulate the balance between eccentric and concentric cardiac growth. *Circ Res* 108:176–183, 2011.
112. van Berlo JH, Elrod JW, Aronow BJ, et al: Serine 105 phosphorylation of transcription factor GATA4 is necessary for stress-induced cardiac hypertrophy in vivo. *Proc Natl Acad Sci U S A* 108:12331–12336, 2011.
113. Kimura TE, Jin J, Zi M, et al: Targeted deletion of the extracellular signal-regulated protein kinase 5 attenuates hypertrophic response and promotes pressure overload-induced apoptosis in the heart. *Circ Res* 106:961–970, 2010.
114. Auger-Messier M, Accornero F, Goonasekera SA, et al: Unrestrained p38 MAPK activation in Dusp1/4 double-null mice induces cardiomyopathy. *Circ Res* 112:48–56, 2013.
115. Liu Q, Sargent MA, York AJ, et al: ASK1 regulates cardiomyocyte death but not hypertrophy in transgenic mice. *Circ Res* 105:1110–1117, 2009.
116. Taniike M, Yamaguchi O, Tsujimoto I, et al: Apoptosis signal-regulating kinase 1/p38 signaling pathway negatively regulates physiological hypertrophy. *Circulation* 117:545–552, 2008.
117. Balijepalli RC, Foell JD, Hall DD, et al: Localization of cardiac L-type Ca(2+) channels to a caveolar macromolecular signaling complex is required for beta(2)-adrenergic regulation. *Proc Natl Acad Sci U S A* 103:7500–7505, 2006.
118. Wu X, Zhang T, Bossuyt J, et al: Local InsP3-dependent perinuclear Ca2+ signaling in cardiac myocyte excitation-transcription coupling. *J Clin Invest* 116:675–682, 2006.
119. Nakayama H, Bodi I, Maillet M, et al: The IP3 receptor regulates cardiac hypertrophy in response to select stimuli. *Circ Res* 107:659–666, 2010.

120. Heineke J, Molkentin JD: Regulation of cardiac hypertrophy by intracellular signalling pathways. *Nat Rev Mol Cell Biol* 7:589–600, 2006.
121. Molkentin JD, Lu JR, Antos CL, et al: A calcineurin-dependent transcriptional pathway for cardiac hypertrophy. *Cell* 93:215–228, 1998.
122. Faul C, Amaral AP, Oskouei B, et al: FGF23 induces left ventricular hypertrophy. *J Clin Invest* 121:4393–4408, 2011.
123. Nakayama H, Chen X, Baines CP, et al: Ca2+- and mitochondrial-dependent cardiomyocyte necrosis as a primary mediator of heart failure. *J Clin Invest* 117:2431–2444, 2007.
124. Nakayama H, Bodi I, Correll RN, et al: Alpha1G-dependent T-type Ca2+ current antagonizes cardiac hypertrophy through a NOS3-dependent mechanism in mice. *J Clin Invest* 119:3787–3796, 2009.
125. Goonasekera SA, Hammer K, Auger-Messier M, et al: Decreased cardiac L-type Ca(2)(+) channel activity induces hypertrophy and heart failure in mice. *J Clin Invest* 122:280–290, 2012.
126. Makarewich CA, Correll RN, Gao H, et al: A caveolae-targeted L-type Ca(2)+ channel antagonist inhibits hypertrophic signaling without reducing cardiac contractility. *Circ Res* 110:669–674, 2012.
127. Heineke J, Auger-Messier M, Correll RN, et al: CIB1 is a regulator of pathological cardiac hypertrophy. *Nat Med* 16:872–879, 2010.
128. Backs J, Backs T, Neef S, et al: The delta isoform of CaM kinase II is required for pathological cardiac hypertrophy and remodeling after pressure overload. *Proc Natl Acad Sci U S A* 106:2342–2347, 2009.
129. He BJ, Joiner ML, Singh MV, et al: Oxidation of CaMKII determines the cardiotoxic effects of aldosterone. *Nat Med* 17:1610–1618, 2011.
130. Joiner ML, Koval OM, Li J, et al: CaMKII determines mitochondrial stress responses in heart. *Nature* 491:269–273, 2012.
131. Li HL, Liu C, de Couto G, et al: Curcumin prevents and reverses murine cardiac hypertrophy. *J Clin Invest* 118:879–893, 2008.
132. Kim Y, Phan D, van Rooij E, et al: The MEF2D transcription factor mediates stress-dependent cardiac remodeling in mice. *J Clin Invest* 118:124–132, 2008.
133. Trivedi CM, Luo Y, Yin Z, et al: Hdac2 regulates the cardiac hypertrophic response by modulating Gsk3 beta activity. *Nat Med* 13:324–331, 2007.
134. Hsu CP, Zhai P, Yamamoto T, et al: Silent information regulator 1 protects the heart from ischemia/reperfusion. *Circulation* 122:2170–2182, 2010.
135. Narayan N, Lee IH, Borenstein R, et al: The NAD-dependent deacetylase SIRT2 is required for programmed necrosis. *Nature* 492:199–204, 2012.
136. Sundaresan NR, Gupta M, Kim G, et al: Sirt3 blocks the cardiac hypertrophic response by augmenting Foxo3a-dependent antioxidant defense mechanisms in mice. *J Clin Invest* 119:2758–2771, 2009.
137. Hang CT, Yang J, Han P, et al: Chromatin regulation by Brg1 underlies heart muscle development and disease. *Nature* 466:62–67, 2010.
138. Guo D, Kassiri Z, Basu R, et al: Loss of PI3Kgamma enhances cAMP-dependent MMP remodeling of the myocardial N-cadherin adhesion complexes and extracellular matrix in response to early biomechanical stress. *Circ Res* 107:1275–1289, 2010.
139. Zhang D, Contu R, Latronico MV, et al: MTORC1 regulates cardiac function and myocyte survival through 4E-BP1 inhibition in mice. *J Clin Invest* 120:2805–2816, 2010.
140. Shende P, Plaisance I, Morandi C, et al: Cardiac raptor ablation impairs adaptive hypertrophy, alters metabolic gene expression, and causes heart failure in mice. *Circulation* 123:1073–1082, 2011.
141. Cheng H, Woodgett J, Maamari M, et al: Targeting GSK-3 family members in the heart: a very sharp double-edged sword. *J Mol Cell Cardiol* 51:607–613, 2011.
142. Lal H, Zhou J, Ahmad F, et al: Glycogen synthase kinase-3alpha limits ischemic injury, cardiac rupture, post-myocardial infarction remodeling and death. *Circulation* 125:65–75, 2012.
143. Portbury AL, Ronnebaum SM, Zungu M, et al: Back to your heart: ubiquitin proteasome system-regulated signal transduction. *J Mol Cell Cardiol* 52:526–537, 2012.
144. Odiete O, Hill MF, Sawyer DB: Neuregulin in cardiovascular development and disease. *Circ Res* 111:1376–1385, 2012.
145. Xie M, Zhang D, Dyck JR, et al: A pivotal role for endogenous TGF-beta-activated kinase-1 in the LKB1/AMP-activated protein kinase energy-sensor pathway. *Proc Natl Acad Sci U S A* 103:17378–17383, 2006.
146. Brown JH, Del Re DP, Sussman MA: The Rac and Rho hall of fame: a decade of hypertrophic signaling hits. *Circ Res* 98:730–742, 2006.
147. Chang L, Zhang J, Tseng YH, et al: Rad GTPase deficiency leads to cardiac hypertrophy. *Circulation* 116:2976–2983, 2007.
148. Kerkela R, Grazette L, Yacobi R, et al: Cardiotoxicity of the cancer therapeutic agent imatinib mesylate. *Nat Med* 12:908–916, 2006.

Abbreviations Used in This Chapter

ABBREVIATION	FULL NAME	NOTE
AngII	Angiotensin II	Hypertrophic agonist
AMPK	Adenosine monophosphate kinase	
ANF	Atrial natriuretic factor	Early response gene
AP-1	Activator protein 1	Transcription factor
$AT_{1a}R$, $AT_{1b}R$	Angiotensin II receptor type Ia or Ib	
Ask-1	Apoptosis signal regulating kinase 1	MAP kinase kinase
ATF-1	Activating transcription factor 1	
B-ARK (GRK2)	β-adrenergic receptor kinase (G-protein receptor kinase 2)	Gβγ dependent, phosphorylates β-adrenergic receptors
BNP	B-type natriuretic peptide	TGF-β superfamily ligands
BMP	Bone morphogenic proteins	
CAD	Caspase associated DNAase	
CaMK	Ca^{2+} calmodulin dependent kinase	
cAMP	Cyclic adenosine monophosphate	
cAMP Kinase	Cyclic 3′,5′-adenosine monophosphate kinase	
CREB	cAMP response element-binding protein	cAMP responsive transcription factor
CREM	Cyclic AMP response element modulator	cAMP responsive transcription factor
CT-1	Cardiotrophin-1	IL-6 family cytokine
DAG	Diacyl glycerol	Endogenous PKC agonist
DISC	Death induced signaling complex	Signaling complex downstream of death receptor
4E-BP	4E-binding protein	
EGF	Epidermal growth factor	
egr-1	Early growth response gene 1	Transcription factor
eIF4F	Eukaryotic initiation factor 4F	Stimulates initiation of translation at a subset of transcripts
ErbB2-4	EGF family tyrosine kinase receptors	Receptors for neuregulins
ET-1	Endothelin 1	
ET_A, ET_B	Endothelin receptors A, B	
ECM	Extracellular matrix	
EGF	Epidermal growth factor	
Elk-1	TCF family transcription factor	
Ets1	TCF family transcription factor	
ERK	Extracellular receptor kinase	MAP kinase
FAK	Focal adhesion kinase	Nonreceptor tyrosine kinase
FGF	Fibroblast growth factor	Growth factor
c-fos	c-fos oncogene	Component of transcription factor AP-1
FoxO	O family of forkhead/winged-helix transcription factors	
Gα, Gβγ	Subunits of heterotrimeric G proteins	
GAP	GTPase activating proteins	
GATA4	GATA binding protein 4	
GDP	Guanosine di-phosphate	
GDF15	Growth differentiation factor 15	TGF-β family protein
GEF	Guanine exchange factor	Activators of small G proteins
gp130	Glycoprotein 130	Receptor for IL-6 family cytokines
GPCR	Heterotrimeric G protein–coupled receptor	

Abbreviations Used in This Chapter—cont'd

ABBREVIATION	FULL NAME	NOTE
Grb2	Growth factor receptor bound protein 2	Adaptor protein linking RTKs and Ras
GRK	G protein receptor kinase	Inhibits G-protein signaling and recruits adaptor proteins to stimulate alternate pathways
GSK3β	Glycogen synthase kinase 3β	Kinase downregulated by hypertrophic stimuli
GTP	Guanosine triphosphate	
HB-EGF	Heparin-binding EGF-like growth factor	
HAT	Histone acetyltransferase	Induces histone acetylation with activation of transcription
HDAC	Histone deacetylase	Represses transcription by inducing histone deacetylation
IGF-1	Insulin-like growth factor	Growth factor
IL-6	Interleukin 6	Cytokine
IP3	Inositol 1,4,5 triphosphate	
ILK	Integrin linked kinase	Serine threonine kinase associated with β-integrin
JAK	Janus activating kinase	Tyrosine kinase activated by gp130
JNK	Jun N terminal kinase	MAP kinase
c-jun	*jun* oncogene	Component of AP-1 transcription factor
KLF-5	Kruppel-like transcription factor	
LIF	Leukemia inhibitory factor	IL-6 cytokine
MADS domain	DNA binding motif	Present in SRF and MEF2 transcription factors
MAPK	Mitogen activated protein kinase	
MAPKK	MAPK kinase	Also known as MEK or MK
MAPKKK	MAPK kinase kinase	Also known as MEKK or MKK
MEF2	Myocyte enhancer factor 2	Transcription factor
MEK-1	MAP kinase kinase 1	Activator of ERK MAPKs
MCIP	Modularity calcineurin-inhibitory proteins	Endogenous inhibitor of calcineurin
MHC	Myosin heavy chain	
miRNAs	MicroRNAs	Endogenous RNAs that inhibit mRNA translation/ enhance degradation
MLC	Myosin light chain	
MLP	Muscle LIM protein	
mTOR	Mechanistic target of rapamycin	Kinase involved in regulation of protein synthesis
c-myc	*myc* oncogene	Transcription factor
NE	Norepinephrine	Catecholamine
Nab1	NGF1a-binding protein	Transcriptional repressor
NFAT	Nuclear factor of activated T cells	Transcription factor
PDK1	Phosphoinositide-dependent kinase 1	Downstream effector of PI3K
PE	Phenylephrine	α-adrenergic agonist
PI3K	Phosphoinositide 3-kinase	
PIP2	Phosphatidyl inositol 4,5-bisphosphate	
PIP3	Phosphatidyl inositol 3,4,5-triphosphate	
PKA	Protein kinase A	
PKB	Protein kinase B	Also known as Akt
PKC	Protein kinase C	
PKD	Protein kinase D	
PLC	Phospholipase C	
PMA	Phorbol 12-myristate 13-acetate	PKC agonist
p53	Tumor suppressor gene	Transcription factor
p70S6K	Ribosomal p70 S6 kinase	Protein kinase involved in protein synthesis
Ras	*ras* oncogene	Small G protein
RTK	Receptor tyrosine kinase	
ROCK	Rho kinases	
RYR	Ryanodine receptor	
SERCA	Sarcoplasmic reticulum Ca^{2+} ATPase	Pumps Ca^{2+} from cytoplasm to sarcoplasmic reticulum
SH2	Src homology domain 2	Binds phosphotyrosine residues
SHP2	SH2 domain-containing cytoplasmic protein tyrosine phosphatase	
siRNAs	Short interfering RNAs	Inhibit mRNA translation
SOCS	Suppressors of cytokine signaling	Endogenous repressor of STATs
c-src	*src* oncogene	Nonreceptor tyrosine kinase
SRF	Serum response factor	Transcription factor
STAT	Signal transducer and activator of transcription	Transcription factor regulated by JAKs
TRPCs	Transient receptor potential channels	Ion channels
TCF/LEF1	T-cell-specific transcription factor/lymphoid enhancer factor 1	Transcription factor
TAK1	TGF-β activated kinase 1	MAPKK activated by TGF-β
TGF-β	Transforming growth factor β	Cytokine
TNF-α	Tumor necrosis factor	Cytokine
TRP	Transient receptor potential channel	Store operated calcium channels
VEGF	Vascular endothelial growth factor	Angiogenic cytokine

2 Cellular Basis for Heart Failure

Adam Nabeebaccus, Can Martin Sag, Ian Webb, and Ajay M. Shah

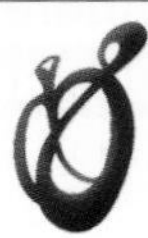

The development of heart failure in the context of chronic disease stresses such as hypertension or myocardial infarction is characterized initially by complex changes in the structure and function of the heart at the molecular (**see also Chapter 1**), cellular, and organ levels. This dynamic process, termed *cardiac remodeling* (**see also Chapter 11**), leads to contractile dysfunction, chamber dilatation, ventricular dyssynchrony, and arrhythmias. At the cellular level, the remodeling heart manifests significant alterations both in the cardiac myocytes and in nonmyocyte cells, such as fibroblasts, endothelial cells, and immune cells. In addition, there are significant changes in the myocardial vasculature and the composition of the extracellular matrix.

Progressive changes in the cardiac myocyte phenotype are a central abnormality in the chronically stressed and failing heart. The phenotype comprises multiple components including cell hypertrophy (**see Chapter 1**) and alterations in calcium handling, sarcomeric function, electrical properties, redox homeostasis, metabolism, energetics, and cell viability that collectively make a major contribution to the global cardiac phenotype. Cardiomyocyte hypertrophy is also observed in physiologic settings (e.g., pregnancy or in athletes), but in this case is not accompanied by detrimental changes such as contractile impairment. This divergence in phenotypes indicates that different components of the cardiomyocyte phenotype are capable of being regulated independently, at least to some extent. Even in a disease setting (e.g., early during pressure overload), the heart may hypertrophy but maintain contractile function (*adaptive* remodeling), whereas with more chronic disease stress it begins to fail. Thus, the overall phenotype may be determined by the balance between potentially adaptive and maladaptive processes that occur within the cardiac myocyte.

In this chapter, we review the main cardiomyocyte cellular alterations that contribute to the pathogenesis of heart failure. We start by discussing the cellular basis for contractile dysfunction, the key cardiac manifestation of heart failure. The contribution of changes in excitation-contraction coupling (particularly calcium handling and sarcomeric function) to contractile dysfunction and arrhythmogenesis is considered. We next discuss several global alterations within cardiomyocytes that also impact on contractile function and cell viability, such as changes in redox homeostasis and signaling, cellular stress responses, and macromolecular and protein turnover. As will become evident, these global processes interact with each other and have complex effects on the remodeling process (e.g., redox homeostasis and signaling modulate excitation-contraction coupling, as well as stress responses). The cardiomyocyte phenotype in the failing heart may also be affected by other cardiac cell types and, in turn, influence those cell types. The role of cardiomyocyte interactions with other cell types—in particular fibroblasts, endothelial cells, and immune/inflammatory cells—is therefore discussed. Finally, we review the role of microRNA-dependent regulation, which often has global effects on cellular signaling pathways in the failing heart. The signaling pathways that underlie the development of myocyte hypertrophy per se are discussed elsewhere in this edition. Likewise, the important role of alterations in myocardial energetics and metabolism, which for example may have a major impact on contractile function during heart failure, is covered in other chapters.

CONTRACTILE DYSFUNCTION

Cardiac myocytes in the failing heart exhibit several abnormalities of contractile function, including a reduction in contractile amplitude and force of contraction, a slowing of contraction and relaxation, an increase in diastolic force, and altered responses to changes in heart rate and β-adrenergic stimulation. Perturbations in both excitation-contraction coupling and sarcomere properties contribute to these abnormalities. We provide a brief overview of

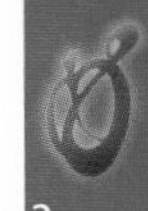

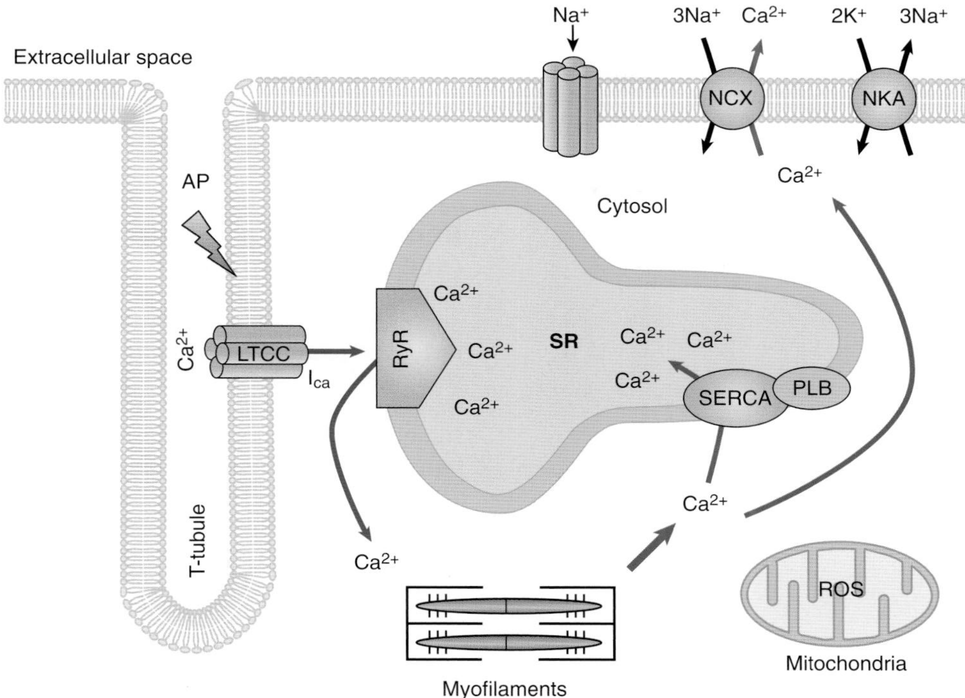

FIGURE 2-1 Normal excitation-contraction coupling. Upon systolic depolarization of the membrane potential, LTCC-mediated Ca^{2+} (I_{Ca}) induces Ca^{2+} release from the SR via the RyR. Ca^{2+} binds to the myofilaments and initiates contraction *(green arrow).* During diastole *(red arrows),* Ca^{2+} is actively taken up into the SR via SERCA2a and also partly extruded to the extracellular space via NCX. *AP,* action potential; *NKA,* Na^+/K^+ ATPase.

normal excitation-contraction coupling and sarcomeric function and then address the distinct abnormalities that occur in heart failure.

Normal Excitation-Contraction Coupling

Physiologic cardiac function requires the coordinated temporal and spatial activation of the heart. At a cellular level, this finely tuned process is regulated mainly by accurately synchronized Ca^{2+} fluxes in every cardiomyocyte (**Figure 2-1**).[1] When an action potential depolarizes the cell, voltage-dependent L-type Ca^{2+} channels (LTCC) located mainly in the transverse tubules (T-tubules) open to generate an inward Ca^{2+} current (I_{Ca}), which induces a localized increase of Ca^{2+} in the "dyadic cleft" in close neighborhood to the Ca^{2+} release or ryanodine receptor channels (RyR2) of the sarcoplasmic reticulum (SR). This trans-sarcolemmal Ca^{2+} influx activates the RyR2 and results in so-called "Ca^{2+}-induced Ca^{2+} release" from the SR, which provides the major component of the increase in cytosolic Ca^{2+} during systole (i.e., the "Ca^{2+} transient"). Intracellular Ca^{2+} concentration increases from approximately 100 nmol/L during diastole to approximately 1 μmol/L during systole and causes myofilament activation and contraction. Repolarization of the membrane potential is induced by inactivation of I_{Ca} and the activation of delayed rectifying K^+ currents. During diastole, Ca^{2+} is removed from the cytosol via two major pathways: (1) the SR Ca^{2+} ATPase (SERCA2a) located in the membrane of the SR, which pumps Ca^{2+} back into the SR lumen; (2) the sarcolemmal Na^+/Ca^{2+} exchanger (NCX1), which transfers Ca^{2+} into the extracellular space. Through these two Ca^{2+} transport mechanisms, $[Ca^{2+}]_i$ decreases to physiologic resting concentrations of approximately 100 nmol/L, allowing the cell to relax and to regain its physiologic diastolic resting cell length.

Impaired Ca^{2+} Handling in Failing Cardiac Myocytes

Prolongation of the action potential duration, depressed force generating capacity, and slowed contraction and relaxation rates are the hallmark functional changes of the failing human heart. Impaired Ca^{2+} handling is a key feature of the failing cardiac myocyte, with great pathophysiologic relevance for the progressive deterioration in contractile function of the failing heart. Distinct alterations in the expression levels, as well as post-translational modifications of important cardiac Ca^{2+}-handling proteins, causatively contribute to systolic and diastolic contractile dysfunction, and to an increased propensity for cardiac arrhythmias.[2] The post-translational modifications that alter the function of key Ca^{2+} handling proteins include alterations in phosphorylation,[3] nitrosylation,[4] oxidation status,[5] and sumoylation.[6] Altered protein phosphorylation occurs secondary to changes in the activity of various kinases (e.g., cAMP-dependent protein kinase [PKA], calcium-calmodulin-dependent kinase II [CaMKII]), as well as perturbations in phosphatase (e.g., protein phosphatase 1 [PP1]) activity.[7]

The failing cardiac myocyte has a significantly diminished amplitude of the systolic Ca^{2+} transient as compared with nonfailing control myocytes (**Figure 2-2**), which is a major factor responsible for the reduced contractile amplitude of the failing cell (*systolic* dysfunction). Failing myocytes typically also exhibit a slowed decay of the Ca^{2+} transient during diastole, which is a major contributor to abnormal (delayed) relaxation. In addition, the normal increase in amplitude of Ca^{2+} transient (and therefore force of contraction) that occurs with faster heart rate is blunted or even reversed in the failing heart (i.e., the normal positive force-frequency relationship [FFR] is converted to a flat or a negative FFR). It is generally accepted that a reduction in the Ca^{2+} content of the SR is a major reason for the diminished amplitude of the systolic Ca^{2+} transient and the abnormal FFR. A decreased SR Ca^{2+} content has been consistently observed in myocytes isolated from failing human and animal hearts, whereas alterations in LTTC-mediated Ca^{2+} influx appear to be less relevant.[1,2] From a mechanistic point of view, a reduction in SR Ca^{2+} content can result either from insufficient diastolic Ca^{2+} refilling (or loading) of the SR or from an increased loss of Ca^{2+} via the RyR2 Ca^{2+} release channels during diastole, and may also be influenced by changes in NCX activity. In fact, all three mechanisms may contribute to the reduction in SR Ca^{2+} content and contractile phenotype of the failing myocyte (**Figure 2-3**).

Decreased "Systolic Ca2+ transient" in failing cardiac myocytes

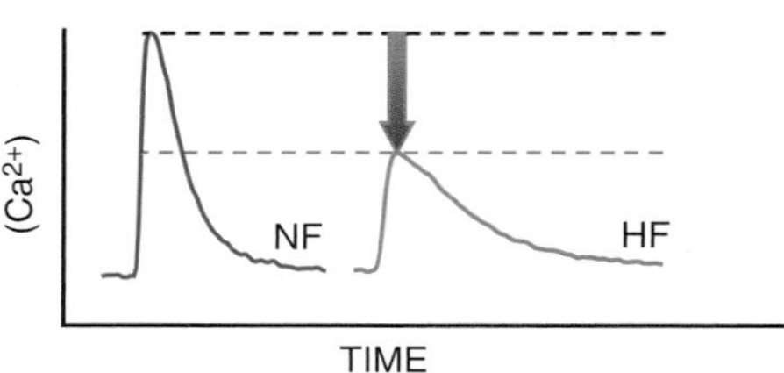

Slowed "Ca2+ transient decline" indicating depressed SR Ca2+ reuptake

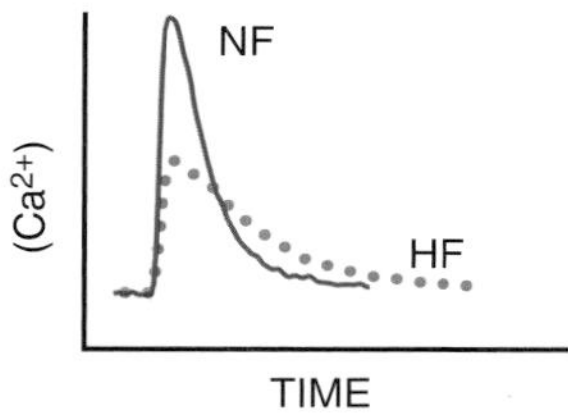

FIGURE 2-2 Representative Ca^{2+} transients of failing and nonfailing cardiac myocytes. In the upper panel, the amplitude of a normal nonfailing (NF) Ca^{2+} transient (blue) is compared to the Ca^{2+} transient that is typically measured in failing myocytes (HF, red). The bottom panel illustrates the slowed Ca^{2+} transient decay kinetics in failing myocytes (red).

Reduced SR Ca^{2+} Reuptake in Heart Failure (see also Chapter 1)

During diastole, SERCA2a pumps Ca^{2+} into the SR lumen and provides a sufficient Ca^{2+} content to be released during the subsequent systolic heartbeat. SERCA2a-dependent diastolic Ca^{2+} uptake into the SR normally dominates over transsarcolemmal Ca^{2+} extrusion via the NCX. SERCA2a is subject to regulation by the phosphoprotein phospholamban (PLB), which upon phosphorylation by CaMKII (at Thr-17) and/or PKA (at Ser-16) releases its inhibitory effect on SERCA2a because of a dissociation of the PLB/SERCA2a complex.[8] SERCA2a protein levels are reduced in failing myocardium, which is paralleled by a reduction in SERCA2a sumoylation,[6] and results in an impairment of diastolic Ca^{2+} reuptake into the SR. Moreover, the levels of PLB are unaltered and its phosphorylation state may be reduced, so that there is greater relative inhibition of SERCA2a by nonphosphorylated PLB, thereby aggravating the impairment of Ca^{2+} reuptake (see Figure 2-3).[9] The decrease in SR Ca^{2+} content results in less Ca^{2+} available for the subsequent systolic Ca^{2+} transient and impairs systolic function.

Decreased SERCA2a expression may also affect diastolic function of the failing heart. If no other mechanism

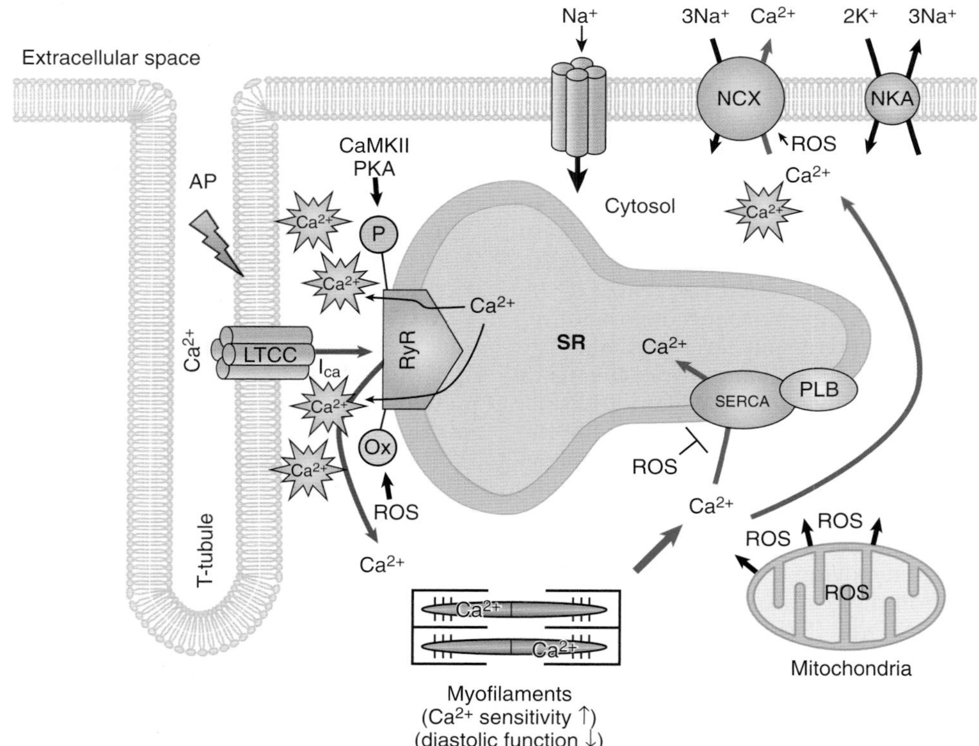

FIGURE 2-3 Abnormalities of cardiac Ca^{2+} handling in heart failure. SR Ca^{2+} content is typically diminished in failing myocytes because of (1) increased diastolic SR Ca^{2+} leak induced by RyR hyperphosphorylation *(orange arrow)* or oxidation *(light blue arrow)*; (2) decreased SR Ca^{2+} reuptake because of reduced SERCA expression; (3) increased NCX expression and activity that removes Ca^{2+} to the extracellular space. Note that increased oxidative stress in heart failure (e.g., because of increased mitochondrial ROS or other sources) can further aggravate these abnormalities. Myofilament dysfunction also contributes to the contractile abnormalities. *AP,* action potential; *NKA,* Na^+/K^+ ATPase.

(such as an increased NCX activity [see later discussion]) compensates for the reduction in SERCA2a function with respect to removal of Ca^{2+} from the cytosol during diastole, then there is diastolic cytosolic Ca^{2+} overload. Myocytes that have increased diastolic Ca^{2+} levels will have persistent low-level myofilament activation at a time when the myofilaments should be fully relaxed, resulting in increased diastolic force and diastolic dysfunction. This failure to relax fully during diastole impairs the filling of the heart and thereby may also worsen systolic dysfunction.[10] Moreover, the abnormally elevated diastolic Ca^{2+} levels may have multiple other effects, such as changes in gene transcription, cell viability, and mitochondrial function through altered activation of Ca^{2+}-dependent kinases (e.g., CaMKII), phosphatases (e.g., calcineurin), mitochondrial enzymes, caspases, and other mechanisms.

In view of these effects on contractile function, as well as other aspects of the failing heart phenotype, restoring SERCA2a function in heart failure might represent a promising therapeutic approach.[11] Experimental studies have shown that adenoviral overexpression of SERCA2a in human cardiomyocytes can improve cardiac contractility because it restores SR Ca^{2+} content and the systolic Ca^{2+} transient, whereas reduced cytosolic Ca^{2+} levels preserve diastolic function. In addition, SERCA2a overexpression was shown to improve myocardial energetics and endothelial function and to have antiarrhythmic effects.[9] The potential clinical relevance of SERCA2a stimulation was suggested in the CUPID trial (Calcium Up-Regulation by Percutaneous Administration of Gene Therapy in Cardiac Disease) in which treatment of heart failure patients with a single infusion of an adeno-associated viral vector delivering SERCA2a versus placebo appeared to improve or stabilize NYHA class and reduce major cardiovascular events and heart failure-related hospitalization.[12] However, larger randomized clinical trials are required to establish the efficacy of such an approach.

Increased NCX Activity in the Failing Heart

The NCX is localized at the cardiomyocyte sarcolemma where, in its "forward mode," it transfers one Ca^{2+} ion into the extracellular space in exchange for three Na^+ ions using the transmembrane gradient for Na^+ (see Figure 2-1). This mechanism is electrogenic because it results in the net movement of one positive charge into the cytosol, and can therefore depolarize the membrane potential and even have arrhythmogenic effects under conditions of spontaneous and localized rises in $[Ca^{2+}]_i$ (see later discussion). NCX expression and activity are found to be increased in human and experimental heart failure, which may have complex functional effects depending upon the mode of NCX activity and stage of heart failure. In the face of downregulated SERCA2a function, enhanced NCX activity competes with SERCA2a for Ca^{2+} elimination during diastole. This may further aggravate the decrease in SR Ca^{2+} content because less cytosolic Ca^{2+} is available for SERCA2a-mediated SR Ca^{2+} loading. However, the increase in NCX function can also partly protect cardiac myocytes against severe diastolic Ca^{2+} overload and diastolic dysfunction. Indeed, an increase in NCX levels in explanted human myocardial samples was found to correlate with a preservation of diastolic function, whereas patients with diastolic dysfunction had decreased NCX levels.[2] On the other hand, NCX activity can contribute to Ca^{2+} overload in settings where there is intracellular Na^+ overload. This is because at high $[Na^+]_i$, NCX switches to a "reverse mode" and pumps out Na^+ in exchange for Ca^{2+}. The increased contribution of NCX-dependent Ca^{2+} influx, as opposed to SR Ca^{2+} release during systole in failing myocytes, has adverse effects on mitochondrial Ca^{2+} uptake (which relies on high Ca^{2+} gradients), and promotes increased mitochondrial reactive oxygen species (ROS) levels because of reduced activity of Ca^{2+}-dependent Krebs cycle dehydrogenases that normally maintain antioxidant reserves.[13] This detrimental mechanism can become further aggravated in a ROS-dependent manner and lead to a vicious cycle of impaired cytosolic and mitochondrial Ca^{2+} fluxes and increased oxidative stress because ROS induce further cytosolic Na^+ overload.[14]

"Leaky" RyR2 Cause Diastolic SR Ca^{2+} Loss in Heart Failure

Diastolic "leak" of Ca^{2+} from the SR due to a pathologic increase in RyR2 open probability is an important mechanism that contributes to the lowering of SR Ca^{2+} content in heart failure. Ca^{2+} leaks from the SR through spontaneous and uncoordinated Ca^{2+} release events or "Ca^{2+} sparks." The expression of RyR2 itself appears to be unchanged in heart failure, but its functional regulation is dramatically altered by complex post-translational modifications. These alterations involve an increase in RyR2 phosphorylation as a result of hyperactive protein kinases, such as CaMKII[15] and PKA,[16] and possibly reduced RyR2 dephosphorylation.[17] An increase in RyR2 oxidation or nitrosylation as a consequence of increased oxidative and nitrosative stress in heart failure may also be important.[5] While transient phosphorylation- and redox-dependent regulation of RyR2 gating may fulfill physiologic functions in healthy myocytes, in the failing myocyte the hyperphosphorylation and/or oxidation of RyR2 leads to severe diastolic SR Ca^{2+} leakage. Furthermore, the coupling of LTCC to RyR is also impaired in heart failure because of T-tubule remodeling, such that some RyR are "orphaned" and contribute to dyssynchronous Ca^{2+} release.[18]

The precise mechanisms of RyR2 hyperphosphorylation and the kinases responsible for this abnormality are important to establish because they may represent therapeutic targets, but are still a matter of debate. Although one laboratory reported strong evidence for a PKA-mediated dysregulation of the RyR2 in heart failure,[3,16] others failed to show an increase in PKA-dependent hyperphosphorylation.[19] There is also evidence for an involvement of CaMKII-dependent RyR2 phosphorylation in inducing SR Ca^{2+} leak.[20] Redox-related dysregulation of RyR2 opening in the failing heart[5] may involve increased ROS produced by mitochondria or other sources such as nicotinamide adenine dinucleotide phosphate (NADPH) oxidases (see also Chapter 8), and is related to the oxidation of specific cysteine residues within the RyR2.[5] Interestingly, both the protein kinases implicated in RyR2 hyperphosphorylation (i.e., CaMKII and PKA) are subject to redox activation,[21,22] so that alterations in the redox milieu of failing myocytes may also exert indirect effects on RyR2. In this regard, it is interesting to note that increased ROS in heart failure also impact adversely on SERCA2a function and other aspects of Ca^{2+} handling in the failing cell (see Figure 2-2).

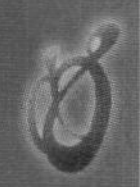

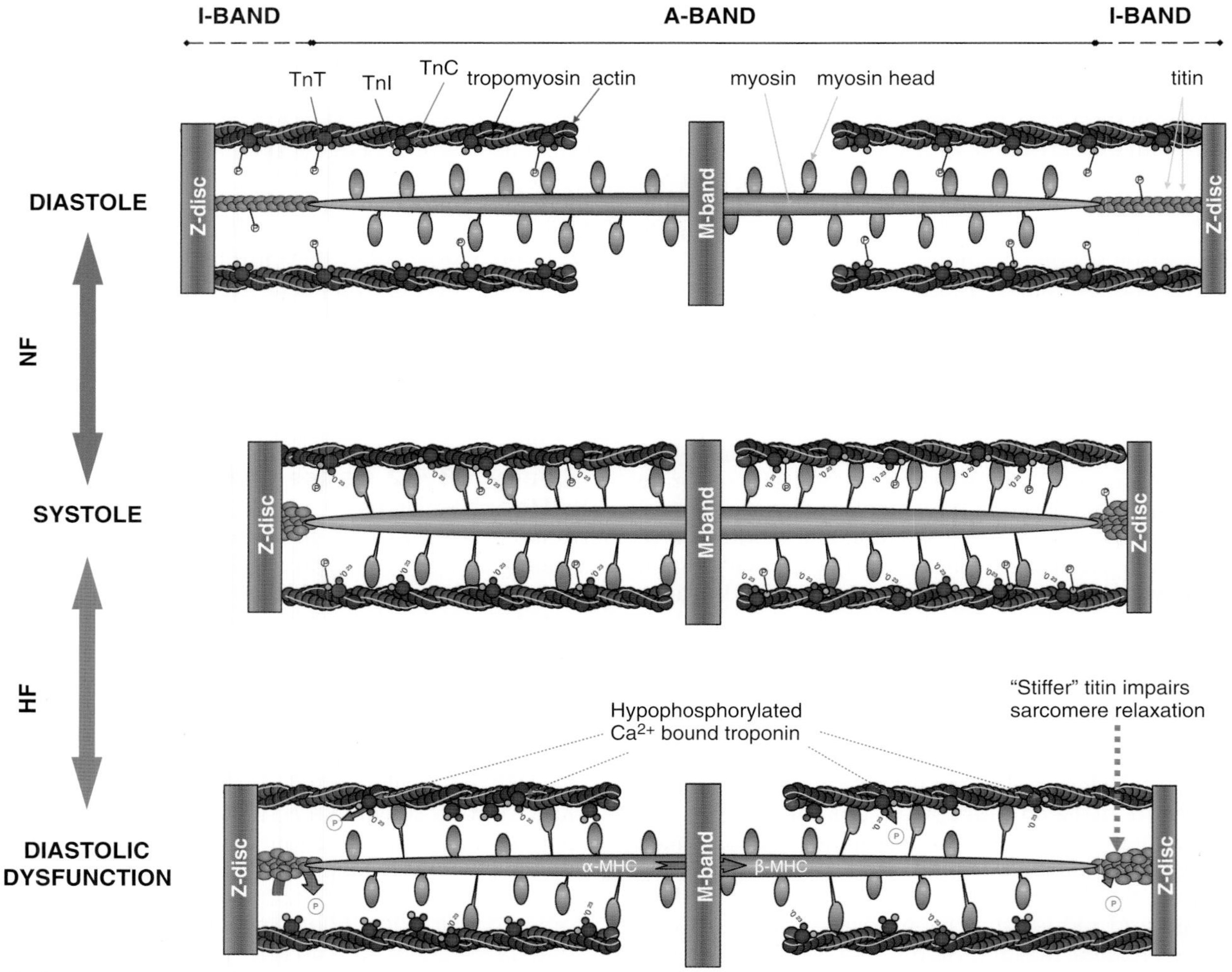

FIGURE 2-4 Main aspects of sarcomeric dysfunction in heart failure. During diastole *(upper panel)*, mechanical interaction of myosin *(light brown)* and actin *(green)* is inhibited by tropomyosin *(yellow)* and troponin I *(gray)*. Titin *(light blue)* is elongated and exerts restraint to diastolic relaxation of the sarcomeres. During systole *(middle panel)*, Ca^{2+} binds to troponin C *(red)*, which causes a conformational change of the tropomyosin-troponin complex *(blue)* and allows the myosin heads to interact with actin. The subsequent sliding movement of myosin and actin relative to each other causes sarcomere shortening and contraction. In heart failure *(HF, bottom panel)*, hypophosphorylation of troponin I and titin results in impaired sarcomere relaxation because of a persistently Ca^{2+}-activated tropomyosin-troponin complex and increased titin-dependent stiffness, respectively. *NF,* nonfailing.

Contribution of Impaired Ca^{2+} Handling to Arrhythmia

Impaired cardiomyocyte Ca^{2+} handling not only leads to systolic and diastolic dysfunction but also contributes to the development of arrhythmias in heart failure. The dysregulation of RyR2 Ca^{2+} release is of particular relevance in this regard.[23-25] The enhanced diastolic SR Ca^{2+} leak in failing cells and the accompanying spatially and temporally uncoordinated increases in intracellular Ca^{2+} may drive the NCX to exchange Ca^{2+} for Na^+, thereby inducing an influx of positive charge (I_{ti}) that partly depolarizes the cell during phase 4 of the action potential (see Figure 2-3). These spontaneous depolarizations of the membrane potential are termed *delayed afterdepolarizations (DAD)* and are arrhythmogenic. Because NCX expression and activity are increased in heart failure, the depolarizing influx of positive charge (I_{ti}) will be greater for any given spontaneous Ca^{2+} release from the SR. Thus, the combination of leaky RyR2 and increased NCX activity synergizes to enhance ventricular arrhythmogenesis. Similar mechanisms may also contribute to the development of atrial fibrillation,[26] the occurrence of which is higher in heart failure. There is a significant potential for feedback among the different ionic mechanisms that contribute to arrhythmogenesis in the failing cardiomyocyte, and therefore the possibility of a self-sustaining vicious cycle of hampered Ca^{2+} and Na^+ handling that contributes to contractile dysfunction and arrhythmia. For example, if the NCX starts to function in reverse mode due to elevated intracellular $[Na^+]$, the resulting increase in Ca^{2+} influx may activate pro-arrhythmogenic kinases such as CaMKII and lead to further arrhythmogenic SR Ca^{2+} leakage through phosphorylation of RyR2.

Sarcomeric Dysfunction in Heart Failure

Cardiac mechanical activity occurs as a result of the interaction between changes in cytosolic Ca^{2+} concentration and the contractile myofilaments (**Figure 2-4**). Contractile function is influenced not only by changes in Ca^{2+} concentration but also by the intrinsic myofilament responsiveness to Ca^{2+}, which is dependent upon the properties of the actomyosin complex and regulatory proteins such as the troponin complex and myosin binding protein C. During diastole, the mechanical interaction between actin and myosin is inhibited by the tropomyosin-troponin complex. When cytosolic Ca^{2+} concentration increases during systole, the binding of Ca^{2+} to troponin C (cTnC) relieves this inhibitory effect and allows actomyosin interaction and contraction to occur. A subsequent decrease in cytosolic Ca^{2+} leads to its release from cTnC and muscle relaxation. Other components of the sarcomere also affect the mechanical properties of heart muscle. In particular, the giant filamentous protein titin—which connects the Z-disc to the M-band and confers significant "elasticity" to the sarcomere—has an important influence on passive muscle stiffness,[27] which in turn is an important determinant of diastolic function.

Significant evidence suggests that alterations in myofilament properties contribute to systolic and diastolic contractile dysfunction in heart failure.[10,28] Perhaps the best known contribution of myofilament properties to contractile changes in the stressed and failing heart is the shift of myosin heavy chain (MHC) from the fast α-MHC to a slower β-MHC isoform. The significantly lower ATPase activity of β-MHC is beneficial in that it is more energetically efficient but at the same time may result in slower relaxation and lower contractility. This isoform shift is a prominent feature in rodent models, where α-MHC is the dominant isoform in healthy myocardium, but may be less important in human heart failure since β-MHC dominates over α-MHC in healthy human ventricular myocardium. Nevertheless, a small impact of such an MHC isoform shift is suggested in failing human ventricular tissue.[10]

A major regulator of myofilament Ca^{2+} sensitivity in the normal heart is the PKA-mediated phosphorylation of troponin I (cTnI), which results in a lower affinity for Ca^{2+} and contributes to faster kinetics of myofilament cross-bridge cycling (i.e., faster contraction and relaxation of myocytes). In the failing heart, PKA-dependent phosphorylation of cTnI is generally decreased (related to reduced β-adrenergic responsiveness) and results in increased myofilament Ca^{2+} sensitivity.[10] The major effect of such an increase in myofilament Ca^{2+} sensitivity is thought to be to impair relaxation and aggravate the slowed kinetics of Ca^{2+} transient decay in the failing myocyte (see Figure 2-4). Similar functional effects on myofilament Ca^{2+} sensitivity have been reported when there is C-terminal truncation of cTnI after myocardial ischemia/reperfusion injury, and these could play a particular role in ischemic heart failure. The phosphorylation of myosin binding protein C is thought to play a role in the physiologic enhancement of rate of contraction and relaxation observed after β-adrenergic stimulation. Therefore, hypophosphorylation of myosin binding protein C may also contribute to contractile dysfunction.[28,29]

Another shift in protein isoform that is reported in failing hearts is a shift from the stiffer (i.e., less elastic) *N2B* titin isoform to a more compliant *N2BA* isoform.[30] It is suggested that this shift may counterbalance the decreased phosphorylation status of titin in the failing human heart,[31] which functionally results in an increased passive stiffness. The underlying defect in titin phosphorylation is thought to be PKA-dependent (as with reduced cTnI and myosin binding protein C phosphorylation),[28] but dysfunctional CaMKII-dependent phosphorylation of titin is also reported.[32] Cyclic GMP-dependent protein kinase (PKG), activated by nitric oxide (NO), may also phosphorylate cTnI and titin and have similar effects to PKA. In heart failure, there is usually a reduction in NO/PKG activity, which promotes increased titin-dependent passive stiffness.[33] Finally, changes in the redox milieu within the failing myocytes may also contribute to contractile dysfunction (e.g., through specific oxidative modifications in titin that lead to increased passive stiffness).[34]

GLOBAL MECHANISMS AFFECTING CARDIOMYOCYTE FUNCTION IN HEART FAILURE

Redox Homeostasis in the Heart (see also Chapter 8)

ROS are generated in cardiac myocytes (as in other cell types) either as a by-product of cellular respiration and metabolism or through specialized enzymes. An important physiologic function of ROS is in redox signaling (i.e., the highly specific, usually reversible oxidation/reduction modification of signaling molecules involved in various homeostatic processes).[35] Redox signaling is tightly regulated in a spatially and temporally confined manner and depends upon appropriate inactivation or scavenging of ROS by cellular antioxidants to terminate the ROS signal. Another critical function of ROS is their involvement in oxidative protein folding in the endoplasmic reticulum (ER). In pathologic settings such as heart failure, physiologic redox signaling pathways may be perturbed or different redox-sensitive signaling pathways may be activated. Altered redox homeostasis in the ER may have a major impact on protein synthesis and stress responses (see later). In addition, an imbalance between ROS production and antioxidant reserves (i.e., oxidative stress) can result in nonspecific detrimental effects due to the irreversible oxidation of macromolecules, membranes, and DNA. Therefore, alterations in redox homeostasis in the failing cardiomyocyte have a profound impact on many aspects of the myocyte phenotype.

Major sources of ROS in failing cardiac myocytes include the mitochondrial electron transport chain (ETC), NADPH oxidase proteins (NOXs), monoamine oxidases, uncoupled NO synthases (NOSs), and xanthine oxidases. Pathophysiologically important ROS species include superoxide, hydrogen peroxide (produced by dismutation of superoxide), hydroxyl ions, and peroxynitrite generated by the reaction of superoxide with NO. Electron leak from the mitochondrial ETC generates superoxide and this becomes quantitatively more important in heart failure as a result of ETC dysfunction, uncoupling, and an impairment of mitochondrial antioxidants. Mitochondrial ROS generation can lead to opening of the mitochondrial permeability transition pore (MPTP) and loss of cell viability. Furthermore, such ROS production may also induce further mitochondrial ROS production, termed *ROS-induced ROS release*.[36] Monoamine oxidases, which catabolize the neurotransmitters noradrenaline and serotonin, have recently been recognized as additional important mitochondrial sources of ROS in the failing heart.[37] Non-mitochondrial ROS sources, such as NOXs and xanthine oxidase, may also stimulate mitochondrial ROS production. Xanthine oxidase-derived ROS may be particularly important in the setting of ischemia-reperfusion.[38] The inhibition of mitochondrial ROS using various mitochondrially targeted agents is considered to be a promising therapeutic approach in heart failure.[39]

NOX proteins are especially important for redox signaling, being the only source that has a primary ROS-generating function. They catalyze electron transfer from NADPH to molecular O_2, thereby generating superoxide and/or hydrogen peroxide. Among seven distinct NOX family members, NOX2 and NOX4 are expressed in cardiomyocytes and other cardiac cells (e.g., endothelial cells, fibroblasts, inflammatory cells).[40-42] Although both isoforms generate ROS, there are significant differences in their structure, activation, and subcellular localization that contribute to important differences in function. NOX2 has been shown to have a physiologic function in stretch-induced excitation-contraction coupling,[43] whereas NOX4 may regulate cardiomyocyte differentiation.[44] The activities of both NOX2 and NOX4 are increased in heart failure, the former mainly as a result of increased activation by stimuli, such as angiotensin II and cytokines, and the latter largely because of increased expression levels. An additional Ca^{2+}-sensitive isoform, NOX5, may be important in the human heart.

NOS enzymes normally catalyze the production of NO from L-arginine. Cardiomyocytes constitutively express neuronal (nNOS) and endothelial (eNOS) isoforms, which have distinct physiologic actions, notably in regulating excitation-contraction coupling and inotropic responsiveness.[45] An inducible iNOS isoform is upregulated in response to cytokine stimulation. During heart failure, NOSs can become "uncoupled" and switch from NO to superoxide generation, resulting in loss of the normal NO-mediated effects, as well as detrimental effects related to ROS production. Partial uncoupling results in the simultaneous generation of NO and superoxide, leading to peroxynitrite production. Uncoupling of NOSs is usually related to a reduction in the availability of the cofactor tetrahydrobiopterin.[45] In the case of eNOS, there additionally is *S*-glutathionylation of specific cysteine residues in the reductase domain.[46] Importantly, both these mechanisms are enhanced by oxidative stress so that NOS uncoupling can often act to amplify ROS generation by other sources.

Alterations in antioxidant balance are an important contributor to altered redox homeostasis in the failing heart. These include changes in antioxidant enzymes, such as superoxide dismutases, catalase, glutathione peroxidase, thioredoxin, peroxiredoxin, glutathione *S*-transferases, and others. A crucial factor for redox homeostasis is the level of NADPH in different cellular compartments, with this nucleotide being required for the regeneration of reduced pools of major cellular antioxidants, such as glutathione, glutaredoxin, and thioredoxin. Therefore, metabolic reactions that generate NADPH have potentially broad impact on the myocyte phenotype. In the mitochondria, the activity of Ca^{2+}-dependent dehydrogenases is important in this regard, and this is inhibited by cytosolic Na^+ overload in heart failure as mentioned earlier.[14] In the cytosol, glucose-6-phosphate dehydrogenase (G6PD) is a key rate-limiting enzyme involved in NADPH production and has been shown to affect cardiomyocyte calcium homeostasis and contractile dysfunction in ischemia-reperfusion.[47] Interestingly, excessively high levels of NADPH and glutathione can be detrimental by inducing so-called reductive stress. In a mouse model of mutant αB-crystallin cardiomyopathy, such reductive stress is associated with abnormal protein folding and the accumulation of protein aggregates in cardiomyocytes.[48]

Altered redox homeostasis affects an extensive range of molecular targets in the failing cardiomyocyte, including kinases, phosphatases, ion transporters and channels, myofilaments, and transcription factors, as reviewed in detail elsewhere.[42] Here we discuss a few examples where the mechanisms of such redox modifications and their impact on the myocyte phenotype have been addressed in sufficient depth to offer the promise of therapeutically tractable targets. Redox dysregulation affects several proteins involved in abnormal excitation-contraction coupling, as discussed earlier. NOX2 appears to be an important ROS source in this regard[43] and may act both through direct oxidation of proteins such as RyR2 and via specific oxidative activation of CaMKII. NOX2 is also implicated in the genesis of atrial fibrillation.[49] Several signaling pathways involved in cardiomyocyte hypertrophy are in part redox-regulated (e.g., the activation of ASK-1, ERK1/2, NF-κB, and Akt). NOX2 is again an important ROS source responsible for such regulation, especially in the setting of increased renin-angiotensin system activation.[50,51] Class II histone deacetylases (HDACs) are key regulators of hypertrophic gene expression, allowing this to occur when they are exported from the cardiomyocyte nucleus. A thioredoxin 1-sensitive pathway for the specific oxidation and subsequent nuclear export of HDAC4 is reported to be important in adrenergic-mediated cardiomyocyte hypertrophy.[52,53] Cardiomyocyte viability may be adversely affected by an altered redox balance (e.g., leading to increased mitochondrial ROS production). In addition, the specific oxidative activation of kinases such as CaMKII has been found to be important.[21] Not all ROS effects are detrimental in the stressed cardiomyocyte. For example, an increase in NOX4 was shown to be cardioprotective during chronic pressure overload by enhancing myocyte HIF1α signaling and leading to a paracrine secretion of the angiogenic peptide vascular endothelial growth factor (VEGF), with a consequent preservation of myocardial capillary density.[54] This underscores the concept that the effects of altered redox homeostasis may vary depending on the ROS source and its subcellular location.

Protein Synthesis, Turnover, Quality Control, and Stress Responses

The dynamic cellular remodeling that occurs in the stressed and failing heart involves substantial changes in protein synthesis and turnover and requires robust quality control mechanisms to ensure the degradation or clearance of abnormal proteins (e.g., misfolded proteins and protein aggregates). Several organelles and systems are important for these functions, including the ER, the ubiquitin-proteosome system, and autophagy. The cell can mount specific stress responses designed to facilitate the maintenance of some of these functions (e.g., the unfolded protein response [UPR] or an enhancement of autophagy). These systems make a major contribution to the cellular phenotype in the failing heart and may represent targets for therapeutic modulation. We next discuss in more detail the role of some of these systems in the failing heart.

The Endoplasmic Reticulum and the Unfolded Protein Response

The cardiac myocyte SR is a specialized ER that is especially important for intracellular Ca^{2+} regulation, and this is known to become dysfunctional in heart failure, as discussed earlier in this chapter. In addition to Ca^{2+} homeostasis, the ER coordinates other important functions such as the correct folding, post-translational modification, and quality control of membrane and secreted proteins, gluconeogenesis, lipid, and

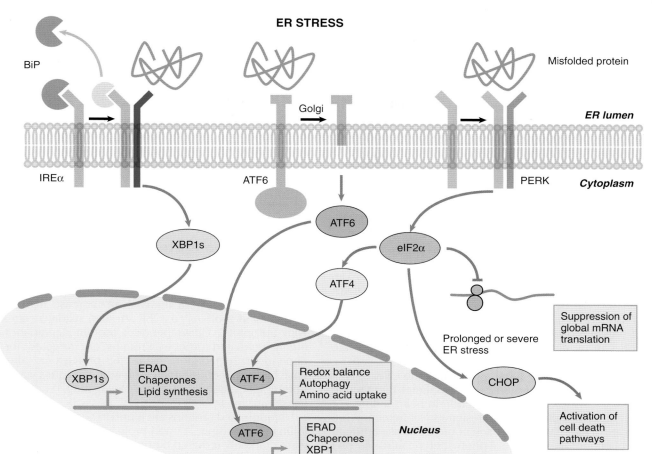

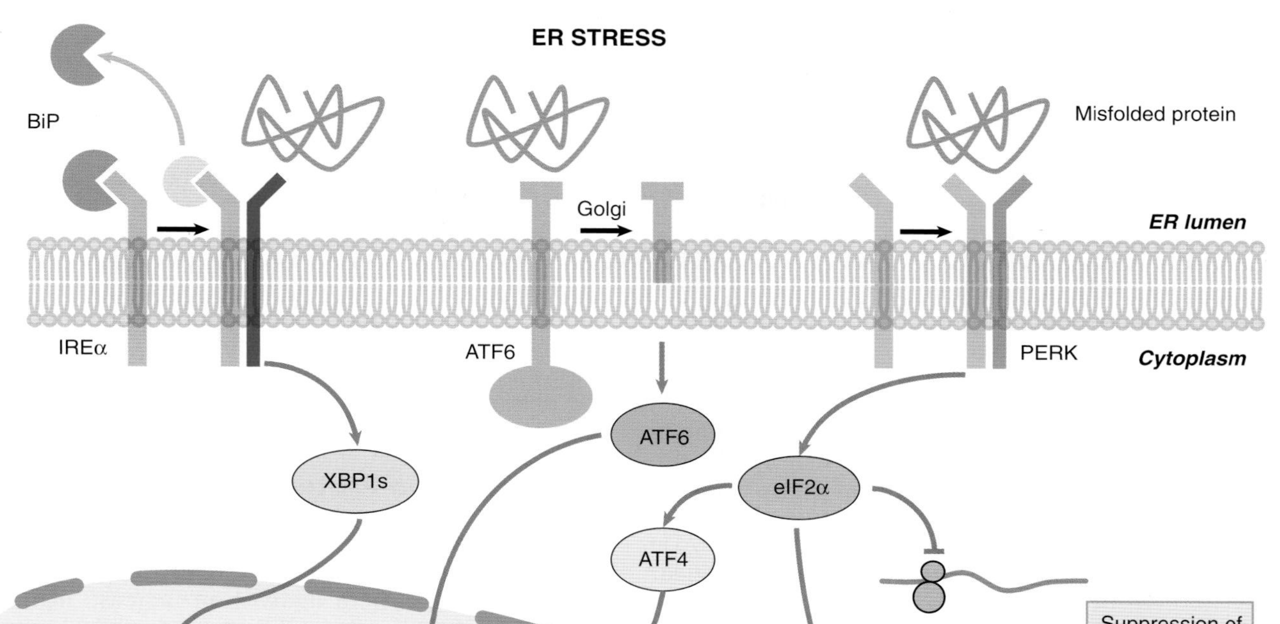

FIGURE 2-5 Endoplasmic reticulum (ER) stress leading to activation of the unfolded protein response. ER stress triggers a set of homeostatic cellular changes termed the *unfolded protein response (UPR)*. This involves the activation of three ER-resident transmembrane proteins: protein kinase RNA-like ER kinase (PERK), inositol-requiring kinase 1 (IRE1), and activating transcription factor 6 (ATF6). ER stress activation of the UPR is an adaptive response to cardiac stress; however, prolonged or more severe stress can lead to the activation of apoptotic pathways and a maladaptive ER stress response. PERK and IRE1 are activated either by dissociation of BiP/GRP78, allowing dimerization and activation by autophosphorylation, or misfolded proteins can directly bind to PERK and IRE1 and cause dimerization and activation. ATF6 is activated through a protease mechanism. Downstream of ATF6 and the transcription factor XBP1s (which is activated by IRE), multiple chaperones and ER-associated degradation (ERAD) proteins are induced, which help to fold proteins and to target misfolded proteins for degradation. In addition, global protein translation is inhibited by PERK-induced phosphorylation of eIF2α, thus reducing protein load to the ER. However, ATF4 translation is upregulated and induces genes involved in adaptive responses (e.g., redox balance, angiogenesis, amino acid uptake, autophagy). Prolonged ER stress can cause ATF4 to activate proapoptotic pathways via C/EBP-homologous protein (CHOP)-mediated signaling.

steroid synthesis.[55] It also interacts with and influences mitochondrial function (e.g., through transfer of Ca^{2+} from the ER). These functions are important in cardiac myocytes as in other cell types, although the distinction and/or overlap between the SR and ER remain poorly defined. The requirement for protein folding, quality control, and related functions in the ER changes significantly in the remodeling heart where there are significant alterations in protein turnover (e.g., due to hypertrophy), metabolism, and energetics. The maintenance of appropriate ER function therefore becomes an important factor in cellular homeostasis.

The ER stress response or unfolded protein response (UPR) is a conserved mechanism that senses the status of ER protein folding by detecting the accumulation of misfolded proteins and inducing a program of changes that affects both the ER and other cellular organelles and processes.[56,57] The UPR encompasses homeostatic mechanisms that include the increased synthesis of chaperones, which assist the refolding of misfolded proteins, inhibition of further protein translation that may aggravate misfolding and ER overload, and the activation of degradation pathways to break down misfolded proteins. Many different stressors can induce the UPR, including glucose or amino acid deprivation, oxidative stress, hypoxia, and ionic imbalance. Induction of the UPR is mediated through three transmembrane ER stress sensors, namely protein kinase RNA-like ER kinase (PERK), inositol-requiring kinase 1 (IRE1), and activating transcription factor 6 (ATF6), that "sense" luminal ER stress and respond by activating specific transcriptional pathways while inhibiting global protein translation (**Figure 2-5**). Such activation of the UPR has the potential to be an adaptive response that restores homeostasis or a detrimental response that triggers cell death pathways, depending upon its strength, duration, and context.

Recent research indicates that the UPR is activated in the ischemic, hypertrophic, and failing heart and contributes to the cellular phenotype through effects on cell protein turnover, metabolism, function, and viability.[55] Myocardial tissue from patients with dilated or ischemic cardiomyopathy shows increased expression of many proteins involved in the UPR, such as the three stress sensors and ER chaperones.[58,59] A similar activation of the UPR is found in animal models of heart failure (e.g., mice subjected to chronic pressure overload or in models of salt-sensitive hypertension and failure).[55,60] The transgenic expression of a mutant KDEL receptor, whose normal function is to retrieve ER chaperones and misfolded proteins with KDEL (Lys-Asp-Glu-Leu) sequences from intracellular compartments, such as the Golgi to the ER, as part of a quality control mechanism, results in dilated cardiomyopathy in a mouse model—indicating the importance of the ER chaperone function.[61] More direct evidence of the role of the UPR in heart failure comes from mouse studies in which heart-specific expression of a dominant negative mutant of ATF6 resulted in adverse cardiac remodeling and heart failure, whereas mice expressing a constitutively active ATF6 had reduced post-MI cardiac remodeling.[62] The activation of an ATF6-dependent gene program by thrombospondin 4 was found to be protective during myocardial injury.[63] ATF6 also seems to protect against acute cardiac stress, such as ischemia-reperfusion injury.[64] These studies suggest that activation of the ATF6 limb of the UPR may be an adaptive response during heart failure. However, there may also be settings where UPR activation is detrimental; for example, during prolonged or severe pressure overload, the PERK/ATF4/CHOP branch of the UPR can be activated, leading to a proapoptotic state and progression of heart failure.[59]

The above data suggest that modulating the UPR, or specific limbs of the UPR, could be a beneficial therapeutic approach to tackle cellular dysfunction in heart failure. For example, approaches could be designed to augment ATF6 activation. An alternative approach could be to use artificial chemical chaperones such as 4-phenylbutyric acid (4-PBA) and tauroursodeoxycholic acid (TUDCA). These have been shown to reduce ER stress and have beneficial effects in models of insulin resistance,[65] and preliminary studies also suggest beneficial effects in mouse models of chronic pressure overload.[66,67]

Autophagy (see also Chapter 1)

Autophagy (self-eating) is an important homeostatic mechanism for the degradation and recycling of various cellular components, including organelles (e.g., mitochondria, ER), macromolecules (e.g., protein aggregates), and lipids.[68] It serves an important quality control function, as well as being a mechanism that generates new building blocks for cellular processes such as energy production and protein, nucleotide, and membrane synthesis (e.g., during starvation).[69] Different forms of autophagy are described, among which macroautophagy (here referred to simply as *autophagy*) is the most prevalent and best studied. The process of autophagy is highly regulated and described in detail elsewhere.[68-70] It is characterized by the formation of double-membraned autophagosomes around damaged organelles or protein aggregates, which then fuse with lysosomes to form autophagolysosomes within which the contents are degraded by lysosomal hydrolases.[70] A family of proteins encoded by autophagy-related (Atg) genes is involved in the different steps of the autophagic process.[70] The mammalian target of rapamycin complex 1 (mTORC1) is a key activator of autophagy in response to "nutrient stress" (e.g., hypoxia or nutrient deprivation).

Increased levels of autophagy are found in human failing hearts, but until recently it has not been clear whether this is detrimental by degrading cellular constituents or a protective quality control mechanism.[71,72] Studies in gene-modified mouse models offer mechanistic data regarding the physiologic and pathologic roles of autophagy in the heart. Mice lacking lysosome-associated membrane protein 2 (LAMP2), which is required for autophagic degradation, develop cardiomyopathy.[73] Similarly, mice with cardiac-specific deficiency of Atg5 develop cardiac dysfunction accompanied by increased levels of ubiquitinated proteins, ER stress, and apoptosis,[74] and die prematurely after about 6 months of age.[75] Furthermore, these animals have an impaired response to imposition of pressure overload, suggesting that autophagy is an adaptive protective mechanism. However, there may some settings in which autophagy could be detrimental.[76]

The Ubiquitin-Proteasome System

The ubiquitin-proteasome system (UPS) is the major cellular system for the degradation of proteins, both as a physiologic pathway (e.g., in various cell signaling responses) and in settings where there is an increase in misfolded or damaged proteins (e.g., ER stress or oxidative stress). As with autophagy, UPS-dependent protein degradation is a highly regulated process. Proteins are targeted for ATP-dependent degradation in the 26S proteasome after they have been poly-ubiquitinated on lysine residues via specific ubiquitin-activating, ubiquitin-conjugating, and ubiquitin ligase enzymes.

Ubiquitinated proteins are found to accumulate in human failing myocardium,[71,77] and proteasomal catalytic activities were markedly reduced compared with nonfailing hearts.[78] However, the functional impact is not clear from these studies. Studies in animal models of heart failure report conflicting findings, with some showing a decrease and others an increase in UPS activity.[77] Of clinical interest, small studies in patients with left ventricular assist devices (LVADs) have reported that proteasomal activity increases in association with the reverse remodeling induced by mechanical unloading, suggesting that the UPS may have a beneficial role perhaps by clearing damaged proteins.[79] Supportive evidence that the removal of damaged proteins is important in the failing heart comes from models of desmin-related cardiomyopathy and of mutations in the chaperone αB-crystallin (CryAB),[80] where the accumulation of protein aggregates appears to be proteotoxic to the heart. Human desmin-related cardiomyopathy can be recapitulated in mice expressing a cardiac-specific $CryAB^{R120G}$ mutant; these animals show evidence of protein aggregation, UPS impairment, and dilated cardiomyopathy.[81]

Coordinated Functions of the UPR, UPS, and Autophagy Systems

The UPR, UPS, and autophagy systems (and other protein degradation systems, such as the calpain pathway, that are not covered here) act in a coordinated manner to regulate protein turnover. The three systems are activated by similar stimuli associated with cardiac stress and heart failure (e.g., oxidative stress, hypoxia, metabolic changes, and Ca^{2+} dysregulation). Alterations in the function of one system often impact on the other systems. For example, ER stress may activate the UPS and autophagy, whereas UPS activation may increase when autophagy is impaired. In addition, these systems have a broader impact on other processes, such as

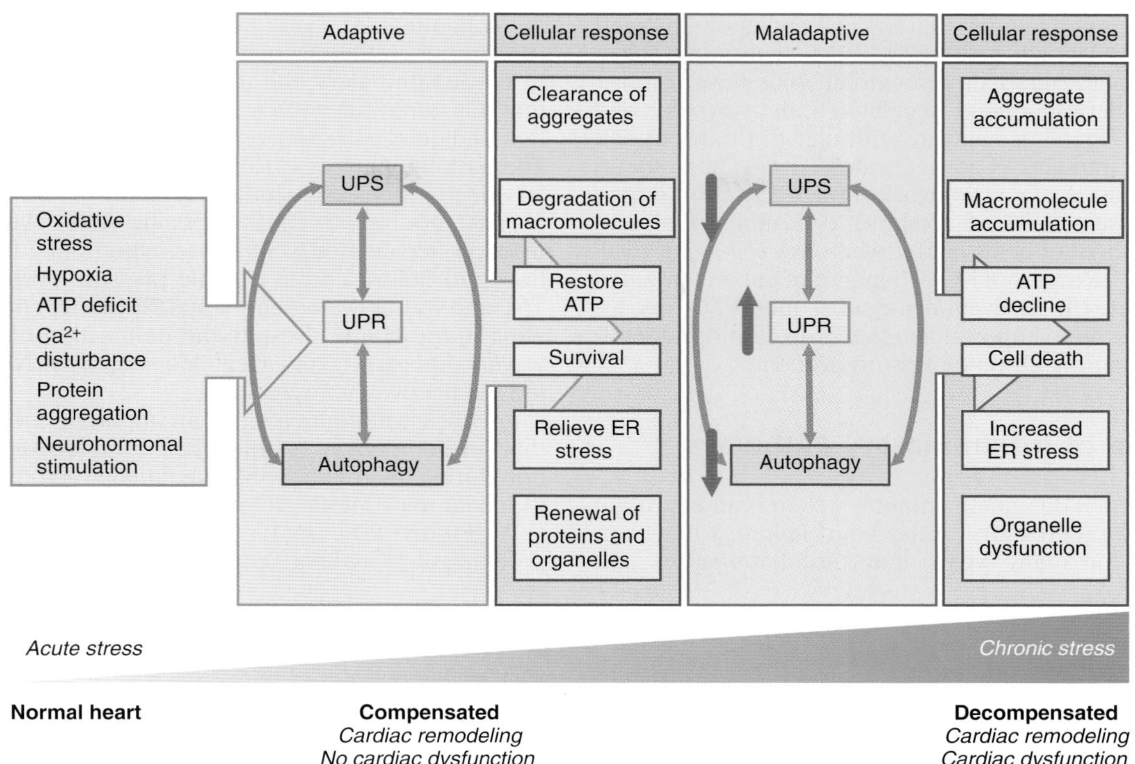

FIGURE 2-6 Coordinated activation of the unfolded protein response (UPR), ubiquitin-proteasome system (UPS), and autophagy systems in response to cardiac stress. Diverse stimuli that result in cardiac stress activate the UPR, autophagy, and UPS systems. Initially these systems serve to reestablish cellular homeostasis and maintain adaptive remodeling and function. Prolonged or more severe stress may override the coordinated and balanced action of these systems and culminate in a maladaptive remodeling process and cardiac dysfunction.

energy metabolism and redox, and ionic homeostasis, and may therefore affect many different aspects of the cellular phenotype in the failing heart. As discussed earlier, appropriate function of these pathways seems to be required for adaptation to chronic cardiac stress and the maintenance of normal cardiac function. On the other hand, an insufficient activation or an excessive activation of these pathways may contribute to maladaptive remodeling and the development of heart failure (**Figure 2-6**).

CARDIOMYOCYTE INTERACTIONS WITH OTHER CELL TYPES

The number of nonmyocytes (e.g., fibroblasts, endothelial cells) in the heart outnumbers the contractile cell population, and interactions between cardiomyocytes and nonmyocytes are important not only physiologically but also in the setting of heart failure. We focus here on intercellular paracrine signaling involving cardiomyocytes during the development of cardiac remodeling and failure.

Paracrine Effects of Endothelial Cells

Coronary microvascular and endocardial endothelial cells are known to exert paracrine effects on cardiomyocytes through the secretion of factors such as nitric oxide (NO), endothelin, and neuregulin, affecting both contractile function and growth.[82,83] NO, for example, modulates myocardial relaxation, the Frank-Starling response, β-adrenergic inotropic responsiveness, and myocardial energetics.[45] Endothelial NO-dependent effects on myocardial function may become impaired during chronic pressure overload and failure (e.g., due to increased endothelial ROS production), and thereby affect contractile function, substrate metabolism, and hypertrophy.[84,85] Endothelial production of endothelin-1 (ET-1) acts as a stimulus for cardiomyocyte hypertrophy during pressure overload.

Paracrine Effects of Fibroblasts

Cardiac fibroblasts are key players not only in fibrosis but also in the regulation of cardiomyocyte hypertrophy. Their phenotype changes in response to stress and they transform into myofibroblasts that secrete cardioactive paracrine factors.[86] Experimental evidence suggests that a significant component of angiotensin II-mediated cardiac hypertrophic effects may be mediated by fibroblast factors, such as ET-1 and TGF-β.[87] Other important growth factors in the paracrine and autocrine interplay between cardiomyocytes and myofibroblasts include fibroblast growth factor-2 (FGF-2), PDGF-A/B, IGF-1, and IL-6 family interleukins, which include leukemia inhibitory factor (LIF) and CT-1. Some of these are cardioprotective, but many act to stimulate fibrosis in the primary "healing" response to injury.

Cardiomyocyte Angiogenic Signaling

There is an important relationship between cardiomyocyte hypertrophy and myocardial capillary density and angiogenesis, especially during chronic pressure overload. Recent experimental work indicates that a matching between capillary density and hypertrophy helps to preserve cardiac contractile function and reduce adverse remodeling. Hypertrophic stimuli induce cardiomyocyte expression of the

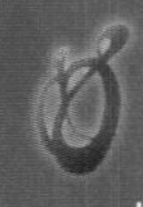

angiogenic growth factors such as VEGF, angiopoietin-2, and platelet-derived growth factor (PDGF), which promote angiogenesis and act to maintain myocardial blood flow.[88] Cardiomyocyte VEGF production is regulated both by hypoxic and nonhypoxic signaling pathways through the transcription factors HIF1 and GATA4, respectively.[89,90] It has been found that an inhibition of cardiomyocyte HIF1 activation during chronic pressure overload promotes decompensation and the development of heart failure, whereas exogenous VEGF is protective.[90] Recently, a NOX4-dependent enhancement of cardiomyocyte HIF1 activation and subsequent VEGF release was identified as an important endogenous cardioprotective mechanism during chronic pressure overload.[91]

Activation of Inflammatory Pathways (see also Chapter 7)

The activation of the innate immune system is an important player in the progression toward heart failure. It has been recognized for many years that proinflammatory and anti-inflammatory cytokines produced within the heart itself under conditions of hemodynamic stress are involved in the inflammatory cell influx into the myocardium, and that this contributes to cardiomyocyte contractile dysfunction and damage, as well as extracellular matrix remodeling. The proinflammatory cytokine tumor necrosis factor (TNF) has been extensively studied in heart failure progression. Mouse models of cardiac-specific TNF overexpression develop accelerated ventricular hypertrophy, fibrosis, dilation, and failure during chronic pressure overload.[92] Both TNF and IL-1 activate detrimental NF-κB-dependent remodeling in the heart.[93] Despite the delineation of these pathways, therapies targeted at cytokines such as TNF-α have not led to effective therapies so far.

Recent studies indicate that an important mechanism for the development of "sterile" (i.e., noninfective) inflammation during heart failure may be damage-associated molecular patterns (DAMPs) released from damaged myocardial cells (**Figure 2-7**). DAMPs consist of released intracellular proteins, such as heat shock proteins, oxidized LDLs, and

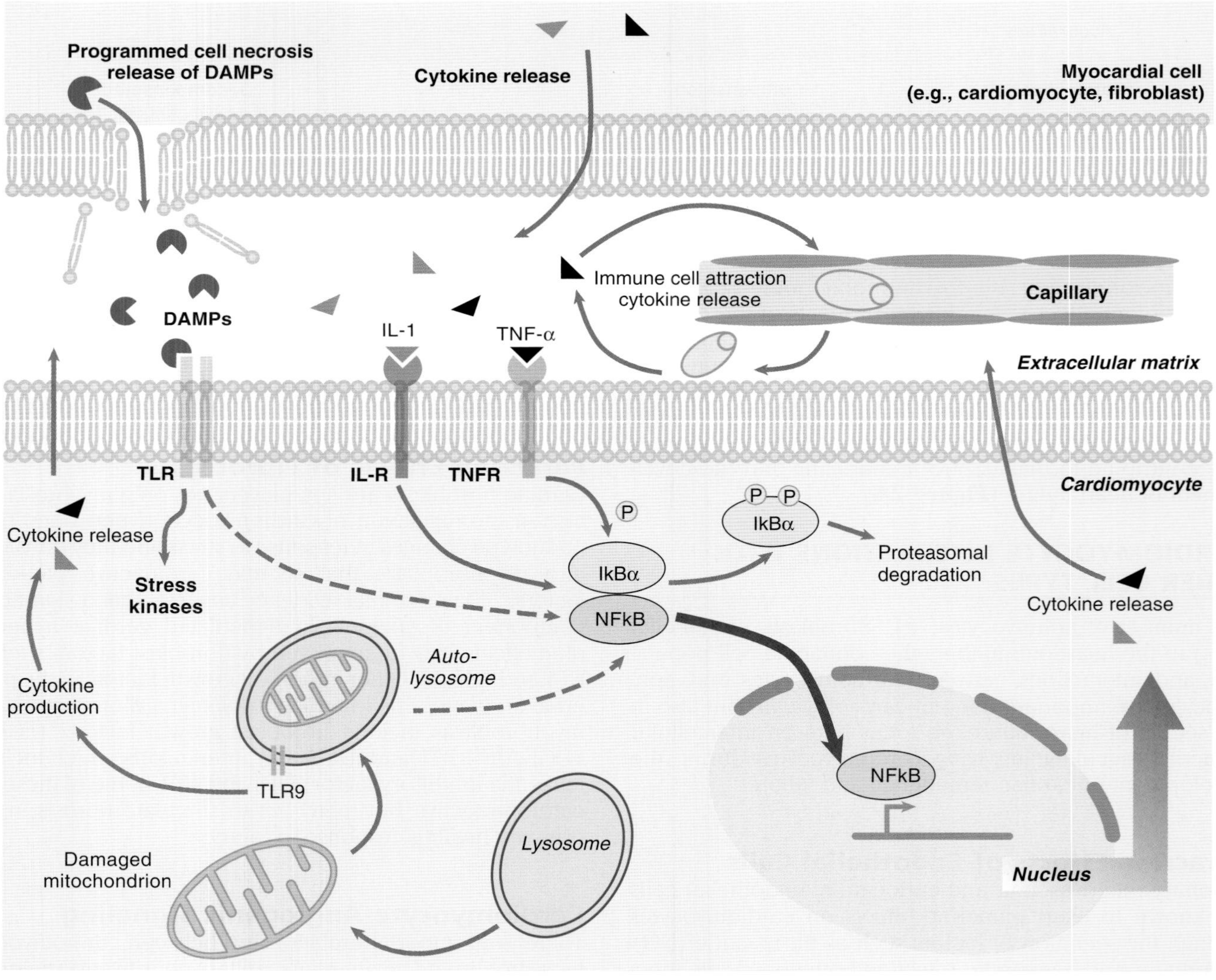

FIGURE 2-7 Overview of the innate immune response in the myocardium during chronic cardiac stress and heart failure. In response to chronic stress, proinflammatory cytokines including IL-1β and TNF-α can be released from myocytes, fibroblasts, or immune cells. They can signal to myocytes, resulting in activation of signaling pathways leading to cardiac remodeling. Activation of the NF-κB pathway promotes further cytokine production, cell death pathway activation, and pro-hypertrophic and fibrotic pathways. Cytokines can trigger cells to undergo programmed necrosis, resulting in the release of damage-associated molecular patterns (DAMPs) that signal via toll-like receptors (TLRs) on the surface of cardiomyocytes to potentiate cytokine production and other stress kinase signaling. Impaired autophagy of damaged mitochondria during cardiac stress can also activate endolysosomal TLR9 through binding to released mitochondrial DNA, thereby triggering proinflammatory cytokine production, macrophage, and immune cell recruitment and further inflammation.

free fatty acids, or extracellular matrix components such as fibronectin.[94] They are recognized by immune cells through cell surface receptors that include toll-like receptors (TLRs) and nucleotide-oligomerization domain (NOD)-like receptors, resulting in the triggering of inflammatory responses.[95] TLRs may also be activated on cardiomyocytes themselves to induce production of cytokines, which then amplify the inflammatory response. Indeed, TLR4 is reported to be upregulated in the failing human heart. Recently, a novel mechanism was reported that links mitochondrial dysfunction, autophagy, and sterile inflammation in the chronic pressure-overloaded heart.[96] Oka and associates discovered that during the process of mitophagy (autophagy of dysfunctional mitochondria) in pressure-overloaded hearts, fragments of mitochondrial DNA may be released that act as stimuli for the activation of cardiomyocyte TLR9 receptors and evoke inflammation. The genetic inactivation of cardiomyocyte DNAse-II, which degrades mitochondrial DNA, resulted in a marked accumulation of mitochondrial DNA in autolysosomes and a profound myocarditis and dilated cardiomyopathy. Importantly, treatment with a TLR9 antagonist could reduce myocardial inflammation both in DNAse-II knockout mice and wild-type mice, suggesting this may be a suitable therapeutic target in heart failure.

MicroRNA-DEPENDENT PATHWAYS

MicroRNAs (miRNAs) are highly conserved endogenous nucleotide segments of noncoding RNA (typically around 22 nucleotides long) that act to regulate the stability and translation of mRNA transcripts. As a general rule, miRNAs function by base pairing with 3′ untranslated regions within a transcript, resulting in gene silencing via translational repression and/or target mRNA degradation. Individual miRNAs can act as "master regulators" of cellular signaling processes through their ability to regulate multiple genes within signaling pathways. As such, they are capable of having a major impact on cellular phenotypes. Recent work in animal models, supported by studies in human tissue, indicates that alterations in miRNA expression have a significant influence on the cardiomyocyte phenotype in the failing heart (**Figure 2-8**).[97,98] Moreover, these effects may extend to an impact on nonmyocyte cells and on cell-cell interactions within the heart.

A large number of miRNAs can influence the cardiomyocyte hypertrophic response to stress, including many that are antihypertrophic (e.g., miR-1, miR-9, miR-26, miR-29, miR-98, miR-133) and others that are pro-hypertrophic (e.g., miR-21, miR-23a, miR-143, miR-199a, miR-199b, miR-208,

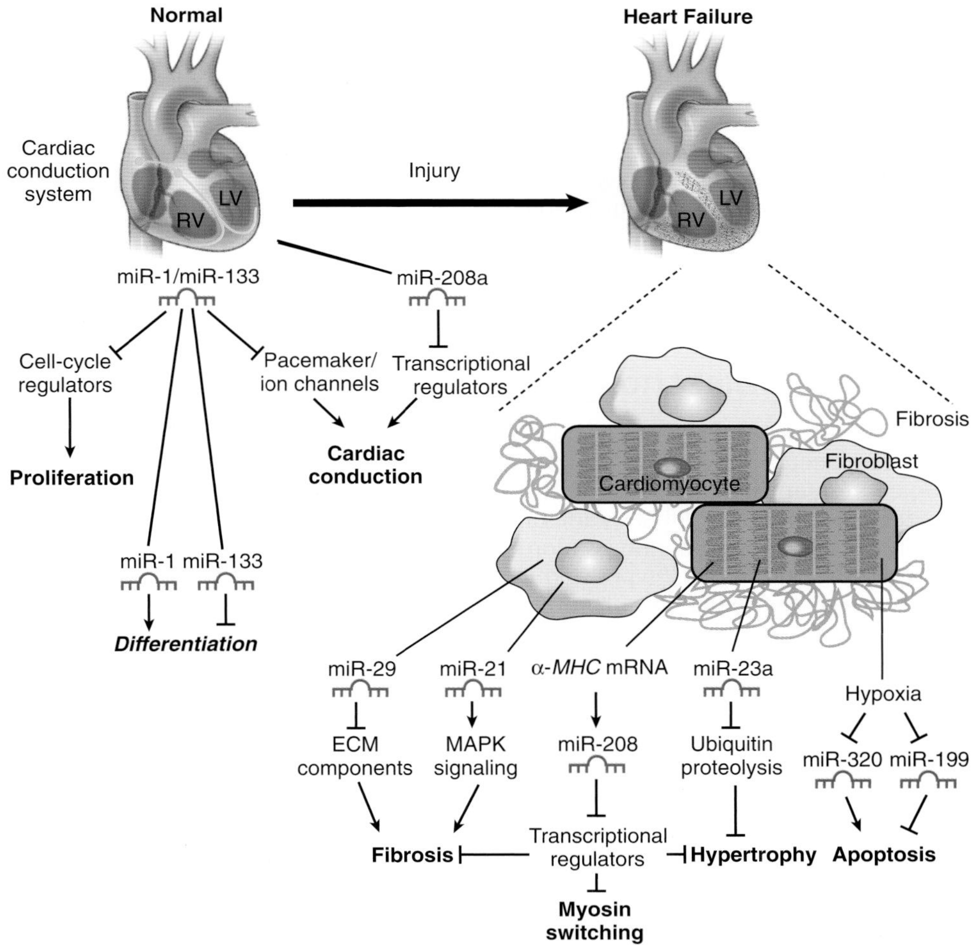

FIGURE 2-8 Functional role of microRNAs in the normal and failing heart. A normal and a hypertrophic/failing heart are shown in schematic form, depicting miRNAs that contribute to normal function or pathologic remodeling. All arrows denote the normal action of each component or process. miR-1 and miR-133 are involved in the development of a normal heart *(left)* by regulating proliferation, differentiation, and cardiac conduction. After cardiac injury *(right),* various miRNAs contribute to pathologic remodeling and the progression to heart failure. miR-29 blocks fibrosis by inhibiting the expression of ECM components, whereas miR-21 promotes. miR-208 controls myosin isoform switching, cardiac hypertrophy, and fibrosis. miR-23a promotes cardiac hypertrophy by inhibiting ubiquitin proteolysis, which itself inhibits hypertrophy. Hypoxia results in the repression of miR-320 and miR-199, which promote and block apoptosis, respectively. *ECM,* extracellular matrix; *LV,* left ventricle; *MAPK,* mitogen-activated protein kinase; *MHC,* myosin heavy chain. *Modified from Small EM, Olson EN: Pervasive roles of microRNAs in cardiovascular biology. Nature 469:336–342, 2011.*

miR-499). Some of these act primarily within nonmyocytes in the remodeling and failing heart (e.g., miR-21 and miR-29 within fibroblasts). Changes in miRNA profiles appear to play an important part in the re-expression of fetal gene profiles in the stressed and failing heart. Interestingly, miRNA transcription may be regulated by certain stress-activated transcription factors (e.g., NFAT, STAT3, SRF), suggesting that global regulatory circuits coordinate the molecular remodeling that underpins the development of the cellular phenotype in the failing heart.[97,98] The specific molecular targets of miRNAs that are altered in heart failure include proteins involved in cardiomyocyte growth, sarcomere function, excitation-contraction coupling, cell-cycle regulation, protein turnover, redox homeostasis, paracrine regulation, fibrosis, inflammation, angiogenesis, and other processes, illustrating the potentially profound effects of these master regulators.

Increases in miRNA expression can in principle be therapeutically targeted (e.g., with antagomirs), and studies in animal models suggest that such approaches offer significant potential.[98] The concept of targeting multiple pathologic components with a single antagomir is intuitively highly attractive but there are significant challenges to overcome, in particular the need to specifically target the heart. In principle, miRNAs could also be delivered as a therapeutic, but again there are challenges with respect to pharmacokinetics, pharmacodynamics, and specific targeting.

miRNAs are also found circulating in the blood in a stable form both in the healthy setting and in diseases. Plasma miRNA profiles change specifically and significantly in different diseases, including heart failure.[99] The pathophysiologic relevance of this finding remains to be established (e.g., do circulating miRNAs facilitate signaling between different cells or tissues or do they simply represent a "spill-over"?). Regardless of the answer to this question, there is great interest in the potential for changes in plasma miRNA profiles to serve as biomarkers for disease diagnosis, prognosis, and/or monitoring.

CONCLUSIONS AND FUTURE DIRECTIONS

Profound alterations in gene and protein expression, molecular regulation, and signaling occur in the cardiomyocytes in a heart under chronic stress and largely underpin the complex changes in cellular phenotype that gradually develop. These changes in cardiomyocyte phenotype, along with associated changes in other cardiac cell types and in the extracellular matrix, play a major role in overall cardiac remodeling and the subsequent development of the multiorgan heart failure syndrome. In this chapter, we have discussed alterations in cardiomyocyte function that contribute to the development of pathologic cardiac remodeling and failure. These include specific abnormalities in cardiac contractile function, as well as global alterations in cellular homeostasis that also impact on the myocyte phenotype. A better understanding of these complex changes offers the potential to identify new therapeutic targets for use in heart failure.

Acknowledgments

The authors' work is supported by the British Heart Foundation; a Fondation Leducq Transatlantic Network of Excellence award; and the Department of Health via a National Institute for Health Research (NIHR) Biomedical Research Centre award to Guy's & St Thomas' NHS Foundation Trust in partnership with King's College London and King's College Hospital NHS Foundation Trust.

References

1. Bers DM: Cardiac excitation-contraction coupling. *Nature* 415:198–205, 2002.
2. Lehnart SE, Maier LS, Hasenfuss G: Abnormalities of calcium metabolism and myocardial contractility depression in the failing heart. *Heart Fail Rev* 14:213–224, 2009.
3. Marx SO, Reiken S, Hisamatsu Y, et al: PKA phosphorylation dissociates FKBP12.6 from the calcium release channel (ryanodine receptor): defective regulation in failing hearts. *Cell* 101:365–376, 2000.
4. Gonzalez DR, Beigi F, Treuer AV, et al: Deficient ryanodine receptor S-nitrosylation increases sarcoplasmic reticulum calcium leak and arrhythmogenesis in cardiomyocytes. *Proc Natl Acad Sci U S A* 104:20612–20617, 2007.
5. Terentyev D, Gyorke I, Belevych AE, et al: Redox modification of ryanodine receptors contributes to sarcoplasmic reticulum Ca2+ leak in chronic heart failure. *Circ Res* 103:1466–1472, 2008.
6. Kho C, Lee A, Jeong D, et al: SUMO1-dependent modulation of SERCA2a in heart failure. *Nature* 477:601–605, 2011.
7. Wittkopper K, Fabritz L, Neef S, et al: Constitutively active phosphatase inhibitor-1 improves cardiac contractility in young mice but is deleterious after catecholaminergic stress and with aging. *J Clin Invest* 120:617–626, 2010.
8. Maier LS, Bers DM: Role of Ca2+/calmodulin-dependent protein kinase (CaMK) in excitation-contraction coupling in the heart. *Cardiovasc Res* 73:631–640, 2007.
9. Kranias EG, Hajjar RJ: Modulation of cardiac contractility by the phospholamban/SERCA2a regulatome. *Circ Res* 110:1646–1660, 2012.
10. Hamdani N, Kooij V, van Dijk S, et al: Sarcomeric dysfunction in heart failure. *Cardiovasc Res* 77:649–658, 2008.
11. Lipskaia L, Chemaly ER, Hadri L, et al: Sarcoplasmic reticulum Ca(2+) ATPase as a therapeutic target for heart failure. *Expert Opin Biol Ther* 10:29–41, 2010.
12. Jessup M, Greenberg B, Mancini D, et al: Calcium Upregulation by Percutaneous Administration of Gene Therapy in Cardiac Disease (CUPID): a phase 2 trial of intracoronary gene therapy of sarcoplasmic reticulum Ca2+-ATPase in patients with advanced heart failure. *Circulation* 124:304–313, 2011.
13. Kohlhaas M, Maack C: Adverse bioenergetic consequences of Na+-Ca2+ exchanger-mediated Ca2+ influx in cardiac myocytes. *Circulation* 122:2273–2280, 2010.
14. Kohlhaas M, Liu T, Knopp A, et al: Elevated cytosolic Na+ increases mitochondrial formation of reactive oxygen species in failing cardiac myocytes. *Circulation* 121:1606–1613, 2010.
15. Ai X, Curran JW, Shannon TR, et al: Ca2+/calmodulin-dependent protein kinase modulates cardiac ryanodine receptor phosphorylation and sarcoplasmic reticulum Ca2+ leak in heart failure. *Circ Res* 97:1314–1322, 2005.
16. Wehrens XH, Lehnart SE, Reiken S, et al: Ryanodine receptor/calcium release channel PKA phosphorylation: a critical mediator of heart failure progression. *Proc Natl Acad Sci U S A* 103:511–518, 2006.
17. Lehnart SE, Wehrens XH, Reiken S, et al: Phosphodiesterase 4D deficiency in the ryanodine-receptor complex promotes heart failure and arrhythmias. *Cell* 123:25–35, 2005.
18. Lyon AR, MacLeod KT, Zhang Y, et al: Loss of T-tubules and other changes to surface topography in ventricular myocytes from failing human and rat heart. *Proc Natl Acad Sci U S A* 106:6854–6859, 2009.
19. Li Y, Kranias EG, Mignery GA, et al: Protein kinase A phosphorylation of the ryanodine receptor does not affect calcium sparks in mouse ventricular myocytes. *Circ Res* 90:309–316, 2002.
20. Sossalla S, Fluschnik N, Schotola H, et al: Inhibition of elevated Ca2+/calmodulin-dependent protein kinase II improves contractility in human failing myocardium. *Circ Res* 107:1150–1161, 2010.
21. Erickson JR, Joiner ML, Guan X, et al: A dynamic pathway for calcium-independent activation of CaMKII by methionine oxidation. *Cell* 133:462–474, 2008.
22. Brennan JP, Bardswell SC, Burgoyne JR, et al: Oxidant-induced activation of type I protein kinase A is mediated by RI subunit interprotein disulfide bond formation. *J Biol Chem* 281:21827–21836, 2006.
23. Sag CM, Wadsack DP, Khabbazzadeh S, et al: Calcium/calmodulin-dependent protein kinase II contributes to cardiac arrhythmogenesis in heart failure. *Circ Heart Fail* 2:664–675, 2009.
24. van Oort RJ, McCauley MD, Dixit SS, et al: Ryanodine receptor phosphorylation by calcium/calmodulin-dependent protein kinase II promotes life-threatening ventricular arrhythmias in mice with heart failure. *Circulation* 122:2669–2679, 2010.
25. Wagner S, Ruff HM, Weber SL, et al: Reactive oxygen species-activated Ca/calmodulin kinase IIdelta is required for late I(Na) augmentation leading to cellular Na and Ca overload. *Circ Res* 108:555–565, 2011.
26. Vest JA, Wehrens XH, Reiken SR, et al: Defective cardiac ryanodine receptor regulation during atrial fibrillation. *Circulation* 111:2025–2032, 2005.
27. Voelkel T, Linke WA: Conformation-regulated mechanosensory control via titin domains in cardiac muscle. *Pflugers Arch* 462:143–154, 2011.
28. van der Velden J: Diastolic myofilament dysfunction in the failing human heart. *Pflugers Arch* 462:155–163, 2011.
29. Chen PP, Patel JR, Rybakova IN, et al: Protein kinase A-induced myofilament desensitization to Ca(2+) as a result of phosphorylation of cardiac myosin-binding protein C. *J Gen Physiol* 136:615–627, 2010.
30. Makarenko I, Opitz CA, Leake MC, et al: Passive stiffness changes caused by upregulation of compliant titin isoforms in human dilated cardiomyopathy hearts. *Circ Res* 95:708–716, 2004.
31. Kruger M, Linke WA: Protein kinase-A phosphorylates titin in human heart muscle and reduces myofibrillar passive tension. *J Muscle Res Cell Motil* 27:435–444, 2006.
32. Hamdani N, Krysiak J, Kreusser MM, et al: Crucial role for Ca2(+)/calmodulin-dependent protein kinase-II in regulating diastolic stress of normal and failing hearts via titin phosphorylation. *Circ Res* 112:664–674, 2013.
33. Kruger M, Kotter S, Grutzner A, et al: Protein kinase G modulates human myocardial passive stiffness by phosphorylation of the titin springs. *Circ Res* 104:87–94, 2009.
34. Grutzner A, Garcia-Manyes S, Kotter S, et al: Modulation of titin-based stiffness by disulfide bonding in the cardiac titin N2-B unique sequence. *Biophys J* 97:825–834, 2009.
35. Forman HJ, Fukuto JM, Torres M: Redox signaling: thiol chemistry defines which reactive oxygen and nitrogen species can act as second messengers. *Am J Physiol Cell Physiol* 287:C246–C256, 2004.
36. Zorov DB, Filburn CR, Klotz LO, et al: Reactive oxygen species (ROS)-induced ROS release: a new phenomenon accompanying induction of the mitochondrial permeability transition in cardiac myocytes. *J Exp Med* 192:1001–1014, 2000.
37. Kaludercic N, Takimoto E, Nagayama T, et al: Monoamine oxidase A-mediated enhanced catabolism of norepinephrine contributes to adverse remodeling and pump failure in hearts with pressure overload. *Circ Res* 106:193–202, 2010.
38. Minhas KM, Saraiva RM, Schuleri KH, et al: Xanthine oxidoreductase inhibition causes reverse remodeling in rats with dilated cardiomyopathy. *Circ Res* 98:271–279, 2006.

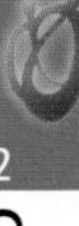

39. Dai DF, Chen T, Szeto H, et al: Mitochondrial targeted antioxidant peptide ameliorates hypertensive cardiomyopathy. *J Am Coll Cardiol* 58:73–82, 2011.
40. Bedard K, Krause KH: The NOX family of ROS-generating NADPH oxidases: physiology and pathophysiology. *Physiol Rev* 87:245–313, 2007.
41. Lassegue B, San Martin A, Griendling KK: Biochemistry, physiology, and pathophysiology of NADPH oxidases in the cardiovascular system. *Circ Res* 110:1364–1390, 2012.
42. Burgoyne JR, Mongue-Din H, Eaton P, et al: Redox signaling in cardiac physiology and pathology. *Circ Res* 111:1091–1106, 2012.
43. Prosser BL, Ward CW, Lederer WJ: X-ROS signaling: rapid mechano-chemo transduction in heart. *Science* 333:1440–1445, 2011.
44. Murray TV, Smyrnias I, Shah AM, et al: NADPH oxidase 4 regulates cardiomyocyte differentiation via redox activation of c-jun protein and the cis-regulation of GATA-4 gene transcription. *J Biol Chem* 288:15745–15759, 2013.
45. Carnicer R, Crabtree MJ, Sivakumaran V, et al: Nitric oxide synthases in heart failure. *Antioxid Redox Signal* 18:1078–1099, 2013.
46. Chen CA, Wang TY, Varadharaj S, et al: S-glutathionylation uncouples eNOS and regulates its cellular and vascular function. *Nature* 468:1115–1118, 2010.
47. Jain M, Brenner DA, Cui L, et al: Glucose-6-phosphate dehydrogenase modulates cytosolic redox status and contractile phenotype in adult cardiomyocytes. *Circ Res* 93:e9–e16, 2003.
48. Rajasekaran NS, Connell P, Christians ES, et al: Human alpha B-crystallin mutation causes oxido-reductive stress and protein aggregation cardiomyopathy in mice. *Cell* 130:427–439, 2007.
49. Kim YM, Guzik TJ, Zhang YH, et al: A myocardial Nox2 containing NAD(P)H oxidase contributes to oxidative stress in human atrial fibrillation. *Circ Res* 97:629–636, 2005.
50. Bendall JK, Cave AC, Heymes C, et al: Pivotal role of a gp91(phox)-containing NADPH oxidase in angiotensin II-induced cardiac hypertrophy in mice. *Circulation* 105:293–296, 2002.
51. Satoh M, Ogita H, Takeshita K, et al: Requirement of Rac1 in the development of cardiac hypertrophy. *Proc Natl Acad Sci U S A* 103:7432–7437, 2006.
52. Ago T, Liu T, Zhai P, et al: A redox-dependent pathway for regulating class II HDACs and cardiac hypertrophy. *Cell* 133:978–993, 2008.
53. Haworth RS, Stathopoulou K, Candasamy AJ, et al: Neurohormonal regulation of cardiac histone deacetylase 5 nuclear localization by phosphorylation-dependent and phosphorylation-independent mechanisms. *Circ Res* 110:1585–1595, 2012.
54. Zhang M, Brewer AC, Schroder K, et al: NADPH oxidase-4 mediates protection against chronic load-induced stress in mouse hearts by enhancing angiogenesis. *Proc Natl Acad Sci U S A* 107:18121–18126, 2010.
55. Doroudgar S, Glembotski CC: New concepts of endoplasmic reticulum function in the heart: programmed to conserve. *J Mol Cell Cardiol* 55:85–91, 2013.
56. Schroder M, Kaufman RJ: The mammalian unfolded protein response. *Annu Rev Biochem* 74:739–789, 2005.
57. Willis MS, Patterson C: Proteotoxicity and cardiac dysfunction–Alzheimer's disease of the heart? *N Engl J Med* 368:455–464, 2013.
58. Sawada T, Minamino T, Fu HY, et al: X-box binding protein 1 regulates brain natriuretic peptide through a novel AP1/CRE-like element in cardiomyocytes. *J Mol Cell Cardiol* 48:1280–1289, 2010.
59. Fu HY, Okada K, Liao Y, et al: Ablation of C/EBP homologous protein attenuates endoplasmic reticulum-mediated apoptosis and cardiac dysfunction induced by pressure overload. *Circulation* 122:361–369, 2010.
60. Okada K, Minamino T, Tsukamoto Y, et al: Prolonged endoplasmic reticulum stress in hypertrophic and failing heart after aortic constriction: possible contribution of endoplasmic reticulum stress to cardiac myocyte apoptosis. *Circulation* 110:705–712, 2004.
61. Hamada H, Suzuki M, Yuasa S, et al: Dilated cardiomyopathy caused by aberrant endoplasmic reticulum quality control in mutant KDEL receptor transgenic mice. *Mol Cell Biol* 24:8007–8017, 2004.
62. Toko H, Takahashi H, Kayama Y, et al: ATF6 is important under both pathological and physiological states in the heart. *J Mol Cell Cardiol* 49:113–120, 2010.
63. Lynch JM, Maillet M, Vanhoutte D, et al: A thrombospondin-dependent pathway for a protective ER stress response. *Cell* 149:1257–1268, 2012.
64. Martindale JJ, Fernandez R, Thuerauf D, et al: Endoplasmic reticulum stress gene induction and protection from ischemia/reperfusion injury in the hearts of transgenic mice with a tamoxifen-regulated form of ATF6. *Circ Res* 98:1186–1193, 2006.
65. Ozcan U, Yilmaz E, Ozcan L, et al: Chemical chaperones reduce ER stress and restore glucose homeostasis in a mouse model of type 2 diabetes. *Science* 313:1137–1140, 2006.
66. Park CS, Cha H, Kwon EJ, et al: The chemical chaperone 4-phenylbutyric acid attenuates pressure-overload cardiac hypertrophy by alleviating endoplasmic reticulum stress. *Biochem Biophys Res Commun* 421:578–584, 2012.
67. Kassan M, Galan M, Partyka M, et al: Endoplasmic reticulum stress is involved in cardiac damage and vascular endothelial dysfunction in hypertensive mice. *Arterioscler Thromb Vasc Biol* 32:1652–1661, 2012.
68. Zhao S, Xu W, Jiang W, et al: Regulation of cellular metabolism by protein lysine acetylation. *Science* 327:1000–1004, 2010.
69. Choi AM, Ryter SW, Levine B: Autophagy in human health and disease. *N Engl J Med* 368:651–662, 2013.
70. Xie Z, Klionsky DJ: Autophagosome formation: core machinery and adaptations. *Nat Cell Biol* 9:1102–1109, 2007.
71. Hein S, Arnon E, Kostin S, et al: Progression from compensated hypertrophy to failure in the pressure-overloaded human heart: structural deterioration and compensatory mechanisms. *Circulation* 107:984–991, 2003.
72. Yan L, Vatner DE, Kim SJ, et al: Autophagy in chronically ischemic myocardium. *Proc Natl Acad Sci U S A* 102:13807–13812, 2005.
73. Tanaka Y, Guhde G, Suter A, et al: Accumulation of autophagic vacuoles and cardiomyopathy in LAMP-2-deficient mice. *Nature* 406:902–906, 2000.
74. Nakai A, Yamaguchi O, Takeda T, et al: The role of autophagy in cardiomyocytes in the basal state and in response to hemodynamic stress. *Nat Med* 13:619–624, 2007.
75. Taneike M, Yamaguchi O, Nakai A, et al: Inhibition of autophagy in the heart induces age-related cardiomyopathy. *Autophagy* 6:600–606, 2010.
76. Zhu H, Tannous P, Johnstone JL, et al: Cardiac autophagy is a maladaptive response to hemodynamic stress. *J Clin Invest* 117:1782–1793, 2007.
77. Tsukamoto O, Minamino T, Okada K, et al: Depression of proteasome activities during the progression of cardiac dysfunction in pressure-overloaded heart of mice. *Biochem Biophys Res Commun* 340:1125–1133, 2006.
78. Predmore JM, Wang P, Davis F, et al: Ubiquitin proteasome dysfunction in human hypertrophic and dilated cardiomyopathies. *Circulation* 121:997–1004, 2010.
79. Day SM: The ubiquitin proteasome system in human cardiomyopathies and heart failure. *Am J Physiol Heart Circ Physiol* 304:11, 2013.
80. Vicart P, Caron A, Guicheney P, et al: A missense mutation in the alphaB-crystallin chaperone gene causes a desmin-related myopathy. *Nat Genet* 20:92–95, 1998.
81. Sanbe A, Osinska H, Saffitz JE, et al: Desmin-related cardiomyopathy in transgenic mice: a cardiac amyloidosis. *Proc Natl Acad Sci U S A* 101:10132–10136, 2004.
82. Brutsaert DL: Cardiac endothelial-myocardial signaling: its role in cardiac growth, contractile performance, and rhythmicity. *Physiol Rev* 83:59–115, 2003.
83. Hsieh PC, Davis ME, Lisowski LK, et al: Endothelial-cardiomyocyte interactions in cardiac development and repair. *Annu Rev Physiol* 68:51–66, 2006.
84. MacCarthy PA, Grieve DJ, Li JM, et al: Impaired endothelial regulation of ventricular relaxation in cardiac hypertrophy: role of reactive oxygen species and NADPH oxidase. *Circulation* 104:2967–2974, 2001.
85. Ruetten H, Dimmeler S, Gehring D, et al: Concentric left ventricular remodeling in endothelial nitric oxide synthase knockout mice by chronic pressure overload. *Cardiovasc Res* 66:444–453, 2005.
86. Weber KT, Sun Y, Bhattacharya SK, et al: Myofibroblast-mediated mechanisms of pathological remodelling of the heart. *Nat Rev Cardiol* 10:15–26, 2013.
87. Koitabashi N, Danner T, Zaiman AL, et al: Pivotal role of cardiomyocyte TGF-beta signaling in the murine pathological response to sustained pressure overload. *J Clin Invest* 121:2301–2312, 2011.
88. Shiojima I, Sato K, Izumiya Y, et al: Disruption of coordinated cardiac hypertrophy and angiogenesis contributes to the transition to heart failure. *J Clin Invest* 115:2108–2118, 2005.
89. Heineke J, Auger-Messier M, Xu J, et al: Cardiomyocyte GATA4 functions as a stress-responsive regulator of angiogenesis in the murine heart. *J Clin Invest* 117:3198–3210, 2007.
90. Sano M, Minamino T, Toko H, et al: p53-induced inhibition of Hif-1 causes cardiac dysfunction during pressure overload. *Nature* 446:444–448, 2007.
91. Schroder K, Zhang M, Benkhoff S, et al: Nox4 is a protective reactive oxygen species generating vascular NADPH oxidase. *Circ Res* 110:1217–1225, 2012.
92. Mann DL: Stress-activated cytokines and the heart: from adaptation to maladaptation. *Annu Rev Physiol* 65:81–101, 2003.
93. Dinarello CA, Simon A, van der Meer JW: Treating inflammation by blocking interleukin-1 in a broad spectrum of diseases. *Nat Rev Drug Discov* 11:633–652, 2012.
94. Lamkanfi M: Emerging inflammasome effector mechanisms. *Nat Rev Immunol* 11:213–220, 2011.
95. Swirski FK, Nahrendorf M: Leukocyte behavior in atherosclerosis, myocardial infarction, and heart failure. *Science* 339:161–166, 2013.
96. Oka T, Hikoso S, Yamaguchi O, et al: Mitochondrial DNA that escapes from autophagy causes inflammation and heart failure. *Nature* 485:251–255, 2012.
97. Da Costa Martins PA, De Windt LJ: MicroRNAs in control of cardiac hypertrophy. *Cardiovasc Res* 93:563–572, 2012.
98. Quiat D, Olson EN: MicroRNAs in cardiovascular disease: from pathogenesis to prevention and treatment. *J Clin Invest* 123:11–18, 2013.
99. Mayr M, Zampetaki A, Willeit P, et al: MicroRNAs within the continuum of postgenomics biomarker discovery. *Arterioscler Thromb Vasc Biol* 33:206–214, 2013.

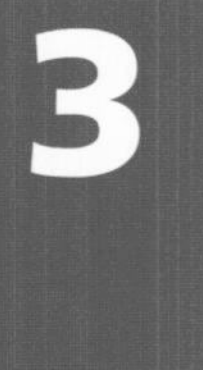

Cellular Basis for Myocardial Regeneration and Repair

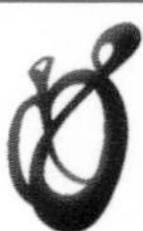

Annarosa Leri, Marcello Rota, Toru Hosoda, and Piero Anversa

OVERVIEW

The traditional view that the reparative ability of the heart is limited by the inability of terminally differentiated cardiomyocytes to undergo cell division after the first weeks of life has been challenged by recent studies that suggest that the heart is capable of limited self-regeneration. Current evidence suggests that there are at least four potential sources of cells that can account for new cardiomyocytes after birth: (1) adult cardiomyocytes (mononucleated) may reenter the cell cycle and divide; (2) bone marrow–derived cardiac stem or progenitor cells that possess the capacity to differentiate into cardiomyocytes may populate the heart after injury; (3) cells that are derived from the embryonic epicardium may give rise to cardiomyocytes; and (4) niches of cardiac stem or cardiac progenitor cells (CPCs) may give rise to cardiomyocytes (**Figure 3-1**). In the following chapter we will focus on the emerging role of CPCs and exogenous progenitor cells in myocardial homeostasis and tissue repair. We will also examine the controversies that have arisen in this field by reviewing the observations that suggest that the heart is a terminally differentiated postmitotic organ and the view that the heart is a self-renewing organ in which myocyte turnover is controlled by resident cardiac stem cells (CSCs). The clinical application of stem cells is presented in Chapter 38.

IS THE HEART A TERMINALLY DIFFERENTIATED POSTMITOTIC ORGAN?

Although there is general agreement that myocyte division is present prenatally and shortly after birth (**Figure 3-2A**), the interpretation of the patterns of myocyte growth postnatally in the adult organ and in the presence of an enhanced workload diverges dramatically (see Figure 3-2B). Despite the ongoing debate, enlarged human myocytes and dividing human myocytes can be found relatively easily in the adult human heart when an appropriate methodology is employed (see Figure 3-2C). However, as will be discussed, the dedifferentiation of cardiomyocytes as a process that is able to reinstitute the proliferative cell phenotype cannot be demonstrated experimentally and is currently a difficult hypothesis to test.

Historically, the foundations for the notion that the heart is a static organ incapable of regeneration were established in the mid-1920s. A significant publication in 1925 claimed that mitotic figures are not detectable in human cardiomyocytes,[1] which thereby had to be considered as cells irreversibly withdrawn from the cell cycle. This work challenged numerous studies published from 1850 to 1911 in which the general belief was that cardiac hypertrophy is the consequence of hyperplasia and hypertrophy of existing myocytes.[2] The 1925 study can be regarded as the one that introduced the concept that the heart is a terminally differentiated postmitotic organ. The impact of this research was enormous, leading generations of pathologists and cardiovascular scientists to adhere to the concept that replicating myocytes are not to be found in the adult myocardium.

The conclusion that new cardiomyocytes cannot be formed in the human heart was dictated by difficulties in identifying mitotic figures in their nuclei. The unrefined methodological approaches and the low level of resolution available 90 years ago histologically made it extremely unlikely to detect chromosomal reorganization and separation. Similarly, the lack of specific markers of karyokinesis precluded the possibility to recognize dividing cells in an organ characterized by differently oriented bundles of cardiomyocytes with distinct volume, length, and shape. The notion that the pool of myocytes present at birth is irreplaceable during the lifespan of the organism gained further support from a series of autoradiographic studies conducted in the 1960s that involved the delivery of tritiated thymidine to the myocardium during postnatal development and pathologic overloads.[2,3] The degree of DNA synthesis in myocyte nuclei was negligible, and this observation, together with the inability to distinguish mitotic images in cardiomyocytes, led to the conviction that the adult heart is composed of a homogeneous population of parenchymal cells that are in a permanent state of growth arrest.

The perception that increases in cell volume constitute the exclusive mechanism of myocyte growth[4] was based on autoradiographic protocols performed using routine tissue

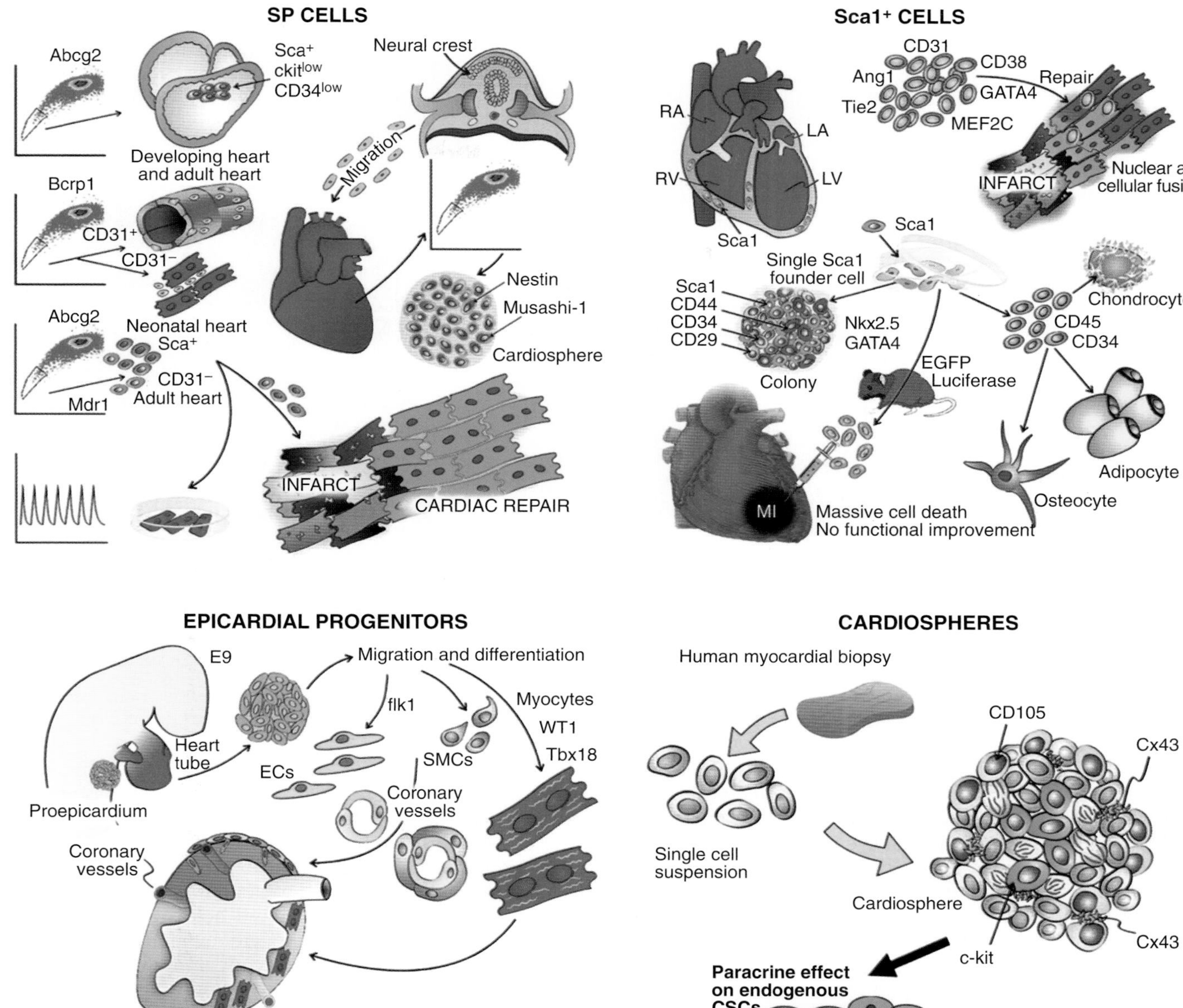

FIGURE 3-1 Classes of cardiac stem cell/progenitor cells. Schematic representation of populations of cardiac-derived stem cells/progenitor cells (see text for details). *From Leri A, Kajstura J, Anversa P: Role of cardiac stem cells in cardiac pathophysiology: a paradigm shift in human myocardial biology. Circ Res 109:941–961, 2011.*

preparations in combination with photographic emulsions, which made it difficult to distinguish important microscopic details.[5] Despite the complexity in defining whether DNA replication or mitosis was restricted to interstitial cells or involved, at times, parenchymal cells, the possibility of myocyte division was acknowledged in the mid-1970s.[4,5] However, the findings fueling the controversy that is not unique to our era began to appear only nearly 15 years later.[2]

Quantitative measurements of myocyte volume and number were performed in human hearts obtained from patients who died as a result of decompensated cardiac hypertrophy and chronic heart failure. In the late 1940s and early 1950s, Linzbach documented that in the presence of a heart weight equal to or greater than 500 g, myocyte proliferation represents the predominant mechanism of increased muscle mass.[6,7] An interesting aspect of this work is that these determinations were all based on two simple but critical parameters that are easily collected in routine histologic sections of the myocardium: myocyte length, assessed by the distance between two nuclei of mononucleated myocytes, and myocyte diameter across the nucleus. Based on a cylindrical shape configuration, myocyte cell volume was computed together with the aggregate volume of the myocyte compartment of the myocardium. The quotient of these two variables yielded the total number of ventricular myocytes. These results were confirmed several years later when more sophisticated techniques were applied.[8,9] In all cases, hearts weighing 500 g or more were characterized by a striking increase in myocyte number that was more prominent than cellular hypertrophy; this adaptation involved both the left and right ventricles.[6-10] Interestingly, polyploidy was considered a critical process of myocardial hypertrophy in humans.[10]

An inherent inconsistency became apparent. Is the adult heart a static organ unable to renew its myocyte

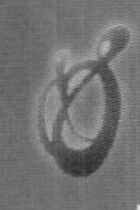

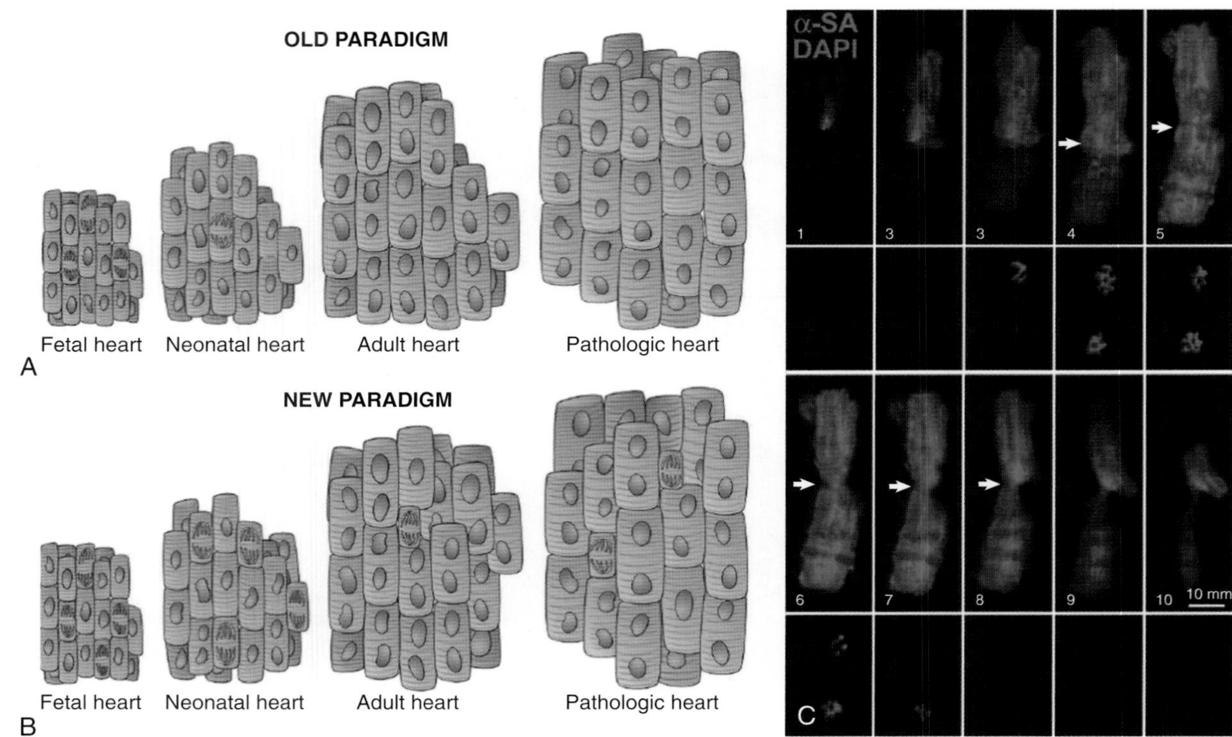

FIGURE 3-2 Mechanisms of myocyte growth. **A,** Schematic representation illustrating a progressive increase in myocyte volume with maturation and cardiac pathology. **B,** Schematic representation of the contribution of myocyte formation and myocyte hypertrophy in the developing and hypertrophied heart. **C,** Optical section reconstruction of a dividing myocyte *(arrows),* 5700 μm^3 in volume, isolated from a 62-year-old normal human female heart. The two sets of telophase chromosomes are illustrated separately. The myocyte cytoplasm is labeled by α-sarcomeric actin *(red).* Nuclei (chromosomes) are stained by DAPI *(blue).*

compartment, or does myocyte regeneration occur with increased workloads? If we assume that cardiomyocytes lack the ability to reenter the cell cycle and replicate, differences in myocyte size would be expected to reflect comparable differences in the size of the organ. However, changes in heart weight and cardiomyocyte volume rarely coincide, challenging the notion that the number of myocytes is an entity that remains largely constant throughout the organ lifespan physiologically and pathologically. This discrepancy has been reported frequently with postnatal maturation, myocardial aging, and cardiac disease states.[2,11] Hearts varying in weight can be composed of myocytes of similar volume, pointing to cardiomyocyte number as the crucial determinant controlling the size of the organ.[12] By necessity, changes in myocyte number are the consequence of two interrelated mechanisms: myocyte death and myocyte formation. The adaptive plasticity of the myocardium cannot be equated to myocyte hypertrophy any longer. Although this seems to be a rather simple biologic conclusion reached on the basis of increased straightforward evidence,[13-22] strong objections persist and publications in high-impact factor journals tend to perpetuate an unsound view of cardiac pathophysiology. Both myocyte death and regeneration are largely ignored, moving the field back to the 1920s.[23-28]

To illustrate the discrepancy between heart weight and myocyte volume, two normal hearts not used for transplantation are compared with two explanted hearts obtained from patients suffering from end-stage ischemic cardiomyopathy. With chronic heart failure (CHF), cardiac weight is 2.2-fold greater than in nonpathologic hearts, and myocyte volume ranges from 3000 to 100,000 μm^3, documenting the high heterogeneity in cell size present in the diseased myocardium. Significant heterogeneity in myocyte volume was also found in normal hearts, but average myocyte size was only 30% larger in ischemic cardiomyopathy (**Figure 3-3**). This modest difference failed to account for the remaining 1.7-fold greater weight of explanted hearts, providing compelling evidence in favor of myocyte regeneration with CHF. Moreover, the variability in myocyte volume in each of the four human hearts argues strongly against the concept that all cardiomyocytes are of comparable age, being present at birth and undergoing cellular hypertrophy with maturation and aging, or following myocardial infarction.

The early morphometric studies have provided the fundamental answer to the question whether myocyte proliferation occurs in the heart.[2] These quantitative findings were not properly appreciated, and the cellular responses implicated in the progression of chronic heart failure were related to defects in the molecular adaptations of the enlarged myocytes, rather than a combination of these with cell growth and cell death, in which myocyte regeneration had a significant role on the structural remodeling of the diseased heart. Alterations in the effector pathways regulating myocyte hypertrophy and contractility were identified and interpreted as the key etiologic factors responsible for the depression in cell mechanics and ventricular performance. But the results in the human heart impose a reexamination of the mechanisms of myocyte growth and division in an attempt to provide novel information for a better understanding of the processes involved in the manifestations of severe ventricular dysfunction.

The critical interaction of cell death and cell renewal is not unique to the heart. Organ mass in prenatal and

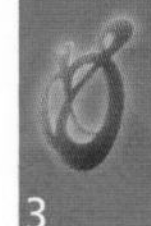

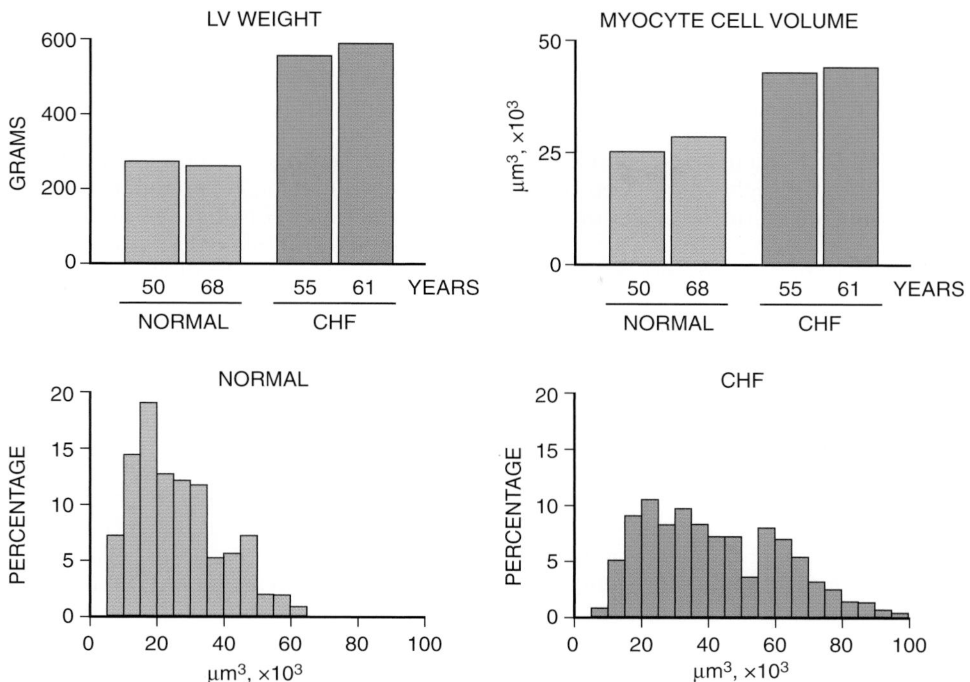

FIGURE 3-3 Left ventricular (LV) weight and myocyte volume. Examples of normal *(blue bars)* and explanted *(red bars)* human hearts. The increase in myocyte volume accounts only in part for the increase in LV mass. A wider distribution of myocyte volumes is found in the failing heart.

postnatal life is controlled by the balance between cell death and cell division, which regulate the number of parenchymal cells within the tissue.[29] With various diseases, cell loss may be compensated by an increase in size of the surviving cells, although this response may become rapidly maladaptive in view of the difficulty of hypertrophied cells to perform efficiently their specialized function.[30] A proficient regenerative outcome depends on the presence of exogenous and/or endogenous stem cells, or on the existence of a pool of constantly cycling parenchymal cells.

The Molecular Basis of the Terminally Differentiated State of Cardiomyocytes

At the dawn of molecular cardiology, a major effort was made to identify the signaling mechanism(s) involved in the irreversible withdrawal of adult cardiomyocytes from the cell cycle and in the acquisition of the terminally differentiated cell phenotype. The premise of this intense search was that myocyte hyperplasia ceases abruptly at birth in rodents and within 3 to 6 months in humans,[31-33] pointing to a major loss in the growth reserve of the myocardium during physiologic postnatal maturation, in adulthood, and with myocardial aging.

Postnatally, the myocardium has to accommodate the increasing demands of the rapidly expanding body mass and the sudden changes in the patterns of blood flow and circulatory resistance that occur shortly after birth. Traditionally, myocyte replication is considered to be restricted mostly to embryonic and fetal life so that the progressive increase in size of the growing organ is viewed to be the result of an increase in volume of preexisting cardiomyocytes formed prenatally. Nearly 20 years ago, the administration of thymidine analogs to mice revealed that two temporally distinct phases of DNA synthesis characterize the prenatal and early postnatal growth of the myocyte compartmemt.[34] The first peak in DNA synthesis was observed in the fetal heart and was attributed to cardiomyocyte proliferation. Conversely, the second phase of DNA synthesis, which was detected 4 days after birth and involved 10% of cardiomyocytes, was arbitrarily associated to binucleation. This claim provided further support to the theory that cardiomyocyte replication is confined to the developing heart and that the network of proteins coordinating cell cycle progression is differentially expressed prenatally and postnatally.

The search for the molecular control of the alleged withdrawal of postnatal cardiomyocytes from the cell cycle resulted in the compilation of an endless list of genes that are known to promote growth arrest in multiple systems. Cessation of myocyte proliferation at birth has been linked to the downregulation of cyclins, cyclin-dependent kinases, and E2F transcription factors,[35] and to the upregulation of the negative modulators of cell cycle progression: Cdkn1a, Cdkn1b, Cdkn1c, and Cdkn2c.[36] Transgenic and knockout mice were developed to document that changes in gene expression overcome the barrier to myocyte renewal at birth but not in adulthood, when myocytes, despite the persistence of the transgene, unexpectedly escape its proproliferative effect and exit from the cell cycle.[36] The normalization of cardiac size and myocyte cell number in adult mice was suggested to be mediated by an increase in cell death to correct for the early postnatal hyperplasia.[36] Importantly, the presence of functional growth factor receptors on the plasma membrane of mature myocytes was postulated to be coupled with the myocyte hypertrophy needed in response to pathologic loads in combination with the reexpression of the fetal gene program.[37]

Based on observations in skeletal myoblasts,[38] the hypothesis was raised that the retinoblastoma (Rb) pocket protein inhibits permanently the transition of cardiomyocytes from the G1 to the S phase of the cell cycle. This claim was supported by the documentation that the expression of hyperphosphorylated inactive Rb is restricted to the neonatal heart when myocyte renewal occurs. Conversely, adult and hypertrophied hearts are characterized by high levels of hypophosphorylated active Rb, which opposes myocyte formation.[39] Similarly, the cell cycle regulators cyclin D1, D2, D3, and A have been found to be highly expressed in the developing heart, undergoing rapid downregulation after birth.[40,41]

Cardiomyocytes collected from normal and failing dog hearts clearly express cyclin D2, cyclin A, cyclin B, cdk2, and cdc2. The kinase activity of these nuclear proteins has also been shown. Cyclin D2 in myocytes increases sevenfold with CHF, and cyclin D2-associated kinase activity increases threefold (**Figure 3-4**). Similarly, cyclin A and cyclin B quantity and activity increase fourfold; cdc2 protein increases eightfold, and cdk2 and cdc2 activity increases threefold and fivefold, respectively.[42] These findings challenge the observations in wild-type and transgenic mice and indicate that cardiomyocytes react to cardiac failure by activating cyclins and cdk, which are coupled with cell regeneration and the recovery of muscle mass.

Replication of Terminally Differentiated Adult Cardiomyocytes

Mitogenic stimulation of terminally differentiated myocytes has been attempted by modulating the expression of various cell cycle regulators.[43-46] The concept that division of mature myocytes may occur by overexpression of cyclin D2, periostin, and neuregulin 1, or by inhibition of p38 MAP kinase is problematic.[47-49] Adult myocytes in animals and humans measure approximately 20,000 to 25,000 μm^3; if these cells were to reenter the cell cycle and divide, they would have to acquire in mitosis a volume of approximately 40,000 to 50,000 μm^3 before two daughter cells of 20,000 to 25,000 μm^3 each are formed. However, dividing cardiomyocytes are typically mononucleated, have a 60% to 80% smaller volume than noncycling myocytes,[18] and show a disorganized contractile apparatus with modest accumulation of myofibrils in the subsarcolemmal region. This pattern of growth is incompatible with the notion that mature cardiomyocytes correspond to a functionally homogeneous pool of cells that, upon need, reenter the cell cycle and divide to generate new parenchymal cells. Myocyte cytokinesis in humans and animals has been shown by the localization of aurora B kinase at the cleavage furrow between the duplicated sets of telophase chromosomes (**Figure 3-5**). Importantly, forced reentry of postmitotic myocytes into the cell cycle results in abortive mitosis and apoptosis.[50] Overexpression of cell cycle genes promotes the progression of cardiomyocytes from G0 to G1 and subsequently to the S phase with synthesis of DNA. However, cells do not traverse the G2/M checkpoint and divide; the arrest in G2/M leads to cellular enlargement, senescence, and death.

Evidence of Myocyte Division in the Human Heart

In the last 15 years, numerous examples of mitotic images in human cardiomyocytes have been documented by immunolabeling and confocal microscopy in acute and chronic ischemic cardiomyopathy,[17,20,22,51] idiopathic dilated cardiomyopathy,[17,22] chronic aortic stenosis with moderate ventricular dysfunction,[18] and myocardial aging.[19,21,22] In early studies, the light microscopic examination of routine histologic sections imposed on the investigators an extensive search for the recognition of occasional dividing myocytes.[52] Because of the low frequency of myocytes in mitosis detected by this inadequate methodology, the possibility was raised that these rare replicating cells reflected actually proliferating interstitial fibroblasts.[3,53] Fibroblasts were described as mobile cells capable of penetrating by several microns the thickness of myocytes, positioning themselves in the central portion of the cytoplasm where myocyte nuclei are typically located. Thus the myocyte nucleus was apparently displaced from its original site, which was now occupied by the "penetrating fibroblast." This interpretation of cardiac cell mitosis fell short[2] on several accounts: the examples of "penetrating" interstitial cells did not show dividing cells, the myocyte nucleus was at its expected position in the middle of the cell, and the electron microscopic preparation suggesting an erroneous interpretation of the identity of the replicating cells showed several artifacts, including the presence of contraction bands produced by inappropriate fixation of the myocardium.[3]

A few comments concerning the multiple markers of the cell cycle may help understanding cardiomyocyte plasticity. The cell cycle can be divided into two gap phases (G1 and G2) separated by a phase of DNA synthesis (S phase), and followed by cell division and cytokinesis (M phase). The transition between these phases is driven by the activity of specific cyclin-dependent kinases (CDKs) bound to their cognate cyclins.[54] BrdU and IdU are thymidine analogs that are incorporated in the DNA of dividing cells during S phase.[55,56] Ki67 is a nuclear protein expressed in late G1, S, G2, prophase, and metaphase, decreasing in anaphase and telophase.[57] Cdc6 and the minichromosome maintenance (MCM) family of proteins are commonly used as indicators of cell multiplication. During S phase, cdc6 recruits MCM and licenses DNA replication, whereas CDKs trigger the initiation of DNA synthesis. Activated MCM promotes the DNA unwinding step, allowing the formation of the replication fork.[58] In late S phase, the dissociation of cdc6 and MCM from chromatin ensures that DNA is replicated only once during a round of division. Subsequently, when the levels of CDKs drop at the completion of mitosis, the restriction on licensing is relieved and a new cell cycle can initiate. Both cdc6 and MCM are downregulated in terminally differentiated and quiescent cells.[58]

Telomerase is a reverse transcriptase that during the cell cycle synthesizes telomeric repeats at the end of chromosomes, preventing loss of DNA.[59] This ribonucleoprotein is present in dividing cells and is not expressed in resting and postmitotic cells. The nuclear co-localization of telomerase and cell cycle proteins represents the structural counterpart of telomerase activity, which has been detected in isolated adult cardiomyocytes.[60-62] Phospho-H3 at Ser 10 is highly expressed in the compacted chromosomes of mitotic cells.[63] This posttranslational modification of H3 promotes the recruitment of chromosomal condensation factors, which are required for normal chromosome assembly and segregation. Depletion of aurora B kinase leads to decreased phospho-H3 so that condensin is not recruited to the DNA and defects in the morphology of chromosomes ensue. Low levels of phospho-H3 are coupled with "dumpy" mitotic figures: sister chromatids do not separate and chromosomes fail to segregate.[64]

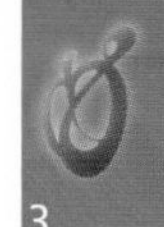

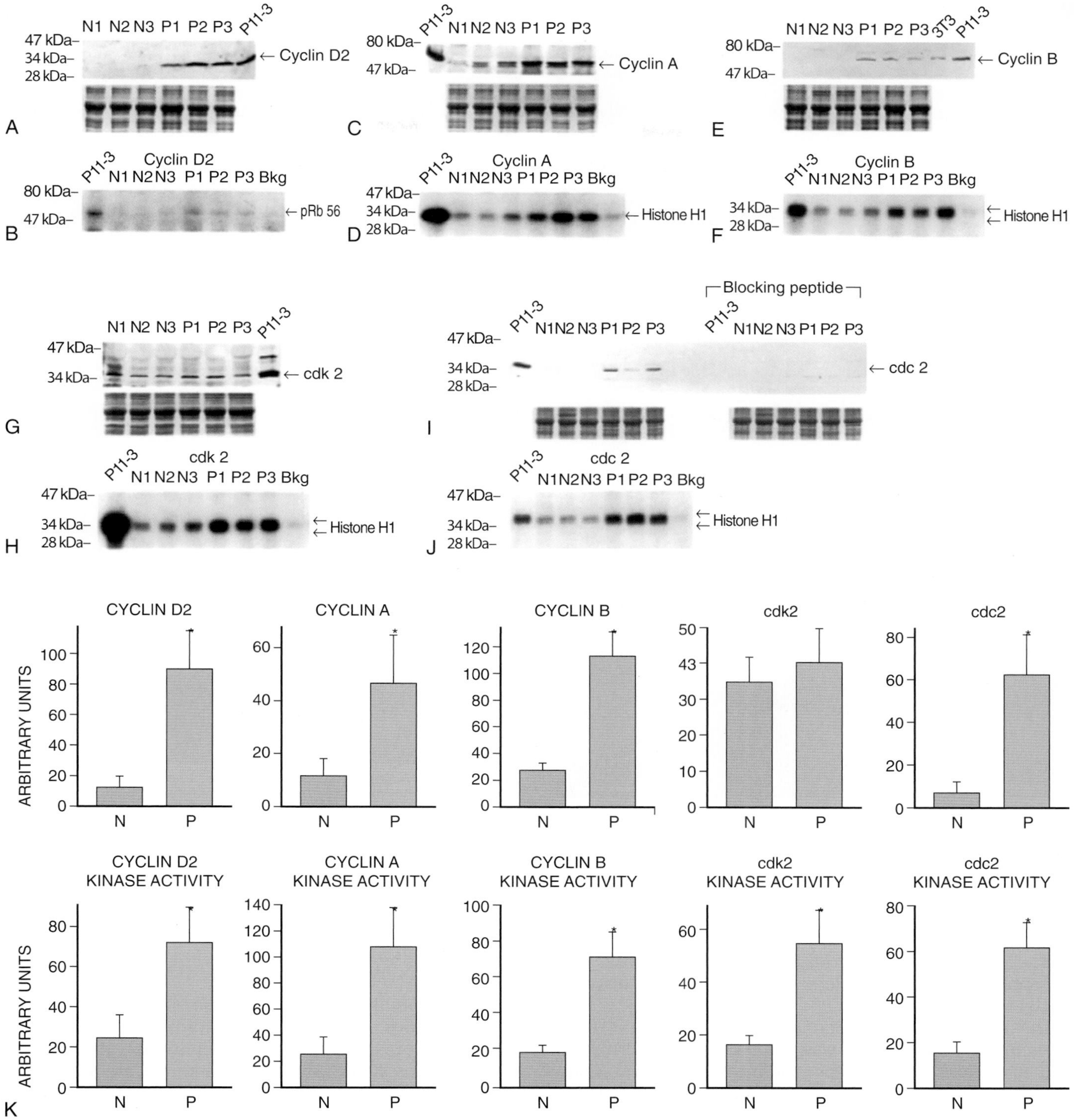

FIGURE 3-4 Molecular indices of myocyte replication. **A-J,** Cyclin D2 **(A)** and cyclin D2-associated kinase activity **(B),** cyclin A protein **(C),** cyclin A-associated kinase activity **(D),** cyclin B protein **(E),** cyclin B-associated kinase activity **(F),** cdk2 protein **(G),** cdk2-associated kinase activity **(H),** cdc2 protein **(I),** and cdc2-associated kinase activity **(J)** in LV myocytes from normal (N) and paced (P) failing hearts. **K,** Quantitative data of cell cycle-related proteins. Data are presented as mean ± SD. *Indicates $P < 0.05$ versus LV myocytes from normal hearts. 3T3 cells and P11-3 cells were used as positive controls. Background kinase activity (Bkg) was obtained after immunoprecipitation with nonimmune rabbit serum. *From Setoguchi M, Leri A, Wang S, et al: Activation of cyclins and cyclin-dependent kinases, DNA synthesis, and myocyte mitotic division in pacing-induced heart failure in dogs. Lab Invest 79:1545–1558, 1999.*

Major advances in the recognition of myocyte replication in the adult human heart have been made by the use of confocal microscopy and immunolabeling, which allow an accurate quantification of mitotic events. These results have strengthened the notion that parenchymal cells are continuously renewed in the human myocardium and myocyte regeneration is markedly enhanced in the failing heart.[17-20,22,51] Similarly, this technology was applied to animal models of the human disease, and dividing myocytes were consistently recognized in tissue sections and isolated cell preparations.[12,46] Cyclins, CDK expression and activity, BrdU or IdU incorporation, and the presence of the

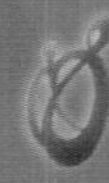

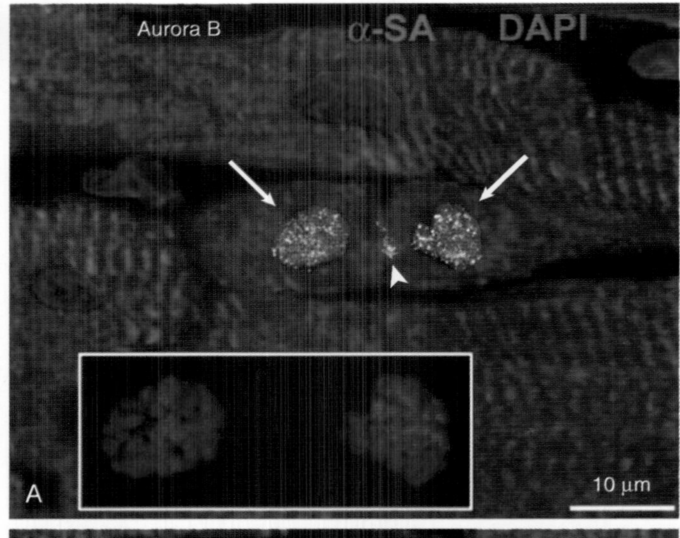

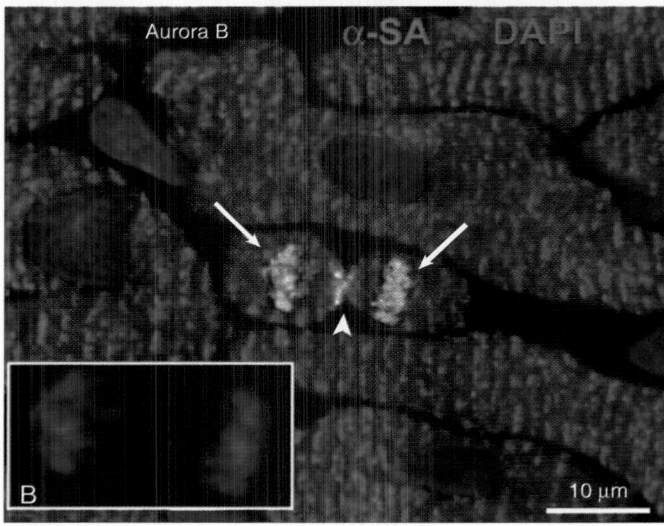

FIGURE 3-5 Myocyte cytokinesis. Dividing human **(A)** and mouse **(B)** mononucleated myocytes. Aurora B kinase is present in both sets of duplicated chromosomes *(white, arrows)* and at the cleavage furrow *(arrowheads)* of the two daughter cells. The mitotic myocyte nuclei are shown separately in the insets. *Panel A from Kajstura J, Gurusamy N, Ogórek B, et al: Myocyte turnover in the aging human heart. Circ Res 107:1374–1386, 2010.*

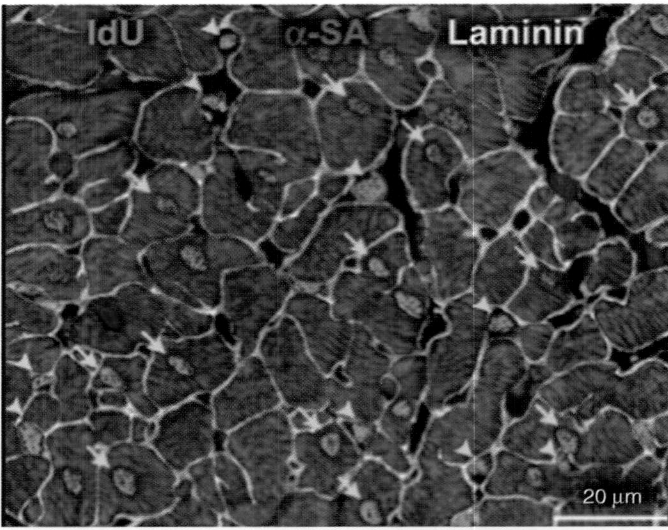

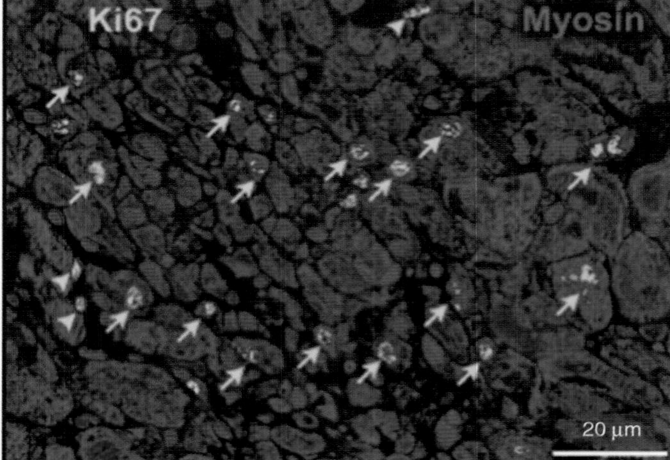

FIGURE 3-6 Markers of myocyte proliferation. *Upper panel,* Several myocyte nuclei *(arrows)* and nonmyocyte nuclei *(arrowheads)* are labeled by IdU *(green).* Myocytes are positive for α-SA *(red).* Laminin *(white)* defines the boundary of myocytes and interstitial cells. *Lower panel,* Cluster of small poorly differentiated myocytes within the hypertrophied human myocardium. Myocytes are labeled by cardiac myosin *(red)* and nuclei by propidium iodide *(blue).* The cell cycle marker Ki67 *(yellow)* labels a large number of myocyte nuclei *(arrows).* Nonmyocyte nuclei *(arrowheads). Upper panel from Kajstura J, Urbanek K, Perl S, et al: Cardiomyogenesis in the adult human heart. Circ Res 107:305–315, 2010; lower panel from Urbanek K, Quaini F, Tasca G, et al: Intense myocyte formation from cardiac stem cells in human cardiac hypertrophy. Proc Natl Acad Sci U S A 100:10440–10445, 2003.*

cell cycle proteins Ki67, MCM5, cdc6, telomerase, and phospho-H3, have been detected repeatedly in myocyte nuclei (**Figure 3-6**).

The distribution of mononucleated and binucleated myocytes in the human heart was defined in the mid-1990s,[65] and these results have been confirmed recently.[22] Aging, cardiac hypertrophy, and ischemic and dilated cardiomyopathy do not change the proportion of these two cell populations, which reach their adult average values at approximately 25 years of age and remain constant thereafter: mononucleated and binucleated myocytes comprise 73% and 27% of the myocardium, respectively.[22,65] The appearance of binucleated myocytes in the adolescent and young adult human heart cannot be explained as the mechanism(s) involved in the preservation of the large quantity of mononucleated cardiomyocytes in adulthood, throughout the aging process, and in the presence of a hemodynamic stress. Whether the fraction of binucleated cardiomyocytes constitutes a pool of older cells predominantly affected by the activation of the apoptotic pathway is a likely possibility. Importantly, these observations indicate that the various indices of myocyte formation, including the expression of the cell cycle proteins Ki67, MCM5, cdc6, cyclin B, phospho-H3, and aurora B kinase, are all markers of myocyte renewal. Similarly, the incorporation of the thymidine analog IdU in myocyte nuclei and the measurement of the myocyte mitotic index are unequivocal documentations of myocyte regeneration in the human heart (**Figure 3-7**).

The recognition of these various markers documents that a pool of cardiomyocytes in the adult heart traverses all the phases of the cell cycle,[18,20-22,51] but does not provide unequivocal evidence of cytokinesis. To address this issue, the presence of the contractile ring between dividing cells and aurora B kinase labeling were searched for in the adult myocardium.[21,22,66] During cell replication, members of the aurora kinase family control various steps ranging from centrosome function to chromosome segregation and

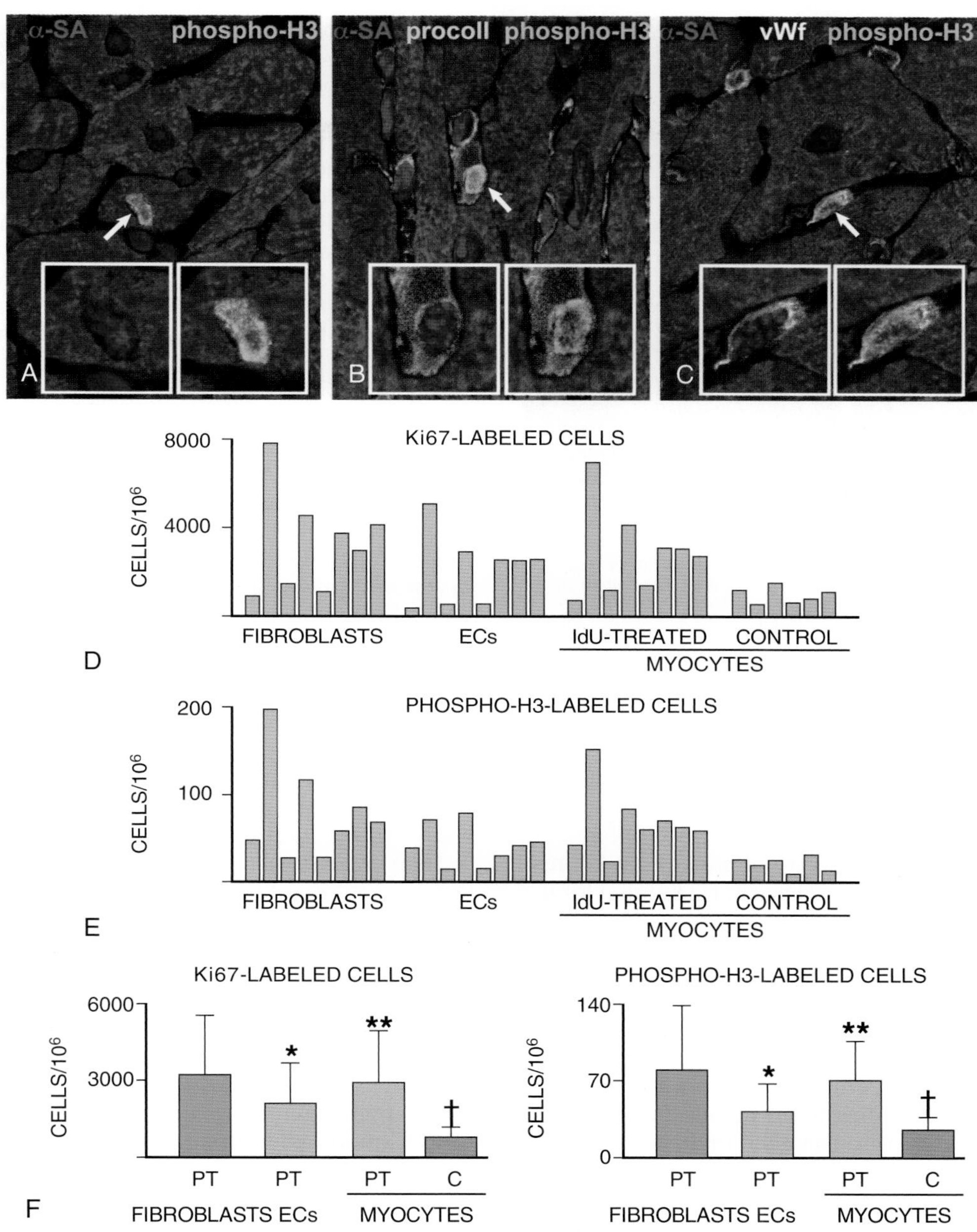

FIGURE 3-7 Cell proliferation. Mitosis in a human myocyte **(A)**, fibroblast **(B)**, and endothelial cell **(C)** is recognized by phospho-H3 labeling *(bright blue, arrows)*. Dividing cells are shown at higher magnification in the insets; DAPI, left insets; phospho-H3, right insets. Percentage of Ki67- **(D)** and phospho-H3-labeled **(E)** fibroblasts, endothelial cells (ECs) and myocytes in patients exposed to IdU. Values for myocytes in six control hearts are also shown. **F**, Comparison of the average values of Ki67 and phospho-H3 in patients (Pt) treated with IdU. *P <0.05 vs. fibroblasts, **P <0.05 vs. ECs, †P <0.05 vs. cardiomyocytes of patients. *C*, Control hearts. *From Kajstura J, Urbanek K, Perl S, et al: Cardiomyogenesis in the adult human heart. Circ Res 107:305–315, 2010.*

cytokinesis. Specifically, aurora B kinase regulates the condensation and cohesion of chromosomes and modulates the assembly and disassembly of the mitotic spindle by promoting the rapid switch in microtubule dynamics in anaphase and telophase.[67] During cytokinesis, the cleavage furrow is generated by contraction of the actinomyosin ring that encircles the cell equator and eventually divides the cytoplasm equally into the two daughter cells. The formation and function of the contractile ring (**Figure 3-8**) is regulated by aurora B kinase (see Figure 3-5), which ensures the phosphorylation of a large complex of proteins and their coordinated activity.[67]

Collectively, these studies have demonstrated that the normal and diseased heart in animals and humans contains a population of dividing cardiomyocytes. These findings, however, left unanswered the question whether proliferating myocytes are transit amplifying cells generated by commitment of endogenous or exogenous stem cells, or constitute a pool of cells that retain the ability to reenter the cell cycle and replicate. The possibility has also been raised that mature myocytes possess a certain degree of developmental plasticity being able to dedifferentiate, acquire a proliferative state, multiply, and form functionally competent cells. Understanding the origin of newly generated myocytes and the mechanisms that regulate cardiac homeostasis offers the extraordinary opportunity to potentiate this naturally occurring process and promote myocardial regeneration following injury.

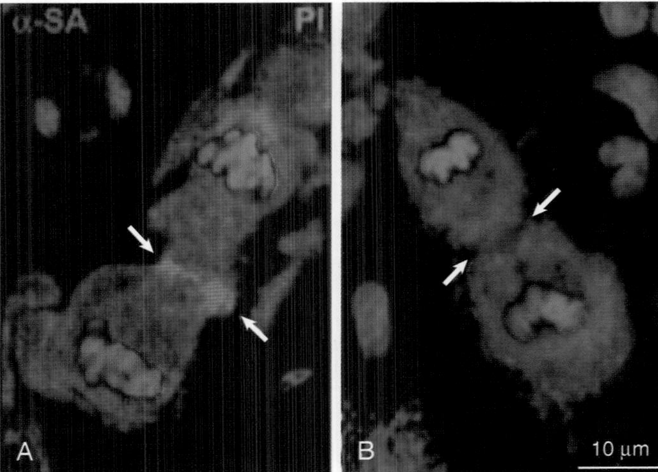

FIGURE 3-8 Critical phases of myocyte division. **A,** Actin accumulation in the region of cytoplasmic division and cell separation (i.e., the contractile ring). α-SA, red. **B,** Myocyte cytokinesis is shown by the combination of labeling of nuclei by propidium iodide *(green fluorescence)* and staining of myocyte cytoplasm by α-SA *(red). From Beltrami AP, Urbanek K, Kajstura J, et al: Evidence that human cardiac myocytes divide after myocardial infarction. N Engl J Med 344:1750–1757, 2001.*

CARDIAC STEM CELLS

Bone Marrow–Derived Stem Cells

Somatic stem cells are present in most if not all adult organs. Tissue-specific adult stem cells are undifferentiated cells characterized by the ability to self-renew and differentiate to yield all specialized cell types of the organ of residence.[12,46] Asymmetric kinetics of growth is essential for the maintenance of the pool of resident stem cells and the formation of an adequate compartment of mature cells. These two processes are maintained in a tight equilibrium during the steady state of organ homeostasis. The mechanism of stem cell activation is dictated by the rate of cell turnover required by the biologic needs of the tissue in which they reside. When parenchymal cells are lost and their number decreases, proliferation signals are generated, and stem cells are induced to leave the niche area and differentiate. In physiologic conditions, the balance between cell death and cell regeneration is highly efficient; cell dropout by normal wear and tear is counteracted by cell renewal to preserve the homeostasis of the organ. Conversely, in the presence of damage, *restitutio ad integrum* does not occur, and healing is associated with scar formation.[68]

The ability of stem cells to continuously replenish the compartment of undifferentiated and lineage-committed cells is a fundamental property of higher organisms with mitotic soma. In these cases, tissues are capable of renewal and repair, and the extent of regeneration positively correlates with animal lifespan.[69] The reduced longevity of lower organisms, including *Caenorhabditis elegans* and *Drosophila,* is linked to the lack of regenerative potential of their postmitotic tissues in adulthood.[69] Dying cells cannot be replaced, resulting in a rapid and progressive decline in organ function. Conversely, cell turnover by proliferation and commitment of resident stem cells is active in mammals, and old injured cells may be restored by new, better functioning cells.

During embryonic-fetal development and physiologic cell turnover in adulthood, cells divide for a predetermined number of rounds, ultimately reaching terminal differentiation and growth arrest. The process of commitment of primitive cells to specialized cells is characterized by a progressive restriction in proliferative and developmental options that culminates in cell cycle withdrawal and acquisition of the mature phenotype.[70] The precise coordination of cell division is required to ensure the production of an appropriate number of lineage committed cells, whereas cell cycle arrest in terminally differentiated cells is critical for tissue architecture and organ function. It is only in their mature state that parenchymal cells exert their highly specific and restricted role critical for the well-being of the entire organism.

A good example of these growth mechanisms is found in the hematopoietic system. The bone marrow can be subdivided into a hematopoietic cell compartment and a stroma composed of mesenchymal stem cells, fibroblasts, adipocytes, and vascular and nervous structures. Hematopoietic stem cells (HSCs), discovered by Till and McCulloch,[71] are the first tissue-specific adult stem cells that have been described, so that stem cells in other adult organs are typically studied based on the characteristics of these blood-forming cells. HSCs were originally identified as clonogenic cells that develop multilineage hematopoietic colonies in the spleen. In addition to the fundamental attributes of self-renewal, clonogenicity, and multipotentiality, HSCs have been defined as units of a hierarchically structured system in which stem cells give rise to oligolineage progenitors that lose self-renewal properties and generate a progeny with restricted differentiating potential.

Stem cell-regulated organs adhere to a model of progressive acquisition of the committed state of stem cells, which undergo maturation into progenitors, precursors, and amplifying cells, and eventually reach terminal differentiation. This hierarchical system of cell growth has been challenged, suggesting that hematopoiesis may be a continuum of transcriptional opportunity. The most primitive HSCs are either constantly cycling at a slow rate, or entering and exiting the cell cycle. These cell cycle passages are accompanied by changes in functional phenotype, including reversible modifications in homing, engraftment, and expression of junctional proteins and cytokine receptors.[72] Stem cell commitment may reflect a functional continuum in which a high level of flexibility characterizes the ability of HSCs to differentiate. Windows of vulnerability for commitment can open and close depending on the phase of the cell cycle. Thus the bone marrow corresponds to a system in which cells continuously shift from the engraftable primitive state to the multifactor responsive progenitor cells. These phenotypic changes occur in both directions and do not coincide with differentiation events. They are dictated by chromatin remodeling and epigenetic mechanisms.[73] HSCs and possibly all adult stem cells should not be viewed as discrete entities but as functional units.[74] These criteria, however, cannot be translated without caveats to solid organs and their resident stem cells.

Cardiac Stem Cells: The Origin of Dividing Myocytes

Several laboratories concur that the heart contains a compartment of primitive cells with the characteristics of stem cells (**Figure 3-9**); however, the identification of the actual CSC, equivalent to the HSC in the bone marrow, has been

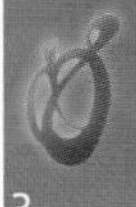

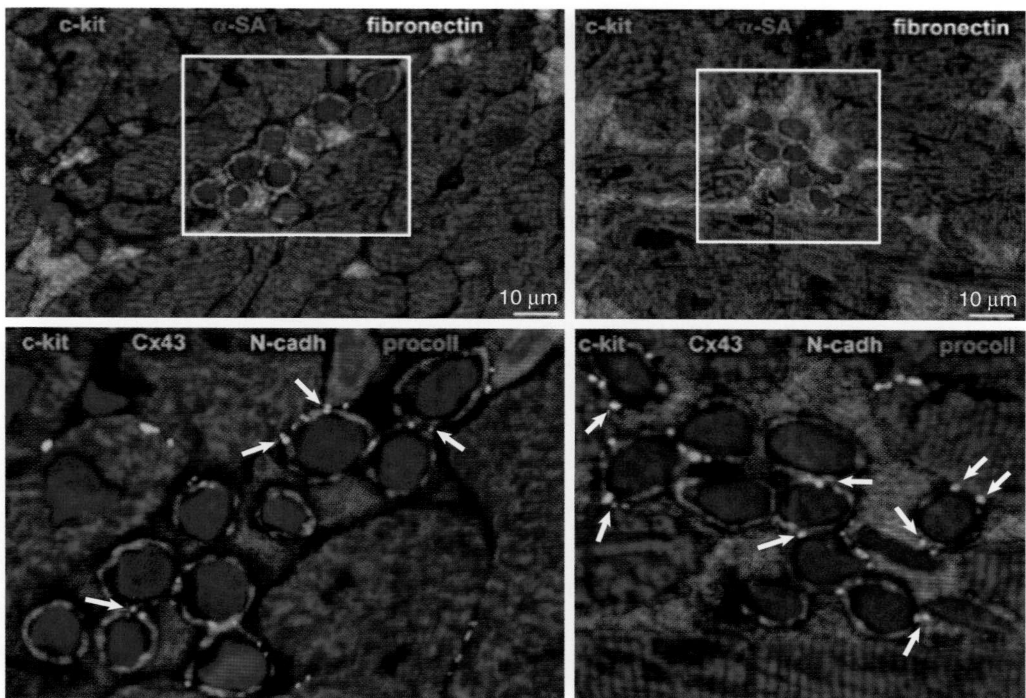

FIGURE 3-9 Myocardial stem cell niches. Sections of human myocardium containing two clusters of c-kit-positive CSCs *(green)* surrounded by fibronectin *(white)*. At higher magnification, connexin 43 (Cx43: *yellow dots, arrows*) and N-cadherin (N-cadh: *bright-blue dots, arrows*) are present between c-kit-positive cells, and between c-kit-positive cells and fibroblasts (procollagen: procoll, *magenta*) and myocytes (α-SA, *red*). *From Bearzi C, Leri A, Lo Monaco F, et al: Identification of a coronary vascular progenitor cell in the human heart. Proc Natl Acad Sci U S A 106:15885–15890, 2009.*

controversial. Stem cells are relatively rare; the frequency of CSCs in humans, one every 30,000 to 40,000 myocardial cells,[12,75] is consistent with that of HSCs in the bone marrow, one every 10,000 to 100,000.[76] The first documentation of resident c-kit-positive CSCs was obtained in rodents 10 years ago.[77] This study adhered to the basic principles required for the recognition of adult stem cells: c-kit-positive CSCs are lineage-negative clonogenic cells that divide symmetrically and asymmetrically and differentiate into cardiomyocytes, and vascular smooth muscle cells (SMCs) and endothelial cells (ECs) in vitro. In vivo, CSCs create myocytes and coronary vessels, forming de novo myocardium. The newly generated myocytes possess the mechanical and electric properties of functionally competent cells, which improve ventricular performance.[77]

Differentiation assays of stem cell clones in vitro have inherent limitations, including the possibility that culture conditions result in the preferential acquisition of a selective cell lineage, masking the full potential of the founder cell. Similarly, the identification of multiple phenotypes in the progeny of transplanted nonclonal stem cell populations does not provide a direct evidence of the multipotentiality of each administered cell. This problem has been overcome by the delivery of clonal CSCs to the injured myocardium; by necessity, all regenerated structures derive from the individual founder cell that underwent amplification ex vivo.[75,78] Following injection into the infarcted myocardium of immunosuppressed rats or immunodeficient mice, clonal human CSCs (hCSCs) divide symmetrically and asymmetrically and generate cardiomyocytes, coronary arterioles, and capillaries (**Figure 3-10**). The human origin of the newly formed structures has been strengthened by the recognition of human sex chromosomes and human

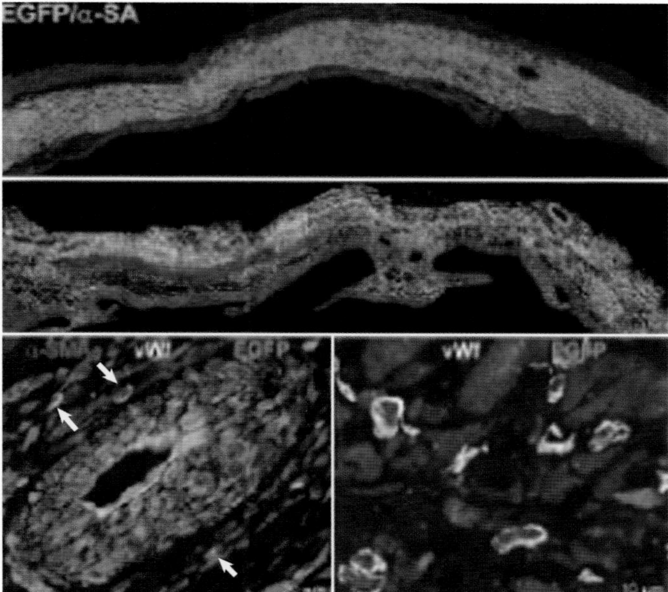

FIGURE 3-10 Myocardial regeneration and hCSC classes. EGFP-tagged hCSCs reconstituted most of the infarcted rat myocardium with newly formed cardiomyocytes *(upper and central:* combination of EGFP and α-SA, *yellowish)*, together with resistance arterioles *(lower left)* and capillary structures *(lower right)*. The arteriole is composed of EGFP-positive smooth muscle cells (SMCs: α-smooth muscle actin, α-SMA, *red*), and EGFP-positive endothelial cells (ECs: von Willebrand factor, vWf, *white*). The capillary profiles are defined by EGFP-positive endothelial cells *(white)*. *From Kajstura J, Bai Y, Cappetta D, et al: Tracking chromatid segregation to identify human cardiac stem cells that regenerate extensively the infarcted myocardium. Circ Res 111:894–906, 2012.*

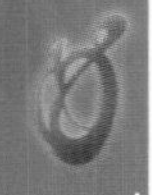

transcripts of genes specific for cardiomyocytes, and vascular ECs and SMCs.[75,77,78]

The fundamental principle of stem cell self-renewal in vivo is established by the serial transplantation assay. This protocol has been used in the last 40 years to test the functional properties of HSCs. The lethally irradiated recipient of a bone marrow transplant is a successful donor for a subsequent serial transplant only if the HSCs from the original donor undergo substantial self-renewal within the primary recipient. This approach has been applied to clonal hCSCs; 2 weeks after infarction and implantation of enhanced green fluorescent protein (EGFP)-labeled hCSCs, the left ventricle of the primary recipient was enzymatically dissociated and cells were double sorted for c-kit and EGFP. Nearly 10,000 hCSCs were recovered from each heart.[78] These cells were delivered immediately to the infarcted region of subsequent recipients. Fifteen days later, human myocytes and coronary vessels were identified, replacing large areas of the infarcted myocardium (**Figure 3-11**). Undifferentiated hCSCs were detected in the secondary recipient, providing further evidence in support of the self-renewal and long-term proliferation in vivo of hCSCs.

However, prolonged passaging in culture may modify the original properties of CSCs, and tissue injury may affect in an unpredictable manner the fate of transplanted CSCs in vivo. Novel protocols have been introduced to document unequivocally that cardiomyocytes and coronary vessels originate from CSCs in the nondamaged heart and during physiologic aging. Viral gene tagging remains the most accurate strategy for the analysis of the growth and multipotency of adult stem cells within their natural environment. Genetic tagging with retroviruses was introduced more than 20 years ago for the characterization of individual HSCs and their progeny.[79] Retroviruses and lentiviruses integrate permanently in the genome of stem cells; the semirandom insertion site of the viral genome is inherited by the population derived from the parental cell and can be amplified by polymerase chain reaction (PCR). The detection of the sites of integration constitutes a unique approach for the documentation of self-renewal and multipotentiality of stem cells in vivo. This methodology has been applied to the bone marrow[79] and the brain,[80] and has been used in the heart.[81]

A lentivirus carrying EGFP was injected in the mouse myocardium in close proximity to the atrial and apical cardiac niches. Six months later, EGFP-labeled CSCs, cardiomyocytes, ECs, and fibroblasts were isolated from the left ventricle and analyzed by PCR. A common integration site was identified in these four cell types, documenting the self-renewal and multipotentiality of CSCs and the clonal origin of the differentiated cell populations. By design, the number of infected CSCs was small; low titer and minimal volume of viral suspension were administered to reduce tissue injury and prevent spreading of viral particles from the atria and apex to the midregion of the left ventricle, where cardiac cell isolation was performed for PCR analysis.[81]

Some limitations in the application of the viral gene tagging protocol to a solid organ such as the heart have to be acknowledged. With respect to studies performed in the bone marrow, serial samples of the transduced progeny via percutaneous endomyocardial biopsies cannot be collected in small animals to establish the long-term repopulating ability of CSCs throughout the lifespan of the organism. Additionally, the restricted number of infected cells, which might be present in endomyocardial biopsies, precludes the

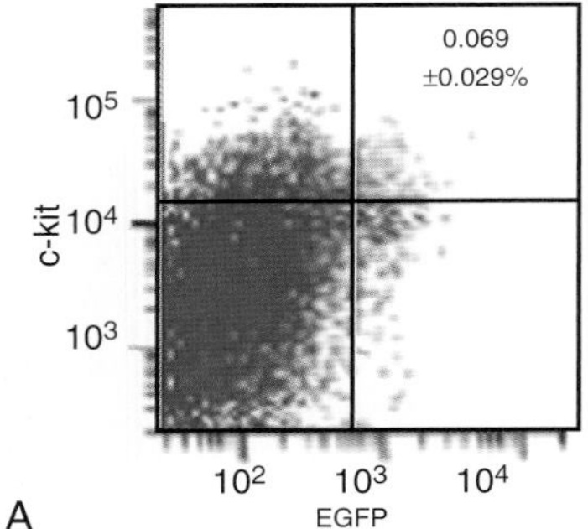

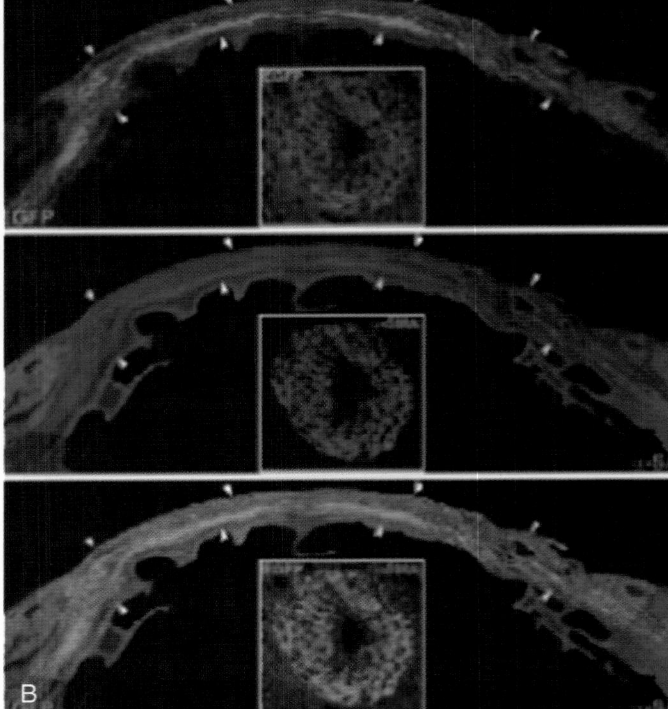

FIGURE 3-11 Serial transplantation of hCSCs. **A,** EGFP-positive hCSCs *(red dots)* isolated after regeneration of the infarcted heart are shown by scatter plot. **B,** Following serial transplantation, a large area of the infarcted myocardium is replaced by EGFP-positive *(upper, green)*, α-SA-positive *(central: red, arrowheads)* cardiomyocytes *(lower: merge, yellowish, arrowheads)*. Coronary vessel *(inset)* composed of SMCs positive for EGFP *(upper, green)*, and α-SMA *(central, red)*; merge *(lower, yellowish)*. *From Kajstura J, Bai Y, Cappetta D, et al: Tracking chromatid segregation to identify human cardiac stem cells that regenerate extensively the infarcted myocardium. Circ Res 111:894–906, 2012.*

transplantation of EGFP-tagged CSCs in secondary and tertiary recipients. Moreover, whether the insertion site confers a selective advantage or disadvantage to the growth of single cells may be easily assessed in blood cells but cannot be established in the heart. However, the stable number of EGFP-positive CSCs detected at the sites of injection over 6 months strongly suggests that atrial and apical CSCs divide asymmetrically, maintaining intact the primitive cell population. Equally important, the CSCs carrying the reporter gene translocated from the site of storage in the atrial and apical niches to the intermediate portion of the ventricular myocardium, where c-kit-positive CSCs and differentiated cardiac cells showed an identical site of integration of the proviral genome. Thus the preservation of the CSC compartment within the niches, together with the formation a myocyte and nonmyocyte progeny, strongly suggests that this class of

CSC corresponds to the pool of long-term repopulating cells in the adult myocardium.

Many of the techniques used for fate mapping of progenitor cells, including EGFP mapping, may lead to an underestimation of the actual number of CSCs.

Viral gene tagging has been used to study the properties of hCSCs.[81] These cells are transduced with the EGFP lentivirus and injected soon after coronary ligation in the region bordering the infarct; 4 to 6 weeks later, EGFP-positive cardiac cells are enzymatically dissociated from the regenerated myocardium and separated into c-kit-positive hCSCs, myocytes, ECs, and fibroblasts. Primers designed for individual integration sites are used to track each clone and its progeny. Several clones can be identified; each PCR product with a unique band length represents distinct clones. Some of the clonal bands present in hCSCs, myocytes, ECs, and fibroblasts have the same molecular weight and a common site of integration, documenting a lineage relationship between hCSCs and cardiac cell progeny. Each random integration site constitutes a distinct clonal marker of the hCSC progeny that arose after cell transplantation.[81] Thus hCSCs self-renew in vivo and generate the various cardiac cell phenotypes, demonstrating that c-kit-positive cells fulfill the criteria of bona fide stem cells.

The identification of resident hCSCs is apparently at variance with the small foci of myocardial regeneration present after acute and chronic infarcts in animals and humans. The limitation that resident hCSCs have in reconstituting myocardium after infarction has been interpreted as the unequivocal documentation of the inability of the adult heart to create cardiomyocytes. However, the inevitable evolution of ischemic injury to scarring characterizes all organs in adult organisms.[68] Although stem cells are present throughout the infarcted myocardium, they follow the same destiny of neighboring cardiomyocytes and die by apoptosis and necrosis.[20,82] The fate of CSCs is comparable to that of the other cells, and myocyte formation by CSCs is predominantly restricted to the viable portion of the infarcted heart.[51]

Importantly, c-kit-positive CSCs are present in the entire ventricular myocardium, although they are preferentially distributed to the atria and apex.[83] CSCs do not express hematopoietic and endothelial cell epitopes, strongly suggesting that they do not originate from the bone marrow but constitute a compartment of resident undifferentiated cells. Moreover, the adult heart typically shows interstitial structures with the architectural organization of stem cell niches. CSCs are functionally coupled to myocytes and fibroblasts by adherens junctions expressing N- and E-cadherin and by gap junctions expressing connexin 43 and 45.[83] Because of these properties, myocytes and fibroblasts appear to operate as supporting cells within the cardiac niches, which provide the necessary, permissive milieu for the long-term residence, survival, and growth of CSCs (**Figure 3-12**). The identification of cardiac niches and the documentation that CSCs have phenotypic characteristics distinct from HSCs offers further evidence in support of the notion that the heart is a self-renewing organ regulated by a stem cell compartment.

Myocardial Progenitor Cells

After the discovery of c-kit-positive CSCs, different classes of progenitor cells have been characterized in the adult heart,[12,46,68] but whether they represent distinct categories of undifferentiated cells with diverse functional import is currently unknown. A variety of surface antigens, transcription factors, and functional assays have been used to define these cell subsets (see Figure 3-1), which include ISL1 progenitors, epicardial progenitors, side population progenitors, Sca1 progenitors, and progenitors generating cardiospheres.

The first identification of myocardial progenitors was based on the ability of stem cells to expel toxic compounds and dyes through an ATP-binding cassette transporter.[84] This property, used initially to isolate side population hematopoietic cells, defines a pool of putative cardiac progenitors that form colonies in semisolid media and differentiate into cardiomyocytes. However, a depletion of side population cells occurs after infarction in mice overexpressing a dominant-negative MEF2C, documenting that side population cells are committed to the myocyte lineage. Although CSCs were not detected, this work introduced the concept of a myocardial stem cell that participates in the response of the heart to ischemic injury.[84]

Several reports document the existence of cardiac side population cells, which are identified based on their ability to extrude dyes.[85-88] These cells have been shown to express multiple surface epitopes; however, only the CD31-negative subset of cardiac side population cells is characterized by a high cardiomyogenic potential (**Figure 3-13**). Different protocols have resulted in the isolation of unrelated Sca1-positive cells; they share the Sca1 antigen, but do not possess the functional properties of stem cells.[89-91] Sca1 identifies a heterogeneous cell population composed of hematopoietic, mesenchymal, endothelial, and possibly CPCs. Monolayered sheets of Sca1-positive cells placed over the necrotic myocardium prevent negative remodeling and improve cardiac function after infarction.[91] This has raised the possibility that cell transplantation acts through the release of humoral factors, activating endogenous CSCs or recruiting bone marrow cells to the infarcted myocardium. In addition, Sca1 cells generate SMCs, ECs, adipocytes, and osteoblasts.

State-of-the-art imaging protocols have been developed to track in vivo the destiny of Sca1-positive cells.[92] These cells were isolated from transgenic mice that constitutively express luciferase and EGFP, enabling in vivo tracking by noninvasive imaging and postmortem identification by immunolabeling.[92] The robust bioluminescence signal at day 2 decays with time (**Figure 3-14**). By (18F)-FDG positron emission tomography scan, the nonviable infarcted portion of the wall was not reduced by cell treatment. Consistently, echocardiographic and MRI measurements did not show functional improvement; an extremely small number of EGFP-positive regenerated myocytes and vessels were found. Poor survival and rapid death of injected cells are common outcomes when neonatal cardiomyocytes, mesenchymal stromal cells, bone marrow mononuclear cells, and human embryonic stem cell–derived cardiomyocytes are adoptively transferred.[68] This phenomenon has prompted the development of novel strategies involving preactivation with growth factors, application of bioengineering methods, and genetic modifications to achieve long-term homing to the injured myocardium.

Collectively, the results with cardiac side population cells and Sca1-positive cells suggest that a small pool of primitive cells, distinct from c-kit-positive CSCs, is present in the myocardium. However, their role in cardiac homeostasis has not been defined, and recent evidence strongly suggests that

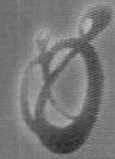

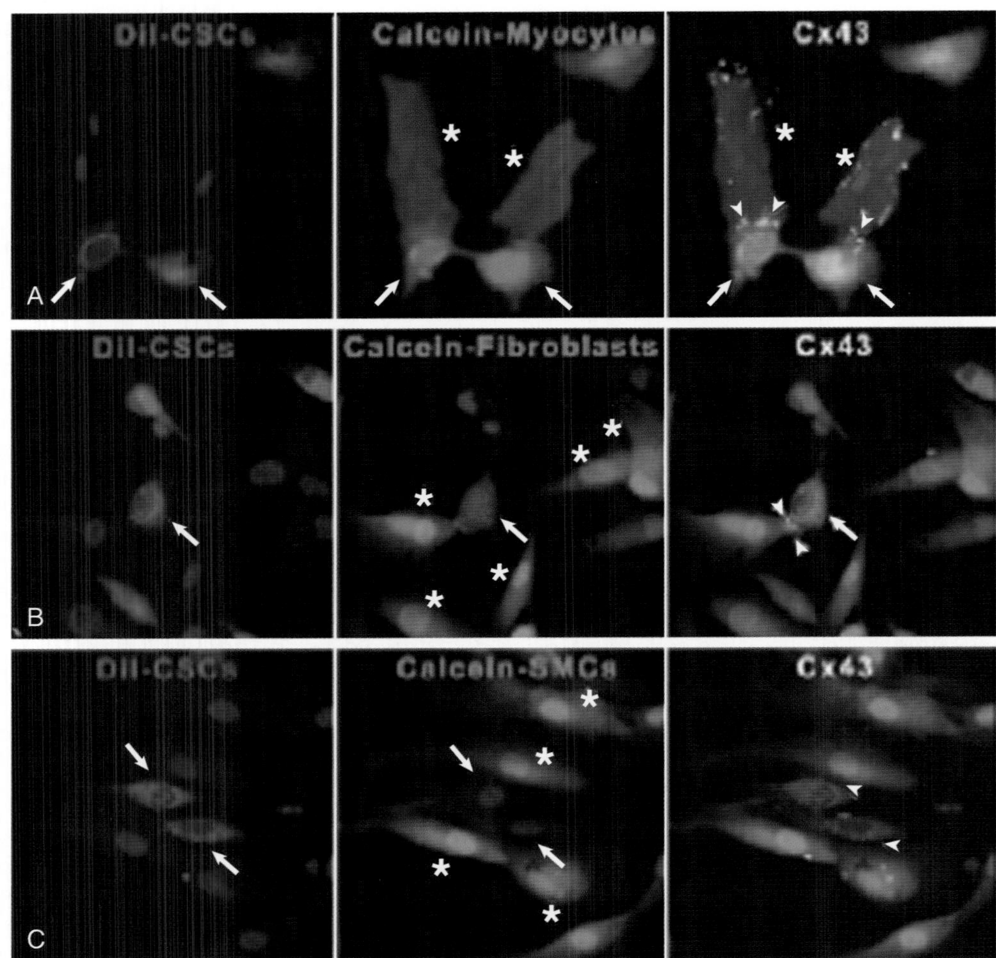

FIGURE 3-12 CSCs and their supporting cells. Supporting cells were identified by dye transfer assay between co-culture of DiI-labeled CSCs *(red)* and unlabeled myocytes, and calcein-labeled ECs, SMCs, and fibroblasts. CSCs generated functional and structural gap junctions with myocytes and fibroblasts but failed to couple with ECs and SMCs. **A,** DiI-labeled *(left panel: red, arrows)* and calcein-labeled *(central panel: green, arrows)* human CSCs were co-cultured with unlabeled adult rat cardiomyocytes, which acquired green fluorescence *(central panel: green, asterisks)*. Cx43 was detected between coupled CSCs and myocytes *(right panel, arrowheads)*. **B,** DiI-labeled human CSCs *(left panel: red, arrow)* were co-cultured with calcein-labeled human fibroblasts *(central panel: green, asterisks)*. Green-fluorescence of calcein was detected in CSCs *(central panel, arrow)* together with red fluorescence of DiI *(right panel: red-green, arrow)*. Cx43 *(white)* was expressed between CSCs and fibroblasts *(right panel, arrowheads)*. **C,** DiI-labeled human CSCs *(left panel: red, arrows)* were co-cultured with calcein-labeled human SMCs *(central panel: green, asterisks)*. Green-fluorescence of calcein was not detected in CSCs *(central panel, arrows)*. Cx43 *(white)* was not expressed between CSCs and SMCs *(right panel, arrowheads)*. ECs behaved as vascular SMCs. *From Bearzi C, Leri A, Lo Monaco F, et al: Identification of a coronary vascular progenitor cell in the human heart. Proc Natl Acad Sci U S A 106:15885–15890, 2009.*

myocyte turnover is almost exclusively regulated by c-kit-positive CSCs in animals[81,83] and humans.[21] Additionally, the extent of myocardial regeneration promoted by the delivery of c-kit-positive CSCs is vastly superior to that associated with the administration of other classes of cardiac progenitors.

The ISL1 transcription factor is associated with the commitment to the myocyte lineage of cardiac cells that have lost their undifferentiated stem cell fate. ISL1 and GATA4 are transcriptional coactivators of the myocyte transcription factor MEF2C.[93] The cardiomyocyte specification dictated by the expression of ISL1 defeats the inclusion of ISL1-positive cells into the category of stem cells. ISL1-positive cells represent myocyte progenitors, which are restricted to the embryonic fetal heart and are no longer present at birth. Lineage tracing studies have led to the recognition that a few myocytes and vascular ECs and SMCs originate from ISL1-positive cardioblasts.[94]

An alternative source of progenitor cells has been identified in the epicardium, which represents an epithelial sheet on the cardiac surface. The epicardium derives from an extracardiac transient structure, the proepicardium, which is located near the venous pole of the developing heart.[95] In avian species, the proepicardium is viewed as the site of origin of hemangioblasts, a pool of immature cells that are considered critical for the development of the coronary circulation. Hemangioblasts migrate from the proepicardium to the avascular heart tube, giving rise first to the epicardial sheet and subsequently to EC and SMC layers of coronary vessels.

Proepicardial cells may not contribute directly to cardiomyogenesis in birds but favor the expansion of myogenic precursors through a paracrine mechanism. In mammals, the identification of an equivalent hemangioblast remains controversial, although a murine hemangioblast has been claimed by in vitro studies of embryonic stem cell differentiation. Cells expressing brachyury and flk1 generate hematopoietic, vascular cells, and, later, myocytes, ECs, and SMCs.[96] Whether brachyury-flk1-positive cells exist in vivo, however, is unknown.

The embryonic fetal epicardium hosts several classes of progenitor cells, uncovering previously unexpected

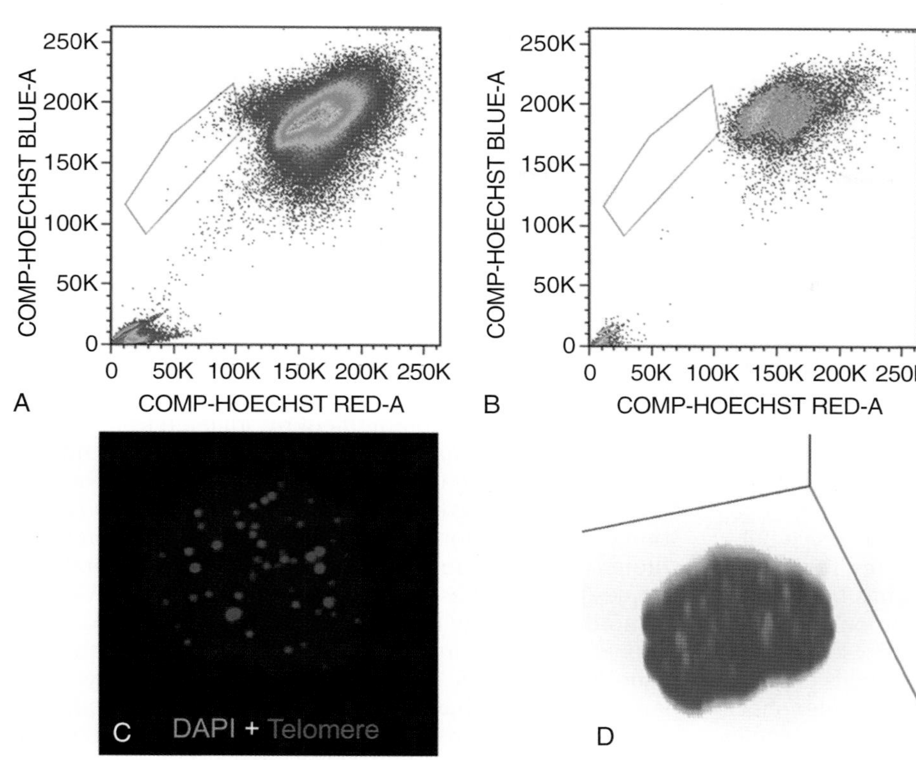

FIGURE 3-13 Cardiac side population cells. **A,** Sheep cardiac side population (sCSP) cells are indicated with a pentagon gate in a FACS profile. **B,** Verapamil-treated sample is used as a negative control for gating. **C,** Q-FISH image at passage 5 exhibits telomere length of 6.9 ± 0.1 kbp of sCSP cells. **D,** 3-D reconstruction of the image shown in panel C. *Courtesy of Dr. Ronglih Liao, Department of Medicine, Brigham and Women's Hospital, Harvard Medical School, Boston, MA.*

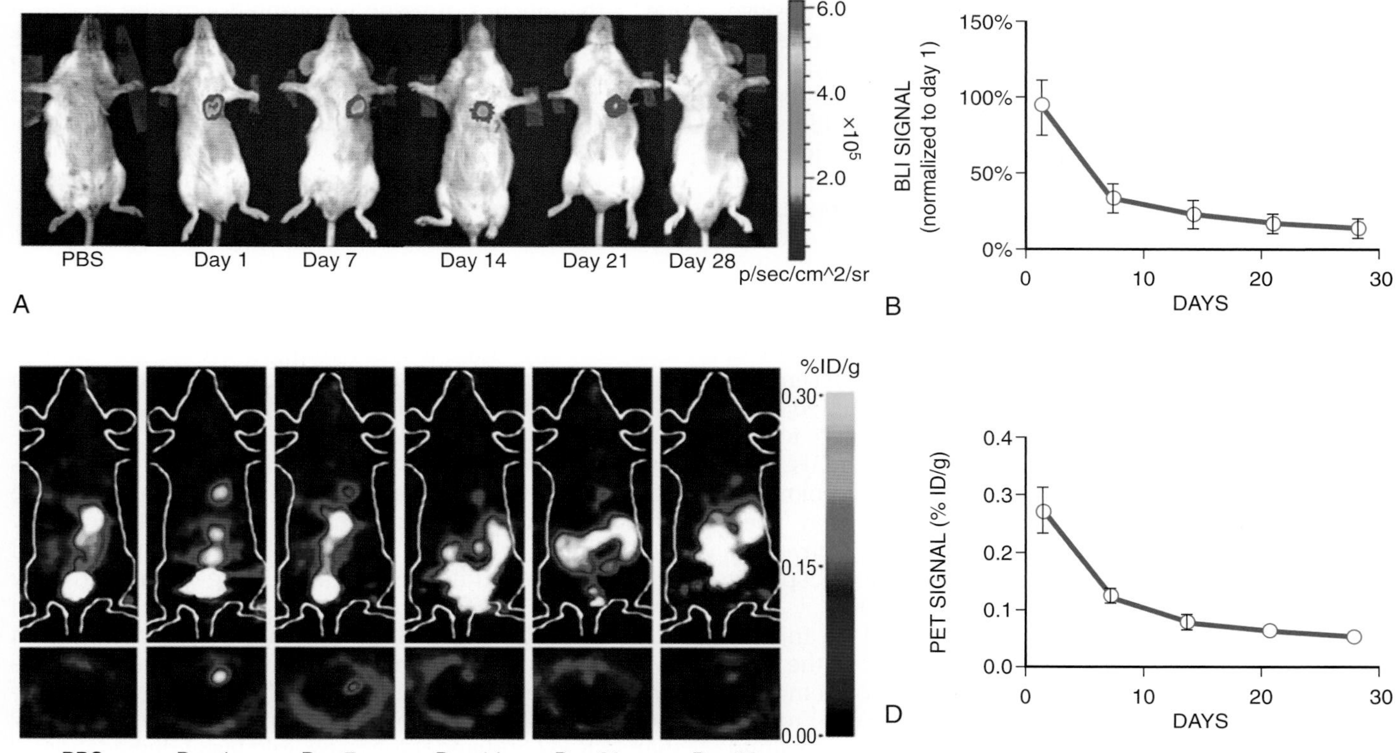

FIGURE 3-14 Temporal kinetics of human cardiac progenitor cell (hCPC) survival in infarcted hearts. **A** and **C,** Longitudinal bioluminescence imaging (BLI) and PET imaging of a representative adult female SCID mouse injected with 1×10^6 hCPCs stably expressing the triple fusion reporter gene. **B** and **D,** Progressive decrease in PET and BLI signal intensity over the 28-day time course. **B,** Normalized to day 1, BLI signals were 22.7 ± 11.5% on day 7, 15.7 ± 7.7% on day 14, and 10.6 ± 5.1% on day 28. **D,** Normalized to day 1, PET signals were 44.7 ± 3.2% on day 7, 22.4 ± 1.6% on day 14, 15.3 ± 1.1% on day 21, and 13.2 ± 0.6% on day 28. *Courtesy of Dr. Joseph C. Wu, Department of Medicine, Division of Cardiology, Stanford School of Medicine, Stanford, CA. From Lan F, Liu J, Narsinh KH, et al: Safe genetic modification of cardiac stem cells using a site-specific integration technique. Circulation 126:S20–S28, 2012.*

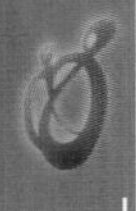

functions of this outer cardiac layer. The epicardial marker WT1 regulates the epithelial-mesenchymal transition.[97] WT1-positive progenitors travel from the proepicardium to the myocardium where they form the epicardium and electrically coupled cardiomyocytes.[98] Moreover, a population of proepicardial Tbx18-positive progenitors may give rise to a substantial fraction of cardiomyocytes.[99]

A pool of c-kit–positive epicardial cells has been identified in the human heart. These cells accumulate in the subepicardial space with ischemic cardiomyopathy.[100] Experimentally, c-kit-positive epicardial cells migrate from the epicardium to the infarct, where they proliferate and differentiate into myocyte precursors and vascular cells.[101] This process is coupled with upregulation of fetal epicardial markers.[101] The recognition of growth factors modulating the behavior of epicardial progenitors may allow their in situ activation, possibly influencing the treatment of the human disease.

The expansion of progenitor cells in nonadhesive substrates leads to the formation of floating spheres. This peculiar form of anchorage-independent growth has been used for the expansion of cardiospheres from endomyocardial biopsies.[102] Cardiospheres contain a core of c-kit-positive primitive cells, several layers of differentiating cells expressing myocyte proteins and connexin 43, and an outer sheet composed of mesenchymal stromal cells. C-kit-positive cells within the aggregates do not correspond to a uniform class of progenitors because of the heterogeneity dictated by the uncommitted or early committed state of the cells, their quiescent or cycling condition, or their migratory properties. This may explain the observed differences in the regenerative potential of single-cell–derived clonal c-kit-positive cells[75,78] and c-kit-positive cells sorted from cardiospheres.

The presence of connexin 43 between more immature and differentiated cells may play a dual role. In undifferentiated progenitors, connexin 43 favors their proliferation, whereas connexin 43 in cells committed to the myocyte phenotype promotes electric coupling with the surrounding cells and the acquisition of functional competence. The presence of gap junctions between uncommitted and differentiated cells within the cardiospheres raises the possibility that the differentiated cells may function as supporting cells. If this were the case, then the cardiospheres would reconstitute in vitro the complex structure of the cardiac niches identified in vivo. Cardiospheres may represent the ideal combination of primitive and early committed cells, but whether the use of cells already committed to the myocyte, EC, and SMC lineages is preferable to the use of a pure population of undifferentiated hCSCs is unknown. Clonal cells have a larger growth reserve but may need more time to acquire the differentiated state. Conversely, committed cells may have a reduced proliferative capacity but may attain the adult phenotype more rapidly.

Collectively, the c-kit-positive CSC identified in animals and humans in our laboratory and others[103-107] is the only one that possesses the fundamental properties of stem cells. All other progenitor cell categories may have some role in myocardial homeostasis and repair, but whether they should be considered additional resident CSCs remains to be demonstrated. This view is supported by the incomplete biologic characterization of these primitive cells and the lack of their prospective clinical implementation in the management of patients affected by acute and chronic heart failure of ischemic and nonischemic origin. Whether these cells may become therapeutically important in the future is open to question, but based on their limited regenerative potential observed in animal models, it seems to be an unlikely possibility.

Proliferation and Dedifferentiation of Cardiomyocytes

As mentioned previously, replicating myocytes are small and mononucleated, suggesting that they might derive from (1) activation and differentiation of stem/progenitor cells (see previous sections); (2) proliferation of preexisting immature myocytes; and (3) dedifferentiation of postmitotic myocytes. The question whether specialized parenchymal cells are the product of stem cell commitment or originate from replication and dedifferentiation of preexisting cells is not unique to the heart, and has been studied in the pancreas.[108,109] Consistently, investigations aiming at the identification of the source of newly formed myocytes in mammals rely on studies performed in amphibians and lower vertebrates.[110] Unquestionably, these organisms are endowed with an extraordinary ability to replace amputated body and organ parts with newly formed structures that resemble the lost tissue. The heart is no exception, and different types of damaging stimuli have been shown to trigger an efficient regenerative response in newts, axolotls, and zebrafish with significant reconstitution of myocardial mass which, however, does not restore the pyramidal shape of the uninjured ventricle.[110] In the adult zebrafish, cardiac regeneration in the absence of scar formation takes place 1 to 2 months after surgical resection of up to 20% of the ventricle.[110] The kinetics of tissue reconstitution in the zebrafish heart is partly conditioned by the type of injury. Disperse ablation of 60% of ventricular cardiomyocytes is repaired within 1 month following tamoxifen injection and activation of the diphtheria toxin, whereas restoration of the cryoinjured apex requires 130 days.[111-113] Damage by cryoinjury is characterized by necrosis of cardiomyocytes and intense inflammatory reaction, mimicking partly the response of the cardiac tissue to ischemic insults. It is noteworthy that the reparative process, although effective, is much slower, emphasizing the complexity of forming new healthy myocardium in the microenvironment of the infarct.[12,46]

In an early study, the DsRed2 fluorescent protein was placed under the control of the cardiac myosin light chain 2 (cmlc2) promoter, resulting in bright labeling of all differentiated myocytes in the intact ventricle.[114] However, following amputation, a large patch of faintly fluorescent cells accumulates at the region of damage and reconstitutes the surgically removed apex of the zebrafish heart. The dimly labeled cells, which are responsible for the initiation and progression of cardiac regeneration, were considered early progenitors.[114] These observations were strengthened in transgenic zebrafish in which EGFP and DsRed2 were driven by the same cmcl2c promoter. The distinct properties of the two fluorescent labels allowed the dynamic analysis of cardiomyogenesis. EGFP folds and fluoresces more rapidly than DsRed2 and undergoes a twofold faster degradation.[115] $EGFP^{pos}$-RFP^{neg} cells correspond to myocytes arisen from undifferentiated precursors at the very early stage of commitment, whereas double-positive cells reflect mature cardiomyocytes. Cells at the amputation edge were uniformly $EGFP^{pos}$-RFP^{neg}, documenting that the newly formed myocytes derive from the commitment of progenitor cells. The absence of EGFP^{neg}-RFP^{pos} cells, which would represent the progeny of mature myocytes, demonstrates that dedifferentiation of postmitotic myocytes is not involved in cardiac regeneration in zebrafish.

Four years later, these conclusions were questioned based on new findings obtained with lineage tracing in a transgenic fish model in which EGFP was driven by the GATA4 promoter.[116] Proliferating cells characterized by massive upregulation of the developmental gene GATA4 are initially located in the subepicardial region and subsequently migrate toward the front of regeneration. GATA4-positive cells may comprise a subset of naturally dormant cardiomyocytes undergoing reactivation of the embryonic-fetal gene program following injury. Importantly, the scarce quantity of contractile proteins, the poor organization of the sarcomeric machinery, and the low mitochondrial density have been interpreted as evidence of the dedifferentiation of mature cells to a more primitive proliferative state.

A comparable regenerative response has been observed after surgical resection of the apex of the left ventricle in the neonatal mouse heart.[117] Again, cardiomyocyte proliferation was evoked as the crucial cellular adaptation supporting the repair process. It is unfortunate, however, that fate-mapping strategies based on promoters encoding myocyte transcription factors and sarcomeric proteins cannot discriminate in vivo the contribution of preexisting myocytes and stem/progenitor cells to the cardiac regenerative process. The GATA4, cmcl2c, and α-MHC promoters are generally considered to be active exclusively in mature myocytes, but CSCs engineered with fluorescent constructs placed under the control of these promoters show transgene protein expression at early stages of cardiogenic lineage commitment.[118] The lack of cell specificity of promoters that are transactivated in three distinct cell populations—postmitotic myocytes, amplifying myocytes, and myocyte precursors—precludes the identification of the mother cell of the replicating myocytes. It has become apparent that a well-organized sarcomeric apparatus physically impedes cytokinesis in the heart of lower and higher vertebrates. However, a partially developed cell may be the end product of stem cell commitment, the daughter cell of dividing preexisting cardiomyocytes, or the consequence of dedifferentiation of postmitotic cells.

The regenerative potential of the neonatal mouse heart has been studied in the more clinically relevant context of ischemic injury.[119,120] A large number of BrdU-positive cardiomyocytes is detected following ligation of the left coronary artery 1 day after birth. Evidence of mitosis and cytokinesis has been obtained by immunolabeling for phospho-H3 and aurora B kinase, respectively. Fate mapping with the fluorescent label driven by the α-MHC promoter has been introduced to claim erroneously that healing in the absence of collagen deposition was essentially independent from stem cells. Again, it was emphasized that dividing myocytes are characterized by rarely detectable striation, a nonsurprising feature of neonatal myocytes in the intact and injured heart. This rapid proliferative response of cardiomyocytes rescued mice with extremely large infarcts; however, the rarely encountered clinical entity of myocardial infarction in newborns is a life-threatening condition with a mortality rate of 90%.[121]

Tissue regeneration in embryos is rapid, efficient, and scar-free. Skin wounds in the mammalian embryo repair with *restitutio ad integrum,* whereas cutaneous lesions in adult mammals result in scarring. The ability of scarless healing is, however, restricted to the early gestation period of the human fetus, less than 24 weeks old.[122] Regardless of the abundance of stem/progenitor cells in the fetal skin throughout prenatal life, the outcome of wounds later during gestation is comparable to that observed postnatally.[122,123] Based on these observations, the properties of the environment surrounding the cutaneous lesions have been defined in the attempt to understand the different response to injury in early and late fetuses. At the site of embryonic-early fetal wounds, the recruitment and infiltration of inflammatory cells, including neutrophils, macrophages, and mast cells are significantly reduced.[124] This process is partly dictated by the distinct growth factor profile of the fetal skin, which is enriched for anti-inflammatory cytokines and poor in profibrotic growth factors.

Deposition of collagen type I and III characterizes the healing process of fetal and adult wounds. However, in early fetal wounds, collagen is distributed in a fine reticular pattern that is comparable to that of the neighboring uninjured tissue. In contrast, postnatal areas of damage display densely arranged bundles of collagen oriented in parallel. Moreover, the ratio of type III to type I collagen is higher in fetal wounds with respect to postnatal lesions.[125] Type III collagen fibers are smaller than type I fibers, which are responsible for higher stiffness and reduced flexibility of the forming tissue, enhancing the biomechanical stress at the site of repair. Collectively, early fetal fibroblasts are programmed to form a more regenerative extracellular matrix, which facilitates the movement, proliferation, and differentiation of stem cells.[122-125] Inefficient migration and homing of progenitor cells to the region of damage is the limiting factor of the ineffective repair response of stem cell-regulated organs in adulthood.[12,46]

Myocyte regeneration occurs acutely after infarction in humans, but it is restricted to the border zone and the distant viable myocardium.[51] This form of cell growth does not result in scarless healing and does not oppose the development of the ischemic myopathy. Similarly, in the old heart, myocyte replication, which is more intense in proximity of areas of fibrosis, does not replace foci of collagen deposition or prevent cavitary dilation and the progressive decline in cardiac function. CSCs accumulate at the sites of active cardiomyogenesis but do not cross the boundary that separates the viable myocardium of the border zone from the necrotic and scarred tissue of the infarct, hindering the reconstitution of the damaged myocardium and the recovery of function. This process is operative in all infarcted organs, including the liver, skin, brain, kidney, and testis. To overcome this obstacle, HGF and IGF-1 have been delivered to the infarcted mouse heart.[82] By creating a chemotactic gradient from the atrial niches to the area of injury, HGF activates the c-Met receptor on the surface membrane of CSCs, promoting their directional migration to the site of the infarct (**Figure 3-15**). IGF-1 favors the successful competition of CSCs with inflammatory cells and fibroblasts present within the necrotic myocardium, preventing the activation of the endogenous cell death program in CSCs.[82]

Cardiomyocyte Dedifferentiation and Fibroblast Reprogramming

Reprogramming, transdifferentiation, transdetermination, and dedifferentiation represent multiple aspects of the same

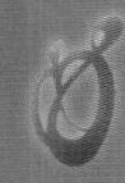

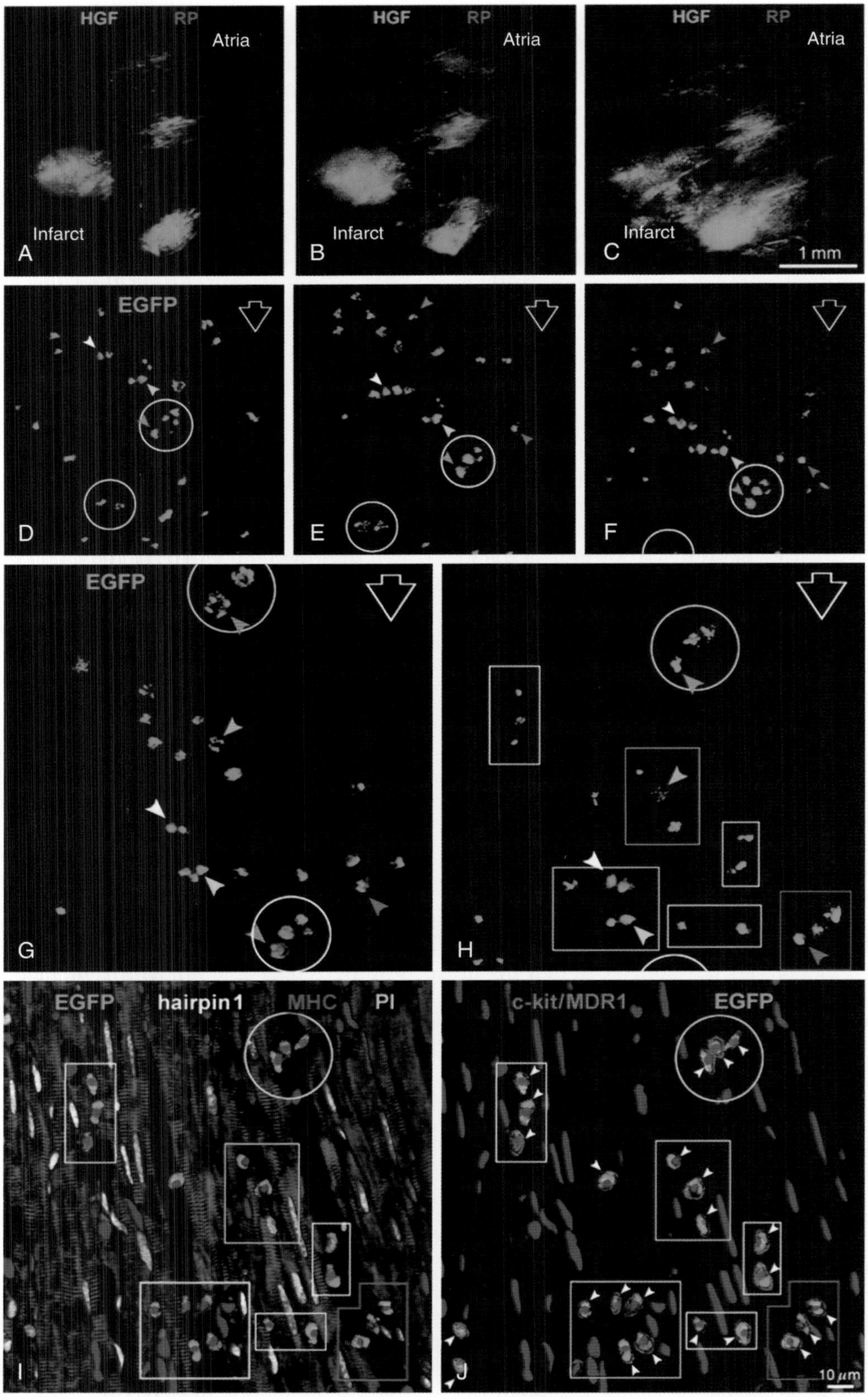

FIGURE 3-15 Growth factor administration and migration of CSCs. **A-C,** Fluorescein-labeled hepatocyte growth factor (HGF) is higher in proximity of the infarct and lower at the atria-ventricular groove (Atria) at 10 **(A),** 30 **(B),** and 60 **(C)** minutes after injection. RP indicates rhodamine particles. **D-H,** Heart perfused with Tyrode-solution. Two-photon microscopy images at the border zone 15 hours after infarct and 10 hours after administration of HGF and IGF-1. Images of the same field were taken 20 minutes apart (**D,** baseline; **E,** 20 minutes; **F,** 40 minutes; **G,** 60 minutes; **H,** 80 minutes). EGFP-positive cells *(green, arrowheads)* moved in the direction of the large open arrows in 80 minutes. White circles **(D)** surround EGFP-positive cells, which were in the field and then progressively disappeared **(F, G,** and **H).** Yellow circle surrounds EGFP-positive cells, which appear in **G** and are in field **H. H, I,** Rectangles and a yellow circle surround EGFP-positive cells detected by 2-photon microscopy (**H;** *green*) and confocal microscopy (**I;** *green*). Green-fluorescence identifies the same EGFP-positive cells **(H** and **I). I,** White-fluorescence corresponds to hairpin-1 labeled apoptotic myocyte-nuclei; EGFP-positive cells within the infarct are viable (hairpin-1-negative). Myocytes are labeled by cardiac myosin, red. **J,** EGFP-positive cells express c-kit-MDR1 *(magenta; arrowheads).*

phenomenon (i.e., the conversion of one cell type into another).[126] Collectively, these cell transformations include the switch from one differentiated cell to another differentiated cell type, the plasticity of stem cells that by crossing tissue boundaries commit to lineages different from those of the organ of origin, and the regression of a mature cell to a proliferative state, or to a primitive unipotent/multipotent progenitor cell. This unexpected biologic flexibility has challenged the view that changes in phenotype could not take place once a cell, through a hierarchical progressive restriction of developmental options, has chosen its fate.

Reprogramming aims to revert somatic differentiated cells into pluripotent cells that have the ability to generate most cell types in the organism. Although reprogramming occurs naturally during fertilization to produce totipotent cells, this process is not a component of the naturally occurring regenerative response. In vitro reprogramming of somatic cells requires complex interventions, including forced overexpression of transcription factors and the introduction of synthetic modified mRNA, recombinant proteins, microRNAs, and minicircle plasmids.[127] In all cases, nuclear reprogramming is coupled with chromatin rearrangements, which are necessary for the acquisition of properties comparable with those of embryonic stem cells. However, a residual epigenetic memory of the original parental source leads to biased differentiation of the biologically modified progeny.[128] Incomplete removal of tissue-specific methylation and aberrant de novo methylation are the molecular bases of this incomplete epigenetic transformation.[128] These currently unresolved molecular and biologic problems raise uncertainties about the possibility to use iPS cells for regenerative purposes. Currently, iPS cells are employed for modeling of diseases induced by genetic mutations and drug screening.

Transdifferentiation may not be a rare event if we consider the nearly infinite number of permutations that occur in each individual during prenatal development and postnatal life. The presence of foreign tissue in ectopic sites (i.e., metaplasia) is more easily recognizable in disease states than under physiologic conditions.[129] This does not exclude the possibility that transdifferentiation might represent a normal aspect of cell turnover, but this process remains one of the most questioned mechanisms of growth and repair in the adult organism. Originally, transdifferentiation was defined as an irreversible switch from one differentiated cell to another differentiated cell type, while transdetermination was defined as the switch in commitment of stem cells toward closely related lineages. However, the term *transdetermination* is rarely used and transdifferentiation or developmental plasticity indicates the process by which adult stem cells are capable of generating mature cells beyond their own tissue boundaries.[129] HSCs are particularly prone to break the law of tissue fidelity and can migrate to sites of injury, repairing damage in various organs, including the heart.[12]

C-kit-positive HSCs injected in the border zone of a myocardial infarct, or mobilized systemically into the circulation with cytokines, lead experimentally to the repair of the necrotic tissue and the formation of functionally competent myocardium.[12,46] These findings and the paucity of newly discovered drugs for the treatment of heart failure have prompted cardiologists to the rapid implementation of cell-based therapy in the management of the infarcted human heart. Shortly after the experimental evidence that HSCs induce myocardial regeneration after infarction, unfractionated mononuclear bone marrow cells and CD34-positive cells have been administered to patients affected by acute and chronic myocardial infarction, dilated cardiomyopathy, and refractory angina. Although the individual outcomes have been inconsistent and variability exists among trials, meta-analyses of pooled data indicate that bone marrow cells (BMC) therapy results in an average 3% to 4% increase in ejection fraction.[130] Reductions in infarct scar size and left ventricular end-systolic volume have been observed, together with small decreases in left ventricular end-diastolic volume. Despite the differences in the type of cells injected, choice of clinical endpoints, methods for the evaluation of cardiac function, and interval between the onset of the cardiac disease and cell infusion, the positive consequences of bone marrow cells have consistently been documented. Importantly, CD34-positive cells exhibit superior efficacy in the preservation of myocardial integrity and function versus unselected circulating mononuclear cells in an experimental model of myocardial infarction.[131] CD34-positive cells have been injected intramyocardially in patients affected by refractory angina, resulting in remarkable improvements in angina frequency and exercise tolerance.[132] Thus far, c-kit-positive HSCs have not been used in clinical trials.

In contrast to transdifferentiation, *dedifferentiation* refers to a regression of a mature cell within its own lineage; this process is typically coupled with the attainment of cell proliferation. Dedifferentiation is considered the natural regenerative response to cardiac injury in zebrafish, newts, and planaria. In mammalian organisms, liver and pancreas regeneration after surgical partial resection are seen as typical examples of cell dedifferentiation.[133] Cell cycle reentry of mature hepatocytes and the reversal of pancreatic duct cells to an immature phenotype constitute the cellular adaptations triggered by the loss of parenchymal mass. Recent reports have emphasized the critical role of myocyte dedifferentiation with amplification of the reprogrammed progeny in the regenerative response of the heart to pathologic stimuli.[134] In addition to the cytoskeletal finding of sarcomeric disorganization, changes in the molecular fingerprint have been considered indicative of myocyte dedifferentiation. However, the lack of structural markers typical of a given cell type is not by itself indicative of the developmental stage of the cell; it impossible to define in vivo whether the cell of interest is undergoing differentiation or whether it is in the process of reverting to an earlier differentiation state.

Myocytes with decreased myofibrils and expansion of the undifferentiated cytoplasm have been found in pathologic cardiac hypertrophy,[18] idiopathic dilated cardiomyopathy,[135] acute myocardial infarction,[51,135] and in the presence of hibernating myocardium. Partial loss in the normal distribution pattern of titin, desmin, and cardiotin has been reported, together with the reexpression of fetal genes, including α-smooth muscle actin, atrial natriuretic peptide, and α-skeletal actin.[135] Dedifferentiation of adult cardiomyocytes has also been claimed following inhibition of p38 MAPK,[47] and myocardial injection of the extracellular matrix component periostin[48] and the growth factor neuregulin.[49]

Recent studies in rodents have shown that intramyocardial injection of transcription factors and miRNAs leads to reprogramming of cardiac fibroblasts into cardiomyocytes, improving cardiac function following myocardial infarction (for review, see reference 136). This process may involve the direct conversion of fibroblasts to the cardiomyocyte fate or the regression to a stem cell phenotype and the subsequent differentiation to the myocyte lineage. These two possibilities were tested in mice expressing yellow fluorescent protein under the control of the Isl1 and Mesp1 promoters. The Isl1 and Mesp1 proteins are transiently expressed in progenitor cells during development. Reprogrammed cardiomyocytes do not show the fluorescent label, suggesting that fibroblasts switch directly to cardiomyocytes without passing through a cardiac progenitor cell state.[137] Induced cardiac-like myocytes are relatively immature, rarely showing action potentials and strong contractility, well-developed sarcomeres, and binucleation, characteristics of adult cardiomyocytes. As emphasized in a recent review,[136] currently unresolved issues include the low efficiency of the reprogramming process, the incomplete conversion to a mature cardiac phenotype, and the long-term stability and integration of reprogrammed cardiomyocytes with native cardiomyocytes.

CONCLUSION AND FUTURE DIRECTIONS

In this chapter we have reviewed the literature that supports the concept that the heart has an endogenous repair system that arises, at least in part, secondary to CPCs and circulating progenitor cells. Nonetheless, several fundamental areas of stem cell research have to be addressed for this field to move forward. One important question involves the identification whether distinct classes of human stem cells condition the efficacy of cardiac repair. Another important question is whether the expression of a single stem cell antigen or a combination of epitopes in CPCs is linked to the formation of a preferential cardiac cell progeny. Similarly, the impact of age, gender, type, and duration of the heart failure on stem cell proliferation and lineage commitment needs to be better understood. Additionally, there is little understanding concerning the difference in the regeneration potential of primitive and partly committed CPCs. Further, an apparent dichotomy exists between our incomplete knowledge of basic mechanisms that regulate stem cell growth, differentiation, and death and the number of patients who have been treated with cells of bone marrow origin. Hopefully ongoing clinical trials (see Chapter 38) will address this important question.

References

1. Karsner HT, Saphir O, Todd TW: The state of the cardiac muscle in hypertrophy and atrophy. *Am J Pathol* 1:351–372, 1925.
2. Anversa P, Kajstura J: Ventricular myocytes are not terminally differentiated in the adult mammalian heart. *Circ Res* 83:1–14, 1998.
3. Soonpaa MH, Field LJ: Survey of studies examining mammalian cardiomyocyte DNA synthesis. *Circ Res* 83:15–26, 1998.
4. Zak R: Development and proliferative capacity of cardiac muscle cells. *Circ Res* 35:17–26, 1974.
5. Spector DL, Goldman RD, Leinwand LA: Light microscopy. In Spector DL, Goldman RD, Leinwand LA, editors: *Cells: light microscopy and cell structure*, Cold Spring Harbor, NY, 1997, Cold Spring Harbor Laboratory Press, pp 94.1–94.53.
6. Linzbach AJ: Mikrometrische und histologische Analyse hypertropher menschlicher Herzen. *Virchow Arch Pathol Anat Physiol* 314:534–594, 1947.
7. Linzbach AJ: The muscle fiber constant and the law of growth of the human ventricles. *Virchows Arch* 318:575–618, 1950.
8. Astorri E, Chizzola A, Visioli O, et al: Right ventricular hypertrophy–a cytometric study on 55 human hearts. *J Mol Cell Cardiol* 2:99–110, 1971.
9. Astorri E, Bolognesi R, Colla B, et al: Left ventricular hypertrophy: a cytometric study on 42 human hearts. *J Mol Cell Cardiol* 9:763–775, 1977.
10. Adler CP, Friedburg H: Myocardial DNA content, ploidy level and cell number in geriatric hearts: post-mortem examinations of human myocardium in old age. *J Mol Cell Cardiol* 18:39–53, 1986.
11. Anversa P, Leri A, Beltrami CA, et al: Myocyte death and growth in the failing heart. *Lab Invest* 78:767–786, 1998.
12. Leri A, Kajstura J, Anversa P: Role of cardiac stem cells in cardiac pathophysiology: a paradigm shift in human myocardial biology. *Circ Res* 109:941–961, 2011.
13. Grajek S, Lesiak M, Pyda M, et al: Hypertrophy or hyperplasia in cardiac muscle. Post-mortem human morphometric study. *Eur Heart J* 14:40–47, 1993.
14. Mallat Z, Tedgui A, Fontaliran F, et al: Evidence of apoptosis in arrhythmogenic right ventricular dysplasia. *N Engl J Med* 335:1190–1196, 1996.
15. Narula J, Haider N, Virmani R, et al: Apoptosis in myocytes in end-stage heart failure. *N Engl J Med* 335:1182–1189, 1996.
16. Olivetti G, Abbi R, Quaini F, et al: Apoptosis in the failing human heart. *N Engl J Med* 336:1131–1141, 1997.
17. Kajstura J, Leri A, Finato N, et al: Myocyte proliferation in end-stage cardiac failure in humans. *Proc Natl Acad Sci U S A* 95:8801–8805, 1998.
18. Urbanek K, Quaini F, Tasca G, et al: Intense myocyte formation from cardiac stem cells in human cardiac hypertrophy. *Proc Natl Acad Sci U S A* 100:10440–10445, 2003.
19. Chimenti C, Kajstura J, Torella D, et al: Senescence and death of primitive cells and myocytes lead to premature cardiac aging and heart failure. *Circ Res* 93:604–613, 2003.
20. Urbanek K, Torella D, Sheikh F, et al: Myocardial regeneration by activation of multipotent cardiac stem cells in ischemic heart failure. *Proc Natl Acad Sci U S A* 102:8692–8697, 2005.
21. Kajstura J, Gurusamy N, Ogórek B, et al: Myocyte turnover in the aging human heart. *Circ Res* 107:1374–1386, 2010.
22. Kajstura J, Rota M, Cappetta D, et al: Cardiomyogenesis in the aging and failing human heart. *Circulation* 126:1869–1881, 2012.
23. Bergmann O, Bhardwaj RD, Bernard S, et al: Evidence for cardiomyocyte renewal in humans. *Science* 324:98–102, 2009.
24. Murry CE, Lee RT: Development biology. Turnover after the fallout. *Science* 324:47–48, 2009.
25. Parmacek MS, Epstein JA: Cardiomyocyte renewal. *N Engl J Med* 361:86–88, 2009.
26. Yi BA, Wernet O, Chien KR: Pregenerative medicine: developmental paradigms in the biology of cardiovascular regeneration. *J Clin Invest* 120:20–28, 2010.
27. Soonpaa MH, Rubart M, Field LJ: Challenges measuring cardiomyocyte renewal. *Biochim Biophys Acta* 1833:799–803, 2013.
28. Senyo SE, Steinhauser ML, Pizzimenti CL, et al: Mammalian heart renewal by pre-existing cardiomyocytes. *Nature* 493:433–436, 2013.
29. Hipfner DR, Cohen SM: Connecting proliferation and apoptosis in development and disease. *Nat Rev Mol Cell Biol* 5:805–815, 2004.
30. Gomer RH: Not being the wrong size. *Nature* 2:48–54, 2001.
31. Pasumarthi KB, Field LJ: Cardiomyocyte cell cycle regulation. *Circ Res* 90:1044–1054, 2002.
32. Field LJ: Modulation of the cardiomyocyte cell cycle in genetically altered animals. *Ann NY Acad Sci* 1015:160–170, 2004.
33. Rakusan K: Assessment of cardiac growth. In Zak R, editor: *Growth of the heart in health and disease*, New York, 1984, Raven Press, pp 25–40.
34. Soonpaa MH, Kim KK, Pajak L, et al: Cardiomyocyte DNA synthesis and binucleation during murine development. *Am J Physiol* 271:H2183–H2189, 1996.
35. Rubart M, Field LJ: Cardiac regeneration: repopulating the heart. *Annu Rev Physiol* 68:29–49, 2006.
36. Trivedi CM, Lu MM, Wang Q, et al: Transgenic overexpression of Hdac3 in the heart produces increased postnatal cardiac myocyte proliferation but does not induce hypertrophy. *J Biol Chem* 283:26484–26489, 2008.
37. Maillet M, van Berlo JH, Molkentin JD: Molecular basis of physiological heart growth: fundamental concepts and new players. *Nat Rev Mol Cell Biol* 14:38–48, 2013.
38. Nadal-Ginard B: Commitment, fusion and biochemical differentiation of a myogenic cell line in the absence of DNA synthesis. *Cell* 15:855–864, 1978.
39. Tam SK, Gu W, Mahdavi V, et al: Cardiac myocyte terminal differentiation. Potential for cardiac regeneration. *Ann N Y Acad Sci* 752:72–79, 1995.
40. Ahuja P, Sdek P, MacLellan WR: Cardiac myocyte cell cycle control in development, disease, and regeneration. *Physiol Rev* 87:521–544, 2007.
41. Yoshizumi M, Lee WS, Hsieh CM, et al: Disappearance of cyclin A correlates with permanent withdrawal of cardiomyocytes from the cell cycle in human and rat hearts. *J Clin Invest* 95:2275–2280, 1995.
42. Setoguchi M, Leri A, Wang S, et al: Activation of cyclins and cyclin-dependent kinases, DNA synthesis, and myocyte mitotic division in pacing-induced heart failure in dogs. *Lab Invest* 79:1545–1558, 1999.
43. Sdek P, Zhao P, Wang Y, et al: Rb and p130 control cell cycle gene silencing to maintain the postmitotic phenotype in cardiac myocytes. *J Cell Biol* 194:407–423, 2011.
44. Zhu W, Hassink RJ, Rubart M, et al: Cell-cycle-based strategies to drive myocardial repair. *Pediatr Cardiol* 30:710–715, 2009.
45. Hassink RJ, Pasumarthi KB, Nakajima H, et al: Cardiomyocyte cell cycle activation improves cardiac function after myocardial infarction. *Cardiovasc Res* 78:18–25, 2008.
46. Anversa P, Kajstura J, Rota M, et al: Regenerating new heart with stem cells. *J Clin Invest* 123:62–70, 2013.
47. Engel FB, Schebesta M, Duong MT, et al: p38 MAP kinase inhibition enables proliferation of adult mammalian cardiomyocytes. *Genes Dev* 19:1175–1187, 2005.
48. Kühn B, del Monte F, Hajjar RJ, et al: Periostin induces proliferation of differentiated cardiomyocytes and promotes cardiac repair. *Nat Med* 13:962–969, 2007.
49. Bersell K, Arab S, Haring B, et al: Neuregulin1/ErbB4 signaling induces cardiomyocyte proliferation and repair of heart injury. *Cell* 138:257–270, 2009.
50. Agah R, Kirshenbaum LA, Abdellatif M, et al: Adenoviral delivery of E2F-1 directs cell cycle reentry and p53-independent apoptosis in postmitotic adult myocardium in vivo. *J Clin Invest* 100:2722–2728, 1997.
51. Beltrami AP, Urbanek K, Kajstura J, et al: Evidence that human cardiac myocytes divide after myocardial infarction. *N Engl J Med* 344:1750–1757, 2001.
52. Quaini F, Cigola E, Lagrasta C, et al: End-stage cardiac failure in humans is coupled with the induction of proliferating cell nuclear antigen and nuclear mitotic division in ventricular myocytes. *Circ Res* 75:1050–1063, 1994.
53. Rubart M, Field LJ: Cardiac regeneration: repopulating the heart. *Annu Rev Physiol* 68:29–49, 2006.
54. Malumbres M, Barbacid M: Cell cycle, CDKs and cancer: a changing paradigm. *Nat Rev Cancer* 9:153–166, 2009.
55. Kajstura J, Urbanek K, Perl S, et al: Cardiomyogenesis in the adult human heart. *Circ Res* 107:305–315, 2010.
56. Cavanagh BL, Walker T, Norazit A, et al: Thymidine analogues for tracking DNA synthesis. *Molecules* 16:7980–7993, 2011.
57. Endl E, Gerdes J: The Ki-67 protein: fascinating forms and an unknown function. *Exp Cell Res* 257:231–237, 2000.
58. Kuipers MA, Stasevich TJ, Sasaki T, et al: Highly stable loading of Mcm proteins onto chromatin in living cells requires replication to unload. *J Cell Biol* 192:29–41, 2011.
59. Martínez P, Blasco MA: Telomeric and extra-telomeric roles for telomerase and the telomere-binding proteins. *Nat Rev Cancer* 11:161–176, 2011.
60. Leri A, Malhotra A, Liew CC, et al: Telomerase activity in rat cardiac myocytes is age and gender dependent. *J Mol Cell Cardiol* 32:385–390, 2000.
61. Leri A, Barlucchi L, Limana F, et al: Telomerase expression and activity are coupled with myocyte proliferation and preservation of telomeric length in the failing heart. *Proc Natl Acad Sci U S A* 98:8626–8631, 2001.
62. Torella D, Rota M, Nurzynska D, et al: Cardiac stem cell and myocyte aging, heart failure, and insulin-like growth factor-1 overexpression. *Circ Res* 94:514–524, 2004.

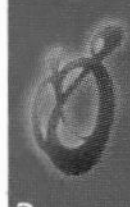

63. Jacobberger JW, Frisa PS, Sramkoski RM, et al: A new biomarker for mitotic cells. *Cytometry A* 73:5–15, 2008.
64. Losada A, Hirano M, Hirano T: Cohesin release is required for sister chromatid resolution, but not for condensin-mediated compaction, at the onset of mitosis. *Genes Dev* 16:3004–3016, 2002.
65. Olivetti G, Cigola E, Maestri R, et al: Aging, cardiac hypertrophy and ischemic cardiomyopathy do not affect the proportion of mononucleated and multinucleated myocytes in the human heart. *J Mol Cell Cardiol* 28:1463–1477, 1996.
66. Urbanek K, Cabral-da-Silva MC, Ide-Iwata N, et al: Inhibition of notch1-dependent cardiomyogenesis leads to a dilated myopathy in the neonatal heart. *Circ Res* 107:429–441, 2010.
67. Hégarat N, Smith E, Nayak G, et al: Aurora A and aurora B jointly coordinate chromosome segregation and anaphase microtubule dynamics. *J Cell Biol* 195:1103–1113, 2011.
68. Leri A, Kajstura J, Anversa P: Cardiac stem cells and mechanisms of myocardial regeneration. *Physiol Rev* 85:1373–1416, 2005.
69. Maier B, Gluba W, Bernier B, et al: Modulation of mammalian life span by the short isoform of p53. *Genes Dev* 18:306–319, 2004.
70. Hsu YC, Pasolli HA, Fuchs E: Dynamics between stem cells, niche, and progeny in the hair follicle. *Cell* 144:92–105, 2011.
71. Becker AJ, McCulloch EA, Till JE: Cytological demonstration of the clonal nature of spleen colonies derived from transplanted mouse marrow cells. *Nature* 197:452–454, 1963.
72. Aliotta JM, Lee D, Puente N, et al: Progenitor/stem cell fate determination: interactive dynamics of cell cycle and microvesicles. *Stem Cells Dev* 21:1627–1638, 2012.
73. Cerny J, Quesenberry PJ: Chromatin remodeling and stem cell theory of relativity. *J Cell Physiol* 201:1–16, 2004.
74. Blau HM, Brazelton TR, Weimann JM: The evolving concept of a stem cell: entity or function? *Cell* 105:829–841, 2001.
75. Bearzi C, Rota M, Hosoda T, et al: Human cardiac stem cells. *Proc Natl Acad Sci U S A* 104:14068–14073, 2007.
76. Shepherd BE, Kiem HP, Lansdorp PM, et al: Hematopoietic stem-cell behavior in nonhuman primates. *Blood* 110:1806–1813, 2007.
77. Beltrami AP, Barlucchi L, Torella D, et al: Adult cardiac stem cells are multipotent and support myocardial regeneration. *Cell* 114:763–776, 2003.
78. Kajstura J, Bai Y, Cappetta D, et al: Tracking chromatid segregation to identify human cardiac stem cells that regenerate extensively the infarcted myocardium. *Circ Res* 111:894–906, 2012.
79. Lemischka IR, Raulet DH, Mulligan RC: Developmental potential and dynamic behavior of hematopoietic stem cells. *Cell* 45:917–927, 1986.
80. Suh H, Consiglio A, Ray J, et al: In vivo fate analysis reveals the multipotent and self-renewal capacities of Sox2+ neural stem cells in the adult hippocampus. *Cell Stem Cell* 1:515–528, 2007.
81. Hosoda T, D'Amario D, Cabral-Da-Silva MC, et al: Clonality of mouse and human cardiomyogenesis in vivo. *Proc Natl Acad Sci U S A* 106:17169–17174, 2009.
82. Urbanek K, Rota M, Cascapera S, et al: Cardiac stem cells possess growth factor-receptor systems that after activation regenerate the infarcted myocardium, improving ventricular function and long-term survival. *Circ Res* 97:663–673, 2005.
83. Urbanek K, Cesselli D, Rota M, et al: Stem cell niches in the adult mouse heart. *Proc Natl Acad Sci U S A* 103:9226–9231, 2006.
84. Hierlihy AM, Seale P, Lobe CG, et al: The post-natal heart contains a myocardial stem cell population. *FEBS Lett* 530:239–243, 2002.
85. Pfister O, Oikonomopoulos A, Sereti KI, et al: Isolation of resident cardiac progenitor cells by Hoechst 33342 staining. *Methods Mol Biol* 660:53–63, 2010.
86. Oyama T, Nagai T, Wada H, et al: Cardiac side population cells have a potential to migrate and differentiate into cardiomyocytes in vitro and in vivo. *J Cell Biol* 176:329–341, 2007.
87. Tomita Y, Matsumura K, Wakamatsu Y, et al: Cardiac neural crest cells contribute to the dormant multipotent stem cell in the mammalian heart. *J Cell Biol* 170:1135–1146, 2005.
88. Pfister O, Oikonomopoulos A, Sereti KI, et al: Role of the ATP-binding cassette transporter Abcg2 in the phenotype and function of cardiac side population cells. *Circ Res* 103:825–835, 2008.
89. Oh H, Bradfute SB, Gallardo TD, et al: Cardiac progenitor cells from adult myocardium: homing, differentiation, and fusion after infarction. *Proc Natl Acad Sci U S A* 100:12313–12318, 2003.
90. Matsuura K, Nagai T, Nishigaki N, et al: Adult cardiac Sca-1-positive cells differentiate into beating cardiomyocytes. *J Biol Chem* 279:11384–11391, 2004.
91. Matsuura K, Honda A, Nagai T, et al: Transplantation of cardiac progenitor cells ameliorates cardiac dysfunction after myocardial infarction in mice. *J Clin Invest* 119:2204–2217, 2009.
92. Lan F, Liu J, Narsinh KH, et al: Safe genetic modification of cardiac stem cells using a site-specific integration technique. *Circulation* 126:S20–S28, 2012.
93. Dodou E, Verzi MP, Anderson JP, et al: Mef2c is a direct transcriptional target of ISL1 and GATA factors in the anterior heart field during mouse embryonic development. *Development* 131:3931–3942, 2004.
94. Moretti A, Caron L, Nakano A, et al: Multipotent embryonic isl1+ progenitor cells lead to cardiac, smooth muscle, and endothelial cell diversification. *Cell* 127:1151–1165, 2006.
95. Ishii Y, Garriock RJ, Navetta AM, et al: BMP signals promote proepicardial protrusion necessary for recruitment of coronary vessel and epicardial progenitors to the heart. *Dev Cell* 19:307–316, 2010.
96. Kattman SJ, Huber TL, Keller GM: Multipotent flk-1+ cardiovascular progenitor cells give rise to the cardiomyocyte, endothelial, and vascular smooth muscle lineages. *Dev Cell* 11:723–732, 2006.
97. Martínez-Estrada OM, Lettice LA, Essafi A, et al: Wt1 is required for cardiovascular progenitor cell formation through transcriptional control of Snail and E-cadherin. *Nat Genet* 42:89–93, 2010.
98. Zhou B, Ma Q, Rajagopal S, et al: Epicardial progenitors contribute to the cardiomyocyte lineage in the developing heart. *Nature* 454:109–113, 2008.
99. Cai CL, Martin JC, Sun Y, et al: A myocardial lineage derives from Tbx18 epicardial cells. *Nature* 454:104–108, 2008.
100. Castaldo C, Di Meglio F, Nurzynska D, et al: CD117-positive cells in adult human heart are localized in the subepicardium, and their activation is associated with laminin-1 and alpha6 integrin expression. *Stem Cells* 26:1723–1731, 2008.
101. Limana F, Zacheo A, Mocini D, et al: Identification of myocardial and vascular precursor cells in human and mouse epicardium. *Circ Res* 101:1255–1265, 2007.
102. Smith RR, Barile L, Cho HC, et al: Regenerative potential of cardiosphere-derived cells expanded from percutaneous endomyocardial biopsy specimens. *Circulation* 115:896–908, 2007.
103. Mohsin S, Siddiqi S, Collins B, et al: Empowering adult stem cells for myocardial regeneration. *Circ Res* 109:1415–1428, 2011.
104. Angert D, Berretta RM, Kubo H, et al: Repair of the injured adult heart involves new myocytes potentially derived from resident cardiac stem cells. *Circ Res* 108:1226–1237, 2011.
105. Sundararaman B, Avitabile D, Konstandin MH, et al: Asymmetric chromatid segregation in cardiac progenitor cells is enhanced by Pim-1 kinase. *Circ Res* 110:1169–1173, 2012.
106. Mohsin S, Khan M, Toko H, et al: Human cardiac progenitor cells engineered with Pim-I kinase enhance myocardial repair. *J Am Coll Cardiol* 60:1278–1287, 2012.
107. Williams AR, Hatzistergos KE, Addicott B, et al: Enhanced effect of combining human cardiac stem cells and bone marrow mesenchymal stem cells to reduce infarct size and to restore cardiac function after myocardial infarction. *Circulation* 127:213–223, 2013.
108. Dor Y, Brown J, Martinez OI, et al: Adult pancreatic beta-cells are formed by self-duplication rather than stem-cell differentiation. *Nature* 429:41–46, 2004.
109. Zhou Q, Brown J, Kanarek A, et al: In vivo reprogramming of adult pancreatic exocrine cells to beta-cells. *Nature* 455:627–632, 2008.
110. Kikuchi K, Poss KD: Cardiac regenerative capacity and mechanisms. *Annu Rev Cell Dev Biol* 28:719–741, 2012.
111. Poss KD, Wilson LG, Keating MT: Heart regeneration in zebrafish. *Science* 298:2188–2190, 2002.
112. Wang J, Panáková D, Kikuchi K, et al: The regenerative capacity of zebrafish reverses cardiac failure caused by genetic cardiomyocyte depletion. *Development* 138:3421–3430, 2011.
113. Kikuchi K, Holdway JE, Werdich AA, et al: Primary contribution to zebrafish heart regeneration by gata4(+) cardiomyocytes. *Nature* 464:601–605, 2010.
114. Lepilina A, Coon AN, Kikuchi K, et al: A dynamic epicardial injury response supports progenitor cell activity during zebrafish heart regeneration. *Cell* 127:607–619, 2006.
115. Baird GS, Zacharias DA, Tsien RY: Biochemistry, mutagenesis, and oligomerization of DsRed, a red fluorescent protein from coral. *Proc Natl Acad Sci U S A* 97:11984–11989, 2000.
116. Kikuchi K, Holdway JE, Werdich AA, et al: Primary contribution to zebrafish heart regeneration by gata4(+) cardiomyocytes. *Nature* 464:601–605, 2010.
117. Porrello ER, Mahmoud AI, Simpson E, et al: Transient regenerative potential of the neonatal mouse heart. *Science* 331:1078–1080, 2011.
118. Bailey B, Izarra A, Alvarez R, et al: Cardiac stem cell genetic engineering using the alphaMHC promoter. *Regen Med* 4:823–833, 2009.
119. Haubner BJ, Adamowicz-Brice M, Khadayate S, et al: Complete cardiac regeneration in a mouse model of myocardial infarction. *Aging (Albany NY)* 4:966–977, 2012.
120. Porrello ER, Mahmoud AI, Simpson E, et al: Regulation of neonatal and adult mammalian heart regeneration by the miR-15 family. *Proc Natl Acad Sci U S A* 110:187–192, 2013.
121. de Vetten L, Bergman KA, Elzenga NJ, et al: Neonatal myocardial infarction or myocarditis? *Pediatr Cardiol* 32:492–497, 2011.
122. Yannas IV, Kwan MD, Longaker MT: Early fetal healing as a model for adult organ regeneration. *Tissue Eng* 13:1789–1798, 2007.
123. Bullard KM, Longaker MT, Lorenz HP: Fetal wound healing: current biology. *World J Surg* 27:54–61, 2003.
124. Colwell AS, Longaker MT, Lorenz HP: Mammalian fetal organ regeneration. *Adv Biochem Eng Biotechnol* 93:83–100, 2005.
125. Leung A, Crombleholme TM, Keswani SG: Fetal wound healing: implications for minimal scar formation. *Curr Opin Pediatr* 24:371–378, 2012.
126. Tosh D, Slack JM: How cells change their phenotype. *Nat Rev Mol Cell Biol* 3:187–194, 2002.
127. Slack JM, Tosh D: Transdifferentiation and metaplasia–switching cell types. *Curr Opin Genet Dev* 11:581–586, 2001.
128. Doi A, Park IH, Wen B, et al: Differential methylation of tissue- and cancer-specific CpG island shores distinguishes human induced pluripotent stem cells, embryonic stem cells and fibroblasts. *Nat Genet* 41:1350–1353, 2009.
129. Leri A, Kajstura J, Anversa P: Identity deception: not a crime for a stem cell. *Physiology (Bethesda)* 20:162–168, 2005.
130. Jeevanantham V, Butler M, Saad A, et al: Adult bone marrow cell therapy improves survival and induces long-term improvement in cardiac parameters: a systematic review and meta-analysis. *Circulation* 126:551–568, 2012.
131. Kawamoto A, Iwasaki H, Kusano K, et al: CD34-positive cells exhibit increased potency and safety for therapeutic neovascularization after myocardial infarction compared with total mononuclear cells. *Circulation* 114:2163–2169, 2006.
132. Losordo DW, Henry TD, Davidson C, et al: Intramyocardial, autologous CD34+ cell therapy for refractory angina. *Circ Res* 109:428–436, 2011.
133. Yanger K, Stanger BZ: Facultative stem cells in liver and pancreas: fact and fancy. *Dev Dyn* 240:521–529, 2011.
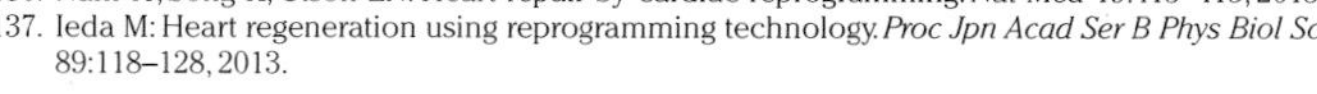
134. Morrisey EE: Rewind to recover: dedifferentiation after cardiac injury. *Cell Stem Cell* 9:387–388, 2011.
135. Kubin T, Pöling J, Kostin S, et al: Oncostatin M is a major mediator of cardiomyocyte dedifferentiation and remodeling. *Cell Stem Cell* 9:420–432, 2011.
136. Nam YJ, Song K, Olson EN: Heart repair by cardiac reprogramming. *Nat Med* 19:413–415, 2013.
137. Ieda M: Heart regeneration using reprogramming technology. *Proc Jpn Acad Ser B Phys Biol Sci* 89:118–128, 2013.

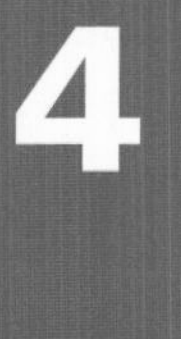

Myocardial Basis for Heart Failure: Role of Cardiac Interstitium

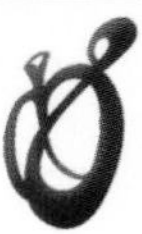

Francis G. Spinale

The term *heart failure (HF)* is not defined by a specific pathologic stimulus but rather the downstream consequence of multifactorial events with the underlying causes being quite diverse, and as such, classification schemes can be problematic. Nevertheless, a categorical description has emerged that encompasses both the HF presentation and key underlying physiologic manifestations.[1-12] Specifically, in patients with a HF presentation whereby quantitative imaging reveals a reduced left ventricular (LV) ejection fraction (EF <50%), this has been assigned the definition of HF with reduced EF (HFrEF [**see also Chapters 17 and 19**]), whereas the same clinical presentation accompanied by a relatively preserved EF (>50%) has been assigned the definition of HF with preserved EF (HFpEF [**see also Chapters 17 and 36**]). In general terms, the pathophysiologic disease states that cause predominant and significant myocardial injury and loss of contractile units, such as ischemic heart disease and the dilated cardiomyopathies, would likely give rise to HFrEF.[13-16] In contrast, HF that arises from an increase in longstanding LV afterload, such as hypertension or aortic valve disease, would be an example that gives rise to HFpEF.[10-12,17] It must be emphasized that in both categorical conditions, the underlying myocardial disease process is not the definition of HF, but only when sufficient to produce clinical symptoms do these definitions apply. In addition, these HF phenotypes are not mutually exclusive and so patients may present with features of both impaired systolic and diastolic function. Nevertheless, for the purposes of focus, the prototypical example of HFrEF as it applies to myocardial infarction (MI) and the dilated cardiomyopathy (DCM), as well as the prototypical example of HFpEF as it applies to hypertensive heart disease (**see also Chapter 23**), will be used in this chapter.

One of the key features of HF irrespective of the category is that changes in LV and myocardial structure and geometry occur and has been generically termed *LV remodeling*. Importantly, there are key features of the LV remodeling process that are present in either HFrEF or HFpEF, and not only hold prognostic relevance but also provide potential clues to the underlying biology unique to each of these HF phenotypes. LV remodeling can be defined as changes in the geometry and function of the LV, which in turn is a summation of cellular and extracellular matrix (ECM) events.[18-22] Moreover, it has become increasingly evident that the myocardial ECM is not a static structure, but rather a dynamic entity that may play a fundamental role in myocardial adaptation to a pathologic stress and thereby facilitate the remodeling process.[23-42] A greater appreciation for the highly complex and dynamic nature of the ECM can be realized by myocardial imaging and direct interrogation of the interstitium and will be discussed in upcoming sections. An example of the complexity of the ECM and the tight interface with respect to tissue structure and function is exemplified by the freeze-etched electron microscopic studies illustrated in **Figure 4-1**.[43] These imaging studies underscore how the ECM environment is tightly coupled to the cell membrane and intracellular structures. In both human and animal studies, it has been reported that alterations in the collagen interface, both in structure and composition, occur within the LV myocardium, which in turn may influence LV geometry.[29-42,44-46] Therefore, identification and understanding of the biologic systems responsible for ECM synthesis and degradation within the myocardium holds particular relevance in the progression of both HFrEF and HFpEF. Accordingly, the purpose of this chapter is fivefold. First, present a brief overview of myocardial ECM structure and biosynthesis. Second, briefly demonstrate how the ECM is altered in specific disease states that give rise to HFrEF (MI, DCM) and HFpEF (pressure overload). Third, present a summation of how measuring dynamic changes in ECM remodeling through either plasma profiling or imaging can provide diagnostic/prognostic utility in HF. Fourth, discuss how increased activation of an interstitial proteolytic system likely contributes to ECM remodeling in CHF. Fifth, examine where the field of ECM biology may be moving in terms of developing therapeutics.

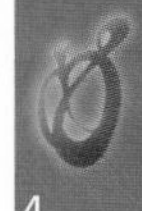

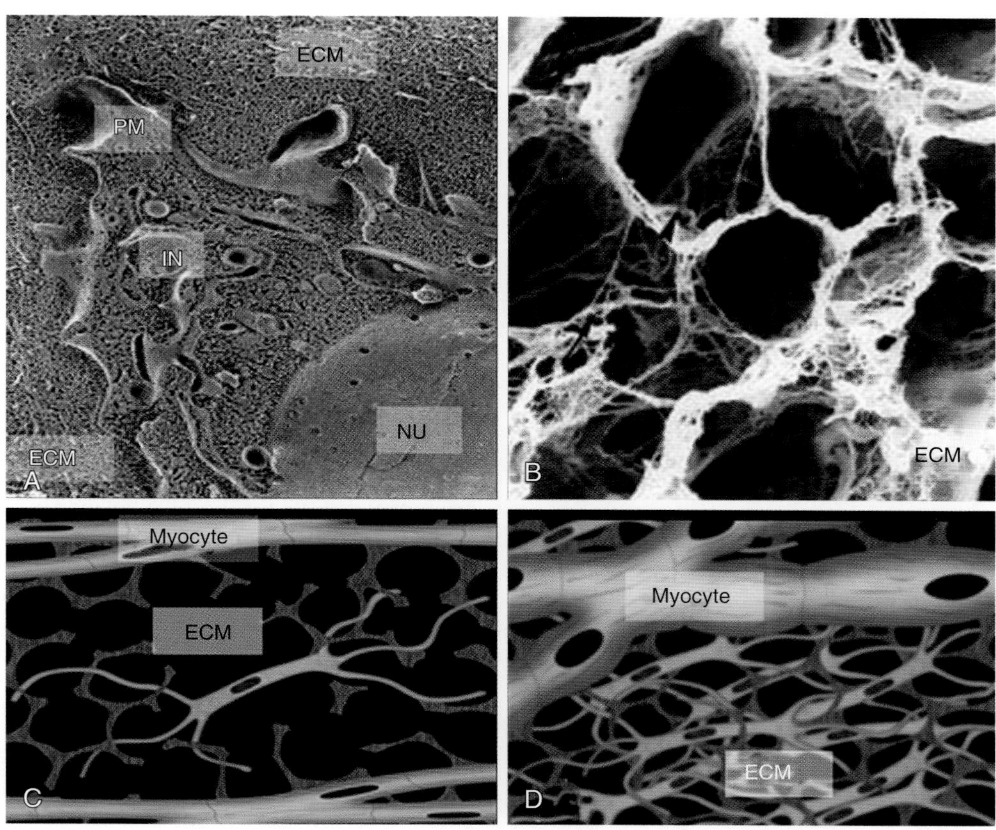

FIGURE 4-1 **A,** An example of the complex nature of the ECM and the tightly coupled interrelationship with the cell membrane and intracellular structures is exemplified in this micrograph of a chondrocyte and the ECM obtained by quick-freeze, deep-etched microscopy.[43] The ECM can be seen to be densely filled with a highly structured architecture that directly interfaces with the plasma membrane (PM), and in turn the intracellular (IN) space. The nuclear pores are evident within the nucleus (NU) and emphasize the tightly coupled arrangement between the nucleus and the ECM. This image reinforces the concept that changes in ECM structure and function will directly affect cellular processes, which include cell function and gene expression. **B,** Sections of myocardium were perfusion fixed and then subjected to maceration digestion and scanning electron microscopy to remove cellular constituents and provide a greater relief of the fibrillar collagen matrix.[237] The fibrillar collagen weave surrounding where individual myocyte profiles existed can be readily appreciated through this process. Moreover, the high degree of complexity of this three-dimensional ECM network can be appreciated. **C,** ECM remodeling entails a number of cellular and interstitial changes in terms of the type of cells within the interstitial space as well as the overall architecture/structure of the ECM. In this example, such as with LV dilation that occurs in volume overload/cardiomyopathies, the eccentric remodeling is accompanied by a loss of ECM integrity and continuous turnover of matrix components, which can facilitate the LV remodeling process. **D,** In pressure overload, growth in both cellular and extracellular constituents occurs, which includes fibroblast proliferation/transdifferentiation and matrix accumulation—both of which can contribute to impaired LV filling and ultimately diastolic dysfunction/failure. ***A,*** *Image courtesy of Dr. Robert Mecham, Washington University School of Medicine.* ***B,*** *Reproduced from Rossi MA: Connective tissue skeleton in the normal left ventricle and in hypertensive left ventricular hypertrophy and chronic chagasic myocarditis. Med Sci Monit 7: 820–832, 2001.*

MYOCARDIAL ECM STRUCTURE AND COMPOSITION

The myocardial ECM contains a fibrillar collagen network, a basement membrane, proteoglycans and glycosaminoglycans, and bioactive signaling molecules. The myocardial fibrillar collagens, such as collagen types I and III, ensure structural integrity of adjoining myocytes, provide the means by which myocyte shortening is translated into overall LV pump function, and is essential for maintaining alignment of myofibrils within the myocyte through a collagen-integrin-cytoskeletal-myofibril relation.[23,25,45-49] While the fibrillar collagen matrix was initially considered to form a relatively static complex, it is now recognized that these structural proteins can undergo rapid degradation and fairly rapid turnover. The complex fibrillar collagen weave that surrounds individual myocytes within the myocardium is demonstrated in Figure 4-1. Collagen fibril formation entails post-translational modification. The carboxy-terminal of the procollagen fibril is cleaved by a proteolytic reaction that results in a conformational change necessary for collagen fibril cross-linking and triple helix formation.[50] A critical step in the proper formation and structural orientation of the fibrillar collagen matrix is collagen cross-linking. Interruption of collagen cross-linking has been clearly demonstrated to alter myocardial ECM structure and in turn LV geometry and function.[51-53] Furthermore, alterations in fibrillar collagen cross-linking have been identified in myocardial samples taken from patients with end-stage HF.[30] Although the newly formed, un–cross-linked collagen fibrils are vulnerable to degradation, the triple helical collagen fiber is resistant to nonspecific proteolysis, and further degradation requires specific enzymatic cleavage. During collagen cross-link formation, the carboxy-terminal peptide is released into the vascular space.[54,55] Collagen type I fiber formation results in the release of a 100-kDa procollagen type I carboxy-terminal propeptide (PIP).[56,57] Similarly, the formation of mature collagen III fibers results in the release of a 42-kDa procollagen peptide (PIIIP) (**Figure 4-2**).[56,58] As will be discussed, a number of associated proteins are necessary for the proper transport, assembly, and stability of the collagen fibril, and monitoring these collagen peptides and associated proteins has been demonstrated to provide diagnostic utility in terms of ECM remodeling and HF progression.

The integrins are a family of transmembrane proteins that serve multiple functions with respect to myocardial

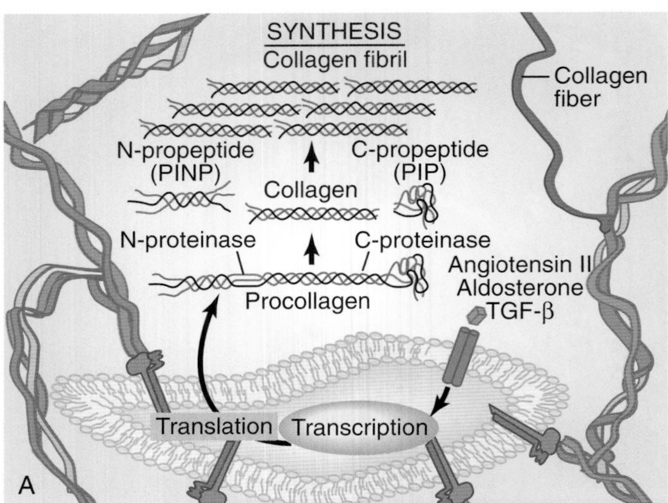

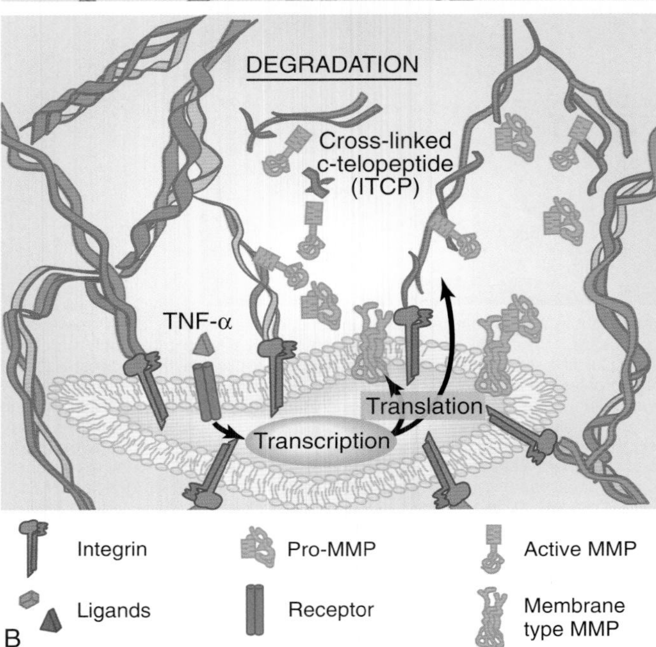

FIGURE 4-2 Collagen synthesis and degradation. **A,** Intracellular signals generated by neurohormonal and/or mechanical stimulation of cardiac fibroblasts results in transcription and translation of nascent collagen proteins, which contain amino-terminal (N-terminal) and carboxy-terminal (C-terminal) propeptides that prevent collagen from assembling into mature fibrils. Once secreted into the interstitium, these propeptides are cleaved by NB and C-proteinases, yielding two procollagen fragments and a mature triple-stranded collagen molecule. In the case of collagen type I, these propeptides are referred to as *N-terminal peptide collagen type I propeptide (PINP)* and *C-terminal peptide type I collagen propeptide (PIP)*. Removal of the propeptide sequences allows the secreted collagen molecule to integrate into growing collagen fibrils, which can then further assemble into collagen fibers. After the collagen fibrils form in the extracellular space, their tensile strength is greatly strengthened by the formation of covalent cross-links between the lysine residues on the collagen molecules. **B,** The degradation of the collagen matrix within the myocardium involves a number of biochemical events involving a number of protease systems. Degradation of collagen fibrils occurs through catalytic cleavage of the three collagen α-chains at a single locus by interstitial collagenase, yielding 36-kDa and 12-kDa collagen telopeptides that maintain their helical structure, and hence are resistant to further proteolytic degradation. The big 36-kDa telopeptide spontaneously denatures into nonhelical gelatin derivatives, which in turn are completely degraded by interstitial gelatinases. The small 12-kDa pyridinoline cross-linked C-terminal telopeptide resulting from the cleavage of collagen type I (ICTP) is found intact in blood, where it appears to be derived from tissues with a stoichiometric ratio of 1 : 1 between the number of collagen type I molecules degraded and that of ITCP released. *From Walsh RA, editor: Molecular mechanisms of cardiac hypertrophy and failure, Boca Raton, Fla, 2005, Taylor and Francis, pp 101–116.*

structure and function.[45,47,48] The integrins form the binding interface, with proteins comprising the basement membrane and therefore directly influencing myocyte growth and geometry. Moreover, the integrins coalesce at important structural sites within the myocyte, called *costameres*, which are composed of cytoskeletal proteins such as alpha-actinin and vinculin, which form a key intracellular support network for contractile protein assembly and maintaining sarcomeric alignment.[45,47,48,59,60] The myocyte costamere is also where the integrins appear to cluster and interdigitate with an intracellular signaling cascade system, such as focal adhesion kinase. Thus disruptions of normal integrin–ECM interactions will likely result in significant changes in myocyte structure and function.

There are a number of extracellular proteins that comprise the basement membrane, such as collagen IV, fibronectin, and laminin. It is the basement membrane that forms the anchoring points for the fibrillar matrix and contact points for other proteoglycans, such as chondroitin sulfate within the ECM. For example, the abundant binding of negatively charged unbranched glycosaminoglycans within chondroitin sulfate results in a molecule with a high osmotic activity.[61] Accordingly, changes in the content and distribution of these proteoglycans will affect hydration within the extracellular space and in turn directly influence myocardial compliance characteristics. Moreover, these highly charged molecules within the ECM result in the formation of a hydrated gel that serves as a reservoir for signaling molecules and bioactive peptides. Therefore, the ECM is an important determinant of extracellular receptor-ligand interactions. Another important function of the myocardial ECM is that it serves as a reservoir for critical biologic signaling molecules that regulate myocardial structure and function. For example, tumor necrosis factor (TNF) is initially a membrane-bound molecule that requires proteolytic processing and release into the interstitial space in order to form ligand complexes with cognate receptors.[62-64] Another example is transforming growth factor-β (TGF), which exists in a latent form bound to the ECM, and requires proteolytic processing within the myocardial interstitium to become a competent signaling molecule.[65-67] TGF signaling produces multiple cellular responses—most importantly, the stimulation of ECM protein synthesis.[68-70] Thus, although this chapter will primarily focus upon the collagen fibrillar network, it is becoming recognized that the myocardial interstitium is a complex environment that contains structural and signaling molecules that directly affect overall myocardial form and function.

THE MYOCARDIAL FIBROBLAST

The most numerous cell type within the LV myocardium is the fibroblast. This is the predominant cell type that is responsible for maintaining ECM homeostasis in terms of collagen synthesis and degradation. This does not imply that the fibroblast is operative in isolation, because significant biomechanical and bioactive signals between the cardiocyte-fibroblast and endothelial cell-fibroblast interactions likely dictate the rate and type of ECM synthesis and degradation. What appears to occur in disease states whereby enhanced fibrosis and/or ECM remodeling occurs is a significant change in the fibroblast phenotype. This process whereby a significant population of phenotypically differentiated fibroblasts arises with ECM remodeling has been termed a *transdifferentiation process*, and the resultant cell type has been defined as the *myofibroblast*.[71-74] However, this does not imply that the normal fibroblast phenotype is extinguished, but rather there is likely increased proliferation of fibroblasts that do not express the myofibroblast phenotype. Thus, in ECM remodeling, there is likely expansion and proliferation of both fibroblasts and myofibroblasts, which in turn will significantly affect the balance between collagen synthesis and degradation. In terms of myocardial ECM remodeling in HFrEF, changes in the synthesis-degradation axis occur, resulting in ECM instability. In contrast, with HFpEF, robust expansion of myofibroblasts occurs, resulting in increased ECM synthesis and accumulation. The specific cell type of origin with respect to the myofibroblast remains unclear and may arise from a stem-cell type, pericyte, or clonal expansion of endogenous fibroblasts. Whatever the case, the myofibroblast is not found in normal LV myocardium but is readily identifiable in the context of LV remodeling. The myofibroblast is typically identified through both cellular constituents and by function.[71-74] Specifically, the mature myofibroblast expresses α smooth muscle actin (SMA), whereas normal fibroblasts do not. In addition, cultured myofibroblasts demonstrate much higher proliferation, margination, invasion, and ECM contractile behavior.

One of the more active areas of research in the cancer field is that of mesenchymal cell transdifferentiation (MET), whereby mesenchymal cells under control of the local environment will transdifferentiate into a proliferative cancer type.[72,74] There are significant similarities in the signaling pathways that are evoked during this mesenchymal transdifferentiation process to that of fibroblast-myofibroblast transdifferentiation.[71-74] Because the myocardial fibroblast is a cell type of mesenchymal origin, it then follows that the expression of specific transcription factors and cell markers would be operative similar to that of MET. There is compelling evidence to suggest that this fibroblast transdifferentiation is accompanied by an intermediate step or cell type, the proto-myofibroblast. This proto-myofibroblast will express unique cell markers, such as a splice variant of fibronectin—the extradomain A (fibronectin ED-A).[71-74] What is clear is that the canonical belief that the fibroblast is a single phenotypic entity must be revisited, and changes in the type, proliferation, and function of subpopulations of fibroblasts likely contribute to specific forms of ECM remodeling, and in turn will influence myocardial form and function with HF.

MYOCARDIAL ECM PROTEOLYTIC DEGRADATION: THE MATRIX METALLOPROTEINASES

The MMPs are a diverse family of zinc-dependent proteases that play a role in normal ECM turnover, as well as in pathologic tissue remodeling processes.[26,27,75-88] Currently, over 25 distinct human MMPs have been identified and characterized. While initially thought to cause only ECM proteolysis, a highly diverse set of biologic functions have been identified, which include cytokine processing and activation of profibrotic signaling molecules.[85-87] Moreover, MMP activity is highly dynamic within the human myocardial ECM. Specifically, using microdialysis techniques coupled with MMP fluorescent substrates, it has been identified that continuous MMP activity exists within the human myocardium under

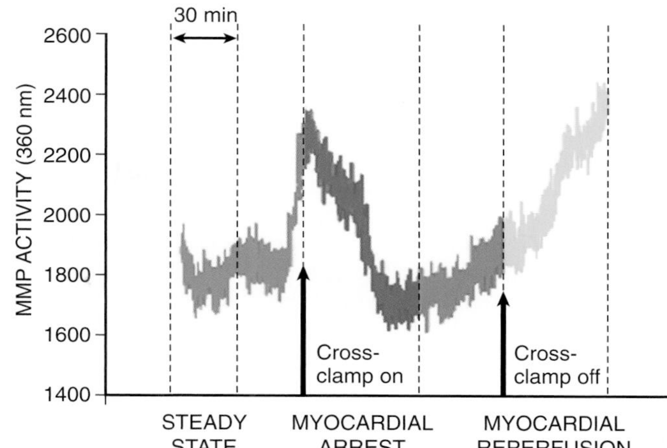

FIGURE 4-3 Although originally considered a static entity, structural and nonstructural proteins and proteases are in a state of constant turnover and can change rapidly and in a dynamic fashion with an imposed cardiovascular stress. In this example, changes in MMP activity were directly measured within the human interstitial space using microdialysis and an MMP-specific fluorescent substrate. Small microdialysis probes are placed in the midmyocardium of patients undergoing elective coronary revascularization, and the fluorescent substrate is infused at microliter volumes, whereby changes in the fluorescence (emission at 360 nm as shown) of the returning fluid from the microdialysis probe will be reflective of interstitial MMP activity. Under steady-state conditions (when artery/vein harvest is ongoing), oscillation in interstitial MMP activity occurs, which is reflective of small continuous changes in proteolytic activity within the myocardial matrix under ambient conditions. With the placement of the aortic cross-clamp and immediate change in LV load, MMP activity increases by approximately 50% and then falls precipitously with induction of cardioplegic arrest and myocardial cooling. However, with removal of the cross-clamp, reperfusion, and resumption of cardiac function, MMP activity increases from steady-state values and continues to rise until the microdialysis probe is removed. *Modified from Spinale FG, Koval CN, Deschamps AM, et al: Dynamic changes in matrix metalloproteinase activity within the human myocardial interstitium during ischemia reperfusion. Circulation 118:S16–23, 2008.*

ambient conditions, which can increase significantly in a matter of seconds (**Figure 4-3**).[88] The MMPs were historically classified into subgroups based upon substrate specificity and/or structure, and an informal nomenclature for some of the individual MMPs arose from these initial substrate studies. However, there is significant overlap in MMP proteolytic substrates and a more rigid numerical classification is now used. Important MMPs in the context of myocardial ECM remodeling include the collagenases, such as MMP-1 and MMP-13; the stromelysins/matrilysins, which include MMP-3/MMP-7; the gelatinases, which include MMP-9 and MMP-2; and the membrane-type MMPs (MT-MMPs). Taken together, once the MMPs are activated, these enzymes can degrade all ECM components, and therefore, it is important that the activity of these enzymes is kept under tight control and interaction.[83,89] The regulation of MMPs can take place at the level of transcription, post-transcription, post-translation, and endogenous inhibition. These levels of control are briefly outlined in the next few paragraphs with examples of how this regulation is operative in the context of myocardial ECM remodeling.

MMP Transcriptional Regulation

The control of gene expression through changes in transcription is an important determinant of MMP tissue levels.[89-94] Studies have identified several consensus sequences for nuclear binding proteins on MMP genes.[90-94] These elements include the tumor response element (TRE), activator protein-1 (AP-1) binding sites, and the polyomavirus

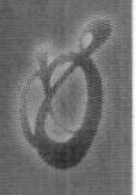

enhancer A-binding protein-3 (PEA-3) sites. The AP-1 and TRE sites bind the dimers of Fos and Jun families, while the members of the Ets family of transcription factors bind to the PEA-3 sites. Although there are similarities among MMP promoters, the promoter of MMP-2 is notably distinct from other members of the MMP family.[90-92] Although most MMP genes contain similar promoter elements, the position of the elements relative to the transcription start site varies among different MMPs, which may partly account for different expression patterns. A clear example of differential MMP transcriptional regulation within the myocardium has been achieved using MMP promoter-reporter constructs.[95,96] For example, the full-length human MMP-2 and MMP-9 promoter has been fused to a reporter and placed into the mouse genome.[95,96] Through this approach, MMP type specific promoter activity can be examined from a spatial and temporal aspect following a pathologic stimulus, such as MI. Representative whole heart mounts for MMP-9 and MMP-2 promoter activity following specific time points post-MI are shown in **Figure 4-4A**. MMP-9 and MMP-2 promoter activity could be readily appreciated following MI induction in these transgenic mice, but the spatial-temporal patterns were different. These studies clearly demonstrate that regulation of MMP promoter activity constitutes an important set point for selective MMP induction within the myocardium.

The potential importance of MMP gene/transcriptional regulation can also be found from clinical studies that have identified variant forms of DNA sequences, polymorphisms, for several of the MMP subtypes.[97-111] The polymorphisms that have been identified thus far often affect the promoter region of the MMP gene, and thereby influence critical steps in the binding of transcription factors or the overall efficiency of transcription. An overview of some of the major polymorphisms reported with respect to MMP-9, -2, -3, and MMP-1, as well as the potential consequences of these alterations in DNA sequences, are summarized in **Table 4-1**. With respect to MMP-9, a variant has been identified that is a single-base substitution between cytosine (C) and thymidine (T).[102-104] The T allele results in a higher relative level of promoter activity when compared to the C allele. The presence of the MMP-9 T allele resulted in increased plasma levels of MMP-9.[102] A naturally occurring variant in the MMP-3 promoter region is the 5A and 6A alleles, which signify a 5 or 6 adenine sequence, respectively. The 5A allele has been associated with increased MMP-3 promoter activity, and in turn, increased relative MMP-3 protein levels.[105-109] In a study performed in over 2800 Japanese patients, the 5A polymorphism was associated with increased risk of MI, particularly in women.[107] Mizon-Gerad and colleagues reported that homozygosity for the 5A allele in patients with nonischemic cardiomyopathy was associated with poor survival rates.[104] In a preliminary clinical study, the addition of a guanine within the MMP-1 promoter region (-1607 1G/2G) was associated within an acceleration of adverse LV myocardial remodeling in patients post-MI.[110,111] While it is possible that additional MMP polymorphisms are likely to be identified, it must be recognized that these MMP genotyping approaches do not provide a clear cause-effect relationship between the MMP system and myocardial matrix remodeling. However, it is intriguing to speculate that these MMP polymorphisms may identify those patients who may be more vulnerable to the adverse matrix myocardial remodeling process and therefore a more rapid progression of HF.

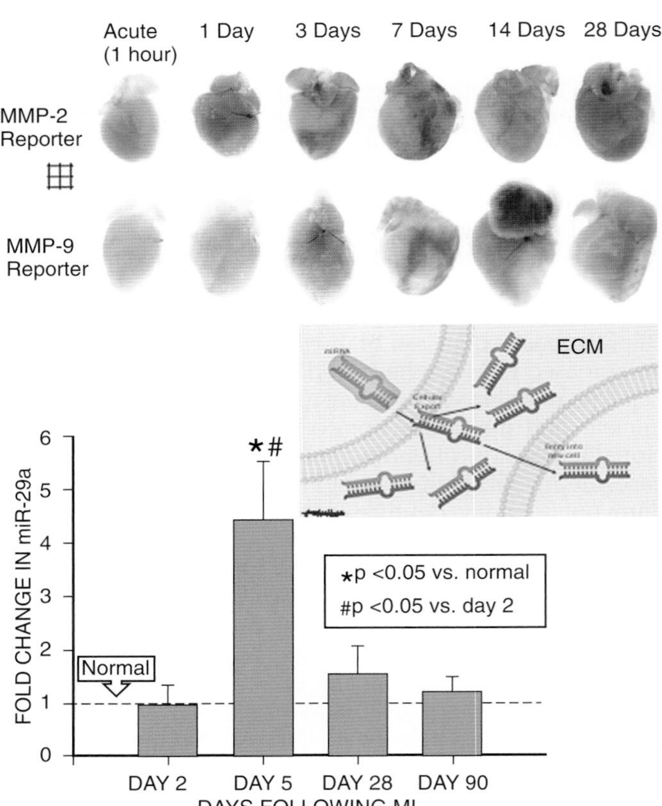

FIGURE 4-4 Specific transcriptional and post-transcriptional events occur following MI, which in turn will contribute specifically to adverse ECM remodeling. *Top:* In this first example, the full-length MMP-2 or MMP-9 promoter was ligated to the β-galactosidase reporter and fused into mice, thereby providing an in vivo index of selective MMP promoter activity. MI was induced in these transgenic constructs and reporter levels visualized at 1 to 28 days post-MI. MMP-2 promoter activity could be readily observed by 3 days post-MI and MMP-9 promoter activity by 7 days post-MI. MMP-2 promoter activity was localized to the MI region and then with longer periods post-MI extended to the border and remote regions. Intense MMP-9 promoter activity could be observed within the area surrounding the MI (border region), which then extended into the remote regions with longer post-MI periods. Scale bar 2 mm × 2 mm square. Figure reproduced from reference 96. *Bottom inset:* A post-transcriptional check point in terms of initiation of protein synthesis is through the binding of transcriptional messenger RNAs by the small non-encoding nucleotides, microRNAs (miRs). One recognized feature of these miRs is that they can be exported into the ECM, and therefore the matrix serves as a potentially important reservoir for miRs. These interstitial miRs can then enter other cells and cell types (i.e., fibroblasts) and thus regulate overall matrix synthesis. *Bottom:* The spillover of miRs from the ECM can be appreciated as these miRs appear in the plasma and have been found to be reasonably stable, thus allowing for serial measurement in patients following MI. In this example, time-dependent changes in plasma miR-29a levels were identified in patients post-MI when compared with referent normal (age-matched, non-MI) subjects. A number of ECM-dependent proteins, such as fibrillar collagens, are regulated by miR-29a, and so these changes in plasma profiles would likely reflect changes in post-transcriptional regulation of the ECM post-MI. *Modified from Zile MR, Mehurg SM, Arroyo JE, et al: Relationship between the temporal profile of plasma microRNA and left ventricular remodeling in patients after myocardial infarction. Circ Cardiovasc Genet 6:614–619, 2011.*

MMP Post-Transcriptional Regulation

The microRNAs directly influence post-transcriptional events through a number of molecular interactions, which include binding to mRNA and interfering with initiation of translation and/or accelerating mRNA degradation. While an area of active research, it is becoming apparent that specific miRs will cause post-transcriptional alterations in functional clusters of proteins that would be relevant to LV remodeling and to the ECM in particular. For example, in a mouse model of MI, changes in relative myocardial miR-29a levels had pronounced and directional effects on ECM remodeling in terms of myocardial fibrosis.[112] Of further

TABLE 4-1 Polymorphisms in MMP Promoters

POLYMORPHISM	BIOLOGIC EFFECT	CLINICAL ASSOCIATION	REFERENCE
MMP-9			
-1562 C/T	Promoter activity	Risk of post-MI remodeling	98, 101-103
		Remodeling in DCM	104
-279 R/Q	Catalytic activity	Remodeling in DCM	101, 104
		Risk of post-MI remodeling	97
		Differing pharmacologic response	99
MMP-2			
-1306 C/T	Promoter activity	Unknown	240
-790 T/G	Transcription factor binding	Coronary artery disease	240
MMP-3			
1171-5A/6A	Promoter activity	Risk of post-MI remodeling	98, 105, 106, 107, 108, 241
1612-5A/6A		LV remodeling in volume overload	
		Remodeling in DCM	100, 105
MMP-1			
-1607 1G/2G	Transcription factor binding	Risk of post-MI remodeling	100, 110, 111
-519-340 A/G-C/T	Promoter activity	Risk of post-MI remodeling	242

Polymorphisms in several MMP promoter sequences have been identified from clinical studies, and the more common variants are outlined on the left. These polymorphisms often entail a single base pair substitution within the promoter locations as indicated. The biologic effects and any clinical associative data associated with these MMP promoter variants have been summarized. The references from which these data were extracted are shown.

DCM, Dilated cardiomyopathy; *LV,* left ventricular; *MI,* myocardial infarction.

relevance to the ECM, miRs can be actively transported into the interstitial space (see Figure 4-4B),[113] and thus a pool of miRs exist within the ECM that can egress to the systemic circulation. Robust and early changes in relative plasma levels of miR-29a have been identified in patients post-MI as shown in Figure 4-4B.[114] More importantly, this past study demonstrated that early changes in plasma miR-29a levels were associated with adverse LV remodeling at 3 months post-MI. This is but one example of what is likely to be a large cluster of miRs that are altered post-MI and may hold prognostic utility in terms of identifying those patients at increased risk for HFrEF, as well as potentially monitoring the progression of this disease process.

MMP Post-Translational Regulation

While the level of MMP synthesis is an important determinant of matrix degradation, the true degradative capacity of the MMPs is dependent upon the activation of the MMP proenzyme. After being synthesized in a latent, proenzyme, or zymogen form, the MMPs are secreted into the extracellular space. For MMP zymogen activation to occur, a sequence of proteolytic events must take place. Thus an important control point or MMP activity is proteolytic cleavage by other enzymes (e.g., serine proteases and other MMP species), or by exposure to certain physical and chemical effectors.[83,84,89] It has been demonstrated that serine proteases, such as plasmin, can generate active MMPs. In addition, MMP activation can also occur at the cell surface involving the MT-MMPs.[115-123] At the cell membrane, MT-MMP is already in an active state, such that it can then activate other MMP species at the cell surface. It has been clearly established that MT1-MMP activates MMP-2, and in fact may be the predominant pathway for MMP-2 activation.[116-121] Moreover, it appears that a very wide proteolytic portfolio for MT1-MMP exists, which would imply that this MMP type may participate in a number of enzymatic and signaling cascades within the myocardial ECM.[85-87] This is likely to hold particular relevance since robust levels of MT1-MMP have been identified within both experimental and clinical forms of HF.*

Endogenous MMP Inhibition

Another important control point of MMP activity is in the inhibition of the activated enzyme by action of a group of specific MMP inhibitors, termed *tissue inhibitors of matrix metalloproteinases (TIMPs)*.[26,27,81-84] There are four known TIMP species, of which TIMP-1 and TIMP-2 are the best characterized. The TIMPs are low-molecular-weight proteins that can complex noncovalently with high efficiency to MMPs in a 1:1 molar ratio. Therefore, these inhibitory proteins are an important endogenous system for regulating MMP activity in vivo. Although the TIMPs are expressed in a variety of cells, TIMP-4 shows a high level of expression in cardiovascular tissue.[125,126] Although a predominant characteristic of the TIMPs is in the inhibition of active enzymes, this is likely to be an oversimplistic view of the function of these proteins. For example, studies have demonstrated TIMPs to be involved in the process of MMP activation, to exhibit growth factor-like properties, and to participate in apoptosis.[127-130] For example, overexpression of TIMP-1,-2,-3,-4 was induced in murine myocardial fibroblasts by adenoviral-mediated transduction.[128] In this study, a number of differential biologic effects were observed by TIMP induction, which included effects on collagen synthesis and apoptosis. These effects were not due to MMP inhibition since pharmacologic MMP inhibition did not recapitulate these effects, therefore indicating a direct action of TIMPs on fibroblast function. Moreover, TIMP-specific effects were observed in which TIMP-2 caused a robust increase in collagen synthesis, whereas TIMP-3 accelerated fibroblast apoptosis. Finally, using transgenic constructs, differential effects of TIMP-3 have been observed in terms of LV remodeling and progression to HF, whether due to MI or pressure overload.[131,132]

*References 20, 21, 29, 40, 123, 124.

These results underscore the highly diverse and complex nature of these proteins that exist within the myocardial interstitium.

HFrEF AND ECM REMODELING—MYOCARDIAL INFARCTION (see also Chapters 11 and 18)

A prolonged ischemic event, with or without reperfusion, causes a cascade of biologic events that can be considered one of a wound healing process and thus the canonical phases of wound healing are often used, which consist of three overlapping phases: inflammation, proliferation, and maturation. The first phase is the acute period in which reactive oxygen species, bioactive signaling molecules, and peptides released from the local environment cause inflammatory cell recruitment and invasion. The initiation of the inflammatory phase is likely due to the release of molecules as a result of myocyte death, and in turn induces the expression of cytokines, such as tumor necrosis factor-α and the interleukins. A more comprehensive examination of cell viability and inflammation is found elsewhere in this text. Some key aspects of the early post-MI inflammatory process include (1) activation of the intracellular transduction pathway, nuclear factor kappa B; (2) induction of a diverse family of chemokines; and (3) neutrophil recruitment and margination. Although initially considered a rather monochromatic cell type in terms of form and function, the macrophages within the MI region appear to be quite heterogeneous and may ultimately influence the magnitude and direction of the localized inflammatory process.[133-137] Although this inflammatory process is critical to initiate a reparative response following myocardial injury, it appears that unlike other sites of tissue injury, the inflammatory response is prolonged within the MI region. The second phase is heralded by proliferation and transdifferentiation of myocardial fibroblasts into myofibroblasts.[138,139] Further, released matrix structural proteins, such as fibrillar collagens, and matrix-integrin-cytoskeletal interactions facilitate contraction of the wound. The third phase of the wound healing process normally results in complete contraction of the wound, apoptosis of the myofibroblasts, and the formation of a relatively acellular scar. However, in the context of post-MI remodeling, this canonical set of events does not necessarily occur. Rather, there is a continued proliferation and transdifferentiation of fibroblasts within the MI and border regions accompanied by a shift in matrix proliferative/degradative pathways within these transformed cells.

Significant changes within the ECM occur during all time points post-MI and likely contribute to the overall adverse LV remodeling process.[22,122,140-142] First, the inflammatory response causes the release of MMPs, as well as other proteases, to degrade the ECM and allow for margination of inflammatory cells.[135,137,142] However, with a persistent inflammatory state, MMP induction will also destabilize the newly formed ECM and the nascent scar. Second, the continued proliferation and altered expression of myofibroblasts within the MI region in terms of the balance between MMP and TIMP levels cause ECM instability and infarct expansion. Specifically, the transformed fibroblast population within the MI region likely results in a shift in the relative balance of MMPs and TIMPs,[22,142] favoring accelerated ECM turnover and a failure of mature scar formation.[22,141,142] Third, a robust expression of "profibrotic" signaling molecules occurs within the myofibroblasts, as well as residual myocyte populations such as TGF, but this does not result in a well-formed ECM.[122,135,140] Specifically, TGF signaling is enhanced within the MI region and causes significantly higher fibrillar collagen transcription[122,136,143]; however, a number of critical post-translational events involving collagen assembly are likely to be defective.[140] For example, a loss of the matricellular protein, secreted protein acidic and rich in cysteine (SPARC), which is involved in procollagen processing to a mature collagen fibril, resulted in impaired collagen maturation and MI scar formation.[144] Further, the interactions of the glycoproteins fibronectin and tenascin C may directly alter cell-ECM interactions, whereby other bioactive molecules, such as osteopontin, can directly influence ECM biosynthesis through a number of signaling pathways. Transmembrane receptors and coreceptors, such as endoglin and syndecan that can modify profibrotic signaling through TGF and other growth factors, also likely play an important role not only in ECM synthesis and degradation but also in terms of myofibroblast transformation. Thus abnormalities in fibroblast phenotype coupled by defects in both ECM synthesis and degradation pathways possibly converge to cause a feed-forward process in terms of MI wall thinning and dyskinesis, increased radial wall stress, and local strain patterns, and ultimately contribute to overall infarct expansion, LV remodeling, and HFrEF. These pathways and processes, as they may relate to the prognosis and diagnosis of HFrEF, are presented in a subsequent section.

HFrEF AND ECM REMODELING—DILATED CARDIOMYOPATHY

DCM constitutes a broad classification of primary myocardial disease states, which contribute to a significant proportion of patients with HFrEF; several chapters within this text examine in detail that there are several animal models of DCM that have identified increased MMPs within the myocardium.[33,36,40,145,146] In the rapid pacing DCM model, increased abundance of several MMP types occurs, with a loss of ECM structural integrity that coincides with the onset of LV remodeling and dilation.[36,40] Moreover, these changes in MMP myocardial levels and LV geometry precede significant alterations in cardiomyocyte contractile function, which underscore the functional importance of MMP-mediated ECM disruption as an early event in this model of DCM. More definitive cause-effect relationships between LV myocardial remodeling and MMP induction have been established through the use of pharmacologic MMP inhibitors.[33,40] For example, MMP inhibition in the pacing DCM model attenuates the degree of LV dilation and dysfunction.[33] In the canine model of ischemic DCM, pharmacologic MMP inhibition attenuates the progression of LV dilation and systolic dysfunction.[147] Thus a contributory mechanism for the LV remodeling that occurs during the experimental form of DCM is MMP induction and heightened MMP activity within the LV myocardium.

A number of studies have examined relative MMP and TIMP expression in end-stage human DCM.[28-32] Uniformly, these past studies have demonstrated an increase in certain MMP species in end-stage human heart failure. One of the first studies was by Gunja-Smith and colleagues in which increased myocardial MMP gelatinolytic activity was reported in DCM.[30] Using immunoblotting procedures,

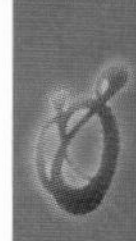

subsequent studies identified several MMP species that were increased in LV myocardial extracts taken from patients with end-stage DCM.[28,29] For example, increased MMP-3 and MMP-9 levels were observed in the DCM myocardial extracts. Although MMP-13 was barely detected in the normal myocardium, a robust immunoreactive signal for MMP-13 was observed in DCM myocardium.[29] Interestingly, MMP-13 has been associated with pathologic remodeling states, such as breast carcinomas.[148,149] The most robust change in MMP types within the DCM myocardium is that of MT1-MMP.[29] A persistent induction and expression of MT1-MMP occurs in DCM fibroblasts when compared with myocardial fibroblasts harvested from nonfailing patients.[150] Li and associates provide evidence to suggest that changes in the MMP/TIMP stoichiometric ratio occur with end-stage DCM disease.[31] In DCM, an absolute reduction in MMP-1/TIMP-1 complex formation has been observed.[29] In a transgenic model of TIMP-3 deletion, a DCM phenotype is reported as a function of age.[131] In DCM patients, chronic unloading of the LV through the use of ventricular assist devices is associated with a reduction in LV chamber dilation and myocardial MMP levels.[41] Taken together, these results suggest that reduced MMP/TIMP complex formation may occur in cardiomyopathic disease states, which in turn would contribute to increased myocardial MMP activity and ECM remodeling.

HFpEF and ECM Remodeling—Hypertensive Heart Disease (see also Chapter 23)

The fundamental milestone in the development and progression of HFpEF is that of concentric LV hypertrophy, which is due to accelerated growth of both the myocyte and ECM compartments. The stimulus for LV hypertrophy is that of a prolonged pressure overload that can arise as a function of hypertension, aortic stenosis, and arterial stiffening as a utility of age.[4,5,8-11] While LV hypertrophy is initially an appropriate adaptive response, continued myocyte growth and expansion of the ECM will eventually lead to fundamental defects in LV diastolic performance. The physiology and pathophysiology of diastolic performance and clinical considerations of HFpEF is the subject of a subsequent chapter. Although a number of active and passive properties of the myocardium are altered in HFpEF, a predominant determinant is change in ECM structure and content. Specifically, increased fibrillar collagen content and the accumulation of other nonstructural ECM proteins are invariable structural events in progressive LV hypertrophy and diastolic dysfunction. The continuous and potentially accelerated accumulation of collagen within the ECM will reduce LV myocardial compliance and thereby impair the passive LV filling phase of diastole and present as a resistance to flow with atrial contraction.[151-154] The summation of these changes in both myocyte and ECM structure and function with progressive LV hypertrophy is a rise in LV filling pressure, and by extension, increased pulmonary capillary wedge pressure (PCWP). The increased PCWP will in turn contribute to higher pulmonary venous pressure and ultimately yield one of the more consistent and severe symptoms associated with HFpEF—exercise intolerance and pulmonary congestion.[155-158] Finally, with persistently increased LV stiffness (both active and passive) and a higher PCWP, left atrial (LA) enlargement occurs, and thus measures of atrial size can also be indicative of worsening LV diastolic function and progression of HFpEF. Clinical studies have demonstrated that both direct and indirect measurements of ECM remodeling, particularly myocardial collagen accumulation, are directly related to increased PCWP, as well as LA volumes.[151-153,155-158]

As shown in **Figure 4-5**, key changes in ECM structure and function include fibroblast proliferation/transdifferentiation, as well as fibrillar collagen accumulation. In pressure overload secondary to aortic stenosis, the significant myocardial collagen accumulation is associated by a concomitant increase in relative myocardial TIMP levels.[159,160] Experimental studies support the concept that diminished myocardial MMP activity can facilitate collagen accumulation in developing hypertrophy.[161,162] In the spontaneously hypertensive rat, the development of compensated hypertrophy is associated with increased myocardial TIMP levels, which would imply reduced MMP activity.[161,162] The changes in myocardial MMP activation are likely to be time dependent and may not be constant throughout the development of pressure overload hypertrophy.[163] Furthermore, using a microdialysis method to directly measure MMP interstitial activity, it was demonstrated that MMP activity is reduced as a function of LV afterload.[44] In a large animal model of progressive aortic stenosis that recapitulated features of HFpEF, changes were induced in MMP and TIMP profiles, which would favor ECM accumulation.[164] In a murine model of LV pressure overload, genetic deletion of MMP-2 reduced the degree of myocardial fibrillar collagen accumulation and improved indices of LV diastolic function.[165] Because the primary mechanism for conversion of pro-MMP-2 to active MMP-2 is through complex formation with MT1-MMP, then induction of this MMP type may be pivotal in the changes in ECM structure and content that occur in HFpEF.[89,166-168] MT1-MMP expression is sensitive to changes in mechanical load, whereby increased wall tension proliferated MT1-MMP promoter activity in vitro.[169] Increased myocardial MT1-MMP expression has been identified in patients with LV pressure overload.[170] In animal models of LV pressure overload, an early and sustained induction of MT1-MMP has been identified.[164,171,172] For example, increased MT1-MMP promoter activity, and subsequently MT1-MMP proteolytic activity, has been reported following the induction of LV pressure overload in mice.[171] The pathways by which MT1-MMP contributes to adverse ECM remodeling likely include facilitating proteolysis of interstitial molecules directly (such as integrins), amplification of active MMP-2 causing ECM instability, and abnormal architecture, as well as through enhancing profibrotic signaling pathways. Specifically, an important proteolytic relationship possibly exists between MT1-MMP and the subsequent activation of the profibrotic signaling molecule TGF,[89,164,165,169,171-174] which would hold particular relevance in the context of LV pressure overload (see Figure 4-5). Competent signaling of TGF requires release from a latency-bound state, binding to the TGF receptor complex, and induction of the transduction elements—Smads. TGF activation through Smads not only will induce fibrillar collagen expression, but will also facilitate fibroblast transformation/transdifferentiation. Thus a likely important proteolytic interaction exists between certain MMP types, such as MT1-MMP, and the TGF signaling axis in terms of ECM accumulation and the progression to HFpEF.

Although certain MMP types, such as MMP-2 and MT1-MMP, appear to be uniformly increased with LV pressure

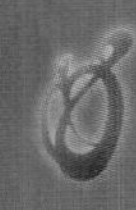

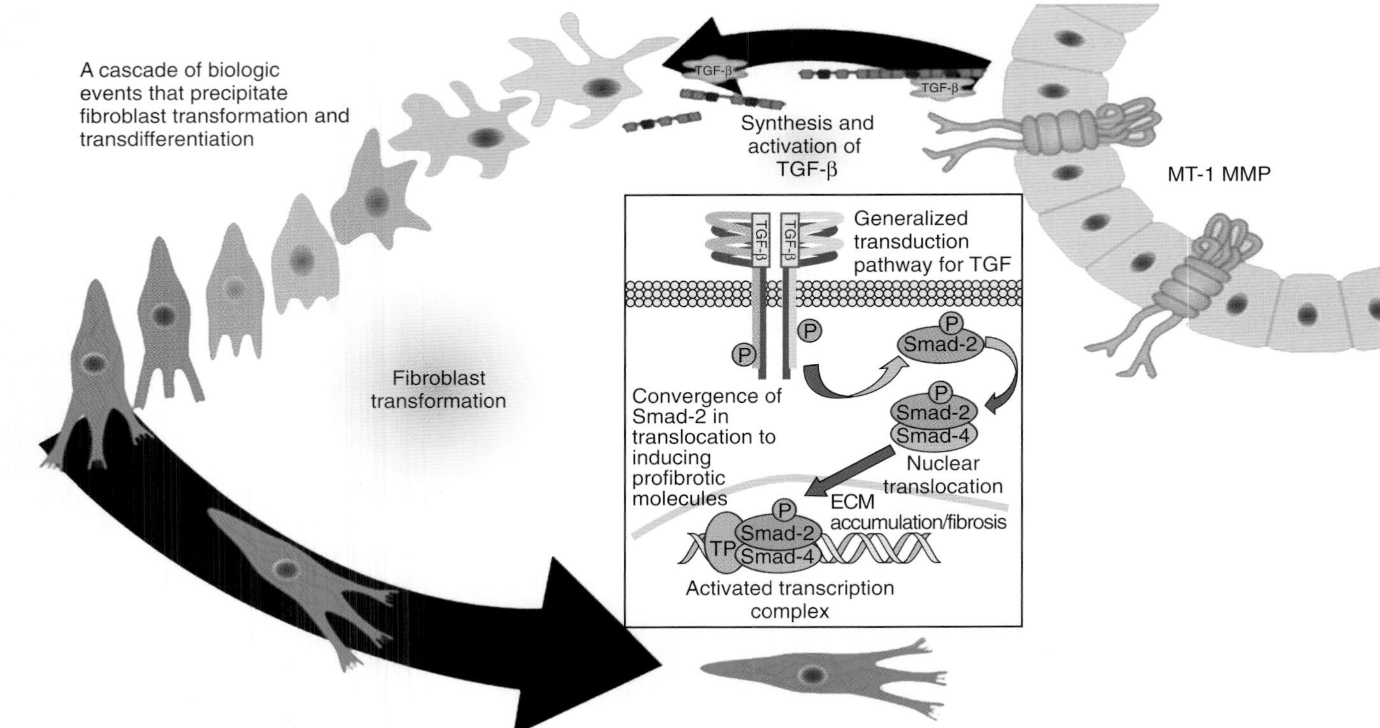

FIGURE 4-5 An important interaction likely exists between ECM proteolytic pathways and profibrotic pathways, particularly in terms of ECM accumulation and fibroblast transformation/transdifferentiation in pressure overload and progression to HFpEF. A specific MT1-MMP recognition sequence exists on the TGF latency binding protein, which will result in the liberation of TGF from a latent state (green protein: TGF latency binding protein). Thus increased MT1-MMP induction that occurs in pressure overload will cause increased liberation of TGF and binding to a transmembrane receptor complex, and ultimately the phosphorylation of receptor transduction elements, the Smad proteins. These ECM-dependent signaling events will cause increased expression of the fibrillar collagens, hence increased collagen accumulation as well as drive TGF-dependent fibroblast transformation/transdifferentiation. Therefore, while MMPs were historically considered to be monotonic in function (i.e., ECM degradation), specific MMP types can facilitate ECM accumulation and changes in fibroblast phenotype, which are both relevant processes in the progression of HFpEF. *For additional details on MT1-MMP and TGF activation, please see Spinale FG, Janicki JS, Zile MR: Membrane associated matrix proteolysis and heart failure. Circ Res 112(1):195–208, 2013.*[238]

overload, other MMP types, such as the interstitial collagenase MMP-13, have been reported to be decreased.[76,160] Other MMP types, such as MMP-1 and MMP-3, appear to be either unchanged or reduced with LV pressure overload.[†] Interestingly, transgenic expression of human MMP-1 in mice (this MMP type is absent in rodents) and induction of LV pressure overload resulted in a relative reduction in myocardial fibrillar collagen content and improved indices of LV function.[178] These findings suggest that the loss of normal constitutive levels of certain MMP types, or failure of an induction of certain MMP types with LV pressure overload, may facilitate abnormal ECM accumulation and adverse myocardial remodeling. This process does not occur in isolation and key matricellular proteins and signaling molecules, such as thrombospondin and osteopontin, are also likely to play a key role in abnormal ECM composition with LV pressure overload and progression to HFpEF. These determinants of ECM regulation with HFpEF are examined further in the context of diagnostic/prognostic potential.

MYOCARDIAL ECM REMODELING IN HEART FAILURE—DIAGNOSTIC POTENTIAL

Chapter 30 is dedicated to biomarker profiling in HF; accordingly, the focus herein will be to examine specific biomarkers that hold relevance to ECM remodeling with particular attention to those that hold diagnostic/prognostic potential. In terms of plasma biomarker profiling with HFrEF and a post-MI etiology, plasma troponin levels and other biomarkers are obviously relevant; thus, it is likely that a specific portfolio of ECM biomarkers will provide specific prognostic information in the post-MI period (**Table 4-2**). For example, past studies have demonstrated that increased plasma levels of collagen peptide fragments occur following MI and in progressive HFrEF.[151,179-181] In keeping with ECM degradation, induction of ECM proteases, such as the MMPs, occur in patients following MI and likely hold predictive value in terms of identifying those patients at greatest risk for the early development of HFrEF (**Figure 4-6**).[151,181-186] For example, the magnitude of plasma MMP-9 levels that occur within the early post-MI period is associated with a greater degree of LV dilation at 6 months post-MI.[183] In a study by Wagner and colleagues, the early increase in MMP-9 levels was associated with an increased risk of the later development of heart failure (odds ratio of 6.5).[182] In a recent report that compiled the results from approximately 60 studies in patients post-MI,[187] those that were most consistently present in prediction models included indices of neurohormonal activation, such as brain natriuretic peptide and indices of ECM degradation, such as MMP-9.[181] Cytokine/chemokine release that would cause the induction of pathways relevant to ECM degradation and fibroblast transformation, as well as the release of matrikines, all occur in patient in the post-MI period.[188-192] Other matrix-related molecules, such as galectin-3, have been associated with determinants of ECM

[†]References 76, 89, 152, 160, 170, 175-177.

TABLE 4-2 Plasma Profiles of Determinants of ECM Remodeling

	SUBJECTS *(N)*	BIOMARKER(S)	PRIMARY OBSERVATION	REFERENCE
Matrix Metabolism	233	PINP, ICTP, PIIINP, MMP-1, TIMP-1	Longitudinal changes in all ECM markers whereby ICTP associated with greater HF symptom progression	179
	1009	PIIINP, MMP-1, TIMP-1, hsCRP, IL-18, IL-10	Indices of increased ECM turnover associated with functional capacity and outcomes	180
	39	MMP-1, TIMP-1 and biopsy	Shift in MMP-1/TIMP-1 balance favoring ECM degradation as evidenced by ECM biopsy histology	151
	Meta-analysis (59 studies)	52 Biomarkers evaluated including determinants of ECM remodeling	Biomarkers most consistently associated with LV remodeling were involved in extracellular matrix turnover, such as collagen propeptides and telopeptides and MMP-9	181
Matrix Protease	109	MMP-2, MMP-9, hsCRP, TNF-α, pro-BNP	Higher plasma MMP-9 levels associated with HF progression	182
	85	Portfolio of MMPs and TIMPs serially examined	A specific cassette of MMPs are increased in plasma following MI and associated with progressive LV remodeling	183
	52	N-BNP, MMP-2, MMP-9	Up to 4 years of follow-up, plasma MMP-9 levels associated with magnitude of LV systolic failure	184
	100	TIMP-1, -2, -4	Early changes in plasma TIMP-4 levels associated with degree of LV dilation at 3 months post-MI	185
	404	TIMP-1, MMP-9, NTproBNP	Changes in MMP-9 associated with adverse post-MI remodeling as defined by LV dilation and TIMP-1 levels demonstrated predictive risk for combined event endpoint (HF/ death)	186

Plasma profiles of determinants of ECM remodeling have been examined in cohorts of patients with HFrEF or at risk for development of HFrEF. This is not intended to be a comprehensive list of studies that have used ECM biomarkers in the clinical context of HFrEF, but to illustrate potential prognostic relevance. In general, indices of ECM degradation/instability were associated with progression of HFrEF.

ECM, Extracellular matrix; *HF,* heart failure; *LV,* left ventricular; *MI,* myocardial infarction.

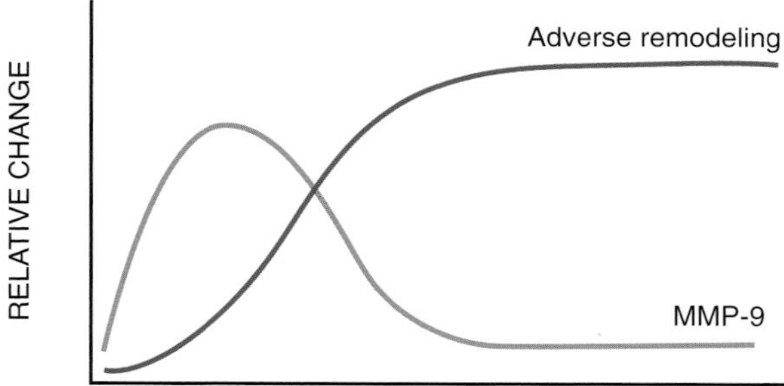

FIGURE 4-6 Significant changes in plasma profiles of MMPs and TIMPs have been reported in patients with ischemic heart disease and developing HFrEF (see Table 4-2) and have been shown to hold prognostic relevance. This schematic summarizes observations in patients following an MI in terms of early changes in MMP-9 levels to subsequent adverse LV remodeling, as defined by significant LV dilation. Early and robust changes in plasma MMP-9 levels (within 3 days of index event) are strongly associated with subsequent post-MI LV dilation at 3 to 6 months. *From Webb CS, Bonnema DD, Ahmed SH, et al: Specific temporal profile of matrix metalloproteinase release occurs in patients after myocardial infarction: relation to left ventricular remodeling. Circulation 114(10):1020–1027, 2006.*

remodeling but not necessarily independently predictive of HFrEF.[193-195] In addition to plasma biomarkers for ECM degradation, increased markers for ECM synthesis have also been identified, which include the TGF coreceptor endoglin and the matrikines tenascin-C, osteopontin, and syndecan-4.[196-201] In large survey studies that included subjects with MI and DCM, plasma levels of MMPs and TIMPs have provided clear prognostic information with respect to cardiovascular events and mortality.[202-205]

Because the ECM likely plays a critical role in the pathophysiology of HFpEF, strategies that can evaluate and quantify changes in this entity hold prognostic relevance. A summary of representative plasma biomarkers that have been evaluated in the context of HFpEF that may hold relevance to ECM remodeling is presented in **Table 4-3**. For example, plasma profiles of peptide fragments of fibrillar collagens (types I and III) have been used in patients with developing and established HFpEF.[‡] The collagen fibril may undergo post-translational modification by enzyme-mediated cross-link reactions as well as nonenzyme-mediated cross-link formation. Of note, nonenzymatic cross-link formation can be mediated by advanced glycation end products (AGEs).[207,208] AGEs bind to specific cell membrane receptors that include RAGE (receptor for AGE). Because increased fibrillar collagen stability can occur through increased RAGE interactions, profiling plasma levels of sRAGE, as well as indices of AGE formation, may hold prognostic/functional relevance in HFpEF.[207,208] A biologically relevant consequence of increased collagen AGEs is reduced susceptibility to MMP-mediated degradation and turnover. Significant and directional changes in the

[‡]References 152, 155, 157, 158, 187, 206.

TABLE 4-3 Plasma Profiles of Determinants of ECM Remodeling in Patients with HFpEF

	SUBJECTS (*N*)	BIOMARKER(S)	PRIMARY OBSERVATION	REFERENCE
Matrix Metabolism	156	MMP-1, TIMP-1, PINP	TIMP-1 levels were highest in patients with elevated PCWP, whereas relative MMP-1 levels were lower and PINP levels higher	155
	171	PICP, PINP, CITP, PIIINP, MMP-1, MMP-2, MMP-9; CTX, serum carboxy-terminal, amino-terminal	A combinatorial predictive model of collagen peptides and MMP-2 levels in patients with indices of worsening diastolic function	183, 184
	880	PICP, ICTP, PIIINP	PICP and ICTP elevated in elderly patients with HF	157
	153	PICP	Collagen I peptide associated with worsening diastolic function	192
	334	PINP, PIIINP, OPN	Stepped increases in procollagen and osteopontin caused incremental increases in the hazard ratio for cardiovascular events	206
	580	AGEs, sRAGE	Indices of AGEs, such as pentosidine and soluble receptor for AGE, increased in plasma in HFpEF and in univariate models associated with clinical outcomes	207
	880	PIP, CITP, PIIINP	CITP specifically associated with worsening HF and hospitalization in patients with HFpEF, but not HFrEF	157
	26	AGEs	Indices of increased AGEs associated with diastolic dysfunction	208
Matrix Protease	103	MMP-2,-9,-13, TIMP-1,-2	Patients with LV hypertrophy and HF demonstrated specific reductions in MMPs and increased TIMP-1.	239
	28	MMP-1	MMP-1 levels reduced in HFpEF	209
	120	TIMP-1	Elevated TIMP-1 associated with reduced early LV filling velocity	210

Plasma profiles of representative determinants of ECM remodeling in patients with HFpEF or at increased risk for HFpEF. This is not a comprehensive list of biomarkers that have been evaluated, but rather is provided to underscore dynamic changes in the balance of key determinants of ECM remodeling, which can be identified through plasma profiling in the context of developing HFpEF.

HF, Heart failure; *LV,* left ventricular; *PCWP,* pulmonary capillary wedge pressure.

plasma profiles of MMPs and TIMPs occur in patients with developing HFpEF and have been shown to hold potential prognostic utility.[76,177,209,210] For example, a specific cassette of MMPs and TIMPs, coupled with NT-BNP, provided significant prediction in terms of patients at risk for development of HFpEF.[177] Other ECM chemokines/matrikines, such as cardiotrophin, have been associated with the development and progression of HFpEF.[211,212]

Although plasma profiling changes in determinants of ECM structure and function likely hold diagnostic and prognostic relevance in terms of HF progression, advanced imaging approaches that target the ECM also will likely play an important role in providing mechanistic insight into this process as well. For example, in a translational imaging study using a labeled MMP radiotracer and hybrid single photon emission computed tomography/computed axial tomography imaging, areas of intense MMP activity could be identified in a post-MI pig model (**Figure 4-7**).[213] Another example of imaging that will likely hold insight into ECM remodeling is through the use of cardiac magnetic resonance imaging (cMRI) and gadolinium contrast.[214,215] Specifically, the use of cMRI delayed gadolinium uptake and T1 mapping has been used to quantify the ECM in patients, whereby the rate of ECM growth was directly associated with adverse outcomes.[215] An example of this cMRI approach in terms of ECM quantitation is shown in **Figure 4-8**. The use of multimodal imaging and advanced algorithms will likely yield important mechanistic insights into ECM remodeling and the progression of both HFrEF and HFpEF as the instrumentation and imaging agents improve.

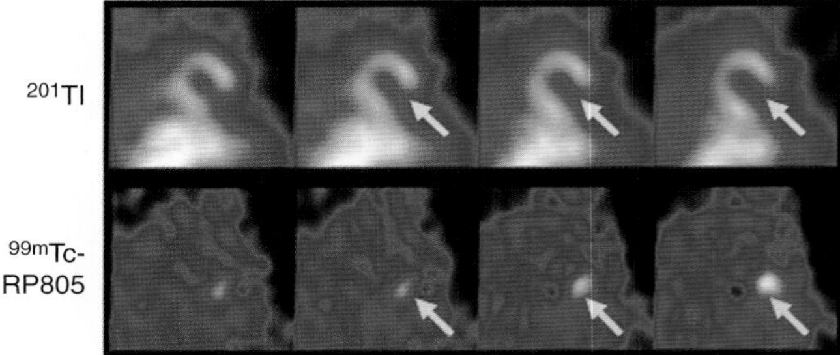

FIGURE 4-7 Molecular imaging approaches coupled with functional measurements will yield important diagnostic insights and identify potential therapeutic targets in HFrEF. In this example, dual-isotope SPECT/CT imaging was performed by injection of thallium (^{201}Tl) and an MMP radiotracer (^{99m}Tc-RP805) in a pig at 2 weeks post-MI. A clear perfusion defect at the site of the MI was evident *(top panel-arrow)* and coregistered with significant MMP radiotracer uptake-indicative of heightened MMP activity. *Modified from Sahul ZH, Mukherjee R, Song J, et al: Targeted imaging of the spatial and temporal variation of matrix metalloproteinase activity in a porcine model of postinfarct remodeling: relationship to myocardial dysfunction. Circ Cardiovasc Imaging 4(4):381–391, 2011.*

FUTURE DIRECTIONS

The ECM and Diagnostics

There is no question that biomarkers will play an ever greater role in identifying the relative risk, presence, and progression of ECM remodeling in both HFrEF and HFpEF. It is also clear that no single biomarker will be sufficient to provide critical insight into the complex ECM remodeling process. What remains to be established and defined is the optimal "cassette" of clinical variables and ECM biomarker measurements, which will provide useful and actionable

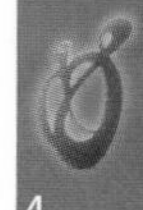

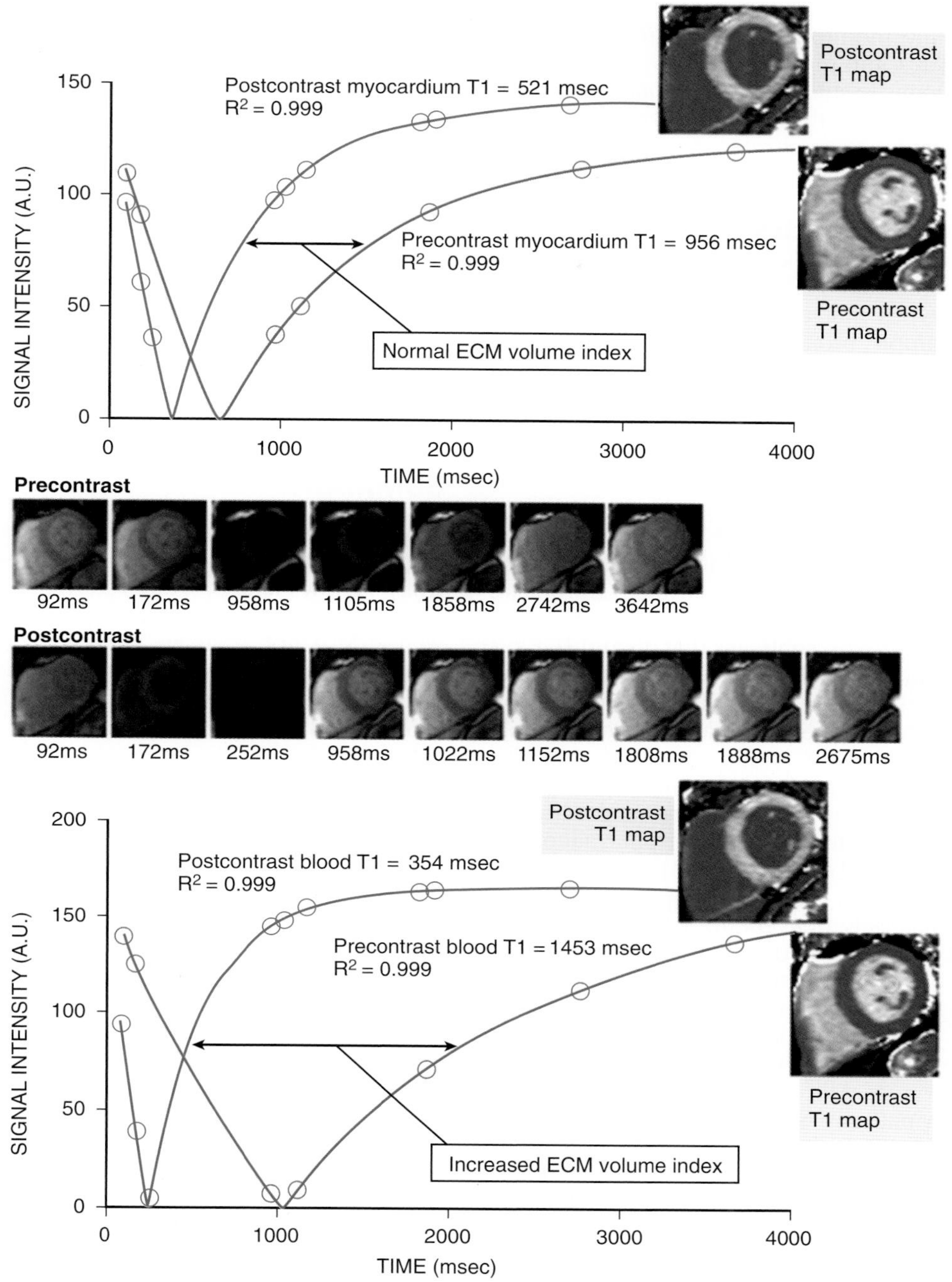

FIGURE 4-8 Cardiac MRI (cMRI) ECM quantitation. **A,** Representative computations for ECM volume index based upon cMRI and gadolinium contrast taken from a referent normal subject. The signal intensities for the myocardium and blood pool (time sequence images shown as thumbnails *[inset]*) were plotted against inversion time, and T1 curves of a region of interest are plotted whereby the shift in the T1 curves following motion and blood pool correction provided an ECM volume index. **B,** Using this approach, patients with increased ECM volume index could be identified, and in this example, an ECM volume index of approximately 23% was recognized. Using Cox regression models, it was demonstrated that increased ECM volume index was a significant risk factor for subsequent mortality, as well as major adverse events. *Adapted from Wong TC, Piehler K, Meier CG, et al: Association between extracellular matrix expansion quantified by cardiovascular magnetic resonance and short-term mortality. Circulation 126(10):1206–1216, 2012.*

predictive value in patients with a high risk for the development of HFrEF or HFpEF. It is most likely that a multimodality approach will be used that is both HF and temporally specific. Indeed, as outlined in previous sections of this chapter, there are important parallels between cancer and the underlying myocardial remodeling process in terms of fibroblast transformation/transdifferentiation and the use of biomarker signatures to define the aggressiveness and potential acceleration of the disease process. For example, the use of markers from several functional domains, such as neurohormonal pathways, indices of cell viability and phenotype, as well as determinants of ECM remodeling, will likely yield a specific cassette of biomarkers that will differentiate HFrEF and HFpEF and also allow "staging" of the underlying myocardial remodeling process. It is further likely that profiling ECM remodeling will entail measurements at the transcriptional, post-transcriptional, and post-translational levels. For example, there is possibly a cluster of miRs that regulate key ECM translational pathways, and profiling these across time would hold prognostic utility in

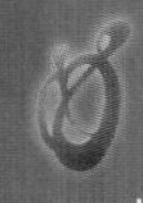

terms of identifying those patients at increased risk for HF, as well as potentially monitoring the progression of this disease process. Thus future translational research that couples basic mechanistic studies of miR function and specific ECM-related targets to that of peripheral profiles of miRs would certainly be of great relevance.

The ECM and Therapeutics

Targeting downstream mediators of ECM remodeling, such as the MMPs, has encountered difficulty in terms of targeting the specific MMP types that are causative in adverse LV remodeling. For example, broad spectrum MMP inhibition demonstrated favorable effects with short-term dosing in large animal models of MI and HFrEF,[142] but concerns regarding systemic toxicity of broad spectrum MMP inhibition and difficulties in dosing strategies yielded equivocal clinical results.[216] Nevertheless, since the role of MMP induction and activation in adverse post-MI remodeling is likely significant, the identification of the specific MMP types and selective MMP inhibitors will remain an important area for research and development. In terms of the activated fibroblasts within the MI region, this appears to be a TGF-dependent process,[122,138-140] and therefore, strategies that disrupt TGF signaling are likely to alter this fibroblast transdifferentiation process.[122,140,217-219] For example, as detailed previously and shown in Figure 4-4, membrane-bound MMPs likely contribute to the activation of TGF within the ECM, and this proteolytic-activation cascade may yield a number of potential targets.[122] In other studies, direct interference with TGF by genetic, neutralizing antibodies or oral pharmacologic inhibitors has demonstrated early favorable results in animal models of HFrEF.[217-220]

The use of biomaterials derived from the ECM or the mimic of a specific composite of the ECM have been the subject of a number of past translational studies with a particular focus upon post-MI remodeling and the progression to HFrEF.[221-227] The predominant approach has been to directly inject these ECM biomaterials into the MI region, whereby interruption of MI wall thinning and changes in local stress-strain patterns have been realized.[221,222,224-226] For example, a purified bovine collagen containing predominantly type I collagen increased LV wall thickness and relative function in a post-MI rat model.[221] Using a polyacrylamide-based hydrogel containing fibroblast growth factor, targeted injections within the MI region in rats improved LV pump function.[223] Initial clinical feasibility studies used injection of an ECM biomaterial seeded with bone marrow cells (MAGNUM trial) and demonstrated that relative MI thickness was augmented up to 1 year post injection.[228] Thus, ECM biomaterials alone or as an adjunctive approach to local pharmacologic or cell-based therapies in the context of post-MI remodeling hold potential therapeutic relevance in the context of developing HFrEF.

Since inappropriate ECM accumulation and structure is a milestone in the progression to HFpEF, strategies that target fibroblast form and function, such as fibroblast transdifferentiation and TGF interference strategies, would be of significance. In addition, directly altering the structure of the ECM with HFpEF will in turn alter LV myocardial stiffness properties and LV diastolic function. Indeed, the changes in fibrillar collagen peptide fragments, indicative of post-translational processing, can be quite dynamic in patients with HFpEF and can be affected by pharmacologic strategies, such as aldosterone receptor antagonists.[229] Another example of the importance of post-translational processing of fibrillar collagen in the context of HFpEF is collagen cross-linking.[230-232] Specifically, the glucose cross-link breaker ALT-711 reduced myocardial stiffness associated with LV hypertrophy. Interestingly, these beneficial effects of this cross-link breaker were not observed in patients with HFrEF.[232] These observations underscore the difference in ECM remodeling between these two HF processes. Moreover, these studies underscore the importance of post-translational steps in the maturation of the collagen fibrillar network in terms of therapeutic targets. Some examples of matricellular proteins that likely play regulatory roles in ECM structure and function, and may hold therapeutic relevance, include SPARC, thrombospondin, osteopontin, and periostin.[122,140,144,217,233-235]

SUMMARY

From the first report of the importance of collagenase by Gross and colleagues[236] regarding the resorption of a tadpole tail, it is now clearly recognized that ECM remodeling plays a critical role in tissue structure and function. The myocardial ECM is not a passive entity, but rather a complex and dynamic microenvironment that represents an important structural and signaling system within the myocardium. Since the last revision of this book chapter, remarkable advancements have been made into our basic understanding and mechanistic role of nonstructural ECM proteins, how the ECM serves as a reservoir for bioactive signaling molecules and miRs, and the interaction of proteolytic enzymes and ECM growth regulation. More importantly, significant advancements have been made in the use of ECM profiling for the purposes of prognosis in both HFrEF and HFpEF. Future translational and clinical research focused upon the molecular and cellular mechanisms that regulate ECM structure and function will likely contribute to an improved understanding of the LV remodeling process in both of these forms of HF, as well as yield important diagnostic and therapeutic targets.

Acknowledgments

Dr. Francis Spinale is supported by the Research Service of the Department of Veterans Affairs. The author wishes to recognize the significant contributions of past MUSC and USC medical and graduate students that participated in our cardiovascular research program over the past two decades. The author wishes to acknowledge Kaelyn Hawkins, Medical University of South Carolina, for constructing the inset of Figure 4-4, as well as Shaun Riffle, USC School of Medicine, for constructing the lower panels of Figure 4-1. The author is grateful to Ashley Sapp, USC School of Medicine, for editorial assistance.

References

1. Ho JE, Gona P, Pencina MJ, et al: Discriminating clinical features of heart failure with preserved vs. reduced ejection fraction in the community. *Eur Heart J* 33(14):1734–1741, 2012.
2. Anderson JL, Adams CD, Antman EM, et al: 2011 ACCF/AHA Focused Update Incorporated Into the ACC/AHA 2007 Guidelines for the Management of Patients With Unstable Angina/Non-ST-Elevation Myocardial Infarction: a report of the American College of Cardiology Foundation/American Heart Association Task Force on Practice Guidelines. *Circulation* 123(18):e426–e579, 2011.
3. Quiñones MA, Greenberg BH, Kopelen HA, et al: Echocardiographic predictors of clinical outcome in patients with left ventricular dysfunction enrolled in the SOLVD registry and trials: significance of left ventricular hypertrophy. Studies of Left Ventricular Dysfunction. *J Am Coll Cardiol* 35(5):1237–1244, 2000.
4. Heart Failure Society of America, Lindenfeld J, Albert NM, et al: HFSA 2010 Executive Summary. *J Card Fail* 16:475–539, 2010.

5. Heart Failure Society of America, Lindenfeld J, Albert NM, et al: HFSA 2010 Comprehensive Heart Failure Practice Guideline. *J Card Fail* 16(6):e1–e194, 2010.
6. Konstam MA, Kramer DG, Patel AR, et al: Left ventricular remodeling in heart failure: current concepts in clinical significance and assessment. *JACC Cardiovasc Imaging.* 4(1):98–108, 2011.
7. Zile MR, Gaasch WH, Anand IS, et al: Mode of death in patients with heart failure and a preserved ejection fraction: results from the Irbesartan in Heart Failure With Preserved Ejection Fraction Study (I-Preserve) trial. *Circulation.* 121(12):1393–1405, 2010.
8. Ahmed A, Rich MW, Fleg JL, et al: Effects of digoxin on morbidity and mortality in diastolic heart failure: the ancillary digitalis investigation group trial. *Circulation* 114:397–403, 2006.
9. Ahmed A, Zile MR, Rich MW, et al: Hospitalizations due to unstable angina pectoris in diastolic and systolic heart failure. *Am J Cardiol* 99:460–464, 2007.
10. Alagiakrishnan K, Banach M, Jones LG, et al: Update on diastolic heart failure or heart failure with preserved ejection fraction in the older adults. *Ann Med* 45(1):37–50, 2013.
11. Ather S, Chan W, Bozkurt B, et al: Impact of noncardiac comorbidities on morbidity and mortality in a predominantly male population with heart failure and preserved versus reduced ejection fraction. *J Am Coll Cardiol* 59(11):998–1005, 2012.
12. Schwartzenberg S, Redfield MM, From AM, et al: Effects of vasodilation in heart failure with preserved or reduced ejection fraction implications of distinct pathophysiologies on response to therapy. *J Am Coll Cardiol* 59(5):442–451, 2012.
13. Weir RA, McMurray JJ, Velazquez EJ: Epidemiology of heart failure and left ventricular systolic dysfunction after acute myocardial infarction: prevalence, clinical characteristics, and prognostic importance. *Am J Cardiol* 97(10A):13F–25F, 2006.
14. Kopecky SL, Gersh BJ: Dilated cardiomyopathy and myocarditis: natural history, etiology, clinical manifestations, and management. *Curr Probl Cardiol* 12(10):569–647, 1987.
15. Rodeheffer RJ: The new epidemiology of heart failure. *Curr Cardiol Rep* 5(3):181–186, 2003.
16. Greenberg B, Quinones MA, Koilpillai C, et al: Effects of long-term enalapril therapy on cardiac structure and function in patients with left ventricular dysfunction. Results of the SOLVD echocardiography substudy. *Circulation* 91(10):2573–2581, 1995.
17. Borlaug BA, Paulus WJ: Heart failure with preserved ejection fraction: pathophysiology, diagnosis, and treatment. *Eur Heart J* 32(6):670–679, 2011.
18. Spinale FG, Mukherjee R, Zavadzkas JA, et al: Cardiac restricted over-expression of membrane type-1 matrix metalloproteinase in mice: effects on myocardial remodeling following myocardial infarction. *J Biol Chem* 285(39):30316–30327, 2010.
19. Spinale FG, Escobar GP, Mukherjee R, et al: Cardiac restricted over-expression of membrane type-1 matrix metalloproteinase in mice: effects on myocardial remodeling with aging. *Circulation Heart Failure* 2(4):351–360, 2009.
20. Mukherjee R, Brinsa TA, Dowdy KB, et al: Myocardial infarct expansion and matrix metalloproteinase inhibition. *Circulation* 107(4):618–625, 2003.
21. King MK, Coker ML, Goldberg A, et al: Selective matrix metalloproteinase inhibition with developing heart failure: effects on left ventricular function and structure. *Circ Res* 92(2):177–185, 2003.
22. Wilson EM, Moainie SL: Region and species specific induction of matrix metalloproteinases occurs with post-myocardial infarction remodeling. *Circ* 107(22):2857–2863, 2003.
23. Burlew BS, Weber KT: Connective tissue and the heart, functional significance and regulatory mechanisms. *Cardiol Clin* 18(3):435–442, 2000.
24. Weber KT, Pick R, Janicki JS, et al: Inadequate collagen tethers in dilated cardiomyopathy. *Am Heart J* 116:1641–1646, 1988.
25. Cluetjens JPM, Verluyten MJA, Smits JFM, et al: Collagen remodeling after myocardial infarction in the rat heart. *Am J Pathol* 147(2):325–338, 1995.
26. Spinale FG: Matrix remodeling and the matrix metalloproteinases: influence on cardiac form and function. *Physiol Rev* 87(4):1285–1342, 2007.
27. Chapman RE, Spinale FG: Extracellular protease activation and unraveling of the myocardial interstitium: critical steps toward clinical applications. *Am J Physiol* 286(1):H1–H10, 2004.
28. Thomas CV, Coker ML, Zellner JL, et al: Increased matrix metalloproteinase activity and selective upregulation in LV myocardium from patients with end-stage dilated cardiomyopathy. *Circulation* 97:1708–1715, 1998.
29. Spinale FG, Coker ML, Heung LJ, et al: A matrix metalloproteinase induction/activation system exists in the human left ventricular myocardium and is upregulated in heart failure. *Circulation* 102:1944–1949, 2000.
30. Gunja-Smith Z, Morales AR, Romanelli R, et al: Remodeling of human myocardial collagen in idiopathic dilated cardiomyopathy: role of metalloproteinases and pyridinoline cross links. *Am J Pathol* 148:1639–1648, 1996.
31. Li YY, Feldman AM, Sun Y, et al: Differential expression of tissue inhibitors of metalloproteinases in the failing human heart. *Circulation* 98:1728–1734, 1998.
32. Spinale FG, Coker ML, Thomas CV, et al: Time dependent changes in matrix metalloproteinase activity and expression during the progression of congestive heart failure: relation to ventricular and myocyte function. *Circ Res* 82:482–495, 1998.
33. Spinale FG, Krombach RS, Coker ML, et al: Matrix metalloproteinase inhibition during developing congestive heart failure in pigs: effects on left ventricular geometry and function. *Circ Res* 85:364–376, 1999.
34. Rohde LE, Ducharme A, Arroyo LH, et al: Matrix metalloproteinase inhibition attenuates early left ventricular enlargement after experimental myocardial infarction in mice. *Circulation* 99:3063–3070, 1999.
35. Creemers E, Davis JN, Parkhurst AM, et al: Deficiency of the tissue inhibitor of matrix metalloproteinase-1 gene exacerbates LV remodeling following myocardial infarction in mice. *Am J Physiol* 284(1):H364–H371, 2003.
36. Coker ML, Thomas CV, Clair MJ, et al: Myocardial matrix metalloproteinase activity and abundance with congestive heart failure. *Am J Physiol* 274(43):H1516–H1523, 1998.
37. Matsumura S, Iwanaga S, Mochizuki S, et al: Targeted deletion or pharmacological inhibition of MMP-2 prevents cardiac rupture after myocardial infarction in mice. *J Clin Invest* 115(3):599–609, 2005.
38. Heymans S, Luttun A, Nuyens D, et al: Inhibition of plasminogen activators or matrix metalloproteinases prevents cardiac rupture but impairs therapeutic angiogenesis and causes cardiac failure. *Nat Med* 5:1135–1142, 1999.
39. Ducharme A, Frantz S, Aikawa M, et al: Targeted deletion of matrix metalloproteinase-9 attenuates left ventricular enlargement and collagen accumulation after experimental myocardial infarction. *J Clin Invest* 106:55–62, 2000.
40. Peterson JT, Hallak H, Johnson L, et al: Matrix metalloproteinase inhibition attenuates left ventricular remodeling and dysfunction in a rat model of progressive heart failure. *Circulation* 103:2303–2309, 2001.
41. Li YY, Feng Y, McTiernan CF, et al: Downregulation of matrix metalloproteinases and reduction in collagen damage in the failing human heart after support with left ventricular assist devices. *Circulation* 104:1147–1152, 2001.
42. Kim HE, Dalal SS, Young E, et al: Disruption of the myocardial extracellular matrix leads to cardiac dysfunction. *J Clin Invest* 106:857–866, 2000.
43. Mecham RP, Heuser J: Three-dimensional organization of extracellular matrix in elastic cartilage as viewed by quick freeze, deep etch electron microscopy. *Connect Tissue Res* 24(2):83–93, 1990.
44. Deschamps AM, Apple KA, Hardin AE, et al: Myocardial interstitial matrix metalloproteinase activity is altered by mechanical changes in LV load: interaction with the angiotensin type 1 receptor. *Circ Res* 96(10):1110–1118, 2005.
45. Ross RS, Borg TK: Integrins and the myocardium. *Circ Res* 88(11):1112–1119, 8, 2001.
46. Stroud JD, Baicu CF, Barnes MA, et al: Viscoelastic properties of pressure overload hypertrophied myocardium: effects of treatment with a serine protease treatment. *Am J Physiol Heart Circ Physiol* 282(6):H232–H235, 2002.
47. Keller RS, Shai SY, Babbitt CJ, et al: Disruption of integrin function in the murine myocardium leads to perinatal lethality, fibrosis, and abnormal cardiac performance. *Am J Pathol* 158:1079–1090, 2001.
48. Hornberger LK, Singhroy S, Cavalle-Garrido T, et al: Synthesis of extracellular matrix and adhesion through beta(1) integrins are critical for fetal ventricular myocyte proliferation. *Circ Res* 87:508–515, 2000.
49. Spinale FG, Tomita M, Zellner JL, et al: Collagen remodeling and changes in LV function during the development and recovery from supraventricular tachycardia. *Am J Physiol* 261:H308–H318, 1991.
50. Nimni ME: Fibrillar collagens: their biosynthesis, molecular structure, and mode of assembly. In Zern MA, Reid LM, editors: *Extracellular matrix*, New York, 1993, Marcel Dekker.
51. Asif M, Egan J, Vasan S, et al: An advanced glycation endproduct cross-link breaker can reverse age related increases in myocardial stiffness. *Proc Natl Acad Sci U S A* 97(6):2809–2813, 2000.
52. Kato S, Spinale FG, Tanaka R, et al: Inhibition of collagen cross-linking: effects on fibrillar collagen and left ventricular diastolic function. *Am J Physiol* 269(38):H863–H868, 1995.
53. Cooper ME: Importance of advanced glycation end products in diabetes-associated cardiovascular and renal disease. *Am J Hypertens* 17(12 Pt 2):31S–38S, 2004.
54. Schuppan D: Connective tissue polypeptides in serum as parameters to monitor antifibrotic treatment in hepatic fibrogenesis. *J Hepatol* 13(Suppl 3):S17–S25, 1991.
55. Erlebacher JA, Weiss JL, Weisfeldt JL, et al: Early dilation of the infarcted segment in acute transmural myocardial infarction: role of infarct expansion in acute left ventricular enlargement. *J Am Coll Cardiol* 4(2):201–208, 1984.
56. Diez J, Laviades C: Monitoring fibrillar collagen turnover in hypertensive heart disease. *Cardiovasc Res* 35:202–205, 1997.
57. Diez J, Panizo A, Gil MJ, et al: Serum markers of collagen type I metabolism in spontaneously hypertensive rats. Relation to myocardial fibrosis. *Circulation* 93:1026–1032, 1996.
58. Diez J, Laviades C, Mayor G, et al: Increased serum concentrations of procollagen peptides in essential hypertension. Relation to cardiac alterations. *Circulation* 91:1450–1456, 1995.
59. Borg TK, Goldsmith EC, Price R, et al: Specialization of the Z line of cardiac myocytes. *Cardiovasc Res* 46:277–285, 2000.
60. Pham CG, Harpf AE, Keller RS, et al: Striated muscle specific beta(1D) integrin and FAK are involved in cardiac myocyte hypertrophic response pathway. *Am J Physiol* 279(6):H2916–H2926, 2000.
61. Kuettner KE, Kimuar JH: Proteoglycans: an overview. *J Cell Biochem* 27:327–336, 1985.
62. Sivasubramanian N, Coker ML, Kurrelmeyer KM, et al: Left ventricular remodeling in transgenic mice with cardiac restricted overexpression of tumor necrosis factor. *Circulation* 104(7):826–831, 2001.
63. Bradham WS, Bozkurt B, Gunasinghe H, et al: Tumor necrosis factor-alpha and myocardial remodeling in progression of heart failure: a current perspective. *Cardiovasc Res* 53(4):822–830, 2002.
64. Fowlkes JL, Winkler MK: Exploring the interface between metalloproteinase activity and growth factor and cytokine bioavailability. *Cytokine Growth Factor Rev* 13(3):277–287, 2002.
65. Annes JP, Munger JS, Rifkin DB: Making sense of latent TGFbeta activation. *J Cell Sci* 116(Pt 2):217–224, 2003.
66. Isogai Z, Ono RN, Ushiro S, et al: Latent transforming growth factor beta-binding protein 1 interacts with fibrillin and is a microfibril-associated protein. *J Biol Chem* 278(4):2750–2757, 2003.
67. Rifkin DB: Latent transforming growth factor-beta (TGF-beta) binding proteins: orchestrators of TGF-beta availability. *J Biol Chem* 280(9):7409–7412, 2005.
68. Bobik A: Transforming growth factor-betas and vascular disorders. *Arterioscler Thromb Vasc Biol* 26(8):1712–1720, 2006.
69. Roberts AB, Sporn MB, Assoian RK, et al: Transforming growth factor type beta: rapid induction of fibrosis and angiogenesis in vivo and stimulation of collagen formation in vitro. *Proc Natl Acad Sci U S A* 83(12):4167–4171, 1986.
70. Leask A, Abraham DJ: TGF-beta signaling and the fibrotic response. *FASEB J* 18(7):816–827, 2004.
71. Järvinen PM, Laiho M: LIM-domain proteins in transforming growth factor β-induced epithelial-to-mesenchymal transition and myofibroblast differentiation. *Cell Signal* 24(4):819–825, 2012.
72. Li J, Bertram JF: Review: Endothelial-myofibroblast transition, a new player in diabetic renal fibrosis. *Nephrology (Carlton)* 15(5):507–512, 2010.
73. Krenning G, Zeisberg EM, Kalluri R: The origin of fibroblasts and mechanism of cardiac fibrosis. *J Cell Physiol* 225(3):631–637, 2010.
74. Goumans MJ, van Zonneveld AJ, ten Dijke P: Transforming growth factor beta-induced endothelial-to-mesenchymal transition: a switch to cardiac fibrosis? *Trends Cardiovasc Med* 18(8):293–298, 2008.
75. Lindsey ML, Escobar GP, Wawrzyniec L, et al: Matrix metalloproteinase-9 gene deletion facilitates angiogenesis following myocardial infarction. *Am J Physiol* 290:232–239, 2006.
76. Ahmed SH, Clark LL, Pennington WR, et al: Matrix metalloproteinases/tissue inhibitors of metalloproteinases: relationship between changes in proteolytic determinants of matrix composition and structural, functional & clinical manifestations of hypertensive heart disease. *Circulation* 113(17):2089–2096, 2006.
77. Dixon JA, Spinale FG: Myocardial remodeling: cellular and extracellular events and targets. *Annu Rev Physiol* 73:47–68, 2011.
78. Turner NA, Porter KE: Regulation of myocardial matrix metalloproteinase expression and activity by cardiac fibroblasts. *IUBMB Life* 64(2):143–150, 2012.
79. Stetler-Stevenson WG: The tumor microenvironment: regulation by MMP-independent effects of tissue inhibitor of metalloproteinases-2. *Cancer Metastasis Rev* 27(1):57–66, 2008.
80. Catania JM, Chen G, Parrish AR: Role of matrix metalloproteinases in renal pathophysiologies. *Am J Physiol Renal Physiol* 292(3):F905–F911, 2007.
81. Verstappen J, Von den Hoff JW: Tissue inhibitors of metalloproteinases (TIMPs): their biological functions and involvement in oral disease. *J Dent Res* 85(12):1074–1084, 2006.
82. Varghese S: Matrix metalloproteinases and their inhibitors in bone: an overview of regulation and functions. *Front Biosci* 11:2949–2966, 2006.
83. Nagase H, Visse R, Murphy G: Structure and function of matrix metalloproteinases and TIMPs. *Cardiovasc Res* 69(3):562–573, 2006.
84. Malemud CJ: Matrix metalloproteinases (MMPs) in health and disease: an overview. *Front Biosci* 11:1696–1701, 2006.
85. Hwang IK, Park SM, Kim SY, et al: A proteomic approach to identify substrates of matrix metalloproteinase-14 in human plasma. *Biochim Biophys Acta* 1702:79–87, 2004.
86. Overall CM, Tam EM, Kappelhoff R, et al: Protease degradomics: mass spectrometry discovery of protease substrates and the CLIP-CHIP, a dedicated DNA microarray of all human proteases and inhibitors. *Biol Chem* 385:493–504, 2004.
87. Woessner JF, Jr, Nagase H: Protein substrates of the MMPs. In *Matrix metalloproteinases and TIMPs*, New York, 2000, Oxford University Press.
88. Spinale FG, Koval CN, Deschamps AM, et al: Dynamic changes in matrix metalloproteinase activity within the human myocardial interstitium during ischemia reperfusion. *Circulation* 118:S16–S23, 2008. PMCID: PMC2663795.
89. Woessner JF, Jr, Nagase H: Activation of the zymogen forms of MMPs. In *Matrix metalloproteinases and TIMPs*, New York, 2000, Oxford University Press.

90. Vincenti MP: The matrix metalloproteinase (MMP) and tissue inhibitor of metalloproteinase (TIMP) genes. In Clark I, editor: *Matrix metalloproteinase protocols*, Totowa, NJ, 2001, Humana Press.
91. Vincenti MP, Brinckerhoff CE: Transcriptional regulation of collagenase (MMP-1, MMP-13) genes in arthritis: integration of complex signaling pathways for the recruitment of gene-specific transcription factors. *Arthritis Res* 4:157–164, 2002.
92. Bergman MR, Cheng S, Honbo N, et al: A functional activating protein 1 (AP-1) site regulates matrix metalloproteinase 2 (MMP-2) transcription by cardiac cells through interactions with JunB-Fra1 and JunB-FosB heterodimers. *Biochem J* 369:485–496, 2003.
93. Siwik DA, Chang DL, Colucci WS: Interleukin-1beta and tumor necrosis factor-alpha decrease collagen synthesis and increase matrix metalloproteinase activity in cardiac fibroblasts in vitro. *Circ Res* 86:1259–1265, 2000.
94. Rangaswami H, Bulbule A, Kundu GC: Nuclear factor-inducing kinase plays a crucial role in osteopontin-induced MAPK/IkappaBalpha kinase-dependent nuclear factor kappaB-mediated promatrix metalloproteinase-9 activation. *J Biol Chem* 279:38921–38935, 2004.
95. Alfonso-Jaume MA, Bergman MR, Mahimkar R, et al: Cardiac ischemia-reperfusion injury induces matrix metalloproteinase-2 expression through the AP-1 components FosB and JunB. *Am J Physiol Heart Circ Physiol* 291(4):H1838–H1846, 2006.
96. Mukherjee R, Mingoia JT, Bruce JA, et al: Selective spatiotemporal induction of matrix metalloproteinase-2 and matrix metalloproteinase-9 transcription after myocardial infarction. *Am J Physiol Heart Circ Physiol* 291(5):H2216–H2228, 2006.
97. Mishra A, Srivastava A, Mittal T, et al: Association of matrix metalloproteinases (MMP2, MMP7 and MMP9) genetic variants with left ventricular dysfunction in coronary artery disease patients. *Clin Chim Acta* 413(19–20):1668–1674, 2012.
98. Wang J, Xu D, Wu X, et al: Polymorphisms of matrix metalloproteinases in myocardial infarction: a meta-analysis. *Heart* 97(19):1542–1546, 2011.
99. Tanner RM, Lynch AI, Brophy VH, et al: Pharmacogenetic associations of MMP9 and MMP12 variants with cardiovascular disease in patients with hypertension. *PLoS ONE* 6(8):e23609, 2011.
100. Velho FM, Cohen CR, Santos KG, et al: Polymorphisms of matrix metalloproteinases in systolic heart failure: role on disease susceptibility, phenotypic characteristics, and prognosis. *J Card Fail* 17(2):115–121, 2011.
101. Horne BD, Camp NJ, Carlquist JF, et al: Multiple-polymorphism associations of 7 matrix metalloproteinase and tissue inhibitor metalloproteinase genes with myocardial infarction and angiographic coronary artery disease. *Am Heart J* 154(4):751–758, 2007.
102. Blankenberg S, Rupprecht HJ, Poirier O, et al: Plasma concentrations and genetic variation of matrix metalloproteinase 9 and prognosis of patients with cardiovascular disease. *Circulation* 107:1579–1585, 2003.
103. Zhang B, Ye S, Herrmann SM, et al: Functional polymorphism in the regulatory region of gelatinase B gene in relation to severity of coronary atherosclerosis. *Circulation* 99(14):1788–1794, 1999.
104. Mizon-Gérard F, de Groote P, Lamblin N, et al: Prognostic impact of matrix metalloproteinase gene polymorphisms in patients with heart failure according to the aetiology of left ventricular systolic dysfunction. *Eur Heart J* 25(8):688–693, 2004.
105. Liu PY, Chen JH, Li YH, et al: Synergistic effect of stromelysin-1 (matrix metallo-proteinase-3) promoter 5A/6A polymorphism with smoking on the onset of young acute myocardial infarction. *Thromb Haemost* 90:132–139, 2003.
106. Terashima M, Akita H, Kanazawa K, et al: Stromelysin promoter 5A/6A polymorphism is associated with acute myocardial infarction. *Circulation* 99(21):2717–2719, 1999.
107. Yamada Y, Ohno Y, Nakashima Y, et al: Prediction and assessment of extrapyramidal side effects induced by risperidone based on dopamine D(2) receptor occupancy. *Synapse* 46(1):32–37, 2002.
108. Beyzade S, Zhang S, Wong YK, et al: Influences of matrix metalloproteinase-3 gene variation on extent of coronary atherosclerosis and risk of myocardial infarction. *J Am Coll Cardiol* 41:2130–2137, 2003.
109. Hirashiki A, Yamada Y, Murase Y, et al: Association of gene polymorphisms with coronary artery disease in low- or high-risk subjects defined by conventional risk factors. *J Am Coll Cardiol* 42(8):1429–1437, 2003.
110. Nojiri T, Morita H, Imai Y, et al: Genetic variations of matrix metalloproteinase-1 and -3 promoter regions and their associations with susceptibility to myocardial infarction in Japanese. *Int J Cardiol* 92(2–3):181–186, 2003.
111. Martin TN, Penney DE, Smith JA, et al: Matrix metalloproteinase-1 promoter polymorphisms and changes in left ventricular volume following acute myocardial infarction. *Am J Cardiol* 94(8):1044–1046, 2004.
112. van Rooij E, Sutherland LB, Thatcher JE, et al: Dysregulation of microRNAs after myocardial infarction reveals a role of miR-29 in cardiac fibrosis. *Proc Natl Acad Sci U S A* 105(35):13027–13032, 2008.
113. Mittelbrunn M, Sánchez-Madrid F: Intercellular communication: diverse structures for exchange of genetic information. *Nat Rev Mol Cell Biol* 13(5):328–335, 2012.
114. Zile MR, Mehurg SM, Arroyo JE, et al: Relationship between the temporal profile of plasma microRNA and left ventricular remodeling in patients after myocardial infarction. *Circ Cardiovasc Genet.* 4(6):614–619, 2011.
115. Sato H, Takino T, Okada Y, et al: A matrix metalloproteinase expressed on the surface of invasive tumour cells. *Nature* 370:61–65, 1994.
116. Osenkowski P, Toth M, Fridman R: Processing, shedding, and endocytosis of membrane type 1-matrix metalloproteinase (MT1-MMP). *J Cell Physiol* 200:2–10, 2004.
117. Lehti K, Valtanen H, Wickstrom SA, et al: Regulation of membrane-type-1 matrix metalloproteinase activity by its cytoplasmic domain. *J Biol Chem* 275:15006–15013, 2000.
118. Remacle AG, Rozanov DV, Baciu PC, et al: The transmembrane domain is essential for the microtubular trafficking of membrane type-1 matrix metalloproteinase (MT1-MMP). *J Cell Sci* 118:4975–4984, 2005.
119. Pavlaki M, Cao J, Hymowitz M, et al: A conserved sequence within the propeptide domain of membrane type 1 matrix metalloproteinase is critical for function as an intramolecular chaperone. *J Biol Chem* 277:2740–2749, 2002.
120. Guo C, Piacentini L: Type I collagen-induced MMP-2 activation coincides with up-regulation of membrane type 1-matrix metalloproteinase and TIMP-2 in cardiac fibroblasts. *J Biol Chem* 278:46699–46708, 2003.
121. Stawowy P, Meyborg H, Stibenz D, et al: Furin-like proprotein convertases are central regulators of the membrane type matrix metalloproteinase-pro-matrix metalloproteinase-2 proteolytic cascade in atherosclerosis. *Circulation* 111:2820–2827, 2005.
122. Spinale FG, Janicki JS, Zile MR: Membrane-associated matrix proteolysis and heart failure. *Circ Res* 112(1):195–208, 2013.
123. Deschamps AM, Yarbrough WM, Squires CE, et al: Trafficking of the membrane type-1 matrix metalloproteinase (MT1-MMP) in ischemia and reperfusion: relation to interstitial MT1-MMP activity. *Circulation* 111(9):1166–1174, 2005.
124. Yarbrough WM, Mukherjee R, Escobar GP, et al: Selective targeting and timing of matrix metalloproteinase inhibition in post-myocardial infarction remodeling. *Circulation* 108:1753–1759, 2003.
125. Greene J, Wang M, Liu YE, et al: Molecular cloning and characterization of human tissue inhibitor of metalloproteinase 4. *J Biol Chem* 271:30375–30380, 1996.
126. Liu YE, Wang M, Greene J, et al: Preparation and characterization of recombinant tissue inhibitor of metalloproteinase 4 (TIMP-4). *J Biol Chem* 272:20479–20483, 1997.
127. Tummalapalli CM, Heath BJ, Tyagi SC: Tissue inhibitor of metalloproteinase-4 instigates apoptosis in transformed cardiac fibroblasts. *J Cell Biochem* 80:512–521, 2001.
128. Lovelock JD, Baker AH, Gao F, et al: Heterogeneous effects of tissue inhibitors of matrix metalloproteinases on cardiac fibroblasts. *Am J Physiol Heart Circ Physiol* 288:H461–H468, 2005.
129. Oelmann E, Herbst H, Zuhlsdorf M, et al: Tissue inhibitor of metalloproteinases 1 is an autocrine and paracrine survival factor, with additional immune-regulatory functions, expressed by Hodgkin/Reed-Sternberg cells. *Blood* 99:258–267, 2002.
130. Guedez L, Stetler-Stevenson WG, Wolff L, et al: In vitro suppression of programmed cell death of B cells by tissue inhibitor of metalloproteinases-1. *J Clin Invest* 102:2002–2010, 1998.
131. Fedak PW, Smookler DS, Kassiri Z, et al: TIMP-3 deficiency leads to dilated cardiomyopathy. *Circulation* 110(16):2401–2409, 2004.
132. Kassiri Z, Oudit GY, Sanchez O, et al: Combination of tumor necrosis factor-alpha ablation and matrix metalloproteinase inhibition prevents heart failure after pressure overload in tissue inhibitor of metalloproteinase-3 knock-out mice. *Circ Res* 97(4):380–390, 2005.
133. Anzai A, Anzai T, Nagai S, et al: Regulatory role of dendritic cells in postinfarction healing and left ventricular remodeling. *Circulation* 125(10):1234–1245, 2012.
134. Dixon JA, Gorman RC, Stroud RE, et al: Mesenchymal cell transplantation and myocardial remodeling after myocardial infarction. *Circulation* 120(11 Suppl):S220–S229, 2009.
135. Frangogiannis NG: Regulation of the inflammatory response in cardiac repair. *Circ Res* 110(1):159–173, 2012.
136. Freytes DO, Kang JW, Marcos-Campos I, et al: Macrophages modulate the viability and growth of human mesenchymal stem cells. *J Cell Biochem* 114(1):220–229, 2013.
137. Ma Y, Halade GV, Zhang J, et al: Matrix metalloproteinase-28 deletion exacerbates cardiac dysfunction and rupture after myocardial infarction in mice by inhibiting m2 macrophage activation. *Circ Res* 112(4):675–688, 2013.
138. Baum J, Duffy HS: Fibroblasts and myofibroblasts: what are we talking about? *J Cardiovasc Pharmacol* 57(4):376–379, 2011.
139. Tomasek JJ, Gabbiani G, Hinz B, et al: Myofibroblasts and mechano-regulation of connective tissue remodelling. *Nat Rev Mol Cell Biol* 3(5):349–363, 2002.
140. Goldsmith EC, Bradshaw AD, Spinale FG: Contributory pathways leading to myocardial fibrosis: moving beyond collagen expression. *Am J Physiol Cell Physiol* 304(5):C393–C402, 2013.
141. Kassiri Z, Defamie V, Hariri M, et al: Simultaneous transforming growth factor beta-tumor necrosis factor activation and cross-talk cause aberrant remodeling response and myocardial fibrosis in Timp3-deficient heart. *J Biol Chem* 284(43):29893–29904, 2009.
142. Spinale FG: Myocardial matrix remodeling and the matrix metalloproteinases: influence on cardiac form and function. *Physiol Rev* 87(4):1285–1342, 2007.
143. Doetschman T, Barnett JV, Runyan RB, et al: Transforming growth factor beta signaling in adult cardiovascular diseases and repair. *Cell Tissue Res* 347(1):203–223, 2012.
144. Schellings MW, Vanhoutte D, Swinnen M, et al: Absence of SPARC results in increased cardiac rupture and dysfunction after acute myocardial infarction. *J Exp Med* 206(1):113–123, 2009.
145. Brower GL, Chancey AL, Thanigaraj S, et al: Cause and effect relationship between myocardial mast cell number and matrix metalloproteinase activity. *Am J Physiol Heart Circ Physiol* 283(2):H518–H525, 2002.
146. Chancey AL, Brower GL, Peterson JT, et al: Effects of matrix metalloproteinase inhibition on ventricular remodeling due to volume overload. *Circulation* 105(16):1983–1988, 2002.
147. Morita H, Khanal S, Rastogi S, et al: Selective matrix metalloproteinase inhibition attenuates progression of left ventricular dysfunction and remodeling in dogs with chronic heart failure. *Am J Physiol Heart Circ Physiol* 290(6):H2522–H2527, 2006.
148. Leeman MF, Curran S, Murray GI: The structure, regulation, and function of human matrix metalloproteinase-13. *Crit Rev Biochem Mol Biol* 37(3):149–166, 2002.
149. Brinckerhoff CE, Rutter JL, Benbow U: Interstitial collagenases as markers of tumor progression. *Clin Cancer Res* 6(12):4823–4830, 2000.
150. Spruill LS, Lowry AS, Stroud RE, et al: Membrane-type-1 matrix metalloproteinase transcription and translation in myocardial fibroblasts from patients with normal left ventricular function and from patients with cardiomyopathy. *Am J Physiol Cell Physiol* 293(4):C1362–C1373, 2007.
151. López B, González A, Querejeta R, et al: Alterations in the pattern of collagen deposition may contribute to the deterioration of systolic function in hypertensive patients with heart failure. *J Am Coll Cardiol* 48(1):89–96, 2006.
152. Martos R, Baugh J, Ledwidge M, et al: Diastolic heart failure: evidence of increased myocardial collagen turnover linked to diastolic dysfunction. *Circulation* 115(7):888–895, 2007.
153. Fomovsky GM, Thomopoulos S, Holmes JW: Contribution of extracellular matrix to the mechanical properties of the heart. *J Mol Cell Cardiol* 48(3):490–496, 2010.
154. Abrahams C, Janicki JS, Weber KT: Myocardial hypertrophy in Macaca fascicularis. Structural remodeling of the collagen matrix. *Lab Invest* 56(6):676–683, 1987.
155. González A, López B, Querejeta R, et al: Filling pressures and collagen metabolism in hypertensive patients with heart failure and normal ejection fraction. *Hypertension* 55(6):1418–1424, 2010.
156. Kasner M, Gaub R, Westermann D, et al: Simultaneous estimation of NT-proBNP on top to mitral flow Doppler echocardiography as an accurate strategy to diagnose diastolic dysfunction in HFNEF. *Int J Cardiol* 149(1):23–29, 2011.
157. Barasch E, Gottdiener JS, Aurigemma G, et al: Association between elevated fibrosis markers and heart failure in the elderly: the cardiovascular health study. *Circ Heart Fail.* 2(4):303–310, 2009.
158. Müller-Brunotte R, Kahan T, López B, et al: Myocardial fibrosis and diastolic dysfunction in patients with hypertension: results from the Swedish Irbesartan Left Ventricular Hypertrophy Investigation versus Atenolol (SILVHIA). *J Hypertens* 25(9):1958–1966, 2007.
159. Fielitz J, Leuschner M, Zurbrugg HR, et al: Regulation of matrix metalloproteinases and their inhibitors in the left ventricular myocardium of patients with aortic stenosis. *J Mol Med* 82:809–820, 2004.
160. Heymans S, Schroen B, Vermeersch P, et al: Increased cardiac expression of tissue inhibitor of metalloproteinase-1 and tissue inhibitor of metalloproteinase-2 is related to cardiac fibrosis and dysfunction in the chronic pressure-overloaded human heart. *Circulation* 112:1136–1144, 2005.
161. Mujumdar VS, Tyagi SC: Temporal regulation of extracellular matrix components in transition from compensatory hypertrophy to decompensatory heart failure. *J Hypertens* 17:261–270, 1999.
162. Li H, Simon H, Bocan TM, et al: MMP/TIMP expression in spontaneously hypertensive heart failure rats; the effect of ACE and MMP inhibition. *Cardiovasc Res* 46:298–306, 2000.
163. Nagatomo Y, Carabello BA, Coker ML, et al: Differential effects of pressure or volume overload on myocardial MMP levels and inhibitory control. *Am J Physiol Heart Circ Physiol* 278:H151–H161, 2000.
164. Yarbrough WM, Mukherjee R, Stroud RE, et al: Progressive induction of left ventricular pressure overload in a large animal model elicits myocardial remodeling and a unique matrix signature. *J Thorac Cardiovasc Surg* 143(1):215–223, 2012.
165. Matsusaka H, Ide T, Matsushima S, et al: Targeted deletion of matrix metalloproteinase 2 ameliorates myocardial remodeling in mice with chronic pressure overload. *Hypertension* 47(4):711–717, 2006.
166. Hadler-Olsen E, Fadnes B, Sylte I, et al: Regulation of matrix metalloproteinase activity in health and disease. *FEBS J* 278(1):28–45, 2011.
167. Clark IM, Swingler TE, Sampieri CL, et al: The regulation of matrix metalloproteinases and their inhibitors. *Int J Biochem Cell Biol* 40(6–7):1362–1378, 2008.

168. Bourboulia D, Stetler-Stevenson WG: Matrix metalloproteinases (MMPs) and tissue inhibitors of metalloproteinases (TIMPs): positive and negative regulators in tumor cell adhesion. *Semin Cancer Biol* 20(3):161–168, 2010.
169. Ruddy JM, Jones JA, Stroud RE, et al: Differential effects of mechanical and biological stimuli on matrix metalloproteinase promoter activation in the thoracic aorta. *Circulation* 120(11 Suppl):S262–S268, 2009.
170. Polyakova V, Hein S, Kostin S, et al: Matrix metalloproteinases and their tissue inhibitors in pressure-overloaded human myocardium during heart failure progression. *J Am Coll Cardiol* 44(8):1609–1618, 2004.
171. Zile MR, Baicu CF, Stroud RE, et al: Pressure overload-dependent membrane type 1-matrix metalloproteinase induction: relationship to LV remodeling and fibrosis. *Am J Physiol Heart Circ Physiol* 302(7):H1429–H1437, 2012.
172. Dai Q, Lin J, Craig T, et al: Estrogen effects on MMP-13 and MMP-14 regulation of left ventricular mass in Dahl salt-induced hypertension. *Gend Med* 5(1):74–85, 2008.
173. Kessenbrock K, Plaks V, Werb Z: Matrix metalloproteinases: regulators of the tumor microenvironment. *Cell* 141(1):52–67, 2010.
174. Gupta V, Grande-Allen KJ: Effects of static and cyclic loading in regulating extracellular matrix synthesis by cardiovascular cells. *Cardiovasc Res* 72(3):375–383, 2006.
175. Marchesi C, Dentali F, Nicolini E, et al: Plasma levels of matrix metalloproteinases and their inhibitors in hypertension: a systematic review and meta-analysis. *J Hypertens* 30(1):3–16, 2012.
176. Mak GJ, Ledwidge MT, Watson CJ, et al: Natural history of markers of collagen turnover in patients with early diastolic dysfunction and impact of eplerenone. *J Am Coll Cardiol* 54(18):1674–1682, 2009.
177. Zile MR, Desantis SM, Baicu CF, et al: Plasma biomarkers that reflect determinants of matrix composition identify the presence of left ventricular hypertrophy and diastolic heart failure. *Circ Heart Fail.* 4(3):246–256, 2011.
178. Foronjy RF, Sun J, Lemaitre V, et al: Transgenic expression of matrix metalloproteinase-1 inhibits myocardial fibrosis and prevents the transition to heart failure in a pressure overload mouse model. *Hypertens Res* 31(4):725–735, 2008.
179. Manhenke C, Orn S, Squire I, et al: The prognostic value of circulating markers of collagen turnover after acute myocardial infarction. *Int J Cardiol* 150(3):277–282, 2011.
180. Radauceanu A, Ducki C, Virion JM, et al: Extracellular matrix turnover and inflammatory markers independently predict functional status and outcome in chronic heart failure. *J Card Fail* 14(6):467–474, 2008.
181. Fertin M, Dubois E, Belliard A, et al: Usefulness of circulating biomarkers for the prediction of left ventricular remodeling after myocardial infarction. *Am J Cardiol* 110(2):277–283, 2012.
182. Wagner DR, Delagardelle C, Ernens I, et al: Matrix metalloproteinase-9 is a marker of heart failure after acute myocardial infarction. *J Card Fail* 12(1):66–72, 2006.
183. Webb CS, Bonnema DD, Ahmed SH, et al: Specific temporal profile of matrix metalloproteinase release occurs in patients after myocardial infarction: relation to left ventricular remodeling. *Circulation* 114(10):1020–1027, 2006.
184. Orn S, Manhenke C, Squire IB, et al: Plasma MMP-2, MMP-9 and N-BNP in long-term survivors following complicated myocardial infarction: relation to cardiac magnetic resonance imaging measures of left ventricular structure and function. *J Card Fail* 13(10):843–849, 2007.
185. Weir RA, Clements S, Steedman T, et al: Plasma TIMP-4 predicts left ventricular remodeling after acute myocardial infarction. *J Card Fail* 16:465–471, 2011.
186. Kelly D, Khan SQ, Thompson M, et al: Plasma tissue inhibitor of metalloproteinase-1 and matrix metalloproteinase-9: novel indicators of left ventricular remodelling and prognosis after acute myocardial infarction. *Eur Heart J* 29(17):2116–2124, 2008.
187. Martos R, Baugh J, Ledwidge M, et al: Diagnosis of heart failure with preserved ejection fraction: improved accuracy with the use of markers of collagen turnover. *Eur J Heart Fail* 11(2):191–197, 2009.
188. Pascual-Figal DA, Manzano-Fernández S, Boronat M, et al: Soluble ST2, high-sensitivity troponin T- and N-terminal pro-B-type natriuretic peptide: complementary role for risk stratification in acutely decompensated heart failure. *Eur J Heart Fail* 13(7):718–725, 2011.
189. Subramanian D, Subramanian V, Deswal A, et al: New predictive models of heart failure mortality using time-series measurements and ensemble models. *Circ Heart Fail.* 4(4):456–462, 2011.
190. Yndestad A, Finsen AV, Ueland T, et al: The homeostatic chemokine CCL21 predicts mortality and may play a pathogenic role in heart failure. *PLoS ONE* 7(3):e33038, 2012.
191. Askevold ET, Nymo S, Ueland T, et al: Soluble glycoprotein 130 predicts fatal outcomes in chronic heart failure: analysis from the Controlled Rosuvastatin Multinational Trial in Heart Failure (CORONA). *Circ Heart Fail.* 6(1):91–98, 2013.
192. Hohensinner PJ, Rychli K, Zorn G, et al: Macrophage-modulating cytokines predict adverse outcome in heart failure. *Thromb Haemost* 103(2):435–441, 2010.
193. Gopal DM, Kommineni M, Ayalon N, et al: Relationship of plasma galectin-3 to renal function in patients with heart failure: effects of clinical status, pathophysiology of heart failure, and presence or absence of heart failure. *J Am Heart Assoc* 1(5):e000760, 2012.
194. Weir RA, Petrie CJ, Murphy CA, et al: Galectin-3 and Cardiac Function in Survivors of Acute Myocardial Infarction. *Circ Heart Fail.* 6(3):492–498, 2013.
195. Gullestad L, Ueland T, Kjekshus J, et al: The predictive value of galectin-3 for mortality and cardiovascular events in the Controlled Rosuvastatin Multinational Trial in Heart Failure (CORONA). *Am Heart J* 164(6):878–883, 2012.
196. Ikemoto T, Hojo Y, Kondo H, et al: Plasma endoglin as a marker to predict cardiovascular events in patients with chronic coronary artery diseases. *Heart Vessels* 27(4):344–351, 2012.
197. Sato A, Hiroe M, Akiyama D, et al: Prognostic value of serum tenascin-C levels on long-term outcome after acute myocardial infarction. *J Card Fail* 18(6):480–486, 2012.
198. Bjerre M, Pedersen SH, Møgelvang R, et al: High osteopontin levels predict long-term outcome after STEMI and primary percutaneous coronary intervention. *Eur J Prev Cardiol* 20(6):922–929, 2013.
199. Georgiadou P, Iliodromitis EK, Kolokathis F, et al: Osteopontin as a novel prognostic marker in stable ischaemic heart disease: a 3-year follow-up study. *Eur J Clin Invest* 40(4):288–293, 2010.
200. Rosenberg M, Zugck C, Nelles M, et al: Osteopontin, a new prognostic biomarker in patients with chronic heart failure. *Circ Heart Fail* 1(1):43–49, 2008.
201. Takahashi R, Negishi K, Watanabe A, et al: Serum syndecan-4 is a novel biomarker for patients with chronic heart failure. *J Cardiol* 57(3):325–332, 2011.
202. Yan AT, Yan RT, Spinale FG, et al: Plasma matrix metalloproteinase-9 level is correlated with left ventricular volumes and ejection fraction in patients with heart failure. *J Card Fail* 12(7):514–519, 2006.
203. Cavusoglu E, Ruwende C, Chopra V, et al: Tissue inhibitor of metalloproteinase-1 (TIMP-1) is an independent predictor of all-cause mortality, cardiac mortality, and myocardial infarction. *Am Heart J* 151:e1101–e1108, 2006.
204. Sundstrom J, Evans JC, Benjamin EJ, et al: Relations of plasma matrix metalloproteinase-9 to clinical cardiovascular risk factors and echocardiographic left ventricular measures: the Framingham Heart Study. *Circulation* 109:2850–2856, 2004.
205. Sundstrom J, Evans JC, Benjamin EJ, et al: Relations of plasma total TIMP-1 levels to cardiovascular risk factors and echocardiographic measures: the Framingham Heart Study. *Eur Heart J* 25:1509–1516, 2004.
206. Krum H, Elsik M, Schneider HG, et al: Relation of peripheral collagen markers to death and hospitalization in patients with heart failure and preserved ejection fraction: results of the I-PRESERVE collagen substudy. *Circ Heart Fail.* 4(5):561–568, 2011.
207. Willemsen S, Hartog JW, van Veldhuisen DJ, et al: The role of advanced glycation end-products and their receptor on outcome in heart failure patients with preserved and reduced ejection fraction. *Am Heart J* 164(5):742–749, e3, 2012.
208. Campbell DJ, Somaratne JB, Jenkins AJ, et al: Diastolic dysfunction of aging is independent of myocardial structure but associated with plasma advanced glycation end-product levels. *PLoS ONE* 7(11):e49813, 2012.
209. Westermann D, Lindner D, Kasner M, et al: Cardiac inflammation contributes to changes in the extracellular matrix in patients with heart failure and normal EF. *Circ Heart Fail.* 4(1):44–52, 2011.
210. Tayebjee MH, Lim HS, Nadar S, et al: Tissue inhibitor of metalloproteinse-1 is a marker of diastolic dysfunction using tissue doppler in patients with type 2 diabetes and hypertension. *Eur J Clin Invest* 35(1):8–12, 2005.
211. López B, Castellano JM, González A, et al: Association of increased plasma cardiotrophin-1 with inappropriate left ventricular mass in essential hypertension. *Hypertension* 50:977–983, 2007.
212. Stahrenberg R, Edelmann F, Mende M, et al: The novel biomarker growth differentiation factor 15 in heart failure with normal ejection fraction. *Eur J Heart Fail* 12(12):1309–1316, 2010.
213. Sahul ZH, Mukherjee R, Song J, et al: Targeted imaging of the spatial and temporal variation of matrix metalloproteinase activity in a porcine model of postinfarct remodeling: relationship to myocardial dysfunction. *Circ Cardiov Imag* 4(4):381–391, 2011.
214. Kramer CM, Sinusas AJ, Sosnovik DE, et al: Multimodality imaging of myocardial injury and remodeling. *J Nucl Med* 51(Suppl 1):107S–121S, 2010.
215. Wong TC, Piehler K, Meier CG, et al: Association between extracellular matrix expansion quantified by cardiovascular magnetic resonance and short-term mortality. *Circulation* 126(10):1206–1216, 2012.
216. Hudson MP, Armstrong PW, Ruzyllo W, et al: Effects of selective matrix metalloproteinase inhibitor (PG-116800) to prevent ventricular remodeling after myocardial infarction: results of the PREMIER (Prevention of Myocardial Infarction Early Remodeling) trial. *J Am Coll Cardiol* 48(1):15–20, 2006.
217. Teekakirikul P, Eminaga S, Toka O, et al: Cardiac fibrosis in mice with hypertrophic cardiomyopathy is mediated by non-myocyte proliferation and requires Tgf-β. *J Clin Invest* 120(10):3520–3529, 2010.
218. Lorts A, Schwanekamp JA, Baudino TA, et al: Deletion of periostin reduces muscular dystrophy and fibrosis in mice by modulating the transforming growth factor-β pathway. *Proc Natl Acad Sci U S A* 109(27):10978–10983, 2012.
219. Huntgeburth M, Tiemann K, Shahverdyan R, et al: Transforming growth factor β_1 oppositely regulates the hypertrophic and contractile response to β-adrenergic stimulation in the heart. *PLoS ONE* 6(11):e26628, 2011.
220. Tan SM, Zhang Y, Wang B, et al: FT23, an orally active antifibrotic compound, attenuates structural and functional abnormalities in an experimental model of diabetic cardiomyopathy. *Clin Exp Pharmacol Physiol* 39(8):650–656, 2012.
221. Dai W, Wold LE, Dow JS, et al: Thickening of the infarcted wall by collagen injection improves left ventricular function in rats: a novel approach to preserve cardiac function after myocardial infarction. *J Am Coll Cardiol* 46(4):714–719, 2005.
222. Dixon JA, Gorman RC, Stroud RE, et al: Targeted regional injection of biocomposite microspheres alters post-myocardial infarction remodeling and matrix proteolytic pathways. *Circulation* 124(11 Suppl):S35–S45, 2011.
223. Garbern JC, Minami E, Stayton PS, et al: Delivery of basic fibroblast growth factor with a pH-responsive, injectable hydrogel to improve angiogenesis in infarcted myocardium. *Biomaterials* 32(9):2407–2416, 2011.
224. Kraehenbuehl TP, Ferreira LS, Hayward AM, et al: Human embryonic stem cell-derived microvascular grafts for cardiac tissue preservation after myocardial infarction. *Biomaterials* 32(4):1102–1109, 2011.
225. Mukherjee R, Zavadzkas JA, Saunders SM, et al: Targeted myocardial microinjections of a biocomposite material reduces infarct expansion in pigs. *Ann Thorac Surg* 86(4):1268–1276, 2008.
226. Tous E, Ifkovits JL, Koomalsingh KJ, et al: Influence of injectable hyaluronic acid hydrogel degradation behavior on infarction-induced ventricular remodeling. *Biomacromolecules* 12(11):4127–4135, 2011.
227. Shuman JA, Zurcher JR, Sapp AA, et al: Localized targeting of biomaterials following myocardial infarction; a foundation to build on. *Trends Cardiovasc Med* 23(8):301–311, 2013.
228. Chachques JC, Trainini JC, Lago N, et al: Myocardial assistance by grafting a new bioartificial upgraded myocardium (MAGNUM clinical trial): one year follow-up. *Cell Transplant* 16(9):927–934, 2007.
229. Zannad F, Alla F, Dousset B, et al: Limitation of excessive extracellular matrix turnover may contribute to survival benefit of spironolactone therapy in patients with congestive heart failure: insights from the randomized aldactone evaluation study (RALES). Rales Investigators. *Circulation* 102(22):2700–2706, 2000.
230. Vaitkevicius PV, Lane M, Spurgeon H, et al: A cross-link breaker has sustained effects on arterial and ventricular properties in older rhesus monkeys. *Proc Natl Acad Sci U S A* 98(3):1171–1175, 2001.
231. Little WC, Zile MR, Kitzman DW, et al: The effect of alagebrium chloride (ALT-711), a novel glucose cross-link breaker, in the treatment of elderly patients with diastolic heart failure. *J Card Fail* 11(3):191–195, 2005.
232. Hartog JW, Willemsen S, van Veldhuisen DJ, et al: Effects of alagebrium, an advanced glycation endproduct breaker, on exercise tolerance and cardiac function in patients with chronic heart failure. *Eur J Heart Fail* 13(8):899–908, 2011.
233. Swinnen M, Vanhoutte D, Van Almen GC, et al: Absence of thrombospondin-2 causes age-related dilated cardiomyopathy. *Circulation* 120(16):1585–1597, 2009.
234. Okamoto H, Imanaka-Yoshida K: Matricellular proteins: new molecular targets to prevent heart failure. *Cardiovasc Ther* 30(4):e198–e209, 2012.
235. Bradshaw AD, Baicu CF, Rentz TJ, et al: Pressure-overload induced alterations in fibrillar collagen content and myocardial diastolic function: role of SPARC in post-synthetic procollagen processing. *Circulation* 119:269–280, 2009.
236. Gross J, Lapiere CM: Collagenolytic activity in amphibian tissues: a tissue culture assay. *Proc Natl Acad Sci U S A* 48:1014–1022, 1962.
237. Rossi MA: Connective tissue skeleton in the normal left ventricle and in hypertensive left ventricular hypertrophy and chronic chagasic myocarditis. *Med Sci Monit* 7:820–832, 2001.
238. Spinale FG, Janicki JS, Zile MR: Membrane associated matrix proteolysis and heart failure. *Circ Res* 112(1):195–208, 2013.
239. Kajimoto K, Madeen K, Nakayama T, et al: Rapid evaluation by lung-cardiac-inferior vena cava (LCI) integrated ultrasound for differentiating heart failure from pulmonary disease as the cause of acute dyspnea in the emergency setting. *Cardiovasc Ultrasound* 10(1):49, 2012.
240. Vasku A, Goldbergová M, Izakovicová Hollá L, et al: A haplotype constituted of four MMP-2 promoter polymorphisms (-1575G/A, -1306C/T, -790T/G and -735C/T) is associated with coronary triple-vessel disease. *Matrix Biol* 22(7):585–591, 2004.
241. Samnegård A, Silveira A, Lundman P, et al: Serum matrix metalloproteinase-3 concentration is influenced by MMP-3-1612 5A/6A promoter genotype and associated with myocardial infarction. *J Intern Med* 258(5):411–419, 2005.
242. Pearce E, Tregouet DA, Samnegård A, et al: Haplotype effect of the matrix metalloproteinase-1 gene on risk of myocardial infarction. *Circ Res* 97(10):1070–1076, 2005.

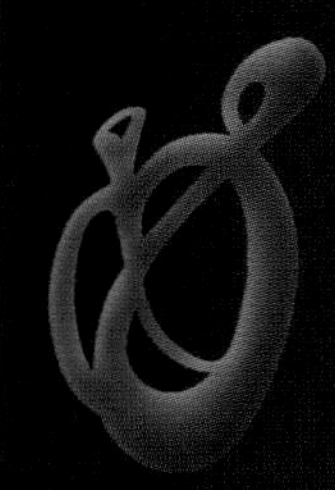

SECTION II

MECHANISMS OF DISEASE PROGRESSION IN HEART FAILURE

5 Molecular Signaling Mechanisms of the Renin-Angiotensin System in Heart Failure

Rajesh Kumar, Kenneth M. Baker, and Jing Pan

THE RENIN-ANGIOTENSIN SYSTEM

The renin-angiotensin system (RAS) is a major determinant of cardiovascular and renal function. RAS inhibitors often provide the first line of treatment for heart failure patients (see Chapter 34). In the simplest form, the RAS consists of a cascade of enzymatic reactions involving three components, angiotensinogen (AGT), renin, and angiotensin-converting enzyme (ACE), which generate angiotensin (Ang) II as the biologically active product. Ang II binds to two types of specific receptors, angiotensin type I (AGTR1) and angiotensin type II (AGTR2). Both receptors belong to the family of seven transmembrane domain, heterotrimeric G protein-coupled receptors (GPCR). The majority of the deleterious actions of Ang II have been attributed to interaction with the AT_1 receptor, which is the predominant receptor in adult tissues, whereas AT_2 generally produces beneficial effects. Several classes of drugs have been developed to block the RAS, either at the level of Ang II synthesis, by inhibiting the enzymatic reactions catalyzed by renin or ACE, or by preventing Ang II interaction with the AGTR1. For the convenience of the reader, a summary table of the abbreviations used is presented at the end of this chapter.

The most proximal component of the RAS, renin, was identified more than 100 years ago by Tigerstedt and Bergman.[1] Discoveries in the past two decades have resulted in characterization of the RAS as both systemic and local or tissue systems.[2] The relative contribution of the systemic versus a local RAS to various cardiovascular pathologies, such as hypertension and heart failure, is still being debated.[3] In addition to categorization, several new aspects of the RAS have been identified, which include novel Ang peptides, enzymes that catalyze synthesis of these peptides, receptors for these novel peptides, and new roles for renin and prorenin.[4] Gender and aging modify susceptibility to cardiovascular diseases, which has been partly attributed to the change in RAS activity or a shift between the traditional deleterious RAS and the novel protective RAS, as have been described below.[5,6]

THE SYSTEMIC RENIN-ANGIOTENSIN SYSTEM

The systemic RAS is also known as the classic, circulatory, or endocrine RAS, with AGT and renin secreted into the circulation from liver and kidneys (juxtaglomerular apparatus), respectively, and the final step of Ang II synthesis occurring in the circulation by the action of ACE (membrane bound on endothelial cells), which results in conversion of the decapeptide Ang I to Ang II (**Figure 5-1**). Ang II modulates vascular tone in response to changes in the blood

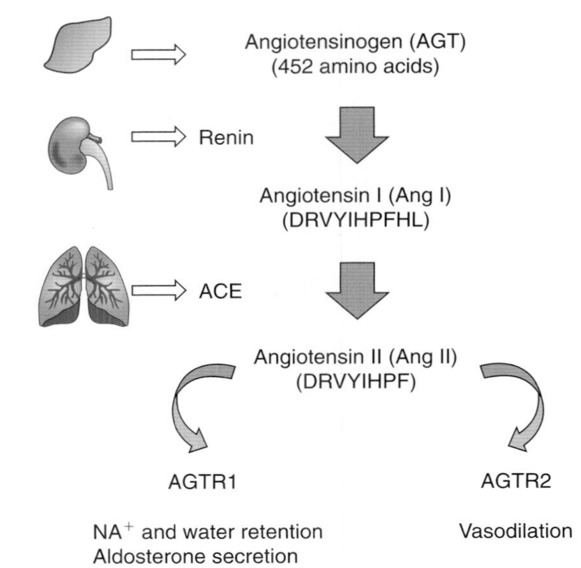

FIGURE 5-1 The systemic renin-angiotensin system. The systemic RAS consists of liver-derived AGT, kidney-derived renin, and endothelium-derived ACE. The latter is particularly abundant in pulmonary endothelial cells. Sequential action of renin and ACE on AGT produces the octapeptide Ang II in the circulation. Ang II acts via binding to AGTR1 and AGTR2, which generally produce opposite effects. AGTR1 is the predominant receptor in adult tissues. The systemic RAS is involved in acute effects to maintain salt and water homeostasis and blood pressure.

pressure and participates in vascular remodeling during vascular injury, hypertension, aneurysm formation, and atherogenesis. Circulating Ang II is taken up by several tissues where it modulates local tissue functions. Circulating AGT and renin also contribute to Ang II synthesis locally at tissue sites, in addition to these components being expressed locally. A recent study has shown that liver-derived AGT is the primary source of renal AGT and Ang II.[7]

Angiotensinogen

AGT is a 485-amino-acid protein with an N-terminal signal peptide, which is cotranslationally removed to yield the 452-amino-acid mature protein, the only known substrate for renin. Though AGT is expressed in multiple tissues, plasma AGT levels are determined primarily by the rate of production by hepatocytes, which constitutively secrete AGT. Recently, adipose tissue has been shown to contribute to about 25% of the circulating AGT, which is important for obesity-induced hypertension in mice.[8,9] Circulating levels of AGT are close to the Michaelis constant for renin; thus a small increase in AGT will increase Ang II synthesis and blood pressure. Several studies in genetically modified mice and rats have demonstrated hypertensive effects of increasing AGT gene copy number or overexpression. AGT occurs in unglycosylated and multiple glycosylated forms, the significance of which is not entirely known.[10] In addition, AGT occurs in reduced and oxidized sulfydryl-bridged forms in a 40:60 ratio in the circulation. The more active oxidized form is increased in preeclamptic maternal circulation.[11] A variety of stimuli regulate circulating levels of AGT, including glucocorticoids, estrogens, thyroid hormone, insulin, and several cytokines.[12] Ang II exerts positive feedback regulation on AGT expression through the AGTR1. Polymorphisms in the AGT gene have been reported, which affect transcriptional regulation of the gene and may provide a genetic mechanism for hypertension.[12]

Renin

Juxtaglomerular cells, in the terminal afferent arteriole of the kidneys, are the major source of circulating renin. Renin is synthesized as pre-prorenin, which is converted into prorenin after removal of the signal peptide during transfer to the endoplasmic reticulum. Prorenin, which is enzymatically inactive, is proteolytically activated by removal of the 43-amino-acid prosegment, to produce renin. The prosegment can also be displaced non-proteolytically, by low pH or binding to the newly discovered prorenin receptor (PRR), to expose the catalytic site.[13] Juxtaglomerular cells constitutively secrete the majority of prorenin; the remainder is targeted to dense core secretory granules, where the prosegment is removed and renin is released in a regulated manner. Recent evidence suggests that collecting ducts, in addition to juxtaglomerular cells, are an important source of circulating prorenin in diabetes.[14] Pregnant women have high levels of circulating prorenin, which is largely from the ovaries.[15] There is no evidence of extrarenal proteolytic conversion of prorenin to renin; thus the physiologic role of circulating prorenin has been uncertain. The PRR, which non-proteolytically activates prorenin and also activates intracellular signaling, might provide clues to the pathophysiologic significance of prorenin.[16]

Renin synthesis and secretion are promoted by low blood pressure, sympathetic stimuli, and prostaglandins and are inhibited by high blood pressure, salt, and volume overload. Ang II also exerts a negative feedback on renin production by the juxtaglomerular cells, which is the reason for the observed reactive rise in renin with RAS blockade.

Angiotensin-Converting Enzyme

Angiotensin-converting enzyme (ACE) is a dicarboxypeptidyl peptidase of 150-180 kDa, which cleaves the two terminal amino acids off of the decapeptide Ang I, a product of the AGT and renin reaction, to form the octapeptide Ang II. Unlike renin, ACE is not specific to a single substrate, but cleaves several peptides, such as bradykinin, substance P, and the tetrapeptide *N*-acetyl-Ser-Asp-Lys-Pro (Ac-SDKP). Some of the beneficial effects of ACE inhibitors have been attributed to prevention of bradykinin and Ac-SDKP degradation. In addition to vascular endothelial cells of lung, retina, and brain, ACE is also highly expressed on the proximal tubular brush border of epithelial cells in the kidneys. While most ACE is anchored to the cell membrane by a C-terminus hydrophobic region, shedding of ACE releases an active enzyme into various body fluids. The extracellular region of ACE contains two homologous and independent catalytic domains, termed *N*- and *C-domains*. An isoform of ACE that contains only the C-domain is expressed in testis, resulting in categorization as somatic and testis ACE. A recent study in genetically modified mice has shown that the C-domain of ACE is the predominant site of Ang I cleavage in vivo.[17] Localization of ACE on endothelial cell membranes generates Ang II in close proximity to vascular smooth muscle, which is important for vasoconstrictive effects of the peptide. In addition to being an important component of the RAS, ACE has roles in multiple physiologic functions that include male fertility,

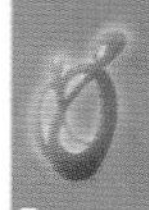

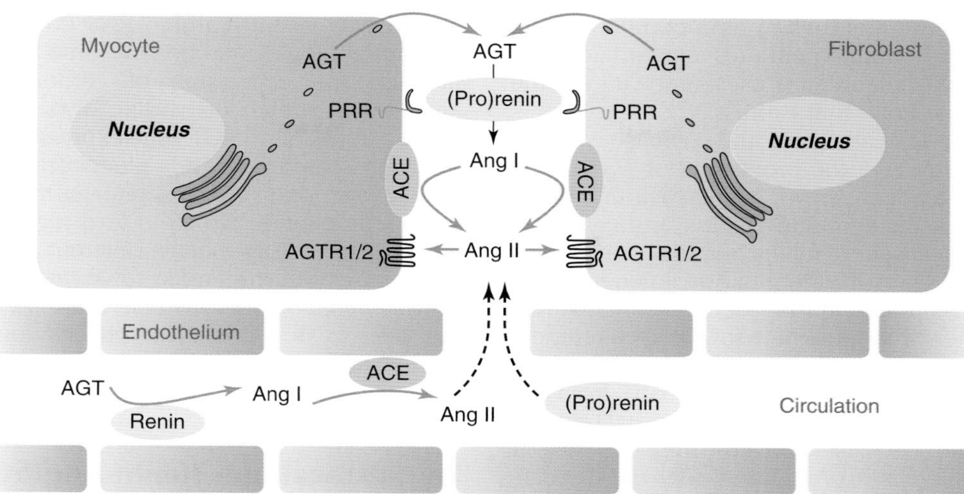

FIGURE 5-2 The cardiac renin-angiotensin system. The cardiac RAS is defined by interstitial Ang II synthesis and direct actions in the heart. A small contribution of circulatory Ang II may also be relevant in addition to the locally synthesized pool. Cardiac cells may also sequester (pro)renin from the circulation. The latter would bind to specific (pro)renin receptors (PRR) on cardiac cells and convert locally produced AGT to Ang I, which is further cleaved to form Ang II by the actions of membrane-bound ACE. Both types of Ang II receptors, AGTR1 and AGTR2, are expressed on cardiac cells. The major effects of Ang II in the heart include cardiac myocyte hypertrophy, cardiac fibroblast proliferation, oxidative stress, and extracellular matrix deposition.

hematopoiesis, MHC class I processing, and resistance to bacterial infection.[18]

THE LOCAL RENIN-ANGIOTENSIN SYSTEM

In the past two decades, it has become evident that several tissues, other than those that contribute to the circulating RAS, express all components of the RAS and generate Ang II locally. This has been most clearly demonstrated in the brain, where circulating components cannot enter because of the blood-brain barrier. The benefits of RAS inhibitors, which cannot be explained solely on the basis of blood pressure reduction, strengthened the concept of local generation and effects of Ang II. Studies using transgenic and knockout animal models (of RAS components) further confirmed the significance of the local RAS in various pathologic conditions. Local RASs have tissue-specific roles and are regulated independently of the circulating system. The major controversy associated with local RASs is in regard to the expression of renin in extrarenal tissues, particularly the heart. However, this has not undermined the concept of a local RAS, as alternative enzymes, such as cathepsins and chymase, have been identified in several tissues that are involved in the conversion of AGT to Ang II. A local RAS has convincingly been demonstrated in the brain, heart, vasculature, kidneys, eyes, pancreas, reproductive organs, and lymphatic and adipose tissues.[2] Recent evidence has indicated that while the circulating RAS exerts acute hemodynamic effects, the tissue RASs are involved in long-term effects of chronic RAS activation associated with target organ damage, such as renal failure and cardiac remodeling.[2] Local system functions of the RAS include cell growth and remodeling in the heart, regulation of blood pressure, central effects on food and water intake, and hormone secretion in the pancreas.[19]

The Cardiac Renin-Angiotensin System

A quantitative study using radiolabeled AGT infusion has shown that more than 90% of cardiac Ang I and 75% of cardiac Ang II are synthesized at cardiac sites (**Figure 5-2**).[20] The RAS precursor components for Ang II biosynthesis are present in both cardiac myocytes and fibroblasts.[21] The interstitial concentration of Ang II in the heart is about 100-fold more than that of plasma, though the myocardial concentration of renin and AGT is only 1% to 4% that of plasma.[22,23] There is debate as to which and in what amount RAS components are synthesized locally or are taken up from the plasma. Much of the controversy surrounds the source of renin in the heart. Active uptake of renin from the plasma, by endothelial cells, cardiomyocytes, and fibroblasts, in addition to de novo synthesis, has been proposed.[24-26] Two uptake mechanisms have been described; one that is mediated by the mannose-6-phosphate receptor and another that is not. The former mainly represents a clearance mechanism of circulating glycosylated prorenin by heart cells, while the latter involves uptake of nonglycosylated prorenin and results in intracellular generation of Ang peptides.[27] Emerging evidence suggests that under specific conditions renin is synthesized in cardiovascular tissues. Renin mRNA has been detected in cardiac atria, ventricles, and primary cultures of neonatal and adult rat ventricular myocytes.[21,28-30] Increased cardiac levels of renin mRNA have been reported in patients following myocardial infarction and in the ventricles of animals with experimental models of infarction.[31] Renin mRNA and protein have been detected in canine cardiac myocytes, the levels of which are upregulated by ventricular-pacing induced cardiac failure.[32] A second renin transcript, lacking the coding region for the secretory signal peptide and termed *Exon 1A renin,* has been detected in the brain, adrenal gland, and heart.[33] Interestingly, Exon 1A renin is the only transcript of renin expressed in the rat heart.[33] The intracellular renin coding mRNA is upregulated in the left ventricle following myocardial infarction.[33] Thus the possibility of two cardiac RASs has been suggested, one the intracardiac RAS, and another an intracellular RAS driven by Exon 1A renin.[27] The local production of AGT and ACE has been clearly demonstrated. AGT mRNA and protein have been detected in cardiac myocytes and fibroblasts in primary cell culture and in vivo.[34-36] ACE has been detected in the heart, with higher amounts in atria compared with the ventricles, and in primary cultures of cardiac myocytes.[28,37-39] Endothelial cells and fibroblasts appear to be the major cell types of the heart that express ACE.

Other enzymes such as cathepsins and chymase can substitute for renin and ACE in the processing of AGT in the heart. Cathepsin D has been shown to increase in cardiac myocytes from failing, paced canine hearts, and cathepsin G was increased in mast cells of failing hearts in humans.[32,40] The role of cathepsin D involvement in Ang II generation is evident in vascular smooth muscle cells (VSMC), where cathepsin D is the predominant aspartic proteinase.[41] Cathepsin D participates in enhanced Ang II synthesis in response to high glucose or a change in VSMC, from the contractile to a synthetic phenotype.[42,43] Cathepsin D cleaves AGT into Ang I, and chymase converts Ang I to Ang II. Chymase is highly specific for Ang I and does not degrade bradykinin and vasoactive intestinal peptide. In myocardial extracts from humans and dogs, chymase accounted for approximately 90% of Ang II forming activity; however, the contribution in intact tissue is not clear.[44,45] In diabetes, Ang II generation appears to be largely chymase-mediated.[29] Dual pathways of Ang II generation, by chymase and ACE, were demonstrated to have an important role in cardiac remodeling, in pressure-overloaded hamster hearts, and in transgenic mice overexpressing human chymase in the heart.[46,47] In addition to Ang II formation, chymase can produce Ang II-independent effects, through conversion of latent to active TGF-β and type I procollagen to collagen.[48] Consistent with an active role of chymase in cardiac remodeling, specific chymase inhibitors have been shown to have protective effects in animal models of myocardial infarction, cardiomyopathy, and tachycardia-induced heart failure. Thus alternative pathways of Ang II synthesis are present in the heart, though it remains unclear in which situations renin-independent or ACE-independent Ang II synthesis occurs.[49]

Cardiac RAS activity is under the control of tissue-specific regulatory influences, differing from that of the systemic RAS. For example, an increase in left ventricular mass produced by abdominal aortic constriction can be prevented by an ACE inhibitor, with no change in afterload.[50] The activity of the cardiac RAS is influenced by several pathophysiologic conditions. Volume and pressure overload increase the expression of cardiac RAS components. Mechanical stretch of cardiac myocytes increases Ang II release from cells.[51] AGT gene expression is increased in the heart by cardiotrophin-1, glucocorticoids, estrogen, and thyroid hormone.[52] Ang II stimulates the production of atrial natriuretic peptide, which in turn regulates renin and AGT mRNA levels.[21] Ang II has a differential effect on renin and AGT expression in cardiac myocytes and fibroblasts, positively regulating the former, while negatively regulating the latter.[51,53] Together, these observations suggest that the cardiac RAS represents a self-sustaining paracrine/autocrine loop, involving both cardiac myocytes and fibroblasts.[54]

The Intracellular Renin-Angiotensin System

In addition to the systemic and local RAS, recent studies have provided evidence of a complete, functional RAS within cells, described as an "intracrine" or intracellular RAS (**Figure 5-3**).[55,56] The intracellular RAS is characterized by the presence of RAS components inside the cell, synthesis of Ang II intracellularly, and actions of Ang II originating from an intracellular location. AGT and renin are generally secreted from the cells in which synthesis occurs. However, recent studies have demonstrated that under certain conditions, cells redistribute AGT and renin, resulting in intracellular synthesis and retention of Ang II.[30] Alternative enzymes, such as cathepsin D and chymase, may substitute for renin and ACE, respectively, in an intracellular system.[43] Studies have shown that participation of alternative mechanisms for Ang II synthesis may depend on the stimulus and cell type.[49,57] Several cells, such as cardiac myocytes, fibroblasts, renal mesangial, and vascular smooth muscle (VSM), have been shown to synthesize intracellular Ang II under hyperglycemic conditions.[30,43,57] Diabetic patients have also been reported to have higher cardiac levels of intracellular Ang II, which are further increased in association with hypertension.[58] In addition to Ang II synthesis, functional intracellular Ang II binding sites have been demonstrated on renal and hepatocyte nuclei and on chromatin.[59-61] Though nuclear Ang II binding sites are AGTR1-like, the nature of chromatin

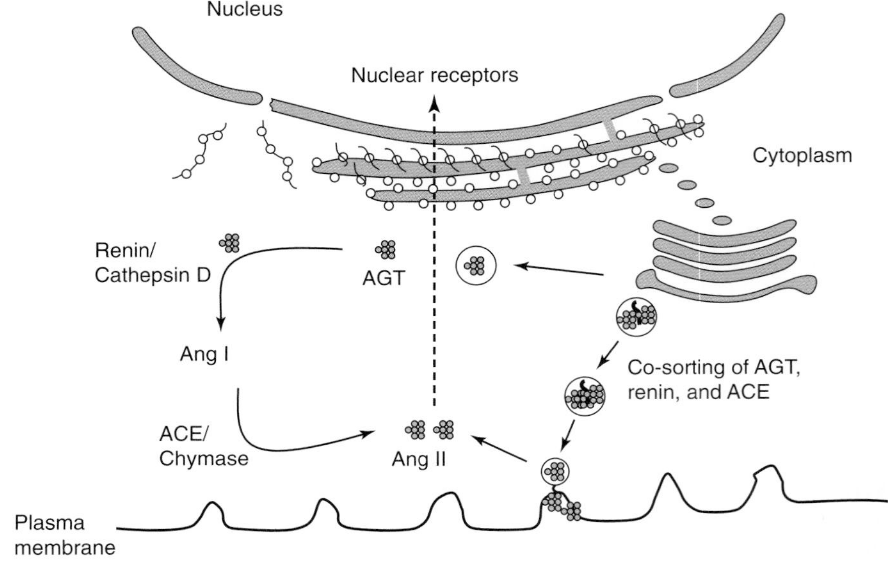

FIGURE 5-3 The intracellular renin-angiotensin system. The intracellular RAS is defined by the synthesis and resultant actions of Ang II inside a cell. The precise intracellular sites of Ang II synthesis and actions are not known. Current evidence suggests that synthesis of Ang II occurs either in secretory vesicles or other cytoplasmic locations, depending on the cell type and nature of the stimulus. Intracellular Ang II likely acts through AGTR1-like receptors on the nuclear envelope, direct chromatin binding, or through unidentified intracellular receptors. Ang II can also likely freely enter the nucleus *(dotted line)*, owing to the small size (8 amino acids). The effects of intracellular Ang II include cell growth, gene expression, extracellular matrix production, and cardiac hypertrophy.

binding is not known. Coupling of chromatin and nuclear membrane Ang II receptors to increased RNA synthesis and gene transcription of AGT, renin, and platelet-derived growth factor (PDGF) has been demonstrated.[62]

Intracellular actions of Ang II have been termed *intracrine* actions.[63] Intracellular production of Ang II in cultured cardiac myocytes and in mouse heart results in hypertrophic cell growth and biventricular hypertrophy, respectively.[64] Microinjection of Ang II into rat VSMC has been shown to increase cytosolic and nuclear Ca^{2+} ($[Ca^{2+}]_i$), which was secondary to an influx of extracellular Ca^{2+}.[65] In addition, intracellular Ang II is associated with diabetes-induced oxidative stress and cardiac fibrosis in rat hearts.[29] Studies on cultured neonatal rat cardiac myocytes have shown that intracellular Ang II upregulates AGT, renin, and AGTR1 receptor through a positive feedback mechanism.[30] Several of the intracrine effects of Ang II are not blocked by angiotensin receptor blockers (ARBs), due either to limited cell penetration of these drugs or to AGTR1-independent mechanisms.[64,66]

The pathophysiologic significance of the intracellular cardiac RAS remains to be determined in the general clinical population.[67] Diabetes is a major stimulus for the activation of the intracellular RAS. Since cardiac myocyte Ang II synthesis in diabetes is chymase dependent and intracellular Ang II effects are not blocked by ARBs, therapeutic modalities, other than ARBs and ACE inhibitors, that would block intracellular synthesis or intracrine effects of Ang II might provide a better outcome in diabetic patients by reducing end-organ damage. However, a renin inhibitor preserved cardiac function equivalent to that by an ARB or ACE inhibitor in an experimental model of type 1 diabetes.[68]

NOVEL ASPECTS OF THE RENIN-ANGIOTENSIN SYSTEM

Ang II has traditionally been considered the only biologically active end product of the RAS. Recent evidence indicates that additional shorter chain angiotensins also serve as effector peptides in this system (**Figure 5-4**). These shorter chain peptides include Ang (1-7), a heptapeptide that lacks the C-terminal phenylalanine of Ang II; Ang III, a heptapeptide lacking the N-terminal aspartate residue; and Ang IV, a hexapeptide, lacking the two N-terminal amino acids. Modulation of the peptide levels and the enzymes that generate these peptides has been associated with cardiovascular regulation, as discussed in the following section. In addition to these peptides, new functions of (pro)renin have been described, which will likely have a significant impact on future therapeutic approaches to cardiovascular diseases. In the last decade, the majority of research in the RAS field has been focused on these novel components of the RAS and their pathophysiologic significance.

Ang (1-7) and ACE2

Ang (1-7) is formed either by the action of neutral endopeptidase on Ang I or by the recently discovered monocarboxypeptidase, ACE2, on Ang II (see Figure 5-4). Ang (1-7) elicits cardiovascular responses, such as antihypertensive, antihypertrophic, antifibrotic, and antithrombotic, that are generally opposite to those mediated by Ang II. The effects of Ang (1-7) may be mediated through direct signaling, as a result of binding to a G protein-coupled receptor, which is a product of the Mas oncogene, or by the modulation of AGTR1 receptor signaling, as a result of heterodimerization of Mas and AGTR1 receptors.[69,70] The Ang (1-7)/Mas receptor signaling includes the PI3K/Akt and ERK pathways that activate downstream effectors, such as NO, FOXO1, and COX-2.[71] Local generation of Ang (1-7) in the myocardium of dogs and elevation of Ang (1-7) in cardiac myocytes, during development of heart failure subsequent to coronary artery ligation, has been reported.[72,73] In addition, increasing Ang (1-7) levels through systemic administration, adenovirus-mediated expression, or transgenic overexpression attenuates cardiac remodeling as a result of Ang II infusion, myocardial infarction, ischemia, isoproterenol treatment, high salt intake, and fructose feeding.[74,75]

ACE2 changes Ang (1-7) levels by converting Ang I into Ang (1-9) and Ang II into Ang (1-7), though the latter is the preferred pathway. ACE2 gene expression is significantly increased in the failing human heart.[76] ACE2-knockout mice have left ventricular dysfunction and wall thinning, along with increased Ang II levels. Similarly, diabetic cardiovascular

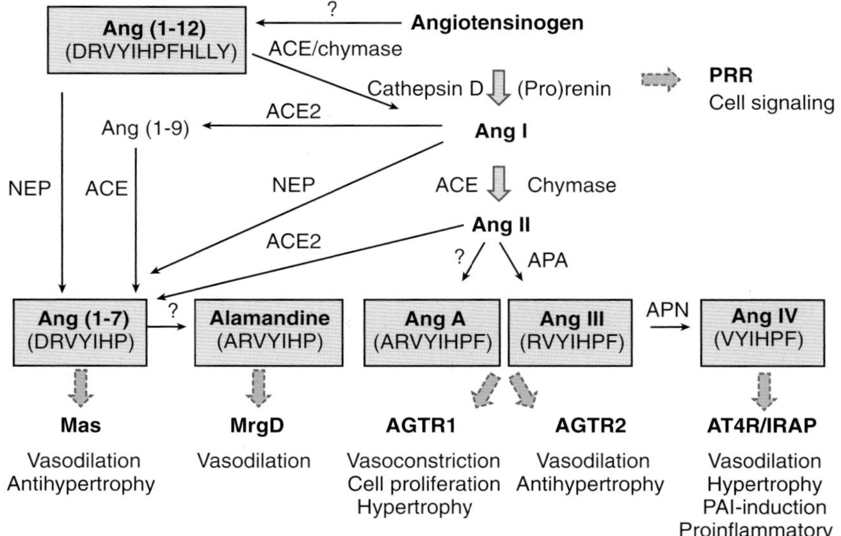

FIGURE 5-4 Novel components of the renin-angiotensin system. The renin and ACE-mediated conversion of AGT to Ang II may also be catalyzed by alternative enzymes, such as cathepsin D and chymase. In addition, AGT is cleaved to Ang (1-12) by an unidentified enzyme. Ang I may be converted to Ang (1-9) by an isoform of ACE, known as ACE2. Ang (1-9) can be converted to Ang (1-7) by ACE. Alternatively, Ang (1-7) can be formed by a direct action of NEP on Ang I and Ang (1-12) or that of ACE2 on Ang II. Ang (1-7) have decarboxylated forms at the first amino acid, called alamandine. Ang (1-7) binds to a specific receptor, which is a product of the Mas oncogene. The effects of Ang (1-7) are beneficial to the cardiovascular system. Alamandine binds to Mas-related GPCR member D (MrgD) and produces vasorelaxation. Ang II can also be further cleaved by APA to produce Ang III or decarboxylated to form Ang A, both of which bind to the same receptors as Ang II and produce similar effects. Some of the renal and brain effects, which were initially thought to be produced by Ang II, require conversion of Ang II to Ang III. Ang III can be further cleaved by APN to form Ang IV, which binds to a specific receptor that was identified as insulin-regulated aminopeptidase (IRAP). Both prorenin and renin bind to the PRR and activate intracellular signaling pathways.

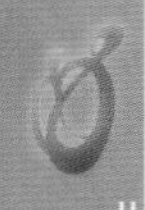

complications are exacerbated in mice lacking ACE2.[77] The ACE and ACE2 double-knockout completely prevents cardiac abnormalities and the increase in Ang II production.[78] Lentiviral-mediated ACE2 overexpression has ameliorator effects on blood pressure and cardiac fibrosis in spontaneously hypertensive rats. Similarly, there is a protective effect on the heart, through preservation of cardiac function, left ventricular wall motion, and contractility, in a myocardial infarction model.[79] In a rat model of type 1 diabetes, adenovirus-mediated ACE2 expression ameliorates cardiac dysfunction.[80] However, transgenic mice with increased cardiac ACE2 expression show a high incidence of sudden death because of ventricular tachycardia and fibrillation, as a result of gap junction remodeling.[81] ACE2 can effectively alter the balance between vasoconstrictive and the cell proliferating effects of Ang II and the vasodilatory and antiproliferating effects of Ang (1-7).[82] The age-dependent cardiomyopathy in ACE2 null mice was related to increased Ang II-mediated oxidative stress and neutrophilic infiltration in the absence of ACE2.[83] Structure-based screening of developmental therapeutic compounds has identified candidates that enhanced ACE2 activity in vitro and reduced blood pressure in spontaneously hypertensive rats.[84] In addition, improvement in cardiac function and reversal of myocardial, perivascular, and renal fibrosis was observed with these compounds. In a significant development toward therapeutic use of modulating the Ang 1-7/Mas pathway, an oral formulation of Ang (1-7) has been developed that shows cardioprotective effects in experimental animals.[85]

Angiotensin III

Angiotensin III (Ang III), also called Ang-(2-8), is generated from Ang II by aminopeptidase A (APA), which cleaves the Asp^1-Arg^2 bond in Ang II (see Figure 5-4). The major physiologic role of Ang III is in the brain, where it has been shown to be more important than Ang II in the central regulation of hypertension, vasopressin release, sympathetic hyperactivity, and cardiac dysfunction postmyocardial infarction.[86,87] Ang III has affinity for AGTR1 and AGTR2 receptors that is comparable with that of Ang II.[86] APA is also highly expressed in kidneys. It was recently shown that renal conversion of Ang II to Ang III is critical for AGTR2-mediated natriuresis and may have a significant role in disorders characterized by Na^+ and fluid retention, such as hypertension and congestive heart failure.[88] Ang III, APA, and aminopeptidase N (APN) could constitute putative therapeutic targets for the treatment of hypertension.[89]

Angiotensin IV

Ang III is metabolized to angiotensin IV (Ang IV) by APN (see Figure 5-4). Ang IV mediates physiologic functions in the central nervous system, which include blood flow regulation, learning and memory.[90] Ang IV binds to a type II integral membrane protein, termed *AT_4R*, which was recently identified as insulin-regulated aminopeptidase (IRAP).[91,92] AT_4R/IRAP is expressed in multiple tissues, including brain, kidneys, blood vessels, and heart. Actions of Ang IV, mediated through the AT_4R receptor, may be related to the activation of several intracellular signaling pathways or by inhibition of the enzymatic activity of IRAP, the physiologic substrates of which include vasopressin.[93] Several studies have suggested a role for Ang IV in cardiovascular diseases, in that Ang IV enhances cell growth in cardiac fibroblasts, endothelial, and VSMC.[90] In VSMC, Ang IV activates the proinflammatory transcription factor NF-κB, which regulates expression of several genes involved in atherogenesis and thrombosis.[94]

Angiotensin (1-12), Angiotensin A, and Alamandine

Recently, Ang (1-12), consisting of N-terminal 12 amino acids of the mature AGT, was identified in human and animal plasma and tissues (see Figure 5-4). Ang (1-12), produced by a yet unidentified enzyme, contributes to Ang II and Ang (1-7) generation in the heart, thereby providing a renin-independent mechanism of RAS activity.[95] In addition to the generation of Ang peptides by enzymatic digestion of AGT, two novel Ang peptides have been identified that are produced as a result of decarboxylation of the first amino acid aspartic acid to alanine. These peptides, Ang A and alamandine, correspond to Ang II and Ang (1-7), respectively (see Figure 5-4).[96,97] It is not known at what step of generation of these peptides the modification occurs. Ang A binds to AGTR1 and AGTR2 and has effects similar to Ang II. Alamandine produces vasorelaxation similar to Ang (1-7), but through binding to the Mas-related GPCR member D. The plasma levels of both peptides are increased in chronic end-stage renal disease patients.

Pro(renin) Receptor

The pro(renin) receptor (PRR), a 350-amino-acid protein, with a single transmembrane domain that is expressed in multiple tissues, including the heart, was cloned in 2002.[13] PRR specifically binds to renin and prorenin. Following binding to the receptor, a conformational change makes prorenin catalytically active, which can produce Ang II locally and therefore available to bind to Ang II receptors. Thus circulating prorenin might contribute significantly to tissue Ang II production.[13] The catalytic efficiency of renin for Ang II generation is also enhanced when bound to PRR. In addition to providing an enhanced capability of local Ang II generation, PRR also mediates intracellular signaling events, which likely contribute to the pathologic effects of RAS activation.[98] PRR activates the p38 MAPK/HSP27 pathway,[98] PI3K, and PLZF (promyelocytic leukemia zinc-finger protein) that represses the expression of PRR itself (**Figure 5-5**).[99] Interestingly, these effects occurred without production of Ang II or stimulation of AGTR1. Recently, it has been demonstrated that PRR can associate with vacuolar H^+-ATPase (v-H^+-ATPase) and is required for canonical Wnt/β-catenin signaling, which has an important role in the development of cardiac hypertrophy, fibrosis, and heart failure.[100,101] These studies suggest that PRR may directly contribute to disease processes, such as hypertension, heart failure, and diabetes mellitus-induced cardiovascular complications.[16]

ANGIOTENSIN II-MEDIATED SIGNALING PATHWAYS IN HEART FAILURE

Angiotensin II Receptors

In mammalian cells, Ang II mediates effects via (at least) two high-affinity plasma membrane receptors, AGTR1 and

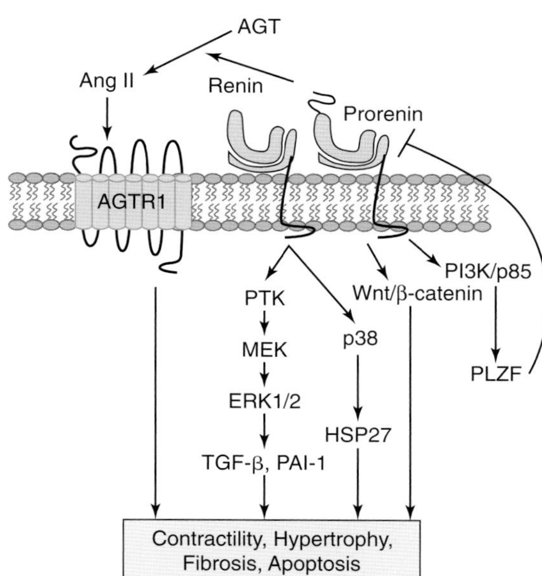

FIGURE 5-5 Intracellular effects of (pro)renin receptors. Binding of renin and/or prorenin to the PRR leads to activation of the enzymatic action of prorenin and enhancement of catalytic activity, resulting in elevated concentrations of Ang II in proximity to the cell surface. Renin and prorenin also independently activate intracellular signaling pathways. Pro(renin) receptor–mediated activation of the MEK/ERK1/2 cascade through tyrosine kinases leads to generation of transforming growth factor-β (TGF-β) and plasminogen activator inhibitor-type 1 (PAI-1), resulting in hypertrophic growth and fibrosis. Pro(renin) receptor–induced activation of p38 MAPK leads to activation of heat shock protein 27 (Hsp27), which is associated with abnormal actin filament dynamics. Activation of these latter pathways is independent of Ang II. *AGT,* Angiotensinogen; *PTK,* protein tyrosine kinase.

AGTR2. The AGTR1 are ubiquitously expressed, were first cloned in 1991,[102] and consist of 359 amino acids with a molecular mass of 41 KDa. Two AGTR1 subtypes have been described in rodents, AT_{1a} and AT_{1b}, with greater than 94% amino acid sequence identity and which have similar pharmacologic properties and tissue distribution. The human AGTR1 gene has been mapped to chromosome 3. The AGTR1 is a glycoprotein, containing extracellular glycosylation sites at the amino terminus (Asn^4) and the second extracellular loop (Asp^{176} and Asn^{188}). The transmembrane domain at the amino-terminal extension and segments in the first and third extracellular loops are responsible for G protein interactions with the receptor. AGTR1 interact with various heterotrimeric G proteins, including Gq/11, Gi/o, Gα12, and Gα13, which couple to distinct signaling cascades. Like most GPCR, AGTR1 are also subject to internalization when stimulated by Ang II, a process dependent on specific residues located on the cytoplasmic tail. Internalization of GPCR involves receptor phosphorylation, which may be mediated, in part, via caveola. Studies have shown that a serine/threonine-rich segment of the carboxy-terminus is essential for phosphorylation and internalization of the receptor and that G protein receptor kinase (GRK)-mediated serine phosphorylation of AGTR1 has an important role in desensitization of the agonist-occupied receptor.[103]

AGTR2 is distinct from AGTR1 in genomic organization, tissue-specific expression, as well as in signaling mechanisms. AGTR2 is encoded by a 363-amino-acid protein with a molecular mass of 41 KDa, but it shares only 34% sequence identity with the AGTR1. Stimulation of AGTR2 by Ang II, in contrast to AGTR1, is not followed by interaction of the activated receptor with β-arrestins and subsequent internalization, suggesting that classic, β-arrestin-mediated mechanisms do not participate in the homologous desensitization of the AGTR2 and that its regulation is different from the AGTR1 and most other GPCR. AGTR2 is highly expressed in fetal tissues, with expression dramatically decreasing after birth, and being restricted to a few organs, including adrenals, kidneys, uterus, ovary, heart, and specialized nuclei in the brain. The expression of AGTR2 in VSMC and endothelial cells can be influenced by diverse pathologic conditions, such as pressure overload and vascular damage.[104] Studies have demonstrated that activation of AGTR2 stimulates vasodilation through bradykinin and B_2 receptor-mediated NO synthesis and cGMP production.[105] The expression of AGTR2 in the heart also increased in response to pathologic stimuli and treatment with ACE inhibitor and AGTR1 blockers; this may result in attenuation of AGTR1-mediated pressor effects and on growth and fibrosis. Transgenic and knockout animal studies have shown contradictory results regarding the role of AGTR2 in cardiac hypertrophy and heart failure.[106] Though chronic activation of AGTR2 by compound 21 (a selective non-peptide AGTR2 agonist) would be predicted to exert beneficial antiremodeling effects on the heart and vasculature, use of compound 21 as an AGTR2 agonist has been questioned.[107] Given its upregulation under pathologic conditions, the AGTR2 remains a promising target for treatment in hypertension, stroke, inflammation, and myocardial fibrosis.

Two other Ang II receptors have been described, AT_3R and AT_4R. The AT_3R is peptide-specific, recognizing mainly Ang II. This subtype does not bind nonpeptide ligands, such as losartan or PD123319 (selective AGTR2 antagonist), and has only been observed in cell lines. The AT_4R, which is distributed in heart, lung, kidney, brain, and liver, binds to Ang IV, but not losartan or PD123319. AT_4R was identified as a specific, high-affinity binding site for the hexapeptide Ang IV (VYIHPF), an insulin-regulated aminopeptidase. Ang IV induces vasorelaxation in various vascular beds, enhances endothelial intracellular calcium release, and increases endothelial nitric oxide synthase (eNOS) activity.[108] Ang IV also stimulates PI3K and phosphatidylinositol-dependent kinase 1 (PDK1) activity and induces phosphorylation of protein kinase B and ERK1/2.[109] These multiple kinase pathways are thought to regulate the cellular proliferative effects of the peptide. Ang IV induces plasminogen activator inhibitor 1 expression in endothelial cells, suggesting a role for Ang IV in fibrinolysis. Ang IV also activates the NF-κB pathway and increases proinflammatory genes in VSMC.[94] Recent studies have shown that Ang IV/AT_4R may counteract Ang II/AGTR1-mediated cardiovascular events, such as blood pressure control, cell growth, and cardiac function.[110,111] These data suggest that this Ang II degradation peptide could participate in the pathogenesis of cardiovascular diseases. However, the overall importance of AT_4R-mediated signaling in cardiovascular diseases needs to be further clarified. In this chapter, our primary focus will be on the signaling pathways mediated by AGTR1 and AGTR2.

AGTR1-Mediated Classic G Protein-Dependent Signaling Pathways

Like other seven-membrane-spanning domain receptor family members, agonist binding to the AGTR1 initiates a multitude of intracellular events. AGTR1 couples to the $Gq/_{11}$ protein, which stimulates phospholipase C (PLC) to generate the second messengers diacylglycerol (DAG) and

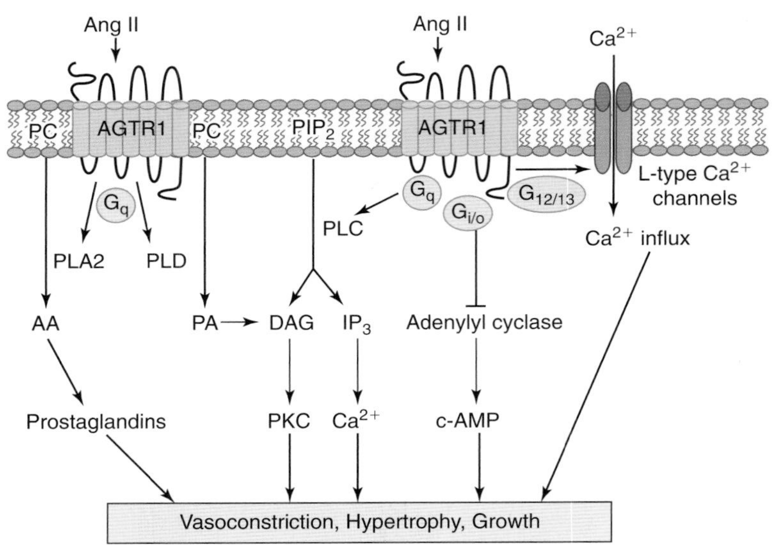

FIGURE 5-6 Classic signal transduction pathways mediated by AGTR1. Binding of Ang II to AGTR1 leads to G protein-coupled activation of PLC (phospholipase C) via Gq, resulting in phosphatidylinositol hydrolysis and formation of IP_3 (inositol trisphosphate) and DAG (diacylglycerol) accumulation. IP_3 mobilizes Ca^{2+} from sarcoplasmic reticular stores and DAG activates PKC (protein kinase C). Both PKC- and calcium-mediated signaling are involved in vasoconstriction and cardiac hypertrophy. AGTR1 couple to $G_{i/o}$ resulting in inhibition of adenylyl cyclase and attenuation of cAMP production, leading to vasoconstriction. Activation of phospholipase A_2 (PLA_2) leads to production of arachidonic acid (AA) and the generation of prostaglandins. AGTR1 coupling to $G_{12/13}$ results in the opening of L-type Ca^{2+} channels and increases the influx of extracellular Ca^{2+}. *PIP2,* Phosphatidylinositol bisphosphate; *PC,* phosphatidylcholine.

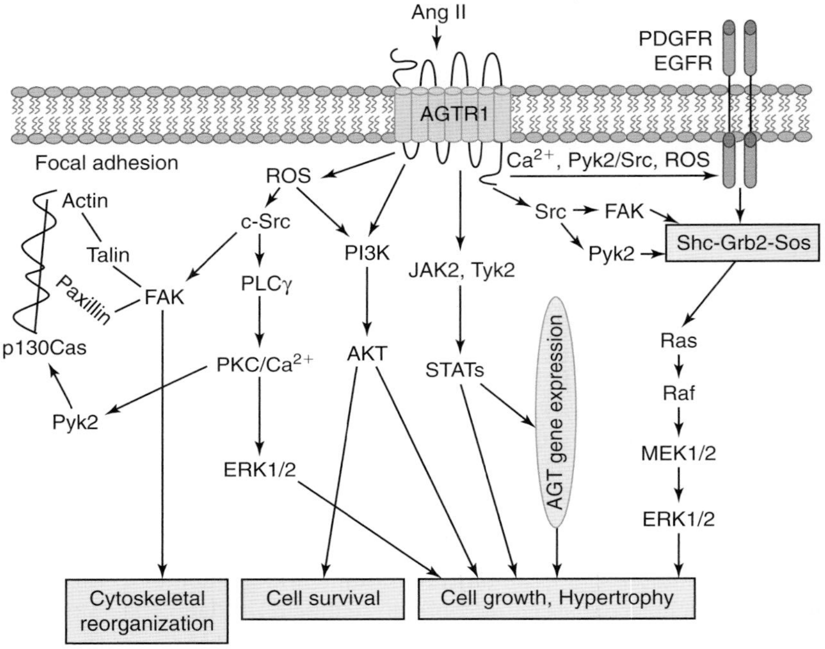

FIGURE 5-7 Ang II induces activation of tyrosine kinases through AGTR1. Ang II influences the activity of receptor tyrosine kinases, such as EGFR (epidermal growth factor receptor) and PDGFR (platelet-derived growth factor receptor). The transactivation event is mediated by several intermediary signaling molecules, including Ca^{2+}, PKC, Pyk2, Src, and reactive oxygen species (ROS). The transactivated EGFR serves as a scaffold for downstream adapters, leading to activation of MAPKs. Ang II also phosphorylates multiple nonreceptor tyrosine kinases, such as JAK-STAT, FAK, Pyk2, p130Cas, and PI3K. Activated tyrosine kinases phosphorylate many downstream targets, which regulate Ang II-induced cellular effects.

inositol trisphosphate (IP_3). DAG activates protein kinase C (PKC) and IP_3 binds to its receptor on sarcoplasmic reticulum, opening a channel that allows calcium efflux into the cytoplasm (see also Chapter 1). Ang II-induced phospholipase D (PLD) activation results in hydrolysis of phosphatidylcholine to choline and phosphatidic acid (PA). PA is rapidly converted to DAG, leading to sustained activation of PKC. Both PKC- and calcium-mediated signaling are involved in vasoconstriction and cardiac hypertrophy.[112,113] Ang II has been shown to phosphorylate and activate phospholipase A_2 (PLA_2), which leads to production of arachidonic acid (AA), the precursor molecule for generation of prostaglandins, and which is involved in the Ang II-induced growth of VSMC and cardiac hypertrophy. AGTR1 also couples to $G_{i/o}$, inhibiting adenylyl cyclase in several target tissues, thereby attenuating the production of the second messenger cAMP and resulting in vasoconstriction. AGTR1 is also involved in the opening of Ca^{2+} channels and an influx of extracellular Ca^{2+} into cells. The activation of L-type Ca^{2+} channels is mediated by AGTR1 coupled to $G_{12/13}$ proteins (**Figure 5-6**).

AGTR1-Mediated Transactivation of Receptor Tyrosine Kinases (see also Chapter 1)

Transactivation of receptor tyrosine kinases (RTKs), by GPCR agonists, is a general phenomenon that has been demonstrated for many unrelated GPCRs and RTKs.[114] It has been reported that Ang II transactivates the epidermal growth factor receptor (EGFR), platelet-derived growth factor receptor (PDGFR), and insulin-like growth factor 1 receptor (IGF-1R) in a variety of cell types, through AGTR1 (**Figure 5-7**).[115,116] Transactivation of EGFR is mediated by several intermediary signaling molecules, including Ca^{2+}, PKC, Pyk2, Src, and reactive oxygen species (ROS).[117] Blocking EGFR kinase activity abolishes Ang II-mediated downstream signaling in VSMC and cardiomyocytes, suggesting that transactivation of EGFR accounts for the majority of growth-promoting responses induced by Ang II.[115,117] Ang II-induced transactivation of the IGF-1 receptor is a critical mediator of PI3K activation.[116] In contrast to EGFR transactivation, Ang II-induced PDGFR transactivation may be ligand independent, requiring an ROS-sensitive kinase distinct from Src or JAK2.[118] Ang II-induced transactivation of the PDGFR has also been shown to contribute to cardiac hypertrophy and vascular remodeling.[119,120]

AGTR1-Mediated Activation of Tyrosine Kinases (see also Chapter 1)

Tyrosine kinases activated by AGTR1 include the Src family kinases, Janus kinases (JAKs), focal adhesion kinase (FAK), Ca^{2+}-dependent tyrosine kinases (e.g., Pyk2), p130Cas, and phosphoinositide 3-OH kinase (PI3K).[121] These AGTR1-regulated tyrosine kinases seem to be required for Ang II effects, such as vasoconstriction, proto-oncogene expression, and protein synthesis. Thus understanding these signaling events mediated by AGTR1 may form the basis for the development of new therapies for cardiovascular diseases.

Src Family Kinases

Studies have demonstrated that Src family kinases, such as c-Src, have an important role in regulation of growth responses induced by Ang II.[122] The Src kinase family consists of at least 14 members, of which the 60-kDa c-Src is a prototype of the cellular members of the Src family kinases (Src, Fyn, Yes, Fgr, Lck, Lyn, Hck, Blk, and Yrk). All Src family members share common functional domains, including an N-terminal myristoylation sequence for membrane targeting, SH2 and SH3 domains for protein binding, and a kinase domain and C-terminal noncatalytic domain. It has been shown that c-Src is activated by $G_{\beta\gamma}$ in an ROS-dependent manner and is involved in activation of a variety of downstream pathways. Src-induced activation of PLCγ, which is a substrate for members of the Src kinase family, promotes release of Ca^{2+} from intracellular stores. Src is also required for Ang II-induced activation of ERK1/2, Pyk2, and several downstream proteins, including FAK, paxillin, JAK2, STAT1, caveolin, and the adapter protein Shc, indicating that activation of Src has a pivotal role in Ang II-mediated cytoskeletal reorganization, focal adhesion formation, cell migration, and growth (see Figure 5-7).

FAK and PYK 2 Activation

FAK and PYK2, also referred to as *cell adhesion kinase, related adhesion focal tyrosine kinase,* or *calcium-dependent protein tyrosine kinase,* are localized prominently within focal adhesions. Activation of FAK and PYK2 has been implicated in the progression of cardiomyocyte hypertrophy and in Ang II-mediated cellular effects.[123,124] As a consequence of association with c-Src, FAK undergoes further tyrosine phosphorylation, resulting in FAK binding to Grb2, Sos, and Ras, leading to ERK1/2 activation. Ang II rapidly induces tyrosine phosphorylation of FAK, allowing for cell adhesion to the extracellular matrix and activation of cytoskeletal proteins, including p130Cas, Pyk2, paxillin, and talin, all of which interact to regulate cell shape and movement. The interaction between p130Cas, Pyk2, and PI3K activates ribosomal $p70^{S6}$ kinase, which has an important role in Ang II-mediated protein synthesis (see Figure 5-7). The activation of Pyk2, a FAK homologue, is dependent on increased intracellular Ca^{2+} and PKC.[125] Since Pyk2 is a candidate to regulate c-Src and links G protein-coupled vasoconstrictor receptors with protein tyrosine kinase-mediated contractile, migratory, and growth responses, it may represent a point of convergence between Ca^{2+}-dependent signaling pathways and protein tyrosine kinase pathways, in cardiovascular cells.

JAK/STAT Activation

The Janus kinase (JAK)-signal transducer and activator of transcription (STAT) pathway is involved in a wide range of distinct cellular processes, including inflammation, apoptosis, cell-cycle regulation, and development. There are four JAK proteins in mammalian cells, JAK1, JAK2, JAK3, and TYK2.[126] JAK proteins, named after the Roman two-faced mythical god Janus, function as cytosolic tyrosine kinases and induce a cascade of phosphorylation steps that result in the activation of STAT proteins. Tyrosine phosphorylation of STATs leads to STAT homo- and heterodimerization and nuclear translocation. In the heart, the JAK-STAT pathway is involved in ischemia/reperfusion injury, hypertrophy, and postpartum cardiomyopathy.[127,128] AGTR1 activates JAK2 and Tyk2, which subsequently activates STAT proteins p91/84 (STAT1), p113 (STAT2), and p92 (STAT3) in the cardiovascular system, and has an important role in Ang II-mediated vascular and cardiac growth, remodeling, and repair.[127] Studies also showed that activation of STAT5A and STAT6 promotes the binding of STATs to the St-domain of AGT, resulting in increases in gene expression.[129] Blockade of AGTR1 signaling or inhibition of JAK2 activation suppresses formation of the STATs/ST-domain complex and reduces gene expression of AGT. These studies support a role for an Ang II autocrine loop in JAK-STAT signaling and cardiac injury. Ang II-induced activation of JAK2 is also an important step in the development of diabetic vascular complications.[130]

Phosphoinositide 3-OH Kinase (see also Chapter 1)

PI3Ks are a family of lipid and protein kinases responsible for the phosphorylation of phosphatidylinositol (PtdIns) at position D3 of the inositol ring. PI3Ks are classified by substrate specificity and subunit organization.[131] Class IA PI3Ks are heterodimeric proteins, each of which consists of a catalytic subunit of 110 to 120 kDa (p110α, β, and δ) and an associated regulatory subunit (p85α and β), that are essential for interaction of these PI3Ks with receptor tyrosine kinases. The class IB PI3K (PI3Kγ) is activated by heterotrimeric G-protein subunits and associates with a p101 adapter required for full responsiveness to $G_{\beta\gamma}$ heterodimers. Class II PI3Ks are distinguished by a carboxy-terminal C2 domain, which is not found in other PI3Ks. Class III PI3K, Vps34, only produces PtdIns3P. PI3Kα, which is activated by RTK, appears to have a critical role in the induction of physiologic cardiac growth, but not pathologic growth, and appears essential for maintaining contractile function in response to pathologic stimuli.[132] PI3Kγ appears to negatively control cardiac contractility through different signaling mechanisms and as a key mediator of NADPH oxidase activation in response to Ang II.[133,134] Akt/PKB has been identified as an important downstream target of PI3K in Ang II-activated cardiomyocytes and VSMC.[135] It regulates protein synthesis by activating p70 S6-kinase and modulates Ang II-mediated Ca^{2+} responses by stimulating Ca^{2+} channel currents. Akt/PKB has also been implicated in promoting cell survival by influencing Bcl-2 and c-Myc expression and inhibiting caspases.

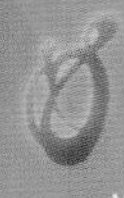

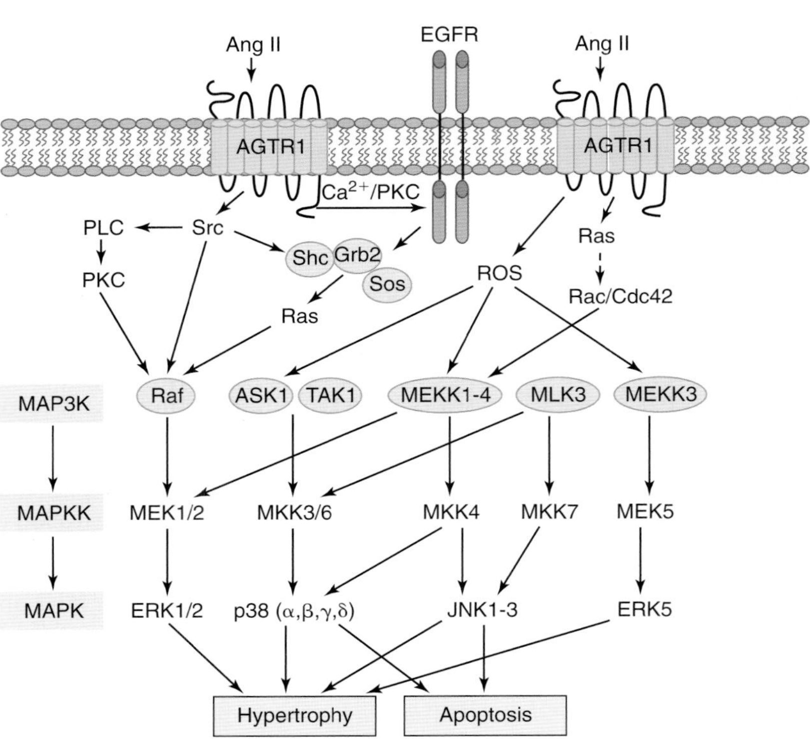

FIGURE 5-8 Schematic diagram of the major MAPK cascades stimulated by AGTR1. The MAKP pathway is a three-module cascade of phosphorylating kinases: MEKK(MAP3K)/MEK(MAPKK)/MAPK. This pathway consists of several subfamilies among which are the ERK, JNK, and p38 MAPK pathways. Each is activated by heterotrimeric G proteins coupled to AGTR1 by Ang II-induced transactivation of EGFR; by small G proteins (such as Ras, cdc42, Rac); by protein kinases (such as Src); by PKC, via activation of PLC; and by ROS.

AGTR1-Mediated Activation of Mitogen-Activated Protein Kinases

Mitogen-activated protein kinase (MAPK) consists of a series of successively acting kinases that function as central regulators of cell growth, differentiation, and transformation. All of the MAPK members are catalytically inactive in resting cells and are activated in response to an appropriate stimulus by phosphorylation on both threonine and tyrosine residues. This phosphorylation is regulated through a dual specificity MAPKK (MAP kinase kinase), which in turn is activated through phosphorylation by a MAPKKK (MAP kinase kinase kinase).[136] Once activated, MAPKs directly phosphorylate a diverse array of cytoplasmic, nuclear, and mitochondrial proteins to modulate gene expression, cellular metabolism, cellular physiology, and cell death.[137] At least four distinctly regulated groups of MAPKs are expressed in mammals: extracellular signal-related kinases (ERK)-1/2, c-Jun N-terminal kinases (JNK1/2/3), p38 proteins (p38α/β/γ/δ), and ERK5, all of which are activated by specific MKKs (**Figure 5-8**). Each MKK can be activated by more than one MEKK, increasing the complexity and diversity of MAPK signaling. Ang II induces phosphorylation of Ras, Raf, and Shc, leading to the activation of MEKKs and MEKs, resulting in tyrosine and threonine phosphorylation of ERK1/2, JNK2, and p38. Ang II-induced activation of ERK1/2 is associated with increased expression of the early response genes c-fos, c-myc, and c-jun, DNA/protein synthesis, cell growth and differentiation, and cytoskeletal organization in cardiovascular cells.[138] The ERK1/2 signaling pathway is involved in mediating the effects of the brain RAS on sympathetic nerve activity in heart failure, suggesting that manipulating brain ERK1/2 signaling could ameliorate the adverse effects of the brain RAS on cardiovascular and renal function during the progression of heart failure.[139] Activation of JNKs by Ang II is involved in regulation of cardiomyocyte and VSMC growth.[140,141] Cardiac-specific activation of p38 MAPK markedly attenuated cardiac contractility.[142] Studies have also demonstrated that p38 activation is preferentially associated with the direct effects of Ang II on cardiac cells, whereas stimulation of ERK and JNK occurs in association with Ang II-induced mechanical stress.[143] These results suggest that MAPKs may provide a novel therapeutic approach to the Ang II-dependent pathophysiology, which accompanies progression of heart failure.

Small GTP-Binding Proteins

The small GTP-binding protein (small G protein) superfamily comprises a multitude of monomeric proteins (over 150 members in humans) that regulate a wide variety of cellular processes, such as cell division, migration, and differentiation. They are structurally classified into at least five families, including the following: Ras (e.g., Ras, Rap, and Ral); Rho (RhoA, Rac1, and cdc42); Rab; Sar1/Arf; and Ran.[144] Small G proteins act as molecular switches, cycling between an active GTP-bound state and an inactive GDP-bound state (**Figure 5-9**). Activated Ras proteins interact with multiple downstream effectors (Raf/MEK1/2/ERK1/2 and PI3K) to regulate gene expression, cell proliferation, differentiation, and survival; the Rho GTPases (RhoA/Rac1/cdc42) regulate cytoskeletal reorganization and gene expression; the Rab and Sar1/Arf families regulate vesicle trafficking; and the Ran family regulates nucleocytoplasmic transport and microtubule organization. Ang II-induced activation of p21 Ras is regulated through activation of the Src family kinases and tyrosine phosphorylation of the adapter protein Shc, with subsequent recruitment of the Grb2-Sos1 complex to the membrane fraction (see Figure 5-8).[145] It has been demonstrated that Rho/Rho kinase-mediated signaling is involved in AGTR1-stimulated cardiovascular cell growth, remodeling, atherosclerosis, and vascular contraction.[146] Rho A is also involved in Ang II-induced activation of NF-κB, which controls the expression of inducible cytokines,

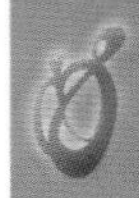

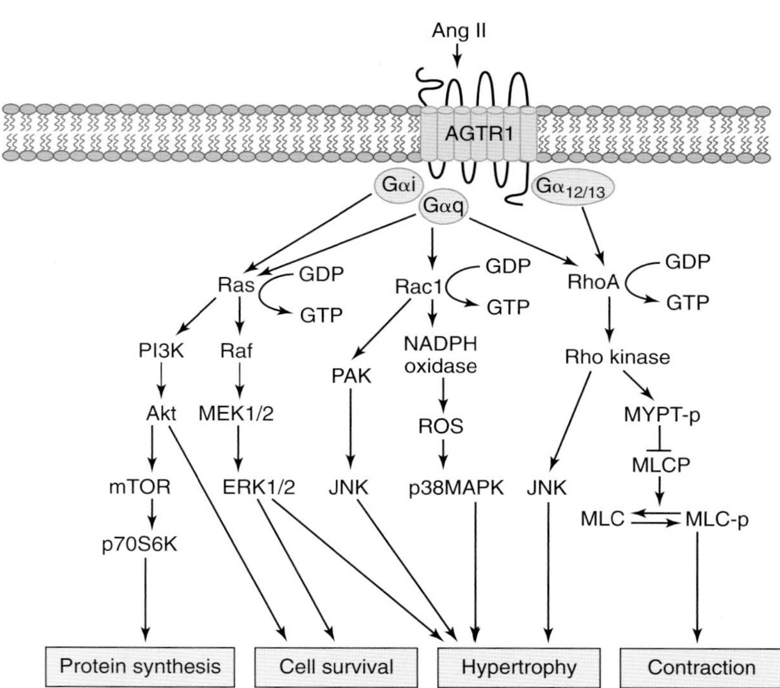

FIGURE 5-9 Regulation of Ang II-induced cellular responses through activation of small GTPases. Ang II stimulates Ras, RhoA, and Rac1 through a process dependent upon activation of a G protein-coupled receptor at the plasma membrane. Small GTPases cycle between a GDP-bound inactive form and a GTP-bound active form. Activated Ras mediated by Gq and Gi regulates the activation of PI3K (phosphatidylinositol-3 kinase) and Raf, the latter being one of the earliest components in the ERK MAPK cascade, which regulates cell survival and cardiac hypertrophy. PI3K modulates cell survival and protein synthesis through Akt and p70S6K. Rac1 activates NADPH oxidase, which in turn regulates generation of ROS. Rac1 also induces the activation of the JNK pathway, through PAK. RhoA regulates cytoskeleton- and hypertrophy-related gene expression, through Rho kinase.

chemokines, cell adhesion molecules, and vasoactive and antiapoptotic proteins important in the cellular stress response.[147] Ang II also activates Rac1, another Rho GTPase, which is an upstream regulator of p21-activated kinase (PAK) and JNK. Rac1 participates in cytoskeletal organization, cell growth, inflammation, and cardiac hypertrophy. It has been demonstrated that Rac-derived superoxide in the cardiovascular system has a diverse array of functions.[148] Rac1 controls intracellular superoxide production by regulating the activity of nicotinamide adenine dinucleotide phosphate (NADPH) oxidase. NADPH oxidase-produced superoxide is an essential mediator of the hypertensive and hypertrophic responses to Ang II.[149] These results suggest that small G proteins of the Rho and Ras families may serve as key components in Ang II/AGTR1-mediated cardiac hypertrophy and heart failure.

Generation of Reactive Oxygen Species (see also Chapter 8)

Accumulating evidence suggests that production of ROS and activation of redox-dependent signaling cascades are critically involved in Ang II-induced actions[150] and have an important role in the development and progression of heart failure, regardless of cause.[151] ROS function as important intercellular second messengers to modulate downstream signaling molecules, such as protein tyrosine phosphatases, protein tyrosine kinases, transcription factors, MAPKs, and ion channels (**Figure 5-10**); they have a physiologic role in vascular tone and cell growth, and a pathophysiologic role in inflammation, ischemia-reperfusion, hypertension, and atherosclerosis. All cardiovascular cell types are capable of producing ROS, and the major enzymatic sources in heart failure are mitochondria, xanthine oxidases, and the nonphagocytic NADPH oxidases (Noxs). NAD(P)H oxidase activity is significantly enhanced and involved in Ang II-induced cardiac and vascular remodeling.[149,152] Studies have demonstrated that mitochondria are the predominant source of ROS and mitochondrial oxidative stress has an important role in Ang II-induced cardiac hypertrophy and heart failure.[153,154] Activation of xanthine oxidase is also involved in Ang II-induced endothelial oxidant stress,[155] and an elevation of xanthine oxidase expression and activity has been documented in end-stage human heart failure.[156] Thus an improved understanding of the specific roles of different ROS sources in redox signaling processes involved in the development of heart failure may result in the development of new therapeutic strategies.

AGTR2-Mediated Intracellular Signaling

Although structurally related to G protein-coupled receptors, AGTR2 displays atypical signal transduction and G protein-coupling mechanisms. It has been shown that AGTR2 mainly couple to intracellular signaling pathways through the pertussis toxin (PTX)-sensitive G proteins $G_i\alpha_2$ and $G_i\alpha_3$.[157] The intracellular signaling pathways of AGTR2 have been studied extensively; however, only a few have been well characterized.[158] We will focus on several signaling pathways (**Figure 5-11**), through which AGTR2 mediates cardiovascular actions.

Activation of Protein Phosphatases and Protein Dephosphorylation

Studies have shown that activation of AGTR2 rapidly induces activation of protein tyrosine phosphatase (PTPase) and serine/threonine phosphatases, resulting in dephosphorylation and inactivation of corresponding tyrosine kinases, and serves to reverse, or counter-regulate, the cell proliferative- and growth-promoting effects mediated by the various protein kinases in response to AGTR1 activation.[159] AGTR2 stimulation results in activation of MAPK phosphatase 1 (MKP-1), SH2 domain-containing phosphatase 1 (SHP-1), and PP2A, thereby inhibiting AGTR1-mediated MAP kinase activation, which is associated with AGTR2-mediated antigrowth and proapoptotic effects. Additionally, the activation

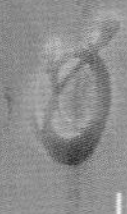

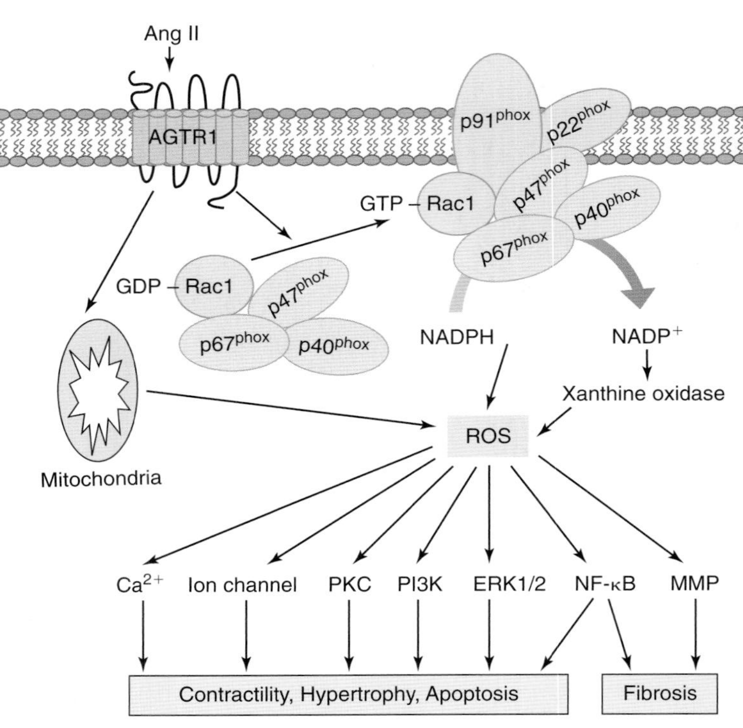

FIGURE 5-10 ROS-mediated signaling in Ang II-induced cardiac remodeling. Major enzymatic sources for intracellular ROS generation in response to Ang II are mitochondria, xanthine oxidases, and the nonphagocytic NADPH oxidases (Noxs). NADPH oxidase is a multisubunit enzyme consisting of gp91phox, p22phox, p47phox, p67phox, and p40phox, which is regulated by Rac1, via AGTR1. Intracellular ROS modify the activity of protein tyrosine kinases (PTK), such as Src, Ras, JAK2, Pyk2, PI3K, and EGFR, as well as MAPKs. ROS also influence gene and protein expression by activating transcription factors, such as NF-κB and activator protein-1 (AP-1). ROS stimulate ion channels, such as plasma membrane Ca^{2+} and K^+ channels, leading to changes in cation concentrations. Activation of these redox-sensitive pathways results in numerous cellular responses, which if uncontrolled, could contribute to the Ang II-induced cardiovascular remodeling process, including cardiac hypertrophy, fibrosis, apoptosis, and impaired heart function.

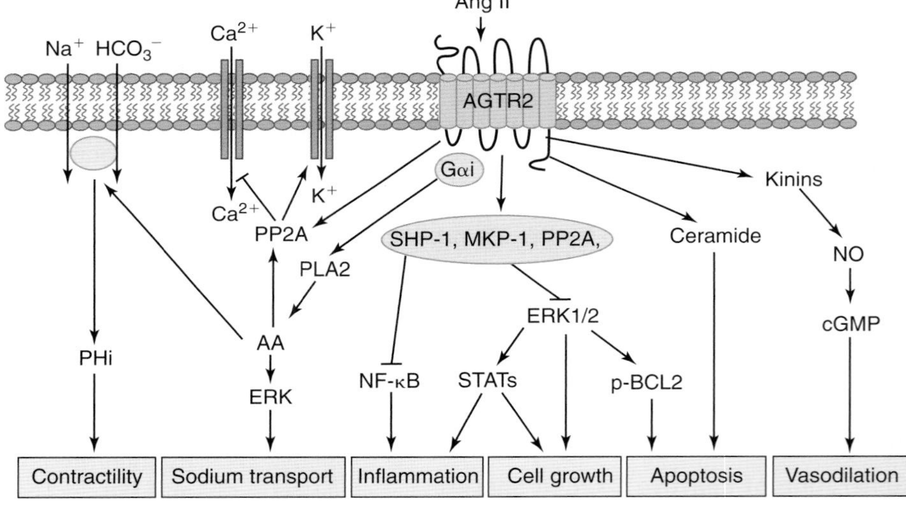

FIGURE 5-11 Signal transduction pathways and physiologic effects of the AGTR2. AGTR2 signaling pathways, include activation of protein phosphatases such as MKP-1, PP2A, and SHP-1, which result in dephosphorylation and inactivation of ERK1/2 and STATs; the NO–cGMP system; and activation of PLA2 (phospholipase A2), which mediates the release of arachidonic acid and contributes to activation of the Na^+/HCO_3^- symporter system and regulation of intracellular pH. PP2A activation also results in the opening of potassium channels and inhibition of T-type Ca^{2+} channels. AGTR2-associated apoptosis is regulated by ceramide-mediated signaling.

of phosphatases is also involved in the anti-inflammatory effect of AGTR2 through inactivation of NF-κB and JAK-STAT signaling pathways.[160,161]

The Nitric Oxide-Cyclic GMP System

Recent studies have shown that activation of AGTR2 by Ang II results in a bradykinin-dependent stimulation of aortic NO release, with subsequent generation of cGMP.[162] The connection between AGTR2 and cGMP/NO has also been made through in vivo studies in cardiovascular tissues. Inhibition of cardiac AGTR2 in hypertrophied heart amplifies the AGTR1-mediated left ventricular growth response, via suppression of cGMP. In stroke-prone spontaneously hypertensive rat, the AGTR2-mediated increase in aortic cGMP was mediated by activation of bradykinin BK2 receptors, which in turn activated NO synthase, leading to NO production.[163] These studies suggest that AGTR2 stimulate production of NO, resulting in an increased formation of the second messenger cGMP. cGMP, in turn, mediates many of the biologic actions of NO, such as vasodilation, natriuresis, and antigrowth, by activating a cGMP-dependent protein kinase. These effects also contribute to the beneficial actions of AGTR1 blockers in the treatment of hypertension.

Stimulation of Phospholipase A2 and Release of Arachidonic Acid

It has been reported that AGTR2 activation is related to Na^+ transport through activation of PLA2 and release of arachidonic acid (AA) and the cytochrome P450-dependent metabolites. This pathway leads to MAPK activation, as well as p21 ras activation, via the tyrosine kinase-Shc-Grb2-Sos pathway.[164,165] AGTR2 have also been reported to mediate sustained AA release in cardiomyocytes, contributing to activation of the Na^+/HCO^- symporter system and regulation of intracellular pH, indicating that AGTR2 is also important for the regulation of intracellular acidosis following injury.[166] These studies provide evidence for an AT_2 signaling pathway, mediated through lipid second messengers.

Sphingolipid-Derived Ceramide

The AGTR2-activated signal transduction pathway associated with apoptosis involves ceramide.[167] Ceramide is a pro-apoptotic second messenger that activates several signaling pathways (PKC, protein phosphatase 1 or 2A, and cathepsin D) that are involved in proapoptotic events, including the suppression of Bcl-2 and activation of caspases.[168] These studies represent the initial observations that may lead to the use of ceramide signaling components as a therapeutic intervention for cardiovascular disease.

Although AGTR2 can couple to multiple signaling molecules in a fashion similar to many other hormone/neurotransmitter G protein-coupled receptors, it is apparent that much additional effort will be necessary to fully establish the various intracellular pathways that are coupled to AGTR2.

SUMMARY AND FUTURE DIRECTIONS

The RAS is a hormonal cascade that regulates cardiovascular, renal, and adrenal function. The circulatory system is important for regulation of fluid and electrolyte homeostasis and arterial pressure. The RAS has also been more recently characterized as a local, self-contained, paracrine, autocrine, and intracrine system. Tissue RASs are likely important in normal physiologic responses, as well as in pathophysiologic states such as hypertension, cardiac hypertrophy, congestive heart failure, and remodeling following myocardial infarction. The intracellular RAS likely does not represent an independent entity, but rather an extension or alternative form of a local RAS, which may be manifested only under select pathophysiologic conditions. This suggests a unique evolutionary role for the intracellular RAS. What remain to be determined are the mechanisms of regulation and actions, and a more precise understanding of the role of the intracellular RAS in (patho)physiology. Several novel components of the RAS, such as ACE2, Ang (1-7), Ang IV, and PRR, have an important role in cardiovascular pathophysiology. Future research will likely target these new components for the development of therapeutic interventions. Though major progress has been made in our understanding of the physiology and pathophysiology of the circulating RAS, it will be important to elucidate more completely the role of tissue RASs in normal physiology and in the pathophysiology of cardiovascular diseases.

References

1. Tigerstedt R, Bergman P: Niere und Kreislauf. *Skand Arch Physiol* 8:223, 1898.
2. Paul M, Poyan Mehr A, Kreutz R: Physiology of local renin-angiotensin systems. *Physiol Rev* 86:747, 2006.
3. Reudelhuber TL, Bernstein KE, Delafontaine P: Is angiotensin II a direct mediator of left ventricular hypertrophy? Time for another look. *Hypertension* 49:1196, 2007.
4. Crowley SD, Coffman TM: Recent advances involving the renin-angiotensin system. *Exp Cell Res* 318:1049, 2012.
5. Conti S, Cassis P, Benigni A: Aging and the renin-angiotensin system. *Hypertension* 60:878, 2012.
6. Hilliard LM, Sampson AK, Brown RD, et al: The "his and hers" of the renin-angiotensin system. *Curr Hypertens Rep* 15:71, 2013.
7. Matsusaka T, Niimura F, Shimizu A, et al: Liver angiotensinogen is the primary source of renal angiotensin II. *J Am Soc Nephrol* 23:1181, 2012.
8. Yiannikouris F, Gupte M, Putnam K, et al: Adipocyte deficiency of angiotensinogen prevents obesity-induced hypertension in male mice. *Hypertension* 60:1524, 2012.
9. Yiannikouris F, Karounos M, Charnigo R, et al: Adipocyte-specific deficiency of angiotensinogen decreases plasma angiotensinogen concentration and systolic blood pressure in mice. *Am J Physiol Regul Integr Comp Physiol* 302:R244, 2012.
10. Campbell DJ, Bouhnik J, Coezy E, et al: Characterization of precursor and secreted forms of human angiotensinogen. *J Clin Invest* 75:1880, 1985.
11. Zhou A, Carrell RW, Murphy MP, et al: A redox switch in angiotensinogen modulates angiotensin release. *Nature* 468:108, 2010.
12. Wu C, Lu H, Cassis LA, et al: Molecular and pathophysiological features of angiotensinogen: a mini review. *North Am Scand J Med Sci* 4:183, 2011.
13. Nguyen G, Delarue F, Burckle C, et al: Pivotal role of the renin/prorenin receptor in angiotensin II production and cellular responses to renin. *J Clin Invest* 109:1417, 2002.
14. Kang JJ, Toma I, Sipos A, et al: The collecting duct is the major source of prorenin in diabetes. *Hypertension* 51:1597, 2008.
15. Sealey JE, Glorioso N, Itskovitz J, et al: Ovarian prorenin. *Clin Exp Hypertens A* 9:1435, 1987.
16. Batenburg WW, Danser AH: (Pro)renin and its receptors: pathophysiological implications. *Clin Sci (Lond)* 123:121, 2012.
17. Fuchs S, Xiao HD, Hubert C, et al: Angiotensin-converting enzyme C-terminal catalytic domain is the main site of angiotensin I cleavage in vivo. *Hypertension* 51:267, 2008.
18. Shen XZ, Ong FS, Bernstein EA, et al: Nontraditional roles of angiotensin-converting enzyme. *Hypertension* 59:763, 2012.
19. Re RN: Tissue renin angiotensin systems. *Med Clin North Am* 88:19, 2004.
20. van Kats JP, Danser AHJ, van Maegen J, et al: Angiotensin production in the heart: a quantitative study with use of radiolabelled angiotensin infusions. *Circulation* 98:73, 1998.
21. Dostal DE, Baker KM: The cardiac renin-angiotensin system: conceptual, or a regulator of cardiac function? *Circ Res* 85:643, 1999.
22. Dell'Italia LJ, Meng QC, Balcells E, et al: Compartmentalization of angiotensin II generation in the dog heart. Evidence for independent mechanisms in intravascular and interstitial spaces. *J Clin Invest* 100:253, 1997.
23. Heller LJ, Opsahl JA, Wernsing SE, et al: Myocardial and plasma renin-angiotensinogen dynamics during pressure-induced cardiac hypertrophy. *Am J Physiol* 274:R849, 1998.
24. Catanzaro DF: Physiological relevance of renin/prorenin binding and uptake. *Hypertens Res* 28:97, 2005.
25. Muller DN, Fischli W, Clozel JP, et al: Local angiotensin II generation in the rat heart: role of renin uptake. *Circ Res* 82:13, 1998.
26. Peters J, Farrenkopf R, Clausmeyer S, et al: Functional significance of prorenin internalization in the rat heart. *Circ Res* 90:1135, 2002.
27. Peters J: Secretory and cytosolic (pro)renin in kidney, heart, and adrenal gland. *J Mol Med* 86:711, 2008.
28. Zhang X, Dostal DE, Reiss K, et al: Identification and activation of autocrine renin-angiotensin system in adult ventricular myocytes. *Am J Physiol* 269:H1791, 1995.
29. Singh VP, Le B, Khode R, et al: Intracellular angiotensin II production in diabetic rats is correlated with cardiomyocyte apoptosis, oxidative stress, and cardiac fibrosis. *Diabetes* 57:3297, 2008.
30. Singh VP, Le B, Bhat VB, et al: High glucose induced regulation of intracellular angiotensin II synthesis and nuclear redistribution in cardiac myocytes. *Am J Physiol Heart Circ Physiol* 293:H939, 2007.
31. Sun Y, Zhang J, Zhang JQ, et al: Renin expression at sites of repair in the infarcted rat heart. *J Mol Cell Cardiol* 33:995, 2001.
32. Barlucchi L, Leri A, Dostal DE, et al: Canine ventricular myocytes possess a renin-angiotensin system that is upregulated with heart failure. *Circ Res* 88:298, 2001.
33. Clausmeyer S, Reinecke A, Farrenkopf R, et al: Tissue-specific expression of a rat renin transcript lacking the coding sequence for the prefragment and its stimulation by myocardial infarction. *Endocrinology* 141:2963, 2000.
34. Singh VP, Le B, Khode R, et al: Intracellular angiotensin II production in diabetic rats is correlated with cardiomyocyte apoptosis, oxidative stress, and cardiac fibrosis. *Diabetes* 57:3297, 2008.
35. Singh VP, Baker KM, Kumar R: Activation of the intracellular renin-angiotensin system in cardiac fibroblasts by high glucose: role in extracellular matrix production. *Am J Physiol Heart Circ Physiol* 294:H1675, 2008.
36. Singh VP, Le B, Bhat VB, et al: High-glucose-induced regulation of intracellular Ang II synthesis and nuclear redistribution in cardiac myocytes. *Am J Physiol Heart Circ Physiol* 293:H939, 2007.
37. Hokimoto S, Yasue H, Fujimoto K, et al: Increased angiotensin converting enzyme activity in left ventricular aneurysm of patients after myocardial infarction. *Cardiovasc Res* 29:664, 1995.
38. Diez J, Panizo A, Hernandez M, et al: Cardiomyocyte apoptosis and cardiac angiotensin-converting enzyme in spontaneously hypertensive rats. *Hypertension* 30:1029, 1997.
39. Dostal DE, Rothblum KN, Conrad KM, et al: Detection of angiotensin I and II in cultured rat cardiac myocytes and fibroblasts. *Am J Physiol* 263:C851, 1992.
40. Jahanyar J, Youker KA, Loebe M, et al: Mast cell-derived cathepsin g: a possible role in the adverse remodeling of the failing human heart. *J Surg Res* 140:199, 2007.
41. Holycross BJ, Saye J, Harrison JK, et al: Polymerase chain reaction analysis of renin in rat aortic smooth muscle. *Hypertension* 19:697, 1992.
42. Hu WY, Fukuda N, Satoh C, et al: Phenotypic modulation by fibronectin enhances the angiotensin II-generating system in cultured vascular smooth muscle cells. *Arterioscler Thromb Vasc Biol* 20:1500, 2000.
43. Lavrentyev EN, Estes AM, Malik KU: Mechanism of high glucose induced angiotensin II production in rat vascular smooth muscle cells. *Circ Res* 101:455, 2007.
44. Balcells E, Meng QC, Johnson WH, Jr, et al: Angiotensin II formation from ACE and chymase in human and animal hearts: methods and species considerations. *Am J Physiol* 273:H1769, 1997.
45. Wolny A, Clozel JP, Rein J, et al: Functional and biochemical analysis of angiotensin II-forming pathways in the human heart. *Circ Res* 80:219, 1997.
46. Li P, Chen PM, Wang SW, et al: Time-dependent expression of chymase and angiotensin converting enzyme in the hamster heart under pressure overload. *Hypertens Res* 25:757, 2002.
47. Chen LY, Li P, He Q, et al: Transgenic study of the function of chymase in heart remodeling. *J Hypertens* 20:2047, 2002.
48. Takai S, Jin D, Miyazaki M: Multiple mechanisms for the action of chymase inhibitors. *J Pharmacol Sci* 118:311, 2012.
49. Kumar R, Boim MA: Diversity of pathways for intracellular angiotensin II synthesis. *Curr Opin Nephrol Hypertens* 18:33, 2009.
50. Bruckshlegel GHS, Jandeleit K, Grimm D, et al: Blockade of renin-angiotensin system in cardiac pressure overload hypertrophy in rats. *Hypertension* 25:250, 1995.
51. Malhotra R, Sadoshima J, Brosius FC, 3rd, et al: Mechanical stretch and angiotensin II differentially upregulate the renin-angiotensin system in cardiac myocytes in vitro. *Circ Res* 85:137, 1999.
52. Fukuzawa J, Booz GW, Hunt RA, et al: Cardiotrophin-1 increases angiotensinogen mRNA in rat cardiac myocytes through STAT3: an autocrine loop for hypertrophy. *Hypertension* 35:1191, 2000.
53. Dostal DE, Booz GW, Baker KM: Regulation of angiotensinogen gene expression and protein in neonatal rat cardiac fibroblasts by glucocorticoid and beta-adrenergic stimulation. *Basic Res Cardiol* 95:485, 2000.
54. Booz GW, Baker KM: *Intracellular signaling and the cardiac renin angiotensin system*, West Sussex, England, 2004, John Wiley & Sons.
55. Kumar R, Singh VP, Baker KM: The intracellular renin-angiotensin system: a new paradigm. *Trends Endocrinol Metab* 18:208, 2007.
56. Kumar R, Yong QC, Thomas CM, et al: Review: intracardiac intracellular angiotensin system in diabetes. *Am J Physiol Regul Integr Comp Physiol* 302:R510, 2012.
57. Singh VP, Baker KM, Kumar R: Activation of the intracellular renin-angiotensin system in cardiac fibroblasts by high glucose: role in extracellular matrix production. *Am J Physiol Heart Circ Physiol* 294:H1675, 2008.

58. Frustaci A, Kajstura J, Chimenti C, et al: Myocardial cell death in human diabetes. *Circ Res* 87:1123, 2000.
59. Booz GW, Conrad KM, Hess AL, et al: Angiotensin-II-binding sites on hepatocyte nuclei. *Endocrinology* 130:3641, 1992.
60. Re RN, Vizard DL, Brown J, et al: Angiotensin II receptors in chromatin fragments generated by micrococcal nuclease. *Biochem Biophys Res Commun* 119:220, 1984.
61. Gwathmey TM, Alzayadneh EM, Pendergrass KD, et al: Review: novel roles of nuclear angiotensin receptors and signaling mechanisms. *Am J Physiol Regul Integr Comp Physiol* 302:R518, 2012.
62. Eggena P, Zhu JH, Clegg K, et al: Nuclear angiotensin receptors induce transcription of renin and angiotensinogen mRNA. *Hypertension* 22:496, 1993.
63. Re RN: The intracellular renin angiotensin system: the tip of the intracrine physiology iceberg. *Am J Physiol Heart Circ Physiol* 293:H905, 2007.
64. Baker KM, Chernin MI, Schreiber T, et al: Evidence of a novel intracrine mechanism in angiotensin II-induced cardiac hypertrophy. *Regul Pept* 120:5, 2004.
65. Haller H, Lindschau C, Erdmann B, et al: Effects of intracellular angiotensin II in vascular smooth muscle cells. *Circ Res* 79:765, 1996.
66. Baker KM, Kumar R: Intracellular angiotensin II induces cell proliferation independent of AT1 receptor. *Am J Physiol Cell Physiol* 291:C995, 2006.
67. Kumar R, Singh VP, Baker KM: The intracellular renin-angiotensin system—implications in cardiovascular remodeling. *Curr Opin Nephrol Hypertens* 17:168, 2008.
68. Thomas CM, Yong QC, Seqqat R, et al: Direct renin inhibition prevents cardiac dysfunction in a diabetic mouse model: comparison with an angiotensin receptor antagonist and angiotensin converting enzyme inhibitor. *Clin Sci (Lond)* 124:529, 2013.
69. Castro CH, Santos RA, Ferreira AJ, et al: Evidence for a functional interaction of the angiotensin-(1-7) receptor Mas with AT1 and AT2 receptors in the mouse heart. *Hypertension* 46:937, 2005.
70. Kostenis E, Milligan G, Christopoulos A, et al: G-protein-coupled receptor Mas is a physiological antagonist of the angiotensin II type 1 receptor. *Circulation* 111:1806, 2005.
71. Passos-Silva D, Verano-Braga T, Santos R: Angiotensin-(1-7): beyond the cardio-renal actions. *Clin Sci (Lond)* 124:443, 2013.
72. Averill DB, Ishiyama Y, Chappell MC, et al: Cardiac angiotensin-(1-7) in ischemic cardiomyopathy. *Circulation* 108:2141, 2003.
73. Wei CC, Ferrario CM, Brosnihan KB, et al: Angiotensin peptides modulate bradykinin levels in the interstitium of the dog heart in vivo. *J Pharmacol Exp Ther* 300:324, 2002.
74. Santos RA, Ferreira AJ, Verano-Braga T, et al: Angiotensin-converting enzyme 2, angiotensin-(1-7) and Mas: new players of the renin-angiotensin system. *J Endocrinol* 216:R1, 2013.
75. McCollum LT, Gallagher PE, Ann Tallant E: Angiotensin-(1-7) attenuates angiotensin II-induced cardiac remodeling associated with upregulation of dual-specificity phosphatase 1. *Am J Physiol Heart Circ Physiol* 302:H801, 2012.
76. Zisman LS, Keller RS, Weaver B, et al: Increased angiotensin-(1-7)-forming activity in failing human heart ventricles: evidence for upregulation of the angiotensin-converting enzyme homologue ACE2. *Circulation* 108:1707, 2003.
77. Patel VB, Bodiga S, Basu R, et al: Loss of angiotensin-converting enzyme-2 exacerbates diabetic cardiovascular complications and leads to systolic and vascular dysfunction: a critical role of the angiotensin II/AT1 receptor axis. *Circ Res* 110:1322, 2012.
78. Crackower MA, Sarao R, Oudit GY, et al: Angiotensin-converting enzyme 2 is an essential regulator of heart function. *Nature* 417:822, 2002.
79. Der Sarkissian S, Grobe JL, Yuan L, et al: Cardiac overexpression of angiotensin converting enzyme 2 protects the heart from ischemia-induced pathophysiology. *Hypertension* 51:712, 2008.
80. Dong B, Yu QT, Dai HY, et al: Angiotensin-converting enzyme-2 overexpression improves left ventricular remodeling and function in a rat model of diabetic cardiomyopathy. *J Am Coll Cardiol* 59:739, 2012.
81. Donoghue M, Wakimoto H, Maguire CT, et al: Heart block, ventricular tachycardia, and sudden death in ACE2 transgenic mice with downregulated connexins. *J Mol Cell Cardiol* 35:1043, 2003.
82. Trask AJ, Averill DB, Ganten D, et al: Primary role of angiotensin-converting enzyme-2 in cardiac production of angiotensin-(1-7) in transgenic Ren-2 hypertensive rats. *Am J Physiol Heart Circ Physiol* 292:H3019, 2007.
83. Oudit GY, Kassiri Z, Patel MP, et al: Angiotensin II-mediated oxidative stress and inflammation mediate the age-dependent cardiomyopathy in ACE2 null mice. *Cardiovasc Res* 75:29, 2007.
84. Hernandez Prada JA, Ferreira AJ, Katovich MJ, et al: Structure-based identification of small-molecule angiotensin-converting enzyme 2 activators as novel antihypertensive agents. *Hypertension* 51:1312, 2008.
85. Marques FD, Ferreira AJ, Sinisterra RD, et al: An oral formulation of angiotensin-(1-7) produces cardioprotective effects in infarcted and isoproterenol-treated rats. *Hypertension* 57:477, 2011.
86. Reaux A, Fournie-Zaluski MC, Llorens-Cortes C: Angiotensin III: a central regulator of vasopressin release and blood pressure. *Trends Endocrinol Metab* 12:157, 2001.
87. Huang BS, Ahmad M, White RA, et al: Inhibition of brain angiotensin III attenuates sympathetic hyperactivity and cardiac dysfunction in rats post-myocardial infarction. *Cardiovasc Res* 97:424, 2013.
88. Padia SH, Kemp BA, Howell NL, et al: Conversion of renal angiotensin II to angiotensin III is critical for AT2 receptor-mediated natriuresis in rats. *Hypertension* 51:460, 2008.
89. Bodineau L, Frugiere A, Marc Y, et al: Orally active aminopeptidase A inhibitors reduce blood pressure: a new strategy for treating hypertension. *Hypertension* 51:1318, 2008.
90. Ruiz-Ortega M, Esteban V, Egido J: The regulation of the inflammatory response through nuclear factor-kappab pathway by angiotensin IV extends the role of the renin angiotensin system in cardiovascular diseases. *Trends Cardiovasc Med* 17:19, 2007.
91. Albiston AL, McDowall SG, Matsacos D, et al: Evidence that the angiotensin IV (AT(4)) receptor is the enzyme insulin-regulated aminopeptidase. *J Biol Chem* 276:48623, 2001.
92. Albiston AL, Fernando RN, Yeatman HR, et al: Gene knockout of insulin-regulated aminopeptidase: loss of the specific binding site for angiotensin IV and age-related deficit in spatial memory. *Neurobiol Learn Mem* 93:19, 2010.
93. Wallis MG, Lankford MF, Keller SR: Vasopressin is a physiological substrate for the insulin-regulated aminopeptidase IRAP. *Am J Physiol Endocrinol Metab* 293:E1092, 2007.
94. Esteban V, Ruperez M, Sanchez-Lopez E, et al: Angiotensin IV activates the nuclear transcription factor-kappaB and related proinflammatory genes in vascular smooth muscle cells. *Circ Res* 96:965, 2005.
95. Ahmad S, Wei CC, Tallaj J, et al: Chymase mediates angiotensin-(1-12) metabolism in normal human hearts. *J Am Soc Hypertens* 7:128, 2013.
96. Jankowski V, Vanholder R, van der Giet M, et al: Mass-spectrometric identification of a novel angiotensin peptide in human plasma. *Arterioscler Thromb Vasc Biol* 27:297, 2007.
97. Lautner RQ, Villela DC, Fraga-Silva RA, et al: Discovery and characterization of alamandine: a novel component of the renin-angiotensin system. *Circ Res* 112:1104, 2013.
98. Saris JJ, 't Hoen PA, Garrelds IM, et al: Prorenin induces intracellular signaling in cardiomyocytes independently of angiotensin II. *Hypertension* 48:564, 2006.
99. Schefe JH, Menk M, Reinemund J, et al: A novel signal transduction cascade involving direct physical interaction of the renin/prorenin receptor with the transcription factor promyelocytic zinc finger protein. *Circ Res* 99:1355, 2006.
100. ter Horst P, Smits JF, Blankesteijn WM: The Wnt/Frizzled pathway as a therapeutic target for cardiac hypertrophy: where do we stand? *Acta Physiol (Oxf)* 204:110, 2012.
101. Cruciat CM, Ohkawara B, Acebron SP, et al: Requirement of prorenin receptor and vacuolar H+-ATPase-mediated acidification for Wnt signaling. *Science* 327:459, 2010.
102. Murphy TJ, Alexander RW, Griendling KK, et al: Isolation of a cDNA encoding the vascular type-1 angiotensin II receptor. *Nature* 351:233, 1991.
103. Ribas C, Penela P, Murga C, et al: The G protein-coupled receptor kinase (GRK) interactome: role of GRKs in GPCR regulation and signaling. *Biochim Biophys Acta* 1768:913, 2007.
104. Jones ES, Vinh A, McCarthy CA, et al: AT2 receptors: functional relevance in cardiovascular disease. *Pharmacol Ther* 120:292, 2008.
105. Batenburg WW, Garrelds IM, Bernasconi CC, et al: Angiotensin II type 2 receptor-mediated vasodilation in human coronary microarteries. *Circulation* 109:2296, 2004.
106. Avila MD, Morgan JP, Yan X: Genetically modified mouse models used for studying the role of the AT2 receptor in cardiac hypertrophy and heart failure. *J Biomed Biotechnol* 2011:141039, 2011.
107. Verdonk K, Durik M, Abd-Alla N, et al: Compound 21 induces vasorelaxation via an endothelium- and angiotensin II type 2 receptor-independent mechanism. *Hypertension* 60:722, 2012.
108. Chen S, Patel JM, Block ER: Angiotensin IV-mediated pulmonary artery vasorelaxation is due to endothelial intracellular calcium release. *Am J Physiol Lung Cell Mol Physiol* 279:L849, 2000.
109. Li YD, Block ER, Patel JM: Activation of multiple signaling modules is critical in angiotensin IV-induced lung endothelial cell proliferation. *Am J Physiol Lung Cell Mol Physiol* 283:L707, 2002.
110. Numaguchi Y, Ishii M, Kubota R, et al: Ablation of angiotensin IV receptor attenuates hypofibrinolysis via PAI-1 downregulation and reduces occlusive arterial thrombosis. *Arterioscler Thromb Vasc Biol* 29:2102, 2009.
111. Yang H, Zeng XJ, Wang HX, et al: Angiotensin IV protects against angiotensin II-induced cardiac injury via AT4 receptor. *Peptides* 32:2108, 2011.
112. Griendling KK, Ushio-Fukai M, Lassegue B, et al: Angiotensin II signaling in vascular smooth muscle. New concepts. *Hypertension* 29:366, 1997.
113. Booz GW, Dostal DE, Singer HA, et al: Involvement of protein kinase C and Ca2+ in angiotensin II-induced mitogenesis of cardiac fibroblasts. *Am J Physiol* 267:C1308, 1994.
114. Natarajan K, Berk BC: Crosstalk coregulation mechanisms of G protein-coupled receptors and receptor tyrosine kinases. *Methods Mol Biol* 332:51, 2006.
115. Eguchi S, Inagami T: Signal transduction of angiotensin II type 1 receptor through receptor tyrosine kinase. *Regul Pept* 91:13, 2000.
116. Zahradka P, Litchie B, Storie B, et al: Transactivation of the insulin-like growth factor-I receptor by angiotensin II mediates downstream signaling from the angiotensin II type 1 receptor to phosphatidylinositol 3-kinase. *Endocrinology* 145:2978, 2004.
117. Saito Y, Berk BC: Transactivation: a novel signaling pathway from angiotensin II to tyrosine kinase receptors. *J Mol Cell Cardiol* 33:3, 2001.
118. Saito S, Frank GD, Mifune M, et al: Ligand-independent trans-activation of the platelet-derived growth factor receptor by reactive oxygen species requires protein kinase C-delta and c-Src. *J Biol Chem* 277:44695, 2002.
119. Kim S, Zhan Y, Izumi Y, et al: In vivo activation of rat aortic platelet-derived growth factor and epidermal growth factor receptors by angiotensin II and hypertension. *Arterioscler Thromb Vasc Biol* 20:2539, 2000.
120. Wang C, Wu LL, Liu J, et al: Crosstalk between angiotensin II and platelet derived growth factor-BB mediated signal pathways in cardiomyocytes. *Chin Med J (Engl)* 121:236, 2008.
121. Yin G, Yan C, Berk BC: Angiotensin II signaling pathways mediated by tyrosine kinases. *Int J Biochem Cell Biol* 35:780, 2003.
122. Touyz RM, He G, Wu XH, et al: Src is an important mediator of extracellular signal-regulated kinase 1/2-dependent growth signaling by angiotensin II in smooth muscle cells from resistance arteries of hypertensive patients. *Hypertension* 38:56, 2001.
123. Qin J, Liu ZX: FAK-related nonkinase attenuates hypertrophy induced by angiotensin-II in cultured neonatal rat cardiac myocytes. *Acta Pharmacol Sin* 27:1159, 2006.
124. Govindarajan G, Eble DM, Lucchesi PA, et al: Focal adhesion kinase is involved in angiotensin II-mediated protein synthesis in cultured vascular smooth muscle cells. *Circ Res* 87:710, 2000.
125. Sabri A, Govindarajan G, Griffin TM, et al: Calcium- and protein kinase C-dependent activation of the tyrosine kinase PYK2 by angiotensin II in vascular smooth muscle. *Circ Res* 83:841, 1998.
126. Aaronson DS, Horvath CM: A road map for those who don't know JAK-STAT. *Science* 296:1653, 2002.
127. Booz GW, Day JN, Baker KM: Interplay between the cardiac renin angiotensin system and JAK-STAT signaling: role in cardiac hypertrophy, ischemia/reperfusion dysfunction, and heart failure. *J Mol Cell Cardiol* 34:1443, 2002.
128. Barry SP, Townsend PA, Latchman DS, et al: Role of the JAK-STAT pathway in myocardial injury. *Trends Mol Med* 13:82, 2007.
129. Guo Y, Mascareno E, Siddiqui MA: Distinct components of Janus kinase/signal transducer and activator of transcription signaling pathway mediate the regulation of systemic and tissue localized renin-angiotensin system. *Mol Endocrinol* 18:1033, 2004.
130. Banes-Berceli AK, Ketsawatsomkron P, Ogbi S, et al: Angiotensin II and endothelin-1 augment the vascular complications of diabetes via JAK2 activation. *Am J Physiol Heart Circ Physiol* 293:H1291, 2007.
131. Walker EH, Perisic O, Ried C, et al: Structural insights into phosphoinositide 3-kinase catalysis and signalling. *Nature* 402:313, 1999.
132. McMullen JR, Shioi T, Zhang L, et al: Phosphoinositide 3-kinase(p110alpha) plays a critical role for the induction of physiological, but not pathological, cardiac hypertrophy. *Proc Natl Acad Sci U S A* 100:12355, 2003.
133. Alloatti G, Montrucchio G, Lembo G, et al: Phosphoinositide 3-kinase gamma: kinase-dependent and -independent activities in cardiovascular function and disease. *Biochem Soc Trans* 32:383, 2004.
134. Kerfant BG, Rose RA, Sun H, et al: Phosphoinositide 3-kinase gamma regulates cardiac contractility by locally controlling cyclic adenosine monophosphate levels. *Trends Cardiovasc Med* 16:250, 2006.
135. Chen QM, Tu VC, Purdon S, et al: Molecular mechanisms of cardiac hypertrophy induced by toxicants. *Cardiovasc Toxicol* 1:267, 2001.
136. Pimienta G, Pascual J: Canonical and alternative MAPK signaling. *Cell Cycle* 6:2628, 2007.
137. Strniskova M, Barancik M, Ravingerova T: Mitogen-activated protein kinases and their role in regulation of cellular processes. *Gen Physiol Biophys* 21:231, 2002.
138. Ravingerova T, Barancik M, Strniskova M: Mitogen-activated protein kinases: a new therapeutic target in cardiac pathology. *Mol Cell Biochem* 247:127, 2003.
139. Wei SG, Yu Y, Zhang ZH, et al: Angiotensin II-triggered p44/42 mitogen-activated protein kinase mediates sympathetic excitation in heart failure rats. *Hypertension* 52:342, 2008.
140. Kim S, Iwao H: Stress and vascular responses: mitogen-activated protein kinases and activator protein-1 as promising therapeutic targets of vascular remodeling. *J Pharmacol Sci* 91:177, 2003.
141. Wang Y, Su B, Sah VP, et al: Cardiac hypertrophy induced by mitogen-activated protein kinase kinase 7, a specific activator for c-Jun NH2-terminal kinase in ventricular muscle cells. *J Biol Chem* 273:5423, 1998.
142. Liao P, Georgakopoulos D, Kovacs A, et al: The in vivo role of p38 MAP kinases in cardiac remodeling and restrictive cardiomyopathy. *Proc Natl Acad Sci U S A* 98:12283, 2001.
143. Pellieux C, Sauthier T, Aubert JF, et al: Angiotensin II-induced cardiac hypertrophy is associated with different mitogen-activated protein kinase activation in normotensive and hypertensive mice. *J Hypertens* 18:1307, 2000.
144. Lezoualc'h F, Metrich M, Hmitou I, et al: Small GTP-binding proteins and their regulators in cardiac hypertrophy. *J Mol Cell Cardiol* 44:623, 2008.
145. Sadoshima J, Izumo S: The heterotrimeric G q protein-coupled angiotensin II receptor activates p21 ras via the tyrosine kinase-Shc-Grb2-Sos pathway in cardiac myocytes. *EMBO J* 15:775, 1996.

146. Jalil J, Lavandero S, Chiong M, et al: Rho/Rho kinase signal transduction pathway in cardiovascular disease and cardiovascular remodeling. *Rev Esp Cardiol* 58:951, 2005.
147. Choudhary S, Lu M, Cui R, et al: Involvement of a novel Rac/RhoA guanosine triphosphatase-nuclear factor-kappaB inducing kinase signaling pathway mediating angiotensin II-induced RelA transactivation. *Mol Endocrinol* 21:2203, 2007.
148. Gregg D, Rauscher FM, Goldschmidt-Clermont PJ: Rac regulates cardiovascular superoxide through diverse molecular interactions: more than a binary GTP switch. *Am J Physiol Cell Physiol* 285:C723, 2003.
149. Harrison DG, Cai H, Landmesser U, et al: Interactions of angiotensin II with NAD(P)H oxidase, oxidant stress and cardiovascular disease. *J Renin Angiotensin Aldosterone Syst* 4:51, 2003.
150. Griendling KK, Ushio-Fukai M: Reactive oxygen species as mediators of angiotensin II signaling. *Regul Pept* 91:21, 2000.
151. Zablocki D, Sadoshima J: Angiotensin II and oxidative stress in the failing heart. *Antioxid Redox Signal* 19:1095, 2013.
152. Nguyen Dinh Cat A, Montezano AC, Burger D, et al: Angiotensin II, NADPH oxidase, and redox signaling in the vasculature. *Antioxid Redox Signal* 19:1110, 2013.
153. Dai DF, Johnson SC, Villarin JJ, et al: Mitochondrial oxidative stress mediates angiotensin II-induced cardiac hypertrophy and Galphaq overexpression-induced heart failure. *Circ Res* 108:837, 2011.
154. Tsutsui H, Kinugawa S, Matsushima S: Mitochondrial oxidative stress and dysfunction in myocardial remodelling. *Cardiovasc Res* 81:449, 2009.
155. Landmesser U, Spiekermann S, Preuss C, et al: Angiotensin II induces endothelial xanthine oxidase activation: role for endothelial dysfunction in patients with coronary disease. *Arterioscler Thromb Vasc Biol* 27:943, 2007.
156. Landmesser U, Spiekermann S, Dikalov S, et al: Vascular oxidative stress and endothelial dysfunction in patients with chronic heart failure: role of xanthine-oxidase and extracellular superoxide dismutase. *Circulation* 106:3073, 2002.
157. Zhang J, Pratt RE: The AT2 receptor selectively associates with Gialpha2 and Gialpha3 in the rat fetus. *J Biol Chem* 271:15026, 1996.
158. Steckelings UM, Kaschina E, Unger T: The AT2 receptor–a matter of love and hate. *Peptides* 26:1401, 2005.
159. Bottari SP, King IN, Reichlin S, et al: The angiotensin AT2 receptor stimulates protein tyrosine phosphatase activity and mediates inhibition of particulate guanylate cyclase. *Biochem Biophys Res Commun* 183:206, 1992.
160. Wu L, Iwai M, Li Z, et al: Regulation of inhibitory protein-kappaB and monocyte chemoattractant protein-1 by angiotensin II type 2 receptor-activated Src homology protein tyrosine phosphatase-1 in fetal vascular smooth muscle cells. *Mol Endocrinol* 18:666, 2004.
161. Horiuchi M, Hayashida W, Akishita M, et al: Stimulation of different subtypes of angiotensin II receptors, AT1 and AT2 receptors, regulates STAT activation by negative crosstalk. *Circ Res* 84:876, 1999.
162. Searles CD, Harrison DG: The interaction of nitric oxide, bradykinin, and the angiotensin II type 2 receptor: lessons learned from transgenic mice. *J Clin Invest* 104:1013, 1999.
163. Gohlke P, Pees C, Unger T: AT2 receptor stimulation increases aortic cyclic GMP in SHRSP by a kinin-dependent mechanism. *Hypertension* 31:349, 1998.
164. Dulin NO, Alexander LD, Harwalkar S, et al: Phospholipase A2-mediated activation of mitogen-activated protein kinase by angiotensin II. *Proc Natl Acad Sci U S A* 95:8098, 1998.
165. Jiao H, Cui XL, Torti M, et al: Arachidonic acid mediates angiotensin II effects on p21ras in renal proximal tubular cells via the tyrosine kinase-Shc-Grb2-Sos pathway. *Proc Natl Acad Sci U S A* 95:7417, 1998.
166. Kohout TA, Rogers TB: Angiotensin II activates the Na+/HCO3- symport through a phosphoinositide-independent mechanism in cardiac cells. *J Biol Chem* 270:20432, 1995.
167. Lehtonen JY, Horiuchi M, Daviet L, et al: Activation of the de novo biosynthesis of sphingolipids mediates angiotensin II type 2 receptor-induced apoptosis. *J Biol Chem* 274:16901, 1999.
168. Pettus BJ, Chalfant CE, Hannun YA: Ceramide in apoptosis: an overview and current perspectives. *Biochim Biophys Acta* 1585:114, 2002.

Abbreviations Used in This Chapter

ABBREVIATION	FULL NAME	ABBREVIATION	FULL NAME
Ang	Angiotensin	MMP	Matrix metallopeptidase
AGT	Angiotensinogen	MKP	Mitogen-activated protein kinase phosphatase
AA	Arachidonic acid	mTOR	Mammalian target of rapamycin
ACE	Angiotensin-converting enzyme	MYPT	Myosin phosphatase
Ac-SDKP	*N*-acetyl-Ser-Asp-Lys-Pro tetrapeptide	NADPH	Nicotinamide adenine dinucleotide phosphate
Akt (PKB)	Protein kinase B	NF-κB	Nuclear factor-kappa B
APA	Aminopeptidase A	NO	Nitric oxide
APN	Aminopeptidase N	PA	Phosphatidic acid
ARBs	Angiotensin receptor blockers	PAI-1	Plasminogen activator inhibitor-1
ASK	Apoptosis signal-regulating kinase	PAK	P21-activated kinases
AGTR1	Angiotensin II type 1 receptor	PC	Phosphatidylcholine
AGTR2	Angiotensin II type 2 receptor	PDGF	Platelet-derived growth factor
Bcl-2	B-cell lymphoma 2	PDGFR	Platelet-derived growth factor receptor
cAMP	Cyclic adenosine monophosphate	PDK1	Phosphoinositide-dependent kinase 1
cGMP	Cyclic guanosine monophosphate	PI3K	Phosphoinositide 3-kinase
COX	Cyclooxygenase	PIP2	Phosphatidylinositol bisphosphate
DAG	Diacylglycerol	PLC	Phospholipase C
EGFR	Epidermal growth factor receptor	PLA2	Phospholipase A2
ERK	Extracellular signal-regulated kinases	PLD	Phospholipase D
FAK	Focal adhesion kinase	PLZF	Promyelocytic leukemia zinc-finger protein
FOXO	Forkhead box-O	PKC	Protein kinase C
Grb2	Growth factor receptor-bound protein 2	PP2A	Protein phosphatase 2A
GPCR	G protein-coupled receptors	Pyk2	Proline-rich tyrosine kinase 2
HSP27	Heat shock protein 27	P38 MAPK	P38 mitogen-activated protein kinase
GEF	Guanine nucleotide exchange factor	p70S6K	p70 ribosomal protein S6 kinase
GDI	Guanosine nucleotide dissociation inhibitor	p130Cas	Crk-associated substrate, 130 kDa
IGFR	Insulin-like growth factor receptor	PtdIns	Phosphatidylinositol
IP_3	Inositol 1,4,5-trisphosphate	PTK	Protein tyrosine kinase
IRAP	Insulin-regulated aminopeptidase	RAS	Renin-angiotensin system
JAK	Janus kinase	RhoA	Ras homolog gene family, member A
JNK	c-Jun N-terminal kinases	ROS	Reactive oxygen species
LV	Left ventricle	Shc	Src homology 2 domain-containing transforming protein
MAPK	Mitogen-activated protein kinase	SHP-1	SH2 domain-containing protein tyrosine phosphatase 1
MEK	MAP kinase kinase	Sos	Son of sevenless
MEKK	MAP kinase kinase kinase	STAT	Signal transducers and activator of transcription
MI	Myocardial infarction	TAK1	Transforming growth factor beta-activated kinase 1
MLC	Myosin light chain	TGF-β	Transforming growth factor β
MLK	Mixed-lineage kinase	VSMC	Vascular smooth muscle cells
M6P-R	Mannose-6-phosphate receptor		

6 Adrenergic Receptor Signaling in Heart Failure

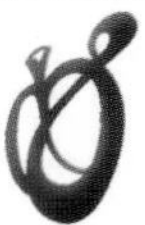

J. David Port, Carmen Sucharov, and Michael R. Bristow

Physiologic and pathophysiologic stresses result in increased myocardial demand that is met by a commensurate increase in cardiac adrenergic drive. To facilitate this increase, the neurotransmitter norepinephrine (NE) is released from adrenergic (sympathetic) nerve endings within the heart. On binding to β-adrenergic receptors, multiple signaling pathways are activated, resulting in increases in heart rate, force of contraction, and rate of relaxation, as well as multiple metabolic adjustments. The result is an immediate increase in cardiac output. In the setting of acute heart failure, adrenergic activation occurs initially in response to hemodynamic overload and/or to an intrinsic reduction in pump function. However, in the setting of chronic heart failure (CHF), a response that is normally physiologic and transient is instead sustained in an attempt to maintain myocardial performance at a homeostatic level. Under these conditions, the initially beneficial adrenergic support mechanisms become maladaptive and contribute directly to the progressive natural history of heart failure.

In this chapter, the long-term consequences of sustained adrenergic activation in CHF from reduced left ventricular ejection fraction (HFrEF), or CHF with systolic dysfunction, will be reviewed. Particular emphasis will be placed on alterations in β-adrenergic signal transduction and gene expression patterns that occur in the failing human heart, and the impact of these changes on myocardial disease progression. Adrenergic receptor pharmacology relevant to heart failure, as well as recent data from transgenic animals and model systems that demonstrate the myopathic potential of individual components of the adrenergic signaling cascade will also be reviewed. Much of this information is likely to be applicable to CHF with preserved left ventricular ejection fraction (HFpEF), but in human heart failure or animal models this form of CHF has not been investigated. Therefore, in this discussion, CHF implies chronic HFrEF.

ROLE OF INCREASED ADRENERGIC DRIVE IN THE NATURAL HISTORY OF HEART FAILURE

In patients with CHF, the adrenergic nervous system is critical to the support of myocardial function. However, its chronic activation contributes concomitantly to progressive myocardial *dys*function. Regardless of the cause, an intrinsic decrease in myocardial function results in activation of afferent signaling from baroreceptors and chemoreceptors to the central nervous system such that efferent cardiac adrenergic nerves release more NE,[1,2] activating β-adrenergic receptors (β-ARs), increasing heart rate, and, depending on degree of functional reserve, increasing myocardial contractility. The increase in contractility favorably affects both systolic and diastolic function and, through the Frank-Starling relationship, mediated by primary and secondary effects on volume expansion, increases cardiac output. As heart failure worsens, adrenergic drive continues to increase in an attempt to compensate for the progressive loss of cardiac function[1,2] (**Figure 6-1**). However, long-term exposure to high concentrations of NE has profoundly adverse effects on myocardial and cardiac myocyte biology[3,4] (**Figure 6-2**). Inhibitors of adrenergic signaling that have demonstrated favorable effects on heart failure natural history include β-blocking agents and inhibitors of the renin-angiotensin-aldosterone system, which indirectly lower adrenergic drive. There is extensive clinical trial literature supporting the use of these classes of agents, as well as definitive guidelines (AHA/ACC) for their optimal administration[5-9] (**see Chapter 34**).

Although the "cardiotoxic" effects of catecholamines, in particular NE, have been recognized for more than a century,[10] we are only just beginning to understand the detailed molecular mechanisms by which these adverse effects occur. Treatment of isolated cardiac myocytes with concentrations of NE equivalent to those in the failing human heart cause dramatic changes in cell morphology, and, within a matter of days, up to a 60% loss of myocyte viability.[3] This effect is mimicked by exposing myocytes to the nonselective β-agonist isoproterenol, an effect that is in turn inhibited pharmacologically by the β-blocker propranolol, suggesting that the acute toxic effects of NE are mediated almost exclusively through β-ARs rather than through α-ARs.[11] As will be described later, of the two most prevalent β-AR subtypes, signaling through the β_1-AR is generally considered to be more biologically harmful than β_2-AR effects.[11,12] This finding is supported by clinical trial data, where differences in β_1-AR blocking doses and enrollment criteria are considered[5,13]; β_1-AR selective blockade[7,14,15] appears equally efficacious as treatment with nonselective β-blockers.[8,15]

As stated above, elevated plasma concentrations of NE, reflecting overflow from adrenergically activated organs including the heart,[2,16,17] are a well-recognized biomarker of CHF.[18] However, as adrenergic activation persists, cardiac NE stores become depleted.[19] Ultimately, other tissue sources of catecholamines (i.e., the adrenal medulla) are stimulated, leading to generalized adrenergic activation and spillover of cardiac-derived NE into the systemic circulation.[2,4] As systemic[18,20] or cardiac[21] NE levels increase, so does mortality in patients with heart failure. These observations have been validated further by evidence from numerous clinical trials of β-blocker therapy, demonstrating reverse remodeling (improved systolic function and decreased left ventricular volumes, typically measured as the ejection fraction)[22,23] and improved survival[7,14] in patients with heart failure who receive β-blocker therapy long term.

It is interesting to note that, in marked contrast to adults with heart failure, β-blocker therapy does not appear to be particularly efficacious in pediatric heart failure patients.[24] Although the findings are somewhat anecdotal, pediatric patients with systolic heart failure appear to respond more favorably than adults to type 3 phosphodiesterase inhibitors.[25] Underlying this difference are markedly different gene expression patterns and adrenergic receptor biology.[26] This is an area of investigation that needs further study.

A recent realization is that *insufficient* adrenergic drive in individuals with CHF can also increase mortality.[5] In contrast to β-blocking agents, sympatholytic agents (agents that lower adrenergic activity) can actually increase mortality, presumably via excessive withdrawal of adrenergic support to the failing heart. In contrast, β-blocking agents are pharmacologically reversible mass-action agents, and in their presence adrenergic support to the failing heart can be accessed if needed simply by increasing cardiac adrenergic drive. One β-blocker in clinical development, bucindolol, is both a nonselective β-blocker and a mild sympatholytic agent.[8,20] When NE lowering from bucindolol is mild, the result is an enhancement of efficacy. In some patients, the degree of sympatholysis can be excessive, obviating any benefit from β-blockade.[20] The sympatholytic effects of bucindolol are under control of prejunctional α_{2C}-adrenergic receptors, and exaggerated/adverse NE lowering can be avoided by not treating patients who have a loss of function α_{2C} polymorphism in combination with a decreased function β_1-AR genetic variant (see later discussion).

Historical studies suggested that one underlying mechanism of NE toxicity involves cAMP-mediated increases in intracellular calcium.[3] Increased formation of the second messenger cAMP leads to activation of protein kinase A (PKA), which in turn phosphorylates a variety of target proteins involved in regulating intracellular calcium, including key targets such as phospholamban (PLB), L-type calcium channels ($CaV_{1.2}$), and ryanodine receptors (RyR2). Enhanced phosphorylation of calcium channels leads to an increased flux of extracellular calcium into the cell

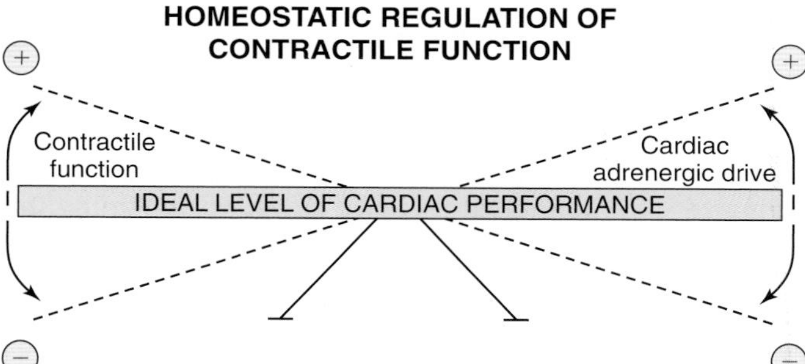

FIGURE 6-1 Homeostatic regulation of contractile function. Adrenergic drive acts as a servo-control regulator of normal cardiac contractile function. When cardiac contractile function is adequate to sustain normal homeostasis, adrenergic drive is low or reduced. In contrast, when contractile function is inadequate to support homeostasis, cardiac adrenergic drive increases to a commensurate degree. *Adapted from Port JD, Bristow MR: Altered β-adrenergic receptor gene regulation and signaling in chronic heart failure. J Mol Cell Cardiol 33:887–905, 2001.*

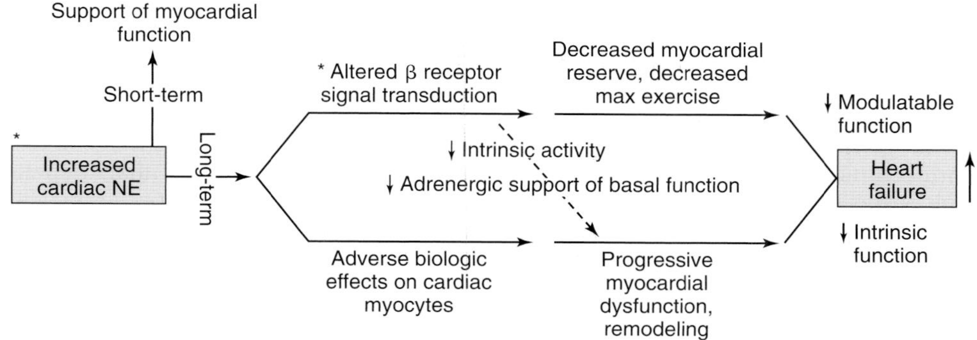

FIGURE 6-2 Role of increased adrenergic drive in the natural history of heart failure. A primary maladaptive response to chronic heart failure is a net increase in cardiac interstitial norepinephrine (NE) concentration, resulting from increased release and/or decreased reuptake. Increased NE results in a second maladaptive response to heart failure, that of altered β-AR signaling. These changes, in combination with the direct adverse biologic effects of catecholamines, result in decreased myocardial reserve and progressive myocardial dysfunction, the ultimate result being decreases in both "modulatable" and intrinsic myocardial function.

activating downstream effectors, including proteases, kinases, and phosphatases. Activation of the β_1-AR subtype also appears to promote increased calcium influx via cAMP-independent mechanisms.[27] β_1-ARs are cAMP-independent activators of CaMKII,[28] a signaling pathway known to have particularly adverse effects on cardiac myocytes.[29] Regardless of the exact mechanism(s) invoked, excessive β-AR stimulation results in oxidative stress and calcium overload, conditions promoting cell death through a number of mechanisms, including necrosis and apoptosis. Long-term adrenergic activation has also been shown to cause changes in the gene expression profile of cardiac myocytes, the general response being activation of the so-called fetal gene program.[30]*

In the failing heart, β-ARs and certain downstream effectors in the β-adrenergic signaling cascade undergo agonist-mediated, time-dependent downregulation and desensitization, presumably in an attempt to withdraw the heart from an excess of deleterious signaling. These changes result in a marked attenuation of the failing heart's ability to respond to either endogenous or exogenous catecholamines. Because of these regulatory changes, the amount of cAMP generated in response to a given amount of adrenergic stimulation is significantly decreased. Evidence for this has been provided through experiments using isolated, denervated preparations of human heart tissue, revealing that failing hearts have a reduced cAMP content compared to nonfailing controls.[31,32] From a clinical standpoint, reduced responsiveness to catecholamines translates into a decrease in myocardial reserve, which is most commonly manifested as an impaired ability to exercise but also means less ability to respond to any form of circulatory stress.

In summary, the role of increased adrenergic drive in the natural history of heart failure is a seemingly paradoxical one. On the one hand, adrenergic activation is essential to meeting the demands of increased physiologic and pathologic stress in the failing heart; on the other hand, chronic adrenergic stimulation is a major contributor to progressive myocardial dysfunction and remodeling that characterizes heart failure. However, from an evolutionary biology standpoint, this situation is entirely plausible; adrenergic mechanisms have evolved to allow reproductive age individuals to cope with and escape from highly stressful short-term situations; they are not particularly well suited to chronic support of the failing heart that typically occurs beyond the reproductive years.

ADRENERGIC RECEPTOR PHARMACOLOGY

As far back as the 1940s, Ahlquist and colleagues[33] recognized that adrenergic receptors could be subdivided into two major classes, α-ARs and β-ARs, both of which are binding sites for the endogenous catecholamines, epinephrine and norepinephrine. Almost 20 years later, Lands and associates,[34] using rank orders of various agonists, proposed that β-ARs could be divided into β_1- and β_2-AR subtypes. A few years later, using selective β_1- and other β-AR antagonists, this classification was confirmed and expanded to include

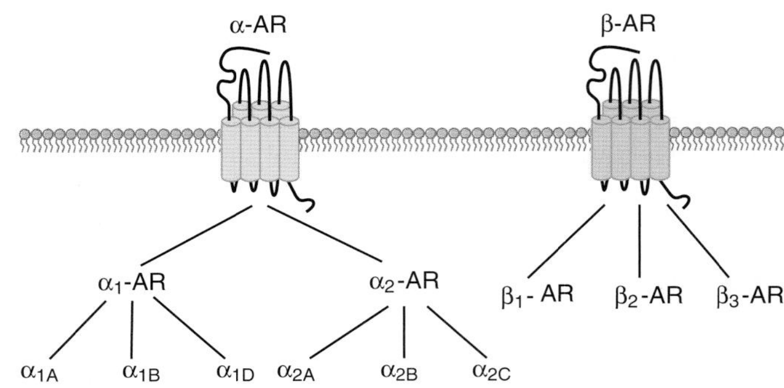

FIGURE 6-3 Adrenergic receptor subtypes. Based on the early work of Alquist et al,[33] adrenergic receptors (AR) were known to fall into two broad classes, alpha (α) and beta (β). Subsequent pharmacologic work by Lands et al[34] served to define subclasses of β-ARs. Molecular biologic work, primarily by Lefkowitz and colleagues,[40-44] led to the precise gene structure of adrenergic receptors and served as the basis for the uncovering of adrenergic receptor polymorphisms and their clinical relevance. The signaling pathways associated with adrenergic receptor subtypes are summarized in Figure 6-5.

an additional β-AR subtype,[35] later named β_3-AR.[36] Building on this basic pharmacology was work in the 1970s and 1980s centered on direct identification of receptors by radioligand binding and the biochemistry of signaling pathways, much of it based on methods and concepts developed by Lefkowitz and colleagues.[37,38]

Based on the groundbreaking biochemical work of Khorana and associates on rhodopsin,[39] subsequent work by Lefkowitz and associates described the molecular cloning of a number of G protein-coupled receptors, including an α_1-, an α_2-, and the β_1- and β_2-ARs.[40-44] Perhaps more than any other previous advance in the field, this knowledge permitted the analysis of adrenergic receptor biology in exquisite detail and allowed for an appreciation of the true complexity of adrenergic receptor signaling, including the definition of a multitude of gene regulatory motifs and the recognition of highly organized multiprotein signaling complexes. The combined work of Lefkowitz and Kobilka on G protein-coupled receptor (GPCR) pharmacology, biochemistry, and molecular biology, as well as Kobilka's subsequent work on GPCR structural biology, resulted in their being awarded the 2012 Nobel Prize in Chemistry.

Relevant to the human heart, there are two major subclasses of α-ARs: α_1- and α_2-. There are several subtypes of α_1-ARs (**Figure 6-3**), all coupled to the Gq/G11 family of G proteins.[45] The Gq pathway is linked to stimulation of phospholipase C (PLC), which promotes phosphoinositide (PIP_2) turnover. The two primary products of this reaction are inositol triphosphate (IP_3), which stimulates the release of intracellular calcium, and diacylglycerol (DAG), which stimulates protein kinase-C (PKC) activity.[46] Increases in intracellular calcium and PKC-mediated phosphorylation of target proteins both activate signaling pathways and gene expression patterns that, depending on the PKC subtype, result in a hypertrophic myocardial phenotype as well as vasoconstriction.[47] Examples of other Gq-coupled receptors whose stimulation also results in a hypertrophic phenotype are the angiotensin II AT1 and endothelin-1 (ET-1) receptors. Each of these receptor pathways represents pharmacologic targets central to the management of heart failure and/or its precursors, such as systemic or pulmonary hypertension.

In contrast to α_1-ARs, α_2-ARs are generally considered to be inhibitory presynaptic or prejunctional neuronal

*The fetal gene program, which is a molecular surrogate for hypertrophy/heart failure, includes downregulation in the gene expression of the fast-contracting α isoform of myosin heavy chain *(MYH6)* and SR Ca^{2+} ATPase *(ATP2A2)*, upregulation of the slow contracting β-MHC isoform *(MYH7)*, and upregulation of ANP *(NPPA)* and BNP *(NPPB)*.

receptors functioning to suppress the release of NE. The potential importance of this function in the setting of heart failure has been emphasized in a study by Small and associates,[48] wherein a naturally occurring "loss of function" polymorphism of the α_{2C}-AR, when present in combination with a "gain of function" polymorphism of the β_1-AR, produced a significantly increased risk of heart failure in certain populations. These and other β-AR polymorphisms, and their relevance to CHF, are discussed in greater detail later.

β-ARs are also subdivided, with three distinct receptor subtypes encoded by separate genes β_1-*(ADRB1)*, β_2-*(ADRB2)*, and β_3-*(ADRB3)*. β_1- and β_2-ARs were first described by agonist[34] or antagonist[35] pharmacologic responses, and then by molecular cloning.[40,41] In contrast, β_3-ARs were first definitively identified by molecular cloning[36] after being classified as beyond the β_1, β_2 paradigm[35] or "atypical"[49] in various organs, as determined by pharmacologic response. β_3-ARs are generally associated with regulation of metabolic rate, modulation of nitric oxide (NO) formation, gut and urinary tract smooth muscle relaxation, and, to a lesser degree, with changes in cardiac contractility.[50] β_3-receptors are expressed at low abundance but are coupled via a NOS/NO/soluble guanylate cyclase/cGMP mechanism to a negative inotropic response in human ventricular myocardium,[51] where they may play a cardioprotective role.[50] In contrast, β_1- and β_2-ARs have the clear functional role of increasing myocardial performance,[5] and both are expressed at a substantial abundance in human ventricular myocardium with β_1-AR density greater than β_2.[52]

By response to catecholamine agonists, β_1- and β_2-ARs, which respond equally well to the full agonist isoproterenol, are distinguished primarily by their affinity for NE. β_1-ARs have 10- to 30-fold greater affinity for NE than β_2-ARs.[13,34] An even greater degree of distinction is achieved through the relative affinities of selective antagonists.[52,53] In the context of heart failure, the most clinically relevant compounds differentiating between β_1- and β_2-ARs are the clinically available β_1-AR selective antagonists metoprolol, bisoprolol, and nebivolol.[5] β_3-ARs are characterized by their relatively low affinity for propranolol[35,49] or the selective β_1-antagonist CGP 20712a,[36] and response to β_3 selective agonists such as BRL 37344[36] or CL316243.[49] Two β-blocking agents in use or development, nebivolol and bucindolol, have β_3-agonist activity that may contribute to their vasodilator properties or possibly to their myocardial effects.[5]

ALTERED β-ADRENERGIC RECEPTOR SIGNAL TRANSDUCTION IN THE FAILING HEART

Downregulation and other forms of desensitization of β_1- and β_2-AR receptor signaling are contributing factors to the contractile dysfunction of failing human heart.[52,53] Heightened adrenergic activation results in decreases in β_1-AR mRNA[54] and protein expression,[52,55] uncoupling of both β_1- and β_2-ARs[56,57] due to receptor phosphorylation[58] from βARK1 (GRK2),[59] or increases in the inhibitory G protein (Gi)[60] (**Figure 6-4**). In nonfailing adult human ventricles, β_1-ARs constitute approximately 70% to 80% of all β-ARs. However, in individuals with heart failure, the β_1-AR is selectively downregulated, resulting in an approximate 60:40 ratio of β_1- to β_2-ARs.[54,61]

Phosphorylation of β-ARs occurs by the G protein-coupled receptor kinase (GRK) family, specifically GRK2, which phosphorylates both β_1- and β_2 receptor subtypes in an agonist occupancy-dependent manner,[62] and GRK5,[63] a kinase of considerable importance linking β_1-ARs to

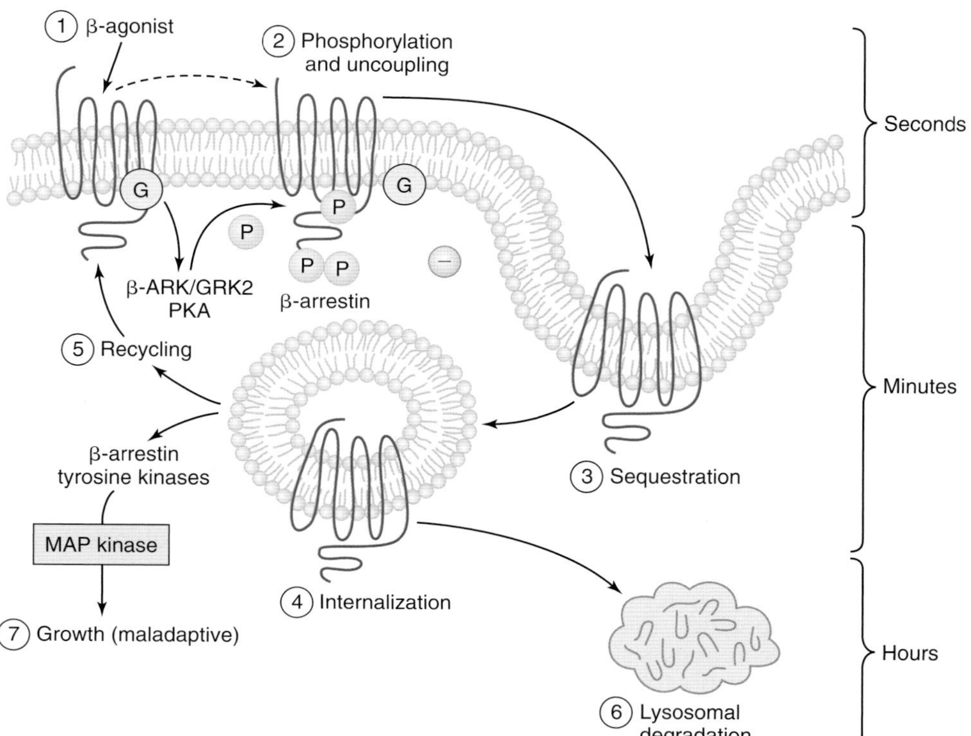

FIGURE 6-4 Mechanisms of β-adrenergic receptor desensitization and internalization. Note links between the internalized receptor complex with growth stimulation via mitogen-activated protein (MAP) kinase. *β-ARK,* β-agonist receptor kinase; *GRK2,* G-coupled receptor kinase; *PKA,* protein kinase A. *Modified from Hein L, Kobilka BK: Adrenergic receptors. From molecular structures to in vivo function. Trends Cardiovasc Med 7:137–145, 1997; and Opie LH: Mechanisms of cardiac contraction and relaxation. In Libby P, Bonow RO, Mann DL, et al, editors: Braunwald's heart disease, Philadelphia, 2008, Elsevier.*

epidermal growth factor receptor (EGFR) transactivation and cardioprotective effects.[64] β-ARs can also be phosphorylated and desensitized by other kinases including PKA and PKC.[65] Therefore, in failing ventricular myocardium both β_1- and β_2-receptor subtypes undergo desensitization, with β_1-ARs exhibiting downregulation, and both β_1- and β_2-ARs uncoupling from PKA signaling. This can be appreciated in vivo by intracoronary infusion studies that eliminate vascular responses from any effect on contractile function, where the contractility effects of the minimally β_1-AR selective compound dobutamine is much more compromised in failing hearts than are the effects of the post receptor acting PDE3 inhibitor milrinone.[66]

The major consequence of β-AR downregulation and desensitization is that for a given level of adrenergic activation, less of the second messenger cAMP is produced. Decreased formation of cAMP in turn leads to diminished activation of PKA. However, decreased PKA activity does not necessarily translate into decreased phosphorylation of all putative PKA substrates. Related to the above, although PKA activity and phospholamban (PLB) phosphorylation[67] are decreased in heart failure, cardiac RyR2s have been shown to be hyperphosphorylated.[68] The net phosphorylation "state" of the RyR and PLB, and thus their activities, is due, at least in part, to their being in separate subcellular A-kinase anchoring protein-scaffolded microdomains. In these discreet microdomains, different phosphodiesterases control cAMP levels and PKA activation, and phosphatase species and activities may also be different. Specifically, in the failing heart there is evidence for the downregulation of phosphatases PP1 and PP2A that are associated with RyR2, as well as to changes in PKA activity.[68,69] Alternatively, recent studies have shown that RyR2 can be phosphorylated by CaMKII,[70] inducing SR calcium leakiness and engendering arrhythmias, an effect that appears to be mediated by cardiac β_1-ARs and the "exchange protein directly activated by cAMP-2," EPAC2.[71]

In contrast to the hyperphosphorylation of RyR2, PKA-mediated phosphorylation of PLB appears to be decreased in CHF,[31] presumably because of reduced cAMP levels in the SERCA II-phospholamban microdomain, as well as to the activation of the phosphatase PP1.[67] PP1 is regulated by protein phosphatase inhibitor I, PPI-1, a protein whose abundance is itself downregulated in heart failure.[72] The reduced PLB phosphorylation results in a greater inhibition of SR Ca^{2+} ATPase (SERCA II), resulting in an impaired ability of the heart to both relax and contract.[73] In contrast, hyperphosphorylation of RyR2 results in defective channel function during excitation-contraction coupling.[74] Together, these changes result in decreased contractility in response to adrenergic stimulation and a propensity for developing arrhythmias.

Substantial evidence from model systems points to significant differences between β_1- and β_2-ARs and their ability to stimulate apoptosis in cardiac myocytes[11] with stimulation of the β_1- but not the β_2-AR pathway, resulting in an increased rate of cardiomyocyte apoptosis. Disruption of β_2-AR coupling to Gi by treatment with pertussis toxin can abrogate the potential protective, antiapoptotic signaling pathways rendering the β_2-AR proapoptotic.[75] Chesley and colleagues[76] have provided evidence to support the supposition that the antiapoptotic effects of β_2-AR are mediated in part by the stimulation of the PI3K and the Akt-PK-D pathways.

In addition to the mechanisms described above, the proapoptotic effect of the β_1-AR pathway may also be due to increased CaMKII activity. Zhu and associates[77] have shown that β_1-AR stimulation results in myocyte apoptosis that is independent of PKA activation, but dependent on CaMKII, suggesting that β_1-AR stimulation may selectively result in CaMKII activation independent of effects on PKA. These studies demonstrate that inhibition of CaMKII, L-type calcium channel phosphorylation, or buffering of intracellular Ca^{2+} results in an attenuation of β_1-AR-mediated apoptosis; conversely, overexpression of CaMKIIδ_c induces apoptosis. More recently, Yoo and colleagues,[78] using transgenic mice with knockouts of β-AR subtypes, have demonstrated that postinfarct, isoproterenol-mediated increases in CaMKII signaling and apoptosis are dependent exclusively on the β_1-AR.

Excessive β_1-AR signaling also activates the fetal gene program[28,30] (**see also Chapter 1**). The change in myosin heavy chain (MHC) isoform expression favoring the low(er) ATPase activity β isoform would be expected to decrease contractile function, as would the downregulation in SERCA II, another adult gene that is considered part of the adult-fetal program. Although the signaling cascades responsible for this activation are complex, CaMKII appears to play a prominent role,[28] and the altered expression of so-called fetal and adult genes appears mediated by β_1- and not β_2-AR stimulation.[28,30] CaMKII activity is upregulated in the failing human heart,[79,80] suggesting that despite the desensitization that occurs in more proximal β_1-receptor signaling steps, adverse signaling through CaMKII may be maintained or even enhanced (**see also Chapter 1**).

As described previously, CaMKII is involved in various pathologic processes in heart failure, including apoptosis, arrhythmias, and changes in gene expression. To gain a better understanding of the role of CaMKII in pathologic cardiac disease, knockout mouse models of CaMKII and a transgenic model overexpressing a CaMKII peptide inhibitor have been generated.[81,82] Mice expressing the inhibitory peptide are resistant to pathologic changes related to β-AR stimulation, and do not exhibit decreases in fractional shortening, increases in heart/body weight, or decreases in left ventricular internal diameter.[83] Different results are obtained in knockout mouse model studies. In response to transverse aortic constriction (TAC) in 6-week-old animals, there is knockout of CaMKIIδ blunted fibrosis as well as reducing heart/body weight ratio, myocyte area, and pathologic changes in gene expression.[84] In an 8-week TAC model, CaMKIIδ downregulation did not prevent the development of pathologic hypertrophy but blunted the transition to heart failure, including chamber dilation, ventricular dysfunction, lung edema, cardiac fibrosis, and apoptosis.[70] However, a 6-week-old CaMKII knockout mouse model of severe thoracic aortic banding showed improved contractility, increased myofilament sensitivity to Ca^{2+}, decreased apoptosis but increased fibrosis. In addition, no improvement in ejection fraction/fractional shortening was observed. The authors also showed that knockout of CaMKII in the setting of severe heart failure may be detrimental due to reduced efficiency of β-AR regulation of contraction and exacerbation of diastolic dysfunction.[82] These studies suggest that although CaMKII is likely to be primarily detrimental, it may also be important for β-AR regulation of contractile function in the failing heart.

In contrast to the general desensitization phenomena exhibited by β_1- and β_2-ARs in failing human ventricular

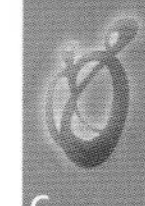

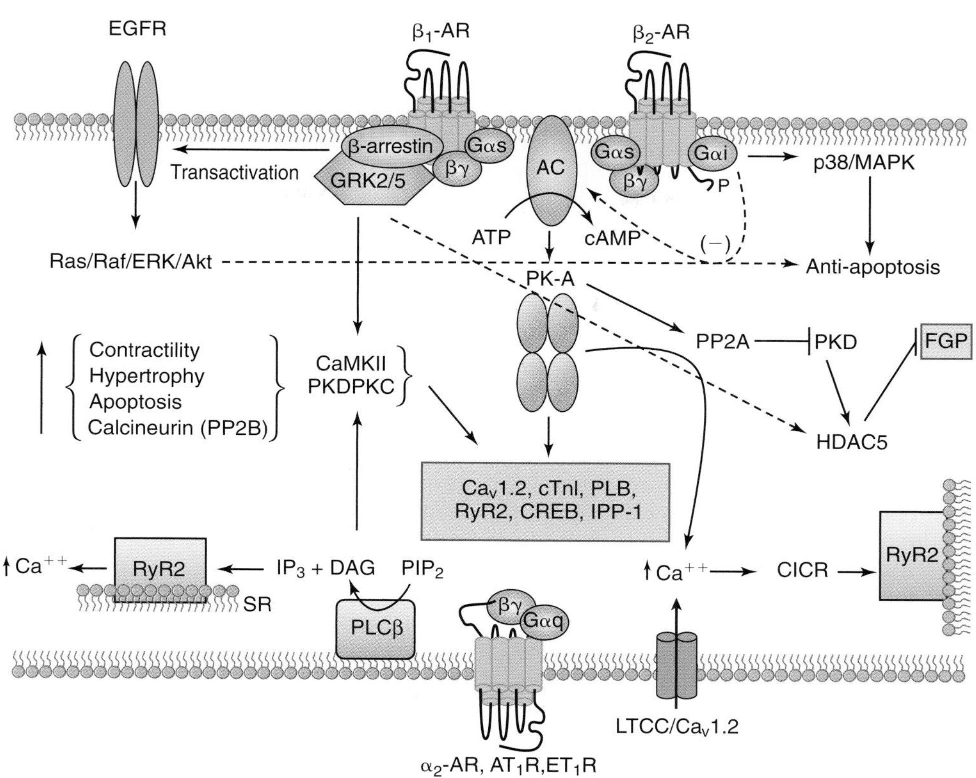

FIGURE 6-5 β-AR myocardial signaling pathways. Catecholamine-mediated stimulation of β_1- and β_2-ARs results in the activation of the stimulatory G protein, Gαs. This activates adenylyl cyclase (AC) increasing production of cyclic AMP (cAMP), resulting in the activation of the serine/threonine kinase, protein kinase A (PKA). PKA phosphorylates multiple downstream targets, including L-type Ca^{++} channels (LTCC, $Ca_v1.2$); modulators of contractile proteins, including troponin I (cTnI); the regulator of sarcoplasmic reticulum (SR) calcium uptake, phospholamban (PLB); the modulator of phosphatase activity, I-PP1; and the transcriptional regulator, CREB. PLB activity is also modulated secondary to phosphorylation by the kinases, CaMKII, PKD, and PKC. PKA increases intracellular calcium concentration, $[Ca^{++}]i$, and contractility by increasing LTCC activity, thereby increasing calcium-induced calcium release (CIRC) via the ryanodine receptor (RyR). PKA phosphorylation of PLB results in the disinhibition of Ca^{++} uptake into the SR by the ATP-dependent calcium pump, SERCA2. In addition to the Gαs/AC/PKA pathway, β_1-ARs activate other signaling pathways, including those of CaMKII and the epidermal growth factor receptor (EGFR). Increased CaMKII activity results in activation of prohypertrophic signaling and the reexpression of the fetal gene program (FGP). Activation of CaMKII also accelerates the rate of myocyte apoptosis. In contrast, β_1-AR stimulation of the EGFR (via GRK5/β-arrestin) appears to be predominantly cardioprotective. The β_1-AR/PKA pathway may be protective via activation of PP2A-mediated dephosphorylation of PKD and a subsequent repression of HDAC5 activity. In distinction to the β_1-AR, the β_2-AR, once phosphorylated by GKRs, couples to the inhibitory G protein, Gαi. This results in direct inhibition of AC activity; via Gβγ signaling, it also results in activation of MAPKs and antiapoptotic pathways. *From Port JD: Beta-adrenergic signaling: complexities and therapeutic relevance to heart failure. Current Signal Transduction Therapy 7:120–131, 2012.*

myocardium, β_3-ARs exhibit upregulation.[85] Because the β_3-AR knockout mouse undergoes excessive remodeling in response to pressure overload,[86] the increased expression of β_3-ARs in the failing human heart may be an adaptive mechanism.

MOLECULAR BASIS OF β-ADRENERGIC RECEPTOR SIGNALING

Canonically, β_1- and the β_2-ARs couple to stimulatory G proteins, Gs, which are composed of two subunits: an α subunit and a βγ-heterodimeric subunit (**Figure 6-5**). Both the α and βγ subunits are competent to signal independently. Gαs is a member of the much larger class of G protein α subunits, of which there are approximately 20 subtypes. Their heterogeneity is a central basis of specificity for G protein-coupled receptor signaling, a subject reviewed in detail elsewhere.[87] Additional layers of signaling diversity are afforded by combinatorial permutations of various βγ-heterodimeric subunits (5 β-subtypes and 11-γ subtypes) with the α subunits.

As a result of agonist stimulation, G protein α and βγ subunits dissociate with the free αs subunit acting to stimulate adenylyl cyclases (AC), for which there are multiple isoforms.[88] In cardiac tissues, the most abundant isoforms are AC V and VI, with the activities of each being feedback inhibited by increases in cytosolic calcium. In turn, adenylyl cyclase stimulation increases production of cAMP that in turn binds to the regulatory subunits of the PKA heterotetramer (two regulatory, and two catalytic subunits). Binding causes the dissociation of the regulatory and catalytic subunits of PKA, with the catalytic subunits proceeding to phosphorylate consensus serine (S) and threonine (T) residues on a broad spectrum of intracellular target proteins. In a number of tissues, including cardiac, PKA, and its targets, are in close approximation because of A-kinase anchoring proteins or AKAPs.[89] An association between the β_2-AR and AKAP79 has been described.[90] Additionally, there is recent clarity as to the scaffolding proteins that interact with β_1-ARs in cardiac tissues.[91] Thus unique interactions between β_1- and β_2-ARs and specific AKAPs and/or other anchoring proteins support the "microdomain" concept of receptor subtype-specific signaling, discussed in greater detail later.

Via the traditional Gαs/adenylyl cyclase pathway, β-AR stimulation results in the phosphorylation by PKA of a number of proteins, including L-type calcium channels (LTCC, $CaV_{1.2}$)[92] and PLB, the primary modulator of the SR-associated ATP-dependent calcium pump, SERCA II, as well as modulatory proteins associated with regulation of the contractile apparatus (e.g., troponin I [TnI]). More directly, however, PKA phosphorylates β-ARs,[93] as well as

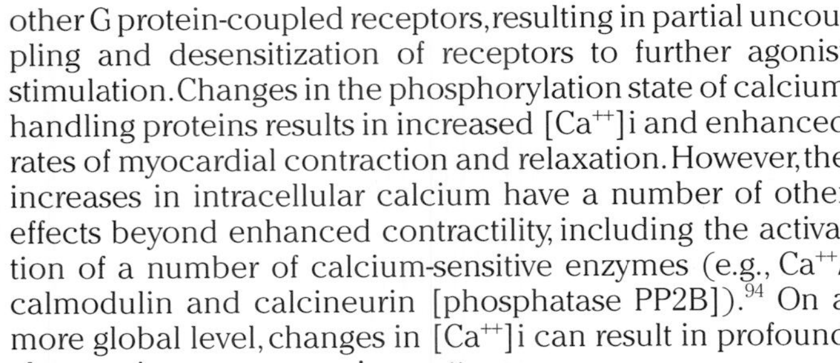

other G protein-coupled receptors, resulting in partial uncoupling and desensitization of receptors to further agonist stimulation. Changes in the phosphorylation state of calcium handling proteins results in increased [Ca^{++}]i and enhanced rates of myocardial contraction and relaxation. However, the increases in intracellular calcium have a number of other effects beyond enhanced contractility, including the activation of a number of calcium-sensitive enzymes (e.g., Ca^{++}/calmodulin and calcineurin [phosphatase PP2B]).[94] On a more global level, changes in [Ca^{++}]i can result in profound changes in gene expression patterns.

It has been known for some time that β_1- and β_2-ARs differ in their efficiency of coupling to adenylyl cyclase and to cAMP production, with the β_2-AR subtype being more efficiently coupled to cAMP production than is the β_1-AR.[53] In trabeculae isolated from the human heart, selective stimulation of contraction by either receptor pathway generally correlates well with receptor abundance.[52,56,57] However, the fact that the β_2-AR produces more cAMP per unit of stimulus does not translate into a greater inotropic potential for β_2-ARs. Rather, these data favor an argument that there is distinct intracellular compartmentalization of cAMP pools produced by β-ARs,[95] with the existence of discrete microdomains of high cAMP concentration in cardiomyocytes. Specifically, in neonatal cardiomyocytes, high concentrations of cAMP are found in the proximity of T tubules and the junctional SR. An argument is also made that diffusion of cAMP outside of these microdomains is quickly curtailed by the action of phosphodiesterases. Support for this notion is the finding that there appears to be close coordination between agonist-stimulated recruitment of phosphodiesterases to the β_2-AR, a process facilitated by interaction with β-arrestins, and the attenuation of signaling.

Recent data indicate that the differential signaling and architecture of β_1- and β_2-ARs appear to be defined in part by a differential association with phosphodiesterases (PDEs),[96] with PDE4 activity preferentially targeting cAMP produced by the β_1-AR, and cAMP produced by the β_2-AR being targeted by multiple subtypes of PDEs. Perhaps counterintuitive to the highly localized responses of β-ARs being dictated by scaffolding proteins is the recent study by Nikolaev and associates,[97] which demonstrated in transgenic mice that isoproterenol-mediated increases in cAMP in cardiac tissues leads to far-reaching cAMP signals for the β_1-AR, whereas β_2-AR-generated cAMP appears to remain locally confined. An excellent recent review, detailing the compartmentalization of β-AR signaling, the interplay of phosphodiesterases, phosphatases, and subtype-specific spaciotemporal patterning, has recently been published by Xiang.[98]

It is becoming increasingly clear that both the β_1-AR and the β_2-AR pathways couple to signaling pathways beyond the "traditional" Gαs/adenylyl cyclase pathway.[99] Perhaps the best example of this diversity of signaling is the finding that the β_2-AR can interact with the inhibitory G protein, Gαi. This is of interest in the setting of CHF for two reasons. As described earlier, increased circulating NE concentrations result in chronic activation of β-ARs. This in turn results in increased βARK activity and an increased phosphorylation state of β-ARs, resulting ultimately in the uncoupling of the receptor from the stimulatory Gαs signaling pathway. It is this phosphorylated form of the β_2-AR that has an increased propensity to couple to the inhibitory Gαi pathway[100] and its downstream effectors, including inhibition of AC and activation of MAPKs. Amplifying this effect is the finding that the abundance of Gαi proteins is significantly elevated in the failing human heart.[101] Thus the increased phosphorylation state of the β_2-AR and the increased abundance of Gαi protein both facilitate increased trafficking of β_2-AR signaling via Gαi-associated pathways. The ramifications of this are potentially significant, particularly in regard to protective, antiapoptotic effects as well as to myocardial growth regulatory effects.

The β_1-AR, although currently thought to be less promiscuous than the β_2-AR in its ability to couple to pathways other than to Gαs, nonetheless does exhibit signaling via additional pathways, as noted previously, to the CaMKII pathway. At least in part, this extra-Gαs coupling, much like that of the β_2-AR, appears to be facilitated by the specificity of the carboxy-terminus PDZ (PSD-95/Dlg/ZO-1) domain of the receptor peptide, which drives the interaction with proteins containing specific PDZ recognition motifs. An excellent review on the general topic of regulation of β-AR signaling by scaffolding proteins has been published by Hall and Lefkowitz.[102] Examples of β_1-AR interacting proteins are PSD-95, MAGI-2, the endophilins (SH3p4/p8/p13), and CNrasGEF, all of which appear to have unique downstream roles. The association of the β_1-AR with PSD-95, which is a neuronal-associated protein, distinctly places the β_1-AR in the proximity of the synapse,[103] a location perhaps even driven by adrenergic innervation. Here, PSD-95 appears to inhibit the internalization of the β_1-AR,[104] an effect that is modulated by the kinase GRK5. Conversely, interaction of the β_1-AR with endophilins appears to negatively modulate Gαs coupling and to promote β_1-AR internalization.[105] A more detailed picture of the β_1-AR SAP97-AKAP79 scaffold at its PSD-95/DLG/ZO1 motif has been demonstrated to be necessary for both PKA-mediated phosphorylation of the β_1-AR, as well as for receptor recycling.[91] This is in contrast to the findings describing the association of the β_1-AR with CNrasGEF (PDZ-GEF1), an effector molecule that activates Ras, and thus growth pathways. In this case, the mechanism of Ras activation is rather unique given that is appears to be via Gαs rather than the well-documented Gβγ signaling pathway (see Figure 6-5).

Additional evidence detailing the importance of PDZ-mediated interactions has been described by Xiang and colleagues.[106] Specifically, mutation of the PDZ motif by disruption of the carboxy-terminus renders the β_1-AR significantly more sensitive to agonist-mediated cell surface downregulation. Further, this deletion of C-terminal amino acids renders the β_1-AR more β_2-AR-like in that it becomes capable of interacting with Gi. Thus even though the β_1-AR[104] and β_2-AR[107] both contain PDZ motifs, the interacting proteins that each couples to via these motifs is unique and is an important basis of different regulatory and signaling properties. To expand this concept, the β_2-AR has been shown to modulate signaling independent of its interactions with G proteins. For example, the β_2-AR appears to couple to at least three other pathways: (1) NHERF, which in turn regulates the function of the Na^+/H^+ exchanger[108]; (2) to a non-PKA-dependent interaction with L-type calcium channels[27,99]; and (3) to the phosphatidylinositol 3′-kinase pathway (PI3K), a pathway associated with the inhibition of apoptosis, and to the PI3K-PTEN pathway, which is relevant to the regulation of both myocardial contractility and cell size and shape.[109]

As alluded to before, β-AR stimulation results in the dissociation of the stimulatory G protein, Gs, into α and βγ subunits, each of which is a signaling entity. A major function of the βγ-heterodimer is to recruit βARKs in proximity to the receptor. By virtue of the lipid-modified (isoprenylation) of the γ subunit, which promotes localization of the βγ subunit to the sarcolemmal membrane, the heterodimer is in position to orchestrate the colocalization of the β-AR with βARK. Protein/protein interaction of the βγ subunit with βARK occurs via a pleckstrin homology (PH) domain.[110] In this way, agonist-dependent, βARK-mediated phosphorylation of β-ARs is an important mode of β-AR desensitization.[62] In addition to playing a scaffolding role, βγ subunits are also signaling molecules in their own right. Downstream targets of signaling include subsets of adenylyl cyclases, PI3K, K^+ channels, and Ras/Raf/MEK/MAPK pathway(s) (see Figure 6-5).

Recently, significant attention has been paid to the specifics of β-AR localization and receptor trafficking. Differential targeting of β-AR subtypes to specific intracellular compartments has been described.[111] Of note is the apparent caveolar colocalization of the β_2-ARs with the inhibitory protein, Gαi, as well as with PKA subunits and with GRK2. What is now becoming clear is that the localization of the β_2-AR to the caveolar compartment is an essential component of its signaling capabilities.[112] In contrast, β_1-ARs, as well as a number of other proteins including Gαs, and ACs V and VI, are not specifically associated with caveolea; instead, these proteins have a more generalized distribution.

An important and newly emergent concept of β-AR signaling is that of the connection between β_1-AR signaling with the cardioprotective effects of the epidermal growth factor receptor (EGFR) pathway. Work from Rockman and colleagues[64,113,114] has shown that GRK5/6-mediated phosphorylation of the β_1-AR targets the association of β-arrestin to the receptor which, in addition to activating MAP kinases, facilitates the activation of matrix metalloproteinases, causing the release of heparin-bound EGF, which then activates the EGFR. Activation of the EGFR leads to activation of Ras/Raf/ERK/Akt and subsequent antiapoptotic, cardioprotective effects (see Figure 6-5).

Recent evidence indicates that the differentiation of β_1- versus β_2-AR signaling extends to the cardiac progenitor cells (CPCs) and their differentiation and survival. Interestingly, β-AR stimulation appears to promote the differentiation of CPCs via β_2-ARs. However, once these cells become committed to a myocyte lineage, they begin to express β_1-ARs. Counteracting the progression, continued β-AR stimulation via β_1-AR leads to a loss of CPCs.[115]

REGULATION OF β-ADRENERGIC RECEPTOR GENE EXPRESSION

Genes encoding β-ARs are regulated at virtually every level, including transcriptional, post-transcriptional/pretranslational, translational, and post-translational. Much like protooncogenes and cytokines, β-ARs can profoundly affect a number of cellular functions affecting cell viability, thus the need for stringent, rapid, and redundant regulatory mechanisms. β-AR expression, at the levels of both mRNA and protein, is the result of a number of independently regulated processes.

At the level of transcriptional regulation, both positive and negative transcriptional regulatory elements exist within the 5′-untranslated regions (UTRs) of β-ARs. Cell culture model systems have provided evidence regarding the effects of a number of transcriptional regulatory pathways starting with the most obvious, that of the direct effects of β-AR stimulation. Increases in cAMP can lead to a transient upregulation of β-AR mRNA via a cAMP-responsive element (CRE)-mediated transcriptional effect. However, it is recognized that in heart failure, at least for the β_1-AR, mRNA and protein are unequivocally downregulated.[58] Therefore, CRE-mediated upregulatory effects are unlikely to be important in the chronic setting. Conversely, β-AR genes have the potential to be negatively regulated by the transcriptional suppressor, ICER (inducible cAMP early repressor). Evidence points to a role for ICER in a pathophysiologic feedback loop, with its upregulation causing a persistent downregulation of PDE3A, a finding associated with increased isoproterenol-mediated cardiomyocyte apoptosis.[116] However, others have not found a downregulation in PDE3 in the failing human heart.[117]

In the cardiac context, a number of other transcriptional regulators of β-AR genes are also known to be important. Most notably, transcriptional regulation of β-AR genes by glucocorticoid- and thyroid hormone-responsive elements can have significant effects via their respective consensus DNA binding elements (e.g., glucocorticoid response element [GREs] and thyroid hormone response element [TREs]).[118,119] In general, glucocorticoids have been associated with causing an upregulation of β_2-ARs and a reciprocal downregulation of β_1-ARs,[118,120] whereas the thyroid hormone has been uniformly associated with upregulation of β-AR expression.[121]

For β-ARs expressed in myocardial tissues, the relationship between mRNA and protein appears to be well preserved.[54] Thus, mechanisms regulating β-AR mRNA abundance likely impact significantly β-AR protein expression. To this end, nucleic acid motifs known as A+U-rich elements, or AREs, found within the 3′ UTRs of several β-ARs, are known to be the target for a number of mRNA-binding proteins associated with changes in mRNA turnover. Previous evidence has confirmed a relationship between agonist-mediated stimulation of β-ARs, production of cAMP, and destabilization of β-AR mRNA, resulting in reduced mRNA and ultimately protein abundance.[122] However, additional evidence points to the role of MAPK pathways as critical regulators of the stability of ARE-containing mRNAs, including those encoding β-ARs.[123] In particular, several proteins associated with mRNA changes in mRNA turnover have been demonstrated to bind to β-AR AREs. These include AUF1/hnRNP D, which is associated with increased mRNA turnover[124]; HuR, which is associated with stabilization of numerous ARE-containing mRNAs[125]; KSRP, which increases turnover of ARE-containing mRNAs, drives muscle cell differentiation, and modulates Wnt/β-catenin and PI3K/AKT signaling[126]; and tristetraprolin (TTP), which is associated with turnover of TNF-α mRNA.[127] How each of these proteins specifically affects β-AR mRNA turnover in the myocardial tissues remains to be explored.[128] However, given the evidence that the homozygous deletion of TTP in transgenic mice results in a dramatic upregulation of TNF-α and a subsequent cardiomyopathy,[129] there is little doubt that these mechanisms are in play.

Other means of post-transcriptional regulation include modulation of translational efficiency that can be controlled by RNA binding proteins and by microRNAs. From the perspective of RNA binding proteins, both HuR and TIAR appear to modulate the β-AR gene expression via their ability to interact with U-rich nucleotide sequences.[130] From the perspective of microRNAs, it is well documented that they change in expression secondary to heart failure[131-134] and to increased β-AR signaling.[135] In turn, several microRNAs are candidates to modulate β-AR expression with miR let-7 being directly shown to do so. Recently, Wang and associates[136] have demonstrated that overexpression of let-7 causes downregulation of the β-AR, as well as an increased association of β_2-AR mRNA with the Ago2/RISC complex. Given the preservation of let-7 binding sites to the β_1-AR, it would be surprising if a similar regulatory pattern were not seen.

MYOPATHIC POTENTIAL OF INDIVIDUAL COMPONENTS OF ADRENERGIC RECEPTOR PATHWAYS

The development and study of transgenic animal models has provided a wealth of information with regard to understanding the role of adrenergic receptor signaling in CHF. This section will summarize a few of the more relevant findings obtained from animal models containing cardiac-targeted overexpression or deletion of various components of adrenergic receptor pathways. The impact of these changes on the development or prevention of cardiomyopathy is discussed.

β_1- and β_2-Adrenergic Receptors

The idea that significant differences exist between β_1- and β_2-AR signaling in the heart has been reinforced by data from a number of transgenic mouse models. One of the more notable initial observations was that overexpression of each receptor subtype can result in strikingly different cardiac phenotypes. As originally reported by Milano and colleagues,[137] overexpression of the wild-type β_2-AR in mice, at relatively high abundance (≈50- to 200-fold), was associated with increased basal AC activity, enhanced contractility, and elevated left ventricular (LV) function. Interestingly, no pathology was apparent in animals up to 4 months of age. In a longer-term study, Liggett and associates[138] reported comparable effects of increased β_2-AR on the myocardium (i.e., enhanced cardiac function from birth); however, this group also noted linear gene dose dependence with regard to the development of cardiomyopathy. Animals expressing more than 60× the background β-AR concentration maintained their hyperdynamic state for more than 1 year without an apparent increase in mortality. In contrast, overexpression of the β_2-AR at approximately 100-fold resulted in progressive cardiac enlargement, the development of heart failure, and premature death occurring at close to 1 year of age. At approximately 350 times the level of wild-type expression, the β_2-AR produced a cardiomyopathy, resulting in premature death in 50% of animals as early as week 25.[138]

Compared with the extremely high levels of β_2-AR expression required to produce myopathic results, wild-type β_1-AR overexpression at relatively low abundance (≈20- to 40-fold) can lead to markedly decreased contractility and LV function, and increased hypertrophy and fibrosis, resulting in progressive myocardial failure and premature death.[139,140] The pathophysiologic mechanism(s) responsible for the detrimental effects of β_1-AR overexpression in these animals are only partially understood. Chronic increases in PKA activity are likely to be a component of the pathology associated with β_1-AR overexpression as overexpression of the catalytic subunit of PKA is, in its own right, cardiomyopathic.[141] However, in the failing heart, cAMP abundance and therefore PKA activity is generally decreased.[31] Thus it is possible or perhaps even likely that β_1-AR-mediated CaMKII activity, which is increased in CHF, underlies the observed pathology.

Initial studies reported an increase in systolic function in young animals overexpressing the β_1-AR, with a progressive decline in LV function occurring with age.[139,140] Interestingly, this appears to occur before any structural alterations, such as fibrosis, which do not become apparent until at least 4 months, depending on level of expression. In this same study,[139] the mechanism of contractile dysfunction was found to involve impaired Ca^{2+} handling in cardiac myocytes, characterized by marked prolongation of intracellular Ca^{2+} transients. Subsequent examination of the expression levels of various sarcoplasmic reticulum (SR) proteins involved in Ca^{2+} release and uptake revealed a modest increase in the expression of SERCA II protein in animals at 2 months of age, and increased phosphorylation of phospholamban at Ser16, a critical regulatory site, was also detected. Collectively, these results indicate that impaired Ca^{2+} handling is likely another a major causal factor in producing early contractile dysfunction in β_1-AR overexpressors, with these changes occurring before the appearance of interstitial fibrosis or other structural alterations.

α_1-Adrenergic Receptors

Both α_{1A} and α_{1B}-ARs are expressed at the protein level in human ventricular myocardium, and neither is downregulated in heart failure.[142] Transgenic animal models that overexpress each subtype have been described. Overexpression of the wild-type α_{1B}-AR results in a dilated cardiomyopathy.[143] In contrast, α_{1A} transgenic cardiac overexpression produces an increase in contractility without hypertrophy.[144] Importantly, double knockout of both α_1 subtypes results in acceleration of remodeling in response to pressure overload,[145] suggesting on balance that α_1-ARs play an adaptive role in maintenance of myocardial chamber integrity. Moreover, of the two subtypes, the α_{1A}-AR appears to be particularly devoid of myopathic potential and is contractility enhancing, at least in rodents, the inference being that selective α_{1A} agonists may have therapeutic potential.[142,144]

G Proteins and Adenylyl Cyclase

As described above, the G proteins involved in adrenergic signaling are several, including Gs and Gi, which modulate AC activity, and Gq, which is linked to activation of PLC. Similar to that observed with the β-ARs, overexpression of each of these downstream signaling components results in a variety of cardiac phenotypes. Transgenic mice overexpressing wild-type Gαs have been described, with this model characterized by having a chronically increased heart rate, enhanced chronotropic and inotropic responses to agonists, altered β-AR density, and an increased frequency of cardiac arrhythmias.[146] Over time, myocardial performance in Gαs-overexpressing animals declines and LV dilation is observed. Likewise, myocyte hypertrophy, apoptosis, and fibrosis become evident with age, and animals die prematurely. In addition, there is evidence that overexpression of Gαs is associated with an increase in L-type Ca^{2+} currents, an effect that appears to be independent of cAMP and AC activation.

From these data, it has been suggested that Gαs may directly regulate the activity of L-type calcium channels. Interestingly, much like transgenic models of β-AR overexpression,[147] the pathophysiologic changes observed with Gαs overexpression can be prevented, and survival improved, through treatment with β-blockers.[148]

Transgenic mice that overexpress Gαq also exhibit a myopathic phenotype characterized by marked myocyte hypertrophy, increased expression of hypertrophy-related genes, and increased fibrosis, ultimately resulting in decreased myocardial contractility.[149] The mechanism of cardiomyopathy appears to involve, at least in part, cross-regulation to β-AR signaling pathways by Gαq or its downstream effectors.[150] Mice that overexpress Gαq exhibit decreased AC activity in response to agonists, which is apparently due to impaired functional coupling of β-ARs to AC, because β-AR density is unchanged when compared to wild-type expression levels. In addition, β-AR stimulation of L-type Ca^{2+} channels is depressed in Gαq overexpressors, and expression levels of Gi are increased, as is PK-C activity. In this model, inhibition of Gαi unexpectedly caused sudden death, suggesting that the change in Gαi expression may be a compensatory mechanism to counteract other detrimental signaling caused by the Gq pathway.

Cardiac-targeted overexpression of a modified Gi-coupled receptor has been reported.[151] Mice that contain this modified receptor reportedly exhibited significant ventricular conduction delays, which can be attenuated by treatment with pertussis toxin, suggesting strongly a Gi-dependent mechanism. Moreover, these animals developed a pronounced dilated cardiomyopathy, resulting in death by 15 weeks of age. These results were the first to suggest a potential causal role for increased Gi signaling in the development and progression of heart failure,[151] and stand in distinction to the notion that the Gi pathway is simply protective, acting to abrogate the deleterious stimulatory effects of the Gαs pathway. In fact, overexpression of the carboxy-terminus of Gαi (GiCT), a peptide construct that inhibits Gi signaling, has been demonstrated to enhance apoptosis associated with ischemia.[152]

In contrast to the above, overexpression of more distal components of the Gs signaling pathways, specifically ACs V or VI, does not appear to cause any form of cardiomyopathy.[153] Agonist-stimulated AC activity is higher in this model, and basal and stimulated PKA activities are also increased; however, these effects translate into modestly enhanced inotropic, lusitropic, or chronotropic function. Further, no long-term histopathologic sequelae or deleterious changes in cardiac function have been noted with AC overexpression.[153] Based on this profile, gene therapy trials using adenovirus-mediated gene transfer of adenylyl cyclases are under consideration.

G-Protein Receptor Kinases

As described above, GRKs are central to modulating β-AR signaling and do so from a variety of perspectives. GRK-mediated phosphorylation of β-ARs desensitize and uncouple the receptors from their signaling pathways, are facilitators of receptor internalization and downregulation, and, as mentioned previously in the case of GRK5, can affect cross-talk between canonical β-AR signaling pathways and other kinase pathways, including those of MAPKs and tyrosine kinases. Worth noting is the extensive work surrounding GRK2, historically described as βARK1. Increased expression and/or activity of GRK2 has been implicated in progression of heart failure and postmyocardial infarction[154] and the use of a GRK2 minipeptide that acts as an inhibitor appears to be of potential therapeutic benefit.[154] The deleterious effects of GRK2 have been linked in part to PKA-mediated phosphorylation of the β_2-AR, leading to Gi-biased signaling,[155] and to prodeath signaling via HSP90 mitochondrial targeting of GRK2.[156]

ADRENERGIC RECEPTOR POLYMORPHISMS AND THEIR IMPORTANCE IN HEART FAILURE NATURAL HISTORY OR THERAPEUTICS

Polymorphisms of many genes, including a number of components of adrenergic receptor signaling pathways and the renin-angiotensin-aldosterone system, have the potential to influence the progression of cardiovascular disease and/or response to individual therapeutic agents. Depending on the genetic variant and the endpoint assessed, variable response may be generalized either to a class of agents (i.e., β-blockers) or delimited to an individual agent.

In groundbreaking work performed by Liggett and collaborators, the effects of polymorphic variants of α- and β-ARs have been shown to have profound effects on receptor signaling and response to pharmacologic agents, and also potentially on clinical outcomes. For more detailed information on the subject, several reviews of adrenergic receptor polymorphisms have been published.[157,158] As with many genes, a number of haplotypes have been described.[159] Further, allele frequencies and combinations of complex haplotypes are not uniform across ethnic and geographic populations.[157,159]

Of particular importance in heart failure, two major polymorphic loci have been identified for the human β_1-AR gene: variants at nucleotide 145 encode either a serine (Ser) or glycine (Gly) variant amino acid at position 49 (Ser49Gly); variants at nucleotide 1165 encode either an arginine (Arg) or Gly variant at amino acid position 389 (Arg389Gly). Data indicate that the minor allele Gly49 variant is significantly more susceptible to agonist-induced downregulation than is the Ser49 variant,[160] even though the two variants do not appear to be different in terms of their ability to couple to stimulation of adenylyl cyclase and production of cAMP. In contrast, the 389 Arg and minor allele Gly variants of the β_1-AR have completely different signal transduction properties.[161,162] The Arg389 variant of the human β_1-AR is much more efficiently coupled to adenylyl cyclase stimulation than is the Gly389 variant,[162] with 3 to 4 times greater signal transduction capacity.[161] The Arg389 variant transduces greater inotropic effects in isolated preparations of both nonfailing and failing human hearts,[161] and has a greater portion of receptors exhibiting constitutive activity.[147,161,162] Perhaps most important, in transfected cells and human ventricular myocardial membranes compared with Gly389, the Arg389 variant has a higher affinity for agonists,[162] including an approximately fivefold greater fraction of receptors in a high-affinity, agonist binding state for NE.[163] This high affinity for NE compared with Gly389, β_2-AR, and β_3-AR means that *the β_1 389Arg AR is the norepinephrine receptor in the human heart.*

For NE binding[163] and inotropic stimulation[161] the Gly389 allele is dominant negative, such that myocardial

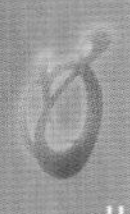

preparations from heterozygotes and Gly homozygotes have similar attenuation of function properties. This means that the genotype frequencies in the general U.S. population are evenly divided between Arg389 homozygous and Gly389 carriers (heterozygotes + Gly389 homozygotes). For historic reasons, the Gly389 variant has been considered to be the wild-type allele, because it was the first to be cloned[41]; however, its frequency in the Caucasian and African American populations of, respectively, approximately 0.27 and 0.42[161] establishes the Arg389 variant as the major allele. The human genome is unique in containing a substantial fraction of Gly389 alleles; all other genomes examined to date are 100% Arg389.[161]

As a follow-up to cell-based studies, transgenic mouse studies—where the β_1-AR Arg389Gly receptor variants have been overexpressed—clearly demonstrate that Arg389 is markedly more pathologic.[135,147] Additionally, Arg389 mice are more pharmacologically responsive to β-blocker therapy,[147] a notion that fits with the increased function receptor variant being able to be suppressed to a greater degree.[161] Interestingly, overexpression of 389Arg or Gly β_1-AR variants results in temporally different gene expression patterns for mRNA[135,147] and miRNA,[135] which when examined temporally appear to vary more quantitatively than qualitatively.[135]

Over the past several years, a number of clinical studies have attempted to associate clinical event and remodeling outcomes to patient β_1-AR 389Arg/Gly genotype.[161,163-166] An example of a study reporting differential reverse remodeling efficacy for carvedilol in patients with β_1-AR Arg389Gly variants was by Chen and colleagues.[167] However, a study by Metra and associates[165] could not confirm this result. Consistent with this finding, a well-designed prospective clinical trial by Sehnert and colleagues[166] found no effect of β_1-AR 389Arg/Gly variants on the primary endpoint of transplant-free survival for heart failure patients receiving either carvedilol or metoprolol. Improvement in reverse remodeling effected by metoprolol treatment in β_1-AR 389Arg homozygotes but not Gly carriers was reported by Terra and associates,[168] but was not confirmed in another study of genotyped heart failure clinic patients.[169] For metoprolol effects on clinical endpoints, in a pharmacogenetic substudy of the MERIT-HF trial, White and associates[170] reported that metoprolol CR/XL did not interact with the β_1-AR Arg389Gly polymorphism for effects on the combined endpoint of mortality or heart failure hospitalization, which was in agreement with metoprolol data from Sehnert and colleagues.[166] From a statistical standpoint, the most robust data on the effects of the β_1-AR Arg389Gly polymorphism on β-blocker clinical effects comes from a large (n = 2460, 765 deaths) heart failure clinic population prospectively followed in an NHLBI genomics study at two large heart failure referral centers.[164] β-blocker treatment occurred in 83%, 90% of whom received carvedilol or metoprolol. There was no evidence of any effect of the β_1-AR Arg389Gly polymorphism on mortality in β-blocker-treated patients, where mortality was lower compared with untreated patients, but only in Caucasians.[164] In marked contrast to these clinical endpoint pharmacogenetic studies investigating the effects of carvedilol and metoprolol CR/XL,[166,170] Liggett and associates[161] demonstrated an effect of β_1-AR 389Arg/Gly variants on mortality and other endpoints for the investigational β-blocker/sympatholytic agent bucindolol, and that this relationship can be modified by the presence or absence of an α_{2C}-AR insertion/deletion polymorphism.[163] Thus for clinical endpoints, differential therapeutic effects of β-blockers by β_1-AR Arg389Gly polymorphism may be agent dependent. The basis for the β_1-AR 389 polymorphism differential effects of bucindolol but not carvedilol or metoprolol may reside in the novel pharmacologic properties of bucindolol, which include promoting inactivation of constitutively active β_1-AR 389Arg receptors[161] and NE lowering.[20,163] The Arg389 β_1-AR variant's much higher affinity for NE compared with its Gly389 counterpart[163] means that NE lowering would have preferentially favorable effects in subjects who are $\beta_1$389 Arg homozygotes.[163]

The effects of the β_1-AR Arg389Gly polymorphism on the risk of developing heart failure and on disease progression have also been investigated. A study by Small and associates[48] investigated the potential synergism between β_1-AR and α_{2C}-AR polymorphisms and uncovered a significantly increased risk of developing heart failure in African American subjects in $\beta_1$389 Arg homozygotes who were also homozygous for the loss of function α_{2C}-AR 322-325 deletion (Del) allele.[48] The β_1-AR Arg389 allele did not appear to be a risk factor for developing heart failure in and of itself,[147] but its presence synergistically increased the risk associated with the α_{2C}-AR Del allele.[163,171] The increased risk of developing heart failure in patients who are $\beta_1$389 Arg and α_{2C} Del combination homozygotes was driven by results in African Americans,[48] who have a 10-fold higher allele frequency for the Del allele.[48,161] These results could not be confirmed in a European population[172] or in a large epidemiologic study in an African American population.[173] The hypothesis for the synergistic risk of the $\beta_1$389Arg and α_{2C} Del homozygous genotype was that based on the loss of tonic inhibition of NE release in adrenergic nerves patients with α_{2C} Del prejunctional receptors would have an increase in adrenergic drive that would then signal through hyperfunctional $\beta_1$389Arg receptors.[48,147] However, in subjects with established CHF the α_{2C} Del polymorphism is not associated with a statistically significant increase in systemic venous NE levels,[171] and so this hypothesis may not be correct.

In the placebo arms of both the BEST[161] and MERIT-HF[170] DNA substudies that examined effects of the β_1-AR Arg389Gly polymorphism on clinical endpoints, there was no evidence of any differences between patients who were Arg homozygous versus those who were Gly carriers. However, in Cresci and colleagues' two-center genomics study,[164] Caucasian patients untreated with β-blockers, who were homozygous for $\beta_1$389 Arg, had an improved survival compared with Gly389 patients. Thus there are mixed reports for the β_1-AR Arg389Gly polymorphism affecting heart failure risk and disease progression, and larger, prospective studies are needed.

A number of polymorphisms have also been described for the human β_2-AR, the best characterized of which is the presence of either a threonine (Thr) or isoleucine (Ile) at amino acid position 164.[174] The allele frequency of the 164 Ile minor allele is quite low (~5%), and only 1% to 5% of the population is heterozygous Thr/Ile. Remarkably, no homozygous Ile/Ile subjects have been identified, possibly because of the myocardial dysfunction and mortality associated with this loss of function polymorphism. Similar to the β_1-AR Arg389 variant, the Thr164 β_2-AR is much more efficiently coupled to adenylyl cyclase activation than is the Ile164 variant.[174] The presence of the Ile164 allele is associated with reduced exercise capacity[175] and reduced transplant-free survival.[176] In a transgenic mouse model system, overexpression of the human β_2-AR Ile164 leads to impaired cardiac function,[174] a finding that recapitulates the observation that this allele is associated with reduced exercise capacity and reduced survival in patients with heart failure.[175] Because of the extremely low Ile164 allele frequency, no intervention studies have been reported for effects in Thr164Ile heterozygotes.

Kaye and associates[177] and Metra and colleagues[165] have reported that a polymorphism of the β_2-AR that affects agonist-mediated downregulation, Gln27Glu, where the Glu allele confers resistance, is associated with a more favorable LVEF response to carvedilol. In terms of effects on clinical endpoints, De Groote and associates[178] reported no effects on mortality in a modest size (n = 444) heart failure clinic population in which 91% were treated with β-blockers.

As described above, one of the major regulators of β-AR signaling is the GRKs. Interestingly, a Gln>Leu41 variant of GRK5 has been shown to be protective against heart failure–associated death or transplantation in an African American population,[164,179] where the Leu allele is approximately 20 times more frequent than in Caucasian populations. The authors speculate that the increased agonist-mediated uncoupling of the β-AR by GRK5-Leu41 is, in essence, the equivalent of "genetic β-blockade."[158,179]

There would seem a high likelihood that beyond what has already been described, other polymorphic variants of adrenergic receptors, other G protein-coupled receptors, and any number of downstream effectors will eventually be described. A significant question that remains to be addressed is whether or not the presence of specific polymorphisms, alone or in combination, are primary factors in the predisposition to, or in the rate of progression of, heart failure. The issue of whether β_1-AR Arg389Gly polymorphisms can alter the clinical response to bucindolol will be answered by prospective Phase 3 clinical trials.

NONCATECHOLAMINE LIGANDS THAT ACTIVATE MYOCARDIAL β-ADRENERGIC RECEPTORS, AND THEIR ROLE IN PRODUCING DILATED CARDIOMYOPATHIES

It does not require a biogenic amine to activate a GPCR; work spanning decades has demonstrated that autoantibodies (AAbs) to the extracellular loops of GPCRs can bind to β_1-[180] and β_2-[181] ARs, and that the consequent signaling[182] can have adverse biologic effects on the myocardium and cardiac myocytes.[183] These AAbs act differently from catecholamine agonists by activating the AR through a different motif.[184] From the standpoint of heart failure, there is no doubt that AAbs to the first and second extracellular loops of the human β_1-AR can produce a dilated cardiomyopathy,[183] and that removal of these AAbs by immunoadsorption[185] can improve myocardial function. Major questions remain as to the incidence of AAbs in dilated or ischemic cardiomyopathies, and their role in a general heart failure population. Some of these questions are being addressed by an ongoing European study called ETiCS.[186]

There are several approaches beyond immunoadsorption to dealing with these AAbs, including the administration of decoy peptides[187] and aptamers that bind to the AAbs with high affinity.[183] Some of these approaches, coupled with a companion diagnostic, may make their way through clinical development over the next several years,[188] and if so will likely be incorporated into the heart failure armamentarium.

SUMMARY AND FUTURE DIRECTIONS

Adrenergic mechanisms are markedly altered in CHF, and exert major effects on the natural history of the clinical syndrome. Adrenergic abnormalities can be classified into two major groups: those that produce a sustained increase in adrenergic drive and those that cause defects or qualitative shifts in β-AR signal transduction. Within each category there is the potential for benefit and harm, and successful therapeutic intervention involves interfering with the harmful components without compromising the beneficial aspects. A pharmacologic concept evolving in this context is that of biased GPCR ligands,[189] and other approaches involving the use of β_1-selective antagonists in combination with a second agent to enhance beneficial adrenergic effects have undergone, or are undergoing, testing.[5]

It should be clear from the scope of this review that adrenergic receptor signaling is far more complex than our naïve supposition that the binding of catecholamines to receptors simply increases the abundance of the second messengers, cAMP and Ca^{++}, thereby affecting an increase in myocardial contractility and heart rate. Although the importance of these functions has not been diminished, adrenergic receptors are now recognized to be important effectors of any number of cellular processes important to cardiac myocyte biology. Undoubtedly, the diversity and complexity of these signaling paradigms will continue to unfold. It is hoped that an increased appreciation of these processes, as well as the recognition that genetic variation is important to both disease progression and to therapeutic response, will lead to advances in heart failure therapeutics.

References

1. Rundqvist B, Elam M, Bergmann-Sverrisdottir Y, et al: Increased cardiac adrenergic drive precedes generalized sympathetic activation in human heart failure. *Circulation* 95(1):169–175, 1997.
2. Esler M, Kaye D, Lambert G, et al: Adrenergic nervous system in heart failure. *Am J Cardiol* 80(11A):7L–14L, 1997.
3. Mann D, Kent R, Parsons B, et al: Adrenergic effects on the biology of the adult mammalian cardiocyte. *Circulation* 85:790–804, 1992.
4. Mann DL: Basic mechanisms of disease progression in the failing heart: the role of excessive adrenergic drive. *Prog Cardiovasc Dis* 41(1 Suppl 1):1–8, 1998.
5. Bristow MR: Treatment of chronic heart failure with beta-adrenergic receptor antagonists: a convergence of receptor pharmacology and clinical cardiology. *Circ Res* 109(10):1176–1194, 2011.
6. Packer M, Bristow MR, Cohn JN, et al: The effect of carvedilol on morbidity and mortality in patients with chronic heart failure. U.S. Carvedilol Heart Failure Study Group. *N Engl J Med* 334(21):1349–1355, 1996.
7. MERIT: Effect of metoprolol CR/XL in chronic heart failure: metoprolol CR/XL Randomised Intervention Trial in Congestive Heart Failure (MERIT-HF) [see comments]. *Lancet* 353(9169):2001–2007, 1999.
8. Investigators B: A trial of the beta-blocker bucindolol in patients with advanced chronic heart failure. *N Engl J Med* 344(22):1659–1667, 2001.
9. Yancy CW, Jessup M, Bozkurt B, et al: 2013 ACCF/AHA Guideline for the Management of Heart Failure: a report of the American College of Cardiology Foundation/American Heart Association Task Force on Practice Guidelines. *Circulation* 128(16):e240–e327, 2013.
10. Ziegler K: Uber die Wirkung intravenoser adrenalin-injektion auf das Gefafssytem und ihre Beziehung zur Arteriosklerose. *Bietrage zur Pathologischen Anatonie* 38:229–254, 1905.
11. Communal C, Singh K, Sawyer DB, et al: Opposing effects of beta(1)- and beta(2)-adrenergic receptors on cardiac myocyte apoptosis : role of a pertussis toxin-sensitive G protein. *Circulation* 100(22):2210–2212, 1999.
12. Communal C, Colucci WS, Singh K: p38 Mitogen-activated protein kinase pathway protects adult rat ventricular myocytes against beta-adrenergic receptor-stimulated apoptosis: evidence for Gi-dependent activation. *J Biol Chem* 275:19395–19400, 2000.
13. Bristow MR, Feldman AM, Adams KF, Jr, et al: Selective versus nonselective beta-blockade for heart failure therapy: are there lessons to be learned from the COMET trial? *J Card Fail* 9(6):444–453, 2003.
14. CIBISII: The Cardiac Insufficiency Bisoprolol Study II (CIBIS-II): a randomised trial [see comments]. *Lancet* 353(9146):9–13, 1999.
15. Poole-Wilson PA, Swedberg K, Cleland JG, et al: Comparison of carvedilol and metoprolol on clinical outcomes in patients with chronic heart failure in the Carvedilol Or Metoprolol European Trial (COMET): randomised controlled trial. *Lancet* 362(9377):7–13, 2003.

16. Swedberg K, Viquerat C, Rouleau J-L, et al: Comparison of myocardial catecholamine balance in chronic congestive heart failure and in angina pectoris without failure. *Am J Cardiol* 54(783–786):1984.
17. Hasking GJ, Esler MD, Jennings GL, et al: Norepinephrine spillover to plasma in patients with congestive heart failure: evidence of increased overall and cardiorenal sympathetic nervous activity. *Circulation* 73(4):615–621, 1986.
18. Cohn JN, Levine TB, Olivari MT: Plasma norepinephrine as a guide to prognosis in patients with chronic congestive heart failure. *N Engl J Med* 311:819–823, 1984.
19. Chidsey CA, Braunwald E, Morrow AG, et al: Myocardial norepinephrine concentrations in man: effects of reserpine and of congestive heart failure. *N Engl J Med* 269:653–659, 1963.
20. Bristow MR, Krause-Steinrauf H, Nuzzo R, et al: Effect of baseline or changes in adrenergic activity on clinical outcomes in the beta-blocker evaluation of survival trial. *Circulation* 110(11):1437–1442, 2004.
21. Brunner-La Rocca HP, Esler MD, Jennings GL, et al: Effect of cardiac sympathetic nervous activity on mode of death in congestive heart failure. *Eur Heart J* 22(13):1136–1143, 2001.
22. Bristow MR, Gilbert EM, Abraham WT, et al: Carvedilol produces dose-related improvements in left ventricular function and survival in subjects with chronic heart failure. MOCHA Investigators. *Circulation* 94(11):2807–2816, 1996.
23. Eichhorn EJ, Bristow MR: Medical therapy can improve the biological properties of the chronically failing heart. A new era in the treatment of heart failure. *Circulation* 94(9):2285–2296, 1996.
24. Shaddy RE, Boucek MM, Hsu DT, et al: Carvedilol for children and adolescents with heart failure: a randomized controlled trial. *JAMA* 298(10):1171–1179, 2007.
25. Ryerson LM, Alexander PM, Butt WW, et al: Rotating inotrope therapy in a pediatric population with decompensated heart failure. *Pediatr Crit Care Med* 12(1):57–60, 2011.
26. Stauffer BL, Russell G, Nunley K, et al: miRNA expression in pediatric failing human heart. *J Mol Cell Cardiol* 57:43–46, 2013.
27. Lader AS, Xiao YF, Ishikawa Y, et al: Cardiac Gsalpha overexpression enhances L-type calcium channels through an adenylyl cyclase independent pathway. *Proc Natl Acad Sci U S A* 95(16):9669–9674, 1998.
28. Sucharov CC, Mariner PD, Nunley KR, et al: A beta1-adrenergic receptor CaM kinase II-dependent pathway mediates cardiac myocyte fetal gene induction. *Am J Physiol Heart Circ Physiol* 291(3):H1299–H1308, 2006.
29. Anderson ME: CaMKII and a failing strategy for growth in heart. *J Clin Invest* 119(5):1082–1085, 2009. PMCID: 2673844.
30. Lowes BD, Gilbert EM, Abraham WT, et al: Myocardial gene expression in dilated cardiomyopathy treated with beta-blocking agents. *N Engl J Med* 346(18):1357–1365, 2002.
31. Bohm M, Reiger B, Schwinger RH, et al: cAMP concentrations, cAMP dependent protein kinase activity, and phospholamban in non-failing and failing myocardium. *Cardiovasc Res* 28(11):1713–1719, 1994.
32. Danielsen W, der Leyen H, Meyer W, et al: Basal and isoprenaline-stimulated cAMP content in failing versus nonfailing human cardiac preparations. *J Cardiovasc Pharmacol* 14(1):171–173, 1989.
33. Ahlquist R: A study of the adrenotropic receptors. *Am J Physiol* 153:586–600, 1948.
34. Lands AM, Arnold A, McAuliff P, et al: Differentiation of receptor systems activated by sympathomimetic amines. *Nature* 214:597–598, 1967.
35. Bristow M, Sherrod TR, Green RD: Analysis of beta receptor drug interactions in isolated rabbit atrium, aorta, stomach and trachea. *J Pharmacol Exp Ther* 171(1):52–61, 1970.
36. Emorine LJ, Marullo S, Briend-Sutren MM, et al: Molecular characterization of the human beta 3-adrenergic receptor. *Science* 245(4922):1118–1121, 1989.
37. Alexander RW, Davis JN, Lefkowitz RJ: Direct identification and characterisation of beta-adrenergic receptors in rat brain. *Nature* 258(5534):437–440, 1975.
38. Williams LT, Snyderman R, Lefkowitz RJ: Identification of beta-adrenergic receptors in human lymphocytes by (-) (3H) alprenolol binding. *J Clin Invest* 57(1):149–155, 1976.
39. Dunn R, McCoy J, Simsek M, et al: The bacteriorhodopsin gene. *Proc Natl Acad Sci U S A* 78(11):6744–6748, 1981. PMCID: 349126.
40. Dixon RA, Kobilka BK, Strader DJ, et al: Cloning of the gene and cDNA for mammalian beta-adrenergic receptor and homology with rhodopsin. *Nature* 321(6065):75–79, 1986.
41. Frielle T, Collins S, Daniel KW, et al: Cloning of the cDNA for the human beta 1-adrenergic receptor. *Proc Natl Acad Sci U S A* 84(22):7920–7924, 1987. PMCID: 299447.
42. Cotecchia S, Schwinn DA, Randall RR, et al: Molecular cloning and expression of the cDNA for the hamster alpha 1-adrenergic receptor. *Proc Natl Acad Sci U S A* 85(19):7159–7163, 1988. PMCID: 282143.
43. Kobilka BK, Dixon RA, Frielle T, et al: cDNA for the human beta 2-adrenergic receptor: a protein with multiple membrane-spanning domains and encoded by a gene whose chromosomal location is shared with that of the receptor for platelet-derived growth factor. *Proc Natl Acad Sci U S A* 84(1):46–50, 1987. PMCID: 304138.
44. Kobilka BK, Matsui H, Kobilka TS, et al: Cloning, sequencing, and expression of the gene coding for the human platelet alpha 2-adrenergic receptor. *Science* 238(4827):650–656, 1987.
45. Rohde S, Sabri A, Kamasamudran R, et al: The alpha(1)-adrenoceptor subtype- and protein kinase C isoform-dependence of norepinephrine's actions in cardiomyocytes. *J Mol Cell Cardiol* 32(7):1193–1209, 2000.
46. Minneman KP: Alpha 1-adrenergic receptor subtypes, inositol phosphates, and sources of cell Ca2. *Pharmacol Rev* 40(2):87–119, 1988.
47. Bowman JC, Steinberg SF, Jiang T, et al: Expression of protein kinase C beta in the heart causes hypertrophy in adult mice and sudden death in neonates. *J Clin Invest* 100:2189–2195, 1997.
48. Small KM, Wagoner LE, Levin AM, et al: Synergistic polymorphisms of beta1- and alpha2C-adrenergic receptors and the risk of congestive heart failure. *N Engl J Med* 347(15):1135–1142, 2002.
49. Cohen ML, Granneman JG, Chaudhry A, et al: Is the "atypical" beta-receptor in the rat stomach fundus the rat beta 3 receptor? *J Pharmacol Exp Ther* 272(1):446–451, 1995.
50. Aragon JP, Condit ME, Bhushan S, et al: Beta3-adrenoreceptor stimulation ameliorates myocardial ischemia-reperfusion injury via endothelial nitric oxide synthase and neuronal nitric oxide synthase activation. *J Am Coll Cardiol* 58(25):2683–2691, 2011. PMCID: 3586978.
51. Gauthier C, Leblais V, Kobzik L, et al: The negative inotropic effect of beta3-adrenoceptor stimulation is mediated by activation of a nitric oxide synthase pathway in human ventricle. *J Clin Invest* 102(7):1377–1384, 1998.
52. Bristow MR, Ginsburg R, Umans V, et al: Beta 1- and beta 2-adrenergic-receptor subpopulations in nonfailing and failing human ventricular myocardium: coupling of both receptor subtypes to muscle contraction and selective beta 1-receptor down-regulation in heart failure. *Circ Res* 59(3):297–309, 1986.
53. Bristow MR, Hershberger RE, Port JD, et al: Beta 1- and beta 2-adrenergic receptor-mediated adenylate cyclase stimulation in nonfailing and failing human ventricular myocardium. *Mol Pharmacol* 35(3):295–303, 1989.
54. Bristow M, Minobe W, Raynolds M, et al: Reduced β1 receptor messenger RNA abundance in the failing human heart. *J Clin Invest* 92:2737–2745, 1993.
55. Brodde OE, Schuler S, Kretsch R, et al: Regional distribution of beta-adrenoceptors in the human heart: coexistence of functional beta 1- and beta 2-adrenoceptors in both atria and ventricles in severe congestive cardiomyopathy. *J Cardiovasc Pharmacol* 8(6):1235–1242, 1986.
56. Bristow MR, Anderson FL, Port JD, et al: Differences in beta-adrenergic neuroeffector mechanisms in ischemic versus idiopathic dilated cardiomyopathy. *Circulation* 84(3):1024–1039, 1991.
57. Brodde OE: Beta 1- and beta 2-adrenoceptors in the human heart: properties, function, and alterations in chronic heart failure. *Pharmacol Rev* 43(2):203–242, 1991.
58. Ungerer M, Bohm M, Elce JS, et al: Altered expression of beta-adrenergic receptor kinase and beta 1-adrenergic receptors in the failing human heart. *Circulation* 87(2):454–463, 1993.
59. Benovic JL, Strasser RH, Caron MG, et al: Beta-adrenergic receptor kinase: identification of a novel protein kinase that phosphorylates the agonist-occupied form of the receptor. *Proc Natl Acad Sci U S A* 83(9):2797–2801, 1986.
60. Feldman AM, Cates AE, Veazey WB, et al: Increase of the 40,000-mol wt pertussis toxin substrate (G protein) in the failing human heart. *J Clin Invest* 82(1):189–197, 1988.
61. Bristow MR, Hershberger RE, Port JD, et al: Beta-adrenergic pathways in nonfailing and failing human ventricular myocardium. *Circulation* 82(2 Suppl):I12–I25, 1990.
62. Pitcher JA, Freedman NJ, Lefkowitz RJ: G protein-coupled receptor kinases. *Annu Rev Biochem* 67:653–692, 1998.
63. Hu LA, Chen W, Premont RT, et al: G Protein-coupled receptor kinase 5 regulates beta 1-adrenergic receptor association with PSD-95. *J Biol Chem* 277(2):1607–1613, 2002.
64. Noma T, Lemaire A, Naga Prasad SV, et al: Beta-arrestin-mediated beta1-adrenergic receptor transactivation of the EGFR confers cardioprotection. *J Clin Invest* 117(9):2445–2458, 2007. PMCID: 1952636.
65. Hausdorff W, Caron M, Lefkowitz R: Turning off the signal: desensitization of β-adrenergic receptor function. *FASEB J* 4:2881–2889, 1990.
66. Colucci WS, Denniss AR, Leatherman GF, et al: Intracoronary infusion of dobutamine to patients with and without severe congestive heart failure. *J Clin Invest* 81:1103–1110, 1988.
67. Schwinger RH, Munch G, Bolck B, et al: Reduced Ca(2+)-sensitivity of SERCA 2a in failing human myocardium due to reduced serine-16 phospholamban phosphorylation. *J Mol Cell Cardiol* 31(3):479–491, 1999.
68. Marx SO, Reiken S, Hisamatsu Y, et al: PKA phosphorylation dissociates FKBP12.6 from the calcium release channel (ryanodine receptor): defective regulation in failing hearts. *Cell* 101(4):365–376, 2000.
69. Marks AR, Marx SO, Reiken S: Regulation of ryanodine receptors via macromolecular complexes: a novel role for leucine/isoleucine zippers. *Trends Cardiovasc Med* 12(4):166–170, 2002.
70. Ling H, Zhang T, Pereira L, et al: Requirement for Ca2+/calmodulin-dependent kinase II in the transition from pressure overload-induced cardiac hypertrophy to heart failure in mice. *J Clin Invest* 119(5):1230–1240, 2009. PMCID: 2673879.
71. Pereira L, Cheng H, Lao DH, et al: Epac2 mediates cardiac beta1-adrenergic-dependent sarcoplasmic reticulum Ca2+ leak and arrhythmia. *Circulation* 127(8):913–922, 2013.
72. Nicolaou P, Hajjar RJ, Kranias EG: Role of protein phosphatase-1 inhibitor-1 in cardiac physiology and pathophysiology. *J Mol Cell Cardiol* 47(3):365–371, 2009. PMCID: 2716438.
73. Koss KL, Kranias EG: Phospholamban: a prominent regulator of myocardial contractility. *Circ Res* 79(6):1059–1063, 1996.
74. Shan J, Betzenhauser MJ, Kushnir A, et al: Role of chronic ryanodine receptor phosphorylation in heart failure and beta-adrenergic receptor blockade in mice. *J Clin Invest* 120(12):4375–4387, 2010. PMCID: 2993577.
75. Communal C, Singh K, Colucci W: Gi protein protects adult rat ventricular myocytes, from β-adrenergic receptor-stimulated apoptosis in vitro. *Circulation* 98(17):I-742, 1998.
76. Chesley A, Lundberg MS, Asai T, et al: The beta(2)-adrenergic receptor delivers an antiapoptotic signal to cardiac myocytes through G(i)-dependent coupling to phosphatidylinositol 3'-kinase. *Circ Res* 87(12):1172–1179, 2000.
77. Zhu W-Z, Wang S-Q, Chakir K, et al: Linkage of beta1-adrenergic stimulation to apoptotic heart cell death through protein kinase A-independent activation of Ca2+/calmodulin kinase II. *J Clin Invest* 111(5):617–625, 2003.
78. Yoo B, Lemaire A, Mangmool S, et al: Beta1-adrenergic receptors stimulate cardiac contractility and CaMKII activation in vivo and enhance cardiac dysfunction following myocardial infarction. *Am J Physiol Heart Circ Physiol* 297:H1377–H1386, 2009.
79. Kirchhefer U, Schmitz W, Scholz H, et al: Activity of cAMP-dependent protein kinase and Ca2+/calmodulin-dependent protein kinase in failing and nonfailing human hearts. *Cardiovasc Res* 42(1):254–261, 1999.
80. Bossuyt J, Helmstadter K, Wu X, et al: Ca2+/calmodulin-dependent protein kinase IIdelta and protein kinase D overexpression reinforce the histone deacetylase 5 redistribution in heart failure. *Circ Res* 102(6):695–702, 2008.
81. Ling H, Gray CB, Zambon AC, et al: Ca2+/Calmodulin-dependent protein kinase II delta mediates myocardial ischemia/reperfusion injury through nuclear factor-kappaB. *Circ Res* 112(6):935–944, 2013. PMCID: 3673710.
82. Cheng J, Xu L, Lai D, et al: CaMKII inhibition in heart failure, beneficial, harmful, or both. *Am J Physiol Heart Circ Physiol* 302(7):H1454–H1465, 2012. PMCID: 3330794.
83. Zhang R, Khoo MS, Wu Y, et al: Calmodulin kinase II inhibition protects against structural heart disease. *Nat Med* 11(4):409–417, 2005.
84. Backs J, Backs T, Neef S, et al: The delta isoform of CaM kinase II is required for pathological cardiac hypertrophy and remodeling after pressure overload. *Proc Natl Acad Sci U S A* 106(7):2342–2347, 2009. PMCID: 2650158.
85. Moniotte S, Kobzik L, Feron O, et al: Upregulation of beta(3)-adrenoceptors and altered contractile response to inotropic amines in human failing myocardium. *Circulation* 103(12):1649–1655, 2001.
86. Moens AL, Leyton-Mange JS, Niu X, et al: Adverse ventricular remodeling and exacerbated NOS uncoupling from pressure-overload in mice lacking the beta3-adrenoreceptor. *J Mol Cell Cardiol* 47(5):576–585, 2009. PMCID: 2761504.
87. Morris AJ, Malbon CC: Physiological regulation of G protein-linked signaling. *Physiol Rev* 79(4):1373–1430, 1999.
88. Defer N, Best-Belpomme M, Hanoune J: Tissue specificity and physiological relevance of various isoforms of adenylyl cyclase. *Am J Physiol* 279(3):F400–F416, 2000.
89. Colledge M, Scott JD: AKAPs: from structure to function. *Trends Cell Biol* 9(6):216–221, 1999.
90. Fraser ID, Cong M, Kim J, et al: Assembly of an A kinase-anchoring protein-beta(2)-adrenergic receptor complex facilitates receptor phosphorylation and signaling. *Curr Biol* 10(7):409–412, 2000.
91. Gardner LA, Naren AP, Bahouth SW: Assembly of an SAP97-AKAP79-cAMP-dependent protein kinase scaffold at the type 1 PSD-95/DLG/ZO1 motif of the human beta(1)-adrenergic receptor generates a receptosome involved in receptor recycling and networking. *Journal of Biological Chemistry* 282(7):5085–5099, 2007.
92. Gao T, Yatani A, Dell'Acqua ML, et al: cAMP-dependent regulation of cardiac L-type Ca2+ channels requires membrane targeting of PKA and phosphorylation of channel subunits. *Neuron* 19(1):185–196, 1997.
93. Benovic JL, Pike LJ, Cerione RA, et al: Phosphorylation of the mammalian beta-adrenergic receptor by cyclic AMP-dependent protein kinase. Regulation of the rate of receptor phosphorylation and dephosphorylation by agonist occupancy and effects on coupling of the receptor to the stimulatory guanine nucleotide regulatory protein. *J Biol Chem* 260(11):7094–7101, 1985.
94. Taigen T, De Windt LJ, Lim HW, et al: Targeted inhibition of calcineurin prevents agonist-induced cardiomyocyte hypertrophy. *Proc Natl Acad Sci U S A* 97(3):1196–1201, 2000.
95. Zaccolo M, Pozzan T: Discrete microdomains with high concentration of cAMP in stimulated rat neonatal cardiac myocytes. *Science* 295(5560):1711–1715, 2002.
96. Richter W, Day P, Agrawal R, et al: Signaling from beta1- and beta2-adrenergic receptors is defined by differential interactions with PDE4. *EMBO J* 27(2):384–393, 2008. PMCID: 2196435.

97. Nikolaev VO, Bunemann M, Schmitteckert E, et al: Cyclic AMP imaging in adult cardiac myocytes reveals far-reaching beta1-adrenergic but locally confined beta2-adrenergic receptor-mediated signaling. *Circ Res* 99(10):1084–1091, 2006.
98. Xiang YK: Compartmentalization of beta-adrenergic signals in cardiomyocytes. *Circ Res* 109:231–244, 2011.
99. Steinberg SF: The molecular basis for distinct beta-adrenergic receptor subtype actions in cardiomyocytes. *Circ Res* 85(11):1101–1111, 1999.
100. Daaka Y, Luttrell LM, Lefkowitz RJ: Switching of the coupling of the beta2-adrenergic receptor to different G proteins by protein kinase A. *Nature* 390(6655):88–91, 1997.
101. Bohm M, Gierschik P, Jakobs KH, et al: Increase of Gi alpha in human hearts with dilated but not ischemic cardiomyopathy. *Circulation* 82(4):1249–1265, 1990.
102. Hall RA, Lefkowitz RJ: Regulation of G protein-coupled receptor signaling by scaffold proteins. *Circ Res* 91(8):672–680, 2002.
103. Shcherbakova OG, Hurt CM, Xiang Y, et al: Organization of beta-adrenoceptor signaling compartments by sympathetic innervation of cardiac myocytes. *J Cell Biol* 176(4):521–533, 2007. PMCID: 2063986.
104. Hu LA, Tang Y, Miller WE, et al: Beta 1-adrenergic receptor association with PSD-95. Inhibition of receptor internalization and facilitation of beta 1-adrenergic recptor interaction with N-methyl-D-aspartate receptors. *J Biol Chem* 275(49):38659–38666, 2000.
105. Tang Y, Hu LA, Miller WE, et al: Identification of the endophilins (SH3p4/p8/p13) as novel binding partners for the beta1-adrenergic receptor. *Proc Natl Acad Sci U S A* 96(22):12559–12564, 1999.
106. Xiang Y, Devic E, Kobilka B: The PDZ binding motif of the beta 1 adrenergic receptor modulates receptor trafficking and signaling in cardiac myocytes. *J Biol Chem* 277(37):33783–33790, 2002.
107. Cao TT, Deacon HW, Reczek D, et al: A kinase-regulated PDZ-domain interaction controls endocytic sorting of the beta2-adrenergic receptor. *Nature* 401(6750):286–290, 1999.
108. Hall RA, Premont RT, Chow CW, et al: The beta2-adrenergic receptor interacts with the Na+/H+-exchanger regulatory factor to control Na+/H+ exchange. *Nature* 392(6676):626–630, 1998.
109. Crackower MA, Oudit GY, Kozieradzki I, et al: Regulation of myocardial contractility and cell size by distinct PI3K-PTEN signaling pathways. *Cell* 110(6):737–749, 2002.
110. Pitcher JA, Touhara K, Payne ES, et al: Pleckstrin homology domain-mediated membrane association and activation of the beta-adrenergic receptor kinase requires coordinate interaction with G beta gamma subunits and lipid. *J Biol Chem* 270(20):11707–11710, 1995.
111. Rybin VO, Xu X, Lisanti MP, et al: Differential targeting of beta -adrenergic receptor subtypes and adenylyl cyclase to cardiomyocyte caveolae. A mechanism to functionally regulate the cAMP signaling pathway. *J Biol Chem* 275(52):41447–41457, 2000.
112. Xiang Y, Rybin VO, Steinberg SF, et al: Caveolar localization dictates physiologic signaling of beta 2-adrenoceptors in neonatal cardiac myocytes. *J Biol Chem* 277(37):34280–34286, 2002.
113. Patel PA, Tilley DG, Rockman HA: Physiologic and cardiac roles of beta-arrestins. *J Mol Cell Cardiol* 46(3):300–308, 2009.
114. Tilley DG, Kim IM, Patel PA, et al: Beta-arrestin mediates beta1-adrenergic receptor-epidermal growth factor receptor interaction and downstream signaling. *J Biol Chem* 284(30):20375–20386, 2009.
115. Khan M, Mohsin S, Avitabile D, et al: Beta-adrenergic regulation of cardiac progenitor cell death versus survival and proliferation. *Circ Res* 112(3):476–486, 2013. PMCID: 3595054.
116. Yan C, Ding B, Shishido T, et al: Activation of extracellular signal-regulated kinase 5 reduces cardiac apoptosis and dysfunction via inhibition of a phosphodiesterase 3A/inducible cAMP early repressor feedback loop. *Circ Res* 100(4):510–519, 2007.
117. Movsesian MA, Smith CJ, Krall J, et al: Sarcoplasmic reticulum-associated cyclic adenosine 5'-monophosphate phosphodiesterase activity in normal and failing human hearts. *J Clin Invest* 88(1):15–19, 1991. PMCID: 295996.
118. Kiely J, Hadcock JR, Bahouth SW, et al: Glucocorticoids down-regulate beta 1-adrenergic-receptor expression by suppressing transcription of the receptor gene. *Biochem J* 302(Pt 2):397–403, 1994.
119. Bahouth SW, Cui X, Beauchamp MJ, et al: Thyroid hormone induces beta1-adrenergic receptor gene transcription through a direct repeat separated by five nucleotides. *J Mol Cell Cardiol* 29(12):3223–3237, 1997.
120. Cornett LE, Hiller FC, Jacobi SE, et al: Identification of a glucocorticoid response element in the rat beta2- adrenergic receptor gene. *Mol Pharmacol* 54(6):1016–1023, 1998.
121. Bahouth SW: Thyroid hormones transcriptionally regulate the beta 1-adrenergic receptor gene in cultured ventricular myocytes. *J Biol Chem* 266(24):15863–15869, 1991.
122. Mitchusson KD, Blaxall BC, Pende A, et al: Agonist-mediated destabilization of human beta1-adrenergic receptor mRNA: role of the 3' untranslated translated region. *Biochem Biophys Res Commun* 252(2):357–362, 1998.
123. Headley VV, Tanveer R, Greene SM, et al: Reciprocal regulation of beta-adrenergic receptor mRNA stability by mitogen activated protein kinase activation and inhibition. *Molecular & Cellular Biochemistry* 258(1-2):109–119, 2004.
124. Pende A, Tremmel KD, DeMaria CT, et al: Regulation of the mRNA-binding protein AUF1 by activation of the beta-adrenergic receptor signal transduction pathway. *Journal of Biological Chemistry.* 271(14):8493–8501, 1996.
125. Ma W-J, Cheng S, Campbell C, et al: Cloning and characterization of HuR, a ubiquitously expressed elav-like protein. *J Biol Chem* 271:8144–8151, 1996.
126. Gherzi R, Trabucchi M, Ponassi M, et al: The RNA-binding protein KSRP promotes decay of beta-catenin mRNA and is inactivated by PI3K-AKT signaling. *PLoS Biol* 5(1):e5, 2006.
127. Lai WS, Carballo E, Strum JR, et al: Evidence that tristetraprolin binds to AU-rich elements and promotes the deadenylation and destabilization of tumor necrosis factor alpha mRNA. *Mol Cell Biol* 19(6):4311–4323, 1999.
128. David Gerecht PS, Taylor MA, Port JD: Intracellular localization and interaction of mRNA binding proteins as detected by FRET. *BMC Cell Biol* 11(1):69, 2010.
129. Taylor GA, Carballo E, Lee DM, et al: A pathogenetic role for TNF alpha in the syndrome of cachexia, arthritis, and autoimmunity resulting from tristetraprolin (TTP) deficiency. *Immunity* 4(5):445–454, 1996.
130. Subramaniam K, Kandasamy K, Joseph K, et al: The 3'-untranslated region length and the AU-rich RNA location modulate RNA-protein interaction and translational control of beta2-adrenergic receptor mRNA. *Mol Cell Biochem* 352:125–141, 2011.
131. Port JD, Walker LA, Polk J, et al: Temporal expression of miRNAs and mRNAs in a mouse model of myocardial infarction. *Physiol Genomics* 43:1087–1095, 2011.
132. Sucharov C, Bristow MR, Port JD: miRNA expression in the failing human heart: functional correlates. *J Mol Cell Cardiol* 45(2):185–192, 2008. PMCID: 2561965.
133. van Rooij E, Sutherland LB, Liu N, et al: A signature pattern of stress-responsive microRNAs that can evoke cardiac hypertrophy and heart failure. *Proc Natl Acad Sci U S A* 103(48):18255–18260, 2006.
134. Condorelli G, Latronico MV, Dorn GW, 2nd: microRNAs in heart disease: putative novel therapeutic targets? *Eur Heart J* 31(6):649–658, 2010. PMCID: 2838683.
135. Dockstader K, Nunley KR, Medway A, et al: Temporal analysis of mRNA and miRNA expression in transgenic mice over expressing Arg- and Gly389 polymorphic variants of the β1-adrenergic receptor. *Physiol Genomics* 43:1294–1306, 2011.
136. Wang WC, Juan AH, Panebra A, et al: MicroRNA let-7 establishes expression of beta2-adrenergic receptors and dynamically down-regulates agonist-promoted down-regulation. *Proc Natl Acad Sci U S A* 108(15):6246–6251, 2011. PMCID: 3076830.
137. Milano CA, Allen LF, Rockman HA, et al: Enhanced myocardial function in transgenic mice overexpressing the beta 2-adrenergic receptor. *Science* 264(5158):582–586, 1994.
138. Liggett SB, Tepe NM, Lorenz JN, et al: Early and delayed consequences of beta(2)-adrenergic receptor overexpression in mouse hearts: critical role for expression level. *Circulation* 101(14):1707–1714, 2000.
139. Engelhardt S, Hein L, Wiesmann F, et al: Progressive hypertrophy and heart failure in beta1-adrenergic receptor transgenic mice. *Proc Natl Acad Sci U S A* 96(12):7059–7064, 1999.
140. Bisognano JD, Weinberger HD, Bohlmeyer TJ, et al: Myocardial-directed overexpression of the human beta(1)-adrenergic receptor in transgenic mice. *J Mol Cell Cardiol* 32(5):817–830, 2000.
141. Antos CL, Frey N, Marx SO, et al: Dilated cardiomyopathy and sudden death resulting from constitutive activation of protein kinase A. *Circ Res* 89(11):997–1004, 2001.
142. Jensen BC, Swigart PM, De Marco T, et al: α1-Adrenergic receptor subtypes in nonfailing and failing human myocardium. *Circ Heart Fail.* 2(6):654–663, 2009. PMCID: 2780440.
143. Lemire I, Ducharme A, Tardif JC, et al: Cardiac-directed overexpression of wild-type alpha1B-adrenergic receptor induces dilated cardiomyopathy. *Am J Physiol Heart Circ Physiol* 281(2):H931–H938, 2001.
144. Lin F, Owens WA, Chen S, et al: Targeted alpha(1A)-adrenergic receptor overexpression induces enhanced cardiac contractility but not hypertrophy. *Circ Res* 89(4):343–350, 2001.
145. O'Connell TD, Ishizaka S, Nakamura A, et al: The alpha(1A/C)- and alpha(1B)-adrenergic receptors are required for physiological cardiac hypertrophy in the double-knockout mouse. *J Clin Invest* 111(11):1783–1791, 2003.
146. Gaudin C, Ishikawa Y, Wight DC, et al: Overexpression of Gs alpha protein in the hearts of transgenic mice. *J Clin Invest* 95(4):1676–1683, 1995.
147. Mialet Perez J, Rathz DA, Petrashevskaya NN, et al: Beta 1-adrenergic receptor polymorphisms confer differential function and predisposition to heart failure. *Nat Med* 9(10):1300–1305, 2003.
148. Asai K, Yang GP, Geng YJ, et al: Beta-adrenergic receptor blockade arrests myocyte damage and preserves cardiac function in the transgenic G(salpha) mouse. *J Clin Invest* 104(5):551–558, 1999.
149. D'Angelo DD, Sakata Y, Lorenz JN, et al: Transgenic Galphaq overexpression induces cardiac contractile failure in mice. *Proc Natl Acad Sci U S A* 94(15):8121–8126, 1997.
150. Dorn GW, 2nd, Tepe NM, Wu G, et al: Mechanisms of impaired beta-adrenergic receptor signaling in G(alphaq)-mediated cardiac hypertrophy and ventricular dysfunction. *Mol Pharmacol* 57(2):278–287, 2000.
151. Redfern CH, Degtyarev MY, Kwa AT, et al: Conditional expression of a Gi-coupled receptor causes ventricular conduction delay and a lethal cardiomyopathy. *Proc Natl Acad Sci U S A* 97(9):4826–4831, 2000.
152. DeGeorge BR, Jr, Gao E, Boucher M, et al: Targeted inhibition of cardiomyocyte Gi signaling enhances susceptibility to apoptotic cell death in response to ischemic stress. *Circulation* 117(11):1378–1387, 2008.
153. Gao MH, Lai NC, Roth DM, et al: Adenylylcyclase increases responsiveness to catecholamine stimulation in transgenic mice. *Circulation* 99(12):1618–1622, 1999.
154. Raake PW, Vinge LE, Gao E, et al: G protein-coupled receptor kinase 2 ablation in cardiac myocytes before or after myocardial infarction prevents heart failure. *Circ Res* 103(4):413–422, 2008. PMCID: 2679955.
155. Zhu W, Petrashevskaya N, Ren S, et al: Gi-biased beta2AR signaling links GRK2 upregulation to heart failure. *Circ Res* 110(2):265–274, 2012. PMCID: 3282829.
156. Chen M, Sato PY, Chuprun JK, et al: Prodeath signaling of G protein-coupled receptor kinase 2 in cardiac myocytes after ischemic stress occurs via extracellular signal-regulated kinase-dependent heat shock protein 90-mediated mitochondrial targeting. *Circ Res* 112(8):1121–1134, 2013.
157. Small KM, McGraw DW, Liggett SB: Pharmacology and physiology of human adrenergic receptor polymorphisms. *Annu Rev of Pharmacol Toxicol* 43:381–411, 2003.
158. Dorn GW, Liggett SB: Mechanisms of pharmacogenomic effects of genetic variation of the cardiac adrenergic network in heart failure. *Mol Pharmacol* 76:466–480, 2009.
159. Small KM, Mialet-Perez J, Liggett SB: Genetic variation within the beta1-adrenergic receptor gene results in haplotype-specific expression phenotypes. *J Cardiovasc Pharmacol* 51(1):106–110, 2008.
160. Rathz DA, Brown KM, Kramer LA, et al: Amino acid 49 polymorphisms of the human beta1-adrenergic receptor affect agonist-promoted trafficking. *J Cardiovasc Pharmacol* 39(2):155–160, 2002.
161. Liggett SB, Mialet-Perez J, Thaneemit-Chen S, et al: A polymorphism within a conserved beta(1)-adrenergic receptor motif alters cardiac function and beta-blocker response in human heart failure. *Proc Natl Acad Sci U S A* 103(30):11288–11293, 2006. PMCID: 1523317.
162. Mason DA, Moore JD, Green SA, et al: A gain-of-function polymorphism in a G-protein coupling domain of the human beta1-adrenergic receptor. *J Biol Chem* 274(18):12670–12674, 1999.
163. O'Connor CM, Fiuzat M, Carson PE, et al: Combinatorial pharmacogenetic interactions of bucindolol and beta1, alpha2C adrenergic receptor polymorphisms. *PLoS ONE* 7(10):e44324, 2012. PMCID: 3468617.
164. Cresci S, Kelly RJ, Cappola TP, et al: Clinical and genetic modifiers of long-term survival in heart failure. *J Am Coll Cardiol* 54(5):432–444, 2009. PMCID: 2749467.
165. Metra M, Covolo L, Pezzali N, et al: Role of beta-adrenergic receptor gene polymorphisms in the long-term effects of beta-blockade with carvedilol in patients with chronic heart failure. *Cardiovasc Drugs Ther* 24(1):49–60, 2010.
166. Sehnert AJ, Daniels SE, Elashoff M, et al: Lack of association between adrenergic receptor genotypes and survival in heart failure patients treated with carvedilol or metoprolol. *J Am Coll Cardiol* 52(8):644–651, 2008.
167. Chen L, Meyers D, Javorsky G, et al: Arg389Gly-beta1-adrenergic receptors determine improvement in left ventricular systolic function in nonischemic cardiomyopathy patients with heart failure after chronic treatment with carvedilol. *Pharmacogenetics & Genomics* 17(11):941–949, 2007.
168. Terra SG, Hamilton KK, Pauly DF, et al: Beta1-adrenergic receptor polymorphisms and left ventricular remodeling changes in response to beta-blocker therapy. *Pharmacogenet Genomics* 15(4):227–234, 2005.
169. Baudhuin LM, Miller WL, Train L, et al: Relation of ADRB1, CYP2D6, and UGT1A1 polymorphisms with dose of, and response to, carvedilol or metoprolol therapy in patients with chronic heart failure. *Am J Cardiol* 106(3):402–408, 2010.
170. White HL, de Boer RA, Maqbool A, et al: An evaluation of the beta-1 adrenergic receptor Arg389Gly polymorphism in individuals with heart failure: a MERIT-HF sub-study. *Eur J Heart Fail* 5(4):463–468, 2003.
171. Bristow MR, Murphy GA, Krause-Steinrauf H, et al: An alpha2C-adrenergic receptor polymorphism alters the norepinephrine-lowering effects and therapeutic response of the beta-blocker bucindolol in chronic heart failure. *Circ Heart Fail* 3(1):21–28, 2010.
172. Metra M, Zani C, Covolo L, et al: Role of beta1- and alpha2c-adrenergic receptor polymorphisms and their combination in heart failure: a case-control study. *Eur J Heart Fail* 8(2):131–135, 2006.
173. Canham RM, Das SR, Leonard D, et al: Alpha2cDel322-325 and beta1Arg389 adrenergic polymorphisms are not associated with reduced left ventricular ejection fraction or increased left ventricular volume. *J Am Coll Cardiol* 49(2):274–276, 2007.
174. Turki J, Lorenz JN, Green SA, et al: Myocardial signaling defects and impaired cardiac function of a human beta 2-adrenergic receptor polymorphism expressed in transgenic mice. *Proc Natl Acad Sci U S A* 93(19):10483–10488, 1996.

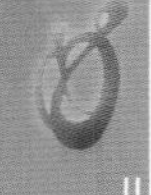

175. Wagoner LE, Craft LL, Singh B, et al: Polymorphisms of the beta(2)-adrenergic receptor determine exercise capacity in patients with heart failure. *Circ Res* 86(8):834–840, 2000.
176. Liggett SB, Wagoner LE, Craft LL, et al: The Ile164 beta2-adrenergic receptor polymorphism adversely affects the outcome of congestive heart failure. *J Clin Invest* 102(8):1534–1539, 1998.
177. Kaye DM, Smirk B, Williams C, et al: Beta-adrenoceptor genotype influences the response to carvedilol in patients with congestive heart failure. *Pharmacogenetics* 13(7):379–382, 2003.
178. de Groote P, Lamblin N, Helbecque N, et al: The impact of beta-adrenoreceptor gene polymorphisms on survival in patients with congestive heart failure. *Eur J Heart Fail* 7(6):966–973, 2005.
179. Liggett SB, Cresci S, Kelly RJ, et al: A GRK5 polymorphism that inhibits beta-adrenergic receptor signaling is protective in heart failure. [see comment]. *Nat Med* 14(5):510–517, 2008.
180. Limas CJ, Goldenberg IF, Limas C: Autoantibodies against beta-adrenoceptors in human idiopathic dilated cardiomyopathy. *Circ Res* 64(1):97–103, 1989.
181. Guillet JG, Lengagne R, Magnusson Y, et al: Induction of a pharmacologically active clonotypic B cell response directed to an immunogenic region of the human beta 2-adrenergic receptor. *Clin Exp Immunol* 89(3):461–467, 1992. PMCID: 1554485.
182. Wallukat G, Fu ML, Magnusson Y, et al: Agonistic effects of anti-peptide antibodies and autoantibodies directed against adrenergic and cholinergic receptors: absence of desensitization. *Blood Press Suppl* 3:31–36, 1996.
183. Haberland A, Wallukat G, Dahmen C, et al: Aptamer neutralization of beta1-adrenoceptor autoantibodies isolated from patients with cardiomyopathies. *Circ Res* 109:986–992, 2011.
184. Jane-wit D, Altuntas CZ, Johnson JM, et al: Beta 1-adrenergic receptor autoantibodies mediate dilated cardiomyopathy by agonistically inducing cardiomyocyte apoptosis. *Circulation* 116(4):399–410, 2007.
185. Muller J, Wallukat G, Dandel M, et al: Immunoglobulin adsorption in patients with idiopathic dilated cardiomyopathy. *Circulation* 101(4):385–391, 2000.
186. Deubner N, Berliner D, Schlipp A, et al: Cardiac beta1-adrenoceptor autoantibodies in human heart disease: rationale and design of the Etiology, Titre-Course, and Survival (ETiCS) Study. *Eur J Heart Fail* 12(7):753–762, 2010.
187. Jahns R, Schlipp A, Boivin V, et al: Targeting receptor antibodies in immune cardiomyopathy. *Semin Thromb Hemost* 36(2):212–218, 2010.
188. Port JD, Bristow MR: Aptamer therapy for heart failure? *Circ Res* 109(9):982–983, 2011.
189. Dewire SM, Violin JD: Biased ligands for better cardiovascular drugs: dissecting G-protein-coupled receptor pharmacology. *Circ Res* 109(2):205–216, 2011.

7 Role of Innate Immunity in Heart Failure

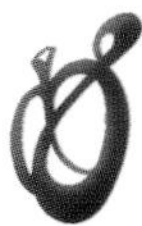

Douglas L. Mann

Although clinicians recognized the pathophysiologic importance of inflammatory mediators in the heart as far back as 1669, the formal recognition that inflammatory mediators were activated in the setting of heart failure did not occur for another three centuries. Since the initial description of inflammatory cytokines in patients with heart failure in 1990,[1] there has been a growing interest in the role that these molecules play in regulating cardiac structure and function, particularly with regard to their potential role in disease progression in heart failure. This interest has expanded recently with the recognition that inflammatory mediators are an integral part of a much larger biologic system referred to as the *innate immune system*. In the present chapter, I will summarize the recent growth of knowledge that has taken place in this field, with a particular emphasis on the biology of proinflammatory cytokines that may play a pathophysiologic role in the progression of heart failure. For the convenience of the reader, a glossary of abbreviations used is presented at the end of Chapter 7.

OVERVIEW OF INNATE IMMUNITY

The adult heart responds to tissue injury by synthesizing a series of proteins that promote homeostasis, either by activating mechanisms that facilitate tissue repair, or alternatively, by upregulating mechanisms that confer cytoprotective responses within the heart. The literature suggests that proinflammatory cytokines serve as the downstream "effectors" of the innate immune system by facilitating tissue repair within the heart. What has been less understood until recently is how these myocardial innate immune responses are coordinated following tissue injury. The relatively recent discovery of a family of receptors termed *Toll-like receptors (TLRs)* and *NOD-like receptors (NLRs)* has greatly increased our understanding of the "upstream" molecular components that regulate the innate immune response.[2] Indeed, knowledge regarding the biology of TLRs has provided important new insights with respect to our understanding of the role of inflammation in health and disease.

TLRs serve as pattern recognition receptors (PRRs) that recognize conserved motifs on pathogens, so-called pathogen-associated molecular patterns (PAMPs). Typical examples of PAMPs include the lipopolysaccharides (LPS) of gram-negative organisms, the teichoic acids of gram-positive organisms, the glycolipids of mycobacterium, the zymosans of yeast, and the double-stranded RNAs of viruses. These PAMPs are unique to these pathogens, and in some cases are required for their virulence. Thus one of the quintessential features of the innate immune system is that it serves as an "early warning system" that enables the host to accurately and rapidly discriminate self from non-self. More recently it has become clear that TLRs also recognize molecular patterns of endogenous host material that is released during cellular injury or death, so-called damage-associated molecular patterns (DAMPs).[3,4] As shown in **Figure 7-1**, DAMPs can be derived from dying or injured cells, damaged extracellular matrix proteins, or circulating oxidized proteins. As will be discussed, the long-term consequences of sustained activation of innate immunity can lead to progressive left ventricular (LV) remodeling and LV dysfunction, thereby contributing to the pathogenesis of heart failure.

EXPRESSION AND REGULATION OF TOLL-LIKE RECEPTORS IN THE HEART

The toll receptor was originally discovered as a protein that was responsible for dorsoventral polarity in the fly. Subsequent studies demonstrated that the human homolog of the *Drosophila* toll protein was sufficient to activate NF-κB–dependent genes in mammalian cells.[5] At the time of this writing, 13 mammalian TLR paralogs have been identified, of which 10 functional TLRs have been identified in humans (functional TLRs 11-13 are only expressed in mice). TLRs 1-6

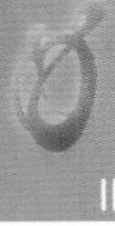

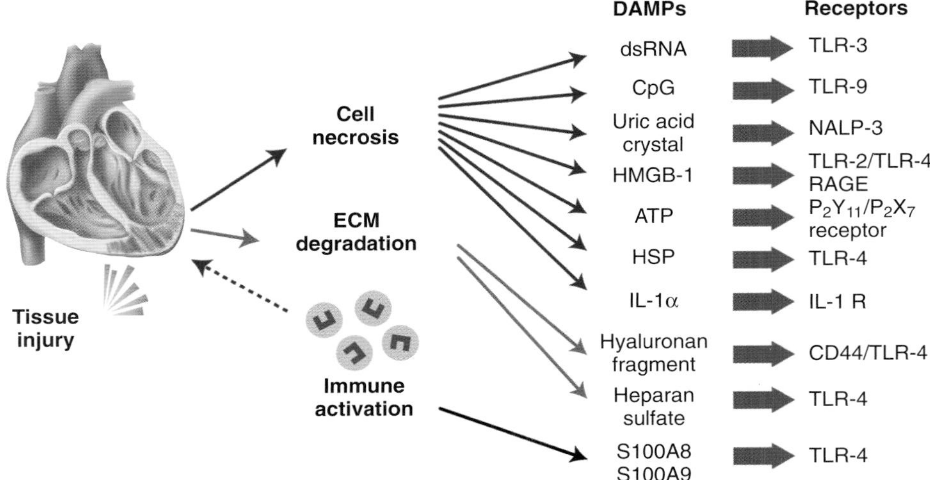

FIGURE 7-1 Damage-associated molecular patterns (DAMPs) are derived from dying cells that release their cytosolic content following myocardial injury, from degradation of the extracellular matrix, as well as by immune cells that become activated following tissue injury. *ATP,* Adenosine triphosphate; *HMGB1,* high mobility box group 1 protein; *HSP,* heat shock protein; *IL-1α,* interleukin-1α; *IL-1R,* interleukin receptor; *NALP,* NACHT, LRR, and PYD domains—containing protein 3 (cryopyrin); *RAGE,* receptor for advanced glycation end products; *TLR,* Toll-like receptor.

are expressed on the cell surface of mammalian cells, whereas TLRs 3, 7, and 9 are expressed in intracellular compartments, primarily endosomes and the endoplasmic reticulum, with the ligand-binding domains facing the lumen of the vesicle. TLR10 is the most recent member of the human TLR receptor family discovered; however, its function and direct ligand are still unknown. Humans also encode a TLR11 gene, but it contains several stop codons and the protein is not expressed.

Messenger RNA for TLRs 1-10 has been identified in the human heart.[6] Of note, the relative expression levels of mRNA for TLRs 2, 3, and 4 are approximately 10-fold higher than TLRs 1 and 5-10.[6] Although expression levels of TLRs have not been identified in human myocytes, TLRs 2, 3, 4, and 6 mRNA have been identified in cardiac myocytes from neonatal rats.[7] Although less is known with regard to the regulation of TLR expression in heart failure, the experimental literature suggests that sustained activation of TLR signaling following cardiac injury is maladaptive and can lead to heart failure. Two studies have shown that TLR4 expression is increased in the hearts of patients with advanced heart failure.[8,9] Moreover, the pattern of TLR4 expression in cardiac myocytes differs in heart failure in that there are focal areas of intense TLR4 staining in failing cardiac myocytes, in contrast to the diffuse pattern of TLR4 staining observed in nonfailing myocytes.[8]

Toll-Like Receptor Signaling Pathways

As shown in **Figure 7-2A**, the signaling pathway that is used by the TLR family of receptors is highly homologous to that of the IL-1 receptor (IL-1R) family (see later discussion). TLRs are type I membrane-spanning receptors that have a leucine-rich repeat extracellular motif and an intracellular signaling motif that is similar to interleukin (IL-1). With the exception of TLR3, all TLRs interact with an adapter protein termed *MyD88 (myeloid differentiation factor 88)* via their toll interleukin receptor (TIR) domains (see Figure 7-2B). MyD88-dependent signaling through TLR2 and TLR4 requires an adapter protein termed *TIRAP (TIR domain-containing adapter protein)* to initiate signaling. When stimulated, MyD88 sequentially recruits IL-1 receptor-associated kinases 4, 1, and 2 (IRAK4, IRAK1, and IRAK2) to the receptor complex. Phosphorylation of IRAK1 on serine/threonine residues by IRAK4 results in recruitment of tumor necrosis receptor-associated factor 6 (TRAF6) to the complex, which is responsible for early responses in response to TLR signaling. More recent studies have suggested an important role for phosphorylation of IRAK2 by IRAK4 in terms of mediating late responses to TLR signaling.[10] Phosphorylated IRAK1 and TRAF6 dissociate from the receptor and form a complex at the plasma membrane with transforming growth factor-activated kinase 1 (TAK1), a mitogen-activated protein kinase kinase kinase, as well as TAK1-binding protein 1 (TAB1) and TAK1-binding proteins 2 or 3 (TAB2 or TAB3), resulting in the phosphorylation of TAB2/3 and TAK1. IRAK1 is degraded at the plasma membrane, and the remaining complex (consisting of TRAF6, TAK1, TAB1, and TAB2 or TAB3) translocates to the cytosol, where it associates with the ubiquitin ligases UBC13 (ubiquitin-conjugating enzyme 13) and UEV1A (ubiquitin-conjugating enzyme E2 variant 1). This leads to the ubiquitylation of TRAF6, which induces the activation of TAK1. TAK1 subsequently phosphorylates IKKα/IKKβ/IKKγ (also known as IKK1, IKK2, and NF-κB essential modulator [NEMO], respectively) and mitogen-activated protein kinase kinase 6 (MP2K6, MKK6, MEK6). The IKK complex then phosphorylates IκB, which leads to its ubiquitylation and subsequent degradation. This allows NF-κB to translocate to the nucleus and induce the expression of its target genes.[11,12]

TLR4 can also signal through a MyD88 independent pathway by recruiting the adapter proteins TRAM (TRIF-related adapter molecule) and TRIF (TIR domain-containing adapter inducing interferon-β) to the receptor complex (see Figure 7-2B). TRIF recruits the noncanonical IKKs, the serine-threonine-protein kinase TANK-binding kinase-1 (TBK1) and IKKε, which phosphorylate the transcription factor interferon regulatory factor 3 (IRF3), thereby inducing interferon-β and costimulatory interferon-inducible genes. TRIF also recruits TRAF6 and RIP-1, which leads to

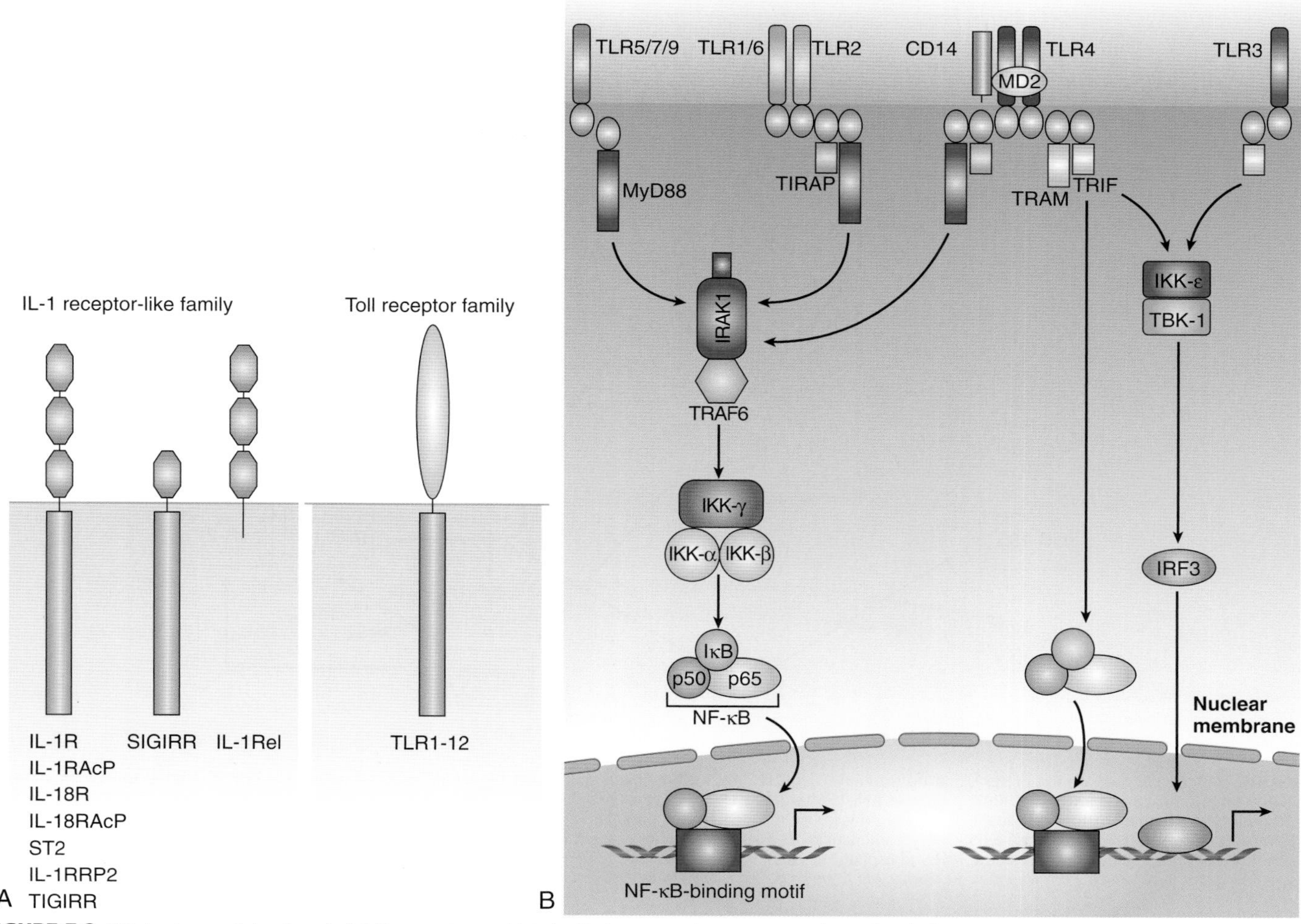

FIGURE 7-2 TLR structure and signaling. **A,** Toll-like receptors and interleukin-1 receptors have a conserved cytoplasmic domain, which is known as the Toll/IL-1-R domain. The TIR domain is characterized by the presence of three highly homologous regions (known as boxes 1, 2, and 3). Despite the similarity of the cytoplasmic domains of these molecules, their extracellular regions differ markedly: TLRs have tandem repeats of leucine-rich regions (known as leucine-rich repeats, LRR), whereas IL-1 Rs have three immunoglobulin (Ig)-like domains. **B,** Stimulation of TLRs triggers the association of MyD88, which in turn recruits IRAK4, thereby allowing the association of IRAK1. IRAK4 then induces the phosphorylation of IRAK1. TRAF6 is also recruited to the receptor complex by associating with phosphorylated IRAK1. Phosphorylated IRAK1 and TRAF6 then dissociate from the receptor and form a complex with TAK1, TAB1, and TAB2 at the plasma membrane *(not shown),* which induces the phosphorylation of TAB2 and TAK1. IRAK1 is degraded at the plasma membrane, and the remaining complex (consisting of TRAF6, TAK1, TAB1, and TAB2) translocates to the cytosol, where it associates with the ubiquitin ligases UBC13 and UEV1A. This leads to the ubiquitylation of TRAF6, which induces the activation of TAK1. TAK1, in turn, phosphorylates both MAP kinases and the IKK complex, which consists of IKK-α, IKK-β, and IKK-γ (also known as IKK1, IKK2, and NEMO, respectively). The IKK complex then phosphorylates IκB, which leads to its ubiquitylation and subsequent degradation. This allows NF-κB to translocate to the nucleus and induce the expression of its target genes. (See table at the end of the chapter for abbreviations.) *Modified from Akira S, Takeda K: Toll like receptor signalling. Nat Rev Immunol 7:499, 2004.*

activation of MAPK and IKKα/IKKβ. These class-specific TLR signaling cascades allow different TLRs to trigger distinct signaling pathways and elicit distinct actions in a cell-specific manner.

TLRs signal by forming homodimers or heterodimers, which allows for approximation of the TIR domains, creating "docking" platforms for recruitment of adapter proteins and kinases that activate downstream signaling cascades. TLR2 and TLR6 are capable of forming heterodimers or homodimers, whereas TLR 3 and 4 signal by forming homodimers. Three general categories of TLR ligands have been identified, including proteins (signal through TLR5), nucleic acids (signal through TLR3, TLR7, TLR9) and lipid-based elements (signal through TLR2, TLR4, TLR6, TLR2/TLR6).[13] Although gram-negative and gram-positive bacteria have been shown, respectively, to signal through TLR4 and TLR2 in the heart, the exact ligands that activate TLR signaling in the heart following tissue injury are not known. As noted previously, TLR receptors are activated by proteins released by DAMPs released by injured and/or dying cells, as well as by fragments of the extracellular matrix (see Figure 7-1).[3,14]

Given the importance TLR signaling, it is not surprising that nature has evolved multiple pathways to negatively regulate TLR signaling. TLR-signaling pathways are negatively regulated by several molecules that are induced following stimulation of TLRs, including IRAK-M (IL-1-receptor-associated kinase M),[15] a nonfunctional IRAK decoy that inhibits the dissociation of the IRAK1-IRAK4 complex from MyD88, thus preventing the formation of IRAK-TRAF6 complexes; SOCS1 (suppressor of cytokine signaling 1), which associates with IRAK1 and negatively modulates TLR signaling; and SHIP-1 (Src homology 2 domain-containing inositol 5-phosphatase 1), a phosphatase that hydrolyzes the 5′ phosphate of PI-3,4-P2, which inhibits PI3 kinase-dependent TLR-MyD88 interactions and NF-kβ activation, and thus negatively regulates TLR signaling.[16] TRIM30α destabilizes the TAK1 complex by promoting the degradation of TAB2 and TAB3,[17] whereas MyD88s (myeloid differentiation primary-response

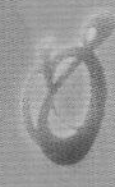

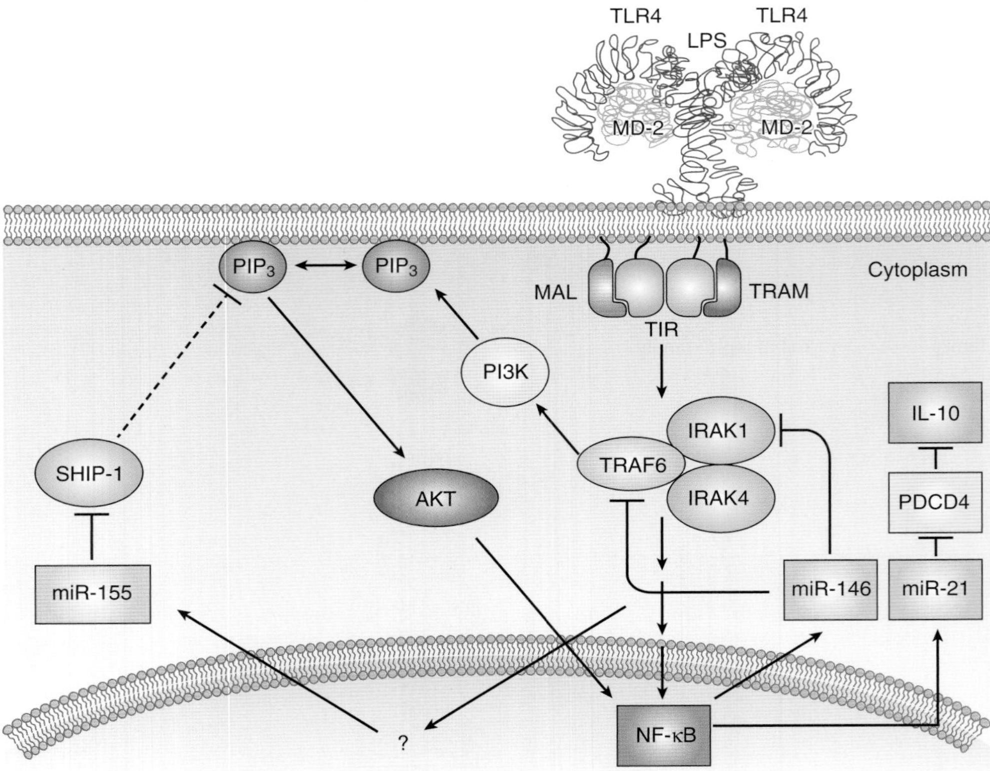

FIGURE 7-3 Negative regulation of TLR signaling through microRNAs. MicroRNAs (miRs) that target the innate immune system have been referred to as *immuno-miRs*. miR-146 targets TRAF6 and interleukin IRAK1, whereas miR-155 targets SHIP-1, which is an inhibitor of NF-κB. miR-21 inhibits PDCD4, which is a transcriptional inhibitor of IL-10, which is anti-inflammatory cytokine IL-10. Increased levels of miR-155 have a proinflammatory effect, whereas increased levels of miR-146 and miR-21 have an anti-inflammatory effect. *Akt,* Protein kinase B (PKB); *IL-10,* interleukin-10; *IRAK,* interleukin-1 receptor-associated kinase; *NF-κB,* nuclear factor kappa-B; *PDCD4,* programmed cell death 4; *PI3K,* phosphatidylinositol-3 kinase; *PIP3,* phosphatidylinositol-3,4,5-triphosphate; *SHIP-1,* SH2-containing inositol 5-phosphatase 1; *TRAF6,* tumor necrosis factor-associated factor 6. *Modified from Hennessy EJ, Parker AE, O'Neill LA: Targeting Toll-like receptors: emerging therapeutics. Nat Rev Drug Discov 9:293, 2010.*

protein 88 short), an alternatively spliced variant of MyD88, blocks the association of IRAK4 with MyD88.SARM (Sterile-α and Armadillo motif containing protein) is a novel adapter protein that specifically blocks TRIF-dependent but not MyD88-dependent signaling.[18] TOLLIP (Toll interacting protein) is thought to maintain immune cells in a quiescent state and/or terminate TLR-mediated signaling, by interacting with the cytoplasmic TIR domains of TLR2 and TLR4 and suppressing IRAK1 phosphorylation. Finally, the TIR (Toll/IL-1R)-domain-containing receptors SIGIRR (single immunoglobulin IL-1 receptor-related molecule) and ST2 have also been shown to negatively regulate TLR signaling. SIGRR interacts transiently with TLR4, IRAK4, and TRAF6, negatively regulating TLR signaling, whereas ST2 sequesters MyD88 and TIRAP, thereby inhibiting NF-κB activation.

Another highly conserved mechanism for regulating innate immunity is being revealed for microRNAs, so-called immuno-miRs, that regulate innate immune gene expression by preventing mRNA translation by promoting mRNA degradation. As illustrated in **Figure 7-3**, several microRNAs negatively regulate TLR signaling, whereas others positively regulate TLR signaling. For example, miR-146 targets TRAF6 and IRAK1, and is upregulated following LPS stimulation, thereby negatively regulating mRNA levels of TRAF6 and IRAK1.[19] miR-155 is also upregulated in response to LPS, and targets SHIP-1, which negatively regulates NF-κB signaling by inhibiting PIP3-dependent signaling.[20] In contrast, LPS increases miR-21 levels, which targets PDCD4, a transcriptional inhibitor of the anti-inflammatory cytokine IL-10, leading to increased levels of IL-10.[21] Thus increased expression of miR-146 or miR-21 negatively regulates innate immune signaling, whereas increased expression of miR-155 positively regulates innate immune signaling. It bears emphasis that these immuno-miRs are expressed in the heart and are differentially regulated in heart failure, with increases in miR-21 and miR-146, and increased expression of miR-155 in some, but not all, studies.

Role of Toll-Like Receptors in Myocardial Disease

Deciphering the role that the innate immune system plays in myocardial disease has been challenging, insofar as it has been difficult to reconcile two sets of conflicting observations, one of which suggests that TLR signaling is beneficial, and the other of which suggests that TLR signaling following ischemic injury is deleterious. Recent "reductionist" studies that have been performed ex vivo, or that have employed chimeric TLR deficient mice that harbor wild-type bone marrow cells, have allowed for a clearer understanding of the central (i.e., myocardial) and peripheral (i.e., bone marrow derived) effects of the innate immune system following ischemic injury. The aggregate data suggest that short-term activation of TLR signaling confers cytoprotective responses within the heart, whereas longer-term TLR signaling is maladaptive and results in the upregulation of

TABLE 7-1 TLR Signaling Modulation of Myocardial Ischemia Reperfusion Injury and Cardiac Remodeling

MICE	INFARCT MODELS	EFFECTS IN KNOCKOUT MICE
TLR2 Signaling		
$TLR2^{-/-}$	I/R (30′ I/60R′)[93]	Smaller infarct sizes, reduced neutrophil recruitment, reduced ROS and cytokines
$TLR2^{-/-}$	Permanent coronary ligation[26]	Improved survival rate, attenuated remodeling, but same infarct sizes at 4 wk
TLR4 Signaling		
C57 BL/10 ScCr C3H/HeJ	I/R (60′ I/24 h R)[25]	Smaller infarct sizes, reduced MPO activity, and complement 3 deposition
C3H/HeJ	I/R (60′ I/120′ R)[23]	Smaller infarct sizes, decreased cardiac expression of TNF, MCP-1, and ILs
C3H/HeJ	I/R (60′ I/24 h R)[24]	Smaller infarct sizes, but no gain in LV function
WT with eritoran	I/R (30′ I/120′ R)[28]	Smaller infarct sizes, reduced pJNK, reduced cytokine expression
C3H/HeJ	Permanent coronary ligation[94]	Reduced LV remodeling, improved systolic function, reduced cytokine expression
C57 BL/10 ScCr	Permanent coronary ligation[29]	Improved LV function on day 6 after infarction, improved survival rate, reduced LV remodeling, and apoptosis at 4 wk
$MyD88^{-/-}$	I/R (30′ I/24 h R)[27]	Smaller infarct sizes, improved LV function, and attenuated cytokine expression and neutrophil recruitment

MPO, Myeloperoxidase; *MCP-1,* monocyte chemoattractant protein-1; *MyD88,* myeloid differentiation primary-response gene 88; *pJNK,* phosphorylated JNK; *ROS,* reactive oxygen species; *TLR,* Toll-like receptor.

Modified from Chao W: Toll-like receptor signaling: a critical modulator of cell survival and ischemic injury in the heart. Am J Physiol Heart Circ Physiol 296:H1–H12, 2009; and Topkara VK, et al: Therapeutic targeting of innate immunity in the failing heart. J Mol Cell Cardiol 51:594–599, 2011.

proinflammatory cytokines and cell adhesion molecules, which leads to activation and recruitment of the "peripheral" neutrophils, monocytes, and dendritic cells to the myocardium, resulting in increased cell death and adverse cardiac remodeling. The sections that follow below will focus on the deleterious long-term effects of activation of innate immunity in the heart.

Toll-Like Receptor Signaling in Ischemia Reperfusion Injury and Myocardial Infarction

TLR-mediated signaling contributes to myocardial damage and adverse cardiac remodeling following ischemia reperfusion injury and/or myocardial infarction. Traditional "loss of function studies" in experimental heart failure models in mice and rats suggest that sustained TLR activation of TLRs is maladaptive and can contribute to LV dysfunction[22] and adverse cardiac remodeling (**Table 7-1**). Mice with a missense mutation of TLR4 or targeted disruption of TLR4,[23-25] TLR2,[26] or MyD88[27] have reduced infarct sizes when compared with wild-type controls. Moreover, mice pretreated with a TLR4 antagonist (eritoran)[28] had reduced nuclear translocation of NF-κB, decreased expression of proinflammatory cytokines (e.g., IL-1, IL-6, TNF), and smaller infarct sizes when compared with vehicle treated animals. Mortality and LV remodeling are reduced in mice with targeted disruption of TLR4 or TLR2.[26,29] Studies performed ex vivo in TLR2-deficient mice suggest that the LV dysfunction that supervenes following I/R is mediated through TLR2-TRAP–mediated upregulation of TNF.

Functional Role of Toll-Like Receptor Signaling in Human Heart Failure

The experimental literature reviewed above suggests that sustained activation of TLR signaling following cardiac injury is maladaptive and can lead to a heart failure phenotype. Unfortunately very little is known with respect to the role of the innate immune system in the failing human heart. To date, two studies have shown that TLR4 expression is increased in the hearts of patients with advanced heart failure.[8,9] Moreover, the pattern of TLR4 expression in cardiac myocytes differs in heart failure in that there are focal areas of intense TLR4 staining in failing cardiac myocytes, in contrast to the diffuse pattern of TLR4 staining observed in nonfailing myocytes.[8] To further clarify the role of innate immunity in the failing heart, we examined the expression profiles of 59 innate immune genes using gene arrays that were from explanted hearts from patients with ischemic cardiomyopathy (ICM), idiopathic dilated cardiomyopathy (DCM), and viral cardiomyopathy (VCM); gene arrays from nonfailing hearts were used as the appropriate controls.[30] Expression data for innate immune signaling genes were analyzed by hierarchical clustering, as well as principal component analysis (PCA), a mathematical modeling procedure that transforms a number of possibly correlated variables into a smaller number of uncorrelated variables that are termed *principal components*.[31] There are two important findings illustrated in the PCA plot shown in **Figure 7-4**. The first is that the numerical values for the PCA plots for nonfailing hearts clustered differently from the numeric values for the PCA plots for the ICM, DCM, and VCM hearts, which tended to cluster together (best observed in Figure 7-4A), suggesting that expression on innate immune genes is different in the failing heart. A second important finding is that the PCA profiles for the ICM patients and DCM patients clustered differently, raising the intriguing possibility that the innate immune system is activated differentially in response to the nature of the pathologic tissue injury pattern. Inspection of Figure 7-4A shows that the PCA plots for VCM patients overlapped those observed in DCM, which is of interest insofar as occult and/or persistent viral myocarditis has been suggested as a potential cause for idiopathic dilated cardiomyopathy.[32] An unsupervised hierarchical clustering analysis of genes that were expressed differently in DCM, ICM, VCM, and nonfailing human hearts confirmed the results of the PCA plots, and showed that there were distinct gene expression profiles for innate immune genes in failing and nonfailing hearts, and that there were distinct gene expression profiles for innate immune genes in ICM and DCM hearts. Although these provisional studies suggest that the innate immune system is activated in human heart failure, it will be important to more precisely determine the expression levels of the different components of the innate immune system, as well as link activation of the innate

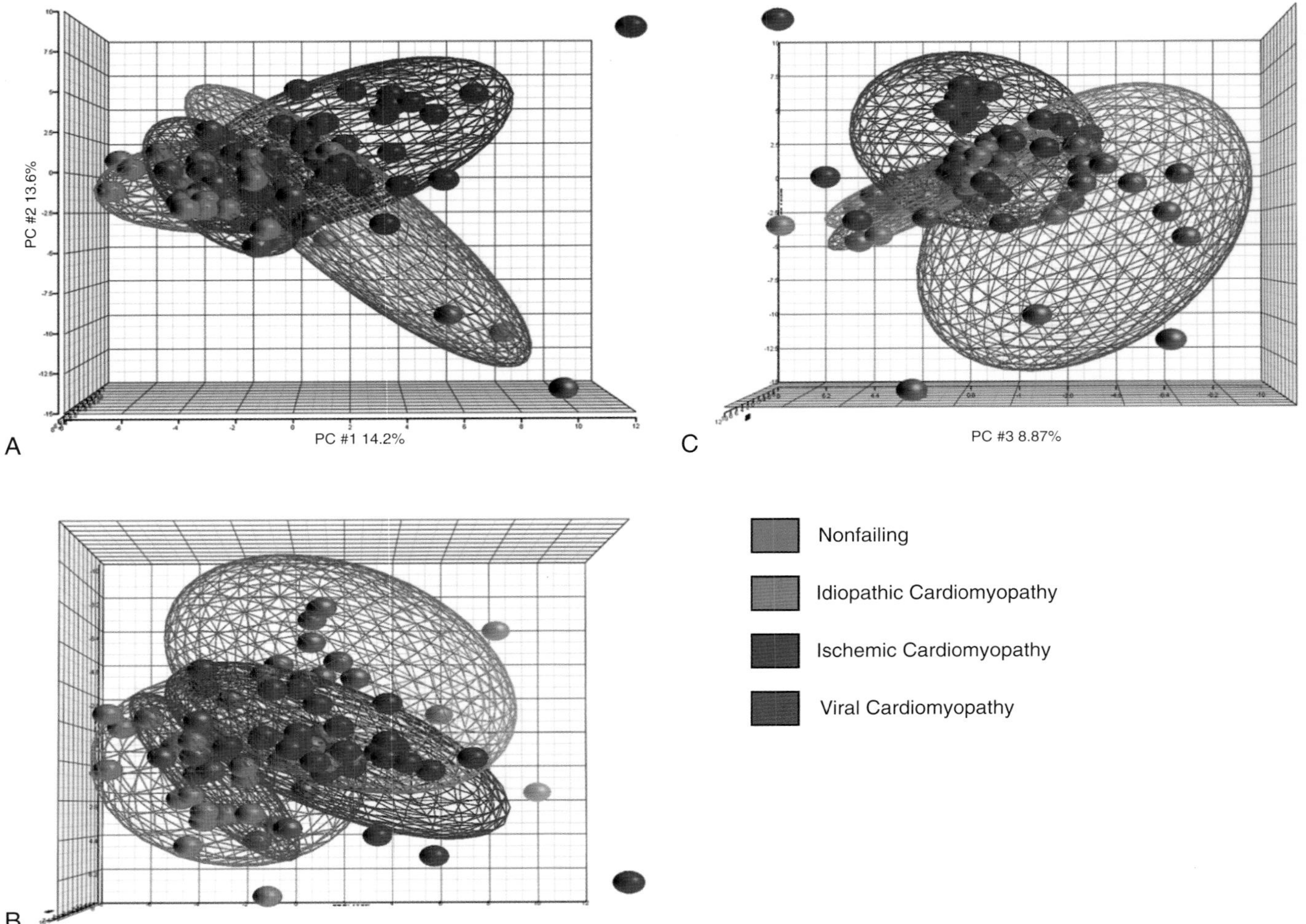

FIGURE 7-4 Principal component analysis of changes in innate immune gene expression in failing and nonfailing human hearts. Innate immune genes were subjected to a principal component analysis (PCA), and the first **(A)**, second **(B)**, and third **(C)** principal components were displayed in a 3-D graphic format. *From Mann DL, Topkara VK, Evans S, et al: Innate immunity in the adult mammalian heart: for whom the cell tolls. Trans Am Clin Climatol Assoc 121:34–50, 2010.*

immune system to the development and progression of heart failure.

PROINFLAMMATORY CYTOKINES

Cytokines are 15-30 kDa proteins that are secreted by cells in response to activation on the innate immune system. Whereas proinflammatory cytokines have traditionally been thought to be produced by the immune cells, it is now widely recognized that cytokines are expressed by a broad variety of nucleated cell types, including cardiac myocytes. Thus from a conceptual standpoint, these molecules should be envisioned as proteins that are produced locally within the myocardium by "cardiocytes" (i.e., cells that reside within the myocardium), in response to one or more different forms of environmental stress. The section that follows will review the biologic properties of the canonical proinflammatory cytokine families, including the tumor necrosis factor (TNF) superfamily (TNFSF), the interleukin-1 family (IL-1F), and the interleukin-6 family.

Tumor Necrosis Factor Superfamily

The tumor necrosis factor (TNF) superfamily consists of 19 well-characterized ligands (TNFSF) and 34 TNF superfamily receptors (TNFRSF). Members of the TNF superfamily of ligands and receptors are expressed in a broad variety of cell types, including myocardial cells.[33] Without exception, all members of the TNF superfamily exhibit proinflammatory activity. Of note, recent studies have identified a potential role for TNF superfamily ligands/receptors in terms of mediating inflammatory responses in the heart, including TNF/TNFR1,TNFR2 (TNFSF2/TNFRSF1A, TNFRSF1B), FasL/Fas (TNFSF6/TNFRSF6), TWEAK (tumor necrosis factor-like weak inducer of apoptosis)/TWEAKR (TNFSF12/TNFRSF12),[34] and RANKL (receptor activator of NF-kB ligand)/RANK (TNFSF11/TNFRSF11A).[35] Cardiac-restricted overexpression of FasL does not lead to a dilated cardiomyopathy,[36] and will not be discussed further herein.

Tumor Necrosis Factor

TNF (TNFSF2), the prototypical member of the TNF superfamily, has a broad variety of pleiotropic biologic capacities. Besides its cytostatic and cytotoxic effects on certain tumor cells, it influences growth, differentiation, and/or function of virtually every cell type investigated, including cardiac myocytes.[37] In most cell types studied, TNF is initially synthesized as a nonglycosylated transmembrane protein of approximately 25 kDa. A 17-kDa fragment is proteolytically cleaved off the plasma membrane of the cell by a membrane-bound

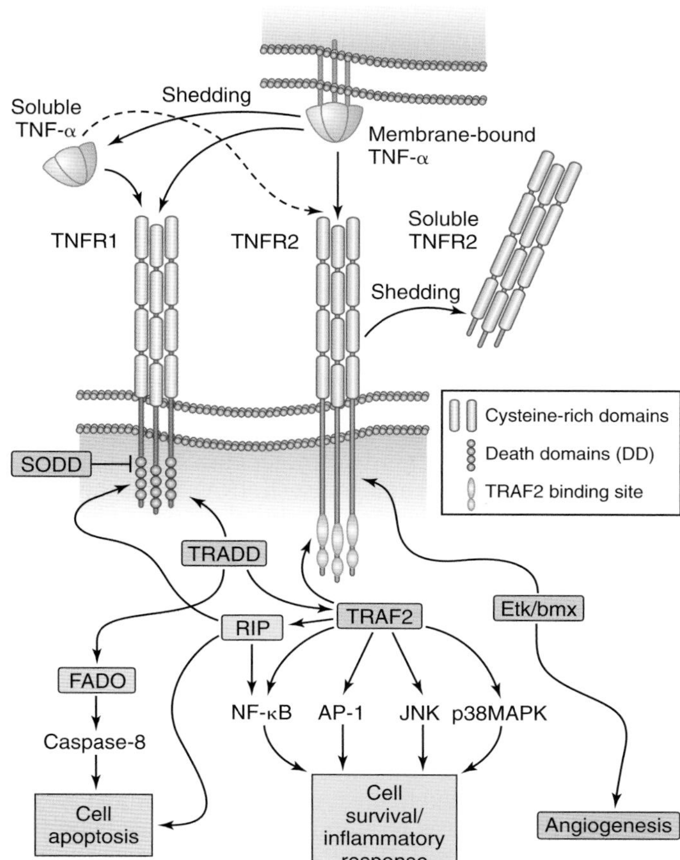

FIGURE 7-5 Overview of TNF signaling. TNF is initially expressed as a functional 26-kDa homotrimeric transmembrane that may be cleaved by a metalloproteinase termed *TACE (TNF-α-converting enzyme [ADAM-17])*. Once TNF is cleaved, it is released into the circulation as a 17-kDa protein that assembles as a functional 60-kDa homotrimer. The function of TNF is relayed by two structurally distinct receptors termed *tumor necrosis factor receptor 1* (TNFR1; TNFRSF1A, p55, CD120a) and *tumor necrosis factor receptor 2* (TNFR2, TNFRSF1B, p75, CD120b). The TNFRs belong to the TNF receptor superfamily, a group of type I transmembrane glycoproteins that are characterized by a conserved homologous cysteine-rich domain in their extracellular region. Both TNFRs can be "shed" (cleaved) from the cell membrane, and are retained in the circulation as circulating "soluble" receptors (referred to as *sTNFR1* and *sTNFR2*, respectively). Both of these soluble receptors retain their ability to bind ligand, as well as to inhibit the biologic activities of TNF. The main structural difference between TNFR1 and TNFR2 is the presence of a death domain (DD) in the cytoplasmic domain of TNFR1. The binding of TNF allows TRADD (TNF receptor-associated death domain protein) to interact with the DD. TRADD is an essential partner of TNFR1 for signal transduction that recruits the downstream adapter molecule FADD (FAS-associated death domain), which initiates the caspase pathway responsible for apoptotic cell death. TRADD can also interact directly with RIP (receptor interacting protein) and TRAF2 (TNF receptor-associated factor 2 protein), which can activate downstream signaling pathways, such as NF-κB, AP-1, c-Jun N-terminal kinase stress kinases (JNK), and p38MAPK. *From Ernandez T, Mayadas TN: Immunoregulatory role of TNFalpha in inflammatory kidney diseases. Kidney Int 76:262–276, 2009.*

enzyme termed *TACE* (*TNF-α convertase [ADAM17]*) to produce the "secreted form," which circulates as a stable 51-kDa TNF homotrimer (**Figure 7-5**). Clinical studies have shown that TNF mRNA and protein are expressed in failing human hearts, but are not detectable in nonfailing hearts.[38]

TNF is initially expressed as a functional 26-kDa homotrimeric transmembrane that may be cleaved by the metalloproteinase termed *TACE* (see Figure 7-5). Once TNF is cleaved, it is released into the circulation as 17-kDa protein that assembles as a functional 60-kDa homotrimer. The function of TNF is relayed by two structurally distinct receptors, termed *tumor necrosis factor receptor 1* (TNFR1; TNFRSF1A, p55, CD120a) and *tumor necrosis factor receptor 2* (TNFR2, TNFRSF1B, p75, CD120b). The TNFRs belong to the TNF receptor superfamily, a group of type I transmembrane glycoproteins that are characterized by a conserved homologous cysteine-rich domain in their extracellular region. Previous studies have identified the presence of both types of TNF receptors in nonfailing[39] and failing human myocardium.[38] Both TNF receptor subtypes have been immunolocalized to the adult human cardiac myocyte, thus providing a potential basis for beginning to understand the signaling pathways that are used by TNF. Although the exact functional significance of TNFR1 and TNFR2 in the heart is not known at present, the majority of the deleterious effects of TNF are coupled to activation of TNFR1,[40] whereas activation of TNFR2 appears to exert protective effects in the heart. Both TNFRs can be shed (cleaved) from the cell membrane, and are retained in the circulation as circulating "soluble" ("s") receptors (referred to as *sTNFR1* and *sTNFR2*, respectively). Both of these soluble receptors retain their ability to bind ligands, as well as to inhibit the biologic activities of TNF. The main structural difference between TNFR1 and TNFR2 is the presence of a death domain (DD) in the cytoplasmic domain of TNFR1. The binding of TNF allows TRADD (TNF receptor-associated death domain protein) to interact with the DD. TRADD is an essential partner of TNFR1 for signal transduction that recruits the downstream adapter molecule FADD (FAS-associated death domain), which initiates the caspase pathway responsible for apoptotic cell death (see also Chapter 2). TRADD can also interact directly with RIP (receptor interacting protein) and TRAF2 (TNF receptor-associated factor 2 protein), which can activate downstream signaling pathways, such as NF-κB, AP-1, c-Jun N-terminal kinase stress kinases (JNK), and p38MAPK.

Tumor Necrosis Factor–Like Weak Inducer of Apoptosis

TNF-like weak inducer of apoptosis (TWEAK, TNFSF12), a member of the TNF superfamily of ligands, is first synthesized as a type II transmembrane protein that is cleaved from the membrane. TWEAK functions primarily as a soluble cytokine with diverse biologic roles, including proinflammatory activity, angiogenesis, regulation of cell survival, and myoblast differentiation/proliferation.[41] TWEAK induces apoptosis indirectly through secondary activation of the TNF/TNFR1 pathway. The expression of TWEAK is relatively low in normal tissues, including the heart, but undergoes dramatic upregulation in the setting of tissue injury. For example, TWEAK is expressed in the border zone of infarcted myocardium, wherein increased angiogenesis is observed, as well as in the nonischemic myocardium remote from the infarct area.[41] Recent studies have suggested that sustained elevated circulating levels of TWEAK, induced via transgenic or adenoviral-mediated overexpression of soluble TWEAK, were sufficient to provoke LV dilation, LV fibrosis, LV dysfunction, as well as increased mortality in mice.[34] Moreover, circulating levels of TWEAK are elevated in patients with nonischemic cardiomyopathy compared to patients with ischemic cardiomyopathy and/or normal controls.[34]

The receptor for TWEAK, TWEAKR (Fn14, TNFSFR12A), is the smallest member of the TNF-receptor family. TWEAKR is a type I transmembrane protein (102 aa) that is expressed both constitutively, as well as in an inducible manner in many tissues including the brain, the kidney, the liver, and the heart.[41] TWEAKR is highly upregulated in the border zone of the heart following left anterior descending artery (LAD) ligation.[41] Both norepinephrine and angiotensin II also strongly upregulate TWEAKR in isolated neonatal cardiomyocytes.[41] TWEAKR contains sequence motifs within the cytoplasmic domain that promote aggregation of a family of adapter proteins termed *TRAF1, 2,* and *3* (tumor necrosis factor-associated factor), which in turn activate intracellular signal transduction cascades, including nuclear factor-κB (NF-κB), and the mitogen-activated protein kinases JNK, p38, and ERK.

Receptor Activator of NF-kB Ligand (RANK Ligand)

Osteoprotegerin (OPG [TNSFR11B]) and the receptor activator of NF-κB ligand (RANKL [TNFSF11]) are two cytokines that have been classically associated with the regulation of bone remodeling. In bone, RANKL activates osteoclasts, and hence bone resorption, after binding to RANK. In contrast, OPG acts as a decoy receptor for RANKL, and thereby inhibits bone resorption. In experimental models of cardiac injury, OPG and RANKL are both increased in direct relation to the severity of heart failure and/or in relation to hemodynamic pressure overload.[35] Studies in rats post myocardial infarction have revealed increased levels of messenger RNA (mRNA) for OPG, RANKL, and RANK within the ischemic zone, and increased protein levels of OPG in the remote zone in fibroblasts and cardiac myocytes.[35] Studies in patients with heart failure have shown that OPG levels are increased in association with worsening NYHA class, LV dysfunction, and elevated levels of B-type natriuretic peptide.[35] Heart failure patients also had increased levels of RANKL; however, increased levels were observed only in patients with NYHA class IV heart failure. Furthermore, there was increased RANK and RANKL immunoreactivity in cardiac myocytes, vascular smooth muscle cells, and endothelial cells in failing human hearts when compared with nonfailing human hearts. Viewed together, these findings suggest a potential role for the RANKL/RANK/OPG axis in heart failure; however, given that both RANKL and its cognate antagonist OPG are both elevated in experimental and clinical heart failure, the clinical significance of this axis remains unclear at present.

Interleukin-1 Family

Although the original IL-1 family (IL-1F) consisted of IL-1α (IL-1 F1) and IL-β (IL-1 F2), the IL-1 family has now expanded to include seven ligands with agonist activity, including IL-1α and IL-1β, IL-18 (IL-1F4), IL-33 (IL-1F11), IL-36α (IL-1F6), IL-36β (IL-1F7), IL-36γ (IL-1F8), three receptor antagonists (IL-1Ra [IL-F3], IL-36Ra [IL-F5], IL-38 [IL-F10]), and an anti-inflammatory cytokine (IL-37 [IL-10]). Members of the IL-1 receptor (IL-1R) family include six receptor chains forming four signaling receptor complexes, two decoy receptors (IL-1R2, IL-18BP), and two negative regulators (TIR8 or SIGIRR [IL-1R8], IL-1RAcPb).[42]

Interleukin-1α and Interleukin-1β

IL-1α (IL-F1) and IL-1β (IL-F2), which are encoded by separate genes, are the "founding" members of the IL-1 family of cytokines. Analogous to TNF, IL-1α and IL-β are responsible for controlling proinflammatory reactions following tissue injury. With the notable exception of IL-1Ra, each member of the IL-1 family is synthesized first as a precursor that does not have a clear signal peptide for processing or secretion. The immature form of IL-1β, pro-IL-1β, is synthesized within mammalian cells as a 31-kD precursor. Processing of IL-1β to a 17-kD "mature" form requires cleavage by interleukin-1 converting enzyme (ICE) or by caspase-1, which is activated by the inflammasome, a multiprotein oligomer consisting of caspase-1, PYCARD, and NALP. Once IL-1β is processed, the mature form is secreted rapidly from the cell. IL-1β is the main form of circulating IL-1. IL-1α is constitutively expressed as membrane-bound protein. For the most part, IL-1α remains intracellular or is retained on the cell membrane, and is therefore not detected in the circulation unless the cell dies and releases its intracellular content. Unlike IL-1α, the inactive or proform of IL-1β is only marginally active. IL-1α and IL-1β both bind to common receptors, which explains the similarity of effects of the two molecules. A third specific ligand, the IL-1 receptor antagonist (IL-1RA), binds the IL-1RI with similar specificity and affinity but does not activate the receptor and trigger downstream signaling, and thus acts as a competitive inhibitor.[43] Similar to TNF, IL-1β appears to be synthesized within the myocardium in response to stressful environmental stimuli, and both IL-1β mRNA and protein have been detected in the hearts of patients with dilated cardiomyopathy.[44]

IL-1α and IL-1β, which are encoded by separate genes, each independently binds the type I IL-1 receptor (IL-1R1). As shown in **Figure 7-6**, the IL-1 receptor accessory protein (IL-1RAcP) is recruited to the type I IL-1 receptor and serves as a coreceptor that is required for signal transduction of IL-1/IL-1RI complexes. IL-1RAcP is required for activation of IL-1R1 by other IL-1 family members, especially IL-18 and IL-33. Whereas early work on the IL-1 receptor (IL-1R) suggested that there was a single receptor, subsequent cross-linking studies have suggested the presence of a low-affinity (80 kDa; IL-1RI) receptor and a higher affinity receptor (68 kDa, IL-1RII), each coded for by a single gene product.[45] The type I receptor (IL-1RI) transduces a signal, whereas the type II receptor (IL- 1RII) binds IL-1α and IL-1β but does not transduce a signal. Indeed, IL-1 RII acts as a sink for IL-1, and has been termed a *decoy receptor*. The extracellular domains of the interleukin receptors or "soluble" portions of the IL-1RI, IL-1RII, and sIL-1RAcP (termed *sIL-1RI, sIL-1RII,* and *sIL-1RAcP,* respectively) circulate in health and disease and function as natural "buffers" that are capable of binding to IL-lα, IL-1β, or IL-1Ra.[46]

The IL-1 receptor/IL-1RAcP complex leads to recruitment of the adapter protein MyD88 (myeloid differentiation primary-response gene 88) to the Toll-IL-1 receptor (TIR) domain of both IL-1RI and IL-1RAcP, leading to phosphorylation of IRAK4, analogous to TLR signaling (see Figure 7-2A). IL-1, IL-1RI, IL-RAcP, MYD88, and IRAK4 form a stable IL-1–induced signaling module, which subsequently phosphorylates IRAK1 and IRAK2 (see Figure 7-6). This is followed by the recruitment and oligomerization of TRAF6, which serves as a ubiquitin E3 ligase that, together with the ubiquitin E2 ligase complex attaches K63-linked polyubiquitin chains to several IL-1–signaling intermediates, including IRAK1 and the adapter proteins TAB 2 and 3 and TAK-1. Ubiquitination of TAK1 promotes its association with TRAF6 and with MEKK3, with the subsequent formation of at least two TAK1 and MEKK3 signaling complexes that activate the NF-κB, c-Jun N-terminal kinase (JNK), and p38 MAPK pathways.[43]

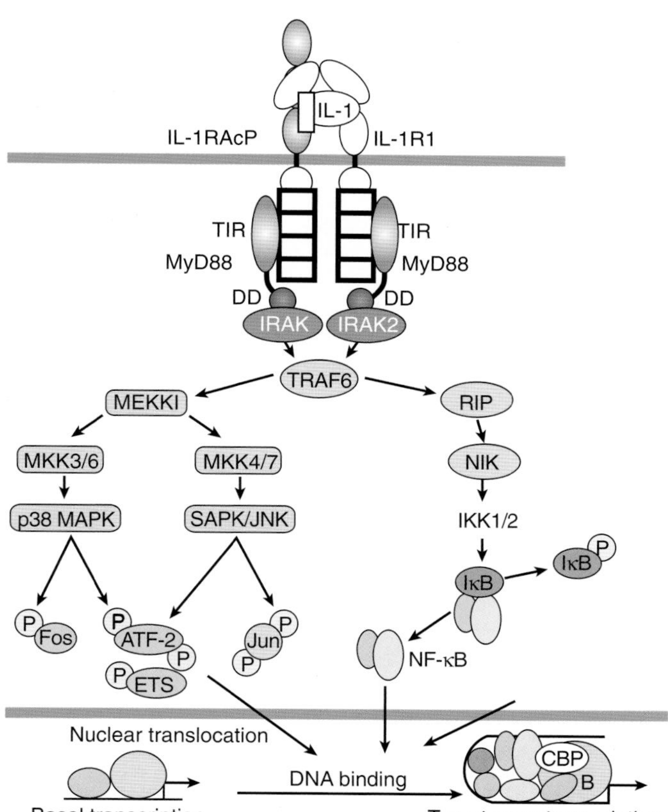

FIGURE 7-6 Intracellular signaling pathways activated by interleukin-1 (IL-1). Binding of IL-1 to the type I IL-1 receptor (IL-1R1) leads to the recruitment of the IL-1R accessory protein (IL-1RAcP). The cytoplasmic Toll/IL-1-receptor (TIR) domains of the receptor recruit MyD88 via its TIR, and the MyD88 death domain (DD) recruits the IL-1 receptor-associated kinases (IRAK and IRAK2) to the receptor complex before being rapidly phosphorylated and degraded. The IRAKs mediate tumor necrosis factor receptor-associated factor 6 (TRAF6) oligomerization, initiating various protein kinase cascades, the major ones of which involve (1) the stress-activated protein kinases, p38 mitogen-activated protein kinase (MAPK), and c-Jun N-terminal kinase (JNK), which lead to activation of activator protein-1 (AP-1) (c-Fos/c-Jun), activating transcription factor-2 (ATF-2), and E Twenty Six (ETS) factors, among other transcription factors; and (2) inhibitor of κB (IκB) kinases 1 and 2 (IKK-1 and IKK-2), which lead to activation of nuclear factor κB (NF-κB). *Modified from Firestein GS: Role of the chondrocyte in cartilage pathology. In Firestein GS, et al, editors: Kelley's textbook of rheumatology, ed 8, Philadelphia, 2008, Saunders, pp 52–55.*

Interleukin-18

Interleukin-18 (IL-18, IL-1F4) is a relatively new member of the IL-1 superfamily.[47] Similar to IL-1β, IL-18 is synthesized as an inactive precursor and is cleaved to its active form by caspase-1. Although IL-18 was initially recognized for its ability to induce interferon-γ (IFN-γ) and its capacity to induce T-helper 1 (Th1) responses, IL-18 was subsequently found to play an important role in LPS-induced hepatotoxicity, which stimulated further study of the role of IL-18 in other settings. Relevant to the present discussion is the recent observation that IL-18 had been shown to be produced in the heart during ischemia reperfusion injury and endotoxemia.[48] Importantly, IL-18 activates NF-κB, which is a transcriptional regulator of many proinflammatory cytokines and cellular adhesion molecules in the heart. In vitro studies have shown that IL-18 increases the production of TNF and IL-1β in murine macrophages and human monocytes and also induces the expression of ICAM-1 and VCAM-1 on endothelial cells and monocytes.[47] In vivo studies have shown that specific blockade of IL-18 using IL-18 binding protein improves contractile function in human atrial tissue following ischemia reperfusion injury,[49] as well as lipopolysaccharide-induced LV dysfunction in experimental animals.[49]

The IL-18 receptor (IL-18R) is related to the IL-1 family of receptors, and is composed of a ligand-binding subunit, I-1Rrp1 and an accessory subunit, AcPL, both of which share sequence homology to the IL-1R family.[50] Moreover, the signal transduction pathways used by IL-1β and IL-18 are similar. In addition, there is a third receptor-like chain, the IL-18 binding protein (IL-18BP), which lacks a transmembrane domain and thus does not signal. IL-18BP is produced constitutively and is secreted, and thus acts as a potent inhibitor of IL-18 activity.

Interleukin-33

As noted above, IL-33 (IL-F11) belongs to the IL-1 superfamily. IL-33 was identified in a search for the ligand for the ST2 receptor (see later discussion). IL-33 induces helper T cells, mast cells, eosinophils, and basophils to produce type II cytokines. The mode by which IL-33 exerts its effect has not been fully established but it probably acts similarly to other members of the IL-1 family. That is, precursor IL-33 is cleaved by caspases and is then released into the interstitium as an active cytokine, where it stimulates signaling in target cells.[51] In the heart, IL-33 is produced by cardiac fibroblasts in response to biomechanical strain. In vitro studies have shown that IL-33 markedly antagonizes angiotensin II and phenylephrine-induced cardiomyocyte hypertrophy; moreover, recombinant IL-33 reduced hypertrophy and fibrosis and improved survival after pressure overload in mice.[52] Thus IL-33 appears to activate a cardioprotective program in the heart.

ST2 is the cognate receptor for IL-33. There are four isoforms of ST2 (sST2 [soluble]), ST2L (membrane bound), ST2V, and ST2LV. The overall structure of ST2L is similar to the structure of the type I IL-1 receptors, which consist of an extracellular domain of three linked immunoglobulin-like motifs, a transmembrane segment, and a TIR (Toll-like interleukin domain) cytoplasmic domain. sST2 lacks a transmembrane and cytoplasmic domains contained within the structure of ST2L and includes a unique 9-amino-acid C-terminal sequence.[51] Whereas ST2L is constitutively expressed primarily in hematopoietic cells, sST2 expression is largely inducible in a variety of cell types, including cells that reside in the heart. Interestingly, high baseline ST2 levels are a significant predictor of cardiovascular death and heart failure (see also Chapter 30) independent of baseline characteristics and NT-proBNP in patients with an ST-segment myocardial infarction.[53] The signaling pathways that are downstream from IL-33/ST2 signaling are still unclear, but may include phosphorylation of extracellular signal-regulated kinase (ERK) 1/2, p38 MAPK, JNKs, and activation of NF-κB. However, the relationship between ST2L and NF-κB activation is a matter of ongoing debate.[51]

Interleukin-6 Family

Based on their functional redundancy, structural similarity, and use of a common signaling receptor, interleukin-6 (IL-6), leukemia inhibitory factor (LIF), cardiotrophin-1 (CT-1), ciliary neurotrophic factor (CNTF), interleukin-11 (IL-11), and oncostatin M (OSM) are considered to represent the IL-6 family of cytokines (**Figure 7-7A**). Inclusion in the IL-6 family is based on a helical cytokine structure and receptor subunit makeup. The IL-6 family of cytokines triggers

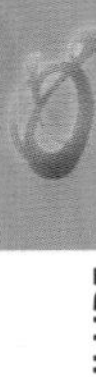

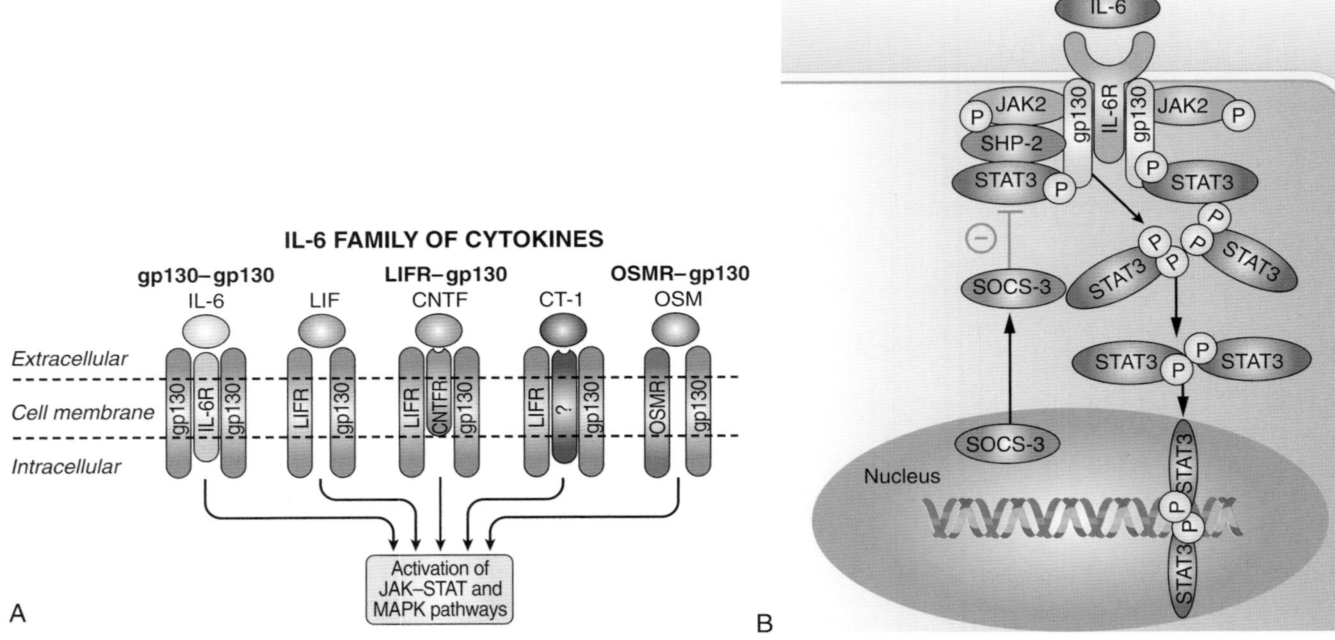

FIGURE 7-7 IL-6 family of cytokines. **A,** Various combinations of receptor subunits and signaling pathways are used by different members of the IL-6 cytokine family. gp130 homodimers associate with specific interleukin (IL) receptors such as the IL-6 receptor (IL-6R) to mediate the actions of IL-6. Leukemia inhibitory factor (LIF) binds to heterodimers of LIF receptor (LIFR) and gp130. LIFR-gp130 heterodimers can also associate with other receptor subunits to bind ciliary neurotrophic factor (CNTF) and cardiotrophin-1 (CT-1). The oncostatin M receptor (OSMR) forms heterodimers with gp130 to bind oncostatin M (OSM). The signal-transducing subunit gp130 is found in all complexes, and is responsible for the intracellular activation of the Janus-activated kinase–signal transducer and activator of transcription (JAK/STAT) and the mitogen-activated protein kinase (MAPK) pathways. **B,** IL-6 stimulation induces the expression of a number of proinflammatory gene products via activation of the JAK/STAT, MAPK, and PI3K signaling cascades. Ligand binding of IL-6 to IL-6R induces dimerization of the gp130 receptor, which activates the associated JAK tyrosine kinases. The JAKs phosphorylate recruitment sites for the STAT proteins and the scaffold protein SHP2, which is linked to MAPK and PI3K signaling cascades. As shown, the SOCS proteins can negatively modulate gp130-mediated JAK-STAT signaling. ***A,*** *Modified from Bauer S, Kerr BJ, Patterson PH: The neuropoietic cytokine family in development, plasticity, disease and injury. Nat Rev Neurosci 8:221–232, 2007;* ***B,*** *Modified from Walters TD, Griffiths AM: Mechanisms of growth impairment in pediatric Crohn's disease. Nat Rev Gastroenterol Hepatol 6:513–523, 2009.*

downstream signaling pathways in multiple cell types, including cardiac myocytes, either through the homodimerization of the gp130 receptor or through the heterodimerization of gp130 with a related transmembrane receptor (see Figure 7-7A). All IL-6 type cytokines potentially activate STAT3, and to a lesser extent STAT1 through their common gp130 subunits. The specificity of cytokine signaling within the IL-6 family is determined by the composition of the cytoplasmic domains associated with the signal-competent receptor complex.[54] For example, IL-6 initiates formation of a signaling receptor complex by binding to an IL-6 receptor (IL-6R), which then heterodimerizes with gp130 to initiate IL-6 signaling. On the other hand LIF, CT-1, and CNTF all transduce signaling events through heterodimerization of LIF receptors (LIFRβ) and gp130. The suppressor of cytokine signaling (SOCS) (also referred to as *cytokine-inducible SH2 proteins [CIS]*) is a family of specific negative regulatory feedback elements of JAK/STAT signaling (see Figure 7-7B). Expression of some SOCS family members is regulated transcriptionally by STATs, thereby acting as a negative feedback loop for JAK-STAT signaling. Both SOCS-1 and SOCS-3 interact with the kinase domain of various JAK proteins, thereby preventing STAT phosphorylation. Previous clinical studies showed that the plasma level of IL-6, CT-1, LIF, and gp130 are elevated in patients with advanced heart failure and that high levels are associated with a poor prognosis for heart failure patients.[55,56]

Interleukin-6

Human IL-6 is produced as a 212-amino-acid precursor and is processed to a 184-amino-acid soluble form following cleavage of a signal sequence during secretion of the mature protein.[57] The mature protein is a 26-kDa glycoprotein,[58] with a number of alternative *N*- and *O*-linked glycosylation sites. IL-6 can be detected in the circulation following gram-negative bacterial infection or TNF infusion, as well as following myocardial stunning,[59] and appears to be secreted in direct response to TNF or IL-1, which are thought to induce IL-6 gene expression by activation of NF-κB.[57] Recently, IL-6 has been shown to exist in the circulation in "chaperoned" complexes of molecular mass 400-500, 150-200, and 25-35 kDa in association with binding proteins that can include soluble IL-6 receptors, anti-IL-6 antibodies, and anti-sIL-6R antibodies, and others. Sustained high levels of different circulating IL-6 complexes are observed in cancer patients subjected to particular active anticancer immunotherapy regimens. However, "chaperoned" IL-6 complexes have not yet been reported in heart failure.[60]

The human IL-6 receptor is a glycoprotein with a molecular mass of 80 kDa. In contrast to the receptors for IL-1 and TNF, the cytoplasmic domain of IL-6 is not necessary for intracellular signaling to occur. Moreover, when bound to its receptor, IL-6 is known to associate with a second membrane glycoprotein with a molecular mass of 130 kDa (gp130). Thus the current evidence suggests that the IL-6R system is composed of two functional chains: an 80-kDa IL-6 binding protein, termed *IL-6R*, and a 130-kDa "docking protein," termed *gp130*, which transmits the intracellular signal.[57] Importantly, IL-6 receptors are expressed with low abundance in adult cardiac myocytes, whereas mice that are deficient in gp130 are embryonically lethal because their hearts do not develop.[61] In contrast, double transgenic mice that have been genetically engineered to overexpress both IL-6 and IL-6R develop substantial concentric hypertrophy.[62]

IL-6 signaling through IL-6/gp130 receptor induces phosphorylation and activation of Janus kinase (JAK) proteins (see Figure 7-7B), which are constitutively associated with the cytoplasmic domains of the gp130 receptor. JAK proteins phosphorylate gp130, creating docking sites for signal transducer and activator of transcription 3 (STAT3) proteins via interaction through their SH2 domains. The STAT proteins are phosphorylated on specific tyrosine residues by the associated JAKs, thereby inducing the formation of parallel STAT dimers (see Figure 7-7B). The STAT dimers dissociate from the receptor and translocate into the nucleus, where they bind to specific DNA sequences and regulate the expression of target genes. Three major signaling pathways have been identified downstream from IL-6/gp130-mediated signaling: JAK-STAT signaling, mitogen-activated protein kinase (MAPK) signaling, and the PI3K/AKT signaling.[56] In the heart, STAT proteins regulate the expression of genes encoding proteins involved in angiogenesis, inflammation, apoptosis, extracellular matrix composition, and cellular signaling.[63] The JAK-STAT pathway has been shown to be involved in ischemia/reperfusion injury, hypertrophy, and postpartum cardiomyopathy.[63,64] Moreover, the JAK-STAT pathway has also been reported to interfere with the renin-angiotensin system (RAS), which is involved in the pathophysiology and progression of hypertrophy and heart failure (see Chapter 5).

Leukemia Inhibitory Factor

Leukemia inhibitory factor (LIF) is a 181-amino-acid glycoprotein that was originally identified as a cytokine that inhibited the proliferation of the murine myeloid leukemic cell line M1, and induced these cells to differentiate into macrophages. There are several forms of LIF; however, the best studied is a secreted and variably glycosylated protein (34-63 kDa) that varies depending on the cell type and context, ranging from proliferation and survival to differentiation and apoptosis. LIF signals, at least in part, through the transmembrane protein gp130 that heterodimerizes with the LIF receptor (LIFR) (see Figure 7-7A). The pleiotropic effects of LIF function may be due, in at least in part, to the integration of the different signaling pathways that can be induced once LIF is combined with its receptor gp130-LIFR.

Analogous to IL-6, LIF signals through JAK-STAT, MAPKs, and the PI3K/AKT pathway.[65] LIF-induced activation of the JAK/STAT pathway is linked to cardiac myocyte cell growth, whereas activation of the MAPK, PI(3)-kinase pathways and the JAK/STAT pathways are linked to cytoprotection.[65] LIF has also been shown to contribute to homing of bone marrow–derived cardiac progenitors in a postinfarct model. The contribution of LIF signaling to contractile function is unclear, with studies suggesting that LIF induces downregulation of the sarcoplasmic reticulum Ca^{2+} ATPase (SERCA) gene and protein expression, whereas others suggest LIF induces increased intracellular Ca^{2+} concentrations in cardiac myocytes secondary to increased L-type Ca^{2+} currents.[65] Whether LIF offers protection to the heart under chronic stress, such as hypertension-induced cardiac remodeling and heart failure, is not known.

Cardiotrophin-1

CT-1 is a 201-amino-acid protein that was originally identified for its ability to induce a hypertrophic growth in neonatal cardiac myocytes.[66] Subsequent studies have shown that CT-1 is synthesized by cardiac myocytes and noncardiac myocytes in response to mechanical stress. Analogous to LIF, the signaling pathways downstream from CT-1 include the JAK/STAT pathway, the MAPK pathway, and the PI3K/AKT pathway.[67] The predominant actions of CT-1 include cytoprotection, cell hypertrophy, cell proliferation, and collagen synthesis. CT-1 exerts a dose-dependent decrease in blood pressure in rats, which is sensitive to nitric oxide synthase inhibition. Although the acute administration of CT-1 had no immediate effect of LV dP/dt, long-term exposure to CT-1 provoked contractile dysfunction in heart tissue engineered from rat cardiac myocytes. Peripheral circulating levels of CT-1 levels increase in relation to worsening NYHA functional class, and correlate with the LV mass index in patients with dilated cardiomyopathy. However, at the time of this writing, it is unclear whether elevated levels of CT-1 are biologic markers (see also Chapter 30) or biologic mediators of worsening heart failure.

Chemokines

Chemokines are a distinct family of cytokines that regulate biologic processes, such as chemotaxis, collagen turnover, angiogenesis, and apoptosis. The chemokine superfamily is divided into four groups (CXC, CX3C, CC, and C) according to the relative positioning of the first two closely paired cysteines of their amino acid sequence. Chemokines exert their effects by interacting with G protein-linked transmembrane receptors, referred to as *chemokine receptors,* that are found on the surfaces of their target cells. A major role of chemokines is the recruitment and activation of specific subpopulations of leukocytes that play a pivotal role in the immune response and inflammation. While chemokine-dependent functions are essential for the control of infection, wound healing, and hematopoiesis, excessive chemokine activation may result in inappropriate inflammation leading to cell death and tissue damage. Studies have shown that circulating levels of CC chemokines are elevated in patients with ischemic and nonischemic heart failure, including macrophage chemoattractant protein-1 (MCP-1), macrophage inflammatory protein-1α (MIP-1α), and RANTES (regulated on activation normally T-cell expressed and secreted). The highest levels of these chemokines were noted in patients with NYHA class IV heart failure.[68] Given that these chemokines can attract inflammatory cells to the heart, they may contribute to disease progression in heart failure.

RATIONALE FOR STUDYING INNATE IMMUNITY IN HEART FAILURE

The interest in understanding the role of innate immunity in heart failure arises from the observation that many aspects of the syndrome of heart failure can be explained by the known biologic effects of proinflammatory cytokines that are downstream for the activation of innate immune receptors (**Table 7-2**). That is, when expressed at sufficiently high concentrations, such as those that are observed in heart failure, cytokines are sufficient to mimic some aspects of the so-called heart failure phenotype, including (but not limited to) progressive LV dysfunction, pulmonary edema, LV remodeling, fetal gene expression, and cardiomyopathy.[69] Thus the "cytokine hypothesis"[70] for heart failure holds that

TABLE 7-2 Effects of Inflammatory Mediators on Left Ventricular Remodeling

Alterations in the Biology of the Myocyte
Myocyte hypertrophy Contractile abnormalities Fetal gene expression
Alterations in the Extracellular Matrix
MMP activation Degradation of the matrix Fibrosis
Progressive Myocyte Loss
Necrosis Apoptosis

heart failure progresses, at least in part, as a result of the toxic effects exerted by endogenous cytokine cascades on the heart and the peripheral circulation. It bears emphasis that the cytokine hypothesis does not imply that cytokines cause "heart failure" per se, but rather that the overexpression of cytokine cascades contributes to disease progression of heart failure. Much like the elaboration of neurohormones, the elaboration of cytokines may represent a biologic mechanism that is responsible for worsening heart failure. Although the deleterious effects of cytokines on myocardial function have received the most attention thus far, it bears emphasis that cytokines may also produce deleterious effects on LV structure (remodeling) and endothelial function. Accordingly, in the following section, we will discuss the studies that form the scientific basis for studying the role of proinflammatory mediators in the failing heart.

Effects of Cytokines on Left Ventricular Function

One of the signatures of proinflammatory cytokines is their ability to depress LV function. The original observation that proinflammatory cytokines were capable of modulating LV function was reported in experimental studies that showed that direct injections of TNF produced hypotension, metabolic acidosis, hemoconcentration, and death within minutes, thus mimicking the cardiac/hemodynamic response seen during endotoxin-induced septic shock.[71] Importantly, the negative inotropic effects of TNF were completely reversible when the TNF infusion was stopped.[69] Subsequent studies in transgenic mice with targeted overexpression of TNF in the cardiac compartment demonstrated that targeted overexpression of TNF results in depressed LV ejection performance that is dependent on TNF "gene dosage."[72,73] At the cellular level, studies in isolated contracting myocytes showed that the negative inotropic effects of TNF were the direct result of alterations in intracellular calcium homeostasis.[74] Treatment with greater than 50 U/mL^{-1} TNF produced a 20% to 30% decrease in the extent of cell shortening (**Figure 7-8A**) and a 40% decrease in peak levels of intracellular calcium (see Figure 7-8B). Moreover, whole cell patch-clamp studies suggested that the decrease in intracellular calcium was not the result of changes in the voltage-sensitive inward calcium current, suggesting that TNF-induced changes in intracellular calcium homeostasis were secondary to alterations in sarcoplasmic reticular handling of calcium.[74]

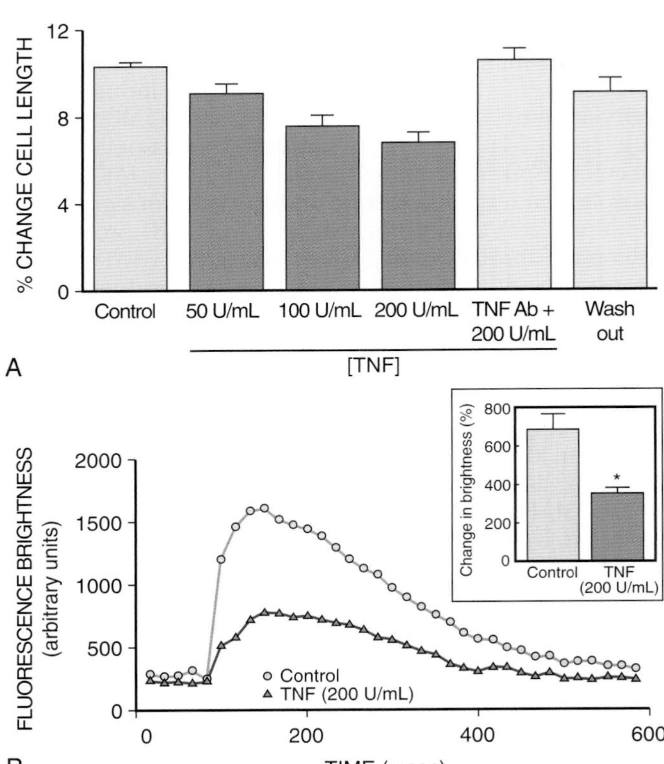

FIGURE 7-8 Effect of TNF on Contractility of Adult Cardiac Myocytes. Panel **A** shows that in comparison with control *(yellow bar)* cells, cardiac myocytes treated with TNF *(purple bars)* developed a concentration-dependent decrease in cell shortening. Pretreatment with a neutralizing anti-TNF antibody *(pink bar)* completely attenuated the effects of 200 U/mL TNF on cell shortening. When the cells were washed free of 200 U/mL TNF and allowed to recover for 45 minutes, the effects of TNF were completely reversible *(pink bar)*. Panel **B** shows a typical time-intensity curve for fluorescence brightness in isolated cardiac myocytes treated with diluent *(circles)* and 200 U/mL TNF-treated *(triangles)*. As shown, the peak level of intracellular fluorescence brightness was reduced strikingly for the cells treated with 200 U/mL TNF. The inset of this figure, which depicts values obtained for group data, shows that there was an approximately 40% decrease in the percent change in peak intensity of fluorescence brightness for the TNF-treated cells. Taken together, panels A and B suggest that TNF produces negative inotropic effects in isolated cardiac myocytes by producing an alteration in intracellular calcium homeostasis. *From Yokoyama T, Vaca L, Rossen RD, et al: Cellular basis for the negative inotropic effects of tumor necrosis factor-alpha in the adult mammalian heart. J Clin Invest 92:2303–2312, 1993.*

Signaling Pathways for the Negative Inotropic Effects of Inflammatory Mediators

With respect to the potential mechanisms for the deleterious effects of TNF on LV function, the literature suggests that TNF modulates myocardial function through at least two different pathways: an immediate pathway that is manifest within minutes and is mediated by activation of the neutral sphingomyelinase pathway,[75] and a delayed pathway that requires hours to days to develop, and is mediated by nitric oxide.[37,76] It has also been suggested recently that TNF and IL-1 produce their negative inotropic effects *indirectly* through activation and/or release of IL-18, which is a recently described member of the IL-1 family of cytokines.[47] Relevant to the present discussion is the observation that specific blockade of IL-18 using the neutralizing IL-18 antibody resulted in a decrease in infarct size in rats subjected to ischemia reperfusion injury.[77] Although the signaling pathways that are responsible for the IL-18–induced negative inotropic effects have not been delineated, it is likely that they will overlap those for IL-1, given that the IL-18 receptor complex uses components of the IL-1 signaling chain, including IL-1R-activating kinase (IRAK) and TNF receptor-associated factor 6 (TRAF6).[47]

Effects of Cytokines on Left Ventricular Structure

Cardiac remodeling contributes to the development and progression of heart failure (see Chapter 11). However, the mechanisms that contribute to the structural changes that underlie progressive cardiac remodeling are only partially understood. As shown in **Table 7-3**, inflammatory mediators have a number of important effects that may play an important role in the process of LV remodeling, including myocyte hypertrophy,[78] alterations in fetal gene expression,[72] degradation of the extracellular matrix,[69,79] as well as progressive myocyte loss through apoptosis.[80] When concentrations of TNF that overlap those observed in patients with heart failure were infused continuously in rats, there was a time-dependent change in LV dimension that was accompanied by progressive degradation of the extracellular matrix.[69] Second, recent studies in transgenic mice with targeted overexpression of TNF have shown that these mice develop progressive LV dilation. For example, Sivasubramanian and colleagues showed that a transgenic mouse line that overexpressed TNF in the cardiac compartment segued from a concentric LV hypertrophy phenotype to a dilated LV phenotype over a 12-week period of observation.[79] Similar findings have also been reported by Kubota and associates[72] and Bryant and colleagues,[81] who observed identical findings with respect to LV dysfunction and LV dilation in transgenic mice with targeted overexpression of TNF in the heart. With respect to the mechanisms that are involved in TNF-induced LV dilation, it has been suggested that TNF-induced activation of matrix metalloproteinases are responsible for this effect.[79] As shown in **Figure 7-9**, there was progressive loss of fibrillar collagen in the hearts of the transgenic mice overexpressing TNF in the cardiac compartment. Subsequent studies suggested that the loss of fibrillar collagen was secondary to increased activation of MMPs. The dissolution of the fibrillar collagen weave that surrounds the individual cardiac myocytes and links the myocytes together would be expected to allow for rearrangement ("slippage") of myofibrillar bundles within the ventricular wall. In addition to TNF, the related TNF superfamily member TWEAK has been shown to have important effects of cardiac remodeling. In a recent study, elevated circulating levels of TWEAK, induced via transgenic or adenoviral-mediated gene expression in mice, resulted in progressive LV remodeling with subsequent severe cardiac dysfunction (**Figure 7-10**) that was independent of TNF signaling. Although the mechanisms for TWEAK-mediated LV dilation have not been fully elucidated, it bears emphasis that TNF superfamily ligands/receptors that provoke a dilated cardiomyopathic phenotype, including TNF, TWEAK, and RANKL, each engage a common scaffolding protein termed *TNF receptor-associated factor 2* (TRAF2; see Figure 7-5). Importantly, TRAF2 engages downstream signal transduction

TABLE 7-3 Deleterious Effects of Inflammatory Mediators in Heart Failure

Left ventricular dysfunction
Pulmonary edema in humans
Cardiomyopathy in humans
Reduced skeletal muscle blood flow
Endothelial dysfunction
Anorexia and cachexia
Receptor uncoupling from adenylate cyclase experimentally
Activation of the fetal gene program experimentally
Cardiac myocyte apoptosis experimentally

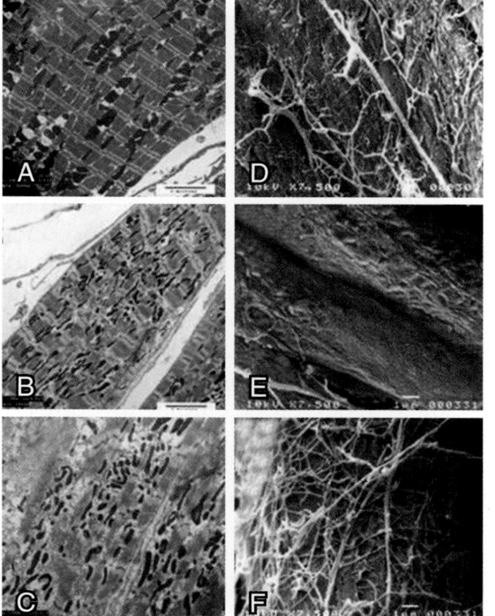

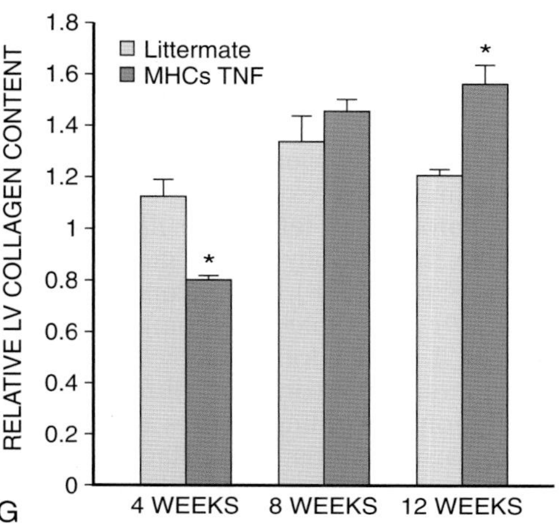

FIGURE 7-9 Effects of sustained proinflammatory cytokine expression on myocardial ultrastructure and collagen content. Panels A-C show representative transmission electron micrographs in littermate controls **(A)** and the TNF transgenic mice at 4 **(B)** and 8 **(C)** weeks of age. The transmission electron micrographs from the littermate control mice at 4 weeks revealed a characteristic linear array of sarcomeres and myofibrils. In contrast, the myofibrils in the 4-week-old TNF transgenic mice were less organized, with loss of sarcomeric registration observed in many of the sections. Panels D-F show representative scanning electron micrographs in littermate controls **(D)** and the TNF transgenic mice at 4 **(E)** and 8 weeks of age **(F).** Panel E shows that there was a significant loss of fibrillar collagen in the TNF transgenic mice at 4 weeks of age when compared with age-matched littermate controls (D). However, as the TNF transgenic mice aged (12 weeks), there was an obvious increase in myocardial fibrillar collagen content. Panel **G** illustrates the myocardial collagen content as determined by picrosirius red staining. There was a loss of myocardial collagen content at 4 weeks of age in the TNF transgenic mice, which was later followed by a progressive increase in myocardial collagen content at 8 and 12 weeks of age. *From Sivasubramanian N, Coker ML, Kurrelmeyer K, et al: Left ventricular remodeling in transgenic mice with cardiac restricted overexpression of tumor necrosis factor. Circulation 104:826–831, 2001.*

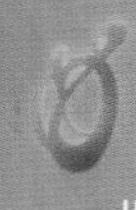

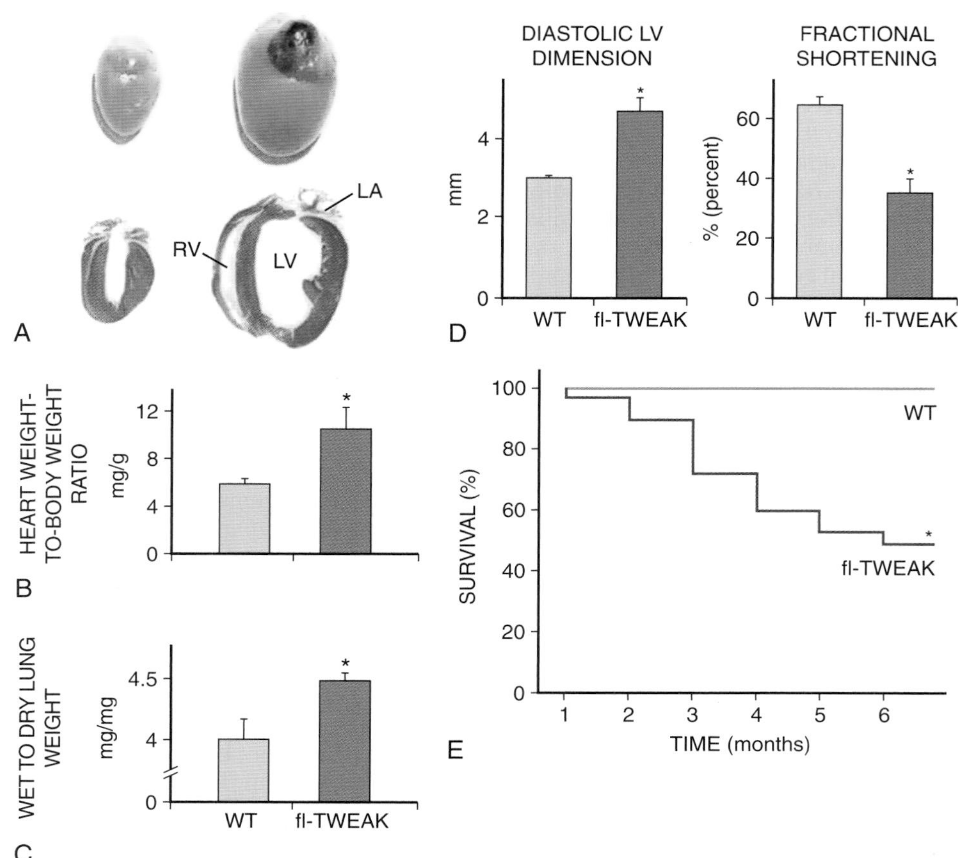

FIGURE 7-10 Effects of TWEAK on LV structure and function. **A,** Representative whole hearts and trichrome-stained longitudinal sections from wild-type and transgenic mice overexpressing a full-length TWEAK construct (fl-TWEAK). *LV,* Left ventricle; *RV,* right ventricle; *LA,* left atrium. **B,** Increased heart weight–to–body weight ratios in fl-TWEAK mice compared with wild-type (WT) mice. **C,** Increased wet-to-dry lung weights in fl-TWEAK mice compared with WT mice. **D,** LV end-diastolic dimension and fractional shortening in WT and fl-TWEAK mice. **E,** Kaplan-Meier survival curves for WT and fl-TWEAK mice demonstrating increased mortality in the fl-TWEAK mice. (* = $P < 0.01$) *Modified from Jain M, Jakubowski A, Cui L, et al: A novel role for tumor necrosis factor-like weak inducer of apoptosis (TWEAK) in the development of cardiac dysfunction and failure. Circulation 119:2058–2068, 2009.*

pathways that have been implicated in the development of a dilated cardiac phenotype, including mitogen-activated protein kinases, NF-κB, and c-jun N-terminal kinases (JNK),[82] suggesting that TRAF2 may coordinate the signaling events that contribute to the changes in LV structure and function that occur during inflammation-induced cardiomyopathy. Indeed, lines of transgenic mice with cardiac restricted overexpression of TRAF2 (MHC-TRAF2_{HC}) develop a dilated cardiac phenotype that overlaps the phenotype observed in transgenic mice overexpressing TNF superfamily ligands, including progressive left ventricular dilation (**Figure 7-11A**), cardiac hypertrophy (see Figure 7-11C), sarcomere disarray (see Figure 7-11F), and adverse cardiac remodeling (increased r/h ratio) that is accompanied by early MMP activation at 4 weeks, followed by increased TIMP expression and increased myocardial fibrosis at 12 weeks of age. Transcriptional profiling studies show that TRAF2 signaling leads to alterations in cardiac myocyte gene expression, which has been associated with the development of heart failure, and that 95% of the genes identified in the hypertrophy/dilated cardiomyopathy pathway were NF-κB dependent.

Cardiac restricted overexpression of TNF has been shown to lead to progressive cardiac myocyte apoptosis and LV wall thinning.[83] Mechanistic studies showed that sustained TNF signaling resulted in activation of the intrinsic cell death pathway, leading to increased cytosolic levels of cytochrome c, Smac/DIABLO, and Omi/HtrA2, and activation of caspases 3 and 9. Targeted overexpression of Bcl-2 blunted activation of the intrinsic pathway and prevented LV wall thinning; however, Bcl-2 only partially attenuated cardiac myocyte apoptosis. Subsequent studies showed that caspase-8 was activated and that Bid was cleaved to t-Bid, suggesting that the extrinsic pathway was activated concurrently.[84] Thus sustained myocardial inflammation leads to activation of multiple cell death pathways that contribute to progressive cardiac myocyte apoptosis and adverse cardiac remodeling.[84] Antagonism of IL-1 signaling by administering anakinra, a recombinant-human IL-1 receptor antagonist, has also resulted in decreased cardiac myocyte apoptosis, decreased LV remodeling, and improved LV function in a rat infarct model.[85] In vitro studies in rat cardiac myocytes demonstrated that anakinra inhibited caspase-1 and -9 activity, and prevented apoptosis in a simulated model of ischemia.[85] From a pathophysiologic standpoint, the increase in LV wall thinning that attends progressive cardiac myocyte apoptosis would be expected to contribute to increased LV wall stress (i.e., afterload mismatch), and hence sustained unfavorable loading conditions of the heart, thereby contributing to progressive cardiac decompensation. Thus excessive activation of proinflammatory cytokines may contribute to LV remodeling through a variety of different mechanisms that involve both the myocyte and nonmyocyte components of the myocardium.

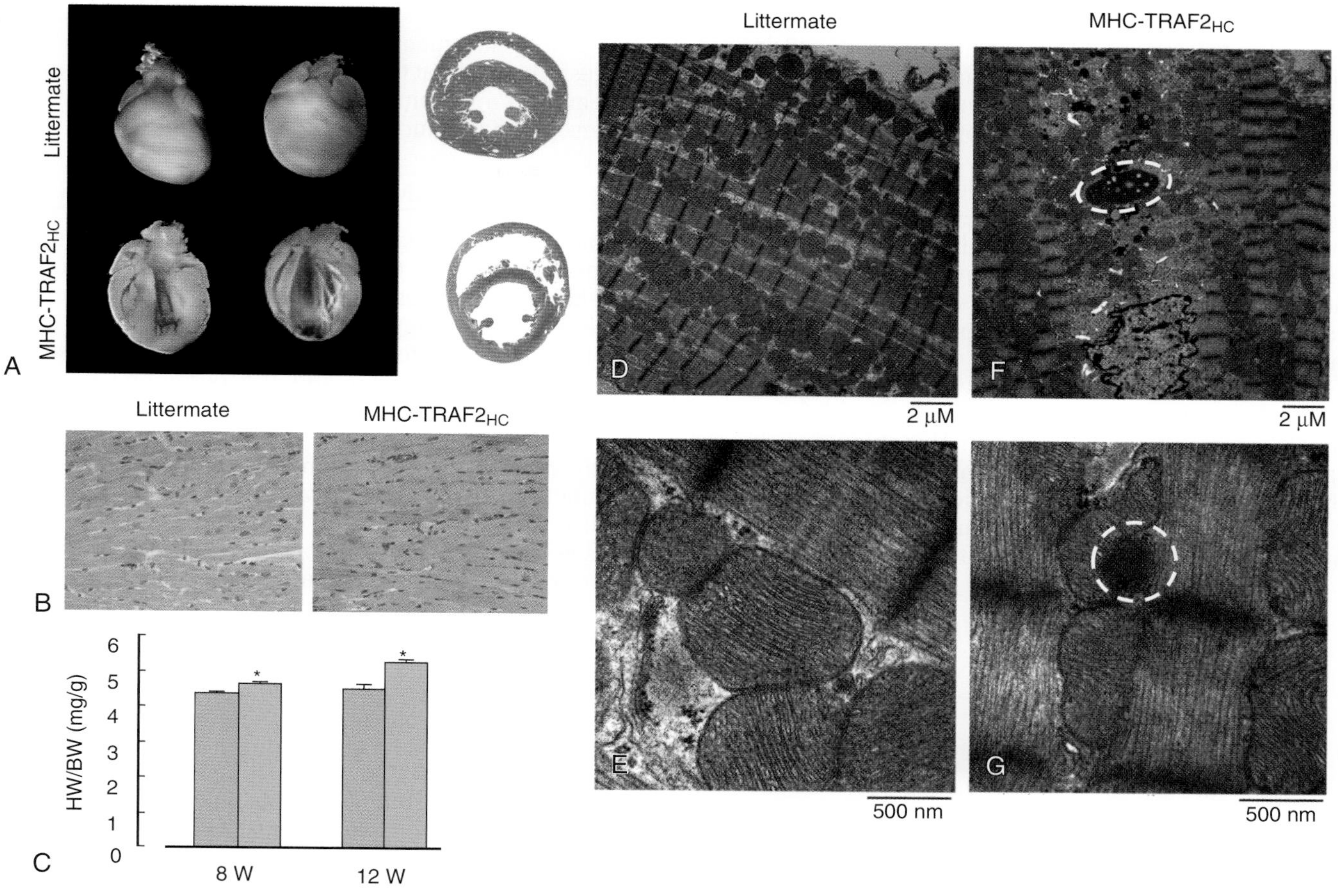

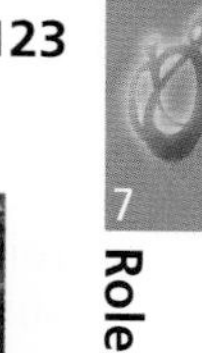

FIGURE 7-11 Characterization of transgenic mice with cardiac-restricted overexpression of TRAF2 (MHC-TRAF2$_{HC}$). **A,** Photographs of whole hearts, coronal and sagittal sections of both LM and MHC-TRAF2$_{HC}$ mouse hearts (12 weeks). **B,** Representative hematoxylin-eosin-stained cross sections at the level of the papillary muscles (400×). **C,** Heart weight–to–body weight ratio (mg/g) of LM and MHC-TRAF2$_{HC}$ at 8 and 12 weeks (n = 6 to 8 mice/group/time point) (* = $P < 0.05$ vs. LM at the indicated time point). **D-G,** Representative transmission electron micrographs from 12-week MHC-TRAF2$_{HC}$ transgenic mice and LM at low (7500×, D, F) and high (60,000×, E, G) magnification. Protein aggregates are enclosed by the circles. *Modified from Divakaran V, Evans S, Topkara VK, et al: Tumor necrosis factor receptor associated factor 2 signaling provokes adverse cardiac remodeling in the adult mammalian heart. Circ Heart Fail 6:535–543, 2013.*

Interactions Between the Renin-Angiotensin System and Proinflammatory Cytokines in Adverse Cardiac Remodeling

Although neurohormonal and cytokine systems have been regarded as functionally distinct biologic systems, recent studies suggest that these two systems can cross-regulate each other, with the result that neurohormonal and cytokine systems may participate in positive feed-forward loops that contribute to adverse cardiac remodeling. Whereas angiotensin II was traditionally viewed as a circulating neurohormone that stimulated the constriction of vascular smooth muscle cells, aldosterone release from the adrenal gland, sodium reabsorption in the renal tubule, and/or as a stimulus for growth of cardiac myocytes or fibroblasts,[86] it is becoming increasingly apparent that angiotensin II provokes inflammatory responses in a variety of different cell and tissue types. For example, angiotensin II activates NF-κB,[87] which is critical for initiating the coordinated expression of the classic components of the myocardial inflammatory response, including increased expression of proinflammatory cytokines, nitric oxide, chemokines, and cell adhesion molecules.[88] Pathophysiologically relevant concentrations of angiotensin II are sufficient to provoke TNF mRNA and protein synthesis in the adult heart through a NF-κB–dependent pathway.[89] **Figure 7-12** shows that treatment with angiotensin II resulted in a rapid increase in TNF mRNA (see Figure 7-12A) and protein synthesis (see Figure 7-12B) in isolated buffer perfused hearts. Stimulation of isolated adult cardiac myocytes with angiotensin II resulted in an approximately 3-fold increase in TNF protein biosynthesis within 1 hour, and an approximately 15-fold increase in TNF protein biosynthesis within 24 hours, suggesting that the increase in TNF biosynthesis in the intact heart was mediated, at least in part, at the level of the cardiac myocyte. The effects of angiotensin II on TNF mRNA and protein synthesis were mediated exclusively through the angiotensin type 1 receptor, insofar as pretreatment with the angiotensin type 1 receptor antagonist losartan completely abolished the effects of angiotensin II on TNF biosynthesis, whereas pretreatment with the angiotensin type 2 receptor antagonist PD123319 had no effect on angiotensin II-induced TNF biosynthesis (see Figure 7-12B). This study further showed that the effects of angiotensin II on TNF myocardial biosynthesis were dependent upon protein kinase C–mediated activation of NF-κB.[89]

There is also increasing evidence that inflammatory mediators are capable of upregulating various components of the renin-angiotensin system in a variety of mammalian tissues, including the heart. As one recent example, studies using transgenic mice with cardiac restricted overexpression of TNF have shown that targeted overexpression of TNF leads to an increase in angiotensin II peptide levels in the

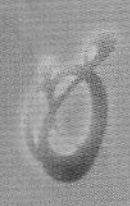

heart.[90] This study serially examined several components of the renin-angiotensin system, including angiotensinogen, renin, angiotensin-converting enzyme (ACE), and angiotensin I and II peptide levels in a transgenic mouse line with cardiac restricted overexpression of TNF. There was a significant increase in ACE mRNA levels and ACE activity, as well as increased angiotensin II peptide levels in the hearts of the TNF transgenic mice relative to littermate controls. Importantly, the expression of renin and angiotensinogen was not increased in the TNF transgenic mice compared with littermate controls. Thus this study suggested that the increased levels of angiotensin II peptide levels in the TNF transgenic mice were principally the result of increased ACE activity, as opposed to increased activation of the more proximal components of the renin-angiotensin system, namely renin and angiotensinogen. This study also showed that activation of the renin-angiotensin system was functionally significant in the TNF transgenic mice. That is, treatment of the TNF transgenic mice from 4 to 8 weeks of age with losartan significantly attenuated cardiac hypertrophy, myocardial fibrosis, and cardiac myocyte apoptosis in the TNF transgenic mice.[90] Taken together, these observations suggest that interactions between the renin-angiotensin system and inflammatory mediators may contribute to adverse cardiac remodeling.

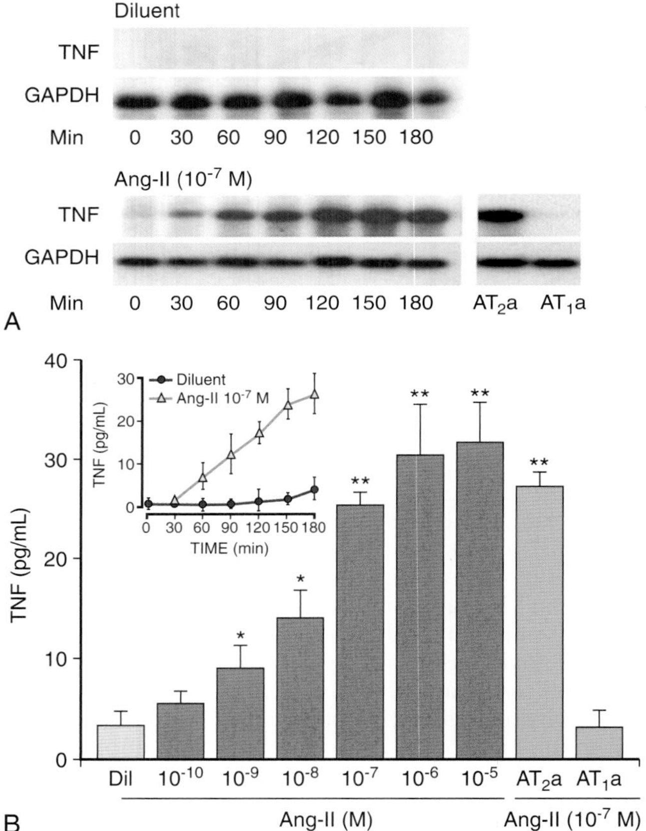

FIGURE 7-12 Angiotensin II-induced myocardial TNF biosynthesis in the adult heart. **A,** TNF mRNA expression (RNase protection assay) was assessed ex vivo in diluent and angiotensin II (10^{-7} M)-treated (0 to 180 min) buffer perfused Langendorff hearts, in the presence or absence of 10^{-6} M PD123319, an AT_2 receptor antagonist (AT_2a), or 10^{-6} M losartan, an AT_1 receptor antagonist (AT_1a). **B,** Myocardial TNF protein production was assessed in the superfusates of the angiotensin II-treated hearts using ELISA, in the presence or absence of PD123319 (10^{-6} M) or losartan (10^{-6} M) pretreatment. The main panel of **B** shows the dose-dependent effects of angiotensin II (10^{-10} M to 10^{-5} M), whereas the inset shows the time course (0 to 180 min) for TNF protein synthesis following stimulation with either diluent *(solid circles)* or 10^{-7} M Ang-II *(open triangles)*. *AT_1a,* AT_1 receptor antagonist (losartan); *AT_2a,* AT_2 receptor antagonist (PD123319). (* = $P < 0.05$ and ** = $P < 0.01$ compared with diluent-treated hearts). *From Kalra D, Sivasubramanian N, Mann DL: Angiotensin II induces tumor necrosis factor biosynthesis in the adult mammalian heart through a protein kinase C-dependent pathway. Circulation 105:2198–2205, 2002.*

CONCLUSION AND FUTURE DIRECTIONS

In this chapter we have focused on the experimental evidence that suggests that activation of the innate immune system with the subsequent elaboration of inflammatory cytokines plays an important role in the progression of heart failure, by virtue of the deleterious effects that these molecules exert on the heart and the peripheral circulation. Indeed, pathophysiologically relevant concentrations of these molecules mimic many aspects of the so-called heart failure phenotype in experimental animals, including LV dysfunction, LV dilation, activation of fetal gene expression, cardiac myocyte hypertrophy and cardiac myocyte apoptosis (see Table 7-3). Thus, analogous to the proposed role for neurohormones, proinflammatory cytokines would appear to represent another distinct class of biologically active molecules that can contribute to heart failure progression. Nonetheless, the early attempts to translate this information to the bedside have not only been disappointing, but have in many instances led to worsening heart failure.[91] While one interpretation of these findings is that inflammatory mediators are not viable targets in heart failure, an alternative point of view is that we simply have not targeted proinflammatory mediators with agents that can be used safely in the context of heart failure, or alternatively, that targeting a single component of the inflammatory cascade is not sufficient in a disease as complex as heart failure. Moreover, it is important to recognize that all currently approved therapies for chronic heart failure, including cardiac resynchronization therapy, have a net beneficial effect on the elaboration of inflammatory mediators.[91] Accordingly, in future studies it may be necessary to use biomarkers to select heart failure patients who have ongoing inflammation despite optimal medical therapy. Indeed a recent consensus statement from the Translation Research Committee of the Heart Failure Association of the European Society of Cardiology suggested that there may not be a common inflammatory pathway that characterizes all of the different forms of heart failure, and that going forward it will be important to design specific anti-inflammatory approaches for different types and stages of heart failure, as well as to determine the specific inflammatory pathways that are activated in different forms of heart failure.[92]

References

1. Levine B, Kalman J, Mayer L, et al: Elevated circulating levels of tumor necrosis factor in severe chronic heart failure. *N Engl J Med* 223:236–241, 1990.
2. Janeway CA, Jr, Medzhitov R: Introduction: the role of innate immunity in the adaptive immune response. *Semin Immunol* 10:349–350, 1998.
3. Gallucci S, Matzinger P: Danger signals: SOS to the immune system. *Curr Opin Immunol* 13:114–119, 2001.
4. Ionita MG, Arslan F, de Kleijn DP, et al: Endogenous inflammatory molecules engage Toll-like receptors in cardiovascular disease. *J Innate Immun* 2:307–315, 2010.
5. Medzhitov R, Preston-Hurlburt P, Janeway CA, Jr: A human homologue of the Drosophila Toll protein signals activation of adaptive immunity. *Nature* 388:394–397, 1997.
6. Nishimura M, Naito S: Tissue-specific mRNA expression profiles of human toll-like receptors and related genes. *Biol Pharm Bull* 28:886–892, 2005.
7. Frantz S, Kelly RA, Bourcier T: Role of TLR-2 in the activation of nuclear factor-kappa B by oxidative stress in cardiac myocytes. *J Biol Chem* 276:5197–5203, 2001.
8. Frantz S, Kobzik L, Kim YD, et al: Toll4 (TLR4) expression in cardiac myocytes in normal and failing myocardium. *J Clin Invest* 104:271–280, 1999.
9. Birks EJ, Felkin LE, Banner NR, et al: Increased toll-like receptor 4 in the myocardium of patients requiring left ventricular assist devices. *J Heart Lung Transplant* 23:228–235, 2004.
10. Lin YC, Chang YM, Yu JM, et al: Toll-like receptor 4 gene C119A but not Asp299Gly polymorphism is associated with ischemic stroke among ethnic Chinese in Taiwan. *Atherosclerosis* 180:305–309, 2005.

11. Frantz S, Ertl G, Bauersachs J: Mechanisms of disease: Toll-like receptors in cardiovascular disease. *Nat Clin Pract Cardiovasc Med* 4:444–454, 2007.
12. Akira S, Takeda K: Toll-like receptor signalling. *Nat Rev Immunol* 4:499–511, 2004.
13. Hennessy EJ, Parker AE, O'Neill LA: Targeting Toll-like receptors: emerging therapeutics? *Nat Rev Drug Discov* 9:293–307, 2010.
14. Bianchi ME: DAMPs, PAMPs and alarmins: all we need to know about danger. *J Leukoc Biol* 81:1–5, 2007.
15. Kobayashi K, Hernandez LD, Galan JE, et al: IRAK-M is a negative regulator of Toll-like receptor signaling. *Cell* 110:191–202, 2002.
16. Sly LM, Rauh MJ, Kalesnikoff J, et al: LPS-induced upregulation of SHIP is essential for endotoxin tolerance. *Immunity* 21:227–239, 2004.
17. Shi M, Deng W, Bi E, et al: TRIM30 alpha negatively regulates TLR-mediated NF-kappa B activation by targeting TAB2 and TAB3 for degradation. *Nat Immunol* 9:369–377, 2008.
18. Carty M, Goodbody R, Schroder M, et al: The human adaptor SARM negatively regulates adaptor protein TRIF-dependent Toll-like receptor signaling. *Nat Immunol* 7:1074–1081, 2006.
19. Taganov KD, Boldin MP, Chang KJ, et al: NF-kappaB-dependent induction of microRNA miR-146, an inhibitor targeted to signaling proteins of innate immune responses. *Proc Natl Acad Sci U S A* 103:12481–12486, 2006.
20. O'Connell RM, Chaudhuri AA, Rao DS, et al: Inositol phosphatase SHIP1 is a primary target of miR-155. *Proc Natl Acad Sci U S A* 106:7113–7118, 2009.
21. Sheedy FJ, Palsson-McDermott E, Hennessy EJ, et al: Negative regulation of TLR4 via targeting of the proinflammatory tumor suppressor PDCD4 by the microRNA miR-21. *Nat Immunol* 11:141–147, 2010.
22. Sakata Y, Dong JW, Vallejo JG, et al: Toll-like receptor 2 modulates left ventricular function following ischemia-reperfusion injury. *Am J Physiol Heart Circ Physiol* 292:H503–H509, 2007.
23. Chong AJ, Shimamoto A, Hampton CR, et al: Toll-like receptor 4 mediates ischemia/reperfusion injury of the heart. *J Thorac Cardiovasc Surg* 128:170–179, 2004.
24. Kim SC, Ghanem A, Stapel H, et al: Toll-like receptor 4 deficiency: smaller infarcts, but no gain in function. *BMC Physiol* 7:5, 2007.
25. Oyama J, Blais C, Jr, Liu X, et al: Reduced myocardial ischemia-reperfusion injury in toll-like receptor 4-deficient mice. *Circulation* 109:784–789, 2004.
26. Shishido T, Nozaki N, Yamaguchi S, et al: Toll-like receptor-2 modulates ventricular remodeling after myocardial infarction. *Circulation* 108:2905–2910, 2003.
27. Feng Y, Zhao H, Xu X, et al: Innate immune adaptor MyD88 mediates neutrophil recruitment and myocardial injury after ischemia-reperfusion in mice. *Am J Physiol Heart Circ Physiol* 295:H1311–H1318, 2008.
28. Shimamoto A, Chong AJ, Yada M, et al: Inhibition of Toll-like receptor 4 with eritoran attenuates myocardial ischemia-reperfusion injury. *Circulation* 114:I270–I274, 2006.
29. Riad A, Jager S, Sobirey M, et al: Toll-like receptor-4 modulates survival by induction of left ventricular remodeling after myocardial infarction in mice. *J Immunol* 180:6954–6961, 2008.
30. Mann DL, Topkara VK, Evans S, et al: Innate immunity in the adult mammalian heart: for whom the cell tolls. *Trans Am Clin Climatol Assoc* 121:34–50, 2010.
31. Ringner M: What is principal component analysis? *Nat Biotechnol* 26:303–304, 2008.
32. Parrillo JE, Cunnion RE, Epstein SE, et al: A prospective randomized controlled trial of prednisone for dilated cardiomyopathy. *N Engl J Med* 321:1061–1068, 1989.
33. Ueland T, Aukrust P, Damas JK, et al: The tumor necrosis factor superfamily in heart failure. *Future Cardiol* 2:101–111, 2006.
34. Jain M, Jakubowski A, Cui L, et al: A novel role for tumor necrosis factor-like weak inducer of apoptosis (TWEAK) in the development of cardiac dysfunction and failure. *Circulation* 119:2058–2068, 2009.
35. Ueland T, Yndestad A, Oie E, et al: Dysregulated osteoprotegerin/RANK ligand/RANK axis in clinical and experimental heart failure. *Circulation* 111:2461–2468, 2005.
36. Nelson DP, Setser E, Hall DG, et al: Proinflammatory consequences of transgenic fas ligand expression in the heart. *J Clin Invest* 105:1199–1208, 2000.
37. Gulick TS, Chung MK, Pieper SJ, et al: Interleukin 1 and tumor necrosis factor inhibit cardiac myocyte β-adrenergic responsiveness. *Proc Natl Acad Sci U S A* 86:6753–6757, 1989.
38. Torre-Amione G, Kapadia S, Lee J, et al: Tumor necrosis factor-α and tumor necrosis factor receptors in the failing human heart. *Circulation* 93:704–711, 1996.
39. Torre-Amione G, Kapadia S, Lee J, et al: Expression and functional significance of tumor necrosis factor receptors in human myocardium. *Circulation* 92:1487–1493, 1995.
40. Ramani R, Mathier M, Wang P, et al: Inhibition of tumor necrosis factor receptor-1-mediated pathways has beneficial effects in a murine model of postischemic remodeling. *Am J Physiol Heart Circ Physiol* 287:H1369–H1377, 2004.
41. Chorianopoulos E, Heger T, Lutz M, et al: FGF-inducible 14-kDa protein (Fn14) is regulated via the RhoA/ROCK kinase pathway in cardiomyocytes and mediates nuclear factor-kappaB activation by TWEAK. *Basic Res Cardiol* 105:301–313, 2010.
42. Garlanda C, Dinarello CA, Mantovani A: The interleukin-1 family: back to the future. *Immunity* 39:1003–1018, 2013.
43. Weber A, Wasiliew P, Kracht M: Interleukin-1 (IL-1) pathway. *Sci Signal* 3:cm1, 2010.
44. Francis SE, Holden H, Holt CM, et al: Interleukin-1 in myocardium and coronary arteries of patients with dilated cardiomyopathy. *J Mol Cell Cardiol* 30:215–223, 1998.
45. Dinarello CA: Interleukin-1. In Thomson A, editor: *The cytokine handbook*, Boston, 1991, Academic Press, pp 47–82.
46. Dinarello CA: Biological basis for interleukin-1 in disease. *Blood* 87:2095–2147, 1996.
47. Dinarello CA: Interleukin-18. *Methods* 19:121–132, 1999.
48. Raeburn CD, Dinarello CA, Zimmerman MA, et al: Neutralization of IL-18 attenuates lipopolysaccharide-induced myocardial dysfunction. *Am J Physiol Heart Circ Physiol* 283:H650–H657, 2002.
49. Pomerantz BJ, Reznikov LL, Harken AH, et al: Inhibition of caspase 1 reduces human myocardial ischemic dysfunction via inhibition of IL-18 and IL-1beta. *Proc Natl Acad Sci U S A* 98:2871–2876, 2001.
50. Born TL, Thomassen E, Bird TA, et al: Cloning of a novel receptor subunit, AcPL, required for interleukin-18 signaling. *J Biol Chem* 273:29445–29450, 1998.
51. Kakkar R, Lee RT: The IL-33/ST2 pathway: therapeutic target and novel biomarker. *Nat Rev Drug Discov* 7:827–840, 2008.
52. Sanada S, Hakuno D, Higgins LJ, et al: IL-33 and ST2 comprise a critical biomechanically induced and cardioprotective signaling system. *J Clin Invest* 117:1538–1549, 2007.
53. Sabatine MS, Morrow DA, Higgins LJ, et al: Complementary roles for biomarkers of biomechanical strain ST2 and N-terminal prohormone B-type natriuretic peptide in patients with ST-elevation myocardial infarction. *Circulation* 117:1936–1944, 2008.
54. Kuropatwinski KK, Imus CD, Gearing D, et al: Influence of subunit combinations on signaling by receptors for oncostatin M, leukemia inhibitory factor, and interleukin-6. *J Biol Chem* 272:15135–15144, 1997.
55. Hartupee J, Mann DL: Positioning of inflammatory biomarkers in the heart failure landscape. *J Cardiovasc Transl Res* 6:485–492, 2013.
56. Fischer P, Hilfiker-Kleiner D: Survival pathways in hypertrophy and heart failure: the gp130-STAT3 axis. *Basic Res Cardiol* 102:279–297, 2007.
57. Hirano T: Interleukin-6. In Thomson A, editor: *The cytokine handbook*, Boston, 1991, Academic Press, pp 169–190.
58. Hirano T, Yasukawa K, Harada H, et al: Complementary DNA for a novel human interleukin (BSF-2) that induces B lymphocytes to produce immunoglobulin. *Nature* 324:73–78, 1986.
59. Finkel MS, Hoffman RA, Shen L, et al: Interleukin-6 (IL-6) as a mediator of stunned myocardium. *Am J Cardiol* 71:1231–1232, 1993.
60. Sehgal PB: Interleukine-6 type cytokines in vivo: regulated bioavailability. *Proc Soc Exp Biol Med* 213:238–247, 1996.
61. Yoshida K, Taga T, Saito M, et al: Targeted disruption of gp130, a common signal transducer for the interleukin 6 family of cytokines, leads to myocardial and hematological disorders. *Proc Natl Acad Sci U S A* 93:407–411, 1996.
62. Hirota H, Yoshida K, Kishimoto T, et al: Continuous activation of gp130, a signal-transducing receptor component for interleukin 6-related cytokines, causes myocardial hypertrophy in mice. *Proc Natl Acad Sci U S A* 92:4862–4866, 1995.
63. Boengler K, Hilfiker-Kleiner D, Drexler H, et al: The myocardial JAK/STAT pathway: from protection to failure. *Pharmacol Ther* 120:172–185, 2008.
64. Hilfiker-Kleiner D, Kaminski K, Podewski E, et al: A cathepsin D-cleaved 16 kDa form of prolactin mediates postpartum cardiomyopathy. *Cell* 128:589–600, 2007.
65. Zouein FA, Kurdi M, Booz GW: LIF and the heart: just another brick in the wall? *Eur Cytokine Netw* 24:11–19, 2013.
66. Pennica D, King KL, Shaw KJ, et al: Expression cloning of cardiotrophin 1, a cytokine that induces cardiac myocyte hypertrophy. *Proc Natl Acad Sci U S A* 92:1142–1146, 1995.
67. Schillaci G, Pucci G, Perlini S: From hypertension to hypertrophy to heart failure: the role of cardiotrophin-1. *J Hypertens* 31:474–476, 2013.
68. Aukrust P, Ueland T, Muller F, et al: Elevated circulating levels of C-C chemokines in patients with congestive heart failure. *Circulation* 97:1136–1143, 1998.
69. Bozkurt B, Kribbs S, Clubb FJ, Jr, et al: Pathophysiologically relevant concentrations of tumor necrosis factor-α promote progressive left ventricular dysfunction and remodeling in rats. *Circulation* 97:1382–1391, 1998.
70. Seta Y, Shan K, Bozkurt B, et al: Basic mechanisms in heart failure: the cytokine hypothesis. *J Cardiac Failure* 2:243–249, 1996.
71. Tracey KJ, Beutler B, Lowry SF, et al: Shock and tissue injury induced by recombinant human cachectin. *Science* 234:470–474, 1986.
72. Kubota T, McTiernan CF, Frye CS, et al: Dilated cardiomyopathy in transgenic mice with cardiac specific overexpression of tumor necrosis factor-alpha. *Circ Res* 81:627–635, 1997.
73. Franco F, Thomas GD, Giroir BP, et al: Magnetic resonance imaging and invasive evaluation of development of heart failure in transgenic mice with myocardial expression of tumor necrosis factor-alpha. *Circulation* 99:448–454, 1999.
74. Yokoyama T, Vaca L, Rossen RD, et al: Cellular basis for the negative inotropic effects of tumor necrosis factor-alpha in the adult mammalian heart. *J Clin Invest* 92:2303–2312, 1993.
75. Oral H, Dorn GW, II, Mann DL: Sphingosine mediates the immediate negative inotropic effects of tumor necrosis factor-alpha in the adult mammalian cardiac myocyte. *J Biol Chem* 272:4836–4842, 1997.
76. Balligand JL, Ungureanu D, Kelly RA, et al: Abnormal contractile function due to induction of nitric oxide synthesis in rat cardiac myocytes follows exposure to activated macrophage-conditioned medium. *J Clin Invest* 91:2314–2319, 1993.
77. Mallat Z, Heymes C, Corbaz A, et al: Evidence for altered interleukin 18 (IL)-18 pathway in human heart failure. *FASEB J* 18:1752–1754, 2004.
78. Yokoyama T, Nakano M, Bednarczyk JL, et al: Tumor necrosis factor-α provokes a hypertrophic growth response in adult cardiac myocytes. *Circulation* 95:1247–1252, 1997.
79. Sivasubramanian N, Coker ML, Kurrelmeyer K, et al: Left ventricular remodeling in transgenic mice with cardiac restricted overexpression of tumor necrosis factor. *Circulation* 2001:826–831, 2001.
80. Krown KA, Page MT, Nguyen C, et al: Tumor necrosis factor alpha-induced apoptosis in cardiac myocytes: involvement of the sphingolipid signaling cascade in cardiac cell death. *J Clin Invest* 98:2854–2865, 1996.
81. Bryant D, Becker L, Richardson J, et al: Cardiac failure in transgenic mice with myocardial expression of tumor necrosis factor-α (TNF). *Circulation* 97:1375–1381, 1998.
82. Gupta S, Sen S: Role of the NF-kappaB signaling cascade and NF-kappaB-targeted genes in failing human hearts. *J Mol Med (Berl)* 83:993–1004, 2005.
83. Engel D, Peshock R, Armstong RC, et al: Cardiac myocyte apoptosis provokes adverse cardiac remodeling in transgenic mice with targeted TNF overexpression. *Am J Physiol Heart Circ Physiol* 287:H1303–H1311, 2004.
84. Haudek SB, Taffet GE, Schneider MD, et al: TNF provokes cardiomyocyte apoptosis and cardiac remodeling through activation of multiple cell death pathways. *J Clin Invest* 117:2692–2701, 2007.
85. Abbate A, Salloum FN, Vecile E, et al: Anakinra, a recombinant human interleukin-1 receptor antagonist, inhibits apoptosis in experimental acute myocardial infarction. *Circulation* 117:2670–2683, 2008.
86. Dostal DE, Baker KM: The cardiac renin-angiotensin system: conceptual, or a regulator of cardiac function? *Circ Res* 85:643–650, 1999.
87. Brasier AR, Jamaluddin M, Han Y, et al: Angiotensin II induces gene transcription through cell-type-dependent effects on the nuclear factor-kappaB (NF-kappaB) transcription factor. *Mol Cell Biochem* 212:155–169, 2000.
88. Luft FC: Workshop: mechanisms and cardiovascular damage in hypertension. *Hypertension* 37:594–598, 2001.
89. Kalra D, Baumgarten G, Dibbs Z, et al: Nitric oxide provokes tumor necrosis factor-alpha expression in adult feline myocardium through a cGMP-dependent pathway. *Circulation* 102:1302–1307, 2000.
90. Flesch M, Hoper A, Dell'Italia L, et al: Activation and functional significance of the renin-angiotensin system in mice with cardiac restricted overexpression of tumor necrosis factor. *Circulation* 108:598–604, 2003.
91. Mann DL: Inflammatory mediators and the failing heart: past, present, and the foreseeable future. *Circ Res* 91:988–998, 2002.
92. Heymans S, Hirsch E, Anker SD, et al: Inflammation as a therapeutic target in heart failure? A scientific statement from the Translational Research Committee of the Heart Failure Association of the European Society of Cardiology. *Eur J Heart Fail* 11:119–129, 2009.
93. Favre J, Musette P, Douin-Echinard V, et al: Toll-like receptors 2-deficient mice are protected against postischemic coronary endothelial dysfunction. *Arterioscler Thromb Vasc Biol* 27:1064–1071, 2007.
94. Timmers L, Sluijter JP, Van Keulen JK, et al: Toll-like receptor 4 mediates maladaptive left ventricular remodeling and impairs cardiac function following myocardial infarction. *Circ Res* 102:257–264, 2007.

Abbreviations Used in This Chapter

ABBREVIATION	FULL NAME
DAMP	Damage-associated molecular pattern
HSP	Heat shock protein
IKK	IκB kinase
IL-1	Interleukin-1
IL-1R	Interleukin-1 receptor
I/R	Ischemia/reperfusion
IRAK	Interleukin-1 receptor-associated kinase
IRAK-M	Interleukin-1 receptor-associated kinase M
IRF3	Interferon regulatory factor 3
LPS	Lipopolysaccharide
MAL	MyD88 adapter-like protein
MAPK	Mitogen-activated protein kinase
MEK	MAP kinase kinase
MEKK	MAP kinase kinase kinase
MyD88	Myeloid differentiation primary response gene 88
MyD88s	MyD88 short
NEMO (IKKγ)	NF-κB essential modulator
NF	Nuclear factor
NF-κB	Nuclear factor kappa B
NIK	NF-κB inducing kinase
PAMP	Pathogen-associated molecular pattern
PDCD4	Programmed cell death 4
PIP_3	Phosphatidylinositol-3,4,5-triphosphate
PRR	Pattern recognition receptor
ROS	Reactive oxygen species
SHIP-1	SH2-containing inositol 5-phosphatase 1
SIGIRR	Single immunoglobulin interleukin-1 receptor-related molecule
TAB	TAK binding protein
TAK1	TGF-β activated kinase 1
TANK	TRAF-family member-associated NF-κB activator
TBK1	TANK binding kinase 1
TGF	Transforming growth factor
TIR	Toll interleukin-1 receptor
TIRAP	TIR domain-containing adapter protein (MAL [MyD88-adapter-like])
TLR	Toll-like receptor
TNF	Tumor necrosis factor
TOLLIP	Toll interacting protein
TRAF6	TNF receptor-associated factor 6
TRAM	TRIF-related adapter molecule (TICAM2)
TRIF	TIR domain-containing adapter inducing IFN-β (TICAM1)
UBC13	Ubiquitin-conjugating enzyme 13
UEV1A	Ubiquitin-conjugating enzyme E2 variant 1

8 Oxidative Stress in Heart Failure

Douglas B. Sawyer, Aaron L. Sverdlov, and Wilson S. Colucci

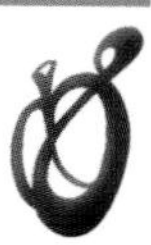

Oxidative stress is increased in heart failure (HF), and experimental studies suggest that this may contribute to structural and functional changes in the heart that are central to both cardiac dysfunction and disease progression. Our understanding of the role of oxidative stress in myocardial dysfunction, though incomplete, continues to grow.

REACTIVE OXYGEN SPECIES AND ANTIOXIDANT SYSTEMS (Figure 8-1)

Reactive Oxygen Species

Reactive oxygen species (ROS) are a by-product of aerobic metabolism, and so the highly metabolically active myocardium is rich in ROS. As in all tissues, ROS are handled in the myocardium by both soluble and enzymatic antioxidant systems. "Oxidative stress" occurs when the production of ROS exceeds the capacity of antioxidant defense systems. ROS cascades begin with the formation of *superoxide anion* (O_2^-) by either enzymatic or nonenzymatic one-electron reduction of molecular oxygen. The unpaired electron in O_2^- is an unstable free radical that reacts with itself and other oxygen-containing species, and directly or indirectly with organic molecules—including lipids, nucleic acids, and proteins—ultimately leading to regulation or disruption of cellular functions. All aerobic organisms, from bacteria to man, have evolved a complex antioxidant defense system of enzymatic and nonenzymatic components to defend against the unavoidable formation of ROS.[1] In parallel there has been the evolution of specific ROS-generating systems that are used both in the immune system, where the toxicity of ROS is exploited to fight infectious organisms,[2] as well as in all cell types where ROS act as signaling intermediates for the purpose of triggering specific intracellular processes.

Primary Antioxidant Systems

Primary antioxidant enzymes, defined here as those that directly interact with ROS, include superoxide dismutases (SOD), catalase, and other peroxidases. These enzymes work in parallel with nonenzymatic antioxidants to protect cells and tissues from ROS. The mitochondrial enzymes manganese superoxide dismutase (MnSOD) and glutathione peroxidase (GPx) appear to be the most important in controlling myocardial levels of O_2^- and H_2O_2. Approximately 70% of the SOD activity in the heart, and 90% of that in the cardiac myocyte, is attributable to *MnSOD (SOD2)*.[3] The remainder consists of *cytosolic Cu/ZnSOD (SOD1)*, with less than 1% contributed by *extracellular SOD (ECSOD, SOD3)*.[4] This is in contrast to other organs where Cu/ZnSOD plays a greater role. The relative importance of MnSOD in the regulation of oxidative stress in the myocardium is highlighted by the demonstration that mice deficient in MnSOD die soon after birth with dilated cardiomyopathy.[5] In contrast, mice deficient in CuZnSOD or ECSOD have no overt myocardial phenotype.[4] As the only SOD located in the mitochondria, MnSOD plays a critical role in the control of mitochondrial ROS generated during normal oxidative phosphorylation (see later discussion). The phenotype of the MnSOD knockout mouse therefore also underscores the importance of the mitochondria as a source of ROS in the myocardium.

H_2O_2, the product of SOD, is handled by catalase and/or one of several GPxs. *Catalase* is expressed in the cytosol, where it is located primarily in peroxisomes (pCAT) and in the mitochondria (mCAT). Catalase contains four porphyrin heme groups that interact with H_2O_2 to facilitate its decomposition to water and oxygen. Transgenic expression of either pCAT or mCAT exerts beneficial effects on cardiac structure and function in a variety of animal HF models,[6,7] suggesting that H_2O_2 is an important oxidant species in the

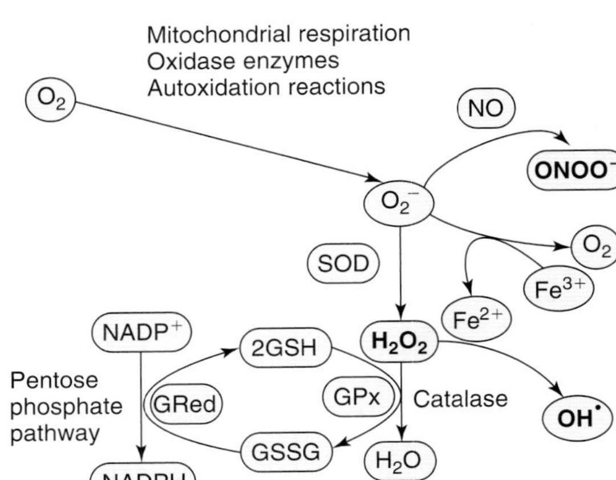

FIGURE 8-1 Reactive oxygen species (ROS) and antioxidant enzyme systems. Enzymatic or nonenzymatic formation of superoxide anion leads to the formation of other ROS *(shown in bold)*. Potentially toxic ROS are removed by the enzymes superoxide dismutase (SOD), glutathione peroxidase (GPx), and catalase. The presence of Fe^{2+} or nitric oxide (NO) can allow the formation of hydroxyl radical ($OH^•$) and peroxynitrite ($ONOO^-$), respectively. These latter reactions are favored when the activity of SOD is decreased. O_2^- can increase the formation of $OH^•$ by reducing Fe^{3+} to Fe^{2+}. Glutathione plays a central role in cellular antioxidant defenses not only as a reducing agent for the action of GPx, but also through direct reactions with ROS. Glutathione is recycled by the enzyme glutathione reductase, which requires NAD(P)H. Thus, indirectly, the pentose phosphate pathway, by supplying NAD(P)H, also plays an important role in antioxidant defenses.

failing heart. Compared with O_2^-, H_2O_2 is longer lasting and able to cross cellular membranes.

Glutathione peroxidases (GPx) are a family of selenium-containing enzymes that catalyze the removal of H_2O_2 through oxidation of reduced glutathione (GSH), which is recycled from oxidized glutathione (GSSG) by the NADPH-dependent glutathione reductase (GRed). GPx-1 is encoded on the nuclear genome but localizes both to the cytosol and mitochondria.

Ancillary Antioxidant Mechanisms

Several enzymes and molecules play a supporting role in regulating oxidative stress and/or the effects of oxidants on targets. The activity of GPx requires stoichiometric quantities of *glutathione* (GSH), and therefore decreased levels of GSH inhibit the activity of GPx. GRed requires NAD(P)H as a reductant to recycle GSSG to GSH. Glutathione is also a direct scavenger of reactive oxygen and nitrogen species. Cells replenish GSH both by de novo GSH synthesis and through the action of glutathione reductase on GSSG. In this context, enzymes in the pentose phosphate pathway and glucose 6-phosphate dehydrogenase (G6PD), the rate-limiting enzyme in this pathway, are ancillary antioxidant enzymes that are critical to cellular antioxidant defenses.[8] In mice chronic GSH depletion causes worse LV function, fibrosis, and survival in response to pressure overload, and GSH supplementation ameliorates the phenotype.[9] Increased oxidative stress lowers the GSH/GSSG ratio, which may thus be used as a measure of myocardial oxidative stress.[10] Unlike the levels of lipid peroxidation products, which can reflect oxidative stress inside and/or outside of the cell, the GSH/GSSG ratio specifically measures intracellular oxidative stress. Other thiol-containing proteins, such as *metallothionein*, have significant antioxidant functions through direct scavenging of ROS, and may play a role in the failing heart.[11] Overexpression of metallothionein suppresses mitochondrial oxidative stress, cardiac apoptosis, and the development of diabetic cardiomyopathy (see also Chapter 16).[12]

Several thiol-containing proteins modulate the effects of ROS. The *thioredoxin (Trx)* system consists of Trx reductase, Trx, peroxiredoxin, and NADPH.[13] This system, like HO-1 and metallothionein, is induced by a variety of oxidative stresses, and Trx levels are increased in the myocardium[14] and blood[15] of patients with HF. Trx exerts an antioxidant effect by scavenging ROS, but also interacts directly with multiple cellular signal transduction pathways, and activates HO-1 and Bcl-2.[16] *Thioredoxin-interacting protein (Txnip)* interacts with Trx via a disulfide bond, decreasing thioredoxin activity and thus increasing oxidative stress.[17]

The *glutaredoxin (Grx)* system is similar in organization and function to the Trx system, but has a much higher selectivity for cysteine thiols that are glutathiolated, and thus may play an important role in the regulation of protein function via glutathionylation.

The *peroxiredoxins* (Prx) are a family of antioxidant enzymes that reduce H_2O_2 and which may also interact with Trx and Grx, from which they accept electrons in order to be active. Although Prxs are abundant, their precise role in the heart remains to be determined.

Heme oxygenase-1 (HO-1) is induced by oxidative stress and serves a cyto-protective function through the breakdown of pro-oxidant heme into equimolar amounts of carbon monoxide, biliverdin/bilirubin, and free ferrous iron. Carbon monoxide and bilirubin exert direct cardioprotective effects via their respective anti-inflammatory and antioxidant actions.[18,19]

Vitamin antioxidants play a role in the control of ROS cascades and the prevention of free radical chain reactions. Vitamin E (α-tocopherol) and vitamin C (ascorbic acid) prevent lipid peroxidation and membrane breakdown. α-Tocopherol is a fat-soluble vitamin that concentrates in cellular membranes. Through the aromatic ring head group, α-tocopherol is able to form a "stable" tocopheryl radical when it reacts with ROS and lipid peroxy radicals. Ascorbic acid reacts with tocopheryl radicals, thereby converting them back to tocopherol. Circulating and tissue levels of α-tocopherol have been used as measures of both antioxidant capacity and oxidative stress.[10]

MARKERS OF OXIDATIVE STRESS IN HUMAN HEART FAILURE

Oxidation products of several organic molecules including lipids, proteins, and nucleic acids have been used to assess oxidative stress in HF (**Table 8-1**). While these methods can individually be criticized for their relative lack of specificity, collectively the data support the conclusion that there is increased systemic and myocardial oxidative stress in patients with HF.

Lipid Oxidation Products

Lipid peroxidation products, such as *malondialdehyde* (MDA)[20] and *4-hydroxy-nonenal*[21] are increased and total thiol levels are decreased in patients with ischemic and nonischemic cardiomyopathy compared with subjects without HF.[22] MDA is an independent predictor of death in patients with chronic HF.[20] *Exhaled pentane,* a volatile lipid peroxidation product, is increased in patients with HF.[23] The *8-isoprostanes* (8-iso-prostaglandin $F_{2\alpha}$) are a family of

TABLE 8-1 Studies of Oxidative Stress Markers in Human Heart Failure

MARKERS	STUDIES	FINDINGS
MDA, Thiols, SOD, GPx	McMurray et al[185]	Increased plasma MDA, decreased plasma thiols in patients with CAD and LV dysfunction
	Belch et al[186]	Increased plasma MDA, decreased plasma thiols in patients with CHF; weak correlation between decreasing thiols and worsening LV function
	McMurray[22]	Increased MDA, decreased plasma thiols in both CAD and non-CAD patients with HF
	Ghatak et al[187]	Increased MDA, and reduced erythrocyte SOD and GPx activities in CHF; weak correlation with LV function; improved by vitamin E administration
	Radovanovic et al[20]	Increased MDA in CHF; MDA predicted death
	Keith et al[188]	Correlated oxidative stress with NYHA clinical class, as well as levels of soluble TNF receptor levels as marker of prognosis
	Maks et al[21]	Plasma unsaturated aldehydes including 4-OH-nonenal were elevated in association with impaired LV contractile function in HF patients
	Polidori et al[189]	Plasma MDA was higher in patients with severe CHF than those with moderate disease
	Campolo et al[190]	Reduced cysteines and MDA were increased in CHF patients
Myeloperoxidase (MPO)	Tang et al[44]	Associated with an increased likelihood of more advanced HF, and predictive of worse long-term clinical outcomes
	Tang et al[46]	MPO predicted development of HF in aging subjects
	Reichlin et al[45]	MPO predicted higher mortality in acute decompensated HF
8-isoprostanes	Mallat et al[26]	Pericardial 8-isoprostanes in patients undergoing open-heart surgery correlated with preoperative NYHA functional class
	Kameda et al[191]	Pericardial 8-isoprostanes correlated with LV end-diastolic volume, and activities of MMP-2 and MMP-9 and gelatinolysis in CAD patients
	Polidori et al[27]	Plasma F2 isoprostanes correlated with antioxidant status and NYHA class
	Nonaka-Sakukawa et al[192]	Urinary 15-Ft-isoprostanes increased in proportion to the severity of CHF, and correlated with plasma BNP and serum IL-6
Paraoxonase-1 (PON-1)	Kim et al[49]	PON-1 activity was reduced in HF
	Tang et al[50]	Indirect measure of PON-1 activity independently predicted high risk of cardiac events in systolic HF
Glutathione *S*-transferase	Andrukhova et al[47]	Serum levels of glutathione *S*-transferase are associated with EF and NYHA class
Breath pentane	Sobotka et al[23]	Increased exhaled pentane in CHF compared with controls; pentane levels reduced by captopril therapy
Pentosidine	Koyama et al[30]	Serum pentosidine was an independent risk factor for cardiac events in patients with HF
Plasma carbonyls	Amir et al[31]	Serum oxidative stress levels increased with NYHA functional class and were associated with higher CRP and BNP
	Radovanovic et al[20]	Increased plasma carbonyls in CHF; carbonyls correlated with echocardiographic remodeling indices
8-hydroxy-2′-deoxyguanosine	Watanabe et al[35]	Correlated with NYHA functional class, left atrial diameter, LV end-diastolic diameters, LV end-systolic diameters, and plasma BNP
	Kono et al[34]	Increased in both the serum and myocardium of patients with HF; reduced with carvedilol therapy
	Pignatelli et al[193]	Serum levels increased in CHF progressively from class I-II to class III-IV; correlated with TNF-α and sCD40L
	Kobayashi et al[36]	Urinary levels correlated with symptoms and functional severity of HF
	Nagayoshi et al[194]	Higher levels in CAD vs. non-CAD HF patients despite same NYHA class
Uric acid	Cicoira et al[195]	Elevated serum uric acid levels correlated with parameters of diastolic dysfunction in HF
	Anker et al[196]	Uric acid predicted mortality in patients with moderate to severe CHF
	Kojima et al[197]	Correlated with Killip's classification and mortality in patients with acute MI
	Sakai et al[37]	Positive transcardiac gradient increased with the severity of HF, and inversely correlated with LVEF
	Kittleson et al[38]	High uric acid was associated with increased cardiac filling pressure and reduced cardiac index; correlated with NT-proBNP
	Ioachimescu et al[198]	An independent predictor of death in patients at high risk of cardiovascular disease
	Manzano et al[39]	Independent predictor of mortality in the SENIORS trial patients with systolic and diastolic HF
	Bishu et al[40]	Elevated levels in acute decompensated HF
Oxidized LDLs	Charach et al[28]	Plasma levels predicted mortality and morbidity in HF patients
PLTP	Chen et al[51]	Higher levels associated with LV systolic function
Biopyrrins	Hokamaki et al[43]	Urinary biopyrrin levels were elevated, and correlated with blood BNP and severity of HF

prostaglandin $F_{2\alpha}$ isomers formed by the peroxidation of arachidonic acid through a noncyclooxygenase-mediated reaction catalyzed by free radicals.[24] In contrast to reactive aldehydes, lipid hydroperoxides, and conjugated dienes, 8-isoprostanes are stabler products of lipid peroxidation and thus may be a more useful indicator of oxidative stress.[25] 8-isoprostanes measured in the pericardial fluid of patients with HF undergoing open heart surgery correlated with increasing New York Heart Association (NYHA) functional class.[26] Plasma and urinary isoprostanes correlate with the clinical severity of HF, antioxidant status, and blood BNP.[27] *Plasma oxidized LDL* (oxLDL), a marker of oxidative stress, is elevated in HF patients and predicts mortality and morbidity independent of conventional factors.[28,29]

Glycoprotein and DNA Products

Oxidation products of glycoproteins and nuclear DNA are increased in patients with HF. Serum *pentosidine*, an advanced glycation end product, is an independent risk factor for cardiac events in patients with HF.[30] Plasma *carbonyls* are increased in patients with more symptomatic HF, and associated with higher CRP and BNP,[31] as well as progressive LV remodeling.[20] *8-hydroxy-2-deoxyguanosine (8-OHdG),* formed when DNA is oxidatively damaged, is increased in myocardium of animals with cardiac hypertrophy[32] and tachycardia-induced cardiomyopathy,[33] and in both the serum and myocardium of patients with HF.[34] Plasma levels of 8-OHdG correlate with NYHA functional class, cardiac function, and several other biomarkers such as plasma BNP, TNF-α, and sCD40L.[35] Urinary 8-OHdG levels correlate with symptoms and functional severity of HF.[36]

Other Oxidative Stress Markers

Uric acid, produced by the ubiquitous ROS-generating xanthine oxidase, is released from the failing human heart in inverse relation to LV ejection fraction.[37] Increased serum uric acid levels are associated with worse hemodynamic function and correlate with plasma NT-proBNP in patients with HF.[38] Uric acid was an independent predictor of mortality in the SENIORS trial, which included patients with both systolic and diastolic HF.[39] Uric acid is elevated in patients presenting with acute decompensated HF.[40] Uric acid is prognostic when due to impaired renal elimination.[41] Small trials of xanthine oxidase inhibitors have shown promise in improving cardiac performance and outcomes in patients with HF.[42]

Biopyrrins are oxidized metabolites of bilirubin, which are increased in HF, probably secondary to hepatic dysfunction and/or increased HO-1 activity. Urinary biopyrrin levels are elevated and correlate with blood BNP and the severity of HF.[43]

Myeloperoxidase (MPO), a peroxidase enzyme abundant in granulocytes, is increased in the circulating blood of patients with HF and is an independent predictor of death, heart transplantation, or HF hospitalization.[44] Among patients with acutely decompensated HF, elevated MPO concentrations are associated with a higher 1-year mortality, even when adjusted for BNP levels.[45] MPO predicts the risk of developing HF in aging individuals.[46]

Glutathione S-transferase P1 participates in the detoxification of ROS and maintenance of the cellular redox state, and is elevated in patients with HF in proportion to systolic dysfunction and functional class.[47]

Paraoxonase-1 (PON-1) is a high-density lipoprotein (HDL)-associated glycoprotein that contributes to the systemic antioxidant activities of HDL.[48] PON-1 is decreased in HF patients[49]; decreased serum arylesterase activity, a measure of diminished antioxidant properties of PON-1, predicts higher risk of long-term adverse cardiac events in patients with systolic HF.[50]

Phospholipid transfer protein (PLTP) modulates lipoprotein metabolism and plays a role in inflammation and oxidative stress. A higher PLTP activity is associated with depressed LV systolic function.[51]

MECHANISMS OF INCREASED OXIDATIVE STRESS IN HEART FAILURE (Figure 8-2)

Increased oxidative stress may occur as a result of the increased generation of ROS, decreased clearance of ROS by various antioxidant systems, or both. Both mitochondria and several enzyme systems that generate O_2^- may produce pathophysiologic amounts of O_2^- in the failing heart.

Oxidases

The *NAD(P)H oxidase (NOX)* family consists of at least five transmembrane enzymes that mediate electron transfer from NAD(P)H to molecular oxygen to generate O_2^-. The NOX-2 isoform was first described in the neutrophil, where it is responsible for the oxidative burst, which produces large amounts of cytotoxic ROS. Other isoforms produce lower levels of ROS that can act as signaling intermediates.[52,53] NOX-2 and NOX-4 are the predominant isoforms in cardiac myocytes, and both have been implicated in mediating hypertrophy.[54,55] NOX-2 is located in the plasma membrane, whereas the localization of NOX-4 is less certain but appears to include the endoplasmic reticulum (ER) and/or mitochondrial membranes. NOX-2 mediates LV hypertrophy and failure in response to activation of the renin-angiotensin system,[53] but not in response to pressure overload.[56] NOX-4 also appears to contribute to oxidative stress and to be involved in mediating cardiac hypertrophy and failure in response to hemodynamic stress, though the data are conflicting.[57,58]

Xanthine oxidoreductase consists of two interconvertible forms, xanthine dehydrogenase and xanthine oxidase, both of which are involved in the conversion of hypoxanthine and xanthine to uric acid. The constitutive xanthine dehydrogenase uses NAD^+ primarily as an electron acceptor, whereas the inducible xanthine oxidase transfers electrons to molecular oxygen, yielding ROS. In addition, xanthine oxidoreductase can generate O_2^- via NADH oxidase activity and produce NO via nitrate and nitrite reductase activities.[59] Thus activation of xanthine oxidoreductase may cause both oxidative and nitrosative stress. The expression of xanthine oxidase is increased in the hearts of rats with HF[60,61] and patients with dilated cardiomyopathy.[62] In animal models of HF, xanthine oxidase inhibitors (e.g., allopurinol, oxypurinol, febuxostat) attenuate the production of ROS, improve cardiac function, decrease LV size, improve β-adrenergic receptor sensitivity, improve myocardial energetic coupling,[63,64] inhibit fetal gene expression, and improve Ca^{2+} handling.[65] In patients with HF, allopurinol reduced plasma MDA, improved endothelium-dependent flow-mediated response,[66,67] reduced myocardial oxygen consumption, and improved myocardial efficiency.[62] In acute and short-term

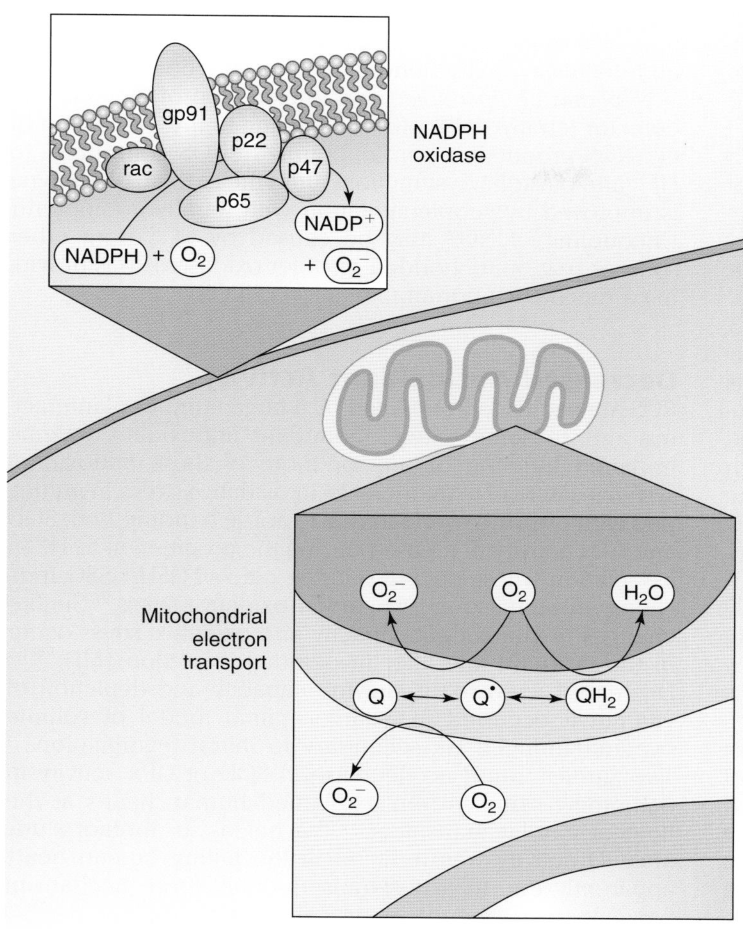

FIGURE 8-2 NAD(P)H oxidases and mitochondria as sources of ROS in the heart. An NAD(P)H oxidase is expressed in cardiac myocytes similar to that found in neutrophils and vascular cells. The oxidase is composed of at least five subunits, with two membrane proteins that comprise the oxidase activity and three cytoplasmic proteins that serve regulatory functions. The complex catalyzes the one-electron reduction of O_2 to O_2^- with NADPH or NADH as a reducing cofactor. The mitochondrial electron transport chain creates a proton-motive force through the transfer of electrons from NADH dehydrogenase (complex I) and succinate dehydrogenase (complex II) to ubiquinone (Q), thereby forming reduced ubiquinone (QH_2). Partially reduced ubiquinone (Q·) is a radical that can reduce O_2 to O_2^-. This oxygen "leakage" is a potentially large source of ROS, and has been implicated in the increased oxidative stress in HF (see text).

human studies, oxypurinol increased LV ejection fraction and reduced LV end-diastolic volume.[68] In a chronic study of patients with systolic HF, a xanthine oxidase inhibitor did not improve the primary composite endpoint (mortality, HF morbidity, or quality of life), but a subgroup analysis suggested that clinical improvement occurred in patients with elevated uric acid and correlated with the treatment-related decrease in uric acid.[69] In rats with pressure overload, the magnitude of improvement in cardiac function with oxypurinol is related to the initial level of xanthine oxidase activity.[70]

Mitochondria

Mitochondria are an important source of myocardial ROS in the failing heart.[71] Under normal circumstances, a small fraction of the electrons entering the electron transport chain "leak" to molecular oxygen forming O_2^-. Under pathologic conditions, the leakage may increase, overwhelming the capacity of the mitochondrial antioxidant system. In dogs with rapid pacing-induced HF, electron paramagnetic resonance (EPR) spectroscopy showed a 2.8-fold increase in the rate of O_2^- formation in a mitochondrial fraction of the heart, thus providing direct evidence for increased mitochondrial ROS generation.[72] There was an approximate 50% decrease in the activity of electron transport complex I, suggesting that increased ROS was due to uncoupling of ETC at complex I. Increased mitochondrial H_2O_2 production was directly demonstrated in mitochondria isolated from *db/db* mice, a model of obesity and type 2 diabetes with a characteristic cardiomyopathy. Increased ROS production was associated with ETC uncoupling, and appeared to be derived from complex I and other complexes.[73]

Indirect support for mitochondrial ROS production comes from studies in transgenic mice that overexpress MnSOD or mCAT in mitochondria. In mice with type 1 diabetes, cross-breeding with MnSOD transgenic mice improved mitochondrial respiration and mass, and ameliorated abnormalities in cardiac structure and function.[74] Likewise, transgenic expression of mCAT improved several aspects of cardiac structure and function in mice with pathologic cardiac remodeling and/or HF due to pressure overload (aortic constriction), systolic failure due to overexpression of Gαq or angiotensin infusion,[6] and ameliorated cardiac aging.[75] Although these studies show that ROS have important adverse effects in the mitochondria, they do not establish the source of the ROS. ROS from nonmitochondrial sources may cause mitochondrial dysfunction and may include ETC electron leakage, leading to further ROS generation (i.e., ROS-mediated ROS release).[76] Further indirect support for mitochondrial ROS is the increase in oxidation products in the mitochondria and damage to mitochondrial DNA.[77] Transgenic overexpression of mitochondrial transcription factor A (TFAM) to increase mitochondrial DNA copy number[78] ameliorates these abnormalities.

Nitric Oxide Synthase

Nitric oxide (NO) is a free radical that can modify the myocardial response to oxidative stress both directly and indirectly. NO is synthesized in the conversion of L-arginine to L-citrulline by a family of nitric oxide synthases (NOS). NO, a free radical gas, is buffered in the cell by reactions with glutathione, and reacts reversibly with sulfhydryl groups of proteins forming *S*-nitrosothiols that can alter protein function.[79] Through chemical reactions with ROS, NO can either *decrease* or *increase* the oxidative stress in a cell or tissue. Under normal circumstances, myocardial NO is produced at low levels by *endothelial NOS (eNOS or NOS3)*. NOS3, which is present in virtually all cell types in the myocardium, including myocytes, fibroblasts, and endothelial cells, is regulated by a calcium-sensitive interaction with calmodulin.[80] *Inducible nitric oxide synthase (NOS2)* is not regulated by Ca^{2+}, and when induced is capable of producing high levels of NO. Though NOS2 is expressed minimally in the normal myocardium, it is induced by exposure to cytokines, hypoxia, and other stimuli in both myocytes and nonmyocytes, leading to a marked increase in the production of NO.[81] NOS2 can catalyze the formation of O_2^-,[82] particularly in the setting of arginine depletion, and may contribute directly to the formation of ROS.[83] The expression and activity of NOS2 are increased in the myocardium of patients with idiopathic and ischemic dilated cardiomyopathies.[84]

Low levels of NO, as are formed by NOS3, may decrease the level of oxidative stress by decreasing the production of O_2^- through inhibition of oxidative enzymes.[85] Through the activation of guanylate cyclase, NO can inhibit signaling and transcription factors that modify myocyte hypertrophic and apoptotic signaling.[86] Mice lacking NOS3 have worse ventricular function late after MI,[87] consistent with the notion that NOS3-derived NO is beneficial for the failing heart. Higher levels of NO increase oxidative stress by reacting with O_2^- to generate *peroxynitrite ($ONOO^-$)*, a free radical that is toxic and longer lived than either NO or O_2^-.[88] $ONOO^-$ can react with many cell constituents, including tyrosine residues of susceptible proteins such as MnSOD, causing irreversible inactivation.[89] Based on the relative rate constants for the reaction of O_2^- with superoxide dismutase (SOD) versus NO, the formation of $ONOO^-$ is favored when the levels of O_2^- and/or NO are high, or the level of SOD is low.

High concentrations of NO can have direct toxic effects on cardiac myocytes in vitro. The cytotoxic effect of cytokines on cardiac myocytes in culture is inhibited by the NOS inhibitor L-NMMA.[90] Cytokine-induced apoptosis can be prevented by either an inhibitor of NOS2 or an SOD-mimetic, thus implicating $ONOO^-$. In mice late post-MI NOS2 expression is increased in the remote myocardium and NOS2 knockout mice have less myocyte apoptosis, improved contractile function, and increased survival.[91] Likewise, in animal models of autoimmune and viral myocarditis, the amount of myocardial injury was reduced by aminoguanidine, an inhibitor of NOS2.[92] Treatment with aminoguanidine also decreased the amount of O_2^- anion formed, suggesting the presence of NOS2-dependent O_2^- production or the inactivation of MnSOD by $ONOO^-$.[93] The divergent effects of NO were revealed when mice with viral myocarditis were treated with L-NAME. A low dose improved survival, HF, and myocardial necrosis, whereas the highest dose worsened survival.[94] Similarly, stretch-induced myocyte apoptosis is inhibited by an NO donor.[95] Potential mechanisms for a protective effect of low NO levels include inhibition of enzymes in the programmed cell death pathway[86] and decreased mitochondrial ROS production.[85]

NOS can be *uncoupled* due to oxidation of the essential cofactor tetrahydrobiopterin,[96] leading to the generation of O_2^-. ROS production from uncoupled eNOS contributes to HF[97] and diastolic dysfunction,[98] and the cardiac phenotype is improved by supplementation with tetrahydrobiopterin. Uncoupling of NOS may be caused by ROS from other sources (e.g., mitochondria or other oxidases), thus providing a mechanism for amplification of ROS.

Decreased Antioxidant Activity

ROS are exquisitely regulated by a large number of interacting and, to some extent, redundant antioxidant systems. Impaired function of one or more of these antioxidant systems can lead to an increase in oxidative stress. In guinea pigs with pressure overload due to aortic banding, both SOD and GPx activity decreased during the progression to HF in association with a decrease in the ratio of GSH/GSSG, indicating an increase in myocardial oxidative stress.[99] Similar changes in antioxidant capacity and oxidative stress occur in the rat heart late after myocardial infarction (MI).[100,101] Decreased antioxidant enzyme capacity and depletion of vitamin E occurred in a large animal model of volume overload-induced HF secondary to mitral regurgitation.[102] Two studies found no decrease in SOD or GPx activity in pathologic samples from explanted human hearts at the time of cardiac transplant[103,104]; whereas in another study, MnSOD activity was reduced in the failing human heart, apparently due to a post-transcriptional level mechanism because mRNA expression was not decreased.[105]

Nonenzymatic Auto-Oxidation

Reactions involving several organic molecules may contribute to the formation of ROS in vivo. Oxidation of norepinephrine and epinephrine to *adrenochrome* and O_2^- has been proposed as a mechanism for myocardial injury in the presence of chronic adrenergic stimulation.[106] Thiol compounds, including cysteine and GSH, can auto-oxidize to form O_2^-, particularly in the presence of transition metals such as iron. The cardiotoxicity of *iron* overload is likely a combination of this plus Fenton chemistry to generate hydroxyl radicals. *Myoglobin* can autoxidize from oxymyoglobin to metmyoglobin with the release of O_2^-.[107]

OXIDATIVE STRESS AND ANTIOXIDANT THERAPY IN ANIMAL MODELS OF HEART FAILURE

Work in animal models has allowed greater insight regarding the sources and consequences of oxidative stress in HF. Studies have been performed in a variety of models of HF and with a range of antioxidant strategies.

Hemodynamic Overload

The aortic constriction model of HF occurs in two phases. In the initial days after constriction there is LV hypertrophy, whereas over the ensuing weeks there is progressive chamber dilation, wall thinning, and systolic failure. Several types of antioxidant intervention have been shown to ameliorate one or both phases of this model.

NOX Transgenic Mice

The NOX-2 and NOX-4 isoforms of NAD(P)H oxidase are predominant in cardiac myocytes.[108] In mice, NOX-2 knockout prevented cardiac hypertrophy and fibrosis caused by chronic sub-pressor infusion of angiotensin,[71,134] suggesting a role in the response to neurohormones. However, NOX-2 knockout did not inhibit the hypertrophic response to pressure overload with aortic constriction.[56,109] NOX-4 appears to modulate the hypertrophic response to pressure overload, although the exact role remains unclear. In one study, NOX-4 knockout mice did better after aortic constriction, and NOX-4 transgenic mice did worse.[57] NOX-4 overexpression was associated with increased mitochondrial ROS and worse mitochondrial function.[57] However, another group using a similar aortic constriction model found that NOX-4 knockout mice developed worse LV failure with aortic constriction, whereas NOX-4 overexpressing animals were protected.[58] These experiments illustrate the complexity of redox systems, which on the one hand can mediate pathophysiologic processes and on the other are essential to normal cellular and defense mechanisms. For example, knockout of both NOX-2 and NOX-4 exacerbated ischemia-reperfusion injury in the heart, suggesting that low-level ROS production by the NOX system is required for activation of protective mechanisms.[110]

NOS3 Knockout and Tetrahydrobiopterin

Aortic constriction causes less LV hypertrophy and fibrosis in NOS3 knockout mice, suggesting that uncoupled NOS3 contributes to myocardial oxidative stress.[111] Likewise, treatment with oral tetrahydrobiopterin (BH4), a cofactor necessary for NOS coupling, re-coupled NOS3, decreased oxidative stress, and decreased both LV hypertrophy and fibrosis.[112]

Thioredoxin and *N*-2-mercaptopropionyl Glycine

N-2-mercaptopropionyl glycine (MPG) is a low-molecular-weight antioxidant analogue of glutathione, which scavenges H_2O_2. Administration of MPG to mice decreased markers of myocardial oxidative stress and myocardial hypertrophy 7 days after aortic constriction.[113] In transgenic mice, cardiac-specific overexpression of a dominant-negative Trx-1 worsened and overexpression of wild-type Trx-1 ameliorated the response to aortic constriction.[32] Consistent with a protective effect of Trx-1, cardiomyocyte-specific knockout of Txnip, which inhibits Trx, protected from early, but not late, pressure overload-induced cardiac dysfunction.[114]

Vitamins E and C, and Resveratrol

In guinea pigs subjected to aortic banding, vitamin E (α-tocopherol) had no effect on LV hypertrophy early after banding, but at late time points prevented the transition to HF.[115] In the same model, vitamin C (ascorbic acid) administration to guinea pigs with aortic banding inhibited LVH.[116] Resveratrol, a naturally occurring polyphenol antioxidant present in grapes, decreased LV hypertrophy and improved diastolic relaxation early after aortic constriction in the rat model.[117]

Mitochondrial Antioxidants

Transgenic overexpression of mCAT[118] or administration of an antioxidant peptide targeted to mitochondria[119] exerts broad beneficial effects in mice with aortic constriction, resulting in less LV hypertrophy and progression to failure. The effects of mCAT were associated with correction of the mitochondrial proteome.[119] Euk-8 is a potent SOD-mimetic, catalase-mimetic, and free radical scavenger.[120] In mice with aortic constriction, Euk-8 decreased LV hypertrophy and progression to failure, and improved survival.[121]

Gαq-Transgenic Mice

The G protein Gαq mediates many of the effects of neurohormones and mechanical strain in cardiac myocytes, and its overexpression in mice leads to pathologic myocardial remodeling that progresses to a severe dilated cardiomyopathy.[122] Myocyte-specific overexpression of catalase that is expressed primarily in the peroxisomes (pCAT) had no effect on the early phenotype of LV dilation and contractile dysfunction at the time of weaning, but prevented the subsequent progression to HF.[7] A key mechanism for improvement in contractile function appeared to be prevention of oxidative post-translational modifications of SERCA at cysteine 674.[123] In another study, overexpression of catalase targeted to the mitochondria (mCAT) prevented progressive adverse remodeling and failure.[6] In the same study, mCAT also alleviated adverse remodeling in response to chronic angiotensin infusion,[6] and the effects in both models were mimicked by an orally administered antioxidant peptide targeted to the mitochondria,[124] thus highlighting the importance of mitochondrial ROS and demonstrating the potential therapeutic utility of this approach.[125]

Anthracyclines

The anthracyclines used in chemotherapy are well known to generate intracellular ROS[126] and induce both myocyte apoptosis and necrosis in a dose-dependent manner.[127] Both NOX-2 and mitochondria-derived ROS have been implicated as potential mediators of these effects.[128,129] The apoptosis, but not necrosis, could be inhibited by the addition of the iron chelator dexrazoxane, which is used clinically in the prevention of anthracycline cardiotoxicity.[130] These results implicate hydroxyl radicals formed via the Fenton reaction in anthracycline-induced apoptosis. Mice treated with doxorubicin exhibit acute cardiac toxicity at 4 days, which is ameliorated in mice with transgenic 60-fold overexpression of pCAT in cardiac myocytes,[131] as is chronic toxicity due to long-term administration of doxorubicin for 10 weeks.[132] Both acute and chronic doxorubicin cardiac toxicity were improved by transgenic overexpression of metallothionein.[133,134] Like metallothionein, Trx exerts a cardioprotective effect in Adriamycin-induced cardiomyopathy.[13]

Diastolic Dysfunction (see also Chapters 10 and 36)

HF with preserved ejection fraction due to diastolic dysfunction is a major cause of HF in *metabolic heart disease (MHD)* and aging. MHD is associated with increased oxidant stress. For example, in diabetic *(db/db)* mice, a model of type 2 diabetes, there are increased levels of MDA and 4-hydroxynonenol (4HNE) in the myocardium, and increased H_2O_2 production by cardiac mitochondria.[73] Mice fed a diet high in fat and sucrose develop obesity, type 2 diabetes, and metabolic syndrome characterized by increased oxidative stress markers (e.g., HNE) in the heart in association with LV fibrosis, hypertrophy, and diastolic dysfunction.[135] In these mice treatment with *resveratrol*, a polyphenol with antioxidant properties, normalized the markers of oxidative stress and improved the cardiac structure and function.[135] Likewise, transgenic overexpression of *HO-1* ameliorated LV dysfunction, myofibril disarray, oxidative stress, inflammation, apoptosis, and autophagy in mice with diabetic cardiomyopathy.[136] *Vitamin E* supplement also improved LV function and decreased myocardial 8-isoprostanes and oxidized glutathione accumulation in rodents with diabetic cardiomyopathy.[137] In *aging mice* transgenic overexpression of either pCAT[138] or mCAT[75] lessened LV hypertrophy and improved LV diastolic function. In addition, pCAT decreased the oxidation of SERCA[138] and mCAT decreased mitochondrial DNA mutations and improved mitochondrial biogenesis.[118] These studies emphasize the central role of oxidative stress in the aging heart.

Other Experimental Models

LV dilation and failure *late post-MI* are related to chronic hemodynamic overload. Although less studied than the aortic constriction model, late post-MI remodeling and failure appear to be ameliorated by antioxidants. The ROS scavenger DMTU prevented both pump dysfunction and chamber dilation in mice post-MI.[144] Probucol decreased the levels of myocardial oxidative stress, preserved myocardial systolic function, and improved animal survival.[143] In rabbits with *pacing-induced* cardiomyopathy, antioxidant vitamins decreased tissue oxidative stress and attenuated cardiac dysfunction.[33]

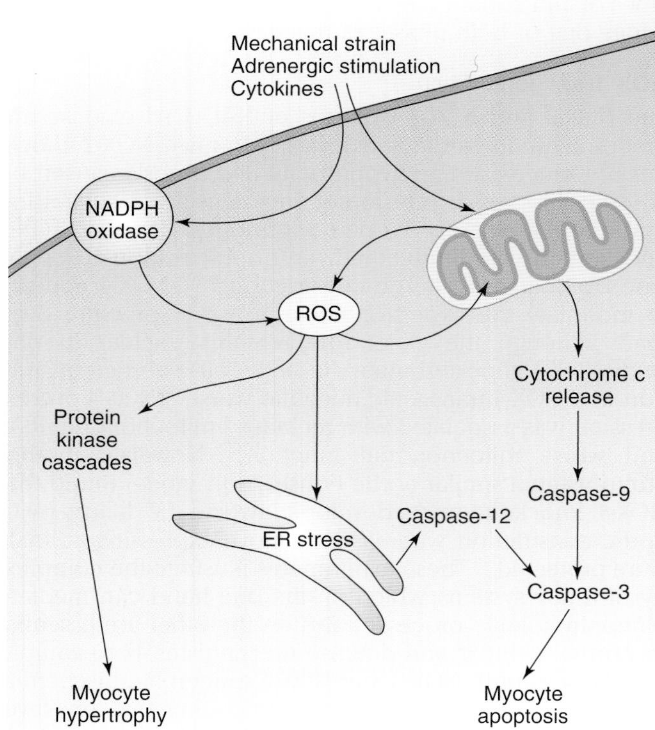

FIGURE 8-3 Schematic presentation of the effects of ROS on myocyte hypertrophy and apoptosis. Through activation of kinase cascades such as MAPK, ROS can induce myocyte hypertrophy. Mitochondrial ROS may be particularly prone to induce apoptosis by stimulating the mitochondrial release of cytochrome c, which is necessary for the activation of caspase cascades. When the ER is overwhelmed by the stress, caspase-12 is released and activates caspase-3 and the final programmed cell death pathway.

MECHANISMS OF ROS-MEDIATED LEFT VENTRICULAR REMODELING AND HEART FAILURE (Figure 8-3)

Left Ventricular Remodeling (see also Chapter 11)

Several mechanisms contribute to myocardial remodeling, including myocyte hypertrophy, myocyte slippage, myocyte apoptosis, and/or alterations in the turnover and properties of the extracellular matrix (**see also Chapter 4**). The stimuli for remodeling include increased wall stress, inflammatory cytokines, and neurohormones, such as catecholamines and angiotensin II. In vitro and in vivo studies have shown that ROS mediate many of the effects of remodeling stimuli, thereby playing an important role in pathologic remodeling.

Myocyte Hypertrophy

A number of stimuli implicated in mediating cardiac remodeling exert pro-hypertrophic actions in ROS-dependent manner.[52] In cardiac myocytes, in vitro partial inhibition of CuZnSOD[139] and exposure to low concentration of exogenous H_2O_2[140] caused myocyte hypertrophy that was inhibited by antioxidants. Likewise, low-amplitude mechanical strain of cardiac myocytes caused amplitude-dependent ROS formation and myocyte hypertrophy, and the hypertrophic effect was inhibited by an SOD-mimetic.[141] Similarly, myocyte hypertrophy stimulated by angiotensin II or TNF-α is mediated by ROS.[142] Myocyte production of angiotensin II and TNF-α has been implicated in the response to mechanical strain.[143] α-Adrenergic receptor stimulation also induces myocyte ROS formation and stimulates myocyte hypertrophy through ROS-dependent pathways.[54] The ROS-mediated hypertrophic effects of these stimuli act via Gαq, NAD(P)H oxidases, and activation of the ras/raf/MEK/ERK signaling cascade (see later discussion), including endothelin, α_1-adrenergic agonists, and mechanical strain.[54,144,145]

Myocyte Death

ROS-mediated *apoptosis and programmed necrosis* contribute to the myocardial failure.[146] In contrast to the growth effects of low levels of ROS generated by specific oxidases and acting via specific signaling systems, ROS-mediated myocyte cell death generally involves higher levels of ROS. For example, whereas partial inhibition of SOD causes myocyte hypertrophy, more complete inhibition causes apoptosis.[139] Low concentrations of exogenous H_2O_2 cause hypertrophy, whereas higher concentrations cause apoptosis.[140,147] In papillary muscle, mechanical strain induces ROS formation and myocyte apoptosis.[95] In cardiac myocytes, in vitro low-amplitude mechanical strain causes myocyte hypertrophy, whereas high-amplitude strain causes apoptosis that is inhibited by SOD-mimetic.[141] As discussed later, myocyte apoptosis may involve regulation of mitochondrial death pathways by the Bcl-2 family proteins. *Programmed necrosis*, which involves similar stimuli as apoptosis, albeit acting via distinct signaling pathways, has also been described in cardiomyocytes.[148]

Interstitial Fibrosis

As discussed in Chapter 4, one mechanism for ventricular chamber dilation is via alterations in the interstitial matrix of the myocardium. Individual ventricular myocytes are mechanically coupled to other cells via interstitial matrix proteins that connect to the sarcomere via integrins and intermediate filaments. Like intracellular proteins, there is a regular turnover of interstitial matrix proteins that is regulated by proteases and the protein synthetic machinery of the cardiac cells. Collagen is the major component of the interstitium that contributes to the structural integrity of the myocardium. Myocardial collagen content is regulated by the balance between synthesis and degradation, the latter primarily due to the action of matrix *metalloproteinases (MMPs)*.[149]

Both cardiac fibroblast collagen synthesis and MMP activity are regulated in part by oxidative stress.[150] Cardiac fibroblasts in primary culture respond to both intracellular and extracellular oxidative stress with decreases in procollagen mRNA expression and collagen synthesis. Moreover, oxidative stress increases fibroblast MMP activity. It is possible that such actions would result in myocyte slippage and chamber dilation, as well as impaired cell-cell mechanical coupling, and thereby contribute to abnormalities in both systolic and diastolic function. Early post-MI, there is increased expression and activity of MMPs, and treatment with an antioxidant (DMTU) reduced the extent of ventricular dilation and suppressed MMP activity.[151]

NOX2 knockout mice have less cardiac fibrosis in response to a variety of stimuli, including angiotensin or aldosterone infusion, pressure overload, or ischemia/infarction.[152,153] In these models NOX2 appears instrumental in activating MMP-2 and MMP-9, the latter via NOX2-dependent CaMKII oxidation. Enhanced expression of extracellular MMP inducer (EMMPRIN), which would lead to MMP-2 activation, has also been demonstrated in response to β-adrenergic stimulation via H_2O_2-dependent activation of JNK.[154]

Molecular and Cellular Mechanisms of ROS-Induced Heart Failure (see also Chapters 1 and 2)

Although ROS have long been known to disrupt cellular function and/or viability via damage to proteins and lipids, and other molecules, it is now recognized that ROS can regulate physiologic protein function by means of *oxidative post-translational modifications (OPTM)*[155] (**Figure 8-4**). Under normal conditions, low physiologic levels of ROS regulate homeostatic functions. However, elevated levels of ROS that are present in the hypertrophied or failing heart have the ability to cause exaggerated signaling that promotes detrimental effects such as hypertrophy, apoptosis, and impaired calcium regulation. The consequences of OPTM likely relate to the specific amino acids modified and the type of modification. For example, a reversible glutathiolation of C674 of SERCA causes activation in response to low levels of ROS, whereas irreversible sulfonylation causes inactivation in response to higher levels of ROS.[156]

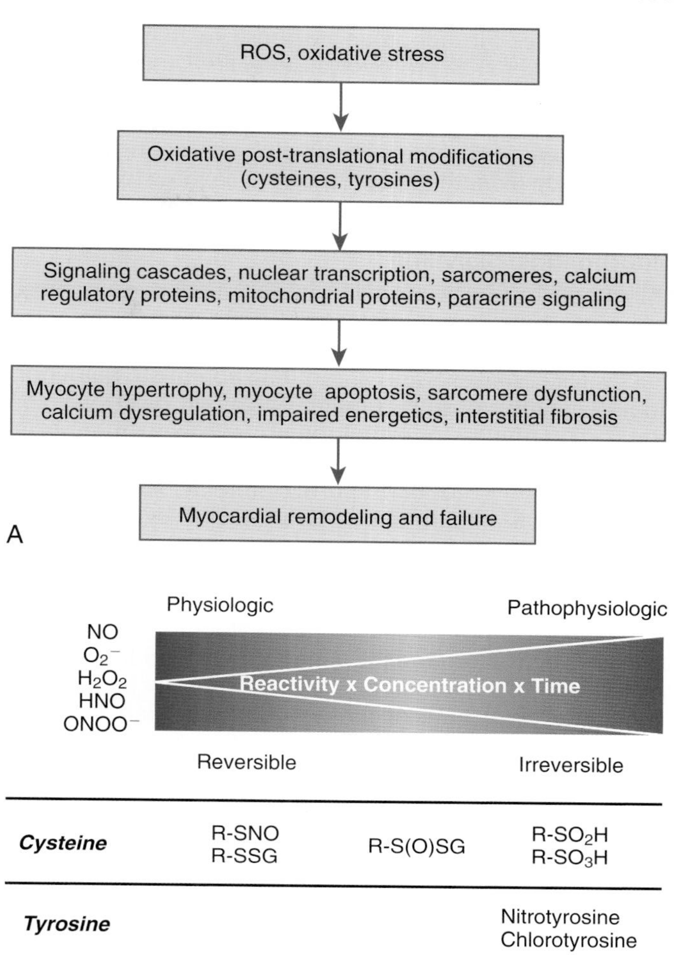

FIGURE 8-4 Oxidative stress in the pathophysiology of heart failure. **A,** Oxidative post-translational modifications (OPTM) of proteins play a central role in transducing the effects of ROS in the myocardium. Increased ROS and oxidative stress lead to OPTM of reactive protein amino acids on key proteins involved in all aspects of cellular function, including intracellular signaling, sarcomere function, calcium regulation, mitochondrial energetics, and paracrine signaling to neighboring cells such as fibroblasts and endothelial cells. **B,** Oxidative post-translational modifications (OPTM) exert a range of effects on protein function from physiologic to pathologic, depending on the target amino acid (e.g., cysteine, tyrosine) and the type (e.g., H_2O_2, $ONOO^-$), intensity (local concentration), and duration of oxidant exposure. In general, oxidant conditions of low intensity that occur under physiologic conditions cause reversible OPTM, such as glutathiolation (R-SSG) of a cysteine thiol. More intense oxidant levels that result from pathologic stimuli lead to irreversible OPTM, such as sulfonylation ($R\text{-}SO_3$) of a cysteine thiol. Reversible OPTM can be modulated by enzyme systems, such as thioredoxin and glutaredoxin, that reduce the OPTM, thereby reversing the effect and restoring normal homeostasis. In contrast, irreversible OPTM typically lead to a permanent decrease (or change) in protein function, are not subject to modulation, and may lead to degradation of the protein, resulting in a further loss of function. The continuous and dynamic nature of oxidant conditions, together with the ability for oxidants to be localized in their actions, allows for a broad spectrum of cellular effects that range from homeostatic to adaptive to maladaptive. Because ROS and protein OPTM are part of normal cellular homeostasis, treatment strategies that cause a global inhibition of ROS may have undesired effects.

Mitogen-Activated Protein Kinases

Many actions of ROS involve activation of one or more stress-responsive protein kinases in the mitogen-activated protein kinase (MAPK) superfamily, which include the *extracellular signal-regulated kinases (ERK)*, the *p38-kinases*, and the *c-Jun N-terminal kinases (JNKs)* that mediate both translational and transcriptional events.[157] The effects of ROS on MAPK signaling appear to be concentration-dependent. Low levels of ROS activate ERK, leading to hypertrophic signaling, whereas higher levels activate the stress-kinases p38 and JNK that are coupled to apoptosis.[140] This pathway can be activated by hypertrophic stimuli such as α-adrenergic receptor stimulation[145] and mechanical strain,[141] leading to oxidation of specific cysteine thiols in Ras and subsequent downstream signaling via the Raf/MEK/ERK. Inhibition of

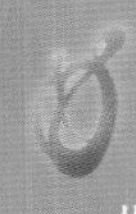

ERK increases the apoptotic response to ROS, suggesting that ERK exerts a pro-survival effect.[147] Apoptosis may involve activation of JNK via ROS-mediated activation of apoptosis signal-regulating kinase 1 (ASK-1).[158-160] ROS-mediated apoptosis may also involve activation of CaMKII via oxidation of methionine residues,[161] leading to apoptosis via p38 kinase.[162]

Mitochondrial Signaling

Mitochondria can be involved in ROS-mediated apoptosis in the heart through the release of cytochrome c from the intermembrane space (see also Chapter 2). Cytochrome c activates caspases 9 and 3, and may potentiate mitochondrial generation of ROS through effects on electron transport.[163] The process of cytochrome c release is modulated by the Bcl-2 family of proteins.[164] Pro-apoptotic members of the Bcl-2 family (Bax, Bad, and Bak) interact with the outer mitochondrial membrane and allow for cytochrome c release and dissipation of the membrane potential through what has been termed the *mitochondrial permeability pore transition*. Antiapoptotic members of the family (e.g., Bcl-2 and Bcl-xL) inhibit Bax-mediated cytochrome c release, caspase-3 activation, and the generation of ROS. In myocytes treated with direct addition of ROS, p53 activity increases in association with translocation of Bax and Bad from the cytosol to the mitochondrial fraction, leading to release of cytochrome c.[165] In contrast, extracellular ROS, and in particular O_2^-, may trigger apoptosis via changes in matrix/integrin interactions.[139]

In addition to being a source of ROS, mitochondria are a target for ROS. Mitochondrial DNA (mtDNA) is very susceptible to ROS damage, in part due to its limited repair activity and the substantial ROS production within the mitochondria in close proximity to mtDNA.[71] Since mtDNA number is a key determinant of gene expression, any reduction or damage to mtDNA may lead to impaired mitochondrial function. In failing myocardium, increased ROS generation was associated with a decrease in mtDNA number with evidence of DNA oxidative damage and impaired mitochondrial function because of decreased ETC activity.[77,166] High levels of oxidative damage to mtDNA can also activate mitochondrial apoptosis pathways.[71]

Endoplasmic Reticulum Stress Response

ROS may exert apoptotic effects via ER stress.[167] The ER is a multifunctional cellular organelle responsible for many cellular functions, including post-translational processing of newly synthesized secretory and membrane proteins, maintenance of calcium homeostasis, and production and storage of macromolecules. A wide range of noxious stimuli, including ROS, hypoxia, ischemia, gene mutation, protein misfolding, and perturbed Ca^{2+} homeostasis, prompt an adaptive process known as the *unfolded protein response* (UPR) that couples the protein load to the folding capacity of the ER.[168] This process promotes the removal of the unfolded proteins to the ubiquitin proteasome for degradation in an attempt to restore cellular homeostasis.[169] If the capacity of UPR to remove unfolded proteins is insufficient, a maladaptive ER overload response (EOR) occurs that is associated with induction of C/EBP homologous protein (CHOP), cleavage of the ER-resident procaspase-12 to active caspase-12, and eventual programmed cell death through the activation of caspases 9 and 3. The UPR and EOR are activated in cardiac hypertrophy and failure.[169-171] Dilated cardiomyopathy occurs in transgenic mice overexpressing a mutant KDEL receptor for ER chaperones that sensitizes the cells to ER stress.[172] The UPR and EOR are activated in an autoimmune cardiomyopathy.[173]

ROS may mediate ER stress/apoptotic signaling via inhibition of antiapoptotic pathways, such as Akt and ARC (apoptosis repressor with caspase recruitment domain). For example, ROS-mediated Akt inactivation is associated with a decrease in pro-survival Bcl proteins[174]; ROS-mediated downregulation of ARC leads to sarcoplasmic reticulum (SR) calcium release with resultant caspase-3 cleavage and apoptosis.[175]

Calcium Handling

Myocytes isolated from the failing heart show markedly abnormal intracellular Ca^{2+} transients along with alterations in the expression and/or activity of Ca^{2+} handling proteins (see also Chapters 1 and 2). ROS can regulate the expression and/or activity of key calcium-regulating proteins.[176] The activity of *sarcoplasmic reticulum Ca^{2+}-ATPase (SERCA)* is decreased in the failing heart and appears to contribute to contractile dysfunction. ROS can decrease SERCA2 activity by decreasing protein expression[139] and by altering protein function due to oxidative post-translational modifications (OPTM).[156] Pathologic levels of ROS are associated with irreversible OPTM of SERCA cysteines and tyrosines that are known to inhibit activity. Sulfonylation of SERCA cysteine 674, which inhibits activity, is present in failing hearts due to transgenic Gαq overexpression,[123] aging,[138] and endotoxemia.[177] Transgenic expression of catalase prevented SERCA OPTM and impairment of calcium and myocyte function in the Gαq[123] and aging[138] mice.

ROS may activate the Na^+/Ca^{2+} exchanger,[178] leading to Ca^{2+} overload,[179] and has been implicated in the pathophysiology of myocardial failing.[180] ROS may also regulate the function of the SR *calcium release channel/ryanodine receptor 2 (RyR2)* and the *voltage-dependent Ca^{2+} channel*.[181,182] Oxidation of RyR2 prolongs opening of the channel leading to increased calcium leak out of the SR leading to SR calcium depletion and cytoplasmic overload.[183]

Impaired Energetics (see also Chapter 16)

In addition to profound effects on calcium regulation, oxidative stress has recently been shown to directly affect cardiac mitochondrial ATP synthesis machinery. In dogs with HF due to dyssynchronous pacing, mitochondrial ATP synthase activity is decreased in association with OPTM of the α-subunit of ATP synthase at cysteine 294.[184]

SUMMARY AND FUTURE DIRECTIONS

Oxidative stress is elevated systemically and in the myocardium of patients with chronic myocardial failure. The cause of increased ROS in this setting is not completely understood, but appears multifactorial including increased production of ROS because of increased metabolic activity, stimulated production by mechanical strain, neurohormonal activation, inflammatory cytokines, as well as decreased antioxidant activity. Based on both in vitro and in vivo studies, it appears likely that increases in oxidative stress contribute to the ventricular remodeling and contractile dysfunction in the failing heart.

ROS exert many effects on myocardial structure and function. It is clear that oxidative stress can trigger a range of responses in myocytes in vitro, and that similar responses may occur in vivo in situations leading to myocardial dysfunction. As in other tissues, oxidative stress can stimulate both the growth and death of cells. The mechanism by which various ROS activate cell signaling pathways remains an area of active investigation, and promises to offer new therapeutic targets for pharmacologic antioxidants.

There remain many unanswered questions about the role of oxidative stress in myocardial failure. In addition, the results of applying preclinical observations to develop therapeutic strategies for patients with HF have been disappointing. In developing therapeutic strategies targeted specifically at oxidative stress, we will need to understand in more detail (1) the relative contributions of decreased antioxidant activity versus increased formation of ROS; (2) the situations in which oxidative and/or nitrosative stress contribute to the pathogenesis of myocardial dysfunction in vivo; (3) the precise ROS involved; and (4) the optimal place in ROS cascades to intervene.

References

1. McCord JM, Fridovich I: Superoxide dismutase. An enzymic function for erythrocuprein (hemocuprein). *J Biol Chem* 244:6049–6055, 1969.
2. Dale DC, Boxer L, Liles WC: The phagocytes: neutrophils and monocytes. *Blood* 112:935–945, 2008.
3. Assem M, Teyssier JR, Benderitter M, et al: Pattern of superoxide dismutase enzymatic activity and RNA changes in rat heart ventricles after myocardial infarction. *Am J Pathol* 151:549–555, 1997.
4. Carlsson LM, Jonsson J, Edlund T, et al: Mice lacking extracellular superoxide dismutase are more sensitive to hyperoxia. *Proc Natl Acad Sci U S A* 92:6264–6268, 1995.
5. Li Y, Huang TT, Carlson EJ, et al: Dilated cardiomyopathy and neonatal lethality in mutant mice lacking manganese superoxide dismutase. *Nat Genet* 11:376–381, 1995.
6. Dai DF, Johnson SC, Villarin JJ, et al: Mitochondrial oxidative stress mediates angiotensin II-induced cardiac hypertrophy and Galphaq overexpression-induced heart failure. *Circ Res* 108(7):837–846, 2011.
7. Qin F, Lennon-Edwards S, Lancel S, et al: Cardiac-specific overexpression of catalase identifies hydrogen peroxide-dependent and independent phases of myocardial remodeling and prevents the progression to overt heart failure in G(alpha)q-overexpressing transgenic mice. *Circ Heart Fail* 3(2):306–313, 2010.
8. Pandolfi PP, Sonati F, Rivi R, et al: Targeted disruption of the housekeeping gene encoding glucose 6-phosphate dehydrogenase (G6PD): G6PD is dispensable for pentose synthesis but essential for defense against oxidative stress. *EMBO J* 14:5209–5215, 1995.
9. Watanabe Y, Watanabe K, Kobayashi T, et al: Chronic depletion of glutathione exacerbates ventricular remodelling and dysfunction in the pressure-overloaded heart. *Cardiovasc Res* 97(2):282–292, 2013.
10. Hill MF, Singal PK: Antioxidant and oxidative stress changes during heart failure subsequent to myocardial infarction in rats. *Am J Pathol* 148:291–300, 1996.
11. Sato M, Sasaki M, Hojo H: Antioxidative roles of metallothionein and manganese superoxide dismutase induced by tumor necrosis factor-alpha and interleukin-6. *Arch Biochem Biophys* 316:738–744, 1995.
12. Cai L: Diabetic cardiomyopathy and its prevention by metallothionein: experimental evidence, possible mechanisms and clinical implications. *Curr Med Chem* 14:2193–2203, 2007.
13. Shioji K, Nakamura H, Masutani H, et al: Redox regulation by thioredoxin in cardiovascular diseases. *Antioxid Redox Signal* 5:795–802, 2003.
14. Nimata M, Kishimoto C, Shioji K, et al: Upregulation of redox-regulating protein, thioredoxin, in endomyocardial biopsy samples of patients with myocarditis and cardiomyopathies. *Mol Cell Biochem* 248:193–196, 2003.
15. Jekell A, Hossain A, Alehagen U, et al: Elevated circulating levels of thioredoxin and stress in chronic heart failure. *Eur J Heart Fail* 6:883–890, 2004.
16. Koneru S, Penumathsa SV, Thirunavukkarasu M, et al: Thioredoxin-1 gene delivery induces heme oxygenase-1 mediated myocardial preservation after chronic infarction in hypertensive rats. *Am J Hypertens* 22:183–190, 2009.
17. Spindel ON, World C, Berk BC: Thioredoxin interacting protein: redox dependent and independent regulatory mechanisms. *Antioxid Redox Signal* 16(6):587–596, 2012.
18. Motterlini R, Gonzales A, Foresti R, et al: Heme oxygenase-1-derived carbon monoxide contributes to the suppression of acute hypertensive responses in vivo. *Circ Res* 83:568–577, 1998.
19. Clark JE, Foresti R, Sarathchandra P, et al: Heme oxygenase-1-derived bilirubin ameliorates postischemic myocardial dysfunction. *Am J Physiol* 278:H643–H651, 2000.
20. Radovanovic S, Savic-Radojevic A, Pljesa-Ercegovac M, et al: Markers of oxidative damage and antioxidant enzyme activities as predictors of morbidity and mortality in patients with chronic heart failure. *J Card Fail* 18(6):493–501, 2012.
21. Mak S, Lehotay DC, Yazdanpanah M, et al: Unsaturated aldehydes including 4-OH-nonenal are elevated in patients with congestive heart failure. *J Card Fail* 6:108–114, 2000.
22. McMurray J, Chopra M, Abdullah I, et al: Evidence of oxidative stress in chronic heart failure in humans. *Eur Heart J* 14:1493–1498, 1993.
23. Sobotka PA, Brottman MD, Weitz Z, et al: Elevated breath pentane in heart failure reduced by free radical scavenger. *Free Rad Biol Med* 14:643–647, 1993.
24. Liu TZ, Stern A, Morrow JD: The isoprostanes: unique bioactive products of lipid peroxidation. An overview. *J Biomed Sci* 5:415–420, 1998.
25. Moore K, Roberts LJ: Measurement of lipid peroxidation. *Free Radic Res* 28:659–671, 1998.
26. Mallat Z, Philip I, Lebret M, et al: Elevated levels of 8-iso-prostaglandin F2alpha in pericardial fluid of patients with heart failure: a potential role for in vivo oxidant stress in ventricular dilatation and progression to heart failure. *Circulation* 97:1536–1539, 1998.
27. Polidori MC, Pratico D, Savino K, et al: Increased F2 isoprostane plasma levels in patients with congestive heart failure are correlated with antioxidant status and disease severity. *J Card Fail* 10:334–338, 2004.
28. Charach G, George J, Afek A, et al: Antibodies to oxidized LDL as predictors of morbidity and mortality in patients with chronic heart failure. *J Card Fail* 15(9):770–774, 2009.
29. Tsutsui T, Tsutamoto T, Wada A, et al: Plasma oxidized low-density lipoprotein as a prognostic predictor in patients with chronic congestive heart failure. *J Am Coll Cardiol* 39:957–962, 2002.
30. Koyama Y, Takeishi Y, Arimoto T, et al: High serum level of pentosidine, an advanced glycation end product (AGE), is a risk factor of patients with heart failure. *J Card Fail* 13:199–206, 2007.
31. Amir O, Paz H, Rogowski O, et al: Serum oxidative stress level correlates with clinical parameters in chronic systolic heart failure patients. *Clin Cardiol* 32:199–203, 2009.
32. Yamamoto M, Yang G, Hong C, et al: Inhibition of endogenous thioredoxin in the heart increases oxidative stress and cardiac hypertrophy. *J Clin Invest* 112:1395–1406, 2003.
33. Shite J, Qin F, Mao W, et al: Antioxidant vitamins attenuate oxidative stress and cardiac dysfunction in tachycardia-induced cardiomyopathy. *J Am Coll Cardiol* 38:1734–1740, 2001.
34. Kono Y, Nakamura K, Kimura H, et al: Elevated levels of oxidative DNA damage in serum and myocardium of patients with heart failure. *Circ J* 70:1001–1005, 2006.
35. Watanabe E, Matsuda N, Shiga T, et al: Significance of 8-hydroxy-2'-deoxyguanosine levels in patients with idiopathic dilated cardiomyopathy. *J Card Fail* 12:527–532, 2006.
36. Kobayashi S, Susa T, Tanaka T, et al: Urinary 8-hydroxy-2'-deoxyguanosine reflects symptomatic status and severity of systolic dysfunction in patients with chronic heart failure. *Eur J Heart Fail* 13(1):29–36, 2011.
37. Sakai H, Tsutamoto T, Tsutsui T, et al: Serum level of uric acid, partly secreted from the failing heart, is a prognostic marker in patients with congestive heart failure. *Circ J* 70:1006–1011, 2006.
38. Kittleson MM, St John ME, Bead V, et al: Increased levels of uric acid predict haemodynamic compromise in patients with heart failure independently of B-type natriuretic peptide levels. *Heart* 93:365–367, 2007.
39. Manzano L, Babalis D, Roughton M, et al: Predictors of clinical outcomes in elderly patients with heart failure. *Eur J Heart Fail* 13:528–536, 2011.
40. Bishu K, Deswal A, Chen HH, et al: Biomarkers in acutely decompensated heart failure with preserved or reduced ejection fraction. *Am Heart J* 164(5):763–770, 2012.
41. Ekundayo OJ, Dell'italia LJ, Sanders PW, et al: Association between hyperuricemia and incident heart failure among older adults: a propensity-matched study. *Int J Cardiol* 142(3):279–287, 2010.
42. Harzand A, Tamariz L, Hare JM: Uric acid, heart failure survival, and the impact of xanthine oxidase inhibition. *Congest Heart Fail* 18(3):179–182, 2012.
43. Hokamaki J, Kawano H, Yoshimura M, et al: Urinary biopyrrins levels are elevated in relation to severity of heart failure. *J Am Coll Cardiol* 43:1880–1885, 2004.
44. Tang WH, Brennan ML, Philip K, et al: Plasma myeloperoxidase levels in patients with chronic heart failure. *Am J Cardiol* 98:796–799, 2006.
45. Reichlin T, Socrates T, Egli P, et al: Use of myeloperoxidase for risk stratification in acute heart failure. *Clin Chem* 56(6):944–951, 2010.
46. Tang WH, Katz R, Brennan ML, et al: Usefulness of myeloperoxidase levels in healthy elderly subjects to predict risk of developing heart failure. *Am J Cardiol* 103(9):1269–1274, 2009.
47. Andrukhova O, Salama M, Rosenhek R, et al: Serum glutathione S-transferase P1 1 in prediction of cardiac function. *J Card Fail* 18(3):253–261, 2012.
48. James RW, Deakin SP: The importance of high-density lipoproteins for paraoxonase-1 secretion, stability, and activity. *Free Rad Biol Med* 37(12):1986–1994, 2004.
49. Kim JB, Hama S, Hough G, et al: Heart failure is associated with impaired anti-inflammatory and antioxidant properties of high-density lipoproteins. *Am J Cardiol* 112(11):1770–1777, 2013.
50. Tang WH, Wu Y, Mann S, et al: Diminished antioxidant activity of high-density lipoprotein-associated proteins in systolic heart failure. *Circ Heart Fail* 4(1):59–64, 2011.
51. Chen X, Sun A, Zou Y, et al: High PLTP activity is associated with depressed left ventricular systolic function. *Atherosclerosis* 228(2):438–442, 2013.
52. Hafstad AD, Nabeebaccus AA, Shah AM: Novel aspects of ROS signalling in heart failure. *Basic Res Cardiol* 108(4):359, 2013.
53. Zhang M, Perino A, Ghigo A, et al: NADPH oxidases in heart failure: poachers or gamekeepers? *Antioxid Redox Signal* 18(9):1024–1041, 2013.
54. Xiao L, Pimentel DR, Wang J, et al: Role of reactive oxygen species and NAD(P)H oxidase in alpha(1)-adrenoceptor signaling in adult rat cardiac myocytes. *Am J Physiol Cell Physiol* 282:C926–C934, 2002.
55. Bendall JK, Cave AC, Heymes C, et al: Pivotal role of a gp91(phox)-containing NADPH oxidase in angiotensin II-induced cardiac hypertrophy in mice. *Circulation* 105:293–296, 2002.
56. Maytin M, Siwik DA, Ito M, et al: Pressure overload-induced myocardial hypertrophy in mice does not require gp91phox. *Circulation* 109(9):1168–1171, 2004.
57. Kuroda J, Ago T, Matsushima S, et al: NADPH oxidase 4 (Nox4) is a major source of oxidative stress in the failing heart. *Proc Natl Acad Sci U S A* 107(35):15565–15570, 2010.
58. Zhang M, Brewer AC, Schroder K, et al: NADPH oxidase-4 mediates protection against chronic load-induced stress in mouse hearts by enhancing angiogenesis. *Proc Natl Acad Sci U S A* 107(42):18121–18126, 2010.
59. Berry CE, Hare JM: Xanthine oxidoreductase and cardiovascular disease: molecular mechanisms and pathophysiological implications. *J Physiol* 555:589–606, 2004.
60. de Jong JW, Schoemaker RG, de Jonge R, et al: Enhanced expression and activity of xanthine oxidoreductase in the failing heart. *J Mol Cell Cardiol* 32:2083–2089, 2000.
61. Engberding N, Spiekermann S, Schaefer A, et al: Allopurinol attenuates left ventricular remodeling and dysfunction after experimental myocardial infarction: a new action for an old drug? *Circulation* 110:2175–2179, 2004.
62. Cappola TP, Kass DA, Nelson GS, et al: Allopurinol improves myocardial efficiency in patients with idiopathic dilated cardiomyopathy. *Circulation* 104:2407–2411, 2001.
63. Ekelund UE, Harrison RW, Shokek O, et al: Intravenous allopurinol decreases myocardial oxygen consumption and increases mechanical efficiency in dogs with pacing-induced heart failure. *Circ Res* 85:437–445, 1999.
64. Amado LC, Saliaris AP, Raju SV, et al: Xanthine oxidase inhibition ameliorates cardiovascular dysfunction in dogs with pacing-induced heart failure. *J Mol Cell Cardiol* 39:531–536, 2005.
65. Minhas KM, Saraiva RM, Schuleri KH, et al: Xanthine oxidoreductase inhibition causes reverse remodeling in rats with dilated cardiomyopathy. *Circ Res* 98:271–279, 2006.
66. Doehner W, Schoene N, Rauchhaus M, et al: Effects of xanthine oxidase inhibition with allopurinol on endothelial function and peripheral blood flow in hyperuricemic patients with chronic heart failure: results from 2 placebo-controlled studies. *Circulation* 105:2619–2624, 2002.
67. Farquharson CA, Butler R, Hill A, et al: Allopurinol improves endothelial dysfunction in chronic heart failure. *Circulation* 106:221–226, 2002.
68. Cingolani HE, Plastino JA, Escudero EM, et al: The effect of xanthine oxidase inhibition upon ejection fraction in heart failure patients: La Plata Study. *J Card Fail* 12:491–498, 2006.
69. Hare JM, Mangal B, Brown J, et al: Impact of oxypurinol in patients with symptomatic heart failure. Results of the OPT-CHF study. *J Am Coll Cardiol* 51:2301–2309, 2008.
70. Kogler H, Fraser H, McCune S, et al: Disproportionate enhancement of myocardial contractility by the xanthine oxidase inhibitor oxypurinol in failing rat myocardium. *Cardiovasc Res* 59:582–592, 2003.
71. Rosca MG, Hoppel CL: Mitochondrial dysfunction in heart failure. *Heart Fail Rev* 18(5):607–622, 2013.
72. Ide T, Tsutsui H, Kinugawa S, et al: Mitochondrial electron transport complex I is a potential source of oxygen free radicals in the failing myocardium. *Circ Res* 85:357–363, 1999.
73. Boudina S, Sena S, Theobald H, et al: Mitochondrial energetics in the heart in obesity-related diabetes: direct evidence for increased uncoupled respiration and activation of uncoupling proteins. *Diabetes* 56(10):2457–2466, 2007.
74. Shen X, Zheng S, Metreveli NS, et al: Protection of cardiac mitochondria by overexpression of MnSOD reduces diabetic cardiomyopathy. *Diabetes* 55(3):798–805, 2006.

75. Dai DF, Chen T, Wanagat J, et al: Age-dependent cardiomyopathy in mitochondrial mutator mice is attenuated by overexpression of catalase targeted to mitochondria. *Aging Cell* 9(4):536–544, 2010.
76. Zinkevich NS, Gutterman DD: ROS-induced ROS release in vascular biology: redox-redox signaling. *Am J Physiol Heart Circ Physiol* 301(3):H647–H653, 2011.
77. Ide T, Tsutsui H, Hayashidani S, et al: Mitochondrial DNA damage and dysfunction associated with oxidative stress in failing hearts after myocardial infarction. *Circ Res* 88:529–535, 2001.
78. Ikeuchi M, Matsusaka H, Kang D, et al: Overexpression of mitochondrial transcription factor a ameliorates mitochondrial deficiencies and cardiac failure after myocardial infarction. *Circulation* 112(5):683–690, 2005.
79. Stamler JS, Simon DI, Osborne JA, et al: S-nitrosylation of proteins with nitric oxide: synthesis and characterization of biologically active compounds. *Proc Natl Acad Sci U S A* 89:444–448, 1992.
80. Michel JB, Feron O, Sacks D, et al: Reciprocal regulation of endothelial nitric-oxide synthase by Ca2+-calmodulin and caveolin. *J Biol Chem* 272:15583–15586, 1997.
81. Singh K, Balligand JL, Fischer TA, et al: Regulation of cytokine-inducible nitric oxide synthase in cardiac myocytes and microvascular endothelial cells. Role of extracellular signal-regulated kinases 1 and 2 (ERK1/ERK2) and STAT1 alpha. *J Biol Chem* 271:1111–1117, 1996.
82. Xia Y, Roman LJ, Masters BS, et al: Inducible nitric-oxide synthase generates superoxide from the reductase domain. *J Biol Chem* 273:22635–22639, 1998.
83. Zimmet JM, Hare JM: Nitroso-redox interactions in the cardiovascular system. *Circulation* 114:1531–1544, 2006.
84. Haywood GA, Tsao PS, von der Leyen HE, et al: Expression of inducible nitric oxide synthase in human heart failure. *Circulation* 93:1087–1094, 1996.
85. Palacios-Callender M, Quintero M, Hollis VS, et al: Endogenous NO regulates superoxide production at low oxygen concentrations by modifying the redox state of cytochrome c oxidase. *Proc Natl Acad Sci U S A* 101:7630–7635, 2004.
86. Mannick JB, Miao XQ, Stamler JS: Nitric oxide inhibits Fas-induced apoptosis. *J Biol Chem* 272:24125–24128, 1997.
87. Feng Q, Song W, Lu X, et al: Development of heart failure and congenital septal defects in mice lacking endothelial nitric oxide synthase. *Circulation* 106:873–879, 2002.
88. Pacher P, Beckman JS, Liaudet L: Nitric oxide and peroxynitrite in health and disease. *Physiol Rev* 87:315–424, 2007.
89. Ischiropoulos H, Zhu L, Chen J, et al: Peroxynitrite-mediated tyrosine nitration catalyzed by superoxide dismutase. *Arch Biochem Biophys* 298:431–437, 1992.
90. Pinsky DJ, Cai B, Yang X, et al: The lethal effects of cytokine-induced nitric oxide on cardiac myocytes are blocked by nitric oxide synthase antagonism or transforming growth factor beta. *J Clin Invest* 95:677–685, 1995.
91. Sam F, Sawyer DB, Xie Z, et al: Mice lacking inducible nitric oxide synthase have improved left ventricular contractile function and reduced apoptotic cell death late after myocardial infarction. *Circ Res* 89:351–356, 2001.
92. Ishiyama S, Hiroe M, Nishikawa T, et al: Nitric oxide contributes to the progression of myocardial damage in experimental autoimmune myocarditis in rats. *Circulation* 95:489–496, 1997.
93. MacMillan-Crow LA, Crow JP, Kerby JD, et al: Nitration and inactivation of manganese superoxide dismutase in chronic rejection of human renal allografts. *Proc Natl Acad Sci U S A* 93:11853–11858, 1996.
94. Mikami S, Kawashima S, Kanazawa K, et al: Low-dose N omega-nitro-L-arginine methyl ester treatment improves survival rate and decreases myocardial injury in a murine model of viral myocarditis induced by coxsackievirus B3. *Circ Res* 81:504–511, 1997.
95. Cheng W, Li B, Kajstura J, et al: Stretch-induced programmed myocyte cell death. *J Clin Invest* 96:2247–2259, 1995.
96. Landmesser U, Dikalov S, Price SR, et al: Oxidation of tetrahydrobiopterin leads to uncoupling of endothelial cell nitric oxide synthase in hypertension. *J Clin Invest* 111(8):1201–1209, 2003.
97. Takimoto E, Kass DA: Role of oxidative stress in cardiac hypertrophy and remodeling. *Hypertension* 49(2):241–248, 2007.
98. Silberman GA, Fan TH, Liu H, et al: Uncoupled cardiac nitric oxide synthase mediates diastolic dysfunction. *Circulation* 121(4):519–528, 2010.
99. Dhalla AK, Singal PK: Antioxidant changes in hypertrophied and failing guinea pig hearts. *Am J Physiol* 266:H1280–H1285, 1994.
100. Hill MF, Singal PK: Antioxidant and oxidative stress changes during heart failure subsequent to myocardial infarction in rats. *Am J Pathol* 148:291–300, 1996.
101. Hill MF, Singal PK: Right and left myocardial antioxidant responses during heart failure subsequent to myocardial infarction. *Circulation* 96:2414–2420, 1997.
102. Prasad K, Gupta JB, Kalra J, et al: Oxidative stress as a mechanism of cardiac failure in chronic volume overload in canine model. *J Mol Cell Cardiol* 28:375–385, 1996.
103. Baumer AT, Flesch M, Wang X, et al: Antioxidative enzymes in human hearts with idiopathic dilated cardiomyopathy. *J Mol Cell Cardiol* 32:121–130, 2000.
104. Dieterich S, Bieligk U, Beulich K, et al: Gene expression of antioxidative enzymes in the human heart: increased expression of catalase in the end-stage failing heart. *Circulation* 101:33–39, 2000.
105. Sam F, Kerstetter DL, Pimental D, et al: Increased reactive oxygen species production and functional alterations in antioxidant enzymes in human failing myocardium. *J Card Fail* 11:473–480, 2005.
106. Singal PK, Dhillon KS, Beamish RE, et al: Myocardial cell damage and cardiovascular changes due to i.v. infusion of adrenochrome in rats. *Br J Exp Pathol* 63:167–176, 1982.
107. Goto T, Shikama K: Autoxidation of native oxymyoglobin from bovine heart muscle. *Arch Biochem Biophys* 163:476–481, 1974.
108. Nabeebaccus A, Zhang M, Shah AM: NADPH oxidases and cardiac remodelling. *Heart Fail Rev* 16(1):5–12, 2011.
109. Byrne JA, Grieve DJ, Bendall JK, et al: Contrasting roles of NADPH oxidase isoforms in pressure-overload versus angiotensin II-induced cardiac hypertrophy. *Circ Res* 93(9):802–805, 2003.
110. Matsushima S, Kuroda J, Ago T, et al: Broad suppression of NADPH oxidase activity exacerbates ischemia/reperfusion injury through inadvertent downregulation of hypoxia-inducible factor-1alpha and upregulation of peroxisome proliferator-activated receptor-alpha. *Circ Res* 112(8):1135–1149, 2013.
111. Takimoto E, Champion HC, Li M, et al: Oxidant stress from nitric oxide synthase-3 uncoupling stimulates cardiac pathologic remodeling from chronic pressure load. *J Clin Invest* 115(5):1221–1231, 2005.
112. Moens AL, Takimoto E, Tocchetti CG, et al: Reversal of cardiac hypertrophy and fibrosis from pressure overload by tetrahydrobiopterin: efficacy of recoupling nitric oxide synthase as a therapeutic strategy. *Circulation* 117(20):2626–2636, 2008.
113. Date MO, Morita T, Yamashita N, et al: The antioxidant N-2-mercaptopropionyl glycine attenuates left ventricular hypertrophy in in vivo murine pressure-overload model. *J Am Coll Cardiol* 39(5):907–912, 2002.
114. Yoshioka J, Imahashi K, Gabel SA, et al: Targeted deletion of thioredoxin-interacting protein regulates cardiac dysfunction in response to pressure overload. *Circ Res* 101(12):1328–1338, 2007.
115. Dhalla AK, Hill MF, Singal PK: Role of oxidative stress in transition of hypertrophy to heart failure. *J Am Coll Cardiol* 28:506–514, 1996.
116. Bell JP, Mosfer SI, Lang D, et al: Vitamin C and quinapril abrogate LVH and endothelial dysfunction in aortic-banded guinea pigs. *Am J Physiol Heart Circ Physiol* 281(4):H1704–H1710, 2001.
117. Juric D, Wojciechowski P, Das DK, et al: Prevention of concentric hypertrophy and diastolic impairment in aortic-banded rats treated with resveratrol. *Am J Physiol Heart Circ Physiol* 292(5):H2138–H2143, 2007.
118. Dai DF, Hsieh EJ, Liu Y, et al: Mitochondrial proteome remodelling in pressure overload-induced heart failure: the role of mitochondrial oxidative stress. *Cardiovasc Res* 93(1):79–88, 2012.
119. Dai DF, Hsieh EJ, Chen T, et al: Global proteomics and pathway analysis of pressure-overload-induced heart failure and its attenuation by mitochondrial-targeted peptides. *Circ Heart Fail* 6(5):1067–1076, 2013.
120. Doctrow SR, Huffman K, Marcus CB, et al: Salen-manganese complexes as catalytic scavengers of hydrogen peroxide and cytoprotective agents: structure-activity relationship studies. *J Med Chem* 45(20):4549–4558, 2002.
121. van Empel VP, Bertrand AT, van Oort RJ, et al: EUK-8, a superoxide dismutase and catalase mimetic, reduces cardiac oxidative stress and ameliorates pressure overload-induced heart failure in the harlequin mouse mutant. *J Am Coll Cardiol* 48(4):824–832, 2006.
122. Dorn GW, Brown JH: Gq signaling in cardiac adaptation and maladaptation. *Trends Cardiovasc Med* 9(1–2):26–34, 1999.
123. Lancel S, Qin F, Lennon SL, et al: Oxidative posttranslational modifications mediate decreased SERCA activity and myocyte dysfunction in Galphaq-overexpressing mice. *Circ Res* 107(2):228–232, 2010.
124. Dai DF, Chen T, Szeto H, et al: Mitochondrial targeted antioxidant peptide ameliorates hypertensive cardiomyopathy. *J Am Coll Cardiol* 58(1):73–82, 2011.
125. Rosca MG, Tandler B, Hoppel CL: Mitochondria in cardiac hypertrophy and heart failure. *J Mol Cell Cardiol* 55:31–41, 2013.
126. Sawyer DB, Fukazawa R, Arstall MA, et al: Daunorubicin-induced apoptosis in rat cardiac myocytes is inhibited by dexrazoxane. *Circ Res* 84:257–265, 1999.
127. Sterba M, Popelova O, Vavrova A, et al: Oxidative stress, redox signaling, and metal chelation in anthracycline cardiotoxicity and pharmacological cardioprotection. *Antioxid Redox Signal* 18(8):899–929, 2013.
128. Zhao Y, McLaughlin D, Robinson E, et al: Nox2 NADPH oxidase promotes pathologic cardiac remodeling associated with doxorubicin chemotherapy. *Cancer Res* 70(22):9287–9297, 2010.
129. Mordente A, Meucci E, Silvestrini A, et al: Anthracyclines and mitochondria. *Adv Exp Med Biol* 385–419, 2012.
130. Speyer JL, Green MD, Kramer E, et al: Protective effect of the bispiperazinedione ICRF-187 against doxorubicin-induced cardiac toxicity in women with advanced breast cancer. *N Engl J Med* 319:745–752, 1988.
131. Kang YJ, Chen Y, Epstein PN: Suppression of doxorubicin cardiotoxicity by overexpression of catalase in the heart of transgenic mice. *J Biol Chem* 271(21):12610–12616, 1996.
132. Kang YJ, Sun X, Chen Y, et al: Inhibition of doxorubicin chronic toxicity in catalase-overexpressing transgenic mouse hearts. *Chem Res Toxicol* 15(1):1–6, 2002.
133. Kang YJ, Chen Y, Yu A, et al: Overexpression of metallothionein in the heart of transgenic mice suppresses doxorubicin cardiotoxicity. *J Clin Invest* 100(6):1501–1506, 1997.
134. Sun X, Zhou Z, Kang YJ: Attenuation of doxorubicin chronic toxicity in metallothionein-overexpressing transgenic mouse heart. *Cancer Res* 61(8):3382–3387, 2001.
135. Qin F, Siwik DA, Luptak I, et al: The polyphenols resveratrol and S17834 prevent the structural and functional sequelae of diet-induced metabolic heart disease in mice. *Circulation* 125(14):1757–1764, S1–S6, 2012.
136. Zhao Y, Zhang L, Qiao Y, et al: Heme oxygenase-1 prevents cardiac dysfunction in streptozotocin-diabetic mice by reducing inflammation, oxidative stress, apoptosis and enhancing autophagy. *PLoS ONE* 8(9):e75927, 2013.
137. Hamblin M, Smith HM, Hill MF: Dietary supplementation with vitamin E ameliorates cardiac failure in type I diabetic cardiomyopathy by suppressing myocardial generation of 8-iso-prostaglandin F2alpha and oxidized glutathione. *J Card Fail* 13:884–892, 2007.
138. Qin F, Siwik DA, Lancel S, et al: Hydrogen peroxide-mediated SERCA cysteine 674 oxidation contributes to impaired cardiac myocyte relaxation in senescent mouse heart. *J Am Heart Assoc* 2(4):e000184, 2013.
139. Siwik DA, Tzortzis JD, Pimental DR, et al: Inhibition of copper-zinc superoxide dismutase induces cell growth, hypertrophic phenotype, and apoptosis in neonatal rat cardiac myocytes in vitro. *Circ Res* 85:147–153, 1999.
140. Kwon SH, Pimentel DR, Remondino A, et al: H(2)O(2) regulates cardiac myocyte phenotype via concentration-dependent activation of distinct kinase pathways. *J Mol Cell Cardiol* 35(6):615–621, 2003.
141. Pimentel DR, Amin JK, Xiao L, et al: Reactive oxygen species mediate amplitude-dependent hypertrophic and apoptotic responses to mechanical stretch in cardiac myocytes. *Circ Res* 89:453–460, 2001.
142. Nakagami H, Takemoto M, Liao JK: NADPH oxidase-derived superoxide anion mediates angiotensin II-induced cardiac hypertrophy. *J Mol Cell Cardiol* 35(7):851–859, 2003.
143. Leri A, Claudio PP, Li Q, et al: Stretch-mediated release of angiotensin II induces myocyte apoptosis by activating p53 that enhances the local renin-angiotensin system and decreases the Bcl-2-to-Bax protein ratio in the cell. *J Clin Invest* 101:1326–1342, 1998.
144. Cheng TH, Shih NL, Chen CH, et al: Role of mitogen-activated protein kinase pathway in reactive oxygen species-mediated endothelin-1-induced beta-myosin heavy chain gene expression and cardiomyocyte hypertrophy. *J Biomed Sci* 12(1):123–133, 2005.
145. Kuster GM, Pimentel DR, Adachi T, et al: Alpha-adrenergic receptor-stimulated hypertrophy in adult rat ventricular myocytes is mediated via thioredoxin-1-sensitive oxidative modification of thiols on Ras. *Circulation* 111(9):1192–1198, 2005.
146. Dorn GW: Apoptotic and non-apoptotic programmed cardiomyocyte death in ventricular remodelling. *Cardiovasc Res* 81(3):465–473, 2009.
147. Aikawa R, Komuro I, Yamazaki T, et al: Oxidative stress activates extracellular signal-regulated kinases through Src and Ras in cultured cardiac myocytes of neonatal rats. *J Clin Invest* 100:1813–1821, 1997.
148. Kung G, Konstantinidis K, Kitsis RN: Programmed necrosis, not apoptosis, in the heart. *Circ Res* 108(8):1017–1036, 2011.
149. Spinale FG, Coker ML, Bond BR, et al: Myocardial matrix degradation and metalloproteinase activation in the failing heart: a potential therapeutic target. *Cardiovasc Res* 46:225–238, 2000.
150. Siwik DA, Pagano PJ, Colucci WS: Oxidative stress regulates collagen synthesis and matrix metalloproteinase activity in cardiac fibroblasts. *Am J Physiol* 280:C53–C60, 2001.
151. Kinugawa S, Tsutsui H, Hayashidani S, et al: Treatment with dimethylthiourea prevents left ventricular remodeling and failure after experimental myocardial infarction in mice: role of oxidative stress. *Circ Res* 87:392–398, 2000.
152. He BJ, Joiner ML, Singh MV, et al: Oxidation of CaMKII determines the cardiotoxic effects of aldosterone. *Nat Med* 17(12):1610–1618, 2011.
153. Johar S, Cave AC, Narayanapanicker A, et al: Aldosterone mediates angiotensin II-induced interstitial cardiac fibrosis via a Nox2-containing NADPH oxidase. *FASEB J* 20(9):1546–1548, 2006.
154. Siwik DA, Kuster GM, Brahmbhatt JV, et al: EMMPRIN mediates beta-adrenergic receptor-stimulated matrix metalloproteinase activity in cardiac myocytes. *J Mol Cell Cardiol* 44(1):210–217, 2008.
155. Kumar V, Calamaras TD, Haeussler D, et al: Cardiovascular redox and ox stress proteomics. *Antioxid Redox Signal* 17(11):1528–1559, 2012.
156. Cohen RA, Adachi T: Nitric-oxide-induced vasodilatation: regulation by physiologic S-glutathiolation and pathologic oxidation of the sarcoplasmic endoplasmic reticulum calcium ATPase. *Trends Cardiovasc Med* 16:109–114, 2006.

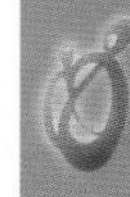

157. Shah AM, Mann DL: In search of new therapeutic targets and strategies for heart failure: recent advances in basic science. *Lancet* 378(9792):704–712, 2011.
158. Remondino A, Kwon SH, Communal C, et al: Beta-adrenergic receptor-stimulated apoptosis in cardiac myocytes is mediated by reactive oxygen species/c-Jun NH2-terminal kinase-dependent activation of the mitochondrial pathway. *Circ Res* 92(2):136–138, 2003.
159. Yamaguchi O, Higuchi Y, Hirotani S, et al: Targeted deletion of apoptosis signal-regulating kinase 1 attenuates left ventricular remodeling. *Proc Natl Acad Sci U S A* 100(26):15883–15888, 2003.
160. Turner NA, Xia F, Azhar G, et al: Oxidative stress induces DNA fragmentation and caspase activation via the c-Jun NH2-terminal kinase pathway in H9c2 cardiac muscle cells. *J Mol Cell Cardiol* 30:1789–1801, 1998.
161. Palomeque J, Rueda OV, Sapia L, et al: Angiotensin II-induced oxidative stress resets the Ca2+ dependence of Ca2+-calmodulin protein kinase II and promotes a death pathway conserved across different species. *Circ Res* 105(12):1204–1212, 2009.
162. Swaminathan PD, Purohit A, Soni S, et al: Oxidized CaMKII causes cardiac sinus node dysfunction in mice. *J Clin Invest* 121(8):3277–3288, 2011.
163. Reed JC: Cytochrome c: can't live with it–can't live without it. *Cell* 91:559–562, 1997.
164. Reed JC, Jurgensmeier JM, Matsuyama S: Bcl-2 family proteins and mitochondria. *Biochim Biophys Acta* 1366:127–137, 1998.
165. von Harsdorf R, Li PF, Dietz R: Signaling pathways in reactive oxygen species-induced cardiomyocyte apoptosis. *Circulation* 99:2934–2941, 1999.
166. Tsutsui H, Ide T, Shiomi T, et al: 8-oxo-dGTPase, which prevents oxidative stress-induced DNA damage, increases in the mitochondria from failing hearts. *Circulation* 104:2883–2885, 2001.
167. Lee Y, Gustafsson AB: Role of apoptosis in cardiovascular disease. *Apoptosis* 14:536–548, 2009.
168. Kaufman RJ: Orchestrating the unfolded protein response in health and disease. *J Clin Invest* 110:1389–1398, 2002.
169. Glembotski CC: The role of the unfolded protein response in the heart. *J Mol Cell Cardiol* 44:453–459, 2008.
170. Okada K, Minamino T, Tsukamoto Y, et al: Prolonged endoplasmic reticulum stress in hypertrophic and failing heart after aortic constriction: possible contribution of endoplasmic reticulum stress to cardiac myocyte apoptosis. *Circulation* 110:705–712, 2004.
171. Mao W, Fukuoka S, Iwai C, et al: Cardiomyocyte apoptosis in autoimmune cardiomyopathy: mediated via endoplasmic reticulum stress and exaggerated by norepinephrine. *Am J Physiol* 293:H1636–H1645, 2007.
172. Hamada H, Suzuki M, Yuasa S, et al: Dilated cardiomyopathy caused by aberrant endoplasmic reticulum quality control in mutant KDEL receptor transgenic mice. *Mol Cell Biol* 24:8007–8017, 2004.
173. Liu J, Mao W, Iwai C, et al: Adoptive passive transfer of rabbit beta1-adrenoceptor peptide immune cardiomyopathy into the Rag2-/- mouse: participation of the ER stress. *J Mol Cell Cardiol* 44:304–314, 2008.
174. Li Q, Ren J: Cardiac overexpression of metallothionein rescues chronic alcohol intake-induced cardiomyocyte dysfunction: role of Akt, mammalian target of rapamycin and ribosomal p70s6 kinase. *Alcohol Alcohol* 41:585–592, 2006.
175. Lu D, Liu J, Jiao J, et al: Transcription factor Foxo3a prevents apoptosis by regulating calcium through the apoptosis repressor with caspase recruitment domain. *J Biol Chem* 288(12):8491–8504, 2013.
176. Wagner S, Rokita AG, Anderson ME, et al: Redox regulation of sodium and calcium handling. *Antioxid Redox Signal* 18(9):1063–1077, 2013.
177. Hobai IA, Buys ES, Morse JC, et al: SERCA Cys674 sulphonylation and inhibition of L-type Ca2+ influx contribute to cardiac dysfunction in endotoxemic mice, independent of cGMP synthesis. *Am J Physiol Heart Circ Physiol* 305(8):H1189–H1200, 2013.
178. Kuster GM, Lancel S, Zhang JM, et al: Redox-mediated reciprocal regulation of SERCA and Na(+)-Ca(2+) exchanger contributes to sarcoplasmic reticulum Ca(2+) depletion in cardiac myocytes. *Free Rad Biol Med* 48(9):1182–1187, 2010.
179. Goldhaber JI, Qayyum MS: Oxygen free radicals and excitation-contraction coupling. *Antioxid Redox Signal* 2:55–64, 2000.
180. Litwin SE, Bridge JH: Enhanced Na(+)-Ca2+ exchange in the infarcted heart. Implications for excitation-contraction coupling. *Circ Res* 81:1083–1093, 1997.
181. Campbell DL, Stamler JS, Strauss HC: Redox modulation of L-type calcium channels in ferret ventricular myocytes. Dual mechanism regulation by nitric oxide and S-nitrosothiols. *J Gen Physiol* 108:277–293, 1996.
182. Xu L, Eu JP, Meissner G, et al: Activation of the cardiac calcium release channel (ryanodine receptor) by poly-S-nitrosylation. *Science* 279:234–237, 1998.
183. Terentyev D, Gyorke I, Belevych AE, et al: Redox modification of ryanodine receptors contributes to sarcoplasmic reticulum Ca2+ leak in chronic heart failure. *Circ Res* 103(12):1466–1472, 2008.
184. Wang SB, Foster DB, Rucker J, et al: Redox regulation of mitochondrial ATP synthase: implications for cardiac resynchronization therapy. *Circ Res* 109(7):750–757, 2011.
185. McMurray J, McLay J, Chopra M, et al: Evidence for enhanced free radical activity in chronic congestive heart failure secondary to coronary artery disease. *Am J Cardiol* 65:1261–1262, 1990.
186. Belch JJ, Bridges AB, Scott N, et al: Oxygen free radicals and congestive heart failure. *Br Heart J* 65:245–248, 1991.
187. Ghatak A, Brar MJ, Agarwal A, et al: Oxy free radical system in heart failure and therapeutic role of oral vitamin E. *Int J Cardiol* 57:119–127, 1996.
188. Keith M, Geranmayegan A, Sole MJ, et al: Increased oxidative stress in patients with congestive heart failure. *J Am Coll Cardiol* 31:1352–1356, 1998.
189. Polidori MC, Savino K, Alunni G, et al: Plasma lipophilic antioxidants and malondialdehyde in congestive heart failure patients: relationship to disease severity. *Free Radic Biol Med* 32:148–152, 2002.
190. Campolo J, De Maria R, Caruso R, et al: Blood glutathione as independent marker of lipid peroxidation in heart failure. *Int J Cardiol* 117:45–50, 2007.
191. Kameda K, Matsunaga T, Abe N, et al: Correlation of oxidative stress with activity of matrix metalloproteinase in patients with coronary artery disease. Possible role for left ventricular remodelling. *Eur Heart J* 24:2180–2185, 2003.
192. Nonaka-Sarukawa M, Yamamoto K, Aoki H, et al: Increased urinary 15-F2t-isoprostane concentrations in patients with non-ischaemic congestive heart failure: a marker of oxidative stress. *Heart* 89:871–874, 2003.
193. Pignatelli P, Cangemi R, Celestini A, et al: Tumour necrosis factor alpha upregulates platelet CD40L in patients with heart failure. *Cardiovasc Res* 78:515–522, 2008.
194. Nagayoshi Y, Kawano H, Hokamaki J, et al: Differences in oxidative stress markers based on the aetiology of heart failure: comparison of oxidative stress in patients with and without coronary artery disease. *Free Radic Res* 43(12):1159–1166, 2009.
195. Cicoira M, Zanolla L, Rossi A, et al: Elevated serum uric acid levels are associated with diastolic dysfunction in patients with dilated cardiomyopathy. *Am Heart J* 143:1107–1111, 2002.
196. Anker SD, Doehner W, Rauchhaus M, et al: Uric acid and survival in chronic heart failure: validation and application in metabolic, functional, and hemodynamic staging. *Circulation* 107:1991–1997, 2003.
197. Kojima S, Sakamoto T, Ishihara M, et al: Prognostic usefulness of serum uric acid after acute myocardial infarction (the Japanese Acute Coronary Syndrome Study). *Am J Cardiol* 96:489–495, 2005.
198. Ioachimescu AG, Brennan DM, Hoar BM, et al: Serum uric acid is an independent predictor of all-cause mortality in patients at high risk of cardiovascular disease: a preventive cardiology information system (PreCIS) database cohort study. *Arthritis Rheum* 58:623–630, 2008.

9 Alterations in Ventricular Function in Systolic Heart Failure

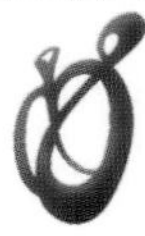

David A. Kass

Systolic cardiac depression is a hallmark of many patients with heart failure. It reflects a fundamental weakness of the pump and thus its inability to deliver sufficient cardiac output at an adequate mean arterial pressure. The failing heart often exhibits major decrements in resting systolic function and the limited reserve that is required for individuals to exercise and perform activities of daily living. The underlying mechanisms are numerous and entail changes in myofilament proteins (**see Chapter 2**) and their interaction with calcium, abnormal calcium cycling[1] into and out of the sarcoplasmic reticulum, altered ion channel function (**see Chapter 1**), mitochondrial and metabolic abnormalities,[2] depressed cell survival signaling, enhanced autophagy and mitophagy,[3] proteasomal dysfunction,[4] protein misfolding stress,[5] redox pathobiology (**see Chapter 8**),[6] and signal transduction.[7] Systolic dysfunction is impacted by more than just abnormal myocytes, because their interaction with the vasculature[8,9] and crosstalk with the interstitial matrix[10-12] play central roles as well.

Direct demonstration of abnormal myocyte function in failing hearts has been achieved using isolated cells in which sarcomere shortening and calcium transients can be measured, or muscle preparations where developed force and length are assessed. Intact and chemically membrane-disrupted (skinned) preparations are also used, the latter to assess changes in myofilament calcium dependence. Results of such studies from numerous experimental models of heart failure and human disease are discussed in detail in **Chapter 2**. For the intact heart, quantitation and analysis of systolic dysfunction is rendered more complex because most measures of systole are also influenced by chamber structure and ambient loading conditions imposed on the heart. As these factors are also abnormal in heart failure, any analysis must take them into consideration.

The ambiguities associated with common assessments of chamber systolic function are not purely of academic interest because they may themselves have contributed to a disappointing history of efforts to improve systolic function in the failing heart. Ejection fraction is neither very specific nor particularly sensitive to changes in underlying contractile function.[13] Thus dosing pharmaceuticals to achieve a given change in ejection fraction (EF) may risk biasing trials toward testing higher doses of medications that ultimately prove disappointing. Furthermore, classification of heart failure based on a parameter such as EF introduces ambiguities. The interpretation of an EF less than 30% in an NYHA class I patient following a myocardial infarction is quite different from that of an individual with class III symptoms associated with dilated cardiomyopathy. For both, the reduced EF largely reflects chamber remodeling/dilation, increasing end-diastolic volume with a preserved stroke volume. However, in one instance, infarct remodeling dominates this decline and the residual myocardium may remain quite compensated and capable of providing adequate cardiac reserve (**see Chapter 11**). In the other example, the myopathy is more homogeneous with little reserve capacity. These two situations may look similar when assessed by conventional parameters such as blood pressure, cardiac output, or EF, yet appear very different when viewed with other mechanical frameworks. The purpose of this chapter is to review the current understanding of the mechanisms underlying systolic depression in cardiac failure, the relationship between properties determined by the muscle and dysfunction assessed in the intact chamber, methods to assess systolic function in the intact heart and the impact that various loading influences have on these measures, the interaction of cardiac function with the arterial loading system (ventricular/arterial interaction), and new approaches to therapeutic targeting of systolic dysfunction. Last, we discuss the contribution of contractile synchrony and effects of artificial resynchronization on systolic function.

CELLULAR AND MOLECULAR DETERMINANTS: A VIEW FROM 30,000 FEET

The greatest advances in understanding of heart failure over the past decade have come from the elucidation of novel

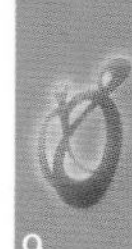

molecular signaling that is involved, and its impact on cellular and organ level pathobiology. Full justice to this topic is a book by itself, but the reader is referred to Chapter 1 for a more comprehensive review. Here, I will provide a brief overview of several key elements involved with systolic failure.

Systolic force generation starts at the level of the actin-myosin cross-bridge, which in turn is coupled via structural proteins to the surface membrane to transduce deformation to net chamber contraction. The contractile proteins themselves can play a central role in systolic depression, both because of genetic mutations that depress the function of the molecular motors[14,15] and by posttranslational changes, particularly of regulatory thin filament proteins that modify contraction.[16,17] Mouse models recapitulating myosin mutations associated with dilated cardiomyopathy have shown weakened power generation and general loss of function in the actin-myosin cross-bridge. Myosin light chain phosphorylation has long been known to regulate smooth muscle tone, and studies now show a major impact on cardiac systolic function and stress responses as well. Mice lacking *Mylk3* (cardiac specific myosin light chain kinase gene) demonstrate marked functional impairment and worsened hypertrophy from pressure overload, whereas those with myocyte-targeted overexpression are protected.[18] Another critical sarcomere protein that impacts systolic function is myosin-binding protein C (MyBP-C).[19] Mutations in MyBP-C are the most common cause of hypertrophic cardiomyopathy. Genetic deletion of functional protein leads to dilated cardiomyopathy[20,21] and the inability of the heart to sustain systolic contraction.[22] Equally important are changes in regulatory thin-filament proteins, such as phosphorylation, redox modulation, or enzymatic cleavage (see Chapter 2). Troponin I and troponin T phosphorylation[16,17] play a role in systolic dysfunction in the failing heart by impacting the sarcomere response to calcium. TnI can also undergo proteolytic truncation associated with the protease calpain. This was first reported in postischemic stunned myocardium, and by itself generates depressed systolic function and chamber dilation.[23] The phosphorylation state of MyBP-C also impacts systolic function, and reduced phosphorylation in animal models and human heart failure may contribute to depressed sarcomere function.[22,24,25] Indeed, while long ignored, the role of the sarcomere as a signal-transduction target of various kinases and phosphatases and other posttranslational changes such as oxidation, nitration, nitrosylation, and glycosylation is now a major area of research.

Heart failure often entails disruption of proteins linking the myofibrils to the cell membrane, a necessary component for transducing force and shortening. Abnormalities in the Z-disk protein muscle limb protein (MLP); plasma membrane sarcoglycan-dystrophin complex; focal adhesion complexes, including vinculin and metavinculin; and nuclear or mitochondrial membrane linking filaments, such as laminin, lamin, and desmin, have all been linked to dilated depressed ventricles.[26,27] Murine models involving these proteins have been reported and are associated with morphogenic abnormalities, congenital defects, and dilated cardiomyopathy.

Systolic dysfunction is also critically dependent upon abnormalities of calcium homeostasis (see Chapters 1 and 2).[28-31] Changes have been described from the level of the voltage-gated calcium channels and sodium-calcium exchanger to altered expression and function of major sarcoplasmic reticular proteins involved with calcium cycling, such as phospholamban and the SR calcium ATPase. Protein stabilization mediated by SUMOylation has also been revealed to play a role in depressed SR Ca^{2+}-ATPase levels.[32] Changes in these and related proteins are presently being explored as potential new therapeutic avenues. A related signaling pathway is the phosphatase inhibitor I-1, which inactivates PP1.[33] I-1 levels decline in heart failure, enhancing PP1 dephosphorylation of phospholamban, contributing to systolic depression. Protein kinase A activates I-1, and downregulation of this pathway in the failing heart may contribute further to this change. Opposite effects occur from protein kinase Cα (e.g., inhibition of I-1, leading to greater dephosphorylation (inactivation) of phospholamban), and upregulation of PKC-α in heart failure is another proposed mechanism of systolic dysfunction.[29,34] Changes in calcium release from the SR have been associated with sustained upregulation of calcium-calmodulin–dependent kinase IIδ and PKA-dependent phosphorylation of the ryanodine receptor to enhance SR calcium leak.[35-38] The precise targeting and responsible kinase remain subjects of some debate.[39] While a prior focus was on the expression levels of key calcium handling proteins, evidence also supports major changes at the posttranslational level, including phosphorylation and oxidation.[40-44] This has tightly linked excitation-contraction coupling with signal transduction mediated by stress response kinases, phosphatases, and transcription factors. These and other changes in calcium handling and myofilament interaction are discussed in more detail elsewhere in this volume.

The molecular signaling changes observed in the failing heart are vast, and as more and more are manipulated by selective genetic gain- and loss-of-function studies, their role in contractile failure has been revealed. As a result, new approaches to treat depressed pump function are now focusing beneath the cell surface to more directly target enzyme and/or gene transcription programs. This work is discussed in more detail earlier in this volume. Two other major contributors to systolic dysfunction that are gaining more and more attention are energetics and metabolism. Abnormalities in mitochondrial function and ATP generation and changes in glucose and fatty acid metabolism in the failing heart have been mechanistically linked to chamber dilation and dysfunction.[45,46] A prime example is the impact of reduced levels of the transcription factor PGC1α, which serves as a master energy regulator.[47,48]

Systolic dysfunction also evolves from changes outside the myocyte, in particular from coupling of the cell to the extracellular matrix and to the vascular supply that surrounds each muscle cell. Signaling via proteins such as p53 and various growth factor signaling cascades are thought to be important in maintaining adequate vasculogenesis to match the increased work and hypertrophy demands in the failing heart, and inadequacy of this matching results in depressed performance. Recent studies have also shown how changes in heart function can occur by gene-targeted manipulation of fibroblasts and vice versa—indicating strong signaling communication between systems.[49] Other studies have shown that selective manipulation of cardiac myocyte transforming growth factor beta receptors has both prominent impact on functional responses to pressure overload, but also impacts fibrosis and angiogenesis.[11] The matricellular protein thrombospondin-4 was recently shown to

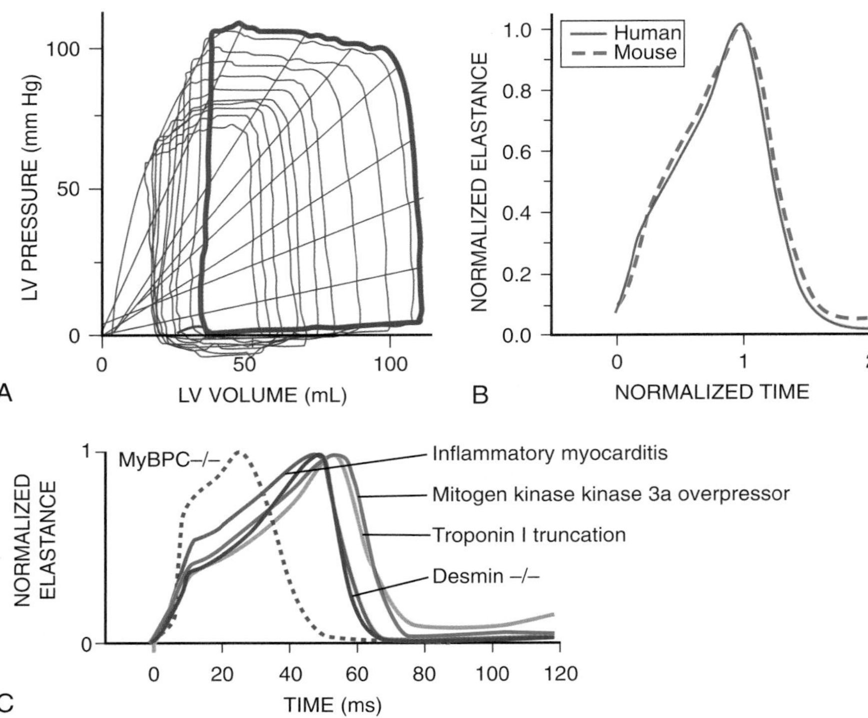

FIGURE 9-1 Time-varying elastance in the human heart. **A,** Generation of time-varying elastance from multiple cardiac cycles. Linear spokes represent isochrones (connecting points on each loop at the same time), and their slope reflects the instantaneous chamber stiffness or elastance achieved at that point in the cycle [Elastance = Pressure/(Volume – Vo)]. The time-varying elastance is the change in this slope throughout the heartbeat (E[t]). **B,** E(t) curves shown normalized to both peak amplitude and time to peak amplitude from the average of greater than 50 human subjects with varying cardiac diseases and from mice. There is remarkable consistency across species in the shape of the waveform, supporting a highly conserved behavior. **C,** The E(t) waveform is also conserved in many experimental models of heart failure regardless of mechanism. Shown here are examples involving a sarcomere protein mutation (troponin I truncation), reduction of intermediate filament expression (desmin gene deletion (–/–)), inflammatory myocarditis, and kinase-dependent disease (MKK3a enhances p38 MAP kinase). A thus far unique example, where the E(t) relation is markedly altered, is in mice lacking myosin-binding protein C (MyBP-C –/–). This results in a very abbreviated time course that declines shortly after opening of the aortic valve, resulting in reduced cardiac output.

play a central role in transducing cardiac stress to the muscle cell in vivo and in muscle,[50] and is also involved with cardioprotective signaling mediated through the ER stress response.[51] Chamber dilation involves the modulation of metalloproteinases and tissue inhibitors of metatalloproteinases (see Chapter 4), with their consequent influence on extracellular matrix remodeling. This is a highly active process and potently contributes to systolic dysfunction.[10,52,53] Myocyte geometry is transformed in the failing heart (longer-thinner in dilated chambers), which plays a role as well.[54] Reversal of chronic dilation and myocyte geometric remodeling with a variety of therapies is often coupled with improved systolic function, though precise cause and effect cannot be determined from these studies.[55]

MEASURING SYSTOLIC FUNCTION—PRESSURE-VOLUME RELATIONS

There are many ways of assessing systolic dysfunction, the most common being changes in fractional shortening or ejection fraction. Other parameters include the ability of the heart to generate maximal power (pressure × flow), the peak rate of rise of pressure (dP/dt_{max}), and the capacity of the heart to generate cardiac output or external stroke work for a given level of preload (end-diastolic volume).[13] Development of such metrics was a major focus of cardiac physiology between 1960 and 1990, and the tools that evolved have largely remained the same since. Among the more powerful tools was the depiction of cardiac contractility by means of plotting simultaneous chamber pressure and cavity volume to derive pressure-volume loops and relations.[56] This framework is now widely used in genetically engineered mouse studies[57] and other experimental models, and has served as a gold standard for defining the pathophysiology of heart failure and therapy advances for several decades.[58,59]

The time course of stiffening or time-varying elastance from human subjects and from mouse hearts is shown in **Figure 9-1**. Data are normalized to the maximal stiffness generated and time to achieve this (adjusting for differences in underlying contractility and heart rate, which are immense among species). The curves define the activation and deactivation process in the heart, and the striking similarity among species suggests this is a fundamental property of the ventricle (see Figure 9-1B).[60] This activation curve is remarkably conserved among patients with various forms of heart disease, or with adrenergic or chronotropic stimulation.[61]

The rise in chamber elastance occurs rapidly at the start of systole during the period of isovolumetric contraction. When the aortic valve opens, the rate of ongoing stiffening during ejection declines but remains largely at a constant rate until the peak is achieved. As a result, about 60% of net cardiac muscle stiffening develops during the process of blood ejection. This pattern is preserved despite a broad range of genetically engineered modifications affecting calcium cycling, sarcomere function, adrenergic signaling, the dystroglycan complex, and signal transduction (see Figure 9-1C).[62] A striking counterexample is provided in mice lacking MyBP-C,[22,62] which display a very abbreviated time course of elastance rise and decline,[22] particularly removing the period during ejection (see Figure 9-1C). MyBP-C binds to myosin (C-terminus)[63,64] and actin[65] (N-terminus, though this is debated[66]), and is thought to impose a restraint on the kinetics of cross-bridge cycling, reducing filament velocity and rate of cross-bridge attachment.[67,68] The latter was identified with acute length perturbation studies, where force redevelopment reflected cross-bridge kinetics.

Several recent novel drugs for heart failure treatment highlight the value of ventricular elastance as a systolic index. One is omecamtiv mecarbil,[69] which stimulates the

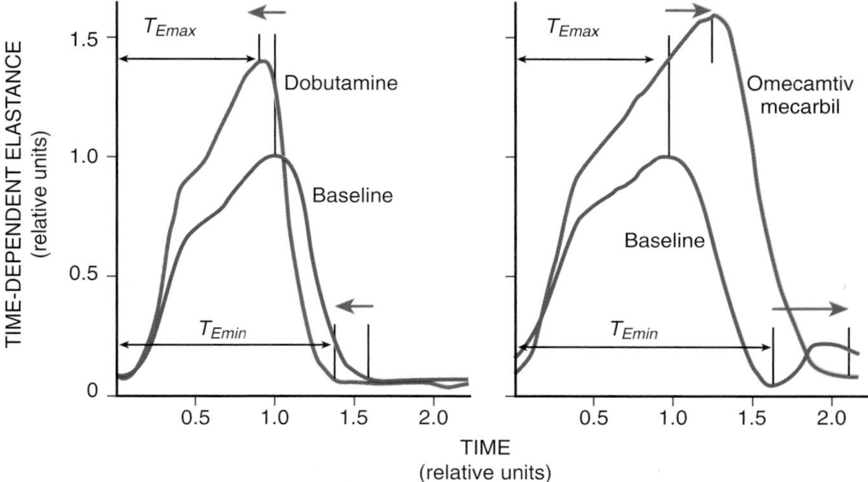

FIGURE 9-2 Time-varying elastance curves in experimental model of heart failure in response to two different types of inotropic stimulation. On the left is the response to the β_1-adrenergic receptor agonist dobutamine, which increases both the magnitude of elastance rise and rate of rise and subsequent decay (e.g., contraction/relaxation kinetics). The kinetic changes are related to targets of protein kinase A phosphorylation induced by the agonist. On the right is the response to the myosin activator omecamtiv mecarbil. A similar augmentation of peak elastance is achieved, but in this case, the myofilament response to calcium increases without any PKA stimulation, and one observed prolonged contraction duration and no acceleration of relaxation. *From Malik FI, Hartman JJ, Elias KA, et al: Cardiac myosin activation: a potential therapeutic approach for systolic heart failure. Science 331:1439–1443, 2011.*

myosin ATPase to increase contraction and has no effect on PKA. Unlike dobutamine, this agent minimally impacts the initial rate of pressure rise (or stiffening) but instead sustains systole longer as stiffening continues (**Figure 9-2**). Another is nitroxyl (HNO), the one-electron reduction of nitric oxide, which has positive inotropic effects independent of PKA, working directly on SR calcium homeostasis and myofilament function via cysteine modification.[70-73] This also impacts elastance more than dP/dt_{max}, in part because it lacks PKA phosphorylation.

Pressure-volume analysis began being applied to human studies of heart disease in the mid-1980s, and has more recently become widely used for assessing cardiac systolic function in basic science investigations conducted in genetically engineered mice.[57,74,75] By this approach, one can derive more accurate and specific quantitations of heart performance than are possible from standard clinical data. **Figure 9-3A** displays human left ventricular (LV) pressure-volume data obtained at rest and during transient reduction of preload volume. The bold loop represents the resting condition, and the labeling depicts end-diastole (point A), isovolumic contraction (point A-B), opening of the aortic valve (point B), ejection (point B-C), isovolumic relaxation (point C-D), opening of the mitral valve and initiation of diastolic filling (point D), and diastolic filling (point D-A). The loop width is stroke volume, the ratio of width to end-diastolic volume is EF, the loop area is external (or stroke) work. When ventricular preload is acutely reduced in the heart, there is a decline in stroke volume and peak pressure per beat (Frank-Starling dependence). Indeed, this set of data could be easily used to generate Frank-Starling curves plotting end-diastolic pressure versus stroke volume or cardiac output. However, one can also determine the ventricular end-systolic elastance by determining the slope of the upper left boundary defined by these loops. This occurs near end-ejection, and the locus of points comprises the end-systolic PV relation (ESPVR). The position and slope of this relation are used to define systolic function. An important feature of the ESPVR is its relative insensitivity to changes in cardiac vascular loading—either preload (sarcomere length or chamber volume) or afterload (force applied to the muscle or cell, or arterial impedance load). In work first conducted in the 1970s and 1980s, isolated and intact hearts demonstrated the utility of the ESPVR for this purpose.[56,76]

Very similar behavior has been demonstrated in intact single myocytes, in which individual cell sarcomere length and force are measured and controlled to generate pseudo force-length loops.[77,78] In one version of this system, cells are coupled to a flexible carbon fiber, and as they develop force, the fiber bends inward. This bending motion can be calibrated to yield force by knowledge of the spring constant of the fiber. Other versions involve a force-transducer attached to a rigid glass or metal fiber. As shown in Figure 9-3B, a picture very similar to that first generated in intact canine and human hearts is revealed, again with a linear end-systolic force-length relation, whose slope is a measure of peak myocyte systolic stiffening. As shown here myocyte end-systolic stiffening is also rather insensitive to the load applied before or during the contraction—so this is not simply a chamber-level phenomenon.

PV analysis facilitates assessment of acute changes in contractility. This is shown by the prototype example in Figure 9-3C, in a patient exposed to the calcium channel blocker verapamil. Indeed, the study from which this figure was taken was among the first to show the impact of this calcium channel blocker on human heart contractility, and the decline in maximal elastance (ESPVR slope shifts downward) is clear.[79] In such acute settings, the rise in end-systolic volume is not accompanied by a change in overall cardiac geometry. However, chronic heart failure involves both contractile changes and remodeling (dilation). An example of this behavior is shown from a study in mice,[80] with the control data shown in solid lines and heart failure data with dotted lines (see Figure 9-3D). The latter display both a depression of the maximal stiffening generated by the heart, but also a marked rightward shift of the entire set of data that indicates structural remodeling/dilation. Patients with dilated cardiomyopathy also typically display both components. In contrast, patients with infarctions that may result in chamber remodeling and a decline in ejection fraction, but have otherwise relatively normal function of the residual wall, will often display peak end-systolic elastances that are similar to a normal heart, but the relation is shifted to the right (higher volumes). As mentioned, geometric formulas can be used to convert pressure-volume into myofibrillar stress and strain[81] to provide a less geometry-dependent parameter (i.e., assess muscle rather than chamber stiffness). However, this is still rather cumbersome and relies on simplifying models. Figure 9-3A also shows a line that slants

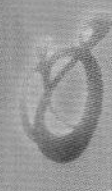

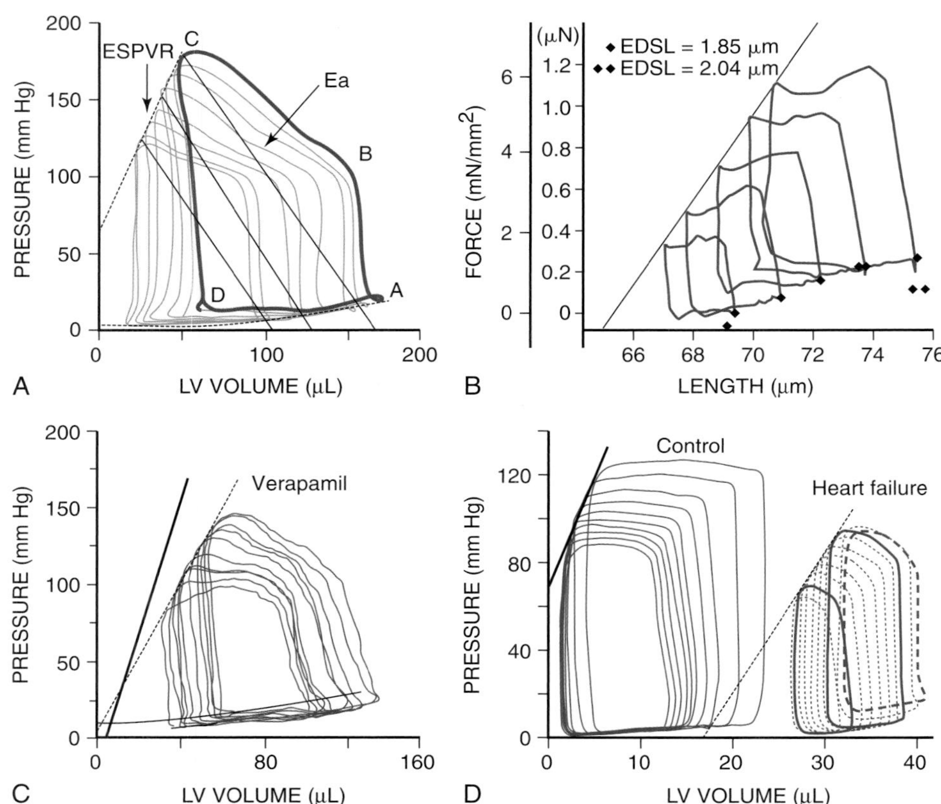

FIGURE 9-3 Pressure-volume (PV) analysis of cardiac function. **A,** Resting *(dark solid loop)* PV loop and multiple cycles derived by varying preload volume in human subjects. Each loop cycle moves counterclockwise in time; (a) end diastole, (b) ejection onset, (c) end systole, (d) onset of diastolic filling. The upper left corners of the set of loops define the end-systolic PV relation (ESPVR), a valuable measure of chamber systolic function, with slope Ees (end-systolic elastance). The group of diagonal lines drawn within several of the beats denotes the arterial load, indexed by their slope (ignoring the negative direction), which is the effective arterial elastance; *Ea,* end-systolic pressure/stroke volume. Ea is similar for each beat despite the decline in preload, a reflection of the fact that the arterial afterload or impedance load is little altered by preload in this range). Ea is a useful measure of ventricular afterload, and the ratio of Ees/Ea is a useful measure of ventricular-vascular interaction. **B,** Similar types of data but obtained from a single cardiac myocyte, with force and sarcomere length measured and controlled to generate "loops." As in the intact heart, there is a time-varying stiffening of the myocyte, and a linear end-systolic force-length dependence. Thus this behavior is intrinsic to the cardiac myocyte. **C,** Prototypical response of ESPVR to a change in contractile state. Data shown are due to acute IV verapamil injection in a human subject.[65] **D,** Example of ventricular remodeling and cardiac systolic depression with sustained cardiac failure. Data in this example were generated using a mouse model of disease (MKK3 overexpression). *B, From Iribe G, Helmes M, Kohl P: Force-length relations in isolated intact cardiomyocytes subjected to dynamic changes in mechanical load. Am J Physiol Heart Circ Physiol 292:H1487–H1497, 2007.*

upward from right to left as a diagonal across each pressure-volume loop. This depicts what is termed the *effective arterial elastance (Ea).*[82-84] Ea is a parameter that incorporates features of the net load imposed on the heart by the arterial vasculature. Ea is equal to the ratio of end-systolic pressure/stroke volume. It is not synonymous with vascular stiffness; indeed its numeric value is mostly influenced by mean arterial resistance (Ea = ESP/SV ≈ R × HR). However, it serves as a useful metric of net ventricular *after*-load—both mean and pulsatile. Unlike arterial pressure, Ea is essentially unaltered even if the filling volume in the heart is changed. This is shown in Figure 9-3A; the slope of each diagonal line (Ea) remains constant despite altered preload. Studies have used this parameter in conjunction with PV relations and Ees to assess mechanisms of inodilator drugs, such as the PDE3 inhibitor amrinone[85] or OPC-18790.[61] As discussed later in this chapter, Ea and Ees are often examined together to quantify heart-vascular coupling.[86-88]

Acute alterations in end-systolic elastance generally reflect changes in contractile function; however, this mechanical property of the chamber is not entirely load-independent, and it may not be the primary reflector of systolic change. The entire relation linking ESPVR is rarely linear in the intact heart, but more often concave downward to the volume axis, giving rise to the frequently observed negative volume-axis intercept of the ESPVR.[89] This means higher slopes (end-systolic elastance, Ees) will occur at lower pressures and lower ones at high pressures. If, for example, a given inotropic stimulation increased pressures while reducing end-systolic volumes, one might observe little apparent change in Ees despite a considerable leftward shift of the relation itself. If the Ees could be measured at the same pressure range as the control state, a higher slope would be observed. Another caveat to interpreting Ees is that this property does not solely reflect contractile properties of the chamber, but is also impacted by chamber geometry and interstitial composition. Chronic elevation of Ees might reflect higher contractility, but it could also be due to wall stiffening from fibrosis, edema, or hypertrophy. A likely example of such changes is the elevation of Ees observed with normal aging.[87,90] In this instance, other "load-insensitive" parameters of systolic function display negligible change, so higher contractility with aging is unlikely to be the cause. Rather, the age-dependent increase in Ees correlates with concomitant rises in diastolic chamber stiffness, so it is more likely structural. Cardiac remodeling associated with chamber hypertrophy is also coupled with a rise in ventricular end-systolic elastance,[91,92] and this can be observed even when myocytes isolated from such hearts display somewhat reduced function.

BEAT-TO-BEAT REGULATION OF SYSTOLIC FUNCTION

There are three primary mechanisms that can regulate beat-to-beat systolic performance of cardiac muscle. These are defined by the dependencies of systolic force on initial sarcomere length, the tension imposed during contraction, and beat frequency. In the intact heart, these components translate to the impact of chamber end-diastolic volume (preload), systemic vascular impedance or wall stress (afterload), and heart rate.

Acute Stretch—The Frank-Starling Effect

Upon being subject to acute stretch, cardiac muscle (or isolated myocytes) displays an immediate rise in force without corresponding changes in intracellular calcium. This is the essence of the multiple loops shown in Figure 9-3A (e.g., during an abrupt change in preload). Initially, the response was attributed to changes in actin-myosin filament overlap, but the marked steepness of the relation between force and length, and its variability with contractile states, made this unlikely.[93] In 1982, Hibberd and Jewell[94] revealed a left shift of the steady-state force-Ca^{2+} relationship with increasing length, both at submaximal and maximal calcium activation, establishing length-dependent Ca^{2+} activation as a central mechanism.

The key remaining question is what generates the change in myofilament-Ca^{2+} dependence with length. A popular theory was that muscle lengthening reduced interfilament spacing between actin and myosin (i.e., stretch in one direction, compressed spacing in the orthogonal one), favoring cross-bridge formation.[95] Stretch extends the I-band region of titin, which spans the sarcomere binding both actin and myosin.[96,97] Sarcomere lengthening might uncoil titin stretching its spring region like a tether, and pull the motor proteins together. Synchrontron x-ray diffraction studies provided support for this mechanism, as did data in which cardiac myocytes were prestretched to varying levels of passive force (pulling out titin) and subsequent length-dependent Ca^{2+}-force responses were found more related to passive force than sarcomere length. Countering the spacing argument are data showing that replacement of cardiac with skeletal TnI (the former but not the latter having PKA phosphorylation sites that when targeted depress Ca^{2+} sensitivity)[95] results in marked opposing changes on interfilament spacing upon PKA stimulation that are uncorrelated with Ca^{2+} sensitivity. Furthermore, reducing lattice spacing by osmotic compression rather than lengthening does not alter Ca^{2+} sensitivity.[95]

Other hypotheses for the Frank-Starling mechanism relate to cooperative filament activation and the notion that bound cross bridges further enhance thin filament activation to facilitate the generation of neighboring cross bridges, either strongly activated cross bridges[98,99] or those more weakly attached.[100] Last, a proline residue at position 144 in slow skeletal TnI becomes a threonine in cTnI, and this appears to confer greater Ca^{2+} sensitivity.[101]

Effect of Systolic Load—The Anrep Effect

The Anrep or slow force response (SFR) is also observed in muscle that is acutely stretched. However, unlike the Frank-Starling change that occurs within one beat without Ca^{2+} change, the SFR is a 25% to 30% additional rise in systolic force over the ensuing 5 to 10 minutes, which is linked to a rise of intracellular calcium.[102-105] The precise source of calcium and whether other mediators are also involved remain under study. Stretch-activated cation channels are well established, though their molecular identity is still the subject of debate. Some propose that members of the non-selective cation transient potential receptor (TRP) channel family play this role. Cardiac muscle expresses several stretch-responsive TRP channels,[106] such as TRPC1, TRPC3, TRPC6, and TRPV1, and they play a role in acute and chronic responses to afterload increase (reviewed in Eder and Molkentin[107]). Seo et al[108] showed the SFR is depressed in myocytes lacking TRPC6 but not TRPC3, and that TRPC6 is required for potent negative modulation of the SFR by protein kinase G. This signaling appears relevant to amplified mechano-sensitivity in models of muscular dystrophy.[108] For TRPC3 and TRPC6, activation can be coupled to $G_{q/11}$ receptor-signaling by DAG stimulation. Channel activity is also mediated by stretch and oxidative stress (for TRPC6), and potentially by depletion of internal Ca^{2+} stores.

An alternative explanation for the SFR attributes Ca^{2+} entry to reverse mode Na^+-Ca^{2+} exchange (NCX) triggered by a rise in intracellular Na^{2+}.[105] This theory also starts with stretch activation of a Gq-receptor, the ETA receptor coupled to AT1 ligand-independent activation, which in turn results in intracellular stimulation of PI3K and Akt.[104] This cascade also involves transactivation of epidermal growth factor receptor (EGFR) to stimulate ERK phosphorylation[109] to activate the surface membrane Na^+/H^+ exchanger to elevate intracellular sodium. Na^+ is exchanged for Ca^{2+} by the NCX, and this leads to the gradual rise in force.[102] It is possible that this mechanism and activation linked to TRP channels are linked, though this remains to be settled. Human cardiac muscle studies tend to support the NHE/NCX pathway.

Effect of Heart Rate

Last, systolic function of cardiac muscle is altered by beat frequency. This occurs within a beat and is due to changes in Ca^{2+} entry into the myocyte and recycling within the sarcoplasmic reticulum.[110] In humans, raising heart rate alone from 70 to 150 min^{-1} increases LV contractility by 100%, and similar ranges are observed in large mammals.[59,111,112] Mice, who operate at a high beat frequency at baseline, have a much smaller change with heart rate.[113] To assess the impact of heart rate on contractility requires measures that are themselves insensitive to load, because chamber filling and effective afterload both vary with frequency (inversely and directly, respectively). One way to do this is by use of Ees or other load-insensitive indexes. The heart rate dependence is markedly blunted in dilated but also hypertrophic cardiac failure, a primary manifestation of abnormal SR calcium handling (see Chapters 1 and 2).[114-117] **Figure 9-4** shows this phenomenon in an intact canine model of dilated heart failure.[117] Two sets of relations are depicted: at rest and after stimulation with the β-adrenergic agonist dobutamine. Contractility was indexed by end-systolic elastance based on pressure-volume analysis. The solid circles show the normal positive dependence of contractility on beat frequency, and solid triangles show its marked depression with heart failure. In the presence of the β-agonist dobutamine, this frequency dependence is augmented in the normal but not failing heart. In controls, the enhanced phosphorylation of the L-type Ca^{2+} channel and phospholamban (among other proteins) increases intracellular calcium, and this is further augmented by a faster frequency (more L-type channel openings, and more internal recycling through the SR) to provide more Ca^{2+} to the myofilaments.[118] By contrast, the failing heart has depressed β-adrenergic signaling and SR function, so this augmentation is depressed. During exercise, both stimulation pathways are relevant, and these data highlight the impact of their loss on contractile reserve in the failing heart.

INTEGRATIVE MEASURES OF SYSTOLIC FUNCTION

At the chamber level, analysis of systolic function generally relies on indirect measures of performance. As already noted, the ability of muscle to stiffen during systole is assessed by Ees and is very useful, though not the most commonly employed index. Many other parameters exist, and can be divided into early isovolumic phase parameters (e.g., dP/dt_{max}, isovolumic contraction time); early-mid ejection phase parameters (e.g., maximal ventricular power, acceleration, velocity of shortening-stress relations); late systolic parameters (e.g., stroke work indexes, end-systolic elastance). To some extent, all are influenced by both intrinsic systolic properties of the sarcomere, by organization of the sarcomere, and muscle fiber into the chamber, and by the loading system to which they are coupled. In this regard, there is no direct measure of contractility—a term that itself remains conceptual rather than physical. Furthermore, not all measures of chamber function index the identical behavior, and there can be striking discrepancies among the measurements. This is less true of human myopathy, but it has been observed in various mouse models with gene targeting.

Chamber systole begins with isovolumetric contraction, and the earliest behavior that can be quantified is the rate of pressure (or force) development by the heart. The maximal rate (dP/dt_{max}) is among the most common and historically used measures of chamber systolic function. Ironically, it is also among the least directly related to physiologically relevant function—i.e., amount of net ejection or work provided during ejection. dP/dt_{max} is depressed in cardiomyopathy, and the absolute level observed in human heart failure is remarkably consistent, being near 1000 mm Hg/sec (normal being near 1600 to 1800 mm Hg/sec). As an index, it has witnessed a remarkable renaissance with the dominance of genetically engineered murine models for studying cardiovascular pathophysiology.

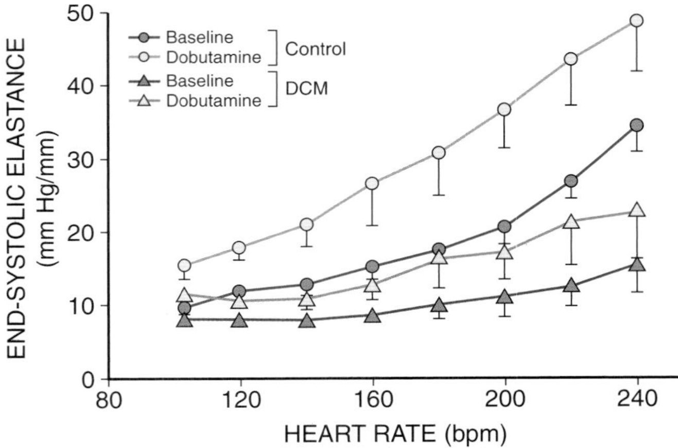

FIGURE 9-4 Force-frequency dependence in intact heart from conscious dog with and without cardiac failure (DCM). The relation is generated in the intact heart, so frequency is presented as heart rate, and contractile force indexed by end-systolic elastance to reduce the potential impact of load-dependent changes. The relation is depressed in cardiac failure. Furthermore, there is an augmentation in the HR-dependent rise in elastance, with concomitant β-adrenergic stimulation provided by dobutamine. This is consistent with an interaction between enhanced calcium transients that are stimulated by the dobutamine and increased intracellular calcium cycling due to higher beat frequency. The interaction of the two mechanisms is also depressed somewhat in cardiac failure. Data are shown as the relative percent increase from resting heart rate. *From Senzaki H, Isoda T, Paolocci N, et al: Improved mechanoenergetics and cardiac rest and reserve function of in vivo failing heart by calcium sensitizer EMD-57033. Circulation 101:1040–1048, 2000.*

dP/dt_{max} is preload dependent in humans and other mammals. This is particularly so in the mouse where changes of even 2 to 3 microliters of end-diastolic volume (10% decline) often result in marked reductions in dP/dt_{max}[113,119] (**Figure 9-5A**). This preload dependence can be minimized by regression of multiple values of dP/dt_{max} versus end-diastolic volume from variably loaded cardiac cycles.[120] While the latter is rarely clinically used because of its complexity, it remains a valuable method to minimize load sensitivity of dP/dt_{max}. dP/dt_{max} is also influenced by internal loading (such as reflected by microfilaments, perhaps titin), extracellular matrix loading (i.e., edema, inflammation, collagen dysregulation), phosphorylation state of MyBP-C, myocyte contractile depression, and the coordination of the chamber walls. Discoordinate contraction associated with bundle branch block depresses dP/dt_{max} acutely even without any primary change in contractile function of the myocytes. This is due to the effect of having part of the wall contract early against a still relaxed portion of the chamber. Pressure rises more slowly as force from one side is dissipated into stretch of the other. Acute increases in dP/dt_{max} associated with biventricular stimulation of a dyssynchronous failing heart occur within a single beat, and similarly do not indicate a change in underlying contractile function, but rather chamber-level consequences of improved coordination of wall contraction.[121,122]

Early midsystolic-ejection parameters are widely used to assess systolic function of the intact chamber. These have been briefly mentioned in the previous section with respect to their derivation from force-velocity behavior. The two most common approaches are preload-adjusted maximal power and stress/rate adjusted circumferential shortening velocity. Maximal power can be assessed from noninvasive-derived aortic flow and arterial pressure data.[123,124] The latter is measured by tonometer or other methods for noninvasive waveform reconstruction. Once obtained, maximal power is normalized to chamber end-diastolic volume (or EDV^2 in dilated failing hearts) to obtain a parameter with relatively little preload and afterload dependence.[125,126] Importantly, its reliability depends upon a relatively high (i.e., arterial level) of afterload and the lack of notable changes in afterload. This limitation can preclude use in the right heart, for example.[127] This index has been applied in a number of clinical studies, including during exercise testing where it displays far more marked sensitivity to contractile function than does the EF.[125] Its advantage in this regard is its simplicity and capacity to be recorded during stress procedures such as exercise. Low levels of reserve power have been shown to predict adverse outcome (need for urgent transplantation or death) in heart failure patients.[128]

The rate-adjusted Vcf-stress relation has also been widely used to index systolic function in animal and human studies. An example of this relation derived from a sequence of

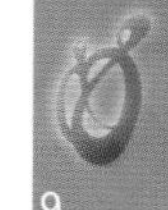

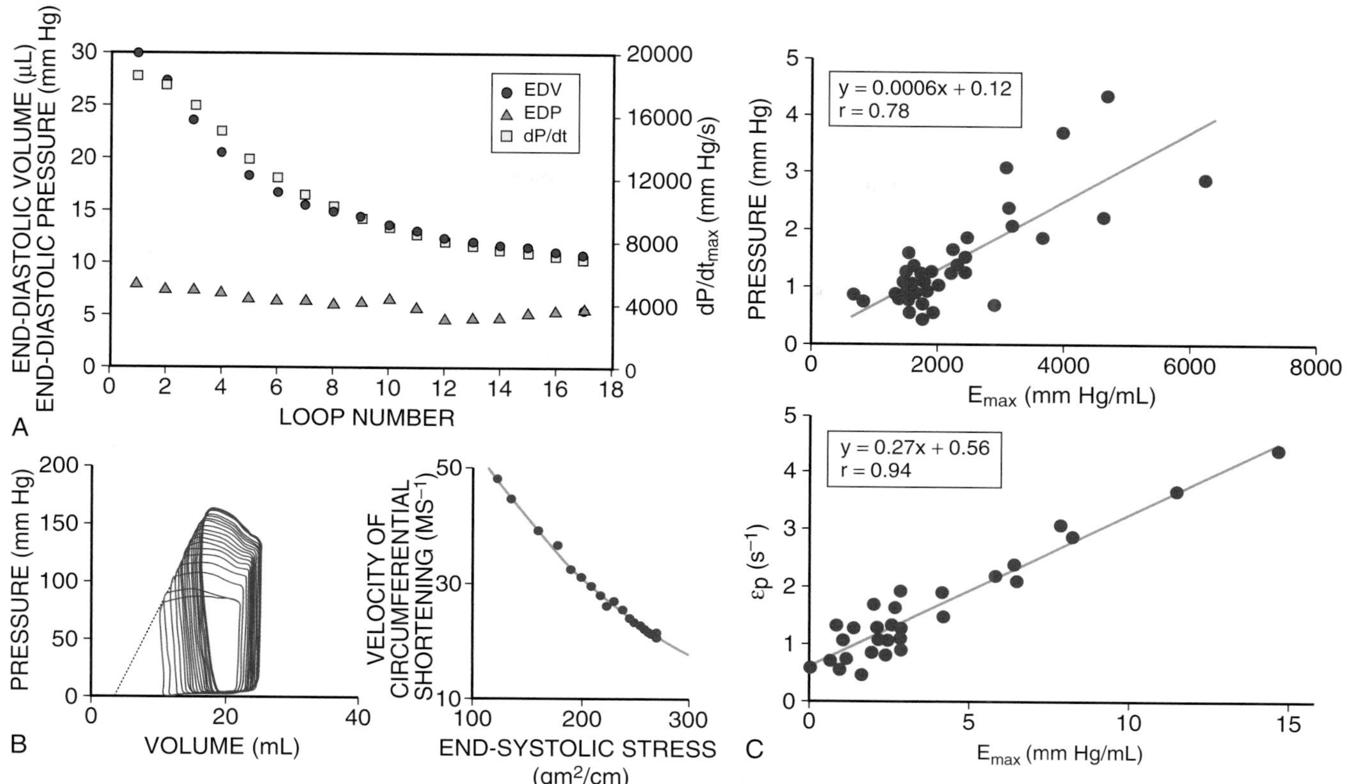

FIGURE 9-5 Indices of contractility in the intact heart. **A,** Preload dependence of dP/dt_{max} in a mouse. Data are derived from a series of cycles at varying preload; beat 0 is at high preload, beat 17 at low preload. Although there is negligible change in end-diastolic pressure for these cycles, preload volume (EDV) declines in direct correlation with dP/dt_{max}. This dramatically shows the marked preload-dependence of dP/dt_{max}, particularly in this species. **B,** Generation of velocity of shortening-stress relations from pressure-volume data at varying afterloads. **C,** Correlation of myocardial strain rate (εp; *y*-axis) or chamber dP/dt_{max} to maximal end-systolic elastance (Emax). Both εp and dP/dt_{max} are commonly used to index contractility. *From Greenberg NL, Firstenberg MS, Castro PL, et al: Doppler-derived myocardial systolic strain rate is a strong index of left ventricular contractility. Circulation 105:99–105, 2002.*

variably afterloaded contractions is shown in Figure 9-5B. Vcf is derived from 2-D mid-chamber level, short axis echocardiographic data, while stress is estimated based on cuff (or invasively measured pressures) and chamber long- and short-axis dimensions and thickness. While many studies have reported individual patient data as a single point—with stress plot on the *x*-axis, and Vcf on the *y*-axis, the actual dependence of each variable on the other depends on chamber preload as well. Furthermore, the stress estimates generally assume homogeneous material wall properties, and may not discriminate between myocyte and extracellular matrix–dependent geometric changes. Still, among parameters, this is relatively unique in attempting to incorporate chamber geometry and derive myocardial properties from chamber-level data.

Tissue Doppler imaging has given rise to strain and strain-rate analysis.[129-132] These approaches essentially quantify myocardial wall motion—much as might be derived from MRI-based tissue tagging methods.[133-135] Actual regional stresses remain unknown, and can influence measured strains and strain rates. Nonetheless, strain rate has been found to correlate with dP/dt_{max} and indices derived from end-systolic pressure-volume relations (see Figure 9-5C),[129] and clearly is prominently influenced by chamber systolic function. In genetic models of hypertrophic cardiomyopathy, tissue Doppler has been used to define early abnormalities of chamber function that precede the evolution of cardiac hypertrophy.[136] Tissue Doppler has been widely employed to index contractile discoordination in patients with cardiac failure and conduction delay.[137,138]

The most commonly used late-systolic parameter is ejection fraction—the chamber translation of fractional shortening. EF is easy to measure, its value is independent of calibration errors of absolute volume assessment (i.e., it is dimensionless), it is moderately sensitive to inotropic changes, and it is rather insensitive to pure alterations in cardiac filling volume (preload). However, EF is highly dependent on arterial impedance load, and so declines can easily reflect both a decrement in underlying myocyte function and reduced shortening because of higher load. This is particularly important in failing hearts where the depressed heart is coupled to high arterial impedance. EF is also heart rate dependent, declining at faster rates. This effect is likely important to the enhancement of EF with chronic β-blockade therapy—in addition to any primary augmentation of underlying systolic function because of the treatment. EF also reflects chamber dilation/remodeling since the denominator (EDV) is increased in such ventricles while the numerator is often near normal range short of severe cardiodepression or restrictive filling. In this sense, the pathophysiologic implication of an acutely reduced EF, which is a strong correlate of other parameters—such as end-systolic elastance or even dP/dt_{max}—may not be present if the mechanism involves chronic chamber remodeling and myocyte depression. Last, EF is not the most sensitive parameter to contractile change.[13]

The Frank-Starling curve remains an important element of systolic analysis, but it is limited because of strong afterload and heart rate dependencies, and ambiguities associated with the use of end-diastolic filling pressure to index preload. The latter is discussed in more detail in a subsequent section. An alternative approach has been to assess relations between cardiac stroke work and preload (preload-recruitable stroke work)—the latter indexed by end-diastolic volume rather than pressure.[139] Stroke work is less afterload dependent than stroke volume, as it incorporates pressure as well, and the SW-EDV relation is both linear and minimally influenced by chamber load, while still reflecting systolic function. A further advantage is that it has units of force, and is therefore chamber-size independent. Values for the slope of this relation are typically between 75 and 90 mm Hg and are very similar between rat, mouse, canine, porcine, and human, and other mammalian ventricles. As with Ees, methods to assess PRSW from single-beat data and noninvasive analysis have been reported.[140]

IMPACT OF PERICARDIAL LOADING ON SYSTOLIC FUNCTION

The intact chamber not only imposes complex filling and ejection loads on the heart during systole to modify its function, but also contains the chambers by a pericardial membrane that couples filling pressures from one chamber to another. While the influence of the pericardium on cardiac diastolic function is long well recognized, its impact on systolic function relations, such as the Frank-Starling relation, has remained underappreciated.[141] However, studies have shown the importance of this interaction for generating the apparent descending limb of the Frank-Starling relation. While increased length and thus sarcomere stretch over 2.4 μ has been suggested to explain a decline in force generated by skeletal muscle because of reduced myofilament overlap, cardiac tissue cannot be stretched to this extent because of the extracellular matrix and cytoskeletal membrane proteins within the myocyte. Yet, cardiac output is often observed to decline with high preloads or conversely increase with preload reduction—leading to the presumption of operation along a descending limb in the failure state. The more likely explanation has been demonstrated by Tyberg et al, and relates to the importance of transmural pressure (not absolute chamber pressure) for determining the net stretch on the heart.[142,143] In patients with dilated cardiomyopathy (DCM), increased end-diastolic pressures may not be associated with elevated transmural pressure because of concomitantly higher extrinsic (pericardial) pressures. With a reduction in preload volume, actual transmural distending pressures have been shown to rise, so that real myocyte stretch is actually increasing rather than declining with the fall in EDP. Plots of CO versus EDP can appear biphasic, whereas those between CO and EDV are linear. This affects any relationship in which filing pressure is used to index the level of chamber preload.

VENTRICULAR-ARTERIAL INTERACTION

An important feature of systolic cardiac function is its dependence on the arterial loading system into which the heart must eject. The interaction of both components ultimately determines systemic variables such as cardiac output, ejection fraction, external work, mechanical efficiency, systolic pressure, and so forth. Depending upon the matching of cardiac and vascular properties, these variables can be optimized or compromised. Furthermore, the interaction of properties of the systolic ventricle and vascular system play a critical role in determining the cardiac output and blood pressure response of the heart failure patient to commonly used therapeutic interventions, such as vasodilators, diuretics, and inotropes. This interaction is also important for understanding the syndrome of cardiac failure with preserved EF. Thus it is useful to both understand how coupling can be studied and the implications for ventricular-arterial interaction in cardiac failure.

Among the more successful methods used to assess ventricular-vascular coupling is the pressure-volume framework, employing the ESPVR and the effective arterial elastance (Ea), which as previously described, indexes arterial properties.[144] As noted in Figure 9-3, E_a is the ratio of end-systolic pressure to stroke volume and its value is dominated by mean arterial resistance and heart rate. It is also influenced by phasic (reactive) loading properties of the arterial system—i.e., properties due to wall compliance, wave reflections, inertance; essentially any property not related to mean resistance. In this description, coupling is generally expressed by a ratio of E_a to the ESPVR slope (i.e., E_a/E_{es}) (**Figure 9-6A**).

Prior studies have shown that when the E_a/E_{es} ratio is near 1.0, there is optimal transfer of energy or work (power or SW) from the heart to arterial system.[145-147] Data obtained in isolated canine hearts first displayed this dependence for both work and cardiac efficiency, and subsequent studies have confirmed similar relations in intact hearts.[148] In normal individuals, the coupling ratio is near 0.8, matching ventricular and arterial properties to yield maximal power, efficiency, and external work. Importantly, this optimally matched condition is maintained during exercise,[147] and may relate to an evolutionary process designed to maintain a minimum relative cardiac/body size ratio.[149]

Work or power output is far from optimal, however, in hearts with depressed contractility and increased vascular loading, typical of the failing dilated heart. Asanoi et al[150] first reported coupling ratios in patients with normal, moderate, and severely depressed LV function. In the patients with reduced EF, ratios rise greater than 3 (see Figure 9-6B), consistent with a decline in cardiac efficiency and effective external work.[88] This relation between heart and artery can play a major role in determining whether a given pharmaceutical intervention will improve chamber function or diminish it. In this example, the DCM patient with high systemic resistance was administered a bolus of intravenous nitroglycerin. The resulting beat-to-beat decline in arterial resistance led to an increase in the width of the pressure-volume loop—increasing stroke volume (and thus cardiac output) by nearly 50% and improving power output. The same intervention in a normal subject would largely reduce work or power output if basal coupling were already near optimal.

Coupling between heart and arterial effective elastance is also central to understanding whether a given intervention is more likely to enhance cardiac output or alternatively influence blood pressures. Dilated cardiomyopathy is typically associated with a depressed maximal chamber elastance (reduced Ees), and this predicts that, for any decline in arterial afterload, the heart will behave principally as a pressure source, providing similar levels of systemic pressure by varying markedly the ejected volume. In contrast, hearts with increased systolic elastance—often observed in hypertrophied syndromes—behave as flow sources, providing similar levels of cardiac output despite

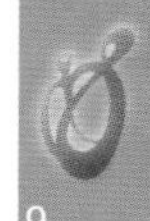

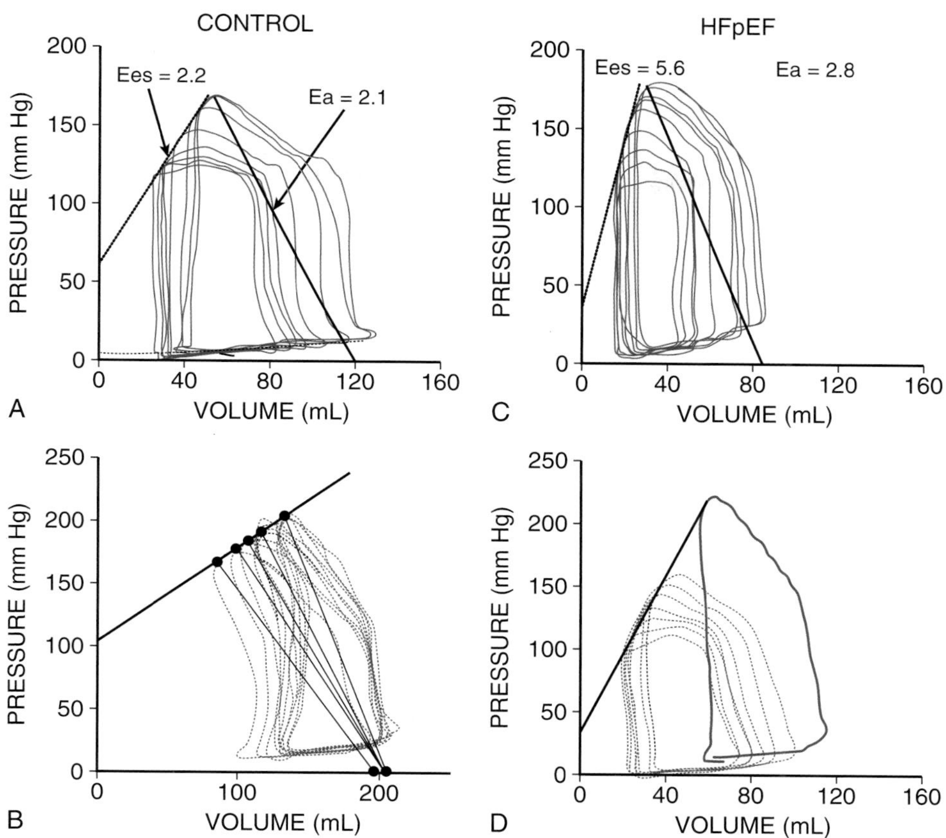

FIGURE 9-6 Ventricular-arterial coupling. **A,** Resting human PV relations showing normal matching between end-systolic elastance (Ees) and arterial elastance (Ea). This matching results in optimized cardiac function and efficiency. **B,** In contrast, the failing heart displays a reduced Ees (depressed systolic function) and elevated Ea (higher afterload), yielding a decline in chamber power output and metabolic efficiency. **C,** Subject with CHF and preserved ejection fraction. In such patients, Ees appears elevated over age/pressure-matched controls, and is accompanied by a further rise in arterial elastance because of reduced vascular distensibility. **D,** This pathophysiology can explain marked increases in blood pressure and cardiac workload with exertion. Shown here is an example subject during isometric hand exercise, with the resting PV loops *(dotted lines)* and stress-response loop as solid. *From Kawaguchi M, Hay I, Fetics B, et al: Combined ventricular systolic and arterial stiffening in patients with heart failure and preserved ejection fraction: implications for systolic and diastolic reserve limitations. Circulation 107:714–720, 2003.*

changes in afterload (or preload), but inducing marked changes in systemic pressures.

The behavior described for a hypertrophic heart may play an important role in the syndrome of cardiac failure with preserved EF (HFpEF).[92] This is still referred to by some as *diastolic heart failure* though the disease reflects far more than that. Nearly half of patients over age 65 who present with symptoms of cardiac failure have an EF that exceeds 50%. While this has been generally taken to mean that systolic function is itself normal, that is not necessarily the case. Differences in wall geometry, such as smaller cavities with ventricular hypertrophy, might otherwise lead to elevated EFs so that an EF of 50% is not in fact normal. Another feature of these individuals is that they can develop exacerbated ventricular end-systolic stiffening—beyond that observed with aging and/or hypertension. Studies in asymptomatic patients of varying ages have revealed that Ees (chamber systolic stiffening) increases in tandem with age-related arterial stiffening.[90] This was demonstrated in a large population study, and intriguingly women developed greater age-dependent increases in both Ees and Ea than men.[87] This may play a contributing role to the higher prevalence of HFpEF in elderly women.

Combined increases in Ees and Ea can potently influence the pressures developed by the heart in response to changes in chamber filling and arterial load. Increased ventricular systolic stiffening means that even small increases or decreases in preload will amplify into marked changes in systolic pressure. This may contribute to the increased diuretic and orthostatic sensitivity in the elderly. In patients with cardiac failure symptoms yet EF greater than 50%, such stiffening is increased further,[92] although studies have shown this is likely related to the presence of systolic hypertension and ventricular hypertrophy, both common features of HFpEF patients.[86,151] The hemodynamic consequence is greater sensitivity of the heart to altered loading, exacerbated blood pressure lability, and potentially increased energetic demand to deliver reserve cardiac output.[92] Indeed, growing evidence supports a central role of limited function reserve in this disease, and these mechanical components likely contribute.[152-154]

Figure 9-6C shows an example of a patient with heart failure and preserved EF, demonstrating the greatly increased stiffening of the ventricle during systole, and increased vascular stiffening. EF may appear normal in such individuals, but this does not necessarily mean that systolic function is normal and the problem resides solely with diastolic abnormalities. Increased chamber systolic stiffening and its impact on ventricular-arterial interaction may play an important pathophysiologic role in symptom lability and hypertension and dysfunction during stress (see Figure 9-6D). Such abnormalities are consistent with the paroxysmal nature of this disorder, frequent flash pulmonary edema associated with hypertension, and sensitivity to preload reduction (diuretics). In this respect, enhanced (as with the more traditional

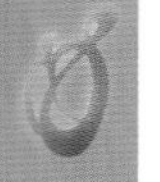

diminished) systolic elastance may be similarly a valuable target for therapeutic intervention.

TREATING SYSTOLIC DYSFUNCTION

Despite a defining role in heart failure for many patients, the amelioration of systolic dysfunction by pharmacotherapy has generally not been a successful therapeutic approach to date (see Chapter 33). The oldest known treatment is digitalis, though the magnitude of contractile stimulation achieved by this agent in human heart failure remains essentially unknown, and it is not potent in experimental models. Acute human treatment has relied on cAMP generation either by stimulation of the β-adrenergic pathway (e.g., dobutamine) or by inhibition of a primary cAMP-targeted phosphodiesterase type 3 (e.g., milrinone). Both ultimately stimulate contraction by cAMP-dependent activation of protein kinase A, targeting calcium handling, and myofilament proteins among other key pathways involved with contractile force generation. Central to this effect is the rise in intracellular calcium involved with contraction. While useful for acute modulation, chronic effects are detrimental,[155] and this has stymied efforts in developing approaches targeting this signaling.

The generation of genetically engineered mice revealed that stimulation of components of this signaling pathway can yield beneficial rather than worsening heart failure outcome. Many of these are now targets for early clinical trials using small molecules and/or gene transfer approaches. One prime example is inhibition of the β-receptor kinase GRK-2, which phosphorylates the β-receptor to suppress signaling and stimulate receptor internalization and desensitization (see Chapter 6). Mutant versions of GRK-2 that lack this kinase activity have been successful in ameliorating various models of heart failure and myocardial infarction in rodents and large mammals.[156,157] Another approach is to target adenylate cyclase. Blockade of AC type 5 is associated with reduced heart failure[158] and improved longevity,[159] though upregulation of the other major isoform, AC-6, has been suggested to ameliorate heart failure.[160] This suggests where and how cAMP is generated is critical and compartmentation of this signaling central to the nature of long-term effects. Controversies persist regarding the precise nature of the alternative signaling with both AC isoforms. Others have focused on deficiencies of the SR proteins such as phospholamban, SERCA2a, and the phosphatase regulator I-1. Gene and/or small molecule clinical studies are under development to test whether upregulation of SERCA2a, for example, can ameliorate systolic dysfunction as it has clearly done in many different experimental animal models.[31,161-163]

Another major area of investigation is in agents that more directly influence the myofilaments to augment their response to a given level of trigger calcium. Referred to as a group as *calcium sensitizers*, this class can have many different targeting mechanisms such as modifying calcium–troponin C interactions or enhancing the myofibrillar ATPase. The theoretical advantages of such agents are several. First, by bypassing the adrenergic system and directly targeting the myofilaments, these drugs should work similarly well in failing as in normal hearts. An example of this behavior is shown in **Figure 9-7A**. In this canine model of heart failure,[117] the dobutamine-stimulated contraction is markedly depressed compared with the normal control response, whereas the response to the sensitizer, EMD-57033, which is thought to target the myosin head to enhance actin attachment, is similar in both conditions. Another feature of these agents is that they can enhance contraction without requiring the level of energy use needed when this occurs via a cAMP-dependent pathway. In this sense, pure

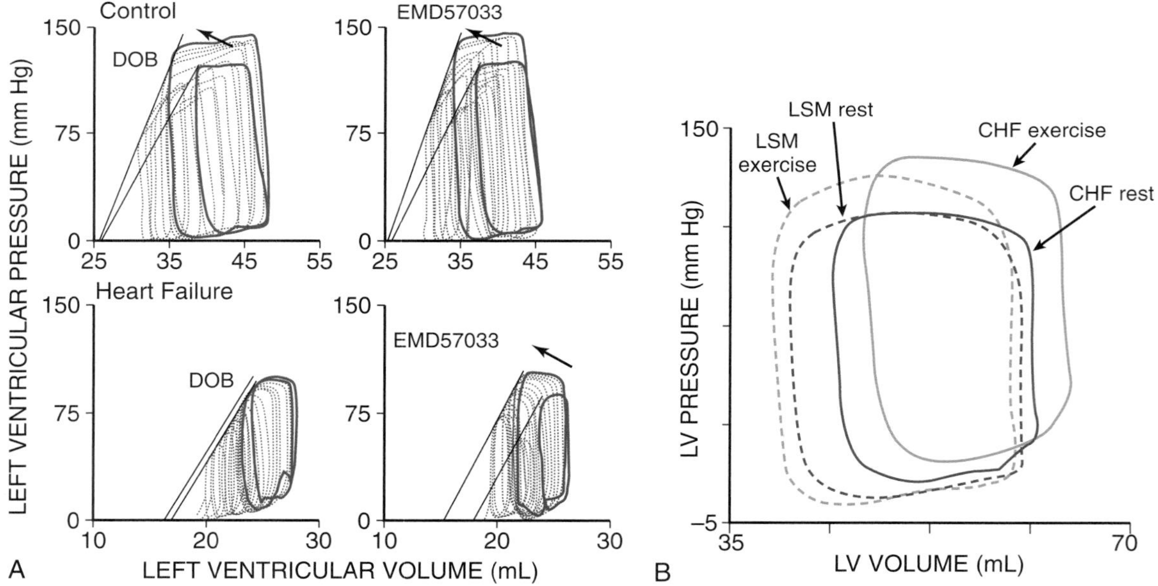

FIGURE 9-7 **A,** Influence of dobutamine (DOB) versus a calcium sensitizer (EMD-57033) on contractile reserve in normal versus failing hearts. In the control hearts *(upper panels)*, both drugs stimulate contractility almost identically, reflected by the leftward shift and slope increase in the end-systolic PV relation. However, in failing hearts *(lower panels)*, the response to dobutamine is markedly depressed, whereas the contractile response to the sensitizer is maintained, consistent with its more distal site of action, directly on the myofilaments. **B,** Enhanced effectiveness from a calcium sensitizer on systolic function during exercise in a canine model of heart failure. The improvement in function reflected by the left shift of the PV loop and increase in its width (stroke volume) is modest in the heart when at rest, but potentiated during exercise. ***A,*** *From Senzaki H, Isoda T, Paolocci N, et al: Improved mechanoenergetics and cardiac rest and reserve function of in vivo failing heart by calcium sensitizer EMD-57033. Circulation 101:1040–1048, 2000.* ***B,*** *From Tachibana H, Cheng HJ, Ukai T, et al: Levosimendan improves LV systolic and diastolic performance at rest and during exercise after heart failure. Am J Physiol Heart Circ Physiol 288:H914–H922, 2005.*

sensitizers should improve cardiac efficiency. Third, their effects on the kinetics of contraction differ from traditional cAMP/PKA-dependent inotropes, in that they have little impact on early rates of contraction (i.e., dP/dt_{max}), but more impact on later phases of systolic function, such as net work, end-systolic elastance, and the duration of systole. This was previously demonstrated for omecamtiv mecarbil in Figure 9-2B. Last, increasing calcium sensitivity means that the impact on systolic function will itself vary with the stimulation of calcium by other means. At rest, calcium activation is reduced, so the impact on rest contractility of the sensitizer is commensurately less. However, with exercise, there are the catecholamine and heart rate–triggered changes that, even while depressed, can still enhance the calcium trigger and thus increase the inotropic effect from the sensitizer. This was nicely demonstrated in an animal study of levosimendan[164] (see Figure 9-7B). Improved systolic function assessed by pressure-volume relations was modest at rest, but much more marked in animals doing treadmill exercise.

One example of a sensitizer is levosimendan, which was originally identified by its interaction with TnC and capacity to enhance myofilament force generation. However, the drug was also shown active in inhibiting phosphodiesterase type 3, which explained some calcium dependence to its effects, and ATP-sensitive potassium channels that likely contributed to systemic vasodilation.[165] Whereas early trials were promising, larger controlled studies were less so.[166] Still, this was not a real test of a pure sensitizer given the complex pharmacology involved. However, several other agents are currently being tested, including a small molecule identified to specifically enhance myofibrillar ATPase activity. This drug, omecamtiv mecarbil, prolongs the systolic period because it increases the probability that a cross bridge will be in the active force-generating state. It does not appear to have any effects on cAMP signaling, and in this sense is one of the purer "calcium-sensitizing" types of agents yet tested.[69,167]

Another novel approach to increasing contractility is the use of nitroxyl, or HNO. This is the reduced form of nitric oxide coupled with hydrogen; the molecule does not dissociate but attaches to thiolates (negatively charged cysteine residues) on selective proteins to modify function.[72,168] The reaction is reversibly controlled by redox state, in that enhancing reducing conditions can block it. HNO was first reported to enhance systolic function in the intact canine heart model of HF, and later cellular mechanisms for this effect have been revealed. These include demonstration of direct enhancement of SR calcium uptake and release,[73] the former related to HNO targeting of C674 in SERCA2a,[169] and at one or more of the three cysteines in phospholamban.[170] HNO also targets the myofilaments with disulfide bonds identified coupling actin and tropomyosin, and myosin heavy chain and myosin light chain-1.[71]

SYSTOLIC EFFECTS OF DYSSYNCHRONY AND RESYNCHRONIZATION (see also Chapter 35)

It has long been recognized that discoordinate cardiac contraction itself reduces the systolic performance of the chamber, and recent developments in therapies to resynchronize contraction have shown this to be a valuable target for heart failure treatment. Conduction disease at or above the atrioventricular (AV) node affects chronotropic competence and effective preload (and left atrial pressure). Both short and excessively long AV delays reduce net LV filling.[171,172] Infranodal conduction delay—commonly left bundle branch block (LBBB) pattern—induces discoordinate contraction.[173-175] DCM hearts, with an LBBB, display early activation of the septal wall with lateral prestretch, followed by markedly delayed lateral contraction with late systolic septal stretch toward the RV. Cardiac discoordination induced by LBBB or RV-ventricular pacing depresses systolic function, increasing the end-systolic volumes at a given pressure (rightward shift of the ESPVR), prolongs isovolumic relaxation,[176-178] and has been coupled to widening of the QRS complex.[178] The energetic cost of contraction can increase relative to effective ejection, because the early activated myocardium largely serves to increase preload on the lateral free wall, leaving the late activated wall to contract at higher stress while wasting work by stretching the more pliable early activated territory.[179-181]

These mechanical effects of discoordinate contraction were the impetus for studies performed over a decade ago in which right ventricular preexcitation was used to treat patients with hypertrophic cardiomyopathy.[182] In such patients, the institution of RV-apex pacing increased end-systolic volumes, reduced dP/dt_{max} and other parameters of systolic function, and importantly in this instance, resulted in a decline in hyperdynamic ejection and thus cavity obliteration. Importantly, this effect did not depend upon the presence of asymmetric hypertrophy—but was equally if not more effective in individuals with concentric LVH associated with symptoms of cardiac failure.[183] **Figure 9-8A** shows time tracings of apical segmental volume in a patient with hypertrophic cardiomyopathy subjected to acute RV apical pacing. Whereas the original data show normal timing of systolic ejection and filling, pacing results in premature contraction of the region, and later restretch (volume increase) during what is still systole. This results in residual systolic volume that is not ejected, so the end-systolic pressure-volume relation shifts rightward (see Figure 9-8B).[91] Though therapeutic generation of ventricular dyssynchrony in patients with septal hypertrophy proved less effective,[184,185] a small single-center trial in patients with concentric LVH and cavity obliteration found benefits from reducing systolic contraction in these patients. Larger controlled trials remain to be done.

The opposite approach—resynchronizing the left ventricle in individuals with dilated cardiomyopathy and underlying basal discoordination because of LBBB—has been far more successful (see Chapter 35). Biventricular pacing or univentricular pacing of the LV lateral free wall can recoordinate contraction and is associated with systolic improvement.[121,122,186-188] Cardiac resynchronization effects manifest abruptly (i.e., rise in dP/dt_{max}, arterial pressure, Figure 9-8C) occurring within one beat, and reflects increased systolic flow. Chronic noninvasive studies have reported sustained responses of similar magnitude.[121] When displayed as ventricular pressure-volume loops, the resynchronization effect can be observed as a widening of the loop (enhanced stroke volume), decline in end-systolic wall stress (left shift of end-systolic pressure-volume point), and increased cardiac work (see Figure 9-8D). Importantly, the latter is not accompanied by increases in energy consumption, but to the contrary, has been shown to be coupled with a decline in energy consumption.[189] Studies have not demonstrated major effects on

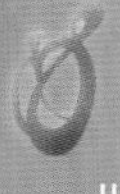

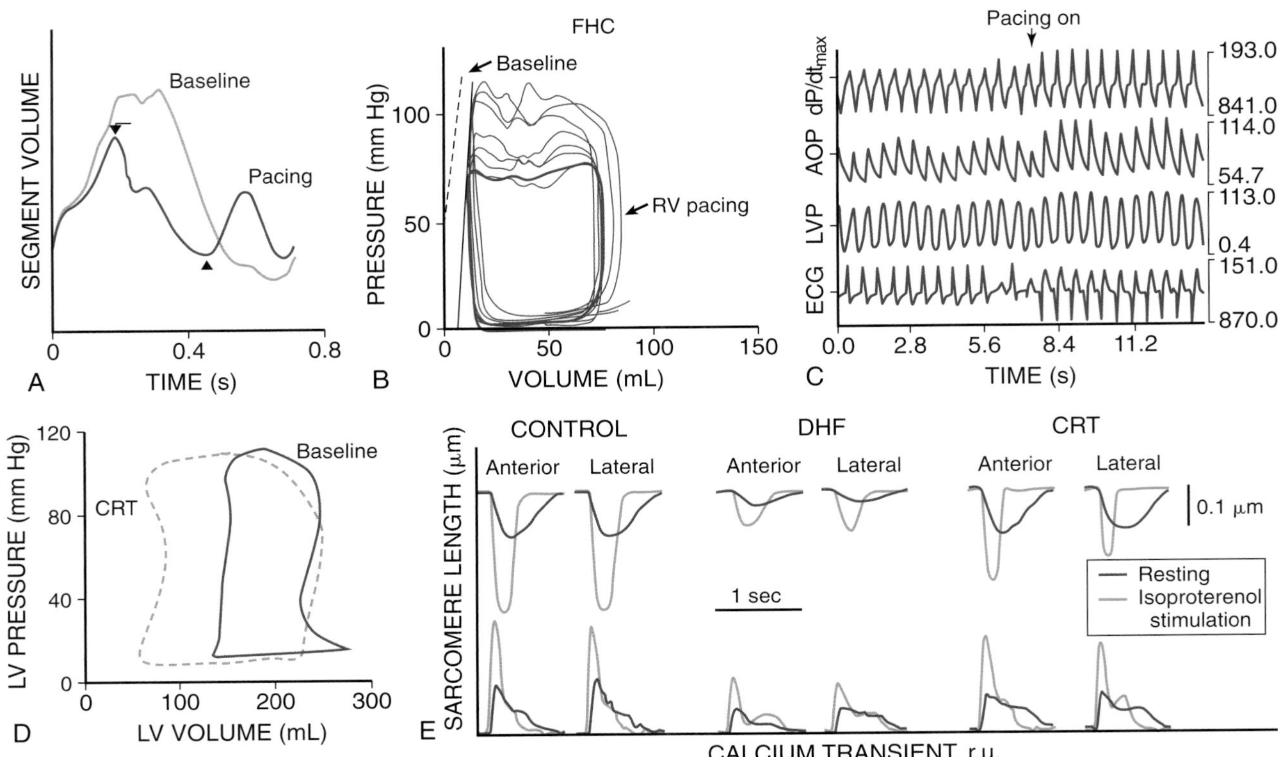

FIGURE 9-8 Impact of ventricular discoordination and resynchronization on chamber systolic function. **A,** Dyssynchrony generated by RV apex pacing in the human ventricle, with local pressure-apical volume loops displayed. The resting condition *(baseline)* shows normal timing of systolic ejection. With early stimulation of this region, shortening occurs at low pressure but is converted to stretch later in systole as the rest of the heart contracts. **B,** Global PV relations during RV apex pacing are compared with sinus controls *(dashed ESPVRs)*. Dyssynchrony results in an increase in end-systolic volume, a rightward shift of the ESPVR, and thus decline in effective systolic function. **C,** Resynchronization in human DCM patient with LBBB. Acute biventricular stimulation enhances dP/dt_{max}, aortic pressure (AOP) and the pulse magnitude, and peak LV pressure (LVP) as shown after the arrow. This effect is near immediate. **D,** Example of pressure-volume loops with resynchronization *(dashed line)* showing enhanced function, increased loop width, and left shift of end-systolic point *(upper left corner)*. This is opposite to the effect in panel B when dyssynchrony was induced by RV-apex pacing. **E,** Myocyte contraction and calcium transients at rest and after adrenergic stimulation. Cells are isolated from hearts with normal function, dyssynchronous heart failure (DHF), or resynchronized heart failure (CRT). DHF cells display markedly depressed rest function and calcium transients, and their responsiveness to isoproterenol (ISO) stimulation is depressed. CRT cells display improvements in both rest and ISO responses for both shortening and calcium transients. These changes are observed in cells obtained throughout the heart, specifically from both early- and late-activated regions. ***B,** From Pak PH, Maughan WL, Baughman KL, et al: Mechanism of acute mechanical benefit from VDD pacing in hypertrophied heart: similarity of responses in hypertrophic cardiomyopathy and hypertensive heart disease. Circulation 98:242–248, 1998.*

diastolic function to date, although there is evidence of reverse cardiac remodeling associated with this therapy.

These initial studies established improvement in systolic function at the chamber level—although, as with acute dyssynchrony, this was likely because of the coordination of contraction and not a primary improvement in myocardial contractility. However, chronic cardiac resynchronization therapy (CRT) treatment enhances rest and systolic reserve function, demonstrated by exercise capacity and the response to increases in heart rate. This has been coupled to upregulation in myocardial gene expression of β_1-receptors, phospholamban, and SERCA2a, among other genes.[190-192] Importantly, new data from animal models of dyssynchronous heart failure and CRT have revealed improvement in resting myocyte function and adrenergic reserve. Myocyte results from canine hearts subjected to either 6 weeks of rapid atrial pacing in the presence of an LBBB (dyssynchronous failure [DHF]) or 3 weeks of this mode followed by 3 weeks of rapid biventricular pacing (CRT) are displayed in Figure 9-8E.[193] Both models involve 6 weeks of tachypacing, a method to induce dilated failure in the mammalian heart. Whereas some global improvement with CRT was observed, overall both groups displayed features of dilated HF. Yet, whereas rest and isoproterenol stimulated sarcomere shortening and calcium transient responses in DHF myocytes were markedly depressed compared with normal controls, myocytes from CRT hearts displayed improvement in both variables under both conditions. The mechanisms include reversal of several abnormalities of cycling regulation, and improved adrenergic signaling cascades, including enhanced suppression of inhibitory G protein and upregulation of both β_1-receptor–coupled signaling and adenylate cyclase activation.[193] Most intriguingly, we also see a reversal of enhanced inhibitory G protein–coupled signaling that is observed in both dyssynchronous and synchronous heart failure. This is reversed by CRT via a mechanism involving the upregulation of regulator of G-protein signaling: RGS2 and RGS3.[194] Another mechanism by which CRT improves systolic function is by enhancing myofilament-calcium sensitivity. As observed in a canine model, this involves the reactivation of glycogen synthase kinase 3-beta, enhancing phosphorylation of several proteins that localize to the the Z-disk and M-band.[195] Thus chronic CRT does enhance systolic function by mechanisms that involve more than chamber-level mechanics. Other studies have revealed potent influences on mitochondrial ATP synthesis,[196] ion channels involved with repolarization and arrhythmia,[197,198] and other features.[199]

SUMMARY

Advances in noninvasive techniques and availability of new systems to directly assess cardiac systolic function have advanced our understanding of its presence and

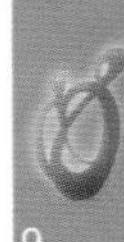

modification by therapies in advanced heart failure. Although central to much heart failure, systolic dysfunction has been difficult to therapeutically target thus far. However, the recent data on cardiac resynchronization showing chronic benefits on function, symptoms, and mortality for a therapy that improves systolic function suggest optimism is warranted. Understanding how CRT functions at the molecular level may indeed provide insights into heart failure in general. Similar optimism stems from recent success in animal models where systolic function is enhanced by gene manipulation of signaling and/or calcium handling distal to the adrenergic receptor. After nearly 15 years of relative inactivity on the inotropy front, new trials now under way may change the way we view improving systole for the failing heart. As these approaches are developed, the assessment of systolic function and its response to therapy should again become an important focus for heart failure researchers and practitioners.

References

1. Marks AR: Calcium cycling proteins and heart failure: mechanisms and therapeutics. *J Clin Invest* 123:46–52, 2013.
2. Bayeva M, Gheorghiade M, Ardehali H: Mitochondria as a therapeutic target in heart failure. *J Am Coll Cardiol* 61:599–610, 2013.
3. Kubli DA, Gustafsson AB: Mitochondria and mitophagy: the yin and yang of cell death control. *Circ Res* 111:1208–1221, 2012.
4. Wang X, Pattison JS, Su H: Posttranslational modification and quality control. *Circ Res* 112:367–381, 2013.
5. Willis MS, Patterson C: Proteotoxicity and cardiac dysfunction—Alzheimer's disease of the heart? *N Engl J Med* 368:455–464, 2013.
6. Shao D, Oka S, Brady CD, et al: Redox modification of cell signaling in the cardiovascular system. *J Mol Cell Cardiol* 52:550–558, 2012.
7. van Berlo JH, Maillet M, Molkentin JD: Signaling effectors underlying pathologic growth and remodeling of the heart. *J Clin Invest* 123:37–45, 2013.
8. Shiojima I, Sato K, Izumiya Y, et al: Disruption of coordinated cardiac hypertrophy and angiogenesis contributes to the transition to heart failure. *J Clin Invest* 115:2108–2118, 2005.
9. Sano M, Minamino T, Toko H, et al: p53-induced inhibition of Hif-1 causes cardiac dysfunction during pressure overload. *Nature* 446:444–448, 2007.
10. Dixon JA, Spinale FG: Myocardial remodeling: cellular and extracellular events and targets. *Annu Rev Physiol* 73:47–68, 2011.
11. Koitabashi N, Danner T, Zaiman AL, et al: Pivotal role of cardiomyocyte TGF-beta signaling in the murine pathological response to sustained pressure overload. *J Clin Invest* 121:2301–2312, 2011.
12. Kakkar R, Lee RT: Intramyocardial fibroblast myocyte communication. *Circ Res* 106:47–57, 2010.
13. Kass DA, Maughan WL, Guo ZM, et al: Comparative influence of load versus inotropic states on indexes of ventricular contractility: experimental and theoretical analysis based on pressure-volume relationships. *Circulation* 76:1422–1436, 1987.
14. Morita H, Nagai R, Seidman JG, et al: Sarcomere gene mutations in hypertrophy and heart failure. *J Cardiovasc Transl Res* 3:297–303, 2010.
15. McNally EM, Golbus JR, Puckelwartz MJ: Genetic mutations and mechanisms in dilated cardiomyopathy. *J Clin Invest* 123:19–26, 2013.
16. Solaro RJ, Henze M, Kobayashi T: Integration of troponin I phosphorylation with cardiac regulatory networks. *Circ Res* 112:355–366, 2013.
17. Solaro RJ, Kobayashi T: Protein phosphorylation and signal transduction in cardiac thin filaments. *J Biol Chem* 286:9935–9940, 2011.
18. Warren SA, Briggs LE, Zeng H, et al: Myosin light chain phosphorylation is critical for adaptation to cardiac stress. *Circulation* 126:2575–2588, 2012.
19. Previs MJ, Beck Previs S, Gulick J, et al: Molecular mechanics of cardiac myosin-binding protein C in native thick filaments. *Science* 337:1215–1218, 2012.
20. Brickson S, Fitzsimons DP, Pereira L, et al: In vivo left ventricular functional capacity is compromised in cMyBP-C null mice. *Am J Physiol Heart Circ Physiol* 292:H1747–H1754, 2007.
21. McConnell BK, Jones KA, Fatkin D, et al: Dilated cardiomyopathy in homozygous myosin-binding protein-C mutant mice. *J Clin Invest* 104:1771, 1999.
22. Nagayama T, Takimoto E, Sadayappan S, et al: Control of in vivo left ventricular contraction/relaxation kinetics by myosin binding protein C: protein kinase A phosphorylation dependent and independent regulation. *Circulation* 116:2399–2408, 2007.
23. Murphy AM, Kogler H, Georgakopoulos D, et al: Transgenic mouse model of stunned myocardium. *Science* 287:488–491, 2000.
24. Nagayama T, Takimoto E, Sadayappan S, et al: Control of in vivo left ventricular [correction] contraction/relaxation kinetics by myosin binding protein C: protein kinase A phosphorylation dependent and independent regulation. *Circulation* 116:2399–2408, 2007.
25. Sadayappan S, Gulick J, Osinska H, et al: A critical function for Ser-282 in cardiac myosin binding protein-C phosphorylation and cardiac function. *Circ Res* 109:141–150, 2011.
26. Arber S, Hunter JJ, Ross J, Jr, et al: MLP-deficient mice exhibit a disruption of cardiac cytoarchitectural organization, dilated cardiomyopathy, and heart failure. *Cell* 88:393–403, 1997.
27. Heydemann A, McNally EM: Consequences of disrupting the dystrophin-sarcoglycan complex in cardiac and skeletal myopathy. *Trends Cardiovasc Med* 17:55–59, 2007.
28. Kranias EG, Bers DM: Calcium and cardiomyopathies. *Subcell Biochem* 45:523–537, 2007.
29. Anderson ME, Brown JH, Bers DM: CaMKII in myocardial hypertrophy and heart failure. *J Mol Cell Cardiol* 51:468–473, 2011.
30. Reuter H, Schwinger RH: Calcium handling in human heart failure—abnormalities and target for therapy. *Wien Med Wochenschr* 162:297–301, 2012.
31. Hulot JS, Senyei G, Hajjar RJ: Sarcoplasmic reticulum and calcium cycling targeting by gene therapy. *Gene Ther* 19:596–599, 2012.
32. Kho C, Lee A, Jeong D, et al: SUMO1-dependent modulation of SERCA2a in heart failure. *Nature* 477:601–605, 2011.
33. Pathak A, del Monte F, Zhao W, et al: Enhancement of cardiac function and suppression of heart failure progression by inhibition of protein phosphatase 1. *Circ Res* 96:756–766, 2005.
34. Braz JC, Gregory K, Pathak A, et al: PKC-alpha regulates cardiac contractility and propensity toward heart failure. *Nat Med* 10:248–254, 2004.
35. Wehrens XH, Lehnart SE, Reiken S, et al: Ryanodine receptor/calcium release channel pka phosphorylation: a critical mediator of heart failure progression. *Proc Natl Acad Sci U S A* 103:511–518, 2006.
36. Marx SO, Marks AR: Dysfunctional ryanodine receptors in the heart: new insights into complex cardiovascular diseases. *J Mol Cell Cardiol* 58:225–231, 2013.
37. Lehnart SE, Wehrens XH, Reiken S, et al: Phosphodiesterase 4D deficiency in the ryanodine-receptor complex promotes heart failure and arrhythmias. *Cell* 123:25–35, 2005.
38. Zhang H, Makarewich CA, Kubo H, et al: Hyperphosphorylation of the cardiac ryanodine receptor at serine 2808 is not involved in cardiac dysfunction after myocardial infarction. *Circ Res* 110:831–840, 2012.
39. Bers DM: Ryanodine receptor S2808 phosphorylation in heart failure: smoking gun or red herring. *Circ Res* 110:796–799, 2012.
40. Lim G, Venetucci L, Eisner DA, et al: Does nitric oxide modulate cardiac ryanodine receptor function? Implications for excitation-contraction coupling. *Cardiovasc Res* 77:256–264, 2008.
41. Terentyev D, Gyorke I, Belevych AE, et al: Redox modification of ryanodine receptors contributes to sarcoplasmic reticulum Ca2+ leak in chronic heart failure. *Circ Res* 103:1466–1472, 2008.
42. Carnicer R, Crabtree MJ, Sivakumaran V, et al: Nitric oxide synthases in heart failure. *Antioxid Redox Signal* 18:1078–1099, 2013.
43. Zhang YH, Casadei B: Sub-cellular targeting of constitutive NOS in health and disease. *J Mol Cell Cardiol* 52:341–350, 2012.
44. Steinberg SF: Oxidative stress and sarcomeric proteins. *Circ Res* 112:393–405, 2013.
45. Rosca MG, Tandler B, Hoppel CL: Mitochondria in cardiac hypertrophy and heart failure. *J Mol Cell Cardiol* 55:31–41, 2013.
46. Kok BP, Brindley DN: Myocardial fatty acid metabolism and lipotoxicity in the setting of insulin resistance. *Heart Fail Clin* 8:643–661, 2012.
47. Schilling J, Kelly DP: The PGC-1 cascade as a therapeutic target for heart failure. *J Mol Cell Cardiol* 51:578–583, 2011.
48. Riehle C, Abel ED: PGC-1 proteins and heart failure. *Trends Cardiovasc Med* 22:98–105, 2012.
49. Thum T, Gross C, Fiedler J, et al: MicroRNA-21 contributes to myocardial disease by stimulating MAP kinase signalling in fibroblasts. *Nature* 456:980–984, 2008.
50. Cingolani OH, Kirk JA, Seo K, et al: Thrombospondin-4 is required for stretch-mediated contractility augmentation in cardiac muscle. *Circ Res* 109:1410–1414, 2011.
51. Lynch JM, Maillet M, Vanhoutte D, et al: A thrombospondin-dependent pathway for a protective ER stress response. *Cell* 149:1257–1268, 2012.
52. Spinale FG, Coker ML, Krombach SR, et al: Matrix metalloproteinase inhibition during the development of congestive heart failure: effects on left ventricular dimensions and function. *Circ Res* 85:364–376, 1999.
53. Spinale FG, Janicki JS, Zile MR: Membrane-associated matrix proteolysis and heart failure. *Circ Res* 112:195–208, 2013.
54. Gerdes AM, Capasso JM: Structural remodeling and mechanical dysfunction of cardiac myocytes in heart failure. *J Mol Cell Cardiol* 27:849–856, 1995.
55. Koitabashi N, Kass DA: Reverse remodeling in heart failure–mechanisms and therapeutic opportunities. *Nat Rev Cardiol* 9:147–157, 2012.
56. Suga H, Sagawa K: Instantaneous pressure-volume relationships and their ratio in the excised, supported canine left ventricle. *Circ Res* 35:117–128, 1974.
57. Pacher P, Nagayama T, Mukhopadhyay P, et al: Measurement of cardiac function using pressure-volume conductance catheter technique in mice and rats. *Nat Protoc* 3:1422–1434, 2008.
58. Kass DA, Midei M, Graves W, et al: Use of a conductance (volume) catheter and transient inferior vena caval occlusion for rapid determination of pressure-volume relationships in man. *Cath Cardiovasc Diag* 15:192–202, 1988.
59. Liu CP, Ting CT, Lawrence W, et al: Diminished contractile response to increased heart rate in intact human left ventricular hypertrophy. Systolic versus diastolic determinants. *Circulation* 88:1893–1906, 1993.
60. Georgakopoulos D, Mitzner WA, Chen CH, et al: Pressure-volume relations in mice by miniaturized impedance-micromanometry. *Circulation* 96:3181, 1997.
61. Senzaki H, Chen CH, Kass DA: Single beat estimation of end-systolic pressure-volume relation in humans: a new method with the potential for non-invasive application. *Circulation* 94:2497–2506, 1996.
62. Palmer BM, Georgakopoulos D, Janssen PM, et al: Role of cardiac myosin binding protein C in sustaining left ventricular systolic stiffening. *Circ Res* 94:1249–1255, 2004.
63. Harris SP, Lyons RG, Bezold KL: In the thick of it: HCM-causing mutations in myosin binding proteins of the thick filament. *Circ Res* 108:751–764, 2011.
64. Flashman E, Watkins H, Redwood C: Localization of the binding site of the C-terminal domain of cardiac myosin-binding protein-C on the myosin rod. *Biochem J* 401:97–102, 2007.
65. Kensler RW, Shaffer JF, Harris SP: Binding of the N-terminal fragment C0-C2 of cardiac MyBP-C to cardiac F-actin. *J Struct Biol* 174:44–51, 2011.
66. Rybakova IN, Greaser ML, Moss RL: Myosin binding protein C interaction with actin: characterization and mapping of the binding site. *J Biol Chem* 286:2008–2016, 2011.
67. Stelzer JE, Dunning SB, Moss RL: Ablation of cardiac myosin-binding protein-C accelerates stretch activation in murine skinned myocardium. *Circ Res* 98:1212–1218, 2006.
68. Tong CW, Stelzer JE, Greaser ML, et al: Acceleration of crossbridge kinetics by protein kinase A phosphorylation of cardiac myosin binding protein C modulates cardiac function. *Circ Res* 103:974–982, 2008.
69. Malik FI, Hartman JJ, Elias KA, et al: Cardiac myosin activation: a potential therapeutic approach for systolic heart failure. *Science* 331:1439–1443, 2011.
70. Flores-Santana W, Salmon DJ, Donzelli S, et al: The specificity of nitroxyl chemistry is unique among nitrogen oxides in biological systems. *Antioxid Redox Signal* 14:1659–1674, 2011.
71. Gao WD, Murray CI, Tian Y, et al: Nitroxyl-mediated disulfide bond formation between cardiac myofilament cysteines enhances contractile function. *Circ Res* 111:1002–1011, 2012.
72. Paolocci N, Katori T, Champion HC, et al: Positive inotropic and lusitropic effects of HNO/NO- in failing hearts: independence from beta-adrenergic signaling. *Proc Natl Acad Sci U S A* 100:5537–5542, 2003.
73. Tocchetti CG, Wang W, Froehlich JP, et al: Nitroxyl improves cellular heart function by directly enhancing cardiac sarcoplasmic reticulum Ca2+ cycling. *Circ Res* 100:96–104, 2007.
74. Georgakopoulos D, Mitzner WA, Chen CH, et al: In vivo murine left ventricular pressure-volume relations by miniaturized conductance micromanometry. *Am J Physiol* 274:H1416–H1422, 1998.
75. Georgakopoulos D, Christe ME, Giewat M, et al: The pathogenesis of familial hypertrophic cardiomyopathy: early and evolving effects from an alpha-cardiac myosin heavy chain missense mutation. *Nat Med* 5:327–330, 1999.
76. Kass DA, Yamazaki T, Burkhoff D, et al: Determination of left ventricular end-systolic pressure-volume relationships by the conductance (volume) catheter technique. *Circulation* 73:586–595, 1986.
77. Nishimura S, Seo K, Nagasaki M, et al: Responses of single-ventricular myocytes to dynamic axial stretching. *Prog Biophys Mol Biol* 97:282–297, 2008.
78. Sugiura S, Nishimura S, Yasuda S, et al: Carbon fiber technique for the investigation of single-cell mechanics in intact cardiac myocytes. *Nat Protoc* 1:1453–1457, 2006.
79. Kass DA, Wolff MR, Ting CT, et al: Diastolic compliance of hypertrophied ventricle is not acutely altered by pharmacologic agents influencing active processes. *Ann Intern Med* 119:466–473, 1993.

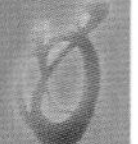

80. Liao P, Georgakopoulos D, Kovacs A, et al: The in vivo role of p38 MAP kinases in cardiac remodeling and restrictive cardiomyopathy. *Proc Natl Acad Sci U S A* 98:12283–12288, 2001.
81. Arts T, Bovendeerd PHM, Prinzen FW, et al: Relation between left ventricular cavity pressure and volume and systolic fiber stress and strain in the wall. *Biophys J* 59:93–102, 1991.
82. Kass DA, Kelly RP: Ventriculo-arterial coupling: concepts, assumptions, and applications. *Ann Biomed Eng* 20:41–62, 1992.
83. Kelly RP, Ting CT, Yang TM, et al: Effective arterial elastance as index of arterial vascular load in humans. *Circulation* 86:513–521, 1992.
84. Sunagawa K, Maughan WL, Burkhoff D, et al: Left ventricular interaction with arterial load studied in isolated canine ventricle. *Am J Physiol* 245:H773–H780, 1983.
85. Kass DA, Grayson R, Marino P: Pressure-volume analysis as a method for quantifying simultaneous drug (amrinone) effects on arterial load and contractile state. *J Am Coll Cardiol* 16:726–732, 1990.
86. Lam CS, Roger VL, Rodeheffer RJ, et al: Cardiac structure and ventricular-vascular function in persons with heart failure and preserved ejection fraction from Olmsted County, Minnesota. *Circulation* 115:1982–1990, 2007.
87. Redfield MM, Jacobsen SJ, Borlaug BA, et al: Age- and gender-related ventricular-vascular stiffening: a community-based study. *Circulation* 112:2254–2262, 2005.
88. Feldman MD, Pak PH, Wu CC, et al: Acute cardiovascular effects of OPC-18790 in patients with congestive heart failure. Time- and dose-dependence analysis based on pressure-volume relations. *Circulation* 93:474–483, 1996.
89. Kass DA, Beyar R, Lankford E, et al: Influence of contractile state on curvilinearity of the in situ end-systolic pressure-volume relations. *Circulation* 79:167–178, 1989.
90. Chen CH, Nakayama M, Nevo E, et al: Coupled systolic-ventricular and vascular stiffening with age implications for pressure regulation and cardiac reserve in the elderly. *J Am Coll Cardiol* 32:1221–1227, 1998.
91. Pak PH, Maughan WL, Baughman KL, et al: Mechanism of acute mechanical benefit from VDD pacing in hypertrophied heart: similarity of responses in hypertrophic cardiomyopathy and hypertensive heart disease. *Circulation* 98:242–248, 1998.
92. Kawaguchi M, Hay I, Fetics B, et al: Combined ventricular systolic and arterial stiffening in patients with heart failure and preserved ejection fraction: implications for systolic and diastolic reserve limitations. *Circulation* 107:714–720, 2003.
93. de Tombe PP, Mateja RD, Tachampa K, et al: Myofilament length dependent activation. *J Mol Cell Cardiol* 48:851–858, 2010.
94. Hibberd MG, Jewell BR: Calcium- and length-dependent force production in rat ventricular muscle. *J Physiol* 329:527–540, 1982.
95. Konhilas JP, Irving TC, de Tombe PP: Myofilament calcium sensitivity in skinned rat cardiac trabeculae: role of interfilament spacing. *Circ Res* 90:59–65, 2002.
96. Irving T, Wu Y, Bekyarova T, et al: Thick-filament strain and interfilament spacing in passive muscle: effect of titin-based passive tension. *Biophys J* 100:1499–1508, 2011.
97. Cazorla O, Wu Y, Irving TC, et al: Titin-based modulation of calcium sensitivity of active tension in mouse skinned cardiac myocytes. *Circ Res* 88:1028–1035, 2001.
98. Fitzsimons DP, Moss RL: Strong binding of myosin modulates length-dependent Ca2+ activation of rat ventricular myocytes. *Circ Res* 83:602–607, 1998.
99. Stelzer JE, Larsson L, Fitzsimons DP, et al: Activation dependence of stretch activation in mouse skinned myocardium: implications for ventricular function. *J Gen Physiol* 127:95–107, 2006.
100. Smith L, Tainter C, Regnier M, et al: Cooperative cross-bridge activation of thin filaments contributes to the Frank-Starling mechanism in cardiac muscle. *Biophys J* 96:3692–3702, 2009.
101. Tachampa K, Wang H, Farman GP, et al: Cardiac troponin I threonine 144: role in myofilament length dependent activation. *Circ Res* 101:1081–1083, 2007.
102. Kockskamper J, von Lewinski D, Khafaga M, et al: The slow force response to stretch in atrial and ventricular myocardium from human heart: functional relevance and subcellular mechanisms. *Prog Biophys Mol Biol* 97:250–267, 2008.
103. von Lewinski D, Stumme B, Fialka F, et al: Functional relevance of the stretch-dependent slow force response in failing human myocardium. *Circ Res* 94:1392–1398, 2004.
104. Cingolani HE, Ennis IL, Aiello EA, et al: Role of autocrine/paracrine mechanisms in response to myocardial strain. *Pflugers Arch* 462:29–38, 2011.
105. Perez NG, de Hurtado MC, Cingolani HE: Reverse mode of the Na+-Ca2+ exchange after myocardial stretch: underlying mechanism of the slow force response. *Circ Res* 88:376–382, 2001.
106. Patel A, Sharif-Naeini R, Folgering JR, et al: Canonical TRP channels and mechanotransduction: from physiology to disease states. *Pflugers Arch* 460:571–581, 2010.
107. Eder P, Molkentin JD: TRPC channels as effectors of cardiac hypertrophy. *Circ Res* 108:265–272, 2011.
108. Seo K, Rainer PP, Lee DI, et al: Hyperactive adverse mechanical stress responses in dystrophic heart are coupled to transient receptor potential canonical 6 and blocked by cGMP-protein kinase G modulation. *Circ Res* 114:823–832, 2014.
109. Villa-Abrille MC, Caldiz CI, Ennis IL, et al: The Anrep effect requires transactivation of the epidermal growth factor receptor. *J Physiol* 588:1579–1590, 2010.
110. Yue DT, Marban E, Wier G: Relationship between force and intracellular Ca2+ in tetanized mammalian heart muscle. *J Gen Physiol* 87:223–242, 1986.
111. Somura F, Izawa H, Iwase M, et al: Reduced myocardial sarcoplasmic reticulum Ca(2+)-ATPase mRNA expression and biphasic force-frequency relations in patients with hypertrophic cardiomyopathy. *Circulation* 104:658–663, 2001.
112. Pieske B, Maier LS, Bers DM, et al: Ca2+ handling and sarcoplasmic reticulum Ca2+ content in isolated failing and nonfailing human myocardium. *Circ Res* 85:38–46, 1999.
113. Georgakopoulos D, Kass D: Minimal force-frequency modulation of inotropy and relaxation of in situ murine heart. *J Physiol* 534:535–545, 2001.
114. Kass DA: Force-frequency relation in patients with left ventricular hypertrophy and failure. *Basic Res Cardiol* 93(Suppl 1):108–116, 1998.
115. Mulieri LA, Hasenfuss G, Leavitt B, et al: Altered myocardial force-frequency relation in human heart failure. *Circulation* 85:1743–1750, 1992.
116. Rossman EI, Petre RE, Chaudhary KW, et al: Abnormal frequency-dependent responses represent the pathophysiologic signature of contractile failure in human myocardium. *J Mol Cell Cardiol* 36:33–42, 2004.
117. Senzaki H, Isoda T, Paolocci N, et al: Improved mechanoenergetics and cardiac rest and reserve function of in vivo failing heart by calcium sensitizer EMD-57033. *Circulation* 101:1040–1048, 2000.
118. Miura T, Miyazaki S, Guth BD, et al: Influence of the force-frequency relation on left ventricular function during exercise in conscious dogs. *Circulation* 86:563–571, 1992.
119. Kass DA, Hare JM, Georgakopoulos D: Murine cardiac function: a cautionary tail. *Circ Res* 82:519–522, 1998.
120. Little WC: The left ventricular dP/dtmax-end-diastolic volume relation in closed-chest dogs. *Circ Res* 56:808–815, 1985.
121. Kass DA, Chen CH, Curry C, et al: Improved left ventricular mechanics from acute VDD pacing in patients with dilated cardiomyopathy and ventricular conduction delay. *Circulation* 99:1567–1573, 1999.
122. Auricchio A, Stellbrink C, Block M, et al: Effect of pacing chamber and atrioventricular delay on acute systolic function of paced patients with congestive heart failure. *Circulation* 99:2993–3001, 1999.
123. Mandarino WA, Pinsky MR, Gorcsan J, III: Assessment of left ventricular contractile state by preload-adjusted maximal power using echocardiographic automated border detection. *J Am Coll Cardiol* 31:861–868, 1998.
124. Borlaug BA, Melenovsky V, Russell SD, et al: Impaired chronotropic and vasodilator reserves limit exercise capacity in patients with heart failure and a preserved ejection fraction. *Circulation* 114:2138–2147, 2006.
125. Sharir T, Feldman MD, Haber H, et al: Ventricular systolic assessment in patients with dilated cardiomyopathy by preload-adjusted maximal power. Validation and noninvasive application. *Circulation* 89:2045–2053, 1994.
126. Nakayama M, Chen CH, Nevo E, et al: Optimal preload-adjustment of maximal ventricular power index varies with cardiac chamber size. *Am Heart J* 136:281–288, 1998.
127. Leather HA, Segers P, Sun YY, et al: The limitations of preload-adjusted maximal power as an index of right ventricular contractility. *Anesth Analg* 95:798–804, 2002. table.
128. Marmor A, Schneeweiss A: Prognostic value of noninvasively obtained left ventricular contractile reserve in patients with severe heart failure. *J Am Coll Cardiol* 29:422–428, 1997.
129. Greenberg NL, Firstenberg MS, Castro PL, et al: Doppler-derived myocardial systolic strain rate is a strong index of left ventricular contractility. *Circulation* 105:99–105, 2002.
130. Suffoletto MS, Dohi K, Cannesson M, et al: Novel speckle-tracking radial strain from routine black-and-white echocardiographic images to quantify dyssynchrony and predict response to cardiac resynchronization therapy. *Circulation* 113:960–968, 2006.
131. Bank AJ, Kelly AS: Tissue Doppler imaging and left ventricular dyssynchrony in heart failure. *J Card Fail* 12:154–162, 2006.
132. Armstrong G, Pasquet A, Fukamachi K, et al: Use of peak systolic strain as an index of regional left ventricular function: comparison with tissue Doppler velocity during dobutamine stress and myocardial ischemia. *J Am Soc Echocardiogr* 13:731–737, 2000.
133. Ozturk C, McVeigh ER: Four-dimensional B-spline based motion analysis of tagged MR images: introduction and in vivo validation. *Phys Med Biol* 45:1683–1702, 2000.
134. Derbyshire JA, Herzka DA, McVeigh ER, et al: Efficient implementation of hardware-optimized gradient sequences for real-time imaging. *Magn Reson Med* 64:1814–1820, 2010.
135. Sampath S, Derbyshire JA, Ledesma-Carbayo MJ, et al: Imaging left ventricular tissue mechanics and hemodynamics during supine bicycle exercise using a combined tagging and phase-contrast MRI pulse sequence. *Magn Reson Med* 65:51–59, 2011.
136. Nagueh SF, Kopelen HA, Lim DS, et al: Tissue Doppler imaging consistently detects myocardial contraction and relaxation abnormalities, irrespective of cardiac hypertrophy, in a transgenic rabbit model of human hypertrophic cardiomyopathy. *Circulation* 102:1346–1350, 2000.
137. Sogaard P, Egeblad H, Kim WY, et al: Tissue Doppler imaging predicts improved systolic performance and reversed left ventricular remodeling during long-term cardiac resynchronization therapy. *J Am Coll Cardiol* 40:723–730, 2002.
138. Yu CM, Chau E, Sanderson JE, et al: Tissue Doppler echocardiographic evidence of reverse remodeling and improved synchronicity by simultaneously delaying regional contraction after biventricular pacing therapy in heart failure. *Circulation* 105:438–445, 2002.
139. Glower DD, Spratt JA, Snow ND, et al: Linearity of the Frank-Starling relationship in the intact heart: the concept of preload recruitable stroke work. *Circulation* 71:994–1009, 1985.
140. Karunanithi MK, Feneley MP: Single-beat determination of preload recruitable stroke work relationship: derivation and evaluation in conscious dogs. *J Am Coll Cardiol* 35:502–513, 2000.
141. Dauterman K, Pak PH, Nussbacher A, et al: Contribution of external forces to left ventricle diastolic pressure: implications for the clinical use of the Frank-Starling law. *Annals Int Med* 122:737–742, 1995.
142. Moore TD, Frenneaux MP, Sas R, et al: Ventricular interaction and external constraint account for decreased stroke work during volume loading in CHF. *Am J Physiol Heart Circ Physiol* 281:H2385–H2391, 2001.
143. Grant DA, Fauchere JC, Eede KJ, et al: Left ventricular stroke volume in the fetal sheep is limited by extracardiac constraint and arterial pressure. *J Physiol* 535:231–239, 2001.
144. Borlaug BA, Kass DA: Ventricular-vascular interaction in heart failure. *Cardiol Clin* 29:447–459, 2011.
145. Burkhoff D, de Tombe PP, Hunter WC, et al: Contractile strength and mechanical efficiency of left ventricle are enhanced by physiological afterload. *Am J Physiol* 260(29):H569–H578, 1991.
146. Sunagawa K, Maughan WL, Sagawa K: Optimal arterial resistance for the maximal stroke work studied in isolated canine left ventricle. *Circ Res* 56:586–595, 1985.
147. Little WC, Cheng CP: Left ventricular-arterial coupling in conscious dogs. *Am J Physiol* 261:H70–H76, 1991.
148. de Tombe PP, Jones S, Burkhoff D, et al: Ventricular stroke work and efficiency both remain nearly optimal despite altered vascular loading. *Am J Physiol* 264:H1817–H1824, 1993.
149. Elzinga G, Westerhof N: Matching between ventricle and arterial load. An evolutionary process. *Circ Res* 68:1495–1500, 1991.
150. Asanoi H, Sasayama S, Kameyama T: Ventriculoarterial coupling in normal and failing heart in humans. *Circ Res* 65:483–493, 1989.
151. Melenovsky V, Borlaug BA, Rosen B, et al: Cardiovascular features of heart failure with preserved ejection fraction versus nonfailing hypertensive left ventricular hypertrophy in the urban Baltimore community: the role of atrial remodeling/dysfunction. *J Am Coll Cardiol* 49:198–207, 2007.
152. Borlaug BA, Olson TP, Lam CS, et al: Global cardiovascular reserve dysfunction in heart failure with preserved ejection fraction. *J Am Coll Cardiol* 56:845–854, 2010.
153. Borlaug BA, Jaber WA, Ommen SR, et al: Diastolic relaxation and compliance reserve during dynamic exercise in heart failure with preserved ejection fraction. *Heart* 97:964–969, 2011.
154. Abudiab MM, Redfield MM, Melenovsky V, et al: Cardiac output response to exercise in relation to metabolic demand in heart failure with preserved ejection fraction. *Eur J Heart Fail* 15:776–785, 2013.
155. Packer M, Carver JR, Rodeheffer RJ, et al: Effect of oral milrinone on mortality in severe chronic heart failure. The PROMISE Study Research Group. *N Engl J Med* 325:1468–1475, 1991.
156. Raake PW, Vinge LE, Gao E, et al: G protein-coupled receptor kinase 2 ablation in cardiac myocytes before or after myocardial infarction prevents heart failure. *Circ Res* 103:413–422, 2008.
157. Kamal FA, Smrcka AV, Blaxall BC: Taking the heart failure battle inside the cell: small molecule targeting of Gbetagamma subunits. *J Mol Cell Cardiol* 51:462–467, 2011.
158. Okumura S, Takagi G, Kawabe J, et al: Disruption of type 5 adenylyl cyclase gene preserves cardiac function against pressure overload. *Proc Natl Acad Sci U S A* 100:9986–9990, 2003.
159. Yan L, Vatner DE, O'Connor JP, et al: Type 5 adenylyl cyclase disruption increases longevity and protects against stress. *Cell* 130:247–258, 2007.
160. Phan HM, Gao MH, Lai NC, et al: New signaling pathways associated with increased cardiac adenylyl cyclase 6 expression: implications for possible congestive heart failure therapy. *Trends Cardiovasc Med* 17:215–221, 2007.
161. Chemaly ER, Hajjar RJ, Lipskaia L: Molecular targets of current and prospective heart failure therapies. *Heart* 99:992–1003, 2013.
162. Kawase Y, Ly HQ, Prunier F, et al: Reversal of cardiac dysfunction after long-term expression of SERCA2a by gene transfer in a pre-clinical model of heart failure. *J Am Coll Cardiol* 51:1112–1119, 2008.
163. Jaski BE, Jessup ML, Mancini DM, et al: Calcium upregulation by percutaneous administration of gene therapy in cardiac disease (CUPID Trial), a first-in-human phase 1/2 clinical trial. *J Card Fail* 15:171–181, 2009.

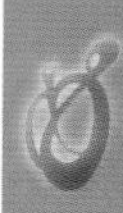

164. Tachibana H, Cheng HJ, Ukai T, et al: Levosimendan improves LV systolic and diastolic performance at rest and during exercise after heart failure. *Am J Physiol Heart Circ Physiol* 288:H914–H922, 2005.
165. Ng TM: Levosimendan, a new calcium-sensitizing inotrope for heart failure. *Pharmacotherapy* 24:1366–1384, 2004.
166. Mebazaa A, Nieminen MS, Packer M, et al: Levosimendan vs dobutamine for patients with acute decompensated heart failure: the SURVIVE Randomized Trial. *JAMA* 297:1883–1891, 2007.
167. Cleland JG, Teerlink JR, Senior R, et al: The effects of the cardiac myosin activator, omecamtiv mecarbil, on cardiac function in systolic heart failure: a double-blind, placebo-controlled, crossover, dose-ranging phase 2 trial. *Lancet* 378:676–683, 2011.
168. Tocchetti CG, Stanley BA, Murray CI, et al: Playing with cardiac "redox switches": the "HNO way" to modulate cardiac function. *Antioxid Redox Signal* 14:1687–1698, 2011.
169. Lancel S, Zhang J, Evangelista A, et al: Nitroxyl activates SERCA in cardiac myocytes via glutathiolation of cysteine 674. *Circ Res* 104:720–723, 2009.
170. Froehlich JP, Mahaney JE, Keceli G, et al: Phospholamban thiols play a central role in activation of the cardiac muscle sarcoplasmic reticulum calcium pump by nitroxyl. *Biochemistry* 47:13150–13152, 2008.
171. Meisner JS, McQueen DM, Ishida Y, et al: Effects of timing of atrial systole on LV filling and mitral valve closure: computer and dog studies. *Am J Physiol* 249:H604–H619, 1985.
172. Brecker SJ, Xiao HB, Sparrow J, et al: Effects of dual-chamber pacing with short atrioventricular delay in dilated cardiomyopathy. *Lancet* 340:1308–1312, 1992.
173. Prinzen FW, Hunter WC, Wyman BT, et al: Mapping of regional myocardial strain and work during ventricular pacing: experimental study using magnetic resonance imaging tagging. *J Am Coll Cardiol* 33:1735–1742, 1999.
174. Wyman BT, Hunter WC, Prinzen FW, et al: Mapping propagation of mechanical activation in the paced heart with MRI tagging. *Am J Physiol* 276:H881–H891, 1999.
175. van der Veen BJ, Al Younis I, Ajmone-Marsan N, et al: Ventricular dyssynchrony assessed by gated myocardial perfusion SPECT using a geometrical approach: a feasibility study. *Eur J Nucl Med Mol Imaging* 39:421–429, 2012.
176. Liu L, Tockman B, Girouard S, et al: Left ventricular resynchronization therapy in a canine model of left bundle branch block. *Am J Physiol Heart CircPhysiol* 282:H2238–H2244, 2002.
177. Park RC, Little WC, O'Rourke RA: Effect of alteration of left ventricular activation sequence on the left ventricular end-systolic pressure-volume relation in closed-chest dogs. *Circ Res* 57:706–717, 1985.
178. Burkhoff D, Oikawa RY, Sagawa K: Influence of pacing site on canine left ventricular contraction. *Am J Physiol* 251:H428–H435, 1986.
179. Baller D, Wolpers HG, Zipfel J, et al: Comparison of the effects of right atrial, right ventricular apex and atrioventricular sequential pacing on myocardial oxygen consumption and cardiac efficiency: a laboratory investigation. *Pacing Clin Electrophysiol* 11:394–403, 1988.
180. Owen CH, Esposito DJ, Davis JW, et al: The effects of ventricular pacing on left ventricular geometry, function, myocardial oxygen consumption, and efficiency of contraction in conscious dogs. *Pacing Clin Electrophysiol* 21:1417–1429, 1998.
181. Prinzen FW, Augustijn CH, Arts T, et al: Redistribution of myocardial fiber strain and blood flow by asynchronous activation. *Am J Physiol* 259:H300–H308, 1990.
182. Fananapazir L, Cannon RO, III, Tripodi D, et al: Impact of dual-chamber permanent pacing in patients with obstructive hypertrophic cardiomyopathy with symptoms refractory to verapamil and beta-adrenergic blocker therapy. *Circulation* 85:2149–2161, 1992.
183. Kass DA, Chen CH, Talbot MW, et al: Ventricular pacing with premature excitation for treatment of hypertensive-cardiac hypertrophy with cavity-obliteration [see comments]. *Circulation* 100:807–812, 1999.
184. Maron BJ, Nishimura RA, McKenna WJ, et al: Assessment of permanent dual-chamber pacing as a treatment for drug-refractory symptomatic patients with obstructive hypertrophic cardiomyopathy. A randomized, double-blind, crossover study (M-PATHY). *Circulation* 99:2927–2933, 1999.
185. Nishimura RA, Trusty JM, Hayes DL, et al: Dual-chamber pacing for hypertrophic cardiomyopathy: a randomized, double-blind, crossover trial. *J Am Coll Cardiol* 29:435–441, 1997.
186. Blanc JJ, Etienne Y, Gilard M, et al: Evaluation of different ventricular pacing sites in patients with severe heart failure: results of an acute hemodynamic study. *Circulation* 96:3273–3277, 1997.
187. Leclercq C, Cazeau S, Le Breton H, et al: Acute hemodynamic effects of biventricular DDD pacing in patients with end-stage heart failure. *J Am Coll Cardiol* 32:1825–1831, 1998.
188. Nelson GS, Curry CW, Wyman BT, et al: Predictors of systolic augmentation from left ventricular preexcitation in patients with dilated cardiomyopathy and intraventricular conduction delay. *Circulation* 101:2703–2709, 2000.
189. Nelson GS, Berger RD, Fetics BJ, et al: Left ventricular or biventricular pacing improves cardiac function at diminished energy cost in patients with dilated cardiomyopathy and left bundle-branch block. *Circulation* 102:3053–3059, 2000.
190. Vanderheyden M, Mullens W, Delrue L, et al: Myocardial gene expression in heart failure patients treated with cardiac resynchronization therapy responders versus nonresponders. *J Am Coll Cardiol* 51:129–136, 2008.
191. Vanderheyden M, Mullens W, Delrue L, et al: Endomyocardial upregulation of beta1 adrenoreceptor gene expression and myocardial contractile reserve following cardiac resynchronization therapy. *J Card Fail* 14:172–178, 2008.
192. Iyengar S, Haas G, Lamba S, et al: Effect of cardiac resynchronization therapy on myocardial gene expression in patients with nonischemic dilated cardiomyopathy. *J Card Fail* 13:304–311, 2007.
193. Chakir K, Daya SK, Aiba T, et al: Mechanisms of enhanced beta-adrenergic reserve from cardiac resynchronization therapy. *Circulation* 119:1231–1240, 2009.
194. Chakir K, Depry C, Dimaano VL, et al: Galphas-biased beta2-adrenergic receptor signaling from restoring synchronous contraction in the failing heart. *Sci Transl Med* 3:100ra88, 2011.
195. Kirk JA, Holewinski RJ, Kooij V, et al: Cardiac resynchronization sensitizes the sarcomere to calcium by reactivating GSK-3β. *J Clin Invest* 124:129–138, 2014.
196. Wang SB, Foster DB, Rucker J, et al: Redox regulation of mitochondrial ATP synthase: implications for cardiac resynchronization therapy. *Circ Res* 109:750–757, 2011.
197. Aiba T, Hasketh GG, Barth AS, et al: Electrophysioloigcal consequences of dyssynchronous heart failure and its restoration by resynchronization therapy. *Circulation* 119:1220–1230, 2009.
198. Aiba T, Tomaselli G: Electrical remodeling in dyssynchrony and resynchronization. *J Cardiovasc Transl Res* 5:170–179, 2012.
199. Barth AS, Chakir K, Kass DA, et al: Transcriptome, proteome, and metabolome in dyssynchronous heart failure and CRT. *J Cardiovasc Transl Res* 5:180–187, 2012.

10 Alterations in Ventricular Function: Diastolic Heart Failure

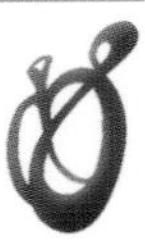

Loek van Heerebeek and Walter J. Paulus

EPIDEMIOLOGY

As discussed in Chapter 17 approximately 20 million people suffer from heart failure (HF) in Europe and the United States. The prevalence of HF continues to rise as a result of the aging of the population, with 80% of HF patients being older than 65 years of age.[1,2] Approximately half of all patients presenting with HF have a normal or near-normal left ventricular ejection fraction (LVEF), which is also referred to as HF with preserved EF (HFpEF), HF with normal EF (HFnEF), or diastolic HF (DHF). HFpEF is increasing in prevalence and is associated with poor outcomes. Moreover, the pathophysiologic mechanisms of HFpEF are incompletely understood, which has contributed to the lack of specific therapeutic strategies (see Chapter 36) to treat HFpEF.[1-3] Whereas the prognosis for patients with HF with reduced EF (HFrEF) or systolic HF (SHF) has improved substantially over the past decades due to modern HF pharmacotherapy,[1-3] similar pharmacologic agents yielded neutral trial results in HFpEF patients as demonstrated for angiotensin-converting enzyme inhibitors,[4] angiotensin receptor blockers,[5,6] aldosterone antagonists,[7] and β-blockers.[8] One of the main reasons for this discrepancy could be the inability of our current therapies to sufficiently address the pathophysiologic mechanisms driving LV remodeling in HFpEF.[9]

DIASTOLIC DYSFUNCTION VERSUS DIASTOLIC HEART FAILURE

The term *diastolic dysfunction* indicates an abnormality of diastolic distensibility, filling, or relaxation of the left ventricle (LV), regardless of whether the EF is normal or abnormal and whether the patient is symptomatic or asymptomatic.[10] After adjustment for established HF risk factors, asymptomatic antecedent LV diastolic dysfunction was associated with increased HF risk in individuals without HF participating in the Framingham Heart Study.[11] Furthermore, in a cross-sectional survey of randomly selected Olmsted County residents, roughly 20% of the population had diastolic LV dysfunction and more than 5% had moderate or severe diastolic dysfunction with normal EF, which was predictive of all-cause mortality even in the absence of clinical HF.[12] The prevalence of diastolic dysfunction increased during 6 years' follow-up of this cohort, whereas diastolic dysfunction was associated with incident HF after adjustment for age, hypertension, diabetes, and coronary artery disease.[13] Thus diastolic dysfunction refers to abnormal mechanical (diastolic) properties of the ventricle and is present in virtually all patients with HF. The term *diastolic heart failure* refers to a clinical syndrome characterized by symptoms or signs of HF, preserved LVEF, and diastolic LV dysfunction.[10] Characteristic symptoms and signs of HF include (exertional) dyspnea, fatigue, peripheral and/or pulmonary edema, orthopnea, hepatomegaly, and raised central venous pressure.[14] The structural remodeling of the heart that is seen in patients with HF is associated with substantial alterations in the systolic and diastolic function of the LV. In HFrEF, the dominant abnormality is a contractile dysfunction with LV enlargement, afterload excess, and reduced EF. In HFpEF, the dominant abnormality is diastolic dysfunction with normal or near-normal LV volume, increased relative wall thickness, preserved EF, abnormal ventricular relaxation and filling, decreased LV suction, increased stiffness, and elevated filling pressures.[10]

SYSTOLIC VERSUS DIASTOLIC HEART FAILURE

It is still debated whether HFpEF and HFrEF represent distinct HF phenotypes.[15] Clinical HF symptoms and signs, exercise intolerance, impaired peak oxygen consumption, and norepinephrine levels are similar between HFpEF and HFrEF patients, despite substantial differences in EF.[16] B-type natriuretic peptide (BNP) levels are elevated in both conditions, although they are elevated to a greater extent in HFrEF.[17] Furthermore, in HFpEF systolic abnormalities also contribute to cardiac dysfunction as evident from subtly but significantly depressed chamber and myocardial contractility, which was associated with a worse outcome in HFpEF patients.[18] In contrast, invasively determined measures of global systolic LV function were preserved in HFpEF,[19] and as diastolic LV dysfunction represents the dominant functional abnormality in HFpEF, it was suggested that "subtle" abnormalities in systolic function are unlikely to be responsible for HF in patients with HFpEF.[10] Moreover, prominent differences in patient demographics, risk factor profile, hemodynamic characteristics, and macroscopic and cardiac myocyte remodeling coupled with disparate responses to similar HF pharmacotherapy would all seem to justify that HFpEF and HFrEF indeed represent distinct HF phenotypes.[20-22]

Distinct Demographic and Cardiovascular Risk Factor Profiles

Numerous studies demonstrate distinct differences between HFpEF and HFrEF patients in demographic and cardiovascular risk factor profiles as HFpEF patients are frequently older, more often female, and have a higher prevalence of hypertension, chronic obstructive pulmonary disease, atrial fibrillation, obesity, and metabolic syndrome.[3,23-27] Diabetes mellitus (DM) demonstrates discordant prevalence rates with either lower,[23] similar,[3,17] or higher[24-26] prevalence in HFpEF compared with HFrEF (see Chapter 16). Conversely, HFrEF patients had a higher heart rate and increased prevalence of coronary artery disease and left bundle branch block.[3,17,24,25]

Left Ventricular and Cardiac Myocyte Remodeling

Myocardial structural remodeling importantly differs between HFpEF and HFrEF patients. Prominent features of HFrEF include LV dilation, eccentric remodeling, lowered LV mass/volume ratio, cardiomyocyte elongation, reduced EF, and decreased contractility.[10,21,28] Conversely, HFpEF is characterized by concentric LV remodeling, concentric hypertrophy, increased LV mass/volume ratio, cardiomyocyte thickening, combined ventricular systolic and arterial stiffening, preserved systolic function and diastolic dysfunction evident from impaired LV relaxation, elevated filling pressures, and increased LV and myocardial stiffness.[10,21,28-31]

Disparate Responses to Similar Pharmacologic Therapy

Current modern evidence-based HF therapy improved the prognosis of patients with HFrEF,[1-3] but not of patients with HFpEF.[4-8] Disparate responses between HFpEF and HFrEF patients to similar pharmacologic HF therapy have also been demonstrated for arterial vasodilators,[32] statins,[33,34] and β-blockers.[35] Because end-systolic elastance is markedly reduced in HFrEF (see Chapter 9), patients with HFrEF respond very favorably to arterial vasodilators with minimal drop in blood pressure and substantial improvement in stroke volume.[30] In contrast, the elevated end-systolic elastance in HFpEF patients leads to more exaggerated drops in blood pressure with vasodilator therapy.[30] For instance, nitroprusside induced a larger drop in systemic arterial pressure and lower enhancement in stroke volume and cardiac output in HFpEF compared with HFrEF patients, suggesting greater vulnerability to preload reduction in HFpEF patients.[32]

A preliminary report suggested statin therapy to lower mortality rates in patients with HFpEF,[33] which contrasts with the neutral outcome of statin therapy in the HFrEF patients of the CORONA trial.[34] β-blocker therapy differentially affected myocardial structural and functional characteristics in HFpEF and HFrEF patients.[35] Effects of β-blocker therapy unique to HFpEF were elevated intrinsic cardiomyocyte stiffness and lower stimulatory G-protein expression, whereas β-blocker therapy reduced inhibitory G-protein expression in HFrEF.[35] Contrasting results have also been reported for the prevention of HFpEF or HFrEF. In hypertensive patients of the ALLHAT (Antihypertensive and Lipid Lowering Treatment to Prevent Heart Attack Trial) study, lisinopril was inferior to chlorthalidone for preventing new-onset HFpEF, but not for new-onset HFrEF.[36] The discordant outcomes of similar pharmacologic therapy in HFpEF and HFrEF suggest that the signal transduction cascades driving myocardial remodeling differ in HFpEF and HFrEF.[14]

Distinct Pathophysiologic Mechanisms Between HFrEF and HFpEF

The pathophysiology of HF in the setting of systolic LV dysfunction is well understood (see Chapter 11).[37] Following myocardial injury inducing cardiomyocyte death, maladaptive changes occur in surviving cardiomyocytes and in the cardiac interstitium, leading to pathologic remodeling of the LV, with dilation and impaired contractility.[37] If these changes are left untreated, they worsen over time, exacerbated by additional injury and by systemic responses to LV systolic dysfunction, notably activation of the sympathetic and renin-angiotensin-aldosterone systems (RAAS).[37] All these responses have detrimental systemic effects, accounting for the clinical manifestations of the syndrome of HF, including the development and worsening of symptoms, declining functional capacity, episodes of decompensation

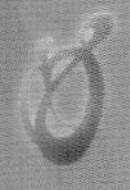

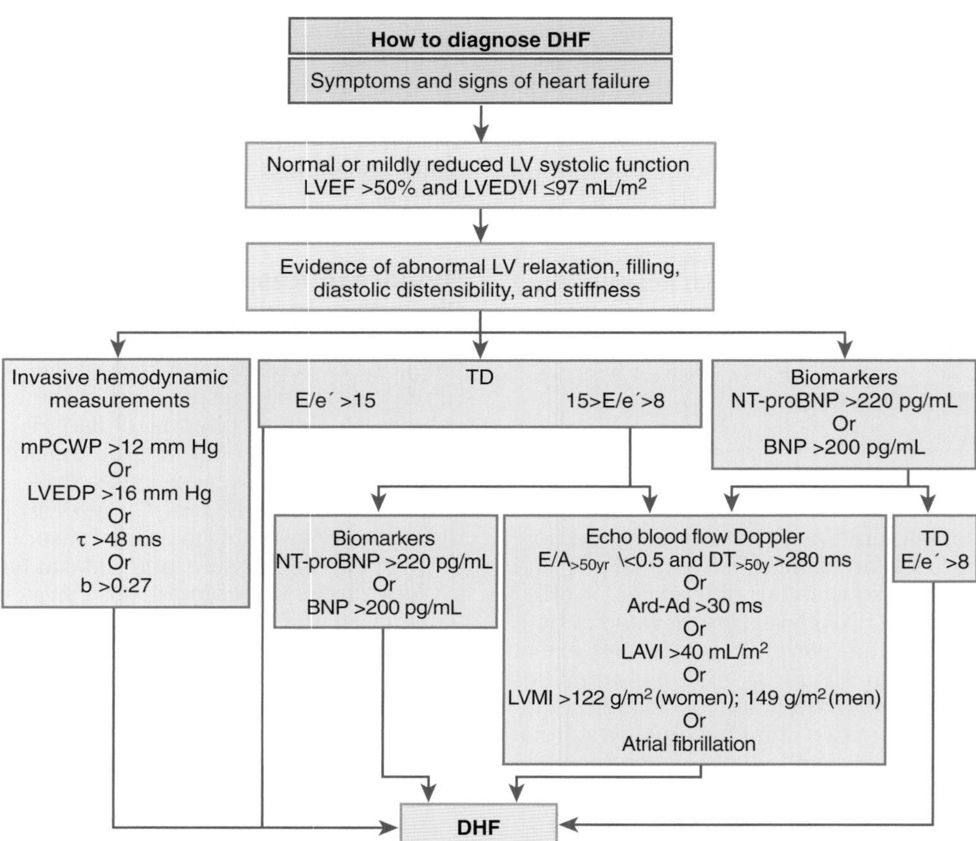

FIGURE 10-1 Diagnostic flowchart on "How to diagnose HFNEF" in a patient suspected of HFpEF. *Ad,* Duration of mitral valve trial wave flow; *Ard,* duration of reverse pulmonary vein atrial systole flow; *b,* constant of left ventricular chamber stiffness; *BNP,* B-type natriuretic peptide; *DT,* deceleration time; *E,* early mitral valve flow velocity; *e′,* velocity of mitral annulus early diastolic motion; *E/A,* ratio of early (E) to late (A) mitral valve flow velocity; *LAVI,* left atrial volume index; *LVEDP,* left ventricular end-diastolic pressure; *LVEDVI,* left ventricular end-diastolic volume index; *LVMI,* left ventricular mass index; *mPCWP,* mean pulmonary capillary wedge pressure; *NT-proBNP,* N-terminal-pro B-type natriuretic peptide; *τ,* time constant of left ventricular relaxation; *TD,* tissue Doppler.

and premature death, usually because of pump failure or ventricular arrhythmia.[37] Conversely, the pathophysiology of HFpEF is incompletely understood, which precludes development of specific therapeutic strategies.

DIAGNOSIS OF HEART FAILURE WITH A PRESERVED EJECTION FRACTION

According to recent recommendations by the European Society of Cardiology, three obligatory conditions need to be satisfied for the diagnosis of HFpEF: (1) presence of signs or symptoms of congestive HF; (2) presence of normal or mildly abnormal LV systolic function, defined as LVEF greater than 50% and LV end-diastolic volume index (LVEDVI) less than 97 mL/m^2, and (3) evidence of diastolic LV dysfunction determined either by invasive measurements or by echocardiography alone or by echocardiography in conjunction with biomarkers (**Figure 10-1**).[14]

The importance of diastolic LV dysfunction for HFpEF was recently emphasized by invasive studies that showed slow LV relaxation and elevated diastolic LV stiffness at rest and exercise.[29,38,39] In patients with HFpEF, invasive pressure-volume loop analysis showed that diastolic stiffness was increased at rest and with exercise, whereas LV end-diastolic pressure (LVEDP) was increased during handgrip exercise, and stroke volume was reduced with a leftward shift of pressure-volume loops during atrial pacing.[38] Similarly, in an another invasive study, HFpEF patients had elevated resting pulmonary artery systolic pressure (PASP) and pulmonary capillary wedge pressure (PCWP) compared with patients with noncardiac dyspnea, whereas LV filling pressures were further increased during exercise by supine bicycle ergometry or arm weight lifting.[39] Exercise-induced elevation in PCWP in HFpEF was confirmed by greater increases in LVEDP and was associated with blunted increases in heart rate, systemic vasodilation, and cardiac output. Exercise-induced pulmonary hypertension was present in 88% of patients with HFpEF and was related principally to elevated PCWP, as pulmonary vascular resistances dropped similarly in both groups. Exercise PASP and PCWP were highly correlated, while exercise PASP of 45 mm Hg or more identified HFpEF with 96% sensitivity and 95% specificity.[39]

Invasive Measurement of Diastolic Function: Relaxation and Chamber Stiffness

Evidence of abnormal LV relaxation, filling, diastolic distensibility, and diastolic stiffness can be acquired invasively during cardiac catheterization.[10,29] Ventricular pressure fall is the hemodynamic manifestation of myocardial relaxation, and the rate of global LV myocardial relaxation is reflected by the exponential course of isovolumic LV pressure fall. Isovolumic relaxation can be quantitated by measuring LV pressure using a high-fidelity micromanometer catheter and calculating the peak instantaneous rate of LV pressure

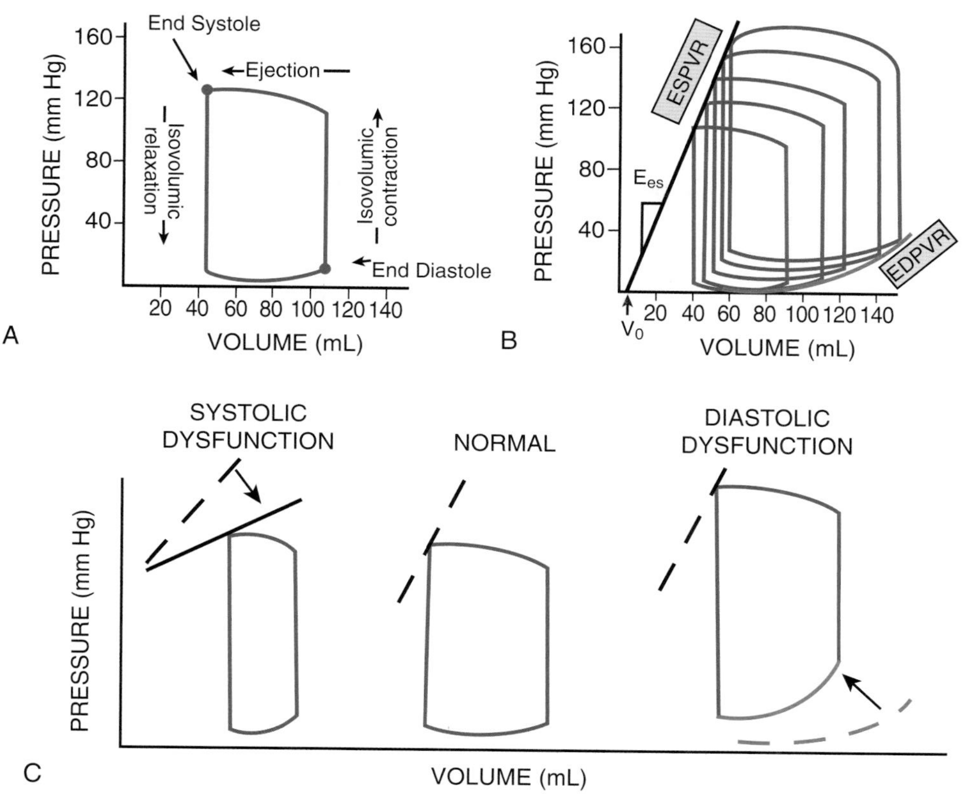

FIGURE 10-2 **A,** The four phases of the cardiac cycle are displayed on the pressure-volume loop, which is constructed by plotting instantaneous pressure versus volume. This loop repeats with each cardiac cycle and shows how the heart transitions from its end-diastolic state to the end-systolic state and back. **B,** With a constant contractile state and afterload, a progressive reduction in ventricular filling pressure causes the loops to shift toward lower volumes at both end systole and end diastole. When the resulting end-systolic pressure-volume points are connected, a reasonably linear end-systolic pressure-volume relationship (ESPVR) is obtained. The linear ESPVR is characterized by a slope (E_{es}) and a volume axis intercept (V_0). In contrast, the diastolic pressure-volume points define a nonlinear end-diastolic pressure-volume relationship (EDPVR). **C,** In systolic dysfunction, contractility is depressed and the ESPVR is displaced downward and to the right; there is diminished capacity to eject blood into a high-pressure aorta. In diastolic dysfunction, chamber stiffness is increased and the EDPVR is displaced up and to the left; there is diminished capacity to fill at low diastolic pressures. The LVEF is low in systolic dysfunction and normal in diastolic dysfunction.

decline, peak -dP/dt, and the time constant of isovolumic LV pressure decline, tau (τ).[29] Tau is the most widely used index to evaluate the rate of LV pressure fall. Tau is inversely related to the rate of LV pressure fall, becoming shorter when LV pressure fall accelerates and longer when LV pressure fall slows such that tau greater than 48 ms represents evidence for delayed relaxation.[29] It remains clinically uncertain if myocardial relaxation can be delayed to such an extent as to cause persistent pressure generation at end-diastole, which could eventually contribute to reduced LV distensibility.[29]

Another invasive approach that can be used to determine LV chamber stiffness and compliance is through measurement of LV pressure volume loops with the use of high-fidelity LV conductance catheters, which simultaneously measure LV pressure and LV volume.[40]

The use of end-systolic and end-diastolic pressure volume relationships derived from measurements of instantaneous LV pressure-volume loops emerged in the 1970s as a comprehensive approach for this purpose.[40] The hemodynamic events occurring during the cardiac cycle are displayed by plotting instantaneous ventricular pressure versus volume (**Figure 10-2A**). Under steady-state conditions and with a constant time interval between beats, this loop is repeated with each contraction. For a given cardiac cycle, there is a single pressure-volume point that coincides with end diastole (which resides at the lower right corner of the loop) and a single pressure-volume point that coincides with end systole (which resides at the upper left corner of the loop).[40] If an intervention is performed that acutely changes the loading conditions on the heart but has no effect on myocardial contractility (e.g., transient inferior vena caval occlusion to reduce preload, administration of phenylephrine to increase afterload), a family of loops is obtained (see Figure 10-2B). The end-systolic and end-diastolic points of these loops delineate two distinct boundaries. The end-diastolic pressure volume relation (EDPVR), constructed by connecting the end-diastolic pressure-volume points of each loop, is nonlinear and defines the passive physical properties of the chamber with the myocardium in its most relaxed state. The end-systolic pressure-volume relation (ESPVR), constructed by connecting the end-systolic pressure-volume points of each loop, defines a reasonably linear relationship that characterizes properties of the chamber with the myocardium in a state of maximal activation at a given contractile state. The ESPVR can be characterized by a slope (E_{es}, end-systolic elastance) and a volume axis intercept (V_0), so that $P_{es} = E_{es}(V_{es} - V_0)$, where P_{es} and V_{es} are end-systolic pressure and volume, respectively.[40] This relationship appears independent of afterloading conditions. Under conditions associated with increased myocardial contractility (e.g., inotropic agents), the slope of E_{es} increases, whereas under conditions associated with decreased contractility (negative inotropic agents), the slope of E_{es} decreases. The ESPVR with slope E_{es} is therefore considered as an index of ventricular contractility.[40]

The EDPVR is intrinsically nonlinear, a characteristic attributed to the different types of structural fibers being stretched in different pressure-volume ranges. In the low pressure-volume range, where there is only a small increase in pressure for a given increment in volume, compliant elastin fibers and myocytes with sarcomeric titin molecules are being stretched and account for stiffness. As volume is increased further to a higher range, pressure rises more steeply as slack lengths of collagen fibers are exceeded and stretch is more strongly resisted by these stiff elements. Therefore, chamber stiffness (the change of pressure for a given change of volume, dP/dV) increases as end-diastolic pressure (or volume) is increased.[40]

An important difference between HFrEF and HFpEF patients resides in these pressure-volume loops, with HFrEF being characterized by decreased contractility and down and rightward displacement of the LV ESPVR (see Figure 10-2C), whereas HFpEF is characterized by preserved global contractility but impaired LV relaxation, elevated filling pressures, and increased stiffness with an up and leftward shift of the LV EDPVR, representing raised LV end-diastolic pressure at any given LV end-diastolic volume (see Figure 10-2C).[10,21,28-31,40] In HFpEF, the LV ESPVR is unaltered or even steeper than in subjects without HF (see Figure 10-2C).[19,28,30,31,40] This steep LV EDPVR in patients with HFpEF seems the most important determinant for impaired exercise tolerance, with deficient early diastolic LV recoil, blunted LV lusitropic or chronotropic response, vasodilator incompetence, and deranged ventriculovascular coupling serving contributory roles.[41] Elevated LV filling pressures constitute the hallmark of diastolic LV dysfunction, and filling pressures are considered elevated when the mean PCWP is greater than 12 mm Hg or when the LVEDP is greater than 16 mm Hg.[14]

Noninvasive Measurement of Diastolic Function: Echocardiography

A comprehensive echocardiographic examination (including imaging and Doppler evaluation) is an important part of the evaluation of all patients with HF (see Chapter 29). Echocardiography provides assessment of the size of the cardiac chambers, LV regional wall motion, and EF, as well as evaluation of valvular function, assessment of the presence of pericardial disease, and an estimation of pulmonary artery pressure.[42-44]

Concentric Left Ventricular Remodeling, Hypertrophy, and Left Atrial Size

A substudy from the largest HFpEF randomized clinical trial to date, the I-PRESERVE trial,[6] demonstrated that LV hypertrophy or concentric remodeling and left atrial (LA) enlargement were present in the majority of HFpEF patients and that both LV mass and LA size were independently associated with an increased risk of morbidity and mortality.[45] Evidence of concentric LV remodeling has important implications for the diagnosis of HFpEF and is regarded as a potential surrogate for direct evidence of diastolic LV dysfunction. Hence, LV hypertrophy and LA enlargement were proposed as contributory evidence for the diagnosis of HFpEF.[14]

Physiology of Diastolic Filling and Compliance

Normal diastolic function allows adequate filling of the heart without an excessive increase in diastolic filling pressure both at rest and with exercise. LV relaxation starts at end systole and LV pressure falls rapidly when the LV expands. This relaxation phase is accompanied by active movement of the mitral annulus away from the apex. The velocity of LV dilation and mitral annular movement during early diastole correlates well with how fast the LV fills and relaxes, respectively.[46,47] Myocardial relaxation continues during early diastole to reach the minimal LV diastolic pressure, and the fall in LV pressure produces an early diastolic pressure gradient from the LA that extends to the LV apex. This accelerates blood out of the LA and produces rapid early diastolic flow that quickly propagates to the apex. Because the diastolic intraventricular pressure gradient pulls blood to the apex, it can be considered a measure of LV suction.[42,43] The lower the early diastolic LV pressure is, the greater the gradient for filling, allowing the heart to fill without requiring elevated LA pressure. Furthermore, the ability to decrease LV early diastolic pressure in response to stress allows an increase in LV stroke volume without much increase in LA pressure.[42] Following filling of the LV, the pressure gradient from the LA to the LV apex decreases and then transiently reverses. The reversed mitral valve pressure gradient decelerates and then stops the rapid flow of blood into the LV in diastole. The time for flow deceleration is determined predominantly by the functional LV chamber stiffness and provides a noninvasive indication of LV diastolic operating stiffness.[42] During the midportion of diastole (diastasis), the pressure in the LA and LV equilibrates and mitral flow nearly ceases. Late in diastole, atrial contraction produces a second LA-to-LV pressure gradient that again propels blood into the LV. After atrial systole, as the LA relaxes, its pressure decreases below LV pressure, causing the mitral valve to begin closing. Normally, early diastole is responsible for the majority of ventricular filling, but with disturbed myocardial relaxation, the rate of early diastolic LV pressure decline is reduced, which increases the time to reach minimal LV diastolic pressure and augments the importance of the contribution of atrial contraction for diastolic filling.[43] As LA pressure increases, the early diastolic filling becomes more dominant despite the impaired myocardial relaxation. Early filling is initiated by the increased LA pressure, which pushes the blood into the LV, instead of the negative LV diastolic pressure, which pulls the blood from the LA by suction. As diastolic function worsens, LA pressure is elevated and myocardial relaxation is impaired at rest. In this stage, most of the diastolic LV filling occurs during early diastole and LA contraction may not be sufficient. In this situation, LA contraction pushes blood back into the pulmonary veins, especially if pulmonary venous diastolic forward flow is already completed at the time of atrial contraction.[42] Various patterns of diastolic dysfunction can occur with normal as well as abnormal ejection fractions (see Chapter 29). It has been well established that diastolic dysfunction and filling pressure can be assessed by 2D, Doppler, and tissue Doppler (TD) (**Figure 10-3**).

Grading of Diastolic Dysfunction

The velocity of mitral annular movement during early diastole, designated as e′ or E′ velocity measured by TD

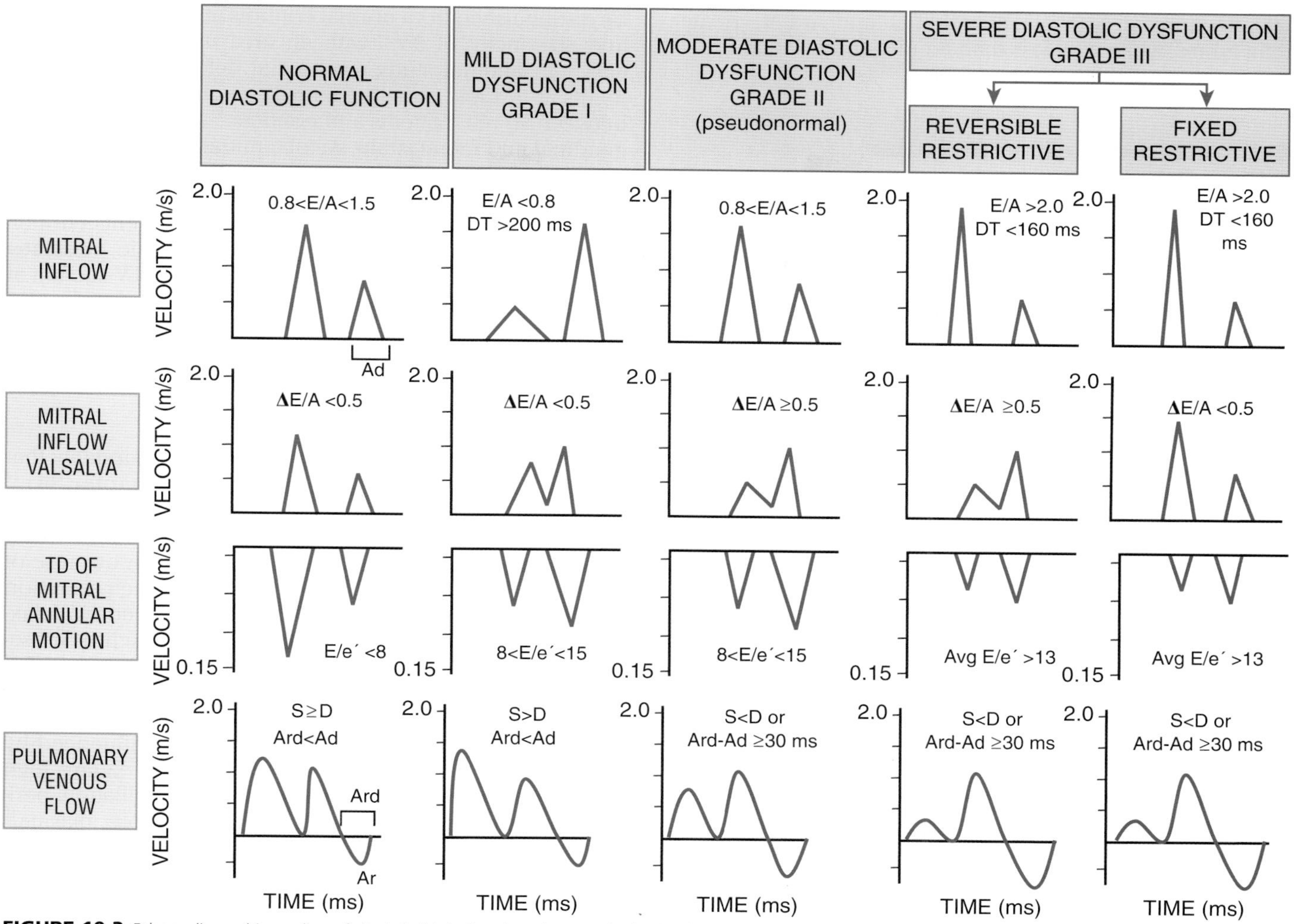

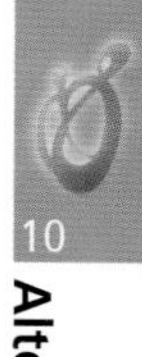

	NORMAL DIASTOLIC FUNCTION	MILD DIASTOLIC DYSFUNCTION GRADE I	MODERATE DIASTOLIC DYSFUNCTION GRADE II (pseudonormal)	SEVERE DIASTOLIC DYSFUNCTION GRADE III: REVERSIBLE RESTRICTIVE	SEVERE DIASTOLIC DYSFUNCTION GRADE III: FIXED RESTRICTIVE
MITRAL INFLOW	0.8<E/A<1.5	E/A <0.8 DT >200 ms	0.8<E/A<1.5	E/A >2.0 DT <160 ms	E/A >2.0 DT <160 ms
MITRAL INFLOW VALSALVA	ΔE/A <0.5	ΔE/A <0.5	ΔE/A ≥0.5	ΔE/A ≥0.5	ΔE/A <0.5
TD OF MITRAL ANNULAR MOTION	E/e′ <8	8<E/e′<15	8<E/e′<15	Avg E/e′ >13	Avg E/e′ >13
PULMONARY VENOUS FLOW	S≥D Ard<Ad	S>D Ard<Ad	S<D or Ard-Ad ≥30 ms	S<D or Ard-Ad ≥30 ms	S<D or Ard-Ad ≥30 ms

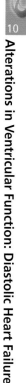

FIGURE 10-3 Echocardiographic grading of diastolic LV dysfunction. *A,* Late mitral valve flow velocity; *Ad,* duration of mitral valve atrial wave flow; *Ar,* reverse pulmonary vein atrial systole flow; *Ard,* duration of reverse pulmonary vein atrial systole flow; *Avg,* average; *D,* pulmonary vein diastolic flow; *DT,* deceleration time; *E,* early mitral valve flow velocity; *e′,* early tissue Doppler mitral annular velocity; *S,* pulmonary vein systolic forward flow.

echocardiography, correlates well with invasive measures of the time constant of myocardial relaxation tau,[46] although it is not entirely governed by relaxation. In healthy young individuals, septal e′ is greater than 10 cm/s and lateral e′ greater than 15 cm/s at rest. These increase with exercise and reflect the ability to achieve a lower minimal LV diastolic pressure to increase early diastolic filling. In individuals with diastolic dysfunction, relaxation or e′ is reduced and remains so in all stages of diastolic dysfunction (see Figure 10-3). Because a normal e′ velocity is unusual in patients with diastolic dysfunction, this parameter is favored in echocardiographic recommendations for assessment of diastolic function. Additional parameters for diastolic function assessment are mitral inflow velocities. Normally, the early diastolic mitral velocity (E) is higher than the late velocity (A) with atrial contraction, so that the E/A ratio is greater than 1. The E velocity is determined mainly by myocardial relaxation and LA pressure. Early stage, or grade 1, diastolic dysfunction is characterized by a lower E than A velocity, prolonged deceleration time (DT), prolonged isovolumic relaxation time (IVRT), higher pulmonary venous systolic than diastolic flow wave (S ≥ D), and reduced e′ (see Figure 10-3).[43,44] Because myocardial relaxation is reduced with aging, this diastolic filling pattern is most common in elderly individuals. As long as necessary filling can be completed during a given diastolic period, there are no clinical symptoms, but diastolic reserve is reduced, and tachycardia or atrial fibrillation compromise diastolic filling significantly. It should be emphasized that filling pressure usually (but not always, especially in the setting of hypertrophy) is normal in patients with grade 1 diastolic dysfunction. The most advanced stage, or grade 3, diastolic dysfunction is characterized by an increased E with short DT (usually <160 ms), decreased A velocity (hence, an E/A ratio ≥ 2), reduced IVRT, a longer duration of reverse pulmonary vein atrial systolic flow than duration of mitral valve atrial flow (Ard-Ad >30 ms), reduced e′ and average E/e′ greater than 13. Because diastolic filling is restricted to early diastole, this stage is also called the *restrictive filling pattern*. LV filling may revert to impaired relaxation with successful therapy in some patients (reversible restrictive), whereas in others, LV filling remains restrictive (fixed restrictive) (see Figure 10-3). Between the early diastolic dysfunction predominated by delayed myocardial relaxation and the late or severe dysfunction predominated by increased filling pressure, as well as delayed relaxation, there is a stage of moderate, or grade 2, diastolic dysfunction where the mitral inflow velocity pattern may look similar to the normal pattern (so-called pseudonormalized), characterized by an E/A ratio of 0.8 to 1.5, which can be decreased by the Valsalva maneuver by

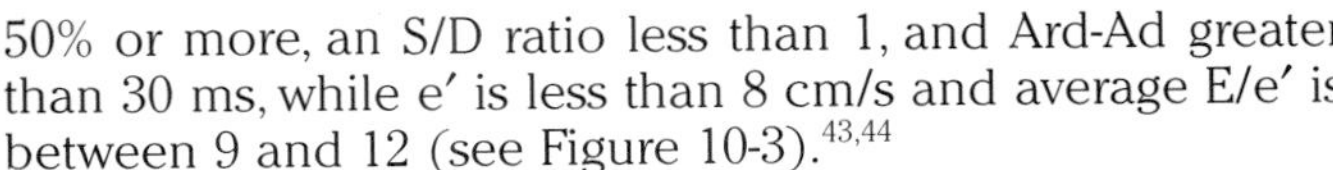

50% or more, an S/D ratio less than 1, and Ard-Ad greater than 30 ms, while e′ is less than 8 cm/s and average E/e′ is between 9 and 12 (see Figure 10-3).[43,44]

Estimation of Left Ventricular Filling Pressures

Earlier it was shown that the E/e′ ratio correlates closely with LV filling pressures.[47] Because E depends on LA driving pressure, LV relaxation kinetics, and age, and e′ depends mostly on LV relaxation kinetics and age, in the E/e′ ratio, effects of LV relaxation kinetics and age are eliminated and the ratio becomes a measure of LA driving pressure or LV filling pressure. A high E/e′ thus represents a high gradient for a low shift in volume. When the ratio E/e′ exceeds 15, LV filling pressures are elevated and when the ratio is lower than 8, LV filling pressures are low.[47] An elevated E/e′ ratio was the best noninvasive measure of diastolic dysfunction for distinguishing patients with HFpEF with invasively proven diastolic dysfunction from normal subjects.[48] The ratio E/e′ is therefore considered diagnostic evidence of the presence of diastolic LV dysfunction if E/e′ is greater than 15, and diagnostic evidence of the absence of HFpEF if E/e′ is less than 8. An E/e′ ratio ranging from 8 to 15 is considered suggestive but nondiagnostic evidence of diastolic LV dysfunction and needs to be implemented with additional echocardiographic measurements or evidence of elevated biomarkers to confirm the diagnosis of HFpEF.[14]

Myocardial Deformation and Strain

The mode of cardiac contraction is determined by the oblique orientation of the myofiber sheets, with subendocardial fibers right-handed oriented and subepicardial fibers left-handed oriented.[43] This geometric fiber orientation induces the characteristic "wringing motion" of the heart around its long axis, characterized by systolic twist and diastolic untwist. Viewed from the apex, the apical portion of the LV normally twists counterclockwise and the basal segment twists clockwise during systole, storing potential energy. LV torsion is the summation of the apical and the basal twisting. The LV untwists immediately after systolic contraction, contributing to generating an intraventricular pressure gradient. Measurement of myocardial twist (or torsion), untwist, and deformation can be determined with a number of techniques of which 2-D speckle tracking echocardiography (STE) from short-axis images of the LV has gained attention. STE is based on tracking myocardial "speckles" from frame to frame in grayscale images. Speckles are very small structures in the image that can be recognized after filtering out noise. STE can be used to determine myocardial velocity, strain (percentage shortening or thickening), and strain rate (rate or speed of myocardial shortening or thickening).[43]

Myocardial strain and strain rate are parameters for the quantification of regional contractility in radial, longitudinal, and circumferential planes and can also be used in the evaluation of diastolic function.[43,44] In both HFpEF and HFrEF patients, with invasively proven elevated LV filling pressures (PCWP >12 mm Hg), LV longitudinal and radial strains were reduced compared with controls, whereas circumferential strain and twist were similar between HFpEF and controls, but lower in HFrEF. Using a cut-off value of global LV longitudinal strain at −16%, HFpEF patients could be distinguished from normal controls at a sensitivity of 95% and specificity of 95%, with an area under the curve of 0.98.[49] In another study, myocardial deformation measurements at rest and on submaximal exercise were compared between HFpEF patients and controls.[50] At rest, systolic longitudinal and radial strain, systolic mitral annular velocities, and apical rotation were lower in HFpEF patients and all failed to rise normally on exercise. Systolic longitudinal functional reserve was also lower in HFpEF patients. Furthermore, HFpEF patients had higher end-diastolic pressures, reduced and delayed untwisting, and reduced LV suction at rest and on exercise. In addition, mitral annular systolic and diastolic velocities, systolic LV rotation, and early diastolic untwist on exercise correlated with peak VO_2 max.[50]

Natriuretic Peptides

Natriuretic peptides (NPs) represent the third modality that can be used in the diagnosis of HFpEF (see Chapter 30).[14] Atrial natriuretic peptide (ANP) and BNP are produced by atrial and ventricular myocardium in response to an increase of atrial or ventricular diastolic stretch because of volume- or pressure-overload conditions and their secretion results in natriuresis, vasodilation, and improved LV relaxation. Cardiac myocytes produce pro-BNP, which is subsequently cleaved in the blood into NT-proBNP and BNP.[51] In HFpEF, NP levels correlate strongly with indices of LV filling pressure as determined by invasive measurements.[52] However, BNP and NT-proBNP levels can be influenced by age, gender, and comorbidities such as kidney failure, high output states, pulmonary embolism, atrial fibrillation, pericardial constriction, and obesity.[51] Furthermore, plasma[17] and myocardial[53] BNP levels are higher in HFrEF than in HFpEF patients, reflecting the higher LV end-diastolic wall stress in HFrEF than in HFpEF. Natriuretic peptides are therefore recommended mainly for exclusion of HFpEF and not for diagnosis of HFpEF. Therefore, when used for diagnostic purposes, natriuretic peptides do not provide diagnostic stand-alone evidence of HFpEF and always need to be implemented with other noninvasive investigations.[14]

LEFT VENTRICULAR DIASTOLIC DYSFUNCTION IN HFpEF

The optimal performance of the LV depends on its ability to cycle between two states: (1) a compliant chamber in diastole that allows the LV to fill from low LA pressure; and (2) a stiff chamber (rapidly rising pressure) in systole that ejects the stroke volume at arterial pressures. Furthermore, stroke volume must increase in response to demand such as exercise, without an increase in LA pressure.[42,43] Determinants of diastolic function include myocardial relaxation and passive properties of the ventricular wall, such as myocardial stiffness, wall thickness, and chamber geometry (**Table 10-1**).[10,28,29] Hence, diastolic dysfunction refers to a disturbance in ventricular relaxation, distensibility, or filling—regardless of whether the LVEF is normal or depressed and whether the patient is symptomatic or asymptomatic.[10]

Relaxation

Myocardial relaxation is the process whereby the myocardium returns after contraction to its unstressed length and force determined by actin-myosin cross-bridge cycling. In

TABLE 10-1 Determinants of Diastolic Function

Myocardial Relaxation
• Load • Inactivation (calcium homeostasis, myofilaments, energetics) • Nonuniformity
Passive Properties of Ventricular Wall
• Myocardial stiffness (cytoskeleton, extracellular matrix) • Wall thickness • Chamber geometry
Other Determinants
• Structures surrounding the left ventricle (pericardium, lungs, right ventricle) • Left atrium, pulmonary veins, and mitral valve • Heart rate

the normal heart, relaxation comprises a major part of ventricular ejection, pressure fall, and the initial part of rapid filling, and with normal load, myocardial relaxation is nearly complete at minimal LV pressure.[28,44] Disturbed myocardial relaxation can result from various mechanisms, including severe or late systolic afterload elevation, nonuniform relaxation due to intraventricular conduction disturbances or myocardial ischemia and disturbed myocardial inactivation.[28]

Effects of Load

Afterload elevations early in the cardiac cycle result in delayed onset and accelerated rate of pressure fall, while a severe or late systolic afterload elevation induces a premature onset and a pronounced slowing of pressure fall. Such slowing might lead to incomplete relaxation and therefore to elevation of filling pressures, a phenomenon that is exacerbated when preload is elevated.[28]

Nonuniform Relaxation

During isovolumic relaxation, reextension of one ventricular segment is accompanied by postsystolic shortening of another segment. The ventricle remains isovolumic but changes its shape and produces intraventricular volume displacement. Asynchronous early segment reextension and regional nonuniformity induce early onset and a slower rate of ventricular pressure fall, and might contribute to the diastolic disturbances observed in coronary heart disease and with intraventricular conduction disturbances.[28]

Myocardial Inactivation

Myocardial inactivation relates to the processes underlying calcium (Ca^{2+}) extrusion from the cytosol and cross-bridge detachment, which is closely related to β-adrenergic signaling. β-adrenergic receptor (β-AR) agonist binding triggers the interaction of guanine nucleotide-binding proteins (G proteins) with adenylyl cyclases to synthesize the second messenger cyclic adenosine monophosphate (cAMP) from ATP. The increase in intracellular cAMP levels activates cAMP-dependent protein kinase A (PKA), which phosphorylates several target proteins involved in Ca^{2+} handling and myofilament contraction (**Figure 10-4**).[54] This affects cardiomyocyte contractility by increasing Ca^{2+} influx through L-type Ca^{2+} channels (LTCC). This Ca^{2+} influx triggers even greater Ca^{2+} release from sarcoplasmic reticulum (SR) Ca^{2+} stores, through ryanodine receptors (Ca^{2+}-induced Ca^{2+} release). The rise in cytosolic Ca^{2+} then induces myofilament activation and consequent muscle contraction. Relaxation is initiated by dissociation of Ca^{2+} from the myofilaments, followed by its reuptake into the SR through phospholamban-regulated SR Ca^{2+}-ATPase (SERCA) and to a limited extent by trans-sarcolemmal Ca^{2+} removal through the sodium-calcium exchanger (NCX).[54,55] The lusitropic effects of PKA result from enhancing diastolic myofilamental Ca^{2+} dissociation through phosphorylation of troponin I (TnI) and cardiac myosin binding protein C, while PKA stimulates Ca^{2+} reuptake through phosphorylation of phospholamban. Furthermore, PKA is known to lower cardiomyocyte stiffness through phosphorylation of the stiff N2B segment of the giant elastic sarcomeric protein titin (for details, see further) (see Figure 10-4).[56,57] In HFrEF, β-adrenergic signaling is depressed as expression of the $β_1$-AR is reduced, whereas the remaining receptors are desensitized.[54] Similar to HFrEF, β-adrenergic signaling is also depressed in HFpEF as evident from downregulated $β_1$-AR expression and reduced SERCA/phospholamban expression ratio.[35]

Myocardial Stiffness

In the absence of endocardial or pericardial disease, the steep LV EDPVR results from increased myocardial stiffness, which is regulated by the extracellular matrix (ECM) and the cardiomyocytes (**Figure 10-5**).[22]

Regulation of Diastolic Stiffness by the Extracellular Matrix

The ECM contributes to passive stiffness in diastole and prevents overstretch, myocyte slippage, and tissue deformation during ventricular filling, whereas ECM components also serve as modulators of growth and tissue differentiation (see Chapter 4).[58] Chronic pressure overload, as occurs in hypertensive heart disease, is associated with excessive collagen deposition, which increases myocardial stiffness.[58] Collagen importantly determines ECM-based stiffness through regulation of its total amount, expression of collagen type I, and degree of collagen cross-linking,[58] which are increased and linked to diastolic LV dysfunction in patients with HFpEF.[59] Myocardial collagen turnover is dynamically modulated by the local RAAS and transforming growth factor β (TGF-β) and through modulation of collagen synthesis and degradation by matrix metalloproteinases (MMPs) and tissue inhibitors of MMPs (TIMPs).[58] In HFpEF, matrix degradation is decreased because of altered expression of MMPs and upregulation of TIMPs.[60,61] Serologic markers of collagen turnover significantly predicted diastolic dysfunction and HFpEF, with MMP2 representing the most sensitive and specific biomarker for the identification of HFpEF.[60] Plasma levels of TIMP-1 also predicted diastolic LV dysfunction and have been proposed as a potential biomarker of HFpEF in hypertensive patients.[61] Distinct expression profiles of MMPs and TIMPs also correspond with unequal patterns of myocardial collagen deposition with mainly interstitial fibrosis in HFpEF and both replacement and interstitial fibrosis in dilated cardiomyopathy.[21] Interestingly, LV endomyocardial biopsy studies demonstrated that one third of HFpEF patients had a normal myocardial collagen volume fraction (CVF), despite similarly elevated LV end-systolic wall stress and LV stiffness modulus when compared with HFpEF patients with raised CVF.[62] In

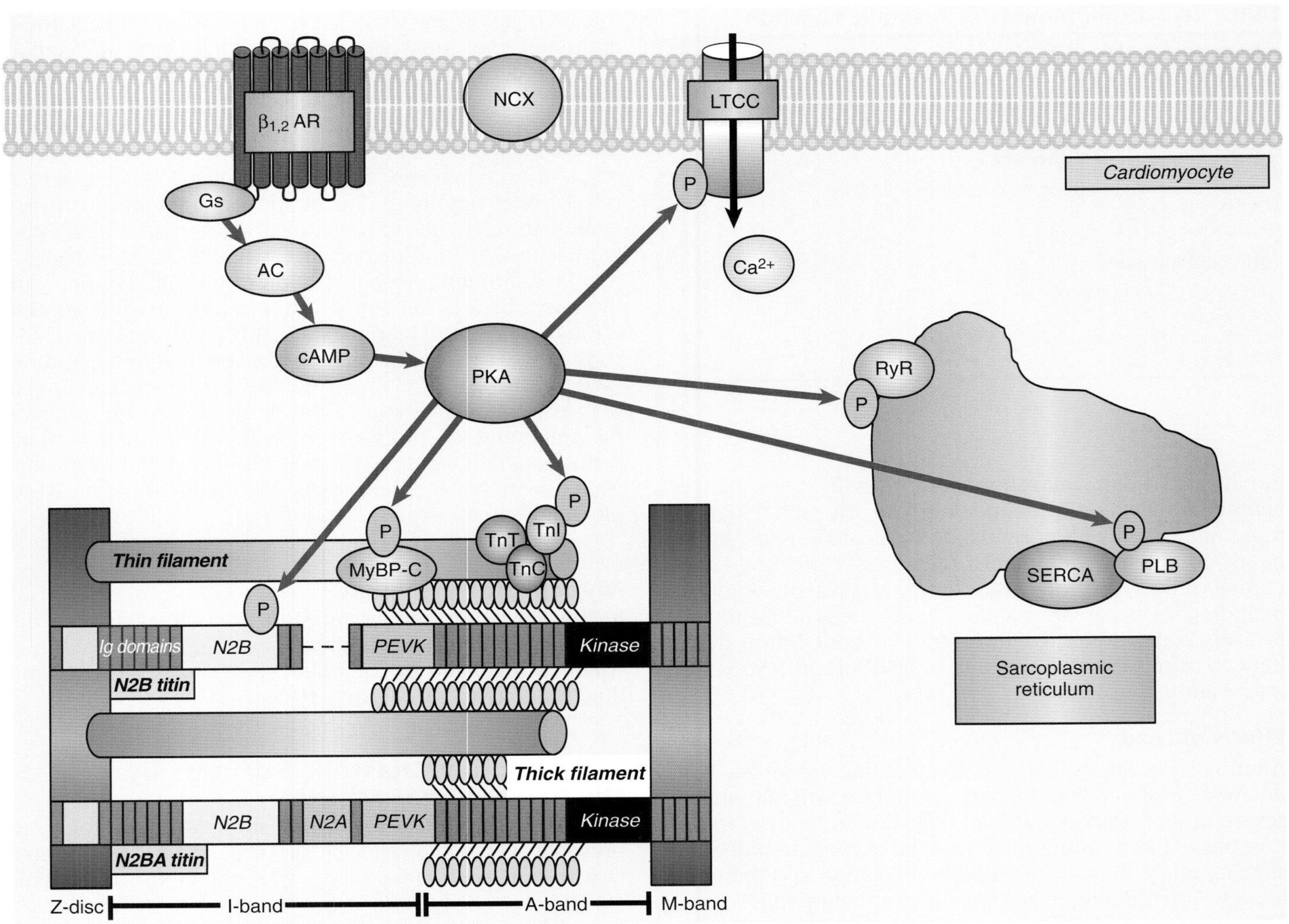

FIGURE 10-4 β-adrenergic signaling and calcium cycling in cardiomyocytes; regulation by PKA. β-adrenergic stimulation triggers the interaction of G proteins with ACs to synthesize cAMP, which stimulates PKA. PKA on its turn enhances inotropic and lusitropic effects in the cardiomyocyte. *AC,* Adenylyl cyclase; *$\beta_{1,2}AR$,* β_1- and β_2-adrenergic receptor; *cAMP,* cyclic adenosine monophosphate; *G_s,* stimulatory G protein; *Ig-domain,* immunoglobulin domains; *MYBP-C,* myosin binding protein C; *N2A,* N2A segment of titin; *N2B,* N2B segment of titin; *NCX,* sodium-calcium exchanger; *P,* phosphorylation; *PEVK,* unique sequence rich in proline, glutamic acid, valine, and lysine; *PLB,* phospholamban; *RyR,* ryanodine receptor; *SERCA,* sarcoplasmic reticulum calcium ATPase; *TnC,* troponin C; *TnI,* troponin I; *TnT,* troponin T.

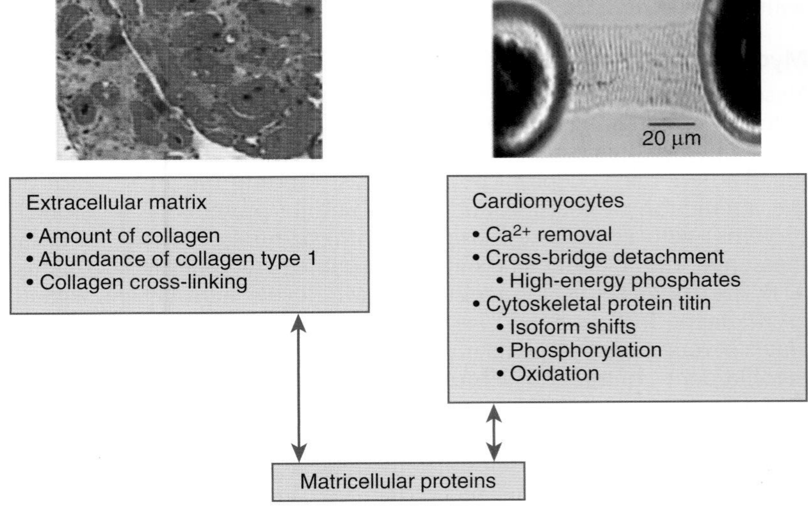

FIGURE 10-5 Extracellular matrix and cardiomyocytes determine myocardial stiffness and interact via matricellular proteins. *Modified from Borlaug BA, Paulus WJ: Heart failure with preserved ejection fraction: pathophysiology, diagnosis and treatment. Eur Heart J 32:670, 2011.*

these patients, high diastolic LV stiffness could unequivocally be attributed to elevated intrinsic cardiomyocyte passive stiffness.[62]

Regulation of Diastolic Stiffness by the Cardiomyocytes

Previous LV endomyocardial biopsy studies conducted force measurements in single, mechanically isolated cardiomyocytes.[21,62] After mechanical isolation, cardiomyocytes were treated with Triton X-100, which disrupts all sarcoplasmic membrane structures, leaving sarcomeric and cytoskeletal structures intact. Subsequently, single "permeabilized" cardiomyocytes were attached with silicone adhesive between a force transducer and piezoelectric motor (**Figure 10-6A**). After adjustment of sarcomere length to 2.2 μm, myocytes were subjected to both relaxing and activating solutions—containing varying Ca^{2+} concentrations—to calculate maximal calcium-activated isometric force. Exposure to a series of solutions with intermediate pCa yields the baseline force-pCa relation. On transfer of the myocyte from relaxing to activating solution, isometric force starts to develop. Once a steady-state force level is reached, the cell is shortened within 1 ms to 80% of its original length (slack test) to determine the baseline of the force transducer. The distance between the baseline and the steady force level is the total force (kN/m^2). Shortly thereafter the cell can be restretched and returned to the relaxing solution, in which a second slack test is performed to determine passive force or resting tension of the cardiomyocyte, which is a measure of intrinsic cardiomyocyte stiffness (kN/m^2) (see Figure 10-6B).[62] In comparative LV endomyocardial biopsy studies, cardiomyocyte passive force was significantly higher in HFpEF than in controls (**Figure 10-7A**)[62] and HFrEF patients (see Figure 10-7B).[21] Moreover, intrinsic cardiomyocyte stiffness correlated with invasive measures of LV stiffness, including LVEDP (see Figure 10-7C), circumferential LV end-diastolic wall stress (σ, kN/m^2) (see Figure 10-7D), and myocardial stiffness modulus (E, kN/m^2) (see Figure 10-7E).[21,62] Interestingly, in vitro administration of PKA acutely lowered passive force only in HFpEF and HFrEF patients (see Figure 10-7B) and not in controls (see Figure 10-7A), whereas the fall in passive force was greatest in HFpEF (see Figure 10-7B).[21,62] Acute lowering of passive force by PKA indicates that increased cardiomyocyte stiffness is partly reversible by stimulating phosphorylation at the sarcomeric protein level. The larger drop in passive force in HFpEF following PKA administration was attributed to a phosphorylation deficit of the giant elastic sarcomeric protein titin, which has numerous phosphorylatable sites and is the main determinant of cardiomyocyte stiffness, passive tension, and myocardial biomechanical stress/stretch signaling.[55,56]

The Giant Elastic Sarcomeric Protein Titin

In the mechanotransduction network of the heart, external force signals (such as those imposed during hemodynamic load) are transmitted from the ECM to the cardiomyocyte cytoskeleton, while at the same time the sarcomeres

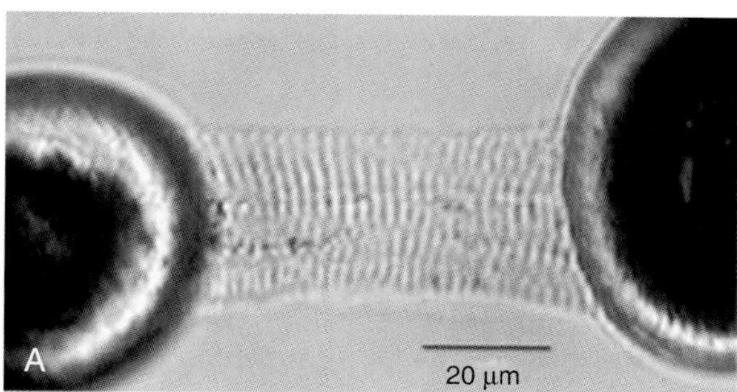

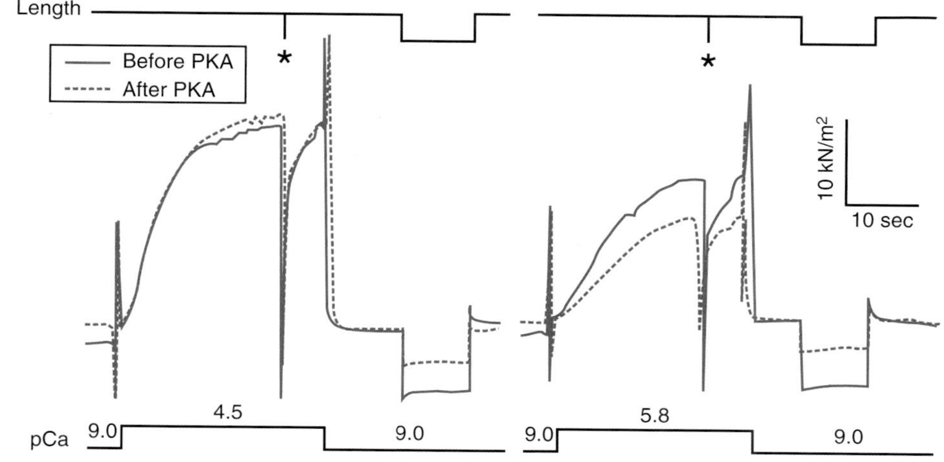

FIGURE 10-6 **A,** Single cardiomyocyte mounted between force transducer and piezoelectric motor. **B,** Contraction-relaxation sequence recorded in single cardiomyocyte before and after PKA treatment during maximal (pCa 4.5) and submaximal (pCa 5.8) activation. *Slack test: see text. *Modified from Borbely A, van der Velden J, Papp Z, et al: Cardiomyocyte stiffness in diastolic heart failure. Circulation 111:774, 2005.*

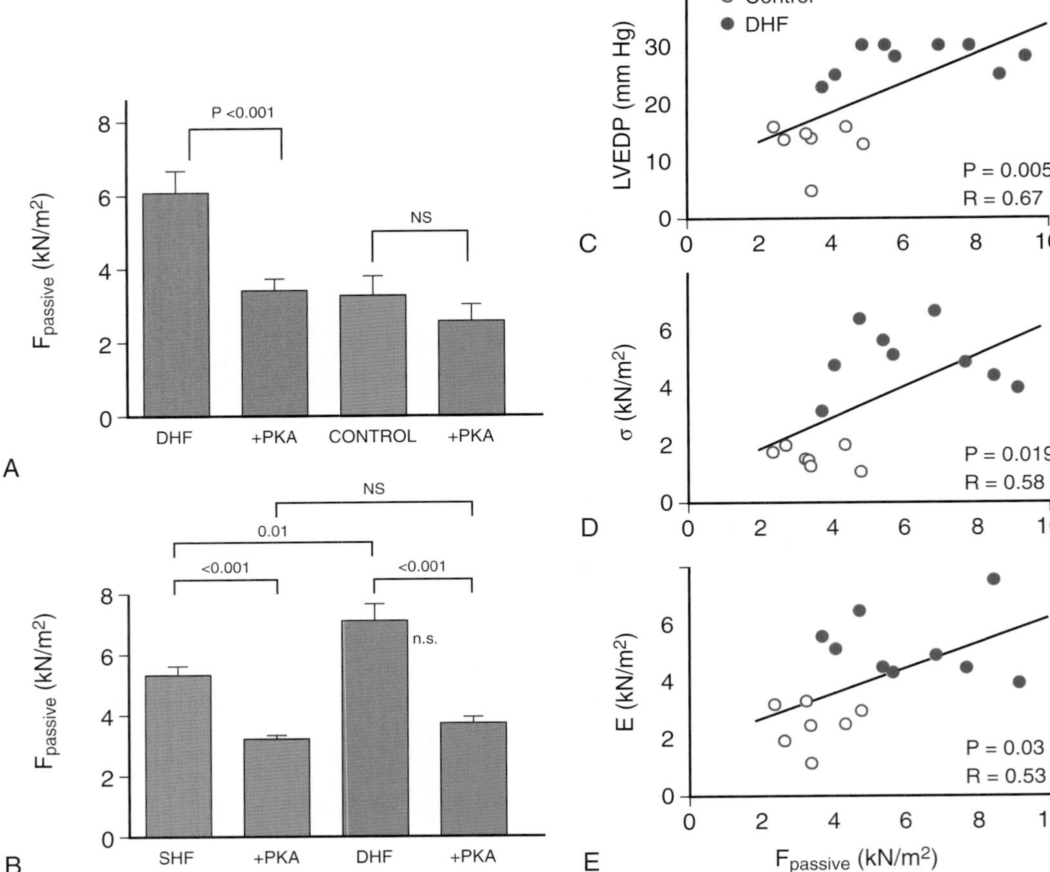

FIGURE 10-7 **A,** PKA treatment reduces cardiomyocyte passive force ($F_{passive}$) of HFpEF patients to values observed in control group at baseline and after PKA treatment. **B,** $F_{passive}$ was higher in HFpEF than in HFrEF; PKA treatment reduced $F_{passive}$ in HFpEF and HFrEF. **C, D,** and **E,** Correlations between $F_{passive}$ of each individual HFpEF patient and LVEDP, σ and E measured at time of cardiac catheterization. *Modified from van Heerebeek L, Borbely A, Niessen HWM, et al: Myocardial structure and function differ in systolic and diastolic heart failure. Circulation 113:1966, 2006; and Borbely A, van der Velden J, Papp Z, et al: Cardiomyocyte stiffness in diastolic heart failure. Circulation 111:774, 2005.*

themselves generate forces, which propagate in the opposite direction. The giant elastic sarcomeric protein titin importantly mediates this bidirectional force transduction and it integrates biomechanical stress/stretch signals to hypertrophy signaling (**Figure 10-8**).[55,56] Titin is the largest protein in the human body and can be considered the backbone of the (half) sarcomere, with its NH_2 terminus anchored at the Z-disk, the elastic spring segment running through the I band, and its longest portion bound to the thick filament, reaching all the way to the M-band (see Figure 10-8).[55,56] Approximately 90% of the mass of the titin molecule is made up of globular domains of the immunoglobulin (Ig) or fibronectin-type III (FN3)-like folds; the remainder is composed of insertions of unique sequences. Nearly all Z-disk and A-band/M-band titin domains are constitutively expressed in the human striated muscle titin-isoforms. Differential splicing occurs mainly in the I-band titin segment, giving rise to the presence of two distinct isoforms in the human heart: the N2B (3000 kDa) and N2BA (≈3200 to 3700 kDa) isoform (see Figure 10-8). Both isoforms have a "proximal" and "distal" Ig-domain region, an "N2B" domain, and a "PEVK" domain, so called for its high content of proline (P), glutamic acid (E), valine (V), and lysine (K) residues. In the N2B titin isoform, many exons coding for Ig domains and unique sequences are skipped, whereas the N2BA isoform contains in addition a "middle-Ig domain" region, an "N2A" domain, and a PEVK segment of variable length. Hence, the N2B isoform represents a shorter, stiffer isoform, whereas N2BA isoforms represent longer, more compliant isoforms.[55,56]

Titin as an Integrator of Sarcomeric Mechanosensory Function

In addition to determining cardiomyocyte passive stiffness, titin is increasingly recognized as a hotspot for protein-protein interactions and a putative mediator of mechanosensory processes. In the following section, a brief overview of just a few of these interactions is depicted.[56,57] A number of titin regions are particularly engaged in protein-protein interactions, including the NH_2-terminal segment at the Z-disk, the elastic I-band part, the COOH-terminal segment within and adjacent to the M-band, and the titin-kinase domain adjacent to the M-band. Various interactions with proteins that shuttle to/from the nucleus suggest that titin signaling is integrated in hypertrophic signaling pathways (**Figure 10-9**).[56,57] The NH_2 terminus of titin is integrated through its Z-disk ligands, telethonin (T-Cap), and α-actinin into a putative mechanosensor complex that may also contain muscle LIM protein (MLP) and perhaps additional proteins. In response to mechanical stress (stretch), MLP is thought to translocate to the nucleus and play a role in

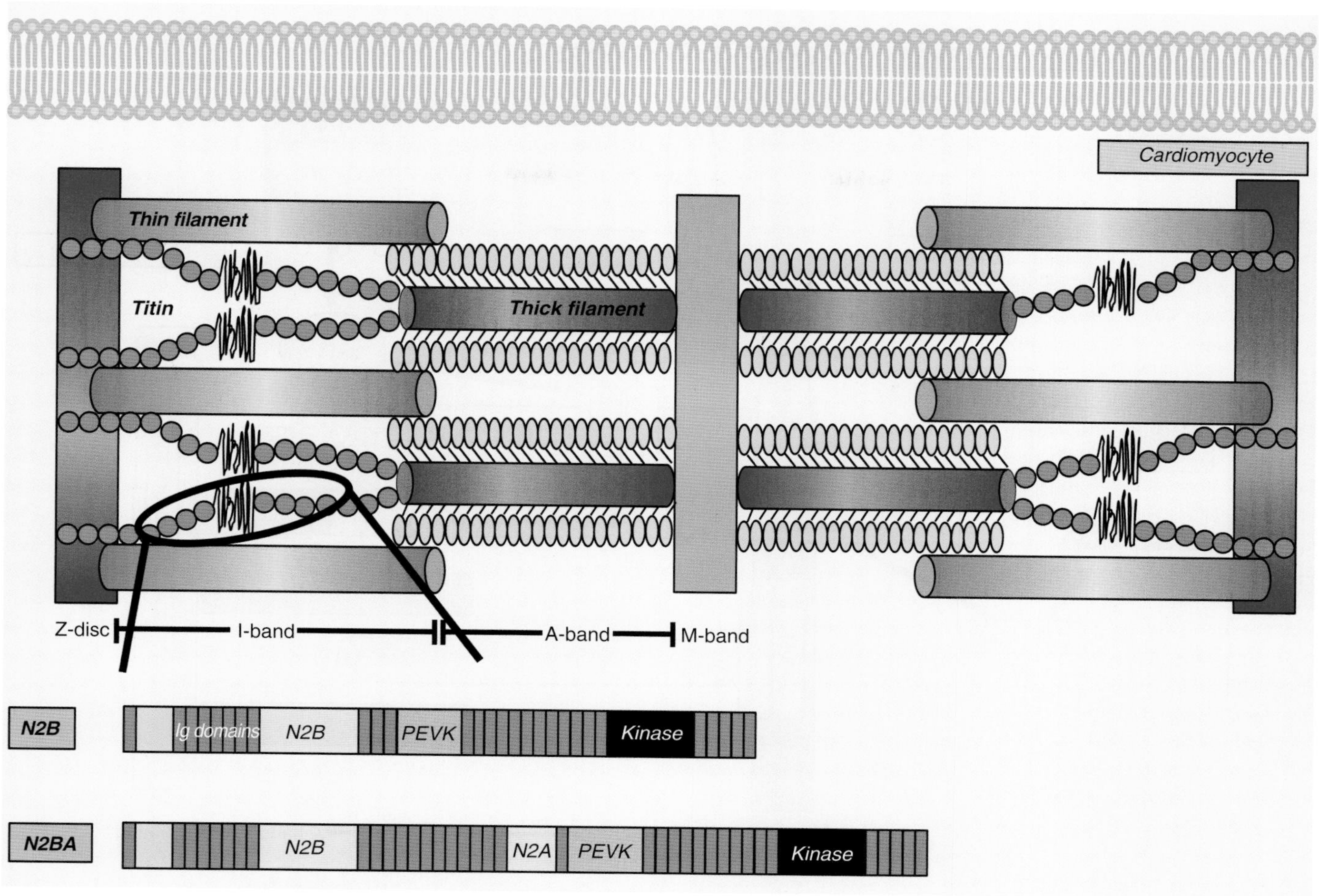

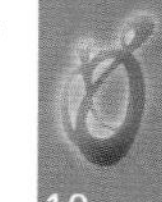

FIGURE 10-8 Schematic of titin in sarcomere. Circled Ps indicate phosphorylatable sites. For details, see text.

regulating myogenic differentiation and hypertrophy (see Figure 10-9).[56,57] Via telethonin/T-Cap binding to calsarcin, the Z-disk titin is tied to the signaling pathway of calcineurin, which initiates—by dephosphorylating nuclear factor of activated T-cells (NFAT)—a hypertrophic gene program, particularly in response to mechanical stress (see Figure 10-9). Other connections involving Z-disk titin substantiate a structural role for that region (e.g., interactions with the two giant muscle proteins, nebulin and obscurin, as well as with γ-filamin, which links titin to integrin and the focal adhesion complex and associated mechanical signaling pathways [see Figure 10-9]).[56,57]

The N2B segment is also involved in protein-protein interactions, such as binding to four-and-a-half-LIM-domain proteins 1 and 2 (FHL1 and 2), which can shuttle to the nucleus and act as transcriptional co-activators.[56,57] The FHLs target metabolic enzymes to the I-band and interact with mitogen-activated protein kinases (MAPKs), whereas FHL1 interacts with G-protein signaling from the G protein–coupled receptor (GPCR), which is stimulated by angiotensin II (AngII) and endothelin-1 (ET-1) (see Figure 10-9).[56,57] Protein-protein interactions also occur preferentially at the center of the sarcomere in the M-band and its close vicinity. Just outside the titin-kinase domain, a stretch of titin domains binds to muscle-specific RING-finger protein (MuRF) 1, which links titin to the proteasomal pathway and to nuclear signaling (see Figure 10-9). MuRF 1 can bind other MuRF isoforms and these proteins can associate with multiple cytoskeletal and signaling molecules mediating energy metabolism, whereas MuRF 1 is thought to inhibit myocardial hypertrophic signaling.[56,57] The titin-kinase is activated by tyrosine phosphorylation and subsequent binding of Ca^{2+}/calmodulin, whereas telethonin/T-cap represents one of the substrates of the titin-kinase. Mechanical stress induces a conformational change in the titin-kinase domain, allowing formation of a signaling complex that links titin to the MuRF pathway, which is mediated by the protein neighbor-of-BRCA1-gene-1 (Nbr1), which targets p62 and MuRF 2 to the titin-kinase. The titin-kinase domain could thus serve a contributory role in biomechanical stress/stretch signaling.[56,57] Finally, the COOH-terminus of titin also cross-links with the thick filament protein and M-band associated proteins, including obscurin, providing mechanical stability and acting as a cross point of biomechanical signaling.[56,57]

Thus titin integrates myocardial biomechanical stress/stretch pathways and hypertrophy signaling, whereas titin functions as a bidirectional spring responsible for early diastolic recoil and late diastolic resistance to stretch with titin-based passive force rising exponentially upon increasing sarcomeric stretch (see Figure 10-8).[56,57] Cardiomyocyte titin-based elasticity can be adjusted through transcriptional and posttranslational modifications.

Transcriptional Titin Isoform Modifications

At the transcriptional level, titin modulates stiffness through shifts in expression of its compliant N2BA and stiff N2B

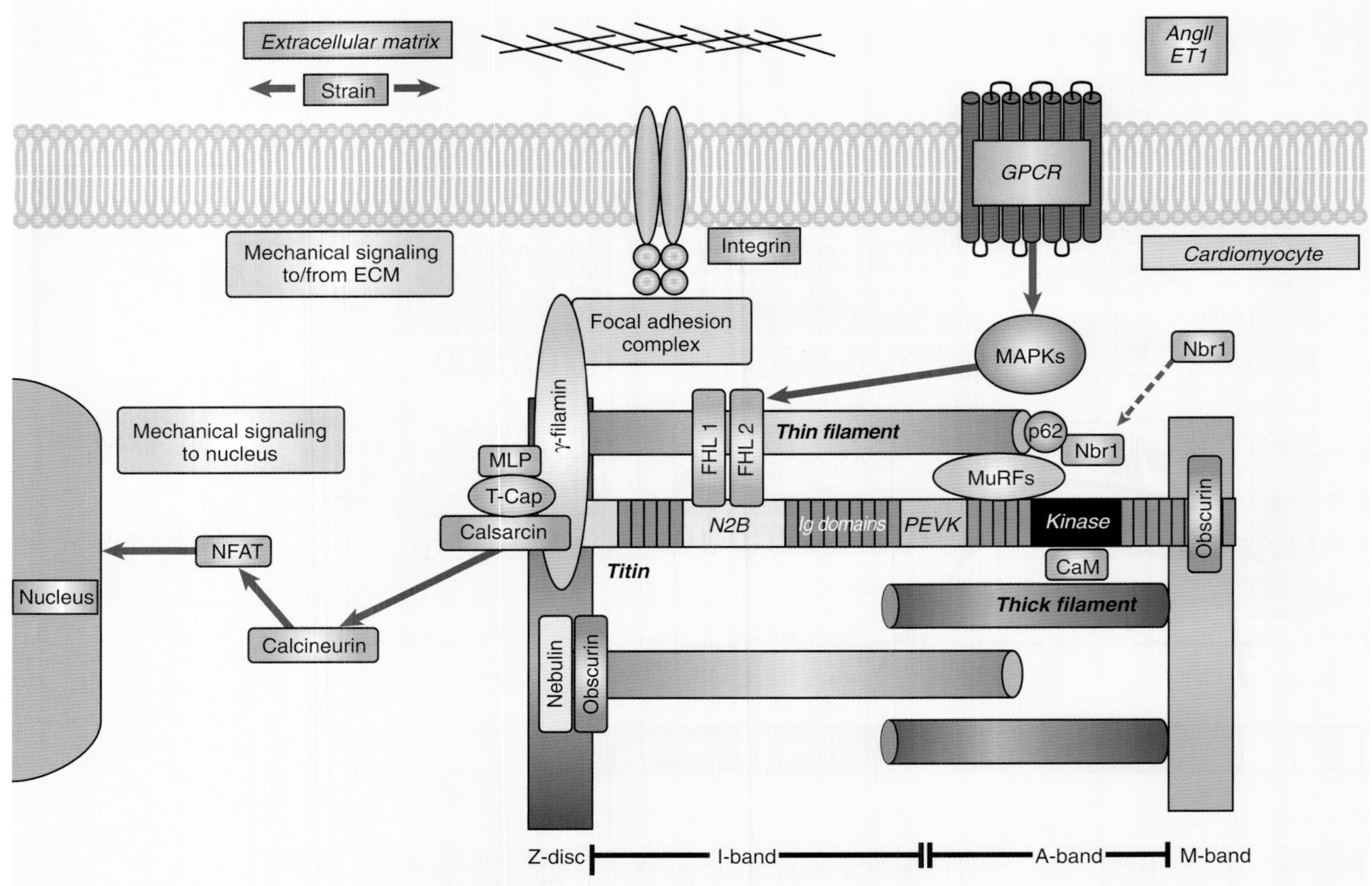

FIGURE 10-9 Links between titin and stress-signaling pathways in the cardiomyocyte (for details, see text). *AngII,* Angiotensin II; *CaM,* Ca^{2+}/calmodulin; *ET-1,* endothelin-1; *FHL1* and *FHL2,* four-and-a-half-LIM-domain protein-1 and -2; *GPCR,* G protein–coupled receptor; *MAPKs,* mitogen-activated protein kinases; *MLP,* muscle LIM protein; *MuRF,* muscle-specific ring finger protein; *Nbr1,* neighbor-of-BRCA-1 gene; *NFAT,* nuclear factor of activated T cells; *T-Cap,* titin-cap (telethonin).

isoforms, which are co-expressed in the normal heart with an N2BA:N2B ratio of approximately 35:65.[56,57] The N2BA:N2B isoform expression ratio is increased in LV endomyocardial biopsies from HFrEF patients,[21] which reduces intrinsic cardiomyocyte stiffness, possibly as a compensatory mechanism initiated in a globally stiffened (fibrotic) environment.[56,57] In contrast, the N2BA:N2B isoform expression ratio is decreased in LV endomyocardial biopsies from HFpEF patients,[21] which can contribute to elevated cardiomyocyte stiffness.[56,57]

Posttranslational Titin Isoform Modifications

Although titin-isoform switching is a confirmed mechanism for adjusting myocardial passive stiffness, phosphorylation-mediated posttranslational modifications of titin represent a means by which titin acutely tunes cardiomyocyte passive stiffness.[56,57] Stimulation of β-AR signaling induces cAMP generation and subsequent activation of PKA, which then phosphorylates a unique sequence of 572 amino acids (N2-Bus) in the stiff N2B segment of titin. PKA-mediated phosphorylation of the N2B segment of titin acutely lowers intrinsic cardiomyocyte stiffness (**Figure 10-10**).[21,62,63] In addition, protein kinase G (PKG), activated upstream by cyclic guanosine monophosphate (cGMP), also phosphorylates the N2-Bus in the stiff N2B segment of titin, thereby acutely lowering cardiomyocyte passive force (see Figure 10-10).[21,53,62,63]

Two additional posttranslational modifications of titin, both increasing titin-based stiffness, include protein kinase C α-mediated phosphorylation of titin's PEVK segment[64] and oxidative stress-induced formation of disulfide bridges in the stiff N2B segment.[65] Contribution by other myofilamentary proteins, such as myosin heavy chain, desmin, actin, troponin T, TnI, and myosin light chain-1 and -2, was recently ruled out,[62,63] suggesting that phosphorylation-mediated posttranslational modification of titin indeed represents the most likely mechanism for acute modulation of intrinsic cardiomyocyte stiffness. Furthermore, contribution to passive force of the thin filament and cross-bridge interaction were ruled out because of unaltered passive force after exposure to gelsolin (which removes the thin filament) and 2,3-butanedione monoxine (which prevents cross-bridge interactions).[63]

The finding of PKG being able to acutely lower intrinsic cardiomyocyte stiffness has received a lot of clinical attention, because myocardial cGMP-PKG signaling crucially regulates cardiovascular physiology and might be amenable for potential therapeutic strategies.

CYCLIC GMP-DEPENDENT SIGNALING IN CARDIOMYOCYTES

The pivotal intracellular second messenger cGMP importantly regulates cardiac contractility, vascular tone, platelet

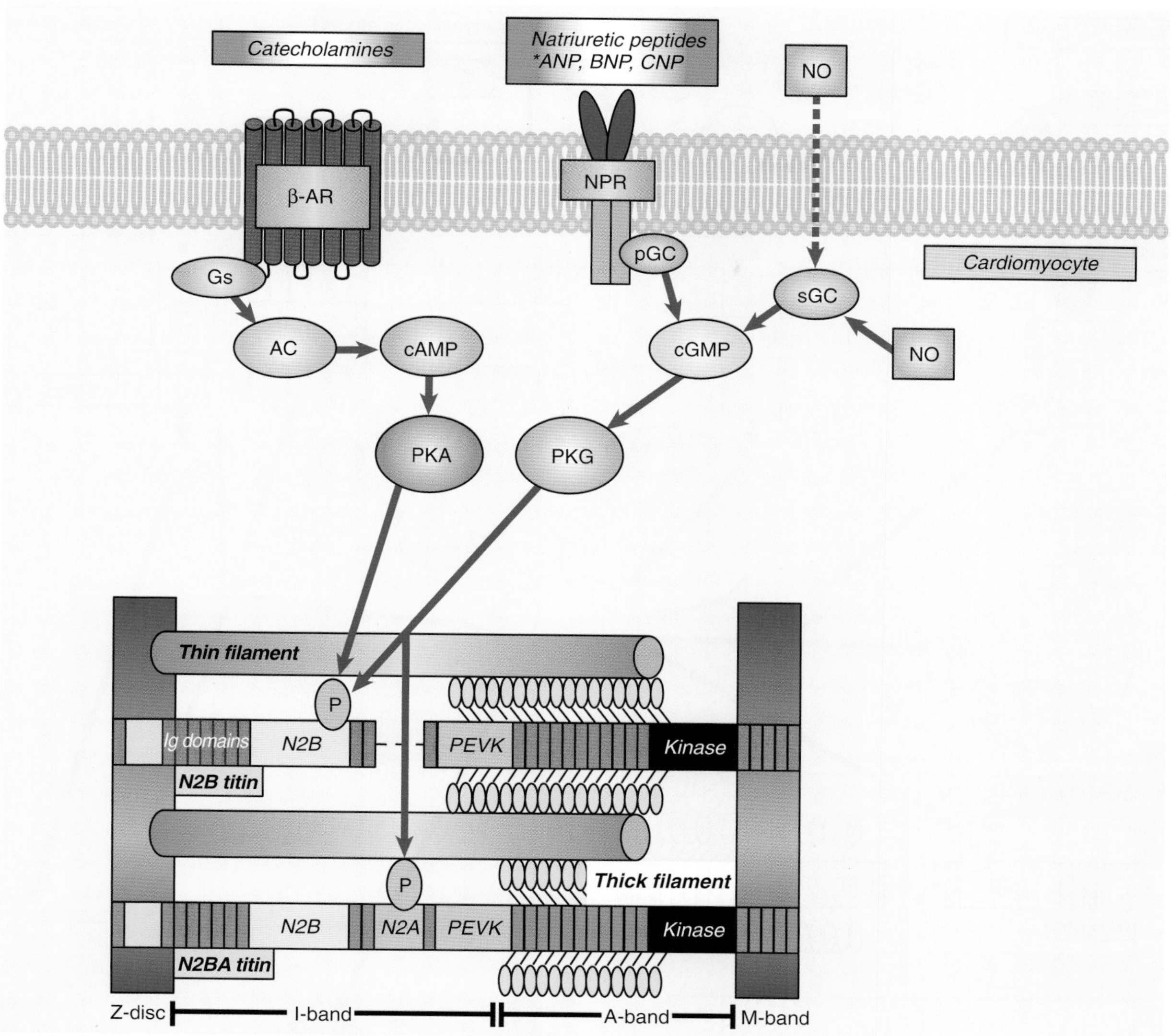

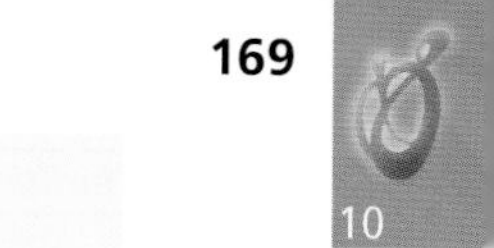

FIGURE 10-10 Cardiomyocyte signaling pathways involved in regulating cardiac titin stiffness. Titin-based stiffness can be modulated by reversible phosphorylation of the N2B segment by both PKA and PKG. Activation of PKA results from stimulation by signaling through the β-adrenergic pathway, which is coupled to the second messenger cAMP. Activation of PKG results from stimulation by the second messenger cGMP. Generation of cGMP results from either activation of sGC by NO or from activation of pGC by NPs. Circled Ps indicate phosphorylatable sites. *AC,* Adenylyl cyclase; *ANP,* atrial natriuretic peptide; *β-AR,* β-adrenergic receptor; *BNP,* B-type natriuretic peptide; *cAMP,* cyclic adenosine monophosphate; *cGMP,* cyclic guanosine monophosphate; *CNP,* C-type natriuretic peptide; *G,* G-stimulatory protein; *Ig,* immunoglobulin domains; *NO,* nitric oxide; *NPR,* natriuretic peptide receptor; *PEVK,* unique sequence rich in proline, glutamic acid, valine, and lysine; *pGC,* particulate guanylate cyclase; *sGC,* soluble guanylate cyclase.

function, mitochondrial function, stress-response signaling, and cardiovascular remodeling (see Chapters 1 and 2).[66,67] Synthesis of cGMP results from either NP-mediated activation of particulate guanylate cyclase (pGC), which is located at the plasma membrane, or from nitric oxide (NO)-mediated activation of soluble guanylate cyclase (sGC) (see Figure 10-10), which is predominantly located in the cytosol, although small sGC plasma membrane fractions have also been identified.[66,67] NO is an ubiquitous intracellular and intercellular signaling molecule generated in a temporally and spatially restricted manner by a family of NO synthases (NOS), including endothelial NOS (eNOS), neuronal NOS (nNOS), and inducible NOS (iNOS).[68] NO is crucially important for diastolic function, while it exerts autocrine and paracrine effects in the heart, depending on where and by which NOS isoform NO is produced. These effects include modulation of contractile function, excitation-contraction coupling, vascular homeostasis and myocardial metabolism through modulation of myocardial substrate use, and through reduction of myocardial oxygen consumption.[68] In healthy individuals, as well as in HFrEF and aortic stenosis (AS) patients, intracoronary administration of NO donors induced an earlier onset of isovolumic LV pressure decay, lowered LV peak systolic, end-systolic, and end-diastolic pressures, and shifted the LV EDPVR rightward.[69] In dilated cardiomyopathy patients, the rightward displacement of the LV EDPVR was accompanied by a significant increase in stroke volume because of improved recruitment of LV preload reserve.[69] Because NO diffusion distances in cardiomyocytes are limited, NO-sGC-cGMP signaling is compartmentalized into functional signalosomes, coupling NO synthesis from eNOS to downstream sGC-cGMP signals.[66-68] The main targets of cGMP include PKG and cGMP-regulated phosphodiesterases (PDEs). cGMP-PKG signaling negatively modulates contractility, accelerates relaxation, improves cardiomyocyte stiffness, and suppresses pro-hypertrophic signaling

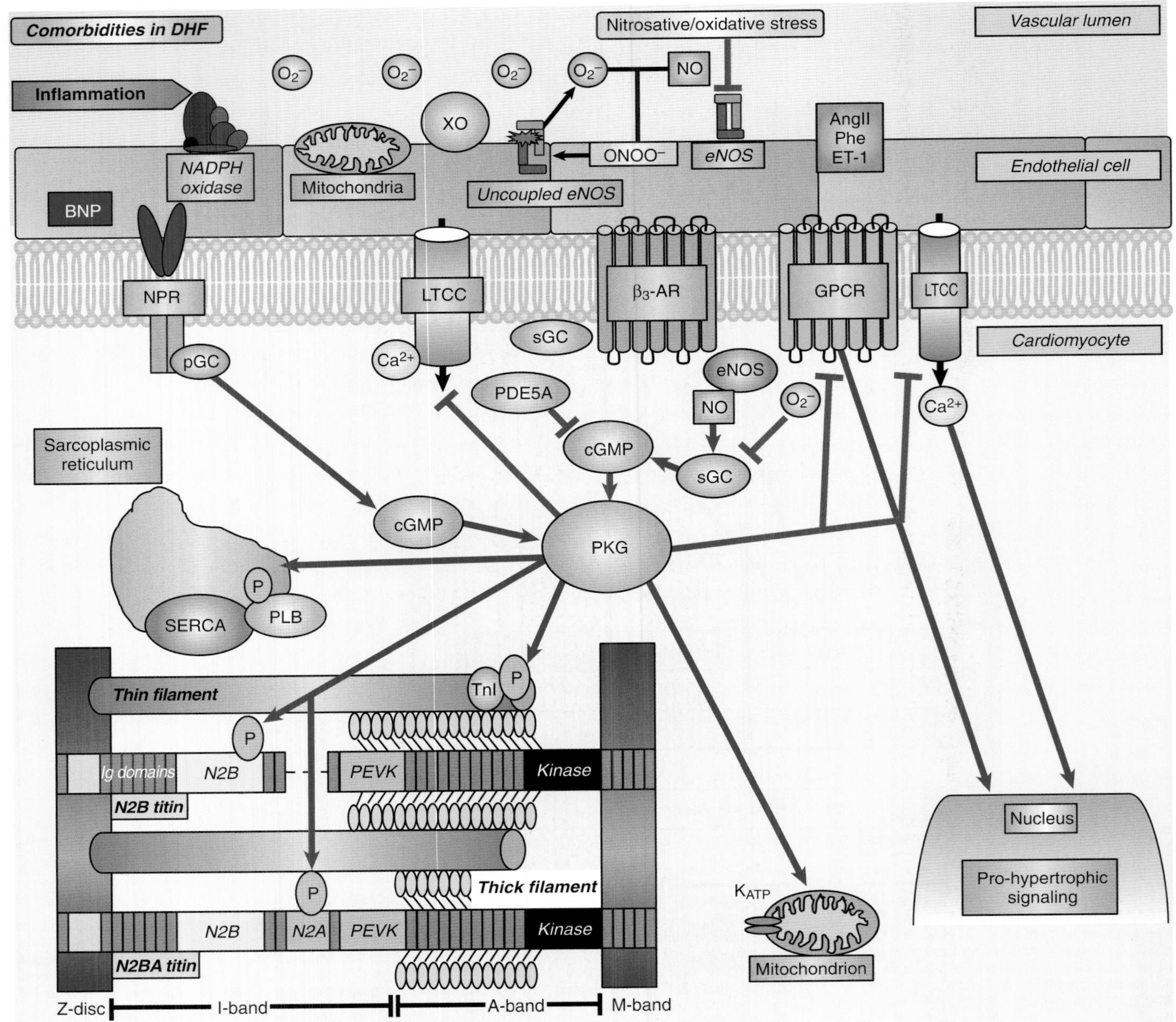

FIGURE 10-11 Comorbidities in HFpEF induce vascular inflammation, endothelial dysfunction, and oxidative stress, causing downregulation of NO-sGC-cGMP-PKG signaling. Superoxide (O_2^-) rapidly reacts with and inactivates NO with formation of peroxynitrite ($ONOO^-$). $ONOO^-$ uncouples eNOS, which then produces O_2^- instead of NO. This results in decreased NO bioavailability and downregulation of NO-sGC-cGMP-PKG signaling. O_2^- also directly inhibits sGC. Within the cardiomyocyte, PKG-mediated phosphorylation importantly regulates intracellular signaling. PKG-mediated phosphorylation of phospholamban, the N2B and N2A segments of titin and TnI, accelerates relaxation and lowers intrinsic cardiomyocyte stiffness and myofilament Ca^{2+} sensitivity, respectively. PKG inhibits pro-hypertrophic signaling pathways through phosphorylation and suppression of GPCRs, LTCC, and TRPC channels. In addition, cGMP-PKG provides cardiac protection in ischemia-reperfusion injury involving mitochondrial K_{ATP} channel regulation. PDE5 specifically hydrolyzes cGMP and thereby offsets cGMP-PKG–mediated signaling. *eNOS,* Endothelial NO synthase; *LTCC,* L-type Ca^{2+} channel; *NADPH oxidase,* nicotinamide adenine dinucleotide phosphate-oxidase; *PDE5,* phosphodiesterase type 5; *Phe,* phenylephrine; *PLB,* phospholamban; *TRPC,* transient receptor potential canonical channel; *XO,* xanthine oxidase.

pathways.[66-68] PKG-mediated phosphorylation of phospholamban, the N2B segment of titin and TnI, accelerates relaxation, lowers cardiomyocyte stiffness, and decreases myofilament Ca^{2+} sensitivity, respectively. Because PKG suppresses signaling through AngII- and ET-1–activated GPCRs, members of the transient receptor potential canonical (TRPC) channels and L-type Ca^{2+} channels, PKG inhibits prominent pro-hypertrophic pathways (**Figure 10-11**).[66,67] Furthermore, the cGMP-PKG pathway has also been implicated in cardiac protection against ischemia-reperfusion injury involving mitochondrial K_{ATP} channel regulation and stress-responsive (survival) signaling cascades (see Figure 10-11).[66] Myocardial cGMP-PKG and cAMP-PKA signaling is offset by PDEs, which hydrolyze cyclic nucleotides (cGMP, cAMP) to the inactive linear form (5′-GMP, 5′-AMP), thereby regulating both the duration and the amplitude of cyclic nucleotide signaling. Of the 11 members of the PDE superfamily, PDE 1 to 5, 8, and 9 are expressed in the heart with individual PDEs exerting differential selectivity for cAMP or cGMP hydrolysis.[66,67] Importantly, the cGMP signal is compartmentalized within a cell so that specific targeted proteins can be regulated by the same "generic" cGMP to exert differential physiologic effects.[66,67] NO-cGMP derived from eNOS is functionally coupled to PDE5, modulating cardiac

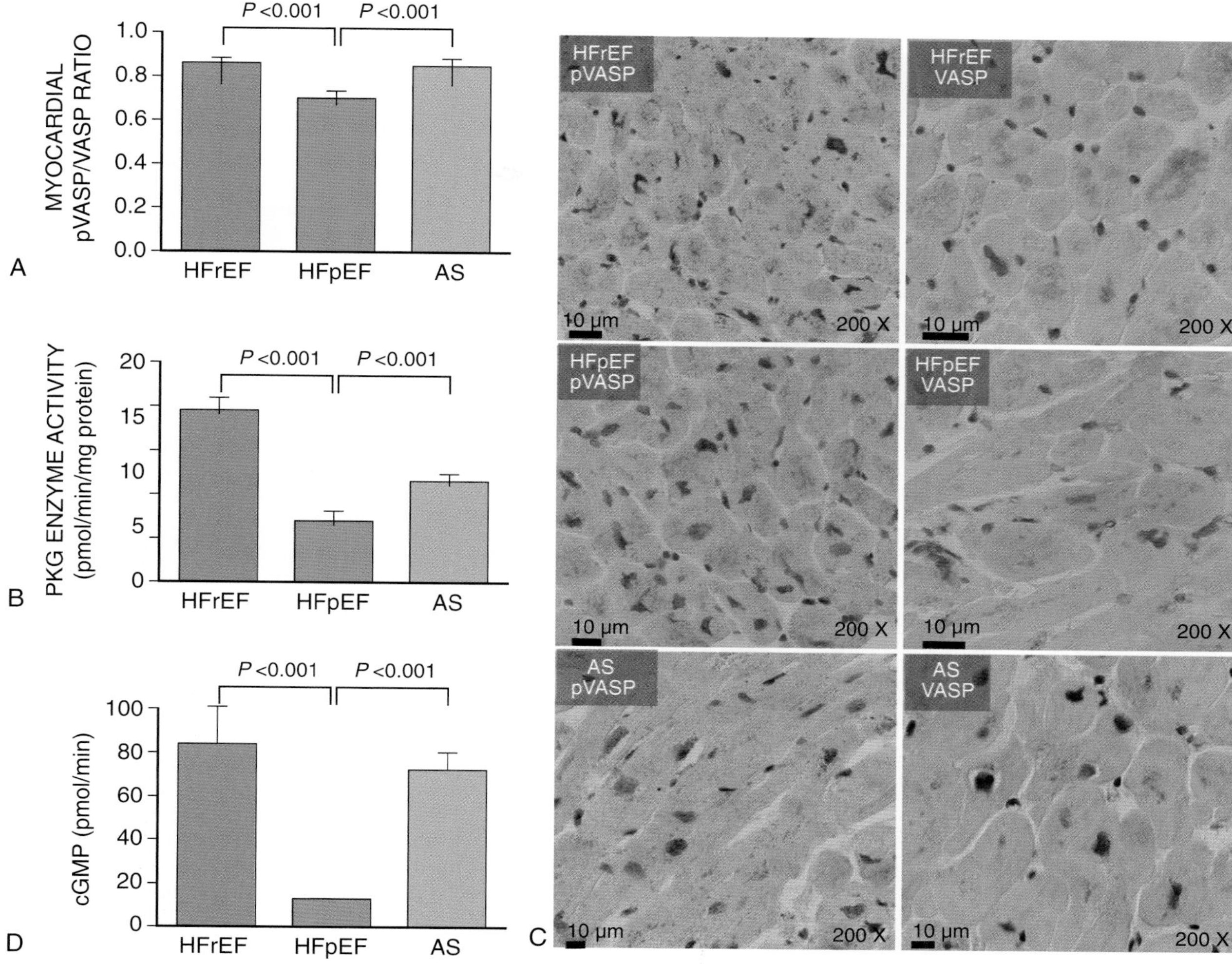

FIGURE 10-12 **A** and **B,** Lower myocardial PKG activity in HFpEF (HFpEF) than in HFrEF (HFrEF) and aortic stenosis (AS) patients. **C,** Representative immunohistochemical images stained for pVASP and VASP in HFpEF, HFrEF, and AS. (The ratio of pVASP/VASP is a marker of PKG activity.) **D,** Lower myocardial cGMP concentration in HFpEF than in HFrEF or in AS. *Modified from van Heerebeek L, Hamdani N, Falcao-Pires I, et al: Low myocardial protein kinase G activity in heart failure with preserved ejection fraction. Circulation 126:830, 2012.*

β-adrenergic–stimulated contractility.[70] Cardiac diastolic function is modified by the NP-pGC pathway similarly to the NO-sGC pathway, with BNP stimulating myocardial relaxation and distensibility.[71]

Myocardial PKG Activity in HFpEF

Acute BNP administration was recently reported to lower diastolic LV stiffness and to increase myocardial titin phosphorylation in an old hypertensive HFpEF dog model[71] but failed to improve clinical endpoints in acutely decompensated HF patients with LVEF of 40% or more.[72] In HFpEF, slow LV relaxation and high diastolic LV stiffness have also been shown to react favorably to raised PKG activity following in vivo administration of the PDE5 inhibitor sildenafil. Sildenafil restored LV relaxation kinetics in mice exposed to transverse aortic constriction (TAC)[73] and reduced diastolic LV stiffness in an old hypertensive dog model through restored titin N2B phosphorylation[71] and in HFpEF patients with pulmonary hypertension.[74] In contrast, in the multicenter, placebo controlled, randomized RELAX trial (Phosphodiesterase-5 Inhibition to Improve Clinical Status and Exercise Capacity in Heart Failure with Preserved Ejection Fraction [see also Chapter 36]), chronic sildenafil treatment did not significantly improve exercise capacity or clinical status in HFpEF patients compared with the placebo, possibly because cGMP levels were not significantly enhanced by sildenafil in the treatment group.[75] In a comparative LV endomyocardial biopsy study, myocardial PKG activity (**Figure 10-12A-C**) and cGMP concentration (see Figure 10-12D) were significantly lower in HFpEF than in HFrEF and AS patients.[53] Reduced myocardial PKG activity and lower cGMP concentration in HFpEF related to elevated cardiomyocyte passive force (**Figure 10-13A**), whereas in vitro administration of PKG acutely lowered cardiomyocyte stiffness in all groups (see Figure 10-13A), with the largest decrement in passive force observed in the HFpEF patients (see Figure 10-13B). HFpEF patients also featured increased myocardial nitrotyrosine levels, indicative of nitrosative/oxidative stress (see Figure 10-13C) (see also Chapter 8).[53]

The reduced PKG activity and lower myocardial cGMP concentration in HFpEF did not result from altered myocardial sGC, PDE5A, or pro-BNP108 expression and was therefore related to the higher nitrosative/oxidative stress observed in HFpEF than in the other conditions.[53] Similarly, in another LV endomyocardial biopsy study, HFpEF patients had exaggerated myocardial fibrosis and inflammation, which were associated with diastolic LV dysfunction and

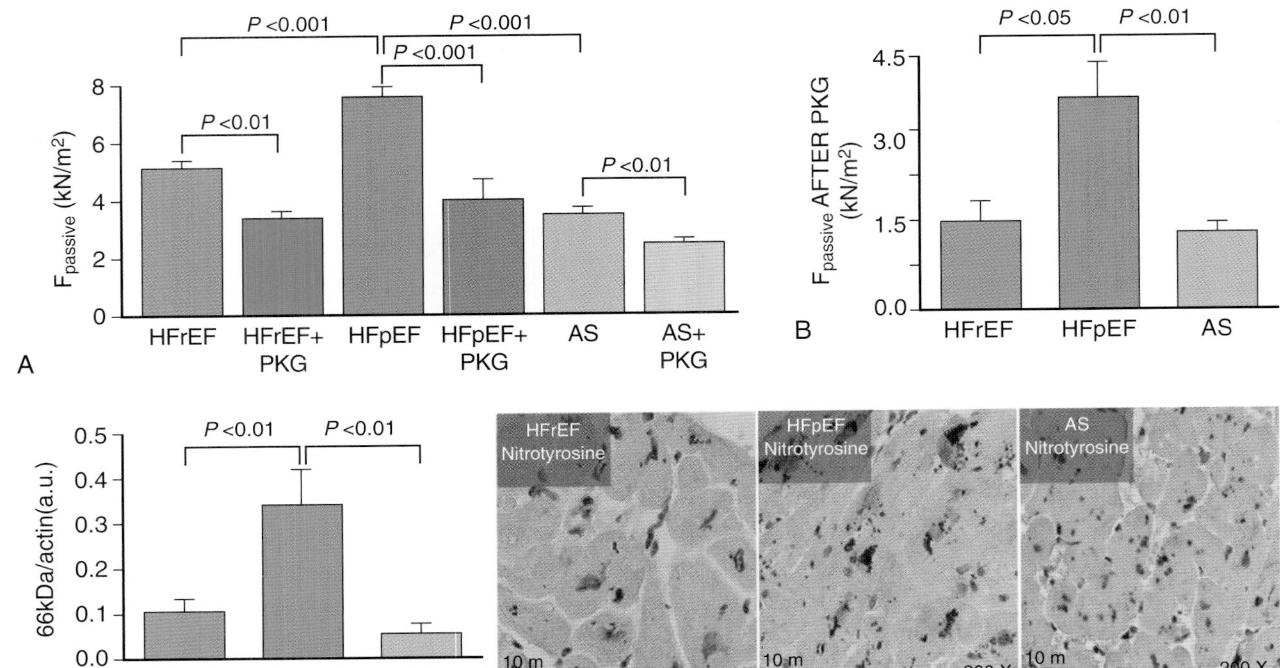

FIGURE 10-13 **A,** Higher cardiomyocyte $F_{passive}$ in HFpEF than in HFrEF or AS with a significant fall in $F_{passive}$ after PKG administration in all three conditions. **B,** Larger fall in cardiomyocyte $F_{passive}$ after PKG administration in HFpEF than in HFrEF or AS. **C,** Higher myocardial nitrotyrosine levels, indicative of nitrosative/oxidative stress in HFpEF than in HFrEF or AS. *Modified from van Heerebeek L, Hamdani N, Falcao-Pires I, et al: Low myocardial protein kinase G activity in heart failure with preserved ejection fraction. Circulation 126:830, 2012.*

with increased oxidative stress compared with controls.[76] Oxidative stress is known to impair NO bioavailability, cGMP-PKG signaling, and NO-based signaling. The latter frequently proceeds through the process of *S*-nitrosylation, which serves as a major effector of NO bioactivity and an important mode of cellular signal transduction.[77-79]

Reduced NO bioavailability, dysregulation of NO-mediated signaling, and increased nitrosative/oxidative stress are firmly implicated in the pathogenesis of HF.[77-79]

Prominent cardiovascular sources of reactive oxygen species (ROS) production include xanthine oxidase, NADPH oxidase, mitochondrial oxidases, and uncoupled NO synthases (see Figure 10-11).[79]

Superoxide rapidly reacts with NO to form peroxynitrite, which impairs NO bioavailability and NO-based signaling. In addition, peroxynitrite oxidizes the essential eNOS cofactor tetrahydrobiopterin, triggering eNOS uncoupling. In its uncoupled form, eNOS generates superoxide instead of NO, thereby augmenting oxidative stress.[77-79] Nitrosative/oxidative stress also directly inhibits sGC activity with subsequent downregulation of cGMP-PKG signaling.[77] Inflammation and oxidative stress have been shown to contribute to HFpEF pathophysiology. In an endomyocardial biopsy study, when compared with controls, HFpEF patients had increased inflammatory cell TGF-β expression, which induces transdifferentiation of fibroblasts into myofibroblasts with high production of collagen and low expression of MMP1, whereas both myocardial collagen and the amount of inflammatory cells correlated with diastolic LV dysfunction.[76] In addition, as compared with asymptomatic hypertensives, HFpEF patients had increased circulating biomarkers of inflammation (interleukin-6 (IL-6), IL-8, monocyte chemoattractant protein 1), of collagen metabolism (aminoterminal propeptide of collagen III, carboxy-terminal telopeptide of collagen I), and of ECM turnover (MMP2 and MMP9).[80] Moreover, the Health ABC study reported inflammatory biomarkers such as IL-6, TNF-α, and CRP to be strongly associated with risk of HFpEF development in older adults.[81]

Hence, in HFpEF reduced myocardial PKG activity and lower cGMP concentration could be associated with upstream nitrosative/oxidative stress-mediated impairment of NO bioavailability. Reduced PKG activity in its turn induces uninhibited stimulation of maladaptive cardiac remodeling and diastolic dysfunction due to deranged Ca^{2+} handling, enhanced cardiomyocyte stiffness, and myofilament Ca^{2+} sensitivity because of hypophosphorylation of titin and TnI (see Figure 10-11).

IMPORTANCE OF COMORBIDITIES IN HEART FAILURE WITH A PRESERVED EJECTION FRACTION

Noncardiac comorbidities are highly prevalent in HFpEF.[26] Of considerable importance are hypertension, overweight/obesity, and diabetes mellitus (DM). All these comorbidities share the ability to induce a systemic inflammatory state.

Hypertension

Arterial hypertension is the most prevalent comorbidity in HFpEF.[27] Although arterial hypertension has been associated with oxidative stress and vascular inflammation,[82] arterial hypertension is usually perceived to induce HFpEF through myocardial afterload excess.[83] However, according to recent registries and large outcome trials,[25,27] arterial hypertension in HFpEF consists of elevated systolic pressure but normal diastolic pressure. In HFpEF, LV cavity dimensions are small and especially in the presence of LV hypertrophy, the LV operates at a favorable Laplace relationship.

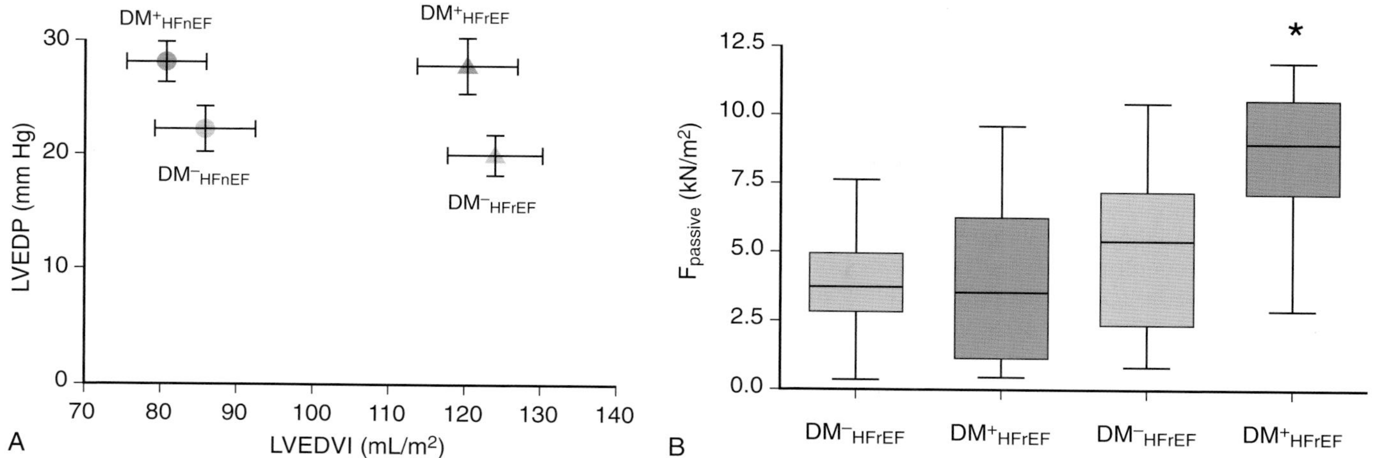

FIGURE 10-14 **A,** LV end-diastolic pressure (LVEDP). LV end-diastolic volume index (LVEDVI) relation in DM^-_{HFrEF}, DM^+_{HFrEF}, DM^-_{HFpEF}, and DM^+_{HFpEF}. Reduced LV end-diastolic distensibility in DM^+_{HFrEF} and DM^+_{HFpEF} patients is evident from higher LVEDP at similar LVEDVI. **B,** $F_{passive}$ is higher in DM^+_{HFpEF} patients. *Modified from van Heerebeek L, Hamdani N, Handoko ML, et al: Diastolic stiffness of the failing diabetic heart: importance of fibrosis, advanced glycation end products, and myocyte resting tension. Circulation 117:43, 2008.*

LV systolic wall stress therefore remains low despite elevated LV systolic pressure.[84]

Some population studies and outcome trials observed a larger contribution to HFpEF development of metabolic comorbidities than of arterial hypertension. In the MONICA registry, LA enlargement was strongly related to obesity, mildly related to age, and unrelated to arterial hypertension.[85] In the ALLHAT trial, which recruited 40,000 patients with arterial hypertension and one additional risk factor, significant baseline characteristics discriminating between in-trial HFrEF or HFpEF development were respectively a history of coronary heart disease favoring HFrEF and a high BMI favoring HFpEF.[36] In contrast, systolic or diastolic blood pressures did not discriminate between in-trial HFrEF or HFpEF development.

Metabolic Risk Factors

Obesity and diabetes mellitus type II (DMII) are strongly related to insulin resistance (IR) and the metabolic syndrome (a constellation of cardiovascular risk factors, including obesity, hypertension, IR, hyperglycemia, dyslipidemia, microalbuminuria, and hypercoagulability). The frequent clustering of these metabolic risk factors causes synergistic adverse effects on myocardial structure and function.[86] The prevalence of DMII, obesity, IR, and metabolic syndrome increases rapidly and is expected to reach pandemic proportions in the next few decades, whereas these metabolic risk factors have all been prospectively identified as precursors of incident HF.[86] Metabolic risk factors are strongly associated with a proinflammatory state, oxidative stress, and endothelial dysfunction,[87] whereas eNOS uncoupling was demonstrated in patients with DM, hypertension, and hypercholesterolemia.[88] Increased markers of endothelial inflammation, such as E-selectin, intercellular adhesion molecule 1, and vascular cell adhesion molecule (VCAM) 1, were demonstrated in metabolic syndrome and obesity, and represent an independent risk factor for subsequent development of DMII.[87] Increased diastolic LV stiffness is recognized as the earliest manifestation of DM-induced LV dysfunction.[89] DM lowers LV diastolic distensibility in both HFpEF and HFrEF patients, as evident from higher LVEDP at similar LVEDVI (**Figure 10-14A**), whereas cardiomyocyte stiffness was higher in HFpEF patients with DM than in HFrEF patients and HFpEF patients without DM (see Figure 10-14B).[90] DM induces diastolic LV dysfunction through numerous mechanisms (**Table 10-2**). DM adversely affects the ECM through enhanced interstitial and perivascular fibrosis, increased expression of collagen type 1, and altered MMP expression. These abnormalities are mediated by hyperglycemia, oxidative stress, and elevated aldosterone and Ang II levels.[91] Hyperglycemia induces oxidative stress via several mechanisms, which include glucose auto-oxidation, activation of

TABLE 10-2 Mechanisms Responsible for Increased LV Diastolic Stiffness in Diabetic Heart Failure

Myocardial fibrosis	Increased production of collagen and profibrotic cytokines Decreased expression of MMPs
AGEs	Increased collagen and ECM cross-linking Activation of AGE receptor-based signaling Increased oxidative stress and impaired calcium homeostasis Endothelial dysfunction and impaired NO bioavailability
Metabolic disturbances	FFA oxidation, lipid accumulation, and lipotoxicity Uncoupling of mitochondrial oxidative phosphorylation
Impaired calcium homeostasis	Reduced activities of calcium handling proteins
Endothelial dysfunction	Increased proinflammatory cytokines, impaired NO bioavailability
Myocardial oxidative stress	Enhanced ROS production, glucose auto-oxidation Activation of polyol pathways Increased FFA and leptin Impaired NO bioavailability
Insulin resistance	Endothelial dysfunction Dysfunctional insulin-based signaling
Impaired NO bioavailability	Endothelial NOS uncoupling Impaired *S*-nitrosylation-based signaling Impaired NO-sGC-cGMP-PKG signaling
Increased cardiomyocyte stiffness	Increased stiff titin N2B expression Titin hypophosphorylation Disruption in titin-based signaling

AGE, Advanced glycation end product; *ECM,* extracellular matrix; *FFA,* free fatty acid; *MMP,* matrix metalloproteinase; *NO,* nitric oxide; *NOS,* NO synthase; *sGC,* soluble guanylate cyclase; *cGMP,* cyclic guanosine monophosphate; *PKG,* protein kinase G; *ROS,* reactive oxygen species.

the polyol pathway, and increased levels of free fatty acid (FFA) and leptin.[92] Furthermore, hyperglycemia induces formation and accumulation of advanced glycation end products (AGEs), which represent modifications of proteins or lipids that become nonenzymatically glycated and oxidized after contact with aldose sugars, resulting in creation of nearly irreversible cross-links.[93] Myocardial AGE deposition augments LV diastolic stiffness through increased collagen production and collagen cross-link formation and activation of specific AGE receptors. AGE receptor activation impairs Ca^{2+} homeostasis, induces profibrotic signaling and endothelial dysfunction, lowers NO bioavailability, and increases oxidative stress and proinflammatory cytokine release.[93]

Additional mechanisms by which DM induces diastolic dysfunction are derangements in cardiac metabolism and cardiomyocyte Ca^{2+} cycling.[94] Substrate metabolism is altered in DM with a shift from glucose use to increased FFA oxidation. This leads to myocardial lipotoxicity, uncoupling of mitochondrial oxidative phosphorylation, and disturbed contraction/relaxation coupling.[94] Because cross-bridge detachment is an energy-consuming process, slow LV relaxation in HFpEF can therefore also result from a myocardial energy deficit. Indeed, recent ^{31}P-MR studies demonstrated reduced myocardial energy reserve in both patients with HFpEF,[95,96] as well as in asymptomatic, normotensive patients with DMII, in whom impaired myocardial bioenergetics correlated with diastolic LV dysfunction.[97] Furthermore, cardiac energetic deficiency relating to diastolic dysfunction was also recently demonstrated in obese compared with normal-weight subjects, both at rest and during inotropic stress with high-dose intravenous dobutamine administration.[98]

Comorbidities in HFpEF: Link to Coronary Microvascular Endothelial Inflammation

Comorbidities were recently shown to be accompanied by a larger deterioration of myocardial function and structure in HFpEF than in arterial hypertension.[99] This finding supports additional deterioration in HFpEF by HF-related mechanisms, such as neuroendocrine activation[100] and lack of high-energy phosphates.[96] Additional involvement of HF-related mechanisms also explains the worse outcome of HFpEF than of comorbidities.[101] The systemic inflammatory state induced by these comorbidities has been shown to be predictive of incident HFpEF, but not of incident HFrEF.[81] Proinflammatory cytokines can be used as markers for risk stratification and prognostication in HF, while inflammatory cytokines elicit endothelial ROS production through activation of NADPH oxidases.[102] Coronary microvascular endothelial inflammation was evident in myocardial biopsies of HFpEF patients from abundant expression of both VCAM and E-selectin, leading to activation and subendothelial migration of circulating leukocytes[76,90] and from increased myocardial nitrotyrosine levels, indicative of nitrosative/oxidative stress.[53,76] Several recent studies emphasized the importance of a deficient systemic vasodilator response for the reduced exercise tolerance of HFpEF patients,[103] and peripheral endothelial dysfunction was recently also identified as an independent predictor of outcome of HFpEF patients.[104] This prognostic implication suggests a causal involvement of endothelial dysfunction in HFpEF.[105] Involvement in HFpEF of cardiac chambers other than the LV also provides a strong argument for a microvascular inflammatory state driving myocardial remodeling. When pulmonary hypertension (PH) secondary to HFpEF (PH-HFpEF) is compared with primary PH, PH-HFpEF patients had higher right atrial (RA) pressures with less RA dilation,[106] consistent with reduced RA compliance in PH-HFpEF. This finding could not be attributed to pulmonary arterial load, because mean pulmonary arterial pressure was similar in both conditions but probably related to the high prevalence of obesity in PH-HFpEF (46% versus 15%). Similarly, in a study that compared HFrEF with HFpEF, PCWP was equally elevated but LA volume significantly smaller in HFpEF than in HFrEF.[32] Finally, the same study assessed right ventricular (RV) systolic performance and found an analogy to LV systolic performance, higher RV end-systolic elastance in HFpEF than in HFrEF.

Structural and Functional Consequences of Inflammation in HFpEF versus HFrEF

Recent insights suggest a new paradigm for HFpEF in which emphasis is shifted from LV afterload excess to comorbidity-driven coronary microvascular inflammation, endothelial dysfunction, and impaired NO-based signaling (**see Chapter 13**). Subsequent downregulation of cGMP-PKG signaling contributes to maladaptive cardiac remodeling and elevated cardiomyocyte stiffness, which in conjunction with fibrosis increases diastolic LV stiffness (**Figure 10-15**).[107] The new HFpEF paradigm substantially differs from the paradigm proposed for HFrEF, where LV remodeling is driven by progressive loss of cardiomyocytes.[37] This loss of cardiomyocytes results from various modalities of cell death, such as exaggerated autophagy, apoptosis, or necrosis, all of which are triggered by oxidative stress present within the cardiomyocyte and usually result from ischemia, infection, or toxicity (**Figure 10-16**).[108] Excessive wall stress because of cardiomyocyte loss shifts the balance in the ECM between collagen deposition and degradation.[109] These alterations within the ECM importantly contribute to LV dilation and eccentric LV remodeling.[109] In HFrEF, replacement of dead cardiomyocytes by collagen creates patchy areas of fibrosis. A comparative analysis of endomyocardial biopsies from HFpEF and HFrEF patients[21,90] indeed showed presence of replacement fibrosis in HFrEF but not in HFpEF. Furthermore, electron-microscopic images of LV myocardium revealed lower myofilamentary density in HFrEF than in HFpEF with some HFrEF cardiomyocytes showing areas of complete myofibrillar loss.[21] These biopsy findings are consistent with cell death occurring in HFrEF but not in HFpEF. Apoptotic cardiomyocyte death mediated by oxidative stress because of upregulated NADPH oxidase activity also appears in late eccentric LV remodeling of TAC mouse models.[110] These studies support a sequence of events whereby myocardial pressure overload initially triggers concentric hypertrophy followed later by eccentric remodeling because of high oxidative stress and cell death. This evolution has also been postulated in human hypertension[111] but seriously questioned by longitudinal cohort studies with sequential cardiac imaging.[112] In these studies, the evolution from concentric to eccentric remodeling appeared to be rare in the absence of interval myocardial infarction. In advanced HFrEF, systemic and coronary endothelial dysfunction is also present and attributed to raised plasma levels of TNF-α and IL-6.[113,114] However, in contrast to HFpEF, the raised plasma levels of TNF-α and IL-6 do not result from preexisting comorbidities, but are reactive to the severity of

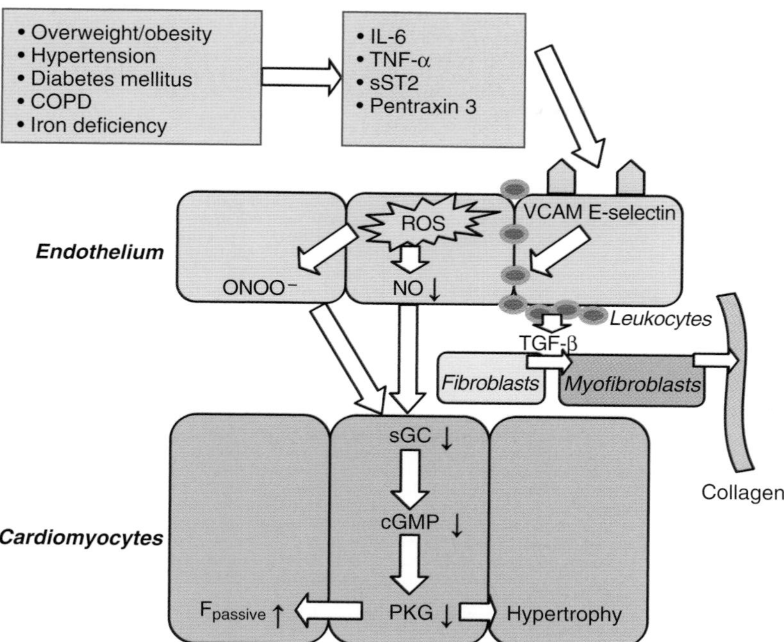

FIGURE 10-15 Comorbidities drive myocardial dysfunction and remodeling in HFpEF. Comorbidities induce a systemic proinflammatory state with elevated plasma levels of IL-6, TNF-α, sST2, and pentraxin 3. Coronary microvascular endothelial cells reactively produce ROS, VCAM, and E-selectin. Production of ROS leads to formation of peroxynitrite ($ONOO^-$) and reduced NO bioavailability, both of which lower sGC activity in adjacent cardiomyocytes. Lower sGC activity decreases cGMP concentration and PKG activity. Low PKG activity raises intrinsic cardiomyocyte stiffness because of hypophosphorylation of titin and removes the brake on pro-hypertrophic stimuli inducing cardiomyocyte hypertrophy. VCAM and E-selectin expression in endothelial cells favors migration into the subendothelium of monocytes. These monocytes release TGF-β. The latter stimulates conversion of fibroblasts into myofibroblasts, which deposit collagen in the interstitial space. *cGMP,* Cyclic guanosine monophosphate; $F_{passive}$, cardiomyocyte passive force; *IL-6,* interleukin 6; *sST2,* soluble ST2; *ROS,* reactive oxygen species; *TGF-β,* transforming growth factor β; *TNF-α,* tumor necrosis factor α; *VCAM,* vascular cell adhesion molecule. *Modified from Paulus WJ, Tschöpe C: A novel paradigm for heart failure with preserved ejection fraction: comorbidities drive myocardial dysfunction and remodeling through coronary microvascular endothelial inflammation. J Am Coll Cardiol 62:263–271, 2013.*

MYOCARDIAL REMODELING IN HFpEF, HFrEF, AND ADVANCED HFrEF

HFpEF

• Overweight/obesity
• Hypertension
• Diabetes mellitus
• COPD
• Iron deficiency

• IL-6
• TNF-α
• sST2
• Pentraxin 3

VCAM E-selectin
ROS
NO ↓
TGF-β
Collagen
sGC ↓
cGMP ↓
PKG ↓
Fpassive ↑
Hypertrophy

HFrEF

Collagen
• Necrosis
• Apoptosis
• Autophagy
ROS
• Ischemia
• Infection
• Toxicity

ADVANCED HFrEF

• IL-6
• TNF-α

VCAM E-selectin
ROS
NO ↓
TGF-β
Collagen
sGC ↓
cGMP ↓
PKG ↓
Fpassive ↑
Hypertrophy
• Necrosis
• Apoptosis
• Autophagy
ROS
• Ischemia
• Infection
• Toxicity

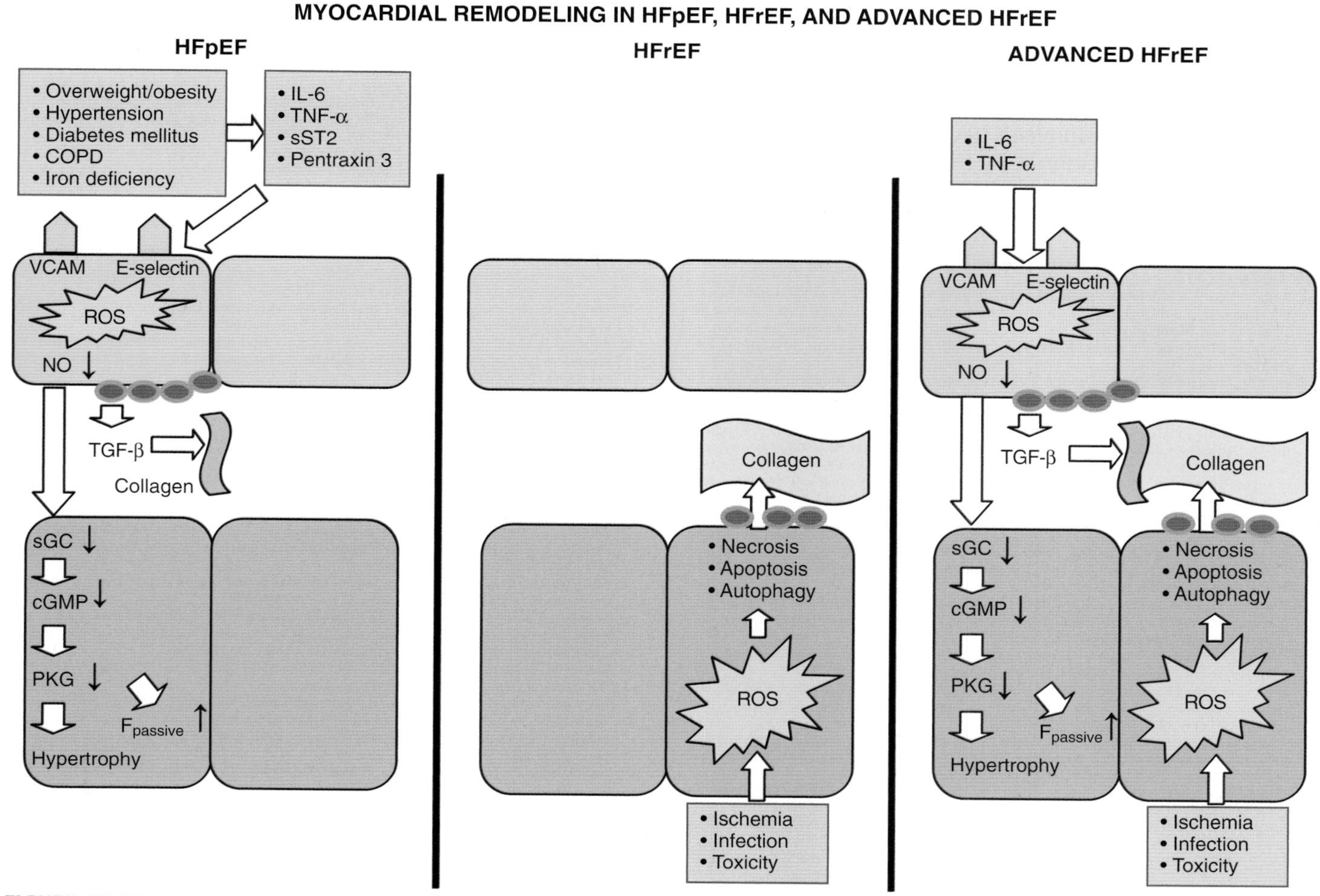

FIGURE 10-16 Myocardial dysfunction and remodeling in HFpEF (HFpEF), HFrEF (HFrEF), and advanced HFrEF. In HFpEF, myocardial dysfunction and remodeling are driven by endothelial oxidative stress. In HFrEF, oxidative stress originates in the cardiomyocytes. In advanced HFrEF both mechanisms get superimposed. *Modified from Paulus WJ, Tschöpe C: A novel paradigm for heart failure with preserved ejection fraction: comorbidities drive myocardial dysfunction and remodeling through coronary microvascular endothelial inflammation. J Am Coll Cardiol 62:263–271, 2013.*

HFrEF as they relate to both New York Heart Association (NYHA) class[113] and depression of LVEF (see Chapter 7).[114] Similar to HFpEF, endothelial dysfunction affects diastolic LV function in advanced HFrEF, as evident from the relation between diastolic LV dysfunction and plasma levels of methylated L-arginine metabolites, which impair NO production by eNOS.[115]

SUMMARY AND FUTURE DIRECTIONS

HFpEF demonstrates an increasing prevalence, and currently approximately 50% of HF patients present with this type of HF. Prognosis of HFpEF is poor and most HFpEF patients die from cardiovascular causes. Especially in HFpEF, pathophysiologic mechanisms and diagnostic and therapeutic strategies remain uncertain, and this is reflected in the lack of improvement of prognosis in HFpEF over the past decennia. Advances in therapeutic strategies are only to be expected when more comprehensive insight has been gained into underlying pathophysiologic mechanisms responsible for development and progression of HFpEF.

HFpEF appears a complex syndrome characterized by maladaptive changes in myocardial and cardiomyocyte structural, functional, and biochemical characteristics, probably induced in a multifactorial fashion by a combination of adverse effects of myocardial inflammation, nitrosative/oxidative stress, endothelial dysfunction, downregulation of NO bioavailability, and NO-mediated signaling, impaired myocardial bioenergetics, disturbed calcium handling, and concentric hypertrophy. Recent translational studies have contributed to improved understanding of HFpEF pathophysiology, and exciting insights providing a potential inroad for novel therapeutic strategies have emerged. Nevertheless, because of the high complexity of HFpEF pathophysiology, continuing translational and clinical research efforts are needed to move this exciting field forward.

References

1. Authors/Task Force Members, McMurray JJ, Adamopoulos S, Anker SD, et al: ESC Guidelines for the diagnosis and treatment of acute and chronic heart failure 2012: The Task Force for the Diagnosis and Treatment of Acute and Chronic Heart Failure 2012 of the European Society of Cardiology. Developed in collaboration with the Heart Failure Association (HFA) of the ESC. *Eur Heart J* 33:1787, 2012.
2. Hunt SA, Abraham WT, Chin MH, et al: American College of Cardiology; American Heart Association Task Force on Practice Guidelines; American College of Chest Physicians; International Society for Heart and Lung Transplantation; Heart Rhythm Society. ACC/AHA 2005 Guideline Update for the Diagnosis and Management of Chronic Heart Failure in the Adult: A Report of the American College of Cardiology/American Heart Association Task Force on Practice Guidelines (Writing Committee to Update the 2001 Guidelines for the Evaluation and Management of Heart Failure): Developed in Collaboration With the American College of Chest Physicians and the International Society for Heart and Lung Transplantation: Endorsed by the Heart Rhythm Society. *Circulation* 112:e154, 2005.
3. Owan TE, Hodge DO, Herges RM, et al: Trends in prevalence and outcome of heart failure with preserved ejection fraction. *N Engl J Med* 355:251, 2006.
4. Cleland JG, Tendera M, Adamus J, et al: The perindopril in elderly people with chronic heart failure (PEP-CHF) study. *Eur Heart J* 27:2338, 2006.
5. Yusuf S, Pfeffer MA, Swedberg K, et al, for the CHARM Investigators and Committees: Effects of candesartan in patients with chronic heart failure and preserved left-ventricular ejection fraction: the CHARM-Preserved Trial. *Lancet* 362:777, 2003.
6. Massie BM, Carson PE, McMurray JJ, et al: I-PRESERVE Investigators. Irbesartan in patients with heart failure and preserved ejection fraction. *N Engl J Med* 359:2456, 2008.
7. Edelmann F, Wachter R, Schmidt AG, et al: Effect of spironolactone on diastolic function and exercise capacity in patients with heart failure with preserved ejection fraction: the Ido-Hfpef randomized controlled trial. *JAMA* 309:781, 2013.
8. Conraads VM, Metra M, Kamp O, et al: Effects of the long-term administration of nebivolol on the clinical symptoms, exercise capacity, and left ventricular function of patients with diastolic dysfunction: results of the ELANDD study. *Eur J Heart Fail* 14:219, 2012.
9. Paulus WJ, van Ballegoij JJ: Treatment of heart failure with normal ejection fraction: an inconvenient truth! *J Am Coll Cardiol* 55:526, 2010.
10. Aurigemma GP, Zile MR, Gaasch WH: Contractile behavior of the left ventricle in diastolic heart failure: with emphasis on regional systolic function. *Circulation* 113:296, 2006.
11. Lam CS, Lyass A, Kraigher-Krainer E, et al: Cardiac dysfunction and noncardiac dysfunction as precursors of heart failure with reduced and preserved ejection fraction in the community. *Circulation* 124:24, 2011.
12. Redfield MM, Jacobsen SJ, Burnett JC, Jr, et al: Burden of systolic and diastolic ventricular dysfunction in the community: appreciating the scope of the heart failure epidemic. *JAMA* 289:194, 2003.
13. Kane GC, Karon BL, Mahoney DW, et al: Progression of left ventricular diastolic dysfunction and risk of heart failure. *JAMA* 306:856, 2011.
14. Paulus WJ, Tschope C, Sanderson JE, et al: How to diagnose diastolic heart failure: a consensus statement on the diagnosis of heart failure with normal left ventricular ejection fraction by the Heart Failure and Echocardiography Associations of the European Society of Cardiology. *Eur Heart J* 28:2539, 2007.
15. De Keulenaer GW, Brutsaert DL: Systolic and diastolic heart failure are overlapping phenotypes within the heart failure spectrum. *Circulation* 123:1996, 2011.
16. Kitzman DW, Little WC, Brubaker PH, et al: Pathophysiological characterization of isolated diastolic heart failure in comparison to systolic heart failure. *JAMA* 288:2144, 2002.
17. Bursi F, Weston SA, Redfield MM, et al: Systolic and diastolic heart failure in the community. *JAMA* 296:2209, 2006.
18. Borlaug BA, Lam CS, Roger VL, et al: Contractility and ventricular systolic stiffening in hypertensive heart disease insights into the pathogenesis of heart failure with preserved ejection fraction. *J Am Coll Cardiol* 54:410, 2009.
19. Baicu CF, Zile MR, Aurigemma GP, et al: Left ventricular systolic performance, function and contractility in patients with diastolic heart failure. *Circulation* 111:2306, 2005.
20. Borlaug BA, Redfield MM: Diastolic and systolic heart failure are distinct phenotypes within the heart failure spectrum. *Circulation* 123:2006, 2011.
21. van Heerebeek L, Borbely A, Niessen HWM, et al: Myocardial structure and function differ in systolic and diastolic heart failure. *Circulation* 113:1966, 2006.
22. Borlaug BA, Paulus WJ: Heart failure with preserved ejection fraction: pathophysiology, diagnosis and treatment. *Eur Heart J* 32:670, 2011.
23. Meta-analysis Global Group in Chronic Heart Failure (MAGGIC): The survival of patients with heart failure with preserved or reduced left ventricular ejection fraction: an individual patient data meta-analysis. *Eur Heart J* 33:1750, 2012.
24. Fonorow GC, Stough WG, Abraham WT, et al: OPTIMIZE-HF Investigators and Hospitals. Characteristics, treatments and outcomes of patients with preserved systolic function hospitalized for heart failure: a report from the OPTIMIZE-HF Registry. *J Am Coll Cardiol* 50:768, 2007.
25. Yancy CW, Lopatin M, Stevenson LW, et al: For the ADHERE Scientific Advisory Committee and Investigators. Clinical presentation, management, and in-hospital outcomes of patients admitted with acute decompensated heart failure with preserved systolic function. A Report from the Acute Decompensated Heart Failure National Registry (ADHERE). *J Am Coll Cardiol* 47:76, 2006.
26. Ather S, Chan W, Bozkurt B, et al: Impact of noncardiac comorbidities on morbidity and mortality in a predominantly male population with heart failure and preserved versus reduced ejection fraction. *J Am Coll Cardiol* 59:998, 2012.
27. McMurray JJV, Carson PE, Komajda M, et al: Heart failure with preserved ejection fraction: clinical characteristics of 4133 patients enrolled in the I-PRESERVE trial. *Eur J Heart Fail* 10:149, 2008.
28. Leite-Moreira AF: Current perspectives in diastolic dysfunction and diastolic heart failure. *Heart* 92:712, 2006.
29. Zile MR, Baicu CF, Gaasch WH: Diastolic heart failure—abnormalities in active relaxation and passive stiffness of the left ventricle. *N Engl J Med* 350:1953, 2004.
30. Borlaug BA, Kass DA: Ventricular-vascular interaction in heart failure. *Heart Fail Clin* 4:23, 2008.
31. Kawaguchi M, Hay I, Tetics B, et al: Combined ventricular systolic and arterial stiffening in patients with heart failure and preserved ejection fraction: implications for systolic and diastolic reserve limitations. *Circulation* 107:714, 2003.
32. Schwartzenberg S, Redfield MM, From AM, et al: Effects of vasodilation in heart failure with preserved or reduced ejection fraction implications of distinct pathophysiologies on response to therapy. *J Am Coll Cardiol* 59:442, 2012.
33. Fukuta H, Sane DC, Brucks S, et al: Statin therapy may be associated with lower mortality in patients with diastolic heart failure: a preliminary report. *Circulation* 112:357, 2005.
34. Kjekshus J, APetrei E, Barrios V, et al, CORONA Group: Rosuvastatin in older patients with systolic heart failure. *N Engl J Med* 357:2248, 2007.
35. Hamdani N, Paulus WJ, van Heerebeek L, et al: Distinct myocardial effects of beta-blocker therapy in heart failure with normal and reduced left ventricular ejection fraction. *Eur Heart J* 30:1863, 2009.
36. Davis BR, Kostis JB, Simpson LM, et al: Heart failure with preserved and reduced left ventricular ejection fraction in the antihypertensive and lipid-lowering treatment to prevent heart attack trial. *Circulation* 118:2259, 2008.
37. McMurray JJ: Clinical practice. Systolic heart failure. *N Engl J Med* 362:228, 2010.
38. Westermann D, Kasner M, Steendijk P, et al: Role of left ventricular stiffness in heart failure with normal ejection fraction. *Circulation* 117:2051, 2008.
39. Borlaug BA, Nishimura RA, Sorajja P, et al: Exercise hemodynamics enhance diagnosis of early heart failure with preserved ejection fraction. *Circ Heart Fail* 3:588, 2010.
40. Burkhoff D, Mirsky I, Suga H: Assessment of systolic and diastolic ventricular properties via pressure-volume analysis: a guide for clinical, translational, and basic researchers. *Am J Physiol Heart Circ Physiol* 289:H501, 2005.
41. Paulus WJ: Culprit mechanism(s) for exercise intolerance in heart failure with normal ejection fraction. *J Am Coll Cardiol* 56:864, 2010.
42. Little WC, Oh JK: Echocardiographic evaluation of diastolic function can be used to guide clinical care. *Circulation* 120:802, 2009.
43. Oh JK, Park SJ, Nagueh SF: Established and novel clinical applications of diastolic function assessment by echocardiography. *Circ Cardiovasc Imaging* 4:444, 2011.
44. Nagueh SF, Appleton CP, Gillebert TC: Recommendations for the evaluation of left ventricular diastolic function by echocardiography. *Eur J Echocardiogr* 10:165, 2009.
45. Zile MR, Gottdiener JS, Hetzel SJ, et al: Prevalence and significance of alterations in cardiac structure and function in patients with heart failure and a preserved ejection fraction. *Circulation* 124:2491, 2011.
46. Oki T, Tabata T, Yamada H, et al: Clinical application of pulsed Doppler tissue imaging for assessing abnormal left ventricular relaxation. *Am J Cardiol* 79:921, 1997.
47. Ommen SR, Nishimura RA, Appleton CP, et al: Clinical utility of Doppler echocardiography and tissue Doppler imaging in the estimation of left ventricular filling pressures: a comparative simultaneous Doppler-catheterization study. *Circulation* 102:1788, 2000.
48. Kasner M, Westermann D, Steendijk P, et al: Utility of Doppler echocardiography and tissue Doppler imaging in the estimation of diastolic function in heart failure with normal ejection fraction: a comparative Doppler-conductance catheterization study. *Circulation* 116:637, 2007.
49. Wang J, Khoury DS, Yue Y, et al: Preserved left ventricular twist and circumferential deformation, but depressed longitudinal and radial deformation in patients with diastolic heart failure. *Eur Heart J* 29:1283, 2008.
50. Tan YT, Wenzelburger F, Lee E, et al: The pathophysiology of heart failure with normal ejection fraction: exercise echocardiography reveals complex abnormalities of both systolic and diastolic ventricular function involving torsion, untwist, and longitudinal motion. *J Am Coll Cardiol* 54:36, 2009.
51. Daniels LB, Maisel AS: Natriuretic peptides. *J Am Coll Cardiol* 50:2357, 2007.
52. Tschöpe C, Kasner M, Westermann D, et al: The role of NT-proBNP in the diagnostics of isolated diastolic dysfunction: correlation with echocardiographic and invasive measurements. *Eur Heart J* 26:2277, 2005.
53. van Heerebeek L, Hamdani N, Falcao-Pires I, et al: Low myocardial protein kinase G activity in heart failure with preserved ejection fraction. *Circulation* 126:830, 2012.
54. Lohse MJ, Engelhardt S, Eschenhagen T: What is the role of beta-adrenergic signaling in heart failure? *Circ Res* 93:896, 2003.
55. Bers DM: Cardiac excitation-contraction coupling. *Nature* 415:198, 2002.

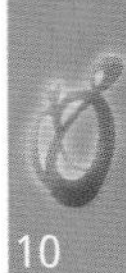

56. Linke WA, Krüger M: The giant protein titin as an integrator of myocyte signaling pathways. *Physiology* 25:186, 2010.
57. Krüger M, Linke WA: Titin-based mechanical signalling in normal and failing myocardium. *J Mol Cell Cardiol* 46:490, 2009.
58. Berk BC, Fujiwara K, Lehoux S: ECM remodeling in hypertensive heart disease. *J Clin Invest* 117:568, 2007.
59. Kasner M, Westermann D, Lopez B, et al: Diastolic tissue Doppler indexes correlate with the degree of collagen expression and cross-linking in heart failure and normal ejection fraction. *J Am Coll Cardiol* 57:977, 2011.
60. Martos R, Baugh J, Ledwidge M, et al: Diagnosis of heart failure with preserved ejection fraction: improved accuracy with the use of markers of collagen turnover. *Eur J Heart Fail* 11:191, 2009.
61. González A, López B, Querejeta R, et al: Filling pressures and collagen metabolism in hypertensive patients with heart failure and normal ejection fraction. *Hypertension* 55:1418, 2010.
62. Borbely A, van der Velden J, Papp Z, et al: Cardiomyocyte stiffness in diastolic heart failure. *Circulation* 111:774, 2005.
63. Borbely A, Falcao-Pires I, van Heerebeek L, et al: Hypophosphorylation of the stiff N2B titin isoform raises cardiomyocyte resting tension in failing human myocardium. *Circ Res* 104:780, 2009.
64. Hidalgo C, Hudson B, Bogomolovas J, et al: PKC phosphorylation of titin's PEVK element. A novel and conserved pathway for modulating myocardial stiffness. *Circ Res* 105:631, 2009.
65. Grützner A, Garcia-Manyes S, Kötter S, et al: Modulation of titin-based stiffness by disulfide bonding in the cardiac titin N2-B unique sequence. *Biophys J* 97:825, 2009.
66. Takimoto E: Cyclic GMP-dependent signaling in cardiac myocytes. *Circ J* 76:1819, 2012.
67. Lee DI, Kass DA: Phosphodiesterases and cyclic GMP regulation in heart muscle. *Physiology* 27:248, 2012.
68. Seddon M, Shah AM, Casadei B: Cardiomyocytes as effectors of nitric oxide signaling. *Cardiovasc Res* 75:315, 2007.
69. Paulus WJ, Bronzwaer JG: Nitric oxide's role in the heart: control of beating or breathing? *Am J Physiol Heart Circ Physiol* 287:H8, 2004.
70. Takimoto E, Champion HC, Belardi D, et al: cGMP catabolism by phosphodiesterase 5A regulates cardiac adrenergic stimulation by NOS3-dependent mechanism. *Circ Res* 96:100, 2005.
71. Bishu K, Hamdani N, Mohammed SF, et al: Sildenafil and BNP acutely phosphorylate titin and improve diastolic distensibility in vivo. *Circulation* 124:2882, 2011.
72. O'Connor CM, Starling RC, Hernandez AF, et al: Effect of nesiritide in patients with acute decompensated heart failure. *N Engl J Med* 365:32, 2011.
73. Takimoto E, Champion HC, Li M, et al: Chronic inhibition of cyclic GMP phosphodiesterase 5A prevents and reverses cardiac hypertrophy. *Nat Med* 11:214, 2005.
74. Guazzi M, Vicenzi M, Arena R, et al: Pulmonary hypertension in heart failure with preserved ejection fraction: a target of phosphodiesterase-5 inhibition in a 1-year study. *Circulation* 124:164, 2011.
75. Redfield MM, Chen HH, Borlaug BA, et al: Effect of phosphodiesterase-5 inhibition on exercise capacity and clinical status in heart failure with preserved ejection fraction: a randomized clinical trial. *JAMA* 309:1268, 2013.
76. Westermann D, Lindner D, Kasner M, et al: Cardiac inflammation contributes to changes in the extracellular matrix in patients with heart failure and normal ejection fraction. *Circ Heart Fail* 4:44, 2011.
77. Münzel T, Gori T, Bruno RM, et al: Is oxidative stress a therapeutic target in cardiovascular disease? *Eur Heart J* 31:2741, 2010.
78. Nediani C, Raimondi L, Borchi E, et al: Nitric oxide/reactive oxygen species generation and nitroso/redox imbalance in heart failure: from molecular mechanisms to therapeutic implications. *Antiox Redox Signal* 14:289, 2011.
79. Hare JM, Stamler JS: NO/redox disequilibrium in the failing heart and cardiovascular system. *J Clin Invest* 115:509, 2005.
80. Collier P, Watson CJ, Voon V, et al: Can emerging biomarkers of myocardial remodelling identify asymptomatic hypertensive patients at risk for diastolic dysfunction and diastolic heart failure? *Eur J Heart Fail* 13:1087, 2011.
81. Kalogeropoulos A, Georgiopoulou V, Psaty BM, et al: Health ABC Study Investigators. Inflammatory markers and incident heart failure risk in older adults: the Health ABC (Health, Aging, and Body Composition) study. *J Am Coll Cardiol* 55:2129, 2010.
82. Cohen RA, Tong X: Vascular oxidative stress: the common link in hypertensive and diabetic vascular disease. *J Cardiovasc Pharmacol* 55:308, 2010.
83. Hart CY, Meyer DM, Tazelaar HD, et al: Load versus humoral activation in the genesis of early hypertensive heart disease. *Circulation* 104:215, 2001.
84. Chirinos JA, Segers P, Gupta AK, et al: Time-varying myocardial stress and systolic pressure-stress relationship: role in myocardial-arterial coupling in hypertension. *Circulation* 119:2798, 2009.
85. Stritzke J, Markus MR, Duderstadt S, et al: The aging process of the heart: obesity is the main risk factor for left atrial enlargement during aging the MONICA/KORA (monitoring of trends and determinations in cardiovascular disease/cooperative research in the region of Augsburg) study. *J Am Coll Cardiol* 54:1982, 2009.
86. Horwich TB, Fonarow GC: Glucose, obesity, metabolic syndrome and diabetes. *J Am Coll Cardiol* 55:283, 2010.
87. Hartge MM, Unger T, Kintscher U: The endothelium and vascular inflammation in diabetes. *Diab Vasc Dis Res* 4:84, 2007.
88. Förstermann U, Münzel T: Endothelial nitric oxide synthase in vascular disease: from marvel to menace. *Circulation* 113:1708, 2006.
89. van Heerebeek L, Somsen A, Paulus WJ: The failing diabetic heart: focus on diastolic left ventricular dysfunction. *Curr Diab Rep* 9:79, 2009.
90. van Heerebeek L, Hamdani N, Handoko ML, et al: Diastolic stiffness of the failing diabetic heart: importance of fibrosis, advanced glycation end products, and myocyte resting tension. *Circulation* 117:43, 2008.
91. Asbun J, Villarreal FJ: The pathogenesis of myocardial fibrosis in the setting of diabetic cardiomyopathy. *J Am Coll Cardiol* 47:693, 2006.
92. Jay D, Hitomi H, Griendling KK: Oxidative stress and diabetic cardiovascular complications. *Free Radic Biol Med* 40:183, 2006.
93. Goldin A, Beckman JA, Schmidt AM, et al: Advanced glycation end products: sparking the development of diabetic vascular injury. *Circulation* 114:597, 2006.
94. Boudina S, Abel ED: Diabetic cardiomyopathy revisited. *Circulation* 115:3213, 2007.
95. Lamb HJ, Beyerbracht HP, van der Laarse A, et al: Diastolic dysfunction in hypertensive heart disease is associated with altered myocardial metabolism. *Circulation* 99:2261, 1999.
96. Phan TT, Abozguia K, Nallur Shivu G, et al: Heart failure with preserved ejection fraction is characterized by dynamic impairment of active relaxation and contraction of the left ventricle on exercise and associated with myocardial energy deficiency. *J Am Coll Cardiol* 54:402, 2009.
97. Diamant M, Lamb HJ, Groeneveld Y, et al: Diastolic dysfunction is associated with altered myocardial metabolism in asymptomatic normotensive patients with well-controlled type 2 diabetes mellitus. *J Am Coll Cardiol* 42:328, 2003.
98. Rider OJ, Francis JM, Ali MK, et al: Effects of catecholamine stress on diastolic function and myocardial energetics in obesity. *Circulation* 125:1511, 2012.
99. Mohammed SF, Borlaug BA, Roger VL, et al: Comorbidity and ventricular and vascular structure and function in heart failure with preserved ejection fraction: a community-based study. *Circ Heart Fail* 5:710, 2012.
100. Bishu K, Deswal A, Chen HH, et al: Biomarkers in acutely decompensated heart failure with preserved or reduced ejection fraction. *Am Heart J* 164:763, 2012.
101. Campbell RT, Jhund PS, Castagno D, et al: What have we learned about patients with heart failure and preserved ejection fraction from DIG-PEF, CHARM-preserved, and I-PRESERVE? *J Am Coll Cardiol* 60:2349, 2012.
102. Gullestad L, Ueland T, Vinge LE, et al: Inflammatory cytokines in heart failure: mediators and markers. *Cardiology* 122:23, 2012.
103. Borlaug BA, Olson TP, Lam CS, et al: Global cardiovascular reserve dysfunction in heart failure with preserved ejection fraction. *J Am Coll Cardiol* 56:845, 2010.
104. Akiyama E, Sugiyama S, Matsuzawa Y, et al: Incremental prognostic significance of peripheral endothelial dysfunction in patients with heart failure with normal left ventricular ejection fraction. *J Am Coll Cardiol* 60:1778, 2012.
105. Lam CS, Brutsaert DL: Endothelial dysfunction: a pathophysiologic factor in heart failure with preserved ejection fraction. *J Am Coll Cardiol* 60:1787, 2012.
106. Thenappan T, Shah SJ, Gomberg-Maitland M, et al: Clinical characteristics of pulmonary hypertension in patients with heart failure and preserved ejection fraction. *Circ Heart Fail* 4:257, 2011.
107. Paulus WJ, Tschöpe C: A novel paradigm for heart failure with preserved ejection fraction: comorbidities drive myocardial dysfunction and remodelling through coronary microvascular endothelial inflammation. *J Am Coll Cardiol* 62:263–271, 2013.
108. Gurusamy N, Das DK: Autophagy, redox signaling, and ventricular remodeling. *Antioxid Redox Signal* 11:1975, 2009.
109. Janicki JS, Brower GL, Gardner JD, et al: The dynamic interaction between matrix metalloproteinase activity and adverse myocardial remodeling. *Heart Fail Rev* 9:33, 2004.
110. Diwan A, Wansapura J, Syed FM, et al: Nix-mediated apoptosis links myocardial fibrosis, cardiac remodeling, and hypertrophy decompensation. *Circulation* 117:396, 2008.
111. Ganau A, Devereux RB, Roman MJ, et al: Patterns of left ventricular hypertrophy and geometric remodeling in essential hypertension. *J Am Coll Cardiol* 27:1201, 1996.
112. Drazner MH: The progression of hypertensive heart disease. *Circulation* 123:327, 2011.
113. Torre-Amione G, Kapadia S, Benedict C, et al: Proinflammatory cytokine levels in patients with depressed left ventricular ejection fraction: a report from the Studies of Left Ventricular Dysfunction (SOLVD). *J Am Coll Cardiol* 27:1201, 1996.
114. Lommi J, Pulkki K, Koskinen P, et al: Haemodynamic, neuroendocrine and metabolic correlates of circulating cytokine concentrations in congestive heart failure. *Eur Heart J* 18:1620, 1997.
115. Wilson Tang WH, Tong W, Shrestha K, et al: Differential effects of arginine methylation on diastolic dysfunction and disease progression in patients with chronic systolic heart failure. *Eur Heart J* 29:2506, 2008.

Alterations in Ventricular Structure: Role of Left Ventricular Remodeling and Reverse Remodeling in Heart Failure

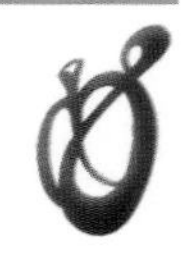

Luigi Adamo and Douglas L. Mann

One of the major conceptual advances in the field of heart failure has been the recognition that heart failure progresses because of the structural changes that occur in the heart in response to hemodynamic, neurohormonal, epigenetic factors, and genetic factors. Although the complex changes that occur in the heart during left ventricular (LV) remodeling have traditionally been described in anatomic terms, the process of LV remodeling arises secondary to changes in biology of the cardiac myocyte, changes in the volume of myocyte and nonmyocyte components of the myocardium, as well as on the geometry and architecture of the LV chamber (**Table 11-1**). Clinical studies have shown that medical and device therapies that reduce heart failure morbidity and mortality also lead to a reversal of LV remodeling, which is characterized anatomically by a return in LV volume and mass toward normal values, as well as a shift in the LV end-diastolic pressure-volume relationship (EDPVR) to the left. These salutary changes represent the summation of a series of integrated biologic changes in cardiac myocyte size and function, as well as modifications in LV structure and organization that are accompanied by shifts of the LV EDPVR toward normal. For want of better terminology, these changes have been referred to collectively as *reverse remodeling*.[1,2] It has also become clear that a small subset of patients whose hearts have undergone reverse remodeling following support with a mechanical left ventricular circulatory assist device (LVAD) are able to be weaned from their LVADs. This latter phenomenon is referred to as *myocardial recovery*.[3] The importance of understanding the biology of LV remodeling, reverse LV remodeling, and myocardial recovery is that it may lead to the identification of novel therapeutic targets for treating/reversing heart failure. In the chapter that follows, we will discuss the changes that occur during the process of LV dilation in heart failure with a reduced ejection fraction. The remodeling that occurs in heart failure with a preserved ejection fraction is discussed in **Chapter 10**.

LEFT VENTRICULAR REMODELING

The term *left ventricular (LV) remodeling* describes the changes in mass, volume, shape, and composition observed in the left ventricle in response to the mechanical (stress and strain) and systemic neurohormonal activation.[4,5] These changes involve both changes in the volume and biology of the cardiac myocyte and changes in the quantity and composition of the extracellular matrix (ECM) that eventually result in changes in the shape of the ventricular chamber. Conceptually, these changes can be envisioned as occurring within the cardiac myocyte, in the ECM, and within the left ventricular chamber.

Alterations in the Biology of the Cardiac Myocyte

The changes that occur in the biology of the failing cardiac myocyte include (1) cell hypertrophy (**see Chapter 2**); (2) loss of myofibrils and changes in excitation-contraction coupling leading to alterations in the contractile properties of the myocyte (**see Chapter 2**); (3) progressive loss and/or disarray of the cytoskeleton; (4) β-adrenergic desensitization (**see Chapter 6**); (5) modifications of myocyte metabolism (**see Chapter 16**); (6) reactivation of fetal genes. Collectively these changes lead to decreased shortening and delayed relaxation of the failing cardiac myocyte.

Two basic patterns of cardiac hypertrophy occur in response to hemodynamic overload (**Figure 11-1**). In pressure overload hypertrophy (e.g., with aortic stenosis or hypertension), the increase in systolic wall leads to the addition of sarcomeres in parallel, an increase in myocyte cross-sectional area, and increased LV wall thickening. This pattern of remodeling has been referred to as *concentric hypertrophy* (see Figure 11-1A) and has been linked with alterations in calcium/calmodulin-dependent protein kinase II-dependent signaling (**Figure 11-2**).[6] In contrast, in

TABLE 11-1 Overview of Left Ventricular Remodeling

Alterations in Myocyte Biology
Excitation contraction coupling
Myosin heavy chain (fetal) gene expression
β-adrenergic desensitization
Hypertrophy
Myocytolysis
Cytoskeletal proteins
Myocardial Changes
Myocyte loss
• Necrosis
• Apoptosis
• Autophagy
Alterations in extracellular matrix
• Matrix degradation
• Myocardial fibrosis
Alterations in Left Ventricular Chamber Geometry
Left ventricular (LV) dilation
Increased LV sphericity
LV wall thinning
Mitral valve incompetence

volume overload hypertrophy (e.g., with aortic and mitral regurgitation), increased diastolic wall stress leads to an increase in myocyte length with the addition of sarcomeres in series, thereby engendering increased LV ventricular dilation). This pattern of remodeling has been referred to as *eccentric hypertrophy* (so-named because of the position of the heart in the chest) or a *dilated phenotype* (see Figure 11-1A) and has been linked with Akt activation (see Figure 11-2).[6] Patients with heart failure classically present with a dilated LV with or without LV thinning. The myocytes from these failing ventricles have an elongated appearance that is characteristic of myocytes obtained from hearts subjected to chronic volume overload. Cardiac myocyte hypertrophy leads to reactivation of portfolios of genes that are normally not expressed postnatally. The reactivation of these fetal genes, the so-called fetal gene program, is also accompanied by decreased expression of a number of genes that are normally expressed in the adult heart. As will be discussed below, activation of the fetal gene program may contribute to the contractile dysfunction that develops in the failing myocyte. As shown in Figure 11-2, the stimuli for the genetic reprogramming of the myocyte include mechanical stretch/strain of the myocyte, neurohormones (e.g., NE, angiotensin II), inflammatory cytokines (e.g., TNF, interleukin-6 [IL-6]), other peptides and growth factors (e.g., ET), and reactive oxygen species (e.g., superoxide, NO). These stimuli occur both locally within the myocardium, where they exert autocrine/paracrine effects, as well as systemically where they exert endocrine effects.

The early stage of cardiac myocyte hypertrophy is characterized morphologically by increases in the number of myofibrils and mitochondria, as well as enlargement of mitochondria and nuclei (**Figure 11-3**). At this stage the cardiac myocytes are larger than normal and have preserved cellular organization. As hypertrophy continues, there is an increase in the number of mitochondria, as well as the addition of new contractile elements in localized areas of the cell. Cells subjected to longstanding hypertrophy show more obvious disruptions in cellular organization, such as markedly enlarged nuclei with highly lobulated membranes, accompanied by the displacement of adjacent myofibrils with loss of the normal registration of the Z bands. The late stage of hypertrophy is characterized by loss of contractile elements (myocytolysis) with marked disruption of Z bands, severe disruption of the normal parallel arrangement of the sarcomeres, accompanied by dilation and increased tortuosity of T tubules.

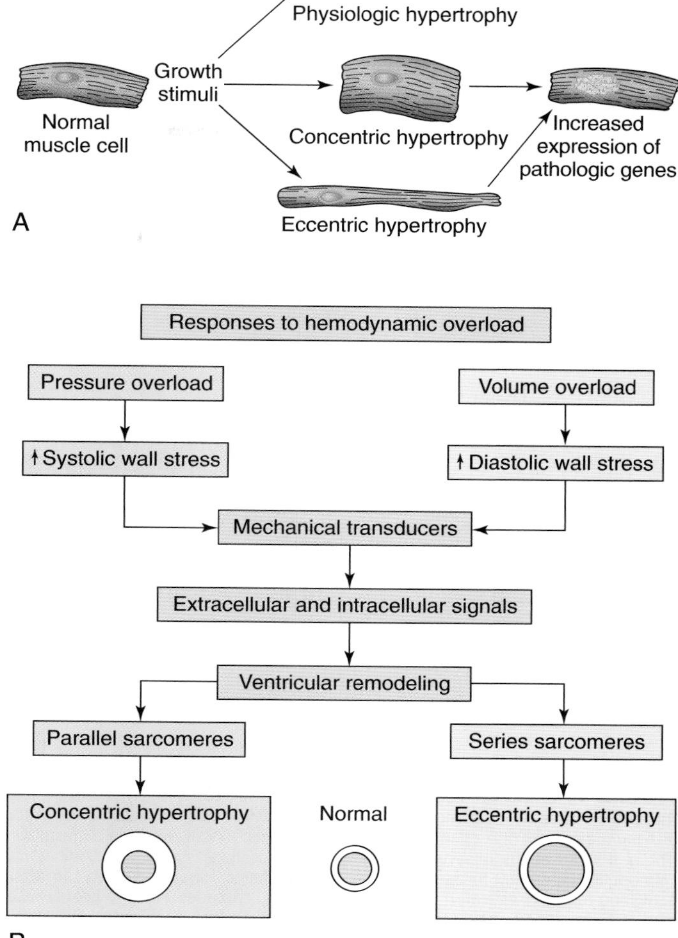

FIGURE 11-1 Patterns of cardiac myocyte hypertrophy. **A,** Morphology of cardiac myocytes in response to hemodynamic pressure and volume overloading. Phenotypically distinct changes in the morphology of myocyte occur in response to the type of hemodynamic overload that is superimposed. When the overload is predominantly due to an increase in pressure, the increase in systolic wall stress leads to the parallel addition of sarcomeres and widening of the cardiac myocytes. When the overload is predominantly due to an increase in ventricular volume, the increase in diastolic wall stress leads to the series addition of sarcomeres, and thus lengthening of cardiac myocytes. **B,** The pattern of cardiac remodeling that occurs in response to hemodynamic overloading depends on the nature of the inciting stimulus. When the overload is predominantly due to an increase in pressure (e.g., with systemic hypertension or aortic stenosis), the increase in systolic wall stress leads to the parallel addition of sarcomeres and widening of the cardiac myocytes, resulting in concentric cardiac hypertrophy. When the overload is predominantly due to an increase in ventricular volume, the increase in diastolic wall stress leads to the series addition of sarcomeres, lengthening of cardiac myocytes, and LV dilation, which is referred to as *eccentric chamber hypertrophy. Modified from Hunter JJ, Chien KR: Signaling pathways for cardiac hypertrophy and failure. N Engl J Med 341:1276, 1999; Colucci WS, editor: Heart failure: cardiac function and dysfunction, ed 2, Philadelphia, 1999, Current Medicine, p 4.2.; and modified from Mann DL: Pathophysiology of heart failure. In Libby PL, Bonow RO, Mann DL, et al, editors: Braunwald's heart disease, ed 8, Philadelphia, 2004, Saunders, pp 541–560.*

Failing human cardiac myocytes also undergo a number of other important changes expected to lead to a progressive loss of contractile function, including decreased

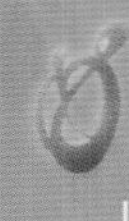

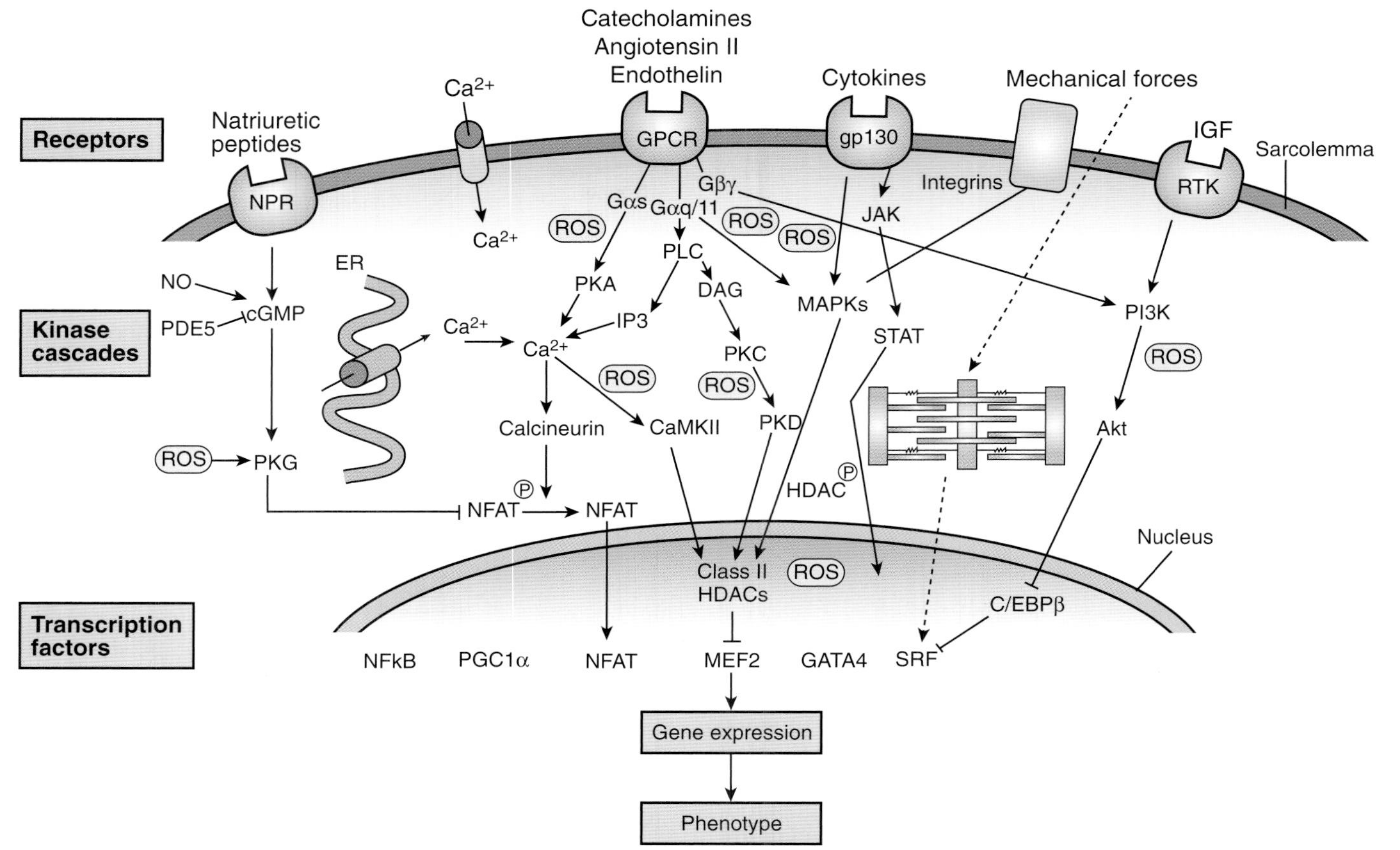

FIGURE 11-2 Cellular signaling pathways in cardiac myocyte hypertrophy. Many signaling pathways have the potential to regulate the growth of cardiac cells acting through an increasingly complex network of intracellular signaling cascades. Agonists for α-adrenergic, angiotensin, and endothelin receptors couple to phospholipase C (PLC) and calcium influx channels by way of G proteins. Activation of PLC results in the generation of two second messengers: inositol triphosphate (IP3) and diacylglycerol (DAG). IP3 causes the release of calcium from intracellular stores, and DAG activates protein kinase C (PKC). Changes in intracellular calcium stores can activate calcium/calmodulin-dependent kinases (CaCMK II), as well as calcineurin, which can affect gene expression in multiple ways. PKC and G proteins can affect gene expression by activating mitogen-activated protein kinase (MAPK) cascades. Histone deacetylase complexes (HDACs) are emerging as important negative regulators of genes involved in cardiac hypertrophy. Cytokines and peptide growth factors, such as insulin-like growth factor (IGF), can be elaborated by various cells within the heart and may act in an autocrine or paracrine manner. These growth factors activate cellular receptors that usually possess tyrosine kinase (RTK) activity and are coupled to a cascade of protein kinase. Mechanical deformation of cardiac myocytes through matrix-integrin interactions can lead to activation or modulation of several signaling pathways, at least in part through autocrine action of released agonists such as angiotensin. Both nitric oxide (NO) and oxidative stress may be induced after stimulation of signaling pathways and modulate the activity of kinase cascades and transcription factors leading to alterations in contractile phenotype, growth, and death in myocytes. *Akt,* Protein kinase; *C/EBPβ,* CCAAT/enhancer binding protein beta; *ER,* endoplasmic reticulum; *GATA4,* GATA binding protein; *gp130,* glycoprotein 130; *GPCR,* G protein–coupled receptor; *HDAC,* histone deacetylases; *JAK,* Janus kinase; *MAPKs,* mitogen-activated protein kinases; *MEF2,* myocyte enhancer facto; *NFAT,* nuclear factor of activated T cells; *NFκB,* nuclear factor kappa B cells; *NPR,* natriuretic peptide receptor; *P,* phosphorylation; *PDE5,* phosphodiesterase type 5; *PGC1α,* peroxisome proliferator-activated receptor gamma, coactivator 1 alpha; *PKA,* protein kinase A; *PKD,* protein kinase D; *PKG,* protein kinase G; *ROS,* reactive oxygen species; *STAT,* signal transducer and activator of transcription; *SRF,* serum response factor. *From Shah AM, Mann DL: In search of new therapeutic targets and strategies for heart failure: recent advances in basic science. Lancet 378:704–712, 2011.*

α-myosin heavy chain gene expression with a concomitant increase in β-myosin heavy chain expression.[7] This is accompanied by alterations in excitation-contraction coupling that have been closely linked to myocardial contractile dysfunction (see Chapter 2). These changes include modification in the abundance of critical Ca^{2+} regulatory proteins including sarcoplasmic endoreticular Ca^{2+} ATPase (SERCA), ryanodine receptor (RyR), L-type calcium channel (LTCC), and sarcolemmal Na^+/Ca^{2+} exchanger (NCX). The cytoskeleton of the myocyte consists of actin, the intermediate filament desmin, the sarcomeric protein titin, and α- and β-tubulin that form microtubules by polymerization. Vinculin, talin, dystrophin, and spectrin represent a separate group of membrane-associated proteins. The failing myocyte shows alterations in cytoskeletal proteins,[8] and in numerous experimental models cytoskeletal and/or membrane-associated proteins have been implicated in the pathogenesis of heart failure. Loss of integrity of the cytoskeleton and its linkage of the sarcomere to the sarcolemma and ECM leads to contractile dysfunction at the myocyte level, as well as at the myocardial level.

In line with all this, when the contractile performance of isolated failing human myocytes was examined under very simple experimental conditions, investigators found that there is an approximately 50% decrease in cell shortening in failing human cardiac myocytes when compared with nonfailing human myocytes.[9]

Alterations in the Myocardium

The alterations that occur in failing myocardium may be categorized broadly into those that occur in the volume of cardiac myocytes, as well as changes that occur in the volume and composition of the extracellular matrix. With respect to the changes that occur in cardiac myocyte component of the myocardium, there is increasing evidence to suggest that progressive myocyte loss may contribute to the development of LV dysfunction and LV remodeling. Necrotic

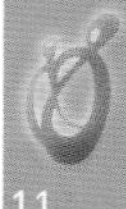

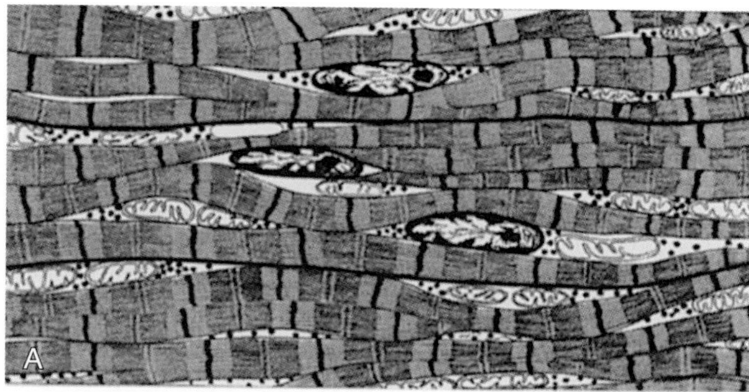

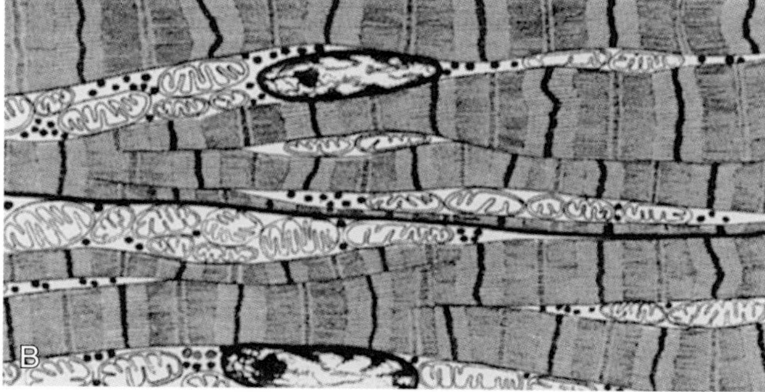

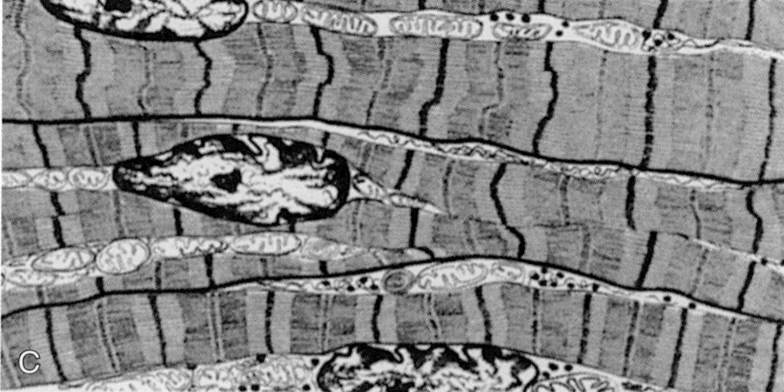

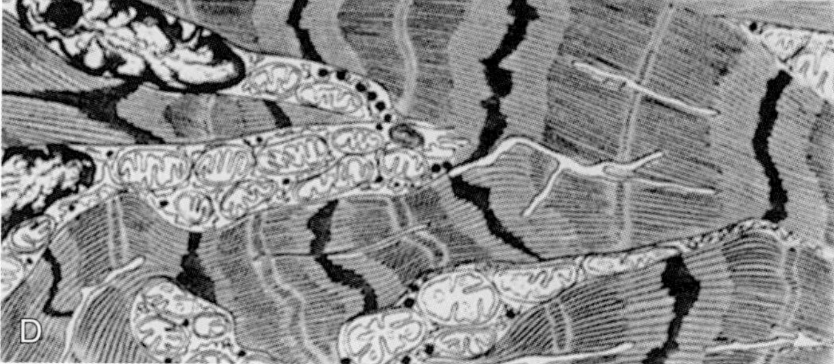

FIGURE 11-3 The early stage of cardiac hypertrophy **(A)** is characterized morphologically by increases in the number of myofibrils and mitochondria, as well as enlargement of mitochondria and nuclei. Muscle cells are larger than normal, but cellular organization is largely preserved. At a more advanced stage of hypertrophy **(B)**, preferential increases in the size or number of specific organelles, such as mitochondria, as well as irregular addition of new contractile elements in localized areas of the cell, result in subtle abnormalities of cellular organization and contour. Adjacent cells may vary in their degree of enlargement. Cells subjected to long-standing hypertrophy **(C)** show more obvious disruptions in cellular organization, such as markedly enlarged nuclei with highly lobulated membranes, which displace adjacent myofibrils and cause breakdown of normal Z-band registration. The early preferential increase in mitochondria is supplanted by a predominance (by volume) of myofibrils. The late stage of hypertrophy **(D)** is characterized by loss of contractile elements with marked disruption of Z bands, severe disruption of the normal parallel arrangement of the sarcomeres, deposition of fibrous tissue, and dilation and increased tortuosity of T tubules. *From Ferrans VJ: Morphology of the heart in hypertrophy. Hosp Pract 18:69, 1983.*

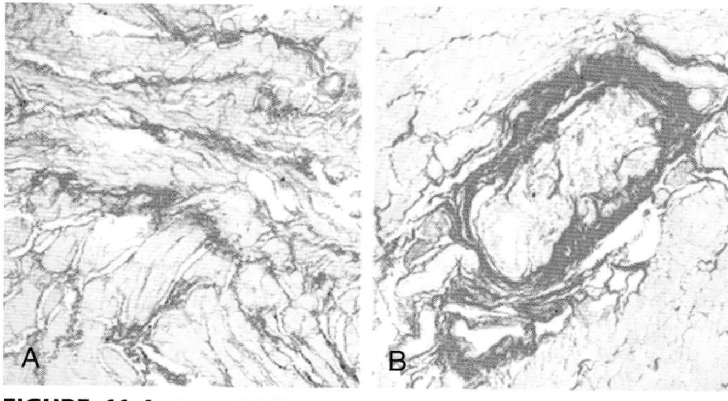

FIGURE 11-4 Myocardial fibrosis. Histologic section of a human myocardial biopsy specimen showing **(A)** interstitial and **(B)** perivascular fibrosis using picrosirius red staining. *Modified from Lopez B, Gonzales A, Varo N, et al: Biochemical assessment of myocardial fibrosis in hypertensive heart disease. Hypertension 38:1222, 2001.*

and apoptotic cell death are discussed in Chapter 2. Whereas the distinction between necrosis and apoptosis is obvious in certain circumstances, the dividing line between these two conditions is often less clear in the failing heart. And indeed, similar mechanisms can operate in both types of cell death. Thus instead of the existence of distinct types of cell death in heart failure, there is likely a continuum of cell death responses that contribute to progressive myocyte loss and disease progression.

Changes within the ECM constitute the second important myocardial adaptation that occurs during cardiac remodeling and include changes in overall collagen content, changes in the relative contents of different collagen subtypes, changes in collagen cross-linking, and modifications of the connections between cells and the ECM via integrins. Studies in failing human myocardium have shown that there is a quantitative increase in collagen I, III, VI, and IV; fibronectin; laminin; and vimentin, and that the ratio of type I collagen to type III collagen is decreased in patients with ischemic cardiomyopathy. Moreover, clinical studies suggest that there is a progressive loss of cross-linking of collagen in the failing heart, as well as loss of connectivity of the collagen network with individual myocytes, which would be expected to result in profound alterations in LV structure and function. Further, loss of cross-linking of the fibrillar collagen has been associated with progressive LV dilation following myocardial injury. The accumulation of collagen can occur on a "reactive" basis around intramural coronary arteries and arterioles (perivascular fibrosis) or in the interstitial space (interstitial fibrosis), and does not require myocyte cell death (**Figure 11-4**). Alternatively, collagen accumulation can occur as a result of microscopic scarring (replacement fibrosis) that develops in response to cardiac myocyte cell necrosis. This scarring or "replacement fibrosis" is an adaptation to the loss of parenchyma and is therefore critical to preserve the structural integrity of the heart. The increased fibrous tissue would be expected to lead to increased myocardial stiffness, which would presumably result in decreased myocardial shortening for a given degree of afterload. In addition, myocardial fibrosis may provide the structural substrate for atrial and ventricular arrhythmias, thus potentially contributing to sudden death. Although the full complement of molecules responsible for fibroblast activation is not known, many of the classical neurohormones (e.g., angiotensin II, aldosterone) and cytokines (ET, transforming growth factor-β [TGF-β], cardiotrophin-1) that are expressed in heart failure are sufficient to provoke fibroblast activation. And indeed, the use of angiotensin-converting enzyme (ACE) inhibitors, β-blockers, and aldosterone receptor antagonists has been associated with a decrease in myocardial fibrosis in experimental heart failure models.[10]

Although the fibrillar collagen matrix was initially considered to form a relatively static complex, it is now recognized that these structural proteins can undergo rapid turnover. As discussed in Chapter 4, one of the more exciting developments with respect to understanding the pathogenesis of cardiac remodeling has been the discovery that a family of collagenolytic enzymes, collectively referred to as *matrix metalloproteinases (MMPs),* are activated within the failing myocardium. Conceptually, disruption of the ECM would be expected to lead to LV dilation and wall thinning as a result of mural realignment (slippage) of myocyte bundles and/or individual myocytes within the left ventricular wall, as well as LV dysfunction as a result of dysynchronous contraction of the LV. Although the precise biochemical triggers that are responsible for activation of MMPs are not known, it bears emphasis that TNF, as well as other cytokines and peptide growth factors that are expressed within the failing myocardium, are capable of activating MMPs. However, the biology of matrix remodeling in heart failure is likely to be much more complex than the simple presence or absence of MMP activation, insofar as degradation of the matrix is also controlled by glycoproteins termed *tissue inhibitors of matrix metalloproteinases (TIMPs),* which are capable of regulating the activation of MMPs by binding to and preventing these enzymes from degrading the collagen matrix of the heart. The TIMP family presently consists of four distinct members, known as TIMP-1, -2, -3, and -4, each of which is constitutively expressed in the heart by fibroblasts, as well as myocytes. TIMPs-1, -2, -3, and -4 are secreted proteins that act as the natural inhibitors of active forms of all MMPs, although the efficiency of MMP inhibition varies among the different members. The extant literature suggests that MMP activation can lead to progressive LV dilation, whereas TIMP expression favors progressive myocardial fibrosis (see Chapter 4).

The histologic modifications of the failing myocardium are not limited to the ECM but also involve significant changes in the relationship between cardiac myocytes and their blood supply. In fact, although cardiac growth and angiogenesis are tightly coordinated during development and physiologic cardiac growth,[11] following hemodynamic overload and/or cardiac injury it is easy to observe a mismatch between cardiac myocyte growth and blood supply that may lead to contractile dysfunction and cell death. This has been especially well documented in patients with dilated cardiomyopathy that have a reduced myocardial capillary density.[12,13] Thus impaired capillary growth may contribute to the development and/or progression of heart failure.

Changes in Left Ventricular Geometry

The changes that occur in the biology of the cardiac myocyte and the myocardium (cardiac myocytes and ECM) lead to progressive LV dilation and increased sphericity of the ventricle. The increase in LV end-diastolic volume, along with LV wall thinning that can occur in some settings, sets the stage for progressive functional *ventricular-afterload mismatch* that contributes further to a decrease in stroke volume. Moreover, the high end-diastolic wall stress might be expected to lead to (1) hypoperfusion of the subendocardium, with resultant ischemia and worsening of LV function; (2) increased oxidative stress with resultant activation of families of genes that are sensitive to free radical generation (e.g., TNF and interleukin-1β); and (3) sustained expression of stretch-activated genes (angiotensin II, endothelin, and TNF) and/or stretch activation of hypertrophic signaling pathways. Increasing LV dilation also results in tethering of the papillary muscles with resultant incompetence of the mitral valve apparatus and functional mitral regurgitation and further hemodynamic overloading of the ventricle.[14]

A second important problem that results from increased sphericity of the ventricle is that the papillary muscles are pulled apart, resulting in incompetence of the mitral valve and the development of "functional mitral regurgitation." Whereas the amount of functional mitral regurgitation was once thought to be mild, the advent of noninvasive imaging modalities has shown that functional mitral regurgitation is clinically significant. Apart from the more obvious problem of loss of forward blood flow, mitral regurgitation presents yet a second problem to the heart insofar as the mitral regurgitation results in further hemodynamic overloading of the ventricle. Taken together, the mechanical burdens that are engendered by LV remodeling might be expected to lead to decreased forward cardiac output, increased LV dilation (stretch), and increased hemodynamic overloading, any or all of which are sufficient to contribute to disease progression independently of the neurohormonal status of the patient. Moreover, the aforementioned changes in LV structure and function might be expected to make the cardiovascular system less responsive to normal homeostatic control mechanisms, such as increased adrenergic drive. Thus alterations in the remodeled ventricle may foster a self-amplifying situation in which worsening neurohormonal activation occurs in response to the inability of the remodeled LV to respond appropriately to these compensatory mechanisms. Moreover, at some point in time it is predictable that the aggregate end-organ changes that occur within the cardiomyopathic ventricle may progress to the point that no amount of neurohormonal stimulation can maintain cardiovascular homeostasis, at which point heart failure may progress independent of the neurohormonal statues of the patient.

Clinical Studies Linking Left Ventricular Remodeling with Untoward Patient Outcomes

Natural history studies have shown that progressive LV remodeling is directly related to future deterioration in LV performance and a less favorable clinical course in patients with heart failure.[15-17] White and colleagues[18] were among the first to demonstrate that LV volume had greater predictive value for survival postinfarction than did LV ejection fraction. These authors measured LV volumes, LV ejection fraction, and severity of coronary arterial occlusions and stenosis at 1 to 2 months after a first or recurrent myocardial infarction. Survivors were followed for a mean of 78 months (range 15 to 165 months). There were 101 cardiac deaths, of which 71 (70%) were sudden (instantaneous or found dead). Multivariate analysis with log rank testing and the Cox proportional hazards model showed that end-systolic volume had greater predictive value for survival than end-diastolic volume or ejection fraction. Interestingly, the severity of coronary occlusions and stenosis showed additional prediction of only borderline significance. Similar findings were reported by St. John Sutton and associates,[19] who studied LV enlargement after myocardial infarction in an echocardiographic substudy of the Survival and Ventricular Enlargement (SAVE) Trial in which patients were randomized to placebo or captopril after an acute myocardial infarction. These investigators found that, irrespective of treatment assignment, baseline left ventricular systolic area and the percent change in LV area were strong predictors of cardiovascular mortality and adverse cardiovascular events. At 1 year, LV end-diastolic and end-systolic areas were significantly larger in the placebo than in the captopril group. Moreover, approximately 25% of the patients who survived 1 year experienced a major adverse cardiovascular event. Relevant to the present discussion, patients who experienced an adverse cardiovascular outcome had a greater than threefold increase in LV cavity size than did patients with an uncomplicated course. In a prospective study of 36 patients with dilated cardiomyopathy, Douglas and associates used two-dimensional echocardiography to study the functional consequences of changes in LV size and shape.[16] In this study nonsurvivors died an average of 11 months after initiation of the study, whereas survivors were followed up for an average of 52 months (range 40-76 months). Survivors had a smaller LV end-diastolic short-axis dimension when compared with nonsurvivors. Moreover, the ratio of short- to long-axis end-diastolic dimensions was more spherical in those with poorer survival (ratio 0.76 versus 0.68, $P < 0.02$). More recently, Vasan and colleagues studied the impact of changes in LV size on mortality in subjects that were followed in the Framingham study.[17] They examined the relation of the LV end-diastolic and end-systolic internal dimensions, as measured by M-mode echocardiography, to the risk of heart failure in subjects who had not sustained a myocardial infarction and who were free of heart failure at the time of enrollment. Data were analyzed using a sex-stratified proportional-hazards regression to assess the association between baseline LV internal dimensions and the subsequent risk of heart failure, after adjusting for age, blood pressure, hypertension treatment, body mass index, diabetes, valve disease, and interim myocardial infarction. Heart failure was diagnosed based on Framingham criteria (two major, or one major and two minor criteria).[20] These investigators found that over an 11-year follow-up period, heart failure developed in approximately 1.6% of the subjects. The risk-factor-adjusted hazard ratio for congestive heart failure was 1.47 (95% confidence interval, 1.25-1.73) for each increment of 1 standard deviation in LV end-diastolic dimension (height indexed). Similar results were obtained using LV end-systolic dimension (hazard ratio = 1.43; 95% confidence interval, 1.24-1.65). Vasan and colleagues concluded that an increase in LV internal dimension is a risk factor for congestive heart failure in men and women who have not had a myocardial infarction. Thus both the increased LV size and LV sphericity are predictive of untoward outcomes in heart failure patients with ischemic and dilated cardiomyopathy.

REVERSE LEFT VENTRICULAR REMODELING

The term *reverse remodeling* was first used to describe the leftward shift in the LV end-diastolic pressure-volume curve of the failing heart following hemodynamic unloading with a ventricular assist device (**Figure 11-5**) or a myocardial wrap with latissimus dorsi muscle.[1,2] An important feature

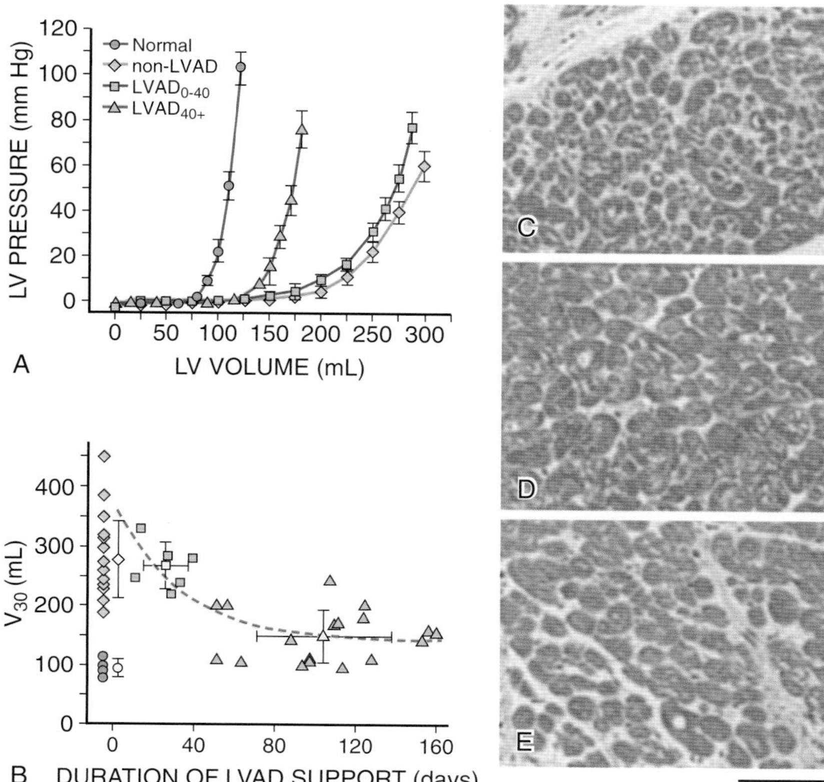

FIGURE 11-5 The ventricular end-diastolic pressure-volume relationship, which is initially shifted far rightward in heart failure, shifts, over time, back toward normal. **A,** Average end-diastolic pressure volume relationships from normal human hearts, from failing hearts not supported with LVAD, hearts supported with an LVAD for less than 40 days, and hearts supported with in LVAD for more than 40 days. **B,** Heart size, indexed by V30, the volume required to achieve an end-diastolic pressure of 30 mm Hg as a function of duration of LVAD support from individual hearts (see insert for symbol key). Also shown are values from normal and failing hearts not supported by LVAD. Underlying the reduction in heart size is regression of cellular hypertrophy. **C,** Cross-section of normal human myocardium. **D,** In chronic heart failure, the myocytes are markedly hypertrophic. **E,** After LVAD support, LV myocardial hypertrophy regresses (individual myocyte cross-sectional area reduced). Increased interstitial fibrosis is also noted. All myocardial samples used for C-E were fixed in an unloaded state. *From Madigan JD, Barbone A, Choudhri AF, et al: Time course of reverse remodeling of the left ventricle during support with a left ventricular assist device. J Thorac Cardiovasc Surg 121:902–908, 2001.*

of the decrease in LV size with reverse remodeling is that the change in LV geometry persisted even if the inciting therapy was abruptly stopped, suggesting that the change in properties reflected intrinsic biologic changes in the LV chamber as opposed to changes in LV volume that occur simply in response to a decrease in LV filling pressure. **Figure 11-6** shows that reverse LV remodeling has been observed in a wide variety of clinical settings, even when the heart failure is quite severe, including viral myocarditis, postpartum cardiomyopathy, or after removal of a cytotoxic agent. A recurring observation in all these clinical studies/observations is that reverse remodeling is associated with an improvement in the clinical manifestations and outcomes in heart failure, raising the interesting possibility that reverse remodeling is linked mechanistically to the observed improved heart failure outcomes. There is also extensive clinical trial-based evidence supporting the potential for reverse remodeling in patients with chronic heart failure who have received device-based and surgical interventions (reviewed in Hellawell and Margulies,[21] and Kramer and associates[22]). As illustrated in Figure 11-6, three major causes of dilated cardiomyopathy are associated with spontaneous recovery of LV function and reverse LV remodeling, including abnormal energetics, inflammation, and toxic insults. The greatest degree of recovery and/or normalization of LV function was observed in cardiomyopathies associated with abnormal energetics, whereas the cardiomyopathies associated with the least degree of recovery and/or normalization of LV function occurred with myocarditis and postpartum cardiomyopathy. Importantly, the percentage of patients with recovery of LV function is greater in more recent clinical studies than in older case series, suggesting the implementation of evidence-based therapies for heart failure has impacted the natural history of the disease. A full discussion of the natural history of the recovery of LV function and reverse LV remodeling are beyond the intended scope of this chapter and are discussed elsewhere in considerable detail.[23]

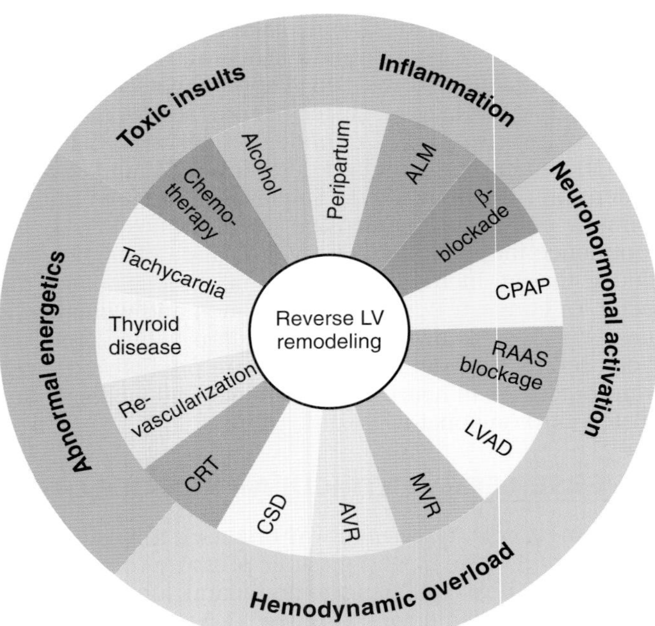

FIGURE 11-6 Reverse LV remodeling in clinical settings. Reverse remodeling is observed in a variety of clinical settings, as shown in the middle ring of the diagram. The segments illustrated in the outermost ring highlight the pathophysiologic processes implicated by reverse remodeling in each particular clinical setting. *ALM,* Acute lymphocytic myocarditis; *AVR,* aortic valve replacement; *CPAP,* continuous positive airway pressure; *CRT,* cardiac resynchronization therapy; *CSD,* cardiac support device; *LVAD,* left ventricular assist device; *MVR,* mitral valve repair/replacement; *RAAS,* renin-angiotensin-aldosterone system. *Modified from Hellawell JL, Margulies KB: Myocardial reverse remodeling. Cardiovasc Ther 20:172–181, 2012; and Mann DL, Barger PM, Burkhoff D: Myocardial recovery: myth, magic or molecular target? J Amer Coll Cardiol 60:2465–2472, 2012.*

Although the precise cellular and molecular mechanisms that are responsible for the return toward normal LV size and shape during reverse remodeling are not completely understood, there is a fairly consistent biologic theme with respect to the parameters that return toward baseline following pharmacologic or device therapy. As shown in **Table 11-2**, there are a series of favorable changes in cardiac myocyte biology, the composition of the myocardium, and the chamber properties of the LV following pharmacologic and device therapies that lead to reverse remodeling.

TABLE 11-2 Cellular and Molecular Determinants of Myocardial Recovery

	β-BLOCKER	ACE INHIBITOR	ARB	ALDOSTERONE ANTAGONISTS	LVAD	CRT
Myocyte Defects						
Hypertrophy	Decreased	Decreased	Decreased	Decreased	Decreased	Decreased
Fetal gene expression	Decreased	Decreased	Decreased	ND	Decreased	Decreased
Myocytolysis	Decreased	ND	ND	ND	Decreased	ND
β-Adrenergic desensitization	Decreased	Decreased	Decreased	ND	Decreased	Decreased
EC coupling	Increased	Increased	Increased	ND	Increased	Increased
Cytoskeletal proteins	ND	ND	ND	Increased	Increased	ND
Myocardial Defects						
Myocyte apoptosis	Decreased	Decreased	Decreased	ND	Decreased	Decreased
MMP activation	Decreased	Decreased	Decreased	Decreased	Decreased	Decreased
Fibrosis	Decreased	Decreased	Decreased	Decreased	Increased*	Decreased
Angiogenesis	Increased	Increased	Increased	Increased	Decreased	Increased
LV Dilation	Decreased	Stabilized	Stabilized	Stabilized	Decreased	Decreased

*With prolonged mechanical support.

ACE, Angiotensin-converting enzymes; *ARB,* angiotensin receptor blockers; *CRT,* cardiac resynchronization therapy; *EC,* excitation-contraction; *LV,* left ventricular; *LVAD,* left ventricular circulatory assist device; *MMP,* matrix metalloproteinases; *ND,* not done.

Alterations in the Biology of the Cardiac Myocyte

Clinical studies from patients undergoing LVAD implantation,[24-29] cardiac resynchronization therapy,[30] or cardiac contractility modulation[31,32] have consistently shown a decrease in cardiac myocyte hypertrophy. Regression of myocyte hypertrophy is accompanied by reversal of many of the changes in myocyte biology that occur during forward LV remodeling, including excitation-contraction coupling, the cytoskeleton, β-adrenergic desensitization, and the fetal gene program. Collectively these changes may explain the significant increase in contractility (maximal calcium saturated force generation) in cardiac myocytes isolated from hearts that have undergone LVAD support, when compared with myocytes isolated before LVAD support.[33]

Fetal Gene Expression

The extant literature suggests that many of the changes in gene expression are reversible with pharmacologic therapies that have been shown to improve patient outcomes. Treatment with ACE inhibitors or angiotensin receptor blockers (ARBs) were associated with an increase in α-MHC and a decrease in β-MHC at the transcriptional level in experimental models of heart failure.[34,35] In patients with dilated cardiomyopathy, β-blockade with metoprolol (selective β_1-blocker) or carvedilol (β_1-, β_2-, and α_1-blocker) inhibited expression of atrial natriuretic peptide (ANP) and β-MHC and restored that of SERCA and α-MHC at the mRNA level (**Figure 11-7**).[36]

Changes in the abnormal gene expression have also been observed with the use of mechanical circulatory assist devices. For example, when gene expression profiling was performed in bridge-to-transplantation patients before and after LVAD support, there was a significant downregulation of β-MHC, α-SKA, and B-type natriuretic peptide (BNP) in patients with nonischemic cardiomyopathy who received LVAD support, whereas no differences were observed in patients with ischemic cardiomyopathy.[37] In a similar study that employed a proprietary gene array platform, there was a global increase in the expression of a variety of sarcomeric genes in the hearts of LVAD-supported ischemic and nonischemic cardiomyopathy patients, whereas β-MHC mRNA expression was downregulated, consistent with the previous reports.[38] In a select cohort of LVAD patients with clinical myocardial recovery leading to device explantation, mechanical unloading resulted in increased protein expression of myosin heavy and light chains, tropomyosin, and troponins I, C, and T.[39] Moreover, chronic hemodynamic unloading with an LVAD significantly reduced the expression of ANP, BNP, and natriuretic peptide receptor-C mRNA in patients with end-stage heart failure.[40] Sequencing-based transcriptomic profiling of changes in the expression levels of myocardial mRNA, microRNA (miRNA), and long noncoding RNAs (lncRNA) before and after mechanical support with a LVAD support, revealed that less than 5% of mRNAs and miRNAs were normalized after LVAD support, whereas approximately 10% on long noncoding RNAs were improved and/or normalized after LVAD support. Further,

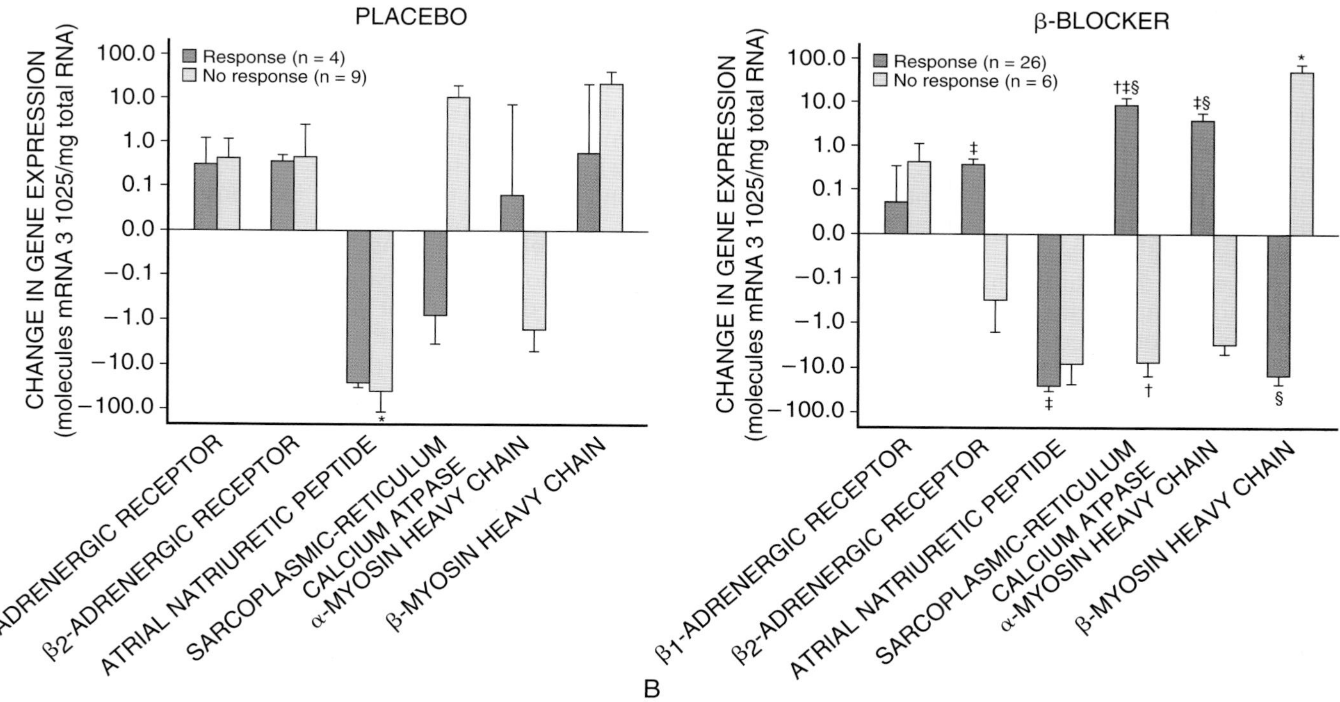

FIGURE 11-7 Changes in fetal gene expression in patients who received β-blockers. **A** and **B,** Changes between baseline and the end of the 6-month study in the abundance of myocardial mRNA for six contractility-regulating or hypertrophy-regulating proteins in patients who received a placebo or β-blocker. The changes in patients who had an improvement in left ventricular ejection fraction by at least five ejection fraction [EF] units were compared with the changes in patients who did not have such a response. Gene expression is shown as molecules of mRNA per microgram of total RNA on a logarithmic scale. The asterisk indicates $P < 0.10$ for the change between the baseline value and the value measured at 6 months by the paired *t*-test, the daggers $P < 0.05$ for the comparison with the placebo group by the test for interaction, the double daggers $P < 0.05$ for the change between the baseline value and the value measured at 6 months by the paired *t*-test, and the section marks $P < 0.05$ for the comparison with patients who did not have a response. Each panel shows the results for patients with complete data for the indicated mRNA and receptor protein measurements. *Modified from Lowes BD, Gilbert EM, Abraham WT, et al: Myocardial gene expression in dilated cardiomyopathy treated with β-blocking agents. N Eng J Med 346:1357, 2002; and Mann DL: Management of patients with a reduced ejection fraction. In Libby PL, Bonow RO, Mann DL, et al, editors: Braunwald's heart disease, ed 8, Philadelphia, 2004, Saunders, pp 611-640.*

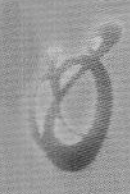

the signature of the expression of long noncoding RNAs, but not mRNAs nor miRNAs, distinguished ischemic from nonischemic heart failure, suggesting a potentially important role for long noncoding RNAs in pathogenesis of heart failure.[41] Left ventricular endomyocardial biopsies obtained from heart failure patients who underwent cardiac resynchronization therapy (CRT) revealed a significant increase in α-MHC and a nonsignificant decrease in β-MHC mRNA levels using quantitative real-time PCR.[42] Vayderheyden and colleagues have demonstrated that CRT resulted in increased expression of α-MHC and BNP mRNA levels, and reduced the expression of β-MHC mRNA in patients who improved clinically.[43] Changes in fetal gene expression were not seen in "nonresponders," defined as failure to improve greater than 1 New York Heart Association (NYHA) functional class score and less than 25% relative increase in EF after 4 months of therapy. In a dog model of heart failure induced by intracoronary microembolization, therapy with a cardiac support device resulted in a return in β-MHC, α-MHC, ANP, and BNP toward values observed in sham-operated animals.[44] Taken together, these data suggest that both drug and device therapies contribute to reversal of the fetal gene program that has been associated with abnormal contractile function of the cardiac myocyte. However, what is not clear from the extant literature is which of the above changes is/are necessary and/or essential for myocardial recovery.

β-Adrenergic Desensitization

As noted above, one of the signatures of advancing heart failure is a reduction in β_1-adrenergic receptor density, isoproterenol-mediated adenylate cyclase stimulation, and isoproterenol-stimulated muscle contraction.[45] β-AR desensitization can be reversed with pharmacologic and device therapies that have been shown to improve patient outcomes. In a substudy of MDC (the Metoprolol in Dilated Cardiomyopathy) trial, treatment with selective β_1-blocker metoprolol resulted in significantly increased total β-receptor density in the heart. Interestingly, carvedilol had no effect on β-adrenergic receptor (β-AR) density despite the fact that it was associated with a marked improvement in myocardial function and a reduction in cardiac adrenergic activity.[46] In a randomized, double-blind, placebo-controlled study, the use of the ACE inhibitor lisinopril resulted in a significant increase in myocardial β-AR density in a subset of heart failure patients with high baseline cardiac adrenergic activity.[47] Normalization of reduced β-adrenergic receptor density and enhanced inotropic responsiveness to isoproterenol have been demonstrated consistently in LVAD-supported failing hearts.[48-50] The enhanced β-adrenergic responsiveness with LVAD support was associated with a decrease in GRK2 protein levels and total GRK activity, but no significant change in GRK5 protein and mRNA levels.[51] Similar findings have been observed following CRT therapy. After 4 months of CRT, β_1-adrenergic receptor expression was significantly upregulated at the transcriptional level in heart failure patients.[52] Treatment with a cardiac support device resulted in increased inotropic responsiveness in a canine model of heart failure.[53]

Excitation-Contraction Coupling

As discussed in Chapter 2, changes in the abundance of critical Ca^{2+} regulatory proteins including sarcoplasmic endoreticular Ca^{2+} ATPase (SERCA), ryanodine receptor (RyR), L-type calcium channel (LTCC), and sarcolemmal Na^+/Ca^{2+} exchanger (NCX) likely play an important role in the contractile dysfunction of the failing cardiac myocyte. In a transgenic mouse model of heart failure overexpressing tropomodulin, treatment with β-blockers resulted in normalization of SERCA and NCX protein levels, as well as LTCC density and function.[54] RyR phosphorylation was unchanged by treatment with β-blockers in this transgenic model. Clinical studies have shown that treatment with β-blockers results in increased myocardial SERCA mRNA and protein content (see Figure 11-7),[36,55] a trend toward a decrease in myocardial PLB and NCX protein content,[55] and reduced PKA-mediated hyperphosphorylation of RyR.[56] Similarly, administration of ACE inhibitors or ARBs in a post-MI rat model of heart failure significantly attenuates the reduction in myocardial SERCA, RYR, and PLB mRNA and protein levels.[57,58] Mechanical unloading with LVAD support has provided the clearest insight into the importance of changes in excitation-contraction coupling during myocardial recovery. As summarized in **Figure 11-8**, the return of contractile function in failing hearts following LVAD-induced unloading is associated with altered gene expression of key Ca^{2+} regulatory proteins, including NCX, SERCA2a, RyR, as well as changes in calcium cycling.[59,60] Moreover, protein kinase A-mediated hyperphosphorylation of RyR was restored to normal in failing hearts following LVAD support.[61] Nonetheless, the significance of some of the reported changes in gene expression is uncertain, insofar as only SERCA2 protein levels increased, whereas protein levels of the RYR and NCX were unchanged following LVAD support.[62] Cardiac resynchronization therapy significantly increased mRNA expression for SERCA2a, RyR, and SERCA/NCX mRNA in heart failure patients.[52] Importantly, improvement in SERCA expression occurred only in patients who clinically responded to CRT.[43] Although treatment with a cardiac support device did not result in changes in SERCA2a and phospholamban expression, treatment with a cardiac support device resulted in increased SERC2A-mediated Ca^{+2} uptake in an experimental model.[63]

Cytoskeletal Proteins

The cytoskeleton of cardiac myocytes consists of actin, the intermediate filament desmin, the sarcomeric protein titin, and α- and β-tubulin that form microtubules by polymerization. Vinculin, talin, dystrophin, and spectrin represent a separate group of membrane-associated proteins. In numerous experimental studies, the role of cytoskeletal and/or membrane-associated proteins has been implicated in the pathogenesis of heart failure insofar as loss of integrity of the cytoskeleton and its linkage of the sarcomere to the sarcolemma and ECM would be expected to lead to contractile dysfunction at the myocyte level, as well as at the myocardial level.

Mechanical unloading with LVAD support also results in restoration of cytoskeletal organization. Vatta and colleagues reported that there was loss of the N-terminal region of dystrophin (which links to the sarcomere through actin) in patients with both ischemic and dilated cardiomyopathy, and that mechanical unloading resulted in increased N-terminal dystrophin expression (**Figure 11-9**).[64] The change in the level of expression of dystrophin was comparable in the RV and the LV after mechanical unloading; however, a greater degree of normalization was achieved in patients treated with pulsatile-flow LVADs than among those treated with continuous-flow LVADs.[65] Mechanical support with an LVAD

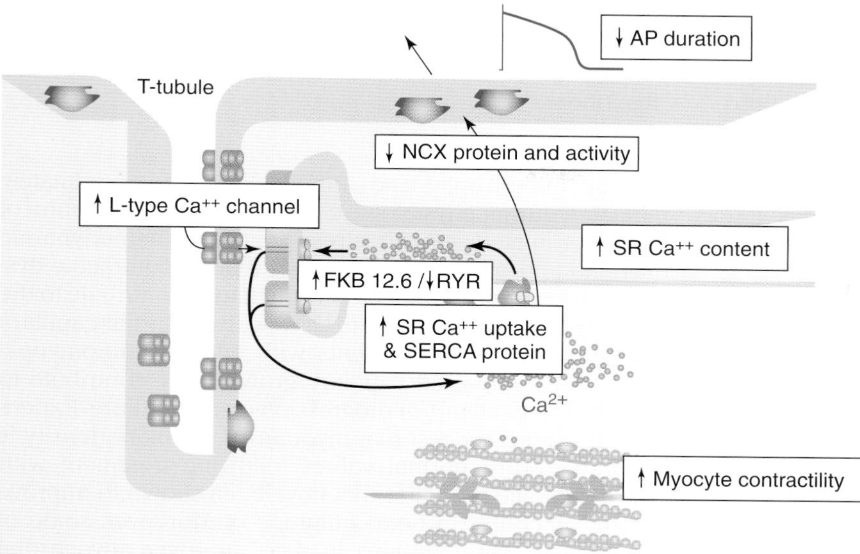

FIGURE 11-8 Summary of changes in excitation-contraction coupling in cardiac myocytes from hearts that have been supported with a left ventricular assist device. As shown, there is an increase in the inward Ca^{++} current through the L-type Ca^{++} channel, a decrease in the levels and activity of the sodium-calcium exchanger (NCX), increased Ca^{++} content of the sarcoplasmic reticulum (SR), decreased activity of the ryanodine receptor (RyR), and decreases in FKB 12.6 levels (a regulatory protein that prevents Ca^{++} release from the RyR). Collectively these changes would be expected to lead to improved myocyte contractility. (Key: The arrows indicate increases [↑] or decreases [↓] in various parameters.) *Modified from Soppa GK, Barton PJ, Terracciano CM, et al: Left ventricular assist device-induced molecular changes in the failing myocardium. Curr Opin Cardiol 23:206–218, 2008.*

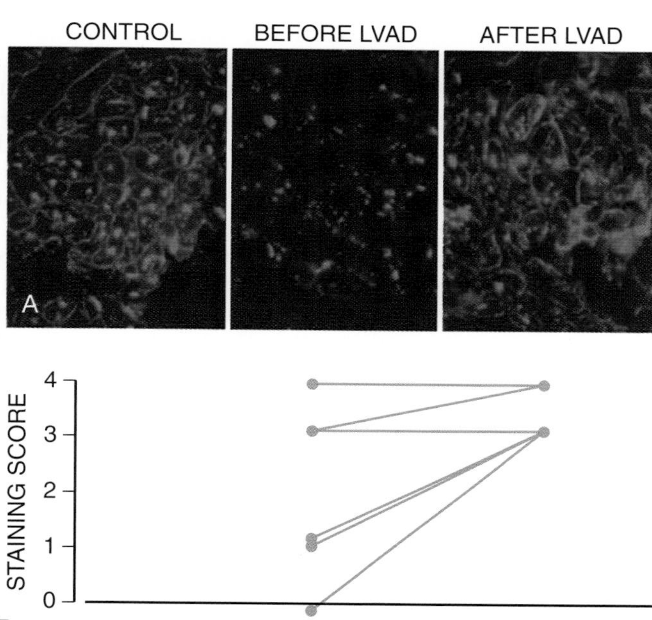

FIGURE 11-9 Effect of LVAD support on dystrophin levels in failing hearts. **A,** Immunohistochemical staining with the N-terminal-specific antibody of myocardial sections from a control sample *(left),* and paired samples from patients with end-stage cardiomyopathy before *(middle)* and after *(right)* LVAD support. Immunostaining for the N-terminal portion of dystrophin was present on the myocyte cell membranes of control hearts, absent in cell membranes from cardiomyopathy, and restored in cardiomyopathic hearts following LVAD support. **B,** Semiquantitative staining scores for N-terminal dystrophin in paired samples, before and after LVAD support. *Modified from Vatta M, Stetson SJ, Perez-Verdia A, et al: Molecular remodeling of dystrophin in patients with end-stage cardiomyopathies and reversal in patients on assistance-device therapy. Lancet 359:936–941, 2002.*

has been reported to increase immunostaining for major sarcomeric proteins, including actin, troponin C, troponin T, tropomyosin, and titin, with a small nonsignificant decrease in myosin,[66] as well as changes in the intracellular distribution of desmin, vinculin, and tubulin, and an increase in desmin protein content, with no change in the content or distribution of α-actinin.[67] Interestingly, in one small study there was a specific pattern of changes in mRNA expression levels for both sarcomeric and nonsarcomeric cytoskeletal proteins in the myocardium (increased β-actin, α-tropomyosin, α_1-actinin, α-filamin A, with decreased troponin T3, α_2-actinin, and vinculin) in patients who were bridged to recovery when compared with heart failure patients who were not supported, suggesting that alterations in cytoskeletal structure might play an important role in and serve as a marker of myocardial recovery (see later discussion).[68]

Collectively the above genomic and proteomic changes would be expected to lead to functional improvements in the failing cardiac myocyte. And indeed, there is a significant increase in contractility (maximal calcium saturated force generation) in cardiac myocytes isolated from hearts that have undergone LVAD support, when compared with myocytes isolated before LVAD support.[33]

Alterations in the Myocardium

In addition to the salutary changes in the biology of the adult cardiac myocyte that occur during reverse remodeling, there are a number of important changes that also occur within the myocardium, including changes in the volume and composition of the ECM, as well as in microvascular density (angiogenesis).

Myocardial Fibrosis

As noted above, both the amount and the organization of the fibrillar collagen are important determinants of myocardial structure and function in the failing heart. β-blockade with metoprolol significantly decreased replacement fibrosis in a dog model of heart failure.[69] Consistent with this finding, treating patients with dilated cardiomyopathy with β-blockers for 4 months resulted in decreased myocardial collagen type I and III mRNA expression in paired myocardial RV biopsy samples.[70] Experimental studies suggest that ACE inhibitors reduce collagen deposition in the failing myocardium in various models of heart failure, and this salutary effect is mediated, at least in part, by kinins.[71,72] Similarly, treatment of patients with ischemic cardiomyopathy with captopril resulted in decreased total collagen content, decreased collagen type III levels, and normalization of the collagen type I:III ratio, when compared with untreated heart failure patients.[73] Angiotensin receptor type I (AT_1) receptor blockers also reduce myocardial collagen content in experimental heart failure models; however, this decrease was not attenuated by blockade of the bradykinin B_2-receptor, suggesting that antagonism of the renin angiotensin system alone is sufficient to reverse myocardial fibrosis.[72] Treatment with eplerenone in a dog model of heart failure significantly attenuated LV collage volume fraction by reducing both interstitial and replacement fibrosis[74] and normalized mRNA and protein expression of MMPs 1, 2, and 9, but had no effect on mRNA levels of TIMP-1 and -2.[75]

Mechanical circulatory support with LVADs also leads to important changes in the ECM and myocardial fibrillar content and organization. There are conflicting reports on the effect of LVAD support on LV myocardial collagen content, with several reports showing increased myocardial collagen content relative to levels observed in failing hearts that have not been supported with LVADs,[76-80] whereas other reports suggest that the collagen volume fraction decreases.[81,82] Although the reason(s) for this discrepancy is not known, it may be related to differences in heart failure etiology, differences in the degree of inotropic and/or pharmacologic support, and the duration of LVAD support. Of note, one report suggests that longer duration of LVAD support results in increased myocardial collagen volume fraction in a time-dependent manner (**Figure 11-10**).[26] Another potential explanation is that collagen content decreased in LVAD-supported patients taking ACE inhibitors and increased in patients not taking ACE inhibitors.[83]

The biologic basis for these changes is suggested by two studies that show that LVAD support resulted in decreased levels of MMP 1 and 9 and increased expression of TIMP-1 and -2, resulting in decreased MMP-1/TIMP-1 ratio (favoring collagen accumulation), and an increase in the ratio of insoluble to total soluble collagen (a measure of collagen cross-linking).[77,78] Moreover, these changes were amplified by concomitant therapy with ACE inhibitors during the period of LVAD support.[84] Serial myocardial biopsies from heart failure patients revealed a significant reduction in the collagen volume fraction following CRT,[30,85] with a significant decrease in MMP-9 levels in the group of patients who underwent reverse remodeling (i.e., "responders").[86]

Angiogenesis

Cardiac hypertrophy and angiogenesis are coordinately regulated during physiologic cardiac growth.[11] Disruption of this coordinated growth stress following hemodynamic overload and/or cardiac injury may lead to contractile dysfunction and cell death, both of which may contribute to the development of heart failure. Of note, myocardial capillary density is reduced in patients with dilated cardiomyopathy.[12,13] Thus impaired capillary growth may contribute to the development and/or progression of heart failure. Experimental studies suggest that myocardial capillary density is restored toward normal values following treatment with pharmacologic therapies that have been shown to improve patient outcomes in heart failure.[69,72,74] Moreover, some of these same therapies also lead to improved myocardial blood flow in patients with heart failure.[87-89] Whether the improved myocardial blood flow is related to increased angiogenesis, altered hemodynamic loading conditions, or both is not known. Analysis of changes in gene expression before and after LVAD support revealed significant alterations in genes that are involved in the regulation of vascular networks, including upregulation of Sprouty-1 and downregulation of neurophilin (VEGF receptor), stromal derived factor-1, FGF9, and endomucin.[90] Sprouty-1 was immunolocalized to the microvasculature, and the upregulation of Sprouty-1 in endothelial cells was associated with a decrease in VEGF-induced endothelial proliferation, which suggests that Sprouty-1 may serve as an intrinsic mediator of cardiac remodeling by regulating angiogenesis.[90] Studies in heart failure patients who underwent CRT revealed increased myocardial capillary density and an improvement in the distribution pattern of myocardial blood flow.[85,91]

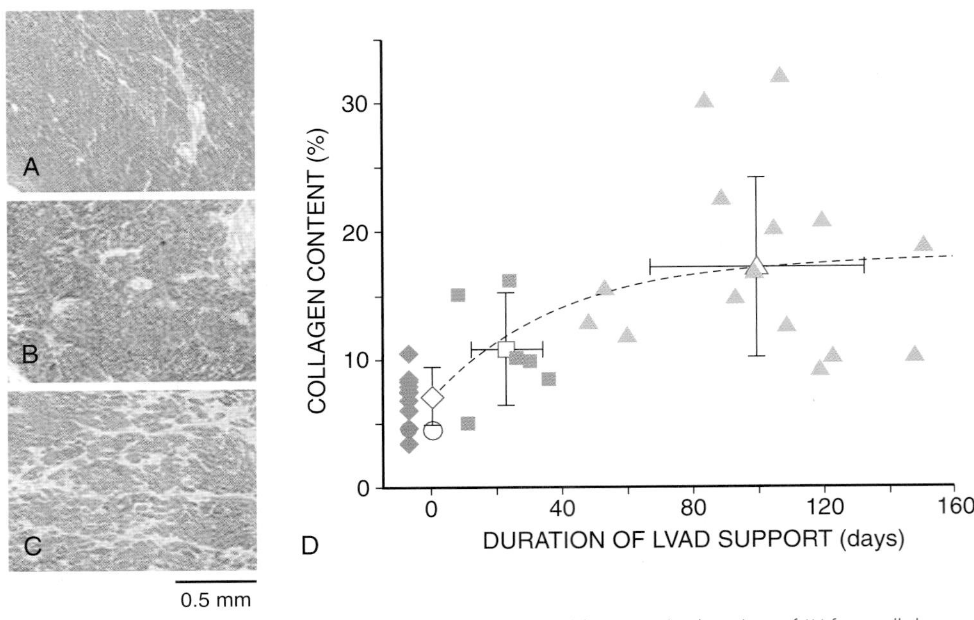

FIGURE 11-10 Effect of the duration of LVAD support on myocardial collagen content. Trichrome-stained sections of LV free wall demonstrating relative myocardial collagen content for **A,** normal **B,** non-LVAD, and **C,** $LVAD_{40+day}$ groups. **D,** Relative myocardial collagen content versus duration of LVAD support *(squares,* $LVAD_{0\text{-}40\ days}$*; triangles,* $LVAD_{40+days}$*; diamonds,* non-LVAD; *circles,* normal. *Modified from Madigan JD, Barbone A, Choudhri AF, et al: Time course of reverse remodeling of the left ventricle during support with a left ventricular assist device. J Thorac Cardiovasc Surg 121:902–908, 2001.*

Changes in Left Ventricular Geometry

As noted previously, clinical studies with ACE inhibitors, β-blockers, aldosterone antagonists, LVADs, and CRT have shown that these treatment modalities lead to return of cardiac myocyte biology toward normal, as well as changes in the ECM that favor increased structural integrity of the heart and reverse remodeling (**Figure 11-11**). In the following section, we will review the literature that shows that drugs and devices that favorably impact clinical outcomes are accompanied by reverse LV remodeling. As illustrated in **Figure 11-12A**, treatment with ACE inhibitors prevented worsening LV remodeling but did not lead to reverse remodeling in a substudy of SOLVD,[92] whereas treatment with β-blockers resulted in decreased LV end-diastolic volumes when compared with the placebo (diuretics and ACE inhibitors) in a substudy of the ANZ (Australia New Zealand) trial (see Figure 11-12B).[93] In an echocardiographic substudy of the Val-HeFT (Valsartan in Heart Failure) trial, treatment with valsartan added to an ACE inhibitor and/or β-blocker significantly resulted in decreased LV internal diastolic diameter (LVIDd)/body surface area from 4 months to greater than 24 months (see Figure 11-12C).[94] Similarly, the addition of spironolactone to candesartan resulted in a significant decrease in LV volume index at 1 year when compared with candesartan alone (see Figure 11-12D).[95]

Device therapies also lead to reverse remodeling of the ventricle. Although pulsatile-flow devices provide a greater degree of ventricular unloading than continuous-flow devices,[96] the continuous-flow LVADs appear to be as effective as pulsatile-flow LVADs with regard to the degree of left ventricular reverse remodeling (see Figure 11-11E).[96,97] As noted previously, the initial clinical experience with mechanical assist devices demonstrated that there were varying degrees of structural and functional recovery of myocyte function that are associated with reverse remodeling. The improvement in LV function was sufficient to allow explantation of the device in approximately 5% to 15% of explanted patients.[98,99] However, although cardiac function improves significantly after device implantation, and although there is cellular recovery and favorable remodeling of the ECM, the degree of clinical recovery is insufficient for device explantation in most patients with chronic heart failure. In the MIRACLE (Multicenter In-Synch Randomized Clinical Evaluation) trial, CRT led to improvements in LVEF, mitral regurgitant area, and LV end-diastolic diameter at 6 months in patients with moderate to severe heart failure and prolonged QRS (see Chapter 35).[100] Similar findings have been reported in the MUSTIC (Multisite Stimulation in Cardiomyopathy) and CARE-HF (Cardiac Resynchronization in Heart Failure) studies, which employed a longer follow-up period (see also Chapter 35).[101,102] Passive cardiac restraint in the Acorn Randomized Trial showed that there was a significant reduction in LV end-diastolic volume over the 12-month course of the study[103] that was

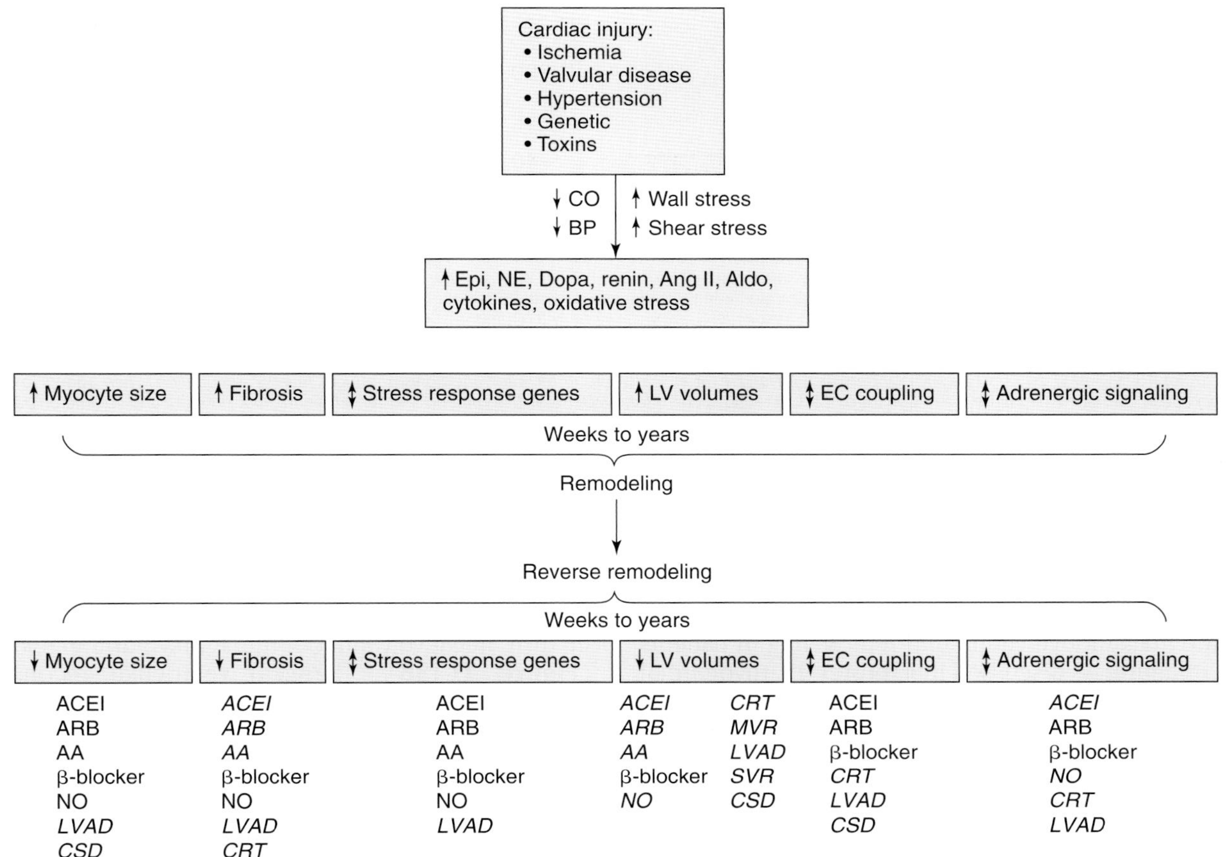

FIGURE 11-11 Structural, molecular, and cellular changes after cardiac injury, leading to remodeling and those therapies that have been shown to contribute to reverse remodeling. Therapies that have been shown in humans to alter the specific reverse remodeling subheadings are bold and italicized. *AA,* Aldosterone antagonists; *ALB,* angiotensin-converting enzyme inhibitor; *Aldo,* aldosterone; *Ang II,* angiotensin II; *ARB,* angiotensin receptor blocker; *BP,* blood pressure; *CO,* cardiac output; *CRT,* cardiac resynchronization; *CSD,* cardiac support device; *Dopa,* dopamine; *EC,* excitation-contraction; *Epi,* epinephrine; *LVADL,* Left ventricular assist device; *MVR,* mitral valve repair; *NE,* norepinephrine; *NO,* nitric oxide; *SVR,* surgical ventricular restoration. *From Mudd JO, Kass DA: Reversing chronic remodeling in heart failure. Expert Rev Cardiovasc Ther 5:585–598, 2007.*

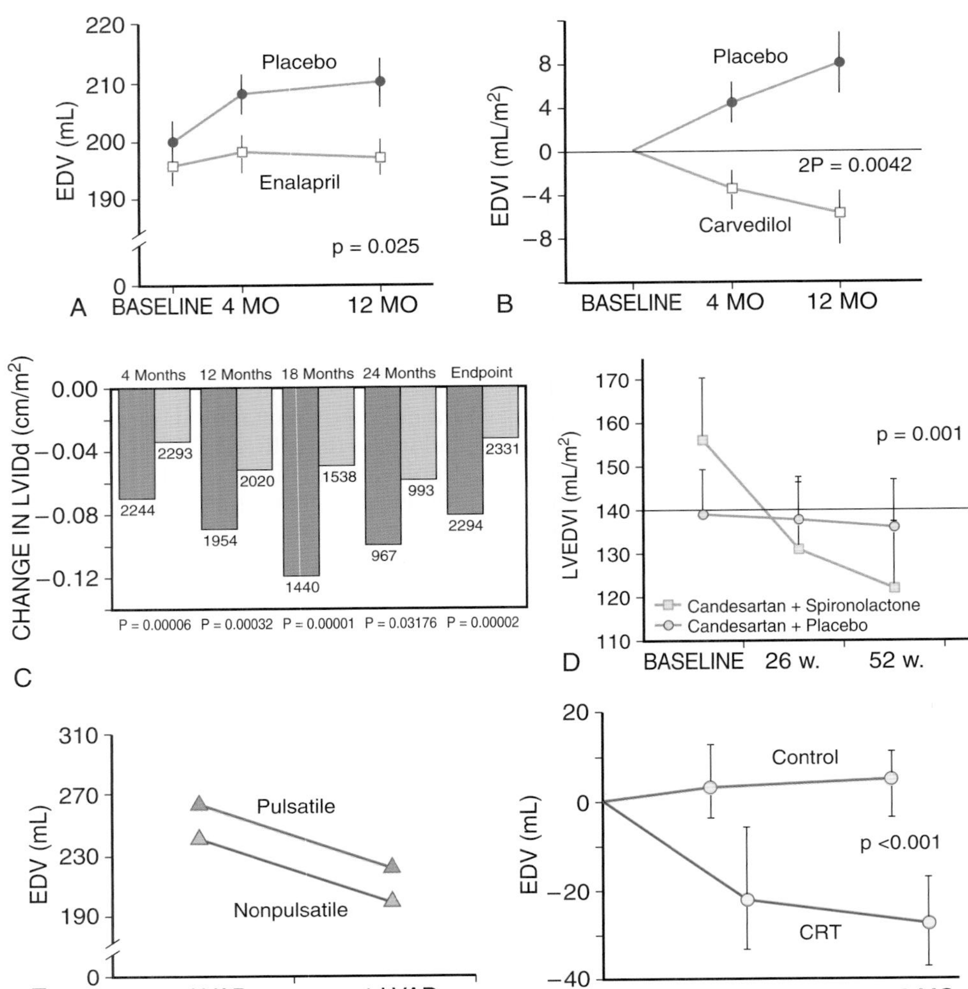

FIGURE 11-12 Reverse cardiac remodeling following pharmacologic and device therapies in patients with heart failure. **A,** Changes in LV end-diastolic volume in the placebo and enalapril-treated patients in SOLVD compared to the placebo. **B,** Changes in LV volume index from baseline during the 12-month follow-up period in the ANZ trial compared to the placebo. **C,** Changes in LV end-diastolic dimension in patients treated with valsartan added to an ACE inhibitor and/or β-blocker significantly resulted in decreased LV internal diastolic diameter (normalized to body surface area [BSA]). **D,** Changes in LV volume index in patients treated with spironolactone and candesartan compared to candesartan alone. **E,** Changes in LV end-diastolic volume in pulsatile versus continuous flow LVADs. **F,** Change in LVEDV at 3 and 6 months after CRT compared to the control group in the MIRACLE trial. ***A-F*** *modified, respectively, from Greenberg B, Quinones MA, Koilpillai C, et al: Circulation 91:2573–2581, 1995; Doughty RN, Whalley GA, Gamble G, et al: Left ventricular remodeling with carvedilol in patients with congestive heart failure due to ischemic heart disease. J Am Coll Cardiol 29:1060–1066, 1998; Wong M, Staszewsky L, Latini R, et al: Valsartan benefits left ventricular structure and function in heart failure: Val-HeFT echocardiographic study. J Am Coll Cardiol 40:970–975, 2002; Chan AK, Sanderson JE, Wang T, et al: Aldosterone receptor antagonism induces reverse remodeling when added to angiotensin receptor blockade in chronic heart failure. J Am Coll Cardiol 50:591–596, 2007; Klotz S, Deng MC, Stypmann J, et al: Left ventricular pressure and volume unloading during pulsatile versus nonpulsatile left ventricular assist device support. Ann Thorac Surg 77:143–149, 2004; and St John Sutton MG, Plappert T, Abraham WT, et al: Effect of cardiac resynchronization therapy on left ventricular size and function in chronic heart failure. Circulation 107:1985–1990, 2003.*

sustained at 3 years in patients with and without concomitant mitral valve surgery.[104]

In addition to the drugs and devices discussed above, a variety of surgical techniques have been introduced to reverse the maladaptive ventricular remodeling in patients with heart failure. As discussed in **Chapter 18**, myocardial revascularization should be considered in patients with evidence of myocardial viability and depressed LV dysfunction. Clinical studies have demonstrated an increase in EF and decrease in left ventricular volume indices in patients with ischemic cardiomyopathy following coronary artery bypass surgery.[105,106] Partial left ventriculectomy, which was a technique developed by Batista in the early 1990s, involves surgical removal of part of the LV to reduce LV volumes. Although an interesting hypothesis, studies ultimately found this technique was ineffective,[107] suggesting that changes in volume alone are not sufficient to allow the heart to recover. One additional explanation that has been provided for the lack of efficacy or partial ventriculectomy is that acute reductions in LV mass are accompanied by unfavorable changes in the diastolic properties of the ventricle, which in turn negatively affects the Frank-Starling relationship (**Figure 11-13B**).[108] Surgical ventricular reconstruction (SVR) of the left ventricle is a specific surgical procedure that was developed for the treatment of LV dysfunction in patients with large akinetic areas of nonviable myocardium secondary to coronary artery disease (**see Chapter 41**). Despite encouraging early results in nonrandomized studies, which showed that SVR could improve patient symptoms and reduce end-diastolic volumes,[109] the NIH-sponsored STICH trial (Surgical Treatment for Ischemic Heart failure) that compared coronary artery bypass grafting (CABG) to CABG with SVR failed to show an improvement in patient symptoms or exercise tolerance or a reduction in the rate of

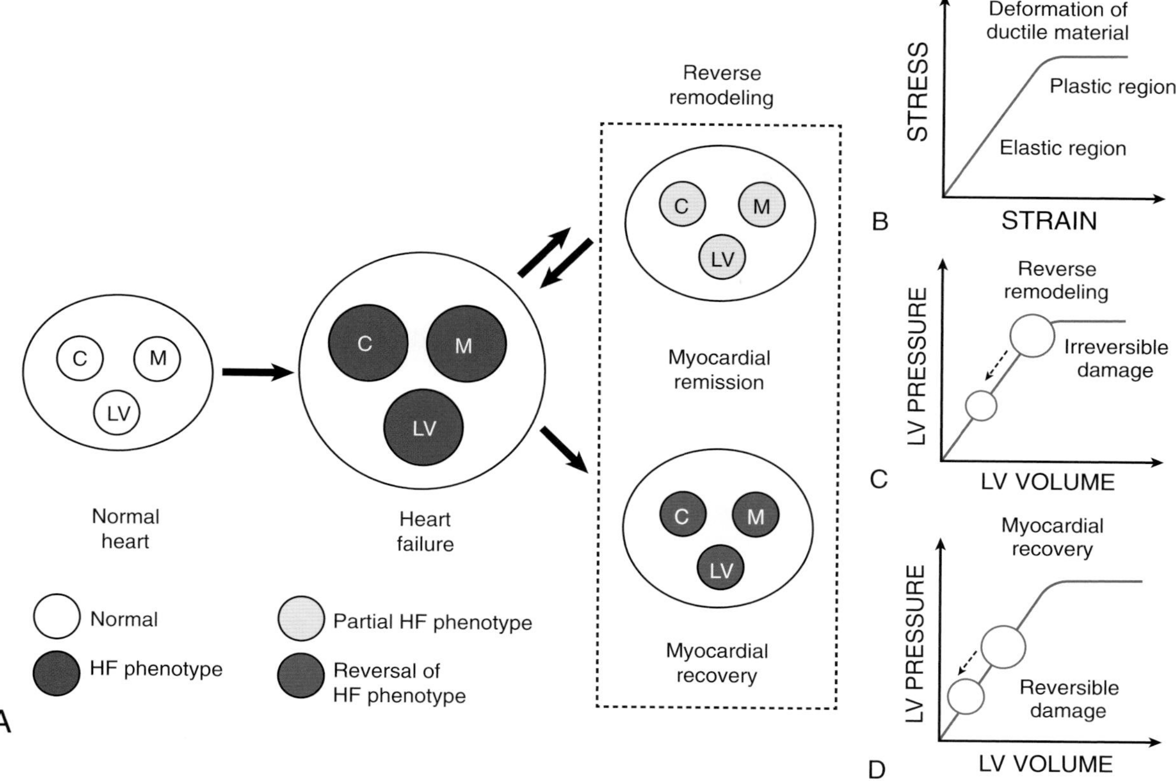

FIGURE 11-13 Myocardial recovery and remission. **A,** Cardiac remodeling arises secondary to abnormalities that arise in the biology of the cardiac myocyte (C), the myocardium (cardiocytes and extracellular matrix [M]), as well as LV geometry (LV), which have collectively been referred to as the *heart failure phenotype*. During reverse remodeling there is a reversal of the abnormalities in the cardiac myocyte, as well as the extracellular matrix, leading to a reversal of the abnormalities in LV geometry. Reverse remodeling can lead to two clinical outcomes (1) myocardial recovery, characterized by freedom from future cardiac events, or (2) myocardial remission, which is characterized by recurrence of heart failure events. **B,** Diagram of a stress-strain curve of a ductile material, illustrating the relationship between an applied force (stress) and deformation (strain). Deformation can lead to reversible changes in a material (elastic deformation) if the properties of the material are not changed, and irreversible changes in a material (plastic deformation). **C,** Hypothetical model of reverse remodeling in heart that has undergone irreversible damage (plastic deformation). **D,** Hypothetical model of reverse remodeling with recovery in heart that has undergone reversible damage (elastic deformation). *Modified from Mann DL, Barger PM, Burkhoff D: Myocardial recovery: myth, magic or molecular target? J Amer Coll Cardiol 60:2465–2472, 2012.*

death or hospitalization for cardiac causes.[106] Various explanations have been provided for the failure of SVR to improve clinical outcomes in STICH, including inappropriate patient selection, lack of a standardized surgical approach, as well as decreased diastolic distensibility from undersizing the LV. Correction of functional mitral regurgitation in patients with ischemic cardiomyopathy was first described by Bolling and colleagues to treat the functional regurgitation that develops in patients with heart failure (Chapter 41). Subsequent studies by this group demonstrated that there were improvements in LV volumes, EF, and sphericity index as assessed over 1 year by echocardiography.[110] And indeed, similar findings were observed in the Acorn trial.[111] However, although mitral valve repair is technically feasible, and has been associated with improved patient quality of life, long-term outcomes have not been shown to confer a mortality benefit for mitral valve annuloplasty as a primary treatment for patients with LV dysfunction.[112]

MYOCARDIAL RECOVERY

Clinical studies have shown that reverse LV remodeling is associated with stabilization of the clinical syndrome of heart failure, and that some patients remain free from future heart failure events, whereas other patients develop recurrent heart failure events over time. Based on the disparate clinical outcomes of reverse remodeling, it has been suggested that the term *myocardial recovery* should be used to describe the normalization of the molecular, cellular, myocardial, and LV geometric changes that are associated with freedom from future heart failure events, whereas the term *myocardial remission* should be used to refer to the normalization of the molecular, cellular, myocardial, and LV geometric changes that provoke cardiac remodeling that are insufficient to prevent the recurrence of heart failure in the face of normal and/or perturbed hemodynamic loading conditions (see Figure 11-13A).[113]

Although the biologic differences between myocardial recovery and myocardial remission are not known, it bears emphasis that in most instances reverse LV remodeling does not lead to a "normal" heart, despite reversal of many aspects of the heart failure phenotype. First, gene expression profiling studies have shown that only approximately 5% of genes that are dysregulated in failing hearts revert back to normal following LVAD support, despite typical morphologic and functional responses to LVAD support.[38,41,114] Second, although maximal calcium-saturated force generation is improved in myocytes following LVAD support, force generation is still less than in myocytes from nonfailing controls, despite reversal of cardiac myocyte hypertrophy.[33] Third, as noted previously, the majority of studies that have examined changes in the ECM following LVAD have suggested that the ECM does not revert to normal on its own and can actually be characterized by increased

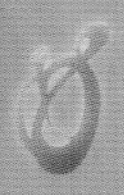

myocardial fibrosis. Moreover, our current understanding of changes in the ECM during LVAD support have focused on ECM content and not on the more fundamental issues of its three-dimensional organization or with the interactions between the collagen matrix and the resident cardiac myocytes, which are likely to be critically important. Fourth, although the LV EDPVRs of LVAD-supported hearts are shifted leftward, and overlap those found in nonfailing ventricles, the ratio of LV wall thickness-to-LV wall radius does not return to normal despite normalization of LV chamber geometry.[115] Rather, this r/h ratio remains elevated at nearly twice normal. This has important implications for LV function, insofar as LV wall stress depends critically on this ratio (Laplace's Law). Given that end-diastolic wall stress represents the load on the cardiac myocyte at the onset of systole, the observation that the r/h ratio is not normalized despite the normalization of LV global chamber properties suggests that the cardiac myocytes in reverse-remodeled ventricles are still exposed to increased physiologic stresses. Whether this represents loss of functioning cardiac myocytes, or failure of the three-dimensional organization of the ECM to revert to normal, is unknown. Thus normalization of the heart failure phenotype during reverse LV remodeling does not necessarily signify that the cellular/molecular biology and physiology of these hearts actually becomes normal, which may explain why reverse remodeling does not invariably lead to freedom from future heart failure events.

Although the potential biologic differences between myocardial recovery and myocardial remission are not known, there are parallels in mechanical engineering science that may help to illuminate potential important differences, as well as to frame future mechanistic discussions. In mechanics, deformation of a material refers to the change in the shape or size of an object due to an applied force. Figure 11-13B shows a representative one-dimensional stress versus strain diagram of a material that is exposed to an increased load. With increasing stress, there is an increase in the length of the material, up until the point when no further changes in length are possible without the material breaking. Importantly, if the material returns to its original state when the load is removed, this is referred to as *elastic deformation*. In contrast, if during the application of stress the mechanical properties of the material are changed irreversibly, such that the object will return only part way to its original shape when the stress is removed, this is referred to as *plastic deformation*. It is sometimes the case that elastic deformation occurs under a certain level of stress and plastic deformation occurs when that stress level is exceeded. Regardless, the important distinction is whether or not the material returns to its original state when the stress is removed. Although precise parallels between cardiac remodeling in heart failure and deformation of solid materials following loading are not appropriate, there could be a parallel between reverse remodeling and plastic deformation, inasmuch as the reverse remodeled heart does not revert completely to normal after cessation of hemodynamic overloading (see Figure 11-13C). Although speculative, it is possible that myocardial recovery is more analogous to elastic deformation in that the recovered heart reverts back to normal after hemodynamic overloading is removed (see Figure 11-13D). Thus, reverse LV remodeling represents a reversal of the heart failure phenotype that occurs in hearts that have undergone irreversible damage, whereas myocardial recovery represents a reversal of the heart failure phenotype that occurs in hearts that have undergone reversible damage (see Figure 11-13C). Although the biologic motifs that separate reversible (elastic) from irreversible (plastic) changes in the heart are not known, it is likely that the progressive loss of cardiac myocytes, as well as the progressive erosion of the native three-dimensional organization of the ECM surrounding the cardiac myocytes will be critical determinants that distinguish between reverse remodeling and myocardial recovery.[4,116] The observation that the great majority of clinical examples of myocardial recovery in the literature occur after transient injury (e.g., viral infection, inflammation, toxic injury) rather than longer standing and/or permanent injury (e.g., myocardial infarction, genetic abnormalities) is consistent with the point of view that the ability of the heart to "recover" is related to the nature of the inciting injury, as well as the extent of underlying myocardial damage that occurs during the resolution of cardiac injury. It is also possible that there are unique biologic changes (e.g., integrin signaling and β-adrenergic signaling) that are associated with myocardial recovery that are not observed in myocardial remission.[117]

SUMMARY AND FUTURE DIRECTIONS

As discussed herein, the failing heart undergoes a number of maladaptive changes in LV structure and function that contribute to disease progression in the clinical syndrome of heart failure. Numerous clinical and epidemiologic studies have also suggested that heart failure is potentially reversible, and that the heart is capable of undergoing favorable reversal of the changes in LV structure and function that are associated with stabilization of the clinical syndrome of heart failure. Although the various components of reverse remodeling have been carefully studied and annotated, it is unclear at present exactly how these changes contribute to restoration of normal LV structure and function. That is, we simply do not understand what the essential biologic "drivers" of myocardial recovery are, nor do we understand how they are coordinated. More importantly, we do not understand why reverse LV remodeling is sometimes associated with freedom from recurrent heart failure events (i.e., myocardial recovery) and why reverse remodeling is sometimes associated with recurrence of heart failure events at a future point in time.[4,116] Indeed, the extant literature does not suggest which of the myriad of changes that occur during reversal of the heart failure phenotype are most important and/or necessary to preserve LV structure and function in the long term. The extant literature suggests that reverse remodeling represents a multilevel (molecular, cellular, anatomic) reversion toward a normal myocardial phenotype and that this reversion of phenotype is accompanied by two different outcomes: namely, myocardial recovery and myocardial remission. Although the reasons for these different outcomes is not at all clear at the time of this writing, one potentially attractive hypothesis is that myocardial remission represents reversal of the heart failure phenotype superimposed upon hearts that have undergone irreversible damage (plastic deformation), whereas myocardial recovery represents reversal of the heart failure phenotype superimposed upon hearts that have not sustained irreversible damage (elastic deformation). Although hypothetical, this formalism can be validated experimentally and clinically, and permits certain predictions with respect to identifying "responders" and

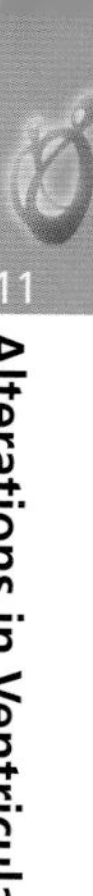

"nonresponders" to medical and device therapies. The quest for elucidating the answers to these questions extends well beyond simple intellectual curiosity about the biology of heart failure, or even selecting the appropriate patients for clinical trials. Indeed, the answer is to provide new heart failure therapies that directly target the phylogenetically conserved pathways that have evolved to repair the myocardium, rather than continuing to target signaling pathways that attenuate remodeling. Given our current lack of understanding about the biology of reverse LV remodeling and the disparate outcomes of remodeling, it is likely that the learning curve will be extremely steep for the foreseeable future.

References

1. Kass DA, Baughman KL, Pak PH, et al: Reverse remodeling from cardiomyoplasty in human heart failure. External constraint versus active assist. *Circulation* 91:2314–2318, 1995.
2. Levin HR, Oz MC, Chen JM, et al: Reversal of chronic ventricular dilation in patients with end-stage cardiomyopathy by prolonged mechanical unloading. *Circulation* 91:2717–2720, 1995.
3. Westaby S, Jin XY, Katsumata T, et al: Mechanical support in dilated cardiomyopathy: signs of early left ventricular recovery. *Ann Thorac Surg* 64:1303–1308, 1997.
4. Mann DL: Mechanisms and models in heart failure: a combinatorial approach. *Circulation* 100:999–1088, 1999.
5. Cohn JN, Ferrari R, Sharpe N: Cardiac remodeling—concepts and clinical implications: a consensus paper from an international forum on cardiac remodeling. Behalf of an International Forum on Cardiac Remodeling. *J Am Coll Cardiol* 35:569–582, 2000.
6. Toischer K, Rokita AG, Unsold B, et al: Differential cardiac remodeling in preload versus afterload. *Circulation* 122:993–1003, 2010.
7. Lowes BD, Minobe W, Abraham WT, et al: Changes in gene expression in the intact human heart. Downregulation of α-myosin heavy chain in hypertrophied, failing ventricular myocardium. *J Clin Invest* 100:2315–2324, 1997.
8. Schaper J, Froede R, Hein ST, et al: Impairment of the myocardial ultrastructure and changes of the cytoskeleton in dilated cardiomyopathy. *Circulation* 83:504–514, 1991.
9. Davies CH, Davia K, Bennett JG, et al: Reduced contraction and altered frequency response of isolated ventricular myocytes from patients with heart failure. *Circulation* 92:2540–2549, 1995.
10. Shafiq MM, Miller AB: Blocking aldosterone in heart failure. *Ther Adv Cardiovasc Dis* 3:379–385, 2009.
11. Hudlicka O, Brown M, Egginton S: Angiogenesis in skeletal and cardiac muscle. *Physiol Rev* 72:369–417, 1992.
12. Karch R, Neumann F, Ullrich R, et al: The spatial pattern of coronary capillaries in patients with dilated, ischemic, or inflammatory cardiomyopathy. *Cardiovasc Pathol* 14:135–144, 2005.
13. Abraham D, Hofbauer R, Schafer R, et al: Selective downregulation of VEGF-A(165), VEGF-R(1), and decreased capillary density in patients with dilative but not ischemic cardiomyopathy. *Circ Res* 87:644–647, 2000.
14. Roche JA, Lovering RM, Bloch RJ: Impaired recovery of dysferlin-null skeletal muscle after contraction-induced injury in vivo. *Neuroreport* 19:1579–1584, 2008.
15. Cohn JN: Structural basis for heart failure: ventricular remodeling and its pharmacological inhibition. *Circulation* 91:2504–2507, 1995.
16. Douglas PS, Morrow R, Ioli A, et al: Left ventricular shape, afterload, and survival in idiopathic dilated cardiomyopathy. *J Am Coll Cardiol* 13:311–315, 1989.
17. Vasan RS, Larson MG, Benjamin EJ, et al: Left ventricular dilation and the risk of congestive heart failure in people without myocardial infarction. *N Engl J Med* 336:1350–1355, 1997.
18. White HD, Norris RM, Brown MA, et al: Left ventricular end-systolic volume as the major determinant of survival after recovery from myocardial infarction. *Circulation* 76:44–51, 1987.
19. St John Sutton MG, Pfeffer MA, Plappert T, et al: Quantitative two-dimensional echocardiographic measurements are major predictors of adverse cardiovascular events after acute myocardial infarction. The protective effects of captopril. *Circulation* 89:68–75, 1994.
20. Ho KK, Pinsky JL, Kannel WB, et al: The epidemiology of heart failure: the Framingham Study. *J Am Coll Cardiol* 22:A6–A13, 1993.
21. Hellawell JL, Margulies KB: Myocardial reverse remodeling. *Cardiovasc Ther* 20:172–181, 2012.
22. Kramer DG, Trikalinos TA, Kent DM, et al: Quantitative evaluation of drug or device effects on ventricular remodeling as predictors of therapeutic effects on mortality in patients with heart failure and reduced ejection fraction: a meta-analytic approach. *J Am Coll Cardiol* 56:392–406, 2010.
23. Givertz MM, Mann DL: Epidemiology and natural history of recovery of left ventricular function in recent onset dilated cardiomyopathies. *Curr Heart Fail Rep* 10:321–330, 2013.
24. Zafeiridis A, Jeevanandam V, Houser SR, et al: Regression of cellular hypertrophy after left ventricular assist device support. *Circulation* 98:656–662, 1998.
25. Baba HA, Grabellus F, August C, et al: Reversal of metallothionein expression is different throughout the human myocardium after prolonged left-ventricular mechanical support. *J Heart Lung Transplant* 19:668–674, 2000.
26. Madigan JD, Barbone A, Choudhri AF, et al: Time course of reverse remodeling of the left ventricle during support with a left ventricular assist device. *J Thorac Cardiovasc Surg* 121:902–908, 2001.
27. Bruckner BA, Stetson SJ, Perez-Verdia A, et al: Regression of fibrosis and hypertrophy in failing myocardium following mechanical circulatory support. *J Heart Lung Transplant* 20:457–464, 2001.
28. Rivello HG, Meckert PC, Vigliano C, et al: Cardiac myocyte nuclear size and ploidy status decrease after mechanical support. *Cardiovasc Pathol* 10:53–57, 2001.
29. Razeghi P, Bruckner BA, Sharma S, et al: Mechanical unloading of the failing human heart fails to activate the protein kinase B/Akt/glycogen synthase kinase-3beta survival pathway. *Cardiology* 100:17–22, 2003.
30. Wang J, Oliveira G, Koerner MM, et al: Cardiac resynchronization therapy induces cellular reverse remodelling in failing human hearts. *Circulation* 114(Suppl II):718, 2006.
31. Butter C, Rastogi S, Minden HH, et al: Cardiac contractility modulation electrical signals improve myocardial gene expression in patients with heart failure. *J Am Coll Cardiol* 51:1784–1789, 2008.
32. Imai M, Rastogi S, Gupta RC, et al: Therapy with cardiac contractility modulation electrical signals improves left ventricular function and remodeling in dogs with chronic heart failure. *J Am Coll Cardiol* 49:2120–2128, 2007.
33. Ambardekar AV, Buttrick PM: Reverse remodeling with left ventricular assist devices: a review of clinical, cellular, and molecular effects. *Circ Heart Fail* 4:224–233, 2011.
34. Brooks WW, Bing OH, Conrad CH, et al: Captopril modifies gene expression in hypertrophied and failing hearts of aged spontaneously hypertensive rats. *Hypertension* 30:1362–1368, 1997.
35. Wang J, Guo X, Dhalla NS: Modification of myosin protein and gene expression in failing hearts due to myocardial infarction by enalapril or losartan. *Biochim Biophys Acta* 1690:177–184, 2004.
36. Lowes BD, Gilbert EM, Abraham WT, et al: Myocardial gene expression in dilated cardiomyopathy treated with beta-blocking agents. *N Engl J Med* 346:1357–1365, 2002.
37. Blaxall BC, Tschannen-Moran BM, Milano CA, et al: Differential gene expression and genomic patient stratification following left ventricular assist device support. *J Am Coll Cardiol* 41:1096–1106, 2003.
38. Rodrigue-Way A, Burkhoff D, Geesaman BJ, et al: Sarcomeric genes involved in reverse remodeling of the heart during left ventricular assist device support. *J Heart Lung Transplant* 24:73–80, 2005.
39. Latif N, Yacoub MH, George R, et al: Changes in sarcomeric and non-sarcomeric cytoskeletal proteins and focal adhesion molecules during clinical myocardial recovery after left ventricular assist device support. *J Heart Lung Transplant* 26:230–235, 2007.
40. Kuhn M, Voss M, Mitko D, et al: Left ventricular assist device support reverses altered cardiac expression and function of natriuretic peptides and receptors in end-stage heart failure. *Cardiovasc Res* 64:308–314, 2004.
41. Yang KC, Yamada KA, Patel AY, et al: Deep RNA sequencing reveals dynamic regulation of myocardial noncoding RNA in failing human heart and remodeling with mechanical circulatory support. *Circulation* 129:1009–1021, 2014.
42. Iyengar S, Haas G, Lamba S, et al: Effect of cardiac resynchronization therapy on myocardial gene expression in patients with nonischemic dilated cardiomyopathy. *J Card Fail* 13:304–311, 2007.
43. Vanderheyden M, Mullens W, Delrue L, et al: Myocardial gene expression in heart failure patients treated with cardiac resynchronization therapy responders versus nonresponders. *J Am Coll Cardiol* 51:129–136, 2008.
44. Rastogi S, Mishra S, Gupta RC, et al: Reversal of maladaptive gene program in left ventricular myocardium of dogs with heart failure following long-term therapy with the Acorn Cardiac Support Device. *Heart Fail Rev* 10:157–163, 2005.
45. Bristow MR, Ginsburg R, Minobe W, et al: Decreased catecholamine sensitivity and β-adrenergic-receptor density in failing human hearts. *N Engl J Med* 307:205–211, 1982.
46. Gilbert EM, Abraham WT, Olsen S, et al: Comparative hemodynamic, left ventricular functional, and antiadrenergic effects of chronic treatment with metoprolol versus carvedilol in the failing heart. *Circulation* 94:2817–2825, 1996.
47. Gilbert EM, Sandoval A, Larrabee P, et al: Lisinopril lowers cardiac adrenergic drive and increases beta-receptor density in the failing human heart. *Circulation* 88:472–480, 1993.
48. Ogletree-Hughes ML, Stull LB, Sweet WE, et al: Mechanical unloading restores beta-adrenergic responsiveness and reverses receptor downregulation in the failing human heart. *Circulation* 104:881–886, 2001.
49. Schnee PM, Shah N, Bergheim M, et al: Location and density of alpha- and beta-adrenoreceptor sub-types in myocardium after mechanical left ventricular unloading. *J Heart Lung Transplant* 27:710–717, 2008.
50. Klotz S, Barbone A, Reiken S, et al: Left ventricular assist device support normalizes left and right ventricular beta-adrenergic pathway properties. *J Am Coll Cardiol* 45:668–676, 2005.
51. Hata JA, Williams ML, Schroder JN, et al: Lymphocyte levels of GRK2 (betaARK1) mirror changes in the LVAD-supported failing human heart: lower GRK2 associated with improved beta-adrenergic signaling after mechanical unloading. *J Card Fail* 12:360–368, 2006.
52. Mullens W, Bartunek J, Wilson Tang WH, et al: Early and late effects of cardiac resynchronization therapy on force-frequency relation and contractility regulating gene expression in heart failure patients. *Heart Rhythm* 5:52–59, 2008.
53. Saavedra WF, Tunin RS, Paolocci N, et al: Reverse remodeling and enhanced adrenergic reserve from passive external support in experimental dilated heart failure. *J Am Coll Cardiol* 39:2069–2076, 2002.
54. Plank DM, Yatani A, Ritsu H, et al: Calcium dynamics in the failing heart: restoration by beta-adrenergic receptor blockade. *Am J Physiol Heart Circ Physiol* 285:H305–H315, 2003.
55. Kubo H, Margulies KB, Piacentino V, III, et al: Patients with end-stage congestive heart failure treated with beta-adrenergic receptor antagonists have improved ventricular myocyte calcium regulatory protein abundance. *Circulation* 104:1012–1018, 2001.
56. Reiken S, Wehrens XH, Vest JA, et al: Beta-blockers restore calcium release channel function and improve cardiac muscle performance in human heart failure. *Circulation* 107:2459–2466, 2003.
57. Guo X, Chapman D, Dhalla NS: Partial prevention of changes in SR gene expression in congestive heart failure due to myocardial infarction by enalapril or losartan. *Mol Cell Biochem* 254:163–172, 2003.
58. Shao Q, Ren B, Saini HK, et al: Sarcoplasmic reticulum Ca2+ transport and gene expression in congestive heart failure are modified by imidapril treatment. *Am J Physiol Heart Circ Physiol* 288:H1674–H1682, 2005.
59. Soppa GK, Barton PJ, Terracciano CM, et al: Left ventricular assist device-induced molecular changes in the failing myocardium. *Curr Opin Cardiol* 23:206–218, 2008.
60. Chen X, Piacentino V, III, Furukawa S, et al: L-type Ca2+ channel density and regulation are altered in failing human ventricular myocytes and recover after support with mechanical assist devices. *Circ Res* 91:517–524, 2002.
61. Marx SO, Reiken S, Hisamatsu Y, et al: PKA phosphorylation dissociates FKBP12.6 from the calcium release channel (ryanodine receptor): defective regulation in failing hearts. *Cell* 101:365–376, 2000.
62. Heerdt PM, Holmes JW, Cai B, et al: Chronic unloading by left ventricular assist device reverses contractile dysfunction and alters gene expression in end-stage heart failure. *Circulation* 102:2713–2719, 2000.
63. Sabbah HN, Sharov VG, Gupta RC, et al: Reversal of chronic molecular and cellular abnormalities due to heart failure by passive mechanical ventricular containment. *Circ Res* 93:1095–1101, 2003.
64. Vatta M, Stetson SJ, Perez-Verdia A, et al: Molecular remodelling of dystrophin in patients with end-stage cardiomyopathies and reversal in patients on assistance-device therapy. *Lancet* 359:936–941, 2002.
65. Vatta M, Stetson SJ, Jimenez S, et al: Molecular normalization of dystrophin in the failing left and right ventricle of patients treated with either pulsatile or continuous flow-type ventricular assist devices. *J Am Coll Cardiol* 43:811–817, 2004.
66. de Jonge N, van Wichen DF, Schipper ME, et al: Left ventricular assist device in end-stage heart failure: persistence of structural myocyte damage after unloading. An immunohistochemical analysis of the contractile myofilaments. *J Am Coll Cardiol* 39:963–969, 2002.
67. Aquila LA, McCarthy PM, Smedira NG, et al: Cytoskeletal structure and recovery in single human cardiac myocytes. *J Heart Lung Transplant* 23:954–963, 2004.

68. Birks EJ, Hall JL, Barton PJ, et al: Gene profiling changes in cytoskeletal proteins during clinical recovery after left ventricular-assist device support. *Circulation* 112:I57–I64, 2005.
69. Morita H, Suzuki G, Mishima T, et al: Effects of long-term monotherapy with metoprolol CR/XL on the progression of left ventricular dysfunction and remodeling in dogs with chronic heart failure. *Cardiovasc Drugs Ther* 16:443–449, 2002.
70. Shigeyama J, Yasumura Y, Sakamoto A, et al: Increased gene expression of collagen Types I and III is inhibited by beta-receptor blockade in patients with dilated cardiomyopathy. *Eur Heart J* 26:2698–2705, 2005.
71. Milanez MC, Gomes MG, Vassallo DV, et al: Effects of captopril on interstitial collagen in the myocardium after infarction in rats. *J Card Fail* 3:189–197, 1997.
72. Liu YH, Yang XP, Sharov VG, et al: Effects of angiotensin-converting enzyme inhibitors and angiotensin II type 1 receptor antagonists in rats with heart failure. Role of kinins and angiotensin II type 2 receptors. *J Clin Invest* 99:1926–1935, 1997.
73. Mukherjee D, Sen S: Alteration of collagen phenotypes in ischemic cardiomyopathy. *J Clin Invest* 88:1141–1146, 1991.
74. Suzuki G, Morita H, Mishima T, et al: Effects of long-term monotherapy with eplerenone, a novel aldosterone blocker, on progression of left ventricular dysfunction and remodeling in dogs with heart failure. *Circulation* 106:2967–2972, 2002.
75. Rastogi S, Mishra S, Zaca V, et al: Effect of long-term monotherapy with the aldosterone receptor blocker eplerenone on cytoskeletal proteins and matrix metalloproteinases in dogs with heart failure. *Cardiovasc Drugs Ther* 21:415–422, 2007.
76. McCarthy PM, Nakatani S, Vargo R, et al: Structural and left ventricular histologic changes after implantable LVAD insertion. *Ann Thorac Surg* 59:609–613, 1995.
77. Li YY, Feng Y, McTiernan CF, et al: Downregulation of matrix metalloproteinases and reduction in collagen damage in the failing human heart after support with left ventricular assist devices. *Circulation* 104:1147–1152, 2001.
78. Klotz S, Foronjy RF, Dickstein ML, et al: Mechanical unloading during left ventricular assist device support increases left ventricular collagen cross-linking and myocardial stiffness. *Circulation* 112:364–374, 2005.
79. Matsumiya G, Monta O, Fukushima N, et al: Who would be a candidate for bridge to recovery during prolonged mechanical left ventricular support in idiopathic dilated cardiomyopathy? *J Thorac Cardiovasc Surg* 130:699–704, 2005.
80. Bruggink AH, van Oosterhout MF, de Jonge N, et al: Reverse remodeling of the myocardial extracellular matrix after prolonged left ventricular assist device support follows a biphasic pattern. *J Heart Lung Transplant* 25:1091–1098, 2006.
81. Bruckner BA, Stetson SJ, Farmer JA, et al: The implications for cardiac recovery of left ventricular assist device support on myocardial collagen content. *Am J Surg* 180:498–501, 2000.
82. Thohan V, Stetson SJ, Nagueh SF, et al: Cellular and hemodynamics responses of failing myocardium to continuous flow mechanical circulatory support using the DeBakey-Noon left ventricular assist device: a comparative analysis with pulsatile-type devices. *J Heart Lung Transplant* 24:566–575, 2005.
83. Klotz S, Burkhoff D, Garrelds IM, et al: The impact of left ventricular assist device-induced left ventricular unloading on the myocardial renin-angiotensin-aldosterone system: therapeutic consequences? *Eur Heart J* 30:805–812, 2009.
84. Klotz S, Danser AH, Foronjy RF, et al: The impact of angiotensin-converting enzyme inhibitor therapy on the extracellular collagen matrix during left ventricular assist device support in patients with end-stage heart failure. *J Am Coll Cardiol* 49:1166–1174, 2007.
85. D'Ascia C, Cittadini A, Monti MG, et al: Effects of biventricular pacing on interstitial remodelling, tumor necrosis factor-alpha expression, and apoptotic death in failing human myocardium. *Eur Heart J* 27:201–206, 2006.
86. Hessel MH, Bleeker GB, Bax JJ, et al: Reverse ventricular remodelling after cardiac resynchronization therapy is associated with a reduction in serum tenascin-C and plasma matrix metalloproteinase-9 levels. *Eur J Heart Fail* 9:1058–1063, 2007.
87. Hara Y, Inoue K, Ogimoto A, et al: Effect of beta-blocker therapy on myocardial perfusion defects in thallium-201 scintigraphy in patients with dilated cardiomyopathy. *Cardiology* 104:16–21, 2005.
88. Akinboboye OO, Chou RL, Bergmann SR: Augmentation of myocardial blood flow in hypertensive heart disease by angiotensin antagonists: a comparison of lisinopril and losartan. *J Am Coll Cardiol* 40:703–709, 2002.
89. de Boer RA, Siebelink HJ, Tio RA, et al: Carvedilol increases plasma vascular endothelial growth factor (VEGF) in patients with chronic heart failure. *Eur J Heart Fail* 3:331–333, 2001.
90. Hall JL, Grindle S, Han X, et al: Genomic profiling of the human heart before and after mechanical support with a ventricular assist device reveals alterations in vascular signaling networks. *Physiol Genomics* 17:283–291, 2004.
91. Knaapen P, van Campen LM, de Cock CC, et al: Effects of cardiac resynchronization therapy on myocardial perfusion reserve. *Circulation* 110:646–651, 2004.
92. Greenberg B, Quinones MA, Koilpillai C, et al: Effects of long-term enalapril therapy on cardiac structure and function in patients with left ventricular dysfunction: results of the SOLVD echocardiography substudy. *Circulation* 91:2573–2581, 1995.
93. Doughty RN, Whalley GA, Gamble G, et al: Left ventricular remodeling with carvedilol in patients with congestive heart failure due to ischemic heart disease. *J Am Coll Cardiol* 29:1060–1066, 1998.
94. Wong M, Staszewsky L, Latini R, et al: Valsartan benefits left ventricular structure and function in heart failure: Val-HeFT echocardiographic study. *J Am Coll Cardiol* 40:970–975, 2002.
95. Chan AK, Sanderson JE, Wang T, et al: Aldosterone receptor antagonism induces reverse remodeling when added to angiotensin receptor blockade in chronic heart failure. *J Am Coll Cardiol* 50:591–596, 2007.
96. Klotz S, Deng MC, Stypmann J, et al: Left ventricular pressure and volume unloading during pulsatile versus nonpulsatile left ventricular assist device support. *Ann Thorac Surg* 77:143–149, 2004.
97. Garcia S, Kandar F, Boyle A, et al: Effects of pulsatile- and continuous-flow left ventricular assist devices on left ventricular unloading. *J Heart Lung Transplant* 27:261–267, 2008.
98. Mancini DM, Beniaminovitz A, Levin H, et al: Low incidence of myocardial recovery after left ventricular assist device implantation in patients with chronic heart failure. *Circulation* 98:2383–2389, 1998.
99. Maybaum S, Mancini D, Xydas S, et al: Cardiac improvement during mechanical circulatory support: a prospective multicenter study of the LVAD Working Group. *Circulation* 115:2497–2505, 2007.
100. St John Sutton MG, Plappert T, Abraham WT, et al: Effect of cardiac resynchronization therapy on left ventricular size and function in chronic heart failure. *Circulation* 107:1985–1990, 2003.
101. Naismith JH, Devine TQ, Brandhuber BJ, et al: Crystallographic evidence for dimerization of unliganded tumor necrosis factor receptor. *J Biol Chem* 270:13303–13307, 1995.
102. Linde C, Leclercq C, Rex S, et al: Long-term benefits of biventricular pacing in congestive heart failure: results from the MUltisite STimulation in cardiomyopathy (MUSTIC) study. *J Am Coll Cardiol* 40:111–118, 2002.
103. Mann DL, Acker MA, Jessup M, et al: Clinical evaluation of the CorCap Cardiac Support Device in patients with dilated cardiomyopathy. *Ann Thorac Surg* 84:1226–1235, 2007.
104. Starling RC, Jessup M, Oh JK, et al: Sustained benefits of the CorCap Cardiac Support Device on left ventricular remodeling: three year follow-up results from the Acorn clinical trial. *Ann Thorac Surg* 84:1236–1242, 2007.
105. Bouchart F, Tabley A, Litzler PY, et al: Myocardial revascularization in patients with severe ischemic left ventricular dysfunction. Long term follow-up in 141 patients. *Eur J Cardiothorac Surg* 20:1157–1162, 2001.
106. Jones RH, Velazquez EJ, Michler RE, et al: Coronary bypass surgery with or without surgical ventricular reconstruction. *N Engl J Med* 360:1705–1717, 2009.
107. Starling RC, McCarthy PM, Buda T, et al: Results of partial left ventriculectomy for dilated cardiomyopathy: hemodynamic, clinical and echocardiographic observations. *J Am Coll Cardiol* 36:2098–2103, 2000.
108. Dickstein ML, Spotnitz HM, Rose EA, et al: Heart reduction surgery: an analysis of the impact on cardiac function. *J Thorac Cardiovasc Surg* 113:1032–1040, 1997.
109. Athanasuleas CL, Buckberg GD, Stanley AW, et al: Surgical ventricular restoration in the treatment of congestive heart failure due to post-infarction ventricular dilation. *J Am Coll Cardiol* 44:1439–1445, 2004.
110. Bach DS, Bolling SF: Improvement following correction of secondary mitral regurgitation in end-stage cardiomyopathy with mitral annuloplasty. *Am J Cardiol* 78:966–969, 1996.
111. Acker MA, Bolling S, Shemin R, et al: Mitral valve surgery in heart failure: insights from the Acorn Clinical Trial. *J Thorac Cardiovasc Surg* 132:568–577, 2006.
112. Wu AH, Aaronson KD, Bolling SF, et al: Impact of mitral valve annuloplasty on mortality risk in patients with mitral regurgitation and left ventricular systolic dysfunction. *J Am Coll Cardiol* 45:381–387, 2005.
113. Mann DL, Barger PM, Burkhoff D: Myocardial recovery: myth, magic or molecular target? *J Amer Coll Cardiol* 60:2465–2472, 2012.
114. Margulies KB, Matiwala S, Cornejo C, et al: Mixed messages: transcription patterns in failing and recovering human myocardium. *Circ Res* 96:592–599, 2005.
115. Barbone A, Oz MC, Burkhoff D, et al: Normalized diastolic properties after left ventricular assist result from reverse remodeling of chamber geometry. *Circulation* 104:I229–I232, 2001.
116. Mann DL, Burkhoff D: Myocardial expression levels of micro-ribonucleic acids in patients with left ventricular assist devices signature of myocardial recovery, signature of reverse remodeling, or signature with no name? *J Am Coll Cardiol* 58:2279–2281, 2011.
117. Birks EJ, Tansley PD, Hardy J, et al: Left ventricular assist device and drug therapy for the reversal of heart failure. *N Engl J Med* 355:1873–1884, 2006.

12 Alterations in the Sympathetic and Parasympathetic Nervous Systems in Heart Failure

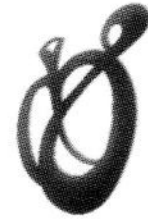

John S. Floras

Of the several identified markers of disease progression and premature mortality in heart failure, disturbances in the adrenergic and vagal regulation of the heart and circulation have received particular attention.[1] Before the prescription of contemporary therapy for heart failure due to left ventricular systolic dysfunction, long-term survival was found to relate inversely to plasma norepinephrine (NE) concentrations, and in a cohort referred for consideration of cardiac transplantation, more specifically to the rate of appearance of NE in the coronary sinus.[2] Diminished tonic and reflex parasympathetic heart rate modulation are also associated with adverse prognosis. However, in many with asymptomatic or mild to moderate symptomatic left ventricular systolic dysfunction plasma NE concentrations and sympathetic nerve firing rates are not elevated.[3,4] These observations raise several questions: (1) what mechanisms account for the presence and variable magnitude of sympathetic activation and parasympathetic withdrawal in heart failure; (2) do these adverse associations between disturbed neurogenic circulatory control and survival reflect causal relationships; and (3) will interventions that inhibit adrenergic activity or augment vagal tone improve outcome?[1]

This chapter primarily summarizes evidence for disturbed autonomic neural regulation of the heart and circulation in human heart failure with reduced left ventricular ejection fraction and mechanisms responsible for this derangement and their relevance to the pathophysiology and contemporary therapy of this relentlessly progressive condition.[1] Heart failure patients with relatively preserved systolic function are less well characterized (**see also Chapter 36**), but the available data also will be reviewed. Reference to animal models will be limited to concepts that have yet to be affirmed in humans.

ASSESSMENT OF SYMPATHETIC AND PARASYMPATHETIC NERVOUS SYSTEM ACTIVITY IN HUMANS

Several distinct yet complementary methods are available for the invasive and noninvasive assessment of specific aspects of sympathetic or parasympathetic function in conscious humans (**Figure 12-1**). Their application has yielded important insights into mechanisms of autonomic dysregulation in heart failure, but none has entered routine clinical practice. Each has specific advantages and limitations in the setting of heart failure.

Catecholamines

Venous plasma NE concentrations relate significantly to outcome in large heart failure trials, but their predictive value for individual patients is low. Measurements obtained at rest provide little indication of the magnitude and duration of sympathetic nerve and adrenal responses to emotional and physical stimuli, such as exercise. These responses are often well differentiated and quite specific to the heart, kidney, or adrenal gland, whereas antecubital venous sampling reflects primarily neurotransmitter release from upstream forearm skeletal muscle. Because of high neuronal and extraneuronal uptake, only a small fraction of NE released from sympathetic vesicles acts on postjunctional adrenoceptors or spills over into plasma. If cardiac output is low, plasma NE concentrations will increase because of reductions in neuronal and extraneuronal clearance. Thus without determining their impact on clearance, the effect of heart failure therapies on neurotransmitter release cannot be deduced with confidence from changes in plasma catecholamine concentrations.[5]

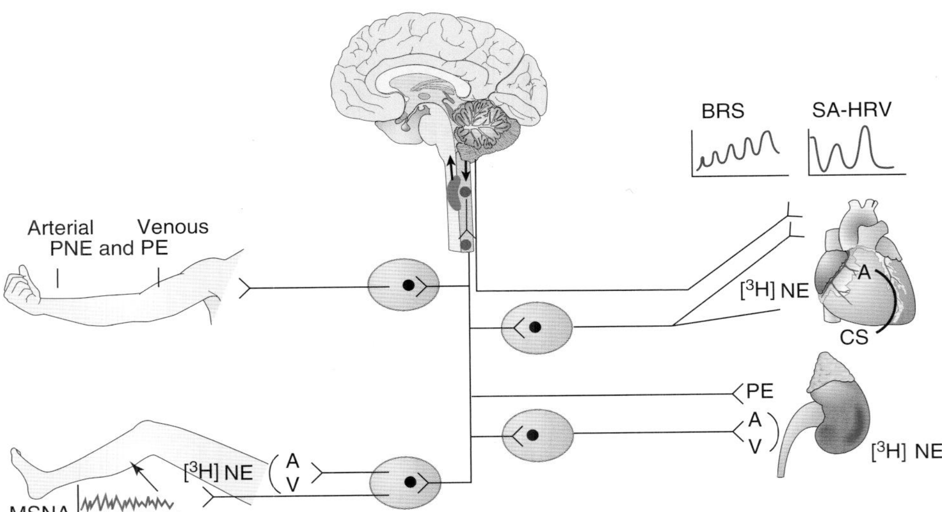

FIGURE 12-1 Assessment of sympathetic and parasympathetic function in humans. Sympathetic function: arterial (A), venous (V), or plasma norepinephrine (PNE) and epinephrine (PE) concentrations *(upper left)*; sympathetic nerve traffic to muscle (MSNA) or skin *(lower left)*; total body norepinephrine ([^{3}H]NE) spillover or regional norepinephrine spillover across the heart (*A*, aorta or arterial; *CS*, coronary sinus) *(upper right)*, kidney *(lower right)*, or leg *(lower left)*; spectral analysis of heart rate variability (SA-HRV) *(upper right)*. Parasympathetic function *(upper right)*: bradycardic response to phenylephrine (baroreflex sensitivity [BRS]) and spectral analysis of heart rate variability (SA-HRV). *From Floras JS: Clinical aspects of sympathetic activation and parasympathetic withdrawal in heart failure. J Am Coll Cardiol 22:72A–84A, 1993, with permission from the American College of Cardiology Foundation.*

The isotopic dilution method overcomes several of these limitations but at increased complexity and cost.[5] Total body NE spillover into plasma is determined from the dilution of tritium-labeled NE during its steady-state infusion in tracer concentrations. If venous effluent from an organ such as the heart, kidney, or brain is collected simultaneously with an arterial sample, the difference in tritium-labeled NE between vein and artery can be used to calculate its local extraction (Extr) by neuronal and extraneuronal transport mechanisms. Organ-specific NE spillover (NES) can then be determined by the equation:

$$NES = [(NEv - NEa) + (NEa \times Extr)] \times PF$$

where NEa and NEv represent arterial and venous concentrations of unlabeled NE, and PF represents plasma flow.

Quantification of norepinephrine metabolites provides additional insight into neuronal and extraneuronal transport. For example, spillover of tritium-labeled dihydroxyphenylglycol (DHPG), the intraneuronal metabolite, provides an index of neuronal NE reuptake and storage.[6,7]

Microneurography

Multifiber or single fiber recording from postganglionic nerves supplying muscular or cutaneous vascular beds provides direct real-time insight into the dynamic nature of sympathetic activity and its reflex control.[8,9] Muscle and skin sympathetic nerves exhibit different discharge characteristics under basal conditions and in response to physical and emotional stimuli. Skin sympathetic nerve activity (SSNA) responds preferentially to noise, touch, or cold and is independent of the cardiac cycle,[10] whereas sympathetic discharge directed at resistance beds in skeletal muscle (MSNA) is entrained by input from arterial and cardiopulmonary mechanoreceptors. MSNA therefore exhibits distinctive pulse-synchronicity, with bursts appearing 1.1 to 1.3 seconds after the preceding R wave of the electrocardiogram.[8] In healthy subjects, MSNA is activated by reductions in diastolic or cardiac filling pressure, exercise, hypoxia, hypercapnia, and arousal from sleep, and is inhibited by lung inflation; a common mechanism appears to influence the strength of resting sympathetic discharge to the heart, kidney, and skeletal muscle. At rest individual values for MSNA correlate with both renal and cardiac NE spillover, and isometric exercise elicits proportionately similar increases in MSNA and cardiac norepinephrine spillover (CNES).[11,12] Such concordance is lost in heart failure.[3]

Baroreflex—Heart Rate Sequences

The arterial baroreflex regulation of heart rate by the parasympathetic and sympathetic nervous systems can be assessed in humans in several ways.[13] Because cardiac cycle length responds much more rapidly to release of acetylcholine than norepinephrine, the normally brisk sinus node response to acute perturbation in blood pressure is mediated primarily by reflex vagal activation or withdrawal. The strength, or gain, of reflex vagal heart rate regulation is determined by quantifying the bradycardic response to a bolus of a vasoconstrictor drug such as phenylephrine or the tachycardic response to nitroprusside- or nitroglycerin-induced hypotension. Longer ("steady-state") infusions of these vasoactive agents evoke competing sympathetic influence. The use of such drugs for this purpose has limitations. Nitrate donors have direct effects on sinoatrial discharge.[14] By causing sustained vasoconstriction or dilation, these drugs distort mechanically baroreceptor nerve endings. Their systemic infusion does not engage specifically the arterial baroreceptor reflex; discharge frequency of mechanoreceptors situated in the atria and pulmonary vasculature also may be altered. Algorithms have been developed to track spontaneous fluctuations in blood pressure and heart rate from continuous noninvasive or invasive recordings, and to identify within these brief sequences concordant changes in systolic blood pressure and the subsequent R–R intervals (inverse of heart rate).[13] Heart rate responses to carotid sinus baroreceptor stimulation by neck suction or unloading by neck pressure have also been studied; aortic arch baroreceptors will elicit counter-regulatory responses to blood pressure changes induced by these maneuvers.

Common to these methods is the construction of a regression equation relating changes in pulse interval (in milliseconds) to changes in systolic blood pressure (in millimeters Hg) of immediately preceding cardiac cycles. The slope of this line estimates the gain of the arterial baroreflex control of heart rate. Values obtained, using the spontaneous sequence method, resemble those derived when blood pressure is altered by bolus administration of vasoactive drugs. Importantly, none of these methods can determine the cause of any impairment of baroreflex sensitivity; responses do not distinguish among altered conduit artery elasticity, changes in the neural transduction of baroreceptor distortion, or altered central processing of afferent input.

Baroreflex—Sympathetic Nerve Sequences

Microneurographic recordings during graded infusions of pressor or vasodilator drugs have been used to evaluate the reflex regulation of central sympathetic outflow.[15] Blood pressure changes induced by such infusions are relatively slow in onset; studies in anesthetized rabbits[16] and conscious humans[17] indicate that the arterial baroreceptors transduce high-frequency oscillations more effectively and at higher gain than low-frequency oscillations.[18] Regression equations synchronizing burst firing to spontaneous changes in diastolic blood pressure also have been used to estimate arterial baroreflex modulation of MSNA.[19]

Heart Rate Variability

Tonic vagal modulation of heart rate may also be estimated by determining its beat-to-beat variation within the time domain (e.g., the standard deviation of all nonectopic pulse intervals occurring within a specified period) or the frequency domain, using spectral analysis, a noninvasive frequency domain method of estimating nonneural and neural (parasympathetic and sympathetic) contributions to short- and long-term oscillations in heart rate.[20]

Algorithms commonly employed to derive power spectra include fast Fourier transformation, autoregression, and coarse-graining spectral analysis (CGSA). Oscillatory autonomic contributions to heart rate variability are superimposed on a broadband nonharmonic fractal signal, most prominent between 0.00003 and 0.1 Hz (i.e., across conventionally defined very low frequencies and extending into the low-frequency spectral range of 0.05 to 0.15 Hz). With CGSA, this nonharmonic power can be quantified by plotting the log of spectral power as a function of the log of frequency (an $1/f^{\beta}$ plot), then extracted, yielding more precise estimates of residual harmonic contributions to low- and high-frequency (0.15 to 0.50 Hz) power.[21] CGSA is therefore particularly useful for studying neural contributions to heart rate variability in heart failure patients, whose harmonic spectral power is both concentrated within the very low- and low-frequency ranges and markedly diminished, relative to the nonharmonic signal.[22]

Because vagal blockade abolishes high-frequency (0.15-0.5 Hz) spectral power, oscillations in heart rate within this band have been attributed to parasympathetic activity, with respiration as its primary rhythmic stimulus. Conversely, because maneuvers known to increase central sympathetic outflow, such as standing, tilt, and exercise, were shown to increase low-frequency (0.05-0.15 Hz) spectral power, whereas decreases were observed during sleep, and after β-blockade or central sympatholysis with clonidine, heart rate fluctuations within this frequency range were initially considered specific representations of sympathetic neural modulation. However, at frequencies below 0.15 Hz, the power spectrum is influenced also by parasympathetic oscillatory input. To address this complexity, the ratio between low- and high-frequency power has been proposed,[20] but not accepted universally, as an estimate of "sympathovagal balance."

Frequency domain analysis should be appreciated primarily for the insight it allows into mechanisms responsible for oscillations in regulatory systems, and for its prognostic value in populations with cardiovascular disease. At best, it provides an estimate of the extent to which parasympathetic and cardiac sympathetic discharge and neurotransmitter release modulate heart rate within these specific frequency bands, but neither the intensity of such neural discharge nor the magnitude of sympathetic outflow directed at the ventricle, kidney, or regional vascular beds.[23]

Cross-Spectral Analysis

Algorithms used to derive power spectra for heart rate can also be applied to blood pressure and respiratory signals. Changes in blood pressure, heart rate, and respiration also reflexively modulate muscle sympathetic nerve discharge. The presence, in normal subjects, of synchronous and concordant changes in low- and high-frequency oscillations in both heart rate and MSNA variability elicited by interventions that raise and lower sympathetic discharge suggest that sympathetic and parasympathetic outflow can be modulated by a shared brainstem mechanism.[24]

Cross-spectral analysis between two variables of interest can be performed to determine their coherence, the influence of input on output power, and the phase delay between these signals.[25] The gain of the transfer function between systolic blood pressure (input) and pulse interval (output) oscillations within the low- or high-frequency regions (α coefficient) is applied as a noninvasive spectral index of the baroreceptor reflex control of heart rate, with the understanding that agreement with values obtained using the vasoactive drug method is weak.[26] The gain of the transfer function between blood pressure (input) and MSNA (output) can be calculated similarly to estimate arterial baroreflex modulation of efferent sympathetic nerve traffic.[25]

Tracer Imaging

Nuclear iodine-123 metaiodobenzylguanidine (^{123}I-MIBG) imaging infers cardiac sympathetic innervation and NE transport and its neural release indirectly from tracer uptake and washout.[27] ^{11}C-metahydroxyephredrine (^{11}C-HED) positron emission tomographic imaging, which has superior spatial resolution, has been applied to assess the homogeneity of left ventricular sympathetic innervation.[28]

SYMPATHETIC ACTIVATION AND PARASYMPATHETIC WITHDRAWAL IN HUMAN HEART FAILURE (see also Chapters 6, 9 and 34)

Heart Failure with Reduced Systolic Function (HFrEF)

Sympathetic Activation

In study cohorts, average plasma NE concentrations, sampled at rest, are elevated in patients with asymptomatic left ventricular dysfunction and increase further upon progression to overt congestive heart failure, but in a substantial proportion of patients with both symptomatic and asymptomatic HFrEF, NE concentrations are similar to those of age-matched control subjects.[1]

In health, approximately 25% of total body NE spillover arises from the kidney and about 2% from the heart.[5] Cardiac NE spillover is elevated in mild heart failure before any obvious increase in total body NE spillover, renal adrenergic drive, or MSNA[3] (**Figures 12-2** and **12-3**). In patients with more advanced left ventricular dysfunction, studied before the advent of contemporary heart failure therapy, NE clearance was a third lower, and total body NE spillover double that of control subjects. Approximately 60% of the latter increase could be attributed to a 2- to 3-fold rise in renal NE spillover, and a 5- to 20-fold elevation in cardiac NE spillover.[5] In the paced-ovine model of heart failure, such preferential activation of cardiac sympathetic nerve traffic benefits from one-third lower resting cardiac than renal burst incidence in healthy sheep, affording much greater augmentation of cardiac sympatho-excitatory capacity in response to progressive reduction in ventricular systolic function.[29] As a consequence, this model has been described as having a cardiac-specific "sympathetic signature;" with the development of heart failure only cardiac sympathetic firing rate increased significantly.[30,31] In human heart failure, both mental stress and cycling exercise have been observed to elicit further increases in cardiac neurotransmitter release

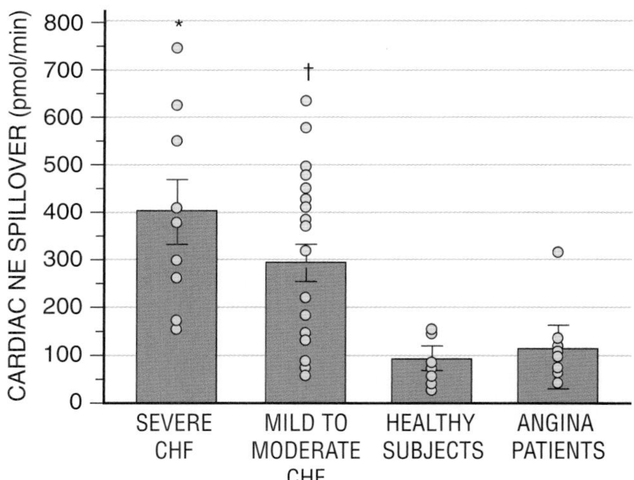

FIGURE 12-2 Individual and mean ± SEM values for cardiac NE spillover in patients with mild to moderate and severe chronic heart failure (CHF), healthy subjects, and patients with stable angina pectoris. *Statistically significant difference ($P < 0.05$) between severe CHF and both control groups. †Statistically significant difference ($P < 0.05$) between mild to moderate CHF and both healthy subjects and angina patients. *From Rundqvist B, Elam M, Bergmann-Sverrisdottir Y, et al: Increased cardiac adrenergic drive precedes generalized sympathetic activation in human heart failure. Circulation 95:169–175, 1997, with permission from the American Heart Association.*

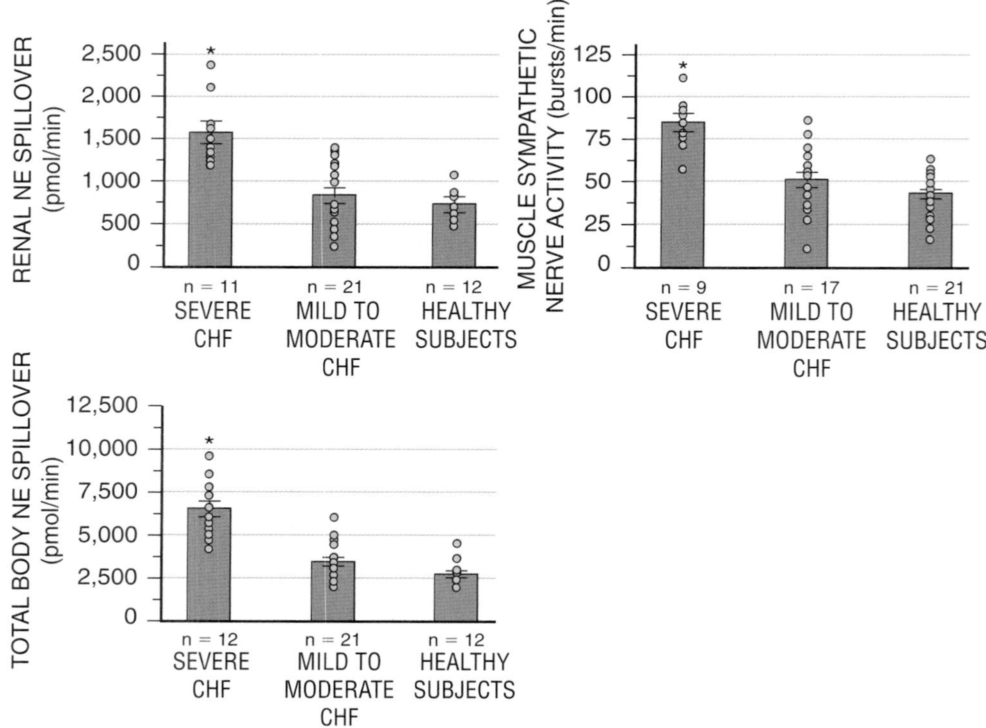

FIGURE 12-3 Individual and mean ± SEM values for renal *(top)* and total body *(middle)* NE spillover and muscle sympathetic nerve activity *(bottom)* in the groups defined in the legend of Figure 12-2. *Statistically significant difference ($P < 0.05$) between severe chronic heart failure (CHF) and both healthy subjects and mild to moderate CHF. *From Rundqvist B, Elam M, Bergmann-Sverrisdottir Y, et al: Increased cardiac adrenergic drive precedes generalized sympathetic activation in human heart failure. Circulation 95:169–175, 1997, with permission from the American Heart Association.*

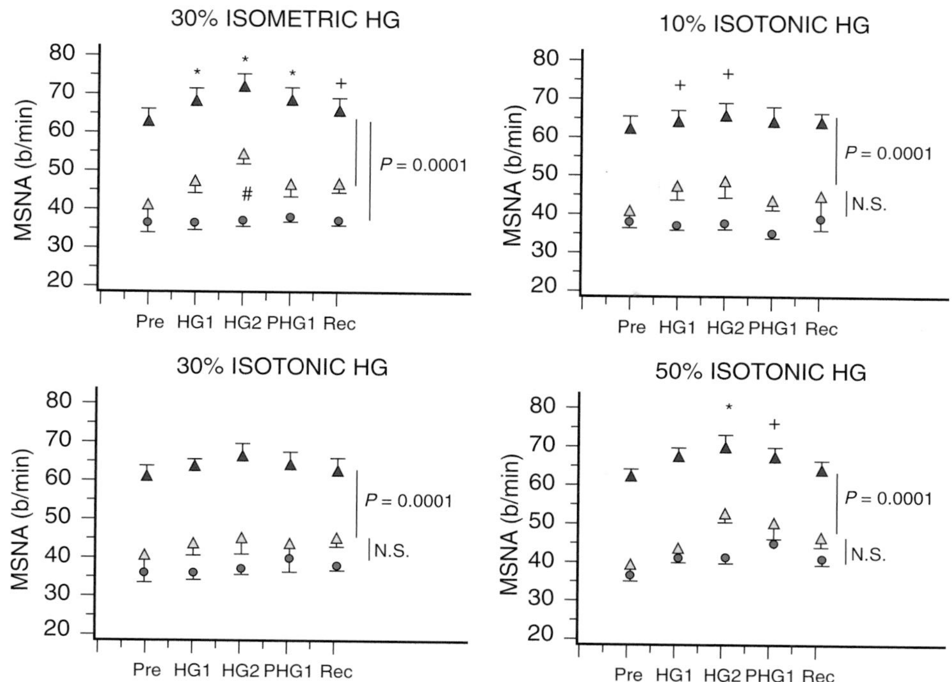

FIGURE 12-4 Muscle sympathetic nerve activity (MSNA) response to handgrip (HG) exercise for peak oxygen uptake ($\dot{V}O_2$ peak) <56% predicted (▲, n = 8HFrEF subjects; >56% predicted (Δ, n = 6) HFrEF subjects; and in normal subjects (●, n = 10). *NS,* Not significant. Stated *P* values refer to the significance level of the main effect of group; **P* <0.05 vs. pre-HG in both HFrEF groups; ⁺*P* <0.05 vs. pre-HG in $\dot{V}O_2$ peak >56% predicted only; #*P* <0.05 vs. $\dot{V}O_2$ peak >56% predicted compared with normal subjects. *From Notarius CF, Atchison DJ, Floras JS: Impact of heart failure and exercise capacity on sympathetic response to handgrip exercise. Am J Physiol Heart Circ Physiol 280:H969–H976, 2001.*

from a high resting baseline, indicating preservation of adrenergic reserve.[32]

In advanced heart failure, plasma epinephrine concentrations also rise, indicating heightened adrenal sympathetic nerve activity and medullary catecholamine release. Under these circumstances, epinephrine, a potent β_2-adrenergic receptor agonist, may be transported into sympathetic nerve terminals and incorporated, along with norepinephrine, into vesicles. Esler and colleagues[33] have documented cardiac epinephrine spillover, averaging 2 ng/min or 2% of the corresponding NE spillover, in untreated congestive heart failure but not healthy subjects. Neuronal release from the gut, liver, lungs, and kidneys, comprising approximately 25% of the total epinephrine plasma appearance rate, also was detected.

To determine whether this increased NE spillover results from greater central sympathetic outflow, or from alterations in its synthesis, release, or reuptake, Leimbach and colleagues recorded MSNA in subjects with moderate to severe HFrEF. Mean sympathetic nerve firing rate correlated with plasma NE concentrations and was significantly elevated as compared with both age-matched and younger subjects with normal ventricular function.[34] The latter observation was replicated subsequently in younger subjects with dilated cardiomyopathy.[35] Single fiber recordings in heart failure patients have demonstrated that these increases result not only from a higher nerve firing probability, but also multiple within-burst discharges and the recruitment of previously silent fibers.[9] Sympathetic discharge to skin, which in contrast to MSNA is not modulated by either high- or low-pressure baroreceptor reflexes, is not increased.[10]

In subjects with mild reduction of left ventricular ejection fraction (down to 40%), group mean values for MSNA burst incidence fall between those of patients with more severe heart failure and healthy control subjects.[15] Once ejection fraction drops below 35%, there is little or no correlation with MSNA burst incidence. Importantly, in many with profound left ventricular systolic dysfunction MSNA remains within the range observed in age-matched control subjects, particularly if their exercise capacity is relatively preserved (**Figure 12-4**).[4] When coupled with the identification in patients with mild to moderate heart failure, by Rundqvist and colleagues, of a selective increase in cardiac NE spillover, without any corresponding increase in mean values for MSNA or total body NE spillover,[3] these findings argue against generalized sympathetic activation as an obligate consequence of HFrEF *per se.*

In the frequency domain, heart failure and age-matched control subjects display similar total MSNA power, harmonic power, nonharmonic power between 0 and 0.5 Hz, and spectral density within the very low- (0-0.05 Hz) and high- (0.15-0.5 Hz) frequency bands. However, low-frequency oscillations in the mean voltage neurogram are diminished markedly or absent, despite near-maximal sympathetic burst incidence, indicating progressive loss of central or reflex modulation of efferent sympathetic traffic as heart failure advances.[25]

Parasympathetic Alterations

Blunted arterial baroreflex control of heart rate is a hallmark of HFrEF. Responses to infusions of both phenylephrine and sodium nitroprusside (expressed either as ms/mm Hg or as beats/min/mm Hg) and to carotid sinus baroreceptor stimulation by neck suction are attenuated. These indices of baroreflex sensitivity for heart rate diminish in proportion to left ventricular systolic dysfunction, New York Heart Association (NYHA) functional symptoms, severity of mitral regurgitation, resting heart rate, blood urea nitrogen,[15,36,37] and the standard deviation of all normal-to-normal pulse

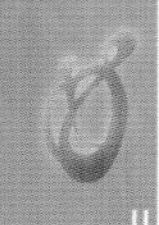

intervals (SDNN), a time domain index of tonic vagal heart rate modulation.[37]

Heart Rate Variability

Loss of vagal heart rate modulation, inversely proportional to the magnitude of sympathetic activation, is evident at the earliest stage of ischemic or dilated cardiomyopathy.[38] For example, soon after the onset of doxorubicin-induced cardiomyopathy high-frequency spectral power decreases, whereas low-frequency spectral power increases in parallel with plasma NE concentration.[39]

Guzzetti and colleagues[40] observed a "predominance" of the low-frequency component of the heart rate power spectrum in NYHA class II patients, but not in class III or IV heart failure. This would be anticipated, because power spectra reflect the fidelity with which postjunctional sinoatrial receptors respond to oscillations in nerve discharge, rather than the intensity of the sympathetic stimulus, and heart rate varies less as failure advances.[23] Saturation or downregulation of cardiac postjunctional β-adrenoceptors and impairment of postsynaptic β-adrenoreceptor signal transduction will decrease sinoatrial responsiveness to neurally released NE. Consequently, low-frequency spectral power is attenuated more often than augmented in HFrEF, and there is an inverse, rather than a direct, relationship between low-frequency spectral power and either discharge frequency of muscle sympathetic nerves or cardiac NE spillover.[41,42] Nonharmonic contributions to the heart rate power spectrum are not attenuated in heart failure, but the complexity of the heart rate signal is reduced in subjects with normal ventricular function, seemingly due to less vagal modulation.[22]

Heart Failure with Preserved Systolic Function (HFpEF) (see also Chapters 10 and 36)

Information as to sympathetic activation in heart failure with preserved ventricular systolic function is sparse. Benedict et al did not detect increased plasma NE concentrations in patients enrolled in the Studies of Left Ventricular Dysfunction (SOLVD) registry who had pulmonary congestion but a left ventricular ejection fraction above 45%.[43] In general, the sympathetic nervous system would not appear to be as activated as it is in heart failure patients with systolic dysfunction,[44] and impairment of cardiac norepinephrine transport function, as assessed using ^{123}I-MIBG imaging,[45] and heart rate variability are not as depressed.[46]

CLINICAL CONSEQUENCES OF AUTONOMIC IMBALANCE

Cardiac

The impact in heart failure of impaired vagal tone on heart rate modulation, regulation of left ventricular performance, and inflammatory pathways has been reviewed in detail.[47] The first manifestation of sympathetic activation is a selective increase in cardiac NE spillover.[3] Cardiac sympathetic activation and vagal withdrawal constitute adaptive mechanisms, engaged to maintain peripheral tissue perfusion in the face of compromised cardiac performance. However, once congestion becomes manifest, the heart is subject to the greatest proportional increase in regional NE spillover, and thus the failing heart is the organ exposed for the longest duration to the greatest magnitude of sympathetic activation. The direct myocardial consequences of such intense cardiac adrenergic drive, which are reviewed in Chapter 6, include myocyte necrosis and apoptosis (see also Chapter 2), fibrosis (see also Chapter 4), decreased β-adrenergic receptor number, diminished $β_1$-adrenoceptor responsiveness to catecholamines and altered β-adrenergic receptor signal transduction, defective calcium regulation by the sarcoplasmic reticulum, induction of proinflammatory cytokine expression, oxidative stress, destruction of sympathetic nerve terminals, and depletion of myocardial NE content.[48] Nonuniform NE depletion and sympathetic denervation disturb the temporal coordination of right and left ventricular contraction and relaxation and alter the dispersion of refractoriness, leading to ventricular dyssynergy and promoting arrhythmogenesis.[28]

Peripheral

Excessive sympathetic drive to arteries, veins, and the kidney exacerbates the hemodynamic derangements of heart failure by increasing both preload and afterload. Stimulation of renal sympathetic nerves activates the renin-angiotensin-aldosterone axis (see also Chapter 5), promotes tubular absorption of sodium and water, decreases glomerular filtration, increases renal vascular resistance, and blunts the renal responsiveness to atrial natriuretic peptide. In young subjects with dilated cardiomyopathy, muscle sympathetic burst frequency at rest correlated directly with resistance to blood flow in the calf, the vascular bed distal to the recording electrode.[35] This observation implicates sympathetically mediated vasoconstriction as an important mechanism for increased afterload in human heart failure. Increased sympathetic outflow may also raise ventricular afterload by decreasing conduit artery compliance.

Exercise

A reduction in exercise capacity, whether due to dyspnea or fatigue, is a common heart failure symptom. A central factor limiting exercise capacity is chronotropic incompetence due to decreased cardiac β-adrenergic receptor density or responsiveness to endogenous catecholamines.[49] Several $β_2$-adrenoceptor polymorphisms associated with impaired exercise performance have been identified.[50]

Augmented neurogenic vasoconstriction has been proposed as one of several peripheral limitations to exercise. In heart failure patients (but not in healthy age-matched control subjects), maximal oxygen uptake during exercise correlates inversely to resting MSNA.[51] Cardiac NE spillover, on the other hand, bears little relation to peak VO_2 in either group.[52] Reductions in blood flow below levels required to meet local metabolic demands during exercise may cause further reflexive increases in central sympathetic outflow by stimulating metaboreceptor afferents in skeletal muscle.[4] In turn, such sympathetic activation could diminish exercise capacity and endothelium-mediated vasodilation.[53] In recent experiments, fibular MSNA was recorded continuously, whereas with the opposite leg subjects performed one-legged cycling without and with resistance. In contrast to healthy controls, whose burst incidence fell, in those with HFrEF exercise increased MSNA; overall there

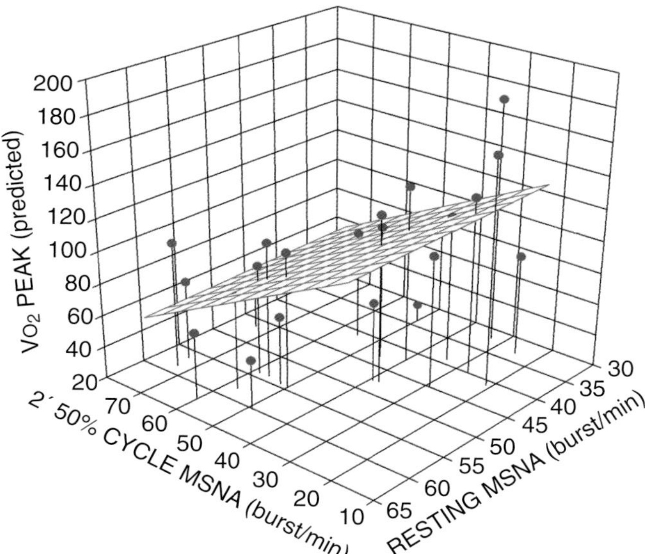

FIGURE 12-5 Relationship between peak oxygen uptake ($\dot{V}O_{2peak}$) and muscle sympathetic nerve activity (MSNA) burst frequency at rest and 2 minutes into one-legged cycling (contralateral limb) at 50% of $\dot{V}O_{2peak}$ in a cohort with and without HFrEF. Three-dimensional graph shows individual data points and regression plane. The slope relating $\dot{V}O_{2peak}$ to exercise-induced MSNA is significant ($P = 0.03$) and remains so when adjusted for baseline MSNA; the slope relating $\dot{V}O_{2peak}$ to resting MSNA is not ($P = 0.93$). *From Notarius CF, Millar PJ, Murai H, et al: Inverse relationship between muscle sympathetic activity during exercise and peak oxygen update in subjects with and without heart failure. J Am Coll Cardiol 63:605–606, 2014, with permission from the American College of Cardiology Foundation.*

was a significant inverse relationship between the maximum MSNA elicited by one-legged exercise and subjects' peak $\dot{V}O_2$ (**Figure 12-5**).[54]

Mortality

Before widespread use of angiotensin-converting enzyme inhibitors and β-adrenoceptor antagonists, the life expectancy of most symptomatic HFrEF patients with venous plasma NE concentrations exceeding 800 pg/mL was less than 1 year.[55] Increased plasma NE concentrations predict also all-cause and cardiovascular mortality of asymptomatic patients with left ventricular systolic dysfunction.[56] This inverse relationship between plasma NE concentrations and survival in symptomatic patients persists despite contemporary therapy, including β-blockade.[57] In a Brazilian study involving 122 heart failure patients, the MSNA also was a significant independent predictor of mortality.[58]

In the pre–β-blocker era, cardiac NE spillover was found to be a particularly potent marker of 1-year mortality of HFrEF patients referred for consideration of transplantation[2] (**Figure 12-6**), but in those now treated chronically with β-adrenoceptor antagonists, renal NE spillover is more closely related to a combined endpoint of death and transplantation.[59]

Estimating cardiac NE stores provides insight into the probable mode of death. In a group of 116 patients with a mean left ventricular ejection fraction of 19%, followed on average for 18 months, those with greater than median estimated cardiac NE stores plus increased cardiac NE spillover had a two- to threefold higher risk of sudden death, whereas patients with depleted myocardial NE stores and high cardiac NE spillover (reflecting chronically increased

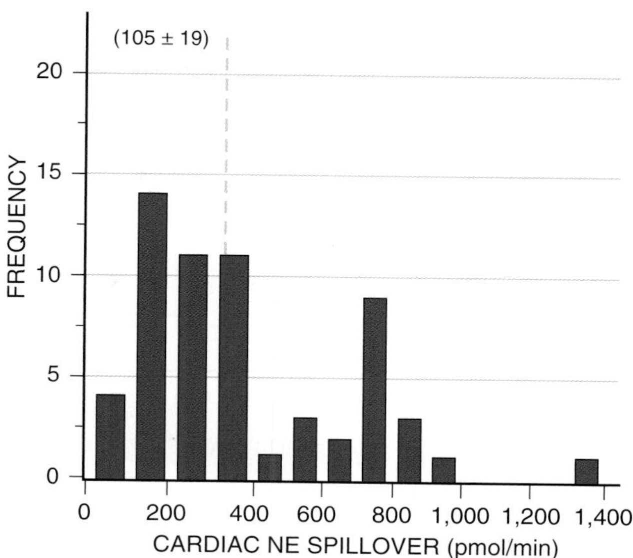

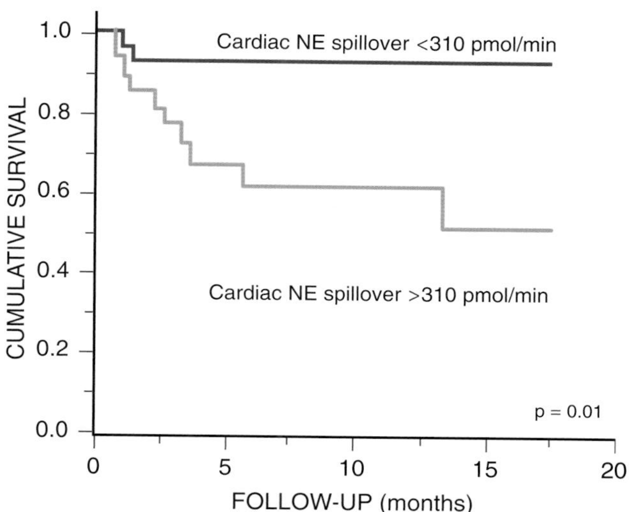

FIGURE 12-6 *Top,* Histogram depicting the frequency distribution of cardiac norepinephrine (NE) spillover rates for patients with HFrEF. Dashed line indicates group median (310 pmol/min). Data above indicate mean cardiac NE spillover rate for healthy subjects, with 95% confidence limits. Cardiac NE spillover was significantly higher in patients with HFrEF (402 ± 37 vs. 105 ± 19 pmol/min; $P < 0.01$). *Bottom,* Survival curves for patients dichotomized by median cardiac NE spillover rate, with reduced survival ($P = 0.01$) in those with the highest values. *Data from Kaye DM, Lefkovitz J, Jennings GL, et al: Adverse consequences of high sympathetic nervous system activity in the failing human heart. J Am Coll Cardiol 26:1257–1263, 1995, with permission from the American College of Cardiology Foundation.*

neurotransmitter turnover and reduced reuptake and storage) had a two- to fourfold higher risk of death from progressive pump failure.[6] Abnormal ^{11}C-HED or ^{123}I-MIBG uptake by ventricular sympathetic nerves also identifies HFrEF patients at increased risk of premature death[27,28,60] (**Figure 12-7**).

Diminished baroreflex sensitivity, loss of heart rate variability, and augmented chemosensitivity to both hypoxia and hypercapnia also are associated with accelerated mortality from progressive myocardial failure and arrhythmias.[1,61-63] An attenuated reflex heart rate response to phenylephrine has similar prognostic implications in patients treated or not treated with β-adrenoceptor antagonists.[37] Loss of complexity in the heart rate signal, as estimated by nonharmonic power-law regression parameters[61] and

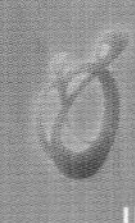

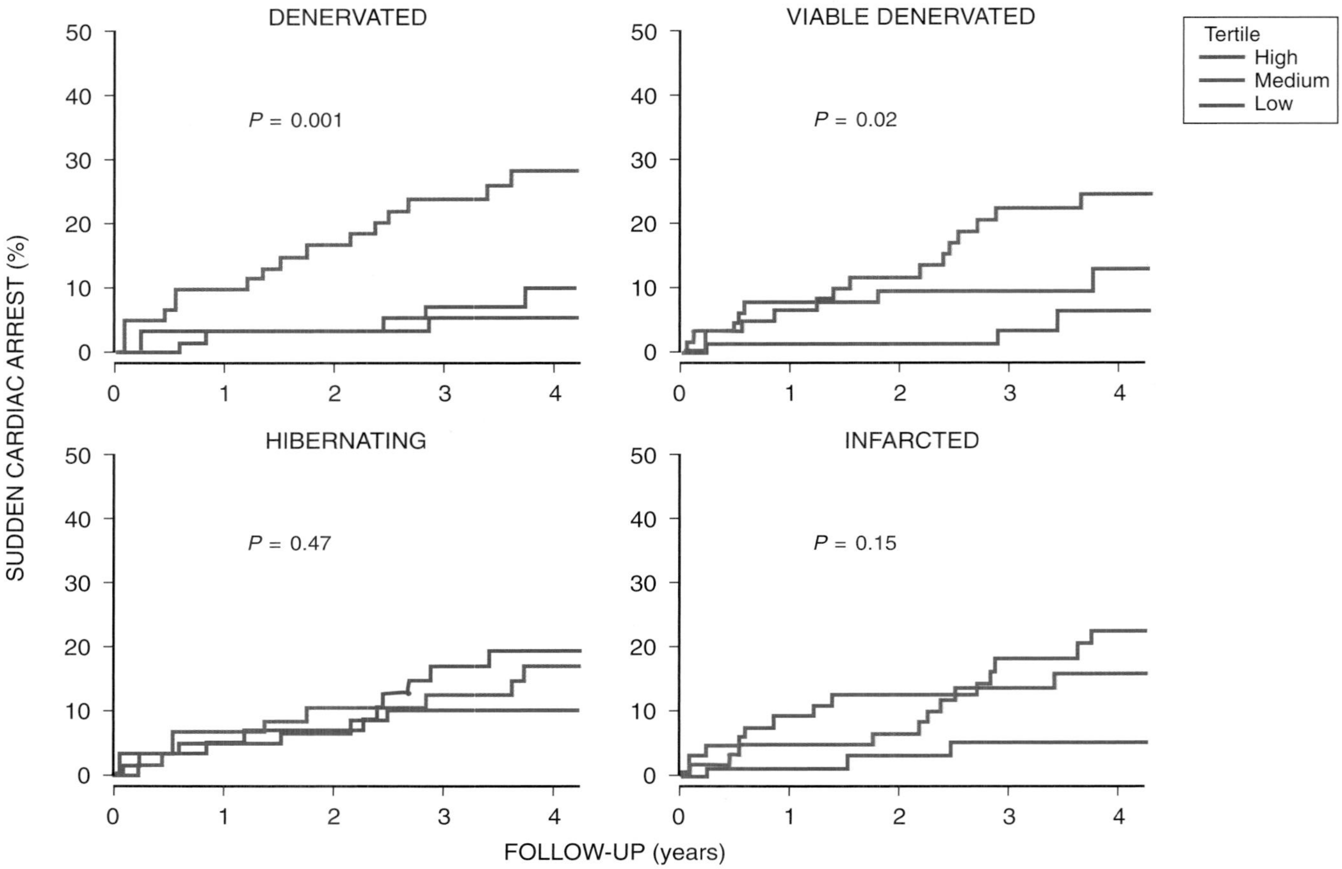

FIGURE 12-7 Kaplan-Meier curves over a median follow-up of 4.1 years demonstrating that myocardial sympathetic denervation (both total volume of denervated myocardium, as well as viable denervated myocardium, *upper panels*), quantified using ^{11}C-HED PET imaging can identify HFrEF patients with ischemic cardiomyopathy at high, medium, and low risk of sudden cardiac death. By contrast, neither hibernating myocardium nor total infarct volume *(lower panels)* identified risk significantly. *From Fallavollita J, Heavey BM, Luisi AJ, et al: Regional myocardial sympathetic denervation predicts the risk of sudden cardiac arrest in ischemic cardiomyopathy. J Am Coll Cardiol 63:141–149, 2014, with permission from the American College of Cardiology Foundation.*

low-frequency harmonic power, appear to be the most sensitive predictors of sudden death.[62]

MECHANISMS OF AUTONOMIC IMBALANCE

Alterations in the neurogenic control of the circulation with the onset and progression of heart failure can arise from one or more elements responsible for the regulation of autonomic tone, such as inhibitory and excitatory input to brainstem vasomotor neurons, cortical modulation of central nervous system integration and catecholamine turnover, and efferent mechanisms determining the release rates of and receptor responsiveness to neurotransmitters (**Figure 12-8**).[1]

Afferent Influences

In healthy subjects, inputs from carotid sinus and aortic arch "arterial high-pressure" and cardiopulmonary "low-pressure" mechanoreceptors provide the principal peripheral inhibitory influences on sympathetic outflow, with discharge from arterial chemoreceptors and muscle "metaboreceptors" providing excitatory information. The efferent vagal component of the baroreceptor heart rate reflex is also subject to arterial baroreceptor afferent input. At rest, healthy individuals display low sympathetic discharge and high heart rate variability. Reflex vagal and sympathoneural responses to acute perturbations in blood pressure are brisk.

Arterial Baroreceptor Reflexes

Arterial baroreceptor nerve discharge is activated by the pressure wave of systole, and diminishes or falls silent during diastole. Systolic stimulation of baroreceptor discharge will increase parasympathetic and decrease efferent sympathetic outflow reflexively. Baroreceptor silence during diastole eliminates the tonic inhibition of efferent sympathetic outflow, permitting a burst of multiunit MSNA.

Because baroreceptor afferent nerve discharge, which governs both sympathetic and vagal efferent limbs of this reflex arc, is less responsive to changes in local distending pressure in experimental models of ventricular systolic dysfunction, the prevailing view had been that arterial baroreflex regulation of vagal and sympathetic outflow in human HFrEF is impaired in parallel. However, assessment of the baroreceptor-heart rate reflex in humans relies upon the indirect estimation of sinoatrial responsiveness to two distinct and differentially regulated autonomic inputs. In heart failure, impaired efferent vagal ganglionic neurotransmission diminishes parasympathetic responsiveness to baroreceptor stimulation,[64] yet myocardial responsiveness to acetylcholine is intact in humans,[65] and in experimental heart failure, augmented.[66] By contrast, cardiac-specific sympathetic neural modulation is attenuated by downregulation or desensitization of β-adrenoceptors, rendering the sinoatrial node less responsive to reflexively elicited changes in neurally released NE.[48] Noncardiac sympathetic efferent responses to arterial baroreflex perturbation upstream of

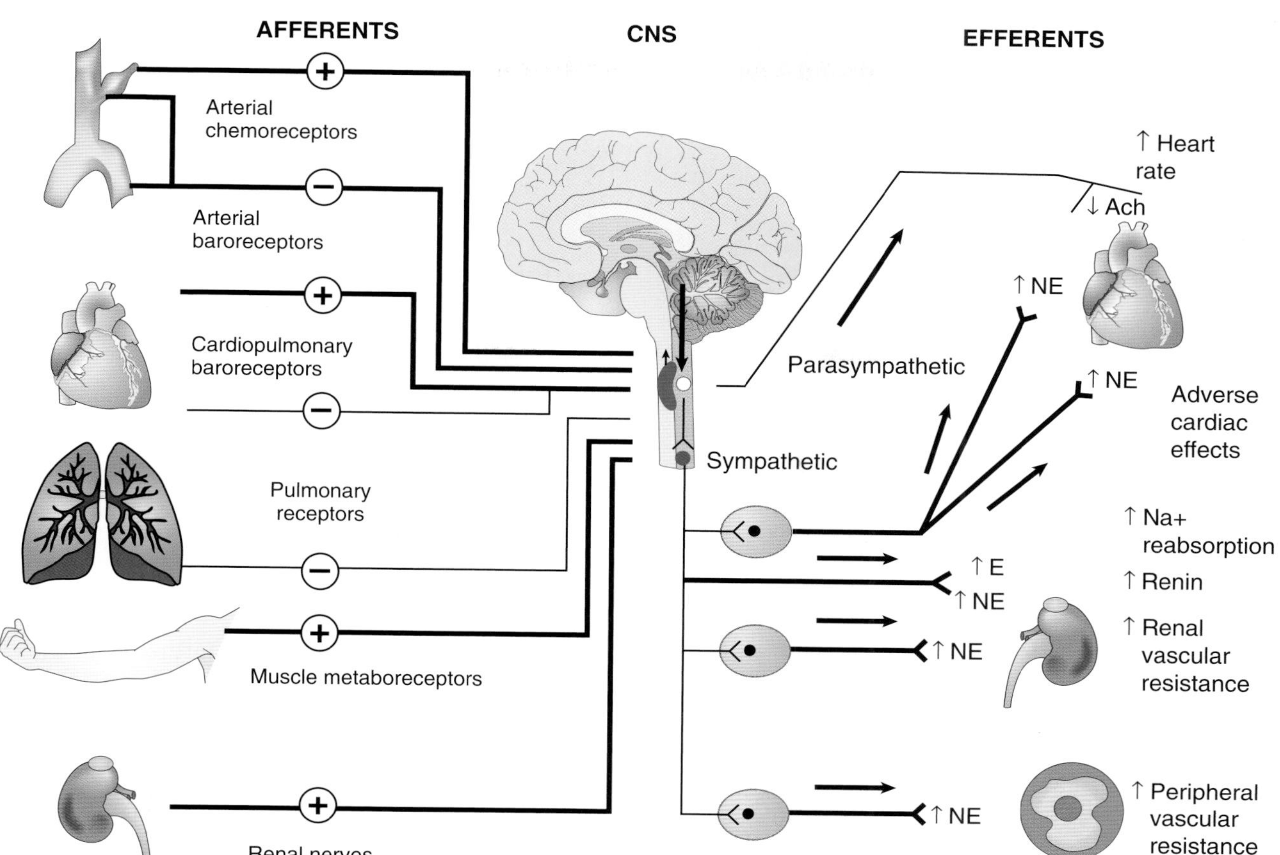

FIGURE 12-8 Updated synthesis illustrating mechanisms involved in the autonomic disturbances of HFrEF. Input from arterial and cardiac mechanoreceptor and chemoreceptor afferents, arterial chemoreceptor, pulmonary stretch receptor, muscle metaboreceptor and mechanoreceptor, and renal afferent nerves converge to modulate sympathetic outflow about a centrally mediated set-point increase involving an angiotensin II-AT_1 receptor-NADPH-superoxide pathway. As systolic dysfunction progresses, input effecting sympatho-inhibition (–) by stimulating ventricular and a population of atrial mechanoreceptor nerve afferents decreases *(thin line),* whereas inhibitory modulation of efferent sympathetic nerve traffic by arterial baroreceptors *(thick line)* is preserved. Efferent vagal heart rate responses to arterial baroreflex perturbations are attenuated *(thin line).* Excitatory (+) afferent input arises from a normally quiescent atrial reflex, activated by increases in cardiac filling pressures; chemically sensitive ventricular afferent nerve endings, triggered by ischemia; augmented sympatho-excitatory input from arterial chemoreceptors; exercising skeletal muscle in heart failure; and renal afferent nerves *(thick lines).* The central set-point for sympathetic outflow *(arrow pointing down)* is raised further by central chemoreceptor sensitization, by sleep apneas, and possibly by obesity. Efferent mechanisms for increased NE spillover include prejunctional facilitation of its release and impaired NE uptake. The time course through which these mechanisms are engaged differs between individuals. Relatively asymptomatic systolic dysfunction is characterized by a selective increase in cardiac NE release, and a reduction in tonic and reflex vagal heart rate modulation. As heart failure advances, there is a generalized increase in sympathetic nerve traffic to the heart, adrenal, kidney, skeletal muscle, and other vascular beds *(thick arrow shafts, thick lines). Ach,* Acetylcholine; *CNS,* central nervous system; *E,* epinephrine; *Na^+,* sodium; *NE,* norepinephrine. *Reproduced with permission of the author.*

the effector target can be measured directly, and specifically, by microneurography. Heart failure, by these several mechanisms, reduces the variability and complexity of heart rate but the variability of blood pressure is similar in patients and age-matched healthy subjects,[22] suggesting relatively preserved modulation of sympathetic outflow in this condition.

Brandle and colleagues[67] found no differences in the time course of changes in hemodynamics and plasma NE concentrations during the development of pacing-induced heart failure in dogs with and without sinoaortic baroreceptor denervation, and concluded that impairment of the arterial baroreflex could not be responsible for sustaining the increase in sympathetic outflow in this experimental model of heart failure. Reports, in heart failure, of significant inverse relationships between stroke work index and MSNA[68] and between cardiac output and cardiac NE spillover[69] suggest that the arterial baroreflex regulation of efferent sympathetic discharge may actually be appropriate, when hemodynamic alterations present in this condition are considered. Grassi and colleagues, using the vasoactive drug method, described an impairment of both limbs of the reflex control of MSNA that worsened with the progression of heart failure.[15] A second study also reported diminished arterial baroflex gain, but unfortunately in this report the mean age of patients was twice that of control subjects.[36] By contrast, Dibner-Dunlap and associates[70] documented similar gains in the arterial baroreflex control of MSNA in healthy and heart failure subjects, whereas reflex responses to stimuli that raised and lowered cardiac filling pressure without affecting systemic blood pressure were markedly attenuated. These investigators concluded that impairment of the cardiopulmonary (not the arterial) baroreflex was the fundamental defect in the regulation of sympathetic outflow in human heart failure[70,71] (see Figure 12-8).

Two autonomic disturbances characteristic of advanced heart failure should be accounted for when interpreting the results of experiments involving vasoactive drugs: (1) muscle sympathetic burst firing is pulse synchronous, and its incidence (i.e., bursts/100 cardiac cycles) approaches

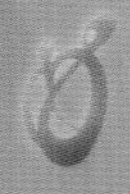

TABLE 12-1 Preserved Arterial Baroreflex Modulation of Sympathetic Activity in Human Heart Failure with Reduced Ejection Fraction

CONCEPT	OBSERVATION
MSNA pulse-synchronicity lost after sinoaortic baroreceptor denervation	Pulse-synchronicity preserved, even in end-stage HF
Pause with decay in DBP after premature beat reflexively increases MSNA burst amplitude, duration, and area; rise in DBP after postextrasystolic beat inhibits MSNA	Extrasystolic augmentation of MSNA amplitude, duration, and area and postextrasystolic suppression replicated in HF; duration or suppression proportional to magnitude of diastolic overshoot
MSNA bursts track previous DBP with 1.2-1.3 s lag	Synchronization of sympathetic neural alternans with pulsus alternans
Frequency domain estimate of arterial BR gain derived by cross-spectral analysis with BP oscillations as stimulus and MSNA oscillations as response	Transfer function gain in HF and healthy subjects similar across all frequency bands; calculated gain highest in high-frequency range
Arterial BR unloading with SNP elicits reflex increase in TNES	Similar reflex increase in TNES in HF and healthy subjects
LV pacing in HF increases DBP	Acute inverse DBP-MSNA relationship immediately upon conversion from RV to LV pacing
Muller maneuver increases acutely intrathoracic aortic and LV transmural pressures	MSNA inhibited similarly in HF and control subjects

BP, Blood pressure; *BR,* baroreceptor reflex; *DBP,* diastolic blood pressure; *HF,* heart failure caused by systolic dysfunction; *LV,* left ventricular; *MSNA,* muscle sympathetic nerve activity; *RV,* right ventricular; *SNP,* sodium nitroprusside; *TNES,* total body norepinephrine spillover.

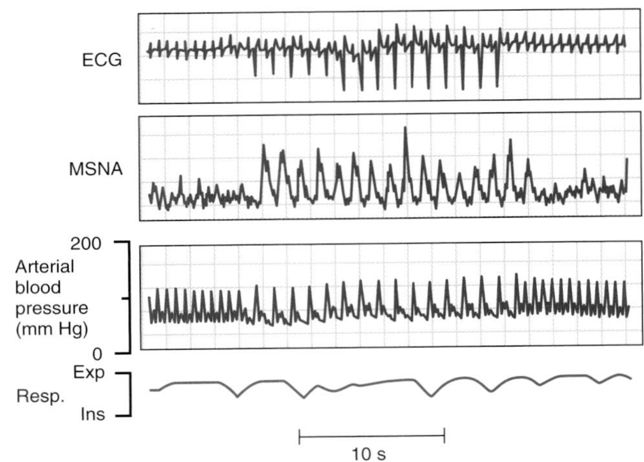

FIGURE 12-9 The electrocardiogram (ECG), mean voltage neurogram for (MSNA), blood pressure, and respiratory excursions in a young man with end-stage heart failure resulting from dilated cardiomyopathy. Paroxysms of ventricular bigeminy result in a doubling of the blood pressure cycle length, a longer diastolic period, and lower diastolic blood pressure. These changes are registered immediately by the arterial baroreceptors and result in a corresponding increase in the duration of the sympathetic burst and a marked increase in burst amplitude. These are reversed with restoration of sinus rhythm.

100%; and (2) the heart rate response to arterial baroreceptor perturbation by phenylephrine or nitroprusside is markedly attenuated. If cardiac frequency hardly changes in response to these interventions, there is little opportunity arithmetically to modify a cardiac frequency-dependent representation of sympathetic nerve firing. If the reported effect of these drug interventions on MSNA burst frequency is reexpressed in terms of cardiac frequency (or as changes in absolute units, rather than as a percentage of baseline values), then the gain of the arterial baroreflex regulation of MSNA is not appreciably impaired.[15,36,72]

Several lines of evidence obtained using different approaches, and summarized in **Table 12-1**, are consistent with the concept that arterial baroreflex modulation of efferent sympathetic outflow is relatively intact in human heart failure[18,25,72-75] (**Figure 12-9**). Further evidence for preserved functionality of the arterial baroreflex arises from recent experiments involving the paced-canine[76] and paced-ovine heart failure models. In the latter, directly recorded cardiac sympathetic nerve activity (CSNA) was significantly increased, and the baroreceptor regulation of heart rate was profoundly impaired, but the arterial baroreflex control of both CSNA and renal sympathetic nerve traffic did not differ from that of normal sheep.[29,77]

In human heart failure, the renal efferent response to arterial baroreceptor unloading behaves differently. In one study, hypotension induced by nitroprusside elicited an 85% increase in renal NE spillover in healthy control subjects, but no net change in heart failure subjects, albeit from a nearly threefold higher baseline.[78] What could not be determined from these experiments is whether the absence of sympatho-excitation represents a ceiling effect (i.e., renal NE spillover cannot be increased further from these high baseline levels), as suggested by the ovine experiments of Ramchandra and colleagues,[29] or the integrated response to the combination of arterial and cardiopulmonary receptor unloading with a concurrent reduction in renal venous pressure. In a more recent study, low-dose nitroglycerin reduced pulmonary artery pressure selectively without altering renal NE spillover in either heart failure or healthy subjects, whereas a higher, hypotensive, dose was accompanied by a significant reduction only in those with systolic dysfunction.[79]

Cardiopulmonary Reflexes

In healthy subjects, cardiopulmonary reflexes, considered conventionally to arise from afferent nerve endings situated in the heart and pulmonary veins, elicit sympathoinhibition and forearm vasodilation when stimulated by increasing cardiac filling pressures, volume, or inotropic state, and sympathoexcitation when unloaded by interventions such as phlebotomy or nonhypotensive lower body negative pressure (LBNP). There is substantial evidence that the latter responses are altered in human heart failure. When Middlekauff and associates[80] performed phlebotomy, the reflex forearm vasoconstrictor response to this stimulus was attenuated in heart failure patients, whereas the renal cortical vasoconstrictor response, as assessed by positron emission tomography, was preserved.

In some patients, lower body negative pressure elicits forearm vasodilation rather than vasoconstriction.[81] Activation of vagal afferents with inhibitory reflex effects on sympathetic outflow as a result of acute increases in ventricular contractile force (possibly due to release of pericardial constraint) has been proposed as a potential mechanism for this paradoxical response. However, sympathetic outflow was not quantified in those experiments. Subsequently, in subjects not receiving angiotensin-converting enzyme inhibition, Dunlap and colleagues reported markedly attenuated reflex MSNA responses to stimuli that raised and lowered cardiac filling pressure without affecting systemic blood pressure.[70] In our laboratory, nonhypotensive LBNP increased total body NE spillover significantly in subjects with normal ventricular systolic function, whereas there was only a trend, not significant, toward higher values in those with impaired ventricular systolic function.[82]

Such impairment would not be sufficient to account for two aspects of sympatho-excitation in HFrEF: (1) a selective increase in cardiac NE spillover in mild to moderate heart failure, without change in total body or renal NE spillover or in MSNA,[3] and (2) the presence of direct correlations, in more advanced heart failure, between MSNA and pulmonary artery or capillary wedge pressure.[34,68] These observations suggest that a reflex that senses the degree of cardiopulmonary volume or pressure overload becomes active in heart failure. Indeed, in the pacing-induced canine model of congestion, Wang and Zucker documented sensitization of cardiac sympathetic afferents responsive to chemical stimulation and speculated that enhancement of this reflex might contribute to increased sympathetic nerve traffic in chronic human heart failure. This cardiac sympathetic afferent reflex was potentiated by acute volume expansion.[83]

Is there evidence in humans for activation, by increased filling pressure, of a cardiac-specific sympatho-excitatory reflex? In HFrEF, there is a significant positive relationship between the pulmonary capillary wedge pressure and cardiac NE spillover.[69] Infusion of sodium nitroprusside in those with secondary pulmonary hypertension lowers cardiac NE spillover in addition to atrial and arterial pressure,[84] as does the brief application of positive airway pressure to reduce atrial and pulmonary venous transmural pressure (simultaneous reductions in intrathoracic aortic arch, and left ventricular transmural pressure should increase sympathetic outflow reflexively[85]). Nonhypotensive LBNP, applied selectively to reduce cardiac filling and pulmonary pressures, decreases cardiac NE spillover in HFrEF, but not in control subjects with normal left ventricular systolic function (**Figure 12-10**).[82] Because this maneuver lowers stroke volume and cardiac output, the reduction in cardiac NE spillover (but not total body NE spillover, which tends to increase) cannot be explained by activation of ventricular mechanoreceptors because of increases in systolic force. Instead, Azevedo and colleagues[82] attributed the sympathoinhibitory response to nonhypotensive LBNP to unloading of low-pressure mechanoreceptor myelinated afferent nerves arising in the heart and lungs that reflexively and selectively excite cardiac adrenergic drive (see Figure 12-8). Saline infusion causes a paradoxical increase in forearm vascular resistance in mild heart failure, an effect not seen in control subjects,[86] suggesting that in humans the efferent limb of this reflex, when stimulated acutely, might not be selective to cardiac sympathetic nerves. Consistent with this concept is our recent identification—in humans with heart failure, relative to controls—of a proportionately greater subpopulation of single unit MSNA discharge responding to lower body positive pressure with paradoxically increased discharge.[87]

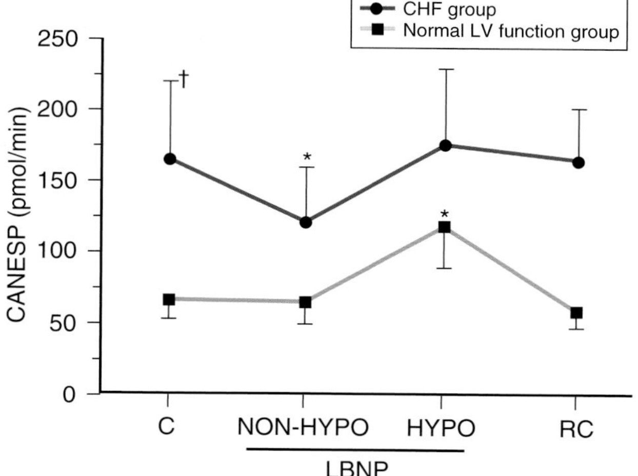

FIGURE 12-10 Cardiac norepinephrine spillover (CANESP) responses to nonhypotensive and hypotensive LBNP. ■, normal LV function group; ●, HFrEF group; *C*, control; *RC*, recovery. $*P < 0.05$ vs. normal LV function group at control. $^{\dagger}P < 0.005$ vs. normal LV function group at control. *Data from Azevedo ER, Newton GE, Floras JS, et al: Reducing cardiac filling pressure lowers cardiac norepinephrine spillover in patients with chronic heart failure. Circulation 101:2053–2059, 2000.*

Increasing the intensity of LBNP to induce systemic hypotension evoked a significant increase in cardiac NE spillover in the control group only (see Figure 12-10).[82] This observation is concordant with the prior description of similar increases in total body NE spillover in HFrEF and healthy subjects, yet attenuation of the reflex increase in cardiac NE spillover in response to a hypotensive infusion of sodium nitroprusside in those with impaired systolic function.[73] Taken together, these findings can be interpreted as indicating that the normal arterial baroreflex-mediated increase in cardiac NE spillover evoked reflexively by a fall in systemic blood pressure is tempered significantly in heart failure by concurrent removal of an excitatory stimulus arising from cardiac sympathetic afferents. If a sympathetic discharge to the heart, kidney, and skeletal muscle were increased in parallel by this stimulus, the consequent increases in renal sodium retention and in systemic afterload could worsen congestion, ventricular systolic function, and exercise performance, and amplify further the efferent discharge from these cardiopulmonary afferents through a positive feedback loop. Recently, in dogs with normal ventricular function, Moore and colleagues identified a pressor reflex, accompanied by increased renal sympathetic nerve firing, stimulated by a selective increase in pulmonary artery pressure.[88] With secondary pulmonary hypertension so prevalent in the heart failure population, this discovery adds to the list of potential sympatho-inhibitory benefits of lowering cardiopulmonary pressure and blood volume.

Thus a large body of present evidence indicates that arterial baroreceptor reflex regulation of muscle and cardiac sympathetic activity is not impaired in human heart failure. Consequently, the higher sympathetic nerve firing rate characteristic of the majority of patients with HFrEF can be considered an appropriate reflex response to alterations in their systemic hemodynamics. The principal defect in baroreceptor regulation of the sympathetic nervous system appears instead to arise from reflexes originating in mechanoreceptors situated within the heart and pulmonary vasculature.[71] In some patients with heart failure, these baroreflex-mediated responses appear sufficient to account for the prevailing level of sympathetic activity, but in many others the contribution of nonbaroreflex-mediated excitatory reflexes or central resetting of sympathetic outflow also must be considered.

Nonbaroreflex Mechanisms

In HFrEF patients, each of age,[89] hypertension,[90] metabolic syndrome,[91] anemia,[92] acute ingestion of a carbohydrate load,[93] and obesity[90,91] has been shown to increase

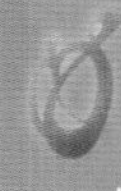

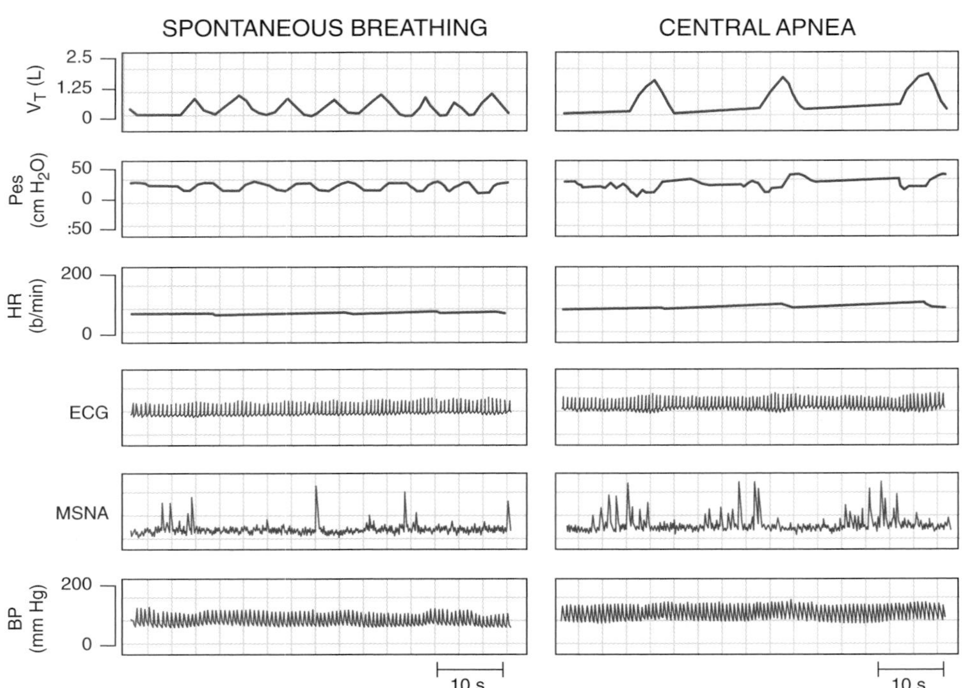

FIGURE 12-11 Tidal volume (V_T), esophageal pressure (Pes), heart rate (HR), the electrocardiogram (ECG), muscle sympathetic nerve activity (MSNA), and blood pressure (BP) in a young patient with dilated cardiomyopathy. Recordings taken during spontaneous breathing and spontaneous episodes of central apnea, while awake and only minutes apart, demonstrate marked activation of central sympathetic outflow and increased BP corresponding to periods of apnea.

independently multiunit MSNA. With respect to the latter, a renal sympatho-excitatory reflex arising from white adipose tissue and involving the paraventricular nucleus has been described recently in rats[94]; whether this "adipose afferent reflex" is functionally important in human obesity remains to be determined.

The presence of atrial fibrillation in heart failure has been reported to increase single-unit MSNA firing frequency and the incidence of multiple firing of single units, inversely proportional to the diastolic pressure nadir during each of the varying cardiac cycle lengths, but not multiunit MSNA[95] or cardiac NE spillover at rest.[96] However, the reflex increase in cardiac NE elicited by head up tilt is attenuated in HFrEF patients with atrial fibrillation.[97]

Pulmonary Stretch Reflexes

Distention of pulmonary stretch receptors by inspiration inhibits reflexively sympathetic outflow. In healthy subjects, breathing frequency correlates positively with MSNA burst frequency, and reflex sympathoneural responses to hypoxia and hypercapnia. This influence of breathing pattern on oscillations in sympathetic discharge is preserved in heart failure patients,[98] in whom decreased tidal volume, high respiratory frequency,[99] and brief periods of apnea elicit marked increases in MSNA (**Figure 12-11**). However, a greater tidal volume is required to inhibit completely MSNA in heart failure patients than in healthy subjects.[98] Rapidly adapting airway vagal sensory receptors, responding to inflation and deflation, are also stimulated by increases in left atrial pressure and extravascular pulmonary fluid volume.[100]

Peripheral Chemoreceptor Reflexes

The contribution of arterial chemoreceptors to sympathetic activation in experimental models of heart failure has been reviewed recently in detail by Schultz and associates.[101] Augmented peripheral chemoreceptor sensitivity to hypoxia is reportedly present in approximately 40% of treated chronic heart failure patients[102,103] (see Figure 12-8). However, in two studies, inhalation of 100% oxygen to suppress peripheral chemoreceptor input had no effect on group mean values for MSNA, suggesting that chemoreceptor-mediated sympatho-excitation may be less prevalent than those studies would suggest.[104,105] Importantly, recent work provides evidence that this disturbance is not generalized to all with impaired systolic function, but specific to those heart failure patients who also are anemic[92] or who have chronic kidney disease.[106] Di Vanna and colleagues[107] described increased MSNA responses to hypoxic (peripheral) and hypercapnic (central) chemoreceptor stimulation in class II-III heart failure patients compared with control subjects. Carotid chemoreceptor reflex-induced sympathetic activation in heart failure may assume greater importance during exercise than in the resting state.[108] Recently, Despas and colleagues reported that in a subset of heart failure patients with increased chemosensitivity, MSNA at rest was elevated and the slope of the relationship between spontaneous changes in diastolic blood pressure and MSNA was attenuated; inhalation of 100% oxygen restored both to values recorded in heart failure patients with normal chemoreceptor responsiveness.[19]

Increased peripheral chemoreceptor sensitivity gives rise to several autonomic disturbances with adverse prognostic implications. These include higher plasma NE concentrations, impaired arterial baroreflex control of heart rate, augmented very low-frequency heart rate and blood pressure spectral power, but loss of low-frequency heart rate variability, the development of periodic oscillations in breathing at very low frequency both during sleep and in the awake state, enhanced ventilatory responses to exercise, and a higher likelihood of developing nonsustained ventricular tachycardia.[102,103]

Myocardial Ischemia and Infarction

Both anterior and inferoposterior wall ischemia elicit sympathoexcitation by stimulating cardiac sympathetic afferent nerves. This reflex is blocked by stellectomy.[109] If arterial blood pressure were to decrease as a consequence of ischemia, unloading of sinoaortic baroreceptors should elicit a further, reflexive, increase in sympathetic outflow. Vagal afferents arising from inferoposterior ventricular segments normally evoke a depressor response, a reflex interrupted by prior myocardial infarction.[110]

Consequently, myocardial ischemia and prior infarction, common in the HFrEF population, could exert via several mechanisms an acute or chronic effect on sympathetic outflow additive to, and independent of, the magnitude of ventricular systolic function. Consistent with this concept, patients with relatively preserved ejection fraction (mean 52%) when evaluated 6 months after uncomplicated myocardial infarction had significantly higher MSNA burst incidence than matched patients with stable coronary artery disease absent prior necrosis or control subjects.[111] Do otherwise clinically similar patients with ischemic and nonischemic cardiomyopathy differ with respect to sympathetic activation? Grassi and colleagues[112] reported virtually identical values for MSNA in patients with ischemic as compared with dilated cardiomyopathy. By contrast, in a second study involving well-matched treated patients with ischemic and nonischemic dilated cardiomyopathy who were 5 to 10 years younger and whose ejection fractions were substantially lower (22% vs. 33% for the Italian group), MSNA was significantly higher in those with an ischemic cardiomyopathy, and in addition, their VO_2 peak was significantly less.[113]

An increase in efferent sympathetic drive will deplete cardiac glycogen stores and stimulate fatty acid oxidation and ketogenesis; blood ketone bodies in heart failure correlate directly with plasma NE concentrations.[114] In advanced nonischemic cardiomyopathy, increased free radical production and a shift from glucose to greater fatty acid oxidation by underperfused myocytes may stimulate sympathoexcitation.[115]

Excitatory Reflexes Arising from Skeletal Muscle

In heart failure, several sympatho-excitatory stimuli arising from skeletal muscle exhibit the capacity to elevate the central set point for sympathetic outflow (see Figure 12-8). These include (1) increases in local venous pressure; (2) a muscle mechanoreflex elicited by passive exercise, present in heart failure but not control subjects; and (3) a muscle metaboreflex elicited by both isotonic and isometric handgrip.[1] In contrast, a sympathoexcitatory reflex, stimulated by adenosine with the participation of the angiotensin AT_1 receptor, is evident in healthy young subjects but not in HFrEF.[116]

Whether because of diminished skeletal muscle mass, impaired tissue perfusion, earlier development of tissue acidosis, or other metabolic derangement, the muscle metaboreflex, which arises primarily from type IV sensory fibers, is activated at a lower workload in heart failure than in age-matched healthy control subjects.[4,117] Using single-unit MSNA recordings, Murai and colleagues[118] observed that handgrip elicited a greater response in heart failure subjects than healthy controls by increasing firing probability. Importantly, the reflex multiunit MSNA response to exercise and postexercise skeletal muscle ischemia, elicited using a maneuver that traps ischemic metabolites in the forearm, is more prominent in heart failure patients with low peak VO_2 than in patients matched for ejection fraction (<20% in both groups) with VO_2 peak greater than 56% of that predicted by their age, sex, weight, and height (see Figure 12-4).[4] This latter finding implies that comparisons between individuals of sympathetic activation obtained only under resting conditions underestimate the magnitude and adverse consequences of sympathetic activation when such heart failure patients are physically active.

Excitatory Reflexes Arising from the Kidney

Renal afferents are predominantly myelinated fibers that discharge in response to increased intrarenal pressure, systemic hypotension, and renal ischemia. The chemoreceptor element is stimulated physiologically by bradykinin, adenosine, urea, and other mediators, resulting in ipsilateral and contralateral renal neural responses. The systemic response elicited is sympatho-excitatory.[119,120] This reflex pathway may assume greater functional importance in HFrEF patients with renal insufficiency or elevated right atrial pressure. In a Japanese cohort involving 101 heart failure patients, renal insufficiency was the only variable that predicted independently MSNA magnitude.[89] In a recent study in which MSNA was significantly greater in those heart failure patients who also had chronic reductions in creatinine clearance, inhalation of 100% oxygen reduced MSNA only in the latter group, indicating an important interaction with the arterial chemoreflex,[106] and in those with "cardiorenal anemia syndrome" with the arterial baroreflex as well.[121]

Sleep-Related Breathing Disorders

Sympathetic outflow, heart rate, stroke volume, and systemic vascular resistance all diminish during normal non–rapid eye movement (non-REM) sleep. Blood pressure typically falls 20% to 25% from average waking levels.[122] Arterial baroreflex vagal control of heart rate is augmented.[123] Paroxysms of sympathetic discharge provoking surges in heart rate and blood pressure occur during rapid eye movement (REM) sleep,[124] but in general REM comprises only 15% of sleep time. Systolic dysfunction itself is associated with briefer sleep duration and interrupted sleep,[125] resulting in a greater integrated daily adrenergic burden. In the contemporary era of drug and device therapy, there is an approximately 50% probability of detecting sleep apnea in a chronic symptomatic HFrEF patient.[126]

By deactivating pulmonary stretch receptors and stimulating peripheral and central chemoreceptors by hypoxia and hypercapnia, each pause in breathing during sleep elicits profound increases in MSNA. Such sympathetic excitation is independent of and in addition to any reflex responses to mechanoreceptor unloading resulting from pump failure or systemic hypotension in heart failure. Inspiratory efforts against a collapsed upper airway, as occurs in obstructive sleep apnea (OSA), will generate extreme negative swings in intrathoracic pressure (i.e., an abrupt increase in left ventricular afterload). Because the failing heart is more sensitive to increases in afterload, obstruction provokes an acute fall in stroke volume and diastolic blood pressure. This unloading of arterial baroreceptors elicits a reflex increase in MSNA of greater intensity in heart failure than in control subjects with normal left ventricular function, who are better able to maintain stable systemic blood pressure in the face of this mechanical stimulus.[127] Arousal from sleep, which terminates an apneic event, is accompanied by a further surge in central sympathetic outflow, a rise in blood pressure above awake levels, and a decrease in heart rate variability because of concurrent reduction in vagal tone.[128] In severely affected patients, these cycles of apnea and arousal recur repeatedly over the course of each night, exposing the failing heart and peripheral circulation during sleep to more NE than is necessary for circulatory homeostasis.

In patients with OSA but normal left ventricular function studied while awake, the after-effects of these nocturnal sympatho-excitatory stimuli include sustained increases in MSNA during wakefulness.[129] Continuous nocturnal and daytime exposure to heightened adrenergic drive represents an important stimulus to chronic hypertension and potentially myocyte dysfunction and heart failure.[128]

Coexisting obesity and hypertension are important clues to the presence of obstructive sleep apnea in patients with left ventricular systolic dysfunction. Grassi and colleagues[90] described higher daytime MSNA in heart failure patients with obesity or hypertension, but did not report the prevalence of sleep apnea in this population. In a study involving 60 heart failure patients, of whom 43 had an apnea-hypopnea index (AHI) of 15 events per hour or more,[130] MSNA during wakefulness was significantly higher in those with sleep apnea. In those with predominantly OSA, MSNA was increased by 11 bursts/100 heartbeats; when OSA was abolished in a subset of such patients by 1 month of continuous positive airway pressure (CPAP), MSNA fell by 12 bursts/100 heartbeats.[130,131] In the absence of sleep apnea, MSNA of treated heart failure patients is not appreciably greater than that of age-matched control subjects (**Figure 12-12**). Such data provide important evidence in human heart failure for convergence, on central sympathetic neurons, of input from two independent sympatho-excitatory influences (heart failure and sleep apnea), which interact to increase MSNA through a process of additive summation[132] (**Figure 12-13**). Mortality rates in patients with untreated OSA and heart failure are greater than those of heart failure patients without OSA,[133] suggesting that this additional OSA-mediated sympatho-excitation has the independent potential to accelerate the progression of systolic dysfunction. Patients with ischemic cardiomyopathy and sleep apnea are at particular risk of premature death.[134]

Over the course of their sleep, some patients transition from predominantly obstructive apnea to mostly central events. This procession is accompanied by prolongation of circulation time and a reduction in P_{CO_2} below the threshold for apnea.[135] These observations suggest that these repetitive increases in left ventricular afterload during airway obstructions cause systolic function to deteriorate over the course of the night, with increased venous return and left ventricular filling pressure stimulating hyperventilation and hypocapnia. Should this pattern progress over a period of months or years, the coexistence of obstructive apnea could predispose heart failure patients to worsening left ventricular systolic function and central sleep apnea (CSA).

Compared with heart failure patients matched for ejection fraction and other clinical characteristics, but without sleep-related breathing disorders, those with CSA have higher nocturnal urinary NE excretion, and increased plasma NE concentrations while awake. The magnitude of such activation is proportional to the frequency of arousal from sleep, and the degree of apnea-related hypopnea.[136] MSNA during wakefulness is also greater in heart failure

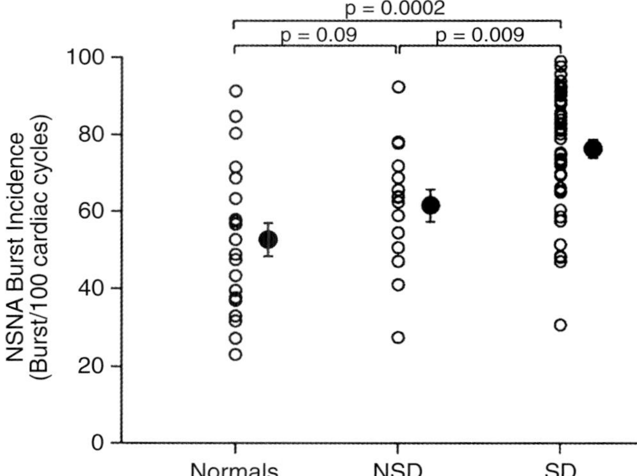

FIGURE 12-12 Scattergrams and means ± standard errors for muscle sympathetic burst incidence (bursts/100 cardiac cycles) in treated HFrEF patients with SD and with no (NSD) sleep-related breathing disorders, as compared with age-matched healthy laboratory controls. Note that MSNA in treated HFrEF patients without sleep apnea is not significantly greater than that of healthy subjects, whereas the coexistence of sleep apnea with heart failure is accompanied by significantly higher MSNA. *From Floras JS: Sympathetic nervous system activation in human heart failure. Clinical implications of an updated model. J Am Coll Cardiol 54:375–385, 2009, with permission of the American College of Cardiology Foundation.*

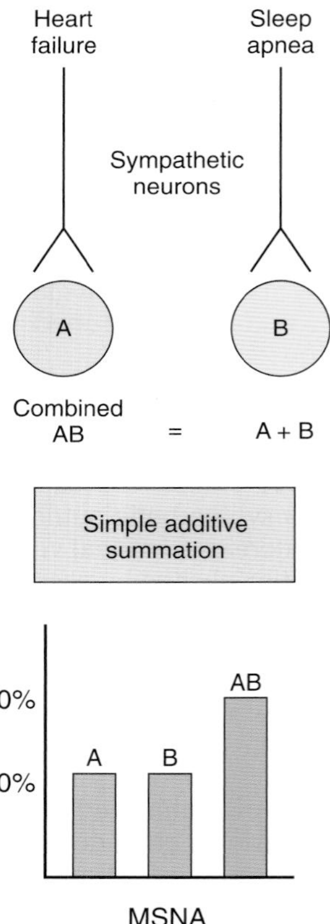

FIGURE 12-13 Convergence of afferent input from two sets of reflexes (in this example, heart failure and sleep apnea), eliciting directionally similar (in this example, excitatory) effects on muscle sympathetic nerve activity (MSNA), may summate and interact centrally through mutual inhibition (redundancy), simple additive summation, or mutual facilitation. The difference in MSNA recorded during wakefulness in heart failure patients with and without obstructive sleep apnea (OSA)[130] is eliminated when OSA is abolished.[131] This finding is consistent with the concept that these two sympatho-excitatory stimuli interact through a process of simple additive summation. *Reproduced with permission of the author. Copyright © 2016 John Floras. All rights reserved.*

patients with, than without, CSA.[130] Mansfield and colleagues[137] reported higher rates of cardiac and total body NE spillover in heart failure patients with CSA than in those without CSA or with OSA, and attributed such differences to greater hemodynamic decompensation in those with CSA. Cardiac washout rate of ^{123}I-MIBG also has been shown to be greater in heart failure patients with central apnea than in those with OSA or without a sleep-related breathing disorder.[138]

As heart failure becomes more symptomatic, ventilatory and sympathetic neural responses to central chemoreceptor stimulation by hypercapnia are augmented[103,107,139] and within-breath sympatho-inhibition is attenuated.[139] An increase in the gain of the central chemoreflex response to CO_2 could assist in establishing the cyclical breathing oscillations characteristic of central sleep apnea; apneas act, in turn, to further stimulate central sympathetic outflow, with exaggerated sympatho-excitation[139] and carryover of high MSNA into the awake state.[130,136] In a recent series, comprising 60 consecutive patients with class I-III heart failure (mean LVEF 31%) receiving contemporary therapy, 47% exhibited increased sensitivity to hypercapnia.[103] Extension of this cohort to 110 consecutive patients, followed a mean of 29 months, reported a 4-year survival of only 49% for those with increased sensitivity to both hypoxia and hypercapnia, as compared with 100% survival in those with normal chemosensitivity.[63]

Central Integration and Interactions

Information arising from baroreceptor and chemoreceptor inputs is integrated within the nucleus tractus solitarius, which then regulates, via projection to the caudal then rostral ventrolateral medullae (VLM), discharge of sympathetic preganglionic neurons in the intermediolateral cell column of the spinal cord. Adjacent respiratory centers, suprabulbar subcortical regions, and a cortical network recently mapped using functional magnetic resonance imaging[140] all interact with brainstem motoneurons to reset the magnitude of central sympathetic outflow to modulate such discharge during both wakefulness and sleep.[141,142]

Experimental Heart Failure Models

Central alterations in the gain of the arterial or cardiopulmonary baroreflex modulation of sympathetic outflow are not accessible to study in humans, but in experimental heart failure models, Zucker's group has documented central augmentation of cardiac sympathetic afferent reflex regulation of renal sympathetic nerve activity, arising from increases in central angiotensin II, decreases in local synthesis of neuronal NO, which exerts sympathoinhibitory actions at several brain sites, generation of reactive oxygen species, and activation of rho kinase. These actions and interactions have important sympatho-excitatory consequences.[143-145]

Angiotensin II inhibits vagal discharge, increases central sympathetic outflow, and interacts with the arterial baroreflex at several sites within and outside the blood-brain barrier.[144,146,147] In dogs without heart failure, the hypotensive response to chronic carotid baroreceptor stimulation is attenuated if angiotensin II is infused concurrently.[148] The cardiac sympathetic afferent reflex in dogs is potentiated by chronic central infusion of angiotensin II[149]; in rats with chronic heart failure, this reflex can be normalized by central administration of antisense oligodeoxynucleotides to AT_1 receptor mRNA.[150] By contrast, in the ovine paced heart failure model, cardiac but not renal sympathetic nerve activity was increased significantly relative to healthy controls; only the former was attenuated by acute intracerebroventricular infusion of losartan.[30] Sympathetically mediated increases in renal renin release in heart failure could therefore generate a positive feedback loop, amplifying sympathetic outflow discharge through these central actions of angiotensin II.

In a rat model of HFrEF, an increase in renal sympathetic outflow and resetting of its regulation by the arterial baroreceptor reflex could be reversed by intracerebroventricular infusion of Fab fragments (to inhibit ouabain-like activity), inhibitors of angiotensin II AT_1 receptor function,[150-152] or an angiotensin-converting enzyme inhibitor[153] and was not observed in transgenic rats deficient in brain angiotensinogen.[154] In a rabbit heart failure model, sympatho-excitation resulted from increased rostral VLM angiotensin AT_1 receptor and NAD(P)H oxidase subunit gene expression with consequent upregulation of superoxide production.[155] This excitatory pathway can be countered by chronic administration of lipophilic statins.[156] Zucker's group has proposed that increased central angiotensin II in heart failure initiates a positive feedback loop involving a reactive oxygen species pathway that may regulate neuronal excitability by modulation of ion channel function. In this model, increased central enhancement of the gain of the cardiac reflex, rather than loss of arterial baroreceptor input,[67] contributes to the increased set point for sympathetic outflow in chronic heart failure.[144]

Central mineralocorticoid receptors also participate in the regulation of sympathetic outflow. In rats with experimental heart failure, intracerebroventricular infusion of spironolactone reduced renal sympathetic nerve firing and augmented its arterial baroreflex regulation.[157] Aldosterone of adrenal origin is capable of stimulating the brain renin-angiotensin system by increasing paraventricular (hypothalamic) nucleus angiotensin AT_1 receptor mRNA, protein, and NAD(P)H oxidase subunit gene expression, and concurrently plasma NE concentrations.[158]

Determining mechanisms by which immune and inflammatory mechanisms initiate centrally mediated sympatho-excitation has been the recent focus of several prominent laboratories. There is now compelling evidence that a bidirectional relationship between the adaptive and innate immune system and the sympathetic nervous system with central neural angiotensin II at its crux is fundamental to the pathophysiology of hypertension.[159,160] There is, in parallel, extensive literature concerning reflex vagal control of immunity.[161] Such interactions are likely to induce similar adrenergic and vagal disturbances in HFrEF.[162] A central cytokine-mediated sympatho-excitatory pathway has been shown active in experimental heart failure. This can be attenuated by anti-inflammatory cytokines,[163] by mineralocorticoid receptor blockade,[164] or by ablation of the forebrain subfornical organ, which lacks a blood-brain barrier.[165]

Clinical Studies

By measuring NE appearance rates in the internal jugular vein, along with those of its lipophilic metabolites, 3-methoxy-4-hydroxyphenylglycol (MHPG) and 3,4-dihydroxyphenylglycol (DHPG), Esler's group has demonstrated significant increases in human heart failure in internal jugular spillover of MHPG, DHPG, epinephrine, and the serotonin metabolite, 5-HIAA,[69,166] and a significant positive correlation between brain NE turnover and cardiac NE spillover.[166] Selective sampling of venous effluent from cortical and subcortical regions detected fourfold higher suprabulbar subcortical turnover of NE in treated heart failure patients than in control subjects.[167] Cortical NE turnover tended to be lower. Furthermore, there was a significant positive correlation between subcortical NE turnover and total body NE spillover in the HRrEF group, an observation consistent with these authors' hypothesis that activation of noradrenergic neurons projecting rostrally from the brainstem mediates sympathetic excitation in heart failure. Because of their participation in arousal, vigilance, and circulatory control in the rat, brain norepinephrine nuclei in the locus coeruleus have received particular attention.[168] Chronic sleep disruption in heart failure (even in the absence of nocturnal breathing disorders)[125] may establish a state of heightened arousal, increasing adrenergic drive as a consequence. In patients with both heart failure and obstructive sleep apnea, there is an inverse relationship between MSNA and a subjective measure of daytime sleepiness.[169]

Efferent Mechanisms

Ganglionic Neurotransmission

The principal defect in the parasympathetic modulation of heart rate in experimental heart failure appears to lie at the level of vagal ganglionic neurotransmission.[64] Conversely, by stimulating sympathetic ganglionic and adrenomedullary neurotransmission, increases in angiotensin II in heart failure could augment NE and epinephrine release.[146]

Prejunctional Mechanisms and Efferent Sympatho-Vagal Interactions

In the hamster model of dilated cardiomyopathy, early increases in cardiac NE turnover, tyrosine hydroxylase and dopamine β-hydroxylase activity, and cardiac dopamine stores are followed by depletion of myocardial NE content and destruction of sympathetic nerve terminals.[48] In a rabbit model of pacing-induced heart failure, ventricular systolic dysfunction and an increase in plasma NE were followed by a reduction in cardiac NE uptake and transporter density, and a subsequent decrease in myocardial β-receptor density, with gradual normalization after pacing ended.[170]

In humans, abnormalities in efferent cardiac sympathetic nerve function assume greater importance as heart failure advances, as reduced NE uptake-1 carrier density would cause transcardiac myocardial extraction to fall, and CNES to increase more than the nerve firing rate and neurotransmitter release. Radio-ligand binding experiments in ventricles derived from patients with class II to IV HFrEF detected a significant decrease of up to 30% in NE uptake-1 carrier density.[171] Isotopic dilution studies have identified reduced efficiency of NE uptake, such that its spillover into the coronary sinus was increased disproportionately more than its neuronal release.[172] Rundqvist and associates[3] calculated the fractional extraction of NE to be 87% in healthy controls, but only 60% in heart failure patients. Abnormalities of cardiac NE imaging kinetics—such as the ^{123}I-MIBG heart/mediastinum uptake ratio and defect score, which can identify individuals at increased risk for malignant ventricular arrhythmias and premature cardiac death[27,173]—improve with chronic β-adrenoceptor blockade,[174] and in patients with heart failure and preserved systolic function, with the angiotensin II AT_1 receptor antagonist, candesartan.[45]

The release of NE from sympathetic nerve endings and the discharge of acetylcholine from vagal nerves also can be augmented or suppressed by endogenous or exogenously administered agonists, acting on a wide variety of prejunctional receptors. NE release from cardiac, intrathoracic, and peripheral sympathetic nerve endings can be facilitated if prejunctional β_2-adrenoceptors are stimulated by its endogenous agonist, epinephrine.[33,175-177] In more advanced heart failure, circulating epinephrine may be transported into sympathetic nerve terminals, incorporated into vesicles along with NE, and released as a cotransmitter[178] with a potential prejunctional sympatho-facilitatory action.[175]

In contrast, α_2-adrenoceptor agonists, such as clonidine, inhibit NE release. Observations concerning the functional importance of such inhibition in human heart failure suggest regional selectivity, with left ventricular[179] but not forearm α_2-adrenoceptors[180] retaining this inhibitory capacity.

Polymorphisms of prejunctional adrenergic receptors might contribute to interindividual variation in NE release. In a retrospective genetic-association study, Small et al[181] detected a 6-fold increase in the risk of developing heart failure in black subjects homozygous for the hypofunctioning prejunctional α_{2C} Del322-325 polymorphism, and a 10-fold increase in those who were also homozygous for the hyperfunctional postjunctional β_1Arg329 receptor. The latter demonstrates greater affinity in vivo for adenylyl cyclase and augmented generation of contractile force in right ventricular trabeculae of nonfailing and failing hearts exposed to isoproterenol.[182] These authors proposed that this increased risk for heart failure resulted from a synergistic enhancement of polymorphisms within these two adrenergic signal-transduction pathways. However, in this initial report, no direct functional data concerning cardiac NE release or postjunctional responsiveness (e.g., heart rate) was provided.[181] By contrast, in healthy subjects, variability in the blood pressure and plasma NE response to the selective α_2-agonist dexmedetomidine was unaffected by this genotype.[183] In a cohort of patients with severe heart failure, Kaye and associates[184] detected no relationship between the α_{2C} Del322-325 or β_2-adrenoceptor polymorphisms and the rate of cardiac NE release. Curiously, the relationship between NE release and heart rate was steeper in β_2-adrenoceptor Arg 16 homozygotes, implying increased postjunctional responsiveness.

Muscarinic M_2 receptors on adrenergic nerve endings also attenuate NE release when stimulated by acetylcholine. In subjects with impaired left ventricular systolic function and increased cardiac adrenergic drive, intracoronary infusion of acetylcholine decreased cardiac NE spillover, an effect not seen in control subjects with normal left ventricular systolic function. Receptor blockade with atropine had no effect in the heart failure group, but increased cardiac NE spillover in control subjects.[185] Conversely, increased NE release from sympathetic nerve endings inhibits acetylcholine release by stimulating prejunctional α_1-adrenoceptors on vagal nerve endings.[186]

Neuregulin-1 signaling has been identified as an important antiadrenergic pathway, requiring eNOS-mediated muscarinic receptor activation. Neuregulin-1 expression initially increases, then decreases with the development of congestive heart failure.[187] In advanced HFrEF, other sympathetic neurotransmitters, such as NPY, also may exert a vagolytic action by inhibiting acetylcholine release.[188,189] In experimental preparations, prejunctional AT_1 receptors have been shown to facilitate neural and adrenal release of catecholamines when stimulated by angiotensin II,[146] but this action has yet to be detected in human HFrEF.[116,190] Circulating activating antibodies against β_1 and/or β_2 adrenoceptors, present in the same patients with dilated cardiomyopathy, can mimic a state of marked sympatho-excitation.[191]

THERAPEUTIC IMPLICATIONS

Parenteral positive inotropic agents were among the earliest therapies for heart failure. Acutely, dobutamine infusion causes a significant reduction in cardiac NE spillover, an effect attributed to reductions in cardiac filling pressures, and activation of ventricular mechanoreceptors.[192] However, the long-term administration of sympathomimetics has been shown consistently to increase mortality, and the application of isotope dilution methodology to heart failure patients disproved the concept that the failing heart required inotropic support to compensate for sympathetic denervation. Use of these agents is now restricted to short-term palliation.

Contemporary autonomic management of heart failure is predicated upon three concepts: (1) in most patients, the magnitude of sympathetic activation exceeds that required to maintain cardiovascular homeostasis; (2) the adrenergic and parasympathetic disturbances of HFrEF are not irreversible; and (3) pharmacologic, behavioral, and device interventions that attenuate sympatho-excitation or augment vagal tone will improve symptoms and prognosis.

Pharmacologic Interventions

Several heart failure therapies counter (directly or indirectly) the adverse effects of excessive cardiac and sympathetic activity or augment vagal tone, or both, yielding improved symptoms or prognosis (see Figure 12-8). β-adrenoceptor antagonists do not alter MSNA,[193] but address the earliest autonomic disturbances identified in HFrEF by shielding the heart from the adverse consequences of sympathetic overactivity by augmenting tonic and reflex heart rate modulation while preserving normal homeostatic oscillations in MSNA,[194] and by attenuating β_1-mediated stimulation of renin. Landmark placebo-controlled trials involving carvedilol, bisoprolol, and metoprolol have demonstrated the symptom, hemodynamic, and mortality benefits of long-term β_1- and nonselective β-blockade for patients with heart failure caused by depressed left ventricular systolic function (see Chapter 34). Unlike metoprolol, carvedilol decreases total body and cardiac NE spillover by a third, presumably because of the blockade of sympathetic prejunctional β_2-adrenoceptors that facilitate neural NE release.[193]

Importantly, β-adrenoceptor blockade does not shield the heart, kidney, or periphery from α-adrenoceptor-mediated vasoconstriction or renal sodium retention (carvedilol's peripheral α-blocking actions diminish over time[195]), or from vasoconstriction caused by neurotransmitters coreleased with norepinephrine such as ATP[196] or neuropeptide Y (NPY), which exerts a more sustained vasoconstrictor response than NE.[197] Myocardial NPY spillover is increased in human HFrEF.[198]

Pharmacologic strategies to restore autonomic balance include sensitization of baroreceptor afferents by digitalis[199,200]; relief of congestion[201] and central sleep apnea[202] through diuresis; countering the central and peripheral sympatho-excitatory and vagolytic effects of angiotensin AT_1 receptor stimulation using angiotensin-converting enzyme inhibitors,[70,203] angiotensin receptor antagonists,[144,204,205] or mineralocorticoid receptor antagonists[206]; and exploiting sympatho-modulatory properties of amiodarone.[207] Importantly, none of these therapies addresses directly nonbaroreflex stimuli to sympathetic nervous system activation, such as skeletal muscle mechano- and metabo-reflexes that augment sympathoneural responses to exercise or the coexistence of sleep-related breathing disorders. Identification of such specific sympatho-excitatory pathophysiology in individual patients affords the opportunity to add, as adjunctive treatment, targeted therapy.

Positing (incorrectly, as indicated earlier) that peripheral sympathetic drive is excessive in all treated HRrEF patients, and that its antagonism will be universally beneficial, more aggressive neurohumoral blockade, or central abolition of sympathetic outflow, or both, has been proposed as a means of further reducing mortality rates. Central sympathetic outflow can be attenuated directly by stimulating α_2 and imidazoline I_1 receptors located within the rostral VLM using either clonidine, an $\alpha_2 + I_1$ receptor agonist, or I_1 agonists such as moxonidine. When given intravenously, 0.1 mg clonidine lowered arterial NE concentrations, cardiac NE spillover, and left ventricular +dP/dt by 47%, 58%, and 15%, respectively,[208] and when administered for 2 months via transdermal patch 0.1 mg of daily clonidine reduced muscle sympathetic burst frequency by 26% and plasma NE concentrations by 47%.[209] However, in both a pilot study[210] and in a large-scale mortality trial[211] there was an excess of deaths in patients allocated moxonidine. In retrospect, this outcome may relate more to the specific aspects of these two trials, than to the validity of the hypothesis that prompted these studies.[74] In many study patients prerandomization NE concentrations were not elevated. The moxonidine dose selected appears to have been sympatho-ablative, perhaps preventing appropriate increases in neurotransmitter release in response to exercise or other stimuli, whereas unpredictable nonadherence would have caused intense rebound surges in NE, heart rate, blood pressure, and ventricular ectopy.[210] When bucindolol was trialed in HFrEF, a marked fall was noted in plasma NE concentration accompanied by an increase in mortality.[212] Although interpreted as "sympatholysis," plasma measurements alone cannot determine whether this reduction resulted from diminished sympathetic outflow, less neural NE release, or increased NE clearance. The hypothesis that targeting directly central sympathetic outflow will improve prognosis is unlikely to be affirmed until a definitive and practical biomarker for sympathetic activation becomes available for routine clinical deployment.

Nonpharmacologic Interventions

HFrEF patients at highest risk because of specific sympatho-excitatory pathophysiology may be offered also personalized intervention designed to diminish sympathetic tone or augment tonic or reflex vagal heart rate modulation, such as by alleviating chronic myocardial ischemia; normalizing elevated cardiac filling pressure[82]; initiating exercise rehabilitation[213,214]; or treating coexisting obstructive sleep apnea.[131,215]

Exercise Training

Several groups have reported beneficial neuromodulatory effects of chronic exercise training in HFrEF heart failure, but the number of subjects studied thus far is small.[213,216] Experimental mechanisms shown to participate in such sympatho-inhibition include mitigation of central neural oxidative stress and angiotensin AT_1 receptor upregulation, normalization of altered nitric oxide metabolism, and GABA- and glutamate-mediated cardiovascular neurotransmission, diminution of peripheral chemosensitivity, reduction of renal sympathetic nerve-mediated sodium and water accumulation retention, and generalized improvement in baroreceptor and chemoreceptor reflex regulation of the heart and circulation.[217] Four months of exercise training reduced the apnea-hypopnea index and the MSNA of HFrEF patients with OSA. It reduced also the MSNA of those with CSA, but had no effect on their apnea-hypopnea index.[218]

Carotid Baroreceptor Stimulation

Demonstration, in human heart failure, that the arterial baroreflex modulation of sympathetic outflow is preserved provides a compelling physiologic rationale to investigate in this condition the autonomic, hemodynamic, and clinical impact of electrical activation of carotid sinus nerves. Recent technical advances permit safe and durable bilateral or unilateral stimulation. In clinical trials involving patients with drug-resistant hypertension, acute stimulation lowered MSNA and blood pressure[219] and increased the relative balance between vagal and sympathetic heart rate modulation[220]; chronic afferent nerve stimulation caused sustained reductions in blood pressure in the majority of treated patients.[221] In dogs with experimental chronic heart failure, carotid baroreceptor activation was accompanied by lower plasma NE and angiotensin II concentrations and significantly longer survival relative to unstimulated control dogs.[76] The ongoing randomized XR-1 study (NCT01471860) is evaluating in NYHA class III patients the effect of 6 months of carotid sinus stimulation, using a novel implantable device, on left ventricular ejection fraction.

Carotid Body Denervation

In both rabbit and rat models of experimental heart failure, carotid body denervation improved autonomic cardiovascular modulation, the density of arrhythmia, and the apnea-hypopnea index.[222,223] When ablation was performed 2 weeks after coronary artery ligation, there was relative preservation of ventricular structure and function; survival improved by approximately 90%.[222] After reviewing extant experimental and clinical literature and preventing genetic sympathetically mediated hypertension with bilateral section of carotid sinus nerves,[224] Paton and colleagues proposed targeting the carotid body of HFrEF patients with increased chemosensitivity as a means of attenuating their sympatho-excitation[225] and sleep-disordered breathing.[226] The future of this line of investigation is at present difficult to predict. A clinical trial (NCT01653821) involving the surgical removal of the carotid body in patients with impaired left ventricular systolic function is currently enrolling participants.

Cardiac Resynchronization Therapy
(see also Chapter 35)

Biventricular pacing has been shown to raise systemic arterial pressure acutely, without affecting central venous pressure, with a resultant fall in MSNA[227] and augmented tonic and reflex vagal heart rate modulation.[228] In an uncontrolled trial, 10 weeks of resynchronization was found in 11 patients to lower mean MSNA by approximately 30%[229]; whether such reduction can be sustained over a longer period has yet to be determined in a randomized controlled trial. In a prospective study in which 45 consecutive patients were restudied 6 months after receiving cardiac resynchronization-defibrillator devices, group mean time domain indices of vagal heart rate modulation and ^{123}I-MIBG estimates of cardiac sympathetic nerve terminal function were improved but in a substantial minority biventricular pacing did not affect ^{123}I-MIBG kinetics, and plasma concentrations of nerve growth factor, a sympathetic neurotrophin, were unchanged.[230] Importantly, the prevalence of obstructive and central sleep apnea is not affected by biventricular pacing; in a cohort of 472 patients screened for sleep-disordered breathing 6 months after cardiac resynchronization-defibrillator implantation, the AHI exceeded 5 events/hr in 80%, and was greater than 15 events/hr in 64%.[231]

Noninvasive Ventilation

There is increasing recognition of the importance of identifying and treating OSA when present in heart failure patients. Conventional pharmacologic approaches to HFrEF have no impact on OSA. By contrast, nocturnal nasal continuous positive airway pressure (CPAP) abolishes upper airway obstruction and four of its sympatho-excitatory consequences: apnea, hypoxia, hypercapnia, and arousal from sleep. In patients with heart failure and obstructive sleep apnea, CPAP reduces nocturnal blood pressure and heart rate, and increases arterial baroreflex modulation of heart rate.[232] Thus the sympatho-inhibitory and vagotonic effects of CPAP during sleep alone may be sufficient to benefit heart failure patients with coexisting OSA. By reducing, when present, right ventricular constraint on left ventricular filling, positive airway pressure acutely increases stroke volume and cardiac output; this in turn should reduce central sympathetic outflow reflexively.

In randomized trials of 1-month duration involving heart failure patients with OSA, nightly use of CPAP abolished apnea; improved left ventricular structure and ejection fraction[215]; lowered systolic blood pressure, heart rate, and MSNA during wakefulness[131,215]; and reduced ventricular ectopy during sleep.[233] A randomized controlled trial involving patients with milder OSA (apnea-hypopnea index >5 events/hr) and a left ventricular ejection fraction less than 55% also observed a significant increase in left ventricular ejection fraction, in conjunction with a reduction in urinary NE excretion after 3 months of CPAP treatment.[234] Data from a nonrandomized observational study involving OSA subjects with HFrEF suggest that abolition of apneas by CPAP may improve survival.[133] In a 3-month randomized trial involving heart failure patients with CSA, the nightly application of CPAP suppressed the apnea-hypopnea index and reduced nocturnal urinary NE by 41% to values similar to those obtained in clinically matched heart failure patients without CSA. CPAP also reduced plasma NE during wakefulness by 22%.[136] In a long-term trial involving 258 heart failure patients with CSA, CPAP did not improve transplant-free survival overall,[235] but this intervention reduced the AHI from 40 to only 20 events per hour. Investigators in this field are encouraged by a post hoc efficacy analysis, which revealed that CPAP improved significantly transplant-free survival of those patients in whom the AHI was suppressed below 15 apneic or hypopneic events per hour, the threshold for recruitment into the CANPAP trial.[236]

Adaptive servo-ventilation (ASV), which provides both end-expiratory pressure support to abolish obstructive apnea and volume or flow-triggered ventilation to counter central apnea, was developed to provide more effective suppression of Cheyne-Stokes respiration.[237] In a randomized trial involving 31 patients, ASV achieved greater compliance, improvement in ejection fraction, and quality of life scores than CPAP, but had no significant impact on overnight urinary NE excretion.[238] In a nonrandomized 6-month comparative study, plasma NE was reduced significantly in those accepting ASV,[239] and in another nonrandomized protocol, cardiac ^{123}I-MIBG kinetics were improved if ASV was used.[240] The hypothesis that treating heart failure patients with either OSA or CSA with ASV will reduce a composite primary endpoint comprising death, cardiac transplantation, left ventricular assist device implantation, and cardiovascular hospitalization is being tested, presently, in a multinational clinical trial (ADVENT-HF NCT01128816).

Vagal Stimulation

Several studies involving cervical vagal nerve stimulation in animal heart failure models have demonstrated less autonomic imbalance, inflammation, and ventricular remodeling and improved survival.[241,242] A clinical multicenter open-label study involving a small series of HFrEF subjects has reported, after 1 year of stimulation, significant improvement in left ventricular ejection fraction (from 21% to 34%), a 9-beat/min reduction in heart rate, and augmented vagal heart rate modulation, but also a substantial number of serious adverse effects, including two device-related and three deaths.[243] The INcrease Of VAgal TonE in CHF (INNOVATE-HF [NCT01037181]) is an ongoing randomized multicenter trial that will assess the impact of chronic vagal pacing on a primary combined endpoint of all-cause mortality and heart failure hospitalization.[244] This and similar studies provide as well an opportunity to test the concept that human immune system function is subject to modulation by the autonomic nervous system.[159,161]

Renal Denervation

That the renal sympathetic nerves play a fundamental role in the pathophysiology, prognosis, and therapy of heart failure is now well established. Renal efferent sympathetics are predominantly unmyelinated fibers innervating the kidney's proximal and distal tubules with catecholamine containing nerve terminals. Exhibiting pulse-synchronous firing, modulated by arterial and atrial baroreceptor reflex input, breathing, muscle contraction, and other stimuli, they increase proportionally to discharge frequency, renin release (β_1-mediated), renal tubular sodium and water reabsorption (α_1-mediated), and renal vascular resistance (α_1-mediated).[245] A randomized controlled trial of heart failure patients requiring high doses of furosemide for clinical stability has revealed the important restraint the renal nerves impose upon both natriuresis and diuresis.[246] In the presence of chronic β-adrenoceptor antagonism, increased renal NE spillover relates inversely to the endpoint risk of early death and transplantation.[59] Accumulation of evidence that renal denervation can reverse the pathologic sodium and water retention of experimental heart failure, cirrhosis, and nephrotic syndrome[245] stimulated the development of percutaneous, nonsurgical methods to interrupt the renal innervation of humans suffering from conditions characterized by inappropriate sympatho-excitation.

Several methods now are available for clinical or research purposes. The greatest cumulative clinical experience, thus far, has been with a radiofrequency generator attached to a 108-cm catheter with a monopolar radiopaque platinum electrode at its distal tip that is advanced sequentially into the renal arteries under fluoroscopic guidance. To assess procedural efficacy, renal NE spillover was assessed in 10 drug-resistant patients enrolled in the initial proof-of-principal hypertension study; they were evaluated before and between 15 and 30 days after the denervation. RNES fell, on average by 47%.[247] A number of investigators are investigating currently the therapeutic potential of denervation as a means of countering renin release and renal sodium retention and attenuating cardiac and skeletal muscle vascular sympathetic excitation in heart failure patients who are not hypotensive. A pilot study of 7 patients with a 6-month follow-up established that denervation could be performed safely, without compromising blood pressure or creatinine.[248] These early findings set the stage for future detailed evaluation of the functional autonomic, renal and hemodynamic consequences of this procedure in this population, longer term trials of its effect on cardiovascular outcome, and comparative effectiveness studies relative to carotid baroreceptor stimulation.[249]

SUMMARY AND FUTURE DIRECTIONS

There has been a major shift in our present conception of how neural circulatory regulation becomes disturbed in heart failure. Mechanisms and processes responsible for the autonomic phenotype of heart failure are more nuanced and patient-specific than initially envisaged. Those with left ventricular systolic dysfunction have in common impaired vagal modulation of heart rate, but differ considerably in the magnitude and mechanisms of their sympathetic activation. Although the set point for central sympathetic outflow is increased in the majority of patients, in a substantial minority of those with asymptomatic or symptomatic left ventricular systolic dysfunction plasma NE concentrations, MSNA and total body NE spillover remain within the range described for control subjects. Therefore, sympathetic activation cannot be considered a defining characteristic of left ventricular systolic dysfunction. Many current therapies for HFrEF attenuate adrenergic drive and augment vagal tone. The therapeutic implication of these findings is that patients without evidence for sympathetic activation are unlikely to benefit from multiple neurohumoral antagonists, or from sympatholytic interventions.

Currently evidence in humans permits five conclusions with respect to mechanoreceptor reflex regulation of heart rate and sympathetic nervous system activity in human HFrEF (see Figure 12-8): (1) the arterial baroreceptor reflex regulation of heart rate by the vagus nerve is impaired; (2) in contrast, the arterial baroreflex regulation of MSNA is rapidly responsive to changes in diastolic blood pressure; (3) pulmonary mechanoreceptor-mediated inhibition of sympathetic outflow is preserved; and (4) cardiopulmonary reflex control of MSNA is blunted. As a consequence, efferent sympathetic outflow to the skeletal muscle is not suppressed by increased cardiac filling pressure. Rather,

(5) elevated filling pressures in heart failure can increase cardiac NE spillover by stimulating a cardiac-specific sympatho-excitatory reflex.[1]

Viewed from this perspective, the heterogeneity and time course of organ-specific sympathetic activation and parasympathetic withdrawal can be considered appropriate to individual hemodynamic profiles, as summarized in **Table 12-2**. As shown, patients will progress from asymptomatic to end-stage HFrEF via different pathways, and at different rates. In some, the initial insult may be a sudden drop in cardiac output and blood pressure, which will reflexively activate the sympathetic nervous and renin-angiotensin systems and decrease vagal tone so as to achieve a state of relative compensation. If, on the other hand, relatively normal stroke volume and blood pressure can be maintained by increases in left ventricular end-diastolic volume, rather than cardiac filling pressure, such patients would be less likely to manifest evidence, at rest, for hemodynamically mediated sympathetic activation. As myocardial contractile performance deteriorates, heart rate will rise through arterial baroreflex-mediated vagal withdrawal and sympathetic activation to maintain cardiac output and systemic arterial pressure. Over time, unloading of arterial baroreceptors by a decline in systolic or pulse pressure will elicit further diminution of cardiac vagal modulation, generalized neurohumoral activation (resulting from reflex increases in sympathetic outflow to the heart, kidney, and skeletal muscle), and loss of low-frequency MSNA spectral modulation, due to impaired neuroeffector transduction. By removing the inhibitory or restraining effect of lung inflation on central sympathetic outflow, pulmonary congestion, altered lung mechanics, and increased work of breathing will cause a further step-up in nerve traffic; indeed, it is those patients with short shallow breaths who display the highest values for MSNA.[99] Other sympatho-excitatory co-morbidities that elevate the set point for central sympathetic outflow or neurotransmitter release above levels required to maintain hemodynamic stability may be present, but with considerable variation from patient to patient.

For heart failure with reduced systolic function, it is now evident that several therapies that modulate sympathetic and vagal outflow or antagonize the postjunctional actions of neurally released and circulating catecholamines also decrease morbidity and prolong survival (**Table 12-3**). Whether there is a causal relationship between such autonomic modulation and improved outcomes; whether patients with heart failure but preserved systolic function exhibit similar alterations in sympathetic and parasympathetic function by these several baroreflex- and nonbaroreflex-mediated mechanisms; and whether a robust and scalable biomarker for sympathetic activation in heart failure can be identified, validated, and commercialized, are three important hypotheses for future investigation.

Large randomized trials evaluating the impact of treating sleep apnea on survival and hospitalization, and small studies examining the effects of cardiovascular conditioning on sympathetic responses to muscle exercise are in progress. A range of additional sympatho-modulatory strategies, acting upon autonomic afferents, or within central sites of cardiovascular autonomic regulation, or upon elements of the efferent sympathetic nervous system are currently within the preclinical or clinical stages of investigation (see Table 12-3). Device-effected autonomic modulation, such as by carotid baroreceptor and vagal nerve stimulation, cardiac

TABLE 12-2 Construct Relating Time Course and Heterogeneity of Autonomic Disturbances in Human Heart Failure with Reduced Ejection Fraction to Hemodynamic and Nonhemodynamic Abnormalities

PRIMARY ABNORMALITY	AUTONOMIC CONSEQUENCE
Acute heart failure with pulmonary congestion and hypotension	Generalized activation of sympathetic and renin-angiotensin-aldosterone systems; parasympathetic withdrawal
Chronic increase in left atrial pressure	Activation of cardiac sympathetic afferents causing reflex increase in efferent cardiac SNA Decrease in tonic ± reflex vagal HR modulation Decreased prejunctional muscarinic receptor-mediated inhibition of NE release
Chronic increase in left ventricular end-diastolic pressure and volume	Reflex inhibition of sympathetic outflow to kidneys, skeletal muscle, and other systemic vascular beds
Chronic exposure to increased cardiac SNA	Impaired cardiac β-mediated signal transduction Increased prejunctional α_1-mediated inhibition of Ach release
Chronic reduction in stroke volume and systemic blood pressure	Impaired arterial baroreflex regulation of HR Reflex sympathetic activation resulting from intact and responsive arterial baroreflex regulation of muscle SNA, total body NE spillover, ± cardiac NE spillover, ± renal NE spillover
Pulmonary congestion	Decreased inhibition of central sympathetic outflow by pulmonary stretch reflexes stimulated by lung inflation Decreased respiratory sinus arrhythmia (vagal)
Chemoreceptor and muscle metaboreceptor activation	Increased muscle SNA Decreased tonic and reflex vagal HR modulation
Coexisting sleep apnea	Increased muscle SNA and decreased vagal HR modulation during sleep Increased daytime plasma NE

Ach, Acetylcholine; *HR,* heart rate; *NE,* norepinephrine; *SNA,* sympathetic nerve activity.

TABLE 12-3 Sympathetic Activation in Heart Failure: Therapeutic Opportunities

Afferent Neural Modulation
Cardiac resynchronization therapy
Carotid baroreceptor reflex activation
Carotid chemoreceptor reflex attenuation
Exercise
Renal denervation
Unloading of cardiopulmonary sympatho-excitatory afferents
Vagal nerve stimulation
Central Neural Action
Centrally acting antagonists, antioxidants, inhibitors, and immune modulators
Treating sleep apnea
Efferent Modulation
Adrenergic receptor blockade
Augmented norepinephrine uptake
Augmented vagal neurotransmission
Prejunctional inhibition of norepinephrine release
Renal denervation

resynchronization therapy, and renal and carotid body denervation, has attracted remarkable interest and considerable resources.[250] It is anticipated that these technologies will be deployed beyond animal and human proof-of-principle studies to thoughtful randomized controlled trials with cardiovascular outcome endpoints. Newer devices for the abolition of central and obstructive sleep apnea, such as adaptive servo-ventilation, have the potential to mitigate or reverse central adaptations to chronic intermittent hypoxia, hypercapnia, and arousal that result in daytime as well as nighttime sympathetic activation and vagal inhibition.

This breadth of therapeutic opportunity holds great promise for patients with heart failure, with both impaired and preserved systolic function currently receiving the full benefits of evidence-based contemporary therapy but, because of persistent sympathetic excitation and impaired vagal heart rate modulation, still at high residual risk for increased morbidity, hospitalization, malign arrhythmias, and premature mortality. That sympathetic nervous system activation is fundamental to the pathogenesis, progression, and prognosis of heart failure has been recognized since the early 1980s, but our understanding of the mechanisms responsible and our translation of this knowledge into new therapies continues to evolve. Proving the efficacy of β-adrenergic therapy for large cohorts of patients with impaired systolic function should not be considered the end of this chapter of heart failure research and innovative therapy, but its beginning.

References

1. Floras JS: Sympathetic nervous system activation in human heart failure: clinical implications of an updated model. *J Am Coll Card* 54:375–385, 2009.
2. Kaye DM, Lefkovits J, Jennings GL, et al: Adverse consequences of high sympathetic nervous activity in the failing human heart. *J Am Coll Cardiol* 26:1257–1263, 1995.
3. Rundqvist B, Elam M, Bergman-Sverrisdottir Y, et al: Increased cardiac adrenergic drive precedes generalized sympathetic activation in human heart failure. *Circ* 95:169–175, 1997.
4. Notarius CF, Atchison DJ, Floras JS: Impact of heart failure and exercise capacity on sympathetic response to handgrip exercise. *Am J Physiol* 280:H969–H976, 2001.
5. Esler M: The 2009 Carl Ludwig Lecture: Pathophysiology of the human sympathetic nervous system in cardiovascular disease: the transition from mechanisms to medical management. *J Appl Physiol* 108:227–237, 2010.
6. Brunner-La Rocca HP, Esler MD, Jennings GL, et al: Effect of cardiac sympathetic nervous activity on mode of death in congestive heart failure. *Eur Heart J* 22:1069–1071, 2001.
7. Eisenhofer G, Esler MD, Meredith IT, et al: Sympathetic nervous function in human heart as assessed by cardiac spillovers of dihydroxyphenylglycol and norepinephrine. *Circ* 85:1775–1785, 1992.
8. Wallin BG, Fagius J: Peripheral sympathetic neural activity in conscious humans. *Ann Rev Physiol* 50:565–576, 1988.
9. Elam M, Macefield V: Multiple firing of single muscle vasoconstrictor neurons during cardiac dysrhythmias in human heart failure. *J Appl Physiol* 91:717–724, 2001.
10. Middlekauff HR, Hamilton MA, Stevenson LW, et al: Independent control of skin and muscle sympathetic nerve activity in patients with heart failure. *Circ* 90:1794–1798, 1994.
11. Wallin BG, Thompson JM, Jennings GL, et al: Renal noradrenaline spillover correlates with muscle sympathetic activity in humans. *J Physiol* 491(Pt 3):881–887, 1996.
12. Wallin BG, Esler MD, Dorward P, et al: Simultaneous measurements of cardiac norepinephrine spillover and sympathetic outflow to skeletal muscle. *J Physiol* 453:59–67, 1992.
13. Parati G, Di Rienzo M, Mancia G: How to measure baroreflex sensitivity: from the cardiovascular laboratory to daily life. *J Hypertens* 19:157–161, 2000.
14. Casadei B, Paterson DJ: Should we still use nitrovasodilators to test baroreflex sensitivity? *J Hypertens* 18:3–6, 2000.
15. Grassi G, Seravalle G, Cattaneo BM, et al: Sympathetic activation and loss of reflex sympathetic control in mild congestive heart failure. *Circ* 92:3206–3211, 1995.
16. Imaizumi T, Sugimachi M, Harasawa Y, et al: Contribution of wall mechanics to the dynamic properties of aortic baroreceptor. *Am J Physiol* 264:H872–H880, 1993.
17. Bath E, Lindblad LE, Wallin GB: Effects of dynamic and static neck suction on muscle nerve sympathetic activity, heart rate and blood pressure in man. *J Physiol* 311:551–564, 1981.
18. Ando S, Dajani HR, Senn BL, et al: Sympathetic alternans. Evidence for arterial baroreflex control of muscle sympathetic nerve activity in congestive heart failure. *Circ* 95:316–319, 1997.
19. Despas F, Lamber E, Vaccaro A, et al: Peripheral chemoreflex activation contributes to sympathetic baroreflex impairment in chronic heart failure. *J Hypertens* 30:753–760, 2012.
20. Task force of the European Society of Cardiology and the North American Society of Pacing and Electrophysiology: Heart rate variability. Standards of measurement, physiological interpretation and clinical use. *Circ* 93:1043–1065, 1996.
21. Yamamoto Y, Hughson RL: Coarse-graining spectral analysis: new method for studying heart rate variability. *J Appl Physiol* 71:1143–1150, 1991.
22. Butler GC, Ando SI, Floras JS: Fractal component of variability of heart rate and systolic blood pressure in congestive heart failure. *Clin Sci* 92:543–550, 1997.
23. Notarius CF, Floras JS: Limitations of the use of spectral analysis of heart rate variability for the estimation of cardiac sympathetic activity in heart failure. *Europace* 3:29–38, 2001.
24. Pagani M, Montano N, Porta A, et al: Relationship between spectral components of cardiovascular variabilities and direct measures of muscle sympathetic nerve activity in humans. *Circ* 95:1441–1448, 1997.
25. Ando S, Dajani HR, Floras JS: Frequency domain characteristics of muscle sympathetic nerve activity in heart failure and healthy humans. *Am J Physiol* 273:R205–R212, 1997.
26. Pitzalis MV, Mastropasqua F, Passantino A, et al: Comparison between noninvasive indices of baroreceptor sensitivity and the phenylephrine method in post-myocardial infarction patients. *Circ* 97:1362–1367, 1998.
27. Jacobson AF, Senior R, Cerqueira MD, et al: Myocardial iodine-123 meta-iodobenzylguanidine imaging and cardiac events in heart failure. Results of the prospective ADMIRE-HF (AdreView Myocardial Imaging for Risk Evaluation in Heart Failure) study. *J Am Coll Card* 55:2212–2221, 2010.
28. Fallavollita JA, Heavey BM, Luisi AJ, et al: Regional myocardial sympathetic denervation predicts the risk of sudden cardiac arrest in ischemic cardiomyopathy. *J Am Coll Cardiol* 63:141–149, 2014.
29. Ramchandra R, Hood SG, Denton DA, et al: Basis for the preferential activation of cardiac sympathetic nerve activity in heart failure. *Proc Natl Acad Sci USA* 106:924–928, 2009.
30. Ramchandra R, Hood SG, Watson AM, et al: Central angiotensin type 1 receptor blockade decreases cardiac but not renal sympathetic nerve activity in heart failure. *Hypertension* 59:634–641, 2012.
31. Osborn JW, Kuroki MT: Sympathetic signatures of cardiovascular disease: a blueprint for development of targeted sympathetic ablation therapies. *Hypertension* 59:545–547, 2012.
32. Kaye DM, Lefkovits J, Cox H, et al: Regional epinephrine kinetics in human heart failure: evidence for extra-adrenal, nonneural release. *Am J Physiol* 269:H182–H188, 1995.
33. Esler M, Eisenhofer G, Chin J, et al: Is adrenaline released by sympathetic nerves in man? *Clin Auton Res* 1:103–108, 1991.
34. Leimbach WN, Wallin BG, Victor RG, et al: Direct evidence from intraneural recordings for increased central sympathetic outflow in patients with heart failure. *Circ* 73:913–919, 1986.
35. Hara K, Floras JS: After-effects of exercise on haemodynamics and muscle sympathetic nerve activity in young patients with dilated cardiomyopathy. *Heart* 75:602–608, 1996.
36. Ferguson DW, Berg WJ, Roach PJ, et al: Effects of heart failure on baroreflex control of sympathetic neural activity. *Am J Cardiol* 69:523–531, 1992.
37. La Rovere MT, Pinna GD, Maestri R, et al: Prognostic implications of baroreflex sensitivity in heart failure patients in the beta-blocking era. *J Am Coll Card* 53:193–199, 2009.
38. Porter TR, Eckberg DL, Fritsch JM, et al: Autonomic pathophysiology in heart failure patients. Sympathetic-cholinergic interrelations. *J Clin Invest* 85:1362–1371, 1990.
39. Nousiainen T, Vanninen E, Jantunen E, et al: Neuroendocrine changes during the elevation of doxorubicin-induced left ventricular dysfunction in adult lymphoma patients. *Clin Sci* 101:601–607, 2001.
40. Guzzetti S, Cogliati C, Turiel M, et al: Sympathetic predominance followed by functional denervation in the progression of chronic heart failure. *Eur Heart J* 16:1100–1107, 1995.
41. Notarius CF, Butler GC, Ando S, et al: Dissociation between microneurographic and heart rate variability estimates of sympathetic tone in normal and heart failure subjects. *Clin Sci* 96:557–565, 1999.
42. Kingwell BA, Thompson JM, Kaye DM, et al: Heart rate spectral analysis, cardiac norepinephrine spillover, and muscle sympathetic nerve activity during human sympathetic nervous activation and failure. *Circ* 90:234–240, 1994.
43. Benedict CR, Weiner DH, Johnson DE, et al: Comparative neurohormonal responses in patients with preserved and impaired left ventricular function. Results of the Studies of Left Ventricular Dysfunction (SOLVD) Registry. *J Am Coll Cardiol* 22:A146–A153, 1993.
44. Hogg K, McMurray J: Neurohumoral pathways in heart failure with preserved systolic function. *Prog Cardiovasc Dis* 47:357–366, 2005.
45. Kasama S, Toyama T, Kumakura H, et al: Effects of candesartan on cardiac sympathetic nerve activity in patients with congestive heart failure and preserved left ventricular ejection fraction. *J Am Coll Cardiol* 45:661–667, 2005.
46. Patel H, Ozdemir BA, Patel M, et al: Impairment of autonomic reactivity is a feature of heart failure whether or not the left ventricular ejection fraction is normal. *Int J Cardiol* 151:34–39, 2011.
47. Olshansky B, Sabbah HN, Hauptman PJ, et al: Parasympathetic nervous system and heart failure: pathophysiology and potential implications for therapy. *Circ* 118:863–871, 2008.
48. Lymperopoulos A, Rengo G, Koch WJ: Adrenergic nervous system in heart failure: pathophysiology and therapy. *Circ Res* 113:739–753, 2013.
49. Colucci WS, Ribeiro JP, Rocco MB, et al: Impaired chronotropic response to exercise in patients with congestive heart failure: role of postsynaptic beta-adrenergic desensitization. *Circ* 80:314–323, 1989.
50. Wagoner LE, Craft LL, Singh B, et al: Polymorphisms of the beta(2)-adrenergic receptor determine exercise capacity in patients with heart failure. *Circ Res* 86:834–840, 2000.
51. Notarius CF, Ando S, Rongen GA, et al: Resting muscle sympathetic nerve activity and peak oxygen uptake in heart failure and normal subjects. *Eur Heart J* 20:880–887, 1999.
52. Notarius CF, Azevedo ER, Parker JD, et al: Peak oxygen uptake is not determined by cardiac norepinephrine spillover in heart failure. *Eur Heart J* 23:800–805, 2001.
53. Santos AC, Alves MJ, Rondon MU, et al: Sympathetic activation restrains endothelium-mediated muscle vasodilation in heart failure patients. *Am J Physiol* 289:H593–H599, 2005.
54. Notarius CF, Millar PJ, Murai H, et al: Inverse relationship between muscle sympathetic activity during exercise and peak oxygen uptake in subjects with and without heart failure. *J Am Coll Cardiol* 63:605–606, 2014.
55. Cohn JN, Levine TB, Olivari MT, et al: Plasma norepinephrine as a guide to prognosis in patients with chronic congestive heart failure. *N Engl J Med* 311:819–824, 1984.
56. Benedict CR, Shelton B, Johnstone DE, et al: Prognostic significance of plasma norepinephrine in patients with asymptomatic left ventricular dysfunction. SOLVD Investigators. *Circ* 94:690–697, 1996.
57. Zugck C, Haunstetter A, Kruger C, et al: Impact of beta-blocker treatment on the prognostic value of currently used risk predictors in congestive heart failure. *J Am Coll Cardiol* 39:1615–1622, 2002.
58. Barretto AC, Santos AC, Munhoz R, et al: Increased muscle sympathetic nerve activity predicts mortality in heart failure patients. *Int J Cardiol* 135:302–307, 2009.
59. Petersson M, Friberg P, Eisenhofer G, et al: Long-term outcome in relation to renal sympathetic activity in patients with chronic heart failure. *Eur Heart J* 26:906–913, 2005.
60. Tamaki S, Yamada T, Okuyama Y, et al: Cardiac iodine-123 metaiodobenzylguanidine imaging predicts sudden cardiac death independently of left ventricular ejection fraction in patients with chronic heart failure and left ventricular systolic dysfunction: results from a comparative study with signal-averaged electrocardiogram, heart rate variability, and QT dispersion. *J Am Coll Card* 53:426–435, 2009.
61. Bigger JT, Steinman RC, Rolnitzky LM, et al: Power law behaviour of RR-interval variability in healthy middle-aged persons, patients with recent acute myocardial infarction, and patients with heart transplants. *Circ* 93:2142–2151, 1996.
62. Galinier M, Pathak A, Fourcade J, et al: Depressed low frequency power of heart rate variability as an independent predictor of sudden death in chronic heart failure. *Eur Heart J* 21:475–482, 2000.
63. Giannoni A, Emdin M, Bramanti F, et al: Combined increased chemosensitivity to hypoxia and hypercapnia as a prognosticator in heart failure. *J Am Coll Card* 53:1975–1980, 2009.
64. Bibevski S, Dunlap ME: Ganglionic mechanisms contribute to diminished vagal control in heart failure. *Circ* 99:2958–2963, 1999.
65. Newton GE, Parker AB, Landzberg JS, et al: Muscarinic receptor modulation of basal and beta-adrenergic stimulated function of the failing human left ventricle. *J Clin Invest* 98:2756–2763, 1996.

66. Dunlap ME, Bibevski S, Rosenberry TL, et al: Mechanisms of altered vagal control in heart failure: influence of muscarinic receptors and acetylcholinesterase activity. *Am J Physiol* 285:H1632–H1640, 2003.
67. Brandle M, Patel KP, Wang W, et al: Hemodynamic and norepinephrine responses to pacing-induced heart failure in conscious sinoaortic-denervated dogs. *J Appl Physiol* 81:1855–1862, 1996.
68. Ferguson DW, Berg WJ, Sanders JS: Clinical and hemodynamic correlates of sympathetic nerve activity in normal humans and patients with heart failure: evidence from direct microneurographic recordings. *J Am Coll Cardiol* 16:1125–1134, 1990.
69. Kaye DM, Lambert GW, Lefkovits J, et al: Neurochemical evidence of cardiac sympathetic activation and increased central nervous system norepinephrine turnover in severe congestive heart failure. *J Am Coll Cardiol* 23:570–578, 1994.
70. Dibner-Dunlap ME, Smith ML, Kinugawa T, et al: Enalaprilat augments arterial and cardiopulmonary baroreflex control of sympathetic nerve activity in patients with heart failure. *J Am Coll Cardiol* 27:358–364, 1996.
71. Dibner-Dunlap ME: Arterial or cardiopulmonary baroreflex control of sympathetic nerve activity in heart failure? *Am J Cardiol* 70:1640–1642, 1992.
72. Floras JS: Arterial baroreceptor and cardiopulmonary reflex control of sympathetic outflow in human heart failure. *Ann NY Acad Sci* 940:500–513, 2001.
73. Newton GE, Parker JD: Cardiac sympathetic responses to acute vasodilation: normal ventricular function versus congestive heart failure. *Circ* 94:3161–3167, 1996.
74. Floras JS: The "unsympathetic" nervous system of heart failure. *Circ* 105:1753–1755, 2002.
75. Grassi G, Seravalle G, Bertinieri G, et al: Sympathetic response to ventricular extrasystolic beats in hypertension and heart failure. *Hypertension* 39:886–891, 2002.
76. Zucker IH, Hackley JF, Cornish KG, et al: Chronic baroreceptor activation enhances survival in dogs with pacing-induced heart failure. *Hypertension* 50:904–910, 2007.
77. Watson AM, Hood SG, Ramchandra R, et al: Increased cardiac sympathetic nerve activity in heart failure is not due to desensitization of the arterial baroreflex. *Am J Physiol* 293:H798–H804, 2007.
78. Al-Hesayen A, Parker JD: Impaired baroreceptor control of renal sympathetic activity in human chronic heart failure. *Circ* 109:2862–2865, 2004.
79. Petersson M, Friberg P, Lambert G, et al: Decreased renal sympathetic activity in response to cardiac unloading with nitroglycerin in patients with heart failure. *Eur J Heart Fail* 7:1003–1010, 2005.
80. Middlekauff HR, Nitzsche EU, Hamilton MA, et al: Evidence for preserved cardiopulmonary baroreflex control of renal cortical blood flow in humans with advanced heart failure. A positron emission tomography study. *Circ* 92:395–401, 1995.
81. Ferguson DW, Thames MD, Mark AL: Effects of propranolol on reflex vascular responses to orthostatic stress in humans: role of ventricular baroreceptors. *Circ* 67:802–807, 1983.
82. Azevedo ER, Newton GE, Floras JS, et al: Reducing cardiac filling pressure lowers cardiac norepinephrine spillover in patients with chronic heart failure. *Circ* 101:2053–2059, 2000.
83. Wang W, Schultz HD, Ma R: Volume expansion potentiates cardiac sympathetic afferent reflex in dogs. *Am J Physiol* 280:H576–H581, 2001.
84. Kaye DM, Jennings GL, Dart AM, et al: Differential effect of acute baroreceptor unloading on cardiac and systemic sympathetic tone in congestive heart failure. *J Am Coll Cardiol* 31:583–587, 1998.
85. Kaye DM, Mansfield D, Aggarwal A, et al: Acute effects of continuous positive airway pressure on cardiac sympathetic tone in congestive heart failure. *Circ* 103:2336–2338, 2001.
86. Volpe M, Tritto C, De Luca N, et al: Failure of atrial natriuretic factor to increase with saline load in patients with dilated cardiomyopathy and mild heart failure. *J Clin Invest* 88:1481–1489, 1991.
87. Millar PJ, Murai H, Morris BL, et al: Microneurogenic evidence in healthy middle-aged humans for a sympathoexcitatory reflex activated by atrial pressure. *Am J Physiol Heart Circ Physiol* 305:H931–H938, 2013.
88. Moore JP, Hainsworth R, Drinhill MJ: Reflexes from pulmonary arterial baroreceptors in dogs: interaction with carotid sinus baroreceptors. *J Physiol* 589(Pt 16):4041–4052, 2011.
89. Oda Y, Joho S, Harada D, et al: Renal insufficiency coexisting with heart failure is related to elevated sympathetic nerve activity. *Auton Neurosci* 155:104–108, 2010.
90. Grassi G, Seravalle G, Quarti-Trevano F, et al: Effects of hypertension and obesity on the sympathetic activation of heart failure patients. *Hypertension* 42:873–877, 2003.
91. Grassi G, Seravalle G, Quart-Trevano F, et al: Excessive sympathetic activation in heart failure with obesity and metabolic syndrome. *Hypertension* 49:535–541, 2007.
92. Franchitto N, Despas F, Labrunee M, et al: Tonic chemoreflex activation contributes to increased sympathetic nerve activity in heart failure—related anemia. *Hypertension* 55:1012–1017, 2010.
93. Scott EM, Greenwood JP, Pernicova I, et al: Sympathetic activation and vasoregulation in response to carbohydrate ingestion in patients with congestive heart failure. *Can J Cardiol* 29:236–242, 2013.
94. Xiong XQ, Chen WW, Han Y, et al: Enhanced adipose afferent reflex contributes to sympathetic activation in diet-induced obesity hypertension. *Hypertension* 60:1280–1286, 2012.
95. Watson-Wright W, Boudreau G, Cardinal R, et al: Beta 1- and beta 2-adrenoreceptor subtypes in canine intrathoracic efferent sympathetic nervous system regulating the heart. *Am J Physiol* 261:R1269–R1275, 1991.
96. Gould PA, Esler MD, Kaye DM: Chronic atrial fibrillation does not influence the magnitude of sympathetic overactivity in patients with heart failure. *Eur Heart J* 24:1657–1662, 2003.
97. Gould PA, Yii M, Esler MD, et al: Atrial fibrillation impairs cardiac sympathetic response to baroreceptor unloading in congestive heart failure. *Eur Heart J* 26:2562–2567, 2005.
98. Goso Y, Asanoi H, Ishise H, et al: Respiratory modulation of muscle sympathetic nerve activity in patients with chronic heart failure. *Circ* 104:418–423, 2001.
99. Naughton MT, Floras JS, Rahman MA, et al: Respiratory correlates of muscle sympathetic nerve activity in heart failure. *Clin Sci* 95:277–285, 1998.
100. Kappagoda CT, Ravi K: The rapidly adapting receptors in mammalian airways and their responses to changes in extravascular fluid volume. *Exp Physiol* 91:647–654, 2006.
101. Schultz HD, Li YL, Ding Y: Arterial chemoreceptors and sympathetic nerve activity: implications for hypertension and heart failure. *Hypertension* 50:6–13, 2007.
102. Ponikowski PP, Chua TP, Anker SD, et al: Peripheral chemoreceptor hypersensitivity: an ominous sign in patients with chronic heart failure. *Circ* 104:544–549, 2001.
103. Giannoni A, Emdin M, Poletti R, et al: Clinical significance of chemosensitivity in chronic heart failure: influence on neurohormonal derangement, Cheyne-Stokes respiration and arrhythmias. *Clin Sci* 114:489–497, 2008.
104. van de Borne P, Oren R, Anderson EA, et al: Tonic chemoreflex activation does not contribute to elevated muscle sympathetic nerve activity in heart failure. *Circ* 94:1325–1328, 1996.
105. Andreas S, Binggeli C, Mohacsi P, et al: Nasal oxygen and muscle sympathetic nerve activity in heart failure. *Chest* 123:322–325, 2003.
106. Despas F, Detis N, Dumonteil N, et al: Excessive sympathetic activation in heart failure with chronic renal failure: role of chemoreflex activation. *J Hypertens* 27:1849–1854, 2009.
107. Di Vanna A, Braga AM, Laterza MC, et al: Blunted muscle vasodilatation during chemoreceptor stimulation in patients with heart failure. *Am J Physiol* 293:H846–H852, 2007.
108. Stickland MK, Miller JD, Smith CA, et al: Carotid chemoreceptor modulation of regional blood flow distribution during exercise in health and chronic heart failure. *Circ Res* 100:1371–1378, 2007.
109. Minisi AJ, Thames MD: Distribution of left ventricular sympathetic afferents demonstrated by reflex responses to transmural myocardial ischemia and to intracoronary and epicardial bradykinin. *Circ* 87:240–246, 1993.
110. Minisi AJ, Thames MD: Effect of chronic myocardial infarction on vagal cardiopulmonary baroreflex. *Circ Res* 65:396–405, 1989.
111. Graham LN, Smith PA, Stoker JB, et al: Time course of sympathetic neural hyperactivity after uncomplicated acute myocardial interaction. *Circ* 106:793–797, 2002.
112. Grassi G, Seravalle G, Bertinieri G, et al: Sympathetic and reflex abnormalities in heart failure secondary to ischaemic or idiopathic dilated cardiomyopathy. *Clin Sci* 101:141–146, 2001.
113. Notarius CF, Spaak J, Morris BL, et al: Comparison of muscle sympathetic activity in ischemic and nonischemic heart failure. *J Card Fail* 13:470–475, 2007.
114. Lommi J, Kupari M, Koskinen P, et al: Blood ketone bodies in congestive heart failure. *J Am Coll Card* 28:665–672, 1996.
115. Tuunanen H, Engblom E, Naum A, et al: Decreased myocardial free fatty acid uptake in patients with idiopathic dilated cardiomyopathy: evidence of relationship with insulin resistance and left ventricular dysfunction. *J Card Fail* 12:644–652, 2006.
116. Wijeysundera HC, Parmar G, Rongen GA, et al: Reflex systemic sympatho-neural response to brachial adenosine infusion in treated heart failure. *Eur J Heart Fail* 13:475–481, 2011.
117. Piepoli MF, Kaczmarek A, Francis DP, et al: Reduced peripheral skeletal muscle mass and abnormal reflex physiology in chronic heart failure. *Circ* 114:126–134, 2006.
118. Murai H, Takamura M, Maruyama M, et al: Altered firing pattern of single-unit muscle sympathetic nerve activity during handgrip exercise in chronic heart failure. *J Physiol* 587:2613–2622, 2009.
119. DiBona GF: Neural control of renal function: cardiovascular implications. *Hypertension* 13:539–548, 1989.
120. Kopp UC: Renorenal reflexes in hypertension. *J Hypertens* 11:765–773, 1993.
121. Franchitto N, Despas F, Labrunee M, et al: Cardiorenal anemia syndrome in chronic heart failure contributes to increased sympathetic nerve activity. *Int J Cardiol* 168:2352–2357, 2013.
122. Floras JS, Sleight P: Ambulatory monitoring of blood pressure. In Sleight P, Jones JV, editors: *Scientific foundations of cardiology*, London, 1983, Heinemann, pp 155–164.
123. Smyth HS, Sleight P, Pickering GW: Reflex regulation of arterial pressure during sleep in man. A quantitative method of assessing baroreflex sensitivity. *Circ Res* 24:109–121, 1969.
124. Somers VK, Dyken ME, Mark AL, et al: Sympathetic-nerve activity during sleep in normal subjects. *N Engl J Med* 328:303–307, 1993.
125. Arzt M, Young T, Finn L, et al: Sleepiness and sleep in patients with both systolic heart failure and obstructive sleep apnea. *Arch Intern Med* 166:1716–1722, 2006.
126. Yumino D, Wang H, Floras JS, et al: Prevalence and physiological predictors of sleep apnea in patients with heart failure and systolic dysfunction. *J Card Fail* 15:279–285, 2009.
127. Bradley TD, Tkacova R, Hall MJ, et al: Augmented sympathetic neural response to simulated obstructive sleep apnoea in human heart failure. *Clin Sci* 104:231–238, 2003.
128. Bradley TD, Floras JS: Obstructive sleep apnoea and its cardiovascular consequences. *Lancet* 373:82–93, 2009.
129. Carlson JT, Hedner J, Elam M, et al: Augmented resting sympathetic activity in awake patients with obstructive sleep apnea. *Chest* 103:1763–1768, 1993.
130. Spaak J, Egri ZJ, Kubo T, et al: Muscle sympathetic nerve activity during wakefulness in heart failure patients with and without sleep apnea. *Hypertension* 46:1327–1332, 2005.
131. Usui K, Bradley TD, Spaak J, et al: Inhibition of awake sympathetic nerve activity of heart failure patients with obstructive sleep apnea by nocturnal continuous positive airway pressure. *J Am Coll Card* 45:2008–2011, 2005.
132. Abboud FM, Thames MD: Interaction of cardiovascular reflexes in circulatory control. In Shepherd JT, Abboud FM, editors: *Handbook of physiology, Section 2: The cardiovascular system; Volume III: Peripheral circulation and organ blood flow, Part 2*, Bethesda, MD, 1983, American Physiological Society, pp 675–753.
133. Wang H, Parker JD, Newton GE, et al: Influence of obstructive sleep apnea on mortality in patients with heart failure. *J Am Coll Card* 49:1625–1631, 2007.
134. Yumino D, Wang H, Floras JS, et al: Relationship between sleep apnoea and mortality in patients with ischaemic heart failure. *Heart* 95:819–824, 2009.
135. Tkacova R, Niroumand M, Lorenzi-Filho G, et al: Overnight shift from obstructive to central apneas in patients with heart failure: role of PCO2 and circulatory delay. *Circ* 103:238–243, 2001.
136. Naughton MT, Benard DC, Liu PP, et al: Effects of nasal CPAP on sympathetic activity in patients with heart failure and central sleep apnea. *Am J Respir Crit Care Med* 152:473–479, 1995.
137. Mansfield D, Kaye D, La Rocca H, et al: Raised sympathetic nerve activity in heart failure and central sleep apnea is due to heart failure severity. *Circ* 107:1396–1400, 2003.
138. Tamura A, Ando S, Goto Y, et al: Washout rate of cardiac iodine-123 metaiodobenzylguanidine is high in chronic heart failure patients with central sleep apnea. *J Card Fail* 16:728–733, 2010.
139. Ueno H, Asanoi H, Yamada K, et al: Attenuated respiratory modulation of chemoreflex-mediated sympathoexcitation in patients with chronic heart failure. *J Card Fail* 10:236–243, 2004.
140. Kimmerly DS, Morris BL, Floras JS: Apnea-induced cortical BOLD-fMRI and peripheral sympathoneural firing response patterns of awake healthy humans. *PLoS One* 8:e82525, 2013.
141. Dampney RAL, Coleman MJ, Fontes MAP, et al: Central mechanisms underlying short- and long-term regulation of the cardiovascular system. *Clin Exp Pharmacol Physiol* 29:261–268, 2009.
142. Silvani A, Dampney RA: Central control of cardiovascular function during sleep. *Am J Physiol Heart Circ Physiol* 305:H1683–H1692, 2013.
143. Gao L, Wang W, Li YL, et al: Superoxide mediates sympathoexcitation in heart failure: roles of angiotensin II and NAD(P)H oxidase. *Circ Res* 95:937–944, 2004.
144. Zucker IH: Novel mechanisms of sympathetic regulation in chronic heart failure. *Hypertension* 48:1005–1011, 2006.
145. Haack KK, Gao L, Schiller AM, et al: Central Rho kinase inhibition restores baroreflex sensitivity and angiotensin II type 1 receptor protein imbalance in conscious rabbits with chronic heart failure. *Hypertension* 61:723–729, 2013.
146. Reid IA: Interactions between ANG II, sympathetic nervous system, and baroreceptor reflexes in regulation of blood pressure. *Am J Physiol* 262:E763–E778, 1992.
147. Potts PD, Hirooka Y, Dampney RA: Activation of brain neurons by circulating angiotensin II: direct effects and baroreceptor-mediated secondary effects. *Neuroscience* 90:581–594, 1999.
148. Lohmeier T, Dwyer T, Hildebrandt D, et al: Influence of prolonged baroreflex activation on arterial pressure in angiotensin hypertension. *Hypertension* 46:1194–1200, 2005.
149. Ma R, Schultz HD, Wang W: Chronic central infusion of ANG II potentiates cardiac sympathetic afferent reflex in dogs. *Am J Physiol* 277:H15–H22, 1999.
150. Zhu GQ, Gao L, Li Y, et al: AT1 receptor mRNA antisense normalizes enhanced cardiac sympathetic afferent reflex in rats with chronic heart failure. *Am J Physiol* 287:H1828–H1835, 2004.
151. DiBona GF, Jones SY, Brooks VL: ANG II receptor blockade and arterial baroreflex regulation of renal nerve activity in cardiac failure. *Am J Physiol* 269:R1189–R1196, 1995.

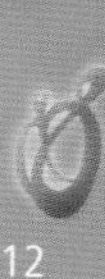

152. Huang BS, Yuan B, Leenen FH: Chronic blockade of brain "ouabain" prevents sympathetic hyper-reactivity and impairment of acute baroreflex resetting in rats with congestive heart failure. *Can J Physiol Pharmacol* 78:45–53, 2000.
153. Francis J, Wei SG, Weiss RM, et al: Brain angiotensin-converting enzyme activity and autonomic regulation in heart failure. *Am J Physiol* 287:H2138–H2146, 2004.
154. Wang H, Huang BS, Ganten D, et al: Prevention of sympathetic and cardiac dysfunction after myocardial infarction in transgenic rats deficient in brain angiotensin. *Circ Res* 94:843, 2004.
155. Gao L, Wang W, Li YL, et al: Sympathoexcitation by central ANG II: roles for AT1 receptor upregulation and NAD(P)H oxidase in RVLM. *Am J Physiol* 288:H2271–H2279, 2005.
156. Millar PJ, Floras JS: Statins and the autonomic nervous system. *Clin Sci (Lond)* 126:401–415, 2014.
157. Francis J, Weiss RM, Wei SG, et al: Central mineralocorticoid receptor blockade improves volume regulation and reduces sympathetic drive in heart failure. *Am J Physiol* 281:H2241–H2251, 2001.
158. Yu Y, Wei SG, Zhang ZH, et al: Does aldosterone upregulate the brain renin-angiotensin system in rats with heart failure? *Hypertension* 51:727–733, 2008.
159. Abboud FM, Harwani SC, Chapleau MW: Autonomic neural regulation of the immune system: implications for hypertension and cardiovascular disease. *Hypertension* 59:755–762, 2012.
160. Harrison DG, Guzik TJ, Lob H, et al: Inflammation, immunity, and hypertension. *Hypertension* 57:132–140, 2011.
161. Pavlov VA, Tracey KJ: The vagus nerve and the inflammatory reflex—linking immunity and metabolism. *Nat Rev Endocrinol* 8:743–754, 2012.
162. Jankowska EA, Ponikowski P, Piepoli MF, et al: Autonomic imbalance and immune activation in chronic heart failure—pathophysiological links. *Cardiovasc Res* 70:434–445, 2006.
163. Yu Y, Zhang ZH, Wei SG, et al: Central gene transfer of interleukin-10 reduces hypothalamic inflammation and evidence of heart failure in rats after myocardial infarction. *Circ Res* 101:304–312, 2007.
164. Kang Y-M, Zhang Z-H, Johnson RF, et al: Novel effect of mineralocorticoid receptor antagonism to reduce proinflammatory cytokines and hypothalamic activation in rats with ischemia-induced heart failure. *Circ Res* 99:758–766, 2006.
165. Wei SG, Zhang ZH, Beltz TG, et al: Subfornical organ mediates sympathetic and hemodynamic responses to blood-borne proinflammatory cytokines. *Hypertension* 62:118–125, 2013.
166. Lambert G, Kaye DM, Lefkovits J, et al: Increased central nervous system monoamine neurotransmitter turnover and its association with sympathetic nervous activity in treated heart failure patients. *Circ* 92:1813–1818, 1995.
167. Aggarwal A, Esler M, Lambert GW, et al: Norepinephrine turnover is increased in suprabulbar subcortical brain regions and is related to whole-body sympathetic activity in human heart failure. *Circ* 105:1031–1033, 2002.
168. Elam M, Yao T, Svensson TH, et al: Regulation of locus coeruleus neurons and splanchnic, sympathetic nerves by cardiovascular afferents. *Brain Res* 290:281–287, 1984.
169. Taranto Montemurro L, Floras JS, Millar PJ, et al: Inverse relationship of subjective daytime sleepiness to sympathetic activity in patients with heart failure and obstructive sleep apnea. *Chest* 142:1222–1228, 2012.
170. Kawai H, Mohan A, Hagen J, et al: Alterations in cardiac adrenergic terminal function and beta-adrenoceptor density in pacing-induced heart failure. *Am J Physiol* 278:H1708–H1716, 2000.
171. Bohm M, La Rosee K, Schwinger RH, et al: Evidence for reduction of norepinephrine uptake sites in the failing human heart. *J Am Coll Cardiol* 25:146–153, 1995.
172. Eisenhofer G, Friberg P, Rundqvist B, et al: Cardiac sympathetic nerve function in congestive heart failure. *Circ* 93:1667–1676, 1996.
173. Boogers MJ, Borleffs CJ, Henneman MM, et al: Cardiac sympathetic denervation assessed with 123-iodine metaiodobenzylguanidine imaging predicts ventricular arrhythmias in implantable cardioverter-defibrillator patients. *J Am Coll Cardiol* 55:2769–2777, 2010.
174. Lotze U, Kaepplinger S, Kober A, et al: Recovery of the cardiac adrenergic nervous system after long-term beta-blocker therapy in idiopathic dilated cardiomyopathy: assessment by increase in myocardial 123I-metaiodobenzylguanidine uptake. *J Nucl Med* 42:49–54, 2001.
175. Floras JS: Epinephrine and the genesis of hypertension. *Hypertension* 19:1–18, 1992.
176. Newton GE, Parker JD: Acute effects of beta 1-selective and nonselective beta-adrenergic receptor blockade on cardiac sympathetic activity in congestive heart failure. *Circ* 94:353–358, 1996.
177. Huang MH, Smith FM, Armour JA: Modulation of in situ canine intrinsic cardiac neuronal activity by nicotinic, muscarinic, and beta-adrenergic agonists. *Am J Physiol* 265:R659–R669, 1993.
178. Johansson M, Rundqvist B, Eisenhofer G, et al: Cardiorenal epinephrine kinetics: evidence for neuronal release in the human heart. *Am J Physiol* 273:H2178–H2185, 1997.
179. Parker JD, Newton GE, Landzberg JS, et al: Functional significance of presynaptic alpha-adrenergic receptors in failing and nonfailing human left ventricle. *Circ* 92:1793–1800, 1995.
180. Aggarwal A, Esler MD, Socratous F, et al: Evidence for functional presynaptic alpha-2 adrenoceptors and their down-regulation in human heart failure. *J Am Coll Cardiol* 37:1246–1251, 2001.
181. Small KM, Wagoner LE, Levin AB, et al: Synergistic polymorphisms of beta1- and alpha 2c-adrenergic receptors and the risk of congestive heart failure. *N Engl J Med* 347:1135–1142, 2002.
182. Liggett SB, Mialet-Perez J, Thaneemit-Chen S, et al: A polymorphism within a conserved beta1-adrenergic receptor motif alters cardiac function and beta-blocker response in human heart failure. *Proc Natl Acad Sci USA* 103:11288–11293, 2006.
183. Kurnik D, Muszkat M, Sofowora GG, et al: Ethnic and genetic determinants of cardiovascular response to the selective alpha-2 adrenoceptor agonist dexmedetomidine. *Hypertension* 51:406–411, 2008.
184. Kaye DM, Smirk B, Finch S, et al: Interaction between cardiac sympathetic drive and heart rate in heart failure: modulation by adrenergic receptor genotype. *J Am Coll Card* 44:2008–2015, 2004.
185. Azevedo ER, Parker JD: Parasympathetic control of cardiac sympathetic activity. Normal ventricular function versus congestive heart failure. *Circ* 100:274–279, 1999.
186. McDonough PM, Wetzel GT, Brown JH: Further characterization of the presynaptic alpha-1 receptor modulating [3H]ACh release from rat atria. *J Pharmacol Exp Ther* 238:612–617, 1986.
187. Lemmens K, Doggen K, De Keulenaer GW: Role of neuregulin-1/ErbB signaling in cardiovascular physiology and disease: implications for therapy of heart failure. *Circ* 116:954–960, 2007.
188. Potter EK: Prolonged non-adrenergic inhibition of cardiac vagal action following sympathetic stimulation: neuromodulation by neuropeptide Y? *Neurosci Lett* 54:117–121, 1985.
189. Smith-White MA, Wallace D, Potter EK: Sympathetic-parasympathetic interactions at the heart in the anaesthetised rat. *J Auton Nerv Syst* 75:171–175, 1999.
190. Goldsmith SR, Hasking GJ, Miller E: Angiotensin II and sympathetic activity in patients with congestive heart failure. *J Am Coll Cardiol* 21:1107–1113, 1993.
191. Magnusson Y, Wallukat G, Waagstein F, et al: Autoimmunity in idiopathic dilated cardiomyopathy. Characterization of antibodies against the beta 1-adrenoceptor with positive chronotropic effect. *Circ* 89:2760–2767, 1994.
192. Al-Hesayen A, Azevedo ER, Newton GE, et al: The effects of dobutamine on cardiac sympathetic activity in patients with congestive heart failure. *J Am Coll Cardiol* 39:1269–1274, 2002.
193. Azevedo ER, Kubo T, Mak S, et al: Nonselective versus selective beta-adrenergic receptor blockade in congestive heart failure differential effects on sympathetic activity. *Circ* 104:2194–2199, 2001.
194. Kubo T, Azevedo ER, Newton GE, et al: Beta-blockade restores muscle sympathetic rhythmicity in human heart failure. *Circ J* 75:1400–1408, 2011.
195. Kubo T, Azevedo ER, Newton GE, et al: Lack of evidence for peripheral alpha(1)-adrenoceptor blockade during long-term treatment of heart failure with carvedilol. *J Am Coll Cardiol* 38:1463–1469, 2001.
196. Rongen GA, Floras JS, Lenders J, et al: Cardiovascular pharmacology of purines. *Clin Sci* 92:13–24, 1997.
197. Clarke J, Benjamin N, Larkin S, et al: Interaction of neuropeptide Y and the sympathetic nervous system in vascular control in man. *Circ* 83:774–777, 1991.
198. Morris MJ, Cox HS, Lambert FW, et al: Region-specific neuropeptide Y overflow at rest and during sympathetic activation in humans. *Hypertension 1997* 29:137–143, 1997.
199. Ferguson DW: Sympathoinhibitory responses to digitalis glycosides in heart failure patients: direct evidence from sympathetic neural recordings. *Circ* 80:65–77, 1989.
200. Newton GE, Tong JH, Schofield AM, et al: Digoxin reduces cardiac sympathetic activity in severe congestive heart failure. *J Am Coll Cardiol* 28:155–161, 1996.
201. Faris R, Flather MD, Purcell H, et al: Diuretics for heart failure. *Cochrane Database Syst Rev* (1):CD003838, 2006.
202. Solin P, Bergin P, Richardson M, et al: Influence of pulmonary capillary wedge pressure on central apnea in heart failure. *Circ* 99:1574–1579, 1999.
203. Grassi G, Cattaneo BM, Seravalle G, et al: Effects of chronic ACE inhibition on sympathetic nerve traffic and baroreflex control of circulation in heart failure. *Circ* 96:1173–1179, 1997.
204. Hikosaka M, Yuasa F, Mimura J, et al: Candesartan and arterial baroreflex sensitivity and sympathetic nerve activity in patients with mild heart failure. *Cardiovasc Pharmacol* 40:875–880, 2002.
205. Ruzicka M, Floras JS, McReynolds AG, et al: Do high doses of AT1-receptor blockers attenuate central sympathetic outflow in humans with chronic heart failure? *Clin Sci* 124:589–595, 2013.
206. Raheja P, Price A, Wang Z: Spironolactone prevents chlorthalidone-induced sympathetic activation and insulin resistance in hypertensive patients. *Hypertension* 60:319–325, 2012.
207. Kaye DM, Dart AM, Jennings GL, et al: Antiadrenergic effect of chronic amiodarone therapy in human heart failure. *J Am Coll Cardiol* 33:1553–1559, 1999.
208. Azevedo ER, Newton GE, Parker JD: Cardiac and systemic sympathetic activity in response to clonidine in human heart failure. *J Am Coll Cardiol* 33:186–191, 1999.
209. Grassi G, Turri C, Seravalle G, et al: Effects of chronic clonidine administration on sympathetic nerve traffic and baroreflex function in heart failure. *Hypertension* 38:286–291, 2001.
210. Swedberg K, Bristow M, Cohn JN, et al: The effects of moxonidine SR, an imidazoline agonist, on plasma norepinephrine in patients with chronic heart failure. *Circ* 105:1797–1803, 2002.
211. Cohn JN, Pfeffer MA, Rouleau J, et al: Adverse mortality effect of central sympathetic inhibition with sustained-release moxonidine in patients with heart failure (MOXCON). *Eur J Heart Fail* 5:659–667, 2003.
212. Bristow MR, Krause-Steinrauf H, Nuzzo R, et al: Effect of baseline or changes in adrenergic activity on clinical outcomes in the beta-blocker evaluation of survival trial. *Circ* 110:1437–1442, 2004.
213. Roveda F, Middlekauff HR, Rondon MU, et al: The effects of exercise training on sympathetic neural activation in advanced heart failure: a randomized controlled trial. *J Am Coll Cardiol* 42:854–860, 2003.
214. Fraga R, Franco FG, Roveda R, et al: Exercise training reduces sympathetic nerve activity in heart failure patients treated with carvedilol. *Eur J Heart Fail* 9:630–636, 2007.
215. Kaneko Y, Floras JS, Usui K, et al: Cardiovascular effects of continuous positive airway pressure in patients with heart failure and obstructive sleep apnea. *N Engl J Med* 348:1233–1241, 2003.
216. Passino C, Severino S, Poletti R, et al: Aerobic training decreases B-type natriuretic peptide expression and adrenergic activation in patients with heart failure. *J Am Coll Cardiol* 47:1835–1839, 2006.
217. Patel KP, Zheng H: Central neural control of sympathetic nerve activity in heart failure folowing exercise training. *Am J Physiol* 302:H527–H537, 2012.
218. Ueno LM, Drager LF, Rodrigues AC, et al: Effects of exercise training in patients with chronic heart failure and sleep apnea. *Sleep* 32:637–647, 2009.
219. Heusser K, Tank J, Engeli S, et al: Carotid baroreceptor stimulation, sympathetic activity, baroreflex function, and blood pressure in hypertensive patients. *Hypertension* 55:619–626, 2010.
220. Wustmann K, Kucera JP, Scheffers I, et al: Effects of chronic baroreceptor stimulation on the autonomic cardiovascular regulation in patients with drug-resistant arterial hypertension. *Hypertension* 54:536, 2009.
221. Alnima T, de Leeuw PW, Tan FES, for the Rheos Pivotol Trial Investigators, et al: Renal responses to long-term carotid baroreflex activation therapy in patients with drug-resistant hypertension. *Hypertension* 61:1334–1339, 2013.
222. Del Rio R, Marcus NJ, Schultz HD: Carotid chemoreceptor ablation improves survival in heart failure: rescuing autonomic control of cardiorespiratory function. *J Am Coll Cardiol* 62:2422–2430, 2013.
223. Marcus NJ, Del Rio R, Schultz EP, et al: Carotid body denervation improves autonomic and cardiac function and attenuates disordered breathing in congestive heart failure. *J Physiol* 592:391–408, 2014.
224. Abdala AP, McBryde FD, Marina N, et al: Hypertension is critically dependent on the carotid body input in the spontaneously hypertensive rat. *J Physiol* 590:4269–4277, 2012.
225. Paton JF, Sobotka PA, Fudim M, et al: The carotid body as a therapeutic target for the treatment of sympathetically mediated diseases. *Hypertension* 61:5–13, 2013.
226. Niewinski P, Janczak D, Rucinski A, et al: Carotid body removal for treatment of chronic systolic heart failure. *Int J Cardiol* 168:2506–2509, 2013.
227. Hamdan MH, Barbera S, Kowal RC, et al: Effects of resynchronization therapy on sympathetic activity in patients with depressed ejection fraction and intraventricular conduction delay due to ischemic or idiopathic dilated cardiomyopathy. *Am J Cardiol* 89:1047–1051, 2002.
228. Gademan MG, van Bommel RJ, Ypenburg C, et al: Biventricular pacing in chronic heart failure acutely facilitates the arterial baroreflex. *Am J Physiol* 295:H755–H760, 2008.
229. Grassi G, Brambilla R, Trevano FQ, et al: Sustained sympathoinhibitory effects of cardiac resynchronization therapy in severe heart failure. *Hypertension* 44:727–731, 2004.
230. Cha YM, Chareonthaitawee P, Dong YX, et al: Cardiac sympathetic reserve and response to cardiac resynchronization therapy. *Circ Heart Fail* 4:339–344, 2011.
231. Bitter T, Westerheide N, Prinz C, et al: Cheyne-Stokes respiration and obstructive sleep apnoea are independent risk factors for malignant ventricular arrhythmias requiring appropriate cardioverter-defibrillator therapies in patients with congestive heart failure. *Eur Heart J* 32:61–74, 2011.

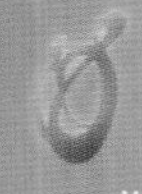

232. Floras JS: Should sleep apnoea be a specific target of therapy in chronic heart failure? *Heart* 95:1041–1046, 2009.
233. Ryan CM, Usui K, Floras JS, et al: Effect of continuous positive airway pressure on ventricular ectopy in heart failure patients with obstructive sleep apnoea. *Thorax* 60:781–785, 2005.
234. Mansfield D, Gollogly NC, Kaye DM, et al: Controlled trial of continuous positive airway pressure in obstructive sleep apnea and heart failure. *Am J Respir Crit Care Med* 169:361–366, 2004.
235. Bradley TD, Logan AG, Kimoff RJ, et al: Continuous positive airway pressure for central sleep apnea and heart failure. *N Engl J Med* 353:2025–2033, 2005.
236. Arzt M, Floras JS, Logan AG, et al: Suppression of central sleep apnea by continuous positive airway pressure and transplant-free survival in heart failure: a post hoc analysis of the Canadian Positive Airway Pressure for Patients with Central Sleep Apnea and Heart Failure Trial (CANPAP). *Circ* 115:3173–3180, 2007.
237. Sharma BK, Bakker JP, McSharry DG, et al: Adaptive servoventilation for treatment of sleep-disordered breathing in heart failure: a systematic review and meta-analysis. *Chest* 142:1211–1221, 2012.
238. Kasai T, Usui Y, Yoshioka T, et al: Effect of flow-triggered adaptive servo-ventilation compared with continuous positive airway pressure in patients with chronic heart failure with coexisting obstructive sleep apnea and Cheyne-Stokes respiration. *Circ Heart Fail* 3:140–148, 2010.
239. Owada T, Yoshihisa A, Yamauchi H: Adaptive servoventilation improves cardiorenal function and prognosis in heart failure patients with chronic kidney disease and sleep-disordered breathing. *J Card Fail* 19:225–232, 2013.
240. Koyama T, Watanabe H, Tamura Y, et al: Adaptive servo-ventilation therapy improves cardiac sympathetic nerve activity in patients with heart failure. *Eur J Heart Fail* 15:902–909, 2013.
241. Li M, Zheng C, Sato T, et al: Vagal nerve stimulation markedly improves long-term survival after chronic heart failure in rats. *Circ* 109:120–124, 2004.
242. Zhang Y, Popovic ZB, Bibevski S, et al: Chronic vagus nerve stimulation improves autonomic control and attenuates systemic inflammation and heart failure progression in a canine high-rate pacing model. *Circ Heart Fail* 2:692–699, 2009.
243. De Ferrari GM, Crilins HJ, Borggrefe M, et al; CardioFit Multicenter Trial Investigators: Chronic vagus nerve stimulation: a new and promising therapeutic approach for chronic heart failure. *Eur Heart J* 32:847–855, 2011.
244. Hauptman PJ, Schwartz PJ, Gold MR, et al: Rationale and study design of the increase of vagal tone in heart failure study: INOVATE-HF. *Am Heart J* 163:954–962, 2012.
245. DiBona GF, Kopp UC: Neural control of renal function. *Physiol Rev* 77:75–197, 1997.
246. Galiwango PJ, McReynolds A, Ivanov J, et al: Activity with ambulation attenuates diuretic responsiveness in chronic heart failure. *J Am Coll Card* 17:797–803, 2011.
247. Krum H, Schlaich M, Whitbourn R, et al: Catheter-based renal sympathetic denervation for resistant hypertension: a multicentre safety and proof-of-principle cohort study. *Lancet* 373:1275–1281, 2009.
248. Davies JE, Manisty CH, Petraco R: First-in-man safety evaluation of renal denervation for chronic systolic heart failure: primary outcome from REACH-Pilot study. *Int J Cardiol* 162:189–192, 2013.
249. Lohmeier TE, Ilescu R, Liu B: Systemic and renal-specific sympathoinhibition in obesity hypertension. *Hypertension* 59:331–338, 2012.
250. Singh JP, Kandala J, Camm AJ: Non-pharmacological modulation of the autonomic tone to treat heart failure. *Eur Heart J* 35:77–85, 2014.

13 Alterations in the Peripheral Circulation in Heart Failure

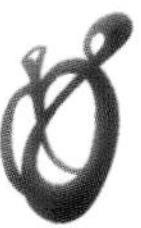

Eduard Shantsila and Gregory Y. H. Lip

The complex pathology of heart failure (HF) can be attributed, at least in part, to important changes that occur in the peripheral circulation. As cardiac output declines, systemic perfusion pressure is maintained predominantly by peripheral vasoconstriction and sodium retention, both of which can be attributed to complex interactions among the autonomic nervous system (**see also Chapter 12**), neurohormonal mechanisms, and the kidney (**see also Chapter 14**). These homeostatic mechanisms tend to preserve circulation to the brain and heart, while decreasing blood flow to the skin, skeletal muscles, splanchnic organs, and kidneys. Impaired circulation of skeletal muscle with a diminished oxygen supply is a major contributor to exercise intolerance and fatigue, a common and sometimes debilitating symptom in patients with HF.[1-3] The sympathetic nervous system is activated very early in the disease process (**see also Chapter 12**), whereas the renin-angiotensin system is usually activated when clinical symptoms develop (**see also Chapter 5**). Vasopressin is released mainly in very advanced stages of chronic HF when systemic perfusion is already threatened. Furthermore, chronic severe HF is associated by an increased endothelial release of locally acting vasoconstricting factors such as endothelin.

These endogenous vasoconstricting factors are counterbalanced in part by endogenous vasodilators.[4-6] In normal individuals, natriuretic peptides attenuate the release of norepinephrine, renin, and vasopressin, as well as their actions on peripheral blood vessels and within the kidneys. In addition, the continuous release of endothelium-derived relaxing factor (nitric oxide) from the endothelium normally counteracts the vasoconstricting factors. In fact, the continuous basal release of nitric oxide keeps the peripheral vasculature in a dilated state. In patients with HF, however, the effects of circulating and locally active vasodilators are attenuated. The release of atrial natriuretic peptide is blunted in chronic HF and the effects of both atrial (ANP) and B-type natriuretic peptide (BNP) lose their ability to suppress the release of renin or dilate peripheral blood vessels. In addition, the vascular availability of nitric oxide is severely diminished in patients with chronic HF.[7] Thus diminished vasodilator forces leave the actions of vasoconstrictors unopposed. It is important to note that the interaction of the sympathetic and renin-angiotensin system even amplifies their vasoconstricting effects. Increased sympathetic activity increases the release of renin and vice versa, and angiotensin enhances the release of both norepinephrine and vasopressin.

PATHOPHYSIOLOGIC INSIGHTS

One of the important insights that has emerged from studies on the peripheral circulation in HF is that endothelial dysfunction plays a significant role in the pathogenesis, symptomatic status, and prognosis in HF. The endothelium is a monolayer of cells that cover the luminal side of the heart and all blood vessels, from the aorta to the capillaries. Historically, the endothelium was considered a relatively inert “border” between the blood and surrounding tissues. However, over the past two decades the endothelial cells, building blocks of the endothelium, were found to exert an extremely diverse range of activities implicated in cardiovascular biology and pathology. Indeed, the endothelium regulates vasomotor function, hemostatic status, the balance of pro- and antioxidant and pro- and anti-inflammatory processes. All these activities are highly relevant to the clinical status of the patients with compromised cardiac function, who are vulnerable to even minor shifts in hemodynamic and homeostatic state.[1-3] Of note, the vast majority of research data in HF has focused on HF with impaired systolic function with less information available on HF with preserved left ventricular ejection fraction.

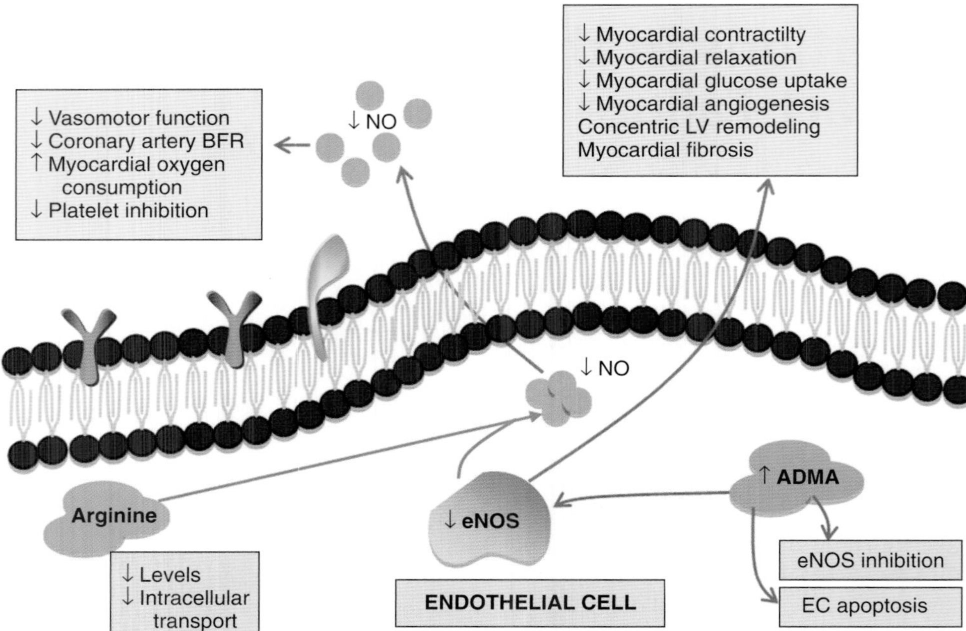

FIGURE 13-1 Mechanisms and effects of vasomotor endothelial function in heart failure. Vasomotor endothelial dysfunction is featured by reduced eNOS expression and NO production. It can also be contributed by diminished arginine availability and its impaired intracellular function, as well as upregulation of the endogenous eNOS inhibitor, ADMA. In HF these abnormalities lead to the reduced coronary blood flow reserve, increased myocardial oxygen consumption, impaired cardiac function, angiogenesis, enhanced cardiac remodeling, and fibrosis. *ADMA,* Asymmetric dimethylarginine; *BFR,* blood flow reserve; *eNOS,* endothelial NO synthase; *LV,* left ventricular; *NO,* nitric oxide.

Although the term *endothelial dysfunction* is used throughout the chapter, there is a continuum from endothelial *activation* to endothelial "dysfunction" and endothelial "damage."[4,5] Endothelial *activation* usually refers to physiologic response to various stimuli (including inflammatory cytokines), such as bleeding and infection, aiming to preserve homeostatic stability of the host (protective changes). Endothelial "activation" may involve increased expression and shedding of some surface adhesion molecules, release of von Willebrand factor, and fibrinolytic factors. A crucial aspect of "activation" is that it is reversible upon cessation of the activating agent(s). In contrast, endothelial *dysfunction* refers to the situations of sustained excessive (e.g., increased reactive oxygen species production) or depressed (e.g., impaired vasodilation) endothelial performance. Given that endothelial "dysfunction" could follow chronic "activation" (for example, by prolonged and inappropriate activation by inflammatory cytokines), there is clear overlap between the two states. In terms of blood flow control, a major pathologic feature of endothelial dysfunction (in the context of cardiovascular disorders) is a functional deficiency of endothelial nitric oxide synthase (eNOS). This leads to the reduced bioavailability of nitric oxide and is usually detected by impaired vasomotor responses. Whereas dysfunction may be reversible, endothelial *damage* refers to the extreme degree of endothelial dysfunction characterized by premature apoptosis/death of endothelial cells. Increased shedding of the circulating endothelial cells and high plasma concentrations of von Willebrand factor are considered markers of endothelial damage. Such damage is unlikely to be reversible.[4]

Although the endothelium serves as a critical regulator of different aspects of vascular biology, such as hemostasis and inflammation, its ability to produce nitric oxide is pivotal for the different endothelial-dependent functions related to the development and progression of HF. In addition to the regulation of the hemodynamics, nitric oxide acts as a potent modulator of myocardial oxygen consumption in the failing heart.[6,7] The reduced availability of nitric oxide in HF stems either from its reduced production by eNOS or accelerated nitric oxide degradation by reactive oxygen species (**Figure 13-1**). Downregulation of constitutively expressed eNOS by the endothelium is a characteristic feature of endothelial dysfunction that can be related to left ventricular (LV) impairment.[8] Paradoxically, the chronic production of nitric oxide by inducible nitric oxide synthase (iNOS) in HF exerts detrimental effects on ventricular contractility and circulatory function.[9]

Mice lacking eNOS have abnormal cardiac nitric oxide production, impaired myocardial glucose uptake, and pathologic concentric left ventricular remodeling, whereas eNOS overexpression reduced severity of HF.[10-12] Reduced eNOS activity leads to the hypertrophic growth of cardiomyocytes in vitro and eNOS deficiency in mice was associated with impaired myocardial angiogenesis.[13,14] Although eNOS mRNA is reduced in left ventricular tissue of patients with end-stage HF, iNOS mRNA is upregulated and associates with impaired myocardial relaxation.[15] iNOS is located primarily and invariably in the endothelium and vascular smooth muscle cells of the myocardial vasculature, and its expression is associated with the condition of HF per se rather than related to HF etiology.[16]

An excess in reactive oxygen species causes endothelial dysfunction by accelerating nitric oxide inactivation (see also Chapter 8). The family of multi-subunit nicotinamide adenine dinucleotide phosphate (NADPH) oxidases is a major contributor to the increase in superoxide anion production and oxidative stress is upregulated in HF.[17] Depression of the endothelial function and eNOS activity may directly lead to increased reactive oxygen species release, thus maintaining a vicious circle of oxidative stress. In a rat model of diastolic HF, the increase in cardiac eNOS expression by the eNOS enhancer, AVE3085 (which is an activator of eNOS transcription), is accompanied by the reduction in NADPH oxidase, as well as attenuation of cardiac hypertrophy, fibrosis, and diastolic dysfunction.[18]

Antioxidant capacity is also diminished in HF. In animal experiments, activity of different superoxide dismutase (SOD) isoforms is present in the failing myocardium while gene transfer of extracellular SOD significantly improves endothelial function.[19-21] Increased xanthine-oxidase and reduced extracellular SOD activity is closely associated with increased vascular oxidative stress in HF patients, indicating increased oxidative burden and loss of vascular oxidative balance as possible contributors to endothelial dysfunction in HF.[22]

There are in vivo and in vitro data for impaired arginine (eNOS substrate) transport in human HF.[23] Additionally, circulating levels of asymmetric dimethylarginine (ADMA, an endogenous inhibitor of eNOS and circulating proinflammatory cytokines) are increased in HF, further contributing to endothelial dysfunction and accelerated apoptosis of endothelial cells.[24] In patients with ischemic chronic HF elevated plasma, ADMA levels tend to be related to higher New York Heart Association (NYHA) functional classes, increased NT-proBNP levels, and worse clinical outcomes.[25] A strong correlation has been demonstrated between eNOS downregulation and endothelial apoptosis.[26] Of some interest, the β-blocker carvedilol suppresses the caspase cascade and excessive human umbilical vein endothelial cell apoptosis induced by the serum from HF patients or addition of tumor necrosis factor α.[27]

Inflammatory changes are common in patients with HF, with numerous studies reporting high concentrations of cytokines (e.g., tumor necrosis factor α and interleukin-6) and C-reactive protein (see also Chapter 7).[28-32] These biomarkers strongly correlate with HF severity and are strongly and independently predictive of mortality.[28,30-33] In animal models, inflammation is not an innocent bystander but is rather an active participant in HF development and progression.[34] A dysfunctional endothelium also facilitates a proinflammatory status in HF by release of inflammatory factors, such as pentraxin 3 (see also Chapter 30). Endothelial activation of nuclear factor-κB, a key proinflammatory transcriptional factor, is more prominent in patients with severe HF undergoing heart transplantation.[35] Of note, pentraxin 3 levels independently predict cardiac death or HF-related rehospitalization.[36] Despite the strong evidence of a detrimental impact of inflammation in HF outcome, data on specific biologic therapies against tumor necrosis factor α (i.e., using etanercept and infliximab) have been generally disappointing (see also Chapter 7).[37,38]

Endothelial Dysfunction in Clinical Heart Failure

Direct evidence of involvement of the endothelial dysfunction in the genesis of hemodynamic abnormalities in HF derives from data on infusion of NG-monomethyl-L-arginine (L-NMMA), an inhibitor of nitric oxide production, to volunteers with HF.[39] Administration of the L-NMMA increases median pulmonary and systemic vascular resistances and arterial pressures, characteristic features of the HF syndrome. Numerous studies have demonstrated peripheral endothelium-dependent vasomotor abnormalities in HF assessed by brachial artery flow-mediated dilation or forearm blood flow changes in response to acetylcholine.[40-42] However, many such studies show weak, if any, correlations between these measures of endothelial dysfunction and clinical parameters of HF severity, cardiac contractility, or wedge pressure.[42-44]

Although the presence of endothelial dysfunction has been uniformly reported in ischemic HF, the evidence is less robust in the case of nonischemic cardiomyopathy. Some data show no evidence of endothelial dysfunction in HF, whereas some reports show a lesser degree of endothelial abnormalities in nonischemic cardiomyopathy compared with systolic HF.[40,45,46] Both endothelial-dependent and endothelial-independent vasodilation have demonstrated HF secondary to valvular heart disease.[47] Although endothelial dysfunction is a feature of HF of any etiology, multiple cardiovascular risk factors and comorbidities common in patients with ischemic HF (e.g., diabetes, systemic atherosclerosis) can contribute to systemic endothelial impairment per se. In contrast, patients with nonischemic HF tend to have more localized endothelial dysfunction limited to the cardiac vasculature. The evidence supporting this concept will be discussed below.

Endothelial Dysfunction of the Coronary Circulation in Heart Failure

Evidence of endothelial dysfunction of coronary arteries is uniformly present in patients with HF of any etiology.[48] Coronary artery endothelial dysfunction appears to play a particular role in nonischemic cardiomyopathy. As opposed to ischemic HF, in which atherosclerosis often affects multiple vascular sites, pathogenic processes in many forms of nonischemic cardiomyopathy are predominantly confined to the heart itself. Under these circumstances, prominent coronary endothelial dysfunction may be seen without any signs of peripheral artery endothelial dysfunction present. In some patients with nonischemic HF, impairment of endothelial function may occur and be attributable to the unmatched circulatory demand related to the failing heart. Of note, in patients with nonischemic left ventricular dysfunction, significant impairment of the endothelial function is evident despite normal epicardial coronary arteries.[49] Profound coronary endothelial dysfunction seen in patients with acute-onset dilated cardiomyopathy suggests early involvement of the endothelium in the pathogenic process.[50]

In ischemic HF, coronary endothelial impairment parallels systemic endothelial dysfunction and involves both resistance and conductance vessels. However, coronary endothelial dysfunction in ischemic HF can vary substantially in its severity, possibly reflecting individual pathologic features of the disease (e.g., inflammatory activity).[51] Pathophysiologic significance of dysfunctional coronary endothelium in ischemic cardiomyopathy is supported by the link between the degree of depression of the coronary blood flow reserve (an index of coronary endothelial dysfunction), magnitude of unfavorable cardiac geometry, and rise in BNP levels.[52,53]

Activity of the coronary endothelium affects both systolic and diastolic cardiac function. Vasomotor capacity of the coronary arteries is predictive of subsequent improvement in left ventricular contractility.[50] The status of coronary endothelium is also independently linked to the impaired cardiac relaxation in patients with preserved systolic function.[54] Also, in patients with ischemic heart disease, coronary endothelial dysfunction predicts progression of the myocardial diastolic dysfunction.[55] The details of molecular mechanisms that link endothelial dysfunction and abnormalities in cardiac contractility and relaxation are still to be understood; however, the altered balance between the generation of nitric oxide and the elimination of nitric oxide in the heart has been shown to be important with respect to the transition from cardiac hypertrophy to HF in experimental animals.[56] Both activity and expression of the normal eNOS in cardiac tissue are reduced while potentially detrimental iNOS is increased in failing human hearts.[56,57] A direct mutual relationship between the coronary endothelial perturbations and pathogenesis of cardiac dysfunction in humans is difficult to establish, and to some extent coronary endothelial dysfunction could still be secondary to the other cardiac pathologic processes.

Systemic Nature of Endothelial Dysfunction in Heart Failure

As was mentioned previously, in most patients with HF, endothelial dysfunction is not confined to a single arterial bed but rather shows a systemic pattern of distribution with peripheral arteries, such as the brachial or radial artery being affected in parallel with the heart vessels. The systemic nature of the endothelial abnormalities spreads beyond the arterial tree itself. Accumulating evidence shows the endothelial dysfunction in systolic HF also involves the venous and capillary endothelium. Endothelium-dependent venodilation is impaired in chronic HF, but particularly so in the acute decompensated phase of the disease.[58] Improvement in vasomotor venous function in patients with decompensated systolic HF is accompanied by increase in exercise tolerance.[58] Animal experiments showed inflammatory activation of the venous endothelial cells secondary to vascular stress and peripheral blood flow congestion typical of HF.[59] However, knowledge of clinical significance of the venous endothelial function in this disorder is limited, and evidence of any independent role of venous endothelial abnormalities in the pathogenesis and prognosis in HF is lacking. It is likely that the bulk of venous endothelial abnormalities may be a consequence rather than a course of HF.[60] Similar to arterial endothelial arterial dysfunction, changes in activity of the venous endothelium appear to vary depending on HF etiology, with no venous endothelial dysfunction evident in patients with chronic nonischemic HF even when the arterial endothelial dysfunction is present.[61]

Resting exhaled nitric oxide, a marker of pulmonary endothelial nitric oxide production, is increased in HF, potentially indicating preserved endothelial function of the pulmonary vessels.[62] Although one may speculate about the possibility that enhanced nitric oxide production may play a role in counterbalancing systemic endothelial dysfunction, this hypothesis seems unlikely. It is not clear whether this increased nitric oxide generation is mediated by eNOS associated with normal endothelial function or iNOS associated with uncontrolled nitric oxide release under conditions of abnormal systemic homeostasis (for example, in sepsis) and responsible for excessive oxidative stress. The fact the patients with HF have reduced ability to increase nitric oxide release by pulmonary arteries during exercise despite enhanced resting nitric oxide production points toward the presence of endothelial dysfunction in the pulmonary vascular system. The presence of systemic endothelial dysfunction in HF is also supported by studies that have demonstrated a defective endothelium-dependent dilatory response of the microvascular bed.[63,64] Microvascular endothelial dysfunction, together with reduced capillary density seen in systolic HF, may significantly contribute to the chronic hypoxia of peripheral tissues, symptoms of fatigue, and poor exercise tolerance.[65]

Chronic dysfunction in the endothelium in HF contributes to the remodeling of peripheral arteries, resulting in the hypertrophy and reduced elastic properties.[66,67] Impaired endothelium-dependent vasodilation correlates with the vascular wall hypertrophy and abnormalities of the local arterial elastic characteristics, such as distensibility and compliance.[67,68] This systemic nature of endothelial dysfunction seen in HF reflects the concept of the endothelium as single unique organ. Nevertheless, this approach also acknowledges significant diversity in phenotype and function of endothelial cells located within different segments of the vascular tree. Further research is still required to provide a holistic view on systemic versus local endothelial disarrangements in the pathophysiology of HF.

ENDOTHELIAL DYSFUNCTION AND CLINICAL OUTCOMES IN HEART FAILURE

Evidence of clinical significance of vasomotor endothelial dysfunction in patients with HF is provided by several prospective outcome studies (**Table 13-1**). All these studies consistently demonstrate an independent relationship between the degree of endothelial dysfunction and the risk of negative outcome. This relationship was true across a population of patients ranging from mild HF (NYHA class I) with relatively preserved cardiac contractility to those with advanced disease (NYHA class IV) with severely depressed left ventricular function.[69,70] Systemic levels of the natural eNOS inhibitor, ADMA, which are elevated in systolic HF, independently predict a reduced effective renal plasma flow.[71] This potentially makes endothelial dysfunction partly responsible for the progressive deterioration of renal function seen in many patients with HF.

Although the severity of vasomotor endothelial dysfunction may vary among patients with ischemic or nonischemic cause of HF, the predictive power of endothelial dysfunction on prognosis does not depend on the HF etiology. Once developed, endothelial dysfunction bears similarly high risk of unfavorable events in both ischemic and nonischemic HF. Moreover, endothelial dysfunction of coronary arteries in patients after cardiac transplantation also independently predicts the risk of future cardiovascular events and death.[72] Endothelial dysfunction may be also accountable for some cases of suboptimal response to cardiac resynchronization therapy. The association of

TABLE 13-1 Endothelial Dysfunction and Clinical Outcomes in Heart Failure

STUDY	STUDY POPULATION	NYHA/EJECTION FRACTION	MEASURE OF ENDOTHELIAL FUNCTION	FOLLOW-UP DURATION	OUTCOME	RESULTS*
Shechter et al[70]	82 (100% IHF)	IV/22 ± 3	FMD	14 mo	Death	HR (median FMD) 2.04; 95% CI 1.09-5.1, $P = 0.03$
de Berrazueta et al[151]	242 (38% IHF)	I-IV/36 ± 13	FBF in response to ACH (VOP)	5 yr	Composite of death, heart attack, angina, stroke, NYHA class IV, or hospitalization due to HF	HR [Exp(B)] 0.67; SE 0.18, $P = 0.01$
Heitzer et al[69]	289 (56% IHF)	I/41 ± 7	FBF in response to ACH (VOP)	4.8 yr	Composite of death from cardiac causes, hospitalization due to HF, heart transplantation	HR 0.96; 95% CI 0.94-0.98, $P = 0.007$
Katz et al[152]	149 (33% IHF)	II-III/25 ± 1	FMD	28 mo	Death or urgent transplantation	HR (1% decrease in FMD) 1.20; 95% CI 1.03-1.45, $P = 0.027$
Katz et al[152]	110 (56% IHF)	II-III/25 ± 1	Exhaled NO production	13 mo	Death or urgent transplantation	HR 1.31; 95% CI 1.01-1.69, $P = 0.04$
Fischer et al[153]	67 (64% IHF)	II-III/47 ± 10	FMD	46 mo	Composite of cardiac death, hospitalization due to HF, or heart transplantation	HR [Exp(B)] 0.665; SE 0.18, $P = 0.01$
Kübrich et al[72]	185 heart transplant recipients (32% IHF)	75 ± 10	Coronary vasomotor function	60 mo	Composite of death, progressive HF, myocardial infarction, percutaneous or surgical coronary revascularization	RR 1.97; CI 1.1-3.6, $P = 0.028$

*For all, endothelial function was an independent predictor of outcome.

ACH, Acetylcholine; *CI,* confidence interval; *FBF,* forearm blood flow; *FMD,* flow-mediated dilation; *HF,* heart failure; *HR,* hazard ratio; *IHF,* ischemic heart failure; *NO,* nitric oxide; *NYHA,* New York Heart Association; *RR,* relative risk; *SE,* standard error; *VOP,* venous occlusion plethysmography.

clinical improvement after cardiac resynchronization therapy and magnitude of endothelium-dependent vasodilation is independent from the factors commonly used to select patients for treatment, such as QRS complex duration, left ventricular ejection fraction, or degree of left ventricular dyssynchrony.[73] Improvement in exercise tolerance after cardiac resynchronization therapy is accompanied by improvements in endothelial vasodilatory capacity, although a causative relationship between the changes cannot be established.[73] Recently, endothelial dysfunction has been shown to be of prognostic significance in patients with HF with preserved ejection fraction.[74,75] However, the clinical significance of the endothelial dysfunction in HF is somewhat limited by relatively small populations of the studied patients, as well as the short- to middle-term duration of follow-up.

Circulating Markers of Endothelial Dysfunction in Heart Failure

The impairment of endothelial function in HF is not limited to vasomotor capacity but apparently affects all the diverse aspects of the endothelial activity, including proinflammatory activation of endothelial cells and failure of the antioxidant defense system (**Figure 13-2**). Among multiple regulatory proteins produced by the endothelium, several have emerged as useful blood markers of endothelial activation or damage. In respect to the HF, increased levels of plasma markers of endothelial activation (e.g., E-selectin) and damage (e.g., von Willebrand factor) are commonly seen (**Table 13-2**). However, most of these studies compared data obtained from patients with HF to those from healthy individuals. Consequently, it is difficult to differentiate precisely the scale to which the endothelial changes are attributable to the HF per se or to comorbidities and risk factors (such as hypercholesterolemia), which are often seen in patients with HF and known to be associated with endothelial perturbation. The influence of comorbidities and risk factors on endothelial function may partly explain why levels of von Willebrand factor and E-selectin do not always correlate with measures of HF severity, such as left ventricular ejection fraction, BNP, HF functional status, or exercise tolerance.[76,77] This viewpoint is also supported by lack of significant differences in parameters of plasma markers of endothelial activation and damage between patients with acute decompensated and chronic HF. Furthermore, increased concentrations of E-selectin and von Willebrand factor in HF were reported in patients with concomitant diabetes but not in diabetes-free patients.[78]

Counts of circulating endothelial cells, another index of endothelial damage, are increased to similar degree in subjects with acute and chronic HF and correlate with other measures of endothelial damage/dysfunction (e.g., levels of von Willebrand factor and E-selectin and flow-mediated dilation).[41,79] In relation to clinical parameters, circulating endothelial cell counts parallel plasma levels of BNP, but not left ventricular contractility or HF functional class.[41,79]

Endothelin-1 is a very powerful vasoconstrictor in which overproduction is related to pathogenesis of various

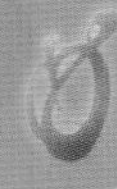

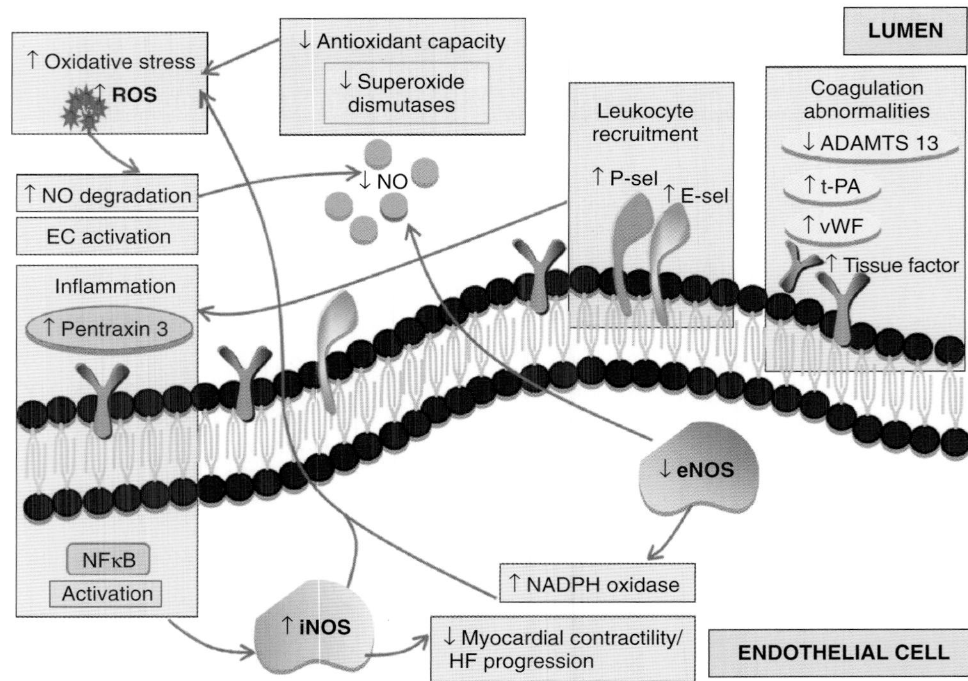

FIGURE 13-2 Diversity of endothelium-related abnormalities in heart failure. Endothelial dysfunction in HF parallels enhanced oxidative stress, which contributes to accelerated NO degradation, and proinflammatory activation of endothelial cells. Activated endothelium produces different inflammatory molecules, such as pentraxin, and also attracts inflammatory cells (leukocytes) in the vascular wall, thus completing the vicious circle on proinflammatory changes. Also dysfunctional endothelium shifts toward a prothrombotic phenotype, associated with increased production of vWF, tissue factor, t-PA, and reduced expression of ADAMTS 13. *EC,* Endothelial cell; *eNOS,* endothelial NO synthase; *E-sel,* soluble E-selectin; *HF,* heart failure; *iNOS,* inducible NO synthase; *NFκB,* nuclear factor κB; *NO,* nitric oxide; *P-sel,* soluble P-selectin; *ROS,* reactive oxygen species; *t-PA;* tissue type plasminogen activator.

TABLE 13-2 Plasma Markers of Endothelial Function in Heart Failure

STUDY	STUDY POPULATION	EF, % (INCLUSION CRITERIA/ ACTUAL)	ETIOLOGY	CONTROLS	MARKER	RESULTS
Kistorp et al[78]	195 CHF with diabetes 147 CHF without diabetes	≤45/30 ± 8 in diabetic group, 30 ± 8 in nondiabetic group	74% IHF in diabetic group, 51% IHF in nondiabetic group	116 healthy	E-selectin vWF	↑ diabetes group ↔ in nondiabetic ↑ diabetes group ↔ in nondiabetic
Chong et al[76]	35 with AHF 40 with CHF	≤40/30 (21-33) in AHF, 30 (29-33) in CHF	63% IHF in AHF group, 83% IHF in CHF group	32 healthy	E-selectin vWF sTM	↑ in AHF and CHF ↔ AHF vs. CHF ↑ in AHF and CHF ↔ AHF vs. CHF ↑ in AHF and CHF ↑ AHF vs. CHF
Vila et al[154]	59 CHF	Not specified	Not specified	59 healthy	vWF thrombospondin-1	↑ ↓
Chong et al[77]	137 CHF	≤45/30 (25-35)	61% IHF	106 healthy	E-selectin vWF	↔ ↔
Chong et al[79]	30 with AHF 30 with CHF	≤40/30 (22-32) in AHF group, 30 (29-34) in CHF	70% IHF in AHF group, 80% IHF in CHF group	20 healthy	E-selectin vWF CECs	↑ in AHF and CHF ↔ AHF vs. CHF ↑ in AHF and CHF ↔ AHF vs. CHF ↑ in AHF and CHF ↔ AHF vs. CHF
Leyva et al[155]	39 CHF	Not specified/22 ± 12 in IHF, 26 ± 16 in DCM	59% IHF	16 healthy	E-selectin	↑ (↔ IHF vs. DCM)
Chong et al[41]	30 CHF	<40/31 (29-35)	77% IHF	20 healthy	vWF sTM CECs	↑ ↔ ↑

↑, Increased; ↓, decreased; ↔, no changes; *AHF,* acute heart failure; *CECs,* circulating endothelial cells; *CHF,* chronic heart failure; *DCM,* dilated cardiomyopathy; *EF,* ejection fraction; *IHF,* ischemic heart failure; *sTM,* soluble thrombomodulin; *vWF,* von Willebrand factor.

cardiovascular diseases.[80] Although produced by endothelial cells, the role of blood endothelin-1 levels—a marker of endothelial dysfunction—has significant limitations. First, its generation is not exclusive to the endothelium and it is also produced by vascular smooth muscle cells.[80] Second, this regulatory protein predominantly acts in a paracrine manner being released toward the location of the vascular smooth muscles rather than to the arterial lumen. Nevertheless, endothelin-1 overexpression is implicated in endothelial dysfunction, and its plasma levels correlate with degree of impairment of the endothelium-mediated vasodilation.[81] Plasma endothelin-1 levels are increased in HF patients and inhibit endothelial activity by stimulation of ADMA production, at least in experimental HF.[82,83] Consequently, increased endothelin-1 activity in HF represents one of the mechanisms responsible for endothelial dysfunction. In experimental work, pharmacologic inhibition of the endothelin-1 pathway significantly improved vasomotor endothelial function.[84] Also, in patients with HF, vasomotor endothelial function improved following administration of small doses of an endothelin A receptor blocker.[85] However, endothelin receptor blockers failed to demonstrate any significant clinical benefits in randomized clinical trials conducted on patients with HF.[86]

PROTHROMBOTIC TRANSFORMATION OF THE ENDOTHELIUM IN HEART FAILURE

Chronic HF confers a considerable prothrombotic risk. The annual incidence of venous thromboembolism is 1.7% to 2.7% in HF compared with about 0.1% in the general population.[87] Although the genesis of prothrombotic risk in HF is multifactorial and includes low cardiac output, dilation of cardiac chambers and stasis of blood in peripheral vascular beds, endothelial damage/dysfunction is considered an important contributor to this process.[86]

The prominent antithrombotic characteristics of healthy endothelial cells are changed dramatically in the dysfunctional endothelium.[86] For example, the abundance of inflammatory cytokines in HF triggers endothelial expression of tissue factor, a trigger of the extrinsic coagulation cascade.[88] Active endothelial production of tissue factor results in downstream activation of factor Xa and leads to cleavage of prothrombin to form thrombin. In acute HF, high tissue factor levels are significantly correlated with inflammatory markers and are highly increased in those who died during the follow-up period.[89] Also, tissue factor is a significant predictor of poor prognosis in chronic HF.[90]

Platelet abnormalities in observed HF are also partly attributable to endothelial impairment.[91] A dysfunctional endothelium triggers expression of platelet-activating factor, which facilitates platelet adhesion to endothelial cells and upregulates production of von Willebrand factor.[92] Dysfunctional endothelial cells release large amounts of von Willebrand factor, further promoting platelet activation and adhesion. Activity of ADAMTS13, a key von Willebrand factor cleaving protease pivotal in the pathogenesis of prothrombotic thrombogenic purpura and hemolytic thrombogenic syndrome, is decreased in HF, being negatively correlated with BNP levels, NYHA class, and endothelial dysfunction.[93] Also, high levels of the tissue type plasmin activator antigen (tPA), predominantly produced by endothelial cells, are independently predictive of a poor prognosis in HF.[94]

TREATMENT OF ENDOTHELIAL DYSFUNCTION IN HEART FAILURE

Pharmaceutical Agents and Endothelial Function

Given the general acceptance of importance of the endothelial dysfunction in pathogenesis and outcome of HF, the endothelium became a target for various therapeutic interventions. Activation of the renin-angiotensin-aldosterone axis seen in HF negatively affects function of endothelial cells and disturbs nitric oxide downstream signaling (**Figure 13-3**).[95] Favorable effects of angiotensin-converting enzyme (ACE) inhibitors on the endothelium in HF are achieved via different mechanisms, including reduction in production of vasoconstrictor prostanoids, upregulation of eNOS, and inhibition of endothelial cell apoptosis (see also Chapter 34).[96-98] The clinical effectiveness of

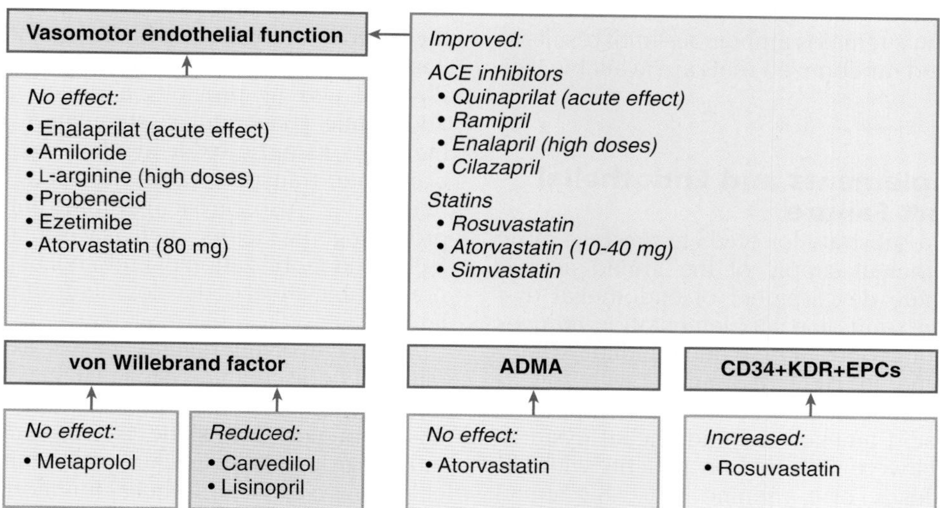

FIGURE 13-3 Effects of therapeutic interventions on characteristics of endothelial function in patients with systolic heart failure. *ACE,* Angiotensin-converting enzyme; *ADMA,* asymmetric dimethylarginine; *EPCs,* endothelial progenitor cells.

inhibitors of the renin-angiotensin-aldosterone system, such as ACE inhibitors or spironolactone, in HF appears to be partly attributable to their beneficial effects on the vascular endothelium.

All published studies uniformly show improvement in endothelium-dependent vasomotor capacity and reduction in the blood levels of von Willebrand factor using neurohormonal antagonists in HF (**Table 13-3**). Several studies, including the African American Heart Failure Trial (A-HeFT), have demonstrated that improvement in morbidity, mortality, and functional status in HF treated by ACE inhibitors was linked to the improvement in endothelial function.[99,100] The capacity of various ACE inhibitors to restore endothelial function may differ significantly and the prescription of higher treatment doses may be required.[101,102] However, the relative impact of the endothelial effects in the overall benefit of such therapy is unclear, and there is little evidence to justify the preference of particular ACE inhibitors based on their endothelial effects.

The majority of reported trials showed that treatment with statins improves endothelial function in HF regardless of its cause (**Table 13-4**). The exact mechanisms of the pleiotropic properties of statins on endothelium are not clear but appear to be independent of their cholesterol-lowering effects.[103] The statins enhance coronary nitric oxide generation in pacing-induced HF and improve endothelial function in normolipidemic patients with HF.[105-108] The cholesterol-independent nature of endothelial responses to statins is further supported by lack of any endothelial effects of ezetimibe, despite similar cholesterol-lowering capacity.[109] It is not clear if statins have any direct specific effect on the endothelial cells to increase their production of nitric oxide. Systemic effects of statins are more likely to be implicated. Antioxidant properties of the statins were also proposed to play a role, but direct mechanistic links between the two processes are difficult to prove, leaving room for debate.[110-112] In the context of lack of evidence from randomized clinical trials to support beneficial effects of statins on outcomes in HF, endothelial dysfunction alone cannot constitute an indication for initiation of statin therapy. Obviously, many patients with HF will still receive statins because of background ischemic heart disease. A number of other medications, such as sildenafil, allopurinol, etanercept, and growth hormone have shown favorable effects on endothelial dysfunction in HF, the clinical utility of such effects remains ambiguous until results of appropriately designed randomized trials are available (see Table 13-3).

Nutritional Supplements and Endothelial Function in Heart Failure

L-Arginine serves as a substrate for eNOS to produce nitric oxide, and an insufficient supply of the amino acid is suggested to contribute development of endothelial dysfunction. Additionally, L-arginine supplementation reduces concentrations of endogenous nitric oxide inhibitor ADMA, known to be elevated in HF.[24] In animals with low L-arginine levels, supplementation with a low, but not high, dose of the amino acid ameliorated endothelial dysfunction. Similarly, results were obtained on patients with HF. Although smaller doses of L-arginine (e.g., 8 g daily) improved endothelial function, such effects were absent in individuals receiving a higher, 20 g daily dose.[113,114] Small to moderate doses of L-arginine significantly improved exercise capacity over a 6-week treatment period in a single placebo-controlled trial study performed in patients with HF.[115] However, longer term effects of L-arginine supplementation and its impact on clinical outcomes in HF remain unclear. Furthermore, administration of higher L-arginine doses in HF was complicated by elevation in urea and aspartate transaminase levels.[114] Accordingly, currently available evidence does not justify routine use of L-arginine supplements in HF.

A similar situation occurs with some other nutritional supplements with favorable effects on endothelial dysfunction in HF. For example, vitamin C intake can increase endothelium-dependent vasodilatory capacity, and it inhibits endothelial cell apoptosis in congestive HF (see Table 13-3).[116] Despite these predominantly short-term benefits, there is no robust evidence for routine supplementation of the diet of HF patients with antioxidant vitamins. Recently, flavanol-rich chocolate improved endothelial function in chronic HF, and its inclusion in a diet may be a suitable option.[117]

Exercise and Endothelial Function in Heart Failure

Regular moderate physical activity has become a crucial part of the healthy lifestyle recommended for patients with HF. Regular physical training in individuals with systolic left ventricular impairment improves HF-related symptoms, exercise capacity, and quality of life and predicts a better prognosis.[118] Ultimately, cumulative analysis of the literature indicates some capacity of regular physical training to delay progression of the disease.[119] The pathophysiologic mechanisms of exercise-mediated benefits in HF are numerous and include inhibition of excessive neurohormonal activation, amelioration of inflammatory responses and oxidative burden, improvement of cardiovascular hemodynamics, and reduction of peripheral vascular resistance.[119] Vascular endothelium plays a prominent role in those processes.

Endothelial cells are capable of sensing vascular flow as changes in sheer stress. The endothelium responds to increase in luminal sheer stress by enhanced production of the nitric oxide followed by relaxation of vascular wall smooth muscles and vasodilation. This process represents the essence of vasomotor function of the endothelium, and it is commonly assessed as arterial flow–mediated dilation. Physical activity provides a direct physiologic stimulus, and gentle (but regular) stimulation of the endothelium increases its nitric oxide synthase expression, accelerates L-arginine transport, and increases basal nitric oxide release.[120-124] Also, physical training enhances generation of proangiogenic factors, such as vascular endothelial growth factor and mobilization of endothelial progenitor cells, with presumable effect of development/remodeling of the vascular tree.[125,126]

Studies involving regular aerobic exercise in both ischemic and nonischemic systolic HF have consistently yielded beneficial effects on systemic endothelial function (**Table 13-5**). In contrast, static exercise confined to isolated muscle groups, such as handgrip training, has limited if any effect on systemic endothelial function.[127] The intensity and modality of the physical activity can affect resulting changes in the endothelial performance. Bouts of high-intensity

TABLE 13-3 Clinical Studies on the Effects of Pharmaceutical Agents and Nutritional Supplements on Endothelial Function in Heart Failure

AUTHOR	STUDY	NUMBER OF HF PATIENTS	EF, %	TREATMENT*	DURATION	RESULTS
Boman et al[156]	R, DB, controlled	267 (53% IHF)	25 ± 7	Carvedilol 25 mg bd or metoprolol 50 mg bd	1 yr	↓vWF by carvedilol ↔vWF by metoprolol
Hornig et al[101]	R, PC	40 (34% IHF)	≈25	Quinaprilat, enalaprilat, IA	Acute effects	↑FMD by quinaprilat ↔FMD by enalaprilat
Hryniewicz et al[157]	R, PC, DB	64 (52% IHF)	25 ± 1	Ramipril 10 mg or sildenafil 50 mg or combination	Acute effects 1-4 hr	↑FMD (with all 3 treatments)
Drakos et al[102]	NR	11		Enalapril 10-30 mg bd	4-8 wk	↑FMD with higher doses
Tavli et al[158]	NR	30 (100% IHF)	25 ± 5	Cilazapril 5 mg	3 days	↑FMD
Gibbs et al[159]	NR	40 (80% IHF)	30	Lisinopril 10 mg od, or BB (bisoprolol 5 mg or carvedilol 25 mg od)	6 mo	↓vWF
Poelzl et al[100]	NR	33 (40% IHF)	≈24	Optimized dose of various ACEI and BB	3 mo	↑FMD in responders defined by improvement in functional capacity
Farquharson et al[160]	R, DB, PC, crossover	10 (100% IHF)	31 ± 6	Spironolactone 50 mg daily	1 mo	↑FBF in response to ACH (VOP)
Macdonald et al[161]	R, DB, PC, crossover	43 (67% IHF)	<25	Spironolactone 12.5-50 mg daily	3 mo	↑FBF in response to ACH (VOP)
Abiose et al[162]	NR	20	24 ± 9	Spironolactone	8 wk	↑FMD
Farquharson et al[163]	R, PC, DB	10 (100% IHF)	20 ± 8	Amiloride 5 mg od	1 mo	↔FBF in response to ACH (VOP)
Belardinelli et al[164]	R, PC, DB	51 (100% IHF)	33 ± 5	Trimetazidine 20 mg tid	4 wk	↑RA response to ACH (US)
Ito et al[165]	NR	12 NIHF	34	Vitamin C 1 g, IV	Acute effects	↔FMD
Hornig et al[166]	PC	15 (20% IHF)	21	Vitamin C 0.25 g, IA; 1 g bd, oral	Acute effects 4 wk	↑FMD
Ellis et al[167]	R, PC, DB, crossover	10		Vitamin C 2 g, IV	Acute effects	↑FMD
Ellis et al[168]	PC	40 NIHF	<35	Vitamin C 2 g, IV; 2 g bd, oral	Acute effects 1 mo	↑FMD
Erbs et al[169]	NR	18 (50% IHF)	25 ± 4	Vitamin C 0.5 g, IA	Acute effects	↑RA response to ACH (US)
George et al[170]	R, PC, DB	30		Allopurinol 300 od or bd	4 wk	↑FBF in response to ACH (VOP) (more with 300 mg bd)
Doehner et al[171]	DB, PC, crossover	14 (79% IHF)	≈23	Allopurinol 300 mg od	1 wk	↑FMD
R[113]	R	40 (40% IHF)	19 ± 3	L-arginine 8 g daily	4 wk	↑FBF in response to ACH (VOP)
Hirooka et al[172]	NR	20 NIHF	≈43	L-arginine 50 mg, IA	Acute effects	↑FBF in response to RH (VOP)
R, PC, DB[114]	R, PC, DB	20 (60% IHF)	21	L-arginine 20 g daily	4 wk	↔FBF in response to ACH (VOP)
Paul et al[173]	R, PC, DB	22 (100% IHF)	27 ± 7	Methyltetrahydrofolate, IV	Acute effects	↔PWA (salbutamol-mediated changes AI) ↓ADMA
Napoli et al[174]	R, DB, PC	16 (31% IHF)	<40	Growth hormone (4 IU, SC every other day)	3 mo	↑FBF in response to ACH (VOP)
Fichtlscherer et al[175]	Controlled	18 (50% IHF)	25 ± 1	Etanercept 25 mg, SC, single dose	7 days	↑FBF in response to ACH (VOP)
Fuentes et al[176]	R, PC, DB	22 (41% IHF)		800 mg magnesium oxide bd	3 mo	↑small artery elasticity index
George et al[170]	R, PC, DB	26		Probenecid 1 g daily	4 wk	↔FBF in response to ACH (VOP)
Patel[177]	NR	19 (100% IHF)	27 ± 2	Dobutamine 3 μg/kg/min, IV	72 h	↑FMD for ≥2 wk
Freimark et al[178]	Controlled	20 (100% IHF)		Dobutamine, 3.5 μg/kg/min, IV, 5 h twice a week	4 mo	↑FMD
Schwarz et al[179]	R, PC	31 NIHF	19 ± 7	GTN 10^{-9} mol/L, IA	20 min or 12 h	↑ FBF in response to ACH (VOP)
Guazzi et al[180]	DB, PC	16 (63% IHF)	≤45	Sildenafil 50 mg	Acute effects	↑FMD

*Oral administration unless indicated otherwise.

ACEI, Angiotensin-converting enzyme inhibitor; *ACH,* acetylcholine; *ADMA,* asymmetric dimethylarginine; *AI,* augmentation index; *BB,* β-blocker; *bd,* twice daily; *DB,* double blind; *EF,* ejection fraction; *FBF,* forearm blood flow; *FMD,* flow-mediated dilation; *GTN,* glyceryl trinitrate; *HF,* heart failure; *IA,* intraarterial; *IHF,* ischemic heart failure; *IU,* international units; *IV,* intravenous; *NIHF,* nonischemic heart failure; *NR,* nonrandomized; *od,* once daily; *PC,* placebo controlled; *PWA,* pulse wave analysis; *R,* randomized; *RA,* radial artery; *RH,* reactive hyperemia; *SC,* subcutaneously; *VOP,* venous occlusion plethysmography; *vWF,* von Willebrand factor.

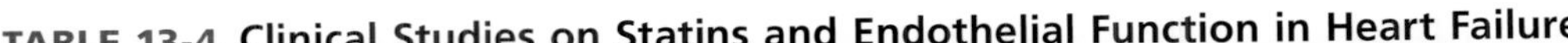

TABLE 13-4 Clinical Studies on Statins and Endothelial Function in Heart Failure

AUTHOR	STUDY	NUMBER OF HF PATIENTS	MEAN EF, %	TREATMENT*	DURATION	RESULTS
Erbs et al[111]	R, PC	42 (27% IHF)	30 ± 1	Rosuvastatin 40 mg od	12 wk	↑FMD ↑CD34/KDR + EPCs
Guonari et al[109]	R, DB, crossover	22 (100% IHF)	30 ± 1	Rosuvastatin 10 mg od or ezetimibe 20 mg od	4 wk	↑FMD with rosuvastatin ↔FMD with ezetimibe
Bleske et al[104]	R, PC, DB	15 NIHF	25 ± 9	Atorvastatin 80 mg	12 wk	↔FMD
Strey et al[181]	R, DB, PC, crossover	23 NIHF	30 ± 8	Atorvastatin 40 mg od	6 wk	↑FMD ↓endothelin-1
Young et al[110]	R, PC, DB	24 (17% IHF)	31 ± 8	Atorvastatin 40 mg od	6 wk	↑FMD ↔ADMA
Castro et al[182]	R, PC	38	27 ± 12	Atorvastatin 20 mg od	8 wk	↑FMD
Strey et al[108]	R, PC, crossover	240 NIHF	<40	Atorvastatin 40 mg od	6 wk	↑FBF in response to ACH (VOP)
Tousoulis et al[107]	R, controlled	38 (66% IHF), cholesterol levels <220 mg/dL	≤35	Atorvastatin 10 mg od	4 wk	↑FBF in response to RH
Tousoulis et al[183]	R, controlled	38 (100% IHF)	≈25	Atorvastatin 10 mg od or atorvastatin 10 mg od plus vitamin E 400 IU/day	4 wk	↑FBF in response to RH in both treatment groups, but more in atorvastatin alone group
Tousoulis et al[184]	R, DB, crossover	22 (100% IHF)		Atorvastatin 10 mg od Atorvastatin 40 mg od	4 wk	↑FMD with 40 mg od only
Landmesser et al[112]	R	20 (33% IHF)	23	Simvastatin 10 mg od or ezetimibe 10 mg od	4 wk	↑RA FMD ↑EPC ("early" EPC colonies) (for both with simvastatin but not ezetimibe)

*Oral administration unless indicated otherwise.

ACH, Acetylcholine; *ADMA,* asymmetric dimethylarginine; *DB,* double blind; *EF,* ejection fraction; *EPC,* endothelial progenitor cell; *FBF,* forearm blood flow; *FMD,* flow-mediated dilation; *HF,* heart failure; *IHF,* ischemic heart failure; *IU,* international units; *KDR,* kinase insert domain receptor; *NIHF,* nonischemic heart failure; *od,* once daily; *PC,* placebo controlled; *R,* randomized; *RA,* radial artery; *RH,* reactive hyperemia; *VOP,* venous occlusion plethysmography.

TABLE 13-5 Exercise and Endothelial Function in Heart Failure

AUTHOR	STUDY DESIGN	HF (N)	MEAN EF, %	EXERCISE PROGRAM	DURATION	RESULTS
Wisloff et al[130]	R, controlled	27 (100% IHF)	29	Treadmill: (i) Aerobic interval training: four 4-minute intervals at 90%-95% PHR, with 3 min active pauses (walking at 50%-70% PHR) (ii) Moderate continuous training (walked at 70%-75% PHR for 47 minutes)—3 dpw	12 wk	↑FMD (more with aerobic interval training than moderate continuous training)
Miche et al[127]	NR	42 (77% IHF)	23	Weekly, cycle ergometer training (3 times), a 6 min walk (twice) and muscle strength training (twice)	4 wk	↔FMD (irrespective of the presence of diabetes)
Sarto et al[126]	NR	22 (64% IHF)	31	Cycle ergometer (55 min)—3 dpw	8 wk	↑CD34+/KDR+ EPC ↑EC-CFU
Bank et al[185]	NR	7	23	Handgrip exercise (30 min)—4 dpw	4-6 wk	↔FBF in response to ACH (↑ in healthy controls)
Parnell et al[121]	Controlled	21 (30% IHF)	22	Walking, light hand weights, and cycling (50%-60% of maximal HR) plus home-base program—3 dpw	8 wk	↑L-arginine transport ↑FBF in response to ACH
Kobayashi et al[186]	R, controlled	28 (46% IHF)	31	Cycle ergometer training (in two 15 min sessions per day)—2-3 tpw	3 mo	↑FMD in tibial arteries ↔FMD in brachial arteries
Linke et al[187]	R, controlled	22 (45% IHF)	25	Cycle ergometer (6 times a day for 10 min, at 70% peak oxygen consumption)	4 wk	↑RAD in response to ACH
Hornig[188]	NR	12	21	Handgrip training (70% of the maximal workload for 30 min)—daily	4 wk	↑RAD in response to ACH
Hambrecht et al[122]	R, controlled	20 (35% IHF)	24	Cycle ergometer (6 times daily for 10 min at 70% PHR)—first 3 wk, followed by twice daily (40 min in total)—5 dpw	6 mo	↑Femoral artery blood flow in response to ACH ↑Basal endothelial NO formation

ACH, Acetylcholine; *dpw,* times per week; *EC-CFU,* endothelial cell colony-forming units; *EF,* ejection fraction; *EPC,* endothelial progenitor cells; *FBF,* forearm blood flow; *FMD,* flow-mediated dilation; *HF,* heart failure; *HR,* heart rate; *IHF,* ischemic heart failure; *KDR,* kinase insert domain receptor; *NO,* nitric oxide; *NR,* nonrandomized; *PHR,* peak heart rate; *R,* randomized; *RAD,* radial artery dilation; *tpw,* times per week.

exercise can lead to acute release of inflammatory cytokines and oxidative stress and thus detrimentally affect endothelial function.[128,129] However, the endothelium does benefit from regular moderate aerobic exercise. Under these conditions, better vasomotor endothelial capacity is reflected by improvement in cardiac contractility and reverse left ventricular remodeling.[130]

GENETIC PREDISPOSITION TO ENDOTHELIAL DYSFUNCTION IN HEART FAILURE

In the Genetic Risk Assessment of Heart Failure (GRAHF) substudy of the African-American Heart Failure Trial, the eNOS genotype differed between white and black patients with HF.[131] In black patients the -786T allele was associated with lower LV ejection fraction.[131] The prevalence of allele Glu298 was significantly higher in HF patients, and the Glu298Glu genotype was associated with an increased prevalence of hypertension.[132] Also HF patients homozygous for eNOS promoter polymorphism (thymidine to cytosine transition [T(-786)C]) were found to have a more advanced cardiac autonomic imbalance (i.e., abnormal heart rate variability).[133] In the GRAHF study, the Glu298Asp polymorphism was associated with reduced effectiveness of fixed-dose combination of isosorbide dinitrate and hydralazine, which only improved the composite score of survival, hospitalization, and quality of life in Glu298Glu allele carriers.[131] Also, poorer event-free survival was confirmed in HF patients with Asp298 variant of eNOS, particularly in those with nonischemic HF.[134]

ENDOTHELIAL PROGENITORS AND ANGIOGENIC FACTORS IN HEART FAILURE

Conflicting reports have been published on the numbers of circulating CD34+ hematopoietic progenitors, with some studies observing reduction or no change in their levels irrespective of HF etiology.[135] HF severity rather than its cause appears to be the main factor affecting levels of CD34+ cells. Indeed, CD34+ cells have been shown to be increased in mild HF and are depressed in severe HF, when compared with HF-free controls.[136] Other studies confirm a significant inverse correlation between CD34+ and CD34+, CD133+ counts, and NYHA functional class, as well as their progressive reduction from NYHA class I-II to NYHA class III HF independent of cause.[137,138]

It is likely that a reduction in CD34+ cell levels is secondary to HF rather than an element of HF pathogenesis itself and is likely to reflect bone marrow depression and anemia common in severe HF. These hypotheses are supported by observations that implantation of ventricular assist devices was associated with a transient increase in CD34+ cells in parallel with a reduction in BNP levels.[139] Also, CD34+ cell numbers in HF are not affected by physical exercise testing and transcoronary transplantation of CD34+ cells into patients with a history of an anterior MI did not have any effect on endothelial function.[140,141] Numbers of "early" endothelial progenitor cells counted in culture are reduced in HF, being inversely related to NYHA class, but not to vascular endothelial growth factor (VEGF), NT-pro-BNP, or C-reactive protein (CRP) levels.[138,142] Migratory activity of such "early endothelial progenitor cells" is significantly impaired in HF (particularly of ischemic etiology), correlates with endothelial dysfunction, and can be normalized by physical exercise.[135,140] Functional impairment of circulating progenitors in HF is also supported by increased numbers of late apoptotic progenitors, particularly in severe HF, which correlated inversely with EF and positively with NYHA class.[143] In 107 patients with chronic HF, "early endothelial progenitor cells" were independent predictors of all-cause mortality.[142] Also, NT-pro-BNP dose-dependently increased the numbers and proliferative and functional capacity of human "early endothelial progenitor cells" in vitro.[144] Systemic BNP administration to mice led to a significant increase in bone marrow Sca-1/Flk-1+ endothelial progenitors and improvement in blood flow and capillary density in the ischemic limbs.[144]

CD34+KDR+ cells seem to be only significantly reduced in patients with very severe HF.[138,140] Indeed, numbers of CD34+KDR+ cells in HF are unaffected by physical exercise or implantation of ventricular assist devices.[139,140] In one randomized study, 3 months' treatment with high doses of rosuvastatin increased CD34+KDR+ cells and their integrative capacity, which paralleled a significant improvement of FMD and ejection fraction.[111] Additionally, the implantation of CD133+ cells in the infarcted zone in seven candidates for cardiac transplantation was associated with NYHA improvement, reduced NT-pro-BNP levels and risk of sudden death, and a significant increase in ejection fraction by 24 months after treatment.[145] However, the last study was small and lacked a control group, and two of the seven patients died during the period of the observation; thus larger controlled trials are essential to draw any robust conclusion on such therapies in HF.

Abnormal levels of angiogenic factors such as angiopoietin-2 and VEGF have been reported in HF patients.[146] VEGF levels are reduced in congestive HF, but upregulated in acute HF.[147,148] VEGF did not independently predict outcome in chronic HF, and a pathophysiologic role of angiogenic factors in human HF is unclear.[90] However, VEGF treatment reduces myocardial apoptosis, promotes capillary growth, and preserves myocardial contractility and prolonged survival in animal studies.[149,150] In summary, the biologic and pathologic roles of altered production of angiogenic factors are still not entirely clear. They may reflect a degree of compensatory angiogenesis in patients with ischemic HF, but it is more plausible that these changes reflect an ongoing process of vascular remodeling in response to the hemodynamic changes. The potential of these pathways as therapeutic targets is still to be determined.

CONCLUSIONS AND FUTURE DIRECTIONS

Endothelial dysfunction is common in patients with systolic HF and is implicated in the pathophysiology of the disease, symptomatic status, and outcome. Endothelial abnormalities in HF are complex and involve apparently all aspects of the activity of the endothelial cells, including their vasomotor, hemostatic, antioxidant, and inflammation related functions. Only scarce data are available on the state of the endothelium in HF with preserved ejection fraction and further research is desirable. There is substantial variability in the pattern of endothelial dysfunction among patients with systolic HF depending on its cause. In patients with ischemic cardiomyopathy, systemic endothelial dysfunction is typically seen within coronary and peripheral arteries, as well as the microvascular bed. In contrast, patients with nonischemic cardiomyopathy show more localized dysfunction of cardiac arteries, which may be present with or without systemic vascular involvement.

There are several pharmaceutical agents and nutritional components with suggested beneficial effects on endothelial function. However, any prognostic benefits of these agents need to have robust evidence from randomized clinical trials before their clinical implementation. At present, none of the existing agents is recommended for use in HF solely based on their endothelial properties. Improvement of endothelial function by regular aerobic physical exercise contributes to overall success of the physical training in HF. However, isolated bouts of extreme physical activity in sedentary patients may have a negative impact on the endothelium by triggering oxidative and inflammatory responses and should be avoided.

Importantly the prognostic significance of endothelial dysfunction in HF has not yet translated effectively to the clinical setting, primarily because of the significant methodologic limitations of its assessment. Indeed, the methods commonly used for research purposes lack standardization and tend to be operator-dependent and sometimes invasive. Increasingly better understanding of molecular mechanisms of endothelial dysfunction in HF will help to identify new targets for future treatments aimed at restoring endothelial function and improved patient outcomes.

References

1. Kubo SH, Rector TS, Bank AJ, et al: Endothelium-dependent vasodilation is attenuated in patients with heart failure. *Circulation* 84:1589–1596, 1991.
2. Katz SD, Biasucci L, Sabba C, et al: Impaired endothelium-mediated vasodilation in the peripheral vasculature of patients with congestive heart failure. *J Am Coll Cardiol* 19:918–925, 1992.
3. Bank AJ, Rector TS, Tschumperlin LK, et al: Endothelium-dependent vasodilation of peripheral conduit arteries in patients with heart failure. *J Card Fail* 1:35–43, 1994.
4. Blann AD, Lip GY: The endothelium in atherothrombotic disease: assessment of function, mechanisms and clinical implications. *Blood Coagul Fibrinolysis* 9:297–306, 1998.
5. Blann AD, Woywodt A, Bertolini F, et al: Circulating endothelial cells. Biomarker of vascular disease. *Thromb Haemost* 93:228–235, 2005.
6. Nakamura R, Egashira K, Arimura K, et al: Increased inactivation of nitric oxide is involved in impaired coronary flow reserve in heart failure. *Am J Physiol Heart Circ Physiol* 281:H2619–H2625, 2001.
7. Arimura K, Egashira K, Nakamura R, et al: Increased inactivation of nitric oxide is involved in coronary endothelial dysfunction in heart failure. *Am J Physiol Heart Circ Physiol* 280:H68–H75, 2001.
8. Heymes C, Vanderheyden M, Bronzwaer JG, et al: Endomyocardial nitric oxide synthase and left ventricular preload reserve in dilated cardiomyopathy. *Circulation* 99:3009–3016, 1999.
9. Calderone A: The therapeutic effect of natriuretic peptides in heart failure; differential regulation of endothelial and inducible nitric oxide synthases. *Heart Fail Rev* 8:55–70, 2003.
10. Tada H, Thompson CI, Recchia FA, et al: Myocardial glucose uptake is regulated by nitric oxide via endothelial nitric oxide synthase in Langendorff mouse heart. *Circ Res* 86:270–274, 2000.
11. Ruetten H, Dimmeler S, Gehring D, et al: Concentric left ventricular remodeling in endothelial nitric oxide synthase knockout mice by chronic pressure overload. *Cardiovasc Res* 66:444–453, 2005.
12. Jones SP, Greer JJ, van Haperen R, et al: Endothelial nitric oxide synthase overexpression attenuates congestive HF in mice. *Proc Natl Acad Sci U S A* 100:4891–4896, 2003.
13. Wenzel S, Rohde C, Wingerning S, et al: Lack of endothelial nitric oxide synthase-derived nitric oxide formation favors hypertrophy in adult ventricular cardiomyocytes. *Hypertension* 49:193–200, 2007.
14. Zhao X, Lu X, Feng Q: Deficiency in endothelial nitric oxide synthase impairs myocardial angiogenesis. *Am J Physiol Heart Circ Physiol* 283:H2371–H2378, 2002.
15. Drexler H, Kastner S, Strobel A, et al: Expression, activity and functional significance of inducible nitric oxide synthase in the failing human heart. *J Am Coll Cardiol* 32:955–963, 1998.
16. Vejlstrup NG, Bouloumie A, Boesgaard S, et al: Inducible nitric oxide synthase (inos) in the human heart: expression and localization in congestive heart failure. *J Mol Cell Cardiol* 30:1215–1223, 1998.
17. Ray R, Shah AM: NADPH oxidase and endothelial cell function. *Clin Sci (Lond)* 109:217–226, 2005.
18. Westermann D, Riad A, Richter U, et al: Enhancement of the endothelial NO synthase attenuates experimental diastolic heart failure. *Basic Res Cardiol* 104:499–509, 2009.
19. Chen Y, Hou M, Li Y, et al: Increased superoxide production causes coronary endothelial dysfunction and depressed oxygen consumption in the failing heart. *Am J Physiol Heart Circ Physiol* 288:H133–H141, 2005.
20. Miller JD, Peotta VA, Chu Y, et al: MnSOD protects against COX1-mediated endothelial dysfunction in chronic heart failure. *Am J Physiol Heart Circ Physiol* 298:H1600–H1607, 2010.
21. Iida S, Chu Y, Francis J, et al: Gene transfer of extracellular superoxide dismutase improves endothelial function in rats with heart failure. *Am J Physiol Heart Circ Physiol* 289:H525–H532, 2005.
22. Landmesser U, Spiekermann S, Dikalov S, et al: Vascular oxidative stress and endothelial dysfunction in patients with chronic heart failure: role of xanthine-oxidase and extracellular superoxide dismutase. *Circulation* 106:3073–3078, 2002.
23. Kaye DM, Ahlers BA, Autelitano DJ, et al: In vivo and in vitro evidence for impaired arginine transport in human heart failure. *Circulation* 102:2707–2712, 2000.
24. Feng Q, Lu X, Fortin AJ, et al: Elevation of an endogenous inhibitor of nitric oxide synthesis in experimental congestive heart failure. *Cardiovasc Res* 37:667–675, 1998.
25. Hsu CP, Lin SJ, Chung MY, et al: Asymmetric dimethylarginine predicts clinical outcomes in ischemic chronic heart failure. *Atherosclerosis* 225:504–510, 2012.
26. Agnoletti L, Curello S, Bachetti T, et al: Serum from patients with severe HF downregulates enos and is proapoptotic: role of tumor necrosis factor-alpha. *Circulation* 100:1983–1991, 1999.
27. Rossig L, Haendeler J, Mallat Z, et al: Congestive HF induces endothelial cell apoptosis: protective role of carvedilol. *J Am Coll Cardiol* 36:2081–2089, 2000.
28. Seta Y, Shan K, Bozkurt B, et al: Basic mechanisms in heart failure: the cytokine hypothesis. *J Card Fail* 2:243–249, 1996.
29. Levine B, Kalman J, Mayer L, et al: Elevated circulating levels of tumor necrosis factor in severe chronic heart failure. *N Engl J Med* 323:236–241, 1990.
30. Torre-Amione G, Kapadia S, Benedict C, et al: Proinflammatory cytokine levels in patients with depressed left ventricular ejection fraction: a report from the studies of left ventricular dysfunction (solvd). *J Am Coll Cardiol* 27:1201–1206, 1996.
31. Tsutamoto T, Hisanaga T, Wada A, et al: Interleukin-6 spillover in the peripheral circulation increases with the severity of heart failure, and the high plasma level of interleukin-6 is an important prognostic predictor in patients with congestive heart failure. *J Am Coll Cardiol* 31:391–398, 1998.
32. Yin WH, Chen JW, Jen HL, et al: Independent prognostic value of elevated high-sensitivity c-reactive protein in chronic heart failure. *Am Heart J* 147:931–938, 2004.
33. Deswal A, Petersen NJ, Feldman AM, et al: Cytokines and cytokine receptors in advanced heart failure: an analysis of the cytokine database from the vesnarinone trial (vest). *Circulation* 103:2055–2059, 2001.
34. Janssen SP, Gayan-Ramirez G, Van den Bergh A, et al: Interleukin-6 causes myocardial failure and skeletal muscle atrophy in rats. *Circulation* 111:996–1005, 2005.
35. Hoare GS, Birks EJ, Bowles C, et al: In vitro endothelial cell activation and inflammatory responses in end-stage heart failure. *J Appl Physiol* 101:1466–1473, 2006.
36. Suzuki S, Takeishi Y, Niizeki T, et al: Pentraxin 3, a new marker for vascular inflammation, predicts adverse clinical outcomes in patients with heart failure. *Am Heart J* 155:75–81, 2008.
37. Mann DL, McMurray JJ, Packer M, et al: Targeted anticytokine therapy in patients with chronic heart failure: results of the randomized etanercept worldwide evaluation (renewal). *Circulation* 109:1594–1602, 2004.
38. Chung ES, Packer M, Lo KH, et al: Randomized, double-blind, placebo-controlled, pilot trial of infliximab, a chimeric monoclonal antibody to tumor necrosis factor-alpha, in patients with moderate-to-severe heart failure: results of the anti-TNF therapy against congestive HF (ATTACH) trial. *Circulation* 107:3133–3140, 2003.
39. Habib F, Dutka D, Crossman D, et al: Enhanced basal nitric oxide production in heart failure: another failed counter-regulatory vasodilator mechanism? *Lancet* 344:371–373, 1994.
40. Tentolouris C, Tousoulis D, Antoniades C, et al: Endothelial function and proinflammatory cytokines in patients with ischemic heart disease and dilated cardiomyopathy. *Int J Cardiol* 94:301–305, 2004.
41. Chong AY, Blann AD, Patel J, et al: Endothelial dysfunction and damage in congestive heart failure: relation of flow-mediated dilation to circulating endothelial cells, plasma indexes of endothelial damage, and brain natriuretic peptide. *Circulation* 110:1794–1798, 2004.
42. Bank AJ, Lee PC, Kubo SH: Endothelial dysfunction in patients with heart failure: relationship to disease severity. *J Card Fail* 6:29–36, 2000.
43. Vittorio TJ, Zolty R, Garg PK, et al: Interdependence of cardiac and endothelial function in patients with symptomatic chronic HF of nonischemic etiology. *Echocardiography* 26:916–921, 2009.
44. Bae JH, Bassenge E, Kim MH, et al: Impact of left ventricular ejection fraction on endothelial function in patients with coronary artery disease. *Clin Cardiol* 27:333–337, 2004.
45. Shah A, Gkaliagkousi E, Ritter JM, et al: Endothelial function and arterial compliance are not impaired in subjects with HF of non-ischemic origin. *J Card Fail* 16:114–120, 2010.
46. Klosinska M, Rudzinski T, Grzelak P, et al: Endothelium-dependent and -independent vasodilation is more attenuated in ischaemic than in non-ischaemic heart failure. *Eur J Heart Fail* 11:765–770, 2009.
47. Nakamura M, Yoshida H, Arakawa N, et al: Endothelium-dependent vasodilatation is not selectively impaired in patients with chronic HF secondary to valvular heart disease and congenital heart disease. *Eur Heart J* 17:1875–1881, 1996.
48. de Jong RM, Blanksma PK, Cornel JH, et al: Endothelial dysfunction and reduced myocardial perfusion reserve in HF secondary to coronary artery disease. *Am J Cardiol* 91:497–500, 2003.
49. Canetti M, Akhter MW, Lerman A, et al: Evaluation of myocardial blood flow reserve in patients with chronic congestive HF due to idiopathic dilated cardiomyopathy. *Am J Cardiol* 92:1246–1249, 2003.
50. Mathier MA, Rose GA, Fifer MA, et al: Coronary endothelial dysfunction in patients with acute-onset idiopathic dilated cardiomyopathy. *J Am Coll Cardiol* 32:216–224, 1998.
51. Bitar F, Lerman A, Akhter MW, et al: Variable response of conductance and resistance coronary arteries to endothelial stimulation in patients with HF due to nonischemic dilated cardiomyopathy. *J Cardiovasc Pharmacol Ther* 11:197–202, 2006.
52. Dini FL, Ghiadoni L, Conti U, et al: Coronary flow reserve in idiopathic dilated cardiomyopathy: relation with left ventricular wall stress, natriuretic peptides, and endothelial dysfunction. *J Am Soc Echocardiogr* 22:354–360, 2009.
53. Stolen KQ, Kemppainen J, Kalliokoski KK, et al: Myocardial perfusion reserve and peripheral endothelial function in patients with idiopathic dilated cardiomyopathy. *Am J Cardiol* 93:64–68, 2004.
54. Elesber AA, Redfield MM, Rihal CS, et al: Coronary endothelial dysfunction and hyperlipidemia are independently associated with diastolic dysfunction in humans. *Am Heart J* 153:1081–1087, 2007.
55. Ma LN, Zhao SP, Gao M, et al: Endothelial dysfunction associated with left ventricular diastolic dysfunction in patients with coronary heart disease. *Int J Cardiol* 72:275–279, 2000.
56. Lapu-Bula R, Ofili E: From hypertension to heart failure: role of nitric oxide-mediated endothelial dysfunction and emerging insights from myocardial contrast echocardiography. *Am J Cardiol* 99:7D–14D, 2007.
57. Ferreiro CR, Chagas AC, Carvalho MH, et al: Expression of inducible nitric oxide synthase is increased in patients with HF due to ischemic disease. *Braz J Med Biol Res* 37:1313–1320, 2004.
58. Rabelo ER, Ruschel K, Moreno H, Jr, et al: Venous endothelial function in heart failure: comparison with healthy controls and effect of clinical compensation. *Eur J Heart Fail* 10:758–764, 2008.
59. Colombo PC, Rastogi S, Onat D, et al: Activation of endothelial cells in conduit veins of dogs with HF and veins of normal dogs after vascular stretch by acute volume loading. *J Card Fail* 15:457–463, 2009.

60. Dworakowski R, Walker S, Momin A, et al: Reduced nicotinamide adenine dinucleotide phosphate oxidase-derived superoxide and vascular endothelial dysfunction in human heart failure. *J Am Coll Cardiol* 51:1349–1356, 2008.
61. Nightingale AK, Blackman DJ, Ellis GR, et al: Preservation of venous endothelial function in the forearm venous capacitance bed of patients with chronic HF despite arterial endothelial dysfunction. *J Am Coll Cardiol* 37:1062–1068, 2001.
62. Funakoshi T, Yamabe H, Yokoyama M: Increased exhaled nitric oxide and impaired oxygen uptake (VO2) kinetics during exercise in patients with chronic heart failure. *Jpn Circ J* 63:255–260, 1999.
63. Andersson SE, Edvinsson ML, Edvinsson L: Cutaneous vascular reactivity is reduced in aging and in heart failure: association with inflammation. *Clin Sci (Lond)* 105:699–707, 2003.
64. Andreassen AK, Gullestad L, Holm T, et al: Endothelium-dependent vasodilation of the skin microcirculation in heart transplant recipients. *Clin Transplant* 12:324–332, 1998.
65. Duscha BD, Kraus WE, Keteyian SJ, et al: Capillary density of skeletal muscle: a contributing mechanism for exercise intolerance in class ii-iii chronic HF independent of other peripheral alterations. *J Am Coll Cardiol* 33:1956–1963, 1999.
66. Naka KK, Tweddel AC, Doshi SN, et al: Flow-mediated changes in pulse wave velocity: a new clinical measure of endothelial function. *Eur Heart J* 27:302–309, 2006.
67. Poelzl G, Frick M, Huegel H, et al: Chronic HF is associated with vascular remodeling of the brachial artery. *Eur J Heart Fail* 7:43–48, 2005.
68. Nakamura M, Sugawara S, Arakawa N, et al: Reduced vascular compliance is associated with impaired endothelium-dependent dilatation in the brachial artery of patients with congestive heart failure. *J Card Fail* 10:36–42, 2004.
69. Heitzer T, Baldus S, von Kodolitsch Y, et al: Systemic endothelial dysfunction as an early predictor of adverse outcome in heart failure. *Arterioscler Thromb Vasc Biol* 25:1174–1179, 2005.
70. Shechter M, Matetzky S, Arad M, et al: Vascular endothelial function predicts mortality risk in patients with advanced ischaemic chronic heart failure. *Eur J Heart Fail* 11:588–593, 2009.
71. Kielstein JT, Bode-Boger SM, Klein G, et al: Endogenous nitric oxide synthase inhibitors and renal perfusion in patients with heart failure. *Eur J Clin Invest* 33:370–375, 2003.
72. Kubrich M, Petrakopoulou P, Kofler S, et al: Impact of coronary endothelial dysfunction on adverse long-term outcome after heart transplantation. *Transplantation* 85:1580–1587, 2008.
73. Akar JG, Al-Chekakie MO, Fugate T, et al: Endothelial dysfunction in HF identifies responders to cardiac resynchronization therapy. *Heart Rhythm* 5:1229–1235, 2008.
74. Akiyama E, Sugiyama S, Matsuzawa Y, et al: Incremental prognostic significance of peripheral endothelial dysfunction in patients with HF with normal left ventricular ejection fraction. *J Am Coll Cardiol* 60:1778–1786, 2012.
75. Matsue Y, Suzuki M, Nagahori W, et al: Endothelial dysfunction measured by peripheral arterial tonometry predicts prognosis in patients with HF with preserved ejection fraction. *Int J Cardiol* 168:36–40, 2013.
76. Chong AY, Freestone B, Patel J, et al: Endothelial activation, dysfunction, and damage in congestive HF and the relation to brain natriuretic peptide and outcomes. *Am J Cardiol* 97:671–675, 2006.
77. Chong AY, Freestone B, Lim HS, et al: Plasma von Willebrand factor and soluble e-selectin levels in stable outpatients with systolic heart failure: the Frederiksberg HF study. *Int J Cardiol* 119:80–82, 2007.
78. Kistorp C, Chong AY, Gustafsson F, et al: Biomarkers of endothelial dysfunction are elevated and related to prognosis in chronic HF patients with diabetes but not in those without diabetes. *Eur J Heart Fail* 10:380–387, 2008.
79. Chong AY, Lip GY, Freestone B, et al: Increased circulating endothelial cells in acute heart failure: comparison with von Willebrand factor and soluble e-selectin. *Eur J Heart Fail* 8:167–172, 2006.
80. Penna C, Rastaldo R, Mancardi D, et al: Effect of endothelins on the cardiovascular system. *J Cardiovasc Med (Hagerstown)* 7:645–652, 2006.
81. Galatius S, Wroblewski H, Sorensen VB, et al: Endothelin and von Willebrand factor as parameters of endothelial function in idiopathic dilated cardiomyopathy: different stimuli for release before and after heart transplantation? *Am Heart J* 137:549–554, 1999.
82. Good JM, Nihoyannopoulos P, Ghatei MA, et al: Elevated plasma endothelin concentrations in heart failure; an effect of angiotensin ii? *Eur Heart J* 15:1634–1640, 1994.
83. Ohnishi M, Wada A, Tsutamoto T, et al: Endothelin stimulates an endogenous nitric oxide synthase inhibitor, asymmetric dimethylarginine, in experimental heart failure. *Clin Sci (Lond)* 103(Suppl 48):241S–244S, 2002.
84. Sakai S, Miyauchi T, Kobayashi M, et al: Inhibition of myocardial endothelin pathway improves long-term survival in heart failure. *Nature* 384:353–355, 1996.
85. Berger R, Stanek B, Hulsmann M, et al: Effects of endothelin a receptor blockade on endothelial function in patients with chronic heart failure. *Circulation* 103:981–986, 2001.
86. Shantsila E, Lip GY: The endothelium and thrombotic risk in heart failure. *Thromb Haemost* 102:185–187, 2009.
87. White RH: The epidemiology of venous thromboembolism. *Circulation* 107:I4–I8, 2003.
88. Kimura C, Oike M: Heparan sulfate proteoglycan is essential to thrombin-induced calcium transients and nitric oxide production in aortic endothelial cells. *Thromb Haemost* 100:483–488, 2008.
89. Padro T, Emeis JJ, Steins M, et al: Quantification of plasminogen activators and their inhibitors in the aortic vessel wall in relation to the presence and severity of atherosclerotic disease. *Arterioscler Thromb Vasc Biol* 15:893–902, 1995.
90. Chin BS, Blann AD, Gibbs CR, et al: Prognostic value of interleukin-6, plasma viscosity, fibrinogen, von Willebrand factor, tissue factor and vascular endothelial growth factor levels in congestive heart failure. *Eur J Clin Invest* 33:941–948, 2003.
91. Celik S, Langer H, Stellos K, et al: Platelet-associated light (tnfsf14) mediates adhesion of platelets to human vascular endothelium. *Thromb Haemost* 98:798–805, 2007.
92. Zimmerman GA, McIntyre TM, Mehra M, et al: Endothelial cell-associated platelet-activating factor: a novel mechanism for signaling intercellular adhesion. *J Cell Biol* 110:529–540, 1990.
93. Gombos T, Mako V, Cervenak L, et al: Levels of von Willebrand factor antigen and von Willebrand factor cleaving protease (adamts13) activity predict clinical events in chronic heart failure. *Thromb Haemost* 102:573–580, 2009.
94. Jug B, Vene N, Salobir BG, et al: Prognostic impact of haemostatic derangements in chronic heart failure. *Thromb Haemost* 102:314–320, 2009.
95. Mollnau H, Oelze M, August M, et al: Mechanisms of increased vascular superoxide production in an experimental model of idiopathic dilated cardiomyopathy. *Arterioscler Thromb Vasc Biol* 25:2554–2559, 2005.
96. Yamamoto E, Kataoka K, Shintaku H, et al: Novel mechanism and role of angiotensin ii induced vascular endothelial injury in hypertensive diastolic heart failure. *Arterioscler Thromb Vasc Biol* 27:2569–2575, 2007.
97. Thai H, Wollmuth J, Goldman S, et al: Angiotensin subtype 1 rreceptor (at1) blockade improves vasorelaxation in HF by up-regulation of endothelial nitric-oxide synthase via activation of the at2 receptor. *J Pharmacol Exp Ther* 307:1171–1178, 2003.
98. Varin R, Mulder P, Tamion F, et al: Improvement of endothelial function by chronic angiotensin-converting enzyme inhibition in HF: role of nitric oxide, prostanoids, oxidant stress, and bradykinin. *Circulation* 102:351–356, 2000.
99. Ferdinand KC: African American HF trial: role of endothelial dysfunction and HF in African Americans. *Am J Cardiol* 99:3D–6D, 2007.
100. Poelzl G, Frick M, Lackner B, et al: Short-term improvement in submaximal exercise capacity by optimized therapy with ACE inhibitors and beta blockers in HF patients is associated with restoration of peripheral endothelial function. *Int J Cardiol* 108:48–54, 2006.
101. Hornig B, Arakawa N, Haussmann D, et al: Differential effects of quinaprilat and enalaprilat on endothelial function of conduit arteries in patients with chronic heart failure. *Circulation* 98:2842–2848, 1998.
102. Drakos SG, Papamichael CM, Alexopoulos GP, et al: Effects of high doses versus standard doses of enalapril on endothelial cell function in patients with chronic congestive HF secondary to idiopathic dilated or ischemic cardiomyopathy. *Am J Cardiol* 91:885–888, 2003.
103. Kjekshus J, Apetrei E, Barrios V, et al: Rosuvastatin in older patients with systolic heart failure. *N Engl J Med* 357:2248–2261, 2007.
104. Bleske BE, Nicklas JM, Bard RL, et al: Neutral effect on markers of heart failure, inflammation, endothelial activation and function, and vagal tone after high-dose HMG-COA reductase inhibition in non-diabetic patients with non-ischemic cardiomyopathy and average low-density lipoprotein level. *J Am Coll Cardiol* 47:338–341, 2006.
105. Trochu JN, Mital S, Zhang X, et al: Preservation of NO production by statins in the treatment of heart failure. *Cardiovasc Res* 60:250–258, 2003.
106. Landmesser U, Engberding N, Bahlmann FH, et al: Statin-induced improvement of endothelial progenitor cell mobilization, myocardial neovascularization, left ventricular function, and survival after experimental myocardial infarction requires endothelial nitric oxide synthase. *Circulation* 110:1933–1939, 2004.
107. Tousoulis D, Antoniades C, Bosinakou E, et al: Effects of atorvastatin on reactive hyperemia and inflammatory process in patients with congestive heart failure. *Atherosclerosis* 178:359–363, 2005.
108. Strey CH, Young JM, Molyneux SL, et al: Endothelium-ameliorating effects of statin therapy and coenzyme q10 reductions in chronic heart failure. *Atherosclerosis* 179:201–206, 2005.
109. Gounari P, Tousoulis D, Antoniades C, et al: Rosuvastatin but not ezetimibe improves endothelial function in patients with heart failure, by mechanisms independent of lipid lowering. *Int J Cardiol* 142:87–91, 2010.
110. Young JM, Strey CH, George PM, et al: Effect of atorvastatin on plasma levels of asymmetric dimethylarginine in patients with non-ischaemic heart failure. *Eur J Heart Fail* 10:463–466, 2008.
111. Erbs S, Beck EB, Linke A, et al: High-dose rosuvastatin in chronic HF promotes vasculogenesis, corrects endothelial function, and improves cardiac remodeling–results from a randomized, double-blind, and placebo-controlled study. *Int J Cardiol* 146:56–63, 2011.
112. Landmesser U, Bahlmann F, Mueller M, et al: Simvastatin versus ezetimibe: pleiotropic and lipid-lowering effects on endothelial function in humans. *Circulation* 111:2356–2363, 2005.
113. Hambrecht R, Hilbrich L, Erbs S, et al: Correction of endothelial dysfunction in chronic heart failure: additional effects of exercise training and oral L-arginine supplementation. *J Am Coll Cardiol* 35:706–713, 2000.
114. Chin-Dusting JP, Kaye DM, Lefkovits J, et al: Dietary supplementation with L-arginine fails to restore endothelial function in forearm resistance arteries of patients with severe heart failure. *J Am Coll Cardiol* 27:1207–1213, 1996.
115. Rector TS, Bank AJ, Mullen KA, et al: Randomized, double-blind, placebo-controlled study of supplemental oral L-arginine in patients with heart failure. *Circulation* 93:2135–2141, 1996.
116. Rossig L, Hoffmann J, Hugel B, et al: Vitamin C inhibits endothelial cell apoptosis in congestive heart failure. *Circulation* 104:2182–2187, 2001.
117. Flammer AJ, Sudano I, Wolfrum M, et al: Cardiovascular effects of flavanol-rich chocolate in patients with heart failure. *Eur Heart J* 33:2172–2180, 2012.
118. Tabet JY, Meurin P, Driss AB, et al: Benefits of exercise training in chronic heart failure. *Arch Cardiovasc Dis* 102:721–730, 2009.
119. Tai MK, Meininger JC, Frazier LQ: A systematic review of exercise interventions in patients with heart failure. *Biol Res Nurs* 10:156–182, 2008.
120. Testa M, Ennezat PV, Vikstrom KL, et al: Modulation of vascular endothelial gene expression by physical training in patients with chronic heart failure. *Ital Heart J* 1:426–430, 2000.
121. Parnell MM, Holst DP, Kaye DM: Augmentation of endothelial function following exercise training is associated with increased L-arginine transport in human heart failure. *Clin Sci (Lond)* 109:523–530, 2005.
122. Hambrecht R, Fiehn E, Weigl C, et al: Regular physical exercise corrects endothelial dysfunction and improves exercise capacity in patients with chronic heart failure. *Circulation* 98:2709–2715, 1998.
123. Varin R, Mulder P, Richard V, et al: Exercise improves flow-mediated vasodilatation of skeletal muscle arteries in rats with chronic heart failure. Role of nitric oxide, prostanoids, and oxidant stress. *Circulation* 99:2951–2957, 1999.
124. Wang J, Yi GH, Knecht M, et al: Physical training alters the pathogenesis of pacing-induced HF through endothelium-mediated mechanisms in awake dogs. *Circulation* 96:2683–2692, 1997.
125. Gustafsson T, Bodin K, Sylven C, et al: Increased expression of VEGF following exercise training in patients with heart failure. *Eur J Clin Invest* 31:362–366, 2001.
126. Sarto P, Balducci E, Balconi G, et al: Effects of exercise training on endothelial progenitor cells in patients with chronic heart failure. *J Card Fail* 13:701–708, 2007.
127. Miche E, Herrmann G, Nowak M, et al: Effect of an exercise training program on endothelial dysfunction in diabetic and non-diabetic patients with severe chronic heart failure. *Clin Res Cardiol* 95(Suppl 1):i117–i124, 2006.
128. Niebauer J, Clark AL, Webb-Peploe KM, et al: Exercise training in chronic heart failure: effects on pro-inflammatory markers. *Eur J Heart Fail* 7:189–193, 2005.
129. Adamopoulos S, Parissis J, Kroupis C, et al: Physical training reduces peripheral markers of inflammation in patients with chronic heart failure. *Eur Heart J* 22:791–797, 2001.
130. Wisloff U, Stoylen A, Loennechen JP, et al: Superior cardiovascular effect of aerobic interval training versus moderate continuous training in HF patients: a randomized study. *Circulation* 115:3086–3094, 2007.
131. McNamara DM, Tam SW, Sabolinski ML, et al: Endothelial nitric oxide synthase (NOS3) polymorphisms in African Americans with heart failure: results from the A-HeFT trial. *J Card Fail* 15:191–198, 2009.
132. Velloso MW, Pereira SB, Gouveia L, et al: Endothelial nitric oxide synthase glu298asp gene polymorphism in a multi-ethnical population with HF and controls. *Nitric Oxide* 22:220–225, 2010.
133. Binkley PF, Nunziatta E, Liu-Stratton Y, et al: A polymorphism of the endothelial nitric oxide synthase promoter is associated with an increase in autonomic imbalance in patients with congestive heart failure. *Am Heart J* 149:342–348, 2005.
134. McNamara DM, Holubkov R, Postava L, et al: Effect of the asp298 variant of endothelial nitric oxide synthase on survival for patients with congestive heart failure. *Circulation* 107:1598–1602, 2003.
135. Kissel CK, Lehmann R, Assmus B, et al: Selective functional exhaustion of hematopoietic progenitor cells in the bone marrow of patients with postinfarction heart failure. *J Am Coll Cardiol* 49:2341–2349, 2007.
136. Nonaka-Sarukawa M, Yamamoto K, Aoki H, et al: Circulating endothelial progenitor cells in congestive heart failure. *Int J Cardiol* 119:344–348, 2007.
137. Fritzenwanger M, Lorenz F, Jung C, et al: Differential number of CD34+, CD133+ and CD34+/CD133+ cells in peripheral blood of patients with congestive heart failure. *Eur J Med Res* 14:113–117, 2009.

138. Valgimigli M, Rigolin GM, Fucili A, et al: CD34+ and endothelial progenitor cells in patients with various degrees of congestive heart failure. *Circulation* 110:1209–1212, 2004.
139. Manginas A, Tsiavou A, Sfyrakis P, et al: Increased number of circulating progenitor cells after implantation of ventricular assist devices. *J Heart Lung Transplant* 28:710–717, 2009.
140. Van Craenenbroeck EM, Beckers PJ, Possemiers NM, et al: Exercise acutely reverses dysfunction of circulating angiogenic cells in chronic heart failure. *Eur Heart J* 31:1924–1934, 2010.
141. Dedobbeleer C, Blocklet D, Toungouz M, et al: Myocardial homing and coronary endothelial function after autologous blood CD34+ progenitor cells intracoronary injection in the chronic phase of myocardial infarction. *J Cardiovasc Pharmacol* 53:480–485, 2009.
142. Michowitz Y, Goldstein E, Wexler D, et al: Circulating endothelial progenitor cells and clinical outcome in patients with congestive heart failure. *Heart* 93:1046–1050, 2007.
143. Geft D, Schwartzenberg S, Rogowsky O, et al: Circulating apoptotic progenitor cells in patients with congestive heart failure. *PLoS ONE* 3:e3238, 2008.
144. Shmilovich H, Ben-Shoshan J, Tal R, et al: B-type natriuretic peptide enhances vasculogenesis by promoting number and functional properties of early endothelial progenitor cells. *Tissue Eng Part A* 15:2741–2749, 2009.
145. Flores-Ramirez R, Uribe-Longoria A, Rangel-Fuentes MM, et al: Intracoronary infusion of CD133+ endothelial progenitor cells improves heart function and quality of life in patients with chronic post-infarct heart insufficiency. *Cardiovasc Revasc Med* 11:72–78, 2010.
146. Chong AY, Caine GJ, Freestone B, et al: Plasma angiopoietin-1, angiopoietin-2, and angiopoietin receptor tie-2 levels in congestive heart failure. *J Am Coll Cardiol* 43:423–428, 2004.
147. Arakawa H, Ikeda U, Hojo Y, et al: Decreased serum vascular endothelial growth factor concentrations in patients with congestive heart failure. *Heart* 89:207–208, 2003.
148. Chin BS, Chung NA, Gibbs CR, et al: Vascular endothelial growth factor and soluble p-selectin in acute and chronic congestive heart failure. *Am J Cardiol* 90:1258–1260, 2002.
149. Friehs I, Barillas R, Vasilyev NV, et al: Vascular endothelial growth factor prevents apoptosis and preserves contractile function in hypertrophied infant heart. *Circulation* 114:I290–I295, 2006.
150. Izumiya Y, Shiojima I, Sato K, et al: Vascular endothelial growth factor blockade promotes the transition from compensatory cardiac hypertrophy to failure in response to pressure overload. *Hypertension* 47:887–893, 2006.
151. de Berrazueta JR, Guerra-Ruiz A, Garcia-Unzueta MT, et al: Endothelial dysfunction, measured by reactive hyperaemia using strain-gauge plethysmography, is an independent predictor of adverse outcome in heart failure. *Eur J Heart Fail* 12:477–483, 2010.
152. Katz SD, Hryniewicz K, Hriljac I, et al: Vascular endothelial dysfunction and mortality risk in patients with chronic heart failure. *Circulation* 111:310–314, 2005.
153. Fischer D, Rossa S, Landmesser U, et al: Endothelial dysfunction in patients with chronic HFis independently associated with increased incidence of hospitalization, cardiac transplantation, or death. *Eur Heart J* 26:65–69, 2005.
154. Vila V, Martinez-Sales V, Almenar L, et al: Inflammation, endothelial dysfunction and angiogenesis markers in chronic HF patients. *Int J Cardiol* 130:276–277, 2008.
155. Leyva F, Anker SD, Godsland IF, et al: Uric acid in chronic heart failure: a marker of chronic inflammation. *Eur Heart J* 19:1814–1822, 1998.
156. Boman K, Jansson JH, Nilsson T, et al: Effects of carvedilol or metoprolol on PAI-1, tPA-mass concentration or von Willebrand factor in chronic heart failure—a COMET substudy. *Thromb Res* 125:e46–e50, 2010.
157. Hryniewicz K, Dimayuga C, Hudaihed A, et al: Inhibition of angiotensin-converting enzyme and phosphodiesterase type 5 improves endothelial function in heart failure. *Clin Sci (Lond)* 108:331–338, 2005.
158. Tavli T, Gocer H: Effects of cilazapril on endothelial function and pulmonary hypertension in patients with congestive heart failure. *Jpn Heart J* 43:667–674, 2002.
159. Gibbs CR, Blann AD, Watson RD, et al: Abnormalities of hemorheological, endothelial, and platelet function in patients with chronic HF in sinus rhythm: effects of angiotensin-converting enzyme inhibitor and beta-blocker therapy. *Circulation* 103:1746–1751, 2001.
160. Farquharson CA, Struthers AD: Spironolactone increases nitric oxide bioactivity, improves endothelial vasodilator dysfunction, and suppresses vascular angiotensin i/angiotensin ii conversion in patients with chronic heart failure. *Circulation* 101:594–597, 2000.
161. Macdonald JE, Kennedy N, Struthers AD: Effects of spironolactone on endothelial function, vascular angiotensin converting enzyme activity, and other prognostic markers in patients with mild HF already taking optimal treatment. *Heart* 90:765–770, 2004.
162. Abiose AK, Mansoor GA, Barry M, et al: Effect of spironolactone on endothelial function in patients with congestive HF on conventional medical therapy. *Am J Cardiol* 93:1564–1566, 2004.
163. Farquharson CA, Struthers AD: Increasing plasma potassium with amiloride shortens the QT interval and reduces ventricular extrasystoles but does not change endothelial function or heart rate variability in chronic heart failure. *Heart* 88:475–480, 2002.
164. Belardinelli R, Solenghi M, Volpe L, et al: Trimetazidine improves endothelial dysfunction in chronic heart failure: an antioxidant effect. *Eur Heart J* 28:1102–1108, 2007.
165. Ito K, Akita H, Kanazawa K, et al: Comparison of effects of ascorbic acid on endothelium-dependent vasodilation in patients with chronic congestive HF secondary to idiopathic dilated cardiomyopathy versus patients with effort angina pectoris secondary to coronary artery disease. *Am J Cardiol* 82:762–767, 1998.
166. Hornig B, Arakawa N, Kohler C, et al: Vitamin C improves endothelial function of conduit arteries in patients with chronic heart failure. *Circulation* 97:363–368, 1998.
167. Ellis GR, Anderson RA, Chirkov YY, et al: Acute effects of vitamin C on platelet responsiveness to nitric oxide donors and endothelial function in patients with chronic heart failure. *J Cardiovasc Pharmacol* 37:564–570, 2001.
168. Ellis GR, Anderson RA, Lang D, et al: Neutrophil superoxide anion–generating capacity, endothelial function and oxidative stress in chronic heart failure: effects of short- and long-term vitamin C therapy. *J Am Coll Cardiol* 36:1474–1482, 2000.
169. Erbs S, Gielen S, Linke A, et al: Improvement of peripheral endothelial dysfunction by acute vitamin C application: different effects in patients with coronary artery disease, ischemic, and dilated cardiomyopathy. *Am Heart J* 146:280–285, 2003.
170. George J, Carr E, Davies J, et al: High-dose allopurinol improves endothelial function by profoundly reducing vascular oxidative stress and not by lowering uric acid. *Circulation* 114:2508–2516, 2006.
171. Doehner W, Schoene N, Rauchhaus M, et al: Effects of xanthine oxidase inhibition with allopurinol on endothelial function and peripheral blood flow in hyperuricemic patients with chronic heart failure: results from 2 placebo-controlled studies. *Circulation* 105:2619–2624, 2002.
172. Hirooka Y, Imaizumi T, Tagawa T, et al: Effects of L-arginine on impaired acetylcholine-induced and ischemic vasodilation of the forearm in patients with heart failure. *Circulation* 90:658–668, 1994.
173. Paul B, Whiting MJ, De Pasquale CG, et al: Acute effects of 5-methyltetrahydrofolate on endothelial function and asymmetric dimethylarginine in patients with chronic heart failure. *Nutr Metab Cardiovasc Dis* 20:341–349, 2010.
174. Napoli R, Guardasole V, Matarazzo M, et al: Growth hormone corrects vascular dysfunction in patients with chronic heart failure. *J Am Coll Cardiol* 39:90–95, 2002.
175. Fichtlscherer S, Rossig L, Breuer S, et al: Tumor necrosis factor antagonism with etanercept improves systemic endothelial vasoreactivity in patients with advanced heart failure. *Circulation* 104:3023–3025, 2001.
176. Fuentes JC, Salmon AA, Silver MA: Acute and chronic oral magnesium supplementation: effects on endothelial function, exercise capacity, and quality of life in patients with symptomatic heart failure. *Congest Heart Fail* 12:9–13, 2006.
177. Patel MB, Kaplan IV, Patni RN, et al: Sustained improvement in flow-mediated vasodilation after short-term administration of dobutamine in patients with severe congestive heart failure. *Circulation* 99:60–64, 1999.
178. Freimark D, Feinberg MS, Matezky S, et al: Impact of short-term intermittent intravenous dobutamine therapy on endothelial function in patients with severe chronic heart failure. *Am Heart J* 148:878–882, 2004.
179. Schwarz M, Katz SD, Demopoulos L, et al: Enhancement of endothelium-dependent vasodilation by low-dose nitroglycerin in patients with congestive heart failure. *Circulation* 89:1609–1614, 1994.
180. Guazzi M, Casali M, Berti F, et al: Endothelium-mediated modulation of ergoreflex and improvement in exercise ventilation by acute sildenafil in HF patients. *Clin Pharmacol Ther* 83:336–341, 2008.
181. Strey CH, Young JM, Lainchbury JH, et al: Short-term statin treatment improves endothelial function and neurohormonal imbalance in normocholesterolaemic patients with non-ischaemic heart failure. *Heart* 92:1603–1609, 2006.
182. Castro PF, Miranda R, Verdejo HE, et al: Pleiotropic effects of atorvastatin in heart failure: role in oxidative stress, inflammation, endothelial function, and exercise capacity. *J Heart Lung Transplant* 27:435–441, 2008.
183. Tousoulis D, Antoniades C, Vassiliadou C, et al: Effects of combined administration of low dose atorvastatin and vitamin E on inflammatory markers and endothelial function in patients with heart failure. *Eur J Heart Fail* 7:1126–1132, 2005.
184. Tousoulis D, Oikonomou E, Siasos G, et al: Dose-dependent effects of short term atorvastatin treatment on arterial wall properties and on indices of left ventricular remodeling in ischemic heart failure. *Atherosclerosis* 227:367–372, 2013.
185. Bank AJ, Shammas RA, Mullen K, et al: Effects of short-term forearm exercise training on resistance vessel endothelial function in normal subjects and patients with heart failure. *J Card Fail* 4:193–201, 1998.
186. Kobayashi N, Tsuruya Y, Iwasawa T, et al: Exercise training in patients with chronic HF improves endothelial function predominantly in the trained extremities. *Circ J* 67:505–510, 2003.
187. Linke A, Schoene N, Gielen S, et al: Endothelial dysfunction in patients with chronic heart failure: systemic effects of lower-limb exercise training. *J Am Coll Cardiol* 37:392–397, 2001.
188. Hornig B, Maier V, Drexler H: Physical training improves endothelial function in patients with chronic heart failure. *Circulation* 93:210–214, 1996.

14 Alterations in Kidney Function Associated with Heart Failure

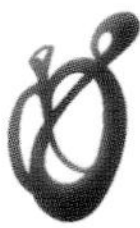

Tamar S. Polonsky and George L. Bakris

The kidney is the major organ responsible for the excretion of waste products and toxins, and also plays a crucial role in the control of fluid, electrolyte, and acid-base homeostasis. In addition, it is the source of renin and erythropoietin and is involved in the formation of vitamin D. Consequently, renal impairment can affect the function of the body in fundamental ways by altering the internal milieu. Although the heart appears to be the main culprit in heart failure (HF), the contributing and disease-modifying role of the kidney has become increasingly recognized in HF. Renal dysfunction can be due to both hemodynamic impairment and preexisting intrinsic renal disease, which can adversely affect cardiac function and contribute to the pathogenesis of cardiovascular disease. Under normal conditions, there is extensive cross-talk between the kidney and the heart to regulate extracellular fluid volume. For example, an increase in atrial pressure normally suppresses release of hormones that promote sodium and water reabsorption, and increases secretion of peptides that promote natriuresis. However, in the setting of HF, the normal mechanisms that control sodium and water balance are overwhelmed by an activation of neurohormonal pathways that lead to increased sympathetic activity, vasoconstriction, and sodium and water reabsorption.[1] Indeed, the kidney contributes to the pathogenesis of HF through increased retention of salt and water in an effort to maintain organ perfusion. However, reduced kidney function as a consequence of reduced cardiac output and reduced renal blood flow is only one component of the complex cardiorenal interaction in HF.[2] Substantial evidence also supports the role of additional pathways, such as neurohormonal mechanisms and venous congestion, in the worsening renal function that is observed in HF.[3]

RENAL REGULATION OF SALT AND WATER HOMEOSTASIS

The kidney controls intravascular volume through the regulation of salt and water excretion. The kidney receives about 25% of the cardiac output and is separated into the cortex, outer medulla, and inner medulla. The single renal nephron (**Figure 14-1**), one of several hundred thousand that make up a kidney, is the basic functional unit of the kidney and includes the glomerulus, which filters the blood delivering plasma ultrafiltrate to the renal tubule for regulation of reabsorption of sodium. The normal glomerulus is impermeable to macromolecules such as albumin, and only in disease states becomes permeable to molecules such as albumin, which when lost in the urine impairs the ability to regulate intravascular volume through reductions in plasma oncotic pressure. The loss of plasma oncotic pressure favors edema formation as occurs in disease states, such as in the nephrotic syndrome, and has been reported in severe HF with increases in renal venous pressure.

Glomerular function is also regulated by glomerular hydrostatic pressure, which is controlled by arterial blood pressure and segmental vascular resistances at the level of pre- and postglomerular vessels (i.e., afferent and efferent arterioles). From the glomerulus, the filtrate flows successively through the proximal tubule, the loop of Henle, the distal tubule, and finally the collecting duct to reach the renal pelvis as urine. The sections of the tubule vary in permeability for water and solutes because of the differential expression of transporters and channels, the activity of which can be affected by hormones and drugs (see Figure 14-1). The proximal tubule is regulated by hormonal and physical factors in the control of sodium reabsorption. The juxtaglomerular apparatus is the location of renin-secreting cells and the macula densa and lies at the junction between the loop of Henle and the distal nephron at which the tubule comes in close proximity to the afferent arteriole. The juxtaglomerular apparatus and macula densa sense alterations in intratubular sodium concentration, which depends on GFR and proximal reabsorption. Increases in sodium concentration to the macula densa and juxtaglomerular apparatus decrease renin secretion, whereas decreases in sodium concentration as a result of decreased

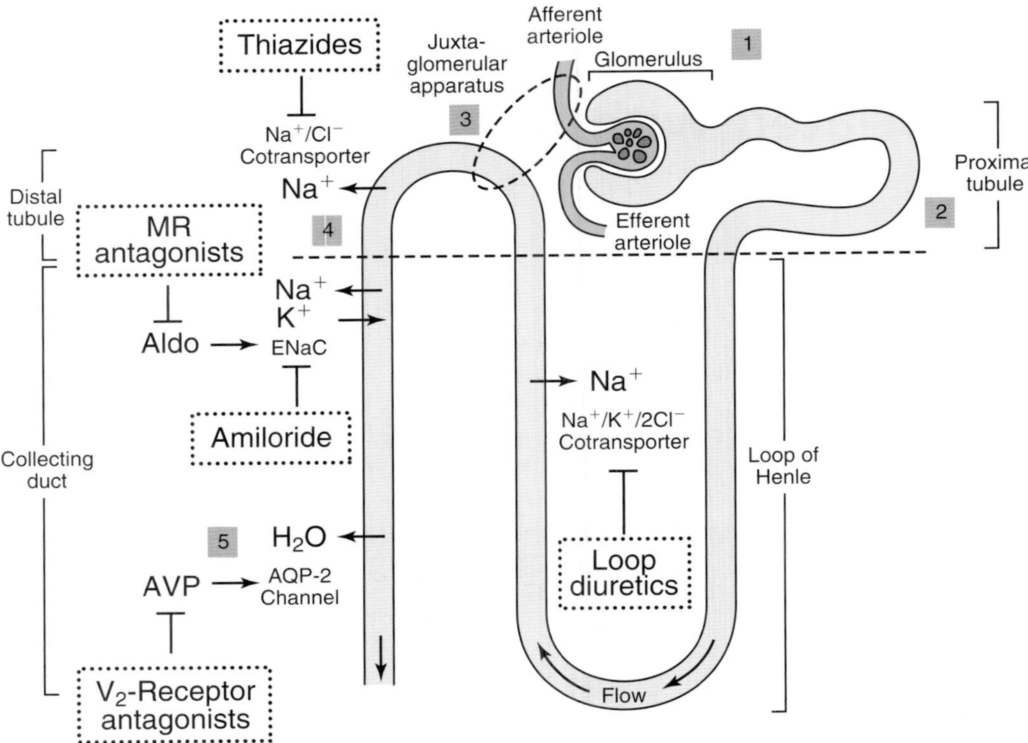

FIGURE 14-1 Schematic of a single nephron with major sites of action of some conventional diuretics and the natriuretic peptides. The juxtaglomerular apparatus, located at the junction of the afferent arteriole and the distal tubule, contains renin secreting cells. Natriuretic peptides have diverse renal actions: they can (1) increase glomerular filtration, (2) oppose proximal reabsorption of sodium by opposing angiotensin II and the sympathetic nervous system, (3) inhibit tubuloglomerular feedback and the secretion of renin, (4) inhibit sodium reabsorption in the distal tubule, and (5) promote free water excretion by opposing arginine vasopressin. *Aldo,* Aldosterone; *AQP-2,* aquaporin 2 water channel; *AVP,* arginine vasopressin; *ENaC,* epithelial sodium channel; *MR,* mineralocorticoid; *V_2-Receptor,* vasopressin 2 receptor. *From Boerrigter G, Costello-Boerrigter L, Burnett JC: Alterations in renal function in heart failure. In Mann DM, editors: Heart failure: a companion to Braunwald's heart disease, ed 2, Philadelphia, 2011, Saunders, p 292.*

GFR or increased proximal reabsorption increase renin release and activate the renin-angiotensin-aldosterone (RAAS) cascade. The loop of Henle is therefore an important segment of the renal nephron and is responsible for reabsorption of sodium through direct alterations in sodium transport, as well as through changes in renal medullary blood flow. The final mediator of renal sodium excretion is the collecting duct, which is under the influence of both natriuretic and antinatriuretic factors. These include aldosterone, which promotes active sodium reabsorption, and arginine vasopressin, which regulates the reabsorption of water. Natriuretic factors, such as the cardiac peptides atrial natriuretic peptide (ANP) and B-type natriuretic peptide (BNP), also act primarily in the distal nephron.

EPIDEMIOLOGY AND IMPACT OF KIDNEY DISEASE IN HEART FAILURE

Decreased glomerular filtration rate (GFR), usually estimated with creatinine-based equations, has emerged as a powerful independent predictor of outcomes in patients with HF (**Figure 14-2**). Importantly, renal dysfunction is commonly seen in both stable patients and those with acute decompensated HF. Ezekowitz and colleagues demonstrated that almost 40% of outpatients with both coronary artery disease and HF have stage 3 or higher chronic kidney disease (CKD), defined as an estimated glomerular filtration (eGFR) less than 60 mL/min/1.73 m^2.[4] The prevalence of stage 3 or higher CKD was as high as 64% among patients admitted for acute decompensated HF.[5] The presence of

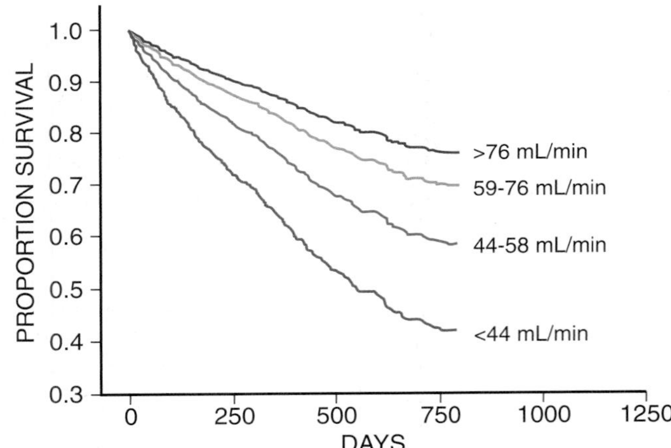

FIGURE 14-2 Proportional relationship of calculated glomerular filtration rate (using the Cockcroft-Gault equation) with mortality in Cox-adjusted survival analysis. Patients had heart failure (New York Heart Association class III or IV, left ventricular ejection fraction <35%) and were enrolled in the Second Prospective Randomized study of Ibopamine on Mortality and Efficacy (PRIME-II) trial, which investigated the oral dopamine agonist ibopamine. *From Boerrigter G, Costello-Boerrigter L, Burnett JC: Alterations in renal function in heart failure. In Mann DM, editor: Heart failure: a companion to Braunwald's heart disease, ed 2, Saunders, 2011, Philadelphia, p 292; and modified from Hillege HL, Girbes AR, de Kam PJ, et al: Renal function, neurohormonal activation, and survival in patients with chronic heart failure. Circulation 102:203–210, 2000.*

CKD is one of the most important prognostic factors for patients with HF, regardless of whether the ejection fraction is preserved or reduced.[6] In a prospective cohort of 754 adults referred to an outpatient HF clinic, a 1% increase in 1-year mortality was seen for every 1 mL/min decrease in

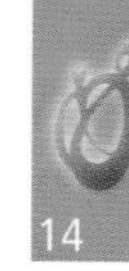

creatinine clearance.[7] Importantly, patients with renal dysfunction experienced the same reduction in mortality from treatment with angiotensin-converting enzyme inhibitors and β-blockers as patients with normal renal function, although they were less likely to receive the medications.

The presence of renal dysfunction is also associated with poor short-term outcomes. Data from the Acute Decompensated HF National Registry (ADHERE) showed that in-hospital mortality increased from 1.9% among patients with normal renal function to 7.6% and 6.5% among patients with renal dysfunction and kidney failure, respectively.[5] Although GFR remained a significant predictor of mortality after adjusting for confounders, the blood urea nitrogen (BUN) level remained the single best predictor. Other investigators have confirmed the usefulness of BUN as a marker of increased risk.[8] In the Acute and Chronic Therapeutic Impact of a Vasopressin Antagonist in Chronic Heart Failure (ACTIV in CHF) trial, patients with a baseline BUN greater than 40 mg/dL experienced an event rate of 30%, whereas patients whose baseline BUN <18 mg/dL had an event rate of 8.6%.[9] It is likely that, in the acute setting, BUN is a marker of neurohormonal activation, which leads to constriction of the afferent arteriole, secretion of vasopressin, and enhanced reabsorption of sodium, water, and urea. These pathways will be discussed in more detail below.

Prognosis of Worsening Renal Function

Worsening kidney function (WKF) among patients admitted with acute decompensated HF is often defined as an increase in creatinine of 0.3 mg/dL or more. As many as one third of patients may experience WKF, which typically occurs in the first 3 to 4 days of admission, but has also been shown to occur in the week after hospital discharge.[10] Risk factors for WKF include baseline creatinine greater than 1.5 mg/dL, diabetes, and pulmonary edema.[11] Data regarding the association of WKF with prognosis have shown varying results. In the Prospective Trial of Intravenous Milrinone for Exacerbations of Chronic Heart Failure (OPTIME-CHF), 12% of participants experienced a greater than 25% decrease in eGFR and 39% experienced a greater than 25% increase in BUN.[12] Every 5 mg/dL increase in BUN (above a 10-mg/dL increase) translated into an additional 8% increase in the risk of 60-day mortality. In the Diuretic Optimization Strategies Evaluation (DOSE) trial, a greater proportion of adults randomized to high-dose diuretics (23%) compared with low-dose (14%) experienced WKF.[13] However, there was no difference in 60-day mortality, suggesting that transient changes in renal function may not have a significant effect on outcomes. Among patients in the placebo arm of the EVEREST trial, those who experienced WKF were also found to have fewer signs of congestion, as measured by body weight, log (brain natriuretic peptide) levels, and blood pressure, suggesting that the WKF reflects arterial underfilling, rather than an intrinsic worsening of renal or cardiac function.[10] Changes in BUN were not reported. Blair and colleagues found that WKF in the postdischarge period was more strongly associated with rehospitalization and cardiovascular mortality than in-hospital WKF (HR 1.87, 1.35-2.58), highlighting the importance of close follow-up once patients leave the hospital.[10] One possible explanation is that patients who develop WKF postdischarge may have a higher degree of neurohormonal activation. The cardiorenal syndrome is discussed in **Chapter 33**.

PATHOPHYSIOLOGY OF RENAL DYSFUNCTION IN HEART FAILURE

The homeostatic association between the heart and kidneys has been appreciated for centuries. When studying "dropsical" patients with congestive heart failure, Withering noted that patients had a brisk diuresis following improved myocardial function with administration of foxglove.[14] In the early phases of HF, the ratio of the glomerular filtration rate to renal blood flow—called the *filtration fraction*—is maintained, and can even be increased. This is largely due to vasoconstrictor peptides, such as arginine vasopressin (AVP), angiotensin II, and norepinephrine (NE) that help maintain GFR by maintaining blood pressure and constriction of the efferent arteriole, resulting in increased intraglomerular capillary pressure (**Figure 14-3**). The section that follows will review normal renal physiology controlling salt and water homeostasis, as well as some of the cardiorenal pathways that are activated in HF that contribute to inappropriate salt and water retention in HF (summarized in **Figure 14-4**).

Peripheral Volume Sensors Affecting Renal Function

Pressure Receptors

Numerous baroreceptors and mechanoreceptors are located in critical areas in the circulatory tree (**see also Chapter 12**), including the carotid sinus, aortic arch, afferent glomerular arterioles in the kidney, and the superior and inferior vena cava.[15-17] The receptors detect alterations in pressure and stretch of the vessel wall. In volume-depleted states, where stretch is decreased, there is a subsequent loss of tonic inhibition of the sympathetic nervous system, which results in increase sympathetic neural tone. The baroreceptors of the carotid body and aortic arch contribute to the antinatriuretic response seen in congestive heart failure. Studies have demonstrated a reduction in urinary output and sodium excretion following volume expansion in the presence of carotid sinus excitation at constant arterial pressures.[18,19]

The atria also possess two types of baroreceptors: (1) type A, located primarily at the entrance of the pulmonary veins, which discharge at the onset of systole and are not affected by volume, and (2) type B, which demonstrate increased activity with atrial filling and increased atrial size.[20,21] The neuronal inputs of the cardiac atria and the carotid body are transmitted to the medulla and hypothalamus through cranial nerves IX and X.[15]

Atrial transmural pressure has a significant influence on kidney function.[22] Experiments in dogs note that decreased atrial wall distention culminated in decreased sodium excretion and urine flow rate by the kidney.[20] In addition, the normal diuretic response to volume expansion was attenuated when atrial wall distention was limited. Other studies examine the interaction between the carotid body and neuronal control of sodium homeostasis. For example, infusion of hypertonic saline increased neural activity along the tracts leading to the hypothalamus and medulla.[21] Conversely, increased left atrial stretch decreased activity of these neural tracts and increased urine flow rate and sodium excretion.[20] Plasma levels of atrial natriuretic peptide (ANP) were increased, whereas AVP and aldosterone levels were decreased.[23] The atria and ventricles have

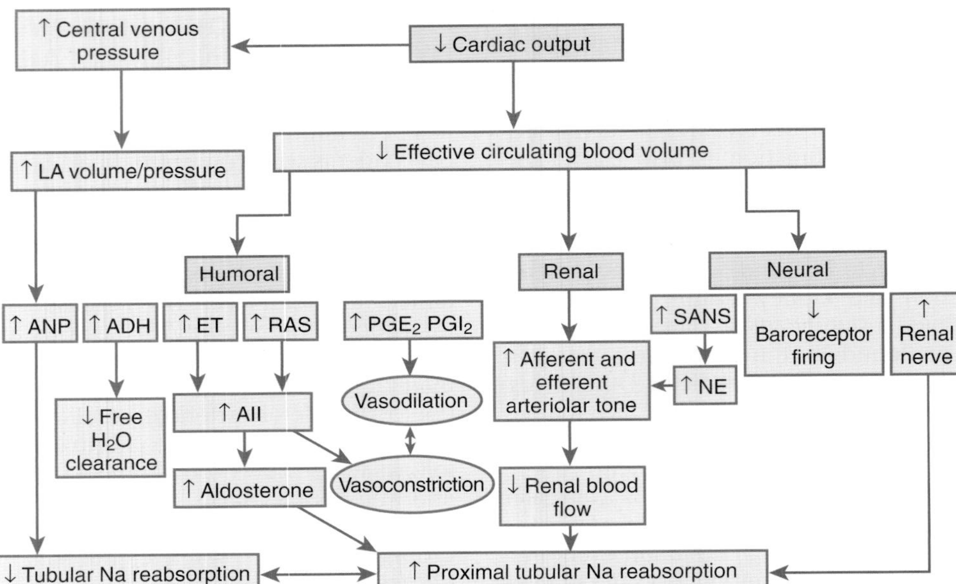

FIGURE 14-3 Intraglomerular changes in heart failure. Glomerular function is regulated by glomerular hydrostatic pressure, which is controlled by arterial blood pressure and segmental vascular resistances at the level of pre- and postglomerular vessels (i.e., afferent and efferent arterioles). In the early phases of HF, the ratio of the glomerular filtration rate to renal blood flow (i.e., the filtration fraction) is maintained largely because of vasoconstrictor peptides such as arginine vasopressin (AVP), angiotensin II, and norepinephrine (NE) that help maintain the glomerular filtration rate (GFR) by maintaining blood pressure and constricting the efferent arteriole, resulting in increased intraglomerular capillary pressure. *AII,* Angiotensin II; *AVP,* arginine vasopressin; *ET,* endothelin; *NE,* norepinephrine.

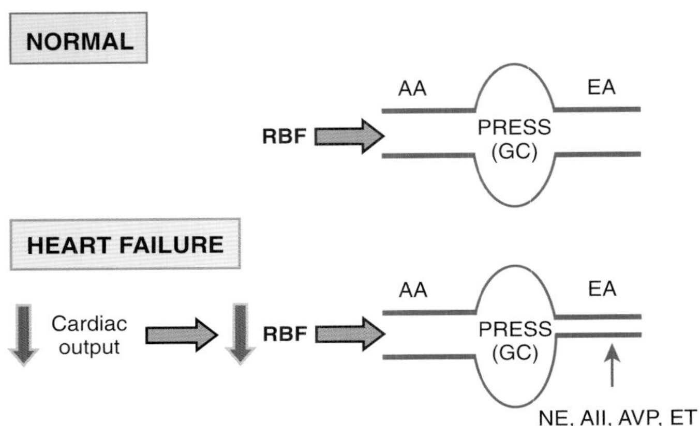

FIGURE 14-4 Overview of the neurohormonal, hemodynamic, and neural changes impacting renal function in heart failure. *AA,* Afferent arteriole; *AII,* angiotensin II; *AVP,* arginine vasopressin; *EA,* afferent arteriole; *ET,* endothelin; *NE,* norepinephrine; PRESS (GC), pressure in the glomerular capsule; *RBF,* renal blood flow.

their own baroreceptors that stimulate secretion of ANP and BNP in response to atrial or ventricular distention. ANP release can stimulate up to a 10-fold increase in sodium excretion.[22] ANP and BNP will be discussed in more detail below.

Renal Baroreceptors

The juxtaglomerular apparatus of the kidney is composed of four basic elements: the terminal portion of the afferent arteriole, the macula densa (a segment of the distal tubule), the extraglomerular mesangial region, and the efferent arteriole at the glomerulus (see Figure 14-1).[24] Because of its location in the nephron, it is very sensitive to changes in volume as well as renal perfusion pressure. The juxtaglomerular apparatus has β_1-adrenoreceptors (see also Chapter 6) and is adrenergically innervated. Sympathetic stimulation or decreases in volume or perfusion pressure can all stimulate the juxtaglomerular apparatus to release renin into the afferent arteriole (see also Chapter 5). Renin then converts angiotensinogen, which is formed in the liver, to angiotensin I. Angiotensin-converting enzyme converts angiotensin I to angiotensin II, which is a potent vasoconstrictor and also stimulates the secretion of aldosterone from the adrenal cortex. Other factors that stimulate the renin-angiotensin-aldosterone system are noted in **Table 14-1**. Most β-blockers can cause several renal hemodynamic alterations, including a decline in renal blood flow and GFR, and a reduction of renin release with a subsequent antinatriuretic response, most prominently with upright posture.[25] The exceptions to these changes are nebivolol and carvedilol.[26,27]

TABLE 14-1 Factors That Inhibit or Stimulate the Renin-Angiotensin-Aldosterone System

INHIBIT ACTIVITY	STIMULATE ACTIVITY
Arginine vasopressin	Activation of renal sympathetic nerves
Angiotensin II	Catecholamines
Salt loading	Hypotension
β-adrenoceptor antagonists	Baroreceptor stimulation
Potassium	Hypoperfusion
Adenosine	Prostaglandin E and I series
Hypocalcemia	Upright posture
Hyperkalemia	Hypovolemia

RENAL SYMPATHETIC INNERVATION

Although initially thought to have little influence on salt and water balance, renal sympathetic nerve activity has been found to be intimately related to body fluid homeostasis. Immunofluorescent electron microscopic and histochemical studies have demonstrated renal nerves in the afferent and efferent arterioles, proximal and distal tubules, ascending limb of the loop of Henle, and the juxtaglomerular apparatus.[28] Dopaminergic receptors have also been found in the tubules and renal nerves.[29] Increased renal sympathetic activity leads to a decrease in renal blood flow and a reduction in urinary sodium excretion. These effects are mediated in part by α_1-adrenoreceptors.[29,30] Renal sympathetic activity is modulated by salt intake. Low-salt diets increase and high-salt diets decrease nerve activity.[28] Increased renal sympathetic nerve activity is documented in states of volume (salt) depletion and contributes to the associated elevation of plasma renin activity, reduction in renal blood flow, and the subsequent antinatriuretic state.[31]

In a study of patients with congestive heart failure, dibenzylchloroethylamine, an α-adrenergic receptor antagonist, was administered intravenously.[32] Despite slight decreases in mean arterial pressure and no significant change in cardiac output, the fractional excretion of sodium was increased without significant changes in renal blood flow or GFR. However, another study in HF patients showed a failure to correct renal hypoperfusion during spinal anesthesia.[33]

Given the recent success of catheter-based renal denervation in resistant hypertension, there is growing interest in applying this technique to patients with heart failure.[34-36] Catheter-based renal denervation involves catheterization of the femoral artery, and then applying radiofrequency energy circumferentially to the endothelium of the distal renal artery. Several studies are currently under way in patients with HF, including the Symplicity-HF (Renal Denervation in Patients with Chronic Heart Failure and Renal Impairment Clinical Trial [NCT01840059]) involving patients with an ejection fraction less than 40% and eGFR 30 to 75 mL/min/m^2. Outcomes will focus on the cardiac and renal responses to denervation, such as left ventricular function, hemodynamics, and renal blood flow at 6 months and 1 year.[35] Another trial, Renal Denervation in Chronic Heart Failure (REACH [NCT01639378]) compares renal denervation with a sham procedure in 100 patients with an ejection fraction less than 40%.[35] The outcomes are symptom status, results of cardiopulmonary exercise testing, arrhythmia burden, and ambulatory blood pressure.

CENTRAL VENOUS PRESSURE AS A DETERMINANT OF RENAL FUNCTION

Human studies from more than 30 years ago highlighted the importance of central venous pressure as a factor in regulating volume status. Many were performed using head-out-of-water immersion, a method of evaluating central venous volume in which study subjects would be immersed in water up to their neck.[37,38] Early studies using head-out-of-water immersion induced a substantial diuresis, which was hypothesized to be secondary to shifting fluid from the limbs to the central circulation and increasing ANP.[39] The resultant increase in central venous pressure then produced atrial distention, a decrease in baroreceptor firing, and an increase in tonic inhibition of the sympathetic nervous system. Early animal models have confirmed the association of central venous pressure with renal function. As early as 1931, Winton used a canine model to demonstrate that urine production decreased substantially at a venous pressure of 20 mm Hg and almost completely stopped at pressure greater than 25 mm Hg.[40] Chronic thoracic vena cava obstruction has been used as a model in dogs to study the association of elevated pressures in HF with renal function.[41] Hemodynamic changes in the dogs included a decrease in cardiac output, GFR, and renal plasma flow.

Studies in patients with HF underscore that central venous pressure may help better identify those who will progress to develop WKF based on cardiac hemodynamic parameters. In the Evaluation Study of Congestive Heart Failure and Pulmonary Artery Catheterization Effectiveness (ESCAPE) trial—a comparison of pulmonary artery catheter-guided treatment for acute heart failure versus clinical assessment—there was no correlation between pulmonary capillary wedge pressure, cardiac index, or systemic vascular resistance with baseline renal function.[42] Right atrial pressure was the only hemodynamic measure that was significantly associated with baseline renal function. In a retrospective analysis of more than 2500 adults who underwent a right heart catheterization, Damman and colleagues found that above a central venous pressure (CVP) of 6 mm Hg, there was a progressive decline in renal function.[43] In a study of 145 patients hospitalized for acute decompensated HF, Mullens and associates found that the mean baseline CVP in patients who developed WKF was significantly higher than those who did not develop WKF (18 ± 7 mm Hg vs. 12 ± 6 mm Hg, P <0.001).[44] Interestingly, the mean cardiac index was higher in those who developed WKF compared with those who did not (2.0 ± 0.8 versus 1.8 ± 0.4 L/min/m^2, P = 0.008), again challenging the notion that renal dysfunction in HF is primarily secondary to poor forward flow.[45]

Research on the association of venous congestion and renal dysfunction has also extended to studies of intra-abdominal pressure (IAP). For example, among 40 consecutive patients admitted with ADHF, 60% had an elevated IAP, defined as 8 mm Hg or more.[46] Of note, none of the patients complained of abdominal symptoms on admission or during therapy. Overall, mean arterial pressure, CVP, pulmonary capillary wedge pressure (PCWP), and cardiac index (CI) were comparable between those with and without an elevated IAP. However, those with an elevated IAP had a higher baseline creatinine (2.3 ± 1.0 mg/dL vs. 1.5 ± 0.8 mg/dL, P <0.009) and at follow-up (1.8 ± 0.8 mg/dL vs. 1.3 ± 0.9 mg/dL, P <0.04). Among the patients with elevated IAP at baseline, improvement in renal function was associated with an improvement in IAP, and not any other hemodynamic measurements.

IMPACT OF NEUROHORMONAL ACTIVATION ON RENAL FUNCTION

Renin-Angiotensin-Aldosterone System

The renin-angiotensin-aldosterone system plays a central role in the maladaptive response of sodium and water reabsorption as HF progresses (see also Chapter 5). Table 14-1 lists the factors that stimulate the renin-angiotensin-aldosterone system. Elevated renin secretion occurs early in the course of heart failure.[47] Circulating levels of renin enzymatically cleave substrate angiotensinogen, subsequently producing angiotensin I (Ang I), which is converted to a potent vasoconstrictor, angiotensin II. Angiotensin II is later converted to Ang III, which then directly stimulates the zona glomerulosa of the adrenal glands to produce aldosterone.

The physiologic effects of Ang II are many and varied. These include stimulation of the central neural centers associated with increased thirst mechanisms, as well as a heightened activity of ganglionic nerves via its effects on the autonomic nervous system. Ang II also serves to increase aldosterone synthesis, thus increasing sodium reabsorption by the kidney, which ultimately may raise arterial pressure and worsen sodium retention, if present. However, normal subjects usually exhibit an escape from the salt-retaining effects of aldosterone within a 3-day period.[48,49] Conversely, in heart failure, this escape phenomenon is not achieved.[50] In addition, these patients have elevated plasma aldosterone levels, which might be secondary to poor hepatic clearance.[51] Despite this fact, spironolactone, the aldosterone antagonist, does not consistently affect sodium or potassium excretion in patients with congestive heart failure.[52] Thus, as renal perfusion declines in concert with decreased cardiac function, loop diuretics are the only effective agents that may be used to achieve a diuresis.

Catecholamines

Catecholamines play an important role in the pathogenesis of HF (see also Chapter 6). Intrarenal circulation is altered when effective circulating volume is reduced and sympathetic tone is increased. Studies by Chidsey and colleagues documented very high plasma norepinephrine (NE) levels in patients with heart failure.[53] More important, elevated plasma NE levels correlate with activation of the sympathetic nervous system, as well as mortality in this patient population.[54] Enhanced sympathetic tone contributes to sodium avidity in several ways. Increased baroreceptor activity causes direct enhancement of proximal tubule sodium reabsorption in the proximal tubule and loop of Henle.[28] Postglomerular capillary pressure falls and oncotic pressure rises, further enhancing proximal tubular reabsorption.

The contribution of dopamine to improvement of cardiac function and maintenance of renal hemodynamics has received considerable attention. Dopamine affects renal hemodynamics by vasodilation of afferent and efferent arterioles and intralobular arteries, thereby enhancing renal blood flow without an increase in glomerular filtration.[55] Note, however, that pure dopaminergic effects are seen at very low concentrations (≈1 mg/min) of dopamine or use of the specific dopamine-1 receptor agonist fenoldopam. Doses greater than 2 mg/min have both α- and β-adrenoreceptor effects.[56] Dopamine inhibits proximal tubule reabsorption of sodium related in part to attenuation of aldosterone secretion.[57] Thus dopamine may be modulating the catecholamine effect in HF and playing a regulatory role on extracellular volume. The National Institutes of Health–sponsored Renal Optimization Strategies Evaluation in Acute Heart Failure and Reliable Evaluation of Dyspnea in the Heart Failure Network (ROSE) study did not show a benefit for low-dose dopamine when compared with a placebo, with respect to the coprimary endpoints of decongestion or renal function, nor other clinical endpoints reflective of clinical outcomes.[57a]

Natriuretic Peptides

The natriuretic peptide system consists of five structurally similar peptides, termed *ANP, urodilantin* (an isoform of ANP), *BNP, C-type natriuretic peptide* (CNP), and *dendroaspis natriuretic peptide* (DNP). ANP, a 28-amino-acid peptide hormone, is produced principally in the cardiac atria, whereas BNP, a 32-amino-acid peptide originally isolated from porcine brain, was later identified as a hormone that was primarily produced in the cardiac ventricles. Both ANP and BNP are secreted in response to increasing cardiac wall tension; however, other factors such as neurohormones (e.g., angiotensin II, ET-1) or physiologic factors (e.g., age, gender, renal function) may also play a role in their regulation. Normally, ANP is stored primarily in the perinuclear granulocytes in cardiac atria, whereas BNP is synthesized in the ventricular myocardium and is not stored in granules. However, under pathologic conditions ANP and BNP can be secreted from both the atria and the ventricles.[58,59]

The biosynthesis, secretion and clearance of BNP differs from ANP, suggesting that these two natriuretic peptides have discrete physiologic and pathophysiologic roles. Whereas ANP is secreted in short bursts in response to acute changes in atrial pressure, the activation of BNP is regulated transcriptionally in response to chronic increases in atrial/ventricular pressure. ANP and BNP are initially synthesized as prohormones that are subsequently proteolytically cleaved, respectively, by corin and furin, to yield large biologically inactive N-terminal fragments (NT-ANP or NT-BNP) and smaller biologically active peptides (ANP or BNP). ANP has a relatively short half-life of approximately 3 min, whereas BNP has a plasma half-life of approximately 20 min. C-type natriuretic peptide (CNP), which is located primarily in the vasculature, is also released as a prohormone that is cleaved into a biologically inactive form (NT-CNP) and a 22-amino-acid biologically active form (CNP). Natriuretic peptides are degraded by neutral endopeptidase 24.11 (neprilysin), which is widely expressed in multiple tissues, where it is often colocalized with angiotensin-converting enzyme (ACE).

Figure 14-5 illustrates the signaling pathway of the natriuretic peptide system. Natriuretic peptides stimulate the production of the intracellular second messenger cGMP via binding to the natriuretic peptide A receptor (NPR-A), which preferentially binds ANP and BNP, and the natriuretic peptide B receptor (NPR-B), which preferentially binds CNP. Both NPR-A and NPR-B receptors are coupled to particulate guanylate cyclase. Activation of NPR-A and NPR-B results in natriuresis, vasorelaxation, inhibition of renin and aldosterone, inhibition, inhibition of fibrosis, and increased lusitropy. The natriuretic peptide C receptor (NPR-C) is not linked to cGMP, and serves as a clearance receptor for the natriuretic peptides. Both ANP and BNP exert several favorable biologic effects in the setting of HF (**Table 14-2**).[60] For example, ANP and BNP have been shown to block sympathetic nervous activity in the cardiovascular system and in the kidney.[61,62] The greatest concentration of receptors in the kidney is found in the glomerulus and medulla.[63] ANP and BNP increase glomerular filtration and prevent sodium reabsorption. The increase in the glomerular filtration rate versus the relatively blunted effect on renal blood flow

TABLE 14-2 Effects of Natriuretic Peptides on the Kidney

DECREASE	INCREASE
Arterial pressure	Glomerular filtration rate
Angiotensin II (inhibits action)	Renal blood flow (transient)
Vasopressin (inhibits action)	Sodium excretion
Renin secretion	Tubular flow rate
Aldosterone secretion	Potassium excretion (minimal)
	Calcium, phosphate, and magnesium excretion

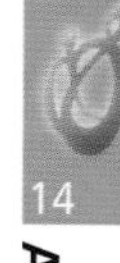

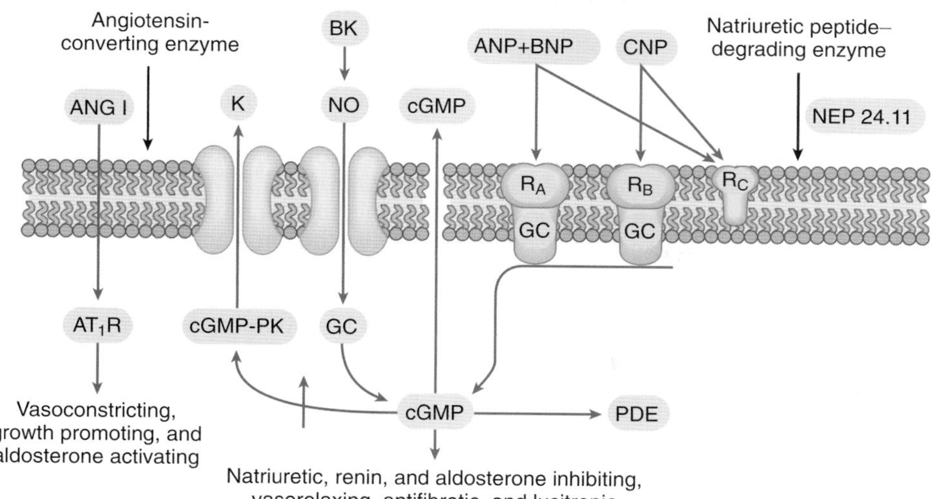

FIGURE 14-5 Cellular actions in signaling of the natriuretic peptide system. *Ang 1,* Angiotensin I; *ANP,* atrial natriuretic peptide; *AT_1R,* angiotensin type 1 receptor; *BK,* bradykinin; *BNP,* B-type natriuretic peptide; *cGMP,* cyclic guanosine monophosphat; *CNP,* C-type natriuretic peptide; *GC,* guanylate cyclase; *K,* potassium; *NEP,* neutral endopeptidase; *PDE,* phosphodiesterase; *PK,* phosphokinase; *R_A,* particulate guanylate cyclase A receptor; *R_C,* particulate guanylate cyclase C receptor. *From Burnett JC, Costello-Boerrigter L, Boerrigter G: Alterations in the kidney in heart failure: the cardiorenal axis in the regulation of sodium homeostasis. In Mann DL, editor: Heart failure: a companion to Braunwald's heart disease, Philadelphia, 2004, Saunders, pp 279–289.*

implies that ANP dilates the afferent arteriole of the nephron while constricting the efferent arteriole, promoting natriuresis.[64] The effects on sodium excretion are mediated by both direct and indirect tubular effects. ANP inhibits tubular salt and water reabsorption that is mediated by angiotensin and vasopressin; a direct inhibition of sodium or chloride transport in the tubules has not been shown.[65] ANP also blunts oxygen consumption in the medullary collecting duct, which may result in direct inhibition of sodium reabsorption. In addition, ANP and BNP have been shown to inhibit the RAAS system. ANP directly inhibits secretion of renin[23,66] and inhibits secretion of aldosterone by acting directly on adrenal cells, and by blocking the stimulatory effects of angiotensin II.[67] BNP has direct lusitropic (relaxing) properties in the myocardium and decreases myocardial fibrosis.[68] Despite the increase in BNP and ANP levels, progressive sodium and water retention develop in heart failure. One potential explanation is that the circulating levels may not be adequate, particularly given the increased sympathetic activity and upregulation of the renin-angiotensin-aldosterone system. Additionally, there may be downregulation of peptide receptors.

There are important differences between ANP and BNP that make BNP more attractive as a biomarker of volume status in HF patients.[69] BNP has a longer plasma half-life than ANP (21 minutes vs. 3 minutes). In addition, BNP levels increase more rapidly and to a higher degree than ANP in response to myocardial stretch. BNP is cleaved from the C-terminal end of its prohormone, pro-BNP. The N-terminal fragment, NT-terminal pro-BNP (NT-proBNP) can also be measured and used as a biomarker. The half-life of NT-proBNP is even longer than that of BNP (25-70 vs. 21 minutes).[70] As discussed in **Chapter 30**, both BNP and NT-proBNP have proven to be valuable biomarkers with respect to diagnosis and prognosis in HF patients.[71-73]

Patients with kidney disease require special consideration when measuring BNP or NT-proBNP levels, because stage 3 or higher CKD is associated with higher concentrations of both hormones.[74] Investigators have therefore sought to determine whether the elevation simply represents decreased clearance of the hormones or increased secretion because of cardiac disease. In a study of 103 non–dialysis-dependent adults with CKD, the plasma BNP level was greater in those with CKD compared to hypertensive controls (28 ± 4 pg/mL vs. 162 ± 21 pg/mL).[75] However, echo measures of volume overload were independent predictors of BNP levels, even after controlling for renal function. Investigators from the Breathing Not Properly Trial found that when they used a BNP cutoff of 200 pg/mL among patients with an eGFR of 59 to 30 (compared to a cutoff of 100 pg/mL for those with normal function), the area under the ROC curve for the diagnosis of HF was 0.81 compared with 0.9 among those with normal renal function.[74]

NT-proBNP levels have a slightly stronger association with eGFR than BNP levels, but they have also been shown to be an independent predictor of outcomes and an indicator of heart failure.[76] For example, in a study of 599 dyspneic patients who presented to the emergency department, patients with kidney disease required higher cutoffs of NT-proBNP for the diagnosis of heart failure compared with patients with normal renal function.[77] Among patients with a GFR less than 60 mL/min/1.73 m^2, a cut point of 1200 pg/mL provided a sensitivity of 89% and a specificity of 72%. Even after adjustment for multiple confounders, including renal function, NT-proBNP remained a significant predictor of mortality.

Nesiritide, a recombinant human BNP, is one of the most studied exogenous peptides (**see also Chapter 33**). Initial randomized controlled trials of nesiritide suggested that it lowered pulmonary capillary wedge pressure more than the placebo but not to intravenous nitroglycerin or standard therapy.[78,79] In the largest study of nesiritide, which included more than 7000 patients in acute heart failure, the drug had a marginal effect on dyspnea, but did not improve 30-day mortality or renal function, compared with the placebo.[80] Clinical studies of exogenous ANP for patients with congestive HF have demonstrated augmented

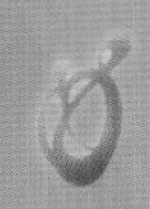

natriuresis and diuresis. However, the effects were small and short-lived.[81] Oral delivery of natriuretic peptides has also been limited, and so efforts to increase bioavailability by blocking its degradation have been ongoing. ANP and BNP are degraded by the enzyme neural endopeptidase, also called *neprilysin*. A new class of drug, angiotensin receptor neprilysin inhibitors (ARNIs), combine inhibition of neprilysin with blockade of the angiotensin receptor.[82] A randomized clinical trial of the ARNI, LSZ696, Prospective comparison of ARNI with ACEI to Determine Impact on Global Mortality and morbidity in Heart Failure trial (PARADIGM-HF [NCT01035255]) is currently under way.[82] The trial is designed to enroll about 8000 patients with an ejection fraction of 35% or less. The primary outcome is cardiovascular mortality or HF hospitalization. Development of renal dysfunction or progression of existing dysfunction is a secondary endpoint.

Arginine Vasopressin

Arginine vasopressin (AVP), also known as antidiuretic hormone (ADH), is a peptide hormone derived from a prehormone precursor that is synthesized in the hypothalamus. It is then transported and stored in the posterior part of the pituitary gland and released in response to multiple mechanisms associated with volume depletion and increased osmolality. In the kidney, AVP facilitates urinary concentration primarily by modulating the passage of water and urea from the collecting ducts into the medullary interstitium.[83,84] Circulating AVP is elevated in many patients with HF, even after correction for plasma osmolality (i.e., nonosmotic release), and may contribute to the hyponatremia that occurs in HF.[85,86] The cellular effects of AVP are mediated mainly by interactions with three types of receptors, termed V_{1a}, V_{2a}, and *V2*. The V_{1a} receptor is the most widespread subtype, and is found in primarily in vascular smooth muscle cells. The V_{1b} receptor has a more limited distribution and is located mainly in the CNS. The V2 receptors are found primarily in the epithelial cells in the renal collecting duct and the thick ascending limb. AVP receptors are members of the G protein–coupled receptors. The V_{1a} receptors mediate vasoconstriction, platelet aggregation, and stimulation of myocardial growth factors.[85,86] As HF progresses, blunting of the baroreceptors (see Chapter 13) results in unopposed secretion of vasopressin, leading to excessive vasoconstriction and adverse hemodynamics.[87] The V_{1b} receptor modulates ACTH secretion from the anterior pituitary, and the V2 receptor mediates antidiuretic effects by stimulating adenyl cyclase to increase the rate of insertion of water-containing channel vesicles into the apical membrane. Because the water channels contain preformed functional water channels, termed *aquaporins*, their localization in the apical membranes in response to V2 stimulation increases the water permeability of the apical membrane, leading to water retention. The "vaptans," vasopressin receptor antagonists with V_{1a} (relcovaptan) or V2 (tolvaptan, lixivaptan) selectivity or non-selective V_{1a}/V2 activity (conivaptan), have been shown to reduce body weight and reduce hyponatremia in patients. The oral vasopressin V2 receptor antagonist tolvaptan has been evaluated in patients with HF in the EVEREST trial (see Chapter 33). Although tolvaptan did improve hyponatremia, there was no significant effect on long-term morbidity and mortality when compared with a placebo.[88]

Prostaglandins

The renal prostaglandin system is implicated in the regulation of renal hemodynamics and renal sodium excretion in congestive heart failure. Plasma levels of prostaglandins (e.g., PGE2 and prostacycline) are elevated in patients with congestive heart failure, especially in those patients with hyponatremia.[89,90] With the exception of PGF2 and thromboxane, the renal prostaglandins are all vasodilators. Additionally, the prostaglandins alter sodium reabsorption at both the thick ascending loop of Henle and the cortical collecting tubule.[91] These actions counteract, at least in part, other hemodynamically active peptides such as AVP, Ang II, and NE.[92]

The importance of prostaglandins as modulators of renal function in patients with HF is exemplified by Dzau and colleagues.[89] In this study, patients with severe HF had PGI2 and PGE2 metabolite levels 3 to 10 times above levels found in normal subjects. The subset of patients with hyponatremia who were challenged with the prostaglandin synthetase inhibitor, indomethacin, had significant decreases in cardiac index along with elevation of pulmonary capillary wedge pressure and systemic vascular resistance.

SUMMARY AND FUTURE DIRECTIONS

The importance of the kidney in HF has been recognized for over a century. As discussed herein, the kidney maintains sodium balance by regulating intravascular volume. Under physiologic conditions, the control of sodium homeostasis by the kidney is regulated by hormones synthesized and released by the heart that act upon the glomerulus and the tubular epithelium to enhance natriuresis and suppress sodium-retaining factors such as aldosterone. However, in HF the cardiorenal axis becomes perturbed, leading to an inappropriate volume expansion of the vascular and extravascular space. Thus far, our enhanced understanding of physiologic and pathophysiologic, biochemical and mechanical mechanisms in which this cardiorenal axis interacts in the maintenance of sodium homeostasis has provided important diagnostic and novel therapeutic opportunities, which may ultimately delay the progression of heart failure.

References

1. Shchekochikhin D, Schrier RW, Lindenfeld J: Cardiorenal syndrome: pathophysiology and treatment. *Curr Cardiol Rep* 15:380–388, 2013.
2. Bock JS, Gottlieb SS: Cardiorenal syndrome: new perspectives. *Circulation* 121:2592–2600, 2010.
3. Lazich I, Bakris GL: Renal hemodynamic changes in heart failure. In Bakris GL, editor: *The kidney in heart failure*, New York, 2012, Springer Science+Business Media, pp 27–38.
4. Ezekowitz J, McAlister FA, Humphries KH, et al: The association among renal insufficiency, pharmacotherapy, and outcomes in 6,427 patients with heart failure and coronary artery disease. *J Am Coll Cardiol* 44:1587–1592, 2004.
5. Heywood JT, Fonarow GC, Costanzo MR, et al: High prevalence of renal dysfunction and its impact on outcome in 118,465 patients hospitalized with acute decompensated heart failure: a report from the ADHERE database. *J Card Fail* 13:422–430, 2007.
6. Hillege HL, Nitsch D, Pfeffer MA, et al: Renal function as a predictor of outcome in a broad spectrum of patients with heart failure. *Circulation* 113:671–678, 2006.
7. McAlister FA, Ezekowitz J, Tonelli M, et al: Renal insufficiency and heart failure: prognostic and therapeutic implications from a prospective cohort study. *Circulation* 109:1004–1009, 2004.
8. Aronson D, Mittleman MA, Burger AJ: Elevated blood urea nitrogen level as a predictor of mortality in patients admitted for decompensated heart failure. *Am J Med* 116:466–473, 2004.
9. Filippatos G, Rossi J, Lloyd-Jones DM, et al: Prognostic value of blood urea nitrogen in patients hospitalized with worsening heart failure: insights from the Acute and Chronic Therapeutic Impact of a Vasopressin Antagonist in Chronic Heart Failure (ACTIV in CHF) study. *J Card Fail* 13:360–364, 2007.
10. Blair JE, Pang PS, Schrier RW, et al: Changes in renal function during hospitalization and soon after discharge in patients admitted for worsening heart failure in the placebo group of the EVEREST trial. *Eur Heart J* 32:2563–2572, 2011.
11. Cowie MR, Komajda M, Murray-Thomas T, et al: Prevalence and impact of worsening renal function in patients hospitalized with decompensated heart failure: results of the prospective outcomes study in heart failure (POSH). *Eur Heart J* 27:1216–1222, 2006.
12. Klein L, Massie BM, Leimberger JD, et al: Admission or changes in renal function during hospitalization for worsening heart failure predict postdischarge survival: results from the

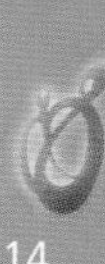

Outcomes of a Prospective Trial of Intravenous Milrinone for Exacerbations of Chronic Heart Failure (OPTIME-CHF). *Circ Heart Fail* 1:25–33, 2008.
13. Felker GM, Lee KL, Bull DA, et al: Diuretic strategies in patients with acute decompensated heart failure. *N Engl J Med* 364:797–805, 2011.
14. Withering W: An account of the foxglove and some of its medical uses: with practical remarks on dropsy and other diseases. Published by Robinsons; London, 1785 [reprint]. *Med Classics* 2:305–326, 1937.
15. Donald DE, Shepherd JT: Reflexes from the heart and lungs: physiological curiosities or important regulatory mechanisms. *Cardiovasc Res* 12:446–469, 1978.
16. Smith HW: Salt and water volume receptors: an exercise in physiologic apologetics. *Am J Med* 23:623–652, 1957.
17. Gilmore JP: Contribution of baroreceptors to the control of renal function. *Circ Res* 14:301–317, 1964.
18. Thames MD, Miller BD, Abboud FM: Baroreflex regulation of renal nerve activity during volume expansion. *Am J Physiol* 243:H810–H814, 1982.
19. Schrier RW, De Wardener HE: Tubular reabsorption of sodium ion: influence of factors other than aldosterone and glomerular filtration rate. 2. *N Engl J Med* 285:1292–1303, 1971.
20. Zucker IH, Share L, Gilmore JP: Renal effects of left atrial distension in dogs with chronic congestive heart failure. *Am J Physiol* 236:H554–H560, 1979.
21. Gauer OH, Henry JP, Behn C: The regulation of extracellular fluid volume. *Annu Rev Physiol* 32:547–595, 1970.
22. Maack T, Camargo MJ, Kleinert HD, et al: Atrial natriuretic factor: structure and functional properties. *Kidney Int* 27:607–615, 1985.
23. Burnett JC, Jr, Granger JP, Opgenorth TJ: Effects of synthetic atrial natriuretic factor on renal function and renin release. *Am J Physiol* 247:F863–F866, 1984.
24. Barajas L: Anatomy of the juxtaglomerular apparatus. *Am J Physiol* 237:F333–F343, 1979.
25. Bakris GL, Wilson DM, Burnett JC, Jr: The renal, forearm, and hormonal responses to standing in the presence and absence of propranolol. *Circulation* 74:1061–1065, 1986.
26. Nikolaidis LA, Poornima I, Parikh P, et al: The effects of combined versus selective adrenergic blockade on left ventricular and systemic hemodynamics, myocardial substrate preference, and regional perfusion in conscious dogs with dilated cardiomyopathy. *J Am Coll Cardiol* 47:1871–1881, 2006.
27. Greven J, Gabriels G: Effect of nebivolol, a novel beta 1-selective adrenoceptor antagonist with vasodilating properties, on kidney function. *Arzneimittelforschung* 50:973–979, 2000.
28. DiBona GF, Sawin LL: Effect of renal nerve stimulation on NaCl and H2O transport in Henle's loop of the rat. *Am J Physiol* 243:F576–F580, 1982.
29. Dinerstein RJ, Jones RT, Goldberg LI: Evidence for dopamine-containing renal nerves. *Fed Proc* 42:3005–3008, 1983.
30. Chapman BJ, Horn NM, Munday KA, et al: Changes in renal blood flow in the rat during renal nerve stimulation: the effects of alpha-adrenergic blockers and a dopaminergic blocker [proceedings]. *J Physiol* 291:64P–65P, 1979.
31. Schrier RW, Humphreys MH, Ufferman RC: Role of cardiac output and the autonomic nervous system in the antinatriuretic response to acute constriction of the thoracic superior vena cava. *Circ Res* 29:490–498, 1971.
32. Gaffney TE, Braunwald E: Importance of the adrenergic nervous system in the support of circulatory function in patients with congestive heart failure. *Am J Med* 34:320–324, 1963.
33. Mokotoff R, Ross G: The effect of spinal anesthesia on the renal ischemia in congestive heart failure. *J Clin Invest* 27:335–339, 1948.
34. Esler MD, Krum H, Sobotka PA, et al: Renal sympathetic denervation in patients with treatment-resistant hypertension (the Symplicity HTN-2 Trial): a randomised controlled trial. *Lancet* 376:1903–1909, 2010.
35. Sobotka PA, Krum H, Bohm M, et al: The role of renal denervation in the treatment of heart failure. *Curr Cardiol Rep* 14:285–292, 2012.
36. Bohm M, Linz D, Urban D, et al: Renal sympathetic denervation: applications in hypertension and beyond. *Nat Rev Cardiol* 10:465–476, 2013.
37. Epstein M, Duncan DC, Fishman LM: Characterization of the natriuresis caused in normal man by immersion in water. *Clin Sci* 43:275–287, 1972.
38. Epstein M, Pins DS, Arrington R, et al: Comparison of water immersion and saline infusion as a means of inducing volume expansion in man. *J Appl Physiol* 39:66–70, 1975.
39. Norsk P, Bonde-Petersen F, Christensen NJ: Catecholamines, circulation, and the kidney during water immersion in humans. *J Appl Physiol* 69:479–484, 1990.
40. Winton FR: The influence of venous pressure on the isolated mammalian kidney. *J Physiol* 72:49–61, 1931.
41. Lifschitz MD, Schrier RW: Alterations in cardiac output with chronic constriction of thoracic inferior vena cava. *Am J Physiol* 225:1364–1370, 1973.
42. Nohria A, Hasselblad V, Stebbins A, et al: Cardiorenal interactions: insights from the ESCAPE trial. *J Am Coll Cardiol* 51:1268–1274, 2008.
43. Damman K, van Deursen VM, Navis G, et al: Increased central venous pressure is associated with impaired renal function and mortality in a broad spectrum of patients with cardiovascular disease. *J Am Coll Cardiol* 53:582–588, 2009.
44. Mullens W, Abrahams Z, Francis GS, et al: Importance of venous congestion for worsening of renal function in advanced decompensated heart failure. *J Am Coll Cardiol* 53:589–596, 2009.
45. Jessup M, Costanzo MR: The cardiorenal syndrome: do we need a change of strategy or a change of tactics? *J Am Coll Cardiol* 53:597–599, 2009.
46. Mullens W, Abrahams Z, Skouri HN, et al: Elevated intra-abdominal pressure in acute decompensated heart failure: a potential contributor to worsening renal function? *J Am Coll Cardiol* 51:300–306, 2008.
47. Packer M: Neurohormonal interactions and adaptations in congestive heart failure. *Circulation* 77:721–730, 1988.
48. Johnson AK, Thunhorst RL: The neuroendocrinology of thirst and salt appetite: visceral sensory signals and mechanisms of central integration. *Front Neuroendocrinol* 18:292–353, 1997.
49. August JT, Nelson DH, Thorn GW: Response of normal subjects to large amounts of aldosterone. *J Clin Invest* 37:1549–1555, 1958.
50. Weber KT: Aldosterone in congestive heart failure. *N Engl J Med* 345:1689–1697, 2001.
51. Cheville RA, Luetscher JA, Hancock EW, et al: Distribution, conjugation, and excretion of labeled aldosterone in congestive heart failure and in controls with normal circulation: development and testing of a model with an analog computer. *J Clin Invest* 45:1302–1316, 1966.
52. Pitt B, Zannad F, Remme WJ, et al: The effect of spironolactone on morbidity and mortality in patients with severe heart failure. Randomized Aldactone Evaluation Study Investigators. *N Engl J Med* 341:709–717, 1999.
53. Chidsey CA, Braunwald E, Morrow AG: Catecholamine excretion and cardiac stores of norepinephrine in congestive heart failure. *Am J Med* 39:442–451, 1965.
54. Cohn JN, Levine TB, Olivari MT, et al: Plasma norepinephrine as a guide to prognosis in patients with chronic congestive heart failure. *N Engl J Med* 311:819–823, 1984.
55. Steinhausen M, Weis S, Fleming J, et al: Responses of in vivo renal microvessels to dopamine. *Kidney Int* 30:361–370, 1986.
56. Lass NA, Glock D, Goldberg LI: Cardiovascular and renal hemodynamic effects of intravenous infusions of the selective DA1 agonist, fenoldopam, used alone or in combination with dopamine and dobutamine. *Circulation* 78:1310–1315, 1988.
57. Krishna GG, Danovitch GM, Beck FW, et al: Dopaminergic mediation of the natriuretic response to volume expansion. *J Lab Clin Med* 105:214–218, 1985.
57a. Chen HH, Anstrom KJ, Givertz MM, et al: Low-dose dopamine or low-dose nesiritide in acute heart failure with renal dysfunction: the ROSE acute heart failure randomized trial. *JAMA* 310:2533–2543, 2013.
58. Yasue H, Obata K, Okumura K, et al: Increased secretion of atrial natriuretic polypeptide from the left ventricle in patients with dilated cardiomyopathy. *J Clin Invest* 83:46–51, 1989.
59. Doyama K, Fukumoto M, Takemura G, et al: Expression and distribution of brain natriuretic peptide in human right atria. *J Am Coll Cardiol* 32:1832–1838, 1998.
60. de Lemos JA, McGuire DK, Drazner MH: B-type natriuretic peptide in cardiovascular disease. *Lancet* 362:316–322, 2003.
61. Brunner-La Rocca HP, Kaye DM, Woods RL, et al: Effects of intravenous brain natriuretic peptide on regional sympathetic activity in patients with chronic heart failure as compared with healthy control subjects. *J Am Coll Cardiol* 37:1221–1227, 2001.
62. Floras JS: Sympathoinhibitory effects of atrial natriuretic factor in normal humans. *Circulation* 81:1860–1873, 1990.
63. Chai SY, Sexton PM, Allen AM, et al: In vitro autoradiographic localization of ANP receptors in rat kidney and adrenal gland. *Am J Physiol* 250:F753–F757, 1986.
64. Fried TA, McCoy RN, Osgood RW, et al: Effect of atriopeptin II on determinants of glomerular filtration rate in the in vitro perfused dog glomerulus. *Am J Physiol* 250:F1119–F1122, 1986.
65. Harris PJ, Thomas D, Morgan TO: Atrial natriuretic peptide inhibits angiotensin-stimulated proximal tubular sodium and water reabsorption. *Nature* 326:697–698, 1987.
66. Scriven TA, Burnett JC, Jr: Effects of synthetic atrial natriuretic peptide on renal function and renin release in acute experimental heart failure. *Circulation* 72:892–897, 1985.
67. Campbell WB, Currie MG, Needleman P: Inhibition of aldosterone biosynthesis by atriopeptins in rat adrenal cells. *Circ Res* 57:113–118, 1985.
68. Tamura N, Ogawa Y, Chusho H, et al: Cardiac fibrosis in mice lacking brain natriuretic peptide. *Proc Natl Acad Sci U S A* 97:4239–4244, 2000.
69. Silver MA, Maisel A, Yancy CW, et al: BNP Consensus Panel 2004: A clinical approach for the diagnostic, prognostic, screening, treatment monitoring, and therapeutic roles of natriuretic peptides in cardiovascular diseases. *Congest Heart Fail* 10:1–30, 2004.
70. Mair J: Biochemistry of B-type natriuretic peptide–where are we now? *Clin Chem Lab Med* 46:1507–1514, 2008.
71. Maisel AS, Krishnaswamy P, Nowak RM, et al: Rapid measurement of B-type natriuretic peptide in the emergency diagnosis of heart failure. *N Engl J Med* 347:161–167, 2002.
72. Doust JA, Pietrzak E, Dobson A, et al: How well does B-type natriuretic peptide predict death and cardiac events in patients with heart failure: systematic review. *BMJ* 330:625, 2005.
73. Hartmann F, Packer M, Coats AJ, et al: Prognostic impact of plasma N-terminal pro-brain natriuretic peptide in severe chronic congestive heart failure: a substudy of the Carvedilol Prospective Randomized Cumulative Survival (COPERNICUS) trial. *Circulation* 110:1780–1786, 2004.
74. McCullough PA, Duc P, Omland T, et al: B-type natriuretic peptide and renal function in the diagnosis of heart failure: an analysis from the Breathing Not Properly Multinational Study. *Am J Kidney Dis* 41:571–579, 2003.
75. Takami Y, Horio T, Iwashima Y, et al: Diagnostic and prognostic value of plasma brain natriuretic peptide in non-dialysis-dependent CRF. *Am J Kidney Dis* 44:420–428, 2004.
76. Hanson ID, McCullough PA: B-type natriuretic peptide: beyond diagnostic applications. In Bakris GL, editor: *The kidney in heart failure*, New York, 2012, Springer Science+Business Media, pp 67–80.
77. Anwaruddin S, Lloyd-Jones DM, Baggish A, et al: Renal function, congestive heart failure, and amino-terminal pro-brain natriuretic peptide measurement: results from the ProBNP Investigation of Dyspnea in the Emergency Department (PRIDE) Study. *J Am Coll Cardiol* 47:91–97, 2006.
78. Colucci WS, Elkayam U, Horton DP, et al: Intravenous nesiritide, a natriuretic peptide, in the treatment of decompensated congestive heart failure. Nesiritide Study Group. *N Engl J Med* 343:246–253, 2000.
79. Intravenous nesiritide vs nitroglycerin for treatment of decompensated congestive heart failure: a randomized controlled trial. *JAMA* 287:1531–1540, 2002.
80. O'Connor CM, Starling RC, Hernandez AF, et al: Effect of nesiritide in patients with acute decompensated heart failure. *N Engl J Med* 365:32–43, 2011.
81. Cody RJ, Atlas SA, Laragh JH, et al: Atrial natriuretic factor in normal subjects and heart failure patients. Plasma levels and renal, hormonal, and hemodynamic responses to peptide infusion. *J Clin Invest* 78:1362–1374, 1986.
82. McMurray JJ, Packer M, Desai AS, et al: Dual angiotensin receptor and neprilysin inhibition as an alternative to angiotensin-converting enzyme inhibition in patients with chronic systolic heart failure: rationale for and design of the Prospective comparison of ARNI with ACEI to Determine Impact on Global Mortality and morbidity in Heart Failure trial (PARADIGM-HF). *Eur J Heart Fail* 15:1062–1073, 2013.
83. Baylis PH: Osmoregulation and control of vasopressin secretion in healthy humans. *Am J Physiol* 253:R671–R678, 1987.
84. Mettauer B, Rouleau JL, Bichet D, et al: Sodium and water excretion abnormalities in congestive heart failure. Determinant factors and clinical implications. *Ann Intern Med* 105:161–167, 1986.
85. Anderson RJ, Cadnapaphornchai P, Harbottle JA, et al: Mechanism of effect of thoracic inferior vena cava constriction on renal water excretion. *J Clin Invest* 54:1473–1479, 1974.
86. Goetz KL, Bond GC, Bloxham DD: Atrial receptors and renal function. *Physiol Rev* 55:157–205, 1975.
87. Russell JA: Vasopressin in vasodilatory and septic shock. *Curr Opin Crit Care* 13:383–391, 2007.
88. Konstam MA, Gheorghiade M, Burnett JC, Jr, et al: Effects of oral tolvaptan in patients hospitalized for worsening heart failure: the EVEREST Outcome Trial. *JAMA* 297:1319–1331, 2007.
89. Dzau VJ, Packer M, Lilly LS, et al: Prostaglandins in severe congestive heart failure. Relation to activation of the renin–angiotensin system and hyponatremia. *N Engl J Med* 310:347–352, 1984.
90. Brown EM, Salzberg DJ: Renal consequences of prostaglandin inhibition in heart failure. In Bakris GL, editor: *The kidney in heart failure*, New York, 2012, Springer Science+Business Media, pp 117–126.
91. Stokes JB: Integrated actions of renal medullary prostaglandins in the control of water excretion. *Am J Physiol* 240:F471–F480, 1981.
92. Yared A, Kon V, Ichikawa I: Mechanism of preservation of glomerular perfusion and filtration during acute extracellular fluid volume depletion. Importance of intrarenal vasopressin-prostaglandin interaction for protecting kidneys from constrictor action of vasopressin. *J Clin Invest* 75:1477–1487, 1985.

Alterations in Skeletal Muscle in Heart Failure

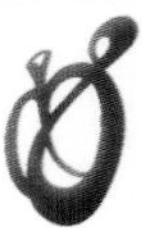

P. Christian Schulze and Michael J. Toth

Dyspnea and fatigue, resulting in diminished exercise tolerance, are among the main factors contributing to decreased social and physical functioning and quality of life for patients with heart failure (HF).[1] There has long been evidence that measures of cardiac function, such as ejection fraction and cardiac output, only poorly correlate with a patient's capacity to exercise, suggesting the involvement of factors other than cardiac insufficiency. Furthermore, many studies of the effects of exercise in patients with HF have failed to demonstrate improvements in cardiac output, stroke volume, or ejection fraction, despite showing gains in exercise capacity and peak oxygen uptake (VO_2).[2] The lack of a close correlation between central hemodynamics and exercise tolerance has led to investigations into alterations in the periphery skeletal muscle. As will be discussed later, the view that alterations in skeletal muscle metabolism, structure, mass, and function play a rate-limiting role in the functional capacity in patients with HF is now broadly accepted. **Figure 15-1** provides a broad hypothetical framework for how factors related to the syndrome of HF (disease-related effectors) diminish skeletal muscle functional capacity (functional phenotypes) and promote exercise intolerance (fatigue and dyspnea) via their effects on skeletal muscle structure and function (skeletal muscle adaptations).

SKELETAL MUSCLE ADAPTATIONS IN HEART FAILURE

The myopathy associated with HF affects both cardiac and skeletal muscle, and encompasses alterations in structure and function in both tissues. Regarding skeletal muscle, the classical model of the myopathy of HF includes a loss of muscle size, strength, and oxidative capacity. More specifically, HF patients experience skeletal muscle atrophy secondary to muscle fiber atrophy, and this loss of muscle quantity may account for a large proportion of the reduction in peak VO_2.[3] Patients also experience muscle weakness,[3] which is caused in part by muscle atrophy, but there are also unique effects of the disease to reduce intrinsic skeletal muscle contractile function.[4] Finally, patients exhibit abnormal skeletal muscle metabolism, with a shift toward glycolytic pathways, changes in mitochondrial function[5,6] and structure,[7] and decreased oxidative enzyme activity.[5] This is due in part to a shift from fatigue-resistant, oxidative type I fibers toward oxidative type II fibers.[8] Altogether, these abnormalities in skeletal muscle structure, function, and cell viability are intimately linked to each other and contribute to the abnormal exercise response, enhanced fatigability, and progressive symptom complex of patients with HF.

SKELETAL MUSCLE ATROPHY

HF patients develop generalized muscle atrophy. Calf muscle volume, assessed by magnetic resonance imaging, revealed reduced muscle volume in patients with HF and significant water and/or fat infiltration.[9] Muscle atrophy develops in patients with severe HF compared with age- and gender-matched controls.[10] However, some studies report normal muscle mass in patients with HF.[11] This disparity may relate to the patients studied, because muscle atrophy may develop secondary to weight loss or inactivity in a subset of the HF population.[12] In general, however, it is widely accepted that HF patients experience some degree of muscle atrophy during the course of the disease.

The mechanisms that mediate skeletal muscle wasting and atrophy have been studied in patients with HF and animal models of cardiac dysfunction. Muscle atrophy occurs during periods of negative muscle protein imbalance, which are due to decreased protein synthesis, increased protein degradation, or both. There is controversy on the impact of clinical status and disease exacerbations on muscle atrophy in HF. The majority of studies have shown no defects in either muscle protein synthesis or breakdown in clinically stable HF patients.[12] It is possible that muscle atrophy initiation and progression are directly linked to episodes of disease exacerbation and hospitalization, which

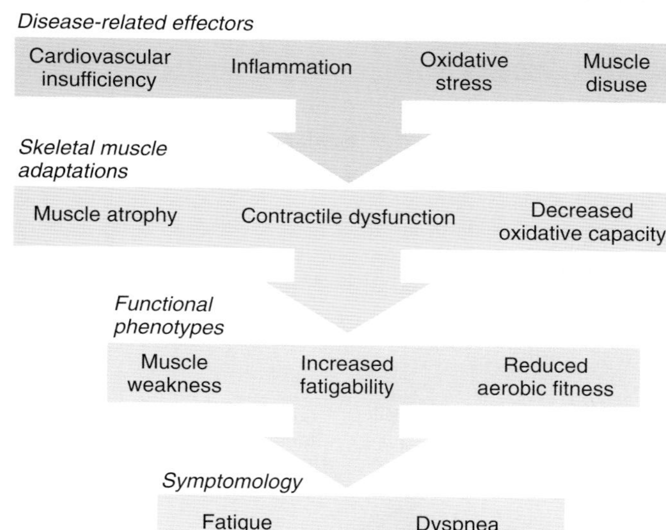

FIGURE 15-1 Broad hypothetical framework for how factors related to the HF syndrome (disease-related effectors) diminish skeletal muscle functional capacity (functional phenotypes) and promote exercise intolerance (fatigue and dyspnea) via their effects on skeletal muscle structure and function (skeletal muscle adaptations).

are accompanied by bed rest, malnutrition, and other factors that may incite atrophy. Unfortunately, no studies have examined patients during acute disease exacerbation to test this postulate or determine what metabolic defects might account for muscle atrophy, although one study has evaluated patients shortly after hospitalization and found evidence for enhanced muscle protein breakdown.[13]

Skeletal muscle atrophy contributes to exercise intolerance in HF patients. Strong correlations have been found between muscle mass and peak V_{O_2}.[3] Moreover, in contrast to nondiseased individuals, in patients with severe HF, the addition of upper arm exercise significantly increases peak V_{O_2}, suggesting the importance of skeletal muscle mass in determining peak V_{O_2} in patients with HF.[14] Thus there is ample evidence supporting a role for muscle atrophy in promoting exercise intolerance. We will now consider the mechanisms underlying this loss of skeletal muscle.

Skeletal Muscle Protein Synthesis and Reduced Anabolic Hormones/Effectors

Skeletal muscle protein synthesis is controlled by mechanoresponsive pathways, paracrine growth factor signaling loops, such as the local insulin-like growth factor-1 (IGF-1) system, but also responds to systemic stimuli including growth hormone, systemic IGF-1, anabolic steroids, and others. The growth hormone (GH)/insulin-like growth factor-1 (GH/IGF-1) axis plays a key role in skeletal muscle growth and differentiation. Low systemic IGF-1 levels have been associated with a reduced leg muscle cross-sectional area and total muscle strength in HF patients.[15] Catabolic syndromes, such as chronic inflammation, sepsis, or cancer, show an altered state of the GH/IGF-1 axis, most probably caused by a peripheral IGF-1 deficiency because of an impaired IGF-1 response to GH, but also abnormal intrahepatic responses to GH.[16] This has been attributed in part to increased serum levels and the local expression of proinflammatory cytokines, such as interleukin-1β (IL-1β) and tumor necrosis factor-α (TNF-α).

In humans with advanced HF and animal models of ischemic cardiomyopathy, reduced local expression of IGF-1 was detected in skeletal muscle compared with controls, accompanied by an increased expression of the IGF-1 receptor in the presence of normal serum levels of IGF-1.[15,17] The serum concentration of the proinflammatory cytokines IL-1β and interleukin-6 (IL-6) were not found to be significantly changed, whereas TNF-α showed a trend toward higher levels in HF. Notably, the local expression of both IL-1β and TNF-α is increased in chronic HF[17,18] and can be reduced by aerobic exercise training.[18] Furthermore, a decreased single muscle fiber CSA in HF has been linked to local expression of IL-1β and impaired expression levels of IGF-1 in skeletal muscle.[17] These results suggest that despite normal serum levels of IGF-1 and proinflammatory cytokines, the local expression of IGF-1 is substantially reduced in HF, indicating a reduction in local anabolic stimuli. Because decreased IGF-1 levels and a reduced muscle fiber CSA correlate with increased levels of IL-1β, these results point toward a cytokine-mediated local catabolic process that is mediated in part through reductions in anabolic hormone expression.

Local expression of IGF-1 in skeletal muscle is mainly regulated by two different mechanisms. The first is GH receptor-dependent,[19] a mechanism that at least in part is impaired in HF-induced weight loss because of a peripheral GH resistance.[20] In addition, skeletal muscle IGF-1 expression is modulated in response to alterations in muscle use, and the expression of IGF-1 increases significantly in response to work overload and passive stretch.[21] In contrast, TNF-α and other cytokines may decrease skeletal muscle expression of IGF-1.[22,23] In addition to its classical role to enhance protein synthesis, IGF-1 has anti-apoptotic effects in various tissues, protecting against cytokine-mediated apoptosis.[24] These findings suggest that IGF-1 may regulate cell survival by modulating both pro- and anti-apoptotic stimuli. Thus the increased rate of skeletal muscle apoptosis in HF[25] may be explained by a decline in local IGF-1 expression. This is suggested by preclinical models, where stimulation of IGF-1 production via GH administration reduces atrophy via reductions in apoptosis.[26]

In male HF patients, deficiencies in circulating total testosterone, dehydroepiandrosterone (DHEA), and IGF-1 are common and correlate with a poor prognosis.[27] Testosterone maintains skeletal muscle mass by increasing fractional muscle protein synthesis. Additionally, testosterone appears to stimulate IGF-1 expression, but the exact molecular pathways are incompletely understood. At supra-physiologic doses, testosterone appears to act through androgen receptor-independent mechanisms. In HF patients, serum levels of free testosterone and DHEA are decreased, and this decrease correlates with HF severity. Perhaps most important, replacement of testosterone improves exercise capacity, muscle strength, and metabolic function.[28]

Finally, insulin resistance is a hallmark of advanced HF (see also Chapter 16). This metabolic abnormality is more pronounced during acute decompensated HF and improves upon cardiac recompensation.[29] Moreover, improved cardiac output through left ventricular assist device placement results in reduced insulin resistance and improved glucose homeostasis in advanced HF (see also Chapter 42).[30] The effects of insulin to promote skeletal muscle anabolism occurs during the daily cycle of feeding and fasting, where it serves to promote postprandial anabolism by reducing

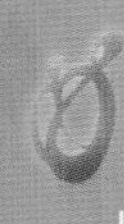

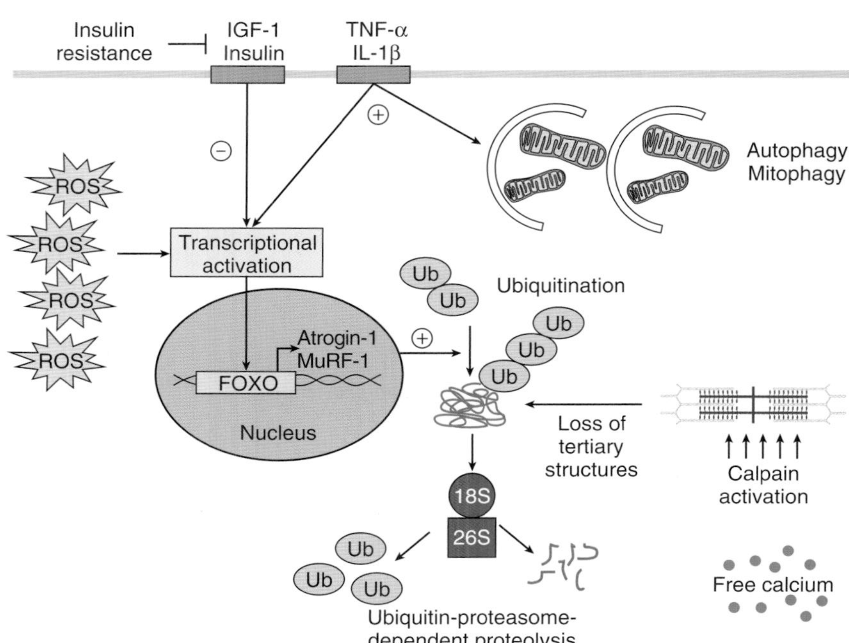

FIGURE 15-2 Regulation of muscle atrophy occurs through several highly conserved pathways of proteolytic changes in skeletal muscle. These are identical for various disease states, as well as disuse and immobilization. The main proteolytic pathway in skeletal muscle is the ATP-dependent degradation of proteins through ubiquitination and action of the 26S proteasome. This pathway is transcriptionally regulated through FOXO transcription factors and expression of atrogenes, such as MuRF-1 and atrogin-1. Activation of calcium-dependent calpains occurs because of increased levels of intracellular calcium released from the sarcoplasmic reticulum (SR). Calpains are primarily responsible for destruction of tertiary structure and subsequent exposure of proteolytic cleavage sites. Finally, lysosomal protein degradation, or autophagy, is a highly regulated process that contributes to the destruction of cellular organelles. All these pathways likely contribute to skeletal muscle atrophy in advanced HF.

skeletal muscle protein breakdown. Recent studies have suggested that HF patients experience impaired suppression of insulin's effects to reduce protein breakdown in response to meal-associated stimuli and that this impaired response was related to circulating IL-6 levels.[31] Thus tissue insulin sensitivity, possibly secondary to immune activation, may contribute to skeletal muscle atrophy.

Skeletal Muscle Protein Breakdown and Increased Catabolic Hormones/Effectors

HF is a catabolic state, with increased levels of various catabolic hormones.[32] Several authors have suggested a role for myostatin in muscle atrophy in patients with advanced HF.[33] Myostatin is a local and circulating factor secreted from skeletal muscle with antianabolic and antihypertrophic actions. In fact, such a mechanism may be operable in patients, because circulating levels of myostatin[34] and other transforming growth factor (TGF) receptor ligands, such as activin,[35] are increased in HF patients.

Whatever might be the proximal hormonal/circulating effector, local skeletal muscle protein breakdown is mediated by several cellular systems that include lysosomal proteases, the ATP-dependent ubiquitin-proteasome system, and the Ca^{2+}-dependent calpain system (**Figure 15-2**). Specifically, the ubiquitin-proteasome system has been implicated in the enhanced protein breakdown of atrophying skeletal muscle in a number of disease models,[36] including chronic HF.[37] Of particular interest is a group of ubiquitin-conjugating enzymes (E3-ligases) that target proteins for degradation by the proteasome. Through transcriptional screening, two E3-ligases, atrogin-1 (also called MFbx-1) and MuRF-1 (muscle ring finger protein-1), have been identified to be highly induced in processes of muscular atrophy of different origin. Gomes and colleagues reported the identification and initial description of an increased expression of atrogin-1, a muscle-specific E3-ligase, following starvation.[38] Through a comparable analysis of genes regulated in atrophying muscle caused by different mechanisms, Bodine and associates identified the same gene (here called MAFbx-1) and, additionally, MuRF-1, another E3-ligase.[39] Through adenovirally mediated overexpression of these genes, their catabolic effects were demonstrated. Further, animals with targeted deletion of MAFbx-1 or MuRF-1 exhibit less muscular atrophy in response to denervation and hindlimb suspension.[38]

Increased atrogin-1 has been reported in other animal models of muscular atrophy induced by immobilization, denervation, hindlimb suspension,[39] starvation,[38] and sepsis.[40] The induction of atrogin-1 expression before muscle weight loss in starvation suggests that the activation of this gene is involved in the development and progression of muscle protein loss.[38] In support of this possibility, overexpression of atrogin-1 in C_2C_{12} myotubes induced atrophy in vitro, whereas muscular atrophy following denervation was prevented in animals with targeted deletion of atrogin-1.[39] Intriguingly, infusion of the proinflammatory cytokine IL-1β induces the expression of atrogin-1[39] and TNF-α increases the ubiquitin-conjugating capacity in myocytes,[41] findings that again support the hypothesis of cytokines as putative mediators of muscular atrophy. Prior studies have shown transcriptional activation of E3-ligases in muscle of animals with left ventricular dysfunction[37] and humans with advanced heart failure,[42] whereas other reports did not show these changes.[43] This might relate to the type of muscle injury and severity of heart failure.[13] However, the exact mechanisms underlying the transcriptional activation of atrogin-1 by IL-1β remain to be elucidated.

Activation of the renin-angiotensin system results in vasoconstriction and elevated skeletal muscle concentration of angiotensin II (Ang II), which increases local oxidative stress, increases muscle proteolysis, and lowers skeletal muscle concentration of IGF-1. These mechanisms may accelerate protein degradation while decreasing protein synthesis. Loss of skeletal muscle mass contributes to muscle reflex alterations in HF.[44] In normal subjects, muscle reflex activation helps raise blood pressure and thereby maintain muscle perfusion during muscle acidosis. In HF, muscle reflex activation occurs at the onset of exercise, resulting in vasoconstriction and limited skeletal muscle perfusion.

SKELETAL MUSCLE CONTRACTILE DYSFUNCTION

Skeletal muscle contractile dysfunction has received relatively minimal attention as a precipitant of functional limitations in the clinical syndrome of HF. Despite this lack of attention, data suggest that HF is associated with marked reductions in skeletal muscle contractility. Skeletal muscle atrophy contributes to this diminished contractile function, but there is evidence for diminished function per unit muscle size (i.e., intrinsic contractile dysfunction). Studies under both static (isometric) and dynamic (isokinetic) conditions suggest intrinsic contractile deficits in HF patients on the order of 15% to 25%.[3,31] This reduction is greater in cachectic versus noncachectic patients[45] and is not corrected by cardiac transplantation.[46] Of note, recent studies have further shown that these decrements in muscle function persist when patients are compared with controls who are matched for habitual physical activity level,[47] arguing that decreased contractility is not a consequence of muscle disuse. Moreover, reduced contractility is not related to impairments in central motor drive or neural transmission.[3,47] Thus there is compelling evidence that HF alters the intrinsic contractile properties of skeletal muscle and that the resulting muscle weakness contributes to exercise intolerance.[3]

Myofilament Contractile Adaptations

Alterations in skeletal muscle contractile function in HF may relate to changes in myofilament protein expression, their function, or both. Regarding the former, adult human skeletal muscle consists of three fiber types, characterized primarily by the type of myosin isoform expressed, and identified based on their differential immunochemistry staining for myosin ATPase. **Table 15-1** details the structural and functional features of these types of muscle fibers. In general, most skeletal muscles contain a mixture of these fiber types, with MHC I (type I) and IIA (type IIA) being predominant and with very few fibers that express only the fastest MHC isoform (MHC IIX [type IIX]). This differs from rodents, which express a fourth fiber type, MHC IIB (type IIB), that is faster and less oxidative than all the other fiber types. There are other contractile proteins whose expression varies by fiber types, but the functional character of each fiber is largely dictated by the type of myosin expressed.

Myofilament Protein Expression

One of the most often cited skeletal muscle adaptions to HF is the shift in fiber type toward a more fast-twitch, glycolytic phenotype, which is reflected by a change in expression of myosin heavy chain (MHC) toward a more fast-twitch isoform (IIA or IIX). The loss of slow-twitch, oxidative fibers has been demonstrated in animal models[48] and humans[8] and has long been held as a mechanism underlying the reduction in aerobic fitness.[8] However, this same phenotype is apparent upon muscle disuse, arguing for the possibility that it may be a by-product of the physical inactivity that accompanies the HF syndrome. Early work that compared MHC expression between HF patients, healthy controls, and stroke patients confined to bed rest for more than 1 year as "inactive" controls argued against this notion.[8] However, it is questionable whether patients who undergo muscle disuse secondary to loss of central neural activation represent the degree of activity restriction that occurs with HF,[49] which is arguably more modest than being bedridden. In fact, studies that have carefully matched HF patients to controls for fitness/activity level have observed no effect of HF to alter MHC isoform expression/fiber type.[43,50]

Discordance between studies finding/not finding a shift in fiber type/MHC expression with HF may be explained by the advent of the use of angiotensin-converting enzyme inhibitors (ACEi) and angiotensin receptor blockers (**see also Chapter 34**), considering that these agents reverse the shift in fiber type back toward a more slow-twitch phenotype.[51] However, more recent studies in human patients have observed this fiber type switch in patients taking ACEi.[52] In fact, studies conducted by the same laboratory in separate cohorts of human patients taking these medications have both observed and not observed changes in muscle fiber type,[43,52] with the only difference between the two cohorts being the activity status of controls. This further highlights the potential modulating role of physical activity on fiber type characteristics in the HF population. Building on this notion, and considering that a similar switch in fiber type from a slow- to a fast-twitch phenotype is emblematic of muscle disuse, the effects of these medications might reflect their ability to improve symptomology and in turn increase physical activity in patients.

In addition to alterations in the expression of specific isoforms of MHC, recent studies have found evidence for a select reduction in the expression of myosin relative to other contractile proteins on the order of 15% to 20% (**Figure 15-3**).[43,52] Mechanical assessments that reflect cross-bridge numbers were similarly reduced,[43] suggesting that these results are not attributable to variation in biochemical extraction of myosin. Moreover, these reductions are similar in magnitude with what has been observed in animal models[48] and have been shown to be related to functional decrements.[52] Importantly, this loss was not related to muscle disuse as suggested by some studies,[53] because patients were matched to controls for physical activity level.[43] Similar patterns of myosin loss have been shown in other clinical conditions (e.g., COPD, critical

TABLE 15-1 The Structural and Functional Features of Muscle Fibers

	Human Fiber Types			*Low Order Mammals*
FIBER TYPE	**TYPE I (RED)**	**TYPE IIA (RED)**	**TYPE IIX (WHITE)**	**TYPE IIB (WHITE)**
Contraction time	Slow	Moderate fast	Fast	Very fast
Oxidative capacity	High	High	Intermediate	Low
Mitochondrial density	High	High	Medium	Low
Glycolytic capacity	Low	High	High	High
Resistance to fatigue	High	Fairly high	Intermediate	Low
Major storage fuel	Triglycerides	Creatine phosphate, glycogen	Creatine phosphate, glycogen	Creatine phosphate, glycogen
Capillary density	High	Intermediate	Low	Low

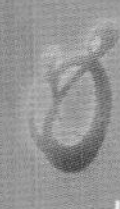

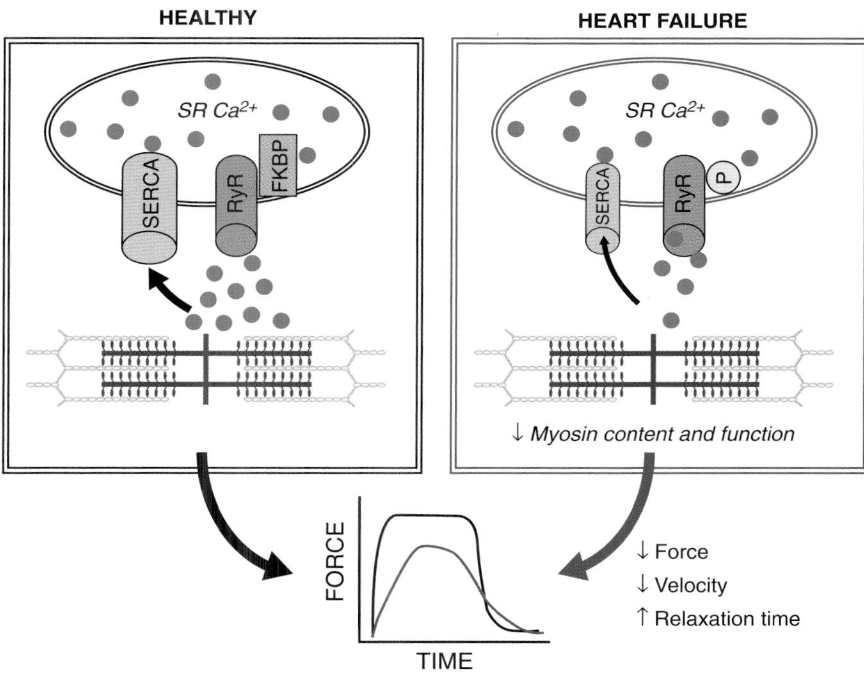

FIGURE 15-3 Effects of HF to decrease skeletal muscle contractile function. HF impairs intracellular Ca^{2+} release, thereby diminishing activation of myofilament proteins and lessening contractile force (lower plateau of the force tracing). Additionally, HF reduces myosin protein expression and myosin-actin cross-bridge function, which likely has the net effect of reducing contractile velocity (ascending limb of the force tracing). Additionally, evidence suggests that HF increases relaxation time (descending limb of the force tracing), possibly secondary to reduced Ca^{2+} reuptake into the sarcoplasmic reticulum (SR). Collectively, these adaptations likely reduce contractile force, velocity, and, in turn, power output, leading to a reduced capacity for physical work. Additionally, adaptations in myofilament function and Ca^{2+} dynamics may contribute to increased fatigability of skeletal muscle.

care myopathy[54,55]), suggesting this may be a common contractile protein adaptation related to some aspect of acute/chronic disease.

Myofilament Protein Function

Several lines of evidence suggest that skeletal muscle contractile protein function is impaired in HF patients, but the exact nature of this effect is in dispute. We will first consider the effect of HF on myofilament protein function.

Preclinical models have generally shown minimal effects of HF on peripheral skeletal muscle myofilament protein function, as assessed in chemically skinned single muscle fibers.[56] In contrast, studies in clinical patients have shown profound reductions (≈30%-50%) in single muscle fiber contractile force per unit of fiber cross-sectional area (i.e., tension).[57] Together with clinical studies showing relationships between whole muscle strength and circulating cytokines in HF patients[58] and similar magnitude reductions in muscle tension with acute and chronic cytokine administration,[59] these results have led to the notion that the immune activation that accompanies HF contributes to exercise intolerance in part through impairment of muscle contractile function. However, recent studies that more carefully matched HF patients to controls for age and physical activity status have found no reduction in tension in single muscle fibers from HF patients.[4] Conflicting results among studies of human muscle fibers may relate to the fact that prior studies have used control populations that differ in age from patients by more than 10 years, and that no account was taken for the physical activity status of the groups.[57] Here again, when the physical inactivity of HF patients is taken into consideration, the effect of the HF syndrome to impact contractile protein force production is lessened.

Despite the absence of an effect on contractile protein force production, HF does alter other aspects of contractile protein function; specifically, the kinetics of the myosin-actin cross-bridge interaction were slowed in HF patients compared with age- and activity-matched controls.[4] Such alterations in the myosin-actin cross-bridge function, although potentially beneficial in maintaining muscle fiber force generating capacity,[4] can have detrimental consequences. A slowing of cross-bridge kinetics would presumably slow contractile velocity,[60] which could in turn reduce muscle power output. Indeed, there is some evidence from preclinical models for reduced contractile velocity with HF.[61] A reduction in the contractile velocity of muscle would contribute to an overall reduction in muscle power output.[47] Thus some proportion of the reduced work capacity of skeletal muscle in HF patients, which would directly influence performance during a peak exercise test, may relate to decreased contractile velocity secondary to impaired cross-bridge function (see Figure 15-3).

Excitation-Contraction Coupling Adaptations

While alterations in myofilament protein function may explain diminished contractile velocity and, in turn, power production, they do not appear to explain reduced force production (i.e., muscle strength). This may be explained instead by impaired excitation-contraction coupling (ECC). More specifically, diminished calcium (Ca^{2+}) release from the sarcoplasmic reticulum (SR) leads to decreased myofilament activation and in turn force production (see Figure 15-3). Additionally, impaired ECC function may partially underlie the fatigue that HF patients report on exertion. In the next section, we review evidence that HF alters the ECC system. Because most of the components of the ECC system intrinsic to skeletal muscle cannot be assessed in humans, this discussion primarily relies on data from animal models.

Most of the research in this field has focused on Ca^{2+} release and reuptake from the SR. Early work in the rat coronary artery ligation model of HF showed that reduced skeletal muscle (extensor digitorum longus; fast-twitch muscle) tension was accompanied by decreased intracellular Ca^{2+} release.[62] Additionally, HF animals were associated with accelerated fatigue rates, as assessed by the decrease in tension following repeated tetanic contractions. Other studies have further suggested that Ca^{2+} uptake may also be impaired in HF, based on diminished expression of the SR Ca^{2+} ATPase (SERCA).[63,64] These seminal results stimulated research in this area because such decrements in Ca^{2+} release and reuptake could underlie greater fatigability in skeletal muscle in HF.

Studies that included slow- (soleus) and fast-twitch muscles/isolated muscle fibers of rats using the same coronary artery ligation model of HF showed conflicting results. Under nonfatigued conditions, there were no decrements in contractile strength with HF, although there was evidence for slowed relaxation times.[65] Interestingly, contrary to the previously mentioned reports of a loss of SERCA protein expression, this study found no effect of HF on SERCA expression, despite the presence of its resultant physiologic phenotype (i.e., slowed relaxation). Moreover, there were no prominent differences between HF and control animals during fatiguing contractions in tension development or intracellular Ca^{2+} levels,[65] although force relaxation was markedly slowed in the slow-twitch soleus muscle. Follow-up studies by this same group, where contractile properties of the soleus muscle were assessed in situ using a protocol that more closely simulated submaximal contractile activity, a reduced relaxation rate was observed in HF animals, which was also accompanied by increased fatigability.[66] Subsequent studies in isolated single muscle fibers have further suggested that increased fatigability in HF animals was not associated with impaired Ca^{2+} release.[67] Instead, the authors assert that impairments in myofilament protein function may develop with fatiguing contraction to produce the reduction in tension. This could potentially be explained by reduced cross-bridge kinetics detailed above,[4] as maneuvers that increase the rate of cross-bridge cycling reduce skeletal muscle fatigue.

More recent studies, also conducted in the rat coronary ligation model of HF, have further supported impaired SR Ca^{2+} release. Ward and associates[68] showed a reduction in the intracellular Ca^{2+} transient in HF animals. Ca^{2+} sparks, which are spontaneous, localized Ca^{2+} release events that play an important role in dictating aggregate intracellular Ca^{2+} release, have smaller amplitude, slower temporal kinetics, and greater spatial spread. In these same studies, the SR Ca^{2+} release channel, the ryanodine receptor, was hyperphosphorylated and had less associated FKBP12 (also known as calstabin). Further work showed that protein kinase A-mediated phosphorylation of the ryanodine receptor causes dissociation of FKBP12, which normally functions to inhibit the channel.[69] This conspiration of changes in ryanodine receptor biochemistry is associated with a "leaky" channel phenotype that has been found in cardiomyocytes in models of HF and is thought to contribute to disease progression.[70] This is significant, because it links the well-known heightened sympathetic nervous system activity in the HF syndrome to the skeletal muscle contractile phenotype. In fact, this leaky channel phenotype may be important for exercise intolerance in HF, because it has been suggested to contribute to fatigue in humans.[71]

Whether similar alterations in intracellular Ca^{2+} dynamics are present in humans with HF is unknown. Using isolated SR vesicles, recent studies have found no alterations in Ca^{2+} release, uptake, or leak in patients compared with controls.[72] Additionally, contrary to animal models, some studies have suggested an upregulation of Ca^{2+} uptake in patients with HF compared with controls,[73] although some studies suggest downregulation of the expression of these proteins.[74] Thus the balance of available evidence, although quite small, suggests that the phenotype of ECC in human HF may not be adequately reflected in available animal models. This could be due to the fact that measurements in human samples are necessarily different from those in animal models. Alternatively, discordant results may be explained by the fact that patients are treated with pharmacologic agents that counteract some of the pathologic Ca^{2+} regulatory alterations (e.g., β-blockers may prevent ryanodine receptor hyperphosphorylation and the resulting calcium release abnormalities). Further work is required to clearly define the ECC phenotype in human HF to determine its contribution to reduced skeletal muscle contractile strength.

DECREASED OXIDATIVE CAPACITY AND METABOLISM

Exercise intolerance, defined subjectively as dyspnea and fatigue upon exertion and clinically as a reduced peak oxygen uptake during an incremental exercise test, is the cardinal symptom of chronic HF. Although this decrement was originally attributed to cardiac insufficiency, work over the past three decades has led to an appreciation of noncardiac, or peripheral, adaptations to HF syndrome that contribute to exercise intolerance.[75] The relative importance of skeletal muscle versus vascular versus neural adaptations that may explain reduced functional capacity in HF patients has been much debated, and the exact admixture of pathophysiologic adaptations contributing to exertional intolerance is likely variable among patients. Instead of offering a resolution to these arguments, we will describe what is known about how HF affects skeletal muscle specifically, with a concentration on what is known about the unique effect of HF syndrome. We focus our efforts mostly on those adaptations confined to skeletal muscle, as Chapter 13 provides an in-depth discussion of the vascular adaptations that occur during HF.

Mitochondrial Adaptations

Much of the early work in this field used phosphorus magnetic resonance spectroscopy (MRS), coupled with isolated limb exercise, to noninvasively monitor inorganic phosphate, phosphocreatine, and ATP levels and cellular pH in skeletal muscle to assess oxidative metabolism. Early studies from a number of laboratories throughout the 1980s and 1990s showed that HF was characterized by intrinsic deficits in skeletal muscle oxidative capacity that yielded disproportionately greater increases in inorganic phosphate and reductions in pH for a given exercise load (**Figure 15-4**). Importantly, these abnormalities were shown to be independent of blood flow,[6] muscle atrophy,[9] and fiber type adaptations,[5] suggesting an intrinsic deficit in oxidative metabolism. At about the same time, ultrastructural studies of skeletal muscle tissue from HF patients showed evidence of significant mitochondrial rarefaction,[7] providing a potential subcellular mechanism underlying the aforementioned

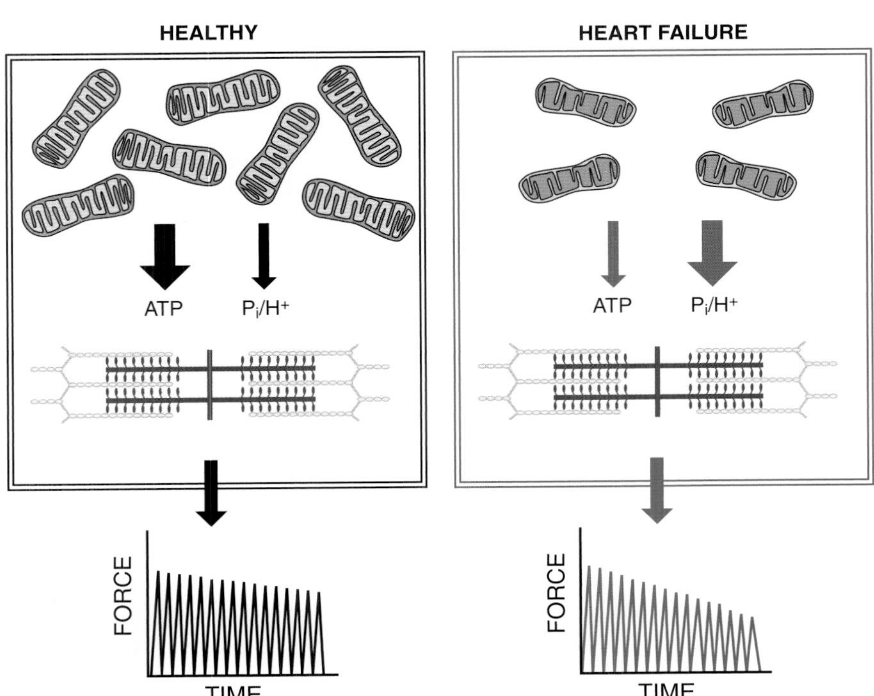

FIGURE 15-4 Effects of HF to impair oxidative capacity and hasten muscle fatigue in skeletal muscle. HF contributes to both structural and functional impairment of skeletal muscle oxidative capacity. HF contributes to quantitative and functional changes in mitochondria, including mitochondrial loss, disrupted ultrastructure (decreased cristae) and reduced capacity for oxidative ATP production. This leads to increased inorganic phosphate levels (Pi), greater acidity, and suboptimal ATP provision during exercise. Increased Pi, reduced pH, and decreased ATP availability would conspire to impair myofilament contractile function. Collectively, these alterations lead to more rapid muscle fatigue during repetitive muscular activity, as indicated by a more rapid reduction in force production (bottom force tracings). Such a reduction in skeletal muscle oxidative capacity would contribute to decreased tissue oxygen utilization and, in turn, reduced whole body peak oxygen consumption.

metabolic derangements identified by MRS. Early studies showing reduced activity of a variety of oxidative enzymes in HF patients[5] further suggested impaired energy metabolism. Collectively, these results implicate impaired oxidative metabolism, and mitochondrial structure/function in particular, in the symptomology of HF. Along with fiber type alterations discussed previously, these energetic abnormalities have become a hallmark of the skeletal muscle myopathy of HF. Additionally, impaired skeletal muscle oxidative metabolism in HF has served as evidence to support the recommendation of aerobic exercise training as an intervention to alleviate exercise intolerance in HF, considering that the primary effect of such exercise to improve aerobic fitness in cardiac populations likely derives from its effects on skeletal muscle oxidative capacity.[76]

A considerable body of research, however, has raised doubts about whether HF, per se, alters skeletal muscle oxidative capacity generally, or mitochondrial content or function specifically. Using magnetic resonance spectroscopy (MRS), Chati and colleagues[77] found no group differences in ATP, inorganic phosphate, or pH during exercise when HF patients were compared with sedentary controls who were recruited to match patients for their low level of physical activity. In contrast, they found that trained control subjects (>14 hr/wk of physical training) showed slower ATP depletion, inorganic phosphate accumulation, and acidification than HF patients or sedentary controls. In another study, which used saponin-skinned muscle fibers, Mettauer and coworkers[50] observed no effect of HF on oxidative metabolism in patients versus sedentary controls (peak Vo_2 <110% of predicted), whereas lower oxidative rates were found in both of these groups compared with active controls (peak Vo_2 >110% of predicted). Finally, Williams and associates,[78] working with isolated mitochondria, showed no differences in ATP production rates between HF patients and sedentary controls (no specification for the designation of "sedentary" was provided). Thus when studying muscle oxidative function using a variety of techniques, from isolated mitochondria to in vivo, these data suggest that a large proportion of the effect of HF on skeletal muscle oxidative capacity may be explained by the chronic physical inactivity that characterizes these patients, rather than the disease process itself. This conclusion should be tempered by the fact that studies have shown defects in oxidative metabolism in forearm muscles, which should not be impacted by muscle disuse,[6] arguing for some contribution from the disease.

Similar questions arise regarding the potential involvement of muscle disuse in the mitochondrial rarefaction observed in HF patients.[7] More recent studies that have matched HF patients and controls for physical activity level did not observe a reduction in mitochondrial content.[79] In fact, the early studies of Drexler and colleagues emphasized that mitochondrial loss is only apparent in patients with later-stage HF, where one might expect more pronounced reductions in physical activity. Arguing against muscle disuse as the precipitant for mitochondrial loss, a recent study has shown mitochondrial rarefaction in HF patients compared with sedentary controls.[80] Thus there is still ambiguity as to whether there is a unique effect of HF on mitochondrial content/morphology. However, from the preceding discussion, it should be apparent that any

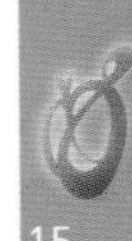

mitochondrial structural abnormalities that might be present have minimal effects on overall mitochondrial function when the effects of physical inactivity are taken into account.

Another consideration that should be factored into this discussion is the effect of medications. Many of the early studies establishing an effect of HF on skeletal muscle oxidative capacity and mitochondrial biology were performed before the widespread use of vasodilator therapy. This point is noteworthy because some studies in preclinical models of ischemic cardiomyopathy (coronary artery ligation model) have shown that initiation of ACEi following coronary infarct can mitigate impaired mitochondrial function related to HF.[81] Thus one reason for the failure of more recent studies to observe an effect of HF on skeletal muscle oxidative capacity may relate to the evolution of HF therapies. Indeed, Drexler and colleagues[7] noted that mitochondrial loss could be largely corrected in patients with treatment that led to sufficient functional improvements. Whether these medications have a unique effect to modulate skeletal muscle oxidative function, or instead derive their benefits from effects on nonmuscle systems that indirectly improve muscle function via reduced disease burden and/or increased physical activity, is not apparent. Arguing against the former, recent studies in preclinical models suggest that ACEi does not modulate skeletal muscle oxidative capacity through alterations in mitochondrial function.[82] Whatever the mechanism, there are clearly effects of HF medications on skeletal muscle oxidative capacity that should be considered when discerning which factors incite decreased aerobic capacity in these patients.

Interventions to improve skeletal muscle oxidative function in HF patients have substantial benefits. HF is characterized by reduced habitual physical activity[49] and acute periods of profound muscle disuse during hospitalization, both of which diminish overall oxidative capacity. Thus aerobic exercise training remains attractive as a means to improve overall functional capacity in HF patients. In fact, some degree of exercise training may be required to remediate the "detraining effects" that the disease imposes on skeletal muscle, because studies have shown that skeletal muscle energetic abnormalities persist after correction of cardiac insufficiency via transplantation.[83] There is substantial evidence that mitochondrial biology and skeletal muscle oxidative capacity can be improved with aerobic training[84,85] and that such improvements can be elicited with relatively low-intensity exercise (40% of peak oxygen uptake).[86] Thus rehabilitation programs that use aerobic exercise training remain an attractive adjunct to classical HF therapeutics to improve functional capacity and quality of life.

Fiber Type Adaptations

Decreased oxidative capacity in HF patients may be a function of disease-related fiber type shifts toward a more fast-twitch, glycolytic phenotype. As addressed previously, these alterations in fiber type, as reflected by alterations in the expression of myosin heavy chain protein, are largely related to muscle disuse rather than a unique effect of the disease process. Regardless of the inciting factor, and beyond its role in dictating skeletal muscle oxidative capacity, fiber type composition plays an important role in determining overall functional capacity, as assessed by peak oxygen consumption.[87] More specifically, lower slow-twitch fiber content is associated with exercise intolerance. In this light, interventions to counter the switch toward a fast-twitch fiber type, such as aerobic exercise, would clearly be beneficial in maintaining and/or improving functional capacity. Indeed, the effect of aerobic training to shift muscle fiber type composition toward a more slow-twitch phenotype in HF patients is well founded.[88] In addition to exercise training, certain HF medications may exert similar beneficial effects on muscle fiber composition. As noted previously, studies in patients[51] have shown that antagonism of angiotensin II via ACEi or angiotensin receptor blockers shifts skeletal muscle fiber composition toward a more slow-twitch phenotype. Commensurate with these shifts in fiber type was an increase in peak aerobic capacity. This provides a potential cellular-level explanation for how medications may alter muscle oxidative capacity and furthermore raises the intriguing possibility that one of the cornerstone therapies for HF may derive some of its beneficial effects, at least in part, from improvements in skeletal muscle abnormalities.

Vascular Adaptations (see also Chapter 13)

Impaired peripheral vascular flow dynamics are only partially explained by reduced cardiac output, and abnormal tissue perfusion through impaired microcirculation constitutes another important disturbance of vascular flow dynamics in HF. This is particularly important in HF, as vascular flow dynamics relate to intrinsic properties of skeletal muscle affecting exercise performance. In oxidative muscle, capillary density is higher in comparison to more glycolytic muscle types. This relates directly to endurance function and exercise performance. Of note, exercise training in normal cohorts, as well as in HF subjects, increases not only muscle function but also skeletal muscle capillary density, which suggests that improved peripheral microcirculatory flow dynamics are linked to improved oxidative function.

Capillary density measured as the ratio of capillaries per muscle fiber shows a consistent reduction in the skeletal muscle of HF patients compared with controls.[7,78,89] This has been linked to reduced exercise tolerance.[89] However, this relationship has been difficult to reproduce in the continuum of clinical stages of patients with HF, suggesting that certain degrees of structural and functional derangements in skeletal muscle are necessary to develop a persistent and significant vascular phenotype. Metabolic changes relating to differences in oxygen use and the ability to extract oxygen from the peripheral circulation, as what might be expected with reduced mitochondria content and function described previously, might in fact be required to promote changes in capillary density. In this context, intrinsic skeletal muscle adaptations may feed back to the vasculature to provoke maladaptive changes.

EFFECTORS OF SKELETAL MUSCLE ADAPTATIONS

Hypoperfusion

Reduced cardiac output and decreased capillary density of skeletal muscle are directly linked.[89] Although cardiac output at rest is only minimally impaired in HF, most changes occur during exercise during a state of increased oxygen demand of the working skeletal muscle. Therefore, the imbalance of oxygen and energy supply to skeletal muscle is in particular impaired during exercise and physical work. While this corresponds to the clinical symptoms of advanced HF, it does not fully explain the underlying mechanisms. Several studies have suggested that impaired cardiac output and pulsatility in advanced HF leads to reduced shear stress in the vascular endothelium and, therefore, to a reduction in shear-released nitric oxide,[90] one of the strongest vasodilators. Further, the chronic activation of the renin-angiotensin-aldosterone system and a hyperadrenergic state in advanced HF favors a vasoconstrictive state of the peripheral vasculature. With that, peripheral hypoperfusion, both at rest and particularly during exercise, is worsened. In turn, the beneficial effects of peripheral vasodilator therapy on improving cardiac output and peripheral perfusion are explained by this phenomenon.

Reduced capillary density, progressive vasodilation, and impaired oxidative metabolism are linked by the molecular response to chronic hypoperfusion and low-grade ischemia. Several studies have confirmed that both in the myocardium and in skeletal muscle, ischemia and ischemia/reperfusion result in a switch toward a more glycolytic metabolism.[91] This is in part explained by the ability of the cell to produce ATP, even in the absence of oxygen, through glycolysis. In contrast, oxidative metabolism requires a sufficient oxygen supply. Although fatty acid oxidation seems to be particularly affected, all other substrates for oxidative metabolism, including glucose, amino acids, and lactate, require oxygen-dependent metabolic steps as part of mitochondrial generation of ATP. Therefore, the increased glycolytic capacity of skeletal muscle in advanced HF might be a direct reflection of impaired tissue oxygenation in combination with other pathomechanisms discussed in this section.

Inflammation (see also Chapter 7)

Although increased levels of circulating cytokines such as TNF-α, IL-6, and IL-1β in chronic disease states are a well-established finding, an increased local expression of proinflammatory cytokines, and their potential role in mechanisms leading to muscular atrophy, has only recently attracted more attention.[15,17,18] Circulating cytokine levels do not reflect tissue levels and their potential activity due to unknown autocrine/paracrine effects, in contrast to the typical endocrine action of circulating hormones/metabolites. Moreover, tissue-specific expression further complicates the analysis of their exact action. It is possible that enhanced local expression of proinflammatory cytokines precedes an increase in circulating levels and, therefore, represents a more sensitive indicator of local skeletal muscle abnormalities in HF.

One possible mechanism leading to an increased local expression of proinflammatory cytokines might be found in an enhanced activation of the transcription factor NF-κB. This transcription factor regulates the expression of proinflammatory cytokines (e.g., TNF-α and IL-1β).[92] Moreover, both cytokines and angiotensin II[93] trigger their local expression by a receptor-mediated activation of NF-κB. The activation of NF-κB occurs in chronic muscle diseases and has been implicated in reduced maturation and regeneration of skeletal muscle.[94] Furthermore, NF-κB regulates the expression of the inducible isoform of the nitric oxide synthase (iNOS), which is overexpressed in skeletal muscle in HF patients[95] and may lead to muscle atrophy[96] and contractile dysfunction.[97]

Oxidative Stress (see also Chapter 8)

Increased oxidant activity can lead to detrimental effects on skeletal muscle structure and function and evolves under conditions where the generation of reactive oxygen/nitrogen species (ROS/RNS) exceeds the capacity of antioxidant systems. Several lines of evidence suggest that HF is accompanied by increased oxidative stress in skeletal muscle, with potential significance for skeletal muscle structure and function.

Studies have shown increased oxidative modification of proteins, lipids, and DNA in animal models[98,99] and humans.[95,100] Whether this is due to increased generation of ROS/RNS or diminished antioxidant activity, however, is uncertain. Studies have shown increased generation of ROS[101] and expression of nitric oxide synthase (NOS)[95,99] and reduced expression of antioxidant systems.[99] The proximal factor contributing to increased oxidative stress in skeletal muscle in HF, however, is unclear. Numerous investigators have suggested that this relates to increased immune activation,[97] and recent studies in animal models have implicated a potential role for increased angiotensin II,[102] but substantiation of any of these mechanisms in humans is lacking.

Elevated skeletal muscle oxidative stress may contribute to both muscle atrophy and dysfunction. Studies have shown that enhanced oxidative stress contributes to muscle atrophy.[103] In fact, recent studies have suggested that increased antioxidant expression in animal models of HF may prevent muscle atrophy.[104] Oxidative modification of proteins important for muscle contraction (e.g., ECC proteins, myofilament proteins[97]) or oxidative metabolism (mitochondrial proteins, creatine kinase) could impair skeletal muscle strength or endurance, leading to exercise intolerance. Indeed, studies in human HF have shown that increased oxidative modification of myofilament proteins is related to reduced exercise capacity.[100] Interestingly, studies in animal models have shown that β-blockers can reduce oxidative protein modifications in HF.[105] Moreover, if angiotensin II contributes to increased skeletal muscle oxidative stress in HF,[102] ACEi and angiotensin receptor blockers may further diminish oxidant activity. This may explain at least part of the effects of these two drugs to alleviate HF symptomology. Additionally, recent studies have shown that aerobic exercise training can increase antioxidant systems and reduce oxidative protein modification,[106] which may in part mediate the beneficial effects of exercise training on exercise tolerance.

Muscle Disuse

Weight-bearing activity is significantly curtailed in HF patients,[49] which may relate to psychological barriers to performing certain activities.[107] Thus one could argue, as we have done throughout this chapter, that a large proportion of the skeletal muscle myopathy of HF actually represents physical inactivity/deconditioning that accompanies the syndrome,[108] rather than a unique effect of the disease. This may seem like an unnecessary distinction, since it is axiomatic that individuals with HF are less active than their healthy counterparts, with physical inactivity frequently being both a cause and a consequence of their underlying heart disease. However, defining which specific skeletal muscle adaptations are directly attributable to the disease process or its sequelae is important for understanding which may be amenable to exercise countermeasures. More specifically, defining which aspect of the skeletal muscle pathology of HF is due to muscle disuse could also help to define the modality that would be most effective at remediating that defect, because much is known about how different training paradigms impact various facets of skeletal muscle biology (e.g., resistance exercise training might be more effective at correcting contractile deficits, whereas aerobic exercise training would be more effective at correcting mitochondrial adaptations/oxidative deficiencies).

It is necessary to further distinguish between acute and chronic muscle disuse, because the magnitude and character of disuse is likely to differ. Acute disuse likely occurs during hospitalization because of acute disease exacerbation or health decline as a result of other comorbidities. Hospitalization for acute HF is often accompanied by protracted bed rest, which is known to lead to dramatic alterations in skeletal muscle. However, with treatment and reambulation, many of these acute adaptations may be remediated. Indeed, even some of the most profound adaptations in skeletal muscle, such as mitochondrial rarefaction, can be largely corrected with successful treatment and reambulation.[7] This is again a necessary distinction because most of the seminal work in this field did not clarify the clinical state of the patients being studied or their proximity to hospitalization. Thus it is unclear to what extent many of the hallmark muscle adaptations to HF represent transient adaptations to factors associated with hospitalization, such as profound muscle disuse, and which are truly attributable to the underlying disease. In contrast, chronic disuse in HF patients represents a drop in normal daily activities on the order of approximately 50%.[49] To what extent such a drop in habitual activity might contribute to the skeletal muscle adaptations observed in HF is unclear, but even short periods of this magnitude of inactivity can affect skeletal muscle in older adults.[109] Thus many of the skeletal muscle adaptations observed in HF patients are likely the result of either acute or chronic reductions in muscle use, rather than any unique effect of the disease process.[108]

CONTRIBUTION OF SKELETAL MUSCLE ADAPTATIONS TO SYMPTOMOLOGY

How do skeletal muscle adaptations contribute to the major symptoms of exercise limitation in HF patients: dyspnea and muscle fatigue? As the earlier discussion of potential precipitating factors should reveal, the skeletal muscle adaptations occurring in any one individual patient are likely to be complex and unique. Thus there is no simple answer to this question, as it will likely be highly variable among patients, as well as within patients throughout the course of the disease. Some generalizations, however, are possible.

In acute HF, much of the symptomology likely occurs secondary to circulatory congestion and cardiac insufficiency. However, there are accompanying alterations in skeletal muscle size and function, characterized by muscle atrophy, contractile dysfunction, and reduced oxidative capacity, which may further lessen exercise tolerance, as all of these adaptations would reduce overall physiologic functional capacity. In other words, any given physical activity would require a greater relative percentage of an individual's physiologic capacity and, accordingly, be more likely to provoke dyspnea and fatigue. Aside from this simple lowering of physiologic capacity, muscle adaptations may contribute to symptomology in ways that have been classically assigned to cardiac contractile dysfunction/circulatory congestion. For instance, increased metabolite generation owing to impaired oxidative capacity, together with enhanced sensory nerve activation (either by mechano- or metabo-receptor hypersensitivity) in skeletal muscle, may increase vasoconstriction and ventilatory drive,[110] which would contribute to muscle fatigue and dyspnea. The precipitating factor for increased sensory nerve stimulation (e.g., metabolic dysfunction in skeletal muscle leading to enhanced metabolite generation and/or effects of acute HF on sensory neurons) is not known, but it is clear that these adaptations in skeletal muscle likely contribute to the symptomology of acute HF.

In chronic HF, the contribution of these skeletal muscle adaptations to symptomology is primarily through their capacity to limit physiologic capacity. For instance, reduced oxidative capacity, owing to reduced mitochondrial content and function, as well as fiber type switching toward a more glycolytic phenotype, contribute to dyspnea and fatigue directly. In the case of the former, metabolic derangements leading to excessive metabolite production (e.g., increased acidity) increase ventilatory drive by activating sensory afferents.[111] Regarding the latter, excessive metabolite generation, such as increased intracellular phosphate levels,[6] decreases myofilament force production,[112] which is the primary physiologic marker of muscular fatigue. These adaptations and others, such as muscle atrophy and weakness, would also contribute to the subjective sensation of fatigue by reducing the overall physiologic capacity and would cause patients to perceive any activity as more demanding. Thus, as can be gleaned from this discussion, there are a large number of possible combinations of skeletal muscle adaptations that can contribute to dyspnea and fatigue in the context of either acute or chronic HF.

SUMMARY AND FUTURE DIRECTIONS

HF is characterized by marked adaptations in skeletal muscle quantity and functionality that contribute to the primary symptoms of fatigue and dyspnea. Many of these adaptations likely result from skeletal muscle disuse that accompanies the syndrome of HF, but heightened inflammation, oxidative stress, and hypoperfusion probably also contribute. Accordingly, exercise training appears to be an effective countermeasure for many of these skeletal muscle adaptations and should be considered as a standard treatment in suitable patients. Various standard HF medications may also counteract some of the skeletal muscle adaptations, raising the intriguing possibility that at least some portion of their clinical benefit derives from their ability to influence skeletal muscle structure and function, either directly or indirectly. Taken together, this evidence solidifies a role for skeletal muscle adaptations in the symptomology of HF.

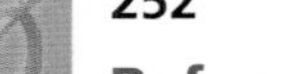

References

1. Downing J, Balady GJ: The role of exercise training in heart failure. *J Am Coll Cardiol* 58(6):561–569, 2011.
2. Belardinelli R, Georgiou D, Cianci G, et al: Exercise training improves left ventricular diastolic filling in patients with dilated cardiomyopathy: clinical and prognostic implications. *Circulation* 91(11):2775–2784, 1995.
3. Harrington D, Anker S, Chua TP, et al: Skeletal muscle function and its relation to exercise tolerance in chronic heart failure. *J Am Coll Cardiol* 30:1758–1764, 1997.
4. Miller MS, VanBuren P, LeWinter MM, et al: Chronic heart failure decreases cross-bridge kinetics in single skeletal muscle fibers from humans. *J Physiol* 588:4039–4053, 2010.
5. Mancini DM, Coyle E, Coggan A, et al: Contribution of intrinsic skeletal muscle changes to ^{31}P NMR skeletal muscle metabolic abnormalities in patients with chronic heart failure. *Circulation* 80:1338–1346, 1989.
6. Massie BM, Conway M, Rajagopalan B, et al: Skeletal muscle metabolism during exercise under ischemic conditions in congestive heart failure: evidence for abnormalities unrelated to blood flow. *Circulation* 78:320–326, 1988.
7. Drexler H, Riede U, Munzel T, et al: Alterations in skeletal muscle in chronic heart failure. *Circulation* 85:1751–1759, 1992.
8. Vescovo G, Serafini F, Facchin L, et al: Specific changes in skeletal muscle myosin heavy chain composition in cardiac failure: differences compared with disuse atrophy as assessed on microbiopsies by high resolution electrophoresis. *Heart* 76:337–343, 1996.
9. Mancini DM, Walter G, Reichek N, et al: Contribution of skeletal muscle atrophy to exercise intolerance and altered skeletal muscle metabolism in heart failure. *Circulation* 85:1364–1373, 1992.
10. Mancini DM, Ferraro N, Tuchler M, et al: Detection of abnormal calf muscle metabolism in patients with heart failure using phosphorus-31 nuclear magnetic resonance. *Am J Cardiol* 62:1234–1240, 1988.
11. Lang CC, Chomsky DB, Rayos G, et al: Skeletal muscle mass and exercise performance in stable ambulatory patients with heart failure. *J Appl Physiol* 82(1):257–261, 1997.
12. Callahan DM, Toth MJ: Skeletal muscle protein metabolism in human heart failure. *Curr Opin Clin Nutr Metab Care* 16:66–71, 2013.
13. Morrison WL, Gibson JNA, Rennie MJ: Skeletal muscle and whole body protein turnover in cardiac cachexia: influence of branched-chain amino acid administration. *Eur J Clin Invest* 18:648–654, 1988.
14. Le Jemtel TH, Padeletti M, Jelic S: Diagnostic and therapeutic challenges in patients with coexistent chronic obstructive pulmonary disease and chronic heart failure. *J Am Coll Cardiol* 49(2):171–180, 2007.
15. Hambrecht R, Schulze PC, Gielen S, et al: Reduction of insulin-like growth factor-I expression in the skeletal muscle of noncachectic patients with chronic heart failure. *J Am Coll Cardiol* 39:1175–1181, 2002.
16. Ng EH, Rock CS, Lazarus DD, et al: Insulin-like growth factor I preserves host lean tissue mass in cancer cachexia. *Am J Physiol* 262(3):R426–R431, 1992.
17. Schulze PC, Gielen S, Adams V, et al: Muscular levels of proinflammatory cytokines correlate with a reduced expression of insulin-like growth factor-I in chronic heart failure. *Basic Res Cardiol* 98:267–274, 2003.
18. Gielen S, Adams V, Mobius-Winkler S, et al: Anti-inflammatory effects of exercise training in the skeletal muscle of patients with chronic heart failure. *J Am Coll Cardiol* 42:861–868, 2003.
19. Loughna PT, Mason P, Bates PC: Regulation of insulin-like growth factor 1 gene expression in skeletal muscle. *Symp Soc Exp Biol* 46:319–330, 2000.
20. Anker SD, Volterrani M, Pflaum CD, et al: Acquired growth hormone resistance in patients with chronic heart failure: implications for therapy with growth hormone. *J Am Coll Cardiol* 38:443–452, 2001.
21. Adams GR: Autocrine/paracrine IGF-I and skeletal muscle adaptation. *J Appl Physiol* 93:1159–1167, 2002.
22. Broussard SR, McCusker RH, Novakofski JE, et al: Cytokine-hormone interactions: tumor necrosis factor-alpha impairs biologic activity and downstream activation of signals of the insulin-like growth factor I receptor in myoblasts. *Endocrinology* 144:2988–2996, 2003.
23. Thissen J-P, Verniers J: Inhibition by interleukin-1β and tumor necrosis factor-α of the insulin-like growth factor I messenger ribonucleic acid response to growth hormone in rat hepatocyte primary culture. *Endocrinology* 138(3):1078–1084, 1997.
24. Mabley JG, Belin V, John N, et al: Insulin-like growth factor I reverses interleukin-1β inhibition of insulin secretion, induction of nitric oxide synthase and cytokine-mediated apoptosis in rat islets of Langerhans. *FEBS Lett* 417(2):235–238, 1997.
25. Adams V, Jiang H, Yu J, et al: Apoptosis in skeletal myocytes of patients with chronic heart failure is associated with exercise intolerance. *J Am Coll Cardiol* 33:959–965, 1999.
26. Dalla Libera L, Ravara B, Volterrani M, et al: Beneficial effects of GH/IGF-1 on skeletal muscle atrophy and function in experimental heart failure. *Am J Physiol* 286:C138–C144, 2004.
27. Aukrust P, Ueland T, Gullestad L, et al: Testosterone: a novel therapeutic approach in chronic heart failure? *J Am Coll Cardiol* 54(10):928–929, 2009.
28. Caminiti G, Volterrani M, Iellamo F, et al: Effect of long-acting testosterone treatment on functional exercise capacity, skeletal muscle performance, insulin resistance, and baroreflex sensitivity in elderly patients with chronic heart failure: a double-blind, placebo-controlled, randomized study. *J Am Coll Cardiol* 54(10):919–927, 2009.
29. Schulze PC, Biolo A, Gopal D, et al: Dynamics in insulin resistance and plasma levels of adipokines in patients with acute decompensated and chronic stable heart failure. *J Card Fail* 17(12):1004–1011, 2011.
30. Chokshi A, Drosatos K, Cheema FH, et al: Ventricular assist device implantation corrects myocardial lipotoxicity, reverses insulin resistance, and normalizes cardiac metabolism in patients with advanced heart failure. *Circulation* 125(23):2844–2853, 2012.
31. Toth MJ, LeWinter MM, Ades PA, et al: Impaired muscle protein anabolic response to insulin and amino acids in heart failure patients: relationships to markers of immune activation. *Clin Sci* 143:467–472, 2010.
32. Saccà L: Heart failure as a multiple hormonal deficiency syndrome. *Circ Heart Fail* 2(2):151–156, 2009.
33. Heineke J, Auger-Messier M, Xu J, et al: Genetic deletion of myostatin from the heart prevents skeletal muscle atrophy in heart failure. *Circulation* 121(3):419–425, 2010.
34. George I, Bish LT, Kamalakkannan G, et al: Myostatin activation in patients with advanced heart failure and after mechanical unloading. *Eur J Heart Fail* 12(5):444–453, 2010.
35. Yndestad A, Ueland T, Øie E, et al: Elevated levels of activin A in heart failure: potential role in myocardial remodeling. *Circulation* 109(11):1379–1385, 2004.
36. Mitch WE, Goldberg AL: Mechanism of muscle wasting: the role of the ubiquitin proteasome pathway. *N Engl J Med* 335:1897–1905, 1996.
37. Schulze PC, Fang J, Kassik KA, et al: Transgenic overexpression of locally acting insulin-like growth factor-1 inhibits ubiquitin-mediated muscle atrophy in chronic left-ventricular dysfunction. *Circ Res* 97(5):418–426, 2005.
38. Gomes MD, Lecker SH, Jago RT, et al: Atrogin-1, a muscle specific F-box protein highly expressed during muscle atrophy. *Proc Natl Acad Sci U S A* 98:14440–14445, 2001.
39. Bodine SC, Latres E, Baumhueter S, et al: Identification of ubiquitin ligases required for skeletal muscle atrophy. *Science* 294:1704–1708, 2001.
40. Wray CJ, Mammen JMV, Hershko DD, et al: Sepsis upregulates the gene expression of multiple ubiquitin ligases in skeletal muscle. *Int J Biochem Cell Biol* 35(5):698–705, 2003.
41. Li YP, Lecker SH, Chen Y, et al: TNF-α increases ubiquitin-conjugating activity in skeletal muscle by up-regulating UbcH2/E220k. *FASEB J* 17(9):1048–1057, 2003.
42. Gielen S, Sandri M, Kozarez I, et al: Exercise training attenuates MuRF-1 expression in the skeletal muscle of patients with chronic heart failure independent of age. *Circulation* 125(22):2716–2727, 2012.
43. Miller MS, VanBuren P, LeWinter MM, et al: Mechanisms underlying skeletal muscle weakness in human heart failure: alterations in single fiber myosin protein content and function. *Circ Heart Fail* 2:700–706, 2009.
44. Piepoli MF, Kaczmarek A, Francis DP, et al: Reduced peripheral skeletal muscle mass and abnormal reflex physiology in chronic heart failure. *Circulation* 114(2):126–134, 2006.
45. Anker SD, Swan JW, Volterrani M, et al: The influence of muscle mass, strength, fatigability and blood flow on exercise capacity in cachectic and non-cachectic patients with chronic heart failure. *Eur Heart J* 18:259–269, 1997.
46. Schaufelberger M, Eriksson BO, Lonn L, et al: Skeletal muscle characteristics, muscle strength and thigh muscle area in patients before and after cardiac transplantation. *Eur J Heart Fail* 3:59–67, 2001.
47. Toth MJ, Shaw AO, Miller MS, et al: Reduced knee extensor function in heart failure is not explained by inactivity. *Int J Cardiol* 143:276–282, 2010.
48. Simonini A, Long CS, Dudley GA, et al: Heart failure in rats causes changes in skeletal muscle morphology and gene expression that are not explained by reduced activity. *Circulation* 79:128–136, 1996.
49. Toth MJ, Gottlieb SS, Goran MI, et al: Daily energy expenditure in free-living heart failure patients. *Am J Physiol* 272:E469–E475, 1997.
50. Mettauer B, Zoll J, Sanchez H, et al: Oxidative capacity of skeletal muscle in heart failure patients versus sedentary or active controls subjects. *J Am Coll Cardiol* 38:947–954, 2001.
51. Vescovo G, Libera LD, Serafini F, et al: Improved exercise tolerance after losartan and enalapril in heart failure: correlation with changes in skeletal muscle myosin heavy chain composition. *Circulation* 98:1742–1749, 1998.
52. Toth MJ, Matthews DE, Ades PA, et al: Skeletal muscle myofibrillar protein metabolism in heart failure: relationship to immune activation and functional capacity. *Am J Physiol* 288:E685–E692, 2005.
53. D'Antona G, Pellegrino MA, Adami R, et al: The effect of ageing and immobilization on structure and function of human skeletal muscle fibres. *J Physiol* 552:499–511, 2003.
54. Larsson L, Li X, Edstrom L, et al: Acute quadriplegia and loss of muscle myosin in patients treated with nondepolarizing neuromuscular blocking agents and corticosteroids: mechanisms at the cellular and molecular levels. *Crit Care Med* 28:34–45, 2000.
55. Ottenheijm CAC, Heunks LMA, Sieck GC, et al: Diaphragm dysfunction in chronic obstructive pulmonary disease. *Am J Respir Crit Care Med* 172:200–205, 2005.
56. De Sousa E, Veksler V, Bigard X, et al: Dual influence of disease and increased load on diaphragm muscle in heart failure. *J Mol Cell Cardiol* 33:699–710, 2001.
57. Szentesi P, Bekedam MA, van Beek-Harmsen BJ, et al: Depression of force production and ATPase activity in different types of humans skeletal muscle fibers from patients with chronic heart failure. *J Appl Physiol* 99:2189–2195, 2005.
58. Cicoira M, Bolger AP, Doehner W, et al: High tumour necrosis factor-alpha levels are associated with exercise intolerance and neurohumoral activation in chronic heart failure patients. *Cytokine* 15:80–86, 2001.
59. Hardin BJ, Campbell KS, Smith JD, et al: TNF-α acts via TNFR1 and muscle-derived oxidants to depress myofibrillar force in murine skeletal muscle. *J Appl Physiol* 104(3):694–699, 2008.
60. Piazzesi G, Reconditi M, Linari M, et al: Skeletal muscle performance determined by modulation of number of myosin motors rather than motor force or stroke size. *Cell* 131(4):784–795, 2007.
61. Coirault C, Guellich A, Barby T, et al: Oxidative stress of myosin contributes to skeletal muscle dysfunction in rats with chronic heart failure. *Am J Physiol* 292:H1009–H1017, 2007.
62. Perreault CL, Gonzalez-Serratos H, Litwin SE, et al: Alterations in contractility and intracellular Ca^{2+} transients in isolated bundles of skeletal muscle fibers from rats with chronic heart failure. *Circ Res* 73:405–412, 1993.
63. Peters DG, Mitchell HL, McCune SA, et al: Skeletal muscle sarcoplasmic reticulum Ca^{2+}-ATPase gene expression in congestive heart failure. *Circ Res* 81:703–710, 1997.
64. Simonini A, Chang K, Yue P, et al: Expression of skeletal muscle sarcoplasmic reticulum calcium-ATPase is reduced in rats with postinfarction heart failure. *Heart* 81:303–307, 1999.
65. Lunde PK, Dahlstedt AJ, Bruton JD, et al: Contraction and intracellular Ca^{2+} handling in isolated skeletal muscle of rats with congestive heart failure. *Circ Res* 88:1299–1305, 2001.
66. Lunde PK, Verburg E, Eriksen M, et al: Contractile properties of *in situ* perfused skeletal muscles from rats with congestive heart failure. *J Physiol* 540:571–580, 2002.
67. Lunde PK, Sejersted OM, Thorud H-MS, et al: Effects of congestive heart failure on Ca2+ handling in skeletal muscle during fatigue. *Circ Res* 98(12):1514–1519, 2006.
68. Ward CW, Reiken S, Marks AR, et al: Defects in ryanodine receptor calcium release in skeletal muscle from post-myocardial infarct rats. *FASEB J* 17:1517–1519, 2003.
69. Reiken S, Lacampagne A, Zhou H, et al: PKA phosphorylation activates the calcium release channel (ryanodine receptor) in skeletal muscle: defective regulation in heart failure. *J Cell Biol* 160:919–928, 2003.
70. Wehrens XH, Lehnart SE, Reiken S, et al: Ryanodine receptor/calcium release channel PKA phosphorylation: a critical mediator of heart failure progression. *Proc Natl Acad Sci U S A* 103(3):511–518, 2006.
71. Bellinger AM, Reiken S, Dura M, et al: Remodeling of ryanodine receptor complex causes "leaky" channels: a molecular mechanism for decreased exercise capacity. *Proc Natl Acad Sci U S A* 105(6):2198–2202, 2008.
72. Munkvik M, Rehn TA, Slettalokken G, et al: Training effects on skeletal muscle calcium handling in human chronic heart failure. *Med Sci Sports Exerc* 42:847–855, 2010.
73. Bekedam MA, van Beek-Harmsen BJ, van Mechelen W, et al: Sarcoplasmic reticulum ATPase activity in type I and II skeletal muscle fibres of chronic heart failure patients. *Int J Cardiol* 133(2):185–190, 2009.
74. Middlekauff HR, Vigna C, Verity MA, et al: Abnormalities of calcium handling proteins in skeletal muscle mirror those of the heart in humans with heart failure: a shared mechanism? *J Card Fail* 18(9):724–733, 2012.
75. Coats AJS: The "muscle hypothesis" of chronic heart failure. *J Mol Cell Cardiol* 28:2255–2262, 1996.
76. Ades PA, Waldmann ML, Meyer WL, et al: Skeletal muscle and cardiovascular adaptations to exercise conditioning in older coronary patients. *Circulation* 94:323–330, 1996.
77. Chati Z, Zannad F, Jeandel C, et al: Physical deconditioning may be a mechanism for the skeletal muscle energy phosphate metabolism abnormalities in chronic heart failure. *Am Heart J* 131:560–566, 1996.
78. Williams AD, Selig S, Hare DL, et al: Reduced exercise tolerance in CHF may be related to factors other than impaired skeletal muscle oxidative capacity. *J Card Fail* 10(2):141–148, 2004.
79. Toth MJ, Miller MS, Ward KA, et al: Skeletal muscle mitochondrial density, gene expression, and enzyme activities in human heart failure: minimal effects of the disease and resistance training. *J Appl Physiol* 112(11):1864–1874, 2012.

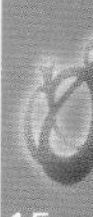

80. Esposito F, Mathieu-Costello O, Shabetai R, et al: Limited maximal exercise capacity in patients with chronic heart failure: partitioning the contributors. *J Am Coll Cardiol* 55(18):1945–1954, 2010.
81. Zoll J, Monassier L, Garnier A, et al: ACE inhibition prevents myocardial infarction-induced skeletal muscle mitochondrial dysfunction. *J Appl Physiol* 101:385–391, 2006.
82. Habouzit E, Richard H, Sanchez H, et al: Decreased muscle ACE activity enhances functional response to endurance training in rats, without change in muscle oxidative capacity or contractile phenotype. *J Appl Physiol* 107(1):346–353, 2009.
83. Stratton JR, Kemp GJ, Daly RC, et al: Effects of cardiac transplantation on bioenergetic abnormalities of skeletal muscle in congestive heart failure. *Circulation* 89:1624–1631, 1994.
84. Minotti JR, Johnson EC, Hudson TL, et al: Skeletal muscle response to exercise training in congestive heart failure. *J Clin Invest* 86:751–758, 1990.
85. Hambrecht R, Niebauer J, Fiehn E, et al: Physical training in patients with stable chronic heart failure: effects on cardiorespiratory fitness and ultrastructural abnormalities of leg muscles. *J Am Coll Cardiol* 25(6):1239–1249, 1995.
86. Belardinelli R, Georgiou D, Scocco V, et al: Low intensity exercise training in patients with chronic heart failure. *J Am Coll Cardiol* 26(4):975–982, 1995.
87. Vescovo G, Serafini F, Libera LD, et al: Skeletal muscle myosin heavy chains in heart failure: correlation between magnitude of the isozyme shift, exercise capacity, and gas exchange measurements. *Am Heart J* 135:130–137, 1998.
88. Hambrecht R, Fiehn E, Yu J, et al: Effects of endurance training on mitochondrial ultrastructure and fiber type distribution in skeletal muscle of patients with stable chronic heart failure. *J Am Coll Cardiol* 29:1067–1073, 1997.
89. Duscha BD, Kraus WE, Keteyian SJ, et al: Capillary density of skeletal muscle: A contributing mechanism for exercise intolerance in class II–III chronic heart failure independent of other peripheral alterations. *J Am Coll Cardiol* 33(7):1956–1963, 1999.
90. Adams V, Yu J, Möbius-Winkler S, et al: Increased inducible nitric oxide synthase in skeletal muscle biopsies from patients with chronic heart failure. *Biochem Mol Med* 61(2):152–160, 1997.
91. Eliason JL, Wakefield TW: Metabolic consequences of acute limb ischemia and their clinical implications. *Sem Vasc Surg* 22(1):29–33, 2009.
92. Barnes PJ, Karin M: Nuclear factor-κB—a pivotal transcription factor in chronic inflammatory diseases. *N Engl J Med* 336(15):1066–1071, 1997.
93. Russell ST, Wyke SM, Tisdale MJ: Mechanism of induction of muscle protein degradation by angiotensin II. *Cell Signal* 18(7):1087–1096, 2006.
94. Guttridge DC, Mayo MW, Madrid LV, et al: NF-kB-induced loss of *myoD* messenger RNA: possible role in muscle decay and cachexia. *Science* 289:2363–2366, 2000.
95. Hambrecht R, Adams V, Gielen S, et al: Exercise intolerance in patients with chronic heart failure and increased expression of inducible nitric oxide synthase in the skeletal muscle. *J Am Coll Cardiol* 33(1):174–179, 1999.
96. Di Marco S, Mazroui R, Dallaire P, et al: NF-κB-mediated myoD decay during muscle wasting requires nitric oxide synthase mRNA stabilization, HuR protein, and nitric oxide release. *Mol Cell Biol* 25(15):6533–6545, 2005.
97. Reid MB, Moylan JS: Beyond atrophy: redox mechanisms of muscle dysfunction in chronic inflammatory disease. *J Physiol* 589(9):2171–2179, 2011.
98. Dalla Libera L, Ravara B, Gobbo V, et al: Skeletal muscle myofibrillar protein oxidation in heart failure and the protective effect of carvedilol. *J Mol Cell Cardiol* 38(5):803–807, 2005.
99. Rush JWE, Green HJ, MacLean DA, et al: Oxidative stress and nitric oxide synthase in skeletal muscles of rats with post-infarction, compensated chronic heart failure. *Acta Physiol Scand* 185(3):211–218, 2005.
100. Vescovo G, Ravara B, Dalla Libera L: Skeletal muscle myofibrillar protein oxidation and exercise capacity in heart failure. *Bas Res Cardiol* 103:285–290, 2008.
101. Tsutsui H, Ide T, Hayashidani S, et al: Enhanced generation of reactive oxygen species in the limb skeletal muscles from a murine infarct model of heart failure. *Circulation* 104:134–136, 2001.
102. Inoue N, Kinugawa S, Suga T, et al: Angiotensin II-induced reduction in exercise capacity is associated with increased oxidative stress in skeletal muscle. *Am J Physiol* 302(5):H1202–H1210, 2012.
103. Powers SK, Kavazis AN, McClung JM: Oxidative stress and disuse muscle atrophy. *J Appl Physiol* 102(6):2389–2397, 2007.
104. Geng T, Li P, Yin X, et al: PGC-1α promotes nitric oxide antioxidant defenses and inhibits FOXO signaling against cardiac cachexia in mice. *Am J Pathol* 178(4):1738–1748, 2011.
105. Libera LD, Ravara B, Gobbo V, et al: Skeletal muscle proteins oxidation in chronic right heart failure in rats: can different beta-blockers prevent it to the same degree? *Int J Cardiol* 143(2):192–199, 2010.
106. Linke A, Adams V, Schulze PC, et al: Antioxidative effects of exercise training in patients with chronic heart failure: increase in radical scavenger enzyme activity in skeletal muscle. *Circulation* 111(14):1763–1770, 2005.
107. Oka RK, Gortner SR, Stotts NA, et al: Predictors of physical activity in patients with chronic heart failure secondary to either ischemic or idiopathic dilated cardiomyopathy. *Am J Cardiol* 77:159–163, 1996.
108. Rehn TA, Munkvik M, Lunde PK, et al: Intrinsic skeletal muscle alterations in chronic heart failure patients: a disease-specific myopathy or a result of deconditioning? *Heart Fail Rev* 17:421–436, 2011.
109. Breen L, Stokes KA, Churchward-Venne TA, et al: Two weeks of reduced activity decreases leg lean mass and induces "anabolic resistance" of myofibrillar protein synthesis in healthy elderly. *J Clin Endocrinol Metab* 98:2604–2612, 2013.
110. Middlekauff HR, Sinoway LI: Increased mechanoreceptor/metaboreceptor stimulation explains the exaggerated exercise pressor reflex seen in heart failure. *J Appl Physiol* 102(1):492–494, 2007.
111. Scott AC, Wensel R, Davos CH, et al: Skeletal muscle reflex in heart failure patients: role of hydrogen. *Circulation* 107(2):300–306, 2003.
112. Pathare N, Walter GA, Stevens JE, et al: Changes in inorganic phosphate and force production in human skeletal muscle after cast immobilization. *J Appl Physiol* 98(1):307–314, 2005.

16 Alterations in Cardiac Metabolism

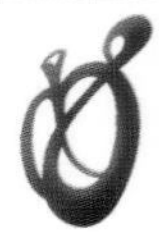

Linda R. Peterson, Joel Schilling, and Heinrich Taegtmeyer

This chapter is based on two broad concepts. *The first concept* considers the heart as an efficient converter of energy. It addresses the hypothesis that defective energy metabolism is a cause for contractile dysfunction of the heart. *The second concept* considers heart failure as a systemic disease in which the heart is affected by the body's metabolic milieu. This chapter covers the entire spectrum, from altered energy metabolism to failure. It also addresses the hypothesis that metabolism not only provides energy for contraction, but also generates signals that regulate cardiac-specific gene programs, including those that the heart manifests in response to different environmental stimuli (**Figure 16-1**).

By definition, energy is the capacity for doing work. The transfer of energy includes adenosine triphosphate (ATP) and phosphocreatine, but it is not limited to energy-rich phosphate compounds. A discussion of myocardial energy metabolism in heart failure should therefore include a brief review of normal energy transfer in the heart, a review of methods used to detect abnormal energy transfer in the heart, and of evolving paradigms on metabolic changes that occur in the failing heart. An inevitable question is whether metabolic derangements are causes or consequences of heart failure. The answer is clear in cases of myocardial ischemia and in the relatively rare cases of genetically determined cardiomyopathies. The answer is less clear in the majority of patients suffering from dilated cardiomyopathies.

Over the years, it has been speculated that the failing heart is "energy starved.[1] "Although ^{31}P-NMR (phosphorus-31 nuclear magnetic resonance) spectroscopy can detect metabolic abnormalities even in asymptomatic patients with cardiomyopathy, the concept of energy starvation has rested primarily on a reductionist approach focusing on some of the final reactions (e.g., the creatine kinase reaction). In this chapter, we use a more inclusive perspective that encompasses consideration of all energy-metabolizing pathways. Such an approach seems justified in light of (1) emerging pharmacologic and surgical strategies directed at shifting substrate flux through specific metabolic pathways, (2) the rapidly emerging concepts of peroxisome proliferator activated receptor signaling in the control of cardiac energy metabolism, and (3) metabolically inducible forms of heart failure.

The complex and highly regulated systems of energy transfer have been the subject of biochemistry studies for most of the past century and provide many likely sites for defective metabolism. In the heart, defective energy metabolism has been characterized best in the case of myocardial ischemia, where the lack of oxygen results in severe impairment of the efficient system of oxidative phosphorylation. Drugs that target specific "bottleneck" reactions in intermediary metabolism of the heart hold the promise of improving cardiac function in ischemic heart disease and in dilated cardiomyopathies. Although conceptually

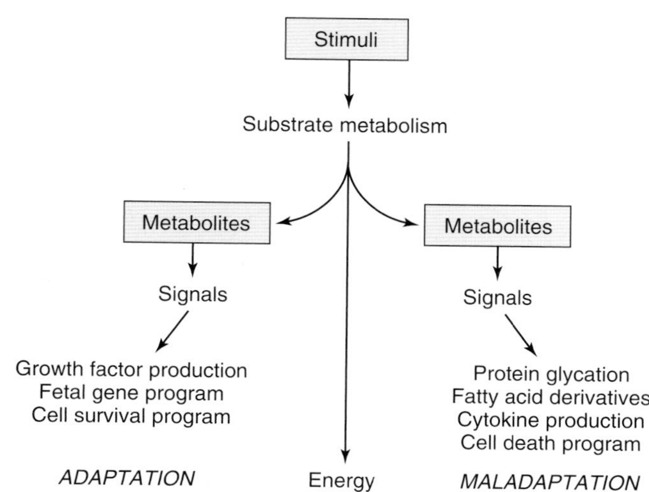

FIGURE 16-1 The pleiotropic role of metabolites in energy metabolism, substrate storage, cell structure, cell signaling, gene expression, and apoptosis (programmed cell death). See text for discussion. *Adapted from Young ME, McNulty P, Taegtmeyer H: Adaptation and maladaptation of the heart in diabetes: Part II. Potential mechanisms. Circulation 105:1861–1870, 2002.*

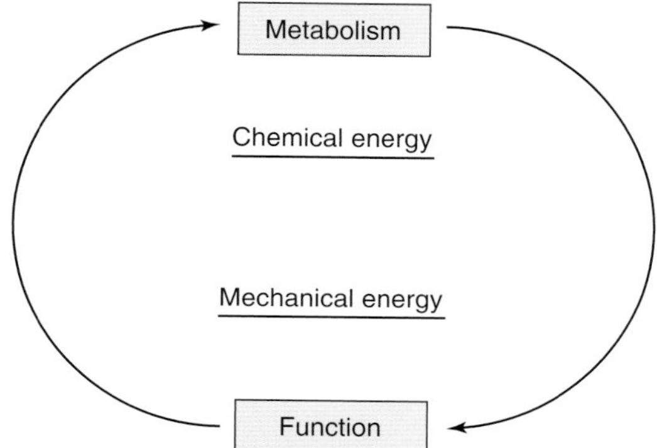

FIGURE 16-2 The metabolic machinery in the heart converts chemical energy into mechanical energy. The tight coupling of energy substrate metabolism and contractile function of the heart underlies a system of high adaptability and efficiency. *Adapted from Taegtmeyer H: Cardiac metabolism as a target for the treatment of heart failure. Circulation 110:894–896, 2004.*

attractive, this concept may be an oversimplification. In the following section, we will see why.

PERSPECTIVES

Metabolism and Function Are Tightly Coupled

Catabolic energy substrate metabolism transfers energy from chemical bonds to ATP, the immediate precursor for conversion to mechanical energy. Heart muscle derives its energy for contraction from the oxidation of a variety of fuels, including glucose, lactate, and especially long-chain fatty acids.[2] When fatty acids are abundant, the myocardium increases fatty acid metabolism, which suppresses glucose metabolism. Conversely, myocardial fatty acid oxidation is suppressed when higher fuel efficiency (from glucose metabolism) is required.[3] Metabolism is an integral part of the heart's physiologic function (**Figure 16-2**). A decrease in energy demand and contractile function (e.g., during sleep or with β-adrenergic receptor blockade) results in a decrease in energy turnover. Conversely, a decrease in energy supply (e.g., during ischemia) results in a decrease in contractile function. Because the heart can store only a small amount of energy (and because energy is the capacity for doing work), it follows that the supply of, and demand for, energy-providing substrates in the heart are finely regulated and need to be in balance. This tight coupling of contractile function and myocardial oxygen consumption in the mammalian heart has been known for over a century. The evidence of this relationship between metabolism and function is seen routinely in the clinical practice of cardiology (e.g., the hearts of patients with a decreased supply of oxygen [ischemia] exhibit decreased contractile function). In simple terms: The prerequisite for normal contractile function is the normal flux of energy, a concept already known to the Ancient Greeks: *παντα ρει*, meaning "all is in flux" (Heraclitus, 540-475 BC).

Heart muscle derives its energy from the oxidative metabolism of fuels. Because the heart is capable of oxidizing a variety of biologic fuels, we have termed it a *metabolic omnivore*.[4] The essence of energy substrate metabolism in the heart is to maintain a dynamic state of equilibrium. Heart muscle burns chemical energy (fuel) and converts it into physical energy (pump function). In doing so, the heart distributes energy in the form of substrates and oxygen to the rest of the body. Hence the concept that heart failure is a disease of impaired energy transfer, beginning and ending with the heart. Hence, when the heart's ability to convert chemical into mechanical energy is impaired for any reason, the consequences of defective energy transfer in the heart affect every organ of the body. The general concept that the failing heart is in an energy-deprived state helps us to understand why in a number of clinical trials inotropic agents failed to produce a beneficial long-term effect. Although these drugs improve symptoms of heart failure, they do so at the expense of cardiac energy expenditure, which can only be expected to worsen cardiac performance.

The Plasticity of Cardiac Metabolism

As mentioned, the heart is able to use multiple different fuels for generation of ATP. Fatty acids (either from free fatty acids or hydrolyzed triglycerides) are the main substrate used and glucose is typically a secondary substrate, but the heart can also use ketone bodies, lactate, and amino acids. One of the main determinants of the heart's substrate choice is substrate availability. Under resting conditions, in the fed and immediate postprandial state, the fuel for respiration is influenced by the composition of the diet, which affects both blood hormone and substrate levels. For example, increases in postprandial plasma glucose and insulin levels increase the heart's glucose uptake and use. During fasting, the main fuel of the heart is fatty acids.[2] During exercise, with increased lactate production, the heart increases lactate and glucose use.[2] Thus there is "plasticity" of the heart's substrate metabolism (i.e., it can readily and rapidly switch substrate preference based on substrate availability under physiologic conditions). Special physiologic conditions also influence substrate choice and a return to the fetal gene program and aging. In the fetal state, the heart predominantly uses glucose rather than fatty acids.[5] Interestingly, the aging heart is also associated most often with predominantly glucose use rather than fatty acid metabolism.[5] As

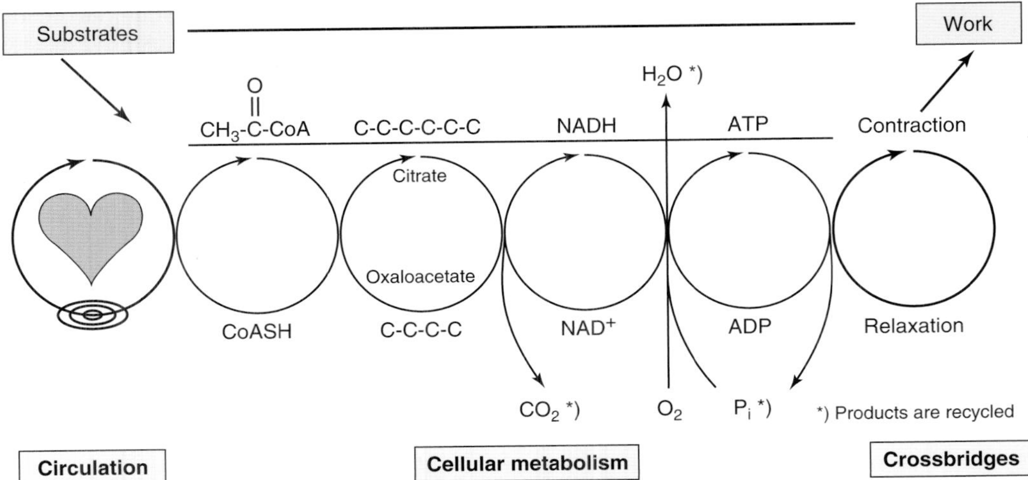

FIGURE 16-3 A series of moiety-conserved cycles underlies the efficient energy transfer from substrates to work. The moiety-conserved cycles can be likened to the wheels of a bicycle and provide a mechanism for immediate response to changes in energy demand. The higher the flux of energy, the greater the rate of turnover of the cycles. The concentration of cycle intermediates (moieties) remains stable over a wide range of energy fluxes. *Adapted from Taegtmeyer H: Tracing cardiac metabolism in vivo: one substrate at a time. J Nucl Med 51:80S–87S, 2010.*

will be discussed later, the failing heart (as a result of idiopathic cardiomyopathy) also predominantly uses glucose, like the fetal and aging heart.

Energy Transfer in the Heart

The heart transforms chemical energy from its substrates into ATP and then uses ATP for cellular function. The heart's demand for ATP is great: it consumes approximately 5 kg of ATP per day or 2 metric tons per year.[2] The main source of ATP is oxidative phosphorylation. The high rate of ATP turnover of the heart is reflected in the heart's high rates of oxygen consumption, the high cellular density of mitochondria, and the high capillary density in heart muscle (2500 capillaries/mm^3 in the heart versus 400 capillaries/mm^3 in red skeletal muscle). Mitochondria in heart muscle are not only more abundant but they also contain a far greater number of cristae (the location of respiratory chain enzymes) than mitochondria of other organs. Classic studies on the ultrastructure of the normal rat myocardium have shown that mitochondria account for 35.8% of myocyte cell volume with a mitochondria/myofibril ratio of 0.75. Mitochondria from failing hearts exhibit decreased respiratory chain function and impaired oxidative reserve.[5]

Although all of the mechanisms by which respiration is coupled to energy expenditure in vivo are not known, the efficacy of oxidative phosphorylation is well established. For example, one mole of glucose yields approximately 36 moles of ATP when fully oxidized, whereas the same amount of glucose yields only 2 moles of ATP when metabolized to lactate under anaerobic conditions. In the context of oxidative metabolism, it is also well established that efficient energy transfer occurs through a series of moiety-conserved cycles (**Figure 16-3**).[6] In the heart, these moiety-conserved cycles begin with the circulation itself, continue with the cyclic metabolic processes in the cell, and end with the cycling of the actin and myosin cross-bridges. Moiety-conserved cycles can be likened to the wheels of a bicycle because these cycles of energy are much more efficient than linear pathways (e.g., anaerobic glycolysis), just as the wheels of a bicycle are a more efficient mechanism for locomotion than the more linear mechanism of walking.[6]

In addition to the concept of interconnected cycles, it is a convenient practice to divide energy transfer into three stages (**Figure 16-4**). Stage 1 involves the uptake of substrates into the cell, their conversion into acetyl-CoA, and oxidation in the Krebs cycle; stage 2 is the final acceptance of electrons from reducing equivalents to molecular oxygen in the respiratory chain, which is coupled to the rephosphorylation of adenosine diphosphate (ADP) to ATP in the proton motive force; and stage 3 is the transfer of energy from the mitochondria to the rest of the cell for contractile and other work. This division of substrate metabolism into stages helps to define sites at which energy transfer may become impaired and to identify potential areas for pharmacologic intervention. In short, each stage can be the site of a metabolic block causing impaired energy transfer and contractile dysfunction. For example, impaired uptake of glucose is a feature of the heart in type 1 diabetes[2]; impaired oxidation of long-chain fatty acids is a feature of lipotoxic heart failure[7]; impaired Krebs cycle flux is a feature of limited cofactor availability for certain dehydrogenases[8]; and impaired respiratory chain flux is a feature of ischemia with a redirection of metabolic fluxes from aerobic to anaerobic metabolism.[9] These concepts will be expanded upon in the section on metabolic adaptation and maladaptation.

Last, it is useful to understand that there are regulatory sites of metabolism, or "pacemaker" enzymes. These are not only targets for the change of metabolic fluxes by physiologic effectors, but also emerging targets for pharmacologic agents. Examples include 5′-AMP-dependent protein kinase (AMPK), which acts like a fuel gauge (i.e., AMPK is the primary sensor of energy charge in the mammalian cell).[5] Most effectors of intracellular ATP depletion are probably mediated through this kinase pathway rather than through direct effects of adenine nucleotides. AMPK promotes glucose uptake and long-chain fatty acid oxidation

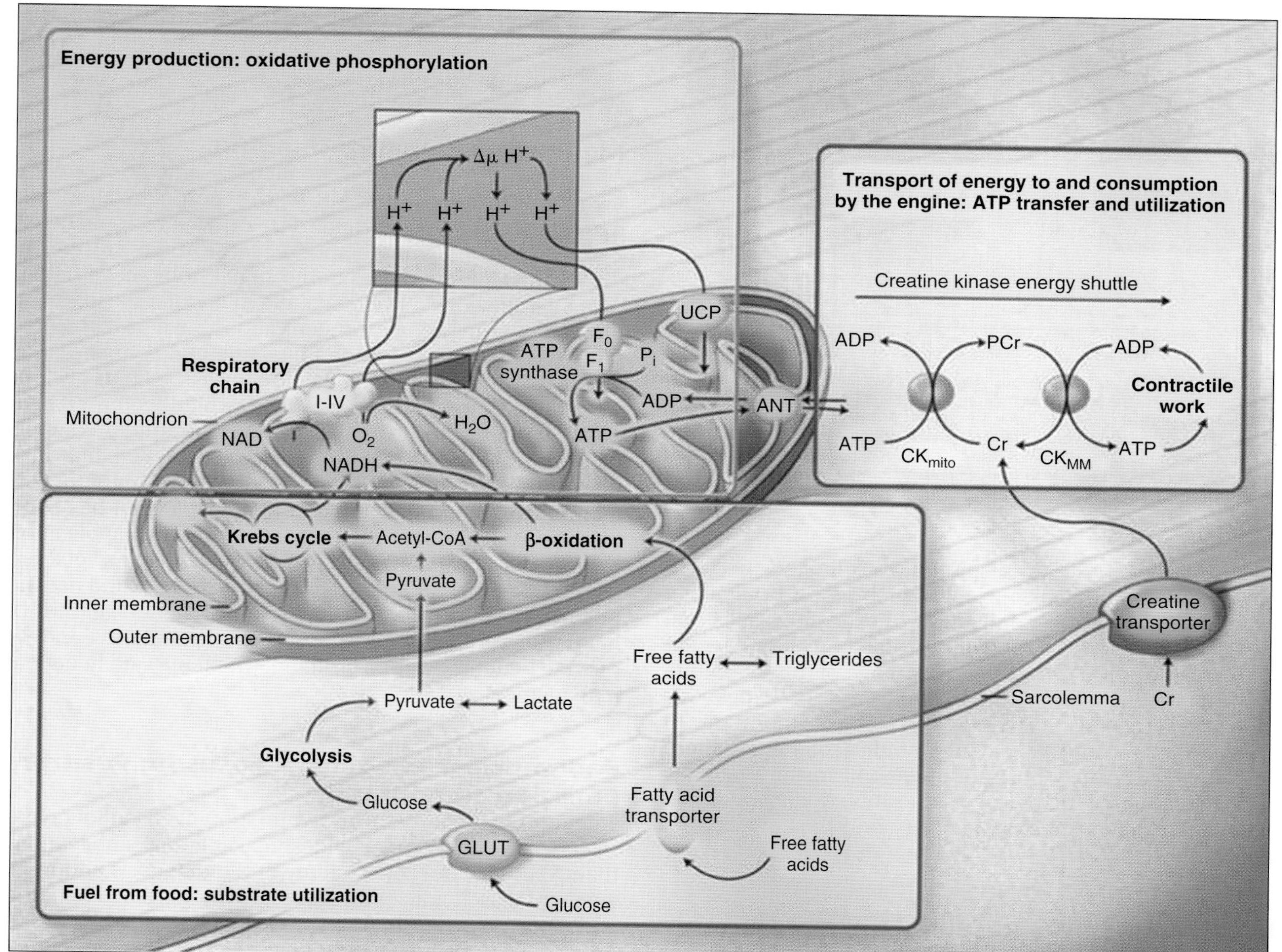

FIGURE 16-4 Energy transfer in the cardiac myocyte occurs in three stages. Each stage may be the site of metabolic derangements causing or accompanying contractile dysfunction of the heart. The first stage is substrate uptake and metabolism *(outlined in red)*. In this stage substrates are broken down by β-oxidation and glycolysis to form acetyl coenzyme A (CoA), from which the Krebs cycle produces NADH and CO_2. The second stage is energy production through oxidative phosphorylation *(outlined in blue)*. Respiratory chain complexes in the mitochondria transfer electrons from NAHD to oxygen. This creates a proton electrochemical gradient ($\Delta\mu$ H^+) across the inner mitochondrial membrane in addition to water and NAD. This gradient drives ATP synthase. Uncoupling proteins (UCPs) use this electrochemical gradient to create heat instead of ATP. The third stage is energy transfer via the creatine kinase shuttle *(outlined in green)*. ATP is transferred to and consumed by myofibrillar ATPase and other reactions. *ANT,* Adenine nucleotide translocase; *CK_{mito},* mitochondrial creatine kinase isoenzyme; *CK_{MM},* myofibrillar creatine kinase isoenzyme; *Cr,* free creatine; *GLUT,* glucose transporter; *PCr,* phosphocreatine; *P_i,* inorganic phosphate. *Reproduced from Neubauer S: The failing heart—an engine out of fuel. N Engl J Med 356:1140–1151, 2007.*

by different mechanisms,[5] and the activity of this kinase can be altered both acutely (e.g., increased workload) and chronically (e.g., ischemia and pressure-overload-induced hypertrophy).[5] In the latter case, partial inhibition of fatty acid oxidation shifts the fuel balance to the energetically more efficient oxidation of glucose.

METHODS FOR DETECTING DEFECTIVE SUBSTRATE METABOLISM IN THE FAILING HEART

Substrate Uptake by Arteriovenous Differences

At the beginning of the past century, the oxygen requirement of the mammalian heart was established by the German physiologist Hans Winterstein. The British physiologist C. Lovatt Evans studied the effect of various mechanical conditions on the gaseous metabolism and efficiency of the mammalian heart. However, it was not until the advent of cardiac catheterization and cannulation of the coronary sinus that the hypothesis of defective energy metabolism in the failing heart could be tested in earnest. The results firmly established that heart muscle derives its energy for contraction from the oxidation of energy-providing substrates and suggested that oxygen consumption is an index of energy production. Despite decreased efficiency of the failing human heart, the results from early studies were disappointing because no qualitative change in substrate metabolism was observed through measurement of arteriovenous (AV) differences.[10] These studies suggested that like the normal human heart, the failing heart under fasting conditions derived about 30% of its energy requirements from carbohydrates, 5% from amino acids, 7% from ketone bodies, and the remaining approximately 58% from fatty acids.[10] However, it should

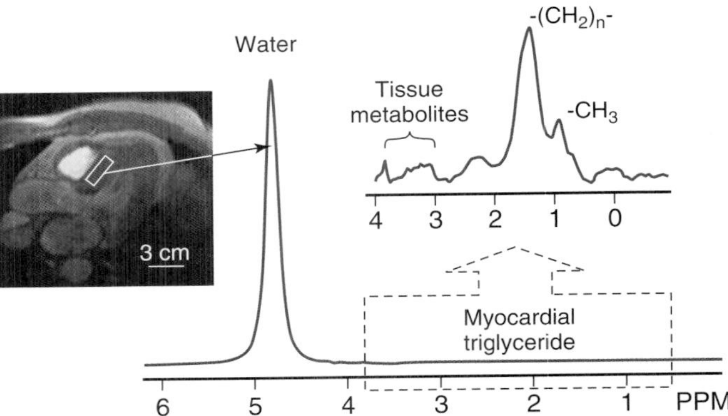

FIGURE 16-5 Magnetic resonance imaging in heart failure. Far left: Magnetic resonance image of the heart showing a region of interest in the ventricular septum. The ^{1}H-NMR spectra generated from the region of interest are next to the MRI image. The largest peak is from water. The myocardial triglyceride peaks have been enlarged. *Reproduced from Szczepaniak LS, Dobbins RL, Metzger GJ, et al: Myocardial triglycerides and systolic function in humans: in vivo evaluation by localized proton spectroscopy and cardiac imaging. Magn Res Med 49:417–423, 2003.*

be noted that these early studies were limited, because they did not use tracer infusions, such as C-13 palmitate, which facilitate the discrimination of *exogenous* substrate use from *endogenous* substrate production. More recent AV balance studies have taken advantage of this technique to evaluate myocardial uptake and use of exogenous versus endogenous substrates. It is also important to note that the early AV balance studies of heart failure did not evaluate substrate metabolism in patients with concomitant diabetes or obesity, which would be expected to affect substrate delivery and thus myocardial substrate use.

Nuclear Magnetic Resonance Spectroscopy

Nuclear magnetic resonance (NMR) spectroscopy of energy-rich phosphates and other biologic compounds detects the magnetic spin of atomic nuclei and is used to monitor changes in metabolic content and enrichment in the intact heart. Commonly used nuclei include ^{1}H, ^{2}H, ^{13}C, ^{15}N, ^{17}O, ^{31}P, ^{23}N, and ^{39}K. ^{31}P-NMR spectroscopy is one of the most commonly used types of NMR spectroscopy, which yields distinct quantitative resonance peaks for monophosphate esters, inorganic phosphates, phosphocreatine, and the three phosphorus atoms of ATP (γ-ATP, α-ATP, and β-ATP). The sizes of these peaks are related to the concentration of these metabolites. ^{1}H-NMR spectroscopy is useful for assessing myocardial lipid retention both in animal models and in humans with heart failure.[11] The spectra generated from ^{1}H-NMR are used to determine intramyocellular triglyceride *deposition* (as opposed to flux). The spectra are acquired from a region of interest in the interventricular septum to avoid contamination from epicardial fat. As shown in **Figure 16-5**, the spectral peak due to water is very large in comparison with the peaks due to myocardial triglycerides. However, the agreement between ^{1}H-NMR spectroscopy measurement of myocardial triglycerides and traditional biochemical methods is very good, and ^{1}H-NMR spectroscopy is reproducible.[11] The amount of myocardial triglyceride deposition correlates with increased ventricular mass, concentric remodeling, and decreased regional systolic function.[11] This noninvasive technique is particularly valuable for the robust myocardial phenotyping of patients with heart failure due to different causes and for monitoring responses to metabolic modulation therapies.

Magnetic Resonance Imaging

A relatively new magnetic resonance (MR) method deserves mention. This method is MR with hyperpolarization and dynamic nuclear polarization (DNP), which dramatically improves signal-to-noise ratios because there are greater than 10,000-fold increases in the signal from active nuclei. Although the concentrations of the metabolic substrate are higher than physiologic concentrations,[12] when ^{13}C-labeled tracers are used in this technique, one can achieve exquisite visualization of biochemical pathways such as glycolysis and the Krebs cycle. Briefly, DNP (which requires a high magnetic field and extremely low temperatures) compels most spins to point in the same direction, resulting in a markedly increased MR signal.[12] A full description of this method is beyond the scope of this chapter but has been recently reviewed by Schroeder et al.[12] The first application in humans was in 2010 in patients with cancer. As yet there are no human heart failure studies, but this method has the potential in the future to improve our understanding of heart failure metabolism with finer granularity and to provide better metabolic profiling, which may aid in patient management.

Radionuclear Imaging: A Focus on Positron Emission Tomography

Tracing metabolic pathways with short-lived radionuclear tracers has found more widespread clinical applications than NMR spectroscopy, mainly in the diagnosis and management of ischemic heart disease. Although single-photon emission computed tomography (SPECT) imaging can be used to evaluate myocardial glucose or fatty acid metabolism, SPECT cannot quantify myocardial metabolism rates, so its utility for measuring metabolism for research has been limited. In contrast, positron emission tomography (PET) can be used to quantify myocardial oxygen and substrate metabolism (**see also Chapter 29**). In general, two types of positron-emitting tracers are used in PET imaging: generator-derived substrate analogs, such as [^{18}F]2-deoxy-2-fluoro-d-glucose (FDG), and cyclotron-derived [^{11}C]-labeled tracers, such as [1-^{11}C]-glucose. The main advantages of generator-produced tracers are that an onsite cyclotron is not needed and the cost is often cheaper than cyclotron-produced tracers. The main advantage of cyclotron-produced tracers is that (in conjunction with compartmental modeling) they can provide more comprehensive information about intracellular myocardial metabolism. (For complete details on all metabolic tracers used or being developed for myocardial metabolic measurements see the recent review.[13]) The most commonly used metabolic tracer is FDG. The method for calculation of myocardial glucose metabolism rates using FDG requires use of a "lumped constant" that represents the ratio of the use of 2-deoxyglucose relative to glucose. The uptake and retention of FDG is linear with time and follows zero-order kinetics. For research purposes, more detailed measurements of metabolism and intracellular fate of substrates is now possible using [1-^{11}C]-labeled glucose, fatty acids, and lactate because of the development of new compartmental models

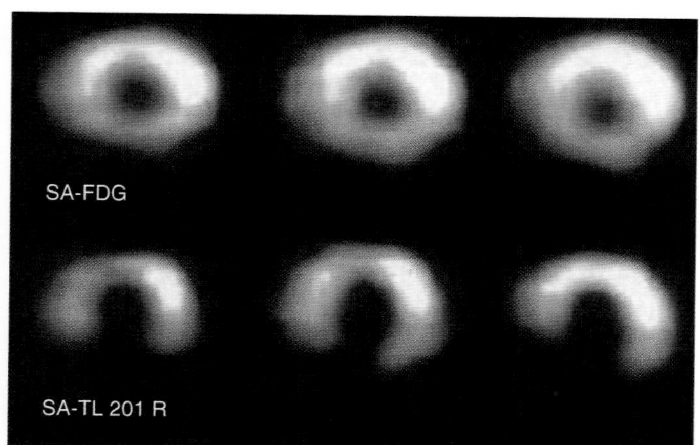

FIGURE 16-6 Assessment of myocardial viability by positron emission tomography. The top short axis positron emission tomography (PET) images show uptake of [^{18}F]2-deoxy-2-fluoro-d-glucose (FDG) in all myocardial segments, consistent with intact glucose metabolism. The bottom images show markedly decreased perfusion in the inferior wall assessed by thallium-201 uptake. Demonstration of enhanced FDG uptake and normal or decreased coronary flow (metabolism/perfusion mismatch) is the current gold standard for identification of potentially reversible contractile dysfunction with revascularization. *Reproduced from Cornel JH, Bax JJ, Fioretti PM, et al: Prediction of improvement of ventricular function after revascularization. 18F-fluorodeoxyglucose single-photon emission computed tomography versus low-dose dobutamine echocardiography. Eur Heart J 18:941–948, 1997.*

that are used in conjunction with the PET-derived time-activity curves from the myocardium and the blood.[13] For example, clearance of labeled long-chain fatty acids is biexponential, suggesting both rapid and slow turnover pools.[13] The size and slope of the exponential components of the ^{11}C time-activity curve reflect immediate and delayed oxidation of labeled fatty acids. Most recently, a methodology designed to measure endogenous triglyceride oxidation in animals using [1-^{11}C] palmitate and three-dimensional PET has shown promise for the potential use of PET for the noninvasive measurement of endogenous triglyceride oxidation.[13]

The most important clinical use for cardiac metabolic PET imaging is the assessment of myocardial viability (**see Chapter 29**). Regional responses in substrate metabolism to myocardial ischemia can be visualized entirely noninvasively. The basis of viability studies is the finding that ischemic, noncontractile, *but viable* myocardium has markedly impaired blood flow yet relatively normal glucose metabolism due to a return to the fetal gene program.[14] Thus demonstration of preserved FDG uptake and normal or decreased coronary flow (metabolism/perfusion mismatch) is the current gold standard for identifying potentially reversible contractile dysfunction with revascularization (**Figure 16-6**).

Transcript Analyses

Another dimension in the evaluation of metabolic disturbances underlying heart failure is the assessment of gene expression in myocardial biopsy samples. With the exception of lipotoxic heart disease (see later discussion) and rare disorders, such as glycogen storage disease, histology and immunocytochemistry have limited usefulness as tools for diagnosing metabolic disturbances of the failing heart. As outlined previously, the use of AV differences, ^{31}P-NMR, and PET have brought to light a number of defects in energy substrate metabolism. These findings are now the basis for further studies examining cardiac gene expression of key regulators in energy substrate metabolism. Moreover, the advent of quantitative RT-PCR and targeted gene expression arrays has facilitated a more complete assessment of metabolic gene expression changes in the failing heart.[15]

Consistent with the observed reduction in fatty acid oxidation capacity in heart failure from dilated cardiomyopathy, the mRNA expression of enzymes that mediate long-chain fatty acid metabolism is downregulated.[16] Similar downregulation in the expression of genes encoding fatty acid oxidation enzymes is observed in animal models of hypertrophy and heart failure.[5]

Many of the genes coding for proteins involved in fatty acid uptake and oxidation are regulated by the nuclear receptor peroxisome proliferator activated receptor α (PPARα).[5] This transcription factor forms a heterodimer with the retinoic X receptor α (RXRα) and complexes with coactivators, most prominently PGC1α.[5] One of the natural ligands for PPARα was recently determined to be 16:0;18:1 glycerol-3-phosphocholine; however, other fatty acid moieties may also be able to activate this nuclear receptor. In animal models of cardiac hypertrophy, gene expression and DNA binding activity of PPARα decrease, as does the expression of various enzymes involved in β-oxidation,[5] suggesting a possible transcriptional mechanism for diminished rates of fatty acid oxidation. These observations are consistent with data demonstrating that PPARα is downregulated in the failing human heart.[5] In addition to PPARα, the heart also expresses high levels of the nuclear receptors PPARβ/δ and estrogen-regulated receptor alpha (ERRα). Although the regulation of these transcription factors in heart failure is less clear, both PPARβ/δ and ERRα upregulate many of the same fatty acid oxidation genes as PPARα.[17] In addition, PPARβ/δ and ERRα are distinct from PPARα in that they induce genes involved in glucose uptake and mitochondrial oxidative phosphorylation, respectively. Mice overexpressing PPARβ/δ in the myocardium are resistant to high-fat diet-induced cardiomyopathy and show increased protection from ischemia reperfusion injury.[17] In contrast, animals with a cardiac-specific deletion of PPARβ/δ develop cardiomyopathy.[18] These data are consistent with the concept that PPARβ/δ-induced transcriptional programs are cardioprotective. ERRα also plays a protective role when the heart is exposed to stresses, such as pressure overload, as evidenced by the rapid development of heart failure in ERRα knockout mice subjected to aortic banding.[19] Recent evidence also suggests that ERRα-regulated pathways are downregulated in humans with heart failure.[20]

In contrast to long-chain fatty acids, the transcriptional regulation of glucose metabolism in heart failure is not as well understood. Late-stage cardiomyopathy is associated with decreased glucose uptake.[1] Recent studies suggest that glucose transporters 1 and 4 are both downregulated in patients with end-stage heart failure at the transcriptional level.[5] In addition, pacing-induced heart failure in a canine model caused decreased mRNA levels of lactate dehydrogenase. In addition, the activities of 3-phosphoglycerate kinase and pyruvate kinase were also downregulated,[5] consistent with an impairment of glucose use in the later stages of heart failure. Thus different causes of heart failure and different levels of severity each appear to affect the heart's substrate metabolism profile.

In addition to changes in transcript levels of enzymes regulating energy substrate metabolism, genes controlling the transfer of high-energy phosphates across the inner mitochondrial membrane also show alterations in the failing heart. For instance, a recent report showed a downregulation of adenine nucleotide translocator 1 (ANT1) in a rodent model of chronic heart failure.[21] In contrast, others have found that hearts from patients with dilated cardiomyopathy have decreased transcript levels of adenine nucleotide translocator 2, whereas adenine nucleotide translocator 1 protein content increased.[22] Overall, these findings suggest that in the failing heart, changes in expression of regulators of energy transfer pathways are likely contributors to the progression of contractile dysfunction.

Transcripts for mitochondrial proteins are also decreased in the failing heart. For instance, in a mouse model of heart failure, mitochondrial DNA-encoded gene transcripts, including the subunits of complex I (ND1, 2, 3, 4, 4L, and 5), complex III (cytochrome b), complex IV (cytochrome oxidase), and rRNA (12S and 16S) are all decreased. These transcriptional changes were accompanied by changes in the enzymatic activity of complexes I, III, and IV.[23] These findings are consistent with other observations of decreased mitochondrial respiration in the failing human heart, and defective mitochondrial structure and function in animal models of heart failure.[5] However, with the exception of certain inherited cardiomyopathies exhibiting mutations for mitochondrial enzymes of long-chain fatty acid metabolism, it still cannot be determined with certainty whether or not mitochondria play a primary role in contributing to heart failure.

The regulation of genes involved in both fatty acid oxidation and mitochondrial oxidative capacity/biogenesis are controlled in large part by the nuclear receptor coactivators PGC-1α and -β.[5] These proteins are highly expressed in the heart where they direct gene expression through interactions with nuclear receptor (PPARα, PPARβ/δ, ERRα) and nonnuclear receptor transcription factors (NRF-1/2, MEF2). The highly inducible nature of these proteins allows them to rapidly reprogram metabolism in response to a variety of stressors. In both human and animal models of hypertrophy, as well as heart failure models of dilated cardiomyopathy, PGC-1 co-activators are downregulated.[24] This is further supported by the observation that mice lacking both PGC-1 isoforms die of heart failure early in life.[25] Thus while a metabolic shift toward glucose metabolism and away from fatty acid metabolism may in some ways be adaptive (e.g., glucose metabolism is more oxygen efficient than fat metabolism), a marked decrease in fatty acid metabolism appears to be maladaptive. The decrease in fatty acid metabolism may be detrimental because the heart can produce more reducing equivalents from fatty acids than from carbohydrates. Thus downregulation of myocardial fatty acid enzymes and fatty acid metabolism may result in reduced energy provision for the failing heart.

Genomic Analysis

Genomic analysis of lipid metabolism enzymes has the potential to contribute to both diagnosis and prognosis in heart failure. At least a dozen separate inherited disorders of mitochondrial fatty acid β-oxidation have been described in humans (**Table 16-1**).[26] The severe clinical manifestations of these inborn errors in human fatty acid oxidizing enzymes include dilated cardiomyopathy and sudden death, underlining the importance of *normal* fatty acid metabolism for *normal* function of the *normal* heart. The most commonly recognized defect is medium-chain acyl-CoA dehydrogenase (MCAD) deficiency. In addition, polymorphisms of the PPARα gene have been shown to influence human left ventricular (LV) growth in response to exercise and hypertension[27] and to modify the response to β-blockers in patients with recent myocardial infarction.[28] Further characterization of the phenotypic impact of polymorphisms within metabolic regulatory proteins has prognostic and therapeutic potential for patients with heart failure.

TABLE 16-1 Defects of Mitochondrial Fatty Acid Oxidation

Fatty acid oxidation defect
Muscular carnitine-palmitoyl transferase (CPT) deficiency (i.e., adult-onset CPT II)
Hepatic CPT I deficiency
MCAD deficiency
LCAD deficiency
ETF deficiency
ETF:QO deficiency
SCAD deficiency
LCHAD deficiency
Carnitine transport defect
2,4-Dienoyl-CoA reductase deficiency
Hepatomuscular CPT (infantile CPT II) deficiency
Carnitine/acylcarnitine translocase deficiency
SCHAD deficiency

CPT, Carnitine palmitoyltransferase; *CPT I,* carnitine palmitoyltransferase I; *CPT II,* carnitine palmitoyltransferase II; *ETF,* electron transfer flavoprotein; *LCAD,* long-chain acyl-CoA dehydrogenase; *LCHAD,* long-chain 3-hydroxyacyl-CoA dehydrogenase; *MCAD,* medium-chain acyl-CoA dehydrogenase; *QO,* ubiquinone oxidoreductase; *SCAD,* short-chain acyl-CoA dehydrogenase; *SCHAD,* short-chain 3-hydroxyacyl-CoA dehydrogenase.

Adapted from Coates PM, Tanaka K: Molecular basis of mitochondrial fatty acid oxidation defects. J Lipid Res 33:1099, 1992.

METABOLIC REMODELING OF THE HUMAN HEART IN NONISCHEMIC HEART FAILURE

Although results in the literature using animal models of heart failure are fairly consistent—there is a metabolic "switch" toward using glucose and away from using fatty acids[5]—results from studies in humans have not been consistent. For example, in one PET study of human idiopathic cardiomyopathy using [^{11}C] palmitate, the mean LV myocardial use of fatty acids was significantly less than that of control subjects.[2] However, in another PET study of both ischemic and nonischemic heart failure patients, myocardial fatty acid use was increased.[2] In an AV balance study of mostly nonischemic (1 ischemic) heart failure patients and controls, there was no significant difference in myocardial fatty acid uptake.[2] In contrast, in a study of hypertrophic cardiomyopathy caused by a particular mutation (Asp175Asn in the α-tropomyosin gene), myocardial oxygen consumption and fatty acid metabolism were increased.[2] Taken together, these studies demonstrate that all human heart failure is not created equally in terms of myocardial substrate metabolism. Different causes lead to different patterns of myocardial metabolic substrate preference, even if decreased function is common to all. This suggests that myocardial metabolic changes observed in heart failure are not solely in response to functional changes. Moreover, it suggests that new treatment strategies aimed at improving myocardial metabolism will have to be individualized to the specific metabolic pattern linked with a specific cause of heart failure.

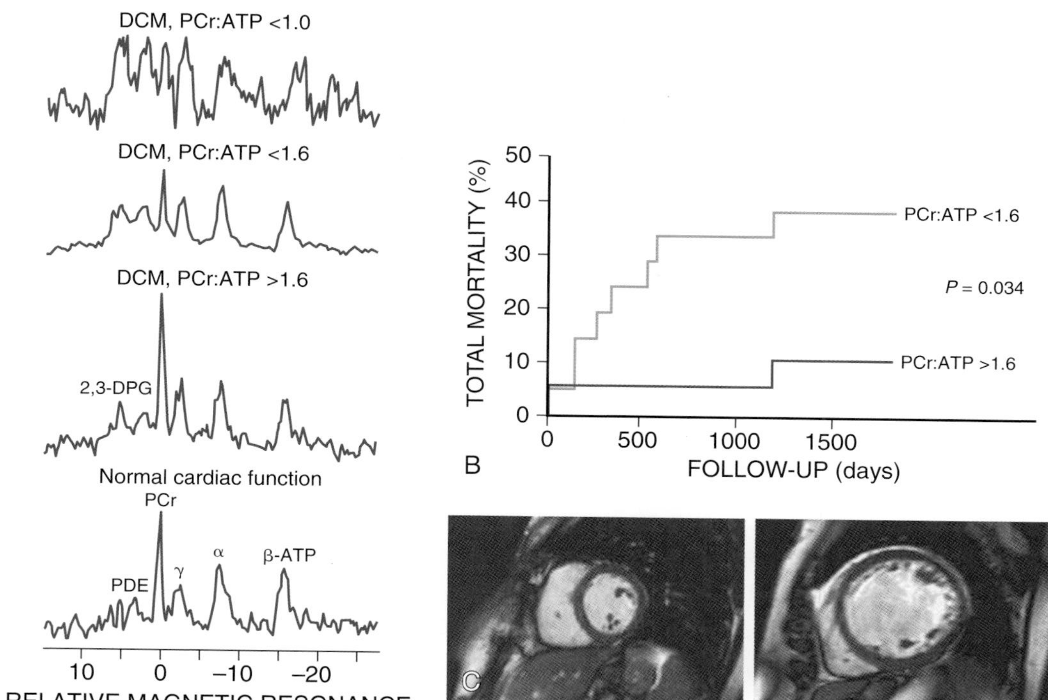

FIGURE 16-7 NMR Spectroscopy in heart failure. **A,** Illustration of a *(top to bottom)* phosphorus-31 nuclear magnetic resonance (^{31}P-NMR) spectra in a normal human, a patient with dilated cardiomyopathy but a favorable phosphocreatine (PCr)/adenosine triphosphate (ATP) ratio of greater than 1.6, a patient with dilated cardiomyopathy and an unfavorable PCr/ATP ratio less than 1.6, and a cardiomyopathy patient with a severely decreased PCr/ATP ratio (<1.0), who died within 7 days after this image was taken. **B,** A Kaplan-Meier analysis showing prognosis differences based on PCr/ATP. **C,** Shows magnetic resonance imaging (MRI) of a normal heart compared with a dilated cardiomyopathy. *Reproduced from Neubauer S: The failing heart—an engine out of fuel. N Engl J Med 356:1140–1151, 2007.*

Along with the changes in substrate metabolism, there are also alterations in myocardial energetics in heart failure. A decrease in the myocardial PCr/ATP ratio occurs relatively early in heart failure and results from a decrease in creatine transporter function, which leads to lower [Cr] and [PCr] levels. A decreased PCr/ATP ratio (<1.6) is a predictor of mortality in patients with dilated cardiomyopathy (**Figure 16-7**).[1] Decreased PCr/ATP ratio is also an early finding in inherited hypertrophic cardiomyopathy (even without frank LV hypertrophy)[29] and in Chagas disease.[30] Heart failure impairs the creatine kinase energy-transfer mechanism, reducing ATP flux rates by approximately 50% in mild to moderate heart failure. ADP concentrations increase in heart failure.[1] A decrease in myocardial ATP level generally only occurs in very advanced heart failure. An overview of the evolution of changes in high-energy phosphate metabolism created by heart failure (along with the changes in myocardial metabolism and oxidative phosphorylation) is illustrated in **Figure 16-8**. Although most clinical ^{31}P-NMR studies of heart failure have measured the PCr/ATP ratio, it is now also possible to quantify concentrations of myocardial phosphometabolites by normalizing their NMR signal to that of a standard of known concentration.[31]

METABOLIC REMODELING OF THE HUMAN HEART UNDER CONDITIONS THAT LEAD TO SECONDARY HEART FAILURE

Perhaps one of the most exciting developments in the field of cardiac metabolism is the recognition that the heart possesses defined mechanisms to adapt to external stress signals. Sustained and/or multiple stressors may also lead to metabolic remodeling and maladaptation of the heart.

Steps Leading to Metabolic Remodeling

Studies carried out in isolated perfused heart preparations have shown that the heart responds to changes in its environment by redirecting substrate fluxes through those pathways that are most appropriate for a given metabolic or physiologic environment. Examples are the suppression of glucose oxidation when there is an oversupply of fatty acids and, conversely, the suppression of long-chain fatty acid oxidation in the presence of high concentrations of glucose and insulin.[32] Conversely, an acute increase in the workload of the heart results in instantaneous mobilization and oxidation of glycogen and a shift from fat to carbohydrates (glucose and lactate) as the main fuel for respiration.[32] As outlined previously, this adaptation can either be acute (alterations in preexisting protein function) or chronic (alterations in gene expression, remodeling), depending upon the intensity and duration of the stimulus.[33] It is reasonable to propose that metabolic adaptation often precedes or parallels functional adaptation of the heart. While this metabolic change may initially be thought of as an adaptation to a stimulus in the short term, it may also have detrimental effects over the long term and lead to contractile dysfunction and failure (maladaptation).

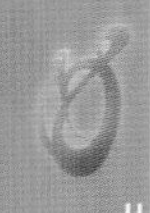

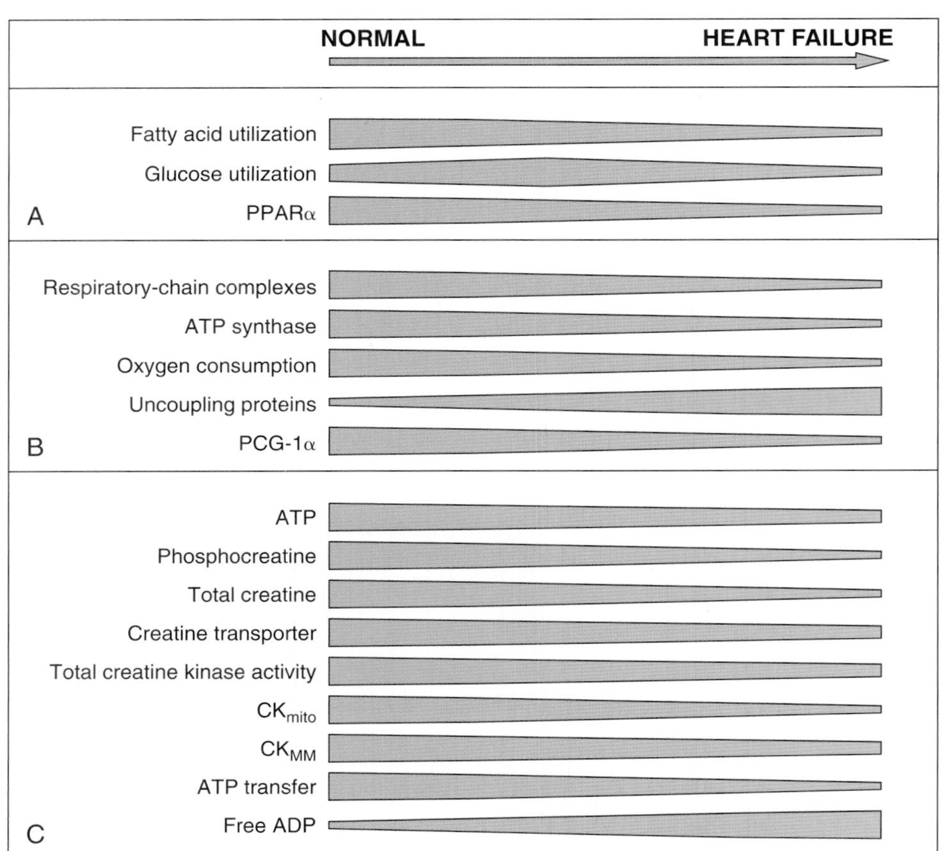

FIGURE 16-8 Cardiac metabolism in heart failure. **A,** Shows the general changes in myocardial substrate metabolism that occur with the development of heart failure (in nondiabetic, nonobese patients). **B,** Shows the heart failure–induced changes in oxidative phosphorylation. There is decreased energy production. **C,** Demonstrates the changes in high-energy phosphate metabolism. *Reproduced from Neubauer S: The failing heart—an engine out of fuel. N Engl J Med 356:1140–1151, 2007.*

Cardiac Hypertrophy in Response to Pressure Overload

The impact of workload on cardiac metabolism, gene expression, and function has been intensely studied. Alterations in workload on the heart have both acute and chronic effects on myocardial metabolism. When the workload is increased, the heart rapidly responds by increasing the flux of carbon through metabolic pathways. In doing so, the heart balances the rates of energy-generating reactions (e.g., oxidative phosphorylation) with that of energy-consuming reactions (e.g., cross-bridge cycling). More specifically, increased workload on the heart rapidly results in increased glucose uptake, glycogenolysis, glycolytic flux, and pyruvate oxidation (whether derived from extracellular glucose, extracellular lactate, or intracellular glycogen), with little effect on fatty acid oxidation.[32]

If the increased workload on the heart is sustained, the heart responds with characteristic alterations in morphology, increased cell size, and gene expression (e.g., reexpression of fetal genes), paralleled by a process of metabolic remodeling. In general terms, the hypertrophied heart increases its reliance on glucose as a fuel, while decreasing fatty acid oxidation.[2] This upregulation of glucose metabolism occurs even before there is an increase in LV mass.[34] Unexpectedly, the heart also responds with an upregulation of glucose metabolism with a sustained *decrease* in workload.[35] It appears that any sustained changes in workload result in similar patterns of metabolic remodeling and in a switch from an energetically less efficient (fatty acids) to an energetically more efficient (glucose) fuel for respiration.

Two important questions arise from these data: (1) What is the mechanism for substrate switching, and (2) why does substrate switching occur? In the past, mechanistic studies of substrate switching have focused on the regulation of the pyruvate dehydrogenase complex (PDC). Recent evidence suggests, however, that the nuclear receptor PPARα plays a key regulatory role in substrate switching.[5] Whereas PDC activity remains relatively unaffected in response to sustained pressure overload, PPARα induces the transcription of multiple genes encoding for proteins involved in fatty acid metabolism. These include fatty acid translocase (FAT/CD36), heart-specific fatty acid binding protein (hFABP), acyl-CoA synthetase I (ACSI), malonyl-CoA decarboxylase (MCD), muscle-specific carnitine palmitoyltransferase I (mCPTI), medium-chain acyl-CoA dehydrogenase (MCAD), and long-chain acyl-CoA dehydrogenase (LCAD). PPARα is itself activated by fatty acids, thereby forming a positive feed-forward mechanism for fatty acid–induced fatty acid oxidation. Pressure overload represses this mechanism by decreasing the expression of PPARα itself and its coactivator, PGC1. PPARα-DNA binding activity is also reduced through covalent modification (phosphorylation) in response to pressure overload. The result is decreased expression of fatty acid metabolizing genes in the hypertrophied heart, and therefore decreased fatty acid oxidation capacity. In addition, several other transcription factors (e.g., Sp1, Coup-TF) known to be activated in the response to pressure overload have been implicated in the repression of fatty acid oxidation genes.[36] What is less clear is the mechanism by which reliance on glucose as a metabolic fuel increases in the hypertrophied heart. One possibility is that the increased glucose oxidation is the result of decreased fatty acid oxidation through a "reverse Randle cycle."[32] In the normal heart, the Randle cycle describes how fatty acids suppress glucose oxidation to a greater extent than glycolysis, and glycolysis to a greater extent than glucose uptake.[32] Conversely, glucose suppresses fatty acid oxidation through a mechanism that involves malonyl-CoA-induced inhibition of the fatty acid transporter protein CPTI in a "reverse Randle cycle."[32] Although rates of glycolysis are increased in the hypertrophied heart, rates of pyruvate oxidation are not increased to the same extent, and insulin's effects on glucose oxidation are attenuated. Thus there is a loss of coordination between glucose oxidation and glycolysis.[2] Other potential factors involved in increased glucose use in response to pressure overload include decreased expression of PDK4 (a PPARα target gene), chronic activation of AMPK, and elevated cytosolic levels of Ca^{2+}.[37]

Why does substrate switching occur in the hypertrophied heart? A classic explanation for this phenomenon is at the energetic level. Glucose is a more efficient energy source compared with fatty acids (i.e., more ATP generated per O_2 consumed). This is particularly important when oxygen demand outstrips oxygen supply, as is the case in ischemia and which may also be the case in the hypertrophied heart. Furthermore, evidence exists suggesting that glycolytically derived ATP is preferentially used by ion channels, the activities of which are increased in the hypertrophied heart. However, the importance of substrate switching during the hypertrophic response has recently been challenged. Mice with a cardiac-specific deletion of acetyl CoA carboxylase 2 (ACC2) produce less malonyl CoA and as a consequence have increased rates of fatty acid oxidation and reduced glucose oxidation. In response to pressure overload, ACC2 knockout mice do not shift substrate use and continue to primarily oxidize FAs. Surprisingly, these mice actually have improved cardiac function in the setting of pressure overload compared with nontransgenic controls.[38] These data argue that metabolic reprograming is not a necessary adaptation for the hypertrophied heart in the setting of pressure overload. In fact, CPT1 haploinsufficient mice, which have reduced fatty acid oxidation at baseline, have accentuated cardiac dysfunction in response to pressure overload.[39] Thus diverting substrate metabolism from fatty acid to glucose in the setting of pressure overload may not be as adaptive as previously thought. Intriguingly, GLUT1 overexpression and increased glucose oxidation can also protect the heart from pressure overload, suggesting that overall myocardial energetics may be more important than the specific substrate that is used.[40] Additional research will be necessary to define the intricacies of crosstalk between glucose and fatty acid oxidation in the hypertrophied heart.

Obesity

Obesity is a well-known risk factor for the development of heart failure, with an estimated 11% to 14% of all cases a result of obesity alone and a much greater percentage linked to obesity plus its frequent comorbidities of diabetes, hypertension, and coronary artery disease (CAD).[41] In morbidly obese patients, overfeeding the heart with energy-providing substrates results in the accumulation of triglycerides in cardiac myocytes and impaired contractile function. This is not a new concept. Virchow observed in his *Cellular Pathology* over 100 years ago that "genuine fatty degeneration (metamorphosis) of the heart is a real transformation of its substance, going on in the interior of the fibers." Although extreme cardiac fatty metamorphosis (adipositas cordis), manifested by a heart so stuffed with lipids that it floats in water is relatively rare, impairment of myocardial triglyceride and fatty acid metabolism on a more modest scale also appears to have deleterious effects on the function of the heart.[42]

Lipotoxicity in a general sense describes the deleterious downstream effects resulting from excessive uptake of fatty acids by the heart. When first described in animal models, however, lipotoxicity referred to a specific pathway in which increased fatty acid uptake exceeded β-oxidation and led to fatty acid *deposition,* ceramide production, increased inducible nitric oxide synthase (iNOS) activity, and apoptosis.[43] Since this initial description, it has been discovered that fatty acid deposition-induced apoptosis may also result from reactive oxygen species generation.[7] Excessive fatty acid *oxidation* may also play a role in the development of obesity-related cardiac dysfunction through pathways that do not result in apoptosis. For example, a study of *db/db* mice showed that increased myocardial fatty acid oxidation precedes contractile dysfunction, suggesting that excessive fatty acid oxidation may contribute to dysfunction. A mouse model with transgenic overexpression of a fatty acid transport protein in the heart also demonstrated increased cardiac fatty acid oxidation, leading to diastolic cardiac dysfunction.[7] It bears emphasis that excessive generation of free radicals secondary to oxidative stress may contribute to alterations in calcium handling and LV dysfunction that is independent of apoptosis-induced LV dysfunction.[7]

In obese humans, there is growing evidence that alterations in myocardial fatty acid metabolism accompany decreased cardiac function. Fat deposition has been demonstrated in pathologic examination of failing human hearts from obese and diabetic patients (**Figure 16-9**).[42] This intramyocardial fat deposition can now be measured in vivo noninvasively, using ^{1}H-NMR as described previously.[11] Fat deposition may be reversible, as shown in one study of obese, diabetic patients placed on a very low-calorie diet, in whom a decrease in myocardial lipid accumulation was accompanied by an improvement in diastolic function.[44] However, the amount of improvement in diastolic function was not related to the amount of change in myocardial steatosis.[44] Thus lipid deposition appears to be a general marker of an altered metabolic milieu and myocardial metabolism that leads to contractile dysfunction rather than a cause of it.[16,44] Obesity and its frequent comorbidity, insulin resistance, also are associated with increased myocardial fatty acid uptake, use, and oxidation, and overall oxygen consumption in asymptomatic young women without frank cardiac systolic dysfunction compared with age-matched controls.[45] Even in these young subjects, increased body mass index was related to impaired LV relaxation.[46] Obesity is also associated with altered high-energy phosphate levels, and this is related to the impairment of diastolic function.[47]

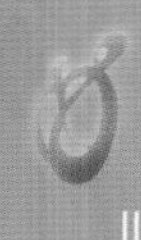

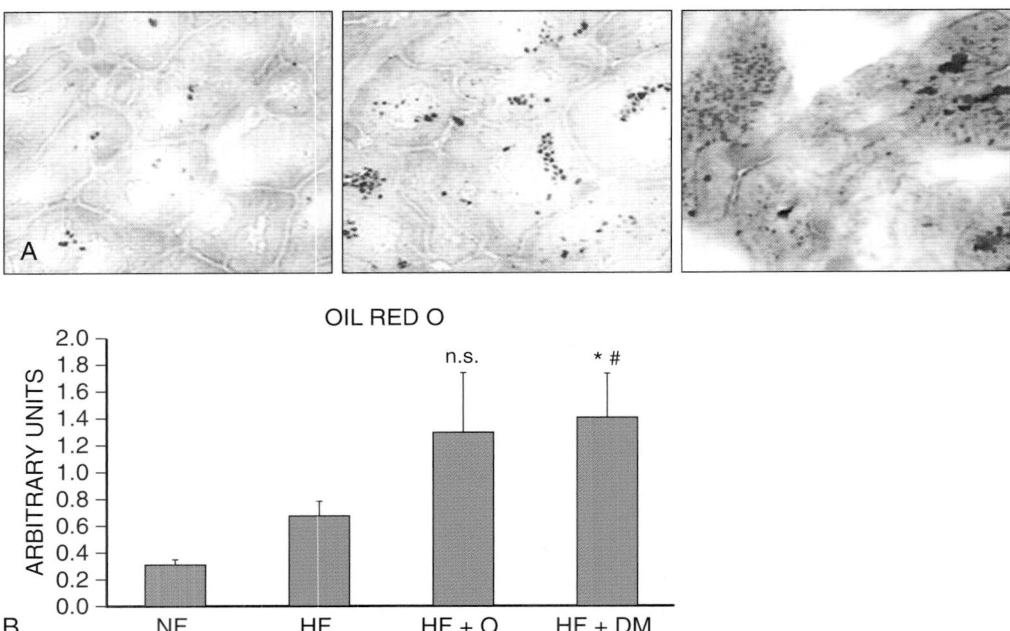

FIGURE 16-9 Cardiac lipotoxicity in heart failure. **A,** *(left to right)* Photomicrographs of low, intermediate, and high lipid accumulation in the myocardium, as stained by Oil Red O. **B,** The amount of intramyocardial triglyceride in explanted hearts from nonfailing (NF) donors not suitable for transplant, nonobese heart failure (HF) patients, obese heart failure patients (HF + O), and diabetic heart failure patients (HF + DM). The patients with diabetes and heart failure had higher intramyocardial fat levels (*$P < 0.05$). *Adapted from Sharma S, Androgue JV, Golfman L, et al: Intramyocardial lipid accumulation in the failing human heart resembles the lipotoxic rat heart. FASEBJ 18:1692–1700, 2004.*

Weight loss can reverse these metabolic and functional abnormalities as it decreases myocardial fatty acid uptake, use, and oxidation, and overall myocardial oxygen consumption.[48] Moreover, the metabolic change that independently predicted the improvement in LV relaxation was the decrease in myocardial oxygen consumption.[48] This suggests that there must be improved coupling between metabolism and function because less oxygen was needed to get better function. This finding also supports the idea that decreased reactive oxygen species generation (accompanying the decreased myocardial oxygen use) may be contributing to the improvement in function. Weight loss has also been associated with improvements in systolic function in humans.[49] The fact that weight loss results in an improvement in diastolic (and sometimes systolic) function also suggests that in humans, apoptosis is not the primary mechanism by which obesity causes heart failure.[49]

Diabetes

Although the question as to whether there is a diabetes-specific cardiomyopathy has been debated for decades, there is increasing evidence that suggests that diabetes has detrimental effects on cardiac function that are not accounted for by coronary or other cardiac disease. The clinical definition of diabetic cardiomyopathy is the presence of diastolic or systolic cardiac dysfunction in a diabetic patient without other obvious causes for cardiomyopathy, such as CAD, hypertension, or valvular heart disease. Typically, LV hypertrophy and diastolic dysfunction are the earliest manifestations of diabetic cardiomyopathy with systolic dysfunction occurring later in the course of disease. Patients with diabetes mellitus have an increased lifetime risk of congestive heart failure and are overrepresented in large heart failure databases. Other evidence for a "diabetic cardiomyopathy" in humans includes a number of morphologic, functional, energetic, and biochemical observations. Moreover, heart disease in general is the leading cause of death among patients with diabetes mellitus. This excess heart disease is observed both in patients with type 1 and type 2 diabetes. Thus the adaptation/maladaptation of the heart in diabetes warrants further discussion.

There are a number of important metabolic alterations in diabetes that are believed to contribute to the development of heart failure (**Figure 16-10**). Glucotoxicity secondary to hyperglycemia has long been considered a central component in the pathogenesis of diabetic cardiomyopathy, and is thought to contribute to cardiac dysfunction through the generation of advanced glycation end products (AGEs) and/or the induction of oxidation. AGEs can modify the function of affected proteins or nucleic acids, but they can also trigger biologic responses via the receptor for AGEs, known as *RAGE*. RAGE is a member of the immunoglobulin superfamily that is expressed on a wide variety of cells, including macrophages, cardiac myocytes, endothelial cells, and smooth muscle cells.[50] RAGE signaling leads to the activation of MAP kinases, PI-3 kinase, rho GTPases, NF-κB, and NADPH oxidase, which triggers inflammatory cytokine production and reactive oxygen species (ROS) generation. Hyperglycemia can also provoke oxidative stress independent of RAGE. The mechanism of ROS generation in this instance is thought to occur via increased glucose flux through the polyol pathway, hexosamine pathway, and mitochondrial oxidative phosphorylation.[50] Importantly, several recent clinical studies have failed to show that aggressive blood glucose control reduces the risk of heart failure in diabetics.[50] Thus abnormal glucose metabolism is only one facet of the pathogenesis of diabetic cardiomyopathy.

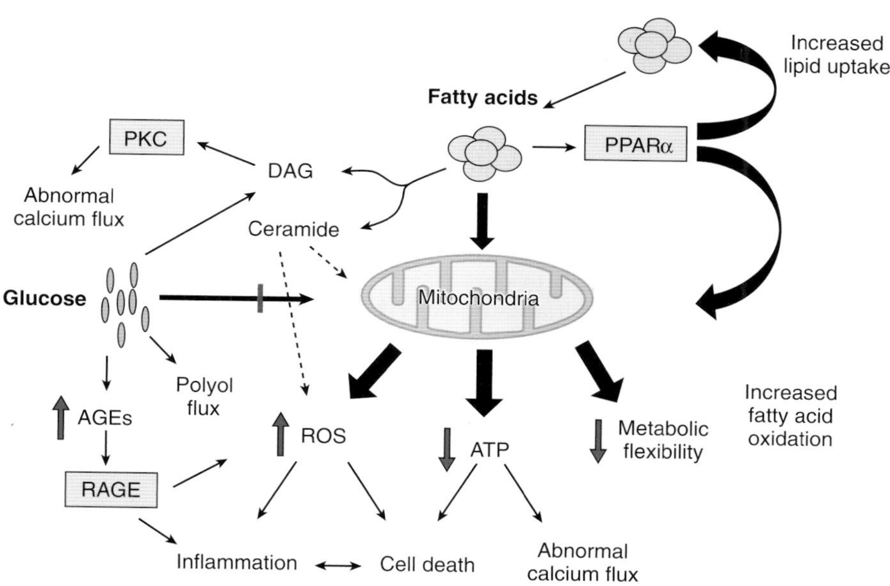

FIGURE 16-10 Pleiotropic effects of diabetes on cardiac myocyte biology. In the diabetic state, excess fatty acids are present inside the cell, leading to excessive mitochondrial fatty acid oxidation, PPARα activation, and the generation of lipid signaling molecules, such as ceramide and DAG. This metabolic reprogramming leads to mitochondrial dysfunction manifested by excess reactive oxygen species (ROS), less efficient adenosine triphosphate (ATP) generation, and loss of metabolic flexibility. Stressed mitochondria also amplify inflammatory and cell death responses. Hyperglycemia can further augment cardiac myocyte toxicity via the formation of advanced glycation end products (AGEs), as well as promoting excess ROS and DAG generation. *Modified from Schilling JD, Mann DL: Diabetic cardiomyopathy: bench to bedside. Heart Fail Clin 8:619–631, 2012.*

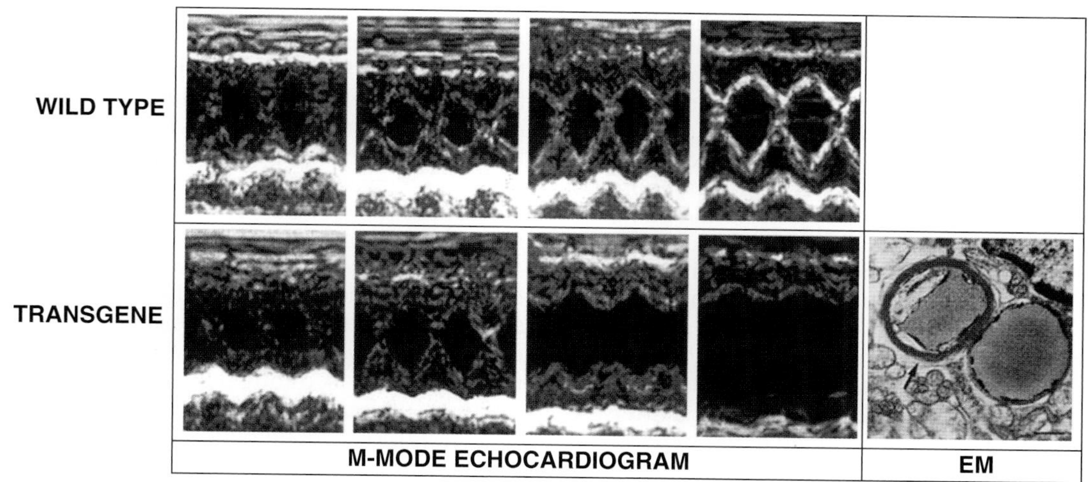

FIGURE 16-11 Cardiac hypertrophy and failure in a mouse heart model of lipotoxicity. The panels are (from *left to right*) serial two-dimensional guided M-mode echocardiographic images obtained from wild-type *(upper panel)* and mice that overexpress long-chain acyl-CoA synthetase *(lower panel)* studied at 2, 3, 4, and 6 weeks of age. Images shown are from a representative pair of age- and sex-matched wild-type transgenic animals. The last panel on the right is a transmission electron micrograph of cardiac tissue from 18-day-old mouse expressing long-chain acyl-CoA synthetase at 15,000× magnification. Numerous lipid droplets are observed in ventricular myocytes. Some droplets at this stage are surrounded by multiple concentric layers of membrane *(arrow)*. *Modified from Chiu HC, Kovacs A, Ford DA, et al: A novel mouse model of lipotoxic cardiomyopathy. J Clin Invest 107:813–822, 2001.*

Diabetes also results in important changes in lipid metabolism that contribute to the development of lipotoxicity. In the diabetic milieu, increased availability of fatty acids is accompanied by increased rates of fatty acid oxidation with a concomitant decrease in glucose metabolism,[7] which may result in loss of metabolic flexibility that is believed to play a crucial role in protecting cardiac myocytes from injury when ATP demand increases and/or substrate availability decreases. The greater reliance on fat oxidation in the diabetic heart is due to activation of PPARα and subsequent induction of PPARα-regulated fatty acid oxidation enzymes.[50] Induction of malonyl coA decarboxylase (MCD) in the heart of a rat model of type I diabetes decreases malonyl-CoA levels (an inhibitor of fatty acyl-CoA entry into the mitochondrion) and increases fatty acid oxidation.[50] Models of type 2 diabetes also demonstrate an increase in myocardial fatty acid oxidation at a young age and lipid accumulation at older ages.[7,43] This increase in fatty acid oxidation and/or lipid accumulation may have direct lipotoxic effects on cardiac function (**Figure 16-11**). The elevation of intracellular fatty acids and lipids have been associated with diabetic cardiomyopathy in rodent models.[43] In this respect, the diabetic heart appears similar to the obese heart, although some studies suggest that the former has even greater fat accumulation.[42] There appear to be multiple mechanisms that contribute to this type of lipid accumulation-related lipotoxicity, including chronically activated PKCs, generation of ROS, and ceramide-induced apoptosis (see Figure 16-10).[50] Other potential factors involved in this diabetic cardiomyopathy include oxidative stress, inflammation, and abnormal calcium handling. These factors and their sequelae will be discussed below.

Oxidative stress secondary to the generation of ROS (see Chapter 8) is routinely observed in various models of diabetic cardiomyopathy. Oxidative stress appears to correlate with lipid delivery and elevated mitochondrial fatty acid oxidation rates, suggesting that mitochondrial-derived free radicals contribute to the oxidative environment in the diabetic heart.[50] However, high rates of fatty acid oxidation do not always lead to excessive ROS generation, implying that other derangements in mitochondrial structure and function must also be involved.[51] Hyperglycemia can also trigger oxidative stress via mitochondrial and nonmitochondrial glucose metabolic pathways.[50] ROS can also be generated by the NAPDH oxidase complex, which is induced by RAGE and PKC activation. Importantly, the NAPDH oxidase system is activated in the diabetic heart.[50] Another factor that may contribute to oxidative stress in diabetes is dysfunction and/or downregulation of ROS scavenging mechanisms.[50] More than likely, these mechanisms act in concert to account for the ROS observed in diabetic cardiomyopathy. The functional consequences of oxidative stress in diabetic cardiomyopathy have also been investigated. Mechanistically, it has been postulated that ROS can cause contractile dysfunction through damage of intracellular organelles and proteins. Consistent with this notion, overexpression of antioxidants, such as superoxide dismutase, catalase, metallothionein, and glutathione peroxidase, can improve contractile function in ex vivo hearts and cardiac myocytes from diabetic mice.[50] However, it should be noted that most of the current data come from STZ models of diabetic heart failure. Whether these findings will translate to other diabetic animal models and humans remains to be determined.

Diabetes also impacts calcium handling in the cardiac myocyte secondary to important alterations in the ryanodine receptor (RyR) and SERCA2A (see also Chapters 1 and 2). The RyR channel is downregulated and hyperphosphorylated in models of type 1 and type 2 diabetes.[50] The hyperphosphorylation of RyR receptors triggers increased SR calcium leak, depleting SR calcium and increasing cytoplasmic calcium during diastole. Concurrently, SERCA2a activity is decreased in diabetes, further exacerbating SR calcium depletion and impairing calcium sequestration during diastole.[50] As a consequence, calcium flux is significantly impaired, resulting in abnormalities in systolic contractility and diastolic relaxation. Interestingly, both oxidative stress and mitochondrial dysfunction have been implicated in impaired calcium flux.[50]

Several protein kinase C (PKC) isoforms are hyperactivated in the diabetic myocardium (see Figure 16-10).[52] The lipid second messenger diacylglycerol (DAG) binds to and activates PKC. In the diabetic heart, DAG levels are elevated as a consequence of enhanced activation of phospholipase C, the enzyme that cleaves phosphatidylinositol 4,5-bisphosphate to form DAG.[50] Hyperactive PKC signaling in the heart can influence calcium handling, ROS generation, and inflammation, all of which can affect cardiac performance. In support of this notion, transgenic mice that overexpress PKCβ in cardiac myocytes develop cardiomyopathy.[50] There is also evidence that PKCβ inhibition can improve the cardiac phenotype of STZ-injected rats.[50] Future investigation will be needed to determine the utility of PKC modulation in other models of diabetic myocardial disease.

CROSSTALK OF METABOLISM WITH CYTOKINE SIGNALING PATHWAYS AND INNATE IMMUNITY

Nitric Oxide: Effects on Metabolism

Nitric oxide (NO) is a modulator of oxidative and nonoxidative cardiac metabolism. In the former case, NO inhibits mitochondrial oxygen consumption through its effects on aconitase, complexes I and II of the electron transport chain, and cytochrome c oxidase, most likely because of a direct interaction of NO with these iron-containing proteins.[53] In addition, exposure of the heart to NO donors has been shown to inhibit oxygen consumption.[5] Conversely, inhibition of nitric oxide synthase (NOS) with L-arginine analogues increases mitochondrial oxygen consumption.[5] Selective NOS isoform knockout mice suggest that NO derived from endothelial NOS, the most highly expressed NOS isoform in the heart, acts as a physiologic inhibitor of mitochondrial oxygen consumption.[54]

NO also affects glucose uptake and glycolytic flux. In contrast to skeletal muscle, NO appears to inhibit cardiac glucose metabolism.[5] Exposure of the heart to NO donors decreases glucose uptake, whereas glucose uptake is stimulated by NOS inhibitors.[5] In addition, eNOS knockout mouse hearts have elevated rates of glucose uptake when perfused ex vivo, compared with wild-type hearts. It has been postulated that these effects of NO are mediated by cGMP. Inhibition of the glycolytic enzyme phosphofructokinase by NO is also due to elevated intracellular cGMP levels and subsequent activation of cGMP-dependent protein kinase (PKG).

In contrast, results of studies regarding the effects of NO on fatty acid metabolism are mixed. Indirect observations suggest that the NO may decrease fatty acid oxidation. For example, activation of acetyl-CoA carboxylase by NO results in increased intracellular levels of malonyl-CoA, an inhibitor of long-chain fatty acyl-CoA transport into the mitochondrion.[5] As mitochondrial fatty acid metabolism is an aerobic process, the inhibition of the mitochondrial electron transport chain components by NO may contribute to inhibition of β-oxidation. However, studies in the dog heart show both an increase in free fatty acid uptake and a decrease in the respiratory quotient (RQ) in response to NO donors, indicative of increased reliance on fatty acid oxidation.[5] This increased reliance on fatty acid oxidation with NO would fit well with the known decrease in glucose metabolism with NO stimulation.

The physiologic relevance of nitric oxide signaling in the myocardium has been underscored by the observation that β-3 adrenergic signaling in the heart activates NO-generating pathways (see also Chapter 6). The activation of β-3 receptors on cardiac myocytes reduces contractility through an NO-dependent mechanism,[55] consistent with the described effects of NO on metabolism. Nebivolol is a third-generation β-blocker that is a highly selective β_1-antagonist, but also a β-3 receptor agonist. This drug produces NO-dependent vasodilation and cardiodepression,[55] which in some circumstances is thought to improve the balance between energy delivery and use. The SENIORs trial investigated this drug in elderly patients with clinical heart failure and demonstrated a significant improvement in clinical outcomes related to therapy with nebivolol (see Chapter 34).[56]

Modulation of Myocardial Metabolism by Proinflammatory Cytokines

In the past decade, it has been suggested that proinflammatory cytokines are involved in the pathogenesis of heart failure.[57] Among these, tumor necrosis factor (TNF) has received special attention (see Chapter 34). Although the precise mechanisms by which TNF-α and other cytokines elicit their effects on contractile function are still not fully understood, activation of neutral sphingomyelinase signaling and uncoupling of β-adrenergic receptors from adenylate cyclase have emerged as potentially important mechanisms. In addition, cytokines have dramatic effects on cardiac energy metabolism.[58] Studies in cardiomyocytes have shown that both TNF and interleukin-1α inhibit mitochondrial respiration and decrease PDC activity.[59] In addition, interleukin-1β increases nonoxidative glucose metabolism and decreases mitochondrial enzyme activity (complex I and complex II).[60] The exact mechanisms by which these cytokines modulate energy substrate metabolism are not known, but may depend on the production of NO, the effects of which were discussed previously.

The impact of inflammatory signaling on myocardial metabolism and function is readily apparent in the syndrome of septic shock. It is now recognized that more than 50% of patients with bacterial sepsis will develop inflammatory-induced transient myocardial dysfunction.[56] The inflammatory cascade responsible for the syndrome of gram-negative sepsis is triggered by the host receptor Toll-like receptor 4 (TLR4), which recognizes bacterial lipopolysaccharide (LPS).[61] In animal models of sepsis, the injection of LPS produces LV dysfunction that is dependent on TLR4 activation.[62] The cardiometabolic effects of LPS include decreased fatty acid oxidation capacity and myocardial triglyceride accumulation.[63] Consistent with these observations, LPS downregulates the expression of genes involved in fatty acid oxidation, including PPARα, ERRα, MCAD, and MCP-1.[64] In addition, the nuclear receptor coactivators PGC-1α and PGC-1β, which regulate fatty acid oxidation and mitochondrial function pathways, are profoundly downregulated during TLR4-induced inflammatory stress. Recently it was shown that cardiac myocyte-specific overexpression of PGC-1β or PPARγ overexpression can restore cardiac fatty acid oxidation capacity and attenuate sepsis-induced cardiac dysfunction.[65,66] Thus alterations in cellular metabolism are a critical component of proinflammatory cytokine-mediated heart failure. These observations also suggest that metabolic-based therapies may have utility for the treatment of septic cardiomyopathy.

The suppression of myocardial fatty acid oxidation pathways by inflammation has been further illustrated in a transgenic mouse with cardiac-specific overexpression of TNF.[67] Similar to the acute model of LPS stimulation, TNF transgenic mice have reduced fatty acid oxidation capacity and downregulation of the genes encoding PGC-1α, PPARα, and many fatty acid oxidation enzymes. In this system, TNF induction of TGF-β was shown to mediate the observed downregulation of PPARα-mediated gene transcription through a Smad3-dependent mechanism. Taken together, it is clear that inflammatory signaling reprograms myocardial metabolism, leading to reduced rates of fatty acid oxidation. In addition to direct relevance to sepsis-induced myocardial dysfunction, the crosstalk between inflammatory and metabolic pathways illustrated by LPS and TNF stimulation models may also be salient to the metabolic reprogramming observed in chronic heart failure, which is often associated with increased inflammation, particularly in end-stage cardiomyopathy.

Modulation of Programmed Cell Death and Cell Survival by Glucose and Fatty Acid Metabolites

Studies have shown that energy metabolism interacts with various pathways regulating programmed cell death and cell survival.[68] There is evidence to suggest that in the heart, metabolites serve as signals for programs of adaptation and maladaptation (see Figure 16-1).[69] For example, the pleiotropic functions of glucose in the heart include a strong cardioprotective component. Provision of glucose during hypoxic stress,[70] overexpression of the glucose transporter GLUT1, and chronic hyperglycemia all reduce cardiac apoptosis.[71,72] With respect to the protective effects of glucose and insulin on cell function of the heart, three observations are of importance. First, in the reperfused heart, insulin itself increases postischemic cardiac power without increasing rates of glucose oxidation during early reperfusion.[73] This suggests that insulin itself improves the efficiency of the heart without a concomitant increase in rates of glucose oxidation and may be tied to the insulin signal transduction in cascade. Key regulators of this pathway are the insulin receptor, insulin receptor substrate (IRS), PI3 kinase, and Akt/protein kinase B.[74] PI3 kinase regulates cardiac growth,[75] while Akt activation reduces cardiomyocyte death and induces cardiac hypertrophy.[76] Downstream from the activation of mTOR and its targets requires hexose 6-phosphate.[77] Akt is antiapoptotic and promotes both glucose uptake and glycogen synthesis.[62] Activation of Akt by insulin affords myocardial protection through the insulin signaling cascade,[63] and it appears that the inhibition of early apoptotic events by Akt is dependent upon the first committed step of glycolysis, and more specifically by the action of hexokinase II, which is bound to the mitochondria.[64] Increased hexokinase activity also protects against acute oxidant-induced cell death.[78]

Deletion of GLUT4 or glucose deprivation, on the other hand, enhances cardiac injury during ischemia.[79,80] Possible mechanisms by which glucose protects the cell from apoptosis include the prevention of intracellular Ca^{2+} accumulation, the activation of Akt,[76] and/or the upregulation of the antiapoptotic protein Bcl-2.[81] Three different pathways have been implicated in this response, including glucose deprivation-induced ATP depletion and stimulation of the mitochondrial death pathway cascade, hypoglycemia-induced oxidative stress and activation of the c-Jun N terminal kinase (JNK)/mitogen-activated protein kinase (MAPK) signaling pathways,[82] and glucose deprivation–induced stabilization of p53 leading to an increase in p53-associated apoptosis.[82]

In contrast to glucose, fatty acids are implicated in the induction of programmed cell death.[83] A study in Zucker diabetic fatty rats found that high levels of myocardial triacylglycerol were associated with increased DNA laddering (a marker of apoptosis).[43] Both myocardial triacylglycerol accumulation and DNA were attenuated by treating the animals with a lipid-lowering drug.[72] One proposed mechanism of lipoapoptosis is the increased synthesis of ceramide from palmitoyl acyl-CoA.[43] Ceramide is a potent inhibitor of complex III of the electron transport chain, and promotes the accumulation of ROS.[84] Ceramide also upregulates iNOS expression, NO production, and peroxynitrite generation. The latter is an inducer of apoptosis.[43] Studies in cell culture have shown that fatty acid–induced apoptosis can also be regulated by ceramide-independent pathways. Other potential pathways appear to be mediated by the generation of ROS and/or lysosomal dysfunction.[85,86]

METABOLIC EFFECTS OF STANDARD HEART FAILURE THERAPIES

Treatment of heart failure patients with standard heart failure medications aimed at blocking the adverse effects of sustained neurohormonal signaling (see Chapter 33) also affects myocardial metabolism and energetics. For example, β-adrenergic blocker treatment leads to a decrease of fatty acid uptake by the heart and overall myocardial oxygen consumption.[87] Although myocardial oxygen consumption decreases, left ventricular performance improves; hence, myocardial efficiency improves with β-blocker therapy.[2] β-blockers likely decrease myocardial fatty acid uptake (and oxygen consumption) because they decrease catecholamine-induced lipolysis, and hence decrease plasma fatty acid availability. There are also some data from an animal model that β-blocker therapy can inhibit myocardial fatty acid use by decreasing carnitine palmitoyl transferase 1 activity.[2] Thus β-adrenergic blockade not only decreases cardiac work, blood pressure, and dp/dt but also changes myocardial substrate metabolism in heart failure.

Angiotensin-converting enzyme (ACE) inhibitor therapy also alters myocardial substrate metabolism and energetics in heart failure. In contrast to β-blockers, however, ACE inhibitors *increase* fatty acid uptake in humans with heart failure.[2] Interestingly, in an animal model of obesity and insulin resistance, ACE inhibitors also improve myocardial insulin responsiveness.[2] Whether this finding extends to those with insulin resistance and heart failure is not yet clear. ACE inhibitor therapy also improves myocardial energetics. ACE inhibitors improve CK flux, which leads to an increase in the heart's capacity for ATP synthesis.[2] This is accompanied by an improvement in cardiac function in the failing heart.[2]

Device therapies may also affect myocardial metabolism in heart failure patients. CRT increases cardiac function without changing overall myocardial oxidative consumption, so overall cardiac efficiency is enhanced.[88] Moreover, oxidative metabolism of the septum and the ratio of the septal/lateral wall oxidation improved with CRT.[88] In addition, myocardial glucose uptake in the septum and the septal/lateral ratio of glucose uptake are improved in the septum after CRT.[89,90]

Treatment of advanced heart failure with left ventricular assist device (LVAD) therapy is now more commonplace for advanced heart failure than in the past. Paradoxically, studies in animal models have shown that in unloaded, atrophic states, the same transcriptional program is activated as in hypertrophy. Metabolically, in atrophy and in hypertrophy the myocardium becomes more reliant on glucose metabolism—similar to the fetal heart. Consistent with those findings, LVAD treatment in humans decreased myocardial total lipid content and potentially toxic lipid intermediates (such as ceramide) and improved ventricular function.[16] The same line of reasoning applies to a reduction in markers of autophagy, which decrease when the failing heart is mechanically unloaded.[91]

METABOLISM AS A TARGET FOR PHARMACOLOGIC INTERVENTION IN HEART FAILURE

The complex and highly regulated network of metabolic pathways provides many potential targets for drug interventions (**Figure 16-12**). Prominent among those are drugs directed at shifting the heart's energy supply from oxidation of fatty acids to the more oxygen-efficient oxidation of glucose. This shift can be brought about by either lowering fatty acid availability in the plasma, by inhibiting fatty acid oxidation, or by direct targeting of mitochondrial metabolism. Last, drugs may be aimed at the restoration of moiety-conserved cycles.

Intravenous Glucose-Insulin-Potassium (GIK)

One of the first myocardial metabolic modulator therapies developed was GIK. The theory behind this treatment is that insulin decreases plasma fatty acid levels and fatty acid uptake by the heart, while increasing glucose uptake and use. Intravenous glucose and potassium are then necessary to maintain glucose and electrolyte stability. GIK was initially tried as a treatment for ischemic heart disease and myocardial infarction.[32] There have been a few small-scale, relatively short-term studies suggesting functional benefits in ischemic cardiomyopathy.[92] For example, GIK may improve wall motion scores, end-systolic ventricular size, and peak systolic velocity in patients with ischemic cardiomyopathy.[92] The feasibility of GIK for the treatment of heart failure, however, is limited, because (1) it is delivered by an intravenous route, (2) the fluid volume given, and (3) the relative difficulty of frequently monitoring blood glucose and potassium levels and adjusting the glucose drip. Thus metabolic modulator therapy that can be given orally is more appealing for the heart failure patient.

Oral Lipid-Lowering Agents

The excessive fatty acid and/or triglyceride delivery to the heart in obesity and diabetes-related heart failure is an attractive target for the development of new treatments. Thiazolidinediones (predominantly PPARγ agonists) reduce plasma lipid levels. However, their use in heart failure is limited because of a "black box warning" of increased cardiovascular events.[2] Another drug, acipimox, known to markedly and acutely decrease plasma free fatty acid levels, *impairs* cardiac output and cardiac efficiency in dilated cardiomyopathy patients.[2] Acipimox also decreases cardiac output (but improves efficiency) in normal healthy controls, but there were far fewer controls studied than patients, so the effect was not statistically significant. However, the results of this study taken together with the fact that the adult human heart normally uses predominantly fatty acids

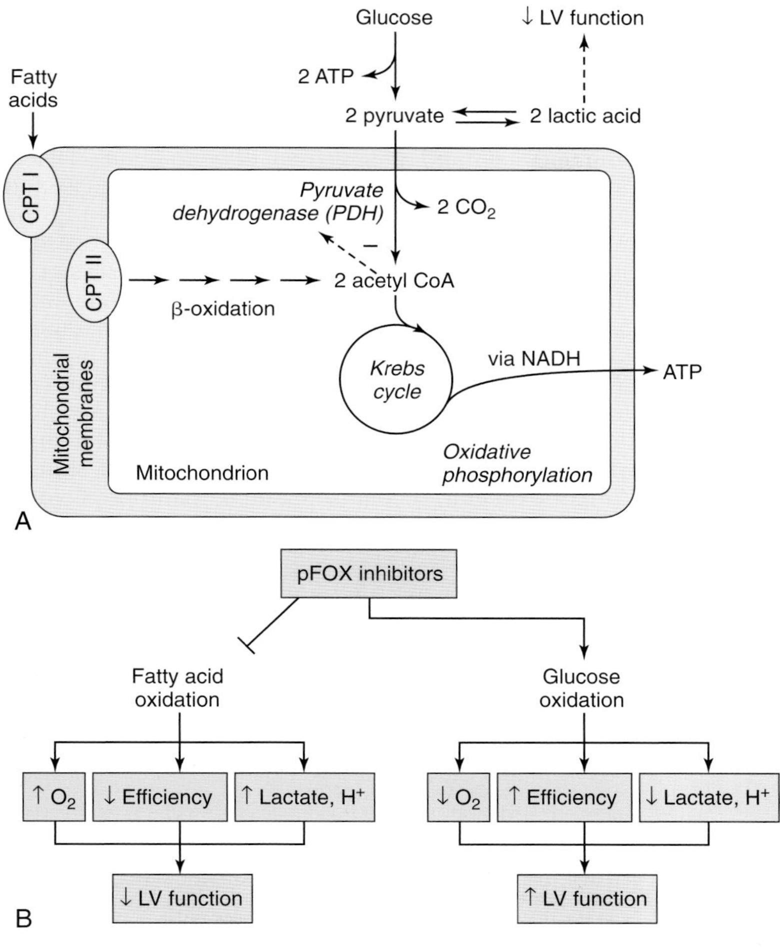

FIGURE 16-12 Metabolic modulation of heart failure. **A,** Metabolic pathway for glucose metabolism and fatty acid oxidation; **B,** Effects of switching metabolism from fatty acid β-oxidation to glucose oxidation (under conditions wherein oxygen supply is rate limiting) using partial inhibitors of fatty acid oxidation (pFOX). *CPT,* Carnitine-palmitoyl transferase. *From Dimmeler S, Mann D, Zeiher AM: Emerging therapies and strategies in the treatment of heart failure. In Libby P, Bonow RO, Mann DL, et al, editors: Braunwald's heart disease, Philadelphia, 2008, Saunders, pp 697–715.*

suggest that the heart needs to be able to use both fatty acids and glucose. Excessive increase *or decrease* in the metabolism of either fuel for prolonged periods of time will likely be detrimental.

Trimetazidine

Unlike the drug therapies listed above, trimetazidine does not primarily decrease plasma fatty acid availability; rather it partially inhibits fatty acid oxidation. Trimetazidine is thought to be cardioprotective because it modulates energy substrate metabolism. Trimetazidine may also have antioxidative properties. Trimetazidine decreases long-chain fatty acid oxidation by inhibition of 3 ketoacyl-CoA thiolase.[2] This decrease in fatty acid oxidation leads to an increase in carbohydrate oxidation. This switch in energy substrate preference results in improved coupling between glycolysis and glucose oxidation, thereby decreasing proton and Na^+ accumulation. There are a few small clinical trials showing that trimetazidine improves heart failure.[2] In one randomized study, those heart failure patients receiving trimetazidine realized improvements in their functional class and LV function. In a PET study, trimetazidine modestly decreased myocardial fatty acid oxidation without changing overall oxygen consumption, implying but not proving an increase in glucose oxidation.[2] However, trimetazidine has limited availability and is not U.S. Food and Drug Administration (FDA)–approved for use in the United States.

Ranolazine

Like trimetazidine, ranolazine belongs to the family of piperazine derivatives, which partially inhibit fatty acid oxidation and hence enhance glucose oxidation.[93] There is also evidence that ranolazine may reduce calcium overload in ischemic myocardium. Activity of PDC, a key regulator of glucose oxidation, increases after ranolazine treatment, most likely due to decreased inhibitory effects of end products of β-oxidation (NADH, acetyl-CoA)[47] or because of changes in the phosphorylation state. There are also data showing that ranolazine improves myocardial efficiency and LV systolic function in animal models of chronic heart failure.[2] To date there are no data on ranolazine's effects on myocardial metabolism in humans with heart failure, so it has no indication for heart failure treatment at present.

Perhexiline

This drug inhibits fatty acid oxidation by inhibiting carnitine-palmitoyl transferase (CPT)-1. Results of studies in humans with heart failure are mixed. In one study of patients with heart failure and angina pain, there were improvements in heart failure symptoms, Vo_2 max, skeletal muscle energetics, and myocardial function.[2] In another study of patients with ischemic cardiomyopathy (but no angina), neither hospital admission rates nor exercise performance improved.[2] Perhexiline is available in Australia and New Zealand. Monitoring plasma drug levels of perhexiline and

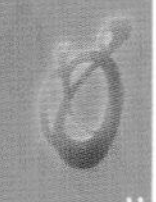

cis-hydroxyperhexiline is recommended to prevent liver and peripheral nerve toxicity.

Propionyl-L-Carnitine

Propionyl-L-carnitine (PLC) has been shown to improve postischemic contractile performance in the heart, presumably through redistribution of long-chain acyl-CoA esters to less toxic intermediates.[94] In the failing heart, PLC may improve energy metabolism by three possible mechanisms. First, PLC provides propionate. As a precursor of succinyl-CoA, propionate may replenish citric acid cycle intermediates.[95] Second, PLC may raise the levels of free CoASH and improves flux through α-ketoglutarate dehydrogenase. Third, PLC may redistribute carnitine levels between cytosol and mitochondria, and improve fatty acid oxidation in the stressed heart.[96] Collectively it appears that PLC (and possibly also carnitine)[97] improves substrate flux, and possibly also contractile function of the heart. Indeed, alterations in substrate metabolism produced by carnitine deficiency result in inadequate ATP production under high workload conditions that cause impaired cardiac contractile performance, and carnitine deficiency may also induce a number of changes in gene expression of key enzymes required for normal cardiac function and metabolism.[98] Chronic cardiomyopathy has been described in children with a defect in carnitine uptake,[99] and systemic carnitine deficiency has been identified as a treatable cardiomyopathy.[100]

SUMMARY AND FUTURE DIRECTIONS

The human heart produces and uses several kilograms of ATP each day. ATP production is linked to a highly regulated system of energy substrate metabolism and is tightly coupled to both oxygen consumption and contractile function of the heart. Intermediary metabolites provide essential signals for pathways of adaptation and maladaptation of the heart to external stimuli (**Figure 16-13**). Because heart failure is a systemic disease that begins and ends with the heart, an appreciation of the principles of myocardial energy metabolism is essential for the understanding of heart failure. Although we already possess a wealth of information on the biochemistry of the heart, we have yet to fully determine how this information can be integrated into the diagnosis and management of heart failure. Defective energy metabolism of the heart is both cause and consequence of heart failure and can be detected in the whole heart by noninvasive methods, or in myocardial biopsy samples by gene or protein expression assays or by biochemical analyses. Pharmacologic and nutritional interventions targeted at the specific myocardial metabolic alterations of particular causes of heart failure hold promise for reversing defective energy metabolism and improving contractile function of the heart. Without an appreciation of the pivotal role of metabolism in the process of adaptation and maladaptation of the heart to external stimuli, we cannot expect to recognize essential pathophysiologic clues to improve future prevention and treatment of heart failure.

Altered environment
(e.g., workload, substrate availability, hormones)
↓
Altered signal transduction
(e.g., AMPK, PI3K, PKC)
↓
Altered metabolism
(e.g., glucose transport, pyruvate oxidation, β-oxidation)
↓
Altered metabolic signals
(e.g., physiologic accumulation of glucose and fatty acid metabolites)
↓
Altered transcription and translation factor activities
(e.g., Sp1, USF1/2, c-myc, eIF2a)
↓
Altered gene and protein expression
(e.g., induction of fetal proteins, growth factors)
↓
Adaptation (which may become maladaptive over time or in particular conditions)

FIGURE 16-13 The sequence of steps leading from altered environment to altered gene and protein expression (see text for details).

References

1. Neubauer S: The failing heart—an engine out of fuel. *N Engl J Med* 356:1140–1151, 2007.
2. Kadkhodayan A, Coggan AR, Peterson LR: A "PET" area of interest: myocardial metabolism in human systolic heart failure. *Heart Fail Rev* 18:567–574, 2013.
3. Hue L, Taegtmeyer H: The Randle cycle revisited: a new head for an old hat. *Am J Physiol Endocrinol Metab* 297:E578–E591, 2009.
4. Taegtmeyer H: Carbohydrate interconversions and energy production. *Circulation* 72:IV1–IV8, 1985.
5. Stanley WC, Recchia FA, Lopaschuk GD: Myocardial substrate metabolism in the normal and failing heart. *Physiol Rev* 85:1093–1129, 2005.
6. Taegtmeyer H: Energy metabolism of the heart: from basic concepts to clinical applications. *Curr Probl Cardiol* 19:59–113, 1994.
7. Peterson LR, Mckenzie CR, Schaffer JE: Diabetic cardiovascular disease: getting to the heart of the matter. *J Cardiovasc Transl Res* 5:436–445, 2012.
8. Russell RR, Taegtmeyer H: Coenzyme a sequestration in rat hearts oxidizing ketone bodies. *J Clin Invest* 89:968–973, 1992.
9. Taegtmeyer H: Metabolic responses to cardiac hypoxia: increased production of succinate by rabbit papillary muscles. *Circ Res* 43:808–815, 1978.
10. Blain JM: Studies in myocardial metabolism. VI. Myocardial metabolism in congestive heart failure. *Am J Med* 820–833, 1956.
11. Szczepaniak LS, Dobbins RL, Metzger GJ, et al: Myocardial triglycerides and systolic function in humans: in vivo evaluation by localized proton spectroscopy and cardiac imaging. *Magn Reson Med* 49:417–423, 2003.
12. Schroeder MA, Clarke K, Neubauer S, et al: Hyperpolarized magnetic resonance: a novel technique for the in vivo assessment of cardiovascular disease. *Circulation* 124:1580–1594, 2011.
13. Peterson LR, Gropler RJ: Radionuclide imaging of myocardial metabolism. *Circ Cardiovasc Imaging* 3:211–222, 2010.
14. Rajabi M, Kassiotis C, Razeghi P, et al: Return to the fetal gene program protects the stressed heart: a strong hypothesis. *Heart Fail Rev* 12:331–343, 2007.
15. Razeghi P, Young ME, Cockrill TC, et al: Downregulation of myocardial myocyte enhancer factor 2c and myocyte enhancer factor 2c-regulated gene expression in diabetic patients with nonischemic heart failure. *Circulation* 106:407–411, 2002.
16. Chokshi A, Drosatos K, Cheema FH, et al: Ventricular assist device implantation corrects myocardial lipotoxicity, reverses insulin resistance, and normalizes cardiac metabolism in patients with advanced heart failure. *Circulation* 125:2844–2853, 2012.
17. Burkart EM, Sambandam N, Han X, et al: Nuclear receptors PPARbeta/delta and PPARalpha direct distinct metabolic regulatory programs in the mouse heart. *J Clin Invest* 117:3930–3939, 2007.
18. Cheng L, Ding G, Qin Q, et al: Cardiomyocyte-restricted peroxisome proliferator-activated receptor-delta deletion perturbs myocardial fatty acid oxidation and leads to cardiomyopathy. *Nat Med* 10:1245–1250, 2004.
19. Huss JM, Imahashi K, Dufour CR, et al: The nuclear receptor erralpha is required for the bioenergetic and functional adaptation to cardiac pressure overload. *Cell Metab* 6:25–37, 2007.
20. Sihag S, Cresci S, Li AY, et al: Pgc-1alpha and erralpha target gene downregulation is a signature of the failing human heart. *J Mol Cell Cardiol* 46:201–212, 2009.
21. Ning XH, Zhang J, Liu J, et al: Signaling and expression for mitochondrial membrane proteins during left ventricular remodeling and contractile failure after myocardial infarction. *J Am Coll Cardiol* 36:282–287, 2000.
22. Dorner A, Schulze K, Rauch U, et al: Adenine nucleotide translocator in dilated cardiomyopathy: pathophysiological alterations in expression and function. *Mol Cell Biochem* 174:261–269, 1997.
23. Ide T, Tsutsui H, Hayashidani S, et al: Mitochondrial DNA damage and dysfunction associated with oxidative stress in failing hearts after myocardial infarction. *Circ Res* 88:529–535, 2001.
24. Schilling J, Kelly DP: The PGC-1 cascade as a therapeutic target for heart failure. *J Mol Cell Cardiol* 51:578–583, 2011.
25. Lamb HJ, Smit JW, Van Der Meer RW, et al: Metabolic MRI of myocardial and hepatic triglyceride content in response to nutritional interventions. *Curr Opin Clin Nutr Metab Care* 11:573–579, 2008.
26. Coaes P, Tanaka K: Molecular basis of mitochondrial fatty acid oxidation defects. *J Lipd Res* 33:1099–1110, 1992.
27. Jamshidi Y, Montgomery H, Hense H, et al: Peroxisome proliferator-activated receptor alpa gene regulates left ventricular growth in response to exercise and hypertension. *Circulation* 105:950–955, 2002.

28. Cresci S, Jones PG, Sucharov CC, et al: Interaction between PPARA genotype and beta-blocker treatment influences clinical outcomes following acute coronary syndromes. *Pharmacogenomics* 9:1403–1417, 2009.
29. Ashrafian H, Redwood C, Blair E, et al: Hypertrophic cardiomyopathy: a paradigm for myocardial energy depletion. *Trends Genet* 19:263–268, 2003.
30. Leme AM, Salemi VM, Parga JR, et al: Evaluation of the metabolism of high energy phosphates in patients with Chagas' disease. *Arq Bras Cardiol* 95:264–270, 2010.
31. El-Sharkawy AM, Gabr RE, Schar M, et al: Quantification of human high-energy phosphate metabolite concentrations at 3 T with partial volume and sensitivity corrections. *NMR Biomed* 26:1363–1371, 2013.
32. Depre C, Vanoverschelde JL, Taegtmeyer H: Glucose for the heart. *Circulation* 99:578–588, 1999.
33. Taegtmeyer H: Genetics of energetics: transcriptional responses in cardiac metabolism. *Ann Biomed Eng* 28:871–876, 2000.
34. Taegtmeyer H, Overturf ML: Effects of moderate hypertension on cardiac function and metabolism in the rabbit. *Hypertension* 11:416–426, 1988.
35. Doenst T, Goodwin GW, Cedars AM, et al: Load-induced changes in vivo alter substrate fluxes and insulin responsiveness of rat heart in vitro. *Metabolism* 50:1083–1090, 2001.
36. Van Bilsen M, Van Der Vusse GJ, Reneman RS: Transcriptional regulation of metabolic processes: implications for cardiac metabolism. *Pflugers Arch* 437:2–14, 1998.
37. Hayashi T, Hirshman MF, Kurth EJ, et al: Evidence for 5'AMP-activated protein kinase mediation of the effect of muscle contraction on glucose transport. *Diabetes* 47:1369–1373, 1998.
38. Kolwicz SCJ, Olson DP, Marney LC, et al: Cardiac-specific deletion of acetyl CoA carboxylase 2 prevents metabolic remodeling during pressure-overload hypertrophy. *Circ Res* 111:728–738, 2012.
39. He L, Kim T, Long Q, et al: Carnitine palmitoyltransferase-1b deficiency aggravates pressure overload-induced cardiac hypertrophy caused by lipotoxicity. *Circulation* 126:1705–1716, 2012.
40. Liao R, Jain M, Cui L, et al: Cardiac-specific overexpression of GLUT1 prevents the development of heart failure attributable to pressure overload in mice. *Circulation* 106:2125–2131, 2002.
41. Kenchaiah S, Evans JC, Levy D, et al: Obesity and the risk of heart failure. *N Engl J Med* 347:305–313, 2002.
42. Sharma S, Adrogue JV, Golfman L, et al: Intramyocardial lipid accumulation in the failing human heart resembles the lipotoxic rat heart. *FASEB J* 18:1692–1700, 2004.
43. Zhou YT, Grayburn P, Karim A, et al: Lipotoxic heart disease in obese rats: implications for human obesity. *Proc Natl Acad Sci U S A* 97:1784–1789, 2000.
44. Hammer S, Snel M, Lamb HJ, et al: Prolonged caloric restriction in obese patients with type 2 diabetes mellitus decreases myocardial triglyceride content and improves myocardial function. *J Am Coll Cardiol* 52:1006–1012, 2008.
45. Peterson LR, Herrero P, Schechtman KB, et al: Effect of obesity and insulin resistance on myocardial substrate metabolism and efficiency in young women. *Circulation* 109:2191–2196, 2004.
46. Peterson LR, Waggoner AD, Schechtman KB, et al: Alterations in left ventricular structure and function in young healthy obese women: assessment by echocardiography and tissue doppler imaging. *J Am Coll Cardiol* 43:1399–1404, 2004.
47. Clarke B, Wyatt KM, McCormack JG: Ranolazine increases active pyruvate dehydrogenase in perfused normoxic rat hearts: evidence for an indirect mechanism. *J Mol Cell Cardiol* 28:341–350, 1996.
48. Lin CH, Kurup S, Herrero P, et al: Myocardial oxygen consumption change predicts left ventricular relaxation improvement in obese humans after weight loss. *Obesity (Silver Spring)* 19:1804–1812, 2011.
49. Ramani GV, Mccloskey C, Ramanathan RC, et al: Safety and efficacy of bariatric surgery in morbidly obese patients with severe systolic heart failure. *Clin Cardiol* 31:516–520, 2008.
50. Schilling JD, Mann DL: Diabetic cardiomyopathy: bench to bedside. *Heart Fail Clin* 8:619–631, 2012.
51. Chambers KT, Leone TC, Sambandam N, et al: Chronic inhibition of pyruvate dehydrogenase in heart triggers an adaptive metabolic response. *J Biol Chem* 286:11155–11162, 2011.
52. Liu X, Wang J, Takeda N, et al: Changes in cardiac protein kinase C activities and isozymes in streptozotocin-induced diabetes. *Am J Physiol* 277:E798–E804, 1999.
53. Stumpe T, Decking UK, Schrader J: Nitric oxide reduces energy supply by direct action on the respiratory chain in isolated cardiomyocytes. *Am J Physiol Heart Circ Physiol* 280:H2350–H2356, 2001.
54. Loke KE, Mcconnell PI, Tuzman JM, et al: Endogenous endothelial nitric oxide synthase-derived nitric oxide is a physiological regulator of myocardial oxygen consumption. *Circ Res* 84:840–845, 1999.
55. Rozec B, Erfanian M, Laurent K, et al: Nebivolol, a vasodilating selective beta(1)-blocker, is a beta(3)-adrenoceptor agonist in the nonfailing transplanted human heart. *J Am Coll Cardiol* 53:1532–1538, 2009.
56. Rudiger A, Singer M: Mechanisms of sepsis-induced cardiac dysfunction. *Crit Care Med* 35:1599–1608, 2007.
57. Kapadia S, Dibbs Z, Kurrelmeyer K, et al: The role of cytokines in the failing human heart. *Cardiol Clin* 16:645–656, 1998.
58. Mann DL, Kneuferman P, Baumgarten G: Cytokines in ischemic heart disease and heart failure. *Dialog Cardiovasc Med* 5:135–146, 2000.
59. Zell R, Geck P, Werdan K, et al: TNF-alpha and il-1 alpha inhibit both pyruvate dehydrogenase activity and mitochondrial function in cardiomyocytes: evidence for primary impairment of mitochondrial function. *Mol Cell Biochem* 177:61–67, 1997.
60. Tatsumi T, Matoba D, Kawahara A, et al: Cytokine-induced nitric oxide production inhibits mitochondrial energy production and impairs contractile function in rat cardiac myocytes. *J Am Coll Cardiol* 35:1338–1346, 2000.
61. Lin WJ, Yeh WC: Implication of toll-like receptor and tumor necrosis factor alpha signaling in septic shock. *Shock* 24:206–209, 2005.
62. Cook SA, Matsui T, Li L, et al: Transcriptional effects of chronic akt activation in the heart. *J Biol Chem* 277:22528–22533, 2002.
63. Jonassen AK, Sack MN, Mjos OD, et al: Myocardial protection by insulin at reperfusion requires early administration and is mediated via akt and P70s6 kinase cell-survival signaling. *Circ Res* 89:1191–1198, 2001.
64. Gottlob K, Majewski N, Kennedy S, et al: Inhibition of early apoptotic events by Akt/pkb is dependent on the first committed step of glycolysis and mitochondrial hexokinase. *Genes Dev* 15:1406–1418, 2001.
65. Schilling J, Lai L, Sambandam N, et al: Toll-like receptor-mediated inflammatory signaling reprograms cardiac energy metabolism by repressing peroxisome proliferator-activated receptor gamma coactivator-1 signaling. *Circ Heart Fail* 4:474–482, 2011.
66. Drosatos K, Drosatos-Tampakaki Z, Khan R, et al: Inhibition of c-jun-N-terminal kinase increases cardiac peroxisome proliferator-activated receptor alpha expression and fatty acid oxidation and prevents lipopolysaccharide-induced heart dysfunction. *J Biol Chem* 286:36331–36339, 2011.
67. Sekiguchi K, Tian Q, Ishiyama M: Inhibition of PPAR-alpha activity in mice with cardiac-restricted expression of tumor necrosis factor: potential role of TGF-beta/smad3. *Am J Physiol Heart Circ Physiol* 292:H1443–H1451, 2007.
68. Depre C, Taegtmeyer H: Metabolic aspects of programmed cell survival and cell death in the heart. *Cardiovasc Res* 45:538–548, 2000.
69. Jackson SP, Tjian R: O-glycosylation of eukaryotic transcription factors: implications for mechanisms of transcriptional regulation. *Cell* 55:125–133, 1988.
70. Malhotra R, Brosius FC: Glucose uptake and glycolysis reduce hypoxia-induced apoptosis in cultured neonatal rat cardiac myocytes. *J Biol Chem* 274:12567–12575, 1999.
71. Zhou L, Huang H, Yuan CL, et al: Metabolic response to an acute jump in cardiac workload: effects on malonyl-CoA, mechanical efficiency, and fatty acid oxidation. *Am J Physiol Heart Circ Physiol* 294:H954–H960, 2008.
72. Zhu P, Lu L, Xu Y, et al: Troglitazone improves recovery of left ventricular function after regional ischemia in pigs. *Circulation* 101:1165–1171, 2000.
73. Doenst T, Richwine RT, Bray MS, et al: Insulin improves functional and metabolic recovery of reperfused working rat heart. *Ann Thorac Surg* 67:1682–1688, 1999.
74. Saltiel AR, Kahn CR: Insulin signalling and the regulation of glucose and lipid metabolism. *Nature* 414:799–806, 2001.
75. Shioi T, Kang PM, Douglas PS, et al: The conserved phosphoinositide 3-kinase pathway determines heart size in mice. *EMBO J* 19:2537–2548, 2000.
76. Matsui T, Tao J, Del Monte F, et al: Akt activation preserves cardiac function and prevents injury after transient cardiac ischemia in vivo. *Circulation* 104:330–335, 2001.
77. Shelton ME, Dence CS, Hwang DR, et al: In vivo delineation of myocardial hypoxia during coronary occlusion using fluorine-18 fluoromisonidazole and positron emission tomography: a potential approach for identification of jeopardized myocardium. *J Am Coll Cardiol* 16:477–485, 1990.
78. Robey RB, Ma J, Santos AV, et al: Regulation of mesangial cell hexokinase activity and expression by heparin-binding epidermal growth factor-like growth factor: epidermal growth factors and phorbol esters increase glucose metabolism via a common mechanism involving classic mitogen-activated protein kinase pathway activation and induction of hexokinase ii expression. *J Biol Chem* 277:14370–14378, 2002.
79. Tian R, Musi N, D'agostino J, et al: Increased adenosine monophosphate-activated protein kinase activity in rat hearts with pressure-overload hypertrophy. *Circulation* 104:1664–1669, 2001.
80. Bialik S, Cryns VL, Drincic A, et al: The mitochondrial apoptotic pathway is activated by serum and glucose deprivation in cardiac myocytes. *Circ Res* 85:403–414, 1999.
81. Schaffer SW, Croft CB, Solodushko V: Cardioprotective effect of chronic hyperglycemia: effect on hypoxia-induced apoptosis and necrosis. *Am J Physiol Heart Circ Physiol* 278:1948–1954, 2000.
82. Moley KH, Mueckler MM: Glucose transport and apoptosis. *Apoptosis* 5:99–105, 2000.
83. Unger RH, Orci L: Diseases of liporegulation: new perspective on obesity and related disorders. *FASEB J* 15:312–321, 2001.
84. Gudz TI, Tserng KY, Hoppel CL: Direct inhibition of mitochondrial respiratory chain complex iii by cell-permeable ceramide. *J Biol Chem* 272:24154–24158, 1997.
85. Schilling JD, Machkovech HM, He L, et al: TLR4 activation under lipotoxic conditions leads to synergistic macrophage cell death through a TRIF-dependent pathway. *J Immunol* 190:1285–1296, 2013.
86. Listenberger LL, Ory DS, Schaffer JE: Palmitate-induced apoptosis can occur through a ceramide-independent pathway. *J Biol Chem* 276:14890–14895, 2001.
87. Beanlands RS, Nahmias C, Gordon E, et al: The effects of beta(1)-blockade on oxidative metabolism and the metabolic cost of ventricular work in patients with left ventricular dysfunction: a double-blind, placebo-controlled, positron-emission tomography study. *Circulation* 102:2070–2075, 2000.
88. Ukkonen H, Beanlands RS, Burwash IG, et al: Effect of cardiac resynchronization on myocardial efficiency and regional oxidative metabolism. *Circulation* 107:28–31, 2003.
89. Nowak B, Sinha AM, Schaefer WM, et al: Cardiac resynchronization therapy homogenizes myocardial glucose metabolism and perfusion in dilated cardiomyopathy and left bundle branch block. *J Am Coll Cardiol* 41:1523–1528, 2003.
90. Neri G, Zanco P, Zanon F, et al: Effect of biventricular pacing on metabolism and perfusion in patients affected by dilated cardiomyopathy and left bundle branch block: evaluation by positron emission tomography. *Europace* 5:111–115, 2003.
91. Kassiotis C, Ballal K, Wellnitz K, et al: Markers of autophagy are downregulated in failing human heart after mechanical unloading. *Circulation* 120:S191–S197, 2009.
92. Khoury VK, Haluska B, Prins J, et al: Effects of glucose-insulin-potassium infusion on chronic ischaemic left ventricular dysfunction. *Heart* 89:61–65, 2003.
93. Zacharowski K, Blackburn B, Thiemermann C: Ranolazine, a partial fatty acid oxidation inhibitor, reduces myocardial infarct size and cardiac troponin t release in the rat. *Eur J Pharmacol* 418:105–110, 2001.
94. Di Lisa F, Menabo R, Siliprandi N: L-propionyl-carnitine protection of mitochondria in ischemic rat hearts. *Mol Cell Biochem* 88:169–173, 1989.
95. Russell RR, Mommessin JI, Taegtmeyer H: Propionyl-L-carnitine-mediated improvement in contractile function of rat hearts oxidizing acetoacetate. *Am J Physiol* 268:H441–H447, 1995.
96. Paulson DJ, Traxler J, Schmidt M, et al: Protection of the ischaemic myocardium by L-propionylcarnitine: effects on the recovery of cardiac output after ischaemia and reperfusion, carnitine transport, and fatty acid oxidation. *Cardiovasc Res* 20:536–541, 1986.
97. Opie LH: Role of carnitine in fatty acid metabolism of normal and ischemic myocardium. *Am Heart J* 97:375–388, 1979.
98. Kaido M, Fujimura H, Ono A, et al: Mitochondrial abnormalities in a murine model of primary carnitine deficiency. Systemic pathology and trial of replacement therapy. *Eur Neurol* 38:302–309, 1997.
99. Stanley CA, Deleeuw S, Coates PM, et al: Chronic cardiomyopathy and weakness or acute coma in children with a defect in carnitine uptake. *Ann Neurol* 30:709–716, 1991.
100. Tripp ME, Katcher ML, Peters HA, et al: Systemic carnitine deficiency presenting as familial endocardial fibroelastosis: a treatable cardiomyopathy. *N Engl J Med* 305:385–390, 1981.

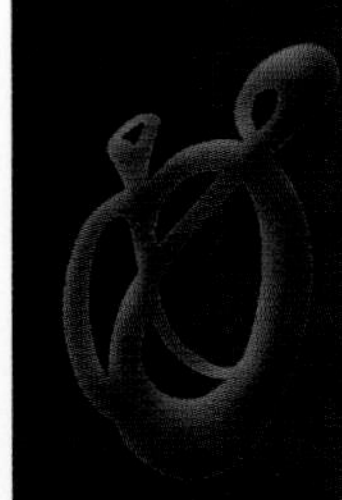

SECTION III

Etiological Basis for Heart Failure

17 Epidemiology of Heart Failure

Andreas P. Kalogeropoulos, Vasiliki V. Georgiopoulou, and Javed Butler

Improved therapies and outcomes of acute cardiac conditions, aging of the population, increasing prevalence of lifestyle-related risk factors, and advances in heart failure (HF) therapy all have led to an ever-increasing prevalence of HF. Because of these trends, HF is currently considered an "epidemic" and a public health priority in developed countries[1-3] and is emerging as major noncommunicable syndrome in developing regions.[4,5] The lack of specific prevention strategies for HF compounds the problem. In the United States, the population prevalence of HF is projected to increase by 23% in the next 20 years.[3]

Heart failure has a high lifetime incidence and serious prognosis, especially after a hospitalization for decompensation. For a middle-aged person, the lifetime risk for HF is estimated at 20% to 30%.[6-8] In recent registries, 1-year mortality after a hospitalization for HF ranges between 25% and 35% and is remarkably consistent across health care systems.[1,2,9,10] Among outpatients, 5-year survival is 50% to 75%.[7,11-13] Heart failure affects quality of life adversely also.[14] From a public health perspective, beyond the direct impact on survival and quality of life, the burgeoning burden imposed on health care systems in terms of resources and costs is another major consideration. The total direct cost of HF in the United States is projected to increase from $21 billion in 2012 to $53 billion in 2030.[3]

PREVALENCE

Estimates and Trends

Age is a major determinant of incidence and prevalence of HF, and therefore, the aging of the population worldwide is expected to have a dramatic impact on the burden of HF. In the United States, prevalence estimates for HF are mainly derived from the National Health and Nutrition Examination Survey (NHANES) (**Figure 17-1**). Based on 2007 to 2010 data, it is estimated that 5.1 million Americans aged 20 years or older have HF[15] and population prevalence for 2012 is estimated at 2.4%.[3] By year 2030, the population prevalence of HF in the United States is projected to reach 3.0%.[3]

Heart failure prevalence is considerably higher among middle-aged or older adults. In the Rotterdam study, a cohort study of approximately 8000 adults aged 55 years or older at inception (1989-1993), the prevalence of HF in the 1998 annual examination was 8.0% in men and 6.0% in women, with a sharp rise with age.[7] The prevalence was 0.9%, 4.0%, 9.7%, and 17.4% in participants age 55 to 64, 65 to 74, 75 to 84, and 85 or older, respectively. In a sample of over 600,000 Medicare beneficiaries in the United States (persons aged 65 years or older) from years 1994 to 2003, the period prevalence of HF was 13.0% among men and 11.5% among women.[16] Importantly, despite decreasing incidence, HF prevalence increased steadily between 1994 and 2000, and this trend was evident among both men and women (**Figure 17-2**).

Prevalence of Preclinical (Stage A and B) Heart Failure (see also Chapter 32)

As with most chronic diseases, HF is usually a progressive condition amenable to preventive interventions at the early stages of the process. To emphasize this concept, the American Heart Association and the American College of Cardiology proposed a model that classifies HF into four stages: stage A, HF risk factors; stage B, asymptomatic cardiac structural or functional abnormalities; stage C, symptomatic HF; and stage D, advanced HF.[17]

Limited prospective data exist on the population prevalence of stages A and B. In a cross-sectional study of over 2000 residents aged 45 years or older in Olmsted County, Minn.,[13] 22% of participants were classified as stage A on the basis of hypertension, diabetes mellitus, obesity, or coronary artery disease (without myocardial infarction [MI]), without abnormal left ventricular (LV) structure or function; 34% were classified as stage B based on electrocardiographic or echocardiographic evidence of prior MI, LV hypertrophy, valvular heart disease, wall-motion abnormality, LV enlargement, and systolic and diastolic dysfunction. Manifest (stage C) and advanced (stage D) HF were present in 12% and 0.2% of participants, respectively (**Figure 17-3**).[13]

Lower prevalence of stage B HF has been reported in cohort studies with more stringent, cardiac imaging-based criteria. In the Dallas Heart study,[18] 284 of 2277 participants (12.5%) aged 30 to 65 years had abnormalities consistent with HF stage B (LV hypertrophy, reduced LV ejection fraction [EF], or prior MI) on cardiac magnetic resonance imaging. Among 296 men (age, 63 ± 11) and 443 women (age, 61 ± 10) in Portugal,[19] stage B, defined as echocardiographic LV hypertrophy, dilation, or systolic dysfunction, was present in 21.6% of men and 21.2% of women. Stage A risk factors were present in 54.4% and 43.8% of men and women, respectively.

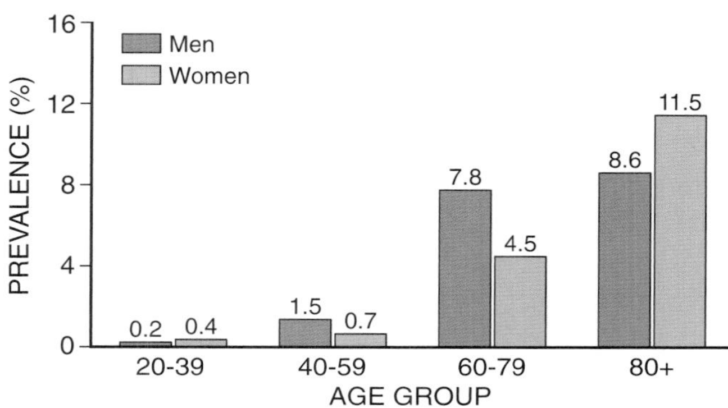

FIGURE 17-1 Prevalence of heart failure by gender and age in the United States. *National Health and Nutrition Examination Survey: 2007-2010.*

INCIDENCE

Contemporary Characteristics and Population Incidence of Heart Failure

Most contemporary data on the characteristics and population incidence of new HF cases come from large health care databases. In a recent study of approximately 12,000 new HF cases identified between 2005 and 2008 among adults enrolled in a major health care plan in the United States, 46% of cases were women and 73% were over age 65.[20] Of note, 52% of cases had preserved (≥50%) EF, and these patients were more likely to be women and older than age 65. Less than 25% of new HF cases had previous acute coronary syndrome or history of revascularization; however,

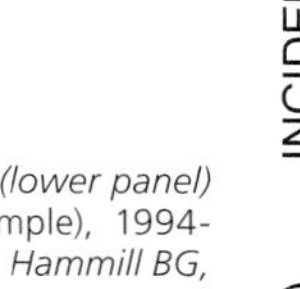

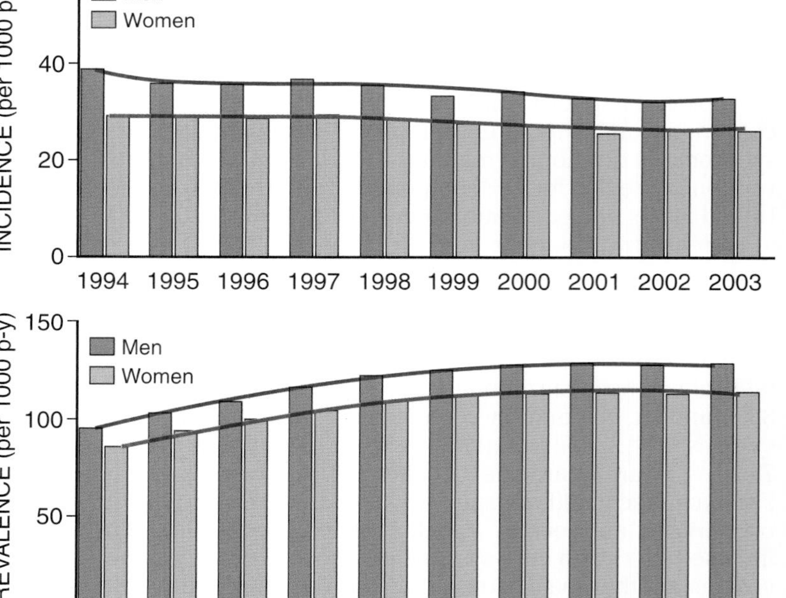

FIGURE 17-2 Incidence *(upper panel)* and prevalence *(lower panel)* of heart failure among Medicare beneficiaries (5% sample), 1994-2003. *p-y,* Person-years. *Data from Curtis LH, Whellan DJ, Hammill BG, et al: Incidence and prevalence of heart failure in elderly persons, 1994-2003. Arch Intern Med 168:418–424, 2008.*

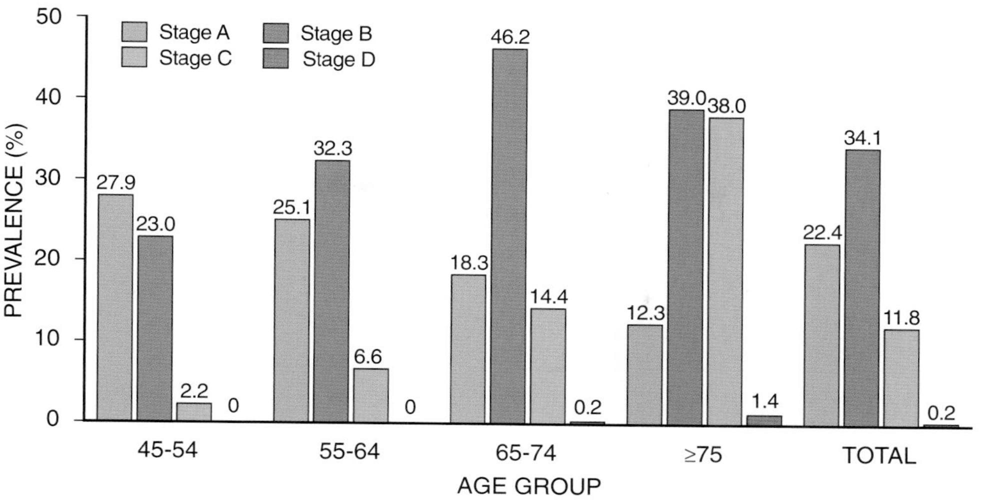

FIGURE 17-3 Prevalence of heart failure stages in Olmsted County, Minn. *Data from Ammar KA, Jacobsen SJ, Mahoney DW, et al: Prevalence and prognostic significance of heart failure stages: application of the American College of Cardiology/American Heart Association heart failure staging criteria in the community. Circulation 115:1563–1570, 2007.*

over 20% had cerebrovascular disease and 30% had atrial fibrillation or flutter. Hypertension was present in 75% and diabetes mellitus in 19%, whereas 35% had concomitant chronic lung disease. Renal dysfunction (estimated glomerular filtration rate <60 mL/min/1.73 m^2) and anemia (hemoglobin <13 g/L in men and <12 g/L in women) were present in over 40% and 30% of cases, respectively. Depression and dementia were present in 16% and 7% of cases, respectively.[20] These data demonstrate a shift from a model where HF was mainly a consequence of coronary artery disease with male preponderance toward a condition of older adults that equally affects both sexes and is accompanied by a complex medical profile.

Among 360,000 adults enrolled in a large, managed care organization in Georgia, the population incidence of HF as determined by administrative data from 2000 to 2005 was 3.9 cases per 1000 patient-years.[21] Incidence was higher in men compared with women (4.2 versus 3.7 per 1000 patient-years); however, among the 4000 new cases, more than 50% were women. Incidence increased dramatically with age, with men demonstrating higher rates before age 75; however, sex-based differences were no longer evident in the 75-year or older age group (**Figure 17-4A**).[21]

Incidence of Heart Failure in Cohort Studies: Impact of Age, Gender, and Race (see also Chapter 37)

In most cohort studies, the incidence of HF reflects the age selection criteria of participants. However, cohort studies provide a clearer picture of gender- and race-related differences in HF incidence, because they are less prone to health care access disparities that may influence estimates obtained from health care databases.

In the Health, Aging, and Body Composition (Health ABC) study, which enrolled over 3000 well-functioning participants aged 70 to 79 years between 1997 and 1998, the incidence of HF over 7 years of follow-up was 15.8 and 11.7 per 1000 person-years in men and women, respectively,[22] reflecting the effect of age on HF incidence. Men and black participants were more likely to develop HF (see Figure 17-4B). In the Atherosclerosis Risk in Communities (ARIC), a population-based study that recruited over 15,000 participants aged 45 to 64 years between 1987 and 1989, the age-adjusted incidence of new HF hospitalizations was 5.7 per 1000 person-years between 1987 and 2002.[23] Although incidence rates were greater for blacks (men, 9.1; women, 8.1) than whites (6.0 and 3.4, respectively) (see Figure 17-4C and D), adjustment for confounders attenuated the difference; hence, the greater HF incidence in blacks could be largely explained by the higher prevalence of risk factors among blacks at cohort inception.[23] Of note, because surveillance for new HF cases was based on hospitalization in both studies, the incidence of HF was likely underestimated in ARIC and Health ABC. In the Rotterdam study (Netherlands), which included surveillance data from outpatient records in addition to hospital discharge records, HF incidence after 7.1 years of follow-up was considerably higher: 17.6 per 1000 in men and 12.5 per 1000 in women, despite a younger population (age 55 or older).[7]

Lifetime Risk of Heart Failure

Several prospective studies have estimated the lifetime risk for HF in the general population. In the Rotterdam study, after accounting for the competing risk of non-HF mortality, the lifetime risk of HF for a person aged 55 years was 30.2% (33.0% for men and 28.5% for women) and declined after age 75.[7] Lifetime HF risks were higher in men than women age 55 to 75 years, but in subjects aged 85 years or older risks were comparable. In a pooled analysis from the Chicago Heart Association Detection Project in Industry and the Cardiovascular Health Study cohorts, lifetime risks for HF at age 45 were 30% to 42% in white men, 20% to 29% in black men, 32% to 39% in white women, and 24% to 46% in black women.[8] Of note, these estimates are higher than those previously reported using data from the Framingham Heart Study.[6]

Trends in Heart Failure Incidence

In population-based cohort studies with longitudinal data from the pre-2000 era, HF incidence in the United States appeared to be stable between the 1970s and the 1990s,

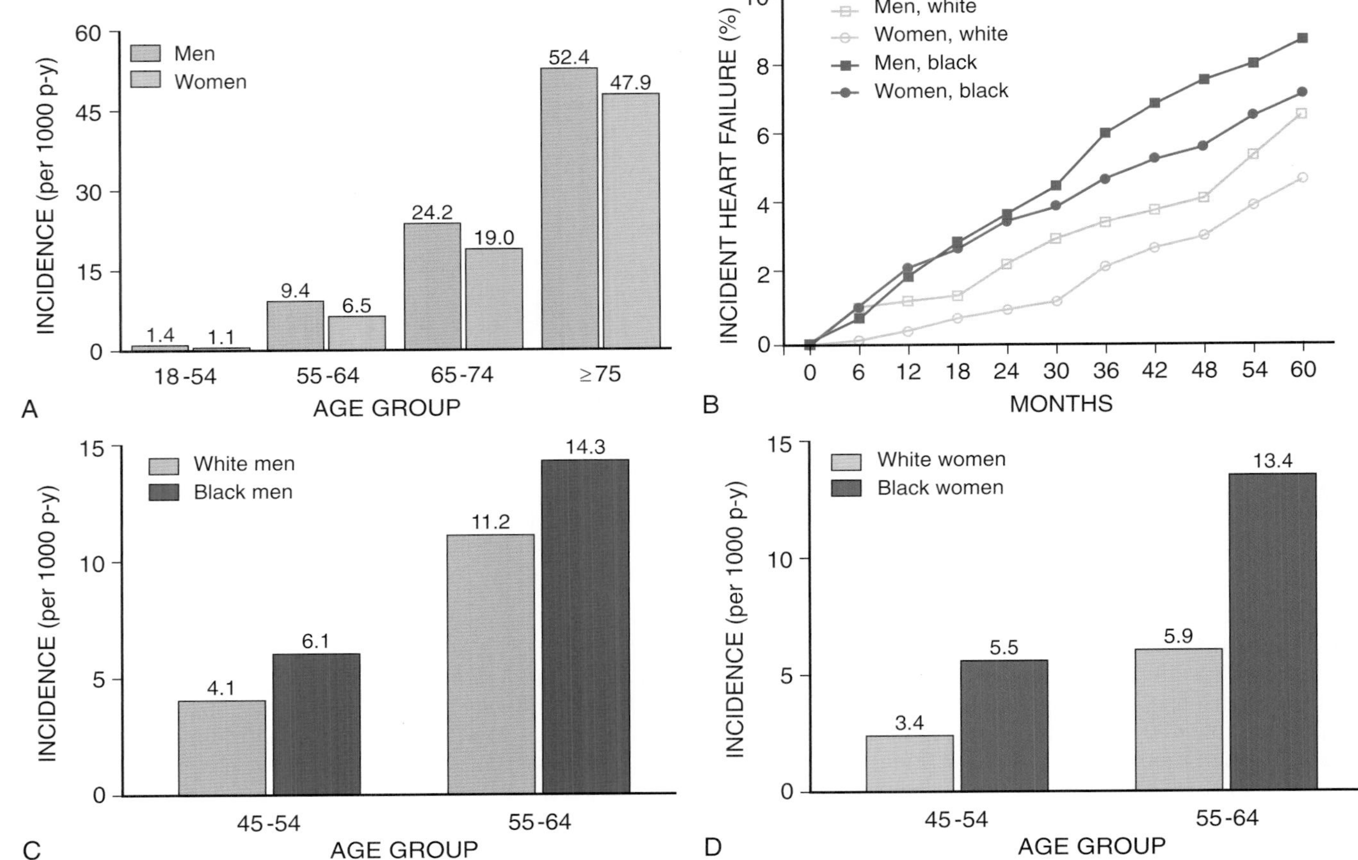

FIGURE 17-4 **A,** Heart failure incidence among adults enrolled in a managed-care organization in Georgia. **B,** Incident heart failure by sex and race in the Health, Aging, and Body Composition study cohort. **C** and **D,** Heart failure incidence by sex, race, and age in the Atherosclerosis Risk in Communities (ARIC) cohort. *p-y,* Person-years. ***A,*** *Data from Goyal A, Norton CR, Thomas TN, et al: Predictors of incident heart failure in a large insured population: a one million person-year follow-up study. Circ Heart Fail 3:698–705, 2010, and personal communication with Dr. Abhinav Goyal;* ***B,*** *Kalogeropoulos A, Georgiopoulou V, Kritchevsky SB, et al: Epidemiology of incident heart failure in a contemporary elderly cohort: the health, aging, and body composition study. Arch Intern Med 169:708–715, 2009;* ***C*** *and* ***D,*** *Data from Loehr LR, Rosamond WD, Chang PP, et al: Heart failure incidence and survival (from the Atherosclerosis Risk in Communities study). Am J Cardiol 101:1016–1022, 2008.*

with a higher incidence among men and increasing average age at diagnosis. However, in recent studies using health care utilization data, the incidence of HF appears to be declining in the 2000s compared to the pre-2000 era, both in the United States and in other westernized countries.

In the Framingham cohort, HF incidence was unchanged between 1970 to 1979 and 1990 to 1999, with approximately 560 new cases per 100,000 person-years in men and 330 in women in the 1990s.[24] The average age at HF diagnosis in 1990 to 1999 was 80 years; in comparison, the average age in 1950 to 1969 was 63 years.[24] Similarly, in the Olmsted County cohort, the incidence of hospitalized HF using the Framingham criteria for diagnosis was estimated at 380 new cases per 100,000 person-years in men and 315 in women in 1996 to 2000, without significant changes from the 1979 to 1984 era.[11] Of note, the Olmsted County study captured new cases using administrative codes during hospitalization, and hence HF incidence was more likely underestimated.

Several studies from administrative databases have consistently reported a recent decline in HF incidence in industrialized countries. In Western Australia, the age-standardized rates (per 100,000) of index hospitalization for HF as a principal diagnosis decreased from 191 to 103 in men and from 130 to 75 in women between 1990 and 2005 (**Figure 17-5A and B**).[1] Although these data might reflect bias secondary to changing approach to new HF cases over time (outpatient vs. inpatient management), the findings are corroborated by a recent study from Canada.[2] In that study, age- and sex-standardized HF incidence decreased from 455 per 100,000 in 1997 to 306 per 100,000 people in 2007, with a comparable decrease in both inpatient and outpatient settings (see Figure 17-5C).[2] In the United States, HF incidence declined from 32 per 1000 person-years in 1994 to 29 per 1000 person-years in 2003 among Medicare beneficiaries (age 65 or older).[16]

Heart Failure after Acute Coronary Syndromes (see also Chapter 18)

Data from the pre-2000 era, when primary percutaneous coronary intervention (PCI) was not standard of care, suggest that the short- and long-term HF incidence after an MI in recent decades has increased, accompanied by a parallel decrease in mortality. In the Framingham Heart Study, the age- and sex-adjusted 30-day incidence of HF after MI rose from 12% in 1970 to 1979 to 19% in 1990 to 1999, whereas 30-day mortality after MI declined from 15% to 3.4%; the 5-year incidence of HF after MI followed similar trends (**Figure 17-6**).[25] Of note, the combined rates of HF and death did not change significantly over time, suggesting that advances in treatment of acute MI have prevented

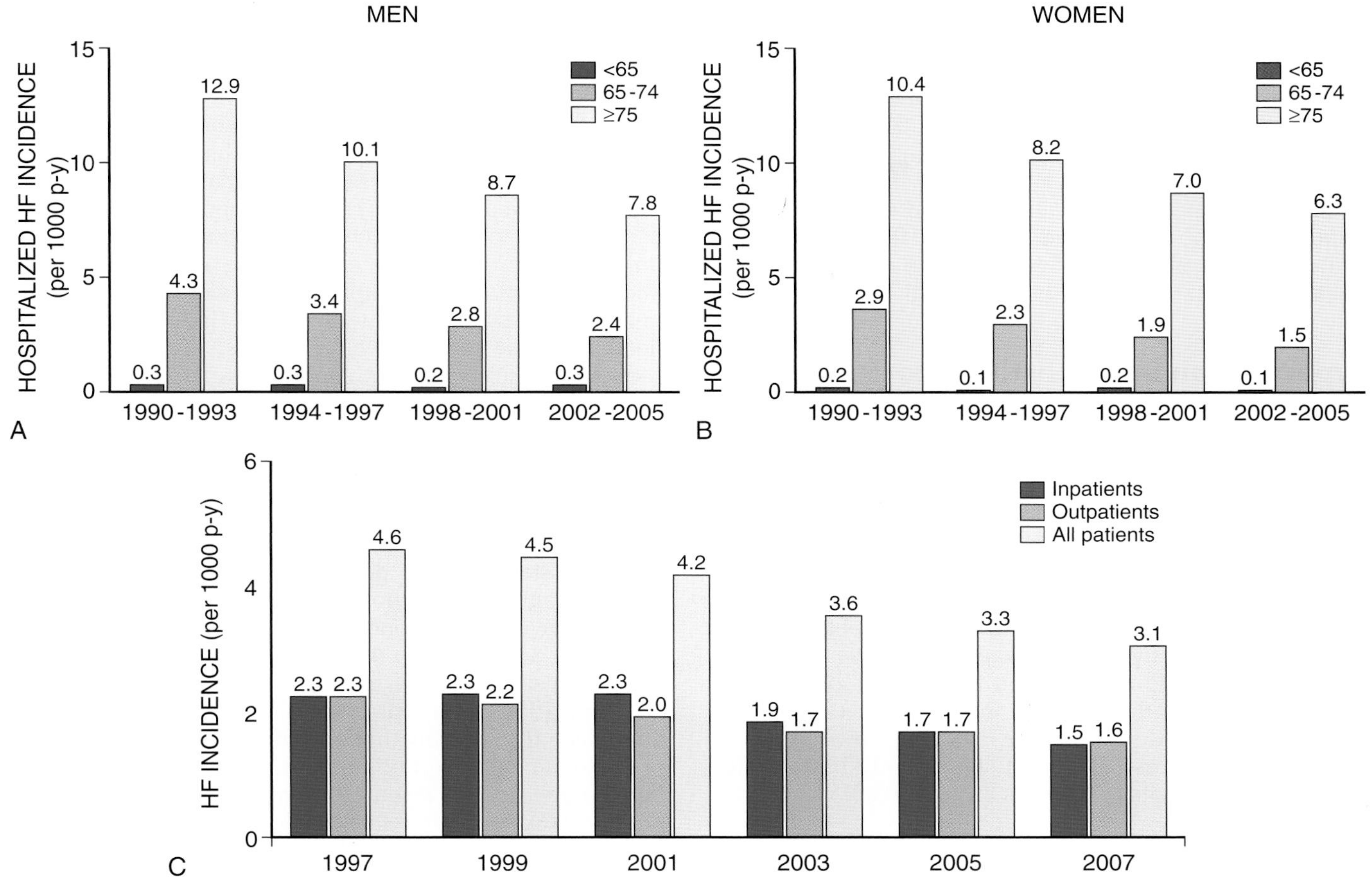

FIGURE 17-5 **A** and **B,** Age-standardized rates of index hospitalization for heart failure as a principal diagnosis in Western Australia between 1990 and 2005. **C,** Age- and sex-standardized heart failure incidence in Ontario, Canada, between 1997 and 2007. *p-y,* Person-years. ***A** and **B,** Data from Teng TH, Finn J, Hobbs M: Heart failure: incidence, case fatality, and hospitalization rates in Western Australia between 1990 and 2005. Circ Heart Fail 3:236–243, 2010;* ***C,** Data from Yeung DF, Boom NK, Guo H, et al: Trends in the incidence and outcomes of heart failure in Ontario, Canada: 1997 to 2007. CMAJ 184:E765–773, 2012.*

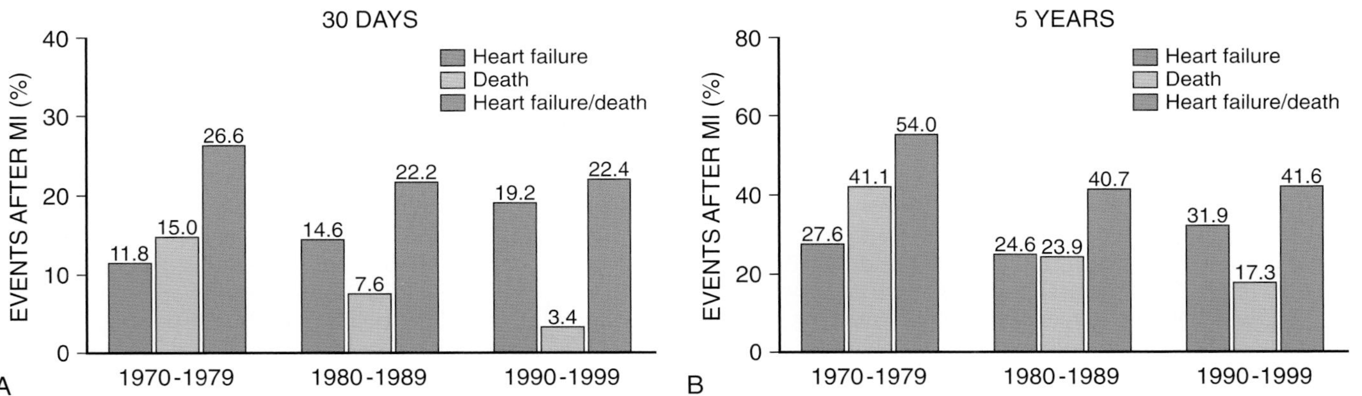

FIGURE 17-6 Temporal trends in **(A)** 30-day and **(B)** 5-year heart failure incidence and mortality after a myocardial infarction in the Framingham Heart Study. *MI,* Myocardial infarction. *Data from Velagaleti RS, Pencina MJ, Murabito JM, et al: Long-term trends in the incidence of heart failure after myocardial infarction. Circulation 118:2057–2062, 2008.*

mortality at the price of increased risk of HF among survivors. These findings are corroborated from a population-based cohort of over 7700 HF-free patients aged 65 years or older hospitalized for a first MI between 1994 and 2000 in Alberta, Canada.[26] During the index hospitalization, 37% of patients were diagnosed with new HF and 13% died. Among HF-free hospital survivors, 71% developed HF by 5 years. Over the study period, the 5-year mortality rate after MI decreased by 28%, whereas the 5-year rate of HF increased by 25%.[26] However, it is important to underline that only 12% of patients received any PCI in this study.

In more contemporary populations, lower HF rates are reported in patients undergoing primary PCI in trial settings compared with unselected populations. In the Harmonizing Outcomes with Revascularization and Stents in Acute Myocardial Infarction (HORIZONS-AMI) trial, 2.6% of patients

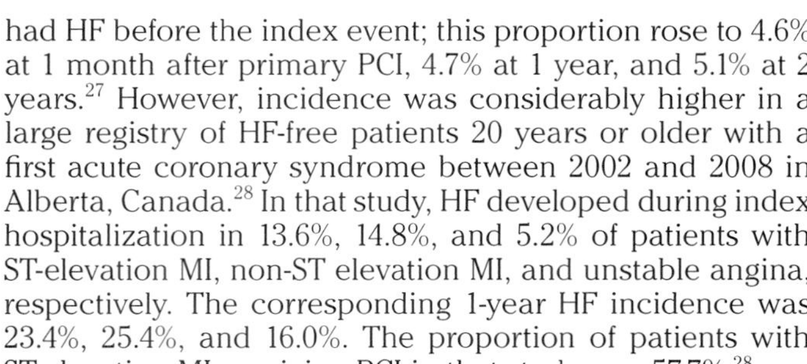
had HF before the index event; this proportion rose to 4.6% at 1 month after primary PCI, 4.7% at 1 year, and 5.1% at 2 years.[27] However, incidence was considerably higher in a large registry of HF-free patients 20 years or older with a first acute coronary syndrome between 2002 and 2008 in Alberta, Canada.[28] In that study, HF developed during index hospitalization in 13.6%, 14.8%, and 5.2% of patients with ST-elevation MI, non-ST elevation MI, and unstable angina, respectively. The corresponding 1-year HF incidence was 23.4%, 25.4%, and 16.0%. The proportion of patients with ST-elevation MI receiving PCI in that study was 57.7%.[28]

Hypertension and Heart Failure (see also Chapter 23)

Along with coronary artery disease, hypertension has the highest population-attributable risk for HF.[22] In the Health ABC study, the 10-year incidence of HF among participants with systolic blood pressure less than 120, 120 to 139, 140 to 159, and 160 mm Hg or more at baseline was 5.9%, 10.5%, 14.8%, and 22.8%, respectively.[29]

African Americans with hypertension are especially vulnerable to development of HF. Among 497 black and 8199 nonblack hypertensive patients aged 55 to 80 years with no history of HF randomly assigned to losartan- or atenolol-based treatment in the Losartan Intervention For Endpoint reduction in hypertension (LIFE) trial, the overall 5-year incidence of HF was 3.0%, with significantly higher rates among black patients (7.0 versus 3.1%; $P < 0.001$).[30]

Diabetes and Heart Failure (see also Chapter 45)

Although coronary artery disease and hypertension have traditionally been considered among the most important modifiable risk factors for HF, recent studies have highlighted the importance of increasingly prevalent metabolic risk factors, including diabetes, glucose intolerance, and insulin resistance for HF development.[31] The association of diabetes with HF risk has been established; importantly, the degree of glycemic control appears to be directly associated with HF risk. In patients with type 2 diabetes enrolled in a large medical care plan in the United States (age, 58 ± 13 years),[32] the crude incidence of new hospitalized HF over a median of 2.2 years was 880 cases per 100,000 patient-years (men: 920; women: 840) and proportional to the glycosylated hemoglobin (HbA_{1c}) levels. In the Swedish national diabetes registry, among 21,000 patients with type 1 diabetes (age, 39 ± 13 years), the incidence of new hospitalized HF was 340 events per 100,000 patient-years.[33] Incidence increased monotonically with HbA_{1c}, with a range of 140 to 520 events per 100,000 patient-years between patients in the lowest (<6.5%) and highest (≥10.5%) categories of HbA_{1c}.[33] Interestingly, a similar association between HbA_{1c} and HF incidence has been reported for older patients (age 45 to 64 at baseline) without diabetes at baseline in the ARIC cohort.[34]

HOSPITALIZED HEART FAILURE (see also Chapter 33)

General Considerations

Hospitalization for decompensated (or "acute") HF, representing largely worsening signs and symptoms among patients with chronic HF, has become the epicenter of intensive research (and debate) both from a therapeutic and a health care perspective in recent years. Hospitalization represents a turning point in the natural history of HF, with a striking increase in mortality and readmission rates afterward. Over the past decade, many therapies have been evaluated in hospitalized HF, but none has proven to reduce mortality or readmission. These disappointing results can be attributed to several factors. Most studies have focused on treatment during the early phase of hospitalization, and the interventions implemented were largely acute, in-hospital, short-term interventions. Interestingly, most deaths in these patients even in the first 30 days occur subsequent to discharge.[35] It is also important to recognize that patients hospitalized with HF represent a heterogeneous group of patients. Finally, the pathophysiologic mechanisms that lead to increased mortality and morbidity after hospitalization for HF are uncertain.

From a health care system perspective, despite efforts to prevent HF hospitalizations, the numbers of HF hospitalizations are staggering in developed economies as populations are aging.[1,36,37] Although more hospitalizations in HF patients have HF as a contributory as opposed to a primary reason for admission,[37] comorbidities can contribute to HF decompensation as well. In the United States, over a million hospitalizations with a primary HF diagnosis are recorded annually.[37] Considering that hospitalizations constitute 80% of the total health expenditure attributable to HF,[3] intensive health care services research is under way in order to identify and tackle system-related factors that contribute to HF admission, albeit with mixed results.[38,39]

Trends in Hospitalization Rates and Total Hospitalizations

Recent reports from the United States and other countries report a decrease in the rate of HF hospitalizations during the past decade, in contrast to previous increasing trends. Despite these favorable trends, the total burden of HF hospitalizations remains largely unchanged secondary to the population aging and increasing prevalence of HF.

The impact of increasing HF prevalence is exemplified by a retrospective cohort study from Western Australia. Although age-standardized rates of index hospitalization for HF as a principal diagnosis decreased between 1990 and 2005, the total number of HF hospitalizations increased during the same period.[1] Similar findings have been recently reported from the United States. Age- and sex-adjusted rates of primary HF hospitalizations decreased steadily from 2001 to 2009, from 566 to 468 per 100,000 people,[37] consistent with a previous report on Medicare beneficiaries.[9] However, the total number of HF-related hospitalizations increased from 3.89 million in 2001 to 4.24 million in 2009.[37] Interestingly, although the number of primary HF hospitalizations decreased from 1.14 million in 2001 to 1.09 million in 2009, hospitalizations with HF as a concomitant diagnosis increased from 2.75 to 3.16 million over the same period.[37]

HEART FAILURE WITH PRESERVED VERSUS REDUCED EJECTION FRACTION

Following the American College of Cardiology and American Heart Association HF guidelines, we refer to HF with preserved and reduced EF as *HFpEF* and *HFrEF*[40]

TABLE 17-1 Relative Proportion of Heart Failure with Preserved and Reduced Ejection Fraction

STUDIES	HFpEF	HFrEF
Cross-sectional HF studies[20,44]	52.0% to 65.0%	35.0% to 48.0%
Hospitalized HF registries[41-43]	36.5% to 47.0%	48.8% to 53.0%
Prospective cohort studies[45,46]	33.4% to 43.0%	56.0% to 64.4%

HF, Heart failure; *HFpEF*, heart failure with preserved ejection fraction; *HFrEF*, heart failure with reduced ejection fraction.

(**Table 17-1**). In Olmsted County, Minn., among 4600 patients from 1987 and 2001, 53% had HFrEF and 47% had HFpEF, when stratified using a definition of ≥ or <50% EF.[41] In the Get With the Guidelines-Heart Failure (GWTG-HF) program, among approximately 111,000 patients between 2005 and 2010, 49.8% had HFrEF (EF <40%), 13.7% borderline EF (EF 40% to 49%), and 36.5% had HFpEF (EF ≥50%); the proportion of HFpEF increased from 33% to 39% over time.[42] In the Organized Program to Initiate Lifesaving Treatment in Hospitalized Patients With Heart Failure (OPTIMIZE-HF) registry, among 41,300 patients, 51.2% were classified as HFpEF (EF ≥40%).[43] Patients with HFpEF were more likely to be older, female, white, and nonischemic. The risk of in-hospital mortality was lower in HFpEF (2.9% vs. 3.9%), but 60 to 90 days mortality and rehospitalization rates were similar. In another study, among 12,000 adults diagnosed with HF between 2005 and 2008, 52% of cases were classified as HFpEF.[20] In a multinational cohort of over 2500 HF outpatients, 65% had HFpEF (EF ≥45%).[44] In the Framingham Heart Study,[45] 457 of 512 participants (89.3%) with a new HF had EF evaluation; 43% had HFpEF (EF >45%) and 56% had HFrEF. In a study from the Netherlands, 33.4% of cases had HFrEF (EF ≤40%) and 64.4% had HFpEF (≥50%).[46]

OUTCOMES

Beyond the effect of known risk factors and comorbid conditions that lead to adverse outcomes among patients with HF, mortality and use of high-cost health care resources (hospital admissions and emergency department visits) are highly dependent on the setting (outpatient vs. inpatient) and sociodemographic factors. Despite significant advances in HF therapy in the past 20 years, mortality and rehospitalization rates have proven difficult to curb,[47] secondary to (1) increasing age of HF patients; (2) diminishing incremental effects of newer treatments as neurohormonal blockade effects reach a plateau; (3) negative results of trials with pharmaceuticals targeting nonneurohormonal pathways; (4) lack of effective treatments for patients with hospitalized HF; and (5) lack of effective treatments for patients with HFpEF. Interestingly, the wealth of data on outcomes of patients hospitalized with HF is not matched by data on HF outpatients.

Effect of Hospitalization for Heart Failure on Outcomes

The dramatic effect of hospitalization on the course of HF has been quantified in an analysis of the Candesartan in Heart failure: Assessment of Reduction in Mortality and morbidity (CHARM) trials data. Among 7572 outpatients with New York Heart Association class II to IV and either HFrEF (EF ≤40%; 63%) or HFpEF (EF >40%; 37%) randomized to placebo or candesartan, 19% had at least one HF hospitalization. Mortality increased after an HF hospitalization, with a hazard ratio of 3.15 (95% confidence interval, 2.83 to 3.50) after adjustment for other predictors of mortality.[48] Repeat HF hospitalizations compounded this effect. Mortality was highest within a month of discharge and declined over time (**Figure 17-7**), lending support to the view that hospitalization for HF represents a prolonged "vulnerable phase" in the natural course of HF.

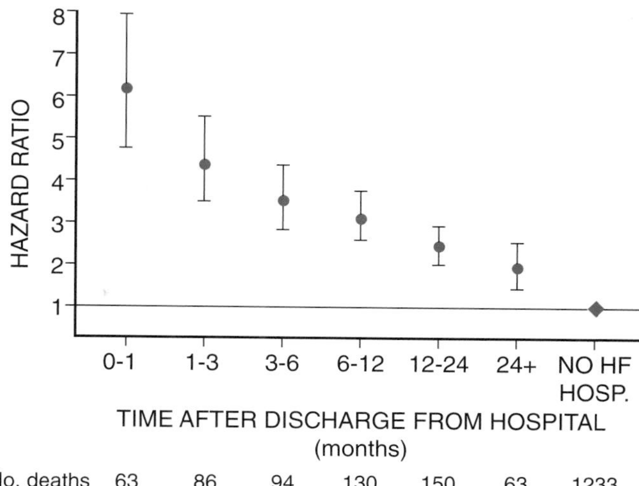

FIGURE 17-7 Adjusted mortality risk after discharge from hospital for a first heart failure-related hospitalization in the Candesartan in Heart failure: Assessment of Reduction in Mortality and morbidity (CHARM) trial program. *From Solomon SD, Dobson J, Pocock S, et al: Influence of nonfatal hospitalization for heart failure on subsequent mortality in patients with chronic heart failure. Circulation 116:1482–1487, 2007.*

Similarly, in the Italian HF registry, 1-year mortality was 24% among patients admitted for HF (19.2% for de novo HF and 27.7% for worsening HF) and 5.9% among outpatients.[10] The corresponding 1-year hospitalization rates were 30.7% for acute and 22.7% for chronic HF.

Contemporary Outcomes and Trends in Outpatients with Heart Failure

Despite relative improvement in HF outcomes over the past 20 years, the absolute mortality and morbidity rates remain unacceptably high. In a longitudinal analysis from Canada, adjusted 1-year mortality decreased from 17.7% in 1997 to 16.2% in 2007 for outpatients.[2] In a study from a single U.S. center, among patients referred for advanced systolic HF, the unadjusted mortality decreased from 20.6% in 1993 to 1998 to 17.8% in 2005 to 2010.[47] Importantly, increasing rates of death from progressive HF have offset reductions in sudden death rates, whereas the rates for heart transplants and mechanical circulatory support increased during the same time.[47] In the Use of Evidence-Based Heart Failure Therapies in the Outpatient Setting (IMPROVE HF) registry, which included data from 167 outpatient cardiology practices in the United States, 2-year mortality was 22.1% among 11,600 patients with available vital status data.[49]

Data suggest that mortality is lower among patients with HFpEF, although the absolute difference is small. In a recent meta-analysis from 7 clinical trials and 24 cohort studies, annual mortality was 12.1% and 14.1% among outpatients

TABLE 17-2 Mortality Rates after Hospitalization for Heart Failure

	ADMINISTRATIVE/REGISTRIES	QUALITY IMPROVEMENT INITIATIVES
In-Hospital		
United States[35,42,43,52]	**National Hospital Discharge Survey:** 10.9% (1980-1984) to 6.5% (2000-2004) **Medicare data:** 8.5% (1993) to 4.3% (2006)	**OPTIMIZE-HF:** HFpEF: 2.9% (2003-2004) HFrEF: 3.9% (2003-2004) **GWTG-HF:** HFpEF: 3.32% (2005) to 2.35% (2010) HFrEF: 3.03% (2005) to 2.83% (2010)
Italy[10]	6.4% (2007-2009)	
Sub-Saharan Africa[54]	4.2% (2007-2010)*	
30-Day		
United States[35,39,56]	**Veterans Affairs:** 7.1% (2002) to 5.0% (2006) **Medicare data:** 12.8% (1993) to 10.7% (2006)	**GWTG-HF:** 11.1% (2006-2007)
Canada[2]	17.3% (1997) to 16.3% (2007)	
Australia[1]	Men: 12.6% (1990) to 8.2% (2005) Women: 12.4% (1990) to 8.7% (2005)	
Scotland[36]	Men: 24.4% (1986) to 16.2% (2003) Women: 20.6% (1986) to 16.9% (2003)	
1-Year		
United States[9,56]	**Veterans Affairs:** 27.7% (2002) to 24.3% (2006) **Medicare data:** 31.7% (1999) to 29.6% (2008)	
Italy[10]	24.0% (2007-2009)	
Canada[2]	35.7% (1997) to 33.8% (2008)	
5-Year		
Scotland[36]	Men: 73.7% (1986) to 65.8% (1999) Women: 69.5% (1986) to 63.6% (1999)	

*Average age, 52 years.

GWTG-HF, Get With the Guidelines-Heart Failure; *HFpEF*, heart failure with preserved ejection fraction; *HFrEF*, heart failure with reduced ejection fraction; *OPTIMIZE-HF*, Organized Program to Initiate Lifesaving Treatment in Hospitalized Patients With Heart Failure.

with HFpEF and HFrEF, respectively.[50] Of note, participants of cohort studies had higher mortality than participants of clinical trials. In a Veterans Affairs database (2000-2002), among 9400 outpatients with available EF data, patients with HFpEF (30% of patients) had lower 2-year mortality compared with HFrEF patients (19.8% vs. 25.5%) and lower HF admission rate, but higher non-HF and similar overall admission rate.[51]

Limited data exist on long-term outcomes among ambulatory HF patients. The majority of evidence suggests that, depending on underlying demographics and comorbid conditions, 50% to 75% of HF outpatients are alive by 5 years.[11-13]

Prognosis of Hospitalized Heart Failure

In the National Hospital Discharge Survey data, in-hospital mortality decreased from 10.9% in 1980 to 1984 to 6.5% in 2000 to 2004 (**Table 17-2**).[52] Among Medicare beneficiaries, length of stay decreased from 8.8 to 6.3 days and in-hospital mortality from 8.5% to 4.3%, between 1993 and 2006.[35] In the GWTG-HF program, in-hospital mortality decreased from 3.32% to 2.35% for HFpEF but remained stagnant for HFrEF between 2005 and 2010.[42] In-hospital mortality was similar between sexes.[53] Higher in-hospital mortality for HFrEF versus HFpEF was seen in OPTIMIZE-HF (3.9% versus 2.9%).[43] In Italy, in-hospital mortality was 6.4% and length of stay was 10 days.[10] In Sub-Saharan Africa, in-hospital mortality was 4.2%, with the length of stay 7 days.[54] In Acute Study of Clinical Effectiveness of Nesiritide in Decompensated Heart Failure (ASCEND-HF) trial, length of stay ranged from 4.9 to 14.6 days across 27 countries.[55] In China, the average length of stay in 2000 was 21.8 days.[5]

Between 1993 and 2006, 30-day mortality among Medicare beneficiaries decreased from 12.8% to 10.7%, but readmission rates increased from 17.2% to 20.1%.[35] In another study, the 30-day mortality after HF admission in 2006 and 2007 was 11.0% among 4460 hospitals.[39] In the Veterans Affairs data, 30-day mortality fell from 7.1% in 2002 to 5.0% in 2006, but the 30-day readmissions for HF increased from 5.6% to 6.1%.[56] In Australia, 30-day mortality decreased from 12.6% to 8.2% in men and 12.4% to 8.7% in women between 1990 and 2005.[1] In Scotland, 30-day mortality fell from 24.4% to 16.2% in men and from 20.6% to 16.9% in women between 1986 and 2003.[36] In Canada, 30-day mortality after admission decreased from 17.3% in 1997 to 16.3% in 2007.[2] In the ASCEND-HF trial, all-cause 30-day readmission ranged from 2.5% to 25.0%, and there was an inverse correlation between country-level length of stay and readmission.[55]

Among Medicare beneficiaries, the risk-adjusted 1-year mortality after HF admission decreased from 31.7% in 1999 to 29.6% in 2008.[9] The risk-adjusted 1-year mortality decreased from 35.7% to 33.8% between 1997 and 2008 in Ontario, Canada.[2] In the Veterans Affairs data, mortality at 1 year decreased from 27.7% in 2002 to 24.3% in 2006.[56] In Scotland, 5-year mortality improved from 73.7% to 65.8% in men and 69.5% to 63.6% in women between 1986 and 1999.[36] From 1987 and 2001 in Rochester, Minn., 5-year mortality was 65% for HFpEF and 68% for HFrEF.[41] In Sweden from 1987 to 2003, 3-year mortality decreased during 1987 to 1995.[57] In the ARIC cohort, overall 5-year mortality following hospitalization for HF was higher in blacks compared with whites, both for men (51.8% vs. 41.2%) and women (46.1% vs. 35.8%).[23]

Reverse Epidemiology in Heart Failure

Higher systolic blood pressure, cholesterol levels, and body mass index are established risk factors for coronary heart disease and HF. However, several studies have now demonstrated that, among patients with established HF, prognosis is worse for those who have lower levels of these risk factors. This phenomenon, termed *reverse epidemiology*, has been described in other chronic disease states and has been attributed to lead-time bias (patients captured during a later, deteriorated status), survival bias (e.g., genetic factors protective against the effects of these risk factors), and HF-induced cachexia (i.e., lower levels of risk factors signify cachexia), among others. Among 867 unselected HF patients (age, 70 ± 13 years, 41% female, 49% EF >40%) in Würzburg, Germany, 34% of the patients died after a median of 1.6 years. Low levels of body mass index, total cholesterol, and systolic blood pressure identified those at the highest mortality risk. Conversely, two or more of these risk factors in the high tertile conferred 51% lower risk (CI, 32% to 65%) compared with subjects with all risk factors in the low tertile.[58]

References

1. Teng T-HK, Finn J, Hobbs M, et al: Heart failure: incidence, case fatality, and hospitalization rates in Western Australia between 1990 and 2005. *Circ Heart Fail* 3:236–243, 2010.
2. Yeung DF, Boom NK, Guo H, et al: Trends in the incidence and outcomes of heart failure in Ontario, Canada: 1997 to 2007. *CMAJ* 184:E765–E773, 2012.
3. Heidenreich PA, Albert NM, Allen LA, et al: Forecasting the impact of heart failure in the United States: a policy statement from the American Heart Association. *Circ Heart Fail* 6:606–619, 2013.
4. Albert MA: Heart failure in the urban African enclave of Soweto: a case study of contemporary epidemiological transition in the developing world. *Circulation* 118:2323–2325, 2008.
5. Jiang H, Ge J: Epidemiology and clinical management of cardiomyopathies and heart failure in China. *Heart* 95:1727–1731, 2009.
6. Lloyd-Jones DM, Larson MG, Leip EP, et al: Lifetime risk for developing congestive heart failure: the Framingham Heart Study. *Circulation* 106:3068–3072, 2002.
7. Bleumink GS, Knetsch AM, Sturkenboom MCJM, et al: Quantifying the heart failure epidemic: prevalence, incidence rate, lifetime risk and prognosis of heart failure The Rotterdam Study. *Eur Heart J* 25:1614–1619, 2004.
8. Huffman MD, Berry JD, Ning H, et al: Lifetime risk for heart failure among white and black Americans: cardiovascular lifetime risk pooling project. *J Am Coll Cardiol* 61:1510–1517, 2013.
9. Chen J, Normand S-LT, Wang Y, et al: National and regional trends in heart failure hospitalization and mortality rates for Medicare beneficiaries, 1998–2008. *JAMA* 306:1669–1678, 2011.
10. Tavazzi L, Senni M, Metra M, et al: Multicenter prospective observational study on acute and chronic heart failure: the one-year follow-up results of IN-HF outcome registry. *Circ Heart Fail* 6:473–481, 2013.
11. Roger VL, Weston SA, Redfield MM, et al: Trends in heart failure incidence and survival in a community-based population. *JAMA* 292:344–350, 2004.
12. Hobbs FDR, Roalfe AK, Davis RC, et al: Prognosis of all-cause heart failure and borderline left ventricular systolic dysfunction: 5 year mortality follow-up of the Echocardiographic Heart of England Screening study (ECHOES). *Eur Heart J* 28:1128–1134, 2007.
13. Ammar KA, Jacobsen SJ, Mahoney DW, et al: Prevalence and prognostic significance of heart failure stages: application of the American College of Cardiology/American Heart Association heart failure staging criteria in the community. *Circulation* 115:1563–1570, 2007.
14. Heo S, Moser DK, Lennie TA, et al: A comparison of health-related quality of life between older adults with heart failure and healthy older adults. *Heart Lung* 36:16–24, 2007.
15. Go AS, Mozaffarian D, Roger VL, et al: Heart disease and stroke statistics–2013 update: a report from the American Heart Association. *Circulation* 127:e6–e245, 2013.
16. Curtis LH, Whellan DJ, Hammill BG, et al: Incidence and prevalence of heart failure in elderly persons, 1994–2003. *Arch Intern Med* 168:418–424, 2008.
17. Hunt SA, American Heart Association Task Force on Practice Guidelines (Writing Committee to Update the 2001 Guidelines for the Evaluation and Management of Heart Failure): ACC/AHA 2005 guideline update for the diagnosis and management of chronic heart failure in the adult: a report of the American College of Cardiology/American Heart Association task force on practice guidelines (writing committee to update the 2001 guidelines for the evaluation and management of heart failure). *J Am Coll Cardiol* 46:e1–e82, 2005.
18. Gupta S, Rohatgi A, Ayers CR, et al: Risk scores versus natriuretic peptides for identifying prevalent stage B heart failure. *Am Heart J* 161:923–930.e2, 2011.
19. Azevedo A, Bettencourt P, Dias P, et al: Population based study on the prevalence of the stages of heart failure. *Heart* 92:1161–1163, 2006.
20. Gurwitz JH, Magid DJ, Smith DH, et al: Contemporary prevalence and correlates of incident heart failure with preserved ejection fraction. *Am J Med* 126:393–400, 2013.
21. Goyal A, Norton CR, Thomas TN, et al: Predictors of incident heart failure in a large insured population: a one million person-year follow-up study. *Circ Heart Fail* 3:698–705, 2010.
22. Kalogeropoulos A, Georgiopoulou V, Kritchevsky SB, et al: Epidemiology of incident heart failure in a contemporary elderly cohort: the health, aging, and body composition study. *Arch Intern Med* 169:708–715, 2009.
23. Loehr LR, Rosamond WD, Chang PP, et al: Heart failure incidence and survival (from the atherosclerosis risk in communities study). *Am J Cardiol* 101:1016–1022, 2008.
24. Levy D, Kenchaiah S, Larson MG, et al: Long-term trends in the incidence of and survival with heart failure. *N Engl J Med* 347:1397–1402, 2002.
25. Velagaleti RS, Pencina MJ, Murabito JM, et al: Long-term trends in the incidence of heart failure after myocardial infarction. *Circulation* 118:2057–2062, 2008.
26. Ezekowitz JA, Kaul P, Bakal JA, et al: Declining in-hospital mortality and increasing heart failure incidence in elderly patients with first myocardial infarction. *J Am Coll Cardiol* 53:13–20, 2009.
27. Kelly DJ, Gershlick T, Witzenbichler B, et al: Incidence and predictors of heart failure following percutaneous coronary intervention in ST-segment elevation myocardial infarction: the HORIZONS-AMI trial. *Am Heart J* 162:663–670, 2011.
28. Kaul P, Ezekowitz JA, Armstrong PW, et al: Incidence of heart failure and mortality after acute coronary syndromes. *Am Heart J* 165:379–85.e2, 2013.
29. Butler J, Kalogeropoulos AP, Georgiopoulou VV, et al: Systolic blood pressure and incident heart failure in the elderly. the cardiovascular health study and the health, ageing and body composition study. *Heart* 97:1304–1311, 2011.
30. Okin PM, Kjeldsen SE, Dahlöf B, et al: Racial differences in incident heart failure during antihypertensive therapy. *Circ Cardiovasc Qual Outcomes* 4:157–164, 2011.
31. Horwich TB, Fonarow GC: Glucose, obesity, metabolic syndrome, and diabetes relevance to incidence of heart failure. *J Am Coll Cardiol* 55:283–293, 2010.
32. Iribarren C, Karter AJ, Go AS, et al: Glycemic control and heart failure among adult patients with diabetes. *Circulation* 103:2668–2673, 2001.
33. Lind M, Bounias I, Olsson M, et al: Glycaemic control and incidence of heart failure in 20,985 patients with type 1 diabetes: an observational study. *Lancet* 378:140–146, 2011.
34. Matsushita K, Blecker S, Pazin-Filho A, et al: The association of hemoglobin a1c with incident heart failure among people without diabetes: the atherosclerosis risk in communities study. *Diabetes* 59:2020–2026, 2010.
35. Bueno H, Ross JS, Wang Y, et al: Trends in length of stay and short-term outcomes among Medicare patients hospitalized for heart failure, 1993–2006. *JAMA* 303:2141–2147, 2010.
36. Jhund PS, Macintyre K, Simpson CR, et al: Long-term trends in first hospitalization for heart failure and subsequent survival between 1986 and 2003: a population study of 5.1 million people. *Circulation* 119:515–523, 2009.
37. Blecker S, Paul M, Taksler G, et al: Heart failure–associated hospitalizations in the United States. *J Am Coll Cardiol* 61:1259–1267, 2013.
38. Hernandez AF, Greiner MA, Fonarow GC, et al: Relationship between early physician follow-up and 30-day readmission among Medicare beneficiaries hospitalized for heart failure. *JAMA* 303:1716–1722, 2010.
39. Heidenreich PA, Hernandez AF, Yancy CW, et al: Get with the guidelines program participation, process of care, and outcome for Medicare patients hospitalized with heart failure. *Circ Cardiovasc Qual Outcomes* 5:37–43, 2012.
40. Yancy CW, Jessup M, Bozkurt B, et al: 2013 ACCF/AHA guideline for the management of heart failure: a report of the American College of Cardiology Foundation/American Heart Association task force on practice guidelines. *J Am Coll Cardiol* 62:e147–e239, 2013.
41. Owan TE, Hodge DO, Herges RM, et al: Trends in prevalence and outcome of heart failure with preserved ejection fraction. *N Engl J Med* 355:251–259, 2006.
42. Steinberg BA, Zhao X, Heidenreich PA, et al: Trends in patients hospitalized with heart failure and preserved left ventricular ejection fraction: prevalence, therapies, and outcomes. *Circulation* 126:65–75, 2012.
43. Fonarow GC, Stough WG, Abraham WT, et al: Characteristics, treatments, and outcomes of patients with preserved systolic function hospitalized for heart failure: a report from the OPTIMIZE-HF registry. *J Am Coll Cardiol* 50:768–777, 2007.
44. Magaña-Serrano JA, Almahmeed W, Gomez E, et al: Prevalence of heart failure with preserved ejection fraction in Latin American, Middle Eastern, and North African regions in the I PREFER Study (identification of patients with Heart Failure and PREserved systolic function: an epidemiological regional study). *Am J Cardiol* 108:1289–1296, 2011.
45. Ho JE, Lyass A, Lee DS, et al: Predictors of new-onset heart failure: differences in preserved versus reduced ejection fraction. *Circ Heart Fail* 6:279–286, 2013.
46. Brouwers FP, de Boer RA, van der Harst P, et al: Incidence and epidemiology of new onset heart failure with preserved vs. reduced ejection fraction in a community-based cohort: 11-year follow-up of PREVEND. *Eur Heart J* 34:1424–1431, 2013.
47. Loh JC, Creaser J, Rourke DA, et al: Temporal trends in treatment and outcomes for advanced heart failure with reduced ejection fraction from 1993–2010: findings from a university referral center. *Circ Heart Fail* 6:411–419, 2013.
48. Solomon SD, Dobson J, Pocock S, et al: Influence of nonfatal hospitalization for heart failure on subsequent mortality in patients with chronic heart failure. *Circulation* 116:1482–1487, 2007.
49. Fonarow GC, Albert NM, Curtis AB, et al: Associations between outpatient heart failure process-of-care measures and mortality. *Circulation* 123:1601–1610, 2011.
50. Meta-analysis Global Group in Chronic Heart Failure (MAGGIC): The survival of patients with heart failure with preserved or reduced left ventricular ejection fraction: an individual patient data meta-analysis. *Eur Heart J* 33:1750–1757, 2012.
51. Ather S, Chan W, Bozkurt B, et al: Impact of noncardiac comorbidities on morbidity and mortality in a predominantly male population with heart failure and preserved versus reduced ejection fraction. *J Am Coll Cardiol* 59:998–1005, 2012.
52. Fang J, Mensah GA, Croft JB, et al: Heart failure-related hospitalization in the U.S., 1979 to 2004. *J Am Coll Cardiol* 52:428–434, 2008.
53. Hsich EM, Grau-Sepulveda MV, Hernandez AF, et al: Sex differences in in-hospital mortality in acute decompensated heart failure with reduced and preserved ejection fraction. *Am Heart J* 163:430–437, 437.e1–3, 2012.
54. Damasceno A, Mayosi BM, Sani M, et al: The causes, treatment, and outcome of acute heart failure in 1006 Africans from 9 countries. *Arch Intern Med* 172:1386–1394, 2012.
55. Eapen ZJ, Reed SD, Li Y, et al: Do countries or hospitals with longer hospital stays for acute heart failure have lower readmission rates? Findings from ASCEND-HF. *Circ Heart Fail* 6:727–732, 2013.
56. Heidenreich PA, Sahay A, Kapoor JR, et al: Divergent trends in survival and readmission following a hospitalization for heart failure in the Veterans Affairs health care system 2002 to 2006. *J Am Coll Cardiol* 56:362–368, 2010.
57. Shafazand M, Schaufelberger M, Lappas G, et al: Survival trends in men and women with heart failure of ischaemic and non-ischaemic origin: data for the period 1987–2003 from the Swedish hospital discharge registry. *Eur Heart J* 30:671–678, 2009.
58. Güder G, Frantz S, Bauersachs J, et al: Reverse epidemiology in systolic and nonsystolic heart failure: cumulative prognostic benefit of classical cardiovascular risk factors. *Circ Heart Fail* 2:563–571, 2009.

Heart Failure as a Consequence of Ischemic Heart Disease

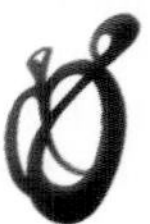

James D. Flaherty, Robert O. Bonow, and Mihai Gheorghiade

Despite significant progress in the prevention and treatment of cardiovascular disease over the past 30 years, national statistics indicate that the incidence and prevalence of heart failure (HF) continue to rise.[1] This has occurred during a time period in which death rates from coronary artery disease (CAD) and stroke have declined. HF and CAD are age-related conditions (the prevalence of HF is 1% between the ages of 50 and 59 years, but 10% above the age of 75 years).[2] The increased survival after myocardial infarction (MI) and advances in medical and device therapies (e.g., β-blockers and implantable cardioverter-defibrillators [ICDs]) for the prevention of sudden cardiac death (SCD) have increased the pool of patients with the potential to develop chronic HF.[3-5]

PREVALENCE OF CORONARY ARTERY DISEASE IN HEART FAILURE

CAD has emerged as the dominant causal factor in HF (**see also Chapter 17**). Survivors of acute MI, even when not complicated by HF, have a relatively high incidence of subsequent HF hospitalization.[6] This is due not only to the initial ventricular insult caused by the MI, but also the progressive nature of CAD (**Figure 18-1**). The Framingham Heart Study suggests that the factors contributing to HF are changing, as evidenced by a decrease in valvular heart disease and left ventricular (LV) hypertrophy, but an increase in MI as a risk factor from 1950 to 1998.[3] In this analysis, the odds of a prior MI as a cause of HF increased by 26% per decade in men and 48% per decade in women. In contrast, hypertension as a cause of HF decreased by 13% per decade in men and 25% in women, and valvular heart disease as a cause of HF decreased by 24% per decade in men and 17% in women.

In the Studies of Left Ventricular Dysfunction (SOLVD) registry, which enrolled 6273 patients, CAD was determined as the underlying cause of chronic HF in approximately 70% of patients, whereas hypertension was invoked as the primary cause in only 7% of cases.[7] Of note, there was a history of hypertension in 43% of patients. There were striking racial differences observed in this registry. HF was considered due to CAD in 73% of Caucasian patients, but only 36% of African American patients (**see also Chapter 37**).

Pooling data from 26 multicenter trials of chronic HF since 1986 with greater than 43,000 patients revealed that 62% carried a diagnosis of CAD[8-33] (**Table 18-1**). This number may actually underestimate the true prevalence of CAD in this population, because in clinical practice and in most studies there is no systemic assessment of coronary artery anatomy. In addition, most of these trials excluded patients with a recent MI, angina, or objective evidence of active ischemia. In a study of 136 patients (<75 years old) hospitalized with de novo HF, a review of the clinical, angiographic, and myocardial perfusion imaging data was used to determine that CAD was the primary cause in greater than 50% of cases.[34] In this study alone, two thirds of all patients who underwent angiography had obstructive CAD (defined as >50% luminal stenosis), although CAD was not considered the primary causal factor in all cases. In a recent analysis of a large U.S. acute HF registry, myocardial ischemia was found to be a leading precipitating factor for hospitalization.[35]

PROGNOSTIC SIGNIFICANCE OF CORONARY ARTERY DISEASE IN HEART FAILURE

The presence of CAD in patients with HF has been shown to be independently associated with a worsened long-term outcome in numerous studies.[36] Atherosclerosis is an important contributing cause of death in HF patients through a variety of mechanisms, including SCD, progressive ventricular failure, MI, renal failure, and stroke. In patients with HF,

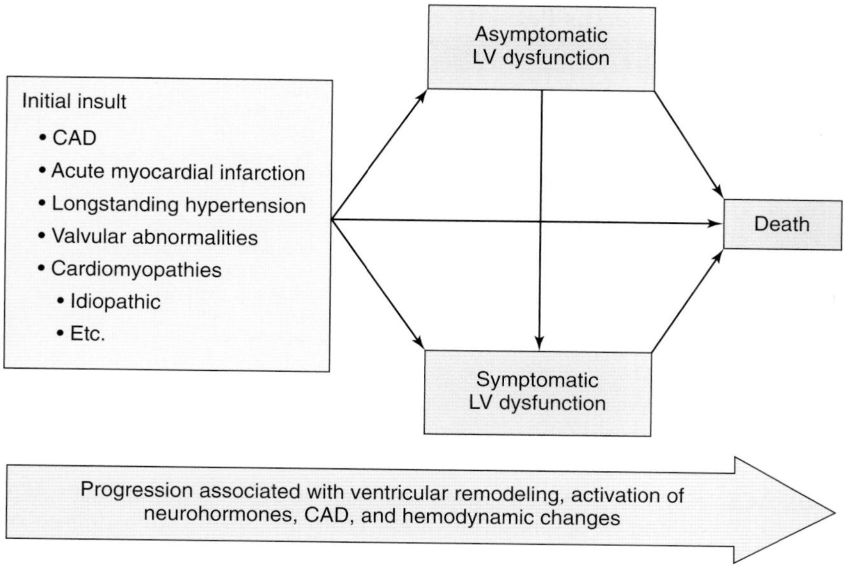

Initial insult
- CAD
- Acute myocardial infarction
- Longstanding hypertension
- Valvular abnormalities
- Cardiomyopathies
  - Idiopathic
  - Etc.

Asymptomatic LV dysfunction

Death

Symptomatic LV dysfunction

Progression associated with ventricular remodeling, activation of neurohormones, CAD, and hemodynamic changes

FIGURE 18-1 Coronary artery disease (CAD) contributes to left ventricular (LV) dysfunction not only during an initial insult (e.g., myocardial infarction) but throughout its progression. In addition, progression of chronic heart failure is associated with ventricular remodeling, activation of neurohormones, and hemodynamic changes.

TABLE 18-1 Prevalence of Coronary Artery Disease (CAD) in 26 Multicenter Chronic Heart Failure Trials Reported by the *New England Journal of Medicine* Since 1986

TRIAL	YEAR	N	CAD
VHEFT-1	1986	642	282
CONSENSUS	1987	253	146
Milrinone	1989	230	115
PROMISE	1991	1088	590
SOLVD-T	1991	2569	1828
VHEFT-2	1991	804	427
SOVLD-P	1992	4228	3518
RADIANCE	1993	178	107
Vesnarinone	1993	477	249
STAT-CHF	1995	674	481
Carvedilol	1996	1094	521
PRAISE	1996	1153	732
DIG	1997	6800	4793
VEST	1998	3833	2236
RALES	1999	1663	907
DIAMOND	1999	1518	1017
Nesiritide	2000	127	58
COPERNICUS	2001	2289	1534
BEST	2001	2708	1587
Val-HeFT	2001	5010	2880
MIRACLE	2002	453	108
COMPANION	2004	1520	842
SCD-HeFT	2005	2521	1310
CARE-HF	2005	813	309
RethinQ	2007	172	90
Dronedarone	2008	627	407
Total		**43,444**	**27,074**

Coronary artery disease was documented to be present in nearly 65% of patients.

the long-term prognosis is directly related to the angiographic extent and severity of CAD.[37,38] This has been demonstrated both in HF patients with LV systolic dysfunction and in those with preserved systolic function.[39]

Recent data suggest that the mechanism of SCD may differ between ischemic and nonischemic HF, with acute coronary events representing the major cause of SCD in patients with CAD.[40,41] In the Assessment of Treatment with Lisinopril and Survival (ATLAS) study, 54% of patients with chronic HF and CAD who died suddenly had autopsy evidence of acute MI.[40] In another autopsy study of 180 patients with known ischemic cardiomyopathy, acute MI was responsible for 57% of the deaths.[41] This study revealed that before autopsy data were available, many deaths as a result of acute MI in patients with HF were misclassified as caused by progressive HF or arrhythmias. In another study of patients with HF and LVSD, 25% of repeat hospitalizations were attributed to acute coronary syndrome (ACS).[42] However, approximately 10% of patients with a history of HF who were subsequently hospitalized for ACS were originally classified as having a nonischemic cause. These findings further emphasize the importance of accurately assessing for the presence of CAD in patients with HF.

PATHOPHYSIOLOGY OF ACUTE HEART FAILURE IN PATIENTS WITH CORONARY ARTERY DISEASE

Underlying Coronary Artery Disease

Patients hospitalized with acute HF differ from patients with chronic ambulatory HF with respect to prognosis and early management (see also Chapter 33).[43] Patients with CAD who develop acute HF do so with either an ACS or a non-ACS presentation. Although the majority of such patients do not have ACS, there is considerable overlap in these two presentations with respect to clinical characteristics (**Table 18-2**) and potential therapies (**Table 18-3**). However, the approach to the patient with ACS has become more standardized in clinical practice guidelines compared with the acute HF patient with a non-ACS presentation. Myocardial injury is common in both, but in ACS patients it is usually the principal cause of HF, whereas in non-ACS patients myocardial injury may be the result of worsening HF. In these latter patients, cardiac troponin levels are frequently elevated in patients with acute HF, representing myocardial injury (see also Chapter 30). These values typically do not reach the established threshold values for ACS, but are still associated with worse outcomes.[44-49]

In acute HF, a high LV diastolic pressure can result in subendocardial ischemia. Excessive neurohormonal activation can exacerbate ischemia via increased cardiac contractility and reduced coronary perfusion because of

TABLE 18-2 Characteristics of Patients with AHFS and CAD versus Patients with ACS Complicated by HF

	AHFS AND CAD	ACS COMPLICATED BY HF
Dyspnea	Common	Common
Chest discomfort	Uncommon	Common
Prior HF	Common	Uncommon
BNP/N-terminal pro-BNP	Elevated	Elevated
Troponin	Normal or elevated*	Usually elevated
Left ventricular systolic function	Normal or depressed	Normal or depressed
Diagnostic testing for CAD† (ischemia/viability/angiography)	Uncommon	Standard (per guidelines)
Myocardial revascularization	Uncommon†	Standard (per guidelines)
Secondary prevention for CAD	Underused	Standard (per guidelines)
In-hospital mortality	Relatively low	Relatively high
Early after-discharge death or rehospitalization	High	High

*Typically low-level elevation.
†During index hospitalization.
ACS, Acute coronary syndrome; *AHFS,* acute heart failure syndrome; *BNP,* B-type natriuretic peptide; *CAD,* coronary artery disease; *HF,* heart failure.

TABLE 18-3 Therapies for AHFS and CAD versus ACS Complicated by HF

	AHFS AND CAD	ACS COMPLICATED BY HF
Immediate Therapies		
Nitrates	Yes	Yes
Antiplatelet agents	Yes	Yes
Anticoagulation	No	Yes
Inotropes	Avoid if possible	Avoid if possible
Statins	Yes	Yes
Renin-Angiotensin System Modulation		
ACE-I or ARB	Yes	Yes
Aldosterone blockade (if LVSD)	Yes	Yes
β-blockers	Yes	Yes
Early angiography/ Revascularization	Yes*	Yes*

*If jeopardized myocardium present (ischemia or viability).
ACE-I, Angiotensin-converting enzyme inhibitor; *ACS,* Acute coronary syndrome; *AHFS,* acute heart failure syndrome; *ARB,* angiotensin receptor blocker; *CAD,* coronary artery disease; *HF,* heart failure; *LVSD,* left ventricular systolic dysfunction.
From Flaherty JD, Bax JJ, De Luca L, et al: Acute heart failure syndromes in patients with coronary artery disease: early assessment and treatment. J Am Coll Cardiol *53:254–263, 2009.*

endothelial dysfunction. In addition, patients with acute HF and CAD often have hibernating or stunned myocardium.[50] Together, all of these factors may result in myocardial injury.

Patients with acute HF and low blood pressure have a much higher mortality compared with patients who are normotensive or hypertensive at the time of admission.[51,52]

Low systemic blood pressure combined with elevated LV diastolic pressure reduces coronary perfusion, and in this setting, the autoregulation between coronary artery perfusion pressure and coronary vasoactive tone may be lost or impaired in patients with obstructive epicardial CAD. This may contribute to myocardial injury (as reflected by cardiac enzyme elevation) and worse outcomes. This may help to explain why patients with acute HF and underlying CAD have a worse outcome than those without CAD and have improved outcomes if they have a history of myocardial revascularization.[48,53]

Acute Coronary Syndromes

Approximately 10% to 20% of patients with ACS have concomitant acute HF and roughly 10% of ACS patients develop HF in-hospital.[54-59] In the EuroHeart Survey II on HF, 42% of all de novo HF cases were due to ACS.[60] Patients with ACS and ST-segment elevation typically have a high degree of myocardial injury. ACS patients with HF but without ST-segment elevation also have significant cardiac enzyme elevation, but a smaller degree of injury.[47] The short-term risk of adverse outcomes in ACS patients with HF is directly proportional to the level of troponin elevation.[61] Most of these patients do not have a history of HF or LVSD.[54,56]

Patients with ACS complicated by HF have markedly increased short- and long-term mortality rates compared with ACS patients without HF.[54-56,61-69] ACS patients who develop HF after the initial presentation have even higher mortality rates.[55,59] The prognosis of ACS complicated by HF is directly related to the Killip class.[55,57,59] Compared with Killip class I patients, patients with an ACS in Killip class II or III HF are four times more likely to die in-hospital.[56,59] The risk goes up to 10-fold for patients with cardiogenic shock (Killip class IV). Among ACS patients who recover from transient HF, the majority develop recurrent HF.[6]

PATHOPHYSIOLOGY OF CHRONIC HEART FAILURE IN PATIENTS WITH CORONARY ARTERY DISEASE AND REDUCED EJECTION FRACTION

HF in the setting of CAD is a heterogeneous condition with several possible factors contributing to clinical manifestations of HF and LVSD and/or diastolic dysfunction. First and foremost, the sequelae of MI, with loss of functioning myocytes, development of myocardial fibrosis, and subsequent LV remodeling, result in chamber dilation and neurohormonal activation that lead to progressive deterioration of the remaining viable myocardium.[70] This is a well-recognized clinical process that can be ameliorated after acute MI by the use of angiotensin-converting enzyme (ACE) inhibitor therapy, β-blocking agents, and myocardial revascularization.[71-74] Second, the majority of patients surviving MI have significant atherosclerotic disease in coronary arteries other than the infarct-related artery.[75] Thus superimposed on the left ventricle with irreversibly damaged myocardium, there is often a considerable degree of jeopardized myocardium served by a stenotic coronary artery either within the infarct zone or remote from the infarcted tissue. This may result in myocardial ischemia/hibernation, contributing to LV dysfunction and the risk of recurrent MI producing further deterioration in LV function

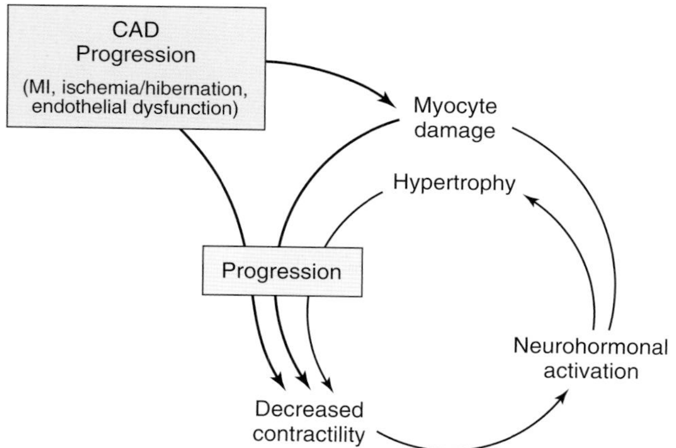

FIGURE 18-2 Progression of coronary artery disease (CAD) leads to decreased contractility, which stimulates neurohormonal activation of chamber remodeling, hypertrophy, and myocyte damage. *MI,* Myocardial ischemia. *Adapted from Gheorghiade M, Bonow RO: Chronic heart failure in the United States: a manifestation of coronary artery disease. Circulation 97:282–289, 1998.*

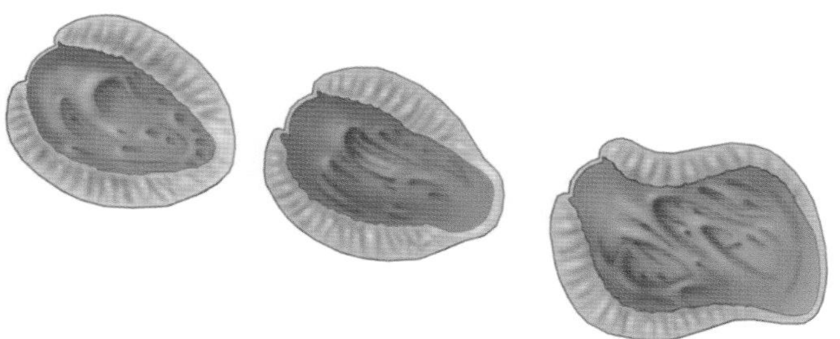

FIGURE 18-3 Remodeling of left ventricle after ST-elevation myocardial infarction (STEMI). *Left,* Apical STEMI (white zone of left ventricle). Over time, the infarct zone elongates and thins. Progressive remodeling of the left ventricle occurs *(center* and *right),* ultimately converting the left ventricle from an oval shape to a spherical shape. Pharmacologic and catheter-based reperfusion strategies for STEMI have a favorable impact on this process by minimizing the extent of myocardial necrosis *(left)* through prompt restoration of flow in the epicardial infarct vessel. *Modified from McMurray JJV, Pfeffer MA, editors: Heart failure updates, London, 2003, Martin Dunitz.*

or SCD. Finally, endothelial dysfunction, a characteristic feature of atherosclerotic CAD, may also contribute importantly and independently to the progression of LV dysfunction (**Figure 18-2**).[76]

Left Ventricular Remodeling (see also Chapter 11)

According to St. John Sutton and Sharpe, LV remodeling is the process by which the left ventricle's size, shape, and function are altered in response to acute and chronic injury or overload, a process that is regulated by mechanical, neurohormonal, and genetic factors (**Figure 18-3**).[70] The severe loss of myocardial cells after acute MI results in an abrupt increase in loading conditions that induces a unique pattern of remodeling involving the infarct zone, the infarct border zone, and the remote noninfarcted myocardium.[70] Myocyte necrosis initiates a process of reparative changes, which consist of dilation, hypertrophy, and the formation of a collagen scar. This process usually continues into the chronic phase until the heart, strengthened by collagen scarring, offsets the dilating forces. Other factors may influence this process, including the location and transmurality of the infarct, the extent of myocardial stunning beyond the initial infarction, infarct-related artery patency, and local trophic factors.[70] Three components participate in this process: the myocytes, the extracellular matrix, and the microcirculation. Postinfarction remodeling has been arbitrarily divided into an early phase (within 72 hours) and a late phase (beyond 72 hours). In patients with transmural MI, the early phase involves expansion of the infarct, with thinning and bulging that may result in ventricular rupture, aneurysm, mitral insufficiency, and ventricular tachyarrhythmias. Late remodeling involves the left ventricle globally and is associated morphologically with dilation, hypertrophy, and myocyte hypertrophy (see Figure 18-3).[70] These processes all may contribute to deterioration in contractile function. In summary, LV remodeling consists of ventricular thinning and dilation in the infarct zone, myocyte hypertrophy in the noninfarct zones, fibrosis, and activation of neurohormones. These processes impact the biology of the cardiac myocyte and nonmyocyte components of the myocardium and contribute independently to the progression of HF.[77]

Myocardial Ischemia

Under basal conditions, episodes of reversible myocardial ischemia caused by a severe coronary artery stenosis superimposed on the left ventricle with depressed systolic function may produce transient worsening of LV function. This exacerbates dyspnea on exertion and fatigue. In many patients, these HF symptoms, stimulated by exercise, represent an anginal equivalent that may occur in the absence of chest pain.

Transient LV dysfunction can aggravate symptoms during stress or spontaneous ischemia in patients with CAD and HF. Ischemia can also produce a rapid and massive increase in the concentration of all three endogenous catecholamines (norepinephrine, epinephrine, dopamine) in the myocardial interstitium, which is mediated by inhibition of neuronal reuptake mechanisms.[78] High myocardial catecholamine concentration may have a deleterious effect on cardiac myocytes.[79-81]

Ischemia may also lead to myocyte apoptosis, which may result in progression of LV dysfunction without a clear ischemic event.[82] This situation also indicates that ischemia from a chronic stenosis can produce substantial myocyte loss in the absence of significant necrosis or fibrosis. Ischemia may also cause an increase in endothelin production that may have a negative effect on LV function.[83] Aggressive medical and surgical interventions designed to ameliorate ischemia appear to have a substantial impact on limiting apoptosis.

Hibernation/Stunning

Episodes of transient myocardial ischemia may cause prolonged LVSD that persists after the ischemic insult itself has resolved. This process is termed *stunning,* which is similar to more severe and protracted myocardial stunning that results from coronary occlusion and reperfusion (**Figure 18-4A**).[84] Recurrent episodes of myocardial ischemia that produce repetitive myocardial stunning may contribute to overall LV dysfunction and HF symptoms.

Another important mechanism for systolic dysfunction with additive effects on LV performance is myocardial hibernation. Once considered a process in which myocardial contraction is downregulated in response to chronic

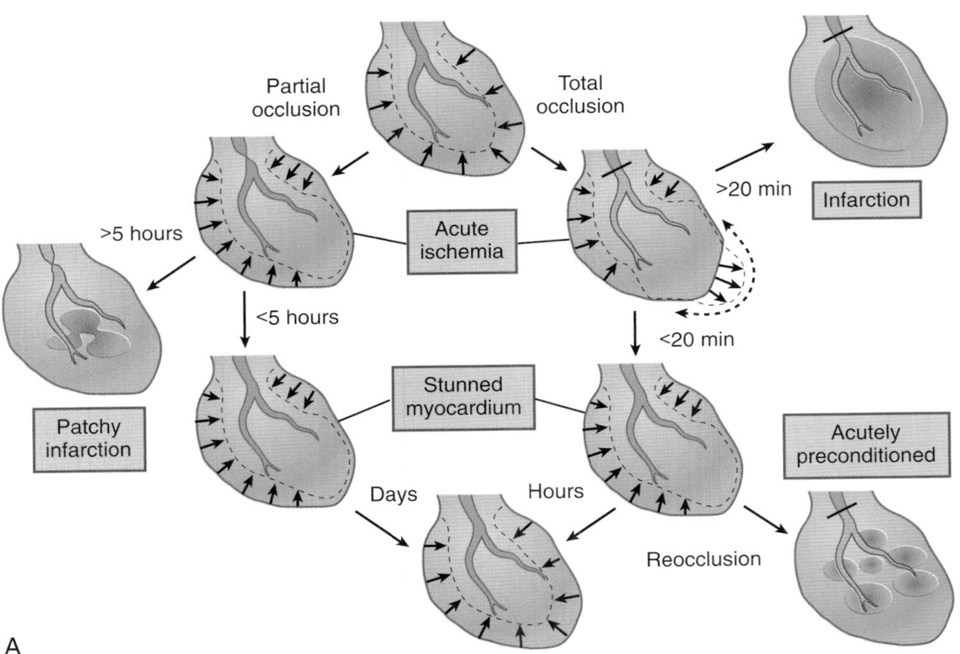

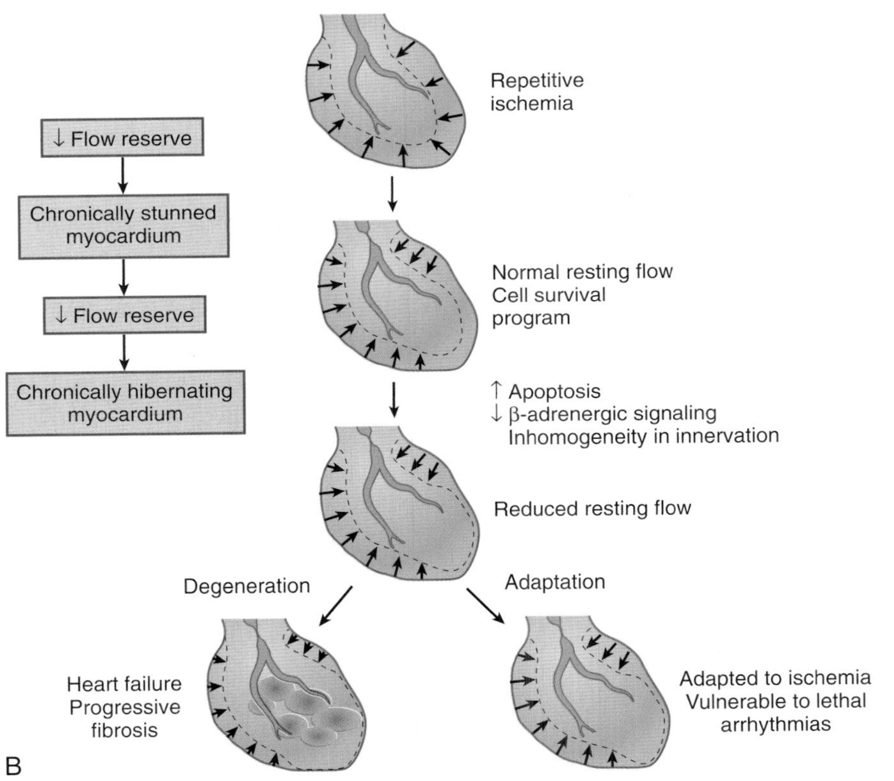

FIGURE 18-4 Effects of ischemia on left ventricular (LV) function and irreversible injury. The ventriculograms illustrate contractile dysfunction *(dashed lines* and *arrows)*. **A,** Consequences of acute ischemia. A brief total occlusion *(right)* or a prolonged partial occlusion (caused by an acute high-grade stenosis, *left*) leads to acute contractile dysfunction proportional to the reduction in blood flow. Irreversible injury begins after 20 minutes following a total occlusion but is delayed for up to 5 hours following a partial occlusion (or with significant collaterals) caused by short-term hibernation. When reperfusion is established before the onset of irreversible injury, stunned myocardium develops and the time required for recovery of function is proportional to the duration and severity of ischemia. With prolonged ischemia, stunning in viable myocardium coexists with subendocardial infarction and accounts for reversible dysfunction. Brief episodes of ischemia preceding prolonged ischemia elicits protection against infarction (acute preconditioning). **B,** Effects of chronic repetitive ischemia on function distal to a stenosis. As stenosis severity increases, coronary flow reserve decreases and the frequency of reversible ischemia increases. Reversible repetitive ischemia initially leads to chronic preconditioning against infarction and stunning (not shown). Subsequently, there is a gradual progression from contractile dysfunction with normal resting flow (chronically stunned myocardium) to contractile dysfunction with depressed resting flow (hibernating myocardium). This transition is related to the physiologic significance of a coronary stenosis and can occur in a time period as short as 1 week or develop chronically in the absence of severe angina. The cellular response during the progression to chronic hibernating myocardium is variable, with some patients exhibiting successful adaptation with little cell death and fibrosis and others developing degenerative changes difficult to distinguish from subendocardial infarction. *From Canty JM: Coronary blood flow and myocardial ischemia. In Libby P, Bonow RO, Mann DL, et al, editors: Braunwald's heart disease, Philadelphia, 2008, Saunders.*

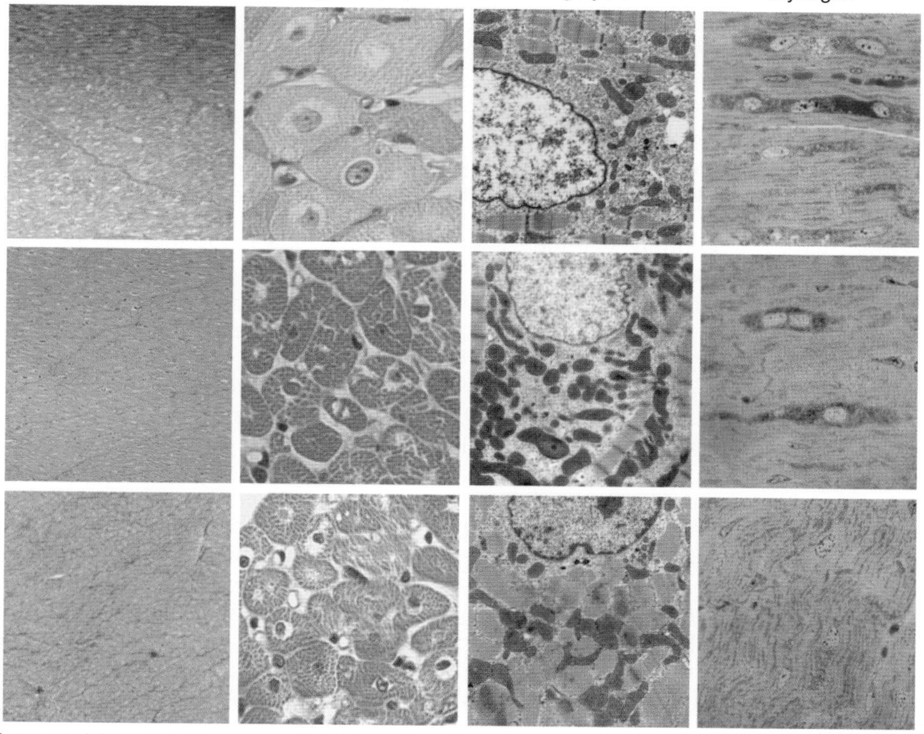

	Reticular collagen	Myocyte hypertrophy	Myolysis	Glycogen
Hibernating LAD				
Normal remote				
Sham				

FIGURE 18-5 Myocyte cellular changes in hibernating myocardium. The increased myocyte loss results in compensatory myocyte cellular hypertrophy in hibernating myocardium. Whereas reticular collagen is regionally increased (about 2%), there is no evidence of infarction. The electron microscopic characteristics of hibernating myocardium demonstrate myofibrillar loss, an increased number of small mitochondria, and increased glycogen content. Although these are markedly different from normal myocardium (sham), biopsies of normal remote, nonischemic segments show similar morphologic changes, indicating that these structural abnormalities are not directly related to ischemia nor are they the cause of regional contractile dysfunction. *LAD,* Left anterior descending artery. *From Canty JM, Fallavollita JA: Hibernating myocardium. J Nucl Cardiol 12:104, 2005.*

reduction in myocardial blood supply,[85-87] the current evidence supports the hypothesis that persistent contractile dysfunction in patients with chronic CAD represents a process of programmed disassembly of contractile elements following repeated episodes of reversible ischemia (see Figure 18-4B).[88-92] Thus rather than a "protective" mechanism, hibernation represents a disadvantageous process that left uncorrected may lead to apoptosis and myocyte loss, replacement fibrosis, graded and reciprocal changes in α- and β-adrenergic receptor density, progressive LVSD, and the risk of ventricular arrhythmias (**Figure 18-5**). This process may affect a substantial number of HF patients. Among patients with HF, CAD, and LVSD, approximately 50% have evidence of viable but dysfunctional myocardium.[93-95]

Diagnosis

Hibernating myocardium should be suspected in all patients with CAD and chronic LV dysfunction of any degree, regional and global.[95] Up to 50% of patients with CAD and chronic LV dysfunction have significant areas of dysfunctional but viable myocardium.[96] Hibernating myocardium can be determined with the use of imaging techniques that detect myocardial contractile reserve, preserved metabolic activity, or cell membrane integrity within the region of dysfunctional myocardium.[74,97-100] Intact perfusion, cell membrane integrity, and intact mitochondria can be evaluated with single photon emission tomography using thallium-201 and/or technetium-99m labeled traces. Preserved glucose metabolism can be assessed by positron emission tomography using F18-fluorodeoxyglucose. Contractile reserve can be unmasked by infusion of low-dose dobutamine during echocardiography. The use of these techniques has been associated with improved survival in patients with chronic HF and significant viability who underwent myocardial revascularization.[97-101]

Cardiac magnetic resonance imaging is also an established technique to assess myocardial viability and the potential for recovery of LV function.[102-104] Resting cine MRI can be used to assess LV end-diastolic wall thickness. An end-diastolic wall thickness less than 5 to 6 mm is a marker of transmural MI and virtually excludes the presence of viable myocardium. In dysfunctional myocardium with preserved end-diastolic wall thickness (6 mm), detection of contractile reserve during low-dose dobutamine infusion confirms the presence of viable myocardium. Gadolinium-based contrast agents have been used to detect nonviable myocardium because these agents accumulate selectively in areas of scar tissue.[102,103] It should be noted that this technique is extremely sensitive in detecting scar tissue (with very high spatial resolution), but the absence of scar tissue does not permit discrimination between normal tissue and hibernating or stunned myocardium.

Clinical Implications

The presence of viable but dysfunctional myocardium can be used to predict a favorable response to myocardial revascularization and pharmacologic therapy.[101,105,106] The restoration of blood flow with revascularization or treatment with agents that improve endothelial function and blood flow, such as statins and β-blockers, may improve contractility in a hibernating area.[105-108] In contrast, agents like dobutamine and milrinone, especially at high doses, may precipitate myocardial necrosis and are associated with worse long-term outcomes in patients with CAD and HF.[109-112] Hibernating myocardium is associated with global alterations in LV volume and shape, not just impairment of underperfused segments.[99] This explains why myocardial revascularization of hibernating territories can promote reverse remodeling globally.[113]

The clinical importance of routine viability testing, however, remains controversial based on the results of the viability testing in the STICH trial described in more detail below.

Endothelial Dysfunction

Available data suggest that the coronary endothelium plays an important role not only in the control of blood flow and vascular patency but also in the physiologic modulation of myocardial structure and function.[114] Thus endothelial dysfunction, an inherent component of the pathophysiology of atherosclerotic CAD, may directly affect ventricular function.[115] According to Bell and associates,[116] the coronary endothelium has numerous physiologic roles including:

- Regulation of vascular tone through the release of mediators such as nitric oxide (NO), prostacyclin, and endothelin
- Maintenance of a permeable barrier to provide for exchange and active transport of substances into the artery wall
- Synthesis and secretion of cytokines and growth factors
- Alterations of lipoproteins in the arterial wall
- Provision of a nonthrombogenic surface and a nonadherence surface for leukocytes
- Maintenance of basement membrane collagen proteoglycans[117]

Endothelial Vasodilators

The endothelial release of NO relaxes vascular smooth muscle cells in association with activation of guanylyl cyclase and increased levels of cyclic glucose monophosphate. NO is the most potent endogenous vasodilator and is responsible for the maintenance of vasovascular tone. NO also inhibits smooth muscle cell proliferation and migration, leukocyte adhesion, and platelet aggregation.[118,119]

Endothelial Vasoconstrictors

The major endothelin-derived vasoconstrictive substances include angiotensin II and endothelin. Angiotensin II is a potent vasoconstrictor that also exerts a variety of effects on vascular structure and function.[120] Studies of angiotensin II indicate the involvement of the renin-angiotensin system in many aspects of vascular homeostasis. Angiotensin II increases the production of plasminogen activator inhibitor type 1, the primary endogenous inhibitor of tissue plasminogen activator, and promotes vascular growth in addition to stimulating the production of other growth factors.[121] Angiotensin II also enhances platelet aggregation, sensitizes the platelets to the effects of direct platelet agonists, and stimulates the production of endothelin.[122] Endothelin is the most potent endogenous vasoconstrictor yet identified and promotes proliferation of smooth muscle cells and secretion of extracellular matrix, which contribute to the formation of atherosclerotic plaque.[123]

Disordered endothelial function in patients with CAD stimulates vasoconstriction, smooth muscle migration and proliferation, increased lipid deposition in the vessel wall, and possibly coronary thrombosis. This promotes myocardial ischemia, which may further contribute directly or indirectly to the progression of LV dysfunction.[115,124-126] The release of endothelin is also increased in failing myocardium.[127] Angiotensin II contributes to the release of endothelin and the excessive degradation of NO.[125] Taken together, these observations make a case for an interplay between the failing myocardium and the coronary endothelium that potentiates the progression of both CAD and LV dysfunction.

Properties of the normal endothelium serve to relax vascular tone, and inhibit smooth muscle growth, platelet aggregation, and leukocyte adhesion. Many drugs that reduce mortality and reinfarction in patients with CAD have the potential to improve endothelial function, including lipid lowering agents, ACE inhibitors, nonselective β-blockers, and aspirin.[128-131] For example, marked reduction of serum cholesterol is associated with a rapid recovery of endothelial function, improvement of myocardial perfusion, and reduction of myocardial ischemia.[132-138] An improvement in tissue perfusion is an important goal in patients with HF in terms of both the peripheral and the coronary circulation.

In summary, endothelial dysfunction may further reduce blood flow, promote progression of coronary atherosclerosis, and have direct negative effects on the myocardial cells and the interstitium.[139,140]

Clinical Manifestations

Reinfarction

Patients with HF and CAD are at increased risk for reinfarction. An analysis of the SOLVD trial found that patients who experienced MI had an approximately twofold higher rate of hospitalization for HF and about a fourfold increase in death compared with patients who did not experience MI.[141] Similarly, an analysis of the Survival and Ventricular Enlargement (SAVE) trial found that patients with evidence of a previous MI before enrollment were at significantly greater risk for cardiovascular death, LV enlargement, or both.[142] In clinical trials, the rate of infarction or reinfarction is relatively low, with a fatal MI rate of 3%.[143] However, in one study, more than half of patients with HF and CAD who died suddenly had autopsy evidence of an acute ischemic event (e.g., coronary clot, recent infarct),[40] suggesting that the number of patients with plaque rupture is not accounted for in clinical trials.

Sudden Cardiac Death

The risk of SCD after MI has significantly declined in recent years.[144] However, the occurrence of HF post-MI is associated with a markedly increased risk of SCD.[144] In several clinical HF trials, SCD accounted for 20% to 60% of deaths, depending on the severity of HF.[145] In the Metoprolol CR/XL Randomised Intervention Trial in Congestive Heart Failure (MERIT-HF), 64% of patients in New York Heart Association (NYHA) class II who subsequently died had SCD compared with 59% of patients in class III and 33% of patients in class IV.[146] Several factors have been implicated in the high rate

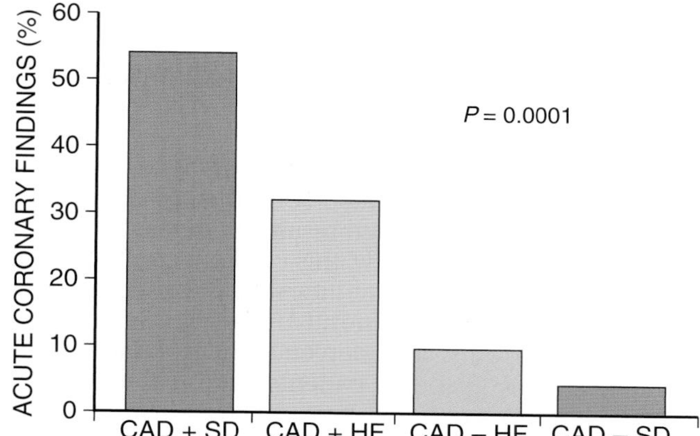

FIGURE 18-6 Relation of acute coronary findings to mode of death and presence of coronary artery disease in the ATLAS trial. Patients with SCD had the highest prevalence of acute coronary findings. +, Presence of CAD; –, absence of CAD. *From Uretsky BF, Thygesen K, Armstrong PW, et al: Acute coronary findings at autopsy in heart failure patients with sudden death: results from the assessment of treatment with lisinopril and survival (ATLAS) trial. Circulation 102:611–616, 2000.*

of SCD in patients with HF. These include subendocardial ischemia, ventricular hypertrophy, stretching of myocytes, a high sympathetic tone, abnormal baroreceptor responsiveness lowering the threshold for a malignant arrhythmia, potassium and magnesium depletion, and coronary artery emboli from atrial or LV thrombi.[145] However, CAD probably contributes directly to SCD.[145] Patients with CAD and systolic HF have dilated hearts, large regions of myocardial scar, and obstructive epicardial coronary stenosis. CAD and its major structural consequences (i.e., plaque rupture, thrombosis, and infarction) constitute the most common structural basis of SCD.[147,148]

Uretsky and colleagues reported the relative importance of an acute coronary event as a trigger for SCD in patients with HF who were studied in the Assessment of Treatment with Lisinopril and Survival (ATLAS) trial, which included 3164 patients with moderate to severe systolic HF.[40] There were 1383 deaths (43.7%) during the follow-up period of 3 to 5 years. An autopsy was performed in only 188 patients, and the postmortem data were available in only 171 patients (12.4% of the total patients who died). Patients who died in this study were older and had both more symptoms and a higher prevalence of CAD than the surviving patients. The patients who died and did not undergo autopsy were similar to those who died and were subjected to autopsy. Acute coronary findings were observed in 54% of the patients with significant CAD who died suddenly (**Figure 18-6**). The ATLAS study was the first to demonstrate that recent coronary events are frequently unrecognized in patients with moderate to advanced HF symptoms who die suddenly, especially in patients with CAD.

Other studies have documented a high frequency of plaque rupture or coronary thrombosis in patients with CAD who suffered SCD.[147,149] However, it should be noted that these studies reported a much higher incidence of ruptured plaque, ranging from 57% to 81%, than the ATLAS autopsy study.[40,147,149] However, the prevalence of clinical acute coronary findings in the same series ranged from 21% to 41%, which was similar to the ATLAS study.[40] Because the autopsy findings reported in ATLAS were based on routine clinical examinations, it is unlikely that the examinations involved the degree of detail necessary to observe ruptured plaque and small thrombi. Therefore, it is possible that the rate of acute coronary events may have been even higher than reported. This study underlines the importance of strategies to prevent and treat acute coronary events to successfully prevent SCD in patients with HF. For example, in the ATLAS trial, two thirds of patients had CAD but only 40% of this group was taking aspirin.[40]

Among patients with HF who receive an ICD for the primary prevention of SCD, those who receive shocks have a markedly increased short-term risk of death compared with those who do not receive shocks. This risk may be much higher in patients with CAD.[150,151] A recent analysis of the Sudden Cardiac Death in Heart Failure Trial (SCD-HeFT) revealed that patients with HF due to CAD who received an appropriate ICD shock had a threefold increased risk of mortality compared with patients with HF and a nonischemic cause who received an appropriate ICD shock. This suggests that among patients with HF, those with CAD can develop fundamental alterations in the underlying arrhythmic substrate that predisposes them to SCD.

CORONARY ARTERY DISEASE AND DIASTOLIC HEART FAILURE (see also Chapter 36)

The vast majority of HF trials conducted over the past 30 years have studied patients with LVSD. However, HF with relatively preserved systolic function is present in approximately half of all patients hospitalized with HF.[152-159] Among patients with HF and preserved systolic function, approximately 60% have documented CAD.[156] Over the past two decades, the relative proportion of patients with HF and preserved systolic function has risen steadily relative to those with LVSD.[153] Patients with HF and preserved systolic function tend to be older than those with HF and LVSD. Thus the relative rise in this category of HF is reflective of an aging population. This rise has also corresponded to increased rates of CAD, hypertension, diabetes, and atrial fibrillation in this population. Among patients hospitalized with HF, the early and long-term risk of death is similar for patients with preserved systolic function and LVSD.[154,157-159] However, patients with HF and preserved systolic function are more likely to die from other cardiac comorbidities, including CAD, rather than progressive HF when compared with patients with HF and LVSD.[160,161]

When systolic function is preserved, it is assumed that the majority of these patients have HF signs and symptoms on the basis of abnormal LV diastolic function.[162] A variety of factors predispose to abnormalities in diastolic functional behavior of the left ventricle and lead to elevating filling pressures, impaired forward output, or both, despite normal systolic function.[163] Myocardial ischemia is one of the leading factors. Pulmonary congestion can be caused by reversible episodes of ischemia, which impair LV relaxation and increase LV filling pressure.[164]

The prognosis in patients with HF and preserved systolic function in the presence of CAD may be directly related to the angiographic burden of CAD. O'Connor and associates demonstrated that patients with HF and preserved systolic function have a worse 5-year survival if they have left main or 3-vessel CAD versus those with 1- to 2-vessel CAD.[42] Similarly, according to the Coronary Artery Surgery Study (CASS) registry, the 6-year survival rate of patients with normal ejection fraction and HF symptoms was 92% in patients with no CAD, 83% in patients with 1- or 2-vessel CAD, and 68% in patients with 3-vessel disease.[165]

There is a need for reappraisal on whether systolic function is truly normal at the time when HF symptoms are present in patients diagnosed with HF and "normal" systolic function. The majority of studies of this syndrome did not report the timing of the evaluation demonstrating normal systolic function relative to the episodes of HF itself.[166] In other studies, the evaluation was performed days to weeks after the episode.[167] Transient ischemia may cause regional systolic dysfunction, which in many patients was severe and extensive enough to cause a brief but profound reduction in global LV function.[167] The pathophysiologic changes in regional and global systolic function form the basis for exercise radionuclide ventriculography and exercise echocardiography as diagnostic tests for myocardial ischemia due to CAD. It may be that many patients with apparently normal systolic function and HF caused by CAD do not have isolated diastolic dysfunction but instead have transient systolic and diastolic dysfunction at the time when myocardial ischemia induces HF symptoms.

DIABETES, HEART FAILURE, AND CORONARY ARTERY DISEASE (see also Chapter 45)

In terms of cardiovascular risk, a diagnosis of diabetes is comparable to a diagnosis of CAD.[168,169] The prevalence of documented CAD in diabetic patients has been shown to be as high as 55%, compared with 2% to 4% for the general population.[170] Diabetic patients with a history of MI have a markedly worse prognosis than individuals with only one of these conditions.[168,169] A significant number of patients with HF have diabetes: 23% in the CONSENSUS trial, 25% in SOLVD, 20% in V-HeFT, 20% in ATLAS, 27% in RESOLVD, 42% in the OPTIMIZE-HF registry, and 44% in the ADHERE registry.[9,11,40,171,172-174] Diabetes is an independent risk factor for the development of HF.[175-177] In the Framingham Heart Study, the relative risk for developing HF in diabetic patients was 3.8 for men and 5.5 for women, respectively, compared with nondiabetic patients.[177] The risk of developing HF in diabetic patients has been directly related to glycemic control.[178,179] In the United Kingdom Prospective Diabetic Study (UKPDS), for each 1% increase in glycosylated hemoglobin level, the risk of HF rose by 12%.[179]

The presence of diabetes in patients with HF is associated with substantially higher mortality rates.[180-189] Several studies suggest that the increased risk in diabetic patients with HF compared with nondiabetic patients with HF is limited to individuals with concomitant CAD.[186-189] Diabetic patients with CAD also have worse outcomes following myocardial revascularization.[190] Derangements associated with diabetes, including hyperglycemia, insulin resistance, dyslipidemia, inflammation, and thrombosis, contribute to the development of hypertension, endothelial cell dysfunction, accelerated atherogenesis, and coronary thrombosis.[190,191] In addition, diabetic patients exhibit more complex and diffuse anatomic patterns of CAD, including more lipid-rich plaques and intracoronary thrombi but less compensatory vascular remodeling.[190,192-194]

Diabetes directly contributes to HF in patients with LVSD, diastolic dysfunction, or both.[195,196] The increased mortality in patients with HF in the presence of diabetes has been observed in patients with either LVSD or preserved systolic function.[182] Ventricular dysfunction in patients with HF and diabetes has been termed *diabetic cardiomyopathy* and is the result of the complex interplay between the sympathetic nervous system and the renin-angiotensin-aldosterone system (RAAS), increased levels of circulation cytokines, alterations in heart rate variability, and increased oxidative stress.[197] Chronic hyperglycemia leads to the glycation of collagen and elevated serum levels of advanced glycation end products, which results in increased myocardial stiffness.[198] Pathologically, this cardiomyopathy is characterized by myocyte atrophy, interstitial fibrosis, increased periodic acid–Schiff (PAS)-positive material, intramyocardial microangiopathy, and depletion of myocardial catecholamines.[199] In diabetic patients with HF and LVSD, myocardial fibrosis and the deposition of advanced glycation end products predominate, whereas in those with HF and preserved systolic function, increased cardiomyocyte resting tension is a more important mechanism.[196]

Therapeutic Options

Recognition that progression of CAD may contribute importantly to progression of HF, in at least a subset of patients, shifts the focus from medical management designed solely to reduce neurohormonal activation and alleviate congestive symptoms to a strategy designed to employ aggressive secondary prevention measures. Those efforts to slow the progression of CAD include attention to reducing the risk of acute coronary events by plaque stabilization, reducing ischemia, and enhancing endothelial function. It is noteworthy that the classes of drugs that have shown conclusively to improve survival in HF-ACE inhibitors, angiotensin receptor blockers (ARBs), β-blockers, and aldosterone antagonists (**see also Chapter 34**), address those factors. The beneficial effects of these drugs may relate as much to their vascular protective effects as to their neurohormonal blocking effects. Patients hospitalized with HF are frequently undertreated for CAD. For example, ACS patients with acute HF are less likely to receive antiplatelet agents, β-blockers, ACE inhibitors, or statins than ACS patients without HF.[42,45,46,51,158] In addition to pharmacologic therapy, myocardial revascularization, surgical therapy, and cardiac device therapy may play an important role in the treatment of patients with HF in the setting of CAD.

Immediate Management of the Hospitalized Patient

The immediate management of acute HF usually occurs in the emergency department (**see also Chapter 33**).[200] There is considerable overlap in the presentation and management of acute HF patients with CAD and ACS versus CAD and non-ACS (see Tables 18-2 and 18-3). In patients with underlying CAD who are not hypotensive, nitrates may provide a rapid reduction of myocardial ischemia and improve coronary perfusion. In patients with severe pulmonary edema, the combination of high-dose nitrates and low-dose diuretics (vs. low-dose nitrates and high-dose diuretics) led to significantly decreased rates of mechanical ventilation and MI.[201] A regimen for acute HF consisting of lower doses of diuretics has been proposed as a method of preserving renal function. In a large acute HF registry, the use of intravenous nitroglycerin or nesiritide was associated with lower in-hospital mortality compared with treatment with dobutamine or milrinone.[202] However, compared with intravenous nesiritide in acute HF patients, of whom greater than 60% had documented CAD, intravenous nitroglycerin has been associated with less deterioration of renal function and a trend toward less mortality at 30 days.[203-204]

Inotropes may be particularly harmful when used in HF patients with CAD. Experimentally, the use of dobutamine in a model of HF with hibernating myocardium led to increased myocardial necrosis.[205] Hospitalized HF patients with troponin elevation have significantly higher in-hospital mortality when inotropes are used.[49] In the Outcomes of a Prospective Trial of Intravenous Milrinone for Exacerbations of Chronic Heart Failure (OPTIME-CHF) trial, use of the phosphodiesterase inhibitor milrinone in patients with CAD was associated with increased postdischarge mortality compared with a placebo.[111] In general, a decrease in coronary perfusion as a result of a decrease in blood pressure and/or an increase in heart rate resulting from inotropes with vasodilator properties, or inotropes used in conjunction with vasodilators, may be particularly deleterious in HF patients with CAD.[112,206]

In a recent series of 112 inotrope-dependent patients with stage D heart failure patients not eligible for transplantation, there was no difference in the adjusted mortality rate observed between those treated with milrinone and those treated with dobutamine.[207]

Long-Term Therapies for the Heart Failure Patient with CAD

Renin-Angiotensin-Aldosterone System Modulators

The RAAS regulates sodium balance, fluid volume, and blood pressure, which has a profound impact on HF and CAD (see also Chapter 5).[208] The use of ACE inhibitors or ARBs is strongly indicated in HF patients with LVSD and is also indicated for the secondary prevention of cardiovascular events in all patients with CAD.[209-211]

Endothelial dysfunction plays a fundamental role in many forms of cardiovascular disease and is the final common pathway through which most cardiovascular risk factors contribute to inflammation and atherosclerosis. Angiotensin II is a powerful vasoconstrictor, and also stimulates smooth muscle cells (hyperplasia), fibroblast proliferation, collagen deposition, inflammation, and thrombosis. All these maladaptations can be mitigated by the use of ACE inhibitors or ARBs.[129,208,212] In the SOLVD and the SAVE trials, the ACE inhibitors enalapril and captopril not only reduced overall mortality in patients with CAD, but also reduced the rate of nonfatal MI and unstable angina.[141,213] In the SAVE trial, a 25% decrease in MI with captopril occurred despite the selection criteria, which excluded patients with residual ischemia who were considered at great risk of reinfarction.[213] The reduction of acute ischemic events would not have been anticipated only on the basis of the hemodynamic or neurohormonal effects of ACE inhibitors. Moreover, in the SOLVD trial, the reduction of unstable angina and MI with enalapril was not evident until more than 6 months after randomization.[141] This suggests that the beneficial effects of enalapril on ischemic events was not due to an immediate effect related to a primary or secondary reduction in LV afterload.

The addition of eplerenone, an aldosterone antagonist, to optimal medical therapy in ACS patients with acute HF and LVSD significantly reduced death and rehospitalization in the Eplerenone Post-Acute Myocardial Infarction Heart Failure Efficacy and Survival Study (EPHESUS) trial (**Figure 18-7**).[104] The reduction in death corresponded with a decrease in SCD, which may be due to the inhibition of myocardial fibrosis.[214]

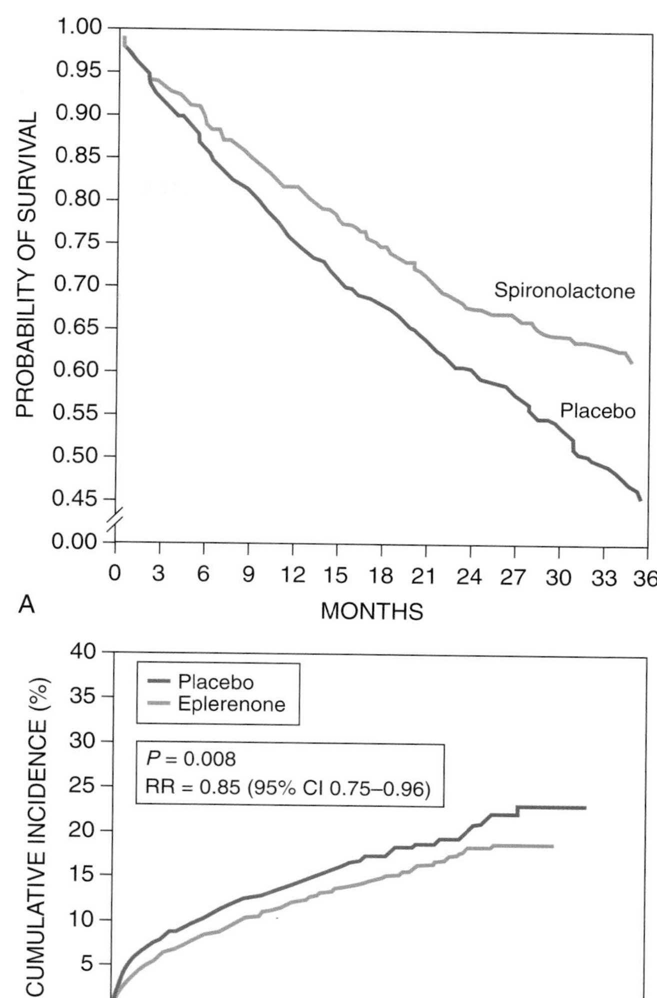

FIGURE 18-7 Trials testing aldosterone antagonists. *EPHESUS*, Eplerenone Post-Acute Myocardial Infarction Heart Failure Efficacy and Survival Study; *RALES*, Randomized Aldactone Evaluation Study; *RR*, relative risk. *Modified from Pitt B, Zannad F, Remme WJ, et al: The effect of spironolactone on morbidity and mortality in patients with severe heart failure. Randomized aldactone evaluation study investigators. N Engl J Med 341:709, 1999; Pitt B, Remme W, Zannad F, et al: Eplerenone, a selective aldosterone blocker, in patients with left ventricular dysfunction after myocardial infarction. N Engl J Med 348:1309, 2003.*

This study was followed by the Eplerenone in Mild Patients Hospitalization and Survival Study in Heart Failure (EMPHASIS-HF),[215] which studied the effects of the eplerenone added to standard therapy in a population of NYHA class II patients with LVSD. Approximately 70% of the patients studied had an ischemic etiology. The addition of eplerenone correlated with a significant reduction in the risk of all-cause death and hospitalization.

Recently, direct renin inhibitors (DRIs) have been added to the armamentarium of RAAS inhibition. These agents effectively suppress angiotensin II and aldosterone levels without the rebound increase in plasma renin activity seen with ACE inhibitors and ARB therapy.[216] The addition of the oral DRI aliskiren to standard therapy in patients with

NYHA class II-IV has been shown to reduce plasma NT-proBNP levels.[217] However, in the Effect of Aliskiren on Postdischarge Mortality and Heart Failure Readmissions Among Patients Hospitalized for Heart Failure (ASTRONAUT) trial, the addition of aliskiren to standard therapy in hospitalized HF patients with LVSD did not reduce CV death or HF hospitalization at 6 months or 12 months postdischarge.[218] Those who received aliskiren had higher rates of hyperkalemia, hypotension, and renal dysfunction. An ongoing trial, the Aliskiren Trial to Minimize OutcomeS in Patients with HEart failuRE (ATMOSPHERE) study, will compare the use of aliskiren both with and against the ACE-I enalapril in a patients with NYHA class II-IV HF and LVSD.[219]

β-Blockers

β-blockers are effective for the reduction of death and rehospitalization in patients with HF and CAD.[98] The continuation or predischarge initiation of β-blockers in patients hospitalized with HF is associated with improved medication adherence and an early survival advantage.[220-222] Patients with viable but dysfunctional myocardium derive greater improvement in LV function and remodeling from β-blocker therapy than those without viability.[96,113]

The improvement in survival with β-blockers in the MERIT-HF and CIBIS II trials was more pronounced in patients with HF and documented CAD than in patients with a presumed nonischemic cause.[145,223] However, improvement in survival was slightly more pronounced in patients with presumed nonischemic HF and mild to moderate HF studied in the U.S. Carvedilol Trials and in patients with severe HF patients studied in the Carvedilol Prospective Randomized Cumulative Survival (COPERNICUS) Trial.[18,19] These differential effects were minor because the reduction in mortality in each of these four trials was less than 30% and there was a nonsignificant difference in mortality benefit between ischemic and nonischemic patients.[224] In MERIT-HF, mortality was slightly higher in diabetic patients with HF who were treated with metoprolol succinate than in nondiabetic patients with HF, while carvedilol showed similar reductions for diabetic and nondiabetic patients in both the U.S. Carvedilol Trials and COPERNICUS. The benefit of carvedilol in CAD patients was later confirmed in post-MI patients in the CAPRICORN study (Carvedilol Post-Infarct Survival Control in LV Dysfunction).[225] In this study of 1959 post-MI patients with a left ventricular ejection fraction (LVEF) of 40% or less, the addition of carvedilol to ACE inhibitor therapy led to a 20% relative reduction in all-cause mortality at a mean follow-up of 1.3 years (**Figure 18-8**).[225] The differences observed with β-blockers in outcomes based on the presence of CAD in HF patients may be due to cause-related differences in pathophysiologic derangements on the β-adrenergic signal transduction pathway.[226] This may also relate to the more severe symptoms of patients enrolled in COPERNICUS, differences in β_1-selectivity versus β_1-nonselectivity, or other pharmacologic differences between β-blocking agents, such as α-blockade, antioxidant effect, and lipophilicity.[227]

Lipid-Lowering Agents

Statin therapy is strongly recommended in patients with CAD.[228] The benefits of statins may be caused by plaque stabilization and improvements in endothelial function. The Cholesterol and Recurrent Events (CARE) trial, which

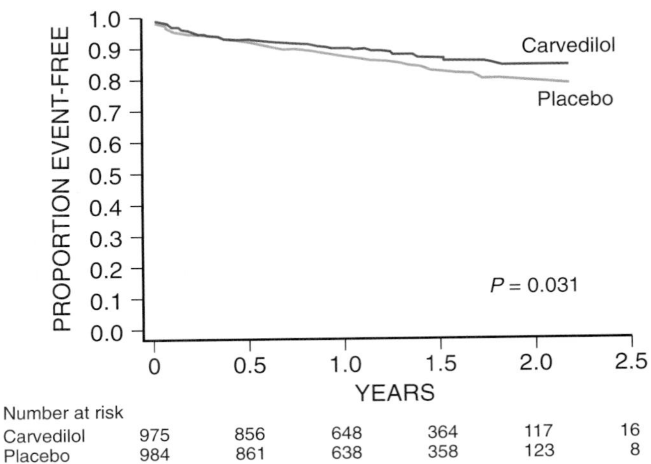

Number at risk						
Carvedilol	975	856	648	364	117	16
Placebo	984	861	638	358	123	8

FIGURE 18-8 Effect of carvedilol on morbidity and mortality in patient with left ventricular dysfunction after acute myocardial infarction in the CAPRICORN study. *From Dargie HJ: Effect of carvedilol on outcome after myocardial infarction in patients with left ventricular dysfunction: the CAPRICORN randomized trial. Lancet 357:1385–1390, 2001.*

demonstrated beneficial effects of pravastatin in patients with mild elevation of serum cholesterol after MI, prospectively randomized a subset of patients with an ejection fraction between 25% and 40%[229]; these patients had similar characteristics to those entered into post-MI ACE inhibitor trials, such as SAVE.[142] Pravastatin significantly decreased cardiac events in this subgroup. Similarly, in the Scandinavian Simvastatin Survival Study (4S), simvastatin decreased the development of HF symptoms after MI; among patients who experienced HF, simvastatin decreased mortality from 32% to 25%.[230] Furthermore, in patients with either stable CAD or ACS, the use of high-dose statin therapy is associated with a decreased risk for HF hospitalization compared with low-dose statin therapy.[231,232]

Dyslipidemia is associated with an increased risk for the development of HF that is independent of its association with MI.[233] This risk has been further linked to individual lipoprotein components, notably the apoB/apoA-1 ratio and triglyceride levels.[234]

In unselected HF patients, the use of statins is associated with lower mortality, including the elderly and patients with preserved systolic function.[235-237] However, the Controlled Rosuvastatin Multinational Trial in Heart Failure (CORONA) showed that rosuvastatin therapy in older patients (60 years or older) with chronic HF and LVSD did not lead to a decrease in all-cause death (**Figure 18-9A**), although there was a reduction in HF hospitalizations.[238] There was also a trend toward fewer coronary events in the patients treated with rosuvastatin. In the Gruppo Italiano per lo Studio della Sopravvievenza nell'Insufficienza Cardiaca Heart Failure (GISSI-HF) trial, the use of rosuvastatin in patients with chronic HF (mean age 68 years, 90% with LVSD, 40% ischemic cause) did not decrease mortality or cardiovascular hospitalization at 4 years (see Figure 18-9B).[239] These data suggest that statin therapy may be important for the prevention of HF and ischemic events in patients with CAD, but may be unable to impact mortality in patients with chronic HF and LVSD.

Fish consumption and dietary supplementation with n-3 polyunsaturated fatty acids (PUFA), in individuals with and without established CAD, is associated with reduced cardiovascular mortality.[176,240,241] In a separate GISSI-HF trial,

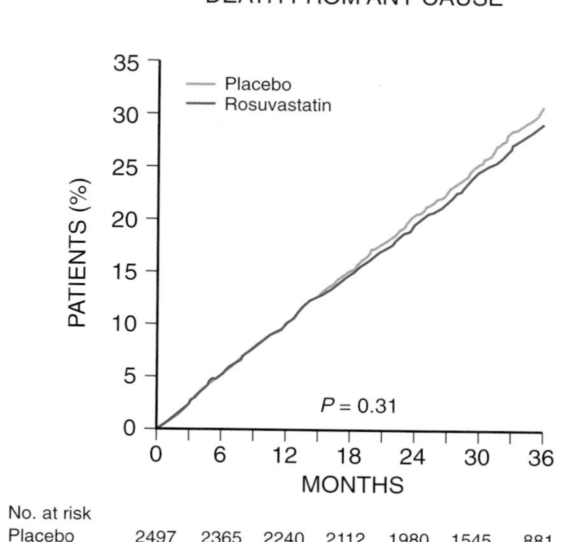

No. at risk

Placebo	2497	2365	2240	2112	1980	1545	881
Rosuvastatin	2514	2379	2260	2139	2018	1566	907

A

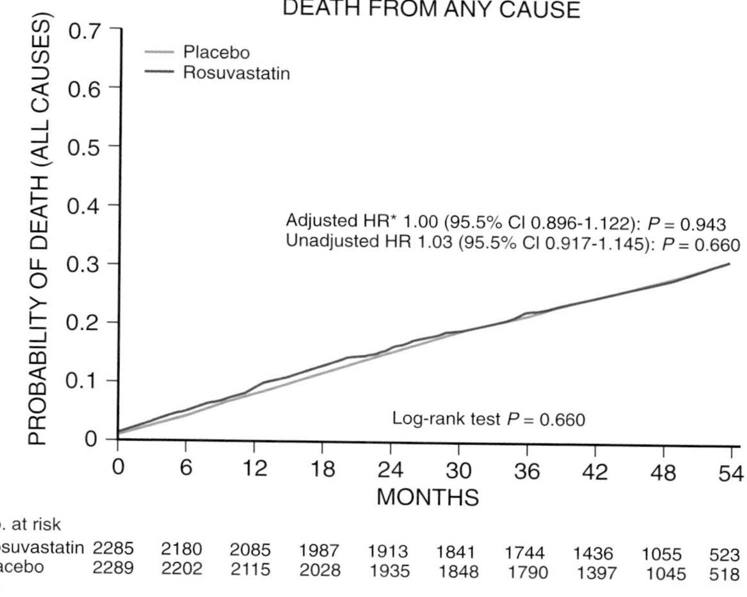

No. at risk

Rosuvastatin	2285	2180	2085	1987	1913	1841	1744	1436	1055	523
Placebo	2289	2202	2115	2028	1935	1848	1790	1397	1045	518

B

FIGURE 18-9 Effect of rosuvastatin on patients with HF. **A,** Effects of rosuvastatin on all-cause death in older patients (60 years of age) with chronic HF and LVSD in the CORONA study. **B,** Effects of rosuvastatin on all-cause death in patients with chronic HF with depressed and preserved systolic function in the GISSI-HF trial. *Estimates were calculated with a Cox proportional hazards model, with adjustments for admission to hospital for heart failure in the previous year, previous pacemaker, sex, diabetes, pathologic Q waves, and angiotensin receptor blockers. *Modified from Kjekshus J, Apetrei E, Barrios V, et al: Rosuvastatin in older patients with systolic heart failure. N Engl J Med 357:2248–2261, 2007; GISSI-HF Investigators: Effect of rosuvastatin in patients with chronic heart failure. Lancet 372:1231–1239, 2008.*

the use of n-3 PUFA in patients with chronic HF (mean age 67 years, 90% with LVSD, 50% ischemic cause) led to a 2% absolute risk reduction in mortality (27% vs. 29% at 4 years, $P = 0.041$) and a similar reduction in cardiovascular hospitalization.[242] It is suspected that n-3 PUFA may exert their beneficial effect via the reduction of arrhythmic events and not ischemic events. As the use of ICD therapy in this trial was low (7%), the impact of this therapy on patients with chronic HF and LVSD with appropriate indications for ICD therapy is unclear.

Antiplatelet and Anticoagulation Therapy

The use of antiplatelet therapy (i.e., aspirin or clopidogrel) is strongly indicated in the presence of CAD for the secondary prevention of cardiovascular events.[243] Dual antiplatelet therapy, clopidogrel added to aspirin, has been shown to be beneficial in ACS patients for the prevention of recurrent ischemic events and was associated with an 18% reduction in subsequent HF.[244] There is experimental evidence that aspirin inhibits the acute arterial and venous vasodilator response to ACE inhibitors in patients with chronic HF.[245] However, there is no prospective evidence that this potential interaction is clinically relevant. Nevertheless, it may be prudent to limit the combination of aspirin and ACE inhibitor therapy in HF patients to those with established CAD.

LVSD is independently associated with an increased risk of ischemic stroke.[246] The use of oral anticoagulation is strongly indicated in HF patients with atrial fibrillation and patients with confirmed or suspected LV thrombus. However, to date, there is a lack of evidence that the use of oral anticoagulation in HF patients without atrial fibrillation has a beneficial effect on cardiovascular events, including embolic stroke.[247,248]

Myocardial Revascularization

The role of surgical management of HF patients with stable CAD has been an area of uncertainty (see also Chapter 41). The three major randomized clinical trials that have compared coronary artery bypass graft surgery with medical management, the Veterans Administration Cooperative Study, the European Coronary Surgery Study, and the Coronary Artery Surgery Study, all excluded patients with heart failure or severe LVSD. Historically, registries and databases have been used to inform decision making for patients with ischemic cardiomyopathy. For example, a report from the Duke database compared coronary artery bypass graft (CABG) surgery versus medical therapy over a 25-year period. Medical therapy was used in 1052 patients and CABG in 339.[72] Unadjusted and adjusted survival (Cox proportional-hazards model) strongly favored CABG after 30 days and at 10 years. This analysis included all groups by extent of CAD, and by different subgroups (**Figure 18-10**). Adjusted overall survival at 1 year, 5 years, and 10 years was 83% versus 74%; 61% versus 37%; and 42% versus 13% for CABG versus medical therapy (all $P < 0.0001$). Other similar analyses in patients with chronic systolic HF and CAD appear to corroborate a protective effect for CABG.[249]

It has been hypothesized that revascularization may improve outcomes in patients with HF and dysfunctional but viable myocardium. In a meta-analysis of greater than 3000 patients with LVSD, revascularization was associated with markedly decreased yearly mortality (3.2% vs. 16.0%, $P < 0.0001$) if viability was present.[101] In patients without hibernating myocardium, revascularization did not improve survival. A different retrospective observational study examined the role of myocardial revascularization in approximately 4000 patients with chronic HF.[250] At 1 year, patients who underwent revascularization had substantially reduced mortality (11.8% vs. 21.6%, HR 0.52, 95% CI 0.47 to 0.58). The survival curves continued to diverge through 7 years of follow-up.

In 2002, the National Institutes of Health initiated funding for the STICH (Surgical Treatment for Ischemic Heart Failure) trial. The STICH trial was a prospective randomized

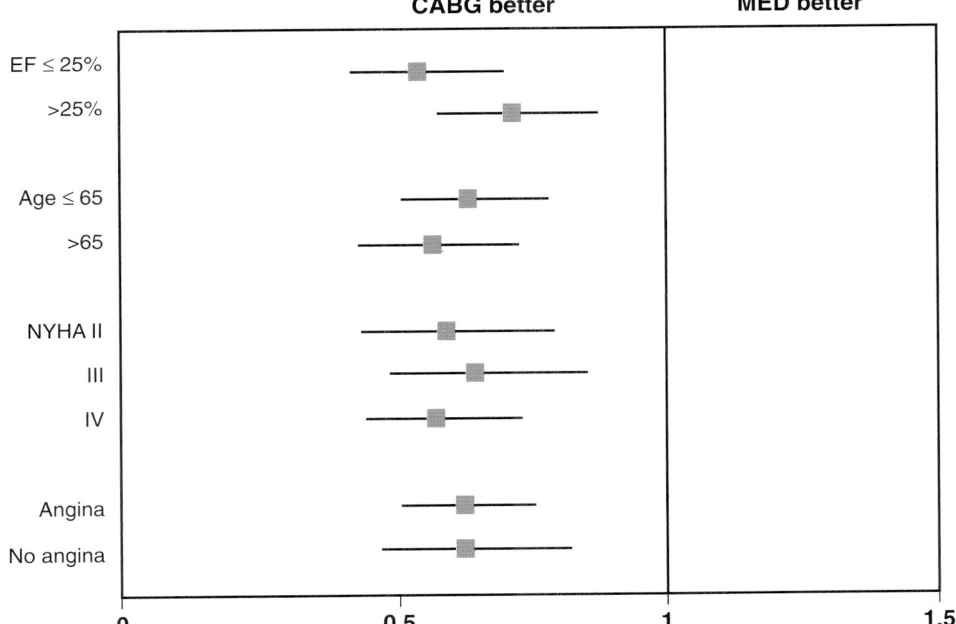

FIGURE 18-10 Subgroup analysis of coronary artery revascularization versus medical therapy in patients with heart failure. Hazard ratios (95% confidence interval) for mortality for a number of baseline characteristics all favored CABG. *CABG,* Coronary artery bypass grafting; *EF,* ejection fraction; *MED,* medical therapy; *NYHA,* New York Heart Association. *Modified from O'Connor CM, Velazquez EJ, Gardner LH, et al: Comparison of coronary artery bypass grafting versus medical therapy on long-term outcome in patients with ischemic cardiomyopathy: a 25-year experience from the Duke cardiovascular disease databank. Am J Cardiol 90:101, 2002.*

study that enrolled more than 2200 patients at approximately 100 centers. Patients with CAD and LVSD amenable to CABG were randomized to combinations of three different treatment strategies: CABG, surgical ventricular reconstruction (SVR), and intensive medical therapy. The trial was designed to address two primary hypotheses: (1) CABG combined with medical therapy improves long-term survival when compared with medical therapy alone; (2) SVR provides an additional long-term survival benefit when combined with CABG and medical therapy.

The results of the second arm of the study were published first.[251] One thousand patients were randomized to CABG alone (499) or CABG with SVR (modified Dor procedure) (501). SVR reduced the end-systolic volume index by 19%, as compared with a reduction of 6% with CABG alone. Cardiac symptoms and exercise tolerance improved from baseline to a similar degree in the two study groups. However, there was no significant difference in a composite of death from any cause and hospitalization for cardiac causes, which was the primary outcome of the trial (**Figure 18-11**). The results from hypothesis 2 of the STICH trial may indicate that a stricter definition of what constitutes an LV aneurysm may need to be applied in future studies of SVR if this procedure is to maintain clinical relevance. Post hoc analyses of the SVR group from STICH suggest a benefit from SVR in patients with smaller preoperative and/or postoperative LV volumes.[252,253]

There are also reports of more refined SVR techniques that may achieve better long-term clinical results.[254]

Meanwhile, the percutaneous placement of a ventricular partitioning device (VPD) represents a novel therapy under development for the treatment of HF in post-MI patient with a low LVEF and anterior wall akinesis or dyskinesis. Early analyses indicate that the placement of a VPD is safe and feasible and may improve hemodynamics and functional capacity.[255] This therapy is currently the subject of a randomized trial in the United States (PARACHUTE IV).[256]

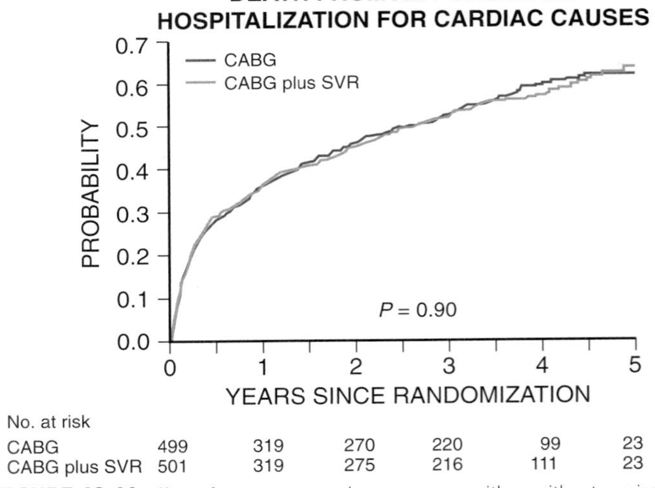

FIGURE 18-11 Effect of coronary artery bypass surgery with or without surgical ventricular reconstruction on all-cause death and hospitalization for cardiac causes in the STICH trial. *Modified from Jones RH, Velazquez EJ, Michler RE, et al: Coronary bypass surgery with or without surgical ventricular reconstruction. N Engl J Med 360:1705–1717, 2009.*

This first arm (hypothesis 1) of the STICH trial randomized 1212 patients with an LVEF of 35% or less and CAD amenable to CABG to medical therapy alone or medical therapy plus CABG. The results of a large subset of patients who underwent myocardial viability testing were reported simultaneously.[257] Overall, there was no survival advantage conferred by CABG over medical therapy alone during the follow-up period in the intention-to-treat analysis (**Figure 18-12A**). However, in a pre-specified analysis, patients who

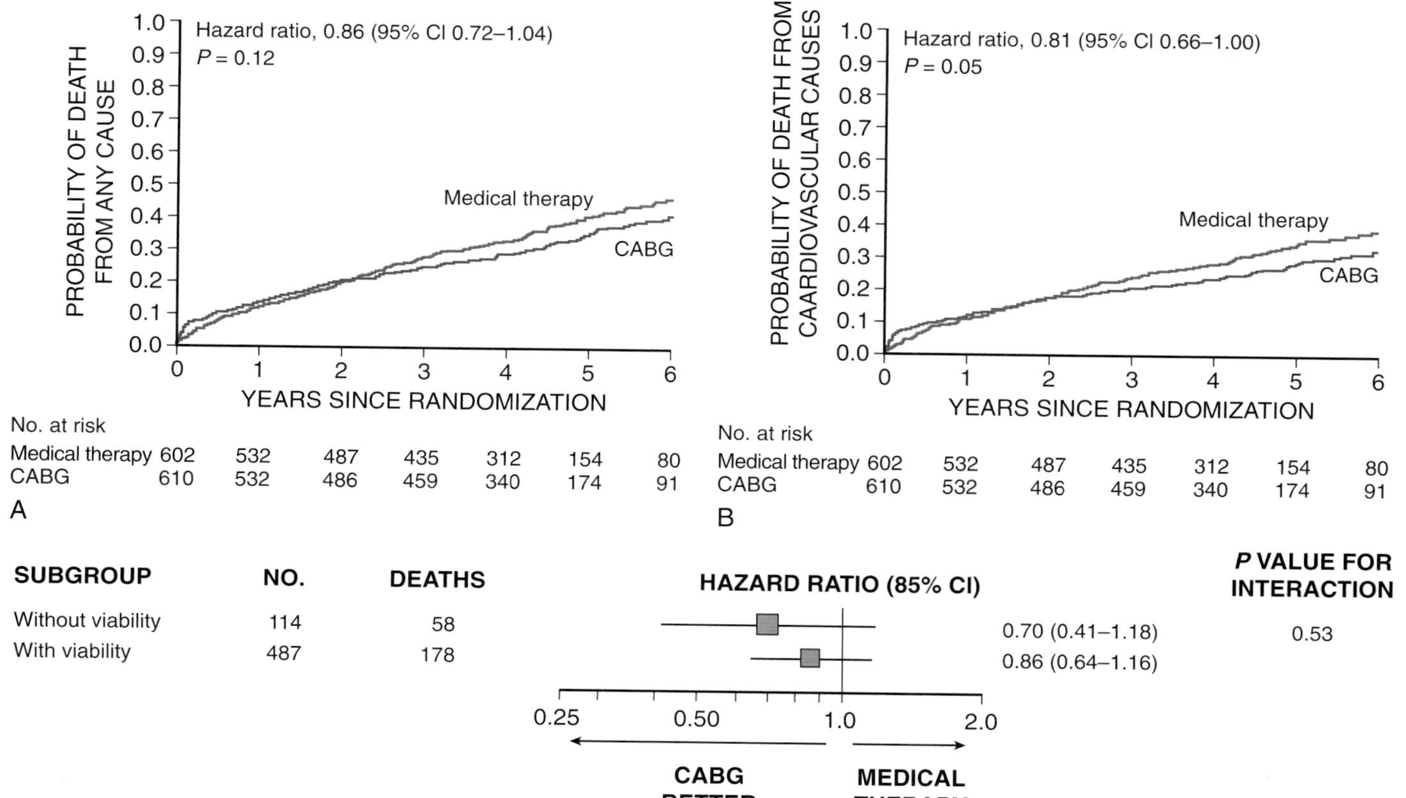

FIGURE 18-12 Influence of coronary artery bypass graft (CABG) on mortality compared with medical therapy alone in the STICH trial. **A,** Per the intention-to-treat analysis, there was not a significant impact of CABG on mortality. **B,** CABG was associated with a decreased risk of death from cardiovascular causes. **C,** After control for baseline variables, there was no significant interaction between viability status and treatment assignment with respect to mortality. *Modified from Velazquez EJ, Lee KL, Deja MA, et al for the STICH Investigators: Coronary artery bypass surgery in patients with left ventricular dysfunction. N Engl J Med 364:1601–1616, 2011; Bonow RO, Maurer G, Lee KL, et al for the STICH Investigators: Myocardial viability and survival in ischemic left ventricular dysfunction. N Engl J Med 364:1617–1625, 2011.*

underwent CABG had significantly less death from cardiovascular causes (see Figure 18-12B). This reduction in cardiovascular death after CABG has been attributed to a decrease in SCD and fatal pump failure events.[258] Nine percent of patients were assigned to but did not undergo CABG, whereas 17% of patients assigned to medical therapy alone crossed over to CABG in the follow-up period. In an as-treated analysis, the hazard ratio for patients who either randomized to CABG or who crossed over to CABG during the first year of follow-up was 0.70 (95% CI 0.58-0.84, P <0.001) compared with those who did not undergo CABG.[259]

The presence of myocardial viability, demonstrated by single-photon emission computed tomography (SPECT) and/or dobutamine echocardiography, in the STICH trial was associated with improved survival. However, this association was not statistically significant after adjustment for other baseline variables (see Figure 18-12C). Furthermore, there was no significant interaction between the presence of viable myocardium and the assigned treatment with respect to mortality, suggesting a limited role for viability testing in treatment selection. Patients with myocardial viability did have a significantly reduced risk for a composite of death or hospitalization (HF 0.59, 95% CI 0.47-0.74), a relationship that remained significant on multivariate analysis (P = 0.003). Overall, this subgroup had more comorbidities and a lower mean LVEF than patients who did not undergo viability testing, implying that it may not be appropriate to extrapolate the results to the entire study population. Also left unanswered is the role of emerging techniques to assess myocardial viability, in particular delayed-enhancement cardiovascular magnetic resonance (CMR) imaging. CMR may have a more powerful role in defining the burden of myocardial scar, which has recently been shown to be indirectly associated with improvement in contractility after revascularization.[260]

STICH largely applies to the outpatient setting as 95% of those who underwent CABG did so on an elective basis. Studies have shown that outcomes in patients with HF in the setting of an ACS are improved by a strategy of early myocardial revascularization.[261] This includes patients with and without ST-segment elevation and those in cardiogenic shock.[262] Despite this, patients with ACS complicated by HF are less likely to undergo revascularization than ACS patients without HF.[6,261] Non-ACS patients hospitalized with acute HF have improved early survival if they have a history of myocardial revascularization, although this a retrospective finding.[47,53] This relationship has been observed in acute HF patients with LVSD or preserved systolic function. These data generate the hypothesis that early revascularization will be beneficial in acute HF patients with ischemia due to CAD. A management strategy for the acute HF failure based on the presence, extent, and severity of CAD could help identify appropriate candidates for optimal medical therapy for CAD and, when indicated, myocardial revascularization (**Figure 18-13**). The performance of in-hospital angiography in patients with acute HF and CAD is associated with

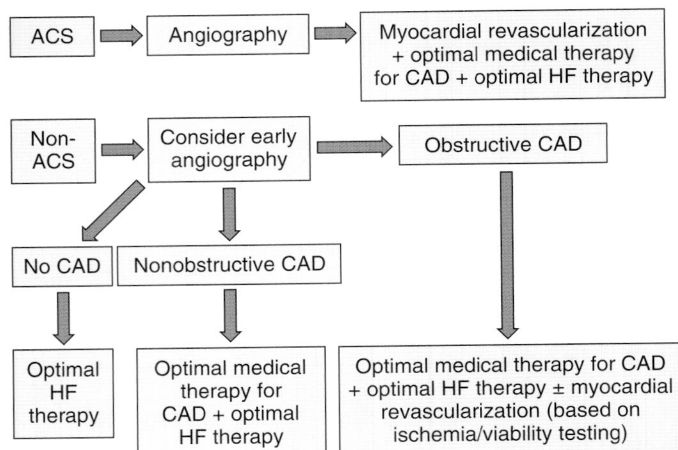

FIGURE 18-13 A proposed algorithm for the management of acute heart failure patients on the basis of presence, extent, and severity of CAD. *For those patients with remote or no history of coronary angiography. *ACS,* Acute coronary syndrome; *CAD,* coronary artery disease; *HF,* heart failure. *From Flaherty JD, Bax JJ, De Luca L, et al: Acute heart failure syndromes in patients with coronary artery disease: early assessment and treatment. J Am Coll Cardiol 53:254–263, 2009.*

an increased use of aspirin, statins, β-blockers, ACE inhibitors, and myocardial revascularization and improved postdischarge outcomes.[263]

CONCLUSIONS

The progression of LV dysfunction, worsening of HF, and death in many patients with CAD may be related to the progressive nature of CAD, in addition to the neurohormonal mechanisms that exacerbate myocardial dysfunction. This progression does not require a discrete coronary event such as an acute MI. Myocardial ischemia or hibernation (or both) may contribute to symptoms of HF. In addition, myocardial hibernation appears to be an unstable process that may progress with time to myocyte loss, apoptosis, and replacement fibrosis, leading to more LV dysfunction. As previously noted, endothelial dysfunction may also lead to progression of myocardial dysfunction. Measures specifically target reduction in the risk of subacute ischemic events and improvement in outcomes.

References

1. Jessup M, Abraham WT, Casey DE, et al: 2009 focused update: ACC/AHF guidelines for the diagnosis and management of heart failure in adults: a report of the American College of Cardiology/American Heart Association task force on practice guidelines. *Circulation* 119:1977–2016, 2009.
2. Ho KK, Pinsky JL, Kannel WB, et al: The epidemiology of heart failure: the Framingham study. *J Am Coll Cardiol* 22:6A–13A, 1993.
3. Levy D, Vasan RS, Benjamin EJ, et al: Temporal trends in heart failure risk factors from 1950-1998. *Circulation* 102(Suppl 2), 2000. II-780 (abstract).
4. Moss AJ, Zareba W, Hall WJ, et al: Prophylactic implantation of a defibrillator in patients with myocardial infarction and reduced ejection fraction. *N Engl J Med* 346:877–883, 2002.
5. Exner DV, Klein GJ, Prystowsky EN: Primary prevention of sudden death with implantable defibrillator therapy in patients with cardiac disease: can we afford to do it? (Can we afford not to?). *Circulation* 104:1564–1570, 2001.
6. Torabi A, Cleland JGF, Khan NK, et al: The timing of development and subsequent clinical course of heart failure after a myocardial infarction. *Eur Heart J* 29:859–870, 2008.
7. Bourassa MG, Gurne O, Bangdiwala SI, et al: Natural history and patterns of current practice in heart failure. The studies of left ventricular dysfunction (SOLVD) investigators. *J Am Coll Cardiol* 22:14A–19A, 1993.
8. Cohn JN, Archibald DG, Ziesche S, et al: Effect of vasodilator therapy on mortality in chronic congestive heart failure. Results of a Veterans Administration cooperative study. *N Engl J Med* 314:1547–1552, 1986.
9. The CONSENSUS Trial Study Group: Effects of enalapril on mortality in severe congestive heart failure. Results of the cooperative North Scandinavian enalapril survival study (CONSENSUS). *N Engl J Med* 316:1429–1435, 1987.
10. DiBianco R, Shabetai R, Kostuk W, et al: A comparison of oral milrinone, digoxin, and their combination in the treatment of patients with chronic heart failure. *N Engl J Med* 320:677–683, 1989.
11. The SOLVD Investigators: Effect of enalapril on survival in patients with reduced left ventricular ejection fractions and congestive heart failure. *N Engl J Med* 325:293–302, 1991.
12. Cohn JN, Johnson G, Ziesche S, et al: A comparison of enalapril with hydralazine-isosorbide dinitrate in the treatment of chronic congestive heart failure. *N Engl J Med* 325:303–310, 1991.
13. Packer M, Carver JR, Rodeheffer RJ, et al: Effect of oral milrinone on mortality in severe chronic heart failure. The PROMISE study research group. *N Engl J Med* 325:1468–1475, 1991.
14. The Studies of Left Ventricular Dysfunction Investigators: Effect of enalapril on mortality and the development of heart failure in asymptomatic patients with reduced left ventricular ejection fractions. *N Engl J Med* 327:685–691, 1992.
15. Packer M, Gheorghiade M, Young JB, et al: Withdrawal of digoxin from patients with chronic heart failure treated with angiotensin-converting-enzyme inhibitors. RADIANCE study. *N Engl J Med* 329:1–7, 1993.
16. Feldman AM, Bristow MR, Parmley WW, et al: Effects of vesnarinone on morbidity and mortality in patients with heart failure. Vesnarinone study group. *N Engl J Med* 329:149–155, 1993.
17. Singh SN, Fletcher RD, Fisher SG, et al: Amiodarone in patients with congestive heart failure and asymptomatic ventricular arrhythmia. Survival trial of antiarrhythmic therapy in congestive heart failure. *N Engl J Med* 333:77–82, 1995.
18. Packer M, Bristow MR, Cohn JN, et al: The effect of carvedilol on morbidity and mortality in patients with chronic heart failure. U.S. carvedilol heart failure study group. *N Engl J Med* 334:1349–1355, 1996.
19. Packer M, O'Connor CM, Ghali JK, et al: Effect of amlodipine on morbidity and mortality in severe chronic heart failure. Prospective randomized amlodipine survival evaluation study group. *N Engl J Med* 335:1107–1114, 1996.
20. The Digitalis Investigation Group: The effect of digoxin on mortality and morbidity in patients with heart failure. *N Engl J Med* 336:525–533, 1997.
21. Cohn JN, Goldstein SO, Greenberg BH, et al: A dose-dependent increase in mortality with vesnarinone among patients with severe heart failure. Vesnarinone trial investigators. *N Engl J Med* 339:1810–1816, 1998.
22. Pitt B, Zannad F, Remme WJ, et al: The effect of spironolactone on morbidity and mortality in patients with severe heart failure. Randomized aldactone evaluation study investigators. *N Engl J Med* 341:709–717, 1999.
23. Torp-Pedersen C, Moller M, Bloch-Thomsen PE, et al: Dofetilide in patients with congestive heart failure and left ventricular dysfunction. Danish investigations of arrhythmia and mortality on dofetilide study group. *N Engl J Med* 341:857–865, 1999.
24. Colucci WS, Elkayam U, Horton DP, et al: Intravenous nesiritide, a natriuretic peptide, in the treatment of decompensated congestive heart failure. Nesiritide study group. *N Engl J Med* 343:246–253, 2000.
25. Packer M, Coats AJ, Fowler MB, et al: Effect of carvedilol on survival in severe chronic heart failure. *N Engl J Med* 344:1651–1658, 2001.
26. The Beta-Blocker Evaluation of Survival Trial Investigators: A trial of the beta-blocker bucindolol in patients with advanced chronic heart failure. *N Engl J Med* 344:1659–1667, 2001.
27. Cohn JN, Tognoni G: A randomized trial of the angiotensin-receptor blocker valsartan in chronic heart failure. *N Engl J Med* 345:1667–1675, 2001.
28. Abraham WT, Fisher WG, Smith AL, et al: Cardiac resynchronization in chronic heart failure. *N Engl J Med* 346:1845–1853, 2002.
29. Bristow MR, Saxon LA, Boehmer J, et al: Cardiac resynchronization therapy with or without an implantable defibrillator in advanced chronic heart failure. *N Engl J Med* 350:2140–2150, 2004.
30. Bardy GH, Lee KL, Mark DB, et al: Amiodarone or an implantable cardioverter-defibrillator for congestive heart failure. *N Engl J Med* 352:225–237, 2005.
31. Cleland JGF, Daubert JC, Erdmann E, et al: The effect of cardiac resynchronization on morbidity and mortality in heart failure. *N Engl J Med* 352:1539–1549, 2005.
32. Beshai JF, Grimm RA, Nagueh SF, et al: Cardiac-resynchronization therapy in heart failure with narrow QRS complexes. *N Engl J Med* 357:2461–2471, 2007.
33. Køber L, Torp-Petersen C, McMurray JJV, et al: Increased mortality after dronedarone therapy for severe heart failure. *N Engl J Med* 358:2678–2687, 2008.
34. Fox KF, Cowie MR, Wood DA, et al: Coronary artery disease as the cause of incident heart failure in the population. *Eur Heart J* 22:228–236, 2001.
35. Fonarow GC, Abraham WT, Albert NM, et al: Factors identified as precipitating hospital admissions for heart failure and clinical outcomes: findings from OPTIMIZE-HF. *Arch Intern Med* 168:847–854, 2008.
36. Follath F, Cleland JG, Klein W, et al: Etiology and response to drug treatment in heart failure. *J Am Coll Cardiol* 32:1167–1172, 1998.
37. Felker GM, Shaw LK, O'Connor CM: A standardized definition of ischemic cardiomyopathy for use in clinical research. *Circulation* 39:210–218, 2002.
38. Bart BA, Shaw LK, McCants BSCB, Jr, et al: Clinical determinants of mortality in patients with angiographically diagnosed ischemic or nonischemic cardiomyopathy. *J Am Coll Cardiol* 30:1002–1008, 1997.
39. O'Connor CM, Gatis WA, Shaw L, et al: Clinical characteristics and long-term outcomes of patients with heart failure and preserved systolic function. *Am J Cardiol* 86:863–867, 2000.
40. Uretsky BF, Thygesen K, Armstrong PW, et al: Acute coronary findings at autopsy in heart failure patients with sudden death: results from the assessment of treatment with lisinopril and survival (ATLAS) trial. *Circulation* 102:611–616, 2000.
41. Orn S, Cleland JGF, Romo M, et al: Recurrent infarction causes the most deaths following myocardial infarction with left ventricular dysfunction. *Am J Med* 118:752–758, 2005.
42. Cleland JGF, Thygesen K, Uretsky BF, et al: Cardiovascular critical event pathways for the progression of heart failure; a report from the ATLAS study. *Eur Heart J* 22:1601–1612, 2001.
43. Flaherty JD, Bax JJ, De Luca L, et al: Acute heart failure syndromes in patients with coronary artery disease: early assessment and treatment. *J Am Coll Cardiol* 53:254–263, 2009.
44. Horwich TB, Patel J, MacLellan WR, et al: Cardiac troponin I is associated with impaired hemodynamics, progressive left ventricular dysfunction, and increased mortality rates in advanced heart failure. *Circulation* 108:833–838, 2003.
45. You JJ, Austin PC, Alter DA, et al: Relation between cardiac troponin I and mortality in acute decompensated heart failure. *Am Heart J* 153:462–470, 2007.
46. Metra M, Nodari S, Parrinello G, et al: The role of plasma biomarkers in acute heart failure: serial changes and independent prognostic value of NT-proBNP and cardiac troponin-T. *Eur J Heart Fail* 9:776–786, 2007.
47. Tavazzi L, Maggioni AP, Lucci D, et al: Nationwide survey on acute heart failure in cardiology ward services in Italy. *Eur Heart J* 27:1207–1215, 2006.
48. Gheorghiade M, Gattis Stough W, Adams KF, Jr, et al: The Pilot Randomized Study of nesiritide versus dobutamine in heart failure (PRESERVD-HF). *Am J Cardiol* 96:18G–25G, 2005.
49. Peacock WF, De Marco T, Fonarow GC, et al: Cardiac troponin and outcome in acute heart failure. *N Engl J Med* 358:2117–2126, 2008.
50. Beohar N, Erdogan AK, Lee DC, et al: Acute heart failure syndromes and coronary perfusion. *J Am Coll Cardiol* 52:13–16, 2008.
51. Gheorghiade M, Zannad F, Sopko G, et al: Acute heart failure syndromes: current state and framework for future research. *Circulation* 112:3958–3968, 2005.
52. Gheorghiade M, Abraham WT, Albert NM, et al: Systolic blood pressure at admission, clinical characteristics, and outcomes in patients hospitalized with acute heart failure. *JAMA* 296:2217–2226, 2006.

53. Rossi JS, Flaherty JD, Fonarow GC, et al: Influence of coronary artery disease and coronary revascularization status on outcomes in patients with acute heart failure syndromes: a report from OPTIMIZE-HF. *Eur J Heart Fail* 10:1215–1223, 2008.
54. Roe MT, Chen AY, Riba AL, et al: Impact of congestive heart failure in patients with non-ST-segment elevation acute coronary syndromes. *Am J Cardiol* 97:1707–1712, 2006.
55. Khot UN, Jia G, Moliterno DJ, et al: Prognostic importance of physical examination for heart failure in non-ST-elevation acute coronary syndromes: the enduring value of Killip classification. *JAMA* 290:2174–2181, 2003.
56. Steg PG, Dabbous OH, Feldman LJ, et al: Determinants and prognostic impact of heart failure complicating acute coronary syndromes: observations from the Global Registry of Acute Coronary Events (GRACE). *Circulation* 109:494–499, 2004.
57. Di Chiara A, Fresco C, Savonitto S, et al: Epidemiology of non-ST elevation acute coronary syndromes in the Italian cardiology network: the BLITZ-2 study. *Eur Heart J* 27:393–405, 2006.
58. Shibata MC, Collinson J, Taneja AK, et al: Long term prognosis of heart failure after acute coronary syndromes without ST elevation. *Postgrad Med J* 82:55–59, 2006.
59. Spencer FA, Meyer TE, Gore JM, et al: Heterogeneity in the management and outcomes of patients with acute myocardial infarction complicated by heart failure: the National Registry of Myocardial Infarction. *Circulation* 105:2605–2610, 2002.
60. Nieminen MS, Brutsaert K, Dickstein K, et al: EuroHeart failure survey II: a survey on hospitalized acute heart failure patients: description of population. *Eur Heart J* 27:2725–2736, 2006.
61. Gattis WA, O'Connor CM, Hasselblad V, et al: Usefulness of an elevated troponin-I in predicting clinical events in patients for acute heart failure and acute coronary syndrome (from the RITZ-4 trial). *Am J Cardiol* 93:1436–1437, 2004.
62. Emanuelsson H, Karlson BW, Herlitz J: Characteristics and prognosis of patients with acute myocardial infarction in relation to occurrence of congestive heart failure. *Eur Heart J* 15:761–768, 1994.
63. O'Connor CM, Hathaway WR, Bates ER, et al: Clinical characteristics and long-term outcome of patients in whom congestive heart failure develops after thrombolytic therapy for acute myocardial infarction: development of a predictive model. *Am Heart J* 133:663–673, 1997.
64. Hasdai D, Topol EJ, Kilaru R, et al: Frequency, patient characteristics, and outcomes of mild-to-moderate heart failure complicating ST-segment elevation acute myocardial infarction: lessons from 4 international fibrinolytic therapy trials. *Am Heart J* 145:73–79, 2003.
65. Ali AS, Rybicki BA, Alam M, et al: Clinical predictors of heart failure in patients with first acute myocardial infarction. *Am Heart J* 138:1133–1139, 1999.
66. Spencer FA, Meyer TE, Goldberg RJ, et al: Twenty year trends (1975-1995) in the incidence, in-hospital and long-term death rates associated with heart failure complicating acute myocardial infarction: a community-wide perspective. *J Am Coll Cardiol* 34:1378–1387, 1999.
67. Wu AH, Parsons L, Every NR, et al: Hospital outcomes in patients presenting with congestive heart failure complicating acute myocardial infarction: a report from the Second National Registry of Myocardial Infarction (NRMI-2). *J Am Coll Cardiol* 40:1389–1394, 2002.
68. Segev A, Strauss BH, Tan M, et al: Prognostic significance of admission heart failure in patients with non-ST-elevation acute coronary syndromes. *Am J Cardiol* 98:470–473, 2006.
69. Haim M, Battler A, Behar S, et al: Acute coronary syndromes complicated by symptomatic and asymptomatic heart failure: does current treatment comply with guidelines? *Am Heart J* 147:859–864, 2004.
70. St. John Sutton MG, Sharpe N: Left ventricular remodeling after myocardial infarction: pathophysiology and therapy. *Circulation* 101:2981–2988, 2000.
71. Sanchez JA, Mentzer RM, Jr: Coronary revascularization in patients with chronic heart failure. *Coron Artery Dis* 9:685–689, 1998.
72. O'Connor CM, Velazquez EJ, Gardner LH, et al: Comparison of coronary artery bypass grafting versus medical therapy on long-term outcome in patients with ischemic cardiomyopathy (a 25-year experience from the Duke cardiovascular disease databank). *Am J Cardiol* 90:101–107, 2002.
73. Challapalli S, Bonow RO, Gheorghiade M: Medical management of heart failure secondary to coronary artery disease. *Coron Artery Dis* 9:659–674, 1998.
74. Ragosta M, Beller GA: The assessment of patients with congestive heart failure as a manifestation of coronary artery disease. *Coron Artery Dis* 9:645–651, 1998.
75. Goldstein JA, Demetriou D, Grines CL, et al: Multiple complex coronary plaques in patients with acute myocardial infarction. *N Engl J Med* 343:915–922, 2000.
76. Gheorghiade M, Bonow RO: Chronic heart failure in the United States: a manifestation of coronary artery disease. *Circulation* 97:282–289, 1998.
77. Mann DL: Mechanisms and models in heart failure: a combinatorial approach. *Circulation* 100:999–1008, 1999.
78. Lameris TW, de Zeeuw S, Alberts G, et al: Time course and mechanism of myocardial catecholamine release during transient ischemia in vivo. *Circulation* 101:2645–2650, 2000.
79. Tomai F, Crea F, Chiariello L, et al: Ischemic preconditioning in humans: models, mediators, and clinical relevance. *Circulation* 100:559–563, 1999.
80. Rona G: Catecholamine cardiotoxicity. *J Mol Cell Cardiol* 17:291–306, 1985.
81. Cruickshank JM, Neil-Dwyer G, Degaute JP, et al: Reduction of stress/catecholamine-induced cardiac necrosis by beta 1-selective blockade. *Lancet* 2:585–589, 1987.
82. Scarabelli T, Stephanou A, Rayment N, et al: Apoptosis of endothelial cells precedes myocyte cell apoptosis in ischemia/reperfusion injury. *Circulation* 104:253–256, 2001.
83. Hiramatsu T, Forbess J, Miura T, et al: Effects of endothelin-1 and endothelin-A receptor antagonist on recovery after hypothermic cardioplegic ischemia in neonatal lamb hearts. *Circulation* 92:II400–II404, 1995.
84. Bolli R: Myocardial "stunning" in man. *Circulation* 86:1671–1691, 1992.
85. Wijns W, Vatner SF, Camici PG: Hibernating myocardium. *N Engl J Med* 339:173–181, 1998.
86. Lim H, Fallavollita JA, Hard R, et al: Profound apoptosis-mediated regional myocyte loss and compensatory hypertrophy in pigs with hibernating myocardium. *Circulation* 100:2380–2386, 1999.
87. Shan K, Bick RJ, Poindexter BJ, et al: Altered adrenergic receptor density in myocardial hibernation in humans: a possible mechanism of depressed myocardial function. *Circulation* 102:2599–2606, 2000.
88. Luisi AJ, Fallavollita JA, Suzuki G, et al: Spatial inhomogeneity of sympathetic nerve function in hibernating myocardium. *Circulation* 106:779–781, 2002.
89. Fallavollita JA, Malm BJ, Canty JM: Hibernating myocardium retains metabolic and contractile reserve despite regional reductions in flow, function, and oxygen consumption at rest. *Circ Res* 92:48–55, 2003.
90. Canty JM, Suzuki G, Banas MK, et al: Hibernating myocardium: chronically adapted to ischemia but vulnerable to sudden death. *Circ Res* 94:1142–1149, 2004.
91. Thijssen VLJL, Borgers M, Lenders MH, et al: Temporal and spatial variations in structural protein expression during the progression from stunned to hibernating myocardium. *Circulation* 110:3313–3321, 2004.
92. Iyer VS, Canty JM: Regional desensitization of β-adrenergic receptor signaling in swine with chronic hibernating myocardium. *Circ Res* 97:789–795, 2005.
93. Auerbach MA, Schoder H, Hoh C, et al: Prevalence of myocardial viability as detected by positron emission tomography in patients with ischemic cardiomyopathy. *Circulation* 99:2921–2926, 1999.
94. Cleland JG, Pennel D, Ray S, et al: The carvedilol hibernation reversible ischaemia trial: marker of success (CHRISTMAS). The CHRISTMAS study steering committee and investigators. *Eur J Heart Fail* 1:191–196, 1999.
95. Challapalli S, Hendel RC, Bonow RO: Clinical profile of patients with congestive heart failure due to coronary artery disease: stunned/hibernating myocardium, ischemia, scar. *Coron Artery Dis* 9:629–644, 1998.
96. Al-Mohammad A, Mahy IR, Norton MY, et al: Prevalence of hibernating myocardium in patients with severely impaired ischemic left ventricles. *Heart* 80:559–564, 1998.
97. Dilsizian V, Bonow RO: Current diagnostic techniques of assessing myocardial viability in patients with hibernating and stunned myocardium. *Circulation* 87:1–20, 1993.
98. Bonow RO: Identification of viable myocardium. *Circulation* 94:2674–2680, 1996.
99. Schinkel AF, Bax JJ, Poldermans D, et al: Hibernating myocardium: diagnosis and patient outcomes. *Curr Probl Cardiol* 32:375–410, 2007.
100. Camici PG, Prasad SK, Rimoldi OE: Stunning, hibernation, and assessment of myocardial viability. *Circulation* 117:103–114, 2008.
101. Allman KC, Shaw LJ, Hachamovitch R, et al: Myocardial viability testing and the impact of revascularization on prognosis in patients with coronary artery disease and left ventricular dysfunction: a meta-analysis. *J Am Coll Cardiol* 39:1151–1158, 2002.
102. Kim RJ, Wu E, Rafael A, et al: The use of contrast-enhanced magnetic resonance imaging to identify reversible myocardial dysfunction. *N Engl J Med* 343:1445–1453, 2000.
103. Bucciarelli-Ducci C, Wu E, Lee DC, et al: Contrast-enhanced cardiac magnetic resonance in the evaluation of myocardial infarction and myocardial viability in patients with ischemic heart disease. *Curr Probl Cardiol* 31:125–168, 2006.
104. Soriano CJ, Ridocci F, Estornell J, et al: Noninvasive diagnosis of coronary artery disease in patients with heart failure and systolic dysfunction of uncertain etiology using late gadolinium-enhanced cardiovascular magnetic resonance. *J Am Coll Cardiol* 45:743–748, 2005.
105. Bello D, Shah DJ, Farah GM: Gadolinium cardiovascular magnetic resonance predicts reversible myocardial dysfunction and remodeling in patients with heart failure undergoing beta-blocker therapy. *Circulation* 108:1945–1953, 2003.
106. Seghatol FF, Shah DJ, Deluzio S, et al: Relation between contractile reserve and improvement in left ventricular function with beta-blocker therapy in patients with heart failure secondary to ischemic or idiopathic dilated cardiomyopathy. *Am J Cardiol* 93:854–859, 2004.
107. McFarlane SI, Muniyappa R, Francisco R, et al: Clinical review 145: pleiotropic effects of statins: lipid reduction and beyond. *J Clin Endocrinol Metab* 87:1451–1458, 2002.
108. Gould KL: New concepts and paradigms in cardiovascular medicine: the noninvasive management of coronary artery disease. *Am J Med* 104:2S–17S, 1998.
109. Schulz R, Guth BD, Pieper K, et al: Recruitment of an inotropic reserve in moderately ischemic myocardium at the expense of metabolic recovery. A model of short-term hibernation. *Circ Res* 70:1282–1295, 1992.
110. Chen C, Li L, Chen LL, et al: Incremental doses of dobutamine induce a biphasic response in dysfunctional left ventricular regions subtending coronary stenoses. *Circulation* 92:756–766, 1995.
111. Felker GM, Benza RL, Chandler AB, et al: Heart failure etiology and response to milrinone in decompensated heart failure: results from the OPTIME-CHF study. *J Am Coll Cardiol* 41:997–1003, 2003.
112. Elkayam U, Tasissa G, Binanay C, et al: Use and impact of inotropes and vasodilator therapy in hospitalized patients with severe heart failure. *Am Heart J* 153:98–104, 2007.
113. Carluccio E, Biagioli P, Alumni G, et al: Patients with hibernating myocardium show altered left ventricular volumes and shape, which revert after revascularization. *J Am Coll Cardiol* 47:969–977, 2006.
114. Azevedo ER, Stewart DJ, Parker JD: Increased extraction of endothelin-1 across the failing human heart. *Am J Cardiol* 88:180–182, A6, 2001.
115. Harrison DG: Endothelial dysfunction in atherosclerosis. *Basic Res Cardiol* 89(Suppl 1):87–102, 1994.
116. Bell DM, Johns TE, Lopez LM: Endothelial dysfunction: implications for therapy of cardiovascular diseases. *Ann Pharmacother* 32:459–470, 1998.
117. Moncada S, Higgs A: The L-arginine-nitric oxide pathway. *N Engl J Med* 329:2002–2012, 1993.
118. Zeiher AM, Drexler H, Saurbier B, et al: Endothelium-mediated coronary blood flow modulation in humans. Effects of age, atherosclerosis, hypercholesterolemia, and hypertension. *J Clin Invest* 92:652–662, 1993.
119. Rubanyi GM: The role of endothelium in cardiovascular homeostasis and diseases. *J Cardiovasc Pharmacol* 22(Suppl 4):S1–S14, 1993.
120. Cody RJ: The integrated effects of angiotensin II. *Am J Cardiol* 79:9–11, 1997.
121. Mehta JL, Li DY, Yang H, et al: Angiotensin II and IV stimulate expression and release of plasminogen activator inhibitor-1 in cultured human coronary artery endothelial cells. *J Cardiovasc Pharmacol* 39:789–794, 2002.
122. Brown NJ, Vaughan DE: Prothrombotic effects of angiotensin. *Adv Intern Med* 45:419–429, 2000.
123. Neylon CB: Vascular biology of endothelin signal transduction. *Clin Exp Pharmacol Physiol* 26:149–153, 1999.
124. Loscalzo J, Vita JA: Ischemia, hyperemia, exercise, and nitric oxide: complex physiology and complex molecular adaptations. *Circulation* 90:2556–2559, 1994.
125. Levin ER: Endothelins. *N Engl J Med* 333:356–363, 1995.
126. Luskutoff DJ, Sawdey M, Mimuro J: Type 1 plasminogen activator inhibitor. *Prog Hemost Thromb* 9:87–115, 1989.
127. Sakai S, Miyauchi T, Sakurai T, et al: Endogenous endothelin-1 participates in the maintenance of cardiac function in rats with congestive heart failure: marked increase in endothelin-1 production in the failing heart. *Circulation* 93:1214–1222, 1996.
128. Kario K, Matsuo T, Hoshide S, et al: Lipid-lowering therapy corrects endothelial cell dysfunction in a short time but does not affect hypercoagulable state even after long-term use in hyperlipidemic patients. *Blood Coagul Fibrinolysis* 10:269–276, 1999.
129. Adams KF, Jr: Angiotensin-converting enzyme inhibition and vascular remodeling in coronary artery disease. *Coron Artery Dis* 9:675–684, 1998.
130. Intengan HD, Schiffrin EL: Disparate effects of carvedilol versus metoprolol treatment of stroke-prone spontaneously hypertensive rats on endothelial function of resistance arteries. *J Cardiovasc Pharmacol* 35:763–768, 2000.
131. Quyyumi AA: Effects of aspirin on endothelial dysfunction in atherosclerosis. *Am J Cardiol* 82:31S–33S, 1998.
132. Gould KL, Martucci JP, Goldberg DI, et al: Short-term cholesterol lowering decreases size and severity of perfusion abnormalities by positron emission tomography after dipyridamole in patients with coronary artery disease. A potential noninvasive marker of healing coronary endothelium. *Circulation* 89:1530–1538, 1994.
133. Eichstadt HW, Eskotter H, Hoffman I, et al: Improvement of myocardial perfusion by short-term fluvastatin therapy in coronary artery disease. *Am J Cardiol* 76:122A–125A, 1995.
134. Van Boven AJ, Jukema JW, Zwinderman AH, et al: Reduction of transient myocardial ischemia with pravastatin in addition to the conventional treatment in patients with angina pectoris. REGRESS study group. *Circulation* 94:1503–1505, 1996.
135. Andrews TC, Raby K, Barry J, et al: Effect of cholesterol reduction on myocardial ischemia in patients with coronary disease. *Circulation* 95:324–328, 1997.

136. Mostaza JM, Gomez MV, Gallardo F, et al: Cholesterol reduction improves myocardial perfusion abnormalities in patients with coronary artery disease and average cholesterol levels. *J Am Coll Cardiol* 35:76–82, 2000.
137. Baller D, Notohamiprodjo G, Gleichmann U, et al: Improvement in coronary flow reserve determined by positron emission tomography after 6 months of cholesterol-lowering therapy in patients with early stages of coronary atherosclerosis. *Circulation* 99:2871–2875, 1999.
138. Segal R, Pitt B, Poole Wilson P, et al: Effects of HMG-CoA reductase inhibitors (statins) in patients with heart failure. *Eur J Heart Fail* 2(Suppl 2):96, 2000.
139. Drexler H: Nitric oxide synthases in the failing human heart: a doubled-edged sword? *Circulation* 99:2972–2975, 1999.
140. Cannon RO, III: Cardiovascular benefit of cholesterol-lowering therapy: does improved endothelial vasodilator function matter? *Circulation* 102:820–822, 2000.
141. Yusuf S, Pepine CJ, Garces C, et al: Effect of enalapril on myocardial infarction and unstable angina in patients with low ejection fractions. *Lancet* 340:1173–1178, 1992.
142. St John SM, Pfeffer MA, Moye L, et al: Cardiovascular death and left ventricular remodeling two years after myocardial infarction: baseline predictors and impact of long-term use of captopril: information from the survival and ventricular enlargement (SAVE) trial. *Circulation* 96:3294–3299, 1997.
143. O'Connor CM, Carson PE, Miller AB, et al: Effect of amlodipine on mode of death among patients with advanced heart failure in the PRAISE trial. Prospective randomized amlodipine survival evaluation. *Am J Cardiol* 82:881–887, 1998.
144. Adabag AS, Therneau TM, Gersh BJ, et al: Sudden death after myocardial infarction. *JAMA* 300:2022–2029, 2008.
145. Stevenson WG, Stevenson LW, Middlekauff HR, et al: Sudden death prevention in patients with advanced ventricular dysfunction. *Circulation* 88:2953–2961, 1993.
146. MERIT-HF Study Group: Effect of metoprolol CR/XL in chronic heart failure: metoprolol CR/XL randomised intervention trial in congestive heart failure (MERIT-HF). *Lancet* 353:2001–2007, 1999.
147. Davies MJ: Anatomic features in victims of sudden coronary death. Coronary artery pathology. *Circulation* 85:119–124, 1992.
148. Zipes DP, Wellens HJ: Sudden cardiac death. *Circulation* 98:2334–2351, 1998.
149. Farb A, Tang AL, Burke AP, et al: Sudden coronary death. Frequency of active coronary lesions, inactive coronary lesions, and myocardial infarction. *Circulation* 92:1701–1709, 1995.
150. Poole JE, Johnson GW, Hellkamp AS, et al: Prognostic importance of defibrillator shocks in patients with heart failure. *N Engl J Med* 359:1009–1017, 2008.
151. Moss AJ, Greenberg H, Case RB, et al: Long-term clinical course of patients after termination of ventricular tachyarrhythmia by an implanted defibrillator. *Circulation* 110:3760–3765, 2004.
152. Cleland JGF, Swedberg K, Follath F, et al: The EuroHeart failure survey programme—a survey on the quality of care among patients with heart failure in Europe: part 1: patient characteristics and diagnosis. *Eur Heart J* 24:442–463, 2003.
153. Owan TE, Hodge DO, Herges RM, et al: Trends in prevalence and outcome of heart failure with preserved ejection fraction. *N Engl J Med* 355:251–259, 2006.
154. Fonarow GC, Gattis Stough W, Abraham WT, et al: Characteristics, treatments and outcomes of patients with preserved systolic function hospitalized with heart failure: a report from OPTIMIZE-HF. *J Am Coll Cardiol* 50:768–777, 2007.
155. Judge KW, Pawitan Y, Caldwell J, et al: Congestive heart failure symptoms in patients with preserved left ventricular systolic function: analysis of the CASS registry. *J Am Coll Cardiol* 18:377–382, 1991.
156. Bhatia RS, Tu JV, Lee DS, et al: Outcome of heart failure with preserved ejection fraction in a population based study. *N Engl J Med* 355:260–269, 2007.
157. Lenzen MJ, Scholte op Reimer WJ, Boersma E, et al: Differences between patients with preserved and a depressed left ventricular function: a report from the EuroHeart Failure Survey. *Eur Heart J* 25:1214–1220, 2004.
158. Tribouilloy C, Rusinaru D, Mahjoub H, et al: Prognosis of heart failure with preserved ejection fraction: a 5 year prospective population-based study. *Eur Heart J* 29:339–347, 2008.
159. Siirilä-Waris K, Lassus J, Melin J, et al: Characteristics, outcomes, and predictors of 1-year mortality in patients hospitalized for acute heart failure. *Eur Heart J* 27:3011–3017, 2006.
160. Shah SJ, Gheorghiade M: Heart failure with preserved ejection fraction. *JAMA* 300:431–433, 2008.
161. Ahmed A, Rich MW, Fleg JL, et al: Effects of digoxin on morbidity and mortality in diastolic heart failure. *Circulation* 114:397–403, 2006.
162. Gandhi SK, Powers JC, Nomeir AM, et al: The pathogenesis of acute pulmonary edema associated with hypertension. *N Engl J Med* 344:17–22, 2001.
163. Grossman W: Diastolic dysfunction in congestive heart failure. *N Engl J Med* 325:1557–1564, 1991.
164. Aroesty JM, McKay RG, Heller GV, et al: Simultaneous assessment of left ventricular systolic and diastolic dysfunction during pacing-induced ischemia. *Circulation* 71:889–900, 1985.
165. Judge KW, Pawitan Y, Caldwell J, et al: Congestive heart failure symptoms in patients with preserved left ventricular systolic function: analysis of the CASS registry. *J Am Coll Cardiol* 18:377–382, 1991.
166. Vasan RS, Benjamin EJ, Levy D: Prevalence, clinical features and prognosis of diastolic heart failure: an epidemiologic perspective. *J Am Coll Cardiol* 26:1565–1574, 1995.
167. Choudhury L, Gheorghiade M, Bonow RO: Coronary artery disease in patients with heart failure and preserved systolic function. *Am J Cardiol* 89:719–722, 2002.
168. Haffner SM, Lehto S, Ronnemaa T, et al: Mortality from coronary heart disease in subjects with type 2 diabetes and in nondiabetic subjects with and without prior myocardial infarction. *N Engl J Med* 339:229–234, 1998.
169. Sowers JR, Epstein M, Frohlich ED: Diabetes, hypertension, and cardiovascular disease: an update. *Hypertension* 37:1053–1059, 2001.
170. Hammond T, Tanguay JF, Bourassa MG: Management of coronary artery disease: therapeutic options in patients with diabetes. *J Am Coll Cardiol* 36:355–365, 2000.
171. Carson P, Johnson G, Fletcher R, et al: Mild systolic dysfunction in heart failure (left ventricular ejection fraction >35%): baseline characteristics, prognosis and response to therapy in the vasodilator in heart failure trials (V-HeFT). *J Am Coll Cardiol* 27:642–649, 1996.
172. McKelvie RS, Yusuf S, Pericak D, et al: Comparison of candesartan, enalapril, and their combination in congestive heart failure: randomized evaluation of strategies for left ventricular dysfunction (RESOLVD) pilot study. The RESOLVD pilot study investigators. *Circulation* 100:1056–1064, 1999.
173. Greenberg BH, Abraham WT, Albert NM, et al: Influence of diabetes on characteristics and outcomes in patients hospitalized with heart failure. *Am Heart J* 154:647–654, 2007.
174. Adams KF, Fonarow GC, Emerman CL, et al: Characteristics and outcomes of patients hospitalized for heart failure in the United States. *Am Heart J* 149:209–216, 2005.
175. Gottdiener JS, Arnold AM, Aurigemma GP, et al: Predictors of congestive heart failure in the elderly. *J Am Coll Cardiol* 35:1628–1637, 2000.
176. He J, Ogden LG, Bazzano LA, et al: Risk factors for congestive heart failure in U.S. men and women. *Arch Intern Med* 161:996–1002, 2001.
177. Kannel WB, Hjortland M, Castelli WP: Role of diabetes in congestive heart failure: the Framingham study. *Am J Cardiol* 34:29–34, 1974.
178. Iribarren C, Karter AJ, Go AS, et al: Glycemic control and heart failure among adult patients with diabetes. *Circulation* 103:2668–2673, 2001.
179. Stratton IM, Adler AI, Neil AW, et al: Association of glycaemia with macrovascular complications of type 2 diabetes. *BMJ* 321:405–412, 2000.
180. Lee DL, Austin PC, Rouleau JL, et al: Predicting mortality among patients hospitalized for heart failure. *JAMA* 290:2581–2587, 2003.
181. Pocock SJ, Wang D, Pfeffer MA, et al: Predictors of mortality and morbidity in patients with chronic heart failure. *Eur Heart J* 27:65–75, 2006.
182. Gustafsson I, Brendorp B, Seibæk M, et al: Influence of diabetes and diabetes-gender interaction on the risk of death in patients hospitalized with congestive heart failure. *J Am Coll Cardiol* 43:771–777, 2004.
183. Bertoni AG, Hundley WG, Massing MW, et al: Heart failure prevalence, incidence, and mortality in the elderly with diabetes. *Diabetes Care* 27:699–703, 2004.
184. Vaur L, Gueret P, Lievre M, et al: Development of congestive heart failure in type 2 diabetes patients with microalbuminuria or proteinuria. *Diabetes Care* 26:855–860, 2003.
185. From AM, Leibson CL, Bursi F, et al: Diabetes in heart failure: prevalence and impact on outcome in the population. *Am J Med* 119:591–599, 2006.
186. Domanski M, Krause-Steinrauf H, Deedwania P, et al: The effect of diabetes on outcomes of patients with advanced heart failure in the BEST trial. *J Am Coll Cardiol* 42:914–922, 2003.
187. Brophy JM, Dagenais GR, McSherry F, et al: A multivariate model for predicting mortality in patients with heart failure and systolic dysfunction. *Am J Med* 116:300–304, 2004.
188. de Groote P, Lamblin N, Mouquet F, et al: Impact of diabetes mellitus on long-term survival in patients with congestive heart failure. *Eur Heart J* 25:656–662, 2004.
189. Dries DL, Sweitzer NK, Drazner MH, et al: Prognostic impact of diabetes mellitus in patients with heart failure according to etiology of left ventricular systolic dysfunction. *J Am Coll Cardiol* 38:421–428, 2001.
190. Flaherty JD, Davidson CJ: Diabetes and coronary revascularization. *JAMA* 293:1501–1508, 2005.
191. Nesto RW: Correlation between cardiovascular disease and diabetes mellitus. *Am J Med* 116(Suppl 5A):11S–22S, 2004.
192. Waller BF, Palumbo PJ, Lie JT, et al: Status of the coronary arteries at necropsy in diabetes mellitus with onset after 30 years. *Am J Med* 69:498–506, 1980.
193. Moreno PR, Murcia AM, Palacios IF, et al: Coronary composition and macrophage infiltration in atherectomy specimens from patient with diabetes mellitus. *Circulation* 102:2180–2184, 2000.
194. Nicholls SJ, Tuzcu EM, Kalidindi S, et al: Effect of diabetes on progression of coronary atherosclerosis and arterial remodeling. *J Am Coll Cardiol* 52:255–262, 2008.
195. MacDonald MR, Petrie MC, Hawkins NM, et al: Diabetes, left ventricular systolic dysfunction and chronic heart failure. *Eur Heart J* 29:1224–1240, 2008.
196. van Heerebeek L, Hamdani N, Handoko L, et al: Diastolic stiffness of the failing diabetic heart. *Circulation* 117:43–51, 2008.
197. Lee TS, Satlsman KA, Ohashi H, et al: Activation of protein kinase C by elevation of glucose concentration: proposal of a mechanism in the development of diabetic vascular complications. *Proc Natl Acad Sci U S A* 86:5141–5145, 1989.
198. Berg TJ, Snorgaard O, Faber J, et al: Serum levels of advanced glycation end products are associated with left ventricular diastolic function in patients with type 1 diabetes. *Diabetes Care* 22:1186–1190, 1999.
199. Grundy SM, Benjamin IJ, Burke GL, et al: Diabetes and cardiovascular disease: a statement for healthcare professionals from the American Heart Association. *Circulation* 100:1134–1146, 1999.
200. Gheorghiade M, Pang PS: Acute heart failure syndromes. *J Am Coll Cardiol* 53:557–573, 2009.
201. Cotter G, Metzkor E, Kaluski E, et al: Randomised trial of high-dose isosorbide dinitrate plus low-dose furosemide versus high-dose furosemide plus low-dose isosorbide dinitrate in severe pulmonary oedema. *Lancet* 351:389–393, 1998.
202. Abraham WT, Adams KF, Fonarow GC, et al: In-hospital mortality in patients with acute compensated heart failure requiring intravenous vasoactive medications: an analysis from the Acute Decompensated Heart Failure Registry (ADHERE). *J Am Coll Cardiol* 46:57–64, 2005.
203. Investigators V.M.A.C.: Intravenous nesiritide vs. nitroglycerin for treatment of decompensated congestive heart failure. *JAMA* 287:1531–1540, 2002.
204. Sackner-Bernstein JD, Skopicki HA, Aaronson KD: Risk of worsening renal function with nesiritide in patients with acutely decompensated heart failure. *Circulation* 111:1487–1491, 2005.
205. Schultz R, Rose J, Martin C, et al: Development of short-term myocardial hibernation. *Circulation* 88:684–695, 1993.
206. Felker GM, Benza RL, Chandler AB, et al: Heart failure etiology and response to milrinone in decompensated heart failure: results from the OPTIME-CHF study. *J Am Coll Cardiol* 41:997–1003, 2003.
207. Gorodeski EZ, Chu EC, Reese JR, et al: Prognosis on chronic dobutamine or milrinone infusions for stage D heart failure. *Circ Heart Fail* 320:320–324, 2009.
208. Schmieder RE: Mechanisms for the clinical benefits of angiotensin II receptor blockers. *Am J Hypertension* 18:720–730, 2005.
209. The Heart Outcomes Prevention Evaluation (HOPE) Study Investigators: Effects of an angiotensin-converting-enzyme inhibitor, ramipril, on cardiovascular events in high-risk patients. *N Engl J Med* 342:145–153, 2000.
210. The EUROPA Investigators: Efficacy of perindopril in reduction of cardiovascular events among patients with stable coronary artery disease: randomised, double-blind, placebo-controlled, multicentre trial. *Lancet* 362:782–788, 2003.
211. The ONTARGET Investigators: Telmisartan, ramipril, or both in patients at high risk for vascular events. *N Engl J Med* 358:1547–1559, 2008.
212. O'Keefe JH, Wetzel M, Moe RR, et al: Should an angiotensin-converting enzyme inhibitor be standard therapy for patients with atherosclerotic disease? *J Am Coll Cardiol* 37:1–8, 2001.
213. Rutherford JD, Pfeffer MA, Moye LA, et al: Effects of captopril on ischemic events after myocardial infarction. Results of the survival and ventricular enlargement trial. SAVE investigators. *Circulation* 90:1731–1738, 1994.
214. Nishioka T, Suzuki M, Onishi K, et al: Eplerenone attenuates myocardial fibrosis in the angiotensin II-induced hypertensive mouse. *J Cardiovasc Pharmacol* 49:261–268, 2007.
215. Zannad F, McMurray JJ, Krum H, et al, EMPHASIS-HF Study Group: Eplerenone in patients with systolic heart failure and mild symptoms. *N Engl J Med* 364:11–21, 2011.
216. Seed A, Gardner R, McMurray J, et al: Neurohumoral effects of the new orally active rennin inhibitor, aliskiren, in chronic heart failure. *Euro J Heart Fail* 9:1120–1127, 2007.
217. McMurray JJ, Pitt B, Latini R, et al: Aliskiren Observation of Heart Failure Treatment (ALOFT) Investigators. Effects of the oral direct renin inhibitor aliskiren in patients with symptomatic heart failure. *Circ Heart Fail* 1:17–24, 2008.
218. Gheorghiade M, Böhm M, Greene SJ, et al, ASTRONAUT Investigators and Coordinators: Effect of aliskiren on postdischarge mortality and heart failure readmissions among patients hospitalized for heart failure: the ASTRONAUT randomized trial. *J Am Coll* 309:1125–1135, 2013.
219. Krum H, Massie B, Abraham WT, et al, ATMOSPHERE Investigators: Direct renin inhibition in addition to or as an alternative to angiotensin converting enzyme inhibition in patients with chronic systolic heart failure: rationale and design of the Aliskiren Trial to Minimize

OutcomeS in Patients with HEart failuRE (ATMOSPHERE) study. *Eur J Heart Fail* 13:107–114, 2011.
220. Gattis WA, O'Connor CM, Gallup DS, et al: Predischarge initiation of carvedilol in patients hospitalized for decompensated heart failure. *J Am Coll Cardiol* 43:1534–1541, 2004.
221. Fonarow GC, Abraham WT, Albert NM, et al: Carvedilol use at discharge in patients hospitalized for heart failure is associated with improved survival. *Am Heart J* 153:82e1–82e11, 2007.
222. Fonarow GC, Abraham WT, Albert NM, et al: Influence of beta-blocker continuation or withdrawal on outcomes in patients hospitalized with heart failure. *J Am Coll Cardiol* 52:190–199, 2008.
223. The CIBIS-II Investigators: The cardiac insufficiency bisoprolol study II (CIBIS-II): a randomised trial. *Lancet* 353:9–13, 1999.
224. Cleland JG, Alamgir F, Nikitin NP, et al: What is the optimal medical management of ischemic heart failure? *Prog Cardiovasc Dis* 43:433–455, 2001.
225. The Capricorn Investigators: Effect of carvedilol on outcome after myocardial infarction in patients with left-ventricular dysfunction: the CAPRICORN randomised trial. *Lancet* 357:1385–1390, 2001.
226. Bristow MR, Anderson FL, Port JD, et al: Differences in beta-adrenergic neuroeffector mechanisms in ischemic versus idiopathic dilated cardiomyopathy. *Circulation* 84:1024–1039, 1991.
227. Bristow MR: Beta-adrenergic receptor blockade in chronic heart failure. *Circulation* 101:558–569, 2000.
228. NCEP Expert Panel: Executive summary of the third report of the national cholesterol education panel (NCEP) expert panel on detection, evaluation, and treatment of high blood cholesterol in adults (adult treatment panel III). *JAMA* 285:2486–2497, 2001.
229. Sacks FM, Pfeffer MA, Moye LA, et al: The effect of pravastatin on coronary events after myocardial infarction in patients with average cholesterol levels. *N Engl J Med* 335:1001–1009, 1996.
230. Kjekshus J, Pedersen TR, Olsson AG, et al: The effects of simvastatin on the incidence of heart failure in patients with coronary heart disease. *J Card Fail* 3:249–254, 1997.
231. Khush KK, Waters DD, Bittner V, et al: Effect of high-dose atorvastatin on hospitalizations for heart failure. *Circulation* 115:576–583, 2007.
232. Scirica BM, Morow DA, Cannon CP, et al: Intensive statin therapy and the risk of hospitalization for heart failure after an acute coronary syndrome in the PROVE IT-TIMI 22 study. *J Am Coll Cardiol* 47:2326–2331, 2006.
233. Velagaleti RS, Massaro J, Vasan RS, et al: Relations of lipid concentrations to heart failure incidence: the Framingham Heart Study. *Circulation* 120:2345–2351, 2009.
234. Holme I, Aastveit AH, Hammar N, et al: Lipoprotein components and risk of congestive heart failure in 84,740 men and women in the Apolipoprotein MOrtality RISk study (AMORIS). *Eur J Heart Fail* 11:1036–1042, 2009.
235. Go AS, Lee WY, Yang J, et al: Statin therapy and risks for death and hospitalization in chronic heart failure. *JAMA* 296:2105–2111, 2006.
236. Foody JM, Shah R, Galusha D, et al: Statins and mortality among elderly patients hospitalized with heart failure. *Circulation* 113:1086–1092, 2006.
237. Fukuta H, Sane DC, Brucks S, et al: Statin therapy may be associated with lower mortality in patients with diastolic heart failure. *Circulation* 112:357–363, 2005.
238. Kjekshus J, Apetrei E, Barrios V, et al: Rosuvastatin in older patients with systolic heart failure. *N Engl J Med* 357:2248–2261, 2007.
239. GISSI-HF Investigators: Effect of rosuvastatin in patients with chronic heart failure. *Lancet* 372:1231–1239, 2008.
240. GISSI-Prevenzione Investigators: Dietary supplementation with n-3 polyunsaturated fatty acids and vitamin E after myocardial infarction. *Lancet* 354:447–455, 1999.
241. Yamagishi K, Iso H, Date C, et al: Fish, n-3 polyunsaturated fatty acids, and mortality from cardiovascular disease in a nationwide community-based cohort of Japanese men and women. *J Am Coll Cardiol* 52:988–996, 2008.
242. GISSI-HF Investigators: Effect of n-3 polyunsaturated fatty acids in patients with chronic heart failure. *Lancet* 372:1223–1230, 2008.
243. Smith SC, Allen J, Blair SN, et al: AHA/ACC guidelines for secondary prevention for patients with coronary and other atherosclerotic vascular disease. *J Am Coll Cardiol* 47:2130–2139, 2006.
244. Yusuf S, Zhao F, Mehta SR, et al: Effects of clopidogrel in addition to aspirin in patients with acute coronary syndromes without ST-segment elevation. *N Engl J Med* 345:494–502, 2001.
245. MacIntrye IM, Jhund PS, McMurray JV: Aspirin inhibits the acute arterial and venous vasodilator response to captopril in patients with chronic heart failure. *Cardiovasc Drugs Ther* 19:261–265, 2005.
246. Hays AG, Sacco RL, Rundek T, et al: Left ventricular systolic dysfunction and the risk of ischemic stroke in a multiethnic population. *Stroke* 37:1715–1719, 2006.
247. Cleland JGF, Findlay I, Jafri S, et al: The warfarin/aspirin study in heart failure. *Am Heart J* 148:157–164, 2004.
248. Cokkinos DV, Haralabopoulos GC, Kostis JB, et al: Efficacy of antithrombotic therapy in chronic heart failure. *Eur J Heart Fail* 8:428–432, 2006.
249. Gheorghiade M, Flaherty JD, Fonarow GC, et al: Coronary artery disease, coronary revascularization, and outcomes in chronic advanced systolic heart failure. *Int J Cardiol* 151:69–75, 2011.
250. Tsuyuki RT, Shrive FM, Galbraith D, et al: Revascularization in patients with heart failure. *Can Med Assoc J* 175:361–373, 2006.
251. Jones RH, Velazquez EJ, Michler RE, et al: Coronary bypass surgery with or without surgical ventricular reconstruction. *N Engl J Med* 360:1705–1717, 2009.
252. Oh JK, Velazquez EJ, Menicanti L, et al, STICH Investigators: Influence of baseline left ventricular function on the clinical outcome of surgical ventricular reconstruction in patients with ischaemic cardiomyopathy. *Eur Heart J* 34:39–47, 2013.
253. Michler RE, Rouleau JL, Al-Khalidi HR, et al, STICH Trial Investigators: Insights from the STICH trial: change in left ventricular size after coronary artery bypass grafting with and without surgical ventricular reconstruction. *J Thorac Cardiovasc Surg* 146:1139–1145, 2013.
254. Sugiki T, Naya M, Manabe O, et al: Effects of surgical ventricular reconstruction and mitral complex reconstruction on cardiac oxidative metabolism and efficiency in nonischemic and ischemic dilated cardiomyopathy. *J Am Coll Cardiol Cardiovasc Imaging* 4:762–770, 2011.
255. Sagic D, Otasevic P, Sievert H, et al: Percutaneous implantation of the left ventricular partitioning device for chronic heart failure: a pilot study with 1-year follow-up. *Eur J Heart Fail* 12:600–606, 2010.
256. Costa MA, Pencina M, Nikolic S, et al: The PARACHUTE IV trial design and rationale: percutaneous ventricular restoration using the parachute device in patients with ischemic heart failure and dilated left ventricles. *Am Heart J* 165:531–536, 2013.
257. Bonow RO, Maurer G, Lee KL, et al, STICH Trial Investigators: Myocardial viability and survival in ischemic left ventricular dysfunction. *N Engl J Med* 364:1617–1625, 2011.
258. Carson P, Wertheimer J, Miller A, et al, for the STICH investigators: Surgical Treatment for Ischemic Heart Failure (STICH) Trial: mode of death results. *J Am Coll Cardiol Heart Failure* 1:399–408, 2013.
259. Velazquez EJ, Lee KL, Deja MA, et al: Coronary-artery bypass surgery in patients with left ventricular dysfunction. *N Engl J Med* 364:1607–1616, 2011.
260. Shah DJ, Kim HW, James O, et al: Prevalence of regional myocardial thinning and relationship with myocardial scarring in patients with coronary artery disease. *JAMA* 309:909–918, 2013.
261. Steg PG, Kerner A, Van de Werf F, et al: Impact of in-hospital revascularization with non-ST-elevation acute coronary syndrome and congestive heart failure. *Circulation* 118:1163–1171, 2008.
262. Hochman JS, Sleeper LA, Webb JS, et al: Early revascularization and long-term survival in cardiogenic shock complicating acute myocardial infarction. *JAMA* 295:2511–2515, 2006.
263. Flaherty JD, Rossi JS, Fonarow GC, et al: Influence of coronary angiography on the utilization of therapies in patients with acute heart failure syndromes: findings from OPTIMIZE-HF. *Am Heart J* 157:1018–1025, 2009.

Heart Failure as a Consequence of Dilated Cardiomyopathy

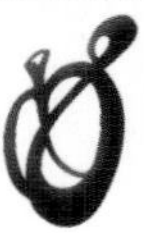

Biykem Bozkurt

DEFINITION

The term *dilated cardiomyopathy* (DCM) refers to a spectrum of heterogeneous myocardial disorders (**Table 19-1**) that are characterized by ventricular dilation and depressed myocardial contractility in the absence of abnormal loading conditions (such as hypertension or valvular disease) or ischemic heart disease sufficient to cause global systolic impairment.[1] The dilated cardiomyopathies constitute the largest group of myopathic disorders that are responsible for systolic heart failure. Indeed, more than 75 specific diseases can produce a dilated cardiomyopathic phenotype. Thus, DCM can be envisioned as the final common pathway for a myriad of cardiac disorders that either damage the heart muscle or, alternatively, disrupt the ability of the myocardium to generate force and subsequently cause chamber dilation.

In clinical practice and recent multicenter trials in heart failure, the cause of heart failure has often been categorized into two categories, ischemic and nonischemic cardiomyopathy, and the term DCM has been interchangeably used with nonischemic cardiomyopathy. Though this approach may be practical, it has certain drawbacks. It fails to recognize that the term *nonischemic cardiomyopathy* may include cardiomyopathies due to volume or pressure overload, such as hypertension or valvular heart disease, which are not conventionally accepted under the definition of DCM.[1] Amyloidosis and other infiltrative cardiomyopathies, which usually present as restrictive cardiomyopathies rather than dilated cardiomyopathies unless end stage, are further discussed in Chapter 20.

EPIDEMIOLOGY OF DILATED CARDIOMYOPATHY

The reported incidence of DCM varies annually about 5 to 8 cases per 100,000 of the population. The true incidence may be underestimated because of underreporting or underdetection of asymptomatic cases of DCM, which may occur in as many as 50% to 60% of heart failure patients. In most multicenter, randomized trials in heart failure, approximately 30% to 40% of the enrolled patients have nonischemic dilated cardiomyopathy. According to the Acute Decompensated Heart Failure National Registry (ADHERE), one of the largest databases on acute heart failure, 47% of the patients admitted to the hospital with heart failure have nonischemic cardiomyopathy.[2] The age-adjusted prevalence of DCM in the United States averages 36 cases per 100,000 population, and DCM accounts for 10,000 deaths annually.[3]

Compared with whites, African Americans have almost a threefold increase in risk for developing DCM. This increased risk for developing DCM in African Americans is not explained by differences in hypertension, cigarette smoking, alcohol use, or socioeconomic factors.[4] Moreover, African Americans have approximately a 1.5- to 2.0-fold higher risk of dying from DCM when compared with age-matched whites with DCM. Although the reason(s) for these differences are not known, there are several potential explanations, including differences in the genetic predisposition, the cause of heart failure, the number of risk factors for development of heart failure, the rate of progression of heart failure, access to medical care, and/or differences in response to therapy.

TABLE 19-1 Causes of Dilated Cardiomyopathy

Idiopathic
Idiopathic dilated cardiomyopathy Idiopathic arrhythmogenic right ventricular dysplasia
Familial (Hereditary)
Autosomal dominant X-chromosomal Polymorphism Other
Toxic
Ethanol Cocaine Adriamycin Catecholamine excess Phenothiazines, antidepressants Cobalt Carbon monoxide Lead Lithium Cyclophosphamide Methysergide Amphetamine Pseudoephedrine/Ephedrine
Inflammatory: Infectious Etiology
Viral (coxsackievirus, parvovirus, adenovirus, echovirus, influenza virus, HIV) Spirochete (leptospirosis, syphilis) Protozoal (Chagas disease, toxoplasmosis, trichinosis)
Inflammatory: Noninfectious Causes
Collagen vascular disease (scleroderma, lupus erythematosus, dermatomyositis, rheumatoid arthritis, sarcoidosis) Kawasaki Hypersensitivity myocarditis
Miscellaneous Acquired Cardiomyopathy
Postpartum cardiomyopathy Obesity
Metabolic/Nutritional
Thiamine Kwashiorkor, pellagra Scurvy Selenium deficiency Carnitine deficiency
Endocrine
Diabetes mellitus Acromegaly Thyrotoxicosis Myxedema Uremia Cushing disease Pheochromocytoma
Electrolyte Imbalance
Hypophosphatemia Hypocalcemia
Physiologic Agents
Tachycardia Heat stroke Hypothermia Radiation
Autoimmune Disorders
Infiltrative Cardiomyopathies (DCM usually after progression from restrictive cardiomyopathy, in end stage)
Cardiac amyloidosis Hemochromatosis
Stress/Catecholamine-Induced Cardiomyopathy

Regarding gender differences, in general, heart failure is more common in men than women. Epidemiologic data suggesting sex-related differences in the occurrence and prognosis of heart failure are conflicting and may be confounded by differing causes of heart failure. One of the challenges in defining gender-specific causes is that hypertension, which represents the major and strongest risk factor for development of heart failure in women, has been categorized under "nonischemic cardiomyopathy" in most large-scale clinical trials. In the Framingham Heart Study, hypertension was the cause of heart failure in 59% of women.[5] There are not many trials reporting specific causes of nonischemic cardiomyopathy in women; therefore, the "true" incidence of dilated cardiomyopathy in women, independent of hypertension, is not well known. One of these few studies was the EuroHeart Failure Survey II (EHFS), in which women had less incidence of dilated cardiomyopathy compared with men.[6]

The prevalence, cause, and prognosis of dilated cardiomyopathy can differ according to the geographic location and sociodemographics of the affected populations. For example, in Western developed countries, dilated nonischemic cardiomyopathy accounts for approximately 30% to 40% of the heart failure population, of which idiopathic cardiomyopathy is the most frequent cause. The prevalence of DCM in Japan appears to be about half,[7] and in Africa and Latin America approximately double that of the Western populations.[8] As populations go through epidemiologic and socioeconomic transitions and health care modifications, the features of DCM will continue to change. Failure of treatment and eradication of AIDS globally and especially in Africa, rising prevalence of ethanol or substance abuse in developing countries, the development of obesity, new metabolic and dietary trends globally, and the success in treatment of protozoal diseases in Latin America will continue to play a dynamic role in the epidemiology of DCM.

NATURAL HISTORY OF DILATED CARDIOMYOPATHY

The natural history of DCM is not well established for two reasons: first, as noted at the outset, DCM represents a heterogeneous spectrum of myocardial disorders that may each progress at different rates[9]; second, the onset of the disease may be insidious, particularly in the case of familial and/or idiopathic dilated cardiomyopathies. Indeed, approximately 4% to 13% of the patients with DCM will present with asymptomatic left ventricular dysfunction and left ventricular dilation. For these patients, the overall prognosis is unclear. However, once DCM patients become symptomatic, the available evidence suggests that the prognosis is relatively poor, with 25% mortality at 1 year and 50% mortality at 5 years (**Figure 19-1**).[10] The cause of death appears to be primarily pump failure in approximately 70% of patients with DCM, whereas sudden cardiac death accounts for approximately 30% of all deaths in patients with DCM. However, it should be recognized that many of the natural history studies of DCM were performed before angiotensin-converting enzyme (ACE) inhibitors and β-blockers were routinely used. More recent studies suggest that the prognosis for patients with DCM may be more favorable, perhaps reflecting earlier diagnosis and better treatment.[11] Furthermore, it should be recognized that approximately 25% of DCM patients with the recent onset of symptoms of heart failure will improve spontaneously, including patients who have been referred for cardiac transplantation.[12] This statement notwithstanding, patients with symptoms lasting more than 3 months who present with severe clinical decompensation generally have less chance of recovery.[12]

As shown in **Table 19-2**, there are a number of other parameters that predict a poor prognosis in patients with DCM, including left and right ventricular enlargement, reduced left and right ventricular ejection fraction (EF), persistent S_3 gallop, right-sided heart failure, elevated left ventricular (LV) filling pressures, moderate to severe mitral regurgitation, pulmonary hypertension, electrocardiogram (ECG) findings of left bundle branch block, recurrent ventricular tachycardia, renal and hepatic dysfunction, elevated levels of B-type natriuretic peptide (BNP), persistently elevated cardiac troponin levels, peak oxygen consumption less than 10 to 12 mL/kg/min, serum sodium less than 137 mmol/L, advanced New York Heart Association class, and age over 64 years.

Ischemic versus Dilated Cardiomyopathy

In general practice and clinical research trials, the term *ischemic cardiomyopathy* is defined as cardiomyopathy due to ischemic heart disease. The classification of cardiomyopathies proposed by the WHO/ISFC Task Force in 1995,[1] however, defines ischemic cardiomyopathy as "a dilated cardiomyopathy with impaired contractile performance not explained by the extent of coronary disease or ischemic damage" reserved for the remodeling process of the noninfarcted myocardium. In this chapter, we will use the term *ischemic cardiomyopathy* defined as cardiomyopathy due to ischemic heart disease rather than the WHO/ISFC Task Force definition.

The existing clinical studies suggest that patients with idiopathic dilated cardiomyopathy have a lower total mortality.[13] In some studies, however, the risk of sudden cardiac death has been reported to be higher in patients with DCM.[13] The differential treatment benefit seen in DCM patients compared with patients with ischemic cardiomyopathy that has been observed in several earlier randomized clinical trials, such as with digoxin[14] or amiodarone,[15] suggest that there may be therapeutic differences between ischemic and nonischemic heart failure. Contrarily, earlier reports of survival benefit with β-blockers[16] or amlodipine[17] in patients with dilated but not ischemic cardiomyopathy have not been reproduced in subsequent large-scale randomized trials, in which the benefit was similar in both the ischemic and nonischemic heart failure patients. This has raised the question whether there truly is a difference in response to treatment according to etiology of heart failure. The absence of a rigorous definition of "nonischemic heart failure" in many studies may account for this discrepancy and make interpretation of the results difficult. Further studies targeting specific causes of heart failure could be particularly important to achieve benefit over and beyond conventional treatment strategies that target heart failure as a single disease entity.

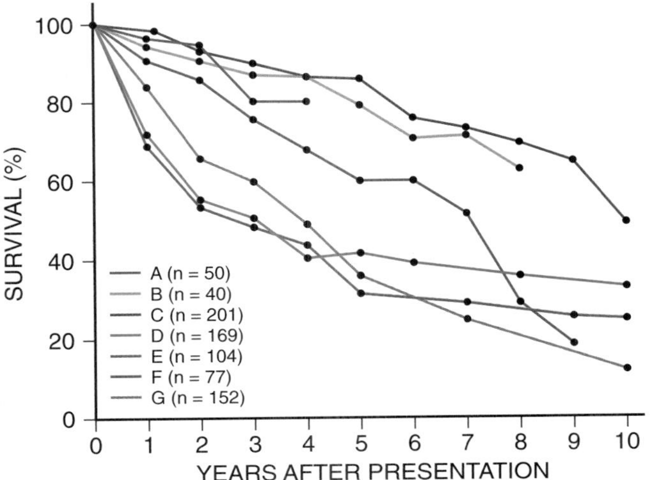

FIGURE 19-1 Survival of patients with idiopathic dilated cardiomyopathy in seven published series (A to G). *n*, Number of patients enrolled. To identify each specific series, please refer to the article by Dec and Fuster.[10] *From Dec GW, Fuster V: Idiopathic dilated cardiomyopathy. N Engl J Med 331:1564–1575, 1994.*

PATHOPHYSIOLOGY

Dilated cardiomyopathy may be viewed as a progressive disorder initiated after an "index event" that either damages the heart muscle, with a resultant loss of functioning cardiac myocytes, or alternatively disrupts the ability of the myocardium to generate force, thereby preventing the heart from contracting normally. This index event may have an abrupt onset, as in the case of acute exposure to toxins, or it may have a gradual or insidious onset, as in the case hemodynamic pressure or volume overloading. It also may be hereditary, as in the case of many of the familial cardiomyopathies. Regardless of the nature of the inciting event, the feature that is common to each of these index events is that they all, in some manner, produce a decline in the pumping capacity of the heart.

The anatomic and pathophysiologic abnormalities that occur in LV remodeling are discussed in Chapter 11. Patients with dilated cardiomyopathy generally present with dilation of all four chambers of the heart (**Figure 19-2**). Despite the fact that there is thinning of the LV wall in patients with DCM, there is massive hypertrophy at the

TABLE 19-2 Factors Predicting a Poor Prognosis in Patients with Dilated Cardiomyopathy

Advanced New York Heart Association class
Recurrent heart failure hospitalizations
Advanced age (>64 years)
Left ventricular enlargement
Right ventricular enlargement
Reduced left and/or right ventricular ejection fraction
Elevated LV filling pressures
Persistent S_3 gallop
Right-sided heart failure
Pulmonary hypertension
Hypotension
Moderate-severe mitral regurgitation
ECG findings of LBBB, persistent tachycardia, wide QRS
Recurrent ventricular tachycardia
Reduced heart rate variability
Late potentials of QRS in signal-averaged EKG
Myocytolysis on endomyocardial biopsy
Elevated levels of neurohormones (BNP, NT-ProBNP)
Elevated levels of proinflammatory cytokines and biomarkers
Elevation of serum cardiac troponin T, troponin I levels
Peak oxygen consumption <10-12 mL/kg/min
Reduced contractile response
Serum sodium <137 mmol/L
Impaired kidney function (elevated creatinine, reduced EGFR)
Impaired liver function (elevated transaminases, elevated bilirubin)

level of the intact heart, as well as at the level of the cardiac myocyte, which has a characteristic elongated appearance that is observed in myocytes obtained from hearts subjected to chronic volume overload (**Figure 19-3**). The coronary arteries are usually normal in DCM, although it should be emphasized that the end-stage "ischemic cardiomyopathies" may also present with a dilated phenotype. The cardiac valves are anatomically normal; however, there is usually LV dilation, global hypokinesis (**Figure 19-4**), tricuspid and mitral annular dilation due to cavity enlargement, distortion of subvalvular apparatus, and stretching of the papillary muscles giving rise to valvular regurgitation. Intracavitary thrombi are common usually in the ventricular apex (**Figure 19-5**).

MYOCARDIAL DISEASES PRESENTING AS DILATED CARDIOMYOPATHY

The most common causes of DCM are genetic, idiopathic, toxic, inflammatory, infectious, or metabolic causes. However, it should be recognized that the exact prevalence of the

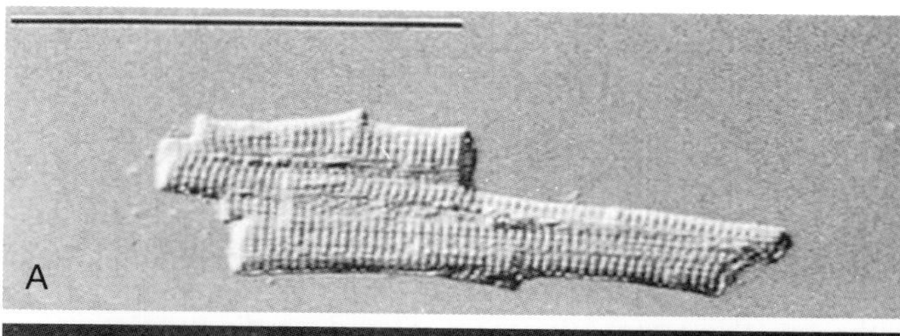

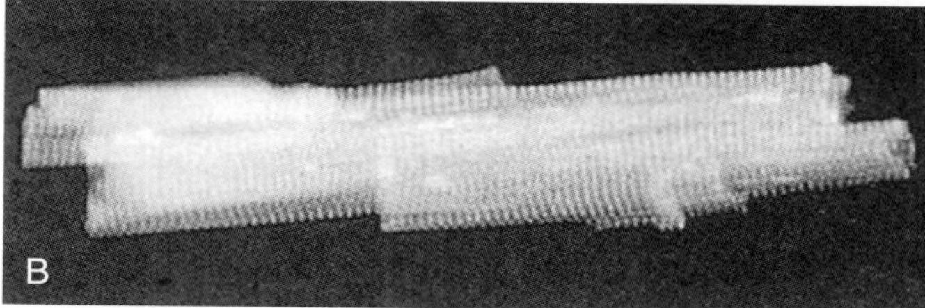

FIGURE 19-3 Cardiac myocyte structure *(top)* in normal myocardium and in dilated cardiomyopathy *(bottom)*. Cardiac myocytes isolated from myocardium from patients with DCM have an elongated shape as the result of the sarcomeres being formed in series. *From Gerdes AM, Kellerman SE, Moore JA, et al: Structural remodeling of cardiac myocytes in patients with ischemic cardiomyopathy. Circulation 86:426–430, 1992.*

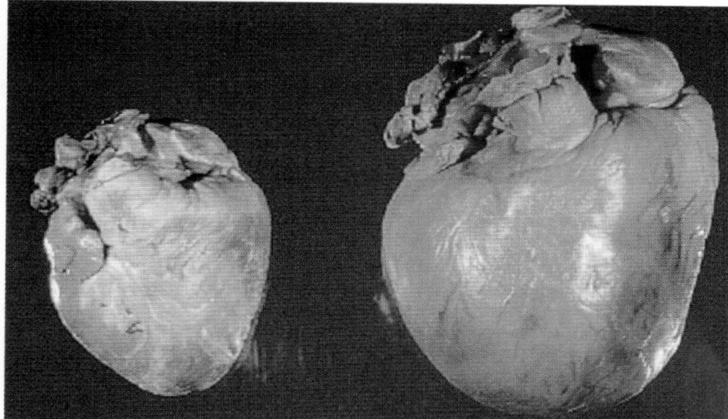

FIGURE 19-2 Pathology of normal heart *(left)* and a dilated cardiomyopathic ventricle *(right)*. The dilated cardiomyopathic ventricle is characterized by enlargement of all four cardiac chambers, and a more spherical shape, in comparison to the normal ventricle. *From Kasper EK, Hruban RH, Baughman KL: Idiopathic dilated cardiomyopathy. In Abelman WH, editor: Atlas of heart diseases: cardiomyopathies, myocarditis and pericardial disease, Philadelphia, 1995, Current Medicine, 3.1–3.18.*

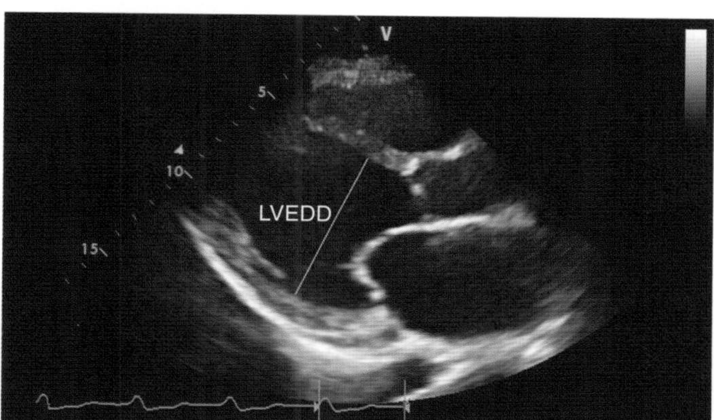

FIGURE 19-4 Left ventricular dilation in dilated cardiomyopathy by transthoracic echocardiography. In this parasternal long-axis image, the LV dimension is measured at the level of the mitral leaflet tips *(white line)*. The LV is severely dilated in this example with a dimension of 7 cm. *LVEDD,* Left ventricular end-diastolic dimension. *Image courtesy of Harris Health System, Houston, TX.*

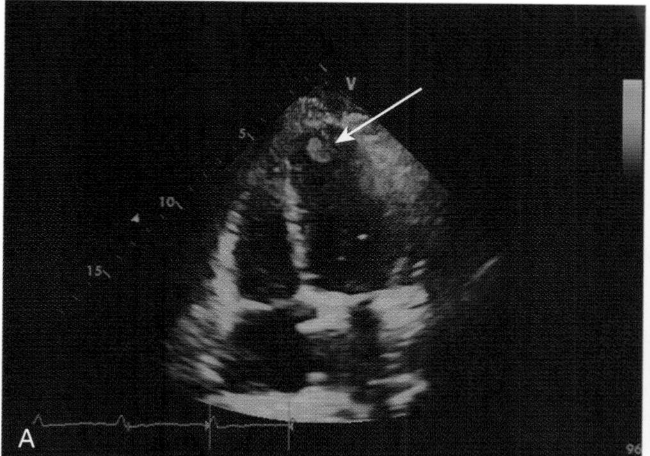

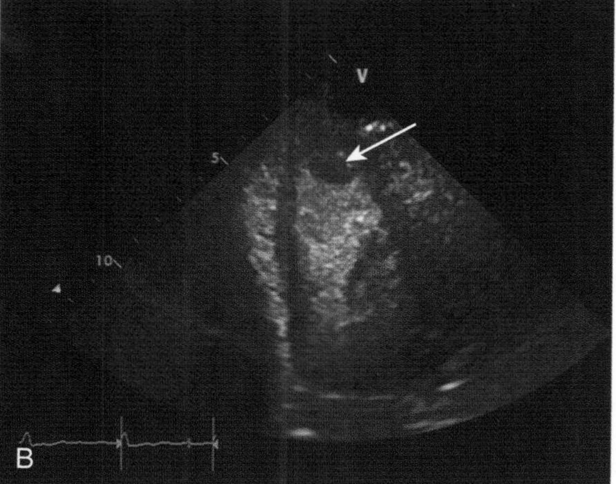

FIGURE 19-5 Left ventricular apical thrombus *(white arrows)* in a patient with dilated cardiomyopathy. Apical four-chamber view without **(A)** and with perfluorocarbon contrast **(B)**, demonstrating a circular mass in the LV apex consistent with thrombus. *Images courtesy of Harris Health System, Houston, TX.*

various forms of dilated cardiomyopathy will vary based on the demographics of the patient population and the ability to identify a specific cause. In the section that follows, we will review the various specific causes that lead to the development of DCM.

Idiopathic Dilated Cardiomyopathy

Although the term *idiopathic dilated cardiomyopathy* has become synonymous with that of *dilated cardiomyopathy* in some heart failure parlance, the term *idiopathic* was originally intended to characterize the subset of DCM patients in whom no known cause for ventricular dilation and depressed myocardial contractility was apparent. However, with increasing sophistication in diagnostic testing, clinicians have become aware that most cases of so-called idiopathic dilated cardiomyopathy may occur as the result of inherited and/or spontaneous mutations of genes that regulate cardiac structure and/or function, such as the genes for cytoskeletal proteins, or in some cases as a consequence of undiagnosed hypertension, autoimmune diseases, toxins (such as cardiotoxic chemotherapy, alcohol, or illicit drugs), or viral myocarditis. Nonetheless, in the context of the present chapter, we use the terminology of idiopathic dilated cardiomyopathy to refer to those patients with DCM whose etiologic cause remains unknown. It is likely that the proportion of patients with idiopathic dilated cardiomyopathy will diminish with increased sophistication in detection of genetic cardiomyopathies and other specific cardiomyopathies.

Familial/Genetic Cardiomyopathies

There is growing evidence that many cases of previously diagnosed "idiopathic" dilated cardiomyopathies have a genetic basis. It is estimated that at least 30% of dilated cardiomyopathy cases are familial or genetic. Such causes, including noncompacted cardiomyopathy; dystrophin, titin-related or other sarcomere, cytoskeleton, nuclear lamina–related genetic cardiomyopathies; X-linked cardiomyopathies, muscular dystrophy–associated cardiomyopathies, other familial dilated cardiomyopathies, and arrhythmogenic right ventricular cardiomyopathy are discussed in detail in Chapter 22.

Cardiomyopathy Due to Cardiotoxins

Alcoholic Cardiomyopathy

Chronic alcoholism is one of the most important causes of dilated cardiomyopathy in the Western world.[18] It is estimated that two thirds of the adult population use alcohol to some extent and more than 10% are heavy users. In the United States, in both sexes and all races, long-term heavy alcohol consumption (of any beverage type) has been quoted as the leading cause of nonischemic dilated cardiomyopathy by some investigators.[18] A large proportion of chronic alcoholics demonstrate impairment of cardiac function. The clinical diagnosis of alcoholic cardiomyopathy can be made when biventricular dysfunction and dilation are persistently observed in a heavy drinker, in the absence of other known causes for myocardial disease. Thus the diagnosis of alcoholic cardiomyopathy remains a diagnosis of exclusion. The prevalence of alcoholic cardiomyopathy is variable and ranges from 23% to 40%. Alcoholic cardiomyopathy most commonly occurs in men 30 to 55 years of age who have been heavy consumers of alcohol for more than 10 years.[18] Women represent approximately 14% of the alcoholic cardiomyopathy cases, but women may be more vulnerable to the development of alcohol-related cardiomyopathy, because it has been reported that alcoholic cardiomyopathy develops in women with a less total lifetime exposure to alcohol compared with men.[18] In all races, death rates due to alcoholic heart muscle disease are greater in men compared with women, and are greater in African American men and women compared with white men and women with alcoholic cardiomyopathy.[18] Even before clinically overt heart failure, LV contractile dysfunction can be demonstrated in alcoholics. Although chronic alcoholic liver disease and heart failure usually are not observed clinically in the same patient, cirrhotic patients may present with asymptomatic LV dysfunction, in which case atrial fibrillation is usually the initial presenting manifestation of cardiac dysfunction. The point at which these abnormalities appear during the course of an individual's lifetime of drinking, such that the abnormalities can be called a dilated cardiomyopathy, is not well established and is highly individualized.

The risk of developing alcoholic cardiomyopathy appears to be related to both the mean daily alcohol intake and the duration of drinking. In general, alcoholic patients consuming greater than 90 g of alcohol a day (approximately seven to eight standard drinks per day) for more than 5 years are at risk for the development of asymptomatic alcoholic cardiomyopathy. On the other hand, mild to moderate alcohol consumption has recently been reported to be protective against development of heart failure in the general population. According to the Framingham Heart Study, moderate alcohol consumption is not associated with increased risk, and in fact appears to be protective against development of congestive heart failure.[19] Similarly, in a prospective cohort study of elderly persons, moderate alcohol consumption was associated with a decreasing risk of heart failure.[20] These paradoxical findings (i.e., alcohol may be protective against development of heart failure in certain populations when used in moderation, but detrimental in others especially when used in excess over longer periods of time, suggest that duration of exposure and individual genetic susceptibility play an important role in pathogenesis). Persistent DCM develops in only 1% to 2% of chronic drinkers, and the role of genetic predisposition or the presence of synergistic cardiovascular factors such as hypertension or arrhythmias in development of alcohol-related cardiomyopathy is not clear at the present time.

Studies in experimental animals have demonstrated that both acute and chronic ethanol administration impairs cardiac contractility. Alcohol results in acute as well as chronic depression of myocardial contractility even when ingested by normal individuals in quantities consumed during social drinking.[21] Compensatory mechanisms, such as vasodilation or sympathetic stimulation, may mask the direct acute myocardial depressant effects of alcohol. Despite the known deleterious effects of alcohol, it has been difficult to produce heart failure in animal models in which ethanol has been administered. Thus the direct causal relationship between alcohol consumption and the development of cardiomyopathy has not been rigorously demonstrated in experimental models, despite the long-recognized clinical relationship between alcohol consumption and the development of DCM. The pathophysiology and progression of alcoholic cardiomyopathy is complex and involves changes in many aspects of myocyte function. The potential mechanisms that have been invoked to explain the depressed myocardial function include the direct toxic effects of alcohol on striated muscle, because most alcoholics have manifestations of skeletal myopathy and cardiomyopathy. Shifts in the relative expression of the contractile proteins, α-myosin heavy chain to β-MHC, have been reported in animal models after exposure to ethanol.[18] Alcohol and its metabolite acetaldehyde can also cause alterations in cellular calcium, magnesium, or phosphate homeostasis. The toxic effects of acetaldehyde or the formation of fatty acid ethyl esters may also impair mitochondrial oxidative phosphorylation. In acute ethanol toxicity free radical damage and/or ischemia may occur, possibly because of increased xanthine oxidase activity or β-adrenergic stimulation, respectively. In addition, ethanol and its metabolites interfere with numerous membrane and cellular functions, such as transport and binding of calcium, mitochondrial respiration, lipid metabolism, myocardial protein synthesis, signal transduction, and excitation-contraction coupling. Both autopsy and endomyocardial biopsy specimens from alcoholic cardiomyopathy patients reveal marked mitochondrial swelling, with fragmentation of cristae, swelling of endoplasmic reticulum, entrance of mitochondria into the nucleus potentially promoting attack of mitochondria by nuclear proteins and the attack of nuclear DNA by proteins of the mitochondrial intermembrane space,[22] cytoskeletal disorganization, and destruction of myofibrils (**Figure 19-6**). Several studies suggest that heavy drinking alters both lymphocyte and granulocyte production and function, raising the possibility that myocardial damage secondary to prolonged alcohol consumption might initiate auto-reactive mechanisms comparable with those observed in viral or idiopathic myocarditis. The point at which the changes in mitochondrial, sarcoplasmic reticulum, contractile protein, and calcium homeostasis culminate in intrinsic cell dysfunction is incompletely understood. There are several early reports that support the role for myocyte loss as a final mechanism underlying alcohol-induced cardiac dysfunction. Application of insulin-like growth factor (IGF)-1 has been reported to attenuate the apoptotic effects of ethanol in primary neonatal myocyte cell cultures.[18]

Recent reports suggest that certain genetic traits influence the occurrence, pathogenesis, and progression of alcoholic cardiomyopathy, which may explain interindividual variations in the sensitivity of the myocardium to alcohol-induced myocardial damage. These include multiple point mutations in the mitochondrial DNA, which have been associated with the occurrence of other cardiomyopathies.[23] In addition, nutritional deficiencies, commonly thiamine deficiency, may play an additive role to the direct myocardial damage of ethanol. Thus the cardiomyopathy that develops following chronic alcohol consumption may be multifactorial in origin.

The management of patients with alcoholic cardiomyopathy begins with total abstinence from alcohol, in addition to the conventional management of heart failure, as described later. There are currently no studies of specific pharmacotherapies in patients with alcoholic cardiomyopathy other than the standard therapy of heart failure; however, there are numerous reports that detail the

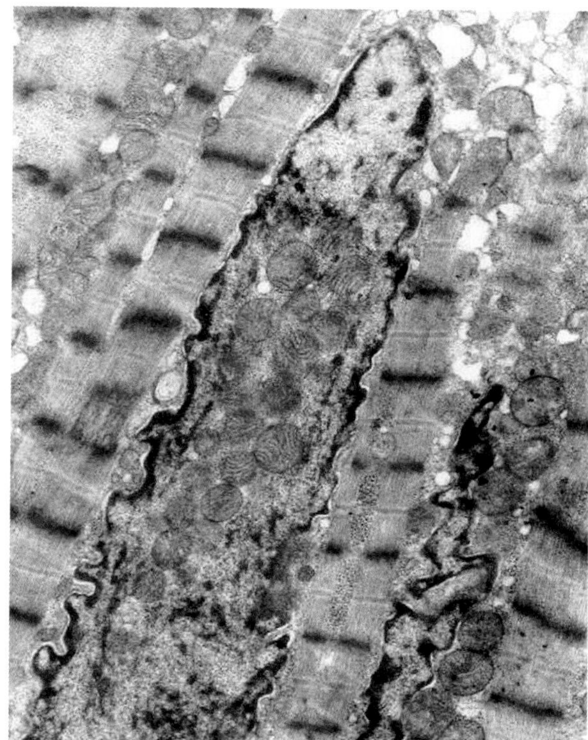

FIGURE 19-6 Electron microscopy of cardiomyocytes of patients with alcoholic cardiomyopathy, revealing the presence of nuclei with mitochondria accumulated in their core, associated with chromatin displacement to periphery of the nucleus. *From Bakeeva LE, Skulachev VP, Sudarikova YV, et al: Mitochondria enter the nucleus (one further problem in chronic alcoholism). Biochemistry (Mosc) 66:1335–1341, 2001.*

reversibility of depressed LV dysfunction after the cessation of drinking.[24] Many heart failure programs limit alcoholic beverage consumption to no more than an alcoholic beverage serving daily for all patients with LV dysfunction, regardless of the cause being alcohol related or not.[25] Even if the depressed LV function does not normalize completely, the symptoms and signs of congestive heart failure improve after abstinence.[24] However, the overall prognosis remains poor, with a mortality of 40% to 50% within 3 to 6 years, if the patient is not abstinent.[18] The survival is significantly lower for patients who continue to drink compared with patients with idiopathic DCM or alcoholic cardiomyopathy patients who abstain.[18]

Cocaine Cardiomyopathy

Long-term abuse of cocaine, a drug that causes postsynaptic nervous system norepinephrine reuptake blockade and possible presynaptic release of dopamine and norepinephrine, may eventuate in dilated cardiomyopathy even without the presence of coronary artery disease, vasculitis, or regional myocardial injury. This has been termed *cocaine-related cardiomyopathy* and perhaps reflects the direct toxicity of the cocaine on the myocardium. In asymptomatic cocaine abusers studied at least 2 weeks after abstinence from the drug, Bertolet and colleagues found that 7% had LV dysfunction. These patients were young and did not have evidence of myocardial infarction or coronary arterial disease.[26] Depressed LV function has been reported in 4% to 9% of asymptomatic cocaine abusers.[27] Similarly, Om and associates reported 18% of cocaine abusers who underwent cardiac catheterization had normal coronary arteries with low EF and global hypokinesia.[28]

The cardiovascular evaluation of a patient abusing cocaine usually reflects the following. The electrocardiogram may reveal increased QRS voltage, early repolarization, ischemic or nonspecific ST-T wave changes, or pathologic Q waves. Episodes of ST elevation may be seen during Holter monitoring. An echocardiogram usually reveals LV hypertrophy, depressed LV ejection fraction, and dilation. Segmental wall motion abnormalities usually suggest myocardial injury; however, as mentioned previously, approximately 18% of patients with cocaine abuse manifest global hypokinesia. Cardiac catheterization in these patients may reveal normal coronaries or mild coronary artery disease not significant enough to explain the extent of myocardial dysfunction. However, accelerated coronary atherosclerosis, coronary vasculitis, coronary spasm, or coronary thrombosis is perhaps a more common finding in cocaine-related heart disease.

Cocaine may produce LV dysfunction through its direct toxic effects on the myocardium, by provoking coronary arterial spasm (and hence myocardial ischemia), and by causing increased release of catecholamines, which may be directly toxic to cardiac myocytes. These effects will decrease myocardial oxygen supply and may increase demand if heart rate and blood pressure rise. The vasoactive effects of cocaine are further complicated with enhanced platelet aggregation, anticardiolipin antibody formation, and endothelial release of potent vasoconstrictors such as endothelin-1. Upregulation of tissue plasminogen activator inhibitors, increased platelet aggregation, and decreased fibrinolysis by cocaine predispose to coronary thrombosis and or microvascular disease.[27] Myocarditis with inflammatory lymphocyte and eosinophils has also been reported in 20% of patients dying of natural or homicidal causes in whom cocaine was detected, raising the possibility of hypersensitivity myocarditis due to cocaine or associated contaminants. Alternatively, the myocarditis may occur directly in response to the necrosis that is caused by the cocaine. Scattered foci of myocyte necrosis, contraction band necrosis, and foci of myocyte fibrosis have been reported in patients with cocaine abuse. Additionally, experimental studies and clinical case reports suggest that cocaine may also cause lethal arrhythmias. Cocaine prolongs repolarization by a depressant effect on potassium current and may generate early afterdepolarizations.[27]

Other than abstinence, very little is known about the treatment of cocaine-induced cardiac dysfunction. Indeed, there are case reports of reversibility of cardiac function after cessation of drug use. In patients who develop cardiomyopathy, the traditional therapy for LV dysfunction is appropriate. Given that some of the toxicity of cocaine is caused by catecholamine excess and/or myocardial ischemia, the use of β-adrenergic blocking agents appears to be a logical treatment, both in terms of preventing further disease progression, as well as for treating the ventricular arrhythmias that are prone to develop in this setting. Two decades ago, the treatment of cocaine-induced cardiovascular effects favored the use of β-blockers, especially propranolol. As the clinical use of propranolol increased, reports of accentuation of cocaine-induced hypertension and myocardial ischemia began to surface, blaming the unopposed α-effects of the β-blockers. Although these reports were isolated, the routine use of propranolol and subsequently all β-adrenergic blockers decreased to the point that β-blockers were considered relatively contraindicated in treating cocaine-induced cardiovascular emergencies. The end result is that an entire generation of potent and selective β-adrenergic blocking agents have been overlooked, both for acute and chronic treatment of cocaine-related cardiac disease, due to the possibility of "unopposed α-effects." The focus of treatment shifted from the cardiovascular effects to combating central nervous system stimulation. As a result, benzodiazepines have been the drug of choice in treating the cerebrovascular and subsequent systemic hyperadrenergic complications of cocaine, and nitroprusside or phentolamine being advocated for peripheral vasodilatory effects. It is now becoming apparent that treatment of cardiovascular effects of cocaine should involve a multifactorial approach to combat both central nervous system and peripheral vasospastic effects of cocaine. In this regard, β-adrenergic blocking agents, especially β-blocking agents with both α- and β-blocking properties such as labetalol or carvedilol, may play an important role in treating cocaine-related cardiomyopathy or chronic heart failure. It should also be noted that β-blockers are not recommended to be used in the acute setting of cocaine-related acute coronary syndrome.

Chemotherapy (see also Chapter 43)

Cardiotoxicity is a well-known side effect of several cytotoxic drugs, especially the anthracyclines, which can lead to long-term morbidity. Anthracyclines, such as doxorubicin (Adriamycin) and daunorubicin, produce cardiac toxicity possibly by increasing oxygen free radical generation, platelet activating factor, prostaglandins, histamine, calcium, and C-13 hydroxy metabolites, or by interfering with the sarcolemmal sodium potassium pump and mitochondrial electron transport chain. The formation of oxygen free radicals that are generated by iron-catalyzed pathways appears to be the most important pathway in the pathogenesis of anthracycline-induced cardiomyopathy as it has been noted that iron-chelating agents that prevent generation of oxygen free radicals, such as dexrazoxane, are cardioprotective. The prognosis for anthracycline-induced cardiomyopathy relates to the time course of treatment and preexisting additional risk factors for myocardial injury, such as radiation, coexisting coronary artery disease, and preexisting cardiac dysfunction. Prior XRT to the heart/mediastinum also increases the risk of doxorubicin-induced cardiomyopathy. In general, patients with anthracycline-induced cardiomyopathy have a worse survival than that seen with idiopathic DCM (**Figure 19-7**). Prevention of anthracycline-induced myocardial damage by use of free radical "scavengers" and antioxidants may reduce cardiotoxicity in some patients. Other chemotherapeutic agents in cancer associated with cardiac toxicity complication are the monoclonal antibody trastuzumab (Herceptin), high-dose cyclophosphamide, taxoids, mitomycin-C, 5-fluorouracil, and the interferons. In contrast to anthracycline-induced cardiac toxicity, trastuzumab-related cardiac dysfunction does not appear to increase with cumulative dose or to be associated with ultrastructural changes in the myocardium and is generally reversible. This topic is discussed in further detail in Chapter 43.

Other Myocardial Toxins

In addition to the classic toxins described previously, as shown in Table 19-1, there are a number of other toxic

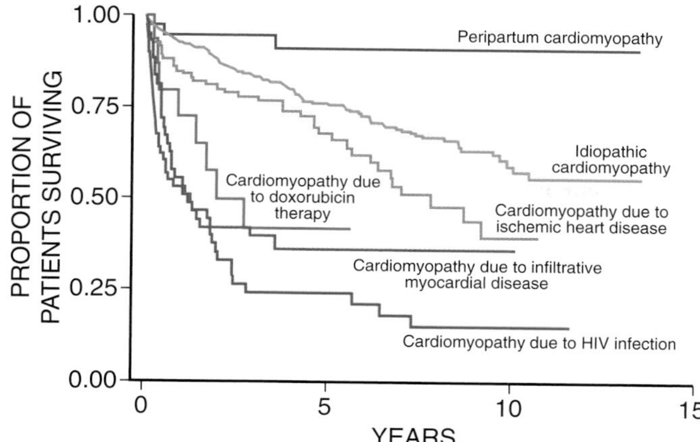

FIGURE 19-7 Survival according to different causes of dilated cardiomyopathy. In a cohort of patients who underwent endomyocardial biopsy as part of an evaluation for heart failure due to unexplained cardiomyopathy, when compared with patients with idiopathic cardiomyopathy, the survival was significantly better in patients with peripartum cardiomyopathy and significantly worse among the patients with cardiomyopathy because of infiltrative myocardial disease, HIV infection, therapy with doxorubicin, and ischemic heart disease. *From Felker GM, Thompson RE, Hare JM, et al: Underlying causes and long-term survival in patients with initially unexplained cardiomyopathy. N Engl J Med 342:1077–1084, 2000.*

agents that may lead to LV dysfunction and heart failure, including amphetamines, cobalt, and catecholamines. One such agent, ephedra, which has been used for the purposes of athletic performance enhancement and weight loss, has been linked to a high rate of serious adverse outcomes, including LV systolic dysfunction, development of heart failure, and cardiac deaths, ultimately resulting in the ban of this agent by the U.S. Food and Drug Administration in the United States. High doses of decongestants, such as pseudoephedrine or ephedrine, have also been implicated in cardiotoxicity and are recommended not to be overused.

INFLAMMATION-INDUCED CARDIOMYOPATHY

Over the past 10 to 15 years there has been increasing evidence that suggests that inflammation and/or inflammatory processes may contribute to the overall pathogenesis of dilated cardiomyopathy (see also Chapter 7). Moreover, there is increasing evidence that biologic properties of inflammatory mediators, such as proinflammatory cytokines, are also sufficient to produce a dilated cardiac phenotype.[29] As will be discussed later, both infectious and noninfectious inflammatory processes may lead to the development of DCM. Although a great many infections and noninfectious processes may impact the myocardium and may transiently lead to systolic dysfunction and congestive symptomatology, the great majority of these infections and noninfectious processes do not lead to the development of DCM. Therefore, in the section that follows, we will focus primarily on those disease states that are considered to lead to DCM.

Infectious Causes

There are a number of infectious diseases that can lead to dilated cardiomyopathy, including viral myocarditis (see Chapter 26), Chagas disease (see Chapter 27), and acquired immunodeficiency syndrome (AIDS), which will be discussed in detail later.

Acquired Immunodeficiency Syndrome

Several investigators have reported that there is an association between acquired immunodeficiency syndrome (AIDS) and dilated cardiomyopathy. Reviews and studies published before the introduction of highly active antiretroviral therapy regimens have correlated the incidence and course of human immunodeficiency virus (HIV) infection in relation to dilated cardiomyopathy in both children and adults. In a long-term echocardiographic follow-up by Barbaro and coworkers,[30] 8% of initially asymptomatic HIV-positive patients were diagnosed with dilated cardiomyopathy during the 60-month follow-up. All patients with dilated cardiomyopathy were in New York Heart Association (NYHA) functional class III or IV. The mean annual incidence rate was 15.9 cases per 1000 patients. The extent of immunodeficiency of the patients, as assessed by the CD4 count, influenced the incidence of dilated cardiomyopathy; specifically, there was a higher incidence among patients with a CD4 count of less than 400 cells per cubic millimeter.

Current hypotheses concerning the pathogenesis of cardiomyopathy associated with infection with the human immunodeficiency virus include infection of myocardial cells with HIV type 1 or co-infection with other cardiotropic viruses, postviral cardiac autoimmunity, autonomic dysfunction, cardiotoxicity from illicit drugs and pharmacologic agents (such as nucleoside analogues and pentamidine), nutritional deficiencies, and prolonged immunosuppression. Recently it has been demonstrated that targeted myocardial expression of HIV transactivator in transgenic mice results in cardiomyopathy and mitochondrial damage,[31] emphasizing the role of the HIV infection itself in AIDS cardiomyopathy. The role of HIV type 1 infection of cardiac myocytes in the development of dilated cardiomyopathy in HIV has not been fully characterized. Even though human myocardial cells are not known to express CD4 cells, an autopsy series of persons dying from AIDS-related illnesses demonstrates histologic evidence of myocarditis in approximately 50% of the patients[32]; by in situ hybridization techniques, HIV nucleic acid sequences were detected in cardiac tissue sections in 27% of the patients who died of AIDS[33] (**Figure 19-8**). Symptomatic heart failure is seen in approximately half of these patients with myocardial involvement. Other than treatment for HIV, the treatment of heart failure in patients with symptomatic HIV cardiomyopathy is the same as the conventional treatment for patients with DCM. The prognosis of HIV cardiomyopathy remains poor, with an over 50% mortality rate in 2 to 3 years[34] (see Figure 19-7).

Noninfectious Causes

Hypersensitivity Myocarditis

Hypersensitivity to a variety of agents may result in allergic reactions that involve the myocardium, characterized by peripheral eosinophilia, and a perivascular infiltration of the myocardium by eosinophils, lymphocytes, and histiocytes. These infiltrates may be occasionally associated with necrosis. A variety of drugs, most commonly the sulfonamides, penicillins, methyldopa, and other agents such as amphotericin B, streptomycin, phenytoin, isoniazid, tetanus

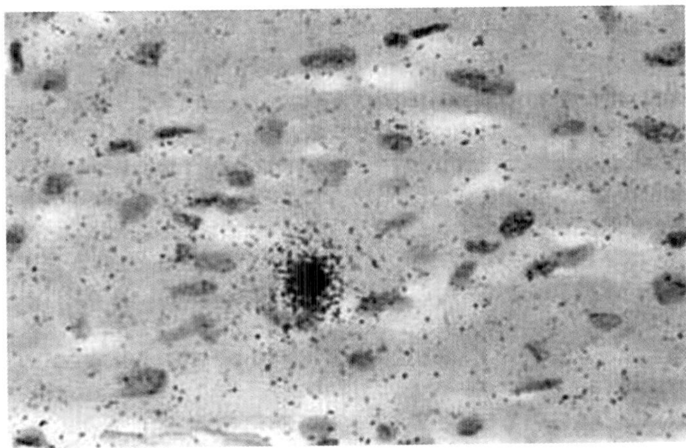

FIGURE 19-8 In situ hybridization of HIV RNA probe in a section of myocardial tissue obtained at autopsy from AIDS patients. Using sulfur-35-labeled ribonucleic acid probes, HIV nucleic acid sequences were detected in cardiac tissue sections. The black grains in the emulsion overlying a presumed cardiac myocyte indicate positive hybridization with HIV nucleic acid sequences. (Counterstained with hematoxylin and eosin, 335×.) *From Grody WW, Cheng L, Lewis W: Infection of the heart by the human immunodeficiency virus. Am J Cardiol 66:203–206, 1990.*

toxoid, hydrochlorothiazide, and chlorthalidone have been reported to cause allergic hypersensitivity myocarditis. Most patients are not clinically ill, but may die suddenly, presumably secondary to an arrhythmia. Hypersensitivity myocarditis is recognized only rarely clinically, but may be sufficient to produce global and/or regional myocardial dysfunction detected by noninvasive methods. This entity is often first diagnosed on postmortem examination, and occasionally on endomyocardial biopsy.[35]

Systemic Lupus Erythematosus

Although a number of cardiac abnormalities have been reported in patients with systemic lupus erythematosus (SLE), the development of DCM is not a prominent manifestation of this disease process. Global LV dysfunction has been reported in 5%, segmental LV wall motion abnormalities in 4%, and right ventricular enlargement in 4% of patients with SLE. In general the abnormalities in cardiac function usually correlate with disease activity. The myocardial involvement is frequently found at autopsy or at endomyocardial biopsy and is less easily detected clinically. The myocardial lesions are characterized by an increase in interstitial connective tissue and myocardial scarring. Recent studies suggest that depolarization abnormalities on signal-averaged EKG, accompanied with echocardiographic evidence of abnormal LV filling, may reflect the presence of myocardial fibrosis and could be a marker of subclinical myocardial involvement in SLE patients.[36] Cardiac involvement may manifest itself by conduction system abnormalities, such as complete atrioventricular heart block. Especially neonatal lupus is characterized by congenital heart block, as well as cardiomyopathy, cutaneous lupus lesions, hepatobiliary disease, and thrombocytopenia.

Scleroderma

The development of DCM is rare in patients with scleroderma. A recent echocardiographic study showed that although there was no difference in LV dimensions or fractional shortening in patients with scleroderma, there was indication of systolic impairment in most patients.[37] A distinctive focal myocardial lesion ranging from contraction band necrosis to replacement fibrosis without morphologic abnormalities of the coronary arteries is noted in approximately half of the patients with scleroderma. This is postulated to be caused by intermittent vascular spasm with intramyocardial Raynaud phenomenon. Thus progressive systemic sclerosis can lead to conduction abnormalities, arrhythmias, heart failure, angina pectoris with normal coronary arteries, myocardial fibrosis, pericarditis, and sudden death. Late contrast enhancement with gadolinium may be used to characterize patchy fibrosis and myocardial edema interspersed with normal myocardium in scleroderma. Cardiac involvement in systemic sclerosis portends an ominous prognosis, and is probably most directly related to the extent of myocardial fibrosis.

Rheumatoid Arthritis

Cardiac involvement in rheumatoid arthritis generally results from the development of myocarditis and/or pericarditis. However, the development of DCM is rare in these patients. In a retrospective study of 172 patients with juvenile rheumatoid arthritis, symptomatic cardiac involvement occurred in 7.6% of patients, including pericarditis, perimyocarditis, and myocarditis. Both myocarditis and pericarditis are regarded as poor prognostic factors in rheumatoid arthritis.[38] Myocardial involvement in rheumatoid arthritis is thought to be secondary to disturbances in the microcirculation secondary to microvasculitis, and occurs in the absence of any clinical symptoms of ECG changes.

Sarcoidosis

Cardiac sarcoidosis is most commonly recognized in patients with systemic or other manifestations of sarcoidosis, and cardiac involvement may occur in isolation and go undetected. Cardiac sarcoidosis may present as asymptomatic LV dysfunction, symptomatic heart failure, atrioventricular block, atrial or ventricular arrhythmia, and sudden cardiac death. Although untested in clinical trials, early use of high-dose steroid therapy may halt or reverse cardiac damage.[39] Cardiac magnetic resonance and cardiac positron emission tomographic scanning can identify cardiac involvement with patchy areas of myocardial inflammation and fibrosis. Cardiac involvement is patchy with granulomas and fibrosis, and endomyocardial biopsy may demonstrate myocardial granulomas characterized by clusters of mononuclear cells and giant cells. In the setting of ventricular tachyarrhythmia, patients may require placement of an implantable cardioverter-defibrillator for primary prevention of sudden cardiac death. Though most present with restrictive cardiomyopathy features with mildly depressed or preserved LV ejection fraction, elevated filling pressures, enlarged atria, and restrictive filling pattern by echocardiography, in advanced stages the cardiac features may progress to dilated cardiomyopathy.

Kawasaki Disease

Kawasaki disease is an acute febrile illness associated with mucosal inflammation, skin rash, and cervical lymphadenopathy. This disease is recognized most often in children less than 4 years of age. Kawasaki disease represents an acute vasculitic syndrome of unknown cause that primarily affects small and medium-sized arteries, including coronary arteries. Coronary arterial aneurysms are seen in 25% to 55% of the acute Kawasaki cases. Of these, 4.7% progress to premature atherosclerotic ischemic heart disease.

Myocardial infarction is noted in approximately 2% of patients, and cardiovascular death is reported in 0.8%. Although the development of DCM is not typical for Kawasaki disease, repetitive infarctions secondary to coronary arterial aneurysms may lead to a dilated cardiomyopathic phenotype.

Peripartum Cardiomyopathy

Peripartum cardiomyopathy (PPCM) is a disease of unknown cause in which severe LV dysfunction occurs during the last trimester of pregnancy or the early puerperium in the absence of an identifiable cause for the cardiac failure other than pregnancy. In the past, the diagnosis of this entity was made on clinical grounds; however, modern echocardiographic techniques have allowed more accurate diagnoses by excluding cases of diseases that mimic the clinical symptoms and signs of heart failure. The former historical diagnostic restriction of the time frame to the last month of pregnancy or first 5 months postpartum for diagnosis has been challenged by observations that almost 20% of the patients developed symptoms of heart failure and were diagnosed with PPCM earlier than the last gestational month.[40] Hence, the more contemporary definition of PPCM is a cardiomyopathy presenting with HF secondary to LV dysfunction toward the end of pregnancy or in the months following delivery, where no other cause of heart failure is found.[41]

The incidence varies geographically. Based on available literature, the incidence of PPCM appears to be 1 in 1000 in South Africa, 1 in 300 in Haiti,[41] and 1 in 3000 to 4000 in the United States.[42] Risk factors for peripartum cardiomyopathy include advanced maternal age, multiparity, obesity, African descent, twinning, pregnancy-induced hypertension or preeclampsia, and long-term tocolysis.

Although its cause remains unknown, most theories have focused on the hemodynamic, inflammatory, oxidative, and immunologic stresses of pregnancy and genetic susceptibility. An immune pathogenesis is supported by the findings of lymphocytic myocarditis on myocardial biopsy, high titers of autoantibodies against selected cardiac tissue proteins in most women with PPCM, fetal microchimerism (fetal cells in maternal blood) in some patients with PPCM, and the fact that multiparity or previous exposure to fetal antigens are significant risk factors.[43] More recent studies have suggested that a defective antioxidant cascade may play a role, specifically implicating the activation of prolactin-cleaving protease cathepsin D and production of proapoptotic derivatives of prolactin, with potentially detrimental cardiovascular actions in the pathophysiology.[44] This concept was supported by the observation that in mice, treatment with bromocriptine, an inhibitor of prolactin secretion, prevented the development of PPCM.[44] Regarding genetic cause, familial clustering of PPCM in certain cases has suggested that a subset of PPCM may be a part of the spectrum of familial DCM, presenting in the peripartum period. However, based on current levels of evidence, genetic testing is not recommended as routine but is currently being done as part of research or individualized assessment.[45]

The prognosis of peripartum cardiomyopathy is related to the recovery of ventricular function. In contrast to patients with idiopathic dilated cardiomyopathy, significant improvement in myocardial function is seen in approximately 50% of patients in the first 6 months after presentation[43] (see Figure 19-7). However, for those patients who do not recover to normal or near normal function, the prognosis is similar to other forms of dilated cardiomyopathy. Cardiomegaly that persists for more than 4 months after diagnosis indicates a poor prognosis.

Diagnosis is based upon the clinical presentation of congestive heart failure and objective evidence of LV systolic dysfunction. Serum BNP or NT-BNP are commonly elevated and electrocardiogram findings may be nonspecific. Sinus tachycardia, atrial fibrillation, atrial flutter, and ventricular tachycardia have been reported in patients with PPCM. Among patients with left ventricular ejection fraction (LVEF) greater than 30% at diagnosis, restoration of normal LVEF is more likely. The left ventricle may not always be dilated; however, an initial LV end-systolic diameter of 5.5 cm or less has been shown to predict recovery of left ventricle function. LV thrombus has been found on initial echocardiography in 10% to 17% of patients, and PPCM is associated with an increased incidence of thromboembolism compared with DCM from other causes. Other imaging modalities, such as cardiac MRI, do not show any specific pattern in PPCM to help differentiate from other causes of cardiomyopathy, although it can give a more accurate measurement of chamber volumes and ventricular function than echocardiography.

For management of PPCM, a multidisciplinary approach involving a cardiologist, obstetrician, intensivist, anesthesiologist, and pediatrician is essential and should be engaged as early as possible. Initial management is similar to that of other forms of nonischemic cardiomyopathy and includes oxygen, fluid restriction, loop diuretics, and/or other diuretics, nitrates, and hydralazine (safe to use during pregnancy), especially for hypertension. ACE inhibitors should be avoided in the second and third trimesters but are safe to use postpartum. β-blockers can be used when not contraindicated during pregnancy, and they can be used postpartum. During pregnancy, β_1 selective agents are preferred because β_2-receptor blockade may have an antitocolytic effect. Inotropic agents can be used in patients with signs of low cardiac output or with persistent congestion despite diuretics/afterload-reducing agents. Anticoagulation is recommended in patients with PPCM, because these patients have a high incidence of LV thrombus, especially patients with an LVEF less than 35%. Heparin (unfractionated and low-molecular-weight) is favored in pregnancy because, unlike warfarin, it does not cross the placenta. Warfarin should be avoided because it is teratogenic in early pregnancy and has a risk of causing fetal cerebral hemorrhage in the second and third trimesters. After delivery, PPCM should be treated according to current guidelines for heart failure. Aggressive use of implantable defibrillators and advances in medical therapy have significantly reduced the risk of sudden death, and all-cause mortality rates. For those patients who remain refractory to conventional pharmacologic therapy, cardiac transplantation and mechanical circulatory support are viable options.

Other treatment strategies summarized in the following paragraph remain investigational. A single nonrandomized study suggested that immunosuppression may benefit women with biopsy-proven myocarditis.[46] The Myocarditis Treatment Trial, however, did not show any benefit of immunosuppressive medications[47] and, given the risks of immunosuppressive therapy, they are currently not widely used. Similarly, the use of intravenous immunoglobulin was associated with an increase in LVEF in a retrospective study,[48] but the placebo-controlled IMAC trial (Controlled Trial of Intravenous Immune Globulin in Recent-Onset Dilated Cardiomyopathy) failed to show a significant improvement with immune globulin treatment of adult patients with recent-onset cardiomyopathy; thus IVIG is not routinely used in PPCM. With recognition of the potential detrimental role of the prolactin cascade, single-center, small studies have studied prolactin blockade with bromocriptine and reported improvement in LVEF and NYHA functional class.[49] The generalizability of these results is unclear given the small sample size, the higher than expected mortality rate in the standard care group, and differences in PPCM characteristics in patients in Africa as compared with those elsewhere. Further studies aimed at clearly establishing the efficacy and safety of bromocriptine are needed before it can be recommended for the treatment of PPCM. Similarly, in a single-center, small study, pentoxifylline—an anti-inflammatory agent—was associated with better LVEF, NYHA class, and survival.[50] The promising role of pentoxifylline in PPCM remains experimental until it is validated by larger scale, placebo-controlled, randomized clinical trials.

PPCM is associated with a high risk of recurrence in subsequent pregnancies, both in patients who have recovery of LV function and in those with persistent LV dysfunction. Patients with PPCM who recover their LV function have a lesser chance of recurrence compared with those with persistent LV dysfunction. The increased deterioration of LV function in subsequent pregnancy in patients with persistent LV dysfunction leads to a worse prognosis (20-30% mortality in subsequent pregnancy), whereas patients with a full recovery of LV function have negligible mortality in subsequent pregnancies. Appropriate counseling regarding subsequent pregnancies and contraception is important, and women with LVEF of less than 25% at diagnosis of PPCM or persistent LV dysfunction should be advised against a subsequent pregnancy. Every subsequent pregnancy in women with PPCM should be managed in high-risk perinatal centers, as subsequent pregnancies are associated with a high risk of recurrence despite recovered LV function.

Autoimmune Mechanisms

There has been increasing evidence suggesting that abnormalities in cellular and humoral immunity may contribute to the overall pathogenesis of dilated cardiomyopathy. Circulating autoantibodies to a variety of cardiac antigens, including G protein–linked receptors (such as those to β_1-adrenoreceptors and muscarinic receptors), mitochondrial antigens, adenosine diphosphate, adenosine triphosphate carrier proteins, and cardiac myosin heavy chain, have been identified in patients with dilated cardiomyopathy. In this regard it is interesting to note that immunization with certain cardiac muscle (but not skeletal) antigens, such as α-myosin heavy chain, can result in the development of a dilated cardiac phenotype in certain susceptible strains of mice. Moreover, a recent meta-analysis has shown that there is increased expression of the antigens of genes located at the major histocompatibility complex (MHC) on chromosome 6, which is the locus that is responsible for regulating immune responses. This study showed that HLA class II antigens such as DR4 or DQw4 were present in 63% of the patients with cardiomyopathy as compared with 26% in the control subjects.[51] Features that support an autoimmune cause in patients who present with myocarditis and DCM include familial aggregation, a weak association with HLA-DR4 haplotype, abnormal expression of HLA class II antigens in cardiac tissue, and detection of organ- and disease-specific cardiac autoantibodies by immunofluorescence and immunoabsorption techniques. Nonetheless, a precise interpretation of the above findings has been complicated by the knowledge that low titers of autoantibodies, which can be part of the normal immunologic repertoire, are not always pathogenic. For example, tissue injury secondary to ischemia or infection may lead to autoantibody production because of alterations of self-antigens or exposure of antigens that are normally sequestered from the immune system. In such situations, the generation of autoantibodies is the result, and not the cause, of the tissue injury. Furthermore, observations about autoimmune responses are generally made in patients with established disease; accordingly, any inferences regarding cause and effect are, invariably, indirect and circumstantial.

ENDOCRINE AND METABOLIC CAUSES OF CARDIOMYOPATHY (see also Chapter 16)

Obesity

Obesity cardiomyopathy is defined as congestive heart failure due entirely or predominantly to obesity. Heart failure in the markedly obese usually develops over a long period of time, and can be directly related to the duration of obesity. Initially the dyspnea and edema in these patients are simply related to alterations in LV compliance, diastolic heart failure with resultant elevated filling pressures. However, with chronicity, some of these patients will develop significant LV hypertrophy and increased LV mass, and some subsequently develop DCM. Although the precise reasons for obesity-related heart failure are not known, it is thought that the excessive adipose accumulation results in an increase in circulating blood volume and subsequently a persistent increase in cardiac output, cardiac work, and systemic blood pressure, which ultimately leads to myocardial failure. Furthermore, there is increased prevalence of hypertension and coronary artery disease in obese patients, which may also contribute to the development of DCM in these patients. Recently, cardiac myocyte injury by lipotoxicity has been implicated as a potential mechanism, especially in individuals with metabolic syndrome and insulin resistance. Cardiac lipotoxicity is hypothesized to arise from an imbalance between fatty acid uptake and use, leading to the inappropriate accumulation of free fatty acids and neutral lipids within cardiomyocytes. This lipid overload causes cellular dysfunction, cell death, and eventual organ dysfunction.[52] Obesity-related hypoventilation and sleep apnea may also contribute to the pathophysiology. A study examining the relation between obesity and heart failure in participants in the Framingham Heart Study[53] reported that after adjustment for established risk factors, there was an increase in the risk of heart failure of 5% for men and 7% for women for each increment of one in body mass index. When compared with subjects with a normal body mass index, obese subjects had a doubling of the risk of heart failure. Obesity

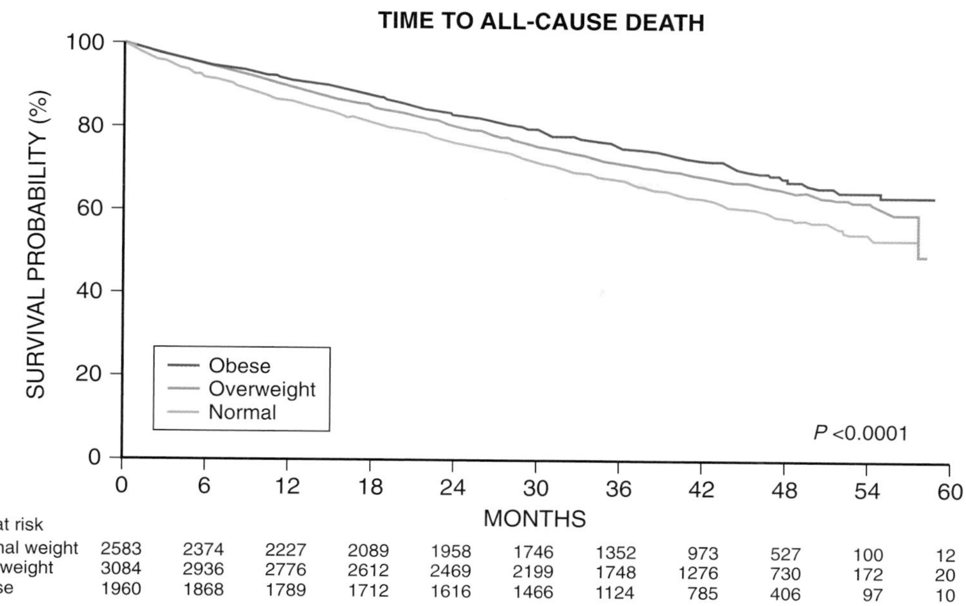

FIGURE 19-9 Kaplan-Meier survival curves by body mass index in the obese, overweight, and normal-weight groups in patients with heart failure. The number of patients at risk for death at each 6-month interval is shown below the figure. *From Bozkurt B, Deswal A: Obesity as a prognostic factor in chronic symptomatic heart failure. Am Heart J 150:1233–1239, 2005.*

alone was estimated to account for 11% of cases of heart failure in men and 14% of those in women.[53] Given the high prevalence of obesity in the past decade, strategies to promote optimal body weight may reduce the population burden of heart failure. In addition to its recognized risk for development of heart failure, intuitively one would anticipate that obesity would adversely affect the outcome of patients with established heart failure. Interestingly, however, there is a recognized paradox with obesity and heart failure, and that is, in patients with established heart failure, obesity is associated with better clinical outcomes[54] (**Figure 19-9**). This paradox, although not clearly understood, may partly be due to comparisons of individuals in a noncatabolic state with the ability to gain weight with individuals who are lean or cachectic because of advanced heart failure; selective survival of different subtypes of obese individuals; earlier detection or misdiagnosis of heart failure in obese patients because of increased prevalence of dyspnea and edema; differences in causes of heart failure in obese (hypertension, diabetes) versus nonobese (coronary artery disease) patients; and the endocrine/paracrine role of the adipose tissue, which may also participate in metabolic turnover or rapid degradation of certain chemokines and neurohormones, including natriuretic peptides. Ongoing studies will provide more insight into the obesity paradox in heart failure.

Although there are anecdotal reports regarding symptomatic improvement following weight reduction in obesity-induced heart failure, large-scale clinical trials on the role of weight loss in heart failure patients with obesity have not yet been performed.[55,56] The safety and efficacy of weight loss drugs, such as orlistat, sibutramine, lorcaserin, or phentermine-topiramate, have not been tested in large-scale trials in cardiac patients. There has been concern against use of sibutramine in heart failure because of reports of development of cardiomyopathy, and this medication is contraindicated in heart failure.[57] In small-scale pilot studies, orlistat appeared to be tolerated and effective in weight loss in heart failure patients with obesity, but ongoing investigations are under way regarding its hepatic safety profile.[58] The safety of lorcaserin, an agonist of the 5-hydroxytryptamine (5-HT, or serotonin) receptor 5-HT2C, in patients with heart failure is unknown; the initial FDA approval includes a provision mandating postmarketing studies to assess for adverse cardiovascular effects. The Food and Drug Administration's approval of phentermine-topiramate combination is indicated for use in adults with a body mass index (BMI) greater than 30 kg/m^2 and at least one weight-related condition such as hypertension, type 2 diabetes, or dyslipidemia, but again safety or efficacy in heart failure is unknown. Similarly there are no large-scale studies on safety or efficacy of weight loss with lifestyle modification with diet or exercise in obese heart failure patients. Because the prevalence of obesity is increasing in the general, as well as in the heart failure, population, examination of obesity and prevention and treatment options will be critical in heart failure patients.

Ephedra, which has been used for the purposes of athletic performance enhancement and weight loss, has been linked to a high rate of serious adverse outcomes, including LV systolic dysfunction, development of heart failure, and cardiac deaths, ultimately resulting in ban of this agent by the FDA in the United States.

Obesity surgery, or bariatric surgery, is recommended for class 2 obesity or above (BMI $\geq$ 35 kg/m^2), and possibly in individuals with a BMI of 30 to 34.9 kg/m^2 when associated with comorbid conditions, such as diabetes, sleep apnea, or systemic hypertension. Although severe heart failure or systolic dysfunction is considered a general contraindication to bariatric surgery, there are a few studies that have investigated its safety and efficacy in obese patients with HF,[56,59] with improvement in LVEF and NYHA functional class. Clearly, further prospective studies are needed to better define which patients can be safely referred for bariatric surgery, optimal surgical techniques, as well as effects on long-term outcomes.

Diabetic Cardiomyopathy

Since its first description in 1972, a considerable amount of experimental, pathologic, epidemiologic, and clinical data have been accumulated to support the existence of "diabetic cardiomyopathy." So far, a large body of literature suggests that the occurrence of diabetic cardiomyopathy is an independent phenomenon from macroangiographic changes in coronary arteries and hypertension. Diabetes is now well recognized as an independent risk factor for the development of heart failure despite correcting for age, hypertension, obesity, hypercholesterolemia, and coronary artery disease. This subject is covered in further detail in Chapter 16 of this textbook.

Hyperthyroidism

Hyperthyroidism has been implicated in causing dilated cardiomyopathy; however, in view of the increased cardiac contractile function of patients with hyperthyroidism, the development of heart failure is unexpected and raises the question whether there truly is a direct causal association between hyperthyroidism and cardiomyopathy. Patients with hyperthyroidism may occasionally have exertional dyspnea or other symptoms and signs of heart failure. Many of these clinical manifestations may be attributed to the direct effects of thyroid hormone on cardiovascular hemodynamics. In most patients with hyperthyroidism, cardiac output is high, and the subnormal response to exercise may be the result of an inability to increase heart rate maximally or to lower vascular resistance further, as normally occurs with exercise. The term *high-output failure* is not appropriate for all cases of cardiomyopathy related to hyperthyroidism, because the ability of the heart to maintain increased cardiac output at rest and with exercise is usually preserved.[60] Occasional patients with severe, longstanding hyperthyroidism have poor cardiac contractility, low cardiac output, and symptoms and signs of heart failure, including a third heart sound and pulmonary congestion. This complex of findings most commonly occurs with persistent sinus tachycardia or atrial fibrillation and is the result of so-called tachycardia-related heart failure. In older patients with heart disease, the increased workload that results from hyperthyroidism may further impair cardiac function and thus result in dilated cardiomyopathy. The presence of ischemic or hypertensive heart disease may compromise the ability of the myocardium to respond to the metabolic demands of hyperthyroidism. Histologic examination usually reveals a nonspecific pattern, including foci of lymphocytic and eosinophilic infiltration, fibrosis, fatty infiltration, and myofibril hypertrophy. Although enhanced adrenergic activity contributes to the hyperdynamic state in hyperthyroidism, β-adrenergic blockade does not fully return the heart rate or contractility to normal, which may suggest a primary cardiac effect of thyroid hormone with contributory effects of catecholamines.[60]

Hypothyroidism

Abnormalities in cardiac systolic and diastolic performance have been reported both in experimental and clinical studies of hypothyroidism; however, the classic findings of myxedema do not usually indicate cardiomyopathy. The most common signs are bradycardia, mild hypertension, a narrowed pulse pressure, and attenuated activity on precordial examination. Pericardial effusions and nonpitting edema (myxedema) can occur in patients with severe, longstanding hypothyroidism. The low cardiac output is caused by bradycardia, a decrease in ventricular filling, and a decrease in cardiac contractility. Systemic vascular resistance may increase by as much as 50%, and diastolic relaxation and filling are slowed.[60] However, heart failure is rare, because the cardiac output is usually sufficient to meet the lowered demand for peripheral oxygen delivery. Positron emission tomographic studies of oxygen consumption in patients with hypothyroidism have revealed that myocardial work efficiency is lower than in normal subjects. From 10% to 25% of patients have diastolic hypertension, which, combined with the increase in vascular resistance, raises cardiac afterload and cardiac work.[60] Abnormal systolic force may improve with thyroid hormone replacement but does not return to normal levels, suggesting the possibility of persistent myocardial dysfunction. Thyroid hormone replacement should be initiated at low doses and titrated slowly because LV failure may be precipitated. Interestingly, patients with heart failure also have low serum tri-iodothyronine concentrations, and the decrease is proportional to the degree of heart failure. Whether such changes in thyroid hormone metabolism contribute to further impairment of cardiovascular function in patients with heart failure is not known.[60]

Acromegaly and Growth Hormone Deficiency

Impaired cardiovascular function has recently been demonstrated to potentially reduce life expectancy both in growth hormone deficiency and excess. Experimental and clinical studies have supported the evidence that growth hormone and insulin-like growth factor-I (IGF-I) are implicated in cardiac development.[61] In most patients with acromegaly, a specific cardiomyopathy, characterized by myocardial hypertrophy with interstitial fibrosis, lymphomononuclear infiltration, and areas of monocyte necrosis, results in biventricular concentric hypertrophy.[61] Myocardial dysfunction is a major cause of morbidity and mortality in acromegaly, and appears to be related to both the severity and duration of growth hormone excess. In contrast, patients with childhood- or adulthood-onset growth hormone deficiency may suffer both from structural cardiac abnormalities, such as narrowing of cardiac walls, and functional impairment, which combine to reduce diastolic filling and impair LV response to peak exercise. In addition, growth hormone deficiency patients may have an increase in vascular intima-media thickness and a higher occurrence of atheromatous plaques, which can further aggravate the hemodynamic conditions and contribute to increased cardiovascular and cerebrovascular risk. Several studies have suggested that the cardiovascular abnormalities can be partially reversed by suppressing growth hormone and IGF-I levels in acromegaly or after growth hormone replacement therapy in growth hormone–deficiency patients.[61] Receptors for both growth hormone and IGF-I are expressed by cardiac myocytes; therefore, growth hormone may act directly on the heart or via the induction of local or systemic IGF-I, while IGF-1 may act by endocrine, paracrine, or autocrine mechanisms. Moreover, experimental studies suggest that growth hormone and IGF-I have stimulatory effects on myocardial contractility, possibly mediated by changes in intracellular calcium handling. Thus, recently, much attention has been focused on the ability of growth hormone to increase cardiac mass, suggesting its possible use in the treatment of chronic heart failure. Initial studies demonstrated that treatment with growth hormone may result in improvement in hemodynamic and clinical status of patients with heart failure; however, two randomized, placebo-controlled studies did not show any significant growth hormone–mediated improvement in cardiac performance in patients with dilated cardiomyopathy, despite significant increases in IGF-I.[62]

NUTRITIONAL CAUSES OF CARDIOMYOPATHY

Thiamine Deficiency

Thiamine serves as a cofactor for several enzymes involved primarily in the carbohydrate catabolism and is found in high concentrations in the heart, skeletal muscle, liver, kidneys, and brain. The most common cause of thiamine deficiency in Western countries is chronic alcoholism and anorexia nervosa; AIDS and pregnancy can account for other rare causes of thiamine deficiency. A state of severe depletion can develop in patients on a strict thiamine-deficient diet in approximately 18 to 21 days. The major manifestations of thiamine deficiency in humans involve the cardiovascular (wet beriberi) and nervous (dry beriberi, or neuropathy and/or Wernicke-Korsakoff syndrome) systems. The cardiovascular signs and symptoms include dyspnea, fatigue, leg edema, and palpitations. Tachycardia is common and there is usually increased jugular venous pressure and warm extremities. Biventricular heart failure is present and the circulation is usually hyperkinetic. Ultimately, circulatory collapse, metabolic acidosis, or shock can develop, at which time the disease has advanced from chronic beriberi to fulminating beriberi heart failure (Shoshin beriberi). Severe lactic acidemia in the presence of a high cardiac output and extremely low oxygen consumption are the classic features of acute fulminant cardiovascular beriberi, which, if unrecognized and untreated, can lead to high cardiac output failure and death. Treatment for beriberi should consist of administration of thiamine along with other conventional treatment of circulatory support and heart failure.

Carnitine Deficiency

L-carnitine and its derivative, propionyl-L-carnitine, are organic amines necessary for oxidation of fatty acids, the deficiency of which may be associated with a syndrome of progressive skeletal myopathy and lipid vacuoles on muscle biopsy. They have also been shown to reduce intracellular accumulation of toxic metabolites during ischemia, demonstrate protective effect on muscle metabolism injuries, inhibit caspases, and decrease the levels of TNF-α and sphingosine, as well as reduce apoptosis of skeletal muscle cells and thus have been implied in the treatment of congestive heart failure. Several metabolic genes, including the muscle carnitine palmitoyl transferase-1, the key enzyme for the transport of long-chain acyl-coenzyme A (acyl-CoA) compounds into mitochondria, are downregulated in the failing human heart.[63] Inhibitors of carnitine palmitoyltransferase I (CPT I), such as etomoxir, have been developed as agents for treating diabetes mellitus. Despite initial promising preclinical and phase II clinical results, a double-blind randomized multicenter clinical trial with etomoxir in heart failure was stopped prematurely, because unacceptably high liver transaminase levels were detected in four patients taking etomoxir.[64]

Selenium Deficiency

Selenium deficiency is associated with cardiomyopathy and congestive heart failure in geographic areas where dietary selenium intake is low.[65] This has been named as the Keshan disease, because of the geographic prevalence of a specific form of dilated cardiomyopathy in northeast China, in which the soil has a low selenium content. Chronic selenium deficiency may also occur in individuals with malabsorption and long-term selenium-deficient parenteral nutrition. Selenium deficiency is implicated in causing cardiomyopathy as a result of the depletion of selenium-associated antioxidant enzymes—selenoenzymes—which protect cell membranes from damage by free radicals. The cardiomyopathy is manifested by insidious onset of congestive heart failure or a complication of sudden death or thromboembolic phenomena. The heart shows biventricular enlargement and histologically exhibits edema, mitochondrial swelling, hyper-contraction bands, widespread myocytolysis, and extensive fibrosis.[65]

HEMATOLOGIC CAUSES OF CARDIOMYOPATHY

Cardiomyopathy Due to Iron Overload: Hemochromatosis and Thalassemia

Iron-overload cardiomyopathy manifests itself as systolic or diastolic dysfunction secondary to increased deposition of iron in the heart and occurs with common genetic disorders, such as primary hemochromatosis and β-thalassemia major.

Hereditary hemochromatosis is an inherited disorder of iron metabolism and is the most common hereditary disease of Northern Europeans, with a prevalence of approximately 5 per 1000. It is an autosomal recessive disorder of iron metabolism characterized by increased iron absorption and deposition in the liver, pancreas, heart, joints, and pituitary gland. Without treatment, death may occur from cirrhosis, primary liver cancer, diabetes, or cardiomyopathy. In 1996, HFE, the gene for hereditary hemochromatosis, was mapped on the short arm of chromosome 6.[66] Two mutations have been implicated in hereditary hemochromatosis: C282Y and H63D, resulting in excessive iron absorption. The former occurs in a homozygous state seen in 75% to 100% of patients. The frequency of the latter mutation, the H63D mutation, is significantly increased in patients with idiopathic dilated cardiomyopathy.[66] The high correlation of the HFE to hemochromatosis has caused it to be considered as a candidate gene for population-based genetic testing for diagnosis and detection of predisposition to hemochromatosis. In addition, mechanisms of iron transport and metabolism are unfolding and are providing clues to the enigma of iron homeostasis and the pathophysiology of iron overload.

The complications of hemochromatosis can be devastating, but its clinical management is simple and effective if the disease is identified early in its progression.

Although the exact mechanism of iron-induced heart failure remains to be elucidated, the toxicity of iron in biologic systems is attributed to its ability to catalyze the generation of oxygen free radicals. It has been shown that chronic iron overload results in dose-dependent increases in myocardial iron burden, decreases in the protective antioxidant enzyme activity, increased free-radical production, and increased mortality.[67] These findings suggest that the mechanism of iron-induced heart dysfunction involves, at least in part, free radical–mediated processes. Myocardial iron deposition is most prominent in and around contractile elements and less common in the conduction system, in contrast to sarcoidosis and amyloidosis in which the pathologic process commonly involves the conduction system.[67] The mechanism by which iron produces cellular dysfunction is not yet clear, because fibrosis may not be prominent. This also implies that the disease process is reversible if the tissue iron concentration can be controlled. Myocardial iron deposits do not occur until other organs, such as the liver, pancreas, and connective tissues, are saturated with iron. Thus the extracardiac manifestations are present before the cardiomyopathy develops.[67]

Iron overload can occur either as a result of inappropriate excess iron absorption, as in the case of hemochromatosis or thalassemia major, or because of multiple transfusions. The most important manifestations of heart disease in hemochromatosis are congestive heart failure and cardiac arrhythmia. During the initial phases of the cardiomyopathy, the hemodynamic profile represents a restrictive pattern. As the severity of cardiomyopathy advances, dilated cardiomyopathy with biventricular enlargement and heart failure ensue. The spectrum of arrhythmia ranges from minor abnormalities on the electrocardiogram to supraventricular arrhythmia, atrioventricular conduction block, and ventricular tachyarrhythmia, presumably due to myocardial dysfunction and iron deposition in the conduction system and AV node. The ECG most commonly shows decreased voltage and nonspecific ST and T wave changes; Q waves are uncommon. Among patients with β-thalassemia major, biventricular dilated cardiomyopathy remains the leading cause of mortality. In some patients, a restrictive type of LV cardiomyopathy or pulmonary hypertension is noted. The clinical course, although variable and occasionally fulminant, is more benign in recent than in older series.

The diagnosis of hemochromatosis is suggested by elevated serum ferritin and an increased ratio of iron to total iron binding capacity (TIBC). The most sensitive screening test for hemochromatosis is saturation of the transferrin with iron; a fasting value greater than 50% is strongly suggestive of the disease. The most definitive test for calculation of iron stores in the body is by measurement of iron concentration by liver biopsy. Magnetic resonance imaging can also be very useful to identify the iron-laden organs and cardiac involvement. Though not required to demonstrate cardiac involvement in every case, endomyocardial biopsy can be useful in assessment of cardiac iron deposition. The echocardiogram usually reveals increased systolic and diastolic ventricular dimensions, and reduced LV ejection fraction.

Before phlebotomy and chelation therapy, survival among patients with hemochromatosis and heart failure was less than 20% in 5 years. The actuarial survival rates of the individuals who are homozygous for the C282Y mutation of the hemochromatosis gene C282Y have been reported to be 95%, 93%, and 66%, respectively, at 5, 10, and 20 years.[68] Similarly, in patients with thalassemia major, cardiac failure is one of the most frequent causes of death. Chelation therapy, including newer forms of oral chelators, such as deferoxamine, and phlebotomy have dramatically improved the outcome of hemochromatosis. Similarly, chelation therapy has improved prognosis in β-thalassemia major both by reducing the incidence of heart failure and by reversing cardiomyopathy. It is important to start therapy early because treatment may prevent or reverse cardiac involvement. Early diagnosis and treatment by phlebotomy before tissue damage has occurred is essential, because lifespan seems to be normal in treated patients but markedly shortened in those who are not. Additionally, genetic counseling with evaluation of first-degree relatives is mandatory.[67] New imaging modalities, especially magnetic resonance imaging, are expected to improve early diagnosis and risk stratification for treatment. By increasing the proportion of patients on optimal chelation, survival in patients with hemachromatosis or β-thalassemia may further improve.

HEMODYNAMIC AND STRESS-INDUCED CARDIOMYOPATHY

Tachycardia-Induced Dilated Cardiomyopathy

The concept that incessant or chronic tachycardia can lead to reversible LV dysfunction is supported both by animal models of chronic pacing, as well as human studies documenting improvement in ventricular function with tachycardia rate or rhythm control. Sustained rapid pacing in experimental animal models can produce severe biventricular systolic dysfunction. In humans, descriptions of reversal of cardiomyopathy with rate or rhythm control of incessant or chronic tachycardias have been reported with atrial tachycardias, accessory pathway reciprocating tachycardias, atrioventricular node reentry, and atrial fibrillation with rapid ventricular responses.[69] Control of the rapid ventricular responses in atrial fibrillation has been shown to improve ventricular function. It should also be noted that in patients with atrial fibrillation and congestive heart failure, a routine strategy of rhythm control does not reduce cardiovascular mortality, but may improve quality of life and LV function when compared with a strategy of rate control alone.[70] The diagnosis of tachycardia-induced cardiomyopathy is usually made following observation of a marked improvement in systolic function after normalization of heart rate. Clinicians should be aware that patients with unexplained systolic dysfunction may have tachycardia-induced cardiomyopathy, and that controlling the arrhythmia may result in improvement and even complete normalization of systolic function.[69] Tachycardia-induced cardiomyopathy may be a more common mechanism of LV dysfunction than recognized, and aggressive treatment of the arrhythmia should be considered.

Stress-Induced Cardiomyopathy

Stress cardiomyopathy is characterized by acute, usually reversible LV dysfunction in the absence of significant coronary artery disease, usually triggered by acute emotional or physical stress.[71] This phenomenon was initially identified

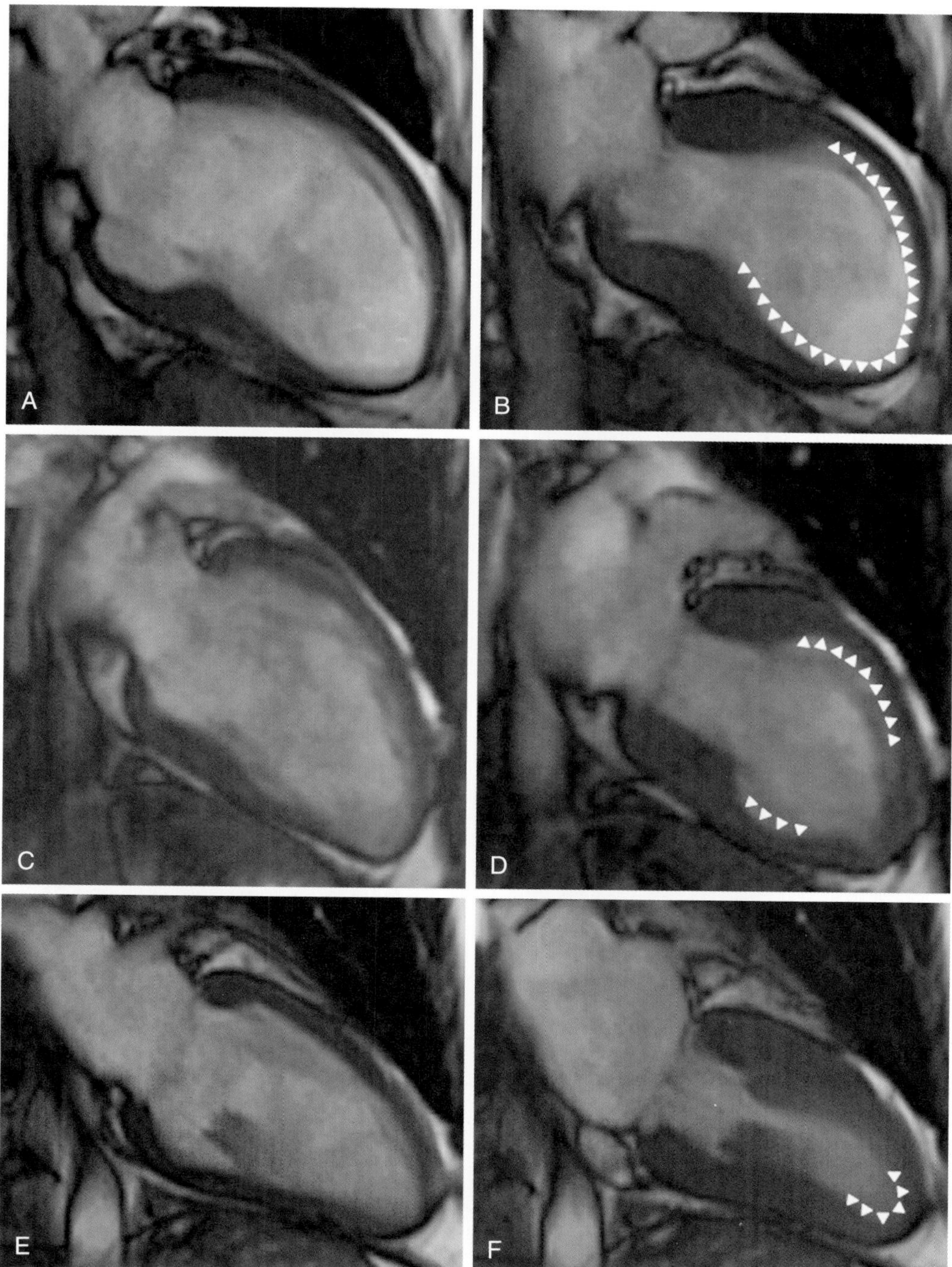

FIGURE 19-10 Diversity of LV contraction patterns in stress cardiomyopathy, as demonstrated by cardiac magnetic resonance imaging in vertical long-axis view **(A, C,** and **E)** diastole; **(B, D,** and **F)** systole. Three types are depicted: (A, B) most common pattern of mid and apical left ventricular (LV) akinesia: Tako-tsubo type *(arrowheads)*; (C, D) mid-LV akinesia *(arrowheads)* with sparing of apical region; and (E, F) apical LV contraction abnormality only *(arrowheads)*. *From Sharkey SW, Windenburg DC, Lesser JR, et al: Natural history and expansive clinical profile of stress (Tako-tsubo) cardiomyopathy. J Am Coll Cardiol 55:333–341, 2010.*

by a distinctive pattern of "apical ballooning," first described in Japan as Tako-tsubo, and often affected postmenopausal women.[72] Most patients have a clinical presentation similar to that of acute coronary syndrome and may have transiently elevated cardiac enzymes such as cardiac troponin. Though apical ballooning is seen in most, other diverse ventricular contraction patterns have been defined by cardiovascular magnetic resonance imaging or by echocardiography[72] (**Figure 19-10**). In the majority, LV function usually returns to normal rapidly, although delayed recovery over 2 months has been described.[73] Despite reversal to normal cardiac function in most cases, stress cardiomyopathy appears to be associated with higher mortality, especially noncardiovascular mortality compared with an age-matched population.[72] Right and/or left ventricular thrombi have been described and are usually associated with embolic events, underlining the importance of anticoagulation in these patients. Although usually benign and rapidly reversible, the clinical spectrum can be heterogeneous. Tako-tsubo cardiomyopathy can occur in either sex, although it occurs most commonly in postmenopausal women. Up to 1.2% of the patients can die in the hospital as a result of cardiogenic shock. Nonfatal recurrence, embolic stroke, or delayed normalization of LVEF can

TABLE 19-3 Specific Treatment Approaches to Dilated Cardiomyopathies

CAUSE OF DCM	SPECIFIC TREATMENT
Alcoholic	Abstinence
Cocaine	Abstinence
Collagen vascular disease	
SLE, RA, sarcoidosis	Steroids, cytotoxic, or immunomodulating agents
Scleroderma	Steroids, Ca channel blockers for Raynaud
Kawasaki disease	IV Immunoglobulin
Viral myocarditis	Prednisone and immunosuppressant therapy for fulminant course
Chagas disease	Benznidazole, nifurtimox
Nutritional deficiency	
Thiamine, selenium, or carnitine deficiency)	Replacement
Hyperthyroidism/hypothyroidism	Achieve euthyroid state
HIV/AIDS	Highly active retroviral therapy, increased CD4 count
Uremia	Dialysis
Pheochromocytoma	Removal of tumor
Tachycardia induced	AV nodal ablation, β-blockers
Stress-induced cardiomyopathy	Management of psychosocial stress
Peripartum cardiomyopathy	Avoid subsequent pregnancy if LV function does not normalize
Chemotherapy-induced cardiomyopathy	Reduce dose or discontinue, avoid cardiotoxic other chemotherapy combinations and XRT, initiate early standard treatment for heart failure

occur, emphasizing the importance of follow-up in these patients. Management needs to be individualized with elimination of psychosocial and cardiac stressors, and initiation of standard guideline-directed medical therapy.

SUMMARY AND FUTURE DIRECTIONS

As noted at the outset, the dilated cardiomyopathies constitute the largest group of myopathic disorders that are responsible for systolic heart failure. Recent advances have allowed for the identification of specific genetic, metabolic, infectious, toxin-induced, nutritional, and hemodynamic causes for dilated cardiomyopathy. Although the current treatment strategies for the dilated cardiomyopathy are similar to those for ischemic cardiomyopathy (**see Chapters 34, 35, and 41**), as illustrated in **Table 19-3**, there are also a number of etiology-specific treatment strategies that clinicians should be consider when treating patients with dilated cardiomyopathy. Although many of these strategies have not been tested in randomized clinical trials, they provide a useful basis for individualizing the care of patients with various etiologies of dilated cardiomyopathy. Further, the observation that reverse remodeling and recovery of LV function are almost exclusively observed in patients with dilated cardiomyopathy (**see also Chapter 11**) raises the intriguing possibility that etiology-specific treatment strategies may one day be developed for various causes of dilated cardiomyopathy.

References

1. Richardson P, McKenna W, Bristow M, et al: Report of the 1995 World Health Organization/International Society and Federation of Cardiology Task Force on the Definition and Classification of cardiomyopathies. *Circulation* 93(5):841–842, 1996.
2. Adams KF, Jr, Fonarow GC, Emerman CL, et al: Characteristics and outcomes of patients hospitalized for heart failure in the United States: rationale, design, and preliminary observations from the first 100,000 cases in the Acute Decompensated Heart Failure National Registry (ADHERE). *Am Heart J* 149(2):209–216, 2005.
3. Manolio TA, Baughman KL, Rodeheffer R, et al: Prevalence and etiology of idiopathic dilated cardiomyopathy (summary of a National Heart, Lung, and Blood Institute workshop. *Am J Cardiol* 69(17):1458–1466, 1992.
4. Dries DL, Exner DV, Gersh BJ, et al: Racial differences in the outcome of left ventricular dysfunction. *N Engl J Med* 340(8):609–616, 1999.
5. Levy D, Larson MG, Vasan RS, et al: The progression from hypertension to congestive heart failure. *JAMA* 275(20):1557–1562, 1996.
6. Nieminen MS, Harjola VP, Hochadel M, et al: Gender related differences in patients presenting with acute heart failure. Results from EuroHeart Failure Survey II. *Eur J Heart Fail* 10(2):140–148, 2008.
7. Miura K, Nakagawa H, Morikawa Y, et al: Epidemiology of idiopathic cardiomyopathy in Japan: results from a nationwide survey. *Heart* 87(2):126–130, 2002.
8. Amoah AG, Kallen C: Aetiology of heart failure as seen from a National Cardiac Referral Centre in Africa. *Cardiology* 93(1–2):11–18, 2000.
9. Felker GM, Thompson RE, Hare JM, et al: Underlying causes and long-term survival in patients with initially unexplained cardiomyopathy. *N Engl J Med* 342(15):1077–1084, 2000.
10. Dec GW, Fuster V: Idiopathic dilated cardiomyopathy. *N Engl J Med* 331(23):1564–1575, 1994.
11. Sugrue DD, Rodeheffer RJ, Codd MB, et al: The clinical course of idiopathic dilated cardiomyopathy. A population-based study. *Ann Intern Med* 117(2):117–123, 1992.
12. Steimle AE, Stevenson LW, Fonarow GC, et al: Prediction of improvement in recent onset cardiomyopathy after referral for heart transplantation. *J Am Coll Cardiol* 23(3):553–559, 1994.
13. Ehlert FA, Cannom DS, Renfroe EG, et al: Comparison of dilated cardiomyopathy and coronary artery disease in patients with life-threatening ventricular arrhythmias: differences in presentation and outcome in the AVID registry. *Am Heart J* 142(5):816–822, 2001.
14. The effect of digoxin on mortality and morbidity in patients with heart failure. The Digitalis Investigation Group. *N Engl J Med* 336(8):525–533, 1997.
15. Singh SN, Fletcher RD, Fisher SG, et al: Amiodarone in patients with congestive heart failure and asymptomatic ventricular arrhythmia. Survival Trial of Antiarrhythmic Therapy in Congestive Heart Failure. *N Engl J Med* 333(2):77–82, 1995.
16. The Cardiac Insufficiency Bisoprolol Study II (CIBIS-II): a randomised trial. *Lancet* 353(9146):9–13, 1999.
17. Packer M, O'Connor CM, Ghali JK, et al: Effect of amlodipine on morbidity and mortality in severe chronic heart failure. Prospective Randomized Amlodipine Survival Evaluation Study Group. *N Engl J Med* 335(15):1107–1114, 1996.
18. Piano MR: Alcoholic cardiomyopathy: incidence, clinical characteristics, and pathophysiology. *Chest* 121(5):1638–1650, 2002.
19. Walsh CR, Larson MG, Evans JC, et al: Alcohol consumption and risk for congestive heart failure in the Framingham Heart Study. *Ann Intern Med* 136(3):181–191, 2002.
20. Abramson JL, Williams SA, Krumholz HM, et al: Moderate alcohol consumption and risk of heart failure among older persons. *JAMA* 285(15):1971–1977, 2001.
21. Lang RM, Borow KM, Neumann A, et al: Adverse cardiac effects of acute alcohol ingestion in young adults. *Ann Intern Med* 102(6):742–747, 1985.
22. Bakeeva LE, Skulachev VP, Sudarikova YV, et al: Mitochondria enter the nucleus (one further problem in chronic alcoholism). *Biochemistry (Mosc)* 66(12):1335–1341, 2001.
23. Teragaki M, Takeuchi K, Toda I, et al: Point mutations in mitochondrial DNA of patients with alcoholic cardiomyopathy. *Heart Vessels* 15(4):172–175, 2000.
24. Pavan D, Nicolosi GL, Lestuzzi C, et al: Normalization of variables of left ventricular function in patients with alcoholic cardiomyopathy after cessation of excessive alcohol intake: an echocardiographic study. *Eur Heart J* 85:535–540, 1987.
25. Yancy CW, Jessup M, Bozkurt B, et al: 2013 ACCF/AHA Guideline for the Management of Heart Failure: A Report of the American College of Cardiology Foundation/American Heart Association Task Force on Practice Guidelines. *Circulation* 128:e240–e327, 2013.
26. Bertolet BD, Freund G, Martin CA, et al: Unrecognized left ventricular dysfunction in an apparently healthy cocaine abuse population. *Clin Cardiol* 13:323–328, 1990.
27. Chakko S, Myerburg RJ: Cardiac complications of cocaine abuse. *Clin Cardiol* 18(2):67–72, 1995.
28. Om A, Warner M, Sabri N, et al: Frequency of coronary artery disease and left ventricle dysfunction in cocaine users. *Am J Cardiol* 69(19):1549–1552, 1992.
29. Bozkurt B, Kribbs S, Clubb FJ, Jr, et al: Pathophysiologically relevant concentrations of tumor necrosis factor-α promote progressive left ventricular dysfunction and remodeling in rats. *Circulation* 97:1382–1391, 1998.
30. Barbaro G, Di Lorenzo G, Grisorio B, et al: Incidence of dilated cardiomyopathy and detection of HIV in myocardial cells of HIV-positive patients. Gruppo Italiano per lo Studio Cardiologico dei Pazienti Affetti da AIDS. *N Engl J Med* 339(16):1093–1099, 1998.
31. Raidel SM, Haase C, Jansen NR, et al: Targeted myocardial transgenic expression of HIV Tat causes cardiomyopathy and mitochondrial damage. *Am J Physiol Heart Circ Physiol* 282(5):H1672–H1678, 2002.
32. Kaul S, Fishbein MC, Siegel RJ: Cardiac manifestations of acquired immune deficiency syndrome: a 1991 update. *Am Heart J* 122:535–544, 1991.
33. Grody WW, Cheng L, Lewis W: Infection of the heart by the human immunodeficiency virus. *Am J Cardiol* 66(2):203–206, 1990.
34. Mayosi BM: Contemporary trends in the epidemiology and management of cardiomyopathy and pericarditis in sub-Saharan Africa. *Heart* 93(10):1176–1183, 2007.
35. Burke AP, Saenger J, Mullick F, et al: Hypersensitivity myocarditis. *Arch Pathol Lab Med* 115(8):764–769, 1991.
36. Paradiso M, Gabrielli F, Masala C, et al: Evaluation of myocardial involvement in systemic lupus erythematosus by signal-averaged electrocardiography and echocardiography. *Acta Cardiol* 56(6):381–386, 2001.
37. Kazzam E, Caidahl K, Hallgren R, et al: Non-invasive assessment of systolic left ventricular function in systemic sclerosis. *Eur Heart J* 12:151–156, 1991.
38. Goldenberg J, Ferraz MB, Pessoa AP, et al: Symptomatic cardiac involvement in juvenile rheumatoid arthritis. *Int J Cardiol* 34:57–62, 1992.
39. Dubrey SW, Falk RH: Diagnosis and management of cardiac sarcoidosis. *Prog Cardiovasc Dis* 52(4):336–346, 2010.
40. Elkayam U, Akhter MW, Singh H, et al: Pregnancy-associated cardiomyopathy: clinical characteristics and a comparison between early and late presentation. *Circulation* 111(16):2050–2055, 2005.
41. Pearson GD, Veille JC, Rahimtoola S, et al: Peripartum cardiomyopathy: National Heart, Lung, and Blood Institute and Office of Rare Diseases (National Institutes of Health) workshop recommendations and review. *JAMA* 283(9):1183–1188, 2000.
42. Mielniczuk LM, Williams K, Davis DR, et al: Frequency of peripartum cardiomyopathy. *Am J Cardiol* 97(12):1765–1768, 2006.
43. Elkayam U, Tummala PP, Rao K, et al: Maternal and fetal outcomes of subsequent pregnancies in women with peripartum cardiomyopathy. *N Engl J Med* 344(21):1567–1571, 2001.
44. Hilfiker-Kleiner D, Kaminski K, Podewski E, et al: A cathepsin D-cleaved 16 kDa form of prolactin mediates postpartum cardiomyopathy. *Cell* 128(3):589–600, 2007.
45. Sliwa K, Hilfiker-Kleiner D, Petrie MC, et al: Current state of knowledge on aetiology, diagnosis, management, and therapy of peripartum cardiomyopathy: a position statement from the Heart Failure Association of the European Society of Cardiology Working Group on peripartum cardiomyopathy. *Eur J Heart Fail* 12(8):767–778, 2010.

46. Midei MG, DeMent SH, Feldman AM, et al: Peripartum myocarditis and cardiomyopathy. *Circulation* 81(3):922–928, 1990.
47. Mason JW, O'Connel JB, Herskowitz A, et al: A clinical trial of immunosuppressive therapy for myocarditis. *N Engl J Med* 333:269–275, 1995.
48. Bozkurt B, Villaneuva FS, Holubkov R, et al: Intravenous immune globulin in the therapy of peripartum cardiomyopathy. *J Am Coll Cardiol* 34(1):177–180, 1999.
49. Sliwa K, Blauwet L, Tibazarwa K, et al: Evaluation of bromocriptine in the treatment of acute severe peripartum cardiomyopathy: a proof-of-concept pilot study. *Circulation* 121(13):1465–1473, 2010.
50. Sliwa K, Skudicky D, Candy G, et al: The addition of pentoxifylline to conventional therapy improves outcome in patients with peripartum cardiomyopathy. *Eur J Heart Fail* 4(3):305–309, 2002.
51. Carlquist JF, Menlove RL, Murray MB, et al: HLA class II (DR and DQ) antigen associations in idiopathic dilated cardiomyopathy. *Circulation* 83:515–522, 1991.
52. Schulze PC: Myocardial lipid accumulation and lipotoxicity in heart failure. *J Lipid Res* 50:2137–2138, 2009.
53. Kenchaiah S, Evans JC, Levy D, et al: Obesity and the risk of heart failure. *N Engl J Med* 347(5):305–313, 2002.
54. Bozkurt B, Deswal A: Obesity as a prognostic factor in chronic symptomatic heart failure. *Am Heart J* 150(6):1233–1239, 2005.
55. Alpert MA, Lambert CR, Panayiotou H, et al: Relation of duration of morbid obesity to left ventricular mass, systolic function, and diastolic filling, and effect of weight loss. *Am J Cardiol* 76(16):1194–1197, 1995.
56. Ristow B, Rabkin J, Haeusslein E: Improvement in dilated cardiomyopathy after bariatric surgery. *J Card Fail* 14(3):198–202, 2008.
57. Sayin T, Guldal M: Sibutramine: possible cause of a reversible cardiomyopathy. *Int J Cardiol* 99(3):481–482, 2005.
58. Beck-da-Silva L, Higginson L, Fraser M, et al: Effect of orlistat in obese patients with heart failure: a pilot study. *Congest Heart Fail* 11(3):118–123, 2005.
59. Ramani GV, McCloskey C, Ramanathan RC, et al: Safety and efficacy of bariatric surgery in morbidly obese patients with severe systolic heart failure. *Clin Cardiol* 31(11):516–520, 2008.
60. Klein I, Ojamaa K: Thyroid hormone and the cardiovascular system. *N Engl J Med* 344(7):501–509, 2001.
61. Colao A, Marzullo P, Di Somma C, et al: Growth hormone and the heart. *Clin Endocrinol (Oxf)* 54(2):137–154, 2001.
62. Osterziel KJ, Strohm O, Schuler J, et al: Randomised, double-blind, placebo-controlled trial of human recombinant growth hormone in patients with chronic heart failure due to dilated cardiomyopathy. *Lancet* 351(9111):1233–1237, 1998.
63. Razeghi P, Young ME, Ying J, et al: Downregulation of metabolic gene expression in failing human heart before and after mechanical unloading. *Cardiology* 97(4):203–209, 2002.
64. Holubarsch CJ, Rohrbach M, Karrasch M, et al: A double-blind randomized multicentre clinical trial to evaluate the efficacy and safety of two doses of etomoxir in comparison with placebo in patients with moderate congestive heart failure: the ERGO (etomoxir for the recovery of glucose oxidation) study. *Clin Sci (Lond)* 113(4):205–212, 2007.
65. Cheng TO: Selenium deficiency and cardiomyopathy. *J R Soc Med* 95(4):219–220, 2002.
66. Mahon NG, Coonar AS, Jeffery S, et al: Haemochromatosis gene mutations in idiopathic dilated cardiomyopathy. *Heart* 84(5):541–547, 2000.
67. Gochee PA, Powell LW: What's new in hemochromatosis. *Curr Opin Hematol* 8(2):98–104, 2001.
68. Wojcik JP, Speechley MR, Kertesz AE, et al: Natural history of C282Y homozygotes for hemochromatosis. *Can J Gastroenterol* 16(5):297–302, 2002.
69. Umana E, Solares CA, Alpert MA: Tachycardia-induced cardiomyopathy. *Am J Med* 114(1):51–55, 2003.
70. Shelton RJ, Clark AL, Goode K, et al: A randomised, controlled study of rate versus rhythm control in patients with chronic atrial fibrillation and heart failure: (CAFE-II Study). *Heart* 95(11):924–930, 2009.
71. Maron BJ, Towbin JA, Thiene G, et al: Contemporary definitions and classification of the cardiomyopathies: an American Heart Association Scientific Statement from the Council on Clinical Cardiology, Heart Failure and Transplantation Committee; Quality of Care and Outcomes Research and Functional Genomics and Translational Biology Interdisciplinary Working Groups; and Council on Epidemiology and Prevention. *Circulation* 113(14):1807–1816, 2006.
72. Sharkey SW, Windenburg DC, Lesser JR, et al: Natural history and expansive clinical profile of stress (tako-tsubo) cardiomyopathy. *J Am Coll Cardiol* 55(4):333–341, 2010.
73. Eitel I, Knobelsdorff-Brenkenhoff F, Bernhardt P, et al: Clinical characteristics and cardiovascular magnetic resonance findings in stress (takotsubo) cardiomyopathy. *JAMA* 306(3):277–286, 2011.

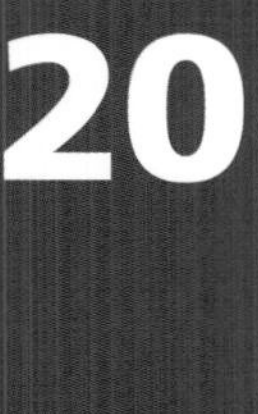

The Restrictive and Infiltrative Cardiomyopathies and Arrhythmogenic Right Ventricular Dysplasia/Cardiomyopathy

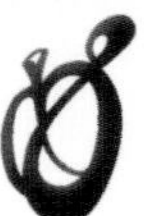

Joshua M. Hare

Cardiomyopathies are diseases of heart muscle that result from a myriad of insults, such as genetic defects, cardiac myocyte injury, or infiltration of myocardial tissues. Thus cardiomyopathies result from insults to both cellular elements of the heart, notably the cardiac myocyte, and processes that are external to cells, such as deposition of abnormal substances into the extracellular matrix. Disorders that lead to the abnormal deposition of noncompliant materials in the myocardium preferentially lead to the restrictive cardiomyopathy phenotype,[1] the prototypic causes being deposition of excessive fibrosis and amyloid proteins.[2] Cardiomyopathies are traditionally defined on the basis of structural and functional phenotypes, notably dilated (characterized primarily by an enlarged ventricular chamber and reduced cardiac performance),[3] hypertrophic (characterized primarily by thickened, hypertrophic ventricular walls and enhanced cardiac performance), and restrictive (characterized primarily by thickened, stiff ventricular walls that impede diastolic filling of the ventricle; cardiac systolic performance is typically close to normal).[1] A fourth, and increasingly appreciated, structural and functional phenotype is a cardiomyopathy that primarily involves the right ventricle—arrhythmogenic right ventricular dysplasia/cardiomyopathy (ARVD/C). This chapter will review the restrictive/infiltrative cardiomyopathies and ARVD/C.

RESTRICTIVE AND INFILTRATIVE CARDIOMYOPATHY

Relative to the dilated (**see Chapter 19**) and hypertrophic (**see Chapter 21**) cardiomyopathies, restrictive cardiomyopathy occurs with lower frequency in the developed world. Specific forms of restrictive cardiomyopathy, such as endomyocardial disease (**Table 20-1**) are important causes of morbidity and mortality common in specific geographic locales, especially in underdeveloped countries.[4-6] The pathophysiologic feature that defines restrictive cardiomyopathy is the increase in stiffness of the ventricular walls, which causes heart failure because of impaired diastolic filling of the ventricle (**see also Chapters 10, 21, and 36**).[7] In early stages of the syndrome, systolic function may be normal, although deterioration in systolic function is usually observed as the disease progresses.[1]

Restrictive cardiomyopathy must be distinguished from constrictive pericarditis, which is also characterized by normal or nearly normal systolic function but abnormal ventricular filling.[1] Differentiation[8] of these two conditions represents a classic diagnostic challenge and is one of significant clinical importance because pericardial constriction may be treated successfully with pericardiectomy.

Approximately 50% of cases of restrictive cardiomyopathy result from specific clinical disorders, whereas the

TABLE 20-1 Classification of Types of Restrictive Cardiomyopathy According to Cause

Myocardial	Storage Disease
Noninfiltrative	Hemochromatosis Fabry disease Glycogen storage disease
Idiopathic cardiomyopathy* Familial cardiomyopathy Hypertrophic cardiomyopathy Scleroderma Pseudoxanthoma elasticum Diabetic cardiomyopathy	**Endomyocardial** Endomyocardial fibrosis* Hypereosinophilic syndrome Carcinoid heart disease Metastatic cancers Radiation* Toxic effects of anthracycline* Drugs causing fibrous endocarditis (serotonin, methysergide, ergotamine, mercurial agents, busulfan)
Infiltrative Amyloidosis* Sarcoidosis* Gaucher disease Hurler disease Fatty infiltration	

*These conditions are more likely than the others to be encountered in clinical practice.

From Kushwaha S, Fallon JT, Fuster V: Restrictive cardiomyopathy. N Engl J Med 336:267, 1997; Hare JM: The dilated and restrictive cardiomyopathies. In Bonow RL, et al, editors: Braunwald's heart disease, ed 9, Philadelphia, 2011, Elsevier, pp 1561–1581.

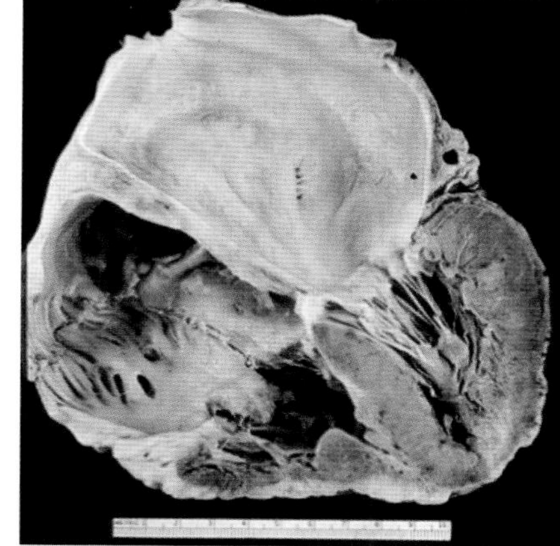
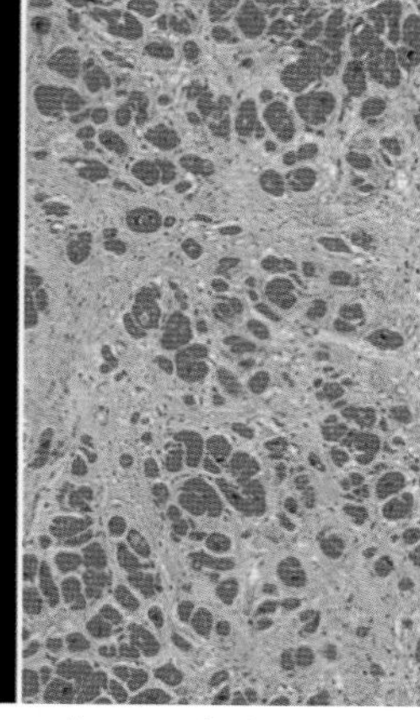

FIGURE 20-1 Pathology of idiopathic restrictive cardiomyopathy in a 63-year-old woman. *Left,* Gross cardiac specimen shown in four-chamber format, demonstrating prominent biatrial enlargement, with normal size ventricles. *Right,* Light microscopy showing marked interstitial fibrosis *(light pink areas).* Hematoxylin and eosin; magnification 120×. *Modified from Ammash NM, Seward JB, Bailey KR, et al: Clinical profile and outcome of idiopathic restrictive cardiomyopathy. Circulation 101:2490, 2000; Hare JM: The dilated and restrictive cardiomyopathies. In Bonow RL, et al, editors: Braunwald's heart disease, ed 9, Philadelphia, 2011, Elsevier, pp 1561–1581.*

remainder represent an idiopathic process. The most common specific cause of restrictive cardiomyopathy is infiltration caused by amyloidosis—there are both acquired and genetic causes of amyloid.[9] Although there are other specific pathologic presentations associated with restrictive cardiomyopathy, their precise etiology often remains obscure. Like dilated cardiomyopathy, there are inflammatory and genetic factors important in the cause of restrictive cardiomyopathy. The identification of specific infiltrative processes may have prognostic and therapeutic implications (**Figure 20-1**).[10] The abnormal diastolic properties of the ventricle are attributable to myocardial fibrosis, infiltration, or scarring of the endomyocardial surface. Myocyte hypertrophy is common, particularly in idiopathic restrictive cardiomyopathy (see Figure 20-1).

Clinical Evaluation

Cardiac Catheterization and Endomyocardial Biopsy

Restrictive Cardiomyopathy versus Constrictive Pericarditis

A classic diagnostic challenge is to differentiate restrictive cardiomyopathy from constrictive pericarditis, which manifests with similar clinical and hemodynamic features. Cardiac catheterization is a key step in this evaluation (see also Chapter 28). Although there is equalization of diastolic pressures in constrictive pericarditis (pressures differ by no more than 5 mm Hg), they may vary to a greater extent in restrictive cardiomyopathy. Pulmonary hypertension is worse in restrictive cardiomyopathy, with systolic pulmonary pressures often exceeding 50 mm Hg. In constrictive pericarditis, the plateau of right ventricular diastolic pressure is usually at least one third of peak systolic pressure; in restrictive cardiomyopathy, this is most often lower. Hemodynamically both conditions have a rapid early diastolic pressure decline followed by a rapid rise and plateau in early diastole, the so-called square root sign. The atrial pressure tracing manifests either a classic square root pattern or an M or W waveform when the x descent is also rapid. Both a and v waves are prominent and frequently have the same amplitude. Right- and left-sided atrial filling pressures are elevated, although in the case of restrictive cardiomyopathy the left ventricular filling pressure typically is 5 mm Hg or more than the right ventricular diastolic pressure. This difference may be accentuated by the Valsalva maneuver, exercise, or a fluid challenge.

Endomyocardial biopsy can also be valuable in the evaluation of these patients to exclude an infiltrative process or cardiomyopathic-appearing myocytes, and received a class IIa recommendation in the guidelines.[11] A normal-appearing biopsy supports the diagnosis of a pericardial process. Surgical exploration is needed far less often, given the availability of biopsy and imaging technology (see later discussion).

Prognosis

Restrictive cardiomyopathy carries a variable prognosis dependent on the cause (**Figure 20-2**). Most often, especially in the case of amyloidosis, it is invariably progressive with an accelerated mortality.[12] A recent longitudinal study of 233 patients revealed the importance of the underlying type of amyloidosis in patient outcome, with patients with transthyretin amyloidosis faring better than those with immunoglobulin-associated amyloidosis (**Figure 20-3**).[9] There is no specific therapy for the idiopathic form of restrictive cardiomyopathy, but intensive fluid and supportive management is required to maintain a patient with a reasonable quality of life. There are ongoing aggressive attempts to devise therapies for secondary forms of restrictive cardiomyopathy tailored to the cause (e.g., iron removal in hemochromatosis or enzyme replacement therapy in Fabry disease).

Clinical Manifestations

Patients with restrictive cardiomyopathy frequently present with exercise intolerance that results from an impaired ability to augment cardiac output during increasing heart rate because of the restriction of diastolic filling. Other notable symptoms are weakness, dyspnea, and edema.

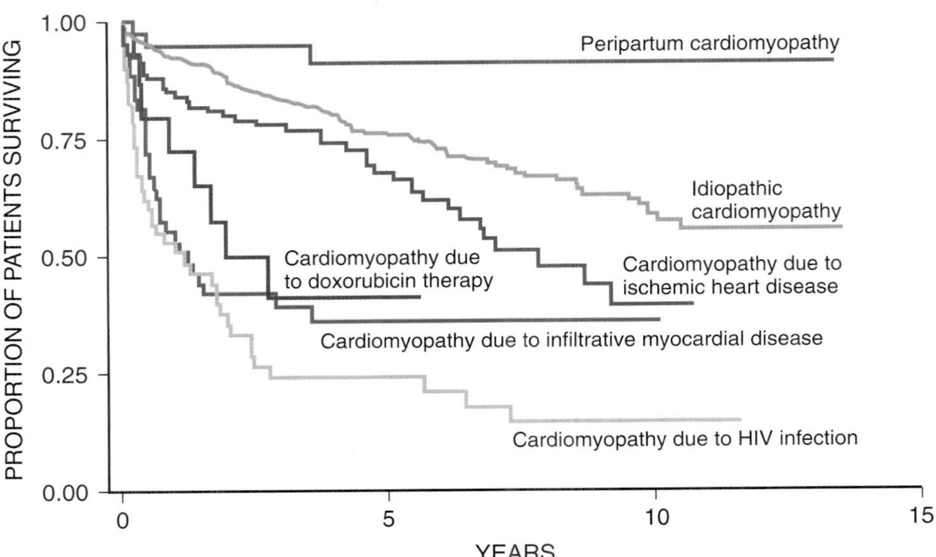

FIGURE 20-2 Adjusted Kaplan-Meier estimates of survival among patients with infiltrative cardiomyopathies. Survival of patients with idiopathic cardiomyopathy is shown for comparison. *Modified from Felker GM, Thompson RE, Hare JM, et al: Underlying causes and long-term survival in patients with initially unexplained cardiomyopathy. N Engl J Med 342:1077, 2000; Hare JM: The dilated and restrictive cardiomyopathies. In Bonow RL, et al, editors: Braunwald's heart disease, ed 9, Philadelphia, 2011, Elsevier, pp 1561–1581.*

Exertional chest pain is reported by some but not all patients. With advancing disease, profound edema occurs that includes peripheral edema, hepatomegaly, ascites, and anasarca. These patients represent the most difficult volume management because of the balance between volume status and hypotension that can result during diuresis because of reduced preload filling of the ventricles. Physical examination is notable for an elevated jugular venous pulse, often with the Kussmaul sign, and a rising jugular pressure during inspiration (because of the restriction to filling). Both S_3 and S_4 gallops are common and the apical pulse is palpable (in contrast to constrictive pericarditis). Patients with restrictive cardiomyopathy are highly prone to developing atrial fibrillation.[1]

Laboratory Studies

Computed tomography and magnetic resonance imaging (MRI) are valuable for differentiating constrictive and restrictive disease. A thickened pericardium supports the diagnosis of pericardial constriction. Other ancillary tests also may be helpful. For example, chest roentgenography may detect pericardial calcification. The electrocardiogram (ECG) may disclose atrial fibrillation. Echocardiography should be routinely performed in patients suspected of restrictive cardiomyopathy or constriction, and may reveal biatrial dilation and increasing wall thickness associated with myocardial infiltration, as well as alterations in the appearance of the myocardium (e.g., speckling). Doppler echocardiography supplemented with tissue Doppler reveals evidence of myocardial relaxation with increased early left ventricular filling velocity, decreased atrial filling velocity, and decreased isovolumetric relaxation time. The latter findings are additionally useful for the discrimination from constrictive disease.[1,13] BNP levels may be used to discriminate between restrictive cardiomyopathy and constrictive disease, with concentrations approximately five times greater in the former compared with the latter.[14]

AMYLOIDOSIS

Etiology and Types

Amyloidosis is a unique disease process that results from tissue deposition of proteins that have a unique secondary structure (twisted β-pleated sheet fibrils) (**Figure 20-4**). Amyloid may be found in almost any organ but does not produce clinically evident disease unless tissue infiltration is extensive. Several classification systems have been used to characterize the different clinical presentations of amyloidosis. *Primary amyloidosis* results from the deposition of portions of immunoglobulin light chain (designated as AL) within tissues. In the vast majority of cases, the excess production of this protein results from a monoclonal expansion of plasma cells in the setting of multiple myeloma. Rarely, a patient with a plasma cell dyscrasia may develop restrictive cardiomyopathy due to deposition of light chains in a nonamyloid manner. Importantly, the latter form of disease may be reversible. Historically, primary amyloidosis occurred from other chronic untreated inflammatory conditions. *Secondary amyloidosis* (also known as *reactive systemic amyloidosis*) results from the excess production of a nonimmunoglobulin protein known as AA.

Familial Amyloidosis

In the past decade, there has been growing recognition that various familial diseases can lead to amyloid deposition in the heart. An autosomal dominant form results from the deposition of a variant form of prealbumin serum carrier termed *transthyretin*. Multiple (>100) point mutations in the transthyretin gene are associated with amyloidosis.[9] Transthyretin amyloidosis usually produces one of three different clinical scenarios—nephropathy, neuropathy, or cardiomyopathy. Isolated cardiomyopathy occurring with older age, associated with the Ile 122 variant, is more common in individuals of African American descent.[15] Given that transthyretin is produced hepatically, liver transplantation may

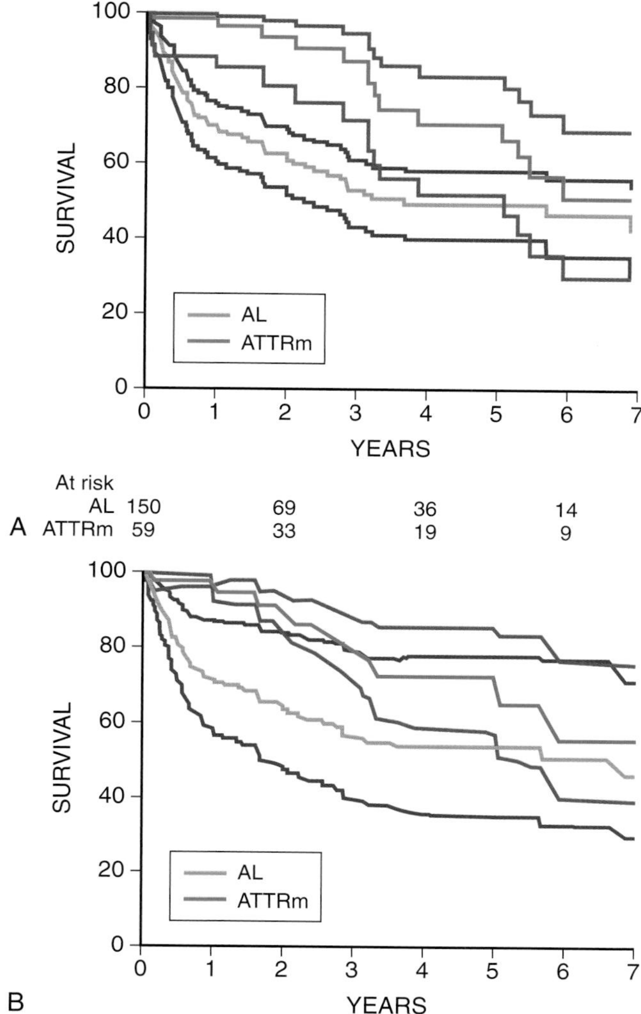

FIGURE 20-3 Variable prognosis in patients with cardiac amyloidosis based upon the specific genotype causing transthyretin deposition before **(A)** and after **(B)** adjustment for renal involvement or insufficiency. *Modified from Rapezzi C, Merlini G, Quarta CC, et al: Systemic cardiac amyloidoses. Disease profiles and clinical courses of the 3 main types. Circulation 120:1203, 2009; Hare JM: The dilated and restrictive cardiomyopathies. In Bonow RL, et al, editors: Braunwald's heart disease, ed 9, Philadelphia, 2011, Elsevier, pp 1561–1581.*

be contemplated in affected individuals who are detected early.

Senile Systemic Amyloidosis

This form of amyloidosis results from amyloid deposition of proteins that are either like atrial natriuretic peptide or transthyretin.[16] This form of amyloidosis is increasing in incidence as the population ages. Although it affects individuals of older age, the prognosis is better than that of AL disease.[16] Deposition of amyloid in the atria and pulmonary vessels is often found at autopsy in octogenarians and may be a risk factor for atrial fibrillation.

Cardiac Amyloidosis

Cardiac amyloidosis is an invariably progressive infiltrative cardiomyopathy that carries a grave prognosis.[12] Cardiac involvement may be present in up to one third of patients with primary amyloidosis resulting from plasma cell dyscrasias. When the heart is studied pathologically, AL protein

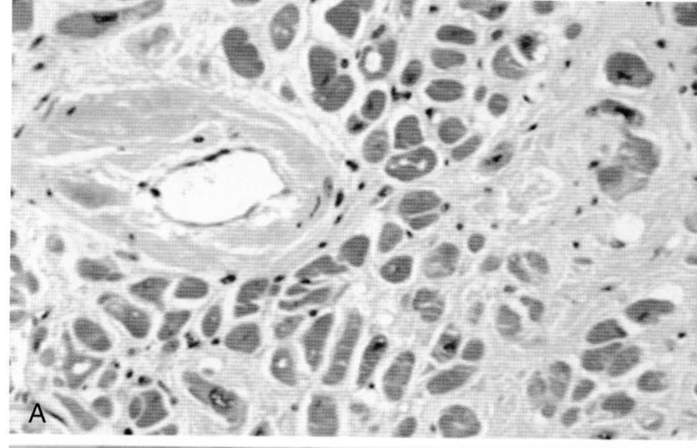

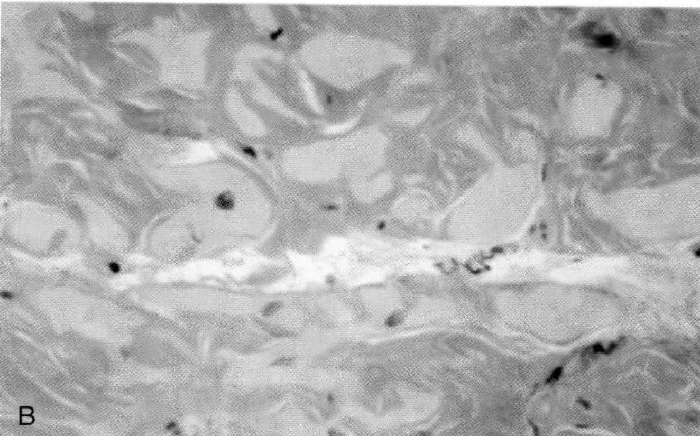

FIGURE 20-4 Histologic phenotype of cardiac amyloidosis. **A,** Endomyocardial biopsy specimen, stained with hematoxylin and eosin, from a patient with cardiac amyloidosis. The amyloid stains light pinkish red and is seen as an amorphous material that separates the darker staining myocytes. **B,** Staining of the tissue from the same patient using sulfated Alcian blue. The amyloid stains turquoise green and the myocytes stain yellow, characteristic of amyloid. *Modified from Falk RH: Diagnosis and management of the cardiac amyloidoses. Circulation 112:2047, 2005; Hare JM: The dilated and restrictive cardiomyopathies. In Bonow RL, et al, editors: Braunwald's heart disease, ed 9, Philadelphia, 2011, Elsevier, pp 1561–1581.*

deposits are present invariably at necropsy even if clinically silent in life. Myocardial infiltration tends to be less with secondary amyloidosis, in which the AA protein deposits tend to be smaller and more perivascular in location, where they are less likely to produce myocardial dysfunction.

Approximately one quarter of patients with transthyretin-induced (familial) amyloidosis experience clinically significant cardiac involvement that is often marked by involvement of the conduction system. Neurologic and/or renal involvement may also predominate in this form of amyloidosis. Patients will typically present with clinical symptoms after the age of 35. In one half of the cases involving deposition of transthyretin, the mode of death is cardiac, either from heart failure or sudden cardiac death. In senile amyloidosis, deposits vary from isolated atrial involvement to extensive ventricular infiltration causing severe restrictive cardiomyopathy. Cardiac amyloidosis is observed more frequently in men than in women and is rare before the age of 40.

Pathology

The term *amyloidosis* was coined by Virchow and means "starchlike." The heart infiltrated with amyloid appears tan and waxy and is rubbery in consistency. The atria are also significantly enlarged (see Figure 20-4). Histologically, amyloid deposits can be detected with Congo red or Sirius red staining and are present between cardiac myocytes.[7,12] Amyloidosis may cause focal thickening of the cardiac valves but infrequently leads to valvular dysfunction. In addition, amyloid may deposit within the media and adventitia of intramural coronary arteries and may cause impairment in coronary perfusion.

Clinical Manifestations

There are four overlapping cardiovascular syndromes that may occur with cardiovascular involvement of amyloidosis: restrictive cardiomyopathy, systolic heart failure, orthostatic hypotension, and presentation with conduction system disease.

Restrictive Cardiomyopathy

Amyloid infiltration and circulating immunoglobulins produce classic restrictive physiology leading to increased diastolic chamber stiffness with a resultant impairment of left ventricular filling. The impairment of chamber filling leads to fluid retention and peripheral edema, hepatomegaly, and elevated jugular venous pressure. Hemodynamic measurements reveal the classic dip and plateau square root sign. One feature differentiating amyloidosis from constrictive pericarditis is the rate of early diastolic filling, which is accelerated in pericardial disease but is diminished in amyloidosis.

Systolic Heart Failure

Although systolic function may be normal early in the disease, it frequently deteriorates late in the disease as the degree of amyloid deposition increases. Deposition of amyloid in the atrium can also lead to atrial arrest, even though the sinus node is fully functional. The loss of atrial transport function may contribute to worsening heart failure, particularly in the face of restrictive cardiac physiology. Patients may also exhibit angina pectoris, although epicardial coronary arteries are normal angiographically. This form of the disease is usually relentlessly progressive.

Orthostatic Hypotension

Approximately 10% of affected individuals will exhibit orthostasis caused by amyloid infiltration of the autonomic nervous system, blood vessels, or both.[17] Infiltration of the heart and adrenal glands may contribute to the pathogenesis of this variant. Renal failure resulting in the nephrotic syndrome and volume retention can worsen the postural hypotension. Patients with amyloidosis frequently experience frank syncope often associated with emotional or physical stress, a phenomenon that may be associated with left ventricular outflow obstruction. Syncope during exertion represents an extremely poor prognosis, with demise likely within 3 months.

Conduction System Disease

Abnormal propagation of cardiac electrical signals is the least common form of amyloidosis and may result in arrhythmias and conduction disturbances. Sudden cardiac death, caused by malignant arrhythmias or conduction block, is an important mode of death. Episodes of syncope may herald more severe events such as sudden cardiac death.

Physical Examination

Most commonly, patients with cardiac amyloidosis present with signs of congestive heart failure. The jugular venous pulse is elevated, often massively, and there are signs of systemic edema with hepatomegaly, ascites, and edema. On auscultation, apical systolic murmurs as a result of mitral regurgitation and S_3 gallops are frequently present, although S_4 is typically absent when there is atrial infiltration with amyloid that leads to impaired atrial contraction. Blood pressure is normal to reduced, and pulse pressure may be quite narrow, consistent with low cardiac output.

Noninvasive Testing

Cardiomegaly is present on chest roentgenography in patients with systolic dysfunction but not in those with restrictive presentations. Pulmonary congestion will be detected if heart failure is present. The electrocardiogram most often reveals low QRS voltage, and bundle branch block and abnormal axis are also common. A pattern of old anterior myocardial infarction may be simulated by diminutive or absent R waves in the right precordial leads, or by inferior Q waves. Amyloid infiltration of the atrium predisposes to atrial fibrillation, and ventricular arrhythmias are also common. Signal-averaged electrocardiography has proved valuable in predicting increased risk for sudden cardiac death. Atrioventricular conduction defects are common, are particularly prominent in familial amyloidosis with polyneuropathy, and may portend a poor prognosis. Electrophysiologic testing is usually necessary to detect significant intrahisian block. Sinus node dysfunction is also common and the ECG may show sick sinus syndrome.

Echocardiography

Echocardiography is quite valuable and reveals increased ventricular wall thickness with small intracavitary chambers, enlarged atria, and a thickened interatrial septum. As noted, systolic function is normal early in the course of the disease, but progressive left ventricular dysfunction ensues with advancing amyloid deposition. The walls of the ventricles often reveal a distinctive appearance with a sparkling and granular texture, most likely resulting from the amyloid deposition itself. The cardiac valves may have a thickened appearance but typically have normal excursion. Pericardial effusions may be present but do not advance to tamponade. Patterns of chamber hypertrophy are on occasion regional, leading to a pattern reminiscent of hypertrophic cardiomyopathy. The echocardiographic appearance of thickened left ventricular walls associated with low voltage on ECG is valuable for differentiation from pericardial disease. Both Doppler echocardiography and radionuclide ventriculography are valuable to evaluate diastolic dysfunction, the degree of which offers prognostic information.

Radionuclide and MRI Cardiac Imaging

Technetium-99m pyrophosphate scintigraphy and other agents that bind to calcium may be valuable for amyloid detection. This tool is frequently strongly positive when amyloidosis is extensive and correlates with the degree of cardiac infiltration; however, false-negative results may occur. Both MRI and indium-labeled antimyosin antibody imaging are useful for the detection of cardiac amyloid involvement. Cardiac MRI has a very high sensitivity for the detection of cardiac amyloid, and may also be valuable in measuring the extent of amyloid deposition in the heart, which may be of significant prognostic importance.[18] There are specialized agents that may detect sympathetic denervation in patients with cardiac amyloidosis.

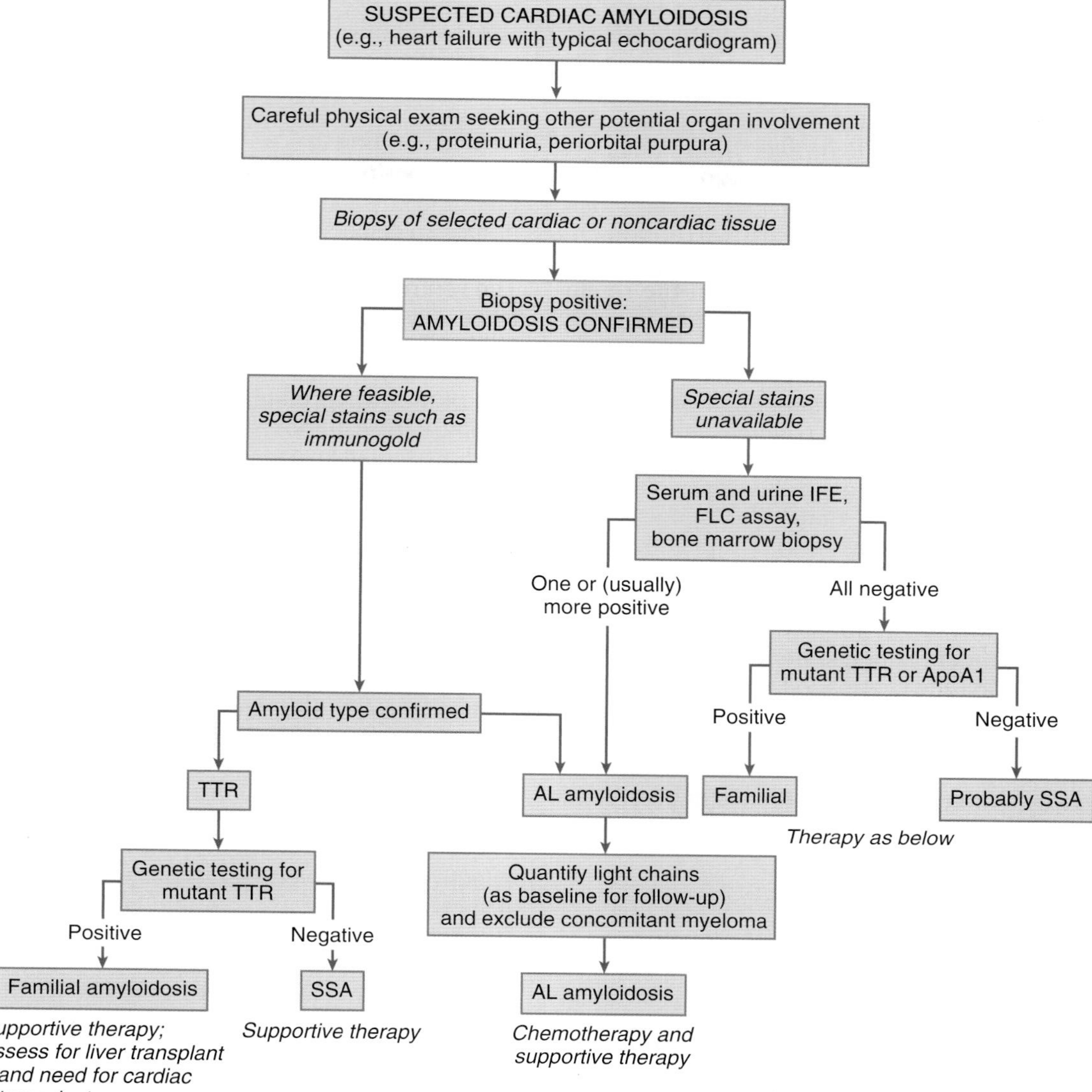

FIGURE 20-5 Flow diagram outlining the evaluation of a patient with suspected cardiac amyloidosis. Clinical evaluation may reveal clues that strengthen the likelihood of amyloidosis, but a tissue diagnosis is mandatory. Although special staining of the biopsy may confirm the type of amyloid, further workup of amyloid (AL) is required to exclude myeloma and to quantify free light chains. If the biopsy stains positive for transthyretin, further testing is needed to determine whether this is a wild-type or mutant transthyretin. *ApoA1,* Apoprotein type A1; *FLC,* free light chain; *IFE,* immunofixation electrophoresis; *SSA,* senile systemic amyloidosis; *TTR,* transthyretin. *From Falk RH: Diagnosis and management of the cardiac amyloidoses. Circulation 112:2047, 2005; Hare JM: The dilated and restrictive cardiomyopathies. In Bonow RL, et al, editors: Braunwald's heart disease, ed 9, Philadelphia, 2011, Elsevier, pp 1561–1581.*

Diagnosis

In the past, systemic amyloidosis was frequently diagnosed at autopsy. However, the increasing awareness and the availability of endomyocardial biopsy now allows for antemortem diagnosis in most patients. Biopsy of alternative tissue locations, such as the abdominal fat pad, the rectum, gingiva, bone marrow, liver, or kidney, is also useful for the detection of systemic amyloidosis. For the diagnosis of cardiac amyloidosis, endomyocardial biopsy performed by an experienced operator is safe and definitive and allows evaluation of the extent of tissue infiltration, which may offer prognostic information.[19] Tissue may be examined by immunohistochemistry to identify specific amyloid proteins, which is increasingly important for targeted therapy. Measurement of circulating serum proteins may also be diagnostically valuable. The importance of seeking the identity of the specific amyloidogenic protein is underscored by a study showing that unsuspected hereditary amyloidosis was detected in almost 10% of patients initially thought to have primary (AL) amyloidosis. Additionally, the specific type of transthyretin amyloidosis has prognostic implications.[9]

Management

Patients with cardiac amyloidosis have few treatment options, although there are ongoing attempts to modify the severe natural history of this disorder (**Figure 20-5**).[20] Approaches for patients with AL amyloidosis involve chemotherapy with alkylating agents alone or in combination with autologous bone marrow stem cell transplantation. Heart transplantation with concomitant autologous bone marrow transplants has been reported with variable degrees of success with a 39%, 4-year survival in one study and 30%,

5-year survival in another, although amyloid is likely to recur in the transplanted heart.[21] Nevertheless, survival rates may exceed those if the patient is left untreated. Moreover, combination bone marrow and cardiac transplantation may offer better survival rates in the future. For patients with transthyretin amyloid, liver transplantation may remove the source of the abnormal amyloidogenic protein.[22] Recently, a reduction in amyloid proteins has been achieved using an RNA interference (RNAi) approach, providing new hope of a method to reduce the protein deposition.[23] No form of therapy is effective in the senile form of amyloidosis, although the clinical course is more benign than in primary amyloidosis.

In terms of conventional cardiac medications, the use of digitalis glycosides requires additional vigilance because patients with cardiac amyloidosis have increased sensitivity to digitalis preparations. Despite this, digitalis glycosides are sometimes useful for successfully controlling the ventricular rate in atrial fibrillation. Calcium-channel antagonists also require caution because their negative inotropic effect has the potential to exacerbate heart failure. Pacemakers are frequently indicated for conduction system disturbances, and implantable cardioverter-defibrillators (ICDs) should be considered for appropriate patients. Perhaps the mainstay of symptom relief in volume overloaded patients is the judicious use of diuretics, which requires very careful titration, in combination with rigorous fluid restriction. Vasodilator agents may also afford symptom relief and enhance diuresis but must be used cautiously to avoid systemic hypotension. Anticoagulation should be considered in the case of atrial standstill or atrial fibrillation.

INHERITED AND ACQUIRED INFILTRATIVE DISORDERS CAUSING RESTRICTIVE CARDIOMYOPATHY

The heritable metabolic disorders resulting from the myocardial accumulation or infiltration of abnormal metabolic products represent an important cause of restrictive cardiomyopathy. These disorders produce classic restrictive cardiomyopathy with diastolic impairment and variable degrees of systolic dysfunction. The heritable metabolic disorders include Fabry disease, Gaucher disease, the glycogenoses, and the mucopolysaccharidoses. Early diagnosis is increasingly important because of the availability, in some cases, of effective enzyme replacement therapy.

Fabry Disease

Fabry disease, or *angiokeratoma corporis diffusum universale,* is an X-linked recessive disorder that results in deficiency of the lysosomal enzyme α-galactosidase A, and the resultant accumulation of glycosphingolipids (most notably globotriaosylceramide) in lysosomes.[24,25] The major clinical features result from the accumulation of glycolipid substrate in the endothelium. More than 160 different mutations are described that have a varying impact, ranging from the absence of α-galactosidase activity to an attenuated level of activity of this enzyme. Patients with absent α-galactosidase activity exhibit widespread systemic manifestations with prominent kidney and cutaneous manifestations, whereas those with an attenuated level of enzyme activity have atypical variants of Fabry disease that may cause isolated myocardial disease. Histologic evaluation of the heart demonstrates diffuse involvement of the myocardium, vascular endothelium, conduction system, and valves—most notably the mitral valve.

Cardiac Findings

Patients with Fabry disease often experience angina pectoris and myocardial infarction caused by the accumulation of lipid species in the coronary endothelium, although epicardial coronary arteries are angiographically normal. The ventricular walls are thickened and have mildly diminished diastolic compliance with normal systolic function. Mild mitral regurgitation may be present. Diastolic abnormalities detected by Doppler echocardiography may be one of the earlier manifestations preceding cardiac hypertrophy. Males almost always present with symptomatic cardiovascular involvement, whereas female carriers may be completely asymptomatic or have only minimal symptoms.[26] Other common features of the disorder include systemic hypertension, congestive heart failure, and mitral valve prolapse. Echocardiography demonstrates increased ventricular wall thickness, which may mimic hypertrophic cardiomyopathy.[24] Whereas echocardiography may not be sufficient to do so, cardiac MRI may be able to differentiate Fabry disease from other infiltrative processes such as amyloidosis.[27,28] The surface ECG may reveal a short PR interval, atrioventricular block, and ST-segment and T wave abnormalities. The endomyocardial biopsy and low plasma α-galactosidase A activity offer a definitive diagnosis, which has therapeutic implications because enzyme replacement therapy for Fabry disease is safe and effective[29]; moreover heart biopsy may be used to monitor response to therapy.[30] Administration of recombinant α-galactosidase A can ameliorate the stores of globotriaosylceramide from the heart and other tissues, leading to symptomatic, clinical, and echocardiographic improvement (**Figure 20-6**).[29,30]

Gaucher Disease

Gaucher disease results from a heritable deficiency of β-glucosidase, which leads to an accumulation of cerebrosides in diffuse organs including spleen, liver, bone marrow, lymph nodes, brain, and heart. Cardiac disease manifests as a stiffened ventricle caused by reduced chamber compliance, leading to impaired cardiac performance. Other manifestations include left ventricular failure and enlargement, hemorrhagic pericardial effusion, and sclerotic, calcified left-sided valves. Gaucher disease is responsive to enzyme replacement therapy, or in more extreme cases, hepatic transplantation; both therapies contribute to reducing tissue infiltration by cerebrosides and can lead to varying degrees of clinical improvement.[31]

Hemochromatosis

Hemochromatosis results from excessive deposition of iron in a variety of parenchymal tissues, notably the heart, liver, gonads, and pancreas. The classic pentad is a symptom complex of heart failure, cirrhosis, impotence, diabetes, and arthritis. The most frequent form of hemochromatosis is inherited as an autosomal recessive disorder that arises from a mutation in the *HFE* gene, which codes for a transmembrane protein that is responsible for regulating iron

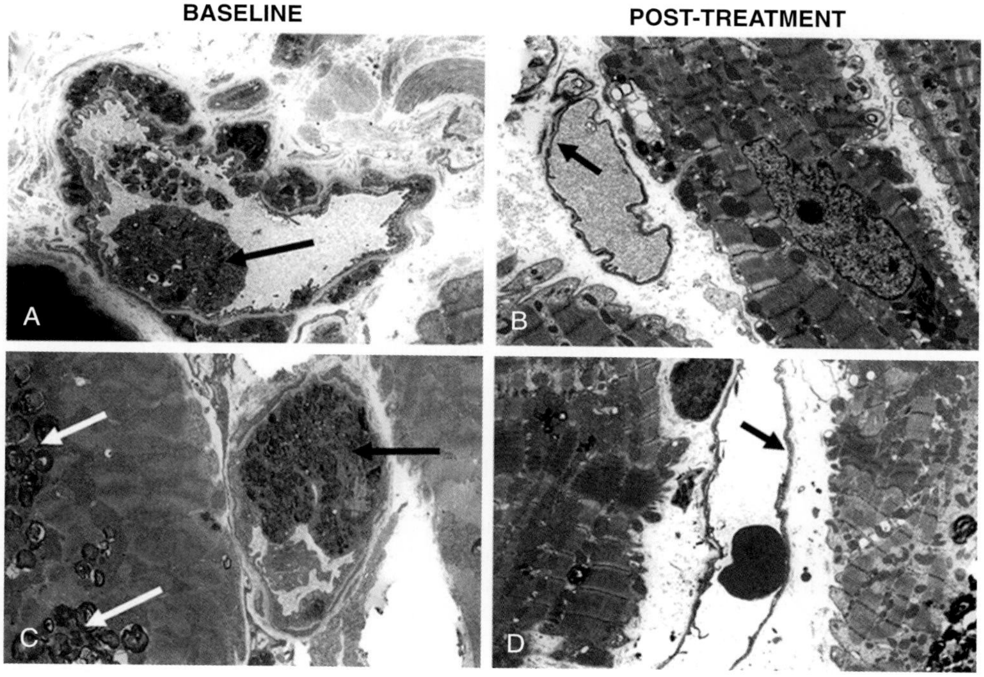

BASELINE POST-TREATMENT

FIGURE 20-6 Electron microscopy demonstrates clearance of GL-3 from cardiac capillaries. **A** and **C,** The substrate accumulates in the endothelial cells of the cardiac capillaries and protrudes into the capillary lumen. **B** and **D,** By 12 months after treatment, the substrate has been cleared from the endothelium. *From Thurberg BL, Fallon JT, Mitchell R, et al: Cardiac microvascular pathology in Fabry disease: evaluation of endomyocardial biopsies before and after enzyme replacement therapy. Circulation 119:2561–2567, 2009; Hare JM: The dilated and restrictive cardiomyopathies. In Bonow RL, et al, editors: Braunwald's heart disease, ed 9, Philadelphia, 2011, Elsevier, pp 1561–1581.*

uptake in the intestine and liver. Hemochromatosis may also arise from ineffective erythropoiesis secondary to a defect in hemoglobin synthesis, as well as from chronic liver disease, or may be acquired as a result of chronic and excessive oral or parenteral intake of iron or blood transfusions.[32]

Iron deposition in the heart is almost always accompanied by varying degrees of infiltration of the liver, spleen, pancreas, and bone marrow, although the degrees of different organ system involvement may not parallel each other. Cardiac involvement produces a mixed pattern of systolic and diastolic dysfunction that is often accompanied by arrhythmias. The severity of hemochromatosis is less and age of onset is later in women because of the menstrual loss of iron. Cardiac toxicity results directly from the free iron moiety in addition to adverse effects of tissue infiltration. Death results most frequently from cirrhosis and hepatocellular carcinoma, whereas cardiac mortality accounts for an additional one third of the mortality and is particularly important in the group of male patients who present at relatively younger ages.

Pathology

Grossly the hearts are dilated and ventricular walls are thickened. Iron deposits locate preferentially in the myocyte sarcoplasmic reticulum, more frequently in ventricular versus atrial cardiomyocytes. Frequently, the conduction system is involved and loss of myocytes with fibrosis is often present. The degree of iron deposition correlates with the extent of myocardial dysfunction.

Clinical Manifestations

Symptoms at presentation vary widely, and some patients are asymptomatic although evidence exists for myocardial involvement. Echocardiography reveals increased left ventricular wall thickness, ventricular dilation, and ventricular dysfunction. Both computed tomography and MRI are useful to detect early subclinical myocardial involvement at a time when therapy is most effective.[33] ECG manifestations occur with advancing cardiac involvement and include ST-segment and T wave abnormalities, and supraventricular arrhythmias.

Clinical and echocardiographic features usually are diagnostic, and endomyocardial biopsy is confirmatory but because of false negativity cannot definitively rule out the diagnosis. Evaluation of iron metabolism may aid in the diagnosis. Plasma iron levels are elevated, total iron-binding capacity is low or normal, and serum ferritin, urinary iron, liver iron, and especially saturation of transferrin are markedly elevated. Management should include repeated phlebotomies and/or treatment with chelating agents such as desferrioxamine. For advanced disease, cardiac transplantation carries acceptable 5- and 10-year survival rates.[34]

Glycogen Storage Disease

Patients with type II, III, IV, and V glycogen storage diseases may have cardiac involvement. However, survival to adulthood is rare with the exception of patients with type III disease (glycogen debranching enzyme deficiency). The most typical cardiac involvement is left ventricular hypertrophy, with electrocardiographic and echocardiographic findings, often with the absence of symptoms. A subset of patients may present with overt cardiac dysfunction, arrhythmias, and presentation of a DCM.

Inflammatory Causes of Infiltrative Cardiomyopathy

Sarcoidosis

Sarcoidosis is a systemic inflammatory condition characterized by the formation of noncaseating granulomas, most commonly involving the lungs, reticuloendothelial system, and skin. Sarcoid has been reported to involve essentially

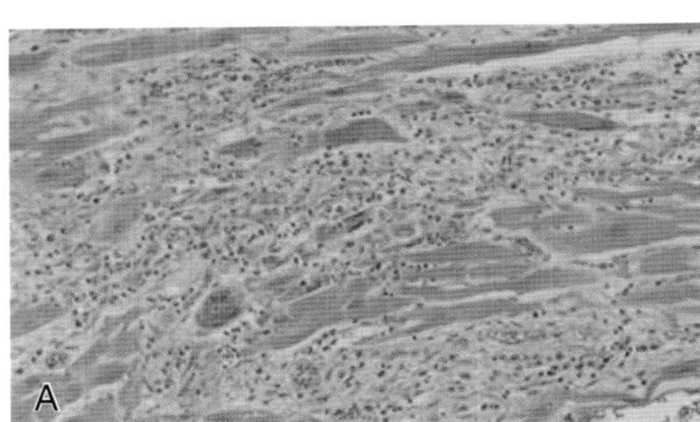

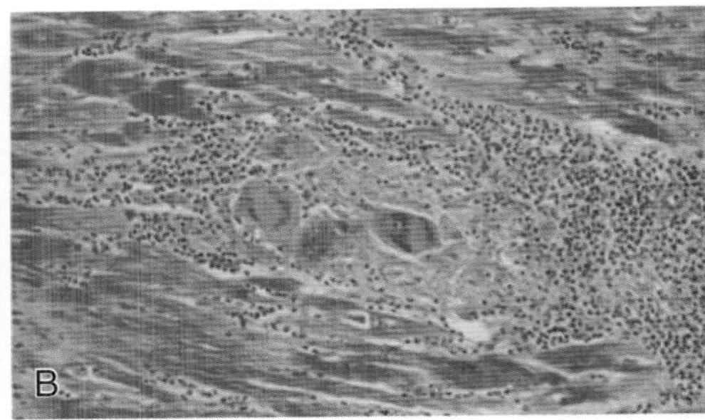

FIGURE 20-7 Sarcoid versus giant cell myocarditis. Giant cell myocarditis **(A)** is characterized by lymphocytic infiltration, myocyte necrosis, and giant cells. Sarcoidosis **(B)** is characterized by the presence of true noncaseating granulomas. *Modified from Hare JM: Etiologic basis of congestive heart failure. In Colucci WS, editor: Atlas of heart failure, ed 5, Philadelphia, 2008, Current Medicine LLC, pp 29–56; Hare JM: The dilated and restrictive cardiomyopathies. In Bonow RL, et al, editors: Braunwald's heart disease, ed 9, Philadelphia, 2011, Elsevier, pp 1561–1581.*

all tissues including the heart, which is recognized in 20% to 30% of autopsies of affected patients. Cardiac impairment may also arise secondary to pulmonary sarcoidosis, in which case extensive pulmonary fibrosis leads to advancing right-sided heart failure. The main clinical manifestations of sarcoid heart disease result from infiltration of the conduction system and myocardium, producing heart block, malignant arrhythmias, heart failure, and sudden cardiac death. Patients with cardiac sarcoidosis may also present with a restrictive cardiomyopathy caused by increased ventricular chamber stiffness.[35]

Pathology

Noncaseating granulomas surrounded by multinucleated giant cells are the diagnostic feature of the disorder and are found in multiple organs. In the heart they infiltrate the myocardium and lead to the formation of fibrotic scars. The condition must be separated from two other inflammatory conditions of the heart—chronic active myocarditis and giant cell myocarditis (see Chapter 26). Giant cell myocarditis, which is characterized by diffuse giant cell inflammation in the absence of discrete granulomas, has a much more fulminant course than cardiac sarcoid (**Figure 20-7**).[11,36] In sarcoidosis, the granulomas may involve discrete areas of the ventricular walls in a patchy fashion, increasing the likelihood of a false-negative endomyocardial biopsy result. Granulomas are most commonly observed in the interventricular septum and left ventricular free wall, and patients with conduction system disease typically have involvement of the basal portion of the interventricular septum. Left ventricular aneurysm formation may occur with extensive transmural free wall involvement. In terms of the coronary anatomy, the large conductance vessels are usually spared, but small coronary artery branches may be involved.

Clinical Manifestations

The clinical manifestations result from infiltration of the conduction system and myocardium. The most devastating presentation is that of sudden death caused by malignant ventricular arrhythmia. Patients may also present with heart block, congestive heart failure, and syncope. Both atrial and ventricular arrhythmias are common.[37] Patients may be asymptomatic despite significant cardiac involvement. Heart failure may result from direct myocardial involvement or cor pulmonale as a result of extensive pulmonary fibrosis. Survival may range from months to years, with the presence of a positive endomyocardial biopsy heralding a grave outcome.[38] An excellent long-term outcome may be achieved with aggressive immunosuppression. Isolated cardiac sarcoid has been reported.

The initial detection of cardiac sarcoidosis often results from the presence of bilateral hilar lymphadenopathy on chest roentgenogram in individuals with clinical or ECG findings suggesting myocardial disease. Endomyocardial biopsy should be performed if available because of the importance of positive findings, but it has a high false-negative rate.[11,38] Multiple imaging modalities assist in assessing diagnosis and prognosis. Echocardiography may demonstrate either global or regional left ventricular dysfunction and rarely may reveal aneurysm formation. Echocardiography is also valuable to evaluate right ventricular hypertrophy and to estimate pulmonary artery systolic pressures. Cardiac MRI is emerging as a highly sensitive and specific test.[39] Other modalities include myocardial nuclear imaging with thallium-201 or technetium-99m, which can reveal segmental perfusion defects because of granulomatous inflammation, and (^{18}F)-fluorodeoxyglucose positron emission tomography, which can reveal focal uptake consistent with sarcoid. Uptake of technetium pyrophosphate, gallium, or labeled antimyosin antibody may also contribute to making the diagnosis.

The *physical examination* may show evidence of extracardiac sarcoid or may be totally normal. An apical systolic murmur as a result of mitral regurgitation is frequently present, often arising from cardiac chamber dilation as opposed to direct papillary muscle infiltration. Murmurs of tricuspid regurgitation, pulmonic regurgitation, and right-sided third heart sounds suggest pulmonary hypertension and cor pulmonale. Both S_3 and S_4 are frequently appreciated.

Electrocardiography typically demonstrates nonspecific findings suggestive of myocardial involvement, with T wave abnormalities commonly present. The ECG is highly valuable to assess the degree of conduction system involvement in terms of intraventricular delays and atrioventricular block. Q waves may be present indicating severe and extensive myocardial replacement and fibrosis. Typical findings on echocardiography include left ventricular dilation with global or regional hypokinesis, right-sided enlargement and hypertrophy, possible left ventricular aneurysm formation, and not infrequently, pericardial effusion. Occasionally, increased echogenicity suggests an infiltrative process.

Management

Sarcoidosis is generally treated with immunosuppression.[11,35] Conduction disturbance, arrhythmias, and myocardial dysfunction may all respond to corticosteroids. Steroids effectively halt the progression of inflammation, and some studies suggest that therapy may offer improved survival. Other drugs that may be of benefit in sarcoidosis include hydroxychloroquine, methotrexate, and cyclophosphamide. It is important to distinguish cardiac sarcoidosis from giant cell myocarditis (see Chapter 26), a much more aggressive disorder that requires intensive immunosuppression and frequently mechanical support or heart transplantation. Whereas antiarrhythmic therapy is often ineffective for controlling malignant arrhythmias, ICD therapy is appropriate for patients at risk for sudden cardiac death. Implantation of a permanent pacemaker is often required in the case of conduction system disease. Heart or heart-lung transplantation should be considered in the case of intractable heart failure, although recurrence of sarcoid may occur in the grafted organ.

Endomyocardial Disease

Definition and Pathogenesis

A common form of restrictive cardiomyopathy found in a geographical location close to the equator is known as endomyocardial disease (EMD). EMD is common in equatorial Africa, and manifests less frequently in South America, Asia, and nontropical countries, including the United States. Two variants are described that, despite similar phenotypes, are likely unique processes, both manifesting as aggressive endocardial scarring obliterating the ventricular apices and subvalvular regions. Endomyocardial fibrosis or Davies disease is the first variant and occurs primarily in tropical regions, and the second, Löffler endocarditis parietalis fibroplastica, or the hypereosinophilic syndrome, is encountered in more temperate zones. Although the pathologic appearance of these two disorders is similar, there are sufficient differences between them, suggesting that they indeed are two distinct entities. Löffler endocarditis is more aggressive and rapidly progresses, affects mainly males, and is associated with hypereosinophilia, thromboemboli, and systemic arteritis; endomyocardial fibrosis occurs in a younger distribution, affects young children, and is only variably associated with eosinophilia.

Differences Between Löffler Endocarditis and Endomyocardial Fibrosis

Overlap between Löffler endocarditis and endomyocardial fibrosis is suggested by the observation that both diseases are attributable to the direct toxic effects of eosinophils in the myocardium. It is suggested that hypereosinophilia (regardless of cause) produces the first phase of EMD, which is characterized by necrosis, intense myocarditis, and arteritis (i.e., Löffler endocarditis). This phase lasts for a period of months and is then followed by a thrombotic stage a year following the initial presentation, in which a nonspecific thickening of the myocardium with a layer of thrombus replaces the inflammatory portion of the myocardium. In the late phase, final healing is achieved by the formation of fibrosis, at which point the clinical features of endomyocardial fibrosis are present. Most of the support for this three-stage pathophysiology, namely necrotic, thrombotic, and fibrotic, comes from autopsy studies. Nonetheless, definitive evidence that each patient passes sequentially through these stages is lacking.

Role of Eosinophils

The mechanisms by which eosinophils participate in the development of cardiac disease is not completely understood. These cells have the capacity to directly infiltrate tissues or release factors that may exert toxicity. The observation that patients with Löffler endocarditis have degranulated eosinophils in their peripheral blood supports the idea that these granules contain cardiotoxic substances capable of causing the necrotic phase of EMD, which leads to the thrombotic and fibrotic phases once the eosinophilia resolves. It is conceivable that this effect may occur only in temperate zones of the world, as the link between eosinophilia and endomyocardial fibrosis is less clear (although parasitic diseases have increased incidence), suggesting that in tropical countries endomyocardial fibrosis may result from a different mechanism. Factors implicated include elevated cerium levels and hypomagnesemia.

Löffler Endocarditis: The Hypereosinophilic Syndrome

In temperate climates, EMD is closely associated with significant hypereosinophilia, which can have several different causes. Hypereosinophilia associated with Löffler endocarditis usually is characterized by eosinophil counts exceeding $1500/mm^3$ for at least 6 months. Most patients with this degree of hypereosinophilia will have cardiac involvement. The eosinophilia may be secondary to leukemia, reactive disorders such as parasite infection, allergies, granulomatous syndromes, hypersensitivity, or neoplastic disorders. In addition, patients with Churg-Strauss syndrome, characterized by asthma or allergic rhinitis and a necrotizing vasculitis, often have cardiac involvement.[40]

Pathology

Hypereosinophilic syndrome involves several organ systems beyond the heart, including the lungs, brain, and bone marrow. Both chambers of the heart are involved and manifest with endocardial thickening of the inflow regions and ventricular apices. Histologically there are variable degrees of eosinophilic myocarditis of the myocardium and subendocardium, thrombosis and inflammation of small intramural coronary vessels, mural thrombosis containing eosinophils, and endocardial fibrotic thickening several millimeters thick.

Clinical Manifestations

Patients with hypereosinophilic syndrome exhibit weight loss, fever, cough, rash, and congestive heart failure. Early in the course of cardiac involvement, patients may be asymptomatic, but with progression in excess of 50%, patients will have overt congestive heart failure and/or cardiomegaly. Murmurs of mitral regurgitation are common. Systemic emboli occur frequently—resulting in neurologic and renal sequelae. Death results from heart failure associated with renal, hepatic, or pulmonary involvement. Sudden cardiac death and syndromes mimicking acute myocardial infarction are described.

Laboratory Examination

Chest roentgenography may demonstrate an enlarged cardiac silhouette accompanied by evidence of pulmonary congestion or less frequently pulmonary infiltrates. Changes on the *electrocardiogram* are nonspecific and include ST-segment and T wave abnormalities. Atrial fibrillation and conduction defects, most notably right bundle branch

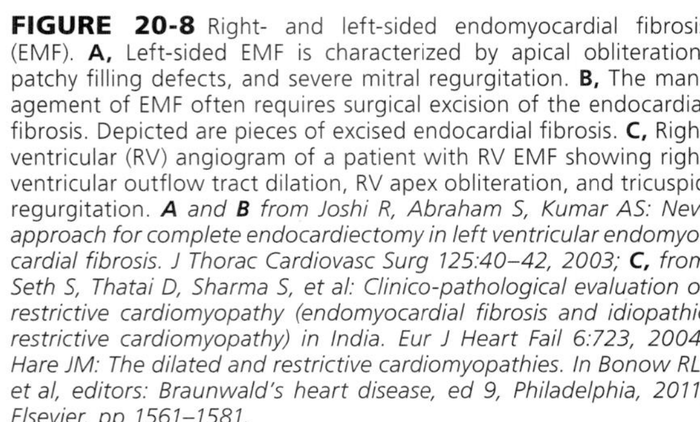

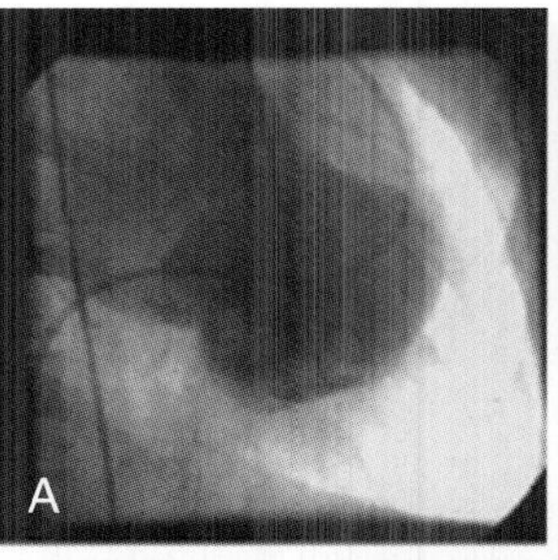

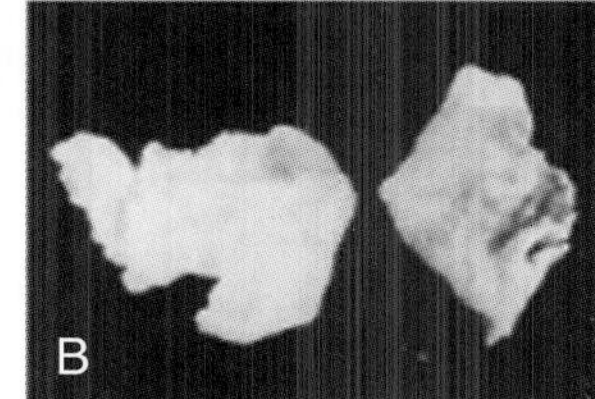

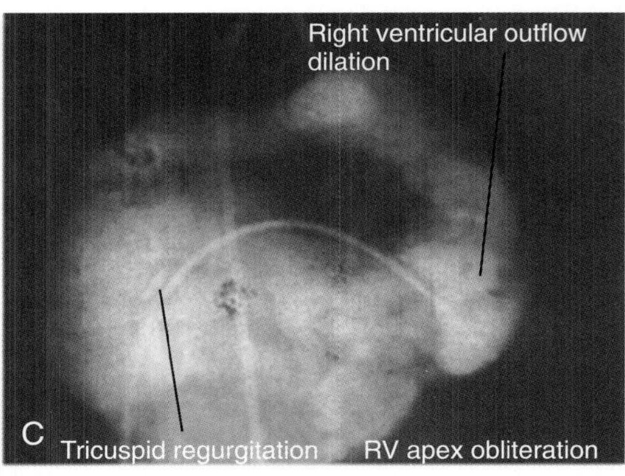

FIGURE 20-8 Right- and left-sided endomyocardial fibrosis (EMF). **A,** Left-sided EMF is characterized by apical obliteration, patchy filling defects, and severe mitral regurgitation. **B,** The management of EMF often requires surgical excision of the endocardial fibrosis. Depicted are pieces of excised endocardial fibrosis. **C,** Right ventricular (RV) angiogram of a patient with RV EMF showing right ventricular outflow tract dilation, RV apex obliteration, and tricuspid regurgitation. ***A** and **B** from Joshi R, Abraham S, Kumar AS: New approach for complete endocardiectomy in left ventricular endomyocardial fibrosis. J Thorac Cardiovasc Surg 125:40–42, 2003; **C,** from Seth S, Thatai D, Sharma S, et al: Clinico-pathological evaluation of restrictive cardiomyopathy (endomyocardial fibrosis and idiopathic restrictive cardiomyopathy) in India. Eur J Heart Fail 6:723, 2004; Hare JM: The dilated and restrictive cardiomyopathies. In Bonow RL, et al, editors: Braunwald's heart disease, ed 9, Philadelphia, 2011, Elsevier, pp 1561–1581.*

block, are often noted. The *echocardiogram* often shows regional thickening of the posterobasal portion of the left ventricular wall, with substantial impairment in the motion of the posterior leaflet of the mitral valve. The apex may be obliterated by thrombus. The atria are often dilated, and there is Doppler ultrasound evidence of atrioventricular regurgitation. As is typical for restrictive cardiomyopathy, systolic function is often normal. Hemodynamic measurements support a restrictive cardiomyopathic appearance with abnormal diastolic filling, secondary to the dense endocardial scarring and reduced size of the ventricular cavity from the organized thrombus. Regurgitation through atrioventricular valves results from involvement of their respective supporting structures. *Cardiac catheterization* reveals markedly elevated ventricular filling pressures, and there may be evidence of tricuspid or mitral regurgitation. A characteristic feature on *angiocardiography* is largely preserved systolic function with obliteration of the apex of the ventricles. *Endomyocardial biopsy* can provide diagnostic confirmation, but is not always positive.

Management

There is a role for both medical and surgical therapy in improving quality and quantity of life in patients with Löffler endocarditis. There is evidence that both corticosteroids and cytotoxic drugs such as hydroxyurea may have an important favorable effect on survival. In refractory patients, treatment with interferon may offer a valuable adjunctive therapy. Routine supportive cardiac therapy with diuretics, neurohormonal blockade, and anticoagulation as indicated is appropriate for management of these patients. Surgical therapy consisting of endocardiectomy and valve replacement or repair appears to provide significant symptomatic palliation once the fibrotic stage of the disease manifests.

Endomyocardial Fibrosis

Endomyocardial fibrosis is a disorder found typically in tropical and subtropical Africa, notably in Uganda, Nigeria, and Mozambique, and as such is a major cause of morbidity and mortality, accounting for 25% of cases of congestive heart failure and death in equatorial Africa.[4,41,42] A recent population-based study in rural Mozambique revealed a prevalence of the disorder, affecting 19.8% of the population.[4] In the latter study, only 48 of 211 patients were symptomatic at the time of detection, and familial occurrence was high.

The disease is increasingly recognized in other tropical and subtropical regions within 15 degrees of the equator including India, Brazil, Colombia, and Sri Lanka.[6] Importantly, it is also recognized in the Middle East, particularly Saudi Arabia.[41] Cardiac dysfunction occurs because of fibrous lesions that affect the inflow of the right and/or left ventricles and that may also involve the atrioventricular valves, thereby producing regurgitant lesions. Endomyocardial fibrosis has increased incidence among the Rwanda tribe of Uganda and in individuals of low socioeconomic status.[5] It has a slight male preponderance, is most common in children[42] and young adults,[4] but has been described in individuals into the sixth decade of life. Although most cases occur in black individuals, there are occasional presentations in white subjects residing in temperate climates. There are rare reports of endomyocardial fibrosis in individuals who have not resided in tropical areas.

Pathology

Endomyocardial fibrosis affects both the right and left ventricles in approximately 50% of patients, purely the left in 40%, and the right ventricle alone in the remaining 10%.[6,41] The typical gross appearance is that of a normal to slightly enlarged heart. The right atrium may be dilated in proportion to the severity of right ventricular involvement. There is often a pericardial effusion, which may be large. The right-sided heart border may be indented because of apical scarring. The hallmark feature of the disorder is fibrotic obliteration of the apex of the affected ventricle(s) (**Figure 20-8**). The fibrosis involves the papillary muscles and chordae tendineae leading to atrioventricular valve distortion and regurgitation. In the left ventricle, the fibrosis extends from the apex to the posterior mitral valve leaflet, usually sparing the anterior mitral leaflet and the ventricular outflow tract. Endocardial calcific deposits can be present, involving diffuse areas of the ventricle. The fibrotic tissue often creates a nidus for thrombus formation, which can be extensive. Atrial thrombi also occur. The process usually does not involve the epicardium, and the coronary artery obstruction is distinctly uncommon.

Histologic Findings

Endomyocardial fibrosis is clearly apparent histologically, presenting as a thick layer of collagen overlying loosely arranged connective tissue.[41] In addition, there are fibrous and granular septations extending into the underlying myocardial tissue. Myocyte hypertrophy is common.[6] Although cellular infiltration is uncommon, interstitial edema is frequently present. Fibroelastosis that is found in the ventricular outflow tracts beneath the semilunar valves often represents a secondary process caused by local trauma. Examination of intramural coronary arteries may show involvement with medial degeneration, the deposition of fibrin, and fibrosis.

Clinical Manifestations

The symptomatic status of patients at presentation relates to which ventricles are involved. Pulmonary congestion signals left-sided involvement, whereas predominantly right-sided disease may mimic restrictive cardiomyopathy and/or constrictive pericarditis. Atrioventricular valve regurgitation is common. The disease may be heralded by an acute febrile illness or may be simply insidious. Endomyocardial fibrosis is a relentless and progressive process, although the time course of decline may vary considerably, with some patients appearing to have periods of stability. Modes of death include progressive heart failure, infection, infarction, sudden cardiac death, and complications of surgery. Atrial fibrillation and ascites are reported to be poor prognostic indicators.[43,44]

Right Ventricular Endomyocardial Fibrosis

In pure or predominant right ventricular involvement, the right ventricular apex is characterized by fibrous obliteration, which may extend to involve the supporting structures of the tricuspid valve, with ensuing tricuspid regurgitation. Patients exhibit an elevated jugular venous pressure, a prominent *v* wave with rapid *y* descent, and a right-sided S_3 gallop. There is prominent hepatomegaly with a pulsatile liver, ascites, splenomegaly, and peripheral edema, but pulmonary congestion is typically absent because of the lack of left-sided involvement. In this regard, pulmonary artery and pulmonary capillary wedge pressures are normal. A large pericardial effusion is often present. The right atrium may be enormously dilated. The *electrocardiogram* often has findings consistent with right-sided enlargement, especially a qR pattern in lead V_1, and supraventricular arrhythmias are common. The *chest roentgenogram* often demonstrates obvious right atrial prominence, a pericardial effusion, and calcification in the walls of the right and, less frequently, the left ventricle. *Echocardiography* demonstrates thickening of the right ventricle with obliteration of the apex, a dilated atrium, hyperechoic endocardial surfaces, and abnormal septal motion in patients with tricuspid regurgitation. On *angiography,* the right ventricular apex is typically not visualized because of fibrous obliteration; tricuspid regurgitation, right atrial enlargement, and filling defects in the right atrium caused by thrombi may be present.

Left Ventricular Endomyocardial Fibrosis

In cases of predominant *left-sided* disease, fibrosis involves the ventricular apex and often the chordae tendineae or the posterior mitral valve leaflet producing mitral regurgitation. The associated murmur may be late systolic, characteristic of a papillary muscle dysfunction murmur, or may be pansystolic. Findings of pulmonary hypertension may be prominent, and an S_3 protodiastolic gallop is frequently present. The *electrocardiogram* usually shows ST-segment and T wave abnormalities, low-voltage QRS complexes if a pericardial effusion is present, or left ventricular hypertrophy. Left atrial abnormality is often noted. As with right-sided involvement, atrial fibrillation is often present and portends a poor prognosis. *Echocardiography* reveals increased endocardial echoreflectivity preserved systolic function, apical obliteration, an enlarged atrium, pericardial effusion of varying size, and Doppler ultrasound evidence of mitral regurgitation. Pulmonary hypertension is typically observed during *cardiac catheterization,* as well as left atrial hypertension and a reduced cardiac index. *Left ventriculography* shows mitral regurgitation, and ventricular filling defects caused by intracavitary thrombi may be present. Coronary *arteriography* usually excludes obstructive epicardial vessel stenoses.

Biventricular Endomyocardial Fibrosis

Biventricular endomyocardial fibrosis is more common than either isolated right- or left-sided disease. The typical clinical presentation of endomyocardial fibrosis (EMF) resembles right ventricular EMF; however, a murmur of mitral regurgitation is indicative of left-sided involvement. Unless left ventricular involvement is extensive, severe pulmonary hypertension is absent and the right-sided findings are the predominant mode of presentation. Approximately 15% of patients will experience systemic embolization and only 2% will have infective endocarditis.

Diagnosis

Detection of endomyocardial fibrosis in individuals from the appropriate geographic area requires typical clinical and laboratory findings, as well as angiography. Eosinophilia is variably present and may result from parasitic infection.[5] Endomyocardial biopsy is diagnostic, but false-positives can occur because of the patchy nature of the disease. Insofar as myocardial biopsy may be complicated by systemic emboli, left-sided myocardial biopsy is contraindicated.

Management

The medical management of endomyocardial fibrosis remains challenging. One third to one half of patients with advanced disease die within 2 years, whereas those who are less symptomatic fare better. The development of atrial fibrillation is a poor prognostic indicator, although symptomatic relief can be achieved with rate control.[43] Heart failure is difficult to control, and diuretics are effective only in early stages of disease, losing efficacy with advanced ascites. Once EMF progresses to severe endocardial fibrosis, surgical resection with atrioventricular valve replacement on affected sides is the treatment of choice.[45] Surgical therapy consisting of endocardiectomy and valve replacement or repair usually results in hemodynamic improvement with reductions in ventricular filling pressure, increased cardiac output, and normalized angiographic appearance. Operative mortality is quite high, between 15% and 25%, and may be lower if valve replacement is not necessary.[46] Fibrosis may recur, although there are case reports of excellent long-term survival.[47-49]

Endocardial Fibroelastosis

Endocardial fibroelastosis (EFE) is a disorder of fetuses and infants of unclear cause that is characterized by deposition of collagen and elastin leading to ventricular hypertrophy and diffuse endocardial thickening. Causes are not completely understood, and there are reports of associations with viral infections (especially mumps), metabolic disorders, autoimmune disease, and congenital left-sided obstructive lesions. Two recent reports implicate mitochondrial disorders and placental insufficiency.[50,51] Like DCM, EFE usually progresses to severe congestive heart failure and subsequent death. The echocardiographic finding of a highly reflective endocardial surface of the ventricular myocardium suggests EFE.

NEOPLASTIC INFILTRATIVE CARDIOMYOPATHY—CARCINOID HEART DISEASE

The carcinoid syndrome results from the metastasis of carcinoid tumors from the gut to the heart.[52] The symptoms include marked cutaneous flushing, diarrhea, bronchoconstriction, and endocardial plaques composed of a unique type of fibrous tissue. The symptom complex is caused in large part by the release of serotonin and other circulating substances secreted by the tumor. Essentially all patients experience diarrhea and flushing, 50% have cardiac lesions detected echocardiographically, and about 25% of the patients have severe right-sided involvement.

Carcinoid tumors originate largely from the gut, with 60% to 90% being found in the small bowel and appendix, and the remainder arising from other regions of the gastrointestinal tract or the bronchi. Carcinoid tumors arising in the ileum pose the greatest risk of metastasis, most likely affecting regional lymph nodes and the liver. The carcinoid tumors arising in the liver affect the heart. The severity of the cardiac lesions is related to the circulating concentrations of serotonin and 5-hydroxyindoleacetic acid (its primary metabolite), which are produced primarily by the carcinoid tumors in the liver. The observation that the right side of the heart is preferentially affected in the carcinoid syndrome reflects inactivation of the circulating toxic substances in the lung; the 5% to 10% of individuals presenting with left-sided lesions are likely to have right-to-left shunts or tumor involvement of the lungs.

Pathology

The characteristic lesions are fibrous plaques involving locations "downstream" of the tricuspid and pulmonic valves, the endocardium, and the intima of the venae cavae, pulmonary artery, and coronary sinus. Both stenotic and regurgitant valvular lesions result from fibrotic distortion originating in plaques.[52] The plaque material appears as a layer of fibrous tissue composed of smooth muscle cells, collagen, and mucopolysaccharides overlying the endocardium, and in some cases extending into the underlying regions. Interestingly, identical pathology results from exposure to the anorectic drugs fenfluramine and dexfenfluramine. Occasionally there is actual metastasis of the tumor to one or both of the ventricles.

Clinical Manifestations

Cardiac murmurs indicating right-sided valve involvement are widely appreciated. A systolic murmur of tricuspid regurgitation along the left sternal border is almost always present and pulmonic valve murmurs of either stenosis or regurgitation may also be present. The *chest roentgenogram* may be either normal or may show cardiac enlargement and pleural effusions or nodules. The pulmonary artery trunk is most often not enlarged, and poststenotic dilation is also absent, differentiating pulmonic involvement from congenital pulmonic stenosis. Although there are no specific changes on the *electrocardiogram* diagnostic of carcinoid heart disease, it is not uncommon to encounter right atrial enlargement without other findings of right ventricular hypertrophy, nonspecific ST-segment and T wave abnormalities, and sinus tachycardia. Patients with advanced disease are likely to have low QRS voltage. *Echocardiography* often reveals tricuspid or pulmonary valve thickening, and enlargement of the right atrium and ventricle; a minority of patients may have a small pericardial effusion. *Cardiac MRI* may offer additional value in evaluating the right side of the heart that may be difficult to image with echocardiography.[53]

Management

For mild congestive heart failure, standard therapy with diuretics and neurohormonal antagonists is appropriate. Both somatostatin analogues and chemotherapy can lead to improved symptoms and possibly enhanced survival, but neither is effective at ameliorating progressive cardiac disease in patients with carcinoid syndrome. A key element of management is relief of stenotic lesions of the tricuspid and pulmonary valves. This may be achieved with either *balloon valvuloplasty* or surgery, both of which can achieve symptomatic relief. Operative mortality is traditionally high, but it has improved significantly in experienced centers.[52]

ARRHYTHMOGENIC RIGHT VENTRICULAR DYSPLASIA/CARDIOMYOPATHY

Arrhythmogenic right ventricular dysplasia/cardiomyopathy (ARVD/C), first described in 1977 by Fontaine and coworkers, is a genetic form of cardiomyopathy characterized prototypically by fibrofatty infiltration of the right ventricle (**Figures 20-9** and **20-10**). ARVD/C accounts for 20% of cases of sudden cardiac death, and, importantly, the prevalence of this condition is higher among young athletes dying suddenly.[54,55]

Presenting Symptoms and Natural History

Patients typically present between the teenage years to their forties, with only 10% falling outside of this age range. The natural history of the disorder is characterized by four phases—a concealed phase in which patients are asymptomatic, a phase characterized by an overt clinical manifestation of an electrical system disturbance, progression to signs and symptoms of right ventricular failure, and finally frank biventricular congestive heart failure. Accordingly, presenting symptoms range from palpitations to syncope and sudden cardiac death. A majority of patients who subsequently experience sudden cardiac death have a history

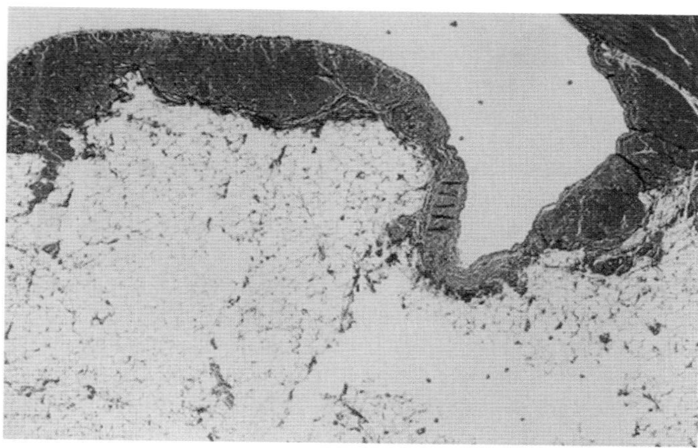

FIGURE 20-9 Arrhythmogenic right ventricular dysplasia/cardiomyopathy (ARVD/C). Histologic appearance of ARVD/C showing fibrosis, adipose infiltration, and myocardial thinning. *Modified from Hare JM: Etiologic basis of congestive heart failure. In Colucci WS, editor: Atlas of heart failure, ed 5, Philadelphia, 2008, Current Medicine LLC, pp 29–56; Hare JM: The dilated and restrictive cardiomyopathies. In Bonow RL, et al, editors: Braunwald's heart disease, ed 9, Philadelphia, 2011, Elsevier, pp 1561–1581.*

of syncope, which thus represents an important prognostic event.[55] Progression to heart failure occurs in the minority of patients, but is the predominant mode of death in individuals who are protected from sudden cardiac death by ICD implantation.

Pathology

Characteristically, a heart affected with ARVD/C exhibits fatty or fibrofatty replacement of the myocardium predominantly affecting the right ventricle. Rarely the process extends to the left ventricles.

Genetics

Several genes and gene loci are associated with ARVD/C, and both autosomal dominant and recessive modes of inheritance are described. Most but not all genes encode for desmosomal proteins.[56] Implicated genes include desmoplakin, junctional plakoglobin (JUP), the cardiac ryanodine receptor, plakophilin-2 (PKP2), and transforming growth factor-b3. JUP mutations are causally implicated in

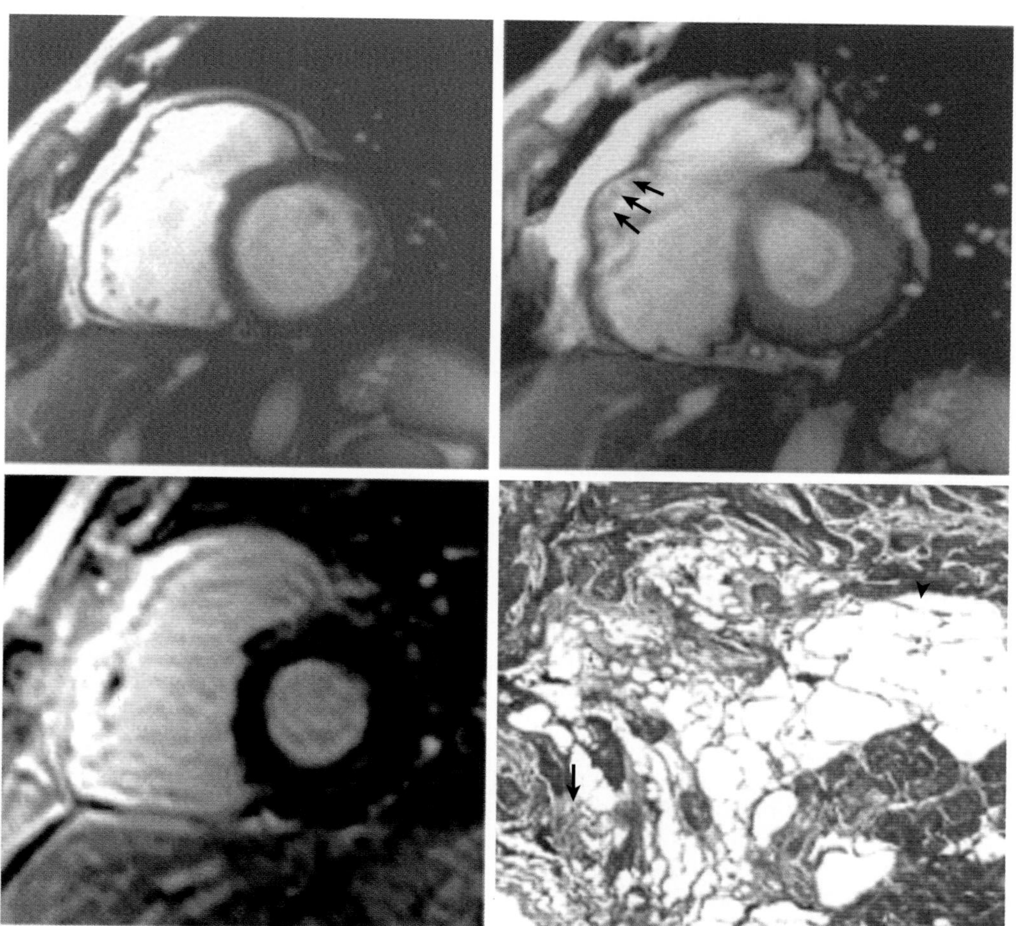

FIGURE 20-10 Arrhythmogenic right ventricular dysplasia/cardiomyopathy (ARVD/C). The *top left* and *right* panels represent the end-diastolic and end-systolic frames of a short-axis cine magnetic resonance image (MRI) showing an area of dyskinesia on right ventricular (RV) free wall characterizing a focal ventricular aneurysm *(arrows).* The *bottom left* panel displays the delayed-enhanced MRI with increased signal intensity within the RV myocardium *(arrows)* at the location of RV aneurysms. The *bottom right* panel shows the corresponding endomyocardial biopsy. Trichrome stain of the right ventricle at high magnification shows marked replacement of the ventricular muscle by adipose tissue. The adipose tissue cells *(arrowhead)* are irregular in size and infiltrate the ventricular muscle. There is also abundant replacement fibrosis *(arrow).* There is no evidence of inflammation. *Modified from Tandri H, Saranathan M, Rodriguez ER, et al: Noninvasive detection of myocardial fibrosis in arrhythmogenic right ventricular cardiomyopathy using delayed-enhancement magnetic resonance imaging. J Am Coll Cardiol 45:98–103, 2005; Hare JM: The dilated and restrictive cardiomyopathies. In Bonow RL, et al, editors: Braunwald's heart disease, ed 9, Philadelphia, 2011, Elsevier, pp 1561–1581.*

Naxos disease, a syndrome characterized by ARVD/C, wooly hair, and palmoplantar ketoderma. Individuals with mutations in PKP2 present at younger ages and are more likely to have malignant arrhythmias.[54] This finding suggests the prognostic importance of genetic testing for ARVD/C. Additionally, immunohistochemical detection of plakoglobin is proposed to be of value in diagnosis.[56]

Diagnosis

A task force has set diagnostic criteria to aid in the study and characterization of ARVD/C. The diagnostic criteria involve features obtained from imaging, ECG, signal-averaged ECG and histologic criteria, as well as a positive family history and a history of arrhythmias.[57] Early diagnosis of ARVD/C remains challenging. Although endomyocardial biopsy may offer valuable diagnostic information, cardiac MRI is emerging as a more definitive diagnostic tool.[58] The main limitation of endomyocardial biopsy is a high false-negative rate because of sampling error and the fact that the right ventricle septum may lack the characteristic histologic changes; however, immunohistochemical detection of plakoglobin may enhance the value of tissue diagnosis.[56] Tandri and colleagues have reported that characterization of the ventricular wall morphology with delayed enhancement gadolinium MRI correlated well with histologic findings, as well as with inducibility of ventricular tachycardia during electrophysiologic testing.[58]

Management

Patients diagnosed with ARVD/C should receive an ICD. Antiarrhythmic therapy is appropriate before ICD insertion, and in some cases after, in patients who have recurrent ICD firings. Use of an ICD can have an enormous clinical impact in reducing the major cause of mortality in affected individuals. It is also recommended that patients receive neurohormonal blockade with angiotensin-converting enzyme inhibitors and β-adrenoreceptor antagonists. In individuals progressing to overt heart failure, management involves the same principles for the treatment of other forms of cardiomyopathy. Consideration of heart transplantation is indicated for patients with overt biventricular failure.

SUMMARY AND FUTURE PERSPECTIVES

Our current understanding of processes leading to restrictive cardiomyopathy remains incomplete as evidenced by the large percentage of patients who are assigned as having idiopathic disease. One of the most challenging cardiovascular disorders and a leading cause of restrictive cardiomyopathy, cardiac amyloidosis, has recently had a potentially important therapeutic advance, that of using RNA interference technology to halt or reduce the deposition of transthyretin amyloid deposition. This exciting new approach heralds an opportunity to treat a disorder with major morbidity and mortality with no current treatment options. The strong genetic basis of restrictive cardiomyopathies and ARVD/C coupled with high throughput technologies will allow for the possibility of widespread genetic testing of affected individuals and their family members. Genetic testing will also facilitate understanding of which patients have a genetic cause of their disease as opposed to a genetic predisposition to an environmental insult. In addition to genetics, measurement of expressed genes (transcriptomics), microRNA abnormalities, and proteins (proteomics) have the potential to aid in understanding cause, prognosis, and individualized responses to therapy (personalized medicine). A key example of the latter is the attempt to identify patients with a viral cause of cardiomyopathy and treat those patients with appropriate antiviral therapy on the one hand, and those without viral infection with immunosuppressive therapy on the other hand. The most recent advance with significant future implications is the observation that the body, including the bone marrow and the heart, possesses reservoirs of endogenous stem cells regulated in stem cell niches—the discovery of these cells and their niches offers new insights into the causes of restrictive cardiomyopathy and may in the future provide a new therapeutic avenue.

References

1. Ammash NM, Seward JB, Bailey KR, et al: Clinical profile and outcome of idiopathic restrictive cardiomyopathy. *Circulation* 101:2490–2496, 2000.
2. Sharma N, Howlett J: Current state of cardiac amyloidosis. *Curr Opin Cardiol* 28:242–248, 2013.
3. Dec GW, Fuster V: Idiopathic dilated cardiomyopathy. *N Engl J Med* 331:1564–1575, 1994.
4. Mocumbi AO, Ferreira MB, Sidi D, et al: A population study of endomyocardial fibrosis in a rural area of Mozambique. *N Engl J Med* 359:43–49, 2008.
5. Rutakingirwa M, Ziegler JL, Newton R, et al: Poverty and eosinophilia are risk factors for endomyocardial fibrosis (Emf) in Uganda. *Trop Med Int Health* 4:229–235, 1999.
6. Seth S, Thatai D, Sharma S, et al: Clinico-pathological evaluation of restrictive cardiomyopathy (endomyocardial fibrosis and idiopathic restrictive cardiomyopathy) in India. *Eur J Heart Fail* 6:723–729, 2004.
7. Hare JM: The etiologic basis of congestive heart failure. In Colucci WS, editor: *Atlas of heart failure*, Philadelphia, 2008, Current Medicine LLC, pp 29–56.
8. Zwas DR, Gotsman I, Admon D, et al: Advances in the differentiation of constrictive pericarditis and restrictive cardiomyopathy. *Herz* 37:664–673, 2012.
9. Rapezzi C, Merlini G, Quarta CC, et al: Systemic cardiac amyloidoses: disease profiles and clinical courses of the 3 main types. *Circulation* 120:1203–1212, 2009.
10. Felker GM, Thompson RE, Hare JM, et al: Underlying causes and long-term survival in patients with initially unexplained cardiomyopathy. *N Engl J Med* 342:1077–1084, 2000.
11. Cooper LT, Baughman KL, Feldman AM, et al, American Heart Association, American College of Cardiology, European Society of Cardiology: The role of endomyocardial biopsy in the management of cardiovascular disease: a scientific statement from the American Heart Association, the American College of Cardiology, and the European Society of Cardiology. *Circulation* 116:2216–2233, 2007.
12. Falk RH: Diagnosis and management of the cardiac amyloidoses. *Circulation* 112:2047–2060, 2005.
13. Ha JW, Ommen SR, Tajik AJ, et al: Differentiation of constrictive pericarditis from restrictive cardiomyopathy using mitral annular velocity by tissue doppler echocardiography. *Am J Cardiol* 94:316–319, 2004.
14. Leya FS, Arab D, Joyal D, et al: The efficacy of brain natriuretic peptide levels in differentiating constrictive pericarditis from restrictive cardiomyopathy. *J Am Coll Cardiol* 45:1900–1902, 2005.
15. Jacobson DR, Pastore RD, Yaghoubian R, et al: Variant-sequence transthyretin (isoleucine 122) in late-onset cardiac amyloidosis in Black Americans. *N Engl J Med* 336:466–473, 1997.
16. Ng B, Connors LH, Davidoff R, et al: Senile systemic amyloidosis presenting with heart failure: a comparison with light chain-associated amyloidosis. *Arch Intern Med* 165:1425–1429, 2005.
17. Wang AK, Fealey RD, Gehrking TL, et al: Patterns of neuropathy and autonomic failure in patients with amyloidosis. *Mayo Clin Proc* 83:1226–1230, 2008.
18. Maceira AM, Joshi J, Prasad SK, et al: Cardiovascular magnetic resonance in cardiac amyloidosis. *Circulation* 111:186–193, 2005.
19. Rahman JE, Helou EF, Gelzer-Bell R, et al: Noninvasive diagnosis of biopsy-proven cardiac amyloidosis. *J Am Coll Cardiol* 43:410–415, 2004.
20. Palladini G, Merlini G: Current treatment of Al amyloidosis. *Haematologica* 94:1044–1048, 2009.
21. Sack FU, Kristen A, Goldschmidt H, et al: Treatment options for severe cardiac amyloidosis: heart transplantation combined with chemotherapy and stem cell transplantation for patients with Al-amyloidosis and heart and liver transplantation for patients with attr-amyloidosis. *Eur J Cardiothorac Surg* 33:257–262, 2008.
22. Delahaye N, Rouzet F, Sarda L, et al: Impact of liver transplantation on cardiac autonomic denervation in familial amyloid polyneuropathy. *Medicine (Baltimore)* 85:229–238, 2006.
23. Coelho T, Adams D, Silva A, et al: Safety and efficacy of RNAi therapy for transthyretin amyloidosis. *N Engl J Med* 369:819–829, 2013.
24. Pieroni M, Chimenti C, De Cobelli F, et al: Fabry's disease cardiomyopathy: echocardiographic detection of endomyocardial glycosphingolipid compartmentalization. *J Am Coll Cardiol* 47:1663–1671, 2006.
25. Sheppard MN, Cane P, Florio R, et al: A detailed pathologic examination of heart tissue from three older patients with Anderson-Fabry disease on enzyme replacement therapy. *Cardiovasc Pathol* 19:293–301, 2010.
26. Glass RB, Astrin KH, Norton KI, et al: Fabry disease: renal sonographic and magnetic resonance imaging findings in affected males and carrier females with the classic and cardiac variant phenotypes. *J Comput Assist Tomogr* 28:158–168, 2004.
27. Imbriaco M, Pisani A, Spinelli L, et al: Effects of enzyme-replacement therapy in patients with Anderson-Fabry disease: a prospective long-term cardiac magnetic resonance imaging study. *Heart* 95:1103–1107, 2009.
28. Thompson RB, Chow K, Khan A, et al: T1 mapping with cardiovascular MRI is highly sensitive for Fabry disease independent of hypertrophy and sex. *Circ Cardiovasc Imaging.* 6:637–645, 2013.
29. Pisani A, Visciano B, Roux GD, et al: Enzyme replacement therapy in patients with Fabry disease: state of the art and review of the literature. *Mol Genet Metab* 107:267–275, 2012.

30. Thurberg BL, Fallon JT, Mitchell R, et al: Cardiac microvascular pathology in Fabry disease: evaluation of endomyocardial biopsies before and after enzyme replacement therapy. *Circulation* 119:2561–2567, 2009.
31. Elstein D, Zimran A: Review of the safety and efficacy of imiglucerase treatment of Gaucher disease. *Biologics.* 3:407–417, 2009.
32. Hoffbrand AV: Diagnosing myocardial iron overload. *Eur Heart J* 22:2140–2141, 2001.
33. Ptaszek LM, Price ET, Hu MY, et al: Early diagnosis of hemochromatosis-related cardiomyopathy with magnetic resonance imaging. *J Cardiovasc Magn Reson* 7:689–692, 2005.
34. Caines AE, Kpodonu J, Massad MG, et al: Cardiac transplantation in patients with iron overload cardiomyopathy. *J Heart Lung Transplant* 24:486–488, 2005.
35. Okura Y, Dec GW, Hare JM, et al: A clinical and histopathologic comparison of cardiac sarcoidosis and idiopathic giant cell myocarditis. *J Am Coll Cardiol* 41:322–329, 2003.
36. Cooper LT, Jr, Hare JM, Tazelaar HD, et al: Usefulness of immunosuppression for giant cell myocarditis. *Am J Cardiol* 102:1535–1539, 2008.
37. Koplan BA, Soejima K, Baughman K, et al: Refractory ventricular tachycardia secondary to cardiac sarcoid: electrophysiologic characteristics, mapping, and ablation. *Heart Rhythm* 3:924–929, 2006.
38. Ardehali H, Howard DL, Hariri A, et al: A positive endomyocardial biopsy result for sarcoid is associated with poor prognosis in patients with initially unexplained cardiomyopathy. *Am Heart J* 150:459–463, 2005.
39. Smedema JP, Snoep G, van Kroonenburgh MP, et al: Evaluation of the accuracy of gadolinium-enhanced cardiovascular magnetic resonance in the diagnosis of cardiac sarcoidosis. *J Am Coll Cardiol* 45:1683–1690, 2005.
40. Pela G, Tirabassi G, Pattoneri P, et al: Cardiac involvement in the Churg-Strauss syndrome. *Am J Cardiol* 97:1519–1524, 2006.
41. Hassan WM, Fawzy ME, Al Helaly S, et al: Pitfalls in diagnosis and clinical, echocardiographic, and hemodynamic findings in endomyocardial fibrosis: a 25-year experience. *Chest* 128:3985–3992, 2005.
42. Marijon E, Ou P: What do we know about endomyocardial fibrosis in children of Africa? *Pediatr Cardiol* 27:523–524, 2006.
43. Barretto AC, Mady C, Nussbacher A, et al: Atrial fibrillation in endomyocardial fibrosis is a marker of worse prognosis. *Int J Cardiol* 67:19–25, 1998.
44. Barretto AC, Mady C, Oliveira SA, et al: Clinical meaning of ascites in patients with endomyocardial fibrosis. *Arq Bras Cardiol* 78:196–199, 2002.
45. Joshi R, Abraham S, Kumar AS: New approach for complete endocardiectomy in left ventricular endomyocardial fibrosis. *J Thorac Cardiovasc Surg* 125:40–42, 2003.
46. Moraes F, Lapa C, Hazin S, et al: Surgery for endomyocardial fibrosis revisited. *Eur J Cardiothorac Surg* 15:309–312, discussion 312–303, 1999.
47. Cherian SM, Jagannath BR, Nayar S, et al: Successful reoperation after 17 years in a case of endomyocardial fibrosis. *Ann Thorac Surg* 82:1115–1117, 2006.
48. Fiore A, Grande AM, Pellegrini C, et al: Long-term survival following surgery for endomyocardial fibrosis. *J Card Surg* 28:675–677, 2013.
49. Mocumbi AO, Falase AO: Recent advances in the epidemiology, diagnosis and treatment of endomyocardial fibrosis in Africa. *Heart* 99:1481–1487, 2013.
50. Corradi D, Tchana B, Miller D, et al: Dilated form of endocardial fibroelastosis as a result of deficiency in respiratory-chain complexes I and IV. *Circulation* 120:e38–e40, 2009.
51. Perez MH, Boulos T, Stucki P, et al: Placental immaturity, endocardial fibroelastosis and fetal hypoxia. *Fetal Diagn Ther* 26:107–110, 2009.
52. Moller JE, Pellikka PA, Bernheim AM, et al: Prognosis of carcinoid heart disease: analysis of 200 cases over two decades. *Circulation* 112:3320–3327, 2005.
53. Bastarrika G, Cao MG, Cano D, et al: Magnetic resonance imaging diagnosis of carcinoid heart disease. *J Comput Assist Tomogr* 29:756–759, 2005.
54. Dalal D, Molin LH, Piccini J, et al: Clinical features of arrhythmogenic right ventricular dysplasia/cardiomyopathy associated with mutations in plakophilin-2. *Circulation* 113:1641–1649, 2006.
55. Dalal D, Nasir K, Bomma C, et al: Arrhythmogenic right ventricular dysplasia: a United States experience. *Circulation* 112:3823–3832, 2005.
56. Asimaki A, Tandri H, Huang H, et al: A new diagnostic test for arrhythmogenic right ventricular cardiomyopathy. *N Engl J Med* 360:1075–1084, 2009.
57. Marcus FI, Zareba W, Calkins H, et al: Arrhythmogenic right ventricular cardiomyopathy/dysplasia clinical presentation and diagnostic evaluation: results from the North American multidisciplinary study. *Heart Rhythm* 6:984–992, 2009.
58. Tandri H, Saranathan M, Rodriguez ER, et al: Noninvasive detection of myocardial fibrosis in arrhythmogenic right ventricular cardiomyopathy using delayed-enhancement magnetic resonance imaging. *J Am Coll Cardiol* 45:98–103, 2005.

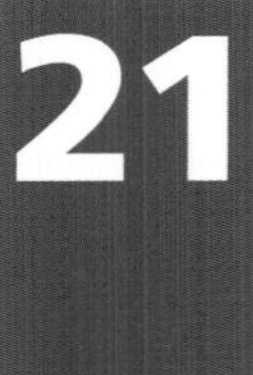

Heart Failure as a Consequence of Hypertrophic Cardiomyopathy

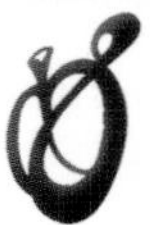

Ali J. Marian

Since the first description of hypertrophic cardiomyopathy (HCM) by the French pathologists Hallopeau and Liouville in the nineteenth century, HCM has intrigued various experts from pathologists to clinicians and more recently geneticists and interventional cardiologists. The continued interest in HCM has largely paralleled technological advances in medicine. Accordingly, HCM was primarily a pathologic entity for the first half of the twentieth century.[1,2] It was largely unrecognized as a clinical entity until the second half of the twentieth century.[3-5] During the latter era, phenotypic description of HCM followed the development of modern diagnostic tools, such as cardiac catheterization and echocardiography. Braunwald and colleagues coined the term *idiopathic hypertrophic subaortic stenosis* (IHSS) in the 1960s and provided the first comprehensive hemodynamic characteristics of left ventricular (LV) outflow tract obstruction in patients with HCM.[6-8] Hence, HCM was mainly recognized as a disease characterized by outflow tract obstruction. The recognition of outflow tract obstruction as a major phenotypic feature of HCM soon led to the description of surgical septal myectomy through a transaortic approach as an effective technique to reduce the outflow tract obstruction, a procedure that is widely known as the Morrow procedure.[9] More recently, Sigwart introduced catheter-based septal ablation typically performed through injection of alcohol into the septal branches of the left anterior descending coronary artery.[10] Surgical myectomy, as well as alcohol septal ablation, are both very effective in reducing the LV outflow tract gradient and improving symptoms.

The widespread use of M mode and two-dimensional echocardiography in the 1970s expanded the phenotypic spectrum of HCM beyond the obstructive form to include concentric LV hypertrophy and asymmetric septal hypertrophy (ASH).[11] Soon Doppler echocardiography emerged as a robust noninvasive method to demonstrate and quantify the LV flow tract obstruction and to characterize cardiac diastolic dysfunction in HCM.[12-14] In recent years tissue Doppler imaging (TDI) has been applied to demonstrate myocardial dysfunction, despite preserved global systolic function, and to show potential utility of TDI in an early and preclinical diagnosis of HCM independent of the expression of cardiac hypertrophy.[15,16]

Seidman and associates discovered the first causal gene for HCM in 1990 and ushered in the era of molecular genetics.[17,18] The discovery was a watershed event because it was soon followed by identification of over a dozen causal genes and several hundred mutations and modifier loci.[19] These advances in the molecular genetic basis of HCM have raised interest in genetic-based screening, diagnosis, and risk stratification. However, it has also become clear that the phenotype in HCM is complex and determined not only by the causal mutations but also by the modifier genes and various other genetic, genomic, and nongenetic factors.

HCM is a relatively benign disease.[20-22] Nevertheless, sudden cardiac death (SCD) has always been the main concern of the patients and physicians alike. The concern is highlighted by the fact that HCM is a major cause of SCD in the young and that SCD often occurs in apparently healthy and asymptomatic individuals.[23,24] The difficult challenge is in appropriate risk stratification and identification of the subgroup of individuals who are at high risk for SCD. The challenge is further compounded not only by the tragic nature of SCD in the apparently healthy and athletic individuals but also by the unproven effectiveness of the conventional pharmacologic interventions. Although such interventions are effective for symptomatic relief, they have not been shown to reduce the risk of SCD. Thus intervention to prevent SCD is primarily limited to the effective use of implantable defibrillators in those who are at high risk for SCD.[25]

Recent experimental data in animal models of HCM have raised the potential utility of new pharmacologic and nonpharmacologic interventions in prevention and regression of cardiac phenotype and possibly reducing the risk of cardiac arrhythmias.[26-28] Large-scale randomized clinical studies are needed to test the potential utility of such new interventions in reversing, attenuating, or preventing cardiac phenotype in HCM, and hence reducing the risk of SCD.

DEFINITION

HCM is a genetic disease of cardiac myocytes. Thus it is primarily a disease of the myocardium. Clinically, HCM is diagnosed by the presence of primary cardiac hypertrophy (i.e., cardiac hypertrophy that cannot be fully explained by the loading conditions, valvular diseases, or other external factors). Typically the LV cavity is normal or even small in size because of concentric hypertrophy, and global LV systolic function is normal or even hyperdynamic.[29] Pathologically, HCM is also defined primarily based on the presence of myocyte disarray, with and without hypertrophy. However, it is not practical to perform endomyocardial biopsy on a routine basis to diagnose HCM. Moreover, diagnostic performance of myocyte disarray, in the absence of cardiac hypertrophy, in an accurate diagnosis of HCM remains to be substantiated.

Diagnostic Challenges

Clinical diagnosis, typically based on the echocardiographic findings of cardiac hypertrophy, is usually straightforward. However, expression of cardiac hypertrophy, the clinical diagnostic hallmark of HCM, is age-dependent. It is typically absent during the first decade of life but its development accelerates during puberty and growth spurt.[30] Left ventricular hypertrophy is expressed in approximately 50% and 75% of those with underlying causal mutations by the third and fifth decades of life, respectively.[31] In about 5% of the cases with the genetic mutations, cardiac hypertrophy, detected by echocardiography, is first expressed after the age of 50 years. The electrocardiogram (ECG) is typically abnormal in those with established HCM. In the familial settings, ECG abnormalities might offer the first clue to identification of the affected family members.

There are a number of clinical diagnostic challenges. The most common is the presence of systemic arterial hypertension, which affects approximately one third of the adult population in the United States. Therefore, it may exist concomitantly in patients with HCM. In the presence of systemic hypertension, mild LV hypertrophy, defined as a maximum LV wall thickness of less than 15 mm, does not offer robust evidence of HCM, because the hypertrophy might be secondary to hypertension alone. On the other end of the spectrum, patients with systemic hypertension might exhibit a disproportionate hypertrophic response, namely exhibiting severe hypertrophy in the presence of mild or controlled systemic hypertension. Such patients who may have an underlying genetic variant(s) might exaggerate the hypertrophic response or a variant that causes HCM. In the latter scenario, systemic hypertension might contribute to phenotypic expression of cardiac hypertrophy in HCM. Conventionally, the presence of uncontrolled systemic hypertension or even valvular abnormalities hampers the firm diagnosis of HCM but should not be considered a definitive exclusion criterion for HCM.

A similar dilemma is often encountered in competitive professional athletes who exhibit significant cardiac hypertrophy, hence necessitating the distinction between pathologic hypertrophy of HCM and physiologic hypertrophy of exercise. Cardiac hypertrophy with a wall thickness of 13 to 15 mm is not uncommon in such athletes. The distinction between physiologic and pathologic hypertrophy is crucial because HCM is the most common discernible cause of SCD in professional athletes and its diagnosis typically forbids athletes from participating in competitive sports. Clinical clues such as the extent, severity, and type of cardiac hypertrophy, hyperdynamic left ventricle, small LV cavity size, presence of outflow tract obstruction, and TDI or cardiac magnetic resonance (CMR) abnormalities of the myocardium could help to differentiate true HCM from other hypertrophic conditions. An ECG might also help to distinguish pathologic and physiologic hypertrophy of athletes. The presence of abnormal Q waves, axis deviation, left atrial enlargement, conduction defects, and severe repolarization abnormalities typically suggests pathologic cardiac hypertrophy.[32]

The clinical diagnosis of HCM based on the presence of primary cardiac hypertrophy is also compounded by the phenocopy conditions, which are diseases that cause gross cardiac hypertrophy and mimic HCM. Phenocopy conditions include various storage diseases, mitochondrial diseases, triplet repeat syndromes, and others.[33,34] The distinction between true HCM and phenocopy conditions is important because their pathogenesis and treatment differ significantly. The clinical distinction, however, is often difficult, because expression of gross cardiac hypertrophy is very similar between true HCM and its phenocopy conditions. Phenotypic features, such as the presence of a hyperdynamic left ventricle and outflow tract obstruction, would favor the diagnosis of true HCM but are not conclusive evidence. In contrast, the presence of depressed global cardiac systolic function, cardiac dilation, conduction defects, or involvement of other organs, such as deafness, neurologic abnormalities, and skeletal myopathy, suggest the possibility of a phenocopy condition. It might be necessary to perform endomyocardial biopsy for histologic examination. Detection of myocyte disarray, which is considered the pathologic hallmark of true HCM, would help to distinguish true HCM from a phenocopy condition. Likewise, specific histologic staining of myocardial sections could help to diagnosis storage diseases. As an example, the phenocopy condition caused by mutations in the $\gamma 2$ subunit of adenosine monophosphate kinase (AMPK) is due to storage of glycogen in the heart.[34-36] The phenotype is characterized by cardiac hypertrophy, conduction defect, and a preexcitation pattern on electrocardiogram. Finally, genetic-based diagnosis might help to provide a clear distinction between true HCM and phenocopy conditions. With advances in the molecular genetic basis of HCM and the phenocopy conditions, one would expect genetic-based screening, under specific circumstances, to provide for a robust distinction between true HCM and its phenocopy. The genetic-based distinction is gaining increasing clinical utility with the development of new specific treatments for HCM and phenocopy conditions.

The shortcomings of the current clinical diagnosis of HCM, which is primarily based on echocardiographic finding of "unexplained" cardiac hypertrophy, have raised the interest in genetic-based diagnosis. Genetic-based diagnosis in the familial setting is expected to provide the opportunity for the preclinical diagnosis of those with the causal mutations. Genetic-based diagnosis not only provides the opportunity for an early diagnosis but could also have considerable implications for early interventions to prevent the evolution of the phenotype, as well as the risk of SCD. However, for the genetic-based diagnosis to supplant the clinical diagnosis of HCM and become routine, further advances in our understanding of the genetic causes of HCM and in the cost of genetic screening would be necessary. A major challenge, particularly in the sporadic cases and in small families, is the distinction between the pathogenic variant and those variants that are either innocuous or simply contribute to expression of the disease but are not the true causal variants. Despite the apparent advantages of genetic-based diagnosis and intervention, phenotypic variability of HCM, even in those with an identical causal mutation, and the complexity of factors that determine the clinical outcome limit the clinical utility of genetic-based risk stratification. Thus clinical decision making in the management of the patients with HCM should comprise all constituents of the determinants of the phenotype, whether genetic, genomic, or environmental.

PREVALENCE

HCM is a relatively common disease with an estimated prevalence of approximately 1:500 in the general population.[37] The estimate was based on the presence of LV wall thickness of 15 mm or greater on an echocardiogram in a relatively young population between the ages of 23 and 35 years. The true prevalence of HCM might be even higher because of the previously discussed diagnostic criteria used to define HCM. Many patients with the causal mutations may express a milder degree of cardiac hypertrophy. Likewise, young individuals with the causal mutations may not yet exhibit the phenotype because of age-dependent expression of the phenotype. Thus prevalence of HCM might be even higher in an older population. Another caveat is the potential presence of concomitant systemic hypertension, which by definition, in most situations, excludes the diagnosis of HCM. The prevalence estimate, however, might include those with the phenocopy conditions, defined as conditions that grossly are similar to HCM but are not true HCM because their pathogenesis differs significantly. The prevalence of phenocopy conditions in those with the clinical diagnosis of HCM is unknown but may comprise a significant number of all cases diagnosed clinically as HCM. Thus, to determine the precise prevalence of true HCM, large-scale genetic studies in conjunction with clinical studies will be needed.

PHENOTYPIC MANIFESTATIONS

Clinical Presentation

Patients with HCM exhibit a diverse array of clinical phenotypes, ranging from a benign asymptomatic course to that of severe diastolic heart failure and SCD. Most patients with HCM are asymptomatic or mildly symptomatic. The most common symptoms are dyspnea, which typically occurs upon exertion; chest pain, which is atypical for being of coronary origin; and palpitations, light-headedness, and less frequently syncope. Syncope is usually due to cardiac arrhythmias and less frequently due to hypotension and autonomic dysfunction. Recurrent syncope often is a major predictor of SCD and merits full evaluation and treatment.[38,39] Supraventricular arrhythmias including atrial fibrillation, as well as ventricular arrhythmias, are the most common cardiac arrhythmias and are important determinants of clinical outcomes.[40,41] Likewise, a small subgroup of patients with HCM exhibits electrocardiographic findings of Wolff-Parkinson-White (WPW) syndrome and therefore may develop AV nodal reciprocating arrhythmias. Presence of the electrocardiographic pattern of preexcitation might suggest a phenocopy condition.[35,36] Atrial fibrillation, which occurs in approximately 20% to 25% of patients, poses significant challenges in the management of patients with HCM.[40,42,43] Not only the rapid heart rate but also the loss of atrial contraction, which in HCM contributes significantly to atrial filling, leads to increased symptoms of heart failure. Atrial fibrillation also increases the risk of stroke and requires anticoagulation.[42]

The annual mortality of patients with HCM is approximately 1% per year.[20-22] Approximately two thirds of patients with HCM have a normal life expectancy and the remainder develop significant symptoms, predominantly as a result of LV outflow tract obstruction, diastolic dysfunction, atrial fibrillation, or ventricular tachycardia.[20,44,45] Serum concentration of NT-ProBNP is a predictor of overall prognosis and heart failure complications in patients with HCM.[46]

Sudden Cardiac Death in Hypertrophic Cardiomyopathy

Despite the heterogeneity of the clinical phenotype, the most pressing issue for the patients, whether symptomatic or not, and physicians is the risk of SCD. The risk is of particular concern in young competitive athletes because HCM is the most common cause of SCD in this group in the United States.[24,47,48] HCM is responsible for approximately half of the cases of SCD in athletes younger than 35 years of age in the U.S. population.[24,48] This is in contrast to Italy where arrhythmogenic right ventricular cardiomyopathy appears to be the most common cause of SCD in professional athletes.[49] In both conditions the death is tragic, because SCD often occurs as the first manifestation of the disease in apparently young healthy individuals.[24] SCD typically occurs during or immediately after exercise and often on the sport field.

There is no reliable predictor of SCD in HCM. However, several clinical, pathologic, and genetic factors have been identified as major risk factors for SCD in patients with HCM, including a previous episode of cardiac arrest, recurrent syncope, severe cardiac hypertrophy, presence of multiple runs of nonsustained ventricular tachycardia or sustained ventricular tachycardia, and a strong family history of SCD.[50-54] The putative risk factors for SCD in patients with HCM are listed in **Table 21-1**. SCD also may occur in the absence of a discernible risk factor but the overall risk is low. In the risk stratification and counseling of patients with HCM for SCD, it is important to consider the global risk, because the positive predictive value of each putative risk marker is relatively low.[52,53] In general, HCM is a relatively benign disease with an estimated annual mortality of about 1% in the adult population but seems to be higher in children, ranging from 2% to 3%.[20,21,55,56]

Morphologic and Functional Features

Cardiac hypertrophy is the quintessential morphologic phenotype of HCM, although the degree of cardiac hypertrophy may be mild and gross hypertrophy may be absent in a small fraction of patients. Likewise, a typical feature of HCM is the asymmetric nature of cardiac hypertrophy, with the predominant involvement of the interventricular septum.

An interventricular septal to posterior wall thickness ratio of greater than 1.3 is considered a major feature of HCM. However, symmetric cardiac hypertrophy involving the interventricular septum and the posterior wall occurs in approximately one third of the cases. In a small group of patients, cardiac hypertrophy is localized to the apex, lateral wall, or posterior wall.[57] Right ventricular involvement is uncommon, variable in severity, and rarely leads to right ventricular outflow tract obstruction.[58] Patients with apical HCM may exhibit the unique phenotype of giant T wave inversion in the precordial leads on an electrocardiogram. Patients with apical HCM may experience significant cardiovascular morbidity but have a relatively benign prognosis with a 15-year survival rate of approximately 95%.[59]

The LV cavity size is usually small or at least not dilated. The LV outflow tract is often narrow. Systolic anterior motion (SAM) of the anterior leaflet of the mitral valve could obstruct the blood flow through the narrow outflow tract and lead to a pressure gradient across the outflow tract. In a small fraction of patients, the mitral valve may have anatomic malposition and/or an elongated anterior leaflet. The left ventricle is typically hyperdynamic and LV ejection fraction, a global index of systolic function, is usually increased or preserved. More sensitive indices of LV regional function such as tissue Doppler velocities show impaired myocardial systolic and diastolic function.[16] The typical feature of HCM is impaired cardiac diastolic function and elevated LV end-diastolic pressure, which is the primary reason for symptoms of heart failure in HCM (**Figure 21-1**). Occasionally the phenotype of HCM (i.e., concentric cardiac hypertrophy with a hyperdynamic left ventricle) evolves into the phenotype of dilated cardiomyopathy (DCM).

Left ventricular outflow tract (LVOT) obstruction at rest is present in approximately 25% of patients with HCM (see Figure 21-1). The obstruction is in part caused by anatomic narrowing of the LVOT because of septal as well as subaortic hypertrophy and in part by dynamic obstruction due to a hyperdynamic left ventricle with a small cavity and SAM of the mitral valve leaflet. LVOT gradient could be provoked using amyl nitrate, exercise, or dobutamine in most patients with HCM. The presence of LVOT obstruction is associated with significant mortality and morbidity in patients with HCM.[60] The LVOT obstruction has characteristic LV systolic pressure peripheral pulse waveforms, with two components of early and late systolic waves, the latter referred to as a *bifid pulse*.

TABLE 21-1 Potential Risk Factors for SCD in Patients with HCM

Established Risk Factors
• Prior episode of cardiac arrest (aborted SCD)
• Family history of SCD (more than one premature SCD)
• Causal mutations, including double mutations
• Modifier genes
• History of syncope
• Sustained and repetitive nonsustained ventricular tachycardia
• Severe cardiac hypertrophy
Probable Risk Factors
• Left ventricular outflow tract obstruction
• Abnormal blood pressure response to exercise
• Severe interstitial fibrosis and myocyte disarray
• Early onset of clinical manifestations (young age)
• Presence of myocardial ischemia

Histopathologic Features

Cardiac myocyte hypertrophy with pleiotropic nuclei is a common histologic feature. However, the histopathologic hallmark of HCM is cardiac myocyte disarray, which is defined as malaligned, distorted, and often short and hypertrophic myocytes oriented in different directions (**Figure 21-2**). Disarray may comprise 20% to 30% of the myocardium as opposed to less than 5% of the myocardium in

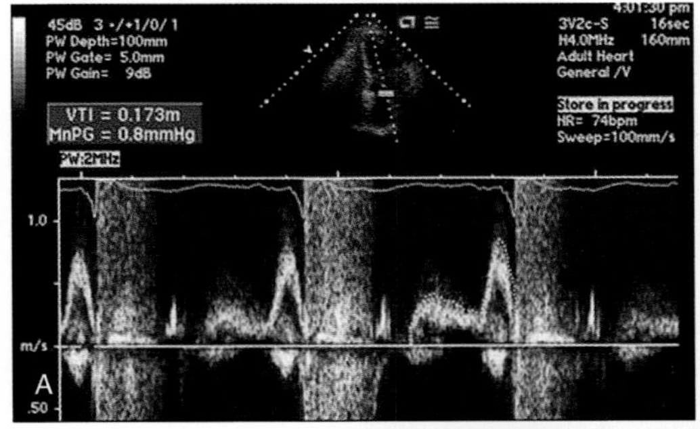

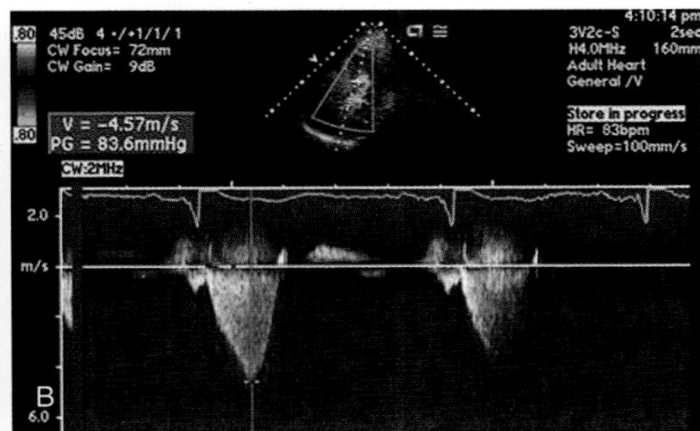

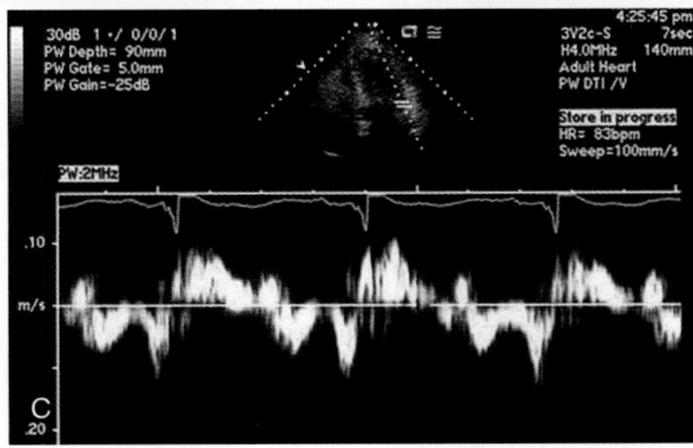

FIGURE 21-1 Echo/Doppler evaluation of cardiac function in a patient with hypertrophic cardiomyopathy (HCM) and severe outflow tract obstruction. **A,** Mitral inflow velocities showing diastolic dysfunction evidenced by decreased E and increased A velocities. **B,** Doppler measurement of left ventricular outflow tract gradient, which is about 80 mm Hg. **C,** Reduced systolic and early diastolic velocities, which are early markers for HCM.

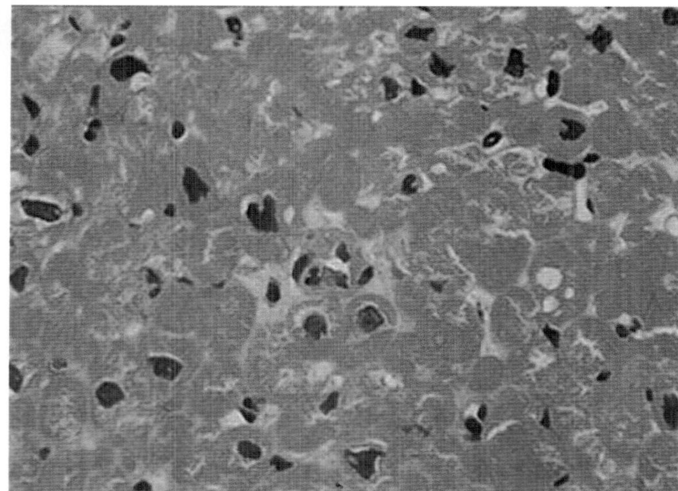

FIGURE 21-2 H&E-stained thin myocardial section from a patient with hypertrophic cardiomyopathy who died suddenly. There is altered myocardial architecture with evidence of myocyte hypertrophy and disarray.

normal hearts.[61] Myocyte disarray might also be found in patients with congenital heart diseases.[62] Myocyte disarray in HCM is commonly found throughout the myocardium but is considered more remarkable in the interventricular septum. Myocyte disarray is associated with the risk of SCD in young patients with HCM.[63]

Interstitial fibrosis is also a common feature of HCM and is associated with cardiac arrhythmias and heart failure.[63,64] Late gadolinium enhancement on CMR images, which is considered a marker for interstitial fibrosis, is present in approximately two thirds of HCM patients.[65] Plasma concentrations of collagens, such as procollagen I and III N-terminal peptides or C-terminal propeptide of type I procollagen, have been used as biomarkers for an early diagnosis of HCM but do not seem to reliably reflect interstitial fibrosis or myocardial collagen content.[66-68] The circulating level of microRNA 29a, a marker for hypertrophy and fibrosis, is also elevated in patients with HCM.[69] Other histopathologic phenotypes include a subaortic thickening of the endocardium, further compromising the outflow tract; thickening of media of intramural coronary arteries; malpositioned mitral valve; and elongated leaflets. Histopathologic phenotypes, such as myocyte disarray, hypertrophy, and interstitial fibrosis, are associated with the risk of SCD, mortality, and morbidity in patients with HCM.

MOLECULAR GENETICS

HCM is a monogenic disease, familial in approximately two thirds of cases and sporadic in the remainder. The mode of inheritance in familial HCM is commonly autosomal dominant.[70] Therefore, 50% of the offspring, males and females equally, will inherit the mutation and hence will develop the disease sometime in life. An autosomal recessive mode of inheritance has also been described.[71] Sporadic cases are caused by inheritance of germline *de novo* mutations from the parents.[72] The causal mutation in a sporadic case will be passed on to the offspring of the affected person in an autosomal dominant fashion.

The pioneering work of Dr. Christine Seidman and colleagues led to identification of the first causal mutation, namely the p.R403Q mutation in the *MYH7* gene encoding the sarcomere protein β-myosin heavy chain (MyHC) protein in families with HCM.[17] The discovery was soon followed by identification of mutations in *TNNT2* and *TPM1* genes, coding for cardiac troponin T, and α-tropomyosin proteins, respectively, in families with HCM. Since then more than a dozen causal genes and several hundred mutations in families with HCM have been identified (**Table 21-2**). These discoveries have shown that HCM is a genetically heterogeneous disease typically caused by rare and private mutations in genes encoding sarcomere proteins. Therefore, HCM is considered a disease of sarcomere proteins (**Figure 21-3**).[73] Perhaps clinically diagnosed HCM could be differentiated into those caused by sarcomere protein mutations, which might be considered true HCM, and HCM caused by mutations in nonsarcomere proteins, which are typically the phenocopy conditions such as glycogen storage disorders.

TABLE 21-2 Causal Genes for HCM

	PROTEIN	PREVALENCE
Established Causal Genes		
MYH7	β-Myosin heavy chain	≈25%
MYBPC	Myosin binding protein-C	≈25%
TNNT2	Cardiac troponin T	≈2-5%
TNNI3	Cardiac troponin I	≈2-5%
TPM1	α-tropomyosin	≈2-5%
MYOZ2	Myozenin 2 (calsarcin 1)	1:250
ACTA1	Cardiac α-actin	<1%
TTN	Titin	<1%
MYL3	Essential myosin light chain	<1%
MYL2	Regulatory myosin light chain	<1%
Likely Causal Genes		
TCAP	Tcap (Telethonin or titin-cap)	Rare
PLN	Phospholamban	Rare
CAV3	Caveolin 3	Rare
MYH6	α-Myosin heavy chain	Rare
MYLK2	Cardiac myosin light peptide kinase	Rare
TNNCI	Cardiac troponin C	Rare
TRIM63	Tripartite motif-containing 63	Rare
JPH2	Junctophilin 2	Rare
FHL1	Four-and-a-half LIM domains protein	Rare
ANKRD1	Ankyrin repeat domain 1	Rare
CASQ2	Calsequestrin 2	Rare
CSRP3	Muscle LIM protein	Rare

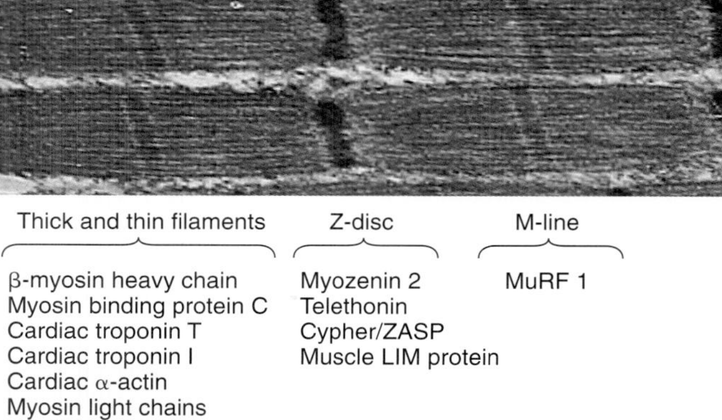

FIGURE 21-3 The vast majority of clinically diagnosed hypertrophic cardiomyopathy is caused by mutations in sarcomeric proteins. Sarcomeres consist of thick and thin filaments and the S disc.

Causal Genes

Causal genes by definition are those that, whenever mutated, cause HCM, albeit with variable penetrance and expressivity. During the past two decades about two thirds of all causal genes for HCM have been identified. The most common causal genes for HCM are *MYH7* and *MYBPC3*, encoding β-MyHC and myosin binding protein C (MyBPC), respectively (see Table 21-2). Each is responsible for approximately 25% of HCM cases.[74-77] Several hundred different mutations in the *MYH7* and *MYBPC3* genes in families and individuals with HCM have been identified. Most *MYH7* mutations are located within the globular head of the β-MyHC, which is the site of ATPase activity, and bind to cardiac α-actin. A few mutations are located in the hinge arm and the rod tail of the β-MyHC.[78,79] Otherwise, there is no obvious predilection toward concentration of the mutations in a specific domain. A noteworthy difference in the *MYH7* and *MYBPC3* mutations is the higher prevalence of insertion/deletion mutations in *MYBPC3*, as opposed to *MYH7*, wherein the vast majority of the mutations are missense mutations. The next most common causal genes are *TNNT2* and *TNNI3*, which encode cardiac troponin T and cardiac troponin I, respectively, with each accounting for approximately 3% to 5% of HCM families.[74,80,81]

There are a large number of uncommon causal genes for HCM, including *TPM1* encoding α-tropomyosin, *ACTC* encoding cardiac α-actin, *TTN* encoding titin, *MYL3* encoding essential myosin light chain, and *MYL2*, which codes for the regulatory myosin light chain.[82-87] The spectrum of causal genes extends beyond the thin and thick filaments of the sarcomere to include genes encoding the Z disc proteins, such as *TCAP* encoding telethonin, *MYOZ2* encoding myozenin 2 or calsarcin 1 and muscle LIM protein (*CSRP3*).[88-90] Finally, mutations in *TNNC1, MYH6, MYLK2, PLN, CAV3,* and *TRIM63* coding for cardiac troponin C, α-MyHC, myosin light chain kinase, phospholamban, caveolin 3, and tripartite motif containing 63 have been reported in patients with HCM (see Table 21-2).[88,91-95] However, most of the latter genes are identified in probands or small families, and hence the causal role of these genes in HCM is less certain.

Most HCM mutations are missense mutations that typically affect a highly conserved amino acid. However, frameshift mutations resulting from an insertion or deletion of one or more nucleotides, as well as splice junction mutations, are also found, more commonly in the *MYBPC3* gene than the other causal genes.[74,76,96] The frameshift mutations typically lead to premature truncation of the protein, which may not be stably expressed.[97] An important point with implications for genetic testing is the low frequency of each causal HCM mutation, and hence most mutations are rare in the population or are "private." Another noteworthy point is the presence of double mutations, which have been reported in a small fraction of patients with HCM but are recognized more often, because systemic screening of many genes is included in genetic analysis.[98,99] A digenic cause of HCM (i.e., two independent mutations causing the disease in a single family) is less certain. Typically one mutation dominates as the causal variant and the second contributes to phenotypic expression of the disease.

An important point in the genetic studies of HCM is the issue of causality, which is often difficult to establish, particularly in sporadic cases or small families whereby the cosegregation of the phenotype with inheritance of the disease cannot be established. It has been stated that "there is no perfect protein," because each protein has a number of polymorphic variants in the population, including nonsynonymous variants. Thus identification of a nonsynonymous variant in an individual with the phenotype is not sufficient to consider the variant as a causal mutation.[100] In accord with this notion, approximately 10% of the general population has one or two rare nonsynonymous variants in genes encoding sarcomere proteins.[101] Nevertheless, the pathogenic variants, which comprise a small fraction of the rare nonsynonymous variants in the population are associated with increased adverse cardiovascular events.[101] To assess the pathogenic role of the variants identified upon genetic screening, several issues have to be considered, the most prominent being cosegregation of the phenotype with inheritance of the variant in the family, whenever applicable. Population frequency of the variant, conservation of the involved amino acid across species, and the biologic and functional effects of variants should be considered.[100,102,103] In the absence of evidence of cosegregation in a family, a functional variant may be considered a "likely disease-causing variant."[102,104] In general, the analogous element of the Koch postulates of causality, partly through experimentation, needs to be fulfilled to consider a variant a disease-causing variant.[102,105]

Modifier Genes

Genetic variants that affect the expression and severity of the phenotype of a single-gene disorder but alone are not sufficient to cause the disease are referred to as the *modifier variants*. Genes containing such variants are referred to as the *modifier genes*. Modifier alleles, unlike causal mutations, are neither necessary nor sufficient to cause HCM. However, when present, they influence phenotypic expression of the disease. In the case of HCM, variants of the modifier genes could influence the severity of cardiac hypertrophy, risk of SCD, and susceptibility to cardiac arrhythmias or heart failure. Modifier genes are partially responsible for the phenotypic variability of HCM.[106] A characteristic feature of HCM is marked phenotypic variability, not only among individuals with different causal mutations, but also among affected members of a given family who share an identical causal mutation (**Figure 21-4**).[106] The influence of the modifier genes on phenotypic expression of HCM is best illustrated in familial HCM, wherein members of the family share an identical causal mutation and yet exhibit significant variation in phenotypic expression.

The interindividual variability in the phenotypic expression of HCM is partially a result of the presence of single-nucleotide polymorphisms or variants (SNPs or SNVs) and structural variants, including copy number variants (CNVs) in the genome. Each genome contains about 4 million SNVs, as compared with the reference genome, and several thousand CNVs.[107,108] Although the CNVs are less frequent in the genome than the SNVs, they affect about three fourths of all variant nucleotides in the genome.[107] These variants, whether SNVs or CNVs, are expected to influence phenotypic expression of HCM, including the severity of cardiac hypertrophy and fibrosis, as well as the risk of SCD.

The modifier genes/variants in HCM are largely unknown. A genome-wide scan in members of a very large family with HCM caused by an insertion mutation in the *MYBPC3* gene led to mapping of five modifier loci that influence

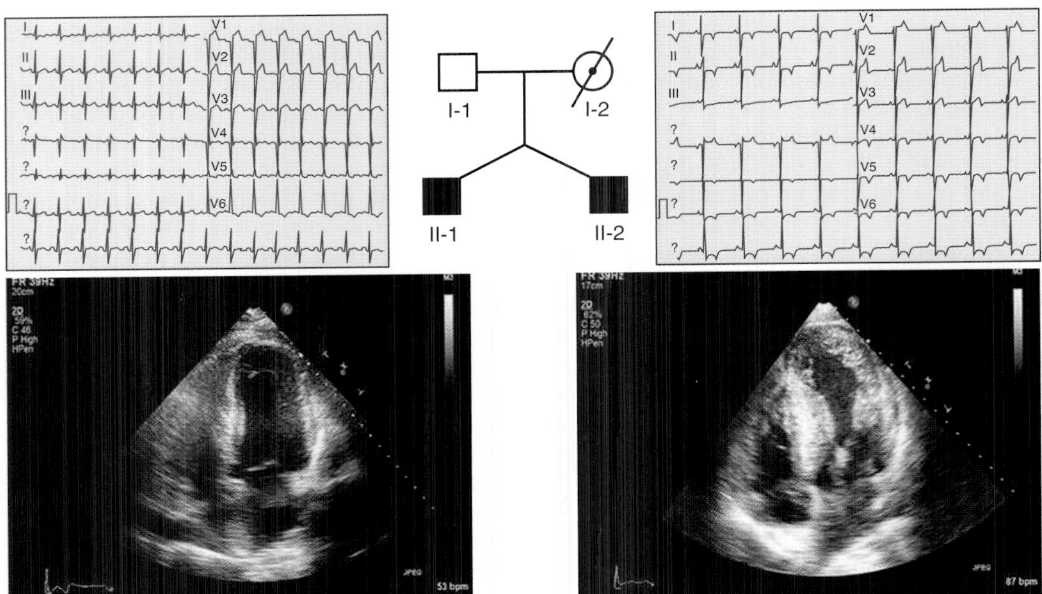

FIGURE 21-4 Phenotypic variability. A truncated pedigree shows twin brothers with hypertrophic cardiomyopathy caused by S48P mutation in *MYOZ2*. There is significant variability in the degree of cardiac hypertrophy on 12-lead electrocardiograms and echocardiograms between the two brothers.

expression of cardiac hypertrophy.[109] The loci, located on 3q26.2 (two separate loci), 10p13, 17q24, and 16q12.2, influenced the magnitude of cardiac hypertrophy in the affected members. The effect sizes of these loci ranged from an approximately 8- to approximately 90-g shift in the LV mass, depending on the heterozygosity or homozygosity of the modifier alleles. The mapped modifier loci encompass several biologically plausible candidate genes, including *GRB2* and *ITGA8*, which have been implicated in modulating cardiac hypertrophy and fibrosis in mice.[110,111] Whether these genes are modifiers of cardiac hypertrophy and fibrosis remains unsettled.

Through candidate gene analysis, several genes have been implicated as the modifiers for cardiac hypertrophy in HCM. Among them is the *ACE*, which encodes the gene for processing angiotensin-I. The insertion/deletion polymorphism in the *ACE*, which is associated with plasma and tissue levels of ACE1,[114] influences the severity of cardiac hypertrophy and the risk of SCD in HCM.[112,113,115] The effect size seems to be modest.[111] *Fhl1* gene encoding 4½ LIM domains protein 1 also has been implicated as a potential modifier of cardiac hypertrophy and function in a mouse model of cardiomyopathy (*Myh6*$^{403/-}$). Transcriptome analysis in this mouse model showed altered 5′ start-site usage of 92 genes, including *Fhl1*. Genetic deletion of *Fhl1* in the background of *Myh6*$^{403/-}$ was associated with worsening of cardiac phenotype.[116] The relevance of these findings to human HCM remains unclear. Overall, given the complexity of the molecular biology of cardiac hypertrophy, a large number of genes are expected to influence phenotypic expression of HCM, each imparting a modest effect on the severity of cardiac hypertrophy or the risk of SCD.

PATHOGENESIS

Identification of the causal genes for HCM has provided the impetus for molecular mechanistic studies to elucidate the molecular pathogenesis of HCM. The precise molecular

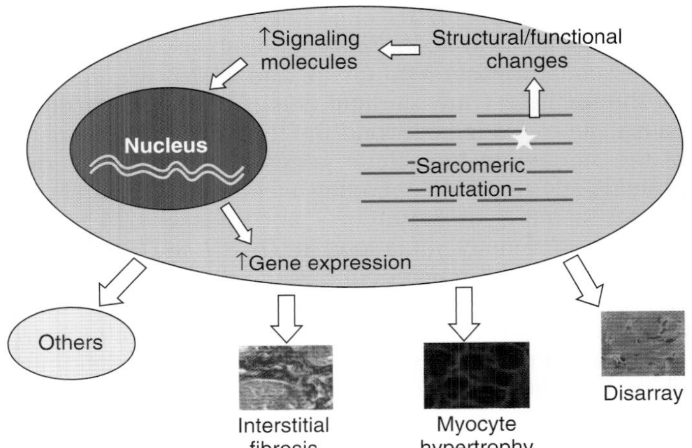

FIGURE 21-5 Pathogenesis of hypertrophic cardiomyopathy (HCM) simplified into three stages of initial structural and functional defects followed by activation of signaling molecules that lead to secondary gene expression, leading to HCM phenotype.

events that link the causal mutations to the clinical or morphologic phenotypes are largely unknown but appear to involve a diverse array of pathways.[117] The link between the genetic mutations and the clinical phenotype could be simplified into three major stages: initial structural and functional defects in the protein encoded by the causal mutation, which affect not only the structure and function of the affected protein but also its interactions with the other proteins (**Figure 21-5**). These initial events of impaired structure, function, and interactions with other proteins are followed by activation of the signaling molecules, which in turn regulate transcriptional programs. Altered transcription and protein expression of a diverse array of genes induce molecular, histologic, and morphologic phenotypes that collectively embody HCM as a clinical phenotype.[117]

The initial functional defects resulting from the mutations are diverse, which is partly reflective of the diversity of the causal genes and mutations and partly the functional diversity of the affected proteins. Among the initial functional defects are altered Ca^{2+} sensitivity of myofibrillar ATPase activity,[118-122] actomyosin cross-bridge kinetics,[123] Ca^{2+} sensitivity of myofibrillar force generation,[124-127] length-dependent activation of sarcomeres,[128] and sarcomere assembly.[129] The initial functional abnormalities impart mechanical, biochemical, and bioenergetic stress on cardiac myocytes and activate a series of stress-responsive signaling molecules that influence gene expression. Consequently, a diverse array of genes are expressed and signaling molecules are activated in response to the causal mutations.[130,131] Myocardial bioenergetic deficit as evidenced by changes in the ratio of cardiac phosphocreatine (PCr) to adenosine triphosphate (ATP) has been implicated as a common intermediary phenotype in HCM.[132-134] Metabolic abnormalities including altered myocardial bioenergetics, however, are common to various forms of cardiac hypertrophy and may be a consequence of cardiac stress.[135,136] Impaired calcium handling also has been observed in patient-specific induced pluripotent stem cells.[137] Other mechanisms may include a direct role for the sarcomere or Z disc proteins in instigating the hypertrophic signaling pathways, such as regulation of the protein phosphatase 2B calcineurin pathway by mutations in the *MYOZ2*.[90,138] Likewise, preferential degradation of the truncated mutant proteins by the ubiquitin-proteasome system (UPS) and targeting of the sarcomere proteins as well as molecules involved in protein synthesis have been implicated in the pathogenesis of HCM.[95,139] The functional defects resulting from the mutant sarcomere proteins are reflected in the whole heart function as evidenced by impaired myocardial contraction and relaxation, which is present before and in the absence of cardiac hypertrophy.[15,140] Thus cardiac hypertrophy and interstitial fibrosis are considered secondary phenotypes resulting from activation of a diverse array of hypertrophic and profibrotic molecules in response to the initial functional defects in the myocytes imparted by the causal mutation. Accordingly, cardiac hypertrophy, the clinical diagnostic phenotype of HCM, and interstitial fibrosis could be potentially reversed upon blockade of the intermediary signaling molecules.

In patients with an autosomal-dominant HCM, only one copy of the causal gene, and hence only half of the sarcomere protein, is expected to be mutated. Therefore, in HCM caused by missense mutations, which encompass most of the cases, the mutant protein is expected to exert a dominant-negative effect to express the phenotype (poison-peptide hypothesis). The variant nucleotide might also affect sub-optimal codon usage and affect expression of the mutant protein.[141] Therefore, the mutant protein might be expressed at a lower level than the wild type (relative haploinsufficiency). A small number of the causal mutations in HCM are splice-junction or frameshift mutations. They lead to expression of truncated proteins that could be degraded by the UPS and hence lead to a null allele status. The effect of such mutations, therefore, is expected to be "haploinsufficiency."[97,139] The molecular event that leads to HCM in haploinsufficiency states remains unclear.

The pathogenesis of myocyte disarray, the pathologic hallmark of HCM, appears to be independent of the pathogenesis of cardiac hypertrophy and fibrosis. Impaired myocyte alignment through the β-catenin-cadherins at the adherens junctions has been implicated as a potential mechanism for myocyte disarray.[28] Alternative possible mechanisms include activation of the signaling pathways involved in myocyte polarity and axis, as well as altered myocardial architecture, by excess extracellular matrix proteins.

Determinants of Cardiac Phenotype in Hypertrophic Cardiomyopathy

The clinical phenotype is the outcome of complex and intertwined interactions between the constituents that contribute to the phenotype. In monogenic diseases such as HCM, the causal mutation is the prerequisite and a major determinant of the phenotype. The phenotype, however, ensues from interactions of the causal mutation with a variety of genetic, genomic, and nongenetic factors (**Figure 21-6**). In a sense, the clinical phenotype of single-gene disorders is a complex phenotype, determined not only by the causal mutation but also by the modifier genes; noncoding RNAs, including long noncoding RNAs; and microRNAs, post-translational modification of proteins, and environmental factors. Although there is considerable information on the significance of each component in influencing cardiac structure and function in general, their roles in affecting expression of the phenotype in HCM are poorly understood. Nevertheless, the complexity of the factors that determine the clinical phenotype points to the limitation of the genotype-phenotype correlation studies in humans with HCM. This point has important clinical implications, as in risk stratification of patients with HCM. It is important to consider all components that contribute to the phenotype in the assessment of the risk of SCD and clinical outcomes. It is equally important to note that the findings in a small subset of patients with HCM, such as association of a mutation with a high risk of SCD in a family, could be restricted to the particular study population and not applicable to the general population of HCM.

Despite the recognized limitations of the genotype-phenotype correlation studies performed in relatively small populations, the causal mutations impart significant impact on the clinical phenotype, including the severity of cardiac hypertrophy and the risk of SCD.[96,142,143] The data suggest that, despite the presence of considerable variability, mutations in *MYH7*, as opposed to those in *MYBPC3*, are

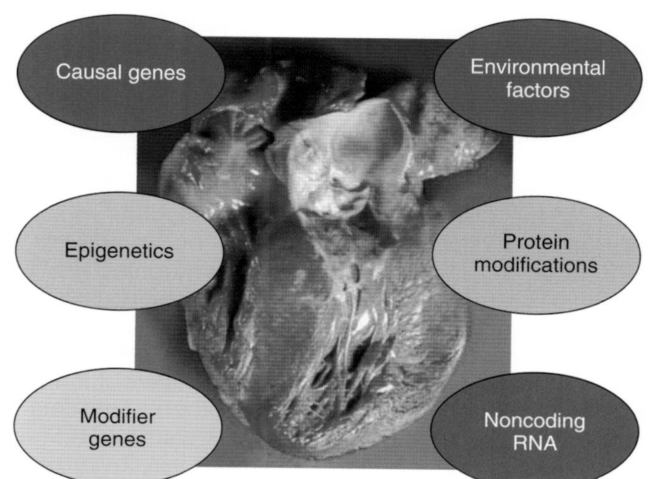

FIGURE 21-6 Major expected determinants of clinical phenotype in patients with hypertrophic cardiomyopathy.

associated with a relatively high penetrance with the expression of significant cardiac hypertrophy relatively early in life.[142] Conversely, mutations in *MYBPC3* generally appear to be associated with a milder degree of cardiac hypertrophy that typically manifests later in life as compared with the *MYH7* mutations.[96] The relatively low penetrance of certain mutations raises an important clinical point in the management of the relatives of patients with HCM, because the normal phenotype in those at risk may reflect the low penetrance. Such individuals may develop the disease later in life.[144] Thus, unless the inheritance of the causal mutation is excluded through genetic screening, those at risk should be evaluated periodically. The prognostic impact of the mutations on the risk of SCD is partly reflective of their effects on the severity of cardiac hypertrophy.[145] It also appears that individuals with mutations leading to premature truncation of the protein exhibit more pronounced phenotypes than those with the missense mutations.[76] Mutations in *TNNT2* and *TNNI3* genes are associated with a relatively milder degree of cardiac hypertrophy but more prominent cardiac myocyte disarray and increased risk of SCD.[146] Nonetheless, no phenotype is specific to a specific gene or mutations, and benign as well as malignant phenotypes have been associated with the common causal genes.[147]

A noteworthy determinant of the clinical phenotype in HCM is the presence of double mutations, whether in *cis* or in *trans*.[74,98,99] Likewise, the presence of concomitant diseases, such as hypertension, could increase the penetrance and accelerate expression and severity of cardiac hypertrophy. The impact of hypertension on the phenotypic expression of HCM mutations might be reflected in the so-called hypertensive hypertrophic cardiomyopathy of the elderly, which is considered a concomitant presence of HCM and systemic arterial hypertension.[148] The impact of heavy physical exercise, particularly isometric exercises, on expression of cardiac hypertrophy and the risk of SCD are speculated based on the observational data but yet to be clarified. One may surmise, because hypertrophy is the secondary response of the heart to the causal mutations, heavy isometric exercise could promote cardiac growth and hence enhance expression of cardiac hypertrophy and consequently the risk of SCD in HCM. Experimental data in a mouse model suggests otherwise.[149] Because HCM is the most common cause of SCD in young competitive athletes, patients with HCM are advised not to participate in competitive or contact sports.[150]

A fascinating feature of mutations in the sarcomere protein is phenotypic plasticity. Accordingly, patients with HCM caused by mutations in *MYH7, TNNT2,* or *TNNI3* genes can develop the phenotype of dilated cardiomyopathy (DCM) or restrictive cardiomyopathy (RCM) during the course of the disease.[151-153] Moreover, mutations in sarcomere proteins could present from the outset with HCM, DCM, RCM, or LV noncompaction syndrome.[154-156] The molecular basis of such phenotypic plasticity is largely unknown but may reflect the topography of the causal mutations imparting different structural and functional effects on the mutant proteins and/or the effects of modifier genes and noncoding RNAs, among others. The data in small rodent models suggest mutations causing HCM are typically associated with enhanced Ca^{2+} sensitivity of the myofibrillar force generation and ATPase activity.[125,157-163] In contrast, mutations leading to DCM are associated with reduced Ca^{2+} sensitivity of the myofibrillar force generation and ATPase activity.[125,157-163] However, differences in the expression levels of MYH6 and MYH7 proteins, two major isoforms of myosin heavy chain in the heart, between humans and rodents might confound the relevance of the findings to HCM.[121,164,165] While MYH7 is the predominant isoform in the human heart (>95% of the total MYH), MYH6 predominates in the mouse heart (>90%).[166,167] MYH7 and MYH6 have considerable differences in the rate of ATPase activity and actomyosin cross-bridge kinetics.[168,169] These differences might influence the relevance of the functional data obtained by imposing a human MYH7 mutation in the mouse MYH6 proteins to human HCM. Functional studies with the mutant human MYH7 or in animals that predominantly express the MYH7 isoform, such as a transgenic rabbit model of HCM, suggest impaired Ca^{2+} sensitivity of myofibrillar ATPase activity.[118,121,164,165] Another putative mechanism for phenotypic plasticity of the sarcomere mutations is differential interactions of the mutant protein with other constituents of the sarcomere. For example, mutations in *TNNT2* that cause the contrasting phenotypes of HCM and DCM in humans, impart differential effects on protein-protein interactions among the constituents of the sarcomeric filaments.[119]

Hypertrophic Cardiomyopathy Phenocopy

A phenocopy is a phenotype that mimics the true phenotype. In the case of HCM, a phenocopy condition will express a phenotype that grossly resembles HCM, mainly "unexplained cardiac hypertrophy," but its cause and pathogenesis differ from the sarcomere HCM. Accordingly, the phenotype of cardiac hypertrophy in the absence of increased loading conditions could occur in a variety of other conditions, such as storage diseases, mitochondrial disorders, and triplet repeat syndromes (**Table 21-3**). The prevalence of phenocopy in patients with the clinical diagnosis of HCM is unclear but is estimated to be around 5% to 10%. The prevalence of phenocopy conditions may be higher in children, probably because of early manifestations of the phenocopy conditions.

The most common HCM phenocopy in children is Noonan syndrome, an uncommon autosomal dominant disorder characterized by dysmorphic facial features, pulmonic stenosis, mental retardation, bleeding disorders, and cardiac hypertrophy. In one report approximately one third of children with the clinical diagnosis of HCM had Noonan syndrome.[170] The known causal genes are protein-tyrosine phosphatase, nonreceptor type 11 *(PTPN11), SOS, KRAS, RAF1,* and *SHOC2* genes, which collectively account for approximately two thirds of the cases.[171-175] Leopard syndrome (lentigines, electrocardiographic conduction abnormalities, ocular hypertelorism, pulmonic stenosis, abnormal genitalia, retardation of growth, and deafness) is an allelic variant of the Noonan syndrome. It is caused primarily by mutations in *RAF1*.[172]

Glycogen storage diseases are relatively common causes of HCM phenocopy. Danon disease is a storage disease caused by mutations in *LAMP2*, which codes for lysosome-associated membrane protein 2.[34] Likewise, mutations in *PRKAG2*, which encode the γ2 regulatory subunit of AMP-activated protein kinase (AMPK) lead to glycogen storage in the heart. The ensuing phenotype is cardiac hypertrophy, as well as AV conduction defects, and a pattern of

TABLE 21-3 HCM Phenocopy Conditions

DISEASE	CAUSAL GENE	PROTEIN
AMPK-mediated glycogen storage	*PRKAG2*	Protein kinase A, γ subunit
Pompe disease	*GAA*	α-1,4-glucosidase (acid maltase)
Anderson-Fabry disease	*GLA*	α-galactosidase A
Danon disease	*LAMP2*	Lysosome-associated membrane protein 2
Myosin VI	*MYO6*	Unconventional myosin 6
Kearns-Sayre syndrome	*MtDNA*	Mitochondrial DNA
Friedreich ataxia	*FRDA*	Frataxin
Myotonic dystrophy	*DMPK* *DMWD*	Myotonin protein kinase
Noonan syndrome	*PTPN11*	Protein tyrosine phosphatase, nonreceptor type 11
	SOS	Son of Sevenless
	RAF1	Murine leukemia viral oncogene homolog 1
	KRAS	Kirsten rat sarcoma virus homolog
Neimann-Pick disease	*NPC*	Neimann-Pick
Refsum disease	*PAHX* (*PHYH*)	Phytanoyl-CoA hydroxylase

preexcitation on the electrocardiogram.[35,36,176,177] The mechanism for cardiac hypertrophy, in addition to increasing glycogen storage in myocytes, also includes cellular proliferation and hypertrophy.[178] Another example of storage diseases mimicking HCM is the Fabry or Anderson-Fabry disease, which is an X-linked lysosomal storage disease.[179,180] The estimated prevalence of Fabry disease in the adult population with a clinical diagnosis of HCM may be as high as 3%.[180] Cardiac phenotype results from the deposits of glycosphingolipids in the heart. Other features of Fabry disease are angiokeratoma, renal insufficiency, proteinuria, neuropathy, transient ischemic attack, stroke, anemia, and corneal deposits.[181,182] The cardiac phenotype includes hypertrophy, which is often indistinguishable from true HCM, high QRS voltage, conduction defects, cardiac arrhythmias, valvular regurgitation, coronary artery disease, myocardial infarction, and aortic annular dilation. Fabry disease is caused by mutations in the *GLA* gene on chromosome Xq22, which encodes the lysosomal hydrolase α-Gal A protein.[181] Mutations lead to deficient activity of α-galactosidase A (α-Gal A), also known as ceramide trihexosidase. Because the causal gene is located on the X chromosome, the disease predominantly affects males and to a lesser extent, female carriers. Fabry disease is diagnosed by the measuring α-Gal A levels and activity in leukocytes. The distinction between true HCM and Fabry disease is important because enzyme replacement therapy using human α-Gal A (agalsidase α) or recombinant human α-Gal A (agalsidase β) is somewhat effective in slowing progression of Fabry disease.[183-185]

Cardiac involvement in triplet repeat syndromes, a group of disorders caused by the expansion of naturally occurring trinucleotide repeats in the genes, includes cardiac hypertrophy, which is usually diagnosed as HCM. The HCM phenocopy is found frequently in patients with Friedreich ataxia, an autosomal recessive neurodegenerative disease caused by expansion of GAA repeat sequences in the intron of *FRDA*.[186] HCM phenocopy in patients with Friedreich ataxia could evolve into DCM. Likewise, cardiac involvement may present as DCM from the outset.

Another important cause of HCM phenocopy is defective mitochondrial oxidative phosphorylation pathways. A prototypic example is Kearns-Sayre syndrome (KSS), which is characterized by a triad of progressive external ophthalmoplegia, pigmentary retinopathy, and cardiac conduction defects.[187] Patients with KSS frequently exhibit cardiac hypertrophy diagnosed as HCM. Various other mitochondrial gene mutations have been associated with HCM. The list of conditions that cause HCM phenocopy is extensive and involves metabolic diseases, such as Refsum disease, glycogen storage disease type II (Pompe disease), Niemann-Pick disease, Gaucher disease, hereditary hemochromatosis, and CD36 deficiency.

MANAGEMENT OF PATIENTS WITH HYPERTROPHIC CARDIOMYOPATHY

Genetic Screening

There is considerable interest in genetic testing for HCM by patients and physicians. The interest stems from potential clinical utility of genetic testing for an accurate diagnosis of HCM, preclinical diagnosis of mutation carriers independent of and before clinical manifestations of the disease, and possibly prognostication, particularly as it regards the risk of SCD. The demand for genetic testing has led to the development of academic and commercial centers for genetic testing of HCM. Clinicians and patients, therefore, need to familiarize themselves with the strengths and limitations of genetic testing and the implications of the findings. Perhaps the most straightforward utility of genetic testing is in familial HCM wherein the causal mutation has already been identified and all members of the family could be tested for inheritance of the causal mutation. Genetic testing in such scenarios could lead to an accurate distinction of those who have or have not inherited the causal mutation. Those who have inherited the causal mutation would be at risk of developing the disease. An early and accurate identification of the mutation carriers in a family could guide the physician for a close monitoring of the individuals at risk and possibly early interventions to prevent or slow evolution of the phenotype. Early pharmacologic interventions in animal models of HCM show the potential to prevent evolution of cardiac phenotype in HCM.[27] Although inheritance of the causal mutation indicates a high likelihood of developing HCM, it does alone not determine the severity of the phenotype. Another implication of genetic testing in familial setting is the accurate identification of those who have not inherited the causal mutation and hence, for practical purposes, are not at risk of developing HCM except in very rare circumstances.

In the most common scenario for genetic testing, neither the causal gene nor the mutation is known. In large families, one may perform linkage analysis and map the causal gene and identify the mutation. The approach, however, is possible in research laboratories only and is expensive. In smaller size families, linkage analysis does not offer sufficient power to map and identify the causal mutation. Thus in small size families and in sporadic cases, one is restricted to the candidate gene approach or whole exome sequencing. The screening is complicated by the allelic and nonallelic heterogeneity of HCM and hence the relatively low prevalence of each causal mutation. In addition, the plethora of SNVs in the genome, including putatively functional variants, further complicates interpretations of the findings.[188] Therefore, the approach mostly focuses on screening of each individual for a panel of causal genes implicated in cardiomyopathies, such as *MYH7, MYBPC3, TNNI3, TNNT2, TPM1*, and *ACTC1*. Typically, the coding regions and the exon-intron boundaries are sequenced to identify the causal mutation. Inclusion of less common causal genes, as well as genes coding for the relatively common phenocopy conditions, is expected to increase the chance of finding the causal mutation slightly. The overall yield of genetic screening at the present time is at about 50%.

One important clinical implication of genetic testing is the distinction between the phenocopy conditions and sarcomere HCM. The distinction is important because the treatment of the two conditions differs significantly and enzyme replacement therapy for many phenocopy conditions has shown beneficial effects, as discussed previously. The utility of genetic testing for prognostication is hindered by the presence of considerable phenotypic variability, including among individuals with identical mutations, and the influence of a large number of determinants of the clinical phenotypes. Accordingly, information garnered through identification of the causal mutation alone in the assessment of the risk of SCD is inadequate but could supplement the clinical data for risk stratification and management of patients with HCM. In this aspect, a comprehensive approach that uses not only the information content of the causal genes and mutations but also encompasses the potential impacts of the double causal mutations and the modifier alleles, as well as the clinical predictors, is necessary to improve risk stratification in patients with HCM.

Management of Risk of Sudden Cardiac Death

The risk of SCD is the primary concern of patients and physicians alike. The risk factors for SCD were discussed previously and are listed in Table 21-1. Pharmacologic treatment has not been shown to reduce the risk of SCD in HCM. In contrast, implantation of AICD is effective in secondary as well as primary prevention of SCD in patients with HCM.[189,190] The specific indication of AICD implantation in various clinical scenarios is less settled and the threshold for intervention varies among different centers. There is a general agreement that patients with a prior episode of cardiac arrest require complete cardiovascular evaluation and AICD implantation. ICD implantation has been shown to be effective in secondary prevention of SCD in HCM.[189] Those patients who are at risk of atherosclerosis are typically evaluated by coronary angiography to detect atherosclerosis followed by appropriate intervention. A family history of premature SCD is an important risk factor for SCD, particularly whenever it occurs in two or more individuals. Whether a family history of premature SCD alone is sufficient for AICD implantation is subject to debate. Given the presence of extensive phenotypic variability, additional risk stratification and hence an individual-based approach is preferable. Recurrent syncope is a major risk factor and necessitates extensive evaluation to determine the cause. In addition to detailed history taking, physical examination, 12-lead ECG, and comprehensive echocardiography, the evaluation should include extended (30-day) cardiac rhythm monitoring, tilt-table testing, whenever autonomic dysfunction and orthostatic hypotension is suspected, and electrophysiologic studies in specific circumstances. Those with sustained or repetitive episodes of nonsustained ventricular tachycardia on Holter or rhythm monitoring are candidates for AICD implantation. AICD is effective in reducing the risk of SCD in those at high risk of SCD.[189]

Severe LV hypertrophy is a major risk factor for SCD and would warrant additional studies to further assess the risk of SCD. Left ventricular outflow tract obstruction, although a major determinant of clinical symptoms, is probably not an indication for routine implantation of an AICD. Those with risk factors for SCD undergoing surgical septal myectomy should be re-evaluated postoperatively, because surgical septal myectomy appears to impart a favorable outcome on the risk of SCD.[191] In contrast, patients with risk factors for SCD undergoing catheter-based alcohol septal ablation probably should also undergo an AICD implantation, because there have been occasional reports of ventricular tachycardia post–catheter-based alcohol septal ablation.[192,193] Finally, the risk of SCD in those who do not have the so-called conventional risk factors is relatively small but not negligible.[194] It is unclear whether interventions to reduce the risk of SCD would be beneficial in the low-risk group.

Exercise testing, including exercise echocardiography, is also used for evaluation and risk stratification of patients with HCM. Patients with impaired exercise tolerance and reduced oxygen consumption have been associated with a high rate of cardiovascular events.[195,196] In contrast, patients who achieve the predicted metabolic equivalent during exercise testing have a low cardiovascular event rate.[197] Similarly, heart rate recovery during the first minute into the recovery period is also associated with long-term outcomes.[197]

Pharmacologic Treatment

Current pharmacologic treatment of patients with HCM is largely empiric and unchanged over the past two decades. A large number of patients with HCM are asymptomatic or minimally symptomatic. Therefore, only periodic clinical and laboratory evaluations that also include assessment of the risk of SCD are recommended. Routine periodic evaluation of such patients should include obtaining a 12-lead ECG, two-dimensional and Doppler echocardiography, and cardiac rhythm monitoring, the latter particularly in those who have risk factors for SCD. The main focus is on the risk of SCD and early intervention, because AICD appears to be effective even in primary prevention of SCD in high-risk patients with HCM.[189] In asymptomatic individuals at low risk of SCD, no intervention is necessary, because none of the existing therapies has been shown to slow or reverse evolution of the cardiac phenotype in HCM. Nevertheless, these patients also require careful and periodic evaluation, because the risk of SCD is not totally negligible.[194]

The cornerstone of pharmacologic treatment of symptomatic patients is β-blockers. β-blockers with intrinsic sympathetic activity are avoided because they could worsen the symptoms. Calcium channel blockers, namely verapamil and diltiazem but not nifedipine, are the agents of choice in those who do not tolerate β-blockers or are added to β-blockers, whenever symptoms persist. However, in patients with LV outflow tract obstruction, the vasodilatory effects of Ca^{2+} channel blockers might precipitate or worsen

LV outflow tract obstruction. Disopyramide, which possesses a negative inotropic effect, is effective in reducing LV outflow tract obstruction and ameliorating symptoms.[198] However, it does not affect overall survival or the risk of SCD.[198] Diuretics are used in those with symptoms of diastolic heart failure, albeit cautiously to avoid volume depletion and precipitation of hypotension. Amiodarone or dronedarone is used primarily for treatment of atrial and ventricular arrhythmias. Patients with new-onset atrial fibrillation are typically treated with electrical cardioversion to restore normal sinus rhythm. In general, patients with severe cardiac hypertrophy or outflow tract obstruction who develop atrial fibrillation develop severe symptoms. It is preferable to convert atrial fibrillation to and maintain such patients in normal sinus rhythm. However, this may prove difficult because of the underlying pathology in HCM. Those with chronic or intermittent atrial fibrillation are anticoagulated to reduce the risk of systemic embolization and stroke. Pharmacologic treatment of such patients includes β-blockers, verapamil and amiodarone, and possibly sotalol and dofetilide. Catheter-based ablation should be considered in HCM patients with atrial fibrillation refractory to medical therapy.

Surgical Myectomy and Catheter-Based Septal Ablation

A subset of patients with HCM remains symptomatic and refractory to medical therapy, some because of severe diastolic heart failure and others because of severe outflow tract obstruction. Those with a significant LV outflow tract obstruction at rest or provoked, and an interventricular septal thickness of 15 mm or greater, are candidates for surgical myectomy or catheter-based alcohol septal ablation. Both approaches are effective in relieving the outflow tract obstruction and improving symptoms.[199-202] Therefore, the choice is largely determined by the presence of concomitant diseases, such as significant valvular lesions and coronary artery disease, which necessitates concomitant surgery and hence preference for surgical myectomy. Likewise, surgical myectomy is more desirable in those at high risk for SCD. In contrast, the presence of comorbidities that increase the surgical risk significantly favors percutaneous interventions. The advantages and disadvantages of these two techniques are summarized in **Table 21-4**.

TABLE 21-4 Comparison of Surgical Myectomy and Ethanol Septal Ablation

	SURGICAL MYECTOMY	ETHANOL SEPTAL ABLATION
Approach	Cardiopulmonary bypass	Cardiac catheterization
Hospital stay	5-7 days	1-2 days
Perioperative mortality	1%-5%	1%-5%
Procedural success	>95%	>85%
Short-term symptomatic relief	Excellent	Excellent
Long-term symptomatic relief	Excellent	Excellent
Long-term safety	Established	Risk of ventricular arrhythmias
Impact on survival	Favorable	Unknown
Septal infarction/fibrosis	None	Present
Recurrence of LVOT gradient	Rare	Uncommon
Repeat procedure	Rare	Uncommon
Atrioventricular block requiring permanent pacemaker	≈2%	10%-20%
Late ventricular arrhythmias	Rare	Uncommon
Postoperative atrial fibrillation	Common	Rare
Significant aortic regurgitation	Infrequent	None
Ventricular septal defect	Rare	None
Correction of concomitant problems	Amenable	NA

LVOT, Left ventricular outflow tract.

Surgical myectomy (myomectomy), which is referred to as the *Morrow procedure*, involves partial resection of the base of the septum through a transaortic approach. It is the procedure of choice in HCM patients who have concomitant coronary artery disease or valvular disorders or have an anatomy that is not amenable to catheter-based septal ablation. It is also preferable in patients at high risk for SCD, as the risk of SCD appears to be low after surgical myectomy.[191] The overall surgical mortality is 1% to 5% but higher in the elderly and those requiring concomitant surgeries, such as coronary artery bypass surgery or valvular repair/replacement.[203,204] The long-term beneficial effects of surgical myectomy in relieving the outflow tract gradient and improving symptoms are well established. The procedure is effective in more than 90% of the patients.[203-206] The recurrence rate and the need for permanent pacemaker implantation are relatively low. Surgical myectomy is also associated with a significant improvement in pulmonary hypertension.[207] Continued postoperative atrial fibrillation and age are independent predictors of long-term clinical outcomes.[206]

Transcatheter alcohol septal ablation is performed by infusing 1 to 3 mL of pure ethanol into the main septal perforators of the left anterior descending artery. It is also very effective in reducing the outflow tract gradient and improving symptoms.[193,208] Infusion of ethanol into the septal branches induces local myocardial necrosis, which is associated with LV remodeling and partial regression of cardiac hypertrophy.[201,208,209] The peri-procedure mortality rate is low. In the largest North American study involving 874 participants, survival estimates at 1, 5, and 9 years after the procedure were 97%, 86%, and 74%, respectively.[201] Likewise, European studies also show a favorable outcome superior after alcohol septal ablation compared with those reported earlier.[69] A major complication is the development of advanced conduction defect requiring permanent pacemaker implantation in 10% to 20% of the patients.[210,211] A prolonged PR interval before the procedure is associated with a higher risk of complete heart block after alcohol septal ablation.[212] Because alcohol septal ablation typically leads to right bundle branch block (RBBB), those with preexisting left bundle branch block (LBBB) are at much higher risk of complete heart block postprocedure. In addition, a small fraction of patients develop late-onset complete heart block after alcohol septal ablation.[212] An uncommon and sometimes late complication of alcohol septal ablation is ventricular arrhythmias, mandating implantation of AICD.[192,193] Likewise, coronary dissection, ventricular septal defect, and pericardial bleed/effusion are rare complications of alcohol septal ablation.[201] Overall, transcoronary septal ablation is a very safe and effective procedure for reduction of LV outflow tract obstruction as well as improvement of symptoms.

Experimental Therapies

The ultimate goal of pharmacologic interventions in human patients with HCM is not only to improve symptoms and reduce the risk of SCD but also to prevent the clinical manifestation of the disease in total. However, current pharmacologic agents have not been shown to reduce mortality, regress cardiac hypertrophy, or prevent the development of the phenotype. Experimental data in animal models of human HCM have raised the potential utility of angiotensin II receptor blockade, 3-hydroxy-3-methyglutaryl-coenzyme A (HMG-CoA) reductase inhibitors (statins), inhibition of mineralocorticoid receptors, and antioxidant *N*-acetylcysteine in prevention, attenuation, and regression of evolving phenotypes in HCM.[26-28,213-215] However, whether the results obtained in animal models caused by specific mutations in the background of relatively homogeneous and under controlled environmental conditions could be extended to humans who have heterogeneous genetic and environmental factors remains to be determined. Three pilot studies have shown potential beneficial effects of the angiotensin II receptor blocker losartan in human patients with HCM.[216-218] The findings suggest a modest reduction in the LV mass, attenuation of late gadolinium enhancement, and improved diastolic function upon treatment with angiotensin II receptor blockers. Two pilot studies with atorvastatin showed no beneficial effect on cardiac mass or function in patients with HCM.[219,220] Large-scale clinical studies in HCM patients genotyped for the causal mutations would be necessary to establish the potential beneficial effects of experimental therapies.

Whereas pharmacologic interventions target specific molecules or pathways involved in the pathogenesis of cardiac phenotype in HCM, selective suppression of the expression of the mutant allele offers an alternative therapeutic approach.[221] A 25% suppression of the mutant transcript levels by an RNAi-based approach was associated with delayed expression of cardiac hypertrophy and fibrosis in a mouse model of HCM.[221] These preliminary findings raise the therapeutic potentials of allele-specific RNAi in the prevention or reversal of cardiac phenotype in HCM.[222] Likewise, several RNA-based approaches that target exon skipping, inclusion, or transsplicing are being investigated for therapeutic applications in animal models of HCM.[223,224]

References

1. Liouville H: Retrecissement cardiaque sous aortique. *Gazette Med Paris* 24:161–165, 1869.
2. Schmincke A: Ueber linkseitige muskulose conusstenosen. *Dtsch Med Wchnschr* 33:2082, 1907.
3. Davies LG: A familial heart disease. *Br Heart J* 14:206–212, 1952.
4. Teare D: Asymmetrical hypertrophy of the heart in young adults. *Br Heart J* 20:1–8, 1958.
5. Brock R, Fleming PR: Aortic subvalvar stenosis; a report of 5 cases diagnosed during life. *Guys Hosp Rep* 105:391–408, 1956.
6. Braunwald E, Ebert PA: Hemodynamic alterations in idiopathic hypertrophic subaortic stenosis induced by sympathomimetic drugs. *Am J Cardiol* 10:489–495, 1962.
7. Braunwald E, Lambrew CT, Rockoff SD, et al: Idiopathic hypertrophic subaortic stenosis. I. A description of the disease based upon an analysis of 64 patients. *Circulation* 30(Suppl 4):3–119, 1964. SUPPL-119.
8. Pierce GE, Morrow AG, Braunwald E: Idiopathic hypertrophic subaortic stenosis. 3. Intraoperative studies of the mechanism of obstruction and its hemodynamic consequences. *Circulation* 30(Suppl 4):152, 1964. SUPPL.
9. Morrow AG, Lambrew CT, Braunwald E: Idiopathic hypertrophic subaortic stenosis. II. Operative treatment and the results of pre- and postoperative hemodynamic evaluations. *Circulation* 30(Suppl 4):120–151, 1964. SUPPL-51.
10. Sigwart U: Non-surgical myocardial reduction for hypertrophic obstructive cardiomyopathy. *Lancet* 346:211–214, 1995.
11. Henry WL, Clark CE, Epstein SE: Asymmetric septal hypertrophy. Echocardiographic identification of the pathognomonic anatomic abnormality of IHSS. *Circulation* 47:225–233, 1973.
12. Boughner DR, Schuld RL, Persaud JA: Hypertrophic obstructive cardiomyopathy. Assessment by echocardiographic and doppler ultrasound techniques. *Br Heart J* 37:917–923, 1975.
13. Joyner CR, Harrison FS, Jr, Gruber JW: Diagnosis of hypertrophic subaortic stenosis with a doppler velocity flow detector. *Ann Intern Med* 74:692–696, 1971.
14. Takenaka K, Dabestani A, Gardin JM, et al: Left ventricular filling in hypertrophic cardiomyopathy: a pulsed doppler echocardiographic study. *J Am Coll Cardiol* 7:1263–1271, 1986.
15. Nagueh SF, Bachinski LL, Meyer D, et al: Tissue doppler imaging consistently detects myocardial abnormalities in patients with hypertrophic cardiomyopathy and provides a novel means for an early diagnosis before and independently of hypertrophy. *Circulation* 104:128–130, 2001.
16. Nagueh SF, McFalls J, Meyer D, et al: Tissue doppler imaging predicts the development of hypertrophic cardiomyopathy in subjects with subclinical disease. *Circulation* 108:395–398, 2003.
17. Geisterfer-Lowrance AA, Kass S, Tanigawa G, et al: A molecular basis for familial hypertrophic cardiomyopathy: a beta cardiac myosin heavy chain gene missense mutation. *Cell* 62:999–1006, 1990.
18. Seidman CE, Seidman JG: Identifying sarcomere gene mutations in hypertrophic cardiomyopathy: a personal history. *Circ Res* 108:743–750, 2011.
19. Marian AJ: Hypertrophic cardiomyopathy: from genetics to treatment. *Eur J Clin Invest* 40:360–369, 2010.
20. Cannan CR, Reeder GS, Bailey KR, et al: Natural history of hypertrophic cardiomyopathy. A population-based study, 1976 through 1990. *Circulation* 92:2488–2495, 1995.
21. Kofflard MJM, ten Cate FJ, van der Lee C, et al: Hypertrophic cardiomyopathy in a large community-based population: clinical outcome and identification of risk factors for sudden cardiac death and clinical deterioration. *J Am Coll Cardiol* 41:987–993, 2003.
22. Cecchi F, Olivotto I, Montereggi A, et al: Hypertrophic cardiomyopathy in tuscany: clinical course and outcome in an unselected regional population. *J Am Coll Cardiol* 26:1529–1536, 1995.
23. Maron BJ: Contemporary insights and strategies for risk stratification and prevention of sudden death in hypertrophic cardiomyopathy. *Circulation* 121:445–456, 2010.
24. Maron BJ, Shirani J, Poliac LC, et al: Sudden death in young competitive athletes. Clinical, demographic, and pathological profiles. *JAMA* 276:199–204, 1996.
25. Maron BJ, Shen WK, Link MS, et al: Efficacy of implantable cardioverter-defibrillators for the prevention of sudden death in patients with hypertrophic cardiomyopathy. *N Engl J Med* 342:365–373, 2000.
26. Patel R, Nagueh SF, Tsybouleva N, et al: Simvastatin induces regression of cardiac hypertrophy and fibrosis and improves cardiac function in a transgenic rabbit model of human hypertrophic cardiomyopathy. *Circulation* 104:317–324, 2001.
27. Senthil V, Chen SN, Tsybouleva N, et al: Prevention of cardiac hypertrophy by atorvastatin in a transgenic rabbit model of human hypertrophic cardiomyopathy. *Circ Res* 97:285–292, 2005.
28. Tsybouleva N, Zhang L, Chen S, et al: Aldosterone, through novel signaling proteins, is a fundamental molecular bridge between the genetic defect and the cardiac phenotype of hypertrophic cardiomyopathy. *Circulation* 109:1284–1291, 2004.
29. Marian AJ: Genetic determinants of cardiac hypertrophy. *Curr Opin Cardiol* 23:199–205, 2008.
30. Maron BJ, Spirito P, Wesley Y, et al: Development and progression of left ventricular hypertrophy in children with hypertrophic cardiomyopathy. *N Engl J Med* 315:610–614, 1986.
31. Charron P, Carrier L, Dubourg O, et al: Penetrance of familial hypertrophic cardiomyopathy. *Genet Couns* 8:107–114, 1997.
32. Sheikh N, Papadakis M, Ghani S, et al: Comparison of ECG criteria for the detection of cardiac abnormalities in elite black and white athletes. *Circulation* 129:1637–1649, 2014.
33. Elliott P, McKenna WJ: Hypertrophic cardiomyopathy. *Lancet* 363:1881–1891, 2004.
34. Arad M, Maron BJ, Gorham JM, et al: Glycogen storage diseases presenting as hypertrophic cardiomyopathy. *N Engl J Med* 352:362–372, 2005.
35. Gollob MH, Green MS, Tang AS, et al: Identification of a gene responsible for familial Wolff-Parkinson-White syndrome. *N Engl J Med* 344:1823–1831, 2001.
36. Blair E, Redwood C, Ashrafian H, et al: Mutations in the gamma(2) subunit of AMP-activated protein kinase cause familial hypertrophic cardiomyopathy: evidence for the central role of energy compromise in disease pathogenesis. *Hum Mol Genet* 10:1215–1220, 2001.
37. Maron BJ, Gardin JM, Flack JM, et al: Prevalence of hypertrophic cardiomyopathy in a general population of young adults. Echocardiographic analysis of 4111 subjects in the CARDIA study. Coronary artery risk development in (young) adults. *Circulation* 92:785–789, 1995.
38. Elliott PM, Poloniecki J, Dickie S, et al: Sudden death in hypertrophic cardiomyopathy: identification of high risk patients. *J Am Coll Cardiol* 36:2212–2218, 2000.
39. Nienaber CA, Hiller S, Spielmann RP, et al: Syncope in hypertrophic cardiomyopathy: multivariate analysis of prognostic determinants. *J Am Coll Cardiol* 15:948–955, 1990.
40. Olivotto I, Cecchi F, Casey SA, et al: Impact of atrial fibrillation on the clinical course of hypertrophic cardiomyopathy. *Circulation* 104:2517–2524, 2001.
41. Monserrat L, Elliott PM, Gimeno JR, et al: Non-sustained ventricular tachycardia in hypertrophic cardiomyopathy: an independent marker of sudden death risk in young patients. *J Am Coll Cardiol* 42:873–879, 2003.
42. Maron BJ, Olivotto I, Bellone P, et al: Clinical profile of stroke in 900 patients with hypertrophic cardiomyopathy. *J Am Coll Cardiol* 39:301–307, 2002.
43. Robinson K, Frenneaux MP, Stockins B, et al: Atrial fibrillation in hypertrophic cardiomyopathy: a longitudinal study. *J Am Coll Cardiol* 15:1279–1285, 1990.
44. Frank S, Braunwald E: Idiopathic hypertrophic subaortic stenosis. Clinical analysis of 126 patients with emphasis on the natural history. *Circulation* 37:759–788, 1968.
45. Maron BJ, Casey SA, Poliac LC, et al: Clinical course of hypertrophic cardiomyopathy in a regional United States cohort. *JAMA* 281:650–655, 1999.
46. Coats CJ, Gallagher MJ, Foley M, et al: Relation between serum N-terminal pro-brain natriuretic peptide and prognosis in patients with hypertrophic cardiomyopathy. *Eur Heart J* 34:2529–2537, 2013.
47. Basavarajaiah S, Shah A, Sharma S: Sudden cardiac death in young athletes. *Heart* 93:287–289, 2007.
48. Maron BJ, Haas TS, Murphy CJ, et al: Incidence and causes of sudden death in U.S. college athletes. *J Am Coll Cardiol* 63:1636–1643, 2014.
49. Corrado D, Basso C, Schiavon M, et al: Screening for hypertrophic cardiomyopathy in young athletes. *N Engl J Med* 339:364–369, 1998.
50. Miller MA, Gomes JA, Fuster V: Risk stratification of sudden cardiac death in hypertrophic cardiomyopathy. *Nat Clin Pract Cardiovasc Med* 4:667–676, 2007.
51. Marian AJ: On predictors of sudden cardiac death in hypertrophic cardiomyopathy. *J Am Coll Cardiol* 41:994–996, 2003.
52. Frenneaux MP: Assessing the risk of sudden cardiac death in a patient with hypertrophic cardiomyopathy. *Heart* 90:570–575, 2004.
53. Elliott PM, Gimeno B, Jr, Mahon NG, et al: Relation between severity of left-ventricular hypertrophy and prognosis in patients with hypertrophic cardiomyopathy. *Lancet* 357:420–424, 2001.
54. O'Mahony C, Jichi F, Pavlou M, et al: A novel clinical risk prediction model for sudden cardiac death in hypertrophic cardiomyopathy (HCM Risk-SCD). *Eur Heart J* 35:2010–2020, 2014.

55. Kofflard MJ, Waldstein DJ, Vos J, et al: Prognosis in hypertrophic cardiomyopathy observed in a large clinic population. *Am J Cardiol* 72:939–943, 1993.
56. Yetman AT, Hamilton RM, Benson LN, et al: Long-term outcome and prognostic determinants in children with hypertrophic cardiomyopathy. *J Am Coll Cardiol* 32:1943–1950, 1998.
57. Klues HG, Schiffers A, Maron BJ: Phenotypic spectrum and patterns of left ventricular hypertrophy in hypertrophic cardiomyopathy: morphologic observations and significance as assessed by two-dimensional echocardiography in 600 patients. *J Am Coll Cardiol* 26:1699–1708, 1995.
58. Malik R, Maron MS, Rastegar H, et al: Hypertrophic cardiomyopathy with right ventricular outflow tract and left ventricular intracavitary obstruction. *Echocardiography* 31:682–685, 2014.
59. Eriksson MJ, Sonnenberg B, Woo A, et al: Long-term outcome in patients with apical hypertrophic cardiomyopathy. *J Am Coll Cardiol* 39:638–645, 2002.
60. Maron MS, Olivotto I, Betocchi S, et al: Effect of left ventricular outflow tract obstruction on clinical outcome in hypertrophic cardiomyopathy. *N Engl J Med* 348:295–303, 2003.
61. Davies MJ, McKenna WJ: Hypertrophic cardiomyopathy–pathology and pathogenesis. *Histopathology* 26:493–500, 1995.
62. Becker AE, Caruso G: Myocardial disarray. A critical review. *Br Heart J* 47:527–538, 1982.
63. Varnava AM, Elliott PM, Mahon N, et al: Relation between myocyte disarray and outcome in hypertrophic cardiomyopathy. *Am J Cardiol* 88:275–279, 2001.
64. Almaas VM, Haugaa KH, Strom EH, et al: Increased amount of interstitial fibrosis predicts ventricular arrhythmias, and is associated with reduced myocardial septal function in patients with obstructive hypertrophic cardiomyopathy. *Europace* 15:1319–1327, 2013.
65. O'Hanlon R, Grasso A, Roughton M, et al: Prognostic significance of myocardial fibrosis in hypertrophic cardiomyopathy. *J Am Coll Cardiol* 56:867–874, 2010.
66. Lombardi R, Betocchi S, Losi MA, et al: Myocardial collagen turnover in hypertrophic cardiomyopathy. *Circulation* 108:1455–1460, 2003.
67. Ho CY, Lopez B, Coelho-Filho OR, et al: Myocardial fibrosis as an early manifestation of hypertrophic cardiomyopathy. *N Engl J Med* 363:552–563, 2010.
68. Ellims AH, Taylor AJ, Mariani JA, et al: Evaluating the utility of circulating biomarkers of collagen synthesis in hypertrophic cardiomyopathy. *Circ Heart Fail* 7:271–278, 2014.
69. Veselka J, Lawrenz T, Stellbrink C, et al: Early outcomes of alcohol septal ablation for hypertrophic obstructive cardiomyopathy: a European multicenter and multinational study. *Catheter Cardiovasc Interv* 84:101–107, 2014.
70. Greaves SC, Roche AH, Neutze JM, et al: Inheritance of hypertrophic cardiomyopathy: a cross sectional and M mode echocardiographic study of 50 families. *Br Heart J* 58:259–266, 1987.
71. Olson TM, Karst ML, Whitby FG, et al: Myosin light chain mutation causes autosomal recessive cardiomyopathy with mid-cavitary hypertrophy and restrictive physiology. *Circulation* 105:2337–2340, 2002.
72. Greve G, Bachinski L, Friedman DL, et al: Isolation of a de novo mutant myocardial beta MHC protein in a pedigree with hypertrophic cardiomyopathy. *Hum Mol Genet* 3:2073–2075, 1994.
73. Thierfelder L, Watkins H, MacRae C, et al: Alpha-tropomyosin and cardiac troponin t mutations cause familial hypertrophic cardiomyopathy: a disease of the sarcomere. *Cell* 77:701–712, 1994.
74. Richard P, Charron P, Carrier L, et al: Hypertrophic cardiomyopathy: distribution of disease genes, spectrum of mutations, and implications for a molecular diagnosis strategy. *Circulation* 107:2227–2232, 2003.
75. Van Driest SL, Jaeger MA, Ommen SR, et al: Comprehensive analysis of the beta-myosin heavy chain gene in 389 unrelated patients with hypertrophic cardiomyopathy. *J Am Coll Cardiol* 44:602–610, 2004.
76. Erdmann J, Raible J, Maki-Abadi J, et al: Spectrum of clinical phenotypes and gene variants in cardiac myosin-binding protein c mutation carriers with hypertrophic cardiomyopathy. *J Am Coll Cardiol* 38:322–330, 2001.
77. Andersen PS, Havndrup O, Bundgaard H, et al: Genetic and phenotypic characterization of mutations in myosin-binding protein C (MYBPC3) in 81 families with familial hypertrophic cardiomyopathy: total or partial haploinsufficiency. *Eur J Hum Genet* 12:673–677, 2004.
78. Marian AJ, Yu QT, Mares A, Jr, et al: Detection of a new mutation in the beta-myosin heavy chain gene in an individual with hypertrophic cardiomyopathy. *J Clin Invest* 90:2156–2165, 1992.
79. Blair E, Redwood C, de Jesus OM, et al: Mutations of the light meromyosin domain of the beta-myosin heavy chain rod in hypertrophic cardiomyopathy. *Circ Res* 90:263–269, 2002.
80. Torricelli F, Girolami F, Olivotto I, et al: Prevalence and clinical profile of troponin t mutations among patients with hypertrophic cardiomyopathy in Tuscany. *Am J Cardiol* 92:1358–1362, 2003.
81. Mogensen J, Murphy RT, Kubo T, et al: Frequency and clinical expression of cardiac troponin I mutations in 748 consecutive families with hypertrophic cardiomyopathy. *J Am Coll Cardiol* 44:2315–2325, 2004.
82. Watkins H, McKenna WJ, Thierfelder L, et al: Mutations in the genes for cardiac troponin t and alpha-tropomyosin in hypertrophic cardiomyopathy. *N Engl J Med* 332:1058–1064, 1995.
83. Olson TM, Doan TP, Kishimoto NY, et al: Inherited and de novo mutations in the cardiac actin gene cause hypertrophic cardiomyopathy. *J Mol Cell Cardiol* 32:1687–1694, 2000.
84. Mogensen J, Klausen IC, Pedersen AK, et al: Alpha-cardiac actin is a novel disease gene in familial hypertrophic cardiomyopathy. *J Clin Invest* 103:R39–R43, 1999.
85. Hayashi T, Arimura T, Itoh-Satoh M, et al: Tcap gene mutations in hypertrophic cardiomyopathy and dilated cardiomyopathy. *J Am Coll Cardiol* 44:2192–2201, 2004.
86. Andersen PS, Havndrup O, Bundgaard H, et al: Myosin light chain mutations in familial hypertrophic cardiomyopathy: phenotypic presentation and frequency in Danish and South African populations. *J Med Genet* 38:E43, 2001.
87. Van Driest SL, Ellsworth EG, Ommen SR, et al: Prevalence and spectrum of thin filament mutations in an outpatient referral population with hypertrophic cardiomyopathy. *Circulation* 108:445–451, 2003.
88. Hayashi T, Arimura T, Ueda K, et al: Identification and functional analysis of a caveolin-3 mutation associated with familial hypertrophic cardiomyopathy. *Biochem Biophys Res Commun* 313:178–184, 2004.
89. Geier C, Perrot A, Ozcelik C, et al: Mutations in the human muscle LIM protein gene in families with hypertrophic cardiomyopathy. *Circulation* 107:1390–1395, 2003.
90. Osio A, Tan L, Chen SN, et al: Myozenin 2 is a novel gene for human hypertrophic cardiomyopathy. *Circ Res* 100:766–768, 2007.
91. Davis JS, Hassanzadeh S, Winitsky S, et al: A gradient of myosin regulatory light-chain phosphorylation across the ventricular wall supports cardiac torsion. *Cold Spring Harb Symp Quant Biol* 67:345–352, 2002.
92. Hoffmann B, Schmidt-Traub H, Perrot A, et al: First mutation in cardiac troponin c, l29q, in a patient with hypertrophic cardiomyopathy. *Hum Mutat* 17:524, 2001.
93. Carniel E, Taylor MR, Sinagra G, et al: Alpha-myosin heavy chain: a sarcomeric gene associated with dilated and hypertrophic phenotypes of cardiomyopathy. *Circulation* 112:54–59, 2005.
94. Minamisawa S, Sato Y, Tatsuguchi Y, et al: Mutation of the phospholamban promoter associated with hypertrophic cardiomyopathy. *Biochem Biophys Res Commun* 304:1–4, 2003.
95. Chen SN, Czernuszewicz G, Tan Y, et al: Human molecular genetic and functional studies identify TRIM63, encoding muscle ring finger protein 1, as a novel gene for human hypertrophic cardiomyopathy. *Circ Res* 111:907–919, 2012.
96. Charron P, Dubourg O, Desnos M, et al: Clinical features and prognostic implications of familial hypertrophic cardiomyopathy related to the cardiac myosin-binding protein c gene. *Circulation* 97:2230–2236, 1998.
97. Rottbauer W, Gautel M, Zehelein J, et al: Novel splice donor site mutation in the cardiac myosin-binding protein-c gene in familial hypertrophic cardiomyopathy. Characterization of cardiac transcript and protein. *J Clin Invest* 100:475–482, 1997.
98. Blair E, Price SJ, Baty CJ, et al: Mutations in cis can confound genotype-phenotype correlations in hypertrophic cardiomyopathy. *J Med Genet* 38:385–388, 2001.
99. Richard P, Isnard R, Carrier L, et al: Double heterozygosity for mutations in the beta-myosin heavy chain and in the cardiac myosin binding protein c genes in a family with hypertrophic cardiomyopathy. *J Med Genet* 36:542–545, 1999.
100. Kapplinger JD, Landstrom AP, Bos JM, et al: Distinguishing hypertrophic cardiomyopathy-associated mutations from background genetic noise. *J Cardiovasc Transl Res* 7:347–361, 2014.
101. Bick AG, Flannick J, Ito K, et al: Burden of rare sarcomere gene variants in the Framingham and Jackson heart study cohorts. *Am J Hum Genet* 91:513–519, 2012.
102. Marian AJ: Causality in genetics: the gradient of genetic effects and back to Koch postulates of causality. *Circ Res* 114:e18–e21, 2014.
103. Watkins H: Assigning a causal role to genetic variants in hypertrophic cardiomyopathy. *Circ Cardiovasc Genet* 6:2–4, 2013.
104. Marian AJ, Belmont J: Strategic approaches to unraveling genetic causes of cardiovascular diseases. *Circ Res* 108:1252–1269, 2011.
105. Marian AJ, Roberts R: On Koch's postulates, causality and genetics of cardiomyopathies. *J Mol Cell Cardiol* 34:971–974, 2002.
106. Marian AJ: Modifier genes for hypertrophic cardiomyopathy. *Curr Opin Cardiol* 17:242–252, 2002.
107. Levy S, Sutton G, Ng PC, et al: The diploid genome sequence of an individual human. *PLoS Biol* 5:e254, 2007.
108. Korbel JO, Urban AE, Affourtit JP, et al: Paired-end mapping reveals extensive structural variation in the human genome. *Science* 318:420–426, 2007.
109. Daw EW, Chen SN, Czernuszewicz G, et al: Genome-wide mapping of modifier chromosomal loci for human hypertrophic cardiomyopathy. *Hum Mol Genet* 16:2463–2471, 2007.
110. Zhang S, Weinheimer C, Courtois M, et al: The role of the GRB2-p38 MAPK signaling pathway in cardiac hypertrophy and fibrosis. *J Clin Invest* 111:833–841, 2003.
111. Bouzeghrane F, Mercure C, Reudelhuber TL, et al: [alpha]8[beta]1 integrin is upregulated in myofibroblasts of fibrotic and scarring myocardium. *J Mol Cell Cardiol* 36:343–353, 2004.
112. Lechin M, Quinones MA, Omran A, et al: Angiotensin-I converting enzyme genotypes and left ventricular hypertrophy in patients with hypertrophic cardiomyopathy. *Circulation* 92:1808–1812, 1995.
113. Marian AJ, Yu QT, Workman R, et al: Angiotensin-converting enzyme polymorphism in hypertrophic cardiomyopathy and sudden cardiac death. *Lancet* 342:1085–1086, 1993.
114. Rigat B, Hubert C, Alhenc-Gelas F, et al: An insertion/deletion polymorphism in the angiotensin I-converting enzyme gene accounting for half the variance of serum enzyme levels. *J Clin Invest* 86:1343–1346, 1990.
115. Tesson F, Dufour C, Moolman JC, et al: The influence of the angiotensin I converting enzyme genotype in familial hypertrophic cardiomyopathy varies with the disease gene mutation. *J Mol Cell Cardiol* 29:831–838, 1997.
116. Christodoulou DC, Wakimoto H, Onoue K, et al: 5'RNA-Seq identifies Fhl1 as a genetic modifier in cardiomyopathy. *J Clin Invest* 124:1364–1370, 2014.
117. Marian AJ: Pathogenesis of diverse clinical and pathological phenotypes in hypertrophic cardiomyopathy. *Lancet* 355:58–60, 2000.
118. Nagueh SF, Chen S, Patel R, et al: Evolution of expression of cardiac phenotypes over a 4-year period in the beta-myosin heavy chain-q403 transgenic rabbit model of human hypertrophic cardiomyopathy. *J Mol Cell Cardiol* 36:663–673, 2004.
119. Lombardi R, Bell A, Senthil V, et al: Differential interactions of thin filament proteins in two cardiac troponin t mouse models of hypertrophic and dilated cardiomyopathies. *Cardiovasc Res* 79:109–117, 2008.
120. Lowey S, Lesko LM, Rovner AS, et al: Functional effects of the hypertrophic cardiomyopathy r403q mutation are different in an alpha- or beta-myosin heavy chain backbone. *J Biol Chem* 283:20579–20589, 2008.
121. Bloemink M, Deacon J, Langer S, et al: The hypertrophic cardiomyopathy myosin mutation r453c alters ATP binding and hydrolysis of human cardiac beta-myosin. *J Biol Chem* 289:5158–5167, 2014.
122. Sommese RF, Sung J, Nag S, et al: Molecular consequences of the r453c hypertrophic cardiomyopathy mutation on human beta-cardiac myosin motor function. *Proc Natl Acad Sci U S A* 110:12607–12612, 2013.
123. Palmer BM, Fishbaugher DE, Schmitt JP, et al: Differential cross-bridge kinetics of FHC myosin mutations R403Q and R453C in heterozygous mouse myocardium. *Am J Physiol Heart Circ Physiol* 287:H91–H99, 2004.
124. Heller MJ, Nili M, Homsher E, et al: Cardiomyopathic tropomyosin mutations that increase thin filament Ca2+-sensitivity and tropomyosin N-domain flexibility. *J Biol Chem* 278:41742–41748, 2003.
125. Szczesna-Cordary D, Guzman G, Zhao J, et al: The e22k mutation of myosin RLC that causes familial hypertrophic cardiomyopathy increases calcium sensitivity of force and ATPase in transgenic mice. *J Cell Sci* 118:3675–3683, 2005.
126. Lang R, Gomes AV, Zhao J, et al: Functional analysis of a troponin I (r145g) mutation associated with familial hypertrophic cardiomyopathy. *J Biol Chem* 277:11670–11678, 2002.
127. Witjas-Paalberends ER, Piroddi N, Stam K, et al: Mutations in MYH7 reduce the force generating capacity of sarcomeres in human familial hypertrophic cardiomyopathy. *Cardiovasc Res* 99:432–441, 2013.
128. Sequeira V, Wijnker PJ, Nijenkamp LL, et al: Perturbed length-dependent activation in human hypertrophic cardiomyopathy with missense sarcomeric gene mutations. *Circ Res* 112:1491–1505, 2013.
129. Wolny M, Colegrave M, Colman L, et al: Cardiomyopathy mutations in the tail of beta-cardiac myosin modify the coiled-coil structure and affect integration into thick filaments in muscle sarcomeres in adult cardiomyocytes. *J Biol Chem* 288:31952–31962, 2013.
130. Hwang JJ, Allen PD, Tseng GC, et al: Microarray gene expression profiles in dilated and hypertrophic cardiomyopathic end-stage heart failure. *Physiol Genomics* 10:31–44, 2002.
131. Lim DS, Roberts R, Marian AJ: Expression profiling of cardiac genes in human hypertrophic cardiomyopathy: insight into the pathogenesis of phenotypes. *J Am Coll Cardiol* 38:1175–1180, 2001.
132. Sieverding L, Jung WI, Breuer J, et al: Proton-decoupled myocardial 31P NMR spectroscopy reveals decreased PCr/Pi in patients with severe hypertrophic cardiomyopathy. *Am J Cardiol* 80:34A–40A, 1997.
133. Jung WI, Dietze GJ: 31p nuclear magnetic resonance spectroscopy: a noninvasive tool to monitor metabolic abnormalities in left ventricular hypertrophy in human. *Am J Cardiol* 83:19H–24H, 1999.

134. Crilley JG, Boehm EA, Blair E, et al: Hypertrophic cardiomyopathy due to sarcomeric gene mutations is characterized by impaired energy metabolism irrespective of the degree of hypertrophy. *J Am Coll Cardiol* 41:1776–1782, 2003.
135. Jung WI, Sieverding L, Breuer J, et al: 31p NMR spectroscopy detects metabolic abnormalities in asymptomatic patients with hypertrophic cardiomyopathy. *Circulation* 97:2536–2542, 1998.
136. Roberts R, Marian AJ: Can an energy-deficient heart grow bigger and stronger? *J Am Coll Cardiol* 41:1783–1785, 2003.
137. Lan F, Lee AS, Liang P, et al: Abnormal calcium handling properties underlie familial hypertrophic cardiomyopathy pathology in patient-specific induced pluripotent stem cells. *Cell Stem Cell* 12:101–113, 2013.
138. Ruggiero A, Chen SN, Lombardi R, et al: Pathogenesis of hypertrophic cardiomyopathy caused by myozenin 2 mutations is independent of calcineurin activity. *Cardiovasc Res* 97:44–54, 2013.
139. Sarikas A, Carrier L, Schenke C, et al: Impairment of the ubiquitin-proteasome system by truncated cardiac myosin binding protein c mutants. *Cardiovasc Res* 66:33–44, 2005.
140. Nagueh SF, Kopelen HA, Lim DS, et al: Tissue doppler imaging consistently detects myocardial contraction and relaxation abnormalities, irrespective of cardiac hypertrophy, in a transgenic rabbit model of human hypertrophic cardiomyopathy. *Circulation* 102:1346–1350, 2000.
141. Zhou M, Guo J, Cha J, et al: Non-optimal codon usage affects expression, structure and function of clock protein FRQ. *Nature* 495:111–115, 2013.
142. Charron P, Dubourg O, Desnos M, et al: Genotype-phenotype correlations in familial hypertrophic cardiomyopathy. A comparison between mutations in the cardiac protein-c and the beta-myosin heavy chain genes. *Eur Heart J* 19:139–145, 1998.
143. Anan R, Greve G, Thierfelder L, et al: Prognostic implications of novel beta cardiac myosin heavy chain gene mutations that cause familial hypertrophic cardiomyopathy. *J Clin Invest* 93:280–285, 1994.
144. Maron BJ, Niimura H, Casey SA, et al: Development of left ventricular hypertrophy in adults in hypertrophic cardiomyopathy caused by cardiac myosin-binding protein c gene mutations. *J Am Coll Cardiol* 38:315–321, 2001.
145. Abchee A, Marian AJ: Prognostic significance of beta-myosin heavy chain mutations is reflective of their hypertrophic expressivity in patients with hypertrophic cardiomyopathy. *J Investig Med* 45:191–196, 1997.
146. Varnava AM, Elliott PM, Baboonian C, et al: Hypertrophic cardiomyopathy: histopathological features of sudden death in cardiac troponin t disease. *Circulation* 104:1380–1384, 2001.
147. Van Driest SL, Ackerman MJ, Ommen SR, et al: Prevalence and severity of "benign" mutations in the beta-myosin heavy chain, cardiac troponin t, and alpha-tropomyosin genes in hypertrophic cardiomyopathy. *Circulation* 106:3085–3090, 2002.
148. Niimura H, Patton KK, McKenna WJ, et al: Sarcomere protein gene mutations in hypertrophic cardiomyopathy of the elderly. *Circulation* 105:446–451, 2002.
149. Konhilas JP, Watson PA, Maass A, et al: Exercise can prevent and reverse the severity of hypertrophic cardiomyopathy. *Circ Res* 98:540–548, 2006.
150. Maron BJ, Fananapazir L: Sudden cardiac death in hypertrophic cardiomyopathy. *Circulation* 85:157–163, 1992.
151. Fujino N, Shimizu M, Ino H, et al: A novel mutation lys273glu in the cardiac troponin t gene shows high degree of penetrance and transition from hypertrophic to dilated cardiomyopathy. *Am J Cardiol* 89:29–33, 2002.
152. Mogensen J, Kubo T, Duque M, et al: Idiopathic restrictive cardiomyopathy is part of the clinical expression of cardiac troponin I mutations. *J Clin Invest* 111:209–216, 2003.
153. Fujino N, Shimizu M, Ino H, et al: Cardiac troponin t arg92trp mutation and progression from hypertrophic to dilated cardiomyopathy. *Clin Cardiol* 24:397–402, 2001.
154. Li D, Czernuszewicz GZ, Gonzalez O, et al: Novel cardiac troponin t mutation as a cause of familial dilated cardiomyopathy. *Circulation* 104:2188–2193, 2001.
155. Klaassen S, Probst S, Oechslin E, et al: Mutations in sarcomere protein genes in left ventricular noncompaction. *Circulation* 117:2893–2901, 2008.
156. Kamisago M, Sharma SD, DePalma SR, et al: Mutations in sarcomere protein genes as a cause of dilated cardiomyopathy. *N Engl J Med* 343:1688–1696, 2000.
157. Yanaga F, Morimoto S, Ohtsuki I: Ca2+ sensitization and potentiation of the maximum level of myofibrillar ATPase activity caused by mutations of troponin t found in familial hypertrophic cardiomyopathy. *J Biol Chem* 274:8806–8812, 1999.
158. Morimoto S, Lu QW, Harada K, et al: Ca(2+)-desensitizing effect of a deletion mutation delta k210 in cardiac troponin t that causes familial dilated cardiomyopathy. *Proc Natl Acad Sci U S A* 99:913–918, 2002.
159. Davis J, Wen H, Edwards T, et al: Allele and species dependent contractile defects by restrictive and hypertrophic cardiomyopathy-linked troponin I mutants. *J Mol Cell Cardiol* 44:891–904, 2008.
160. Chang AN, Harada K, Ackerman MJ, et al: Functional consequences of hypertrophic and dilated cardiomyopathy-causing mutations in alpha-tropomyosin. *J Biol Chem* 280:34343–34349, 2005.
161. Burton D, Abdulrazzak H, Knott A, et al: Two mutations in troponin I that cause hypertrophic cardiomyopathy have contrasting effects on cardiac muscle contractility. *Biochem J* 362:443–451, 2002.
162. Bottinelli R, Coviello DA, Redwood CS, et al: A mutant tropomyosin that causes hypertrophic cardiomyopathy is expressed in vivo and associated with an increased calcium sensitivity. *Circ Res* 82:106–115, 1998.
163. Bing W, Knott A, Redwood C, et al: Effect of hypertrophic cardiomyopathy mutations in human cardiac muscle alpha-tropomyosin (asp175asn and glu180gly) on the regulatory properties of human cardiac troponin determined by in vitro motility assay. *J Mol Cell Cardiol* 32:1489–1498, 2000.
164. Lowey S, Lesko LM, Rovner AS, et al: Functional effects of the hypertrophic cardiomyopathy r403q mutation are different in an alpha- or beta-myosin heavy chain backbone. *J Biol Chem* 283:20579–20589, 2008.
165. Lowey S, Bretton V, Gulick J, et al: Transgenic mouse alpha- and beta-cardiac myosins containing the r403q mutation show isoform-dependent transient kinetic differences. *J Biol Chem* 288:14780–14787, 2013.
166. Lowes BD, Gilbert EM, Abraham WT, et al: Myocardial gene expression in dilated cardiomyopathy treated with beta-blocking agents. *N Engl J Med* 346:1357–1365, 2002.
167. Lompre AM, Schwartz K, d'Albis A, et al: Myosin isoenzyme redistribution in chronic heart overload. *Nature* 282:105–107, 1979.
168. Schwartz K, Lecarpentier Y, Martin JL, et al: Myosin isoenzymic distribution correlates with speed of myocardial contraction. *J Mol Cell Cardiol* 13:1071–1075, 1981.
169. Holubarsch C, Goulette RP, Litten RZ, et al: The economy of isometric force development, myosin isoenzyme pattern and myofibrillar ATPase activity in normal and hypothyroid rat myocardium. *Circ Res* 56:78–86, 1985.
170. Nugent AW, Daubeney PEF, Chondros P, et al: Clinical features and outcomes of childhood hypertrophic cardiomyopathy: results from a national population-based study. *Circulation* 112:1332–1338, 2005.
171. Tartaglia M, Mehler EL, Goldberg R, et al: Mutations in PTPN11, encoding the protein tyrosine phosphatase SHP-2, cause Noonan syndrome. *Nat Genet* 29:465–468, 2001.
172. Pandit B, Sarkozy A, Pennacchio LA, et al: Gain-of-function RAF1 mutations cause Noonan and LEOPARD syndromes with hypertrophic cardiomyopathy. *Nat Genet* 39:1007–1012, 2007.
173. Tartaglia M, Pennacchio LA, Zhao C, et al: Gain-of-function SOS1 mutations cause a distinctive form of Noonan syndrome. *Nat Genet* 39:75–79, 2007.
174. Carta C, Pantaleoni F, Bocchinfuso G, et al: Germline missense mutations affecting KRAS isoform b are associated with a severe Noonan syndrome phenotype. *Am J Hum Genet* 79:129–135, 2006.
175. Cordeddu V, Di Schiavi E, Pennacchio LA, et al: Mutation of SHOC2 promotes aberrant protein N-myristoylation and causes Noonan-like syndrome with loose anagen hair. *Nat Genet* 41:1022–1026, 2009.
176. Gollob MH, Seger JJ, Gollob TN, et al: Novel PRKAG2 mutation responsible for the genetic syndrome of ventricular preexcitation and conduction system disease with childhood onset and absence of cardiac hypertrophy. *Circulation* 104:3030–3033, 2001.
177. Arad M, Benson DW, Perez-Atayde AR, et al: Constitutively active AMP kinase mutations cause glycogen storage disease mimicking hypertrophic cardiomyopathy. *J Clin Invest* 109:357–362, 2002.
178. Kim M, Hunter RW, Garcia-Menendez L, et al: Mutation in the gamma2-subunit of AMP-activated protein kinase stimulates cardiomyocyte proliferation and hypertrophy independent of glycogen storage. *Circ Res* 114:966–975, 2014.
179. Chimenti C, Pieroni M, Morgante E, et al: Prevalence of Fabry disease in female patients with late-onset hypertrophic cardiomyopathy. *Circulation* 110:1047–1053, 2004.
180. Sachdev B, Takenaka T, Teraguchi H, et al: Prevalence of Anderson-Fabry disease in male patients with late onset hypertrophic cardiomyopathy. *Circulation* 105:1407–1411, 2002.
181. Brady RO, Schiffmann R: Clinical features of and recent advances in therapy for Fabry disease. *JAMA* 284:2771–2775, 2000.
182. Desnick RJ, Brady R, Barranger J, et al: Fabry disease, an under-recognized multisystemic disorder: expert recommendations for diagnosis, management, and enzyme replacement therapy. *Ann Intern Med* 138:338–346, 2003.
183. Eng CM, Guffon N, Wilcox WR, et al: Safety and efficacy of recombinant human alpha-galactosidase a–replacement therapy in Fabry's disease. *N Engl J Med* 345:9–16, 2001.
184. Schiffmann R, Murray GJ, Treco D, et al: Infusion of alpha-galactosidase a reduces tissue globotriaosylceramide storage in patients with Fabry disease. *Proc Natl Acad Sci U S A* 97:365–370, 2000.
185. Wilcox WR, Banikazemi M, Guffon N, et al: Long-term safety and efficacy of enzyme replacement therapy for Fabry disease. *Am J Hum Genet* 75:65–74, 2004.
186. Meyer C, Schmid G, Gorlitz S, et al: Cardiomyopathy in Friedreich's ataxia—assessment by cardiac MRI. *Mov Disord* 22:1615–1622, 2007.
187. Karpati G, Carpenter S, Larbrisseau A, et al: The Kearns-Shy syndrome. A multisystem disease with mitochondrial abnormality demonstrated in skeletal muscle and skin. *J Neurol Sci* 19:133–151, 1973.
188. Marian AJ: Challenges in medical applications of whole exome/genome sequencing discoveries. *Trends Cardiovasc Med* 22:219–223, 2012.
189. Maron BJ, Spirito P, Shen WK, et al: Implantable cardioverter-defibrillators and prevention of sudden cardiac death in hypertrophic cardiomyopathy. *JAMA* 298:405–412, 2007.
190. Maron BJ, Spirito P, Ackerman MJ, et al: Prevention of sudden cardiac death with implantable cardioverter-defibrillators in children and adolescents with hypertrophic cardiomyopathy. *J Am Coll Cardiol* 61:1527–1535, 2013.
191. McLeod CJ, Ommen SR, Ackerman MJ, et al: Surgical septal myectomy decreases the risk for appropriate implantable cardioverter defibrillator discharge in obstructive hypertrophic cardiomyopathy. *Eur Heart J* 28:2583–2588, 2007.
192. McGregor JB, Rahman A, Rosanio S, et al: Monomorphic ventricular tachycardia: a late complication of percutaneous alcohol septal ablation for hypertrophic cardiomyopathy. *Am J Med Sci* 328:185–188, 2004.
193. Sorajja P, Valeti U, Nishimura RA, et al: Outcome of alcohol septal ablation for obstructive hypertrophic cardiomyopathy. *Circulation* 118:131–139, 2008.
194. Spirito P, Autore C, Formisano F, et al: Risk of sudden death and outcome in patients with hypertrophic cardiomyopathy with benign presentation and without risk factors. *Am J Cardiol* 113:1550–1555, 2014.
195. Peteiro J, Bouzas-Mosquera A, Fernandez X, et al: Prognostic value of exercise echocardiography in patients with hypertrophic cardiomyopathy. *J Am Soc Echocardiogr* 25:182–189, 2012.
196. Sorajja P, Allison T, Hayes C, et al: Prognostic utility of metabolic exercise testing in minimally symptomatic patients with obstructive hypertrophic cardiomyopathy. *Am J Cardiol* 109:1494–1498, 2012.
197. Desai MY, Bhonsale A, Patel P, et al: Exercise echocardiography in asymptomatic HCM: exercise capacity, and not LV outflow tract gradient predicts long-term outcomes. *JACC Cardiovasc imaging* 7:26–36, 2014.
198. Sherrid MV, Barac I, McKenna WJ, et al: Multicenter study of the efficacy and safety of disopyramide in obstructive hypertrophic cardiomyopathy. *J Am Coll Cardiol* 45:1251–1258, 2005.
199. Agarwal S, Tuzcu EM, Desai MY, et al: Updated meta-analysis of septal alcohol ablation versus myectomy for hypertrophic cardiomyopathy. *J Am Coll Cardiol* 55:823–834, 2010.
200. Alam M, Dokainish H, Lakkis NM: Hypertrophic obstructive cardiomyopathy-alcohol septal ablation vs. myectomy: a meta-analysis. *Eur Heart J* 30:1080–1087, 2009.
201. Nagueh SF, Groves BM, Schwartz L, et al: Alcohol septal ablation for the treatment of hypertrophic obstructive cardiomyopathy. A multicenter North American registry. *J Am Coll Cardiol* 58:2322–2328, 2011.
202. Sorajja P, Ommen SR, Holmes DR, Jr, et al: Survival after alcohol septal ablation for obstructive hypertrophic cardiomyopathy. *Circulation* 126:2374–2380, 2012.
203. Schonbeck MH, Brunner-La Rocca HP, Vogt PR, et al: Long-term follow-up in hypertrophic obstructive cardiomyopathy after septal myectomy. *Ann Thorac Surg* 65:1207–1214, 1998.
204. Schulte HD, Bircks WH, Loesse B, et al: Prognosis of patients with hypertrophic obstructive cardiomyopathy after transaortic myectomy. Late results up to twenty-five years. *J Thorac Cardiovasc Surg* 106:709–717, 1993.
205. McCully RB, Nishimura RA, Tajik AJ, et al: Extent of clinical improvement after surgical treatment of hypertrophic obstructive cardiomyopathy. *Circulation* 94:467–471, 1996.
206. Desai MY, Bhonsale A, Smedira NG, et al: Predictors of long-term outcomes in symptomatic hypertrophic obstructive cardiomyopathy patients undergoing surgical relief of left ventricular outflow tract obstruction. *Circulation* 128:209–216, 2013.
207. Geske JB, Konecny T, Ommen SR, et al: Surgical myectomy improves pulmonary hypertension in obstructive hypertrophic cardiomyopathy. *Eur Heart J* 35:2032–2039, 2014.
208. van Dockum WG, ten Cate FJ, ten Berg JM, et al: Myocardial infarction after percutaneous transluminal septal myocardial ablation in hypertrophic obstructive cardiomyopathy: evaluation by contrast-enhanced magnetic resonance imaging. *J Am Coll Cardiol* 43:27–34, 2004.
209. Nagueh SF, Lakkis NM, Middleton KJ, et al: Changes in left ventricular diastolic function 6 months after nonsurgical septal reduction therapy for hypertrophic obstructive cardiomyopathy. *Circulation* 99:344–347, 1999.

210. Chang SM, Nagueh SF, Spencer WH, 3rd, et al: Complete heart block: determinants and clinical impact in patients with hypertrophic obstructive cardiomyopathy undergoing non-surgical septal reduction therapy. *J Am Coll Cardiol* 42:296–300, 2003.
211. Talreja DR, Nishimura RA, Edwards WD, et al: Alcohol septal ablation versus surgical septal myectomy: comparison of effects on atrioventricular conduction tissue. *J Am Coll Cardiol* 44:2329–2332, 2004.
212. Axelsson A, Weibring K, Havndrup O, et al: Atrioventricular conduction after alcohol septal ablation for obstructive hypertrophic cardiomyopathy. *J Cardiovasc Med* 15:214–221, 2014.
213. Lim DS, Lutucuta S, Bachireddy P, et al: Angiotensin II blockade reverses myocardial fibrosis in a transgenic mouse model of human hypertrophic cardiomyopathy. *Circulation* 103:789–791, 2001.
214. Marian AJ, Senthil V, Chen SN, et al: Antifibrotic effects of antioxidant N-acetylcysteine in a mouse model of human hypertrophic cardiomyopathy mutation. *J Am Coll Cardiol* 47:827–834, 2006.
215. Teekakirikul P, Eminaga S, Toka O, et al: Cardiac fibrosis in mice with hypertrophic cardiomyopathy is mediated by non-myocyte proliferation and requires TGF-beta. *J Clin Invest* 120:3520–3529, 2010.
216. Araujo AQ, Arteaga E, Ianni BM, et al: Effect of losartan on left ventricular diastolic function in patients with nonobstructive hypertrophic cardiomyopathy. *Am J Cardiol* 96:1563–1567, 2005.
217. Yamazaki T, Suzuki J, Shimamoto R, et al: A new therapeutic strategy for hypertrophic nonobstructive cardiomyopathy in humans. A randomized and prospective study with an angiotensin II receptor blocker. *Int Heart J* 48:715–724, 2007.
218. Shimada YJ, Passeri JJ, Baggish AL, et al: Effects of losartan on left ventricular hypertrophy and fibrosis in patients with nonobstructive hypertrophic cardiomyopathy. *JACC Heart Fail* 1:480–487, 2013.
219. Bauersachs J, Stork S, Kung M, et al: HMG CoA reductase inhibition and left ventricular mass in hypertrophic cardiomyopathy: a randomized placebo-controlled pilot study. *Eur J Clin Invest* 37:852–859, 2007.
220. Nagueh SF, Lombardi R, Tan Y, et al: Atorvastatin and cardiac hypertrophy and function in hypertrophic cardiomyopathy: a pilot study. *Eur J Clin Invest* 40:976–983, 2010.
221. Jiang J, Wakimoto H, Seidman JG, et al: Allele-specific silencing of mutant Myh6 transcripts in mice suppresses hypertrophic cardiomyopathy. *Science* 342:111–114, 2013.
222. Roberts R: Specific RNA inhibition of causal alleles: a potential therapy for familial hypertrophic cardiomyopathy. *Circ Res* 114:751–753, 2014.
223. Mearini G, Stimpel D, Kramer E, et al: Repair of Mybpc3 MRNA by 5'-trans-splicing in a mouse model of hypertrophic cardiomyopathy. *Mol Ther Nucleic Acids* 2:e102, 2013.
224. Gedicke-Hornung C, Behrens-Gawlik V, Reischmann S, et al: Rescue of cardiomyopathy through U7snRNA-mediated exon skipping in Mybpc3-targeted knock-in mice. *EMBO Mol Med* 5:1060–1077, 2013.

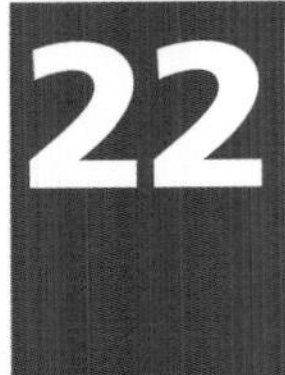

Heart Failure as a Consequence of Genetic Cardiomyopathy

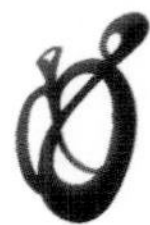

Daniel P. Judge

The genetic contributions to heart failure are numerous and remarkably heterogeneous, extending from the monogenic forms of cardiomyopathy to more common polygenic diseases, such as hypertension (**see also Chapter 23**), coronary atherosclerosis, and myocardial infarction (**see also Chapter 18**). For the monogenic diseases, the responsible mutations are rare but carry a very high pathogenic burden. The polygenic conditions typically include DNA variants that are common in healthy populations, imparting only a small pathogenic effect. For all of these conditions, both genetic factors and environmental stimuli likely work in synergy to cause heart disease. This chapter will focus on the monogenic disorders, such as familial dilated, hypertrophic, restrictive, and arrhythmogenic forms of cardiomyopathy, and their progression to heart failure.

In considering the genetic aspects of heart failure, one should contemplate not only the underlying cause of a familial form of cardiomyopathy, but also the pattern of familial segregation, or more specifically consider who else in the family is at risk of developing heart failure.[1] One should also recognize syndromic features of disorders that include familial cardiomyopathy. Genetic testing is an important aspect of the evaluation for familial cardiomyopathy, and it should be preceded by genetic counseling by a trained counselor. From a research perspective, improved understanding of the genetic basis for familial forms of cardiomyopathy should help to develop better treatments.

The following clinical scenario highlights many of these aspects. A 30-year-old man was referred for genetic evaluation of dilated cardiomyopathy. He was healthy as a child and young adult, participating in high school and college sports (baseball), although he described himself as a "toe walker." He developed transient hemiparesis 1 year previously, and his evaluation included an echocardiogram, which showed severe LV dilation with normal wall thickness, ejection fraction of 20%, and normal valves. Evaluation for the cause of his dilated cardiomyopathy showed no discernible coronary disease, and his laboratory testing was otherwise normal.

His family history is shown in the pedigree in **Figure 22-1**. There was no antecedent history of DCM, heart failure, or sudden cardiac death in prior generations. His first child was a son, who died at age 3 days with dilated cardiomyopathy on autopsy and a normal karyotype. His surviving son was age 3 years with left ventricular (LV) dilation (Z score >2.0, normalized for age and body size) with normal ejection fraction and valves. The son's serum creatine kinase level was normal, but the father's creatine kinase level was approximately 800 U/L, and he had calf pseudohypertrophy. This raised concern for several different forms of muscular dystrophy, which include dilated cardiomyopathy. The male-to-male transmission excludes X-linked disorders. Notably, a mutation in *LMNA* encoding the nuclear envelope protein lamin A/C, could cause this condition. *LMNA* mutations are associated with high rates of sudden death and systemic manifestations.[2] Such a mutation may influence decisions about implantable cardioverter-defibrillator (ICD) placement and arrhythmia risk in the proband and family members.[3]

After genetic counseling, clinical genetic testing was performed in the proband *(arrow)* using a panel of genes in which mutations cause DCM. His has a heterozygous substitution of a highly conserved arginine with a proline at codon 1909 in exon 39 of *MYH7*, encoding cardiac β-myosin heavy chain (β-MHC) (**Figure 22-2**). This mutation was present in the proband's living son with LV dilation, and it was also identified in DNA from the deceased son, which was stored at the time of his death. It was a de novo mutation, not present in either of the proband's parents, further supporting its pathogenicity. Mutations in β-MHC typically cause either hypertrophic cardiomyopathy or dilated cardiomyopathy, but alterations of the C-terminus (exons 30-40) also cause Laing distal skeletal myopathy.[4-6]

CLINICAL PRESENTATIONS

People with familial forms of cardiomyopathy typically do not have overt symptoms until they have advanced dysfunction with very low cardiac output fairly late in the course of

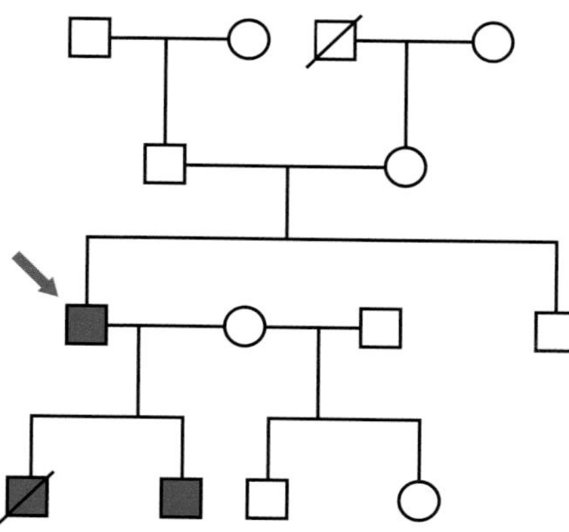

FIGURE 22-1 Pedigree for the 30-year-old man with dilated cardiomyopathy. The proband is highlighted with a red arrow. Circles represent females, and squares represent males; blue shading indicates those with dilated cardiomyopathy. A diagonal line through a square or circle indicates an individual who is deceased.

***MYH7* p.Arg1909Pro**

Human	FRKVQHELDEAEERADIAESQVNKLRAK
Macaque	FRKVQHELDEAEERADIAESQVNKLRAK
Gorilla	FRKVQHELDEAEERADIAESQVNKLRAK
Pig	FRKVQHELDEAEERADIAESQVNKLRAK
Cow	FRKVQHELDEAEERADIAESQVNKLRAK
Horse	FRKVQHELDEAEERADIAESQVNKLRAK
Chicken	FRKVQHELDEAEERADMAESQVNKLRAR
Rat	FRKVQHELDEAEERADIAESQVNKLRAK
Mouse	FRKVQHELDEAEERADIAESQVNKLRAK
Xenopus	YKKLQHELDDAQERADIAESQVNKLRSK
Zebrafish	FRKIQHDLDEAEERADMAESQVNKLRVR

FIGURE 22-2 Conservation of the mutated amino acid. Arginine (Arg or R) at codon 1909 is highly conserved among different species. Amino acids are shown with their single-letter abbreviations, and the position of the mutation is highlighted with red text. Substitution of this position with a proline (Pro or P) inserts a nonpolar neutral amino acid where normally there would be a polar amino acid that is strongly basic.

their disease. When cardiac function abruptly declines, as with acute ischemic or inflammatory injury to the heart, the sudden elevation of ventricular filling pressures usually causes prominent symptoms. With gradual loss of ventricular systolic function, physiologic compensation due to neurohormonal activation causes progressive dilation of the heart and initial preservation of the stroke volume. Yet this same process of neurohormonal activation eventually becomes pathologic, contributing to greater LV dilation and loss of force.

The prevalence of familial dilated cardiomyopathy (see also Chapter 19) is often underestimated.[7] Though sometimes considered rare, careful assessment of the first-degree relatives of individuals with otherwise unexplained dilated cardiomyopathy for the same condition has repeatedly shown 20% to 35% with familial DCM.[7,8] One study considered family members with LV enlargement greater than 112% of the size predicted on the basis of body surface area and normal systolic function as affected, and they reported a prevalence of familial DCM of 48% in a cohort that was previously considered to be idiopathic.[9] With this in mind, the ACC/AHA/ASE guidelines for the use of echocardiography provide a class I recommendation for evaluation of first-degree relatives (parents, siblings, and children) of people with unexplained DCM.[10]

The genetic forms of cardiomyopathy are typically categorized based on the appearance of the heart. Because of pioneering research identifying its genetic basis, hypertrophic cardiomyopathy (HCM) is now usually well recognized as a familial condition.[6] In contrast, nonischemic dilated cardiomyopathy (DCM) can be caused by numerous other factors.[11] Accordingly, familial DCM is less well recognized when it occurs. Incomplete pedigrees, age-dependent onset of symptoms, de novo mutations, recessive inheritance, and low penetrance are all factors contributing to failed recognition of familial forms of cardiomyopathy.[1] The phrase "heart attack" is a commonly used lay term that infers coronary thrombosis or occlusion, but it may otherwise refer to arrhythmic sudden death in the context of familial cardiomyopathy. Thus when discussing family history with individuals with idiopathic cardiomyopathy, it is important to clarify whether "heart attack" or sudden death occurred in the context of known coronary disease or extensive coronary atherosclerotic risk factors. If an autopsy was performed, it should be able to discern ischemic and nonischemic forms of heart failure. Familial cardiomyopathy also includes restrictive cardiomyopathy (RCM) and left ventricular noncompaction cardiomyopathy (LVNC). Once again, incomplete pedigrees, age-dependent onset of symptoms, de novo mutations, recessive inheritance, and low penetrance all contribute to failed recognition of familial forms of these rare cardiomyopathies. Both RCM and LVNC may overlap with DCM and HCM, and they may be missed without careful imaging. Arrhythmogenic right ventricular dysplasia/cardiomyopathy (ARVD/C) is another rare form of familial cardiomyopathy that is becoming better characterized with regard to its genetic basis over the past few years.[12] Heart failure appears to be less common among individuals with ARVD/C than other forms of cardiomyopathy.[13,14]

The most easily recognized pattern of inheritance is autosomal dominant, but autosomal recessive, X-linked, and matrilinear (mitochondrial) patterns also occur. In X-linked forms of cardiomyopathy, female carriers may manifest the condition, although typically later and less severely than affected men. A familial trait like cardiomyopathy does not need to affect a large number of people in the family. In fact, recessive, X-linked, or de novo dominant forms of cardiomyopathy can appear without a clear family history to alert health care providers to its underlying basis. Simply the presence of a single similarly affected family member allows for the diagnosis of familial cardiomyopathy.[15] A family history of early and unexplained sudden death, typically below the age of 35 years, may also be considered as a criterion for the diagnosis of familial cardiomyopathy.[15,16]

FINDINGS THAT INDICATE A GENETIC FORM OF CARDIOMYOPATHY

Although the family history and phenotypic characterization of family members who are at risk of inheriting the same genetic disorder are the best way to recognize inherited forms of cardiomyopathy, some additional features may help to make this diagnosis on initial presentation (**Table 22-1**). Because the heart and skeletal muscles both contain several of the same protein components, an individual with concomitant heart failure and skeletal myopathy almost certainly has a monogenic condition that explains both findings. Skeletal myopathy may be subtle, consisting of asymptomatic elevation of the serum creatine

TABLE 22-1 Noncardiac Findings Suggesting a Genetic Form of Cardiomyopathy

ORGAN	MANIFESTATION	CONSIDER
HEENT	Dysmorphic appearance	Chromosomal abnormality, *LMNA* mutation
	Blindness or unexplained loss of vision	Mitochondrial disorder
	Deafness or premature presbycusis	Mitochondrial disorder
	Unexplained corneal keratopathy	Fabry disease
	Retinopathy	Danon disease
Adipose	Lipodystrophy	*LMNA* mutation
Skin	Angiokeratomas	Fabry disease
	Palmoplantar keratodermas	Naxos, Carvajal, ARVC
	Hypohidrosis	Fabry disease
Central nervous system	Developmental delay	Chromosomal disorder
		Danon disease
		Mitochondrial disorder
		Presenilin mutation
Peripheral nervous system	Peripheral neuropathy	Fabry disease
		TTR amyloidosis
Skeletal muscle	Reduced strength, tone, or bulk	Cardioskeletal myopathy
	Pseudohypertrophy	Cardioskeletal myopathy
	Unexplained elevation of serum creatine kinase	Cardioskeletal myopathy

ARVC, Arrhythmogenic right ventricular cardiomyopathy; *HEENT,* heads/eyes/ears/nose/throat.

kinase level or abnormalities in muscle bulk (pseudohypertrophy or muscle hypotrophy).

Mitochondrial disorders typically include cardiomyopathy, in addition to skeletal myopathy, blindness or loss of vision, early hearing loss, developmental delay, seizures, or short stature. Elevation of the resting lactic acid level in blood without hypoperfusion also suggests a mitochondrial disorder and should prompt further evaluation for systemic manifestations.

There are several forms of glycogen- and lysosomal-storage diseases with cardiac manifestations. These are recessive or X-linked disorders with loss-of-function mutations in enzymes, and they result in excessive production and deposition of intermediate metabolites.

Fabry Disease

Mutations in *GLA* encoding α-galactosidase A cause X-linked Fabry disease (or Anderson-Fabry disease).[17] Johannes Fabry in Germany and William Anderson in England simultaneously first reported this condition in 1898.[18,19] The constellation of hypertrophic cardiomyopathy, renal dysfunction, peripheral neuropathy, hypohidrosis, and angiokeratomas of the skin should raise concern for Fabry disease, but it can also occur with isolated cardiac involvement.[20] Corneal opacity (keratopathy) also occurs in Fabry disease, and it may be indistinguishable from amiodarone-induced corneal disease.[21]

The age of onset for Fabry disease depends on gender and the type of mutation. Males with complete absence of α-galactosidase A enzyme activity typically have their initial symptoms during late childhood.[17] Males who have partial enzyme activity often present later in life with HCM, and often without systemic features. Clinical manifestations in women with a heterozygous *GLA* mutation range from asymptomatic to the full spectrum seen in affected men.[17] Since the responsible gene is on the X chromosome, male-to-male transmission of HCM in a family makes Fabry-associated HCM unlikely.

A clinical suspicion of Fabry disease can be confirmed by measurement of serum α-galactosidase A enzyme activity or by *GLA* genetic testing. In one study, 90 probands with HCM underwent genetic analysis; 31/90 (34%) had sarcomere mutations and 3/90 (3%) had *GLA* mutations.[22] None of these individuals had systemic features of Fabry disease. The inclusion of this gene in large panels for genetic evaluation of cardiomyopathies should help to increase recognition of Fabry disease, particularly with isolated cardiac involvement.

The availability of replacement enzyme infusions for Fabry disease should lead to consideration of this condition in anyone with unexplained HCM.[23] One study showed that treatment of affected individuals with recombinant human α-galactosidase A slowed progression to a composite endpoint, including cardiac, renal, and cerebrovascular complications or death, when compared with the placebo.[24] The development of recombinant α-galactosidase A for the treatment of Fabry disease highlights the possibility of similar targeted therapy for related enzyme deficiencies.

Danon Disease

Danon and colleagues reported another X-linked glycogen storage disease with cardiomyopathy.[25] Phenotypic manifestations include cardiac hypertrophy with loss of systolic function, skeletal myopathy, developmental delay, and retinopathy. Loss-of-function mutations in *LAMP2,* encoding a lysosome-associated membrane protein, cause this condition, although enzyme replacement therapy is not currently available.[26]

One report highlighted the rapid progression and early mortality in a very small cohort of children (six males and one female aged 7-17 years) with *LAMP2* mutations.[27] Four died from heart failure, one died from ventricular fibrillation refractory to defibrillator shocks, and one underwent cardiac transplantation with mean age of 21 years for these endpoints.[27] In a much larger cohort of 82 individuals with Danon disease from 36 separate families, in addition to 63 previously reported cases (145 people with this condition), another group more comprehensively characterized the natural history of this rare disorder.[28] In this report, the average ages of first symptom, cardiac transplantation, and death were 12.1, 17.9, and 19.0 years in men and 27.9, 33.7, and 34.6 years in women, respectively. Cardiac transplantation (see Chapter 40) appropriately addresses heart failure when it progresses to advanced stages, but progressive disease in other organ systems will occur in that context.[29]

Transthyretin Cardiac Amyloidosis (see also Chapter 20)

Cardiac amyloidosis may be suspected based on discordance between imaging studies with concentric ventricular hypertrophy and electrocardiograms with low ECG voltage.[30] Light chain (AL) amyloid is the most common form, with associated monoclonal gammopathy due to underlying plasma cell dyscrasias or multiple myeloma. Mutations in *TTR*, encoding transthyretin, are the most common form of inherited cardiac amyloidosis.[30] From a diagnostic perspective, suspicion of cardiac amyloidosis should not be dismissed in the absence of a monoclonal gammopathy, because familial forms of amyloid and senile transthyretin amyloid occur without gammopathy. Senile transthyretin amyloid (without *TTR* mutation) is typically only found in the heart, and a cardiac biopsy is required to make the diagnosis.

Transthyretin is a carrier protein in the blood, binding to thyroid hormone and retinol binding protein. Investigating the increased prevalence of isolated cardiac amyloidosis among African Americans, Jacobson and colleagues reviewed 52,370 autopsies in Los Angeles.[31] In this cohort, 136 cases of cardiac amyloidosis were identified among those age 60 years or older. A greater proportion of African Americans was affected in every age group, with a ratio of blacks to whites of approximately 8:1 for the ages 60 to 69. The ratio was greatest (13:1) for ages 70 to 79. The ratio decreased in later decades because of an increase in cardiac amyloidosis among whites. Further analysis showed that 23% of the affected African Americans had a *TTR* mutation substituting an isoleucine for valine at position 122 (Val122Ile).[31] Approximately 3.5% to 4% of African Americans carry this mutation in heterozygosity or homozygosity, and its presence is associated with a higher frequency of heart failure and mortality after age 70 years.[32] The high prevalence of this allele among individuals with black African ancestry and the concomitantly high prevalence of heart failure with preserved ejection fraction (HFPEF) among older individuals suggest that many older patients with black African ancestry and HFPEF may have unrecognized transthyretin cardiac amyloidosis.

In a combined analysis from both Mayo Clinic and Johns Hopkins, among 143 people with biopsy-proven cardiac amyloidosis, 57% had transthyretin-type amyloid and 43% had light chain disease, although this analysis likely reflects the bias of these tertiary referral centers.[33] Mass spectrometry analysis of biopsies with amyloid can definitively ascertain the cause of amyloidosis.[33] Because transthyretin is mostly produced by the liver, amyloidosis caused by *TTR* mutations may be treated by liver transplantation, which is optimal only if used early in the course of the disease.[30] Several new medication strategies are under investigation, including medications to stabilize the soluble transthyretin tetramer or to decrease its production.[34,35]

Arrhythmogenic Right Ventricular Cardiomyopathy

Arrhythmogenic right ventricular cardiomyopathy (ARVC) is a genetic disorder characterized by a right ventricular fibrofatty scar and prominent ventricular arrhythmias.[12] In one U.S. study of 100 affected individuals, the median age at presentation was 26 years, with postmortem diagnosis in 31%.[36] The original description of this condition and subsequent diagnostic criteria focused on cardiomyopathies that predominantly (or exclusively) involved the RV.[37,38] More recently, overlap with left ventricular involvement is expanding the diagnosis to include all forms of arrhythmogenic cardiomyopathy.[39,40] Naxos disease and Carvajal syndrome are two similar recessive disorders that also involve palmoplantar keratodermas and wooly hair.[41,42] Noncardiac involvement in ARVC is quite rare.

The most frequent manifestation of ARVC is ventricular tachyarrhythmia, and once the condition is recognized with institution of appropriate antiarrhythmic therapies, the development of heart failure is uncommon.[36] The largest reported series of cardiac transplant for ARVC reported 18 patients with this condition who all had left ventricular involvement.[14] Most received transplants for heart failure rather than for refractory arrhythmia, and transplants occurred at an average age of 40 years.

Approximately 50% of individuals with ARVC have a mutation in a component of the cardiac desmosome.[43] Immunohistochemical analysis for plakoglobin is consistently reduced in ARVC hearts, in contrast with HCM, DCM, ischemic cardiomyopathy, and control hearts.[44] Notably, cardiac sarcoid is commonly on the differential diagnosis for ARVC, and reduced plakoglobin immunoreactivity is quite similar in sarcoid as in ARVC.[45]

Left Ventricular Noncompaction Cardiomyopathy

Left ventricular noncompaction cardiomyopathy (LVNC), which is also known as LV hypertrabeculation, has been described as a "new form of heart failure," but this likely reflects improved imaging technologies that have increased its recognition.[46] Early reports of this condition describe marked sinusoids in the ventricles with associated cardiac dysfunction and arrhythmias.[47-49] LVNC is frequently associated with other cardiac malformations, with craniofacial abnormalities, and with concomitant skeletal myopathy.[47,48,50,51] Because of high resolution cardiac imaging, such as cardiac MRI and improved echocardiography, defined criteria have been developed.[52,53] Briefly summarized, the noncompacted endocardial layer has to be thicker than the compacted epicardial layer, with a ratio of noncompacted/compacted of 2 or more, with prominent and excessive trabeculations, and deep recesses filled with blood from the ventricular cavity. The incidence of thromboembolic complications appears higher in LVNC than in other forms of cardiomyopathy.[52,53]

LVNC is well recognized as a genetic form of cardiomyopathy, although the range of different genes in which mutations occur is similar to the remarkable heterogeneity in familial DCM. Its presence in a young male suggests Barth syndrome, which also causes neutropenia, skeletal myopathy, and abnormal mitochondria.[54] As in most other forms of cardiomyopathy, mutations of the cardiac sarcomere can cause LVNC.[55] If dysmorphic features or cognitive impairment is present, one should consider chromosomal abnormalities.[56,57]

GENETIC CAUSES OF CARDIOMYOPATHIES

Because of overlap among the etiologies of these phenotypes, including dilated, hypertrophic, restrictive, noncompaction, and right ventricular, the next section will be subdivided by etiology rather than specific cardiac morphologies. A list of genes with mutations known to cause cardiomyopathy in humans is shown in **Table 22-2**.

TABLE 22-2 Genes with Mutations Known to Cause Cardiomyopathy

ENCODED PROTEIN'S CELLULAR LOCATION/FUNCTION	GENE	DCM	HCM	RCM	ARVD/C	LVNC
Sarcomere/myofilament or Z-disc	*ACTC*	+	+	−	−	+
	ACTN2	+	+	−	−	−
	ANKRD1	+	+	−	−	−
	BAG3	+	−	+	−	−
	CSRP3	+	+	+	−	−
	MYBPC3	+	+	−	+	+
	MYH6	+	+	−	−	−
	MYH7	+	+	+	+	+
	MYL2	−	+	−	−	−
	MYL3	−	+	−	−	−
	MYLK2	−	+	−	−	−
	MYOZ2	+	+	−	−	−
	MYPN	+	+	+	−	−
	NEBL	+	−	−	−	−
	NEXN	+	+	−	−	−
	TCAP	+	+	−	−	−
	TNNC1	+	+	−	−	−
	TNNT2	+	+	+	−	+
	TNNI3	+	+	+	−	−
	TPM1	+	+	−	−	+
	TTN	+	+	−	+	−
	TCAP	+	+	−	−	−
Cytoskeleton	*DES*	+	−	+	+	−
	DMD	+	−	−	−	−
	DTNA	−	−	−	−	+
	LDB3	+	+	−	−	+
	PDLIM3	+	−	−	−	−
	SGCD	+	−	−	−	−
	VCL	+	+	−	−	−
Calcium regulation	*CAV3*	+	−	−	−	−
	JPH2	−	+	−	−	−
	PLN	+	−	−	+	−
	PSEN1	+	−	−	−	−
	PSEN2	+	−	−	−	−
	RYR2	−	−	−	+	−
Nuclear envelope	*EMD*	+	−	−	−	−
	ILK	+	−	−	−	−
	LAMA4	+	−	−	−	−
	LAP2	+	−	−	−	−
	LMNA	+	+	+	+	+
	TMEM43	+	−	−	+	−
Ion channel	*SCN5A*	+	−	−	−	−
	ABCC9	+	−	−	−	−
Transcription factor or regulator of transcription	*EYA4*	+	−	−	−	−
	GATAD1	+	−	−	−	−
	NKX2-5	+	−	−	−	−
	PRDM16	−	−	−	−	+
	RBM20	+	−	−	−	−
Desmosome	*DSP*	−	−	−	+	−
	DSG2	−	−	−	+	−
	DSC2	−	−	−	+	−
	JUP	−	−	−	+	−
	PKP2	−	−	−	+	−
Mitochondria	*ANT1*	+	+	−	−	−
	FKRP	+	−	−	−	−
	FXN	−	+	+	−	−
	ND1	−	+	−	−	+
	tRNA	+	−	−	−	+
	TAZ	−	+	−	−	+
Storage disease	*GLA*	−	+	−	−	−
	LAMP2	−	+	−	−	−
	PRKAG2	−	+	−	−	−
	TTR	−	+	−	+	−

Sarcomere Mutations

The cardiac sarcomere is the primary subunit in myocytes used for generation of force (**Figure 22-3**). Mutation in a gene encoding any component of the sarcomere can cause cardiomyopathy. Phenotypic manifestations related to sarcomere mutations include DCM, HCM, RCM, and LVNC, and there is also a report of *MYH7* mutation mimicking ARVD/C.[4,6,58-60] Oddly, prediction of the morphologic consequence for the left ventricle by any particular sarcomere mutation is not currently feasible, although phenotypes remain consistent for each individual mutation. Most missense substitutions in sarcomere genes are predicted to cause loss of function, although gain-of-function mutations would cause heterogeneity among individual subcellular units, and this could cause disease. In addition to mediating both contraction and relaxation of the heart, additional functions of the sarcomere and its network of associated proteins include integration, regulation, and coordination of cardiac signaling,[61,62] sensation and response to reactive oxygen species within the heart,[63] and modulation of ubiquitination and autophagy.[64] With such central roles in cardiac function and homeostasis, it is not surprising that sarcomere dysfunction causes heart failure.

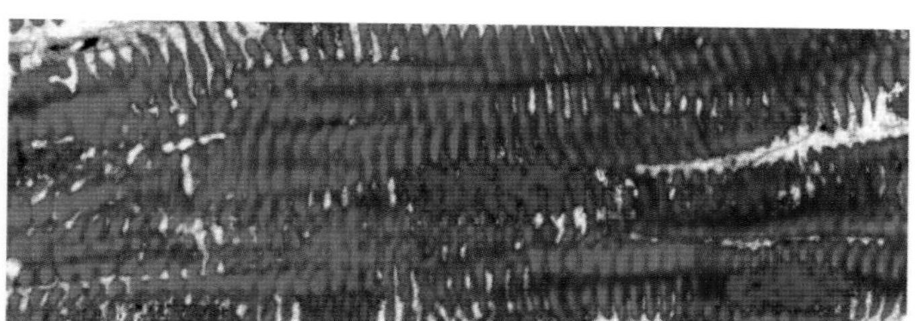

FIGURE 22-3 The cardiac sarcomeres make up myofibrils, which are highlighted in this image with immunostaining for cardiac troponin T *(red),* a component of the sarcomeres. Nuclei are stained with DAPI *(blue)* and wheat germ agglutinin *(white)* binds to the plasma membrane to demonstrate cell boundaries.

Clinical Implications

Pathogenic heterozygous mutations tend to be sufficient to cause disease, and the presence of more than 1 mutation tends to worsen its severity within families.[65] The diversity of phenotypes associated with sarcomere mutations limits the applicability of generalizations regarding sarcomere mutations. Among patients with HCM and mutations in *TNNT2* or *TNNI3,* encoding cardiac troponin T and cardiac troponin I, respectively, the likelihood of arrhythmia appears to be greater than that predicted by LV wall thickness. Regarding mutations in *TPM1,* encoding α-tropomyosin, one group has reported a wide range of onset and severity within families sharing the same mutation.[66] Because of the long history of investigation of genes encoding most elements of the cardiac sarcomere, clinical laboratories typically have a large number of variants from which to ascertain the likelihood of pathogenicity, and this increases the feasibility of using sarcomere mutation analysis among patients with all types of inherited cardiomyopathy.

Cytoskeletal Mutations

The cardiac cytoskeleton includes a large number of proteins that are responsible for the transmission of force, which is generated by the contractile elements of the sarcomere (**Figure 22-4**). Dystrophin was the first cytoskeletal element that was recognized with mutations in association with dilated cardiomyopathy among patients with Duchenne and Becker muscular dystrophies.[67,68] Subsequently, dystrophin gene mutations were identified in patients with X-linked DCM,[69] which suggested that other forms of familial DCM could be inherited through mutations affecting the

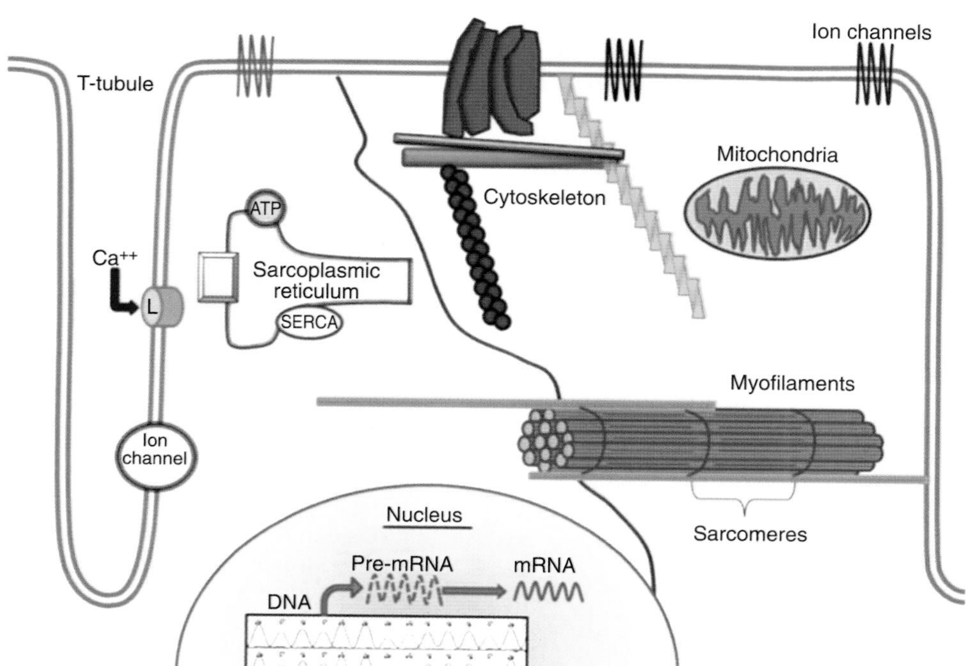

FIGURE 22-4 Diagram of a cardiomyocyte. Mutations can occur in the genes encoding elements of the cardiac sarcomere, the cytoskeletal proteins, those involved with calcium uptake into and release from the sarcoplasmic reticulum, the nuclear envelope, the cardiac ion channels, factors involved with DNA transcription into pre-mRNA and its splicing into mRNA, and mitochondria.

cytoskeletal complex. Broadly interpreted, the cardiac cytoskeleton includes sarcoglycans, other associated glycoproteins, the basal lamina, and the intermediate filaments that link the sarcomeric Z-discs to the sarcolemma cell membrane. If the mutated gene encoding a cytoskeletal element is exclusively or predominantly expressed in the heart, then the phenotype should be isolated DCM. If the mutated cytoskeletal element is also present in skeletal muscle, then skeletal muscle weakness may also be present. More examples of genes encoding cytoskeletal elements that can be mutated in cardiomyopathy are listed in Table 22-2.

Clinical Implications

As in the example regarding dystrophin, many cytoskeletal proteins are present in both heart and skeletal muscle. Certain myofibrillar proteins, such as desmin, are much more abundant in heart than skeletal muscle, and the range of skeletal muscle dysfunction is quite large.[70] Among the cytoskeletal components with mutations resulting in cardiomyopathy, desmin is one in which arrhythmia can be a prominent feature, and recognition of a definite mutation in this gene should prompt earlier consideration for an ICD among affected individuals.[71,72]

Mutations Altering Calcium Handling

Calcium is one of the most important cations for the relationship between electrical activation and mechanical function of cardiomyocytes, and it is intricately regulated[73] (see Figure 22-4). Accordingly, disruption or mutation of any of the regulatory components can result in either electrical or mechanical cardiac disease. When the mutation results primarily in mechanical dysfunction, it is likely that arrhythmia is also a consequence. For example, *PLN* encoding phospholamban is a gene in which mutations cause several forms of cardiomyopathy, and arrhythmia is prominent in this setting.[74] Phospholamban is a negative regulator of the sarcoplasmic reticulum calcium-ATPase, and loss-of-function mutations might be predicted to cause improved cardiac function. However, the disruption of excitation-contraction coupling instead causes DCM or ARVD/C.[74,75] Mutations in the cardiac ryanodine receptor (encoded by *RYR2*) typically cause catecholaminergic polymorphic ventricular tachycardia without structural heart disease, although at least one report ties mutations in this gene to ARVD/C.[76]

Clinical Implications

Because of the intricate connection between calcium handling and arrhythmia, people with a mutation that alters cardiomyocyte calcium regulation should be evaluated closely for arrhythmia, regardless of their EF or severity of structural heart disease. Although there is not typically skeletal muscle disease with alterations in the cardiac calcium regulatory genes, one report highlights the possibility of overlap between DCM and Alzheimer dementia due to *PSEN1* or *PSEN2* mutations.[77]

Nuclear Envelope Mutations

Present in every nucleated cell, the nuclear envelope has emerged over the past few years as far more than a passive structural membrane to encapsulate the nuclear contents. Several reports help to identify the role of the nuclear envelope components in the organization of chromatin, regulation of signaling and gene expression, nuclear-cytoplasmic transport, cell division, and aging.[78-82] Mutations in genes encoding elements of the nuclear envelope have a broad range of phenotypes, prominently including dilated cardiomyopathy, cardiac conduction disease, and heart failure.[83] Systemic manifestations include skeletal myopathy (limb girdle muscular dystrophy type 1b and Emery-Dreifuss muscular dystrophy), partial lipodystrophy, premature aging, Charcot-Marie-Tooth disease, malignancy, and mandibuloacral dysplasia.[84-91]

LMNA is the most frequent nuclear envelope gene with mutations causing cardiovascular disease.[83,92] *LMNA* encodes two isoforms, lamin A and lamin C (sometimes called lamin A/C), and mutations in this gene cause dysmorphic nuclei (**Figure 22-5**). People with *LMNA* mutations have higher rates of sudden death and worse cumulative survival than those with DCM without *LMNA* mutations.[2,93,94] Although the mechanisms for development of cardiac disease due to alterations of the nuclear envelope are not well known, a recent report demonstrated a role for lamin A/C and emerin in regulating nuclear translocation and downstream signaling of a mechanosensitive transcription factor, MKL1, which is important in cardiovascular development and function.[95]

Clinical Implications

Phenotypic features among patients with DCM that suggest a possible nuclear envelope mutation include unexplained elevation of creatine kinase, muscle weakness, cardiac conduction disease, frequent ventricular arrhythmias, or a family history of early sudden death. Recognition of a gene mutation that predisposes to life-threatening arrhythmia should prompt earlier use of implantable cardioverter-defibrillators.[3]

Ion Channel Mutations

Cardiac ion channel (see Figure 22-4) mutations are most commonly recognized to cause inherited disorders of arrhythmia, such as long-QT syndrome and Brugada syndrome.[96] Chronic tachycardia or cardiac arrest in that setting can cause a secondary form of structural cardiomyopathy, and rarely, mutations in ion-channel genes can cause a primary form of cardiomyopathy. Phospholamban is a regulator of the SERCA2a channel, and mutations have been reported in several different forms of cardiomyopathy, although somewhat surprisingly, heterozygous loss-of-function mutations in the SERCA2a gene do not cause impairment in cardiac performance.[97] Following a hypothesis that mutations in another regulator of myocyte calcium flux, the regulatory SUR2A subunit of the cardiac K_{ATP} channel encoded by *ABCC9*, could cause cardiomyopathy, investigators evaluated 323 individuals with unexplained DCM for mutations in this gene.[98] They identified two probands with functional alterations, establishing that cardiac ion channel mutations can rarely cause DCM. Similarly, *SCN5A* encodes the $Na_V1.5$ cardiac sodium channel, and mutations in this gene cause type 3 long-QT and Brugada syndromes, as well as atrial fibrillation.[99,100] Investigation of a large family segregating DCM with prominent arrhythmia (atrial fibrillation, impaired automaticity, and conduction delay) led to linkage to chromosome 3p, and subsequently to a missense mutation in *SCN5A*.[101] These investigators subsequently looked

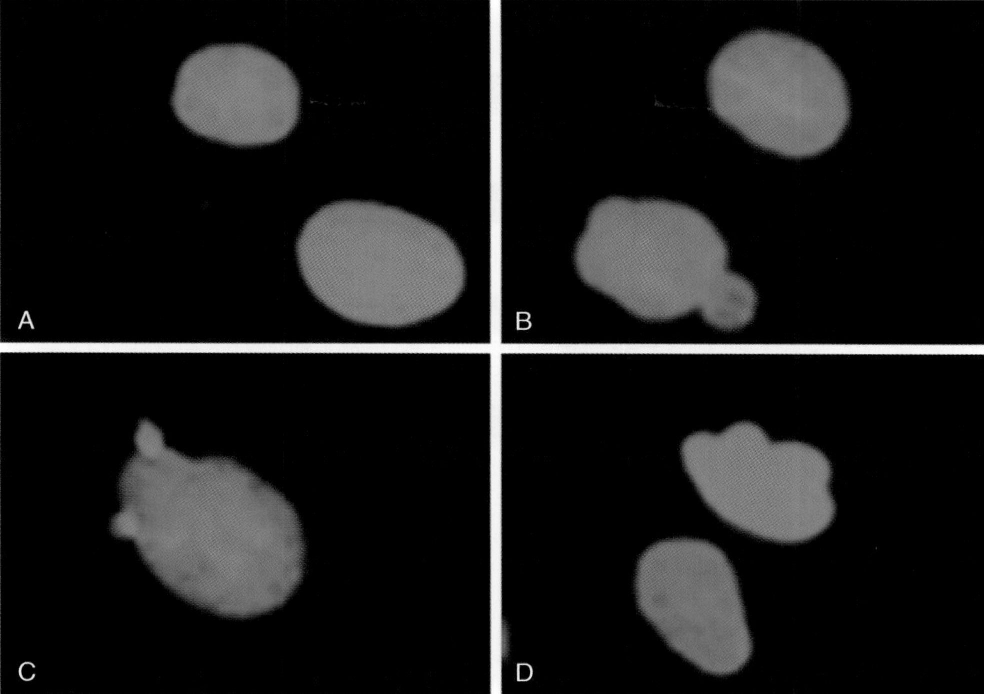

FIGURE 22-5 Dysmorphic nuclei due to an *LMNA* mutation. Immunohistochemical staining for lamin A. Normal nuclei are shown in panel **A,** with dysmorphic nuclei in panels **B, C,** and **D.** The heterozygous *LMNA* mutation is p.Asp300Gly, and it causes cardiomyopathy with accelerated cardiovascular aging. *From Kane MS, Lindsay ME, Judge DP, et al: LMNA-associated cardiocutaneous progeria: an inherited autosomal dominant premature aging syndrome with late onset. Am J Med Genet A 161A:1599–1611, 2013.*

for mutations in this gene among a cohort of 156 unrelated probands with DCM and identified that 4 (2.5%) also had a mutation in *SCN5A*.[101]

Clinical Implications

Recognition of a mutation in *SCN5A* should prompt greater scrutiny for arrhythmia because of its association with long-QT and Brugada syndromes, as well as atrial fibrillation. Importantly, certain drugs can prolong the QT interval, and they should be avoided among individuals with a mutation in an ion channel. Mice with knockout mutation in *Kir6.2*, encoding another element of the K_{ATP} channel, are prone to heart failure, arrhythmia, and sudden death, which are preventable by calcium channel blockers.[102] While it is premature to recommend similar treatment for people with rare mutations affecting the K_{ATP} channel with cardiomyopathy, it holds promise.

Transcription and Splicing Factor Mutations

Cardiac transcription factor mutations typically cause congenital malformations of the heart, although cardiomyopathy can also occur. For example, *NKX2-5* mutations cause congenital cardiac malformations and cardiomyopathy.[103] Using a traditional positional cloning approach in a large family segregating DM with sensorineural hearing loss, investigators found linkage to chromosome 6q23–q24, and subsequently identified mutations in *EYA4*, encoding eyes-absent-4, a transcription factor.[104] In addition, mutations in *RBM20*, encoding a ribonucleic acid binding protein that regulates titin splicing, cause familial DCM with prominent arrhythmia.[105]

Clinical Implications

When mutations in a transcription factor gene that is associated with congenital malformations are identified, careful assessment for subtle or overt cardiac malformations should be performed in the proband and relatives who are at risk of inheriting the mutation. *RBM20* mutations, in particular, are associated with high rates of sudden cardiac death.

Desmosome Mutations

Desmosomes form cell junctions, and alterations in their components are associated with both cardiomyopathy and dermatologic disorders. Homozygous mutations in *JUP*, encoding junction plakoglobin, cause a recessive form of arrhythmogenic cardiomyopathy, wooly hair, and palmoplantar keratoderma called *Naxos syndrome*.[41] Similarly, recessive mutations in *DSP*, encoding desmoplakin, cause a related disorder called *Carvajal syndrome*.[106] Since both desmoplakin and plakoglobin are components of the cardiac desmosomes, investigation next turned to mutations in other components in arrhythmogenic forms of cardiomyopathy or ARVD/C. The most prevalent gene with mutations underlying this phenotype is *PKP2* encoding plakophilin-2.[107] Other desmosome gene mutations are noted in Table 22-2 and shown schematically in **Figure 22-6**. The phenotypes that result from desmosome mutations include RV, LV, and biventricular cardiomyopathy.

There are several possible mechanisms whereby mutations in a component of the cardiac desmosome cause cardiomyopathy.[12] A simple structural model predicts that loss of cell adherence leads to apoptosis and scarring within the ventricle, particularly at sites with greatest stress

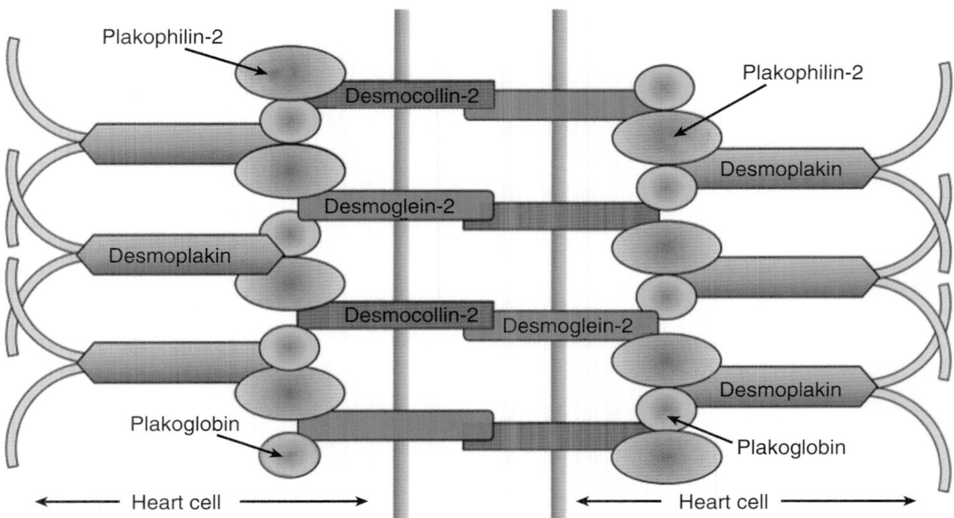

FIGURE 22-6 The cardiac desmosome is composed of transmembrane cadherins (desmocollins and desmogleins), armadillo proteins (plakoglobin and plakophilins), and plakins, such as desmoplakin. Mutations in these proteins disrupt the desmosome complex and cause arrhythmogenic forms of cardiomyopathy.

in response to exercise. A landmark publication demonstrated that disruption of the desmosome complex causes plakoglobin to accumulate in the nucleus, where it competes with β-catenin for its downstream activation, thereby decreasing canonical Wnt/β-catenin signaling.[108] However, this model does not account for the identical phenotype that results from plakoglobin deficiency. Loss of desmosomes may disrupt other cell junction complexes, and it also affects the sodium channel complex, which contributes to arrhythmia.[109] Recently, investigation of induced cardiomyocytes derived from patients with desmosome mutations helped to identify an important role for abnormal activation of the peroxisome proliferator-activated receptor gamma (PPAR-gamma) pathway in this condition.[110]

Clinical Implications

A few important factors should be taken into account for patients with desmosome gene mutations. First, penetrance of mutations in these genes seems lower, with one study showing that only 31% of first-degree relatives of probands with ARVD/C and a *PKP2* mutation also met diagnostic criteria, with wide intrafamilial variability among mutation carriers.[111] Another study showed that rare missense variation in these genes is commonly seen in control populations.[112] In the setting of a clear pathogenic mutation with cardiomyopathy, careful assessment for arrhythmia should be performed on a regular basis, particularly in those who do not yet have an ICD. Among patients with ARVD/C, a history of extensive athletic activity is common, and in a retrospective analysis, exercise increases age-related penetrance and risk of arrhythmia in desmosome mutation carriers.[113]

Mitochondrial Mutations

Heart muscle requires high levels of energy to maintain its constant requirement for delivering oxygen throughout the body. Production of energy relies heavily on mitochondria (see Figure 22-4), and dysfunction of the mitochondria contributes to heart failure. Heart failure is associated with a shift in the substrate for mitochondrial function, with a decline in fatty acid oxidation and a proportional increase in the oxidation of glucose in advanced phases.[114] Mitochondrial mutations that cause inherited forms cardiomyopathy may occur with an isolated cardiac phenotype, but more often these mutations have multifaceted manifestations, including the involvement of many other tissues in which mitochondrial function is important for producing energy. Additional phenotypes that may be found in mitochondrial disorders include skeletal muscle disease, blindness, premature hearing loss, diabetes, encephalopathy, and seizures.[115] They may occur due to nuclear DNA mutations encoding components of the mitochondria, or in the approximately 16,600 nucleotides that comprise the mitochondrial DNA (mtDNA). If due to mtDNA mutation, then transmission to the next generation can only occur through female carriers. Differences in disease severity or age at presentation may be due to heteroplasmy, or variation in the percentage of the mtDNA in which the mutation occurs. If the mtDNA mutation is homoplasmic, then the entire content of the mtDNA is mutant.

Mitochondrial disorders can cause HCM, DCM, or LV noncompaction, with or without systemic manifestations.[116-118] When cardiomyopathy occurs in isolation, it can be difficult to recognize a mitochondrial cause without molecular genetic testing. Cardiomyopathy in Friedreich ataxia usually begins with concentric (nonobstructive) LV hypertrophy, with eventual loss of systolic function. The hypertrophy appears to be caused by a combination of fibrosis and marked proliferation of mitochondria with an associated loss of contractile elements.[119] Barth syndrome, another mitochondrial disorder, is an X-linked mitochondrial condition in which males typically present in infancy or childhood with DCM or LV noncompaction, associated with skeletal myopathy and neutropenia.[120]

Many treatment trials of mitochondrial forms of cardiomyopathy have focused on antioxidants. In addition to generating ATP, the mitochondria produce reactive oxygen species, such as superoxide and hydrogen peroxide, and mitochondrial dysfunction increases electron leakage from the mitochondrial transport chain.[121] To date, clinical trials for antioxidants, such as coenzyme Q10 and idebenone, have been not been convincing and these strategies remain experimental.[122]

Clinical Implications

Recognition of a mitochondrial form of cardiomyopathy is clinically important for several reasons. First, systemic manifestations should be assessed in organs in which mitochondrial production of energy is important, such as skeletal muscles, vision, and hearing. Once a nuclear versus mtDNA mutation is recognized, there will likely be important implications for risk assessment in family members. Although antioxidant treatments have greater appeal for mitochondrial disorders than in other forms of heart failure, a clear benefit from treatment with these medications is not yet known.

GENETIC TESTING

Research investigating the genetic basis of cardiomyopathy over the past 20 years has been remarkably successful. Traditional linkage studies initially facilitated the recognition of several genes in which mutations cause different forms of cardiomyopathy, and candidate-based studies, exome analysis, and whole genome association techniques have subsequently elucidated many other genes involved with these conditions. Improvements in the costs and efficiency of technologies applied to DNA sequencing have helped to bring genetic testing from the research benches to clinical applications. Today, the clinical use of genetic testing is gaining greater recognition for its value. Determination of a responsible gene mutation can help to support the clinical diagnosis, to identify individuals who are at risk of syndromic or extracardiac manifestations, to recognize those within the family who are at highest risk of developing cardiomyopathy, and for family planning.

Several different sets of guidelines for the clinical use of genetic testing for inherited cardiac disease have been published.[3,123-125] In this context, some common themes have emerged, such as recommendations for genetic counseling in conjunction with genetic testing. Genetic testing should include genetic counseling, typically by master's-trained counselors. A typical genetic counseling evaluation would include assessment of the pedigree, including the pattern of inheritance and determination of those who are at risk of cardiomyopathy.[126] Discussion of genetic testing should include the testing options that are available, the possible outcomes of these tests including uncertain or unexpected results, communication of results to family members, and the costs of such testing. Most physicians are not trained in helping patients deal with issues such as guilt arising from passing on a genetic predisposition to cardiomyopathy to their children.

Some experts recommend targeted analysis of the top few genes in which mutations occur, in an effort to minimize unnecessary genetic sequencing and to lower costs. This approach also simplifies the process and decreases the likelihood of finding nonpathogenic variation in genes that are included in larger sequencing panels. Others recommend larger panels since the costs are declining and the additional data may help to determine other genetic factors contributing to a disorder such as cardiomyopathy in which there is reduced penetrance. One should decide between these two approaches based on availability and costs, as well as the feasibility of discerning pathogenicity of multiple variants based on cosegregation within the family, if there are several individuals with cardiomyopathy and DNA available for testing.

Looking to the future, the costs of DNA sequencing are rapidly declining, and we are learning the extent and potential pathogenicity of human genetic variation through large web-based platforms.[127] Because genotypes do not change, assessment of DNA sequence may soon become a standard aspect of primary care. For now, the use of genetic analysis is best if handled through highly specialized centers with expertise and familiarity with these topics.

References

1. Judge DP: Use of genetics in the clinical evaluation of cardiomyopathy. *JAMA* 302:2471–2476, 2009.
2. Taylor MRG, et al: Natural history of dilated cardiomyopathy due to lamin A/C gene mutations. *J Am Coll Cardiol* 41:771–780, 2003.
3. Ackerman MJ, et al: HRS/EHRA expert consensus statement on the state of genetic testing for the channelopathies and cardiomyopathies. *Heart Rhythm* 8:1308–1339, 2011.
4. Kamisago M, et al: Mutations in sarcomere protein genes as a cause of dilated cardiomyopathy. *N Engl J Med* 343:1688–1696, 2000.
5. Lamont P, Wallefeld W, Davis M, et al: Clinical utility gene card for: Laing distal myopathy. *Eur J Hum Genet* 19(3), 2011.
6. Geisterfer-Lowrance AA, et al: A molecular basis for familial hypertrophic cardiomyopathy: a beta cardiac myosin heavy chain gene missense mutation. *Cell* 62:999–1006, 1990.
7. Michels VV, et al: The frequency of familial dilated cardiomyopathy in a series of patients with idiopathic dilated cardiomyopathy. *N Engl J Med* 326:77–82, 1992.
8. Grunig E, et al: Frequency and phenotypes of familial dilated cardiomyopathy. *J Am Coll Cardiol* 31:186–194, 1998.
9. Baig MK, et al: Familial dilated cardiomyopathy: cardiac abnormalities are common in asymptomatic relatives and may represent early disease. *J Am Coll Cardiol* 31:195–201, 1998.
10. Cheitlin MD, et al: ACC/AHA/ASE 2003 guideline update for the clinical application of echocardiography: summary article: a report of the American College of Cardiology/American Heart Association Task Force on Practice Guidelines. *Circulation* 108:1146–1162, 2003.
11. Felker GM, et al: Underlying causes and long-term survival in patients with initially unexplained cardiomyopathy. *N Engl J Med* 342:1077–1084, 2000.
12. Awad MM, Calkins H, Judge DP: Mechanisms of disease: molecular genetics of arrhythmogenic right ventricular dysplasia/cardiomyopathy. *Nat Clin Pract Cardiovasc Med* 5:258–267, 2008.
13. Dalal D, et al: Clinical features of arrhythmogenic right ventricular dysplasia/cardiomyopathy associated with mutations in plakophilin-2. *Circulation* 113:1641–1649, 2006.
14. Tedford RJ, et al: Cardiac transplantation in arrhythmogenic right ventricular dysplasia/cardiomyopathy. *J Am Coll Cardiol* 59:289–290, 2012.
15. Mestroni L, et al: Guidelines for the study of familial dilated cardiomyopathies. Collaborative Research Group of the European Human and Capital Mobility Project on Familial Dilated Cardiomyopathy. *Eur Heart J* 20:93–102, 1999.
16. McKenna WJ, et al: Diagnosis of arrhythmogenic right ventricular dysplasia/cardiomyopathy. Task Force of the Working Group Myocardial and Pericardial Disease of the European Society of Cardiology and of the Scientific Council on Cardiomyopathies of the International Society and Federation of Cardiology. *Br Heart J* 71:215–218, 1994.
17. Desnick RJ, et al: Fabry disease, an under-recognized multisystemic disorder: expert recommendations for diagnosis, management, and enzyme replacement therapy. *Ann Intern Med* 138:338–346, 2003.
18. Fabry J: Ein beitrag zur kenntnis der purpura haemorrhagica nodularis (Purpura papulosa hemorrhagica Hebrae). *Arch Dermatol Syph* 43:187, 1898.
19. Anderson W: A case of angiokeratoma. *Brit J Derm* 10:113, 1898.
20. Chimenti C, et al: Prevalence of Fabry disease in female patients with late-onset hypertrophic cardiomyopathy. *Circulation* 110:1047–1053, 2004.
21. Bloomfield SE, David DS, Rubin AL: Eye findings in the diagnosis of Fabry's disease. Patients with renal failure. *JAMA* 240:647–649, 1978.
22. Havndrup O, et al: Fabry disease mimicking hypertrophic cardiomyopathy: genetic screening needed for establishing the diagnosis in women. *Eur J Heart Fail* 12:535–540, 2010.
23. Desnick RJ, Banikazemi M: Fabry disease: clinical spectrum and evidence-based enzyme replacement therapy. *Nephrol Ther* 2(Suppl 2):S172–S185, 2006.
24. Banikazemi M, et al: Agalsidase-beta therapy for advanced Fabry disease: a randomized trial. *Ann Intern Med* 146:77–86, 2007.
25. Danon MJ, et al: Lysosomal glycogen storage disease with normal acid maltase. *Neurology* 31:51–57, 1981.
26. Nishino I, et al: Primary LAMP-2 deficiency causes X-linked vacuolar cardiomyopathy and myopathy (Danon disease). *Nature* 406:906–910, 2000.
27. Maron BJ, et al: Clinical outcome and phenotypic expression in LAMP2 cardiomyopathy. *JAMA* 301:1253–1259, 2009.
28. Boucek D, Jirikowic J, Taylor M: Natural history of Danon disease. *Genet Med* 13:563–568, 2011.
29. Van Der Starre P, et al: Late profound muscle weakness following heart transplantation due to Danon disease. *Muscle Nerve* 47:135–137, 2013.
30. Falk RH: Diagnosis and management of the cardiac amyloidoses. *Circulation* 112:2047–2060, 2005.
31. Jacobson DR, et al: Variant-sequence transthyretin (isoleucine 122) in late-onset cardiac amyloidosis in black Americans. *N Engl J Med* 336:466–473, 1997.
32. Buxbaum J, et al: Significance of the amyloidogenic transthyretin Val 122 Ile allele in African Americans in the Arteriosclerosis Risk in Communities (ARIC) and Cardiovascular Health (CHS) Studies. *Am Heart J* 159:864–870, 2010.
33. Maleszewski JJ, et al: Relationship between monoclonal gammopathy and cardiac amyloid type. *Cardiovasc Pathol* 22:189–194, 2013.
34. Coelho T, et al: Tafamidis for transthyretin familial amyloid polyneuropathy: a randomized, controlled trial. *Neurology* 79:785–792, 2012.
35. Coelho T, et al: Safety and efficacy of RNAi therapy for transthyretin amyloidosis. *N Engl J Med* 369:819–829, 2013.
36. Dalal D, et al: Arrhythmogenic right ventricular dysplasia: a United States experience. *Circulation* 112:3823–3832, 2005.
37. Marcus FI, et al: Right ventricular dysplasia: a report of 24 adult cases. *Circulation* 65:384–398, 1982.
38. McKenna WJ, et al: Diagnosis of arrhythmogenic right ventricular dysplasia/cardiomyopathy. *Br Heart J* 71:215–218, 1994.
39. Marcus FI, et al: Diagnosis of arrhythmogenic right ventricular cardiomyopathy/dysplasia: proposed modification of the task force criteria. *Circulation* 121:1533–1541, 2010.

40. Thiene G, Marcus F: Arrhythmogenic cardiomyopathy: a biventricular disease in search of a cure. *Heart Rhythm* 10:290–291, 2013.
41. McKoy G, et al: Identification of a deletion in plakoglobin in arrhythmogenic right ventricular cardiomyopathy with palmoplantar keratoderma and woolly hair (Naxos disease). *Lancet* 355:2119–2124, 2000.
42. Carvajal-Huerta L: Epidermolytic palmoplantar keratoderma with woolly hair and dilated cardiomyopathy. *J Am Acad Dermatol* 39:418–421, 1998.
43. den Haan AD, et al: Comprehensive desmosome mutation analysis in North Americans with arrhythmogenic right ventricular dysplasia/cardiomyopathy. *Circ Cardiovasc Genet* 2: 428–435, 2009.
44. Asimaki A, et al: A new diagnostic test for arrhythmogenic right ventricular cardiomyopathy. *N Engl J Med* 360:1075–1084, 2009.
45. Asimaki A, et al: Altered desmosomal proteins in granulomatous myocarditis and potential pathogenic links to arrhythmogenic right ventricular cardiomyopathy. *Circ Arrhythm Electrophysiol* 4:743–752, 2011.
46. Towbin JA: Left ventricular noncompaction: a new form of heart failure. *Heart Fail Clin* 6:453–469, viii, 2010.
47. Chenard J, Samson M, Beaulieu M: Embryonal sinusoids in the myocardium: report of a case successfully treated surgically. *Can Med Assoc J* 92:1356–1359, 1965.
48. Jenni R, et al: Persisting myocardial sinusoids of both ventricles as an isolated anomaly: echocardiographic, angiographic, and pathologic anatomical findings. *Cardiovasc Intervent Radiol* 9:127–131, 1986.
49. Dusek J, Ostadal B, Duskova M: Postnatal persistence of spongy myocardium with embryonic blood supply. *Arch Pathol* 99:312–317, 1975.
50. Chin TK, Perloff JK, Williams RG, et al: Isolated noncompaction of left ventricular myocardium. A study of eight cases. *Circulation* 82:507–513, 1990.
51. Finsterer J: Cardiogenetics, neurogenetics, and pathogenetics of left ventricular hypertrabeculation/noncompaction. *Pediatr Cardiol* 30:659–681, 2009.
52. Oechslin EN, Attenhofer Jost CH, Rojas JR, et al: Long-term follow-up of 34 adults with isolated left ventricular noncompaction: a distinct cardiomyopathy with poor prognosis. *J Am Coll Cardiol* 36:493–500, 2000.
53. Stacey RB, Andersen MM, St Clair M, et al: Comparison of systolic and diastolic criteria for isolated LV noncompaction in CMR. *JACC Cardiovasc Imaging* 6:931–940, 2013.
54. Bleyl SB, et al: Neonatal, lethal noncompaction of the left ventricular myocardium is allelic with Barth syndrome. *Am J Hum Genet* 61:868–872, 1997.
55. Probst S, et al: Sarcomere gene mutations in isolated left ventricular noncompaction cardiomyopathy do not predict clinical phenotype. *Circ Cardiovasc Genet* 4:367–374, 2011.
56. Blinder JJ, et al: Noncompaction of the left ventricular myocardium in a boy with a novel chromosome 8p23.1 deletion. *Am J Med Genet A* 155A:2215–2220, 2011.
57. Beken S, et al: A neonatal case of left ventricular noncompaction associated with trisomy 18. *Genet Couns* 22:161–164, 2011.
58. Roberts JD, Veinot JP, Rutberg J, et al: Inherited cardiomyopathies mimicking arrhythmogenic right ventricular cardiomyopathy. *Cardiovasc Pathol* 19:316–320, 2009.
59. Kaski JP, et al: Idiopathic restrictive cardiomyopathy in children is caused by mutations in cardiac sarcomere protein genes. *Heart* 94:1478–1484, 2008.
60. Klaassen S, et al: Mutations in sarcomere protein genes in left ventricular noncompaction. *Circulation* 117:2893–2901, 2008.
61. Frank D, Frey N: Cardiac Z-disc signaling network. *J Biol Chem* 286:9897–9904, 2011.
62. Krüger M, Linke WA: The giant protein titin: a regulatory node that integrates myocyte signaling pathways. *J Biol Chem* 286:9905–9912, 2011.
63. Sumandea MP, Steinberg SF: Redox signaling and cardiac sarcomeres. *J Biol Chem* 286: 9921–9927, 2011.
64. Portbury AL, Willis MS, Patterson C: Tearin' up my heart: proteolysis in the cardiac sarcomere. *J Biol Chem* 286:9929–9934, 2011.
65. Girolami F, et al: Clinical features and outcome of hypertrophic cardiomyopathy associated with triple sarcomere protein gene mutations. *J Am Coll Cardiol* 55:1444–1453, 2010.
66. Lakdawala NK, et al: Familial dilated cardiomyopathy caused by an alpha-tropomyosin mutation: the distinctive natural history of sarcomeric dilated cardiomyopathy. *J Am Coll Cardiol* 55:320–329, 2010.
67. Koenig M, et al: Complete cloning of the Duchenne muscular dystrophy (DMD) cDNA and preliminary genomic organization of the DMD gene in normal and affected individuals. *Cell* 50:509–517, 1987.
68. Malhotra SB, et al: Frame-shift deletions in patients with Duchenne and Becker muscular dystrophy. *Science* 242:755–759, 1988.
69. Muntoni F, et al: Deletion of the dystrophin muscle-promoter region associated with X-linked dilated cardiomyopathy. *N Engl J Med* 329:921–925, 1993.
70. Judge DP: Phenotypic diversity arising from a single mutation. *Heart Rhythm* 6:1584–1585, 2009.
71. Goldfarb LG, Dalakas MC: Tragedy in a heartbeat: malfunctioning desmin causes skeletal and cardiac muscle disease. *J Clin Invest* 119:1806–1813, 2009.
72. Otten E, et al: Desmin mutations as a cause of right ventricular heart failure affect the intercalated disks. *Heart Rhythm* 7:1058–1064, 2010.
73. Venetucci L, Denegri M, Napolitano C, et al: Inherited calcium channelopathies in the pathophysiology of arrhythmias. *Nat Rev Cardiol* 9:561–575, 2012.
74. Schmitt JP, et al: Dilated cardiomyopathy and heart failure caused by a mutation in phospholamban. *Science* 299:1410–1413, 2003.
75. van der Zwaag PA, et al: Phospholamban R14del mutation in patients diagnosed with dilated cardiomyopathy or arrhythmogenic right ventricular cardiomyopathy: evidence supporting the concept of arrhythmogenic cardiomyopathy. *Eur J Heart Fail* 14:1199–1207, 2012.
76. Tiso N, et al: Identification of mutations in the cardiac ryanodine receptor gene in families affected with arrhythmogenic right ventricular cardiomyopathy type 2 (ARVD2). *Hum Mol Genet* 10:189–194, 2001.
77. Li D, et al: Mutations of presenilin genes in dilated cardiomyopathy and heart failure. *Am J Hum Genet* 79:1030–1039, 2006.
78. Osorio FG, et al: Nuclear envelope alterations generate an aging-like epigenetic pattern in mice deficient in Zmpste24 metalloprotease. *Aging Cell* 9:947–957, 2010.
79. Anderson DJ, Hetzer MW: Nuclear envelope formation by chromatin-mediated reorganization of the endoplasmic reticulum. *Nat Cell Biol* 9:1160–1166, 2007.
80. Speese SD, et al: Nuclear envelope budding enables large ribonucleoprotein particle export during synaptic Wnt signaling. *Cell* 149:832–846, 2012.
81. Malhas A, Saunders NJ, Vaux DJ: The nuclear envelope can control gene expression and cell cycle progression via miRNA regulation. *Cell Cycle* 9:531–539, 2010.
82. Gómez-Baldó L, et al: TACC3-TSC2 maintains nuclear envelope structure and controls cell division. *Cell Cycle* 9:1143–1155, 2010.
83. Fatkin D, et al: Missense mutations in the rod domain of the lamin A/C gene as causes of dilated cardiomyopathy and conduction-system disease. *N Engl J Med* 341:1715–1724, 1999.
84. Bonne G, et al: Mutations in the gene encoding lamin A/C cause autosomal dominant Emery-Dreifuss muscular dystrophy. *Nat Genet* 21:285–288, 1999.
85. Muchir A, et al: Identification of mutations in the gene encoding lamins A/C in autosomal dominant limb girdle muscular dystrophy with atrioventricular conduction disturbances (LGMD1B). *Hum Mol Genet* 9:1453–1459, 2000.
86. Cao H, Hegele RA: Nuclear lamin A/C R482Q mutation in Canadian kindreds with Dunnigan-type familial partial lipodystrophy. *Hum Mol Genet* 9:109–112, 2000.
87. Eriksson M, et al: Recurrent de novo point mutations in lamin A cause Hutchinson-Gilford progeria syndrome. *Nature* 423:293–298, 2003.
88. Kane MS, et al: LMNA-associated cardiocutaneous progeria: an inherited autosomal dominant premature aging syndrome with late onset. *Am J Med Genet A* 161A:1599–1611, 2013.
89. De Sandre-Giovannoli A, et al: Homozygous defects in LMNA, encoding lamin A/C nuclear-envelope proteins, cause autosomal recessive axonal neuropathy in human (Charcot-Marie-Tooth disorder type 2) and mouse. *Am J Hum Genet* 70:726–736, 2002.
90. Novelli G, et al: Mandibuloacral dysplasia is caused by a mutation in LMNA-encoding lamin A/C. *Am J Hum Genet* 71:426–431, 2002.
91. Nagano A, et al: Emerin deficiency at the nuclear membrane in patients with Emery-Dreifuss muscular dystrophy. *Nat Genet* 12:254–259, 1996.
92. van Tintelen JP, et al: High yield of LMNA mutations in patients with dilated cardiomyopathy and/or conduction disease referred to cardiogenetics outpatient clinics. *Am Heart J* 154:1130–1139, 2007.
93. van Berlo JH, et al: Meta-analysis of clinical characteristics of 299 carriers of LMNA gene mutations: do lamin A/C mutations portend a high risk of sudden death? *J Mol Med* 83:79–83, 2005.
94. Meune C, et al: Primary prevention of sudden death in patients with lamin A/C gene mutations. *N Engl J Med* 354:209–210, 2006.
95. Ho CY, Jaalouk DE, Vartiainen MK, et al: Lamin A/C and emerin regulate MKL1-SRF activity by modulating actin dynamics. *Nature* 497:507–511, 2013.
96. Priori SG: The fifteen years of discoveries that shaped molecular electrophysiology: time for appraisal. *Circ Res* 107:451–456, 2010.
97. Mayosi BM, et al: Heterozygous disruption of SERCA2a is not associated with impairment of cardiac performance in humans: implications for SERCA2a as a therapeutic target in heart failure. *Heart* 92:105–109, 2006.
98. Bienengraeber M, et al: ABCC9 mutations identified in human dilated cardiomyopathy disrupt catalytic KATP channel gating. *Nat Genet* 36:382–387, 2004.
99. Remme CA, Wilde AA, Bezzina CR: Cardiac sodium channel overlap syndromes: different faces of SCN5A mutations. *Trends Cardiovasc Med* 18:78–87, 2008.
100. Ruan Y, Liu N, Priori SG: Sodium channel mutations and arrhythmias. *Nat Rev Cardiol* 6:337–348, 2009.
101. Olson TM, et al: Sodium channel mutations and susceptibility to heart failure and atrial fibrillation. *JAMA* 293:447–454, 2005.
102. Yamada S, et al: Protection conferred by myocardial ATP-sensitive K+ channels in pressure overload-induced congestive heart failure revealed in KCNJ11 Kir6.2-null mutant. *J Physiol* 577:1053–1065, 2006.
103. Pashmforoush M, et al: Nkx2–5 pathways and congenital heart disease: loss of ventricular myocyte lineage specification leads to progressive cardiomyopathy and complete heart block. *Cell* 117:373–386, 2004.
104. Schonberger J, et al: Mutation in the transcriptional coactivator EYA4 causes dilated cardiomyopathy and sensorineural hearing loss. *Nat Genet* 37:418–422, 2005.
105. Guo W, et al: RBM20, a gene for hereditary cardiomyopathy, regulates titin splicing. *Nat Med* 18:766–773, 2012.
106. Norgett EE, et al: Recessive mutation in desmoplakin disrupts desmoplakin-intermediate filament interactions and causes dilated cardiomyopathy, woolly hair and keratoderma. *Hum Mol Genet* 9:2761–2766, 2000.
107. Gerull B, et al: Mutations in the desmosomal protein plakophilin-2 are common in arrhythmogenic right ventricular cardiomyopathy. *Nat Genet* 36:1162–1164, 2004.
108. Garcia-Gras E, et al: Suppression of canonical Wnt/beta-catenin signaling by nuclear plakoglobin recapitulates phenotype of arrhythmogenic right ventricular cardiomyopathy. *J Clin Invest* 116:2012–2021, 2006.
109. Delmar M: Desmosome-ion channel interactions and their possible role in arrhythmogenic cardiomyopathy. *Pediatr Cardiol* 33:975–979, 2012.
110. Kim C, et al: Studying arrhythmogenic right ventricular dysplasia with patient-specific iPSCs. *Nature* 494:105–110, 2013.
111. Dalal D, et al: Penetrance of mutations in plakophilin-2 among families with arrhythmogenic right ventricular dysplasia/cardiomyopathy. *J Am Coll Cardiol* 48:1416–1424, 2006.
112. Kapplinger JD, et al: Distinguishing arrhythmogenic right ventricular cardiomyopathy/dysplasia-associated mutations from background genetic noise. *J Am Coll Cardiol* 57:2317–2327, 2011.
113. James CA, et al: Exercise increases age-related penetrance and arrhythmic risk in arrhythmogenic right ventricular dysplasia/cardiomyopathy associated desmosomal mutation carriers. *J Am Coll Cardiol* 62:1290–1297, 2013.
114. Davila-Roman VG, et al: Altered myocardial fatty acid and glucose metabolism in idiopathic dilated cardiomyopathy. *J Am Coll Cardiol* 40:271–277, 2002.
115. Chinnery PF: Mitochondrial disorders overview. *GeneReviews* 1993.
116. Obayashi T, et al: Point mutations in mitochondrial DNA in patients with hypertrophic cardiomyopathy. *Am Heart J* 124:1263–1269, 1992.
117. Li YY, Maisch B, Rose ML, et al: Point mutations in mitochondrial DNA of patients with dilated cardiomyopathy. *J Mol Cell Cardiol* 29:2699–2709, 1997.
118. Zaragoza MV, Brandon MC, Diegoli M, et al: Mitochondrial cardiomyopathies: how to identify candidate pathogenic mutations by mitochondrial DNA sequencing, MITOMASTER and phylogeny. *Eur J Hum Genet* 19:200–207, 2011.
119. Vyas PM, et al: A TAT–Frataxin fusion protein increases lifespan and cardiac function in a conditional Friedreich's ataxia mouse model. *Hum Mol Genetics* 21:1230–1247, 2012.
120. Spencer CT, et al: Cardiac and clinical phenotype in Barth syndrome. *Pediatrics* 118:e337–e346, 2006.
121. Bratic A, Larsson NG: The role of mitochondria in aging. *J Clin Invest* 123:951–957, 2013.
122. Koopman WJ, Willems PH, Smeitink JA: Monogenic mitochondrial disorders. *N Engl J Med* 366:1132–1141, 2012.
123. Hershberger RE, et al: Genetic evaluation of cardiomyopathy—a Heart Failure Society of America practice guideline. *J Card Fail* 15:83–97, 2009.
124. Gollob MH, et al: Recommendations for the use of genetic testing in the clinical evaluation of inherited cardiac arrhythmias associated with sudden cardiac death: Canadian Cardiovascular Society/Canadian Heart Rhythm Society joint position paper. *Can J Cardiol* 27:232–245, 2011.
125. Ingles J, et al: Guidelines for genetic testing of inherited cardiac disorders. *Heart Lung Circ* 20:681–687, 2011.
126. Judge DP, Johnson NM: Genetic evaluation of familial cardiomyopathy. *J Cardiovasc Trans Res* 2:144–154, 2008.
127. Johnston JJ, Biesecker LG: Databases of genomic variation and phenotypes: existing resources and future needs. *Hum Mol Genet* 22:R27–R31, 2013.

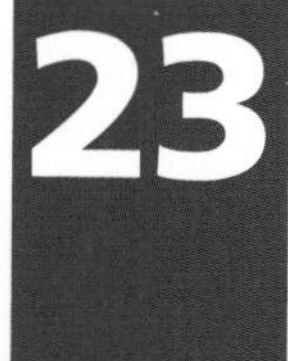

Heart Failure as a Consequence of Hypertension

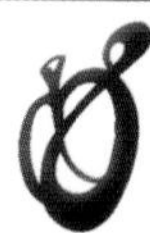

Florian Rader and Ronald G. Victor

INTRODUCTION: DEFINITION AND IMPACT

Hypertension (HTN) affects over 1 billion people worldwide and is the most prevalent risk factor for the development of heart failure[1-3] (see also Chapter 17). Despite some improvements in the treatment and control of hypertension,[4] the societal burden of hypertensive heart disease in an aging population has increased and heart failure—one major manifestation of hypertensive heart disease—continues to be the most frequent hospital admission diagnosis in the United States.[5] The term *hypertensive heart disease* encompasses a disease spectrum ranging from clinically silent structural remodeling, such as left ventricular hypertrophy (LVH), to the development of clinical symptoms—often decades later—such as heart failure. **Figure 23-1** shows a diagram of the progression and cardiovascular complications of hypertensive heart disease.

The human heart is a highly adaptive organ that responds to pressure overload with recruitment of contractile elements to maintain normal left ventricular systolic wall stress: myocyte hypertrophy leads to increased relative wall thickness (i.e., concentric LVH).[6] Although LVH can precede the clinical diagnosis of hypertension,[7] it is considered to be the inciting event in the development of hypertensive heart disease. Complex neurohumoral stimulation accompanies chronic hypertension and eventually leads to cardiomyocyte dysfunction, pathologic increases in cardiac extracellular matrix (i.e., fibrosis) and disturbance of intramyocardial microvasculature. Left ventricular diastolic dysfunction, left atrial enlargement, and atrial arrhythmias are early clinical signs of hypertensive heart disease (see also Chapter 36). The development of ischemic events as a result of hypertension is a common but not obligatory intermediate disease stage that can accelerate the progression of hypertensive heart disease.[8-10] Finally, increases in left ventricular dimensions, worsening of systolic performance and ventricular arrhythmias indicate severe or end-stage disease.[11,12]

LVH is a potent cardiovascular risk factor, independent of the degree of blood pressure elevation or other comorbidities.[13-15] Regression of LVH even in advanced stages of hypertensive heart disease with medical treatment improves prognosis and thus may be an important therapeutic target.[16]

This chapter provides an overview of the diagnosis, epidemiology, molecular mechanisms, and the treatment of hypertensive heart disease.

LEFT VENTRICULAR HYPERTROPHY

Epidemiology

As described previously, LVH is a compensatory mechanism to adapt to higher left ventricular work demands, including pressure load. The threshold between adaptive (healthy) and maladaptive (pathologic) hypertrophy is not clearly defined and therefore makes an estimation of pathologic LVH difficult on a population level. In the Multi-Ethnic Study of Atherosclerosis (MESA), a study of middle-aged and older men and women without a diagnosis of cardiovascular disease (including a diagnosis of hypertension), 11% met the criteria for LVH by cardiac MRI.[17] In the Dallas Heart Study, which included both hypertensive and normotensive persons 30 to 67 years of age, the overall prevalence of LVH by cardiac MRI was 9.4%, but was higher in participants with elevated systolic blood pressure (BP).[18] These prevalence rates are some of the most reliable estimates for the general adult population, because they stem from population-based samples with cardiac MRI for the detection of LVH. In contrast, the estimates of LVH prevalence among hypertensives varies markedly among studies, depending on the testing modality (e.g., electrocardiography [ECG] vs. echo vs. cardiac magnetic resonance imaging [MRI]), the LVH diagnostic criteria, and importantly the demographics and comorbidity profile of the study population. In a pooled analysis of studies using ECG as the diagnostic test, the reported prevalence of LVH ranged from 0.6% to 40% (average 24% in men and 16% in women).[19] In another study, pooled analysis of studies using echocardiography for the detection of LVH showed less variable prevalence estimates, ranging from 36% to 41% among patients with hypertension.[20]

Ethnic Differences

In most population-based studies, non-Hispanic (NH) black individuals have a much greater prevalence of LVH compared with their NH white counterparts.[18,21,22] Specifically, in the Hypertension Genetic Epidemiology Network Study (HyperGEN),[23] middle-aged black adults with hypertension had 2.5-fold greater odds for LVH by echocardiography even after adjustment for cardiovascular risk factors and body surface area. In the Dallas Heart Study, young and middle-aged black adults, which included both normotensives and hypertensives, had 1.8-fold greater odds of LVH by cardiac MRI after adjustment for systolic BP, body mass, age, gender, history of diabetes, and socioeconomic status.[18] The cause of this much greater propensity for LVH in blacks is unknown, but could be from earlier onset,[24,25] less nocturnal dipping,[26-28] and greater severity of hypertension.[4] However, the fact that the greater odds for LVH in blacks increased to 2.3-fold in the subgroup of hypertensives and that the prevalence of LVH was only increased in blacks if they were either in the prehypertensive or hypertensive range of systolic BP suggests genetic predisposition of blacks to develop LVH in response to pressure overload as discussed later (see section on genetic factors in LVH). MESA compared left ventricular mass indexed with body surface area between NH whites, NH blacks, and Hispanic of Mexican, Caribbean, and South/Central American origin. Hypertension was much more common in NH blacks than all other groups. However, LVH (defined as >95th percentile of cumulative distribution separately for men and women) was more common in all Hispanic subgroups than NH whites, but was as frequently observed in Hispanics as in NH blacks.[29] Similarly increased prevalence of LVH in Hispanics and NH blacks compared with NH whites have also been observed in chronic kidney disease.[30] In the Northern Manhattan Study, a tri-ethnic community cohort of NH white, NH black, and Hispanic participants found that both Hispanics and blacks had worse echo-derived left ventricular diastolic indices than whites. However, these differences were not related to left ventricular mass or hypertension, but rather to cardiovascular comorbidities and socioeconomic factors.[31]

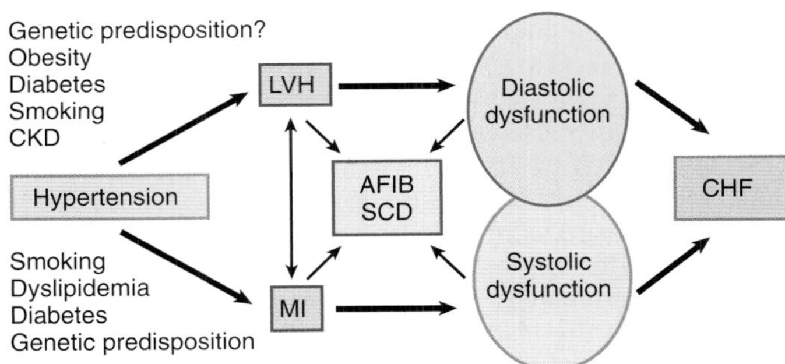

FIGURE 23-1 Risk factors and the progression of hypertensive heart disease and its complications. *AFIB,* Atrial fibrillation; *CHF,* congestive heart failure; *CKD,* chronic kidney disease; *LVH,* left ventricular hypertrophy; *MI,* myocardial infarction; *SCD,* sudden cardiac death.

Gender Differences

In general, men have greater left ventricular mass indexed to body surface area than women. Therefore, different threshold values have been established for the diagnosis of LVH in men and women. Using these different thresholds for the diagnosis of LVH, men tend to have a greater incidence of LVH, even after adjustment for other characteristics thought of as risk factors for LVH.[18,23,32]

Risk Factors for Left Ventricular Hypertrophy

Besides the aforementioned demographic determinants of LVH, many other clinical risk factors have been identified. Not surprisingly, blood pressure tracks left ventricular mass in a linear fashion. However, single office blood pressure measurements are only weakly associated with left ventricular mass (**Figure 23-2**),[33] whereas 24-hour ambulatory blood pressure—a better measure of hemodynamic burden on the left ventricle—is much more closely linked to left ventricular mass.[34] Another explanation for the weak correlation of blood pressure measurements and left ventricular mass are nonhemodynamic (i.e., neurohumoral) stimuli to myocardial muscle growth, which are discussed in the next section of this chapter. Epidemiologic studies have identified the following risk factors for LVH: In the MESA study of adults without clinical cardiovascular disease, left ventricular mass was independently associated with current smoking and diabetes and more recently, even impaired glucose tolerance in persons without diabetes was a risk factor for LVH after adjustment for obesity.[35,36] Sleep-disordered breathing has also been identified as a determinant of greater left ventricular mass,[37] which is likely related to a greater prevalence of nocturnal hypertension and sympathetic nerve activation[38] in these individuals.[39] Closely linked to sleep apnea is body mass index and subscapular

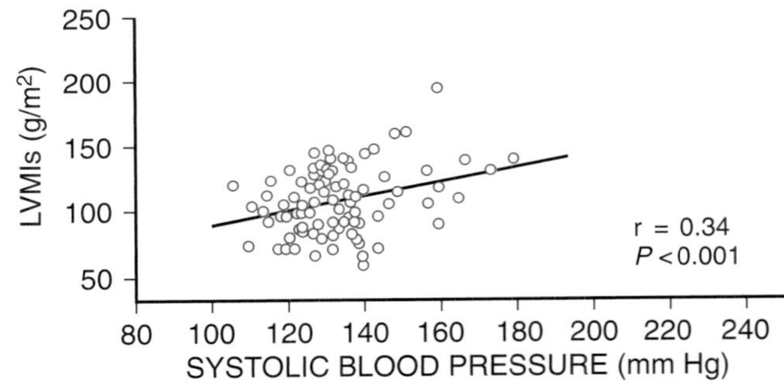

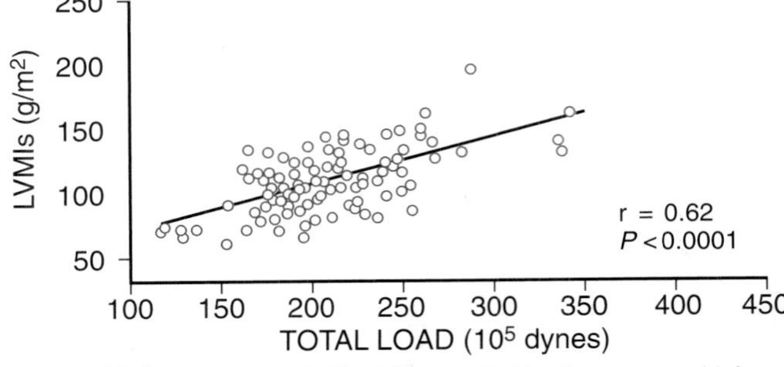

FIGURE 23-2 Correlation of office/clinic systolic blood pressure and left ventricular load with left ventricular mass indexed to body surface area. The correlation is less than perfect, suggesting that office/clinic blood pressure is not the only determinant of left ventricular hypertrophy. *LVMI,* Left ventricular mass index. *From Ganau A, Devereux RB, Pickering TG, et al: Relation of left ventricular hemodynamic load and contractile performance to left ventricular mass in hypertension. Circulation 81:25–36, 1990.*

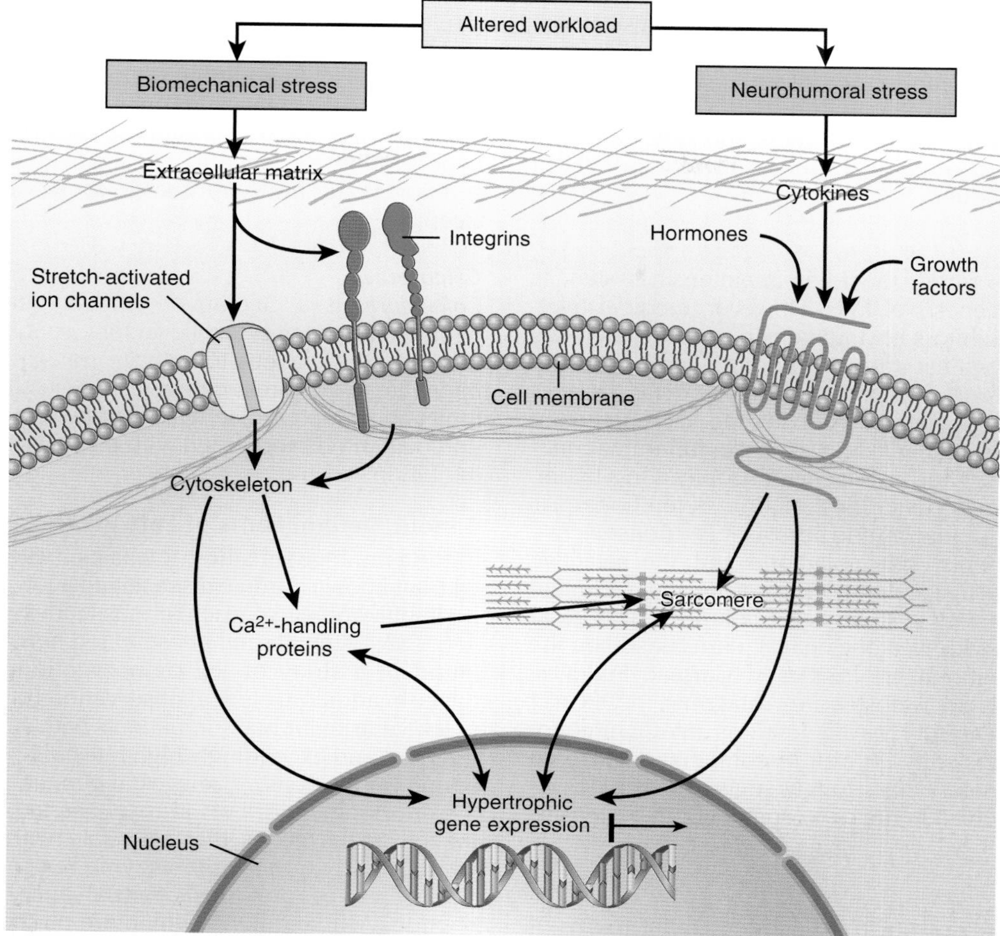

FIGURE 23-3 Hemodynamic and neurohumoral stimuli and pathways leading to myocyte hypertrophy. Both mechanical and neurohumoral stress in hypertension stimulate local release of paracrine substances, which signal hypertrophic gene expression and sarcomere hypertrophy. *From Hill JA, Olson EN: Cardiac plasticity. N Engl J Med 358:1370–1380, 2008.*

skin fold thickness, which was associated with greater left ventricular mass in the Coronary Artery Risk Development in Young Adults (CARDIA) study and in MESA.[40,41] Chronic kidney disease is closely linked to LVH, even when renal functions are only mildly abnormal.[42] The combination of black race and chronic kidney disease is associated with a staggering LVH prevalence of 70%.[43]

Pathophysiologic Mechanisms

Macroscopically, LVH is an increase of myocardial muscle mass. However, on a cellular level, increases in muscle mass not only consist of increases in cardiomyocyte protein and recruitment of contractile elements, but also other cell types, such as fibroblasts, vascular smooth muscle cells, and endothelial cells, undergo changes that contribute to an altered extracellular matrix (i.e., the connective tissue) (see also Chapter 4). **Figure 23-3** depicts the complex interplay between mechanical (hemodynamic) and neurohumoral stress and key pathways for stimulating hypertrophic gene expression.[44] The inability of the myocardial microvasculature to keep up with myocyte growth is a key aspect in the genesis of hypertensive heart disease. Although our understanding of underlying mechanisms remains incomplete, decades of research have identified several molecular mechanisms, as recently reviewed by Cacciapuoti,[45] and genetic factors that influence the development of hypertensive heart disease.

Importance of Hemodynamic Burden

As mentioned previously, the correlation between office/clinic blood pressure and left ventricular mass is less than perfect (see Figure 23-2).[46] There are several explanations for this finding: (1) Office blood pressure is not a reliable surrogate for hemodynamic burden; 24-hour ambulatory blood pressure correlates much better.[34] (2) Neither office nor 24-hour ambulatory blood pressure monitoring provides information on lifetime hemodynamic burden—onset and progression of hypertension. (3) Neurohumoral stimulation linked to the development of LVH may differ between hypertensive individuals. (4) A genetic propensity for LVH may exist in some and be absent in other hypertensive patients. Racial/ethnic differences in the probability of developing LVH strongly suggest (but do not prove) a genetic component and are discussed separately.

Molecular Mechanisms

Renin-Angiotensin-Aldosterone System

(see also Chapter 5)

Local release of angiotensin II causes G-protein and Rho-protein activations, increasing protein synthesis in myocardial cells, and collagen synthesis in fibroblasts.[47-50]

Overexpression of angiotensin II in transgenic mice causes pressure-independent LVH.[51] Angiotensin II may also stimulate paracrine endothelin-1 release from fibroblasts.[52] Clinical evidence for the importance of renin-stimulation and angiotensin II in the development of LVH comes from the fact that angiotensin receptor blockers and ACE inhibitors are the most effective medical therapy to reduce LVH in hypertensive individuals.[53]

Aldosterone

As previously described, the renin-angiotensin system is important in the genesis of LVH. However, medical treatment with ACE inhibitors or angiotensin receptor blockers does not protect against effects from circulating aldosterone (i.e., aldosterone escape).[54] Cardiomyocytes express mineralocorticoid receptors.[55] Aldosterone itself has been shown to cause vascular[56] and cardiac inflammation,[57] myocardial fibrosis,[58] and cardiac hypertrophy.[59] In a hypertensive model of endothelial dysfunction, eplerenone prevented cardiac inflammation and fibrosis.[60] The nonselective aldosterone antagonist spironolactone and the selective aldosterone antagonist eplerenone provide clear clinical benefit in patients with systolic heart failure,[61,62] less clear benefit in patients with diastolic heart failure (based on the results of the Treatment of Preserved Cardiac Function Heart Failure With an Aldosterone Antagonist [TOPCAT] trial),[63,64] and decrease LVH as efficiently as an ACE inhibitor and even more efficiently if given in combination with an ACE inhibitor.[65] These data strongly suggest that aldosterone is directly involved in the development of hypertensive heart disease.

Endothelin-1

Endothelin has been shown to induce hypertrophy in animal models and this phenotype can be suppressed by a pharmacologic endothelin-1 receptor blocker.[52,66,67] Direct evidence of endothelin-1 from human studies is lacking. As mentioned previously, there is an interplay between angiotensin II and endothelin-1.[52]

Heat-Shock Proteins

A group of intracellular proteins, which become more abundant in cells exposed to thermal or other forms of stress, regulate nuclear transcription factors. One of these is nuclear factor kappa B (NF-κB), which is increased in a pressure-overload model in the rat and can be suppressed by either gene therapy with a viral vector or an antioxidant substance. As a result, the hypertrophic response to pressure overload was markedly attenuated in treated animals.[68] Furthermore, in mice with cardiomyocyte-restricted expression of an NF-κB superrepressor gene, both angiotensin II and isoproterenol-induced hypertrophic response and the expression of hypertrophic markers, such as β-myosin heavy chain and natriuretic peptides, are reduced.[69] The proteasome inhibitor PS-519, known to suppress NF-κB, prevented isoproterenol-induced LVH if given before and during isoproterenol infusion and caused regression of LVH in those animals, which already had isoproterenol-induced LVH.[70]

G Proteins

Many substances involved in the hypertrophic response to pressure and stress, including phenylephrine, angiotensin II, and endothelin-1, bind to myocyte membrane receptors that activate G protein and small subforms of G proteins (i.e., Rho proteins). These proteins regulate transcription and have been shown to be involved in phenylephrine-induced LVH.[71] In addition, in transgenic mice that overexpress the carboxyl-terminal peptide of the G protein and thus inhibit normal G-protein activation, the slope of the hypertrophic response to increased left ventricular pressure overload from transverse aortic banding was less steep.[72]

Calcineurin

Calcineurin is a calcium-dependent phosphatase, which dephosphorylates cytosolic factors, enabling them to translocate to the nucleus to activate transcription. Transgenic mice that overexpress calcineurin or its transcription factor targets develop cardiac hypertrophy and failure. This phenotype can be suppressed with pharmacologic calcineurin inhibition.[73]

Genetic Determinants of Left Ventricular Hypertrophy

In the Framingham study, it was estimated that in patients without known cardiac disease and a low risk factor profile, heritability of left ventricular mass index was between 0.24 and 0.32.[74] A much higher estimated heritability of 0.59 was found in a study of 182 monozygotic and 194 dizygotic twins. In addition, clinical observations of a large variability of left ventricular mass in patients with similar office blood pressure and exceedingly high rates of LVH in certain race/ethnic populations,[18,23] suggest a genetic predisposition for the development of LVH in response to pressure overload. Indeed, some genes that associate with LVH have been identified: (1) *Corin* is the enzyme responsible for the processing of the preforms of atrial and B-type natriuretic peptide (ANP and BNP), which are protective against LVH. Corin knockout mice develop hypertension and cardiac hypertrophy.[74] Mutations of the corin I555(P568) gene were exclusive to African Americans in multiethnic samples with an allelic prevalence of 6% to 12%.[75] Its association with an increased prevalence of hypertension and LVH in African Americans has been demonstrated in 3 independent population-based samples.[75] (2) *Protein C* overexpression causes progressive LVH and diastolic dysfunction in animals. (3) Bradykinin-2 receptor gene polymorphism, specifically the 9bp receptor gene deletion is associated with greater left ventricular mass in subjects undergoing physical training.[76] (4) ACE gene polymorphism is also associated with both greater tissue and plasma ACE levels, as well as greater probability for LVH.[77,78]

CLASSIFICATION AND DIAGNOSIS OF HYPERTENSIVE HEART DISEASE

Hypertensive heart disease is classified using a combination of structural and functional criteria. Two distinct entities are excluded from these classifications and therefore not discussed in this section: (1) physiologic hypertrophy as seen in pregnant women or athletes: moderate adaptive increases of left ventricular internal dimensions and left ventricular muscle mass, but with normal relative wall thickness (0.32-0.42)[79] and normal Doppler-derived left ventricular filling parameters; and (2) genetic or acquired hypertrophic cardiomyopathies: pressure-independent left ventricular wall thickening due to sarcomere-protein mutations as seen in familial hypertrophic cardiomyopathy or protein/glycolipid deposits as seen in amyloidosis or Fabry disease.

Clinical Presentation/Functional Classes

The onset of symptomatic heart failure and especially hospitalization for heart failure is an important indicator for poor outcomes and a high mortality rate, both in heart failure with preserved ejection fraction (HFpEF) and heart failure with depressed left ventricular systolic function. Therefore, considering symptoms in the classification of hypertensive heart disease is extremely important.[80]

Class I: Subclinical diastolic dysfunction without LVH: Asymptomatic patients with abnormal left ventricular relaxation/stiffness by Doppler echocardiography, a common finding in individuals older than 65 years of age.[81]

Class II: LVH

- **IIA:** with normal or mildly abnormal functional capacity (New York Heart Association Class I)
- **IIB:** with abnormal functional capacity (New York Heart Association Class II or greater)

Class III: Heart failure with preserved ejection fraction: clinical signs and symptoms of cardiac decompensation (i.e., dyspnea, pulmonary edema) from increased left atrial pressure.

Class IV: Heart failure with depressed ejection fraction

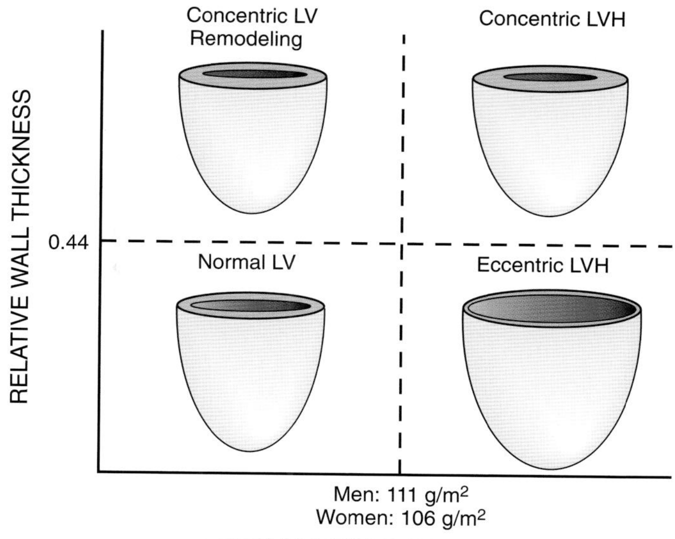

FIGURE 23-4 Anatomic classification of hypertensive heart disease. Pressure overload of the left ventricle initiates concentric remodeling as compensatory mechanism, followed by frank increase in left ventricular mass above cutoff values for left ventricular hypertrophy. Left ventricular dilation with increased left ventricular mass occurs at an advanced stage of decompensation. *LV,* Left ventricle; *LVH,* left ventricular hypertrophy. *Adapted from Ganau A, Devereux RB, Roman MJ, et al: Patterns of left ventricular hypertrophy and geometric remodeling in essential hypertension. J Am Coll Cardiol 19:1550–1558, 1992.*

Anatomic Classification of Left Ventricular Hypertrophy

The anatomic classification proposed by Ganau and colleagues (1992)[33] is based on echocardiographic measurements of left ventricular geometry and left ventricular muscle mass. Left ventricular geometry is determined by *relative wall thickness (RWT)* calculated as doubling the width of the left ventricular inferolateral wall and divided by the left ventricular end-diastolic internal diameter in end diastole. An RWT of 0.44 or more is diagnostic for concentric LVH, whereas an RWT less than 0.44 with increased left ventricular mass is indicative of eccentric remodeling. This category can be further distinguished from physiologic hypertrophy, which is characterized by mild increases of left ventricular mass and an RWT between 0.32 and 0.44.[79] Left ventricular mass is best calculated according to the modified Simpson rule and most commonly indexed to body surface area.[82] **Figure 23-4** depicts the four anatomic classes of left ventricular mass and geometry.

Class I: Normal left ventricle
Class II: Concentric remodeling without hypertrophy
Class III: Concentric LVH
Class IV: Eccentric LVH

Diagnostic Criteria for Left Ventricular Hypertrophy

LVH, the increase in left ventricular myocardial mass beyond defined cutoffs, can be diagnosed by ECG, echocardiography, or cardiac MRI. Although cardiac MRI is the most accurate and precise method for determining left ventricular mass, the preferred method is echocardiography, because it is more widely available than cardiac MRI, while providing increased sensitivity compared with ECG.[83] ECG is a reasonable cost-conscious alternative to the more expensive testing modalities, especially in the asymptomatic hypertensive patient with a low index of suspicion for hypertensive heart disease in whom an echocardiogram is not necessarily indicated.[84] A clear limitation to the usefulness of screening for LVH irrespective of the testing modality is the fact that awareness of the presence or absence of LVH typically has little impact on physician behavior in the treatment of hypertension.[85]

Electrocardiography

Among the many published ECG criteria for the diagnosis of LVH shown in **Table 23-1**, the Cornell criteria appear to be both reasonably sensitive and highly prognostic for cardiovascular events.[86] The sensitivity can be improved by using several ECG criteria in conjunction (i.e., Romhilt-Estes score, Perugia criteria). It is important to recognize that the sensitivity and specificity of ECG for the diagnosis of LVH depends on the LVH severity among the study populations.

Echocardiography

Echocardiography is the preferred testing modality for the diagnosis of LVH. The use of the calculated left ventricular mass index provides both greater sensitivity and specificity for the diagnosis of LVH than linear measurements of the left ventricular septum or posterior wall.[87] Of note, three-dimensional echocardiography may be equally accurate and reproducible as cardiac MRI—the current gold standard for detecting LVH—but is not widely used in clinical practice.[88,89] For determination of LVH, left ventricular mass is calculated using the formula:

$$\text{left ventricular mass} = 0.8 \times \left(1.04 \times \left[(\text{LVIDd} + \text{PWTd} + \text{SWTd})^3 - (\text{LVIDd})^3\right]\right) + 0.6\ \text{g}$$

TABLE 23-1 Definition, Sensitivity, and Specificity of Some ECG Criteria for Left Ventricular Hypertrophy

ECG CRITERIA	DIAGNOSTIC CUTOFF	SENSITIVITY	SPECIFICITY
R in aVL	≥1.1 mV	11	97
Sokolow-Lyon voltage[191] S in V_1 + R in V_5 or V_6	≥3.5 mV	13	93
Cornell voltage[192] S in V_3 + R in aVL	>2.8 mV (men) >2.0 mV (women)	19	97
Romhilt-Estes score[193]	**Total of ≥5 points**	16	96
Components:			
1. Any of these: R or S in limb leads ≥ 20; S in V1 or V2 ≥ 30; R in V5 or V6 ≥ 30	3 points		
2. ST-T vector opposite to QRS with digitalis	1 point		
ST-T vector opposite to QRS without digitalis	3 points		
3. Left atrial enlargement in V_1	3 points		
4. Left-axis deviation	2 points		
5. QRS duration ≥ 0.09 s	1 point		
6. Intrinsicoid deflection in V_5 or V_6 >0.05 s	1 point		
Perugia criteria[194]	**≥1 of the following criteria**	36	90
Components:			
1. S in V_3 + R in aVL	>2.4 mV (men) >2.0 mV (women)		
2. LV strain (ST-T vector opposite to QRS)	Present		
3. Romhilt-Estes score	≥5 points		

ECG, Electrocardiography.

TABLE 23-2 LVH Severity by Echocardiogram-Derived Left Ventricular Mass Indexed by Body Surface Area[82]

SEVERITY	LVMI IN MEN g/m²	LVMI IN WOMEN g/m²
Mild LVH	103 to 116	89 to 100
Moderate LVH	117 to 130	101 to 112
Severe LVH	≥131	≥113

LVH, Left ventricular hypertrophy; *LVMI*, left ventricular mass index.

and indexed to body surface area; the latter is calculated according to Du Bois or Mosteller.[82,90] LVIDd indicates left ventricular internal diameter in diastole; PWTd, posterior wall thickness in diastole; SWTd, septal wall thickness in diastole; and LVIDd, left ventricular internal diameter in diastole. The severity of LVH is graded by the left ventricular mass index as shown in **Table 23-2**.

Cardiac Magnetic Resonance Imaging

Estimation of left ventricular mass by two-dimensional echocardiography is based on linear measurements with the assumption that the left ventricle is geometrically a prolate ellipsoid of revolution, which is oftentimes inaccurate. In contrast, cardiac MRI permits estimation of left ventricular mass by direct three-dimensional tracing without any geometric assumptions. As a result, cardiac MRI has been shown to be twice as precise than two-dimensional echocardiography in determining left ventricular mass, with a 93% lower interstudy variability, and is therefore considered the gold standard.[91,92] However, higher cost, less availability, and poorer tolerability continue to limit its broad use as a screening test for LVH in hypertensive patients.

COMPLICATIONS OF HYPERTENSIVE HEART DISEASE

Heart Failure with Preserved Ejection Fraction (see also Chapter 36)

Hypertension is the most prevalent cause for heart failure.[1] Left ventricular remodeling in response to pressure overload and neurohumoral stimulation causes left ventricular structural geometric changes, which are initially adaptive but later in the course of hypertensive heart disease maladaptive evidence of left ventricular decompensation. Diastolic dysfunction—abnormal left ventricular relaxation and filling—occurs typically much earlier than systolic dysfunction.[93,94]

Diastolic function is noninvasively determined by echocardiography (see also Chapter 29). The diastolic phase of the cardiac cycle consists of four distinct components: (1) *isovolumic relaxation,* which starts at closure of the aortic valve and ends with the opening of the mitral valve; (2) *passive filling of the left ventricle;* after opening of the mitral valve there is rapid filling of the left ventricle propelled by the pressure gradient between the left atrium and left ventricle (i.e., pulsed Doppler-derived E wave); (3) *diastasis:* when the pressure gradient between the left ventricle and the left atrium approaches zero, flow across the mitral valve is equal to pulmonary vein inflow, which is limited by left ventricular pressure and compliance; (4) *atrial contraction* (i.e., pulsed Doppler-derived A wave). Qualitative and quantitative evaluation of these four diastolic measures by Doppler echocardiography is essential to determine diastolic function and to noninvasively estimate left ventricular filling pressures. Other echocardiographic surrogates of diastolic function are left atrial enlargement—a prevalent feature of hypertensive heart disease,[95] pulmonary vein flow pattern, and pulmonary arterial pressure. A detailed description of the evaluation of left ventricular diastology

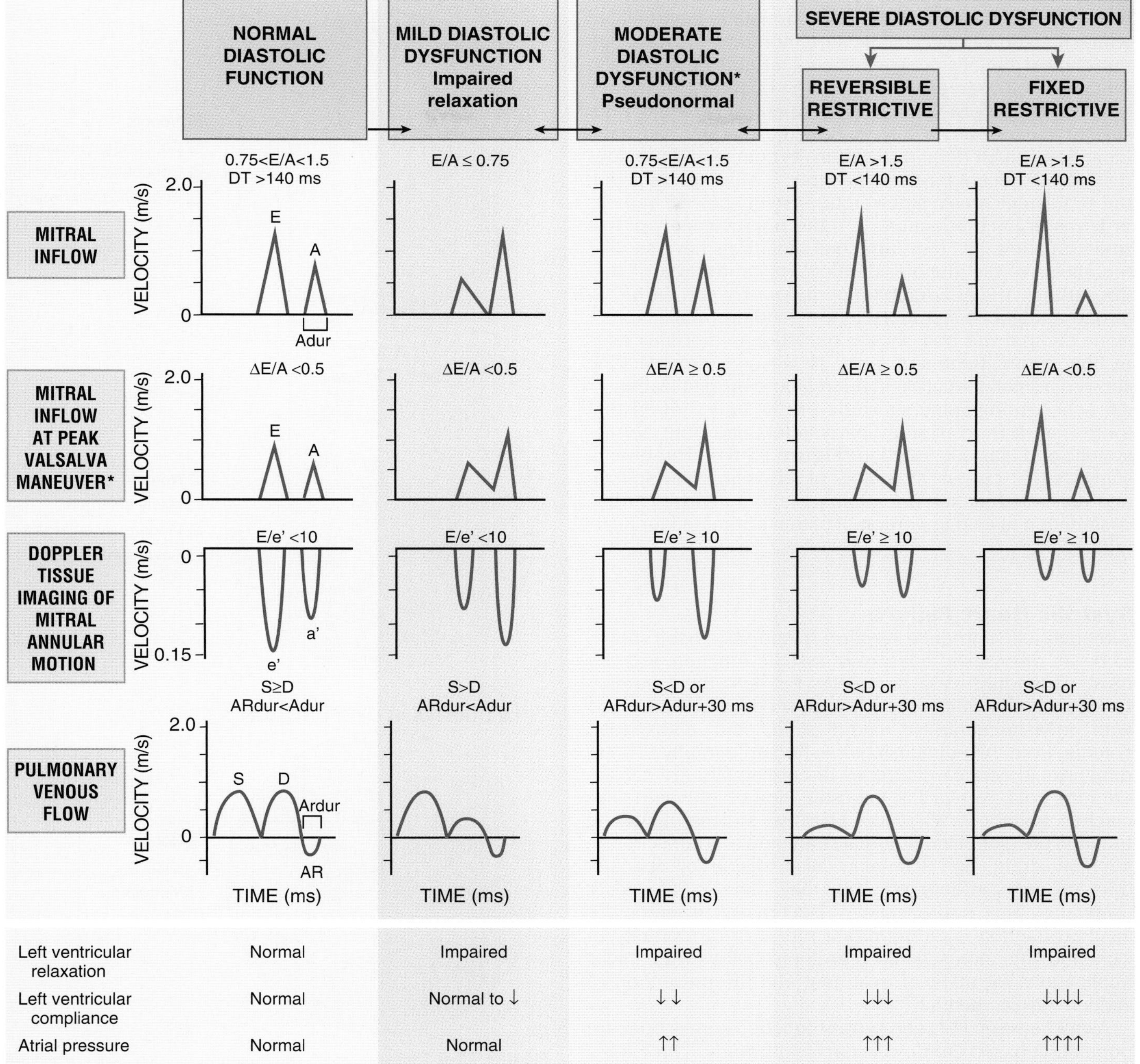

	Normal	Mild	Moderate	Reversible restrictive	Fixed restrictive
Left ventricular relaxation	Normal	Impaired	Impaired	Impaired	Impaired
Left ventricular compliance	Normal	Normal to ↓	↓↓	↓↓↓	↓↓↓↓
Atrial pressure	Normal	Normal	↑↑	↑↑↑	↑↑↑↑

FIGURE 23-5 Classification of diastolic function by Doppler/tissue, Doppler echocardiography, and correlating left ventricular and left atrial abnormalities. *A*, Late mitral inflow velocity during atrial contraction; *AR*, pulmonary vein flow reversal during atrial contraction; *ARdur* and *Adur*, duration of AR or A; *D*, diastolic component of pulmonary vein flow; *DT*, early mitral inflow deceleration time; *E*, early mitral inflow velocity; *e'*, early annular velocity by tissue Doppler; *S*, systolic component of pulmonary vein flow. *From Redfield MM, Jacobson SJ, Burnett JC et al: Burden of systolic and diastolic ventricular dysfunction in the community: appreciating the scope of the heart failure epidemic. JAMA 289:194–202, 2003.*

is beyond the scope of this chapter. **Figure 23-5** summarizes echocardiography-derived grading of diastolic dysfunction, using Doppler-derived measurement of the early and late mitral inflow and pulmonary vein patterns, tissue Doppler-derived atrioventricular annulus velocities, and color Doppler-derived mitral inflow propagation velocity.[96] Strain and strain rate can be assessed with echocardiography or MRI and promise to be useful determinants of both left ventricular diastolic and systolic function. The association of some common measures of diastolic function with incident cardiovascular events, including heart failure, has been well established.[97-99]

Heart failure with preserved ejection fraction (HFpEF) is a major public health concern. Sixty percent of patients admitted for heart failure have normal left ventricular ejection fraction.[100] HFpEF is linked to older age, female gender, diabetes, obesity, chronic kidney disease, hypertension, and coronary artery disease,[101] and thus with an aging population, hospital admissions for heart failure, especially HFpEF, are increasing.[102] Even after adjustment for other cardiovascular risk factors, which are common in patients with HFpEF, this common form of heart failure is associated with a marked increase in all-cause mortality.[96,102] Although the clinical benefit of several medical and device-based therapies has been established in the treatment of systolic heart failure, HFpEF remains a therapeutic challenge. After several randomized trials, no specific therapy has been identified, which definitively alters its course and provides a mortality benefit for these patients.[103] Although targeting the renin-angiotensin-aldosterone system showed benefits in terms of LVH reduction,[104-106] and improvements of diastolic function,[107-109] four large outcome trials have studied the effects of the angiotensin blockers candesartan[110] and irbesartan,[111] the ACE inhibitor perindopril,[112] and the aldosterone antagonist spironolactone (pending publication).[63] None of them was able show a reduction in mortality rates in the active treatment arm. However, spironolactone showed a small reduction in heart failure hospitalizations.[63] An echocardiographic substudy of this trial showed that more than a third of study participants had both normal systolic and diastolic function (**Figure 23-6**).[64] This finding suggests that current indicators of left ventricular systolic and diastolic function are inadequate to diagnose cardiac dysfunction in a large portion of patients admitted for heart failure.

Systolic Heart Failure

Although left ventricular ejection fraction has been shown to be an insensitive measure of systolic function, it is the most commonly used parameter for describing cardiac function in clinical practice. It is most commonly assessed with measurements of end-diastolic and end-systolic volume from two-dimensional echocardiography. Three-dimensional echocardiography or cardiac MRI are considered the gold standard in the estimation of left ventricular ejection fraction.[88,89,91,92] More sensitive indices of systolic function are global longitudinal strain, radial strain, circumferential strain, and left ventricular torsion by speckle-tracking echocardiography, but they are not yet widely used (see also Chapter 29).[113-116] Decreased left ventricular ejection fraction is an important predictor of mortality in ischemic and nonischemic cardiomyopathy, with major implications for medical treatment and the prevention of sudden cardiac death.[117,118]

A link between LVH and systolic function comes from the population-based Cardiovascular Health Study.[119] Increased LV mass indexed to body surface area was a strong predictor of depressed left ventricular function after an average of 4.9 years of follow-up independent of age, baseline blood pressure, diabetes, coronary artery disease, and Q waves or atrial fibrillation on baseline ECG. This finding suggests that LVH is a direct or indirect—via ischemic events—predecessor of systolic deterioration in hypertensive heart disease. In patients with LVH, even minimal increases in natriuretic peptides and cardiac troponin may identify malignant subgroups with a high risk for progression to systolic heart failure and cardiovascular death.[120] The treatment of systolic heart failure, including medical therapies, device-based therapies, and prevention of sudden cardiac death are beyond the scope of this chapter and are described in the pertinent chapters of this book. It should be noted here, that reduction of LVH with medical therapy also improves systolic left ventricular function.[121,122]

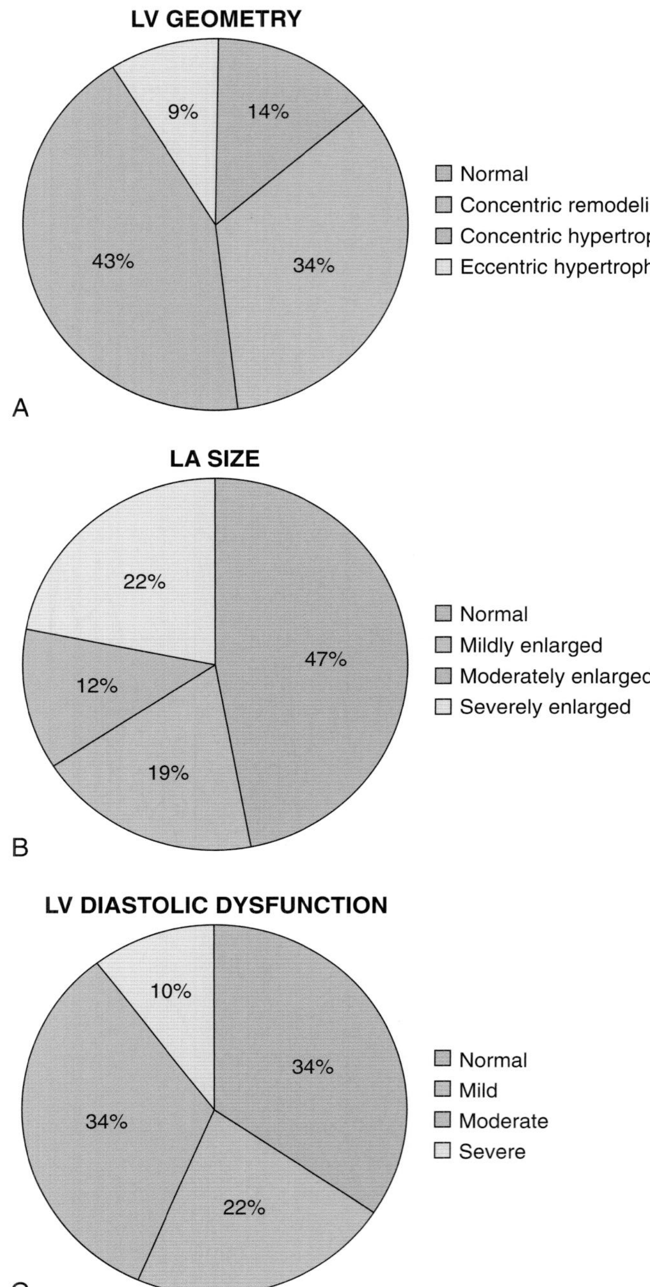

FIGURE 23-6 Distribution of left ventricular geometry, left atrial size, and diastolic function among patients with HFpEF in the TOPCAT trial. **A** and **B** indicate that almost half of HFpEF patients do not meet criteria for left ventricular hypertrophy and have normal left atrial size (a sensitive marker of diastolic dysfunction); **C** indicates that over one third of HFpEF patients have normal diastolic function by Doppler-echocardiography. This is evidence for the heterogeneity of HFpEF as a clinical entity. *HFpEF,* Heart failure with preserved ejection fraction; *LA,* left atrium; *LV,* left ventricular. *From Shah AM, Shah SJ, Anand IS, et al: Cardiac structure and function in heart failure with preserved ejection fraction: baseline findings from the echocardiographic study of the Treatment of Preserved Cardiac Function Heart Failure with an Aldosterone Antagonist trial. Circ Heart Fail 7:104–115, 2014.*

Myocardial Ischemia (see also Chapter 18)

Convincing evidence exists that both hypertension and LVH are potent risk factors for coronary heart disease. In the Framingham study, LVH was an important determinant of coronary artery disease in older participants.[123] Similarly, in the Coronary Artery Risk Development in Young Adults (CARDIA) study, LV mass by echocardiography was independently associated with coronary calcium in young adults.[124] Thus, hypertension, especially when accompanied by LVH, appears to cause progressive coronary plaque buildup to the point where the disease leads to cardiovascular events. Furthermore, LVH is not only associated with stable coronary artery disease from progressive arterial narrowing but also increases the risk of acute coronary plaque rupture.[125] In addition to macrovascular ischemia from epicardial coronary artery disease, microvascular ischemia is a hallmark of LVH and leads to cardiac complications. Therapeutic implications of microvascular blood flow disturbances are discussed in the last section of this chapter (Treatment Targets and the J Curve Debate). Microvascular angina in the absence of obstructive epicardial coronary artery disease is now an established clinical entity and seems to be more common in women.[126,127] From a mechanistic point of view, both microvascular and macrovascular ischemia are key factors in the development of hypertensive heart disease and perpetuate its progression.[9]

Atrial Fibrillation (see also Chapter 35)

Atrial fibrillation is the most common supraventricular arrhythmia, with a prevalence ranging from 0.1% in individuals younger than 55 years old to 10% in octogenarians.[128] Like hypertensive heart disease and diastolic dysfunction, atrial fibrillation is closely linked to older age, hypertension, obesity, and diabetes. Hypertension is the most prevalent modifiable risk factor for atrial fibrillation on a population level.[129,130] The severity of diastolic dysfunction[131,132] and the degree of left atrial enlargement[131,133] both correlate with the incidence rate of atrial fibrillation. Increased left atrial pressure load from chronic hypertension and diastolic dysfunction causes similar changes in the atrial myocardium as previously described in the ventricular myocardium in the development of LVH (see Pathophysiologic Mechanism section). Myocyte hypertrophy, interstitial fibrosis, and cell loss change structural and electrophysiologic properties and lead to zones of conduction slowing and micro-reentrant circuits (i.e., "rotors") that perpetuate atrial fibrillation.[134-137] In animal models, pressure overload from aortic banding, angiotensin II infusion, and 5/6 nephrectomy, a model of chronic kidney disease, all caused left atrial fibrosis and increased atrial fibrillation inducibility.[138] Oxidative stress and inflammation appear to be centrally involved, because pharmacologic antioxidants suppress both left atrial fibrosis and atrial fibrillation inducibility in these animal models.[138] Important clinical sequelae of atrial fibrillation are thromboembolism and worsening heart failure, both from loss of atrial systole in preload-dependent stiff left ventricles and from deterioration of systolic function from persistently elevated heart rates (i.e., tachycardia-mediated cardiomyopathy).[139] Atrial fibrillation has also been associated with an increased risk of mortality independent of the presence or absence of hypertensive heart disease.[140,141] In addition, new-onset atrial fibrillation increases the risk for sudden cardiac death in patients with LVH.[142] Therefore, the prevention of atrial fibrillation may improve outcomes in hypertensive heart disease. This question has been asked in one large observational[143] and two post hoc analyses of randomized studies.[144,145] In these studies, subjects who received an angiotensin receptor blocker had a significant (19% to 37%) relative risk reduction for new-onset atrial fibrillation compared with control subjects. In contrast, in a large randomized trial for the prevention of recurrent (not new-onset) atrial fibrillation as the primary outcome, assignment to the angiotensin receptor blocker valsartan was ineffective.[146]

Sudden Cardiac Death (see also Chapter 35)

Patients with LVH have greater incidence of ventricular premature beats and ventricular tachycardia,[147-149] irrespective of the cause of LVH.[150] Sudden cardiac death, which is most frequently caused by sustained ventricular tachyarrhythmias, is among the leading causes of death worldwide,[151,152] and has been linked to LVH in large epidemiologic studies and registries.[10,11,14,123,153] In the Framingham study, there was a 1.45-fold increase in sudden cardiac death risk for every 50-g increase in left ventricular mass.[11] Although the mechanisms are not well understood, the arrhythmogenic substrate for sudden cardiac death may be subendocardial ischemia, interstitial fibrosis, increased sympathetic tone, increased tissue catecholamine levels, repolarization delay (i.e., prolongation of the QT interval), increased incidence of early afterdepolarizations, and a genetic predisposition of channelopathies in patients with LVH.[12,154] Because of the strong association between LVH and sudden cardiac death, the former may be a viable treatment target to prevent the latter. Indeed, regression of LVH decreased the incidence of sudden cardiac death in two large studies.[7,155] In the Losartan Intervention for Endpoint reduction in Hypertension (LIFE) study, sudden cardiac death occurred at similar rates in both the atenolol and losartan treatment arms. However, absence of on-treatment LVH by Cornell voltage-duration product criteria on ECG was associated with a 66% risk reduction for incident sudden cardiac death, even after adjustment for demographic and clinical characteristics. Given these and other encouraging results, it has been speculated that LVH could increase the accuracy in the prediction of sudden cardiac death and thus make implantation of implantable cardioverter-defibrillators more cost-effective.[12]

All-Cause Mortality

LVH is a potent cardiovascular risk factor, independent of the degree of blood pressure (BP) elevation or other comorbidities.[13-15] In the Framingham study, adults older than 40 years of age without apparent cardiovascular disease underwent echocardiography for determination of left ventricular mass. During a mean follow-up of 4 years, for each 50-g increase in left ventricular mass the relative risk for all-cause mortality increased by 49% in men (adjusted relative risk [aRR] 1.49, confidence interval [CI] 1.14 to 1.94) and doubled in women (aRR 2.01, CI 1.44 to 2.81).[14] In patients who are treated for hypertension, LVH carries a much greater risk for cardiovascular death. In an observational study of 280 patients with essential hypertension, after a mean follow-up period of over 10 years, cardiovascular death occurred in 14% of individuals with LVH compared with 0.5% of individuals without LVH (P <0.0001).[15] Conversely, in the Losartan Intervention For Endpoint Reduction in Hypertension (LIFE) study, absence of in-treatment LVH was associated with a markedly reduced risk for all-cause mortality (multivariable adjusted hazard ratio 0.36, CI 0.23-0.59, P <0.001) (**Figure 23-7**).[16] Left ventricular mass by echocardiography (not ECG) and age, not gender or blood pressure, were the only independent predictors of cardiovascular events. Across the range of left ventricular geometry, concentric LVH was associated with the greatest risk. Interestingly, an obesity paradox appears to exist for the association of LVH with all-cause mortality in women. In a large retrospective study of over 26,000 women with normal systolic left ventricular function who underwent echocardiography in a large academic center, abnormal left ventricular geometry was more common in obese than nonobese individuals. Although LVH—concentric more so than eccentric hypertrophy—was associated with increased all-cause mortality in both obese and nonobese individuals, this increase in mortality was much less dramatic in obese individuals compared with nonobese women (**Figure 23-8**).[156]

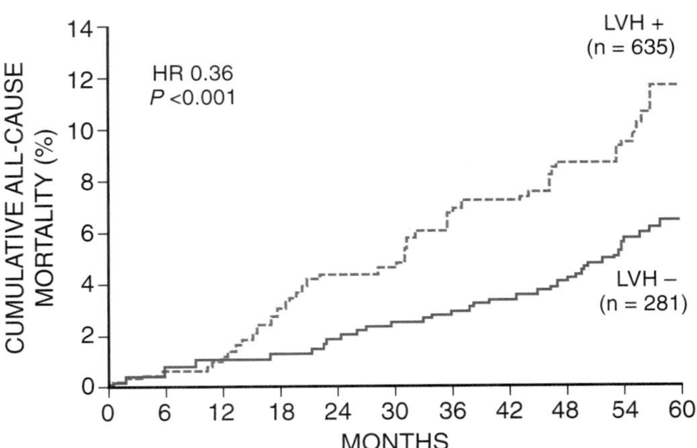

FIGURE 23-7 Prognostic significance of LVH during treatment of hypertension from the echocardiography substudy of the LIFE trial. Hypertensive patients who never had LVH have a markedly lower rate of all-cause mortality than hypertensive patients with LVH. *HR*, Hazard ratio; *LVH*, left ventricular hypertrophy. *Adapted from Devereux RB, Wachtell K, Gerdts E, et al: Prognostic significance of left ventricular mass change during treatment of hypertension. JAMA 292:2350–2356, 2004.*

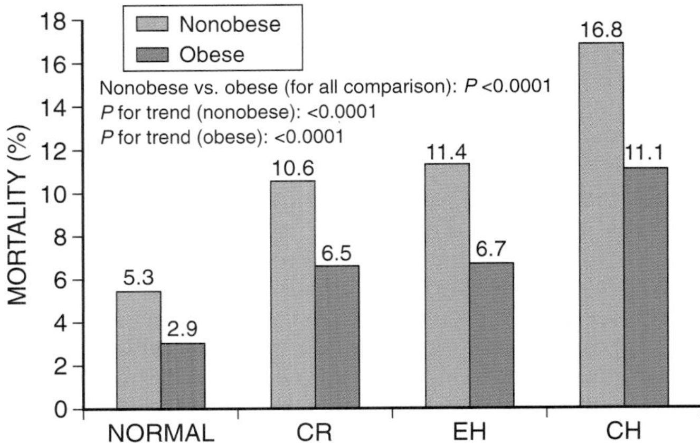

FIGURE 23-8 Left ventricular geometry and risk of death among obese and nonobese women—another obesity paradox. Eccentric and especially concentric left ventricular hypertrophy is associated with increased mortality risk in both obese and nonobese women. However, the gradient is much steeper in nonobese women. *CH*, Concentric hypertrophy; *CR*, concentric remodeling; *EH*, eccentric hypertrophy. *From Patel DA, Lavie CJ, Artham SM, et al: Effects of left ventricular geometry and obesity on mortality in women with normal ejection fraction. Am J Cardiol 113:877–880, 2014.*

TREATMENT

General Considerations and Left Ventricular Hypertrophy Regression (see also Chapter 32)

Although lifestyle modifications and medical treatment are associated with both regression of LVH and improvements in cardiovascular outcomes in hypertensive heart disease, prevention of maladaptive LVH is arguably the most effective approach to reducing cardiovascular complications in chronic hypertension. Especially in high-risk groups with a propensity to developing LVH—such as African Americans and to a lesser degree Hispanics[18,23,29]—early detection and aggressive treatment are key.[157] Once a diagnosis of LVH has been made, the cardiovascular prognosis is less favorable when compared with hypertensive persons without LVH (see Figure 23-7).[16] However, the temporal changes in left ventricular mass while on antihypertensive medical therapy predict the incidence of cardiovascular events, and therefore LVH itself is an important treatment target. Weight loss[158] (and bariatric surgery),[159] dietary salt restriction,[160,161] and treatment of obstructive sleep apnea with continuous positive airway pressure[162] are potential nonpharmacologic approaches for LVH regression and improvement in left ventricular diastolic function, all of which are associated with only modest reductions of blood pressure—the most important determinant of LVH regression. Although blood pressure reduction is essential, there appear to be some differences independent of blood pressure reduction between antihypertensive drug classes. Although some meta-analyses suggest that ACE inhibitors are more effective in reducing left ventricular mass,[163,164] a more recent meta-analysis suggested a possible superiority of angiotensin receptor blockers in reducing left ventricular mass compared with other drug classes.[165] In another analysis[53] of 146 treatment arms of 80 double-blind, randomized controlled trials, after adjustment for treatment duration and change in blood pressure, angiotensin receptor blockers reduced left ventricular mass on average by 13% (95% confidence interval [CI] 8% to 18%), calcium channel blockers by 11% (95% CI 9% to 13%), ACE inhibitors by 10% (95% CI 8% to 12%), diuretics by 8% (95% CI 5% to 10%), and β-blockers by 6% (95% CI 3% to 8 %). When drug classes were statistically compared regarding their effect on left ventricular mass reduction, angiotensin receptor blockers, ACE inhibitors, and calcium channel blockers were more effective than β-blockers. In other studies, the direct renin inhibitor aliskirin[106] has been shown to reduce left ventricular mass, whereas vasodilators (such as hydralazine and minoxidil), α-blockers, and central sympatholytics (such as clonidine) may have no effect on left ventricular mass.[166] A possible explanation for the lack of left ventricular mass reduction in vasodilators may be reflex sympathetic activation,[167] and in central sympatholytics their short half-life and rebound hypertension.[168] The mechanisms leading to differential effects of the aforementioned drug classes, however, are not well established. What has been established is that regression of LVH while on treatment reduces cardiovascular events, including death, myocardial infarction, congestive heart failure, and stroke.[7,169-173] Despite normalization of blood pressure, LVH does not always regress, suggesting that some of the changes in the development of LVH are irreversible and that left ventricular pressure overload is not the only hypertrophic stimulus in some patients.

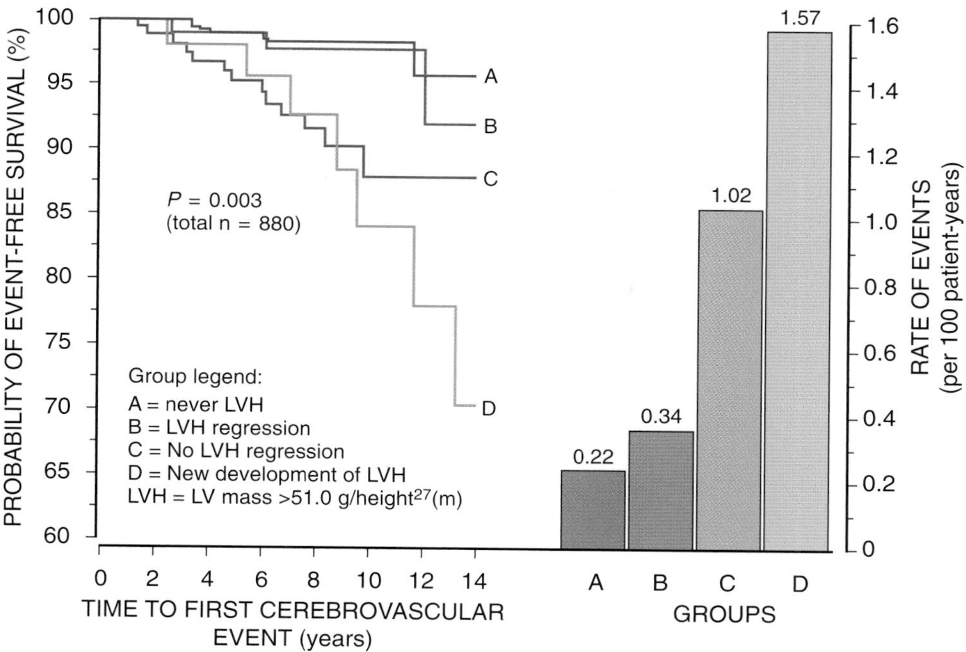

FIGURE 23-9 Dynamic changes of left ventricular mass and risk of stroke. Patients who never had LVH *(blue curve)* and patients who have on-treatment regression of LVH *(red curve)* had a similar risk of stroke during up to 14 years of follow-up, whereas those whose LVH did not regress *(green curve)* or those who developed LVH while on treatment *(orange curve)* had the highest risk of stroke. *LV,* Left ventricular; *LVH,* left ventricular hypertrophy. *From Verdecchia P, Angeli F, Gattobigio R, et al: Regression of left ventricular hypertrophy and prevention of stroke in hypertensive subjects. Am J Hypertens 19:493–499, 2006.*

Whether or not LVH regresses has important prognostic implications, especially for incident stroke. Patients who never had LVH and those whose LVH regresses while on treatment appear to have a similar risk for stroke, whereas those patients whose LVH does not regress or patients who develop LVH while on treatment are at much higher risk for a cerebrovascular event (**Figure 23-9**).[173] It should be briefly noted here that catheter-based renal denervation, which may or may not reliably lower blood pressure,[174,175] also has been reported to reduce left ventricular mass.[176]

Treatment Targets and the J Curve Debate

As discussed in the previous section, it has been well established that lowering blood pressure with medications in patients with hypertension prevents future complications from hypertensive heart disease. What is less clear is the blood pressure threshold for initiation of antihypertensive therapy or the treatment target for lowering blood pressure, which provide the most benefit in the prevention of cardiovascular events. A blood pressure of 140/90 mm Hg is a reasonable threshold/target recommended for most patients in recent hypertension guidelines,[177,178] although some guidelines recommend more lenient thresholds in elderly patients[179] or more stringent thresholds in high-risk patients, such as African Americans.[157] There is little evidence supporting blood pressure thresholds below 140/90 mm Hg, and there is some evidence that such thresholds may be harmful. First observational data suggesting an increase in myocardial infarction in patients whose diastolic BP was reduced to less than 90 mm Hg was reported by Stewart[180] and later Cruickshank and colleagues.[181,182] This phenomenon was termed *J curve* and describes the decrease of cardiovascular events with lowering of elevated blood pressure down to a threshold point of blood pressure below which mortality increases progressively. Polese and associates[183] demonstrated that lowering of diastolic BP to less than 90 mm Hg with intravenous nitroprusside causes a progressive fall in coronary sinus blood flow in hypertensive patients with LVH, whereas reduction of diastolic BP to less than 70 mm Hg had no effect on coronary sinus flow in hypertensive patients without LVH. This finding suggests that (rapid) lowering of BP in patients with hypertensive heart disease may be deleterious, especially in patients with LVH (**Figure 23-10**). Whether the same principle applies to chronic treatment of hypertension, however, is unknown. One explanation for this finding is that an abnormal myocardial microvasculature, which does not keep up with the left ventricular hypertrophic response to pressure overload and neurohumoral stimulation, loses the ability to maintain coronary blood flow with acute drops in blood pressure.

Clinical evidence in favor of the J curve comes from post hoc analyses of randomized clinical trials. In the INVEST (International Verapamil SR/T Trandolapril) trial of hypertensive patients with established coronary artery disease, the incidence of cardiovascular death decreased progressively in patients whose diastolic BP was lowered from 120 mm Hg to 80 to 89 mm Hg and then increased progressively in those with achieved diastolic BP below 80 mm Hg (see Figure 23-10).[184] The J curve was less pronounced in patients who had undergone coronary revascularization and much more pronounced for diastolic than systolic BP and for MI rather than stroke, consistent with the notion that the coronaries are only perfused diastole so that diastolic BP constitutes coronary perfusion pressure. In the large Ongoing Telmisartan Alone and in Combination with Ramipril Trial (ONTARGET) trial of patients who had very high cardiovascular risk but were not all hypertensive, lowering of blood pressure reduced the incidence of cardiovascular events with treatment (ramipril, telmisartan, or both) down to a threshold of 125/72, below which an increase in cardiovascular events was observed.[185] In the PRoFESS (Prevention Regimen for Effectively Avoiding Second Strokes) trial of secondary stroke prevention with telmisartan (vs. placebo), the risk of a second stroke (or cardiovascular events) gradually declined when systolic BP was reduced from a baseline of 150 mm Hg or more to either 130 to 139 mm Hg or 120 to 129 mm Hg but increased again when it was reduced below 120 mm Hg.[186]

Although this observational evidence on the existence of a J curve phenomenon is concerning and should be considered in the treatment of hypertensive heart disease, several counterarguments have been proposed and weaken the clinical significance of this debate, as recently reviewed by Verdecchia and colleagues[187]: (1) Post hoc observational analysis loses the intended balance of baseline characteristics in the original randomized design such that patients with the lowest achieved BP sometimes were the sickest to begin with, leading to *reverse causality* (i.e., patients with the most advanced illness—whether severe heart failure or cancer—and thus the highest mortality rates had lower blood pressure rather than aggressive antihypertensive therapy causing cardiovascular death from diastolic ischemia). The fact that in some papers the J-shaped association of lower blood pressure is eliminated or at least reduced by multivariate analyses supports this hypothesis. (2) Most observational data on the J curve suffer from low sample size in the low blood pressure range and thus have wide confidence margins (see arrow in **Figure 23-11**).[184] In clinical practice, too low blood pressure is rarely a problem, but uncontrolled high blood pressure oftentimes is. (3) Diastolic J curves have been seen in post hoc analyses even in placebo arms of randomized trials, because low diastolic BP is characteristic of elderly patients with isolated systolic hypertension, which carries a high risk of cardiovascular events. (4) A post hoc analysis of the diastolic subgroup of INVEST did not show a J curve in cardiovascular events but did show a systolic J curve for all-cause mortality, which argues against treatment-induced ischemia.[188] (5) Another post hoc analysis of the persons with diabetes subgroup of ONTARGET showed a progressive reduction in stroke risk down to achieved systolic BP of 110 mm Hg with no evidence of a J curve, and there was no J curve for myocardial infarction and cardiovascular events from lowering systolic blood pressure below 130 mm Hg but also no benefit.[189] (6) In the Action to Control Cardiovascular Risk in Diabetes (ACCORD) trial,[190] patients with diabetes randomized to more intense blood pressure control (achieved systolic blood pressure 119 mm Hg) compared with less intense blood pressure control (achieved systolic blood pressure 133 mm Hg) had no benefit, but also no harm (i.e., absence of a J curve) regarding cardiovascular events, but more hypotensive events and acute renal insufficiency.

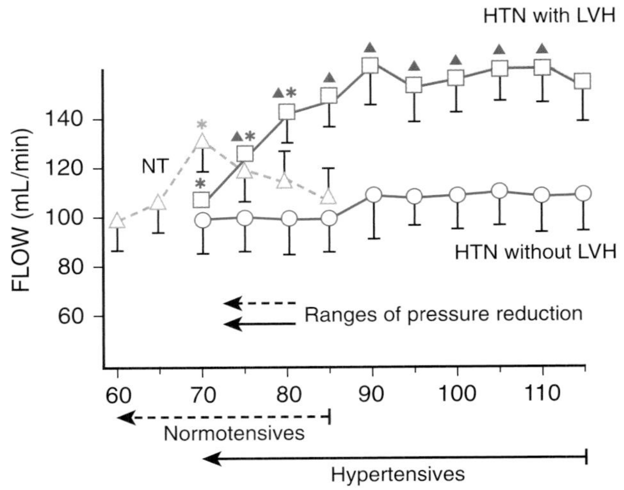

FIGURE 23-10 Coronary blood flow during acute blood pressure reduction. In normotensive patients and hypertensive patients without LVH, coronary blood flow is maintained despite acute blood pressure reduction with nitroprusside. In contrast, in hypertensive patients with LVH, coronary blood flow decreases when coronary perfusion pressure falls below 90 mm Hg. *HTN,* Patients with hypertension; *LVH,* left ventricular hypertrophy; *NT,* patients with normotension. *Adapted from Polese A, De Cesare N, Montorsi P, et al: Upward shift of the lower range of coronary flow autoregulation in hypertensive patients with hypertrophy of the left ventricle. Circulation 83:845–853, 1991.*

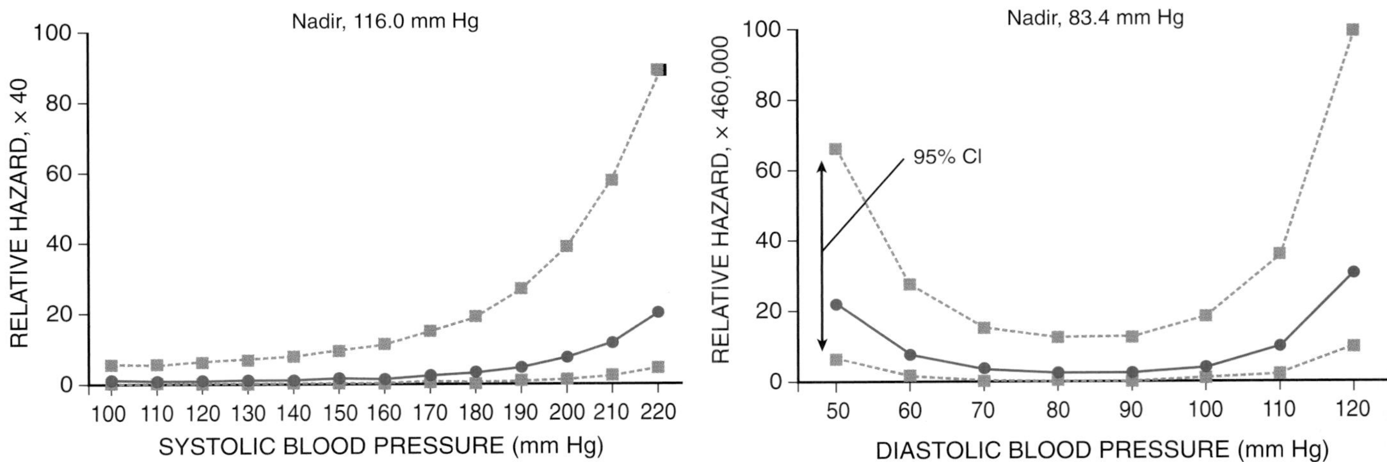

FIGURE 23-11 Observational evidence for the existence of a J curve in the treatment of hypertension. These data indicate that lowering of diastolic blood pressure *(right panel, blue line)* decreases the risk for death down to a nadir of 83 mm Hg, below which mortality increases. Note the large confidence interval *(black arrow)* of diastolic blood pressure due to small patient numbers on both ends of the blood pressure range, making these estimates less stable. A J curve was not seen with lowering of systolic blood pressure *(left panel, blue line)* and was less pronounced after adjustment for patient characteristics (not shown). *Adapted from Messerli FH, Mancia G, Conti R, et al: Dogma disputed: can aggressively lowering blood pressure in hypertensive patients with coronary artery disease be dangerous? Ann Intern Med 144:884–893, 2006.*

References

1. Levy D, Larson MG, Vasan RS, et al: The progression from hypertension to congestive heart failure. *JAMA* 275:1557–1562, 1996.
2. Writing Group Members, Roger VL, Go AS, et al: Executive summary: heart disease and stroke statistics—2012 update: a report from the American Heart Association. *Circulation* 125:188–197, 2012.
3. Whitworth JA, World Health Organization, International Society of Hypertension Writing Group: 2003 World Health Organization (WHO)/International Society of Hypertension (ISH) statement on management of hypertension. *J Hypertens* 21:1983–1992, 2003.
4. Guo F, He D, Zhang W, et al: Trends in prevalence, awareness, management, and control of hypertension among United States adults, 1999 to 2010. *J Am Coll Cardiol* 60:599–606, 2012.
5. Liu L, An Y, Chen M, et al: Trends in the prevalence of hospitalization attributable to hypertensive diseases among United States adults aged 35 and older from 1980 to 2007. *Am J Cardiol* 112:694–699, 2013.
6. Gaasch WH, Zile MR: Left ventricular structural remodeling in health and disease: with special emphasis on volume, mass, and geometry. *J Am Coll Cardiol* 58:1733–1740, 2011.
7. Levy D, Salomon M, D'Agostino RB, et al: Prognostic implications of baseline electrocardiographic features and their serial changes in subjects with left ventricular hypertrophy. *Circulation* 90:1786–1793, 1994.
8. Zabalgoitia M, Berning J, Koren MJ, et al: Impact of coronary artery disease on left ventricular systolic function and geometry in hypertensive patients with left ventricular hypertrophy (the LIFE study). *Am J Cardiol* 88:646–650, 2001.
9. Drazner MH: The progression of hypertensive heart disease. *Circulation* 123:327–334, 2011.
10. Kannel WB, Gordon T, Castelli WP, et al: Electrocardiographic left ventricular hypertrophy and risk of coronary heart disease. The Framingham study. *Ann Intern Med* 72:813–822, 1970.
11. Haider AW, Larson MG, Benjamin EJ, et al: Increased left ventricular mass and hypertrophy are associated with increased risk for sudden death. *J Am Coll Cardiol* 32:1454–1459, 1998.
12. Stevens SM, Reinier K, Chugh SS: Increased left ventricular mass as a predictor of sudden cardiac death: is it time to put it to the test? *Circ Arrhythm Electrophysiol* 6:212–217, 2013.
13. Gosse P, Cremer A, Vircoulon M, et al: Prognostic value of the extent of left ventricular hypertrophy and its evolution in the hypertensive patient. *J Hypertens* 30:2403–2409, 2012.
14. Levy D, Garrison RJ, Savage DD, et al: Prognostic implications of echocardiographically determined left ventricular mass in the Framingham Heart Study. *N Engl J Med* 322:1561–1566, 1990.
15. Koren MJ, Devereux RB, Casale PN, et al: Relation of left ventricular mass and geometry to morbidity and mortality in uncomplicated essential hypertension. *Ann Intern Med* 114:345–352, 1991.
16. Devereux RB, Wachtell K, Gerdts E, et al: Prognostic significance of left ventricular mass change during treatment of hypertension. *JAMA* 292:2350–2356, 2004.
17. Jain A, Tandri H, Dalal D, et al: Diagnostic and prognostic utility of electrocardiography for left ventricular hypertrophy defined by magnetic resonance imaging in relationship to ethnicity: the Multi-Ethnic Study of Atherosclerosis (MESA). *Am Heart J* 159:652–658, 2010.
18. Drazner MH, Dries DL, Peshock RM, et al: Left ventricular hypertrophy is more prevalent in blacks than whites in the general population: the Dallas Heart Study. *Hypertension* 46:124–129, 2005.
19. Cuspidi C, Rescaldani M, Sala C, et al: Prevalence of electrocardiographic left ventricular hypertrophy in human hypertension: an updated review. *J Hypertens* 30:2066–2073, 2012.
20. Cuspidi C, Sala C, Negri F, et al: Prevalence of left-ventricular hypertrophy in hypertension: an updated review of echocardiographic studies. *J Hum Hypertens* 26:343–349, 2012.
21. Kizer JR, Arnett DK, Bella JN, et al: Differences in left ventricular structure between black and white hypertensive adults: the Hypertension Genetic Epidemiology Network study. *Hypertension* 43:1182–1188, 2004.
22. Rodriguez CJ, Sciacca RR, Diez-Roux AV, et al: Relation between socioeconomic status, race-ethnicity, and left ventricular mass: the Northern Manhattan study. *Hypertension* 43:775–779, 2004.
23. Kizer JR, Arnett DK, Bella JN, et al: Differences in left ventricular structure between black and white hypertensive adults: the Hypertension Genetic Epidemiology Network study. *Hypertension* 43:1182–1188, 2004.
24. Wang X, Poole JC, Treiber FA, et al: Ethnic and gender differences in ambulatory blood pressure trajectories: results from a 15-year longitudinal study in youth and young adults. *Circulation* 114:2780–2787, 2006.
25. Selassie A, Wagner CS, Laken ML, et al: Progression is accelerated from prehypertension to hypertension in blacks. *Hypertension* 58:579–587, 2011.
26. Ogedegbe G, Spruill TM, Sarpong DF, et al: Correlates of isolated nocturnal hypertension and target organ damage in a population-based cohort of African Americans: the Jackson Heart Study. *Am J Hypertens* 26:1011–1016, 2013.
27. Wang X, Poole JC, Treiber FA, et al: Ethnic and gender differences in ambulatory blood pressure trajectories: results from a 15-year longitudinal study in youth and young adults. *Circulation* 114:2780–2787, 2006.
28. Profant J, Dimsdale JE: Race and diurnal blood pressure patterns. A review and meta-analysis. *Hypertension* 33:1099–1104, 1999.
29. Rodriguez CJ, Diez-Roux AV, Moran A, et al: Left ventricular mass and ventricular remodeling among Hispanic subgroups compared with non-Hispanic blacks and whites: MESA (Multi-ethnic Study of Atherosclerosis). *J Am Coll Cardiol* 55:234–242, 2010.
30. Ricardo AC, Lash JP, Fischer MJ, et al: Cardiovascular disease among Hispanics and non-Hispanics in the chronic renal insufficiency cohort (CRIC) study. *Clin J Am Soc Nephrol* 6:2121–2131, 2011.
31. Russo C, Jin Z, Homma S, et al: Race/ethnic disparities in left ventricular diastolic function in a triethnic community cohort. *Am Heart J* 160:152–158, 2010.
32. Salton CJ, Chuang ML, O'Donnell CJ, et al: Gender differences and normal left ventricular anatomy in an adult population free of hypertension. A cardiovascular magnetic resonance study of the Framingham Heart Study Offspring cohort. *J Am Coll Cardiol* 39:1055–1060, 2002.
33. Ganau A, Devereux RB, Roman MJ, et al: Patterns of left ventricular hypertrophy and geometric remodeling in essential hypertension. *J Am Coll Cardiol* 19:1550–1558, 1992.
34. Devereux RB, Pickering TG, Harshfield GA, et al: Left ventricular hypertrophy in patients with hypertension: importance of blood pressure response to regularly recurring stress. *Circulation* 68:470–476, 1983.
35. Heckbert SR, Post W, Pearson GD, et al: Traditional cardiovascular risk factors in relation to left ventricular mass, volume, and systolic function by cardiac magnetic resonance imaging: the Multiethnic Study of Atherosclerosis. *J Am Coll Cardiol* 48:2285–2292, 2006.
36. Shah RV, Abbasi SA, Heydari B, et al: Insulin resistance, subclinical left ventricular remodeling, and the obesity paradox: MESA (Multi-Ethnic Study of Atherosclerosis). *J Am Coll Cardiol* 61:1698–1706, 2013.
37. Chami HA, Devereux RB, Gottdiener JS, et al: Left ventricular morphology and systolic function in sleep-disordered breathing: the Sleep Heart Health Study. *Circulation* 117:2599–2607, 2008.
38. Spaak J, Egri ZJ, Kubo T, et al: Muscle sympathetic nerve activity during wakefulness in heart failure patients with and without sleep apnea. *Hypertension* 46:1327–1332, 2005.
39. Ramos AR, Jin Z, Rundek T, et al: Relation between long sleep and left ventricular mass (from a multiethnic elderly cohort). *Am J Cardiol* 112:599–603, 2013.
40. Gardin JM, Siscovick D, Anton-Culver H, et al: Sex, age, and disease affect echocardiographic left ventricular mass and systolic function in the free-living elderly. The Cardiovascular Health Study. *Circulation* 91:1739–1748, 1995.
41. Turkbey EB, McClelland RL, Kronmal RA, et al: The impact of obesity on the left ventricle: the Multi-Ethnic Study of Atherosclerosis (MESA). *JACC Cardiovasc Imaging* 3:266–274, 2010.
42. Moran A, Katz R, Jenny NS, et al: Left ventricular hypertrophy in mild and moderate reduction in kidney function determined using cardiac magnetic resonance imaging and cystatin C: the multi-ethnic study of atherosclerosis (MESA). *Am J Kidney Dis* 52:839–848, 2008.
43. Peterson GE, de Backer T, Gabriel A, et al: Prevalence and correlates of left ventricular hypertrophy in the African American Study of Kidney Disease Cohort Study. *Hypertension* 50:1033–1039, 2007.
44. Hill JA, Olson EN: Cardiac plasticity. *N Engl J Med* 358:1370–1380, 2008.
45. Cacciapuoti F: Molecular mechanisms of left ventricular hypertrophy (LVH) in systemic hypertension (SH)—possible therapeutic perspectives. *J Am Soc Hypertens* 5:449–455, 2011.
46. Ganau A, Devereux RB, Pickering TG, et al: Relation of left ventricular hemodynamic load and contractile performance to left ventricular mass in hypertension. *Circulation* 81:25–36, 1990.
47. Aoki H, Izumo S, Sadoshima J: Angiotensin II activates RhoA in cardiac myocytes: a critical role of RhoA in angiotensin II-induced premyofibril formation. *Circ Res* 82:666–676, 1998.
48. Dzau VJ: Tissue renin-angiotensin system in myocardial hypertrophy and failure. *Arch Intern Med* 153:937–942, 1993.
49. Sadoshima J, Xu Y, Slayter HS, et al: Autocrine release of angiotensin II mediates stretch-induced hypertrophy of cardiac myocytes in vitro. *Cell* 75:977–984, 1993.
50. Cuspidi C, Ciulla M, Zanchetti A: Hypertensive myocardial fibrosis. *Nephrol Dial Transplant* 21:20–23, 2006.
51. Mazzolai L, Nussberger J, Aubert JF, et al: Blood pressure-independent cardiac hypertrophy induced by locally activated renin-angiotensin system. *Hypertension* 31:1324–1330, 1998.
52. Harada M, Itoh H, Nakagawa O, et al: Significance of ventricular myocytes and nonmyocytes interaction during cardiocyte hypertrophy: evidence for endothelin-1 as a paracrine hypertrophic factor from cardiac nonmyocytes. *Circulation* 96:3737–3744, 1997.
53. Klingbeil AU, Schneider M, Martus P, et al: A meta-analysis of the effects of treatment on left ventricular mass in essential hypertension. *Am J Med* 115:41–46, 2003.
54. Struthers AD, MacDonald TM: Review of aldosterone- and angiotensin II-induced target organ damage and prevention. *Cardiovasc Res* 61:663–670, 2004.
55. Messaoudi S, Gravez B, Tarjus A, et al: Aldosterone-specific activation of cardiomyocyte mineralocorticoid receptor in vivo. *Hypertension* 61:361–367, 2013.
56. Rocha R, Rudolph AE, Frierdich GE, et al: Aldosterone induces a vascular inflammatory phenotype in the rat heart. *Am J Physiol Heart Circ Physiol* 283:H1802–H1810, 2002.
57. Sun Y, Zhang J, Lu L, et al: Aldosterone-induced inflammation in the rat heart: role of oxidative stress. *Am J Pathol* 161:1773–1781, 2002.
58. Robert V, Silvestre JS, Charlemagne D, et al: Biological determinants of aldosterone-induced cardiac fibrosis in rats. *Hypertension* 26:971–978, 1995.
59. Qin W, Rudolph AE, Bond BR, et al: Transgenic model of aldosterone-driven cardiac hypertrophy and heart failure. *Circ Res* 93:69–76, 2003.
60. Tsukamoto O, Minamino T, Sanada S, et al: The antagonism of aldosterone receptor prevents the development of hypertensive heart failure induced by chronic inhibition of nitric oxide synthesis in rats. *Cardiovasc Drugs Ther* 20:93–102, 2006.
61. Pitt B, Zannad F, Remme WJ, et al: The effect of spironolactone on morbidity and mortality in patients with severe heart failure. Randomized Aldactone Evaluation Study Investigators. *N Engl J Med* 341:709–717, 1999.
62. Pitt B, Remme W, Zannad F, et al: Eplerenone, a selective aldosterone blocker, in patients with left ventricular dysfunction after myocardial infarction. *N Engl J Med* 348:1309–1321, 2003.
63. Desai AS, Lewis EF, Li R, et al: Rationale and design of the treatment of preserved cardiac function heart failure with an aldosterone antagonist trial: a randomized, controlled study of spironolactone in patients with symptomatic heart failure and preserved ejection fraction. *Am Heart J* 162:966–972, e10, 2011.
64. Shah AM, Shah SJ, Anand IS, et al: Cardiac structure and function in heart failure with preserved ejection fraction: baseline findings from the echocardiographic study of the treatment of preserved cardiac function heart failure with an aldosterone antagonist trial. *Circ Heart Fail* 7:104–115, 2014.
65. Pitt B, Reichek N, Willenbrock R, et al: Effects of eplerenone, enalapril, and eplerenone/enalapril in patients with essential hypertension and left ventricular hypertrophy: the 4E-left ventricular hypertrophy study. *Circulation* 108:1831–1838, 2003.
66. Masaki T, Kimura S, Yanagisawa M, et al: Molecular and cellular mechanism of endothelin regulation. Implications for vascular function. *Circulation* 84:1457–1468, 1991.
67. Ichikawa KI, Hidai C, Okuda C, et al: Endogenous endothelin-1 mediates cardiac hypertrophy and switching of myosin heavy chain gene expression in rat ventricular myocardium. *J Am Coll Cardiol* 27:1286–1291, 1996.
68. Li Y, Ha T, Gao X, et al: NF-kappaB activation is required for the development of cardiac hypertrophy in vivo. *Am J Physiol Heart Circ Physiol* 287:H1712–H1720, 2004.
69. Freund C, Schmidt-Ullrich R, Baurand A, et al: Requirement of nuclear factor-kappaB in angiotensin II- and isoproterenol-induced cardiac hypertrophy in vivo. *Circulation* 111:2319–2325, 2005.
70. Stansfield WE, Tang RH, Moss NC, et al: Proteasome inhibition promotes regression of left ventricular hypertrophy. *Am J Physiol Heart Circ Physiol* 294:H645–H650, 2008.
71. Clerk A, Sugden PH: Small guanine nucleotide-binding proteins and myocardial hypertrophy. *Circ Res* 86:1019–1023, 2000.
72. Akhter SA, Luttrell LM, Rockman HA, et al: Targeting the receptor-Gq interface to inhibit in vivo pressure overload myocardial hypertrophy. *Science* 280:574–577, 1998.
73. Molkentin JD, Lu JR, Antos CL, et al: A calcineurin-dependent transcriptional pathway for cardiac hypertrophy. *Cell* 93:215–228, 1998.
74. Post WS, Larson MG, Myers RH, et al: Heritability of left ventricular mass: the Framingham Heart Study. *Hypertension* 30:1025–1028, 1997.
75. Dries DL, Victor RG, Rame JE, et al: Corin gene minor allele defined by 2 missense mutations is common in blacks and associated with high blood pressure and hypertension. *Circulation* 112:2403–2410, 2005.
76. Brull D, Dhamrait S, Myerson S, et al: Bradykinin B2BKR receptor polymorphism and left-ventricular growth response. *Lancet* 358:1155–1156, 2001.
77. Schunkert H, Hense HW, Holmer SR, et al: Association between a deletion polymorphism of the angiotensin-converting-enzyme gene and left ventricular hypertrophy. *N Engl J Med* 330:1634–1638, 1994.
78. Hernandez D, Lacalzada J, Rufino M, et al: Prediction of left ventricular mass changes after renal transplantation by polymorphism of the angiotensin-converting-enzyme gene. *Kidney Int* 51:1205–1211, 1997.
79. Gaasch WH, Zile MR: Left ventricular structural remodeling in health and disease: with special emphasis on volume, mass, and geometry. *J Am Coll Cardiol* 58:1733–1740, 2011.
80. Iriarte M, Murga N, Sagastagoitia D, et al: Classification of hypertensive cardiomyopathy. *Eur Heart J* 14(Suppl J):95–101, 1993.

81. Nagueh SF, Appleton CP, Gillebert TC, et al: Recommendations for the evaluation of left ventricular diastolic function by echocardiography. *J Am Soc Echocardiogr* 22:107–133, 2009.
82. Lang RM, Bierig M, Devereux RB, et al: Recommendations for chamber quantification: a report from the American Society of Echocardiography's Guidelines and Standards Committee and the Chamber Quantification Writing Group, developed in conjunction with the European Association of Echocardiography, a branch of the European Society of Cardiology. *J Am Soc Echocardiogr* 18:1440–1463, 2005.
83. Devereux RB: Is the electrocardiogram still useful for detection of left ventricular hypertrophy? *Circulation* 81:1144–1146, 1990.
84. American College of Cardiology Foundation Appropriate Use Criteria Task Force, American Society of Echocardiography, American Heart Association, et al: ACCF/ASE/AHA/ASNC/HFSA/HRS/SCAI/SCCM/SCCT/SCMR 2011 Appropriate Use Criteria for Echocardiography. A Report of the American College of Cardiology Foundation Appropriate Use Criteria Task Force, American Society of Echocardiography, American Heart Association, American Society of Nuclear Cardiology, Heart Failure Society of America, Heart Rhythm Society, Society for Cardiovascular Angiography and Interventions, Society of Critical Care Medicine, Society of Cardiovascular Computed Tomography, and Society for Cardiovascular Magnetic Resonance Endorsed by the American College of Chest Physicians. *J Am Coll Cardiol* 57:1126–1166, 2011.
85. Hackam DG, Shojania KG, Spence JD, et al: Influence of noninvasive cardiovascular imaging in primary prevention: systematic review and meta-analysis of randomized trials. *Arch Intern Med* 171:977–982, 2011.
86. Cuspidi C, Facchetti R, Bombelli M, et al: Accuracy and prognostic significance of electrocardiographic markers of left ventricular hypertrophy in a general population: findings from the Pressioni Arteriose Monitorate E Loro Associazioni population. *J Hypertens* 32:921–928, 2014.
87. Devereux RB, Casale PN, Hammond IW, et al: Echocardiographic detection of pressure-overload left ventricular hypertrophy: effect of criteria and patient population. *J Clin Hypertens* 3:66–78, 1987.
88. van den Bosch AE, Robbers-Visser D, Krenning BJ, et al: Comparison of real-time three-dimensional echocardiography to magnetic resonance imaging for assessment of left ventricular mass. *Am J Cardiol* 97:113–117, 2006.
89. Qin JX, Jones M, Travaglini A, et al: The accuracy of left ventricular mass determined by real-time three-dimensional echocardiography in chronic animal and clinical studies: a comparison with postmortem examination and magnetic resonance imaging. *J Am Soc Echocardiogr* 18:1037–1043, 2005.
90. Mosteller RD: Simplified calculation of body-surface area. *N Engl J Med* 317:1098, 1987.
91. Grothues F, Smith GC, Moon JC, et al: Comparison of interstudy reproducibility of cardiovascular magnetic resonance with two-dimensional echocardiography in normal subjects and in patients with heart failure or left ventricular hypertrophy. *Am J Cardiol* 90:29–34, 2002.
92. Bottini PB, Carr AA, Prisant LM, et al: Magnetic resonance imaging compared to echocardiography to assess left ventricular mass in the hypertensive patient. *Am J Hypertens* 8:221–228, 1995.
93. Fouad FM, Slominski JM, Tarazi RC: Left ventricular diastolic function in hypertension: relation to left ventricular mass and systolic function. *J Am Coll Cardiol* 3:1500–1506, 1984.
94. Aeschbacher BC, Hutter D, Fuhrer J, et al: Diastolic dysfunction precedes myocardial hypertrophy in the development of hypertension. *Am J Hypertens* 14:106–113, 2001.
95. Cuspidi C, Rescaldani M, Sala C: Prevalence of echocardiographic left-atrial enlargement in hypertension: a systematic review of recent clinical studies. *Am J Hypertens* 26:456–464, 2013.
96. Redfield MM, Jacobsen SJ, Burnett JC, Jr, et al: Burden of systolic and diastolic ventricular dysfunction in the community: appreciating the scope of the heart failure epidemic. *JAMA* 289:194–202, 2003.
97. Aurigemma GP, Gottdiener JS, Shemanski L, et al: Predictive value of systolic and diastolic function for incident congestive heart failure in the elderly: the cardiovascular health study. *J Am Coll Cardiol* 37:1042–1048, 2001.
98. Schillaci G, Pasqualini L, Verdecchia P, et al: Prognostic significance of left ventricular diastolic dysfunction in essential hypertension. *J Am Coll Cardiol* 39:2005–2011, 2002.
99. de Simone G, Izzo R, Chinali M, et al: Does information on systolic and diastolic function improve prediction of a cardiovascular event by left ventricular hypertrophy in arterial hypertension? *Hypertension* 56:99–104, 2010.
100. Hogg K, Swedberg K, McMurray J: Heart failure with preserved left ventricular systolic function; epidemiology, clinical characteristics, and prognosis. *J Am Coll Cardiol* 43:317–327, 2004.
101. Mohammed SF, Borlaug BA, Roger VL, et al: Comorbidity and ventricular and vascular structure and function in heart failure with preserved ejection fraction: a community-based study. *Circ Heart Fail* 5:710–719, 2012.
102. Owan TE, Hodge DO, Herges RM, et al: Trends in prevalence and outcome of heart failure with preserved ejection fraction. *N Engl J Med* 355:251–259, 2006.
103. Galderisi M: Diagnosis and management of left ventricular diastolic dysfunction in the hypertensive patient. *Am J Hypertens* 24:507–517, 2011.
104. Muller-Brunotte R, Kahan T, Lopez B, et al: Myocardial fibrosis and diastolic dysfunction in patients with hypertension: results from the Swedish Irbesartan Left Ventricular Hypertrophy Investigation versus Atenolol (SILVHIA). *J Hypertens* 25:1958–1966, 2007.
105. Mattioli AV, Zennaro M, Bonatti S, et al: Regression of left ventricular hypertrophy and improvement of diastolic function in hypertensive patients treated with telmisartan. *Int J Cardiol* 97:383–388, 2004.
106. Solomon SD, Appelbaum E, Manning WJ, et al: Effect of the direct renin inhibitor aliskiren, the angiotensin receptor blocker losartan, or both on left ventricular mass in patients with hypertension and left ventricular hypertrophy. *Circulation* 119:530–537, 2009.
107. Mizuta Y, Kai H, Mizoguchi M, et al: Long-term treatment with valsartan improved cyclic variation of the myocardial integral backscatter signal and diastolic dysfunction in hypertensive patients: the echocardiographic assessment. *Hypertens Res* 31:1835–1842, 2008.
108. Solomon SD, Janardhanan R, Verma A, et al: Effect of angiotensin receptor blockade and antihypertensive drugs on diastolic function in patients with hypertension and diastolic dysfunction: a randomised trial. *Lancet* 369:2079–2087, 2007.
109. Yip GW, Wang M, Wang T, et al: The Hong Kong diastolic heart failure study: a randomised controlled trial of diuretics, irbesartan and ramipril on quality of life, exercise capacity, left ventricular global and regional function in heart failure with a normal ejection fraction. *Heart* 94:573–580, 2008.
110. Yusuf S, Pfeffer MA, Swedberg K, et al: Effects of candesartan in patients with chronic heart failure and preserved left-ventricular ejection fraction: the CHARM-Preserved Trial. *Lancet* 362:777–781, 2003.
111. Massie BM, Carson PE, McMurray JJ, et al: Irbesartan in patients with heart failure and preserved ejection fraction. *N Engl J Med* 359:2456–2467, 2008.
112. Cleland JG, Tendera M, Adamus J, et al: The perindopril in elderly people with chronic heart failure (PEP-CHF) study. *Eur Heart J* 27:2338–2345, 2006.
113. Cho GY, Marwick TH, Kim HS, et al: Global 2-dimensional strain as a new prognosticator in patients with heart failure. *J Am Coll Cardiol* 54:618–624, 2009.
114. Wang J, Khoury DS, Yue Y, et al: Preserved left ventricular twist and circumferential deformation, but depressed longitudinal and radial deformation in patients with diastolic heart failure. *Eur Heart J* 29:1283–1289, 2008.
115. Park SJ, Miyazaki C, Bruce CJ, et al: Left ventricular torsion by two-dimensional speckle tracking echocardiography in patients with diastolic dysfunction and normal ejection fraction. *J Am Soc Echocardiogr* 21:1129–1137, 2008.
116. Kosmala W, Plaksej R, Strotmann JM, et al: Progression of left ventricular functional abnormalities in hypertensive patients with heart failure: an ultrasonic two-dimensional speckle tracking study. *J Am Soc Echocardiogr* 21:1309–1317, 2008.
117. Moss AJ, Zareba W, Hall WJ, et al: Prophylactic implantation of a defibrillator in patients with myocardial infarction and reduced ejection fraction. *N Engl J Med* 346:877–883, 2002.
118. Bardy GH, Lee KL, Mark DB, et al: Amiodarone or an implantable cardioverter-defibrillator for congestive heart failure. *N Engl J Med* 352:225–237, 2005.
119. Drazner MH, Rame JE, Marino EK, et al: Increased left ventricular mass is a risk factor for the development of a depressed left ventricular ejection fraction within five years: the Cardiovascular Health Study. *J Am Coll Cardiol* 43:2207–2215, 2004.
120. Neeland IJ, Drazner MH, Berry JD, et al: Biomarkers of chronic cardiac injury and hemodynamic stress identify a malignant phenotype of left ventricular hypertrophy in the general population. *J Am Coll Cardiol* 61:187–195, 2013.
121. Trimarco B, De Luca N, Ricciardelli B, et al: Cardiac function in systemic hypertension before and after reversal of left ventricular hypertrophy. *Am J Cardiol* 62:745–750, 1988.
122. Perlini S, Muiesan ML, Cuspidi C, et al: Midwall mechanics are improved after regression of hypertensive left ventricular hypertrophy and normalization of chamber geometry. *Circulation* 103:678–683, 2001.
123. Levy D, Garrison RJ, Savage DD, et al: Left ventricular mass and incidence of coronary heart disease in an elderly cohort. The Framingham Heart Study. *Ann Intern Med* 110:101–107, 1989.
124. Gardin JM, Iribarren C, Detrano RC, et al: Relation of echocardiographic left ventricular mass, geometry and wall stress, and left atrial dimension to coronary calcium in young adults (the CARDIA study). *Am J Cardiol* 95:626–629, 2005.
125. Heidland UE, Strauer BE: Left ventricular muscle mass and elevated heart rate are associated with coronary plaque disruption. *Circulation* 104:1477–1482, 2001.
126. Brush JE, Jr, Cannon RO, 3rd, Schenke WH, et al: Angina due to coronary microvascular disease in hypertensive patients without left ventricular hypertrophy. *N Engl J Med* 319:1302–1307, 1988.
127. Bairey Merz CN: Women and ischemic heart disease paradox and pathophysiology. *JACC Cardiovasc Imaging* 4:74–77, 2011.
128. Roger VL, Go AS, Lloyd-Jones DM, et al: Executive summary: heart disease and stroke statistics—2012 update: a report from the American Heart Association. *Circulation* 125:188–197, 2012.
129. Fuster V, Ryden LE, Cannom DS, et al: ACCF/AHA/HRS focused updates incorporated into the ACC/AHA/ESC 2006 guidelines for the management of patients with atrial fibrillation: a report of the American College of Cardiology Foundation/American Heart Association Task Force on practice guidelines. *Circulation* 123:e269–e367, 2011.
130. Kannel WB, Wolf PA, Benjamin EJ, et al: Prevalence, incidence, prognosis, and predisposing conditions for atrial fibrillation: population-based estimates. *Am J Cardiol* 82:2N–9N, 1998.
131. Tsang TS, Gersh BJ, Appleton CP, et al: Left ventricular diastolic dysfunction as a predictor of the first diagnosed nonvalvular atrial fibrillation in 840 elderly men and women. *J Am Coll Cardiol* 40:1636–1644, 2002.
132. Rosenberg MA, Gottdiener JS, Heckbert SR, et al: Echocardiographic diastolic parameters and risk of atrial fibrillation: the Cardiovascular Health Study. *Eur Heart J* 33:904–912, 2012.
133. Patton KK, Ellinor PT, Heckbert SR, et al: N-terminal pro-B-type natriuretic peptide is a major predictor of the development of atrial fibrillation: the Cardiovascular Health Study. *Circulation* 120:1768–1774, 2009.
134. Dun W, Boyden PA: Aged atria: electrical remodeling conducive to atrial fibrillation. *J Interv Card Electrophysiol* 25:9–18, 2009.
135. Liu XK, Jahangir A, Terzic A, et al: Age- and sex-related atrial electrophysiologic and structural changes. *Am J Cardiol* 94:373–375, 2004.
136. Finet JE, Rosenbaum DS, Donahue JK: Information learned from animal models of atrial fibrillation. *Cardiol Clin* 27:45–54, viii, 2009.
137. Burstein B, Nattel S: Atrial fibrosis: mechanisms and clinical relevance in atrial fibrillation. *J Am Coll Cardiol* 51:802–809, 2008.
138. Takahashi N, Kume O, Wakisaka O, et al: Novel strategy to prevent atrial fibrosis and fibrillation. *Circ J* 76:2318–2326, 2012.
139. Gopinathannair R, Sullivan R, Olshansky B: Tachycardia-mediated cardiomyopathy: recognition and management. *Curr Heart Fail Rep* 6:257–264, 2009.
140. Piccini JP, Hammill BG, Sinner MF, et al: Incidence and prevalence of atrial fibrillation and associated mortality among Medicare beneficiaries, 1993–2007. *Circ Cardiovasc Qual Outcomes* 5:85–93, 2012.
141. Strait JB, Lakatta EG: Aging-associated cardiovascular changes and their relationship to heart failure. *Heart Fail Clin* 8:143–164, 2012.
142. Okin PM, Bang CN, Wachtell K, et al: Relationship of sudden cardiac death to new-onset atrial fibrillation in hypertensive patients with left ventricular hypertrophy. *Circ Arrhythm Electrophysiol* 6:243–251, 2013.
143. Wachtell K, Lehto M, Gerdts E, et al: Angiotensin II receptor blockade reduces new-onset atrial fibrillation and subsequent stroke compared to atenolol: the Losartan Intervention For End Point Reduction in Hypertension (LIFE) study. *J Am Coll Cardiol* 45:712–719, 2005.
144. Ducharme A, Swedberg K, Pfeffer MA, et al: Prevention of atrial fibrillation in patients with symptomatic chronic heart failure by candesartan in the Candesartan in Heart failure: Assessment of Reduction in Mortality and morbidity (CHARM) program. *Am Heart J* 152:86–92, 2006.
145. Maggioni AP, Latini R, Carson PE, et al: Valsartan reduces the incidence of atrial fibrillation in patients with heart failure: results from the Valsartan Heart Failure Trial (Val-HeFT). *Am Heart J* 149:548–557, 2005.
146. GISSI-AF Investigators, Disertori M, Latini R, et al: Valsartan for prevention of recurrent atrial fibrillation. *N Engl J Med* 360:1606–1617, 2009.
147. Messerli FH, Ventura HO, Elizardi DJ, et al: Hypertension and sudden death. Increased ventricular ectopic activity in left ventricular hypertrophy. *Am J Med* 77:18–22, 1984.
148. McLenachan JM, Henderson E, Morris KI, et al: Ventricular arrhythmias in patients with hypertensive left ventricular hypertrophy. *N Engl J Med* 317:787–792, 1987.
149. Levy D, Anderson KM, Savage DD, et al: Risk of ventricular arrhythmias in left ventricular hypertrophy: the Framingham Heart Study. *Am J Cardiol* 60:560–565, 1987.
150. Spacek R, Gregor P: Ventricular arrhythmias in myocardial hypertrophy of various origins. *Can J Cardiol* 13:455–458, 1997.
151. Chugh SS, Reinier K, Teodorescu C, et al: Epidemiology of sudden cardiac death: clinical and research implications. *Prog Cardiovasc Dis* 51:213–228, 2008.
152. Fishman GI, Chugh SS, Dimarco JP, et al: Sudden cardiac death prediction and prevention: report from a National Heart, Lung, and Blood Institute and Heart Rhythm Society Workshop. *Circulation* 122:2335–2348, 2010.

153. Turakhia MP, Schiller NB, Whooley MA: Prognostic significance of increased left ventricular mass index to mortality and sudden death in patients with stable coronary heart disease (from the Heart and Soul Study). *Am J Cardiol* 102:1131–1135, 2008.
154. Wolk R: Arrhythmogenic mechanisms in left ventricular hypertrophy. *Europace* 2:216–223, 2000.
155. Wachtell K, Okin PM, Olsen MH, et al: Regression of electrocardiographic left ventricular hypertrophy during antihypertensive therapy and reduction in sudden cardiac death: the LIFE Study. *Circulation* 116:700–705, 2007.
156. Patel DA, Lavie CJ, Artham SM, et al: Effects of left ventricular geometry and obesity on mortality in women with normal ejection fraction. *Am J Cardiol* 113:877–880, 2014.
157. Flack JM, Sica DA, Bakris G, et al: Management of high blood pressure in Blacks: an update of the International Society on Hypertension in Blacks consensus statement. *Hypertension* 56:780–800, 2010.
158. MacMahon SW, Wilcken DE, Macdonald GJ: The effect of weight reduction on left ventricular mass. A randomized controlled trial in young, overweight hypertensive patients. *N Engl J Med* 314:334–339, 1986.
159. Cuspidi C, Rescaldani M, Tadic M, et al: Effects of bariatric surgery on cardiac structure and function: a systematic review and meta-analysis. *Am J Hypertens* 27:146–156, 2014.
160. du Cailar G, Fesler P, Ribstein J, et al: Dietary sodium, aldosterone, and left ventricular mass changes during long-term inhibition of the renin-angiotensin system. *Hypertension* 56:865–870, 2010.
161. Ferrara LA, de Simone G, Pasanisi F, et al: Left ventricular mass reduction during salt depletion in arterial hypertension. *Hypertension* 6:755–759, 1984.
162. Koga S, Ikeda S, Nakata T, et al: Effects of nasal continuous positive airway pressure on left ventricular concentric hypertrophy in obstructive sleep apnea syndrome. *Intern Med* 51:2863–2868, 2012.
163. Dahlof B, Pennert K, Hansson L: Reversal of left ventricular hypertrophy in hypertensive patients. A metaanalysis of 109 treatment studies. *Am J Hypertens* 5:95–110, 1992.
164. Schmieder RE, Martus P, Klingbeil A: Reversal of left ventricular hypertrophy in essential hypertension. A meta-analysis of randomized double-blind studies. *JAMA* 275:1507–1513, 1996.
165. Fagard RH, Celis H, Thijs L, et al: Regression of left ventricular mass by antihypertensive treatment: a meta-analysis of randomized comparative studies. *Hypertension* 54:1084–1091, 2009.
166. Gottdiener JS, Reda DJ, Massie BM, et al: Effect of single-drug therapy on reduction of left ventricular mass in mild to moderate hypertension: comparison of six antihypertensive agents. The Department of Veterans Affairs Cooperative Study Group on Antihypertensive Agents. *Circulation* 95:2007–2014, 1997.
167. Lin MS, McNay JL, Shepherd AM, et al: Increased plasma norepinephrine accompanies persistent tachycardia after hydralazine. *Hypertension* 5:257–263, 1983.
168. Hunyor SN, Hansson L, Harrison TS, et al: Effects of clonidine withdrawal: possible mechanisms and suggestions for management. *Br Med J* 2:209–211, 1973.
169. Okin PM, Devereux RB, Jern S, et al: Regression of electrocardiographic left ventricular hypertrophy during antihypertensive treatment and the prediction of major cardiovascular events. *JAMA* 292:2343–2349, 2004.
170. Pierdomenico SD, Lapenna D, Cuccurullo F: Regression of echocardiographic left ventricular hypertrophy after 2 years of therapy reduces cardiovascular risk in patients with essential hypertension. *Am J Hypertens* 21:464–470, 2008.
171. Mathew J, Sleight P, Lonn E, et al: Reduction of cardiovascular risk by regression of electrocardiographic markers of left ventricular hypertrophy by the angiotensin-converting enzyme inhibitor ramipril. *Circulation* 104:1615–1621, 2001.
172. Kizer JR, Dahlof B, Kjeldsen SE, et al: Stroke reduction in hypertensive adults with cardiac hypertrophy randomized to losartan versus atenolol: the Losartan Intervention For Endpoint reduction in hypertension study. *Hypertension* 45:46–52, 2005.
173. Verdecchia P, Angeli F, Gattobigio R, et al: Regression of left ventricular hypertrophy and prevention of stroke in hypertensive subjects. *Am J Hypertens* 19:493–499, 2006.
174. Esler MD, Krum H, Schlaich M, et al: Renal sympathetic denervation for treatment of drug-resistant hypertension: one-year results from the Symplicity HTN-2 randomized, controlled trial. *Circulation* 126:2976–2982, 2012.
175. Brinkmann J, Heusser K, Schmidt BM, et al: Catheter-based renal nerve ablation and centrally generated sympathetic activity in difficult-to-control hypertensive patients: prospective case series. *Hypertension* 60:1485–1490, 2012.
176. Brandt MC, Mahfoud F, Reda S, et al: Renal sympathetic denervation reduces left ventricular hypertrophy and improves cardiac function in patients with resistant hypertension. *J Am Coll Cardiol* 59:901–909, 2012.
177. Krause T, Lovibond K, Caulfield M, et al: Management of hypertension: summary of NICE guidance. *BMJ* 343:d4891, 2011.
178. Mancia G, Fagard R, Narkiewicz K, et al: 2013 ESH/ESC Guidelines for the management of arterial hypertension: the Task Force for the management of arterial hypertension of the European Society of Hypertension (ESH) and of the European Society of Cardiology (ESC). *J Hypertens* 31:1281–1357, 2013.
179. James PA, Oparil S, Carter BL, et al: 2014 Evidence-Based Guideline for the Management of High Blood Pressure in Adults: Report From the Panel Members Appointed to the Eighth Joint National Committee (JNC 8). *JAMA* 311:507–520, 2014.
180. Stewart IM: Relation of reduction in pressure to first myocardial infarction in patients receiving treatment for severe hypertension. *Lancet* 1:861–865, 1979.
181. Cruickshank JM, Thorp JM, Zacharias FJ: Heart attacks and lowering of blood pressure. *Lancet* 1:1154, 1987.
182. Cruickshank JM, Thorp JM, Zacharias FJ: Benefits and potential harm of lowering high blood pressure. *Lancet* 1:581–584, 1987.
183. Polese A, De Cesare N, Montorsi P, et al: Upward shift of the lower range of coronary flow autoregulation in hypertensive patients with hypertrophy of the left ventricle. *Circulation* 83:845–853, 1991.
184. Messerli FH, Mancia G, Conti CR, et al: Dogma disputed: can aggressively lowering blood pressure in hypertensive patients with coronary artery disease be dangerous? *Ann Intern Med* 144:884–893, 2006.
185. Mancia G, Schumacher H, Redon J, et al: Blood pressure targets recommended by guidelines and incidence of cardiovascular and renal events in the Ongoing Telmisartan Alone and in Combination With Ramipril Global Endpoint Trial (ONTARGET). *Circulation* 124:1727–1736, 2011.
186. Ovbiagele B, Diener HC, Yusuf S, et al: Level of systolic blood pressure within the normal range and risk of recurrent stroke. *JAMA* 306:2137–2144, 2011.
187. Verdecchia P, Angeli F, Mazzotta G, et al: Aggressive blood pressure lowering is dangerous: the J-curve: con side of the argument. *Hypertension* 63:37–40, 2014.
188. Cooper-DeHoff RM, Gong Y, Handberg EM, et al: Tight blood pressure control and cardiovascular outcomes among hypertensive patients with diabetes and coronary artery disease. *JAMA* 304:61–68, 2010.
189. Redon J, Mancia G, Sleight P, et al: Safety and efficacy of low blood pressures among patients with diabetes: subgroup analyses from the ONTARGET (ONgoing Telmisartan Alone and in combination with Ramipril Global Endpoint Trial). *J Am Coll Cardiol* 59:74–83, 2012.
190. ACCORD Study Group, Cushman WC, Evans GW, et al: Effects of intensive blood-pressure control in type 2 diabetes mellitus. *N Engl J Med* 362:1575–1585, 2010.
191. Sokolow M, Lyon TP: The ventricular complex in left ventricular hypertrophy as obtained by unipolar precordial and limb leads. 1949. *Ann Noninvasive Electrocardiol* 6:343–368, 2001.
192. Casale PN, Devereux RB, Alonso DR, et al: Improved sex-specific criteria of left ventricular hypertrophy for clinical and computer interpretation of electrocardiograms: validation with autopsy findings. *Circulation* 75:565–572, 1987.
193. Romhilt DW, Estes EH, Jr: A point-score system for the ECG diagnosis of left ventricular hypertrophy. *Am Heart J* 75:752–758, 1968.
194. Schillaci G, Verdecchia P, Borgioni C, et al: Improved electrocardiographic diagnosis of left ventricular hypertrophy. *Am J Cardiol* 74:714–719, 1994.

24 Heart Failure as a Consequence of Valvular Heart Disease

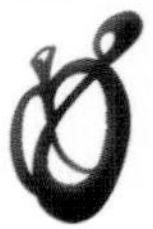

Blase A. Carabello

Valvular heart disease is emerging as a progressively more common cause of congestive heart failure. Demographic data from New York City demonstrate that while admissions as a result of coronary artery disease have fallen over the past decade, admissions for the treatment of valvular heart disease have progressively increased.[1] This has occurred primarily because valvular heart disease in Western culture today is often a consequence of aging and our population is getting older. Although the incidence of valve disease caused by rheumatic fever has fallen dramatically, both aortic stenosis and mitral regurgitation have increased with the aging population. A persistent background incidence of infective endocarditis adds additional cases of both aortic and mitral insufficiency.

All valvular heart diseases impart a hemodynamic load on the left and/or right ventricles. If this load is severe and acute, or severe and prolonged, it causes heart failure and death. The importance of valvular disease is further heightened because proper recognition and management of these diseases removes the hemodynamic overload and can either prevent or reverse the heart failure syndrome, a situation rare in the realm of heart failure where most diseases that cause it confer persistent systolic and/or diastolic dysfunction.

On the following pages, each valvular heart disease will be addressed regarding mechanisms by which acute and chronic hemodynamic overload leads to heart failure, the medical and surgical options for treating heart failure, and proper timing of intervention to prevent heart failure from occurring or at least from becoming permanent.

AORTIC INSUFFICIENCY

Acute Aortic Insufficiency

Acute severe aortic insufficiency, such as might occur due to perforation of an aortic leaflet by infective endocarditis, is usually a surgical emergency. The hemodynamics of acute aortic insufficiency are demonstrated in **Figure 24-1**.[2] Although the clinician is accustomed to finding a myriad of hyperdynamic signs produced by chronic aortic insufficiency, these are usually absent in acute disease. In chronic aortic insufficiency, eccentric hypertrophy allows the ventricle to generate increased total stroke volume to help compensate for the regurgitant volume. This large total stroke volume is ejected into the aorta where it produces a widened pulse pressure and a hyperdynamic circulation responsible for Corrigan pulse, de Musset sign, Quincke pulse, etc. However, in acute disease, left ventricular dilation has not developed and thus acute aortic insufficiency causes little increase in total stroke volume, a sudden fall in forward output, and a fall in systemic blood pressure. At the same time, backward flow into the left ventricle stretches sarcomeres toward their maximum. This volume overload does allow the ventricle to generate increased force by the Frank Starling mechanism, but also exposes the unprepared small ventricle to a large increase in diastolic pressure. Although the lungs are partially protected by this increased pressure by preclosure of the mitral valve, the ventricle is not. The driving gradient for generating coronary blood flow is the aortic diastolic pressure minus the left ventricular (LV) filling pressure, which compresses the endocardium, preventing coronary inflow. As can be seen in **Figure 24-2**, these pressures may become equal midway through diastole, reducing coronary blood flow, in turn leading to myocardial ischemia and worsening muscle function.[3] Although unproven, it is likely that it is this sequence of events that often generates a rapid downhill course so that a patient with acute aortic insufficiency can go from mild decompensation to death within hours. Medical therapy is often to no avail. Vasodilators, which might help to increase forward flow, further decrease blood pressure, leading to worsening myocardial perfusion. Pressor agents, some of which increase blood pressure by causing vasoconstriction, are also likely to worsen the amount of regurgitation severely limiting the usefulness of

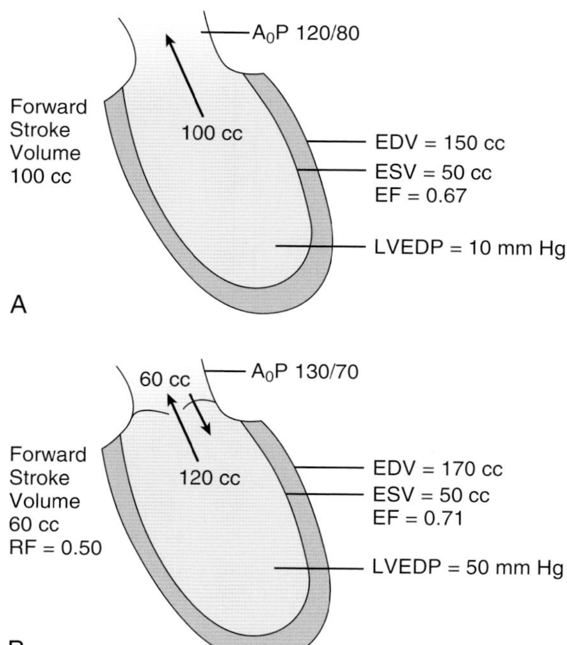

FIGURE 24-1 **A,** Normal physiology. **B,** Pathophysiology of acute aortic regurgitation. In response to acute volume overload, end-diastolic volume (EDV) increases modestly, allowing for a modest increase in total stroke volume. This small increase widens pulse pressure only slightly. The regurgitant volume is summed with that returning from the pulmonary veins, causing left ventricular volume overload. This overload on the unprepared left ventricle causes a large increase in left ventricular end-diastolic pressure (LVEDP). At the same time, forward stroke volume is reduced. Thus all the manifestations of heart failure are present even though myocardial function is normal. *AoP,* Aortic pressure; *EF,* ejection fraction; *ESV,* end-systolic volume; *RF,* regurgitant fraction. *Reprinted from Carabello BA: Hemodynamic determinants of prognosis. In Cohn LH, DiSesa VJ, editors: Aortic regurgitation: medical and surgical management (Cardiothoracic Surgery Series, vol 2). New York, 1986, Marcel Dekker, pp 90–91.*

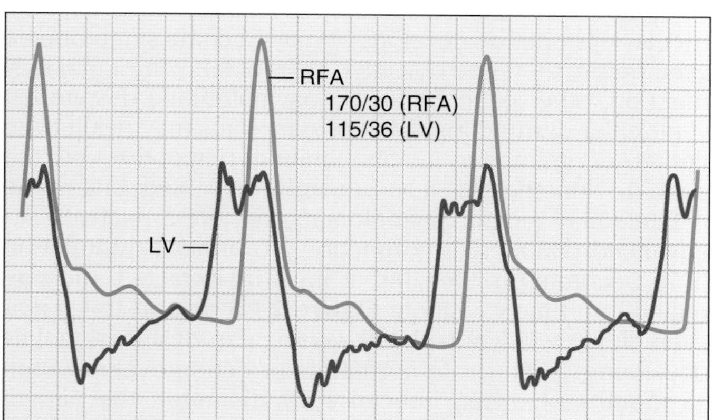

FIGURE 24-2 Hemodynamic effects of aortic regurgitation. End-diastolic aortic and ventricular pressure become equal in mid-diastole, a point at which there can be no significant coronary blood flow. *LV,* Left ventricle; *RFA,* right femoral artery. *Reprinted from Carabello BA, Gazes PC: Cardiology pearls, ed 2, Philadelphia, 2001, Hanley & Belfus, pp 199–200.*

these agents. Agents that increase heart rate can help by decreasing the time for aortic run-off, but these drugs also increase myocardial oxygen consumption, potentially worsening ischemia. Intra-aortic balloon pumping is obviously contraindicated and ineffective because diastolic inflation of the balloon dramatically worsens the amount of aortic insufficiency. Thus in acute aortic insufficiency, acute severe volume overload forces the operation of the left ventricle to the high right-hand side of the pressure volume relationship, leading to pulmonary congestion. The sharp reduction in forward output further compounds the heart failure syndrome. Reduced output diminishes systemic blood pressure, leading to reflex vasoconstriction and in turn worsening regurgitation.

The therapy for this syndrome requires aggressive action. As indicated previously, although it is often hoped that medical therapy may stabilize the patient and give more time for antibiotics (in infective endocarditis) to become effective, continued hemodynamic deterioration usually occurs despite medical therapy. Even the mildest symptoms and signs of heart failure, such as slight orthopnea or tachycardia unexplained by the patient's fever, should be taken as an early warning that aortic valve replacement should be imminent.[4] It should be recognized that despite the worry that replacement valve may become infected, this worry is usually not justified even in mechanical valves where the reinfection rate is less than 10%.[5] The reinfection rate with homographs may even lower, but whereas some advocate the homograft as the valve of choice in treating endocarditis,[6] others have questioned whether this is still the case.[7]

Chronic Aortic Insufficiency

Common causes of chronic aortic insufficiency include annulo-aortic ectasia, Marfan syndrome, rheumatic heart disease, and endocarditis (that was not severe enough to require immediate valve replacement). In chronic aortic insufficiency, volume overload leads to the development of eccentric hypertrophy, where sarcomeres laid down in series increase the length of individual myocytes. Increased myocyte length leads to increased left ventricular volume, allowing total stroke volume to increase. This mechanism may be quite effective, allowing the patient with even severe chronic aortic insufficiency to be totally asymptomatic. Indeed, young patients who have developed the disease from endocarditis can often engage in sports activities (although this is contraindicated if there is substantial left ventricle dilation) without symptoms. At the same time, increased ventricular size allows the regurgitant volume to be accommodated at a lower filling pressure, thus relieving or preventing the symptoms of congestion that are seen in acute aortic insufficiency when the ventricle is small (**Figure 24-3**).[2] Accordingly, severe aortic insufficiency may be extremely well compensated with a normal forward output and normal filling pressure. As noted previously, the large stroke volume produced in aortic insufficiency causes a wide pulse pressure and systolic hypertension. Thus there is an element of increased afterload seen in aortic insufficiency that is not present in mitral insufficiency.[8] This increased afterload leads to an element of concentric hypertrophy in addition to the eccentric hypertrophy generated by the volume overload.[9] Concentric hypertrophy helps to normalize systolic wall stress allowing ejection fraction to be normal. However, as the disease progresses, this mechanism may become inadequate to normalize stress; wall stress increases and ejection fraction is reduced.[10] At this time, symptoms may develop, because the systolic dysfunction engendered by increased systolic wall stress places the ventricle on a higher portion of its operating pressure-volume relationship. In addition, the concentric hypertrophy that develops diminishes diastolic function,

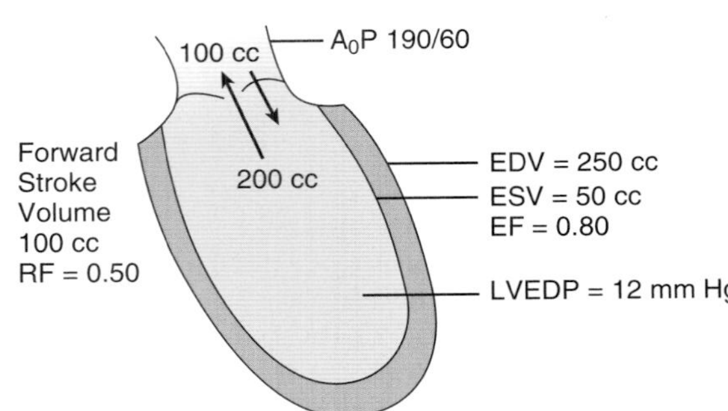

FIGURE 24-3 Pathophysiology of chronic compensated aortic regurgitation. Compared with Figure 24-1B, eccentric hypertrophy has developed, allowing a large increase in end-diastolic volume (EDV), increasing total stroke volume and in turn returning forward stroke volume toward normal. The larger ventricle can now accommodate the volume overload at much lower left ventricular end-diastolic pressure (LVEDP). The large total stroke volume results in a widened pulse pressure, which is responsible for many of the signs of chronic aortic regurgitation. *AoP,* Aortic pressure; *EF,* ejection fraction; *ESV,* end-systolic volume; *RF,* regurgitant fraction. *From Carabello BA: Hemodynamic determinants of prognosis. In Cohn LH, DiSesa VJ, editors: Aortic regurgitation: medical and surgical management (Cardiothoracic Surgery Series, vol 2). New York, 1986, Marcel Dekker, pp 90–91.*

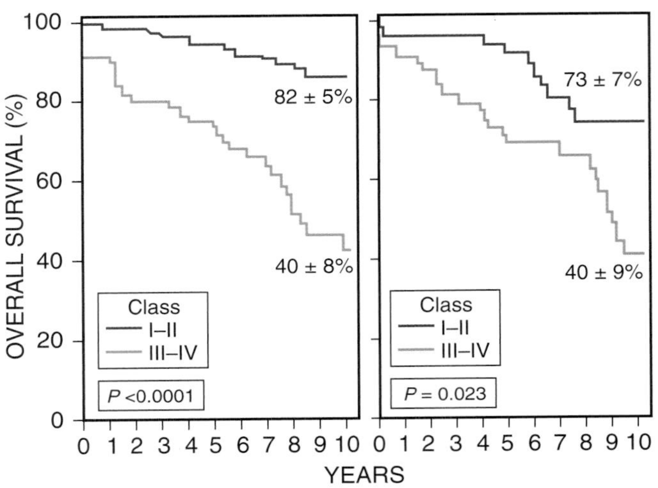

FIGURE 24-4 The importance of symptoms. Whether ejection fraction was normal *(left panel)* or reduced *(right panel),* survival in patients with aortic regurgitation was most influenced by symptom severity. *From Klodas E, Enriquez-Sarano M, Tajik AJ, et al: Optimizing timing of surgical correction in patients with severe aortic regurgitation: role of symptoms. JACC 30:746–752, 1997.*

further contributing to the syndrome of heart failure. Apart from the abnormal loading that helps generate the heart failure syndrome, muscle dysfunction may also intervene. The mechanisms of myocardial dysfunction are not yet well worked out for aortic insufficiency. However, it is known that coronary blood flow, especially to the endocardium, is reduced in these patients. Thus ischemia, especially during exercise, may contribute to the syndrome.[11] In an important rabbit model of aortic insufficiency, increased extracellular matrix deposition leads to increased myocardial stiffness and to myocyte destruction, thus contributing both to diastolic and systolic dysfunction.[12] In patients with aortic insufficiency, increased fibrosis and decreased myosin content in the myocardium has also been detected and both obviously could lead, respectively, to diastolic and systolic dysfunction.[13]

MANAGEMENT OF HEART FAILURE IN AORTIC INSUFFICIENCY

Avoidance of Heart Failure

Aortic insufficiency is a mechanical problem that places an overload on the myocardium. This mechanical problem can be corrected by valve replacement or occasionally by valve repair. Close surveillance of the patient with aortic insufficiency allows for the timing of this correction to occur before irreversible muscle damage has developed and also in time to allow for a potentially normal life expectancy following valve replacement. Further, as surgical techniques and prosthetic valves have improved, their risk has diminished, making earlier timing of surgery progressively more attractive because as risk diminishes, benefit increases.

Once even mild symptoms of congestive heart failure develop into chronic aortic insufficiency, prognosis worsens, as shown in **Figure 24-4**.[14] Although it seems intuitive that the symptoms from valvular heart disease would have the same implications as those from other types of heart disease, the higher risk of prosthetic valves and surgery decades ago generated a strategy of withholding surgery until it was inevitable. Typically, patients were not operated upon until their symptoms were far advanced. However, once the detrimental cascade of congestive heart failure has been initiated, a downhill course can be expected until that cascade is halted. Fortunately, in valvular heart disease, the cascade can be reversed and prognosis restored to normal. Thus even mild symptoms are an indication for mechanical intervention in this disease, especially in light of improved modern surgical techniques.

Asymptomatic Left Ventricular Dysfunction

Although many patients develop symptoms when left ventricular dysfunction develops or may become symptomatic even before there are objective signs of left ventricular dysfunction, other patients remain asymptomatic despite left ventricular dysfunction. Lack of symptoms may result from denial or unknown factors limiting perception by the patient. Nonetheless, it is generally accepted that some patients may remain asymptomatic despite a relatively far advanced contractile dysfunction. To prevent dysfunction from becoming irreversible, it must be detected and corrected in a timely fashion. **Figure 24-5** demonstrates that even if fairly advanced left ventricular dysfunction has developed, it returns to normal if correction occurs within 15 months of onset.[15] Because by definition the patient under consideration is asymptomatic, the clinician needs a tool other than patient complaint to alert him or her that dysfunction is developing. Currently, echocardiographic surveillance is the standard technique for early detection of left ventricular dysfunction. Several studies have examined echocardiographic markers associated with poor versus good outcome following surgery. These can be summarized most simply as stating that when ejection fraction falls below 0.50 or when end-systolic dimension exceeds 50 to 55 mm, postsurgical outcome is reduced.[16] Presumably, these markers of poor outcome indicate that left ventricular dysfunction is becoming irreversible and therefore are an indication for mechanical relief from the volume and pressure overload. B-type natriuretic peptide (BNP), which is released when there is a need for preload reserve to

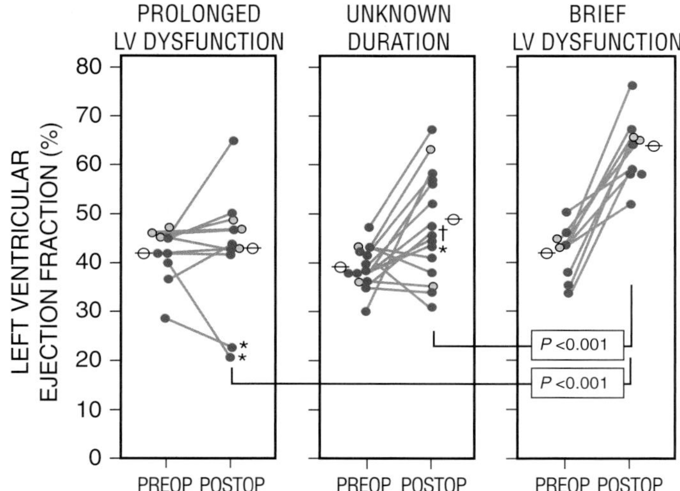

FIGURE 24-5 The effects of the duration of left ventricular dysfunction on the recovery of function after valve replacement. If ejection fraction was reduced for 15 months or less before surgery *(far right panel)*, ejection fraction improved; improvement was less likely *(far left panel)* if ejection fraction had been depressed for longer periods. *From Bonow RO, Rosing DR, Maron BJ, et al: Reversal of left ventricular dysfunction after aortic valve replacement for chronic aortic regurgitation: influence of duration of preoperative left ventricular dysfunction. Circulation 70:570–579, 1984.*

maintain cardiac output, is increased in some patients with aortic regurgitation (AR). In one study, BNP greater than 130 pg/mL predicted a poorer outcome independent of standard echo parameters and may become a useful tool if these data are confirmed in additional studies.[17]

Following surgery, ejection fraction usually improves if it was reduced preoperatively. As noted, this is especially true if correction of the mechanical lesion is provided within 15 months of the onset of LV dysfunction. Improvement in systolic function is predicated upon a fall in afterload as both the pressure and radius terms of the Laplace equation (stress = pressure × radius/2× thickness) are reduced following surgery and also due to improved myocardial function.[10] Improved diastolic function following surgery is predicated upon a reduction in collagen content and an improvement in myosin content.[18]

Medical Therapy

Because aortic insufficiency increases left ventricular afterload, afterload-reducing agents have been used in an attempt to forestall the onset of LV dysfunction. In a controlled study, nifedipine compared to digoxin forestalled the need for surgery as indicated by the development of symptoms or LV dysfunction by 2 to 3 years.[19] However, a more recent study randomized patients to receive nifedipine versus a true placebo (instead of digoxin) and employed a third arm, enalapril.[20] It found no benefit to vasodilator use. Thus the AHA/ACC Guidelines for the management of valvular heart disease reduced the indication for vasodilator use in aortic insufficiency from a class 1 indication (beneficial) to a class 2b indication (uncertain benefit).[16] However, in the patient with heart failure due to aortic insufficiency in whom surgery cannot be performed, standard heart failure therapy should be initiated.

It has generally been held that β-blockers were contraindicated in aortic insufficiency. It was thought that slowing the heart rate would increase the period during which regurgitation could occur, worsening the volume overload. However, a recent report suggests that some patients with severe aortic insufficiency actually benefitted from β-blockade.[21] In a retrospective study, aortic insufficiency patients taking β-blockers had improved survival compared with those who were not receiving them. Most had heart failure, and the presence of coronary disease and hypertension did not account for β-blockade benefit. Although this finding goes against current wisdom and must be confirmed, it may be that the beneficial effects of β-blockade in heart failure in general outweigh the negative potential of increasing the diastolic leak in aortic insufficiency. It should also be noted that paradoxically, the β-blockade group actually had slightly faster heart rates than the unblocked group and it was the group with the fastest heart rates that benefitted most from β-blockade.

Likewise, agents that block the renin-angiotensin system that are effective in treating heart failure have also been administered to AR patients. In an observational study of 2266 AR patients, those receiving angiotensin-converting enzyme inhibitors (ACEI) or receptor blockers (ARB) had significantly fewer heart failure events and improved survival compared with patients not receiving these agents.[22] The data are encouraging but must be confirmed by a prospective randomized trial.

Far Advanced Left Ventricular Dysfunction

The question often arises, "Has left ventricular dysfunction ever become so far advanced that surgery is impossible?" As indicated in Figure 24-5, even patients with a very low ejection fraction may benefit from aortic valve replacement, especially if the left ventricular dysfunction has been of short duration. Thus no specific ejection fraction provides a cutoff that prohibits surgery, although as demonstrated in **Figure 24-6**, low ejection fraction negatively impacts the prognosis.[23] It does seem logical that, because one of the major mechanisms of improvement following surgery is reduction in afterload, the absence of afterload excess preoperatively is a bad prognostic sign. Thus in the patient with severe aortic insufficiency and a reduced ejection fraction, who also has low rather than elevated systolic blood pressure, outcome may be reduced. The exact prognosis in such patients awaits further study.

MITRAL REGURGITATION

Acute Mitral Regurgitation

In acute mitral regurgitation such as might occur with rupture of a chorda tendina, there is the sudden opening of a new pathway for ejection from the left ventricle. This pathway produces two unwanted consequences leading to congestive heart failure. First, there is volume overload of the unprepared left atrium and left ventricle as the regurgitant flow is summed with flow returning from the pulmonary veins. This volume overload acutely raises left atrial and left ventricular diastolic pressures, leading to pulmonary congestion and dyspnea. At the same time, forward cardiac output is reduced by the amount of flow lost to regurgitation. As shown in **Figure 24-7**, there is partial compensation for this insult because the volume overload stretches existing sarcomeres in the left ventricle to their maximum, thus increasing end-diastolic volume and the pumping capacity of the left ventricle.[24] Also, the reduced

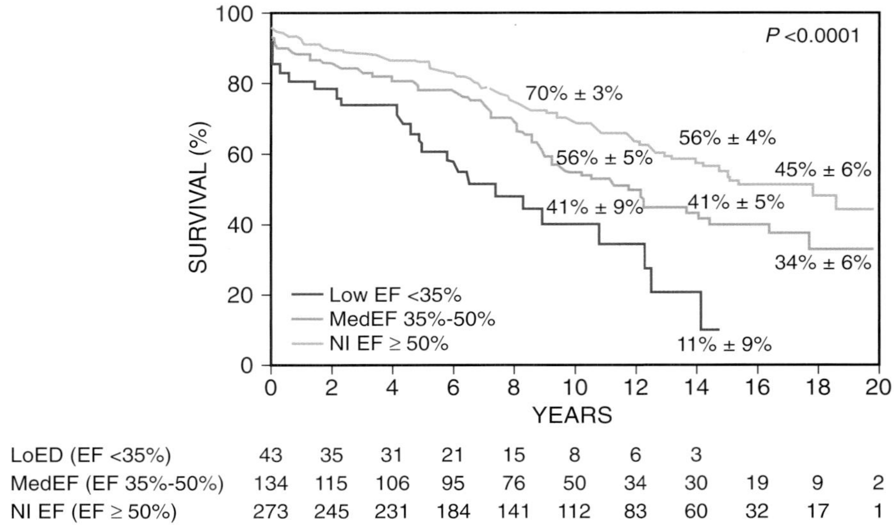

FIGURE 24-6 Postoperative survival for patients with aortic insufficiency is plotted according to preoperative ejection fraction (EF). *From Chaliki HP, Mohty D, Avierinos JF, et al: Outcomes after aortic valve replacement in patients with severe aortic regurgitation and markedly reduced left ventricular function. Circulation 106:2687–2693, 2002.*

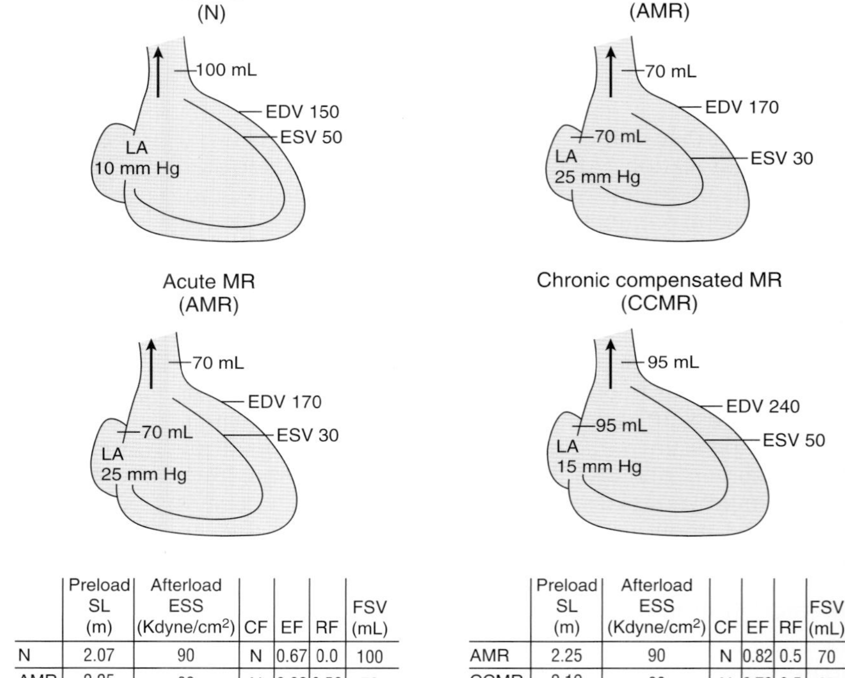

	Preload SL (m)	Afterload ESS (Kdyne/cm²)	CF	EF	RF	FSV (mL)
N	2.07	90	N	0.67	0.0	100
AMR	2.25	60	N	0.82	0.50	70

	Preload SL (m)	Afterload ESS (Kdyne/cm²)	CF	EF	RF	FSV (mL)
AMR	2.25	90	N	0.82	0.5	70
CCMR	2.19	60	N	0.79	0.5	95

FIGURE 24-7 Normal physiology *(upper left panel)* is compared with that of acute mitral regurgitation (MR) *(bottom left panel)* and chronic compensated mitral regurgitation *(bottom right panel).* In acute MR, volume overload increases end-diastolic volume (EDV), whereas the new pathway for ejection into the left atrium (LA) reduces afterload, in turn reducing end-systolic volume. These factors increase total stroke volume but not enough to compensate for that which is lost to regurgitation; thus forward stroke volume is reduced. The volume overload on the small left atrium and left ventricle increase left atrial pressure, leading to pulmonary congestion. In chronic compensated MR, eccentric hypertrophy develops, allowing an increase in both total and forward stroke volumes; the now-enlarged left-sided chambers accommodate the volume overload at lower filling pressure. *CF,* Contractile function; *EF,* ejection fraction; *ESS,* end-systolic stress; *ESV,* end-systolic volume; *FSV,* forward stroke volume; *RF,* regurgitant fraction; *SL,* sarcomere length. *From Carabello B: Mitral regurgitation: basic pathophysiologic principles. Mod Concepts Cardiovasc Dis 57:53–58, 1988.*

afterload created by the new ejection pathway into the relatively low pressure of the left atrium enhances ejection and reduces end-systolic volume. Increased end-diastolic volume and decreased end-systolic volume increase total stroke volume, in part compensating for that which is lost to regurgitation. However, this increase is inadequate to normalize forward stroke volume. In this case, LV contractile function is normal; ejection fraction is markedly increased because of the favorable loading conditions on the left ventricle, yet all of the hemodynamic and clinical facets of congestive heart failure are present. If the regurgitant lesion is severe, reduced forward stroke volume leads to lower blood pressure while at the same time the patient develops pulmonary edema. In such patients, arterial vasodilators may allow for a preferential increase in forward flow while diminishing regurgitant flow, in turn improving the hemodynamic situation.[25] However, if hypotension is already present, vasodilators cannot be used because they may further lower blood pressure. In such cases, intra-aortic balloon pumping is used to maintain mean arterial pressure while reducing afterload and increasing forward stroke volume until surgical correction of the defect can be performed.

If the acute regurgitation is less severe, it may be attended by only mild symptoms that can be treated successfully with diuretics. Currently at issue is what constitutes the best management of patients who have been rendered asymptomatic by relatively minimal medical therapy. As shown in Figure 24-7, eccentric cardiac hypertrophy may develop over time, allowing for normalization of forward stroke volume. At the same time, atrial and ventricular chamber enlargement can accommodate the regurgitant volume, resulting in normal filling pressure and relieving the symptoms of pulmonary congestion. Such patients may remain asymptomatic for months or years, thereby avoiding cardiac surgery. However, one study has found that a few such patients rendered asymptomatic by medical therapy may have been at risk for sudden death although asymptomatic.[26,27] Thus whether successful medical therapy is in fact beneficial or whether it simply masks potential risk for sudden death awaits further study.

Chronic Mitral Regurgitation

It appears that moderate mitral regurgitation can be tolerated for years or perhaps indefinitely. In studies of patients undergoing mitral valve replacement for mitral regurgitation, regurgitant fraction almost always exceeds 50%.

In a dog model of mitral regurgitation that causes myocardial dysfunction, there is almost complete recovery of function if mitral valve repair reduces regurgitant fraction to less than 35%.[28] Thus it seems that it requires a regurgitant fraction of between 40% and 50% to create and maintain left ventricular dysfunction. Figure 24-7 demonstrates that the major compensatory mechanism for mitral regurgitation is the development of eccentric cardiac hypertrophy. Here, individual myocytes add sarcomeres in series so that the individual cell becomes longer, increasing ventricular volume. In addition, the volume overload causes sarcomere stretch, increasing preload. Thus increased preload, together with normal contractile function of an enlarged left ventricle, allows for increased total stroke volume, increasing forward stroke volume toward normal. At the same time, enlargement of the left atrium and left ventricle allows for accommodation of the regurgitant volume at fairly normal filling pressure. In this compensated phase of mitral regurgitation, patients might be entirely asymptomatic even during vigorous activities. It should be noted, however, that such patients may have activation of the adrenergic nervous system, which can maintain both contractile and pump function at normal levels despite concealed intrinsic muscle dysfunction.[29,30]

If mitral regurgitation is severe, eventually muscle dysfunction occurs. Although mitral regurgitation was once believed to be well tolerated for prolonged periods of time, it is now evident that most patients with severe mitral regurgitation develop adverse clinical events within 5 years of recognition of severe disease.[31,32] The mechanisms of this dysfunction are now being worked out. In both an experimental model of mitral regurgitation and in humans, at the papillary muscle level there is a loss of contractile proteins and contractile elements that obviously reduces muscle function.[33] The second cause of the muscle dysfunction that develops is a shift in the force-frequency relationship such that the muscle develops less force, with peak force developing at a slower heart rate than normal. These changes imply that abnormalities in calcium handling are the source of the dysfunction.[34]

In addition, the hypertrophy that occurs in mitral regurgitation is both adaptive and maladaptive. It is adaptive because it allows the chamber to pump an increase in total volume. It is maladaptive because as volume increases, the radius term in the Laplace equation also increases, thereby increasing both systolic and diastolic stress. Although mitral regurgitation is usually viewed as a lesion that reduces left ventricular afterload (and it does in acute mitral regurgitation), as the radius increases, afterload returns first to normal and then even to higher than normal levels when left ventricular dysfunction develops. This abnormality of chamber geometry further contributes to left ventricular dysfunction in chronic mitral regurgitation.[35]

Besides the changes in chamber geometry noted previously, the hypertrophy that develops in mitral regurgitation seems to be qualitatively different from that occurring in pressure overload. In left ventricular pressure overload, hypertrophy accrues primarily by an increase in synthesis of contractile proteins.[36] However, in both canine and lapine models of mitral regurgitation, hypertrophy seems to accrue not by an increase in synthesis but rather by a diminution in degradation rate.[37] These changes would mean that the contractile proteins in mitral regurgitation are turning over more slowly and thus are older than normal, which could in some way be implicated in the muscle dysfunction that accrues.

Reversal of Left Ventricular Dysfunction in Mitral Regurgitation

Both in humans and dogs, correction of mitral regurgitation can lead to an improvement in contractility.[38,39] This improvement is presumably time-dependent, although it is not clear at what point the ventricular dysfunction is irreversible. Of interest, much of the left ventricular dysfunction that develops in experimental mitral regurgitation also can be corrected by initiation of β-blockade.[40] The benefits of β-blockade are now not surprising in view of their usefulness in treating the contractile dysfunction of dilated cardiomyopathy. Presumably, overactivation of the adrenergic nervous system leads to myocardial damage, and this damage can be corrected by protecting the myocardium from catecholamines. Reports of benefit in humans are accumulating. A recent report shows that β-blockade decreased stroke work but increased stroke volume, potential mechanisms by which β-blockade could be beneficial.[41] An observational study of almost 900 mitral regurgitation patients found improved survival for patients receiving β-blockers compared with those not receiving them.[42] In a small randomized trial of asymptomatic patients with severe mitral regurgitation and normal LV function, β-blockade prevented LV dysfunction from occurring.[43]

Strategies for Detection and Correction of Congestive Heart Failure in Chronic Primary Mitral Regurgitation

Once even mild symptoms of congestive heart failure develop in the patient with chronic mitral regurgitation, prognosis is impaired.[44,45] Thus it seems clear that mitral valve repair or replacement should be performed at the onset of symptoms. There is no evidence that medical therapy at this point in the disease is beneficial, although no human trials of either β-blockers or ACE inhibitors have been performed in a scale large enough to know whether these therapies might be of benefit.

As with aortic regurgitation, patients with mitral regurgitation may develop left ventricular dysfunction without developing symptoms. Once ejection fraction declines below 60%[46] or once the left ventricle is unable to contract to an end-systolic dimension of 40 mm,[47] prognosis worsens (**Figure 24-8**). A recent study suggests even more aggressive "triggers" for surgery, with prognosis worsening when EF falls below 0.64 and when end-systolic dimension increases to greater than 37 mm.[48]

In protecting the patient with mitral valve regurgitation from congestive heart failure, it is crucial that during surgery all, or at least part, of the mitral valve apparatus and its natural connections be preserved.[49-52] It is clear that the mitral valve apparatus contributes substantially to left ventricular contraction and to maintaining the shape of the left ventricle. If the apparatus is destroyed, there is a substantial and irreversible decline in the ejection performance following surgery.[50] Even if a prosthetic valve is inserted, the posterior connections between the papillary muscles, the chordae, and the posterior leaflet can be maintained and this amount of preservation is beneficial to the outcome.[52] In light of this evidence it is gratifying that the mitral valve repair rate is improving in the United States to approximately 70% today. However, there is substantial variation in the repair rate from institution to institution, with some institutions reporting a 95% repair rate, whereas some surgeons still perform no repairs at all.[53]

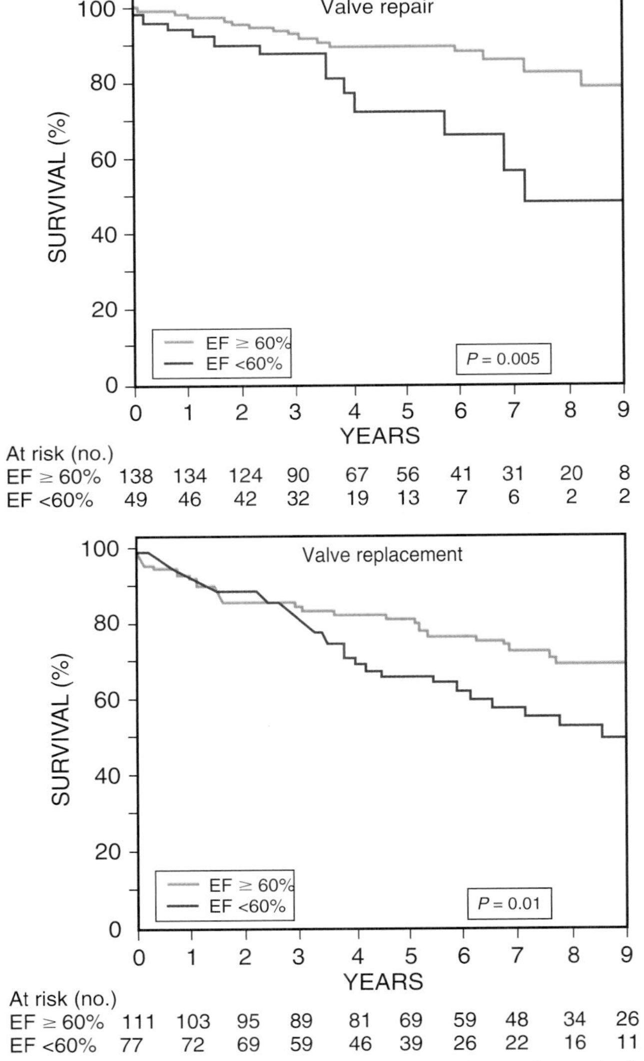

FIGURE 24-8 Survival following mitral valve surgery for mitral regurgitation. Whether repair or replacement is done, survival is excellent as long as the preoperative ejection fraction (EF) exceeds 0.60. *From Enriquez-Sarano M, Tajik AJ, Schaff HV, et al: Echocardiographic prediction of survival after surgical correction of organic mitral regurgitation. Circulation 90:830–837, 1994.*

Secondary Mitral Regurgitation

As systolic function worsens in patients with ischemic or dilated cardiomyopathy, ventricular dilation and wall motion abnormalities frequently lead to mitral incompetence. As such virtually all patients with secondary mitral regurgitation (SMR) have heart failure and should undergo standard medical therapy for that condition. Patients with conduction disease causing further wall motion abnormalities may benefit from cardiac resynchronization therapy that reduces MR and may enhance survival.[54,55] It seems clear that in SMR the burden of volume overload caused by regurgitation is added to the already serious problem of the primary disease. The presence of functional MR worsens the prognosis of heart failure.[56] But what is not certain is whether the MR is the cause of the worsened prognosis or simply a marker of poorer LV function. A recent study of over 1200 heart failure patients found that the presence of SMR contributed independently to mortality risk.[57] However, it has been extremely difficult to demonstrate that mechanical correction of SMR improves the prognosis. In a seminal study, surgical correction of mitral regurgitation using a simple ring angioplasty substantially decreased the amount of mitral regurgitation, had a 70% one-year survival rate, and significantly reduced cardiac volumes while improving ejection fraction.[58] However, follow-up of these patients found no survival benefit compared with medical therapy.[59] Other studies also have found little or no benefit to correcting MR in the face of severe heart failure.[60,61] However, a recent observational study did suggest improved survival following mitral surgery for patients with SMR.[62]

Strategies to control mitral regurgitation less invasively have been conceived and are currently undergoing early phase testing. Most promising is the MitraClip, which clips the two leaflets together in their midsection, reducing SMR.[63,64] The clip is inserted through a transseptal approach during which the leaflets are grasped and clipped together causing a "bow tie" or "figure of 8" mitral orifice. The device has the advantage of avoiding surgery but often results in significant residual MR. The device is now approved in the United States for inoperable patients. Randomized trials are under way to test whether such therapy can reduce mortality and hospitalizations for patients with SMR.

AORTIC STENOSIS

Acute Aortic Stenosis

The occurrence of acute aortic stenosis is limited to the sudden malfunction of a prosthetic aortic valve in which thrombus or other material prevents the valve leaflets from opening properly. Unlike chronic aortic stenosis where the obstruction to outflow develops gradually, allowing the left ventricle time for hypertrophic compensation, in acute aortic stenosis sudden obstruction increases afterload and impairs left ventricle ejection. Depending on the severity of the obstruction, the amount of impairment may range from mild to catastrophic. The only satisfactory therapy is immediate release of the obstruction by replacing the prosthesis, or if a clot is the cause of the obstruction, thrombolytic agents have been used safely for dissolution of a thrombus on the aortic valve.[65]

Chronic Aortic Stenosis

Little hemodynamic consequence develops as the aortic valve becomes narrowed from its normal aperture to one half its normal orifice area. However, further narrowing creates progressive obstruction to left ventricular outflow, resulting in a pressure gradient between the left ventricle and aorta. This gradient represents the additional pressure work that the left ventricle must perform to drive blood past the stenotic valve. It is generally agreed that an adaptive response to this pressure overload is the development of concentric left ventricular hypertrophy.[66,67] Examining the Laplace equation, when pressure in the numerator is increased, it can be offset by increased wall thickness in the denominator. Thus, even though there is an increase in left ventricular pressure, wall stress can remain normal and afterload on an individual muscle fiber can be maintained in the normal range despite the presence of aortic stenosis.

However, although left ventricular hypertrophy is adaptive in some cases of aortic stenosis, it is maladaptive in others. Even if the amount of hypertrophy that develops is just enough to offset the increased left ventricular pressure, the increased wall thickness requires a higher filling pressure to distend the ventricle to a given volume than if thickness were normal. Although the characteristics of the muscle in concentric hypertrophy can be normal, increased thickness mandates diastolic dysfunction. In addition, as the pressure overload becomes more severe and more prolonged, collagen content of the myocardium increases, further increasing ventricular stiffness and decreasing diastolic function.[68,69]

With regard to systole, as noted previously, the amount of hypertrophy that develops may exactly offset the pressure overload to maintain normal stress. However, in some patients, especially men, the amount of hypertrophy is not adequate to normalize wall stress; wall stress rises and ejection fraction is depressed.[67,70,71] In other patients, especially older women, the amount of hypertrophy that develops appears to be in excess of what is needed to normalize stress. Stress becomes subnormal and ventricular function becomes supernormal at the chamber level.[72] However, although systolic function is normal, or even supernormal, diastolic function is compromised. Recently attention has been called to another pattern of muscle distribution in aortic stenosis: concentric remodeling.[73,74] In such patients there is an increase in wall thickness with a decrease in LV radius so that stress normalization occurs without an increase in LV mass. However, such patients also have reduced stroke volume because LV end-diastolic volume is reduced. This may cause the symptoms of low-output heart failure with a normal ejection fraction.[75] Because stroke volume generates the transvalvular pressure gradient, gradient is low in such cases, potentially misleading the physician to underestimate the severity of the AS. Often patients with this LVH pattern have reduced LV function at the myocardial level despite preserved EF, and the prognosis may be worsened.[76]

Irrespective of the effects of hypertrophy in normalizing or failing to normalize wall stress, left ventricular muscle function eventually declines. The cellular mechanisms leading to the transition from compensated to decompensated left ventricular hypertrophy remain a topic of intense investigation.[77] Several mechanisms have been delineated but none entirely explains the left ventricular dysfunction that is present. In concentric hypertrophy, especially that which has been acquired in adults, coronary blood flow to the subendocardium is reduced during activity.[78] Thus it is likely that subendocardial ischemia plays a role in the left ventricular dysfunction of aortic stenosis, although there is little evidence that ischemia is present at rest. In the case of aortic stenosis, where persistently high wall stress has been created by inadequate hypertrophy, there is a densification of the microtubules compromising a portion of the cytoskeleton of the heart.[79] Densified tubules act as internal stents that increase internal load on the myocytes, inhibiting left ventricular contraction. In other circumstances, abnormalities in calcium handling appear to be part of the mechanism causing contractile dysfunction. Finally, although many believe in a gradual transition from normal to compensated hypertrophy to hypertrophy with failure, this concept has recently been challenged. Buermans and colleagues found genetic expression differed in animals with hypertrophy destined to develop failure from those that remained compensated very early in the course of hypertrophy, well before failure developed.[80] These data suggest diverging pathways to decompensated versus compensated hypertrophy rather than one transitioning to the other.

TREATMENT OF THE HEART FAILURE OF AORTIC STENOSIS

Heart failure in aortic stenosis responds well only to aortic valve replacement (AVR). In almost all cases of aortic stenosis complicated by heart failure, afterload mismatch plays at least a partial role in causing left ventricular dysfunction.[71] By replacing the valve, left ventricular pressure overload is reduced, afterload is reduced, and ejection fraction improves. Even patients with severely reduced preoperative ejection fraction can have the ejection fraction return to normal following aortic valve replacement. This is especially true if the mean transvalvular gradient exceeds 40 mm Hg. In patients with reduced ejection fraction and a transvalvular gradient of less than 30 mm Hg, output and gradient are reduced because of severe muscle dysfunction.[70] Although in many cases this dysfunction is irreversible and prognosis is poor,[81-84] recent studies have demonstrated an advantage to aortic valve replacement even in this group of patients, especially if they demonstrate inotropic reserve preoperatively (**Figure 24-9**).[85] However, although operative risk is high in patients lacking inotropic reserve, even those patients who survive surgery may have a dramatic improvement in LV function.[86] Additionally, it appears that those patients with the most severely stenotic valves are the ones who benefit the most from valve replacement. A conundrum has been that at rest, two different groups appear to exist even though each has a similar valve area.[87,88] In one group, there is mild stenosis but a myopathic ventricle from another cause is unable to open the valve completely. In this case the cardiomyopathy is primary and the mild stenosis does not constitute the major pathophysiologic problem. In such cases, it is unlikely that aortic valve replacement will be helpful, although this hypothesis is virtually untested. This group does relatively well with

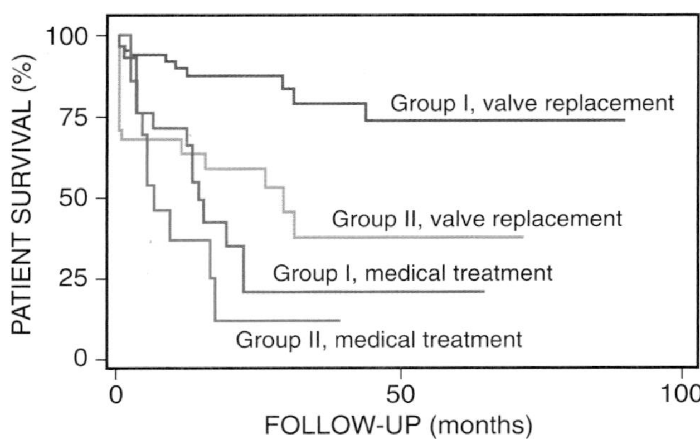

FIGURE 24-9 Postoperative outcome for aortic stenosis patients with low preoperative ejection fraction and low transvalvular gradient is demonstrated. Group I patients demonstrated preoperative inotropic reserve during dobutamine infusion, whereas group II patients did not. An obvious advantage to surgical intervention in group I patients is demonstrated. *From Monin JL, Quere JP, Monchi M, et al: Low-gradient aortic stenosis: operative risk stratification and predictors for long-term outcome: a multicenter study using dobutamine stress hemodynamics. Circulation 108:319–324, 2003.*

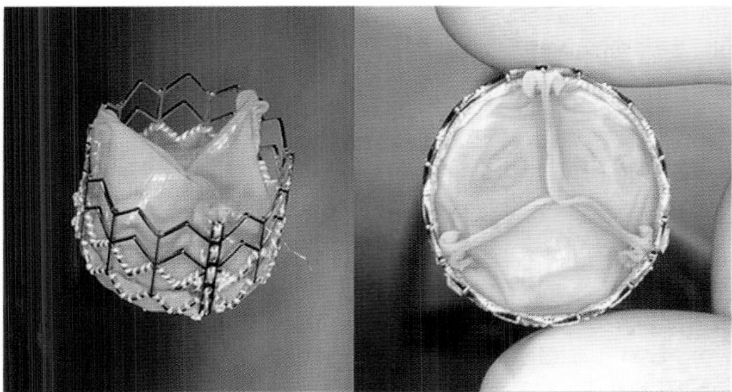

FIGURE 24-10 The SAPEIN transcatheter aortic prosthesis is mounted on a balloon-expandable stainless steel stent that is placed in the subcoronary position. The trileaflet bovine pericardial prosthesis is attached to the stent and treated with an anticalcification treatment. The stent has a polyethylene terephthalate fabric skirt that decreases perivalvular leaks. *From Zajarias A, Cribier AG: Outcomes and safety of percutaneous aortic valve replacement. J Am Coll Cardiol 53:1829–1836, 2009.*

medical therapy.[89] In other cases where severe stenosis has led to left ventricular dysfunction, valve replacement appears warranted.[85,86] The two groups can be divorced by increasing cardiac output either with exercise or pharmacologically. If output increases and the gradient fails to increase proportionally, the valve area increases substantially; it is these patients who are likely to do better with medical rather than surgical therapy.[90] In other cases where gradient increases proportionally with the output, there is likely severe aortic stenosis, and it is this group with low ejection fraction and low gradient that is most likely to benefit from the aortic valve replacement.

Although aortic valve replacement is the only effective therapy for aortic stenosis, many patients with the disease have acquired so many comorbidities as they have aged that aortic valve replacement is too risky to perform. However, development of percutaneous valve replacement has expanded the availability of aortic valve replacement for patients too infirm to undergo surgery or for patients at high surgical risk[91-93] (**Figure 24-10**). The PARTNERS study was a clinical randomized trial comparing transcatheter AVR (TAVR) with medical therapy in inoperable patients in one arm and TAVR to standard AVR in high-risk but operable patients. TAVR reduced mortality compared with medical therapy by 40% and was noninferior to surgical AVR in the high-risk group. Because TAVR has excellent hemodynamics, it has also provided a substantial improvement in EF in low EF patients.[93]

MITRAL STENOSIS

Mitral stenosis inhibits left ventricular filling by preventing decompression of the left atrium during diastole. In turn, left atrial pressure and pulmonary venous pressure are elevated, leading to pulmonary congestion. These changes in left ventricular and left atrial loading cause heart failure (diminished cardiac output and increased pulmonary venous pressure), yet in most cases left ventricular muscle function in mitral stenosis is normal.[94] However, in some cases of aggressive rheumatic fever (the usual cause of mitral stenosis), myocarditis and depressed left ventricular function may ensue.[95]

Interestingly, about a third of patients with mitral stenosis have reduced left ventricular ejection performance. In most cases, this accrues from abnormal loading of the left ventricle.[94] Reduced forward output initiates reflex vasoconstriction, in turn increasing left ventricular afterload, a cause for reduced ejection performance. At the same time, inhibition of left ventricular inflow prevents the use of preload reserve to overcome the afterload access, and ejection fraction remains depressed. However, after mitral valve commissurotomy ejection fraction often returns to normal, indicating that it was abnormalities in loading that were primarily responsible for the preprocedure left ventricular dysfunction.

Left ventricular filling is primarily driven by an early transmitral gradient in diastole. This gradient accrues (1) from ventricular suction as the restoring forces created by systolic compression of the ventricle are released in diastole, and (2) from increased left atrial pressure as the atrium fills following mitral valve closure in systole. In mitral stenosis, however, obstruction to inflow into the left ventricle reduces left ventricular filling. The obstruction is compensated in part by an increased pressure head delivered by the right ventricle. Thus mitral stenosis leads to pulmonary hypertension. In addition to the mitral gradient, pulmonary vasoconstriction develops, further increasing pulmonary artery pressure.[96] Eventually pulmonary hypertension leads to right ventricular dysfunction, which clearly worsens the outcome in mitral stenosis; thus surgery should be timed before the onset of severe pulmonary hypertension.

The issue of right ventricular contractile function in mitral stenosis has not been resolved. Pulmonary hypertension in experimental animals induces right ventricular muscle dysfunction. However, studies of right ventricular function in mitral stenosis in humans have not confirmed muscle dysfunction,[97] but it must be pointed out that ventricular loading on the right ventricle has been extremely difficult to study. The shape of the right ventricle has defied easy expression of wall stress used to calculate afterload. Thus stress-strain relations used to analyze left ventricular function have been difficult to employ in estimating right ventricular function.

Therapy

Ultimately the only satisfactory therapy for the treatment of mitral stenosis is relief of the obstruction at the mitral valve. In cases of mild disease with mild symptoms, diuretics alone may be sufficient to lower left atrial pressure and render the patient asymptomatic. There is no evidence that this type of therapy results in either sudden death or increased mortality. β-blockers and calcium channel blockers have been used to slow heart rate, increasing diastolic filling time in an effort to lower LA pressure. However, these therapies have been of only marginal benefit because their negative inotropic effects tend to increase LV filling pressure. Thus LA pressure remains high despite a smaller transmitral gradient.[98,99] Once the symptoms of mitral stenosis advance beyond New York Heart Association (NYHA) class II or if asymptomatic pulmonary hypertension develops, surgical outcome worsens. Thus mechanical correction of the lesion should take place before symptoms become far advanced or before pulmonary hypertension has been well established. In most cases, balloon valvulotomy produces a durable improvement in the orifice area with enhanced postoperative diastolic function and a rapid decline in pulmonary artery pressure toward normal.[100-102] In cases where valvulotomy is impossible, mitral valve replacement produces a similar benefit.

TRICUSPID REGURGITATION

Most cases of tricuspid regurgitation (TR) are secondary to right ventricular pressure overload induced either from left ventricular disease or from pulmonary parenchymal or pulmonary artery disease. However, occasionally tricuspid regurgitation is primary, due to either tricuspid valve endocarditis, or motor vehicle accidents where sudden deceleration and chest impact injure the valve. It is clear that severe TR leads to right-sided heart failure that compromises survival.[103] Recent animal studies indicate that tricuspid regurgitation, unlike mitral regurgitation, does not cause intrinsic muscle dysfunction.[104] Rather, tricuspid regurgitation increases systemic venous pressure, leading to the symptoms of right ventricular failure. Presumably, in some way, differences in loading between the right ventricle in tricuspid regurgitation and the left ventricle in mitral regurgitation are responsible for the differences in myocyte adaptation to the volume overload of each chamber. However, these differences have made it hard to define benchmarks of RV function that define the best timing for tricuspid surgery. Currently tricuspid valve repair is performed when there are intractable symptoms of right heart failure.

Because most TR is secondary to left-sided heart disease or to lung disease, the usual therapy for tricuspid regurgitation is to improve the primary disease responsible for it. Thus, if left-sided failure has resulted in pulmonary hypertension and secondary tricuspid regurgitation, improvement in left-sided failure will result in reduced pulmonary pressure, reducing the tricuspid regurgitation. Likewise, improvement in lung disease may reduce pulmonary pressure, improving TR.

CONCLUSION

Valvular heart disease accounts for only about 5% of all cases of congestive heart failure. However, because this group of diseases is easily recognized and reversed, it should be a focus of the clinician's attention. Proper timing of surgical intervention is crucial in managing this group of illnesses, and the burgeoning improvement in surgical practice has pushed this timing earlier and earlier in the course of these diseases. The advent of percutaneous devices may advance the timing of mechanical intervention yet further and already has made therapy available to patients considered too risky for a standard surgical approach.

References

1. Borer JS, Isom OW, editors: *Pathophysiology, evaluation and management of valvular heart diseases. The epidemiology of valvular heart disease: an emerging public health problem. Adv Cardiol*, vol 39, Basel, 2002, Karger, pp 1–6.
2. Carabello BA: Aortic regurgitation: hemodynamic determinants of prognosis, Chapter 3. In Cohn LH, DiSesa VJ, editors: *Aortic regurgitation: medical and surgical management*, New York, 1986, Marcel Dekker, pp 87–106.
3. Carabello BA, Gazes PC: *Cardiology pearls*, ed 2, 2001, Hanley & Belfus, pp 199–200.
4. Larbalestier RI, Kinchia NM, Aranki SF, et al: Acute bacterial endocarditis—optimizing surgical results. *Circulation* 86([Suppl 2]2):II-68–II-74, 1992.
5. al Jubair K, al Fagih MR, Ashmeg A, et al: Cardiac operations during active endocarditis. *J Thorac Cardiovasc Surg* 104:487–490, 1992.
6. Musci M, Weng Y, Hubler M, et al: Hemograft aortic root replacement in native or prosthetic active infective endocarditis: twenty-year single-center experience. *J Thorac Cardiovasc Surg* 139:665–673, 2010.
7. Jassar AS, Bavaria JE, Szeto WY, et al: Graft selection for aortic root replacement in complex active endocarditis: does it matter? *Ann Thorac Surg* 93(2):480–487, 2012.
8. Wisenbaugh T, Spann JF, Carabello BA: Differences in myocardial performance and load between patients with similar amounts of chronic aortic versus chronic mitral regurgitation. *J Am Coll Cardiol* 3:916–923, 1984.
9. Feiring AJ, Rumberger JA: Ultrafest computed tomography analysis of regional radius-to-wall thickness ratios in normal and volume-overloaded human left ventricle. *Circulation* 85:1423–1432, 1992.
10. Taniguchi K, Nakano S, Kawashima Y, et al: Left ventricular ejection performance, wall stress, and contractile state in aortic regurgitation before and after aortic valve replacement. *Circulation* 82:798–807, 1990.
11. Gascho JA, Mueller TM, Eastham C, et al: Effect of volume-overload hypertrophy on the coronary circulation awake dogs. *Cardiovasc Res* 16(5):288–292, 1982.
12. Borer JS, Truter SL, Herrold EM, et al: The cellular and molecular basis of heart failure in regurgitant valvular diseases: the myocardial extracellular matrix as a building block for future therapy. *Adv Cardiol* 39:7–14, 2002.
13. Schwarz F, Flameng W, Schaper J, et al: Myocardial structure and function in patients with aortic valve disease and their relation to postoperative results. *Am J Cardiol* 41:661–669, 1978.
14. Klodas E, Enriquez-Sarano M, Tajik AJ, et al: Optimizing timing of surgical correction in patients with severe aortic regurgitation: role of symptoms. *JACC* 30(3):746–752, 1997.
15. Bonow RO, Rosing DR, Maron BJ, et al: Reversal of left ventricular dysfunction after aortic valve replacement for chronic aortic regurgitation: influence of duration of preoperative left ventricular dysfunction. *Circulation* 70:570–579, 1984.
16. American College of Cardiology/American Heart Association Task Force on Practice Guidelines; Society of Cardiovascular Anesthesiologists; Society for Cardiovascular Angiography and Interventions; Society of Thoracic Surgeons, Bonow RO, Carabello BA, et al: ACC/AHA 2006 guidelines for the management of patients with valvular heart disease: a report of the American College of Cardiology/American Heart Association Task Force on Practice Guidelines (writing committee to revise the 1998 Guidelines for the Management of Patients With Valvular Heart Disease): developed in collaboration with the Society of Cardiovascular Anesthesiologists: endorsed by the Society of Cardiovascular Angiography and Interventions and the Society of Thoracic Surgeons. *Circulation* 114(5):e84–e231, 2006.
17. Pizarro R, Bazzino OO, Oberti PF, et al: Prospective validation of the prognostic usefulness of B-type natriuretic peptide in asymptomatic patients with chronic severe aortic regurgitation. *J Am Coll Cardiol* 58(16):1705–1714, 2011.
18. Krayenbuehl HP, Hess OM, Monrad ES, et al: Left ventricular myocardial structure in aortic valve disease before, intermediate, and late after aortic valve replacement. *Circulation* 79(4):744–755, 1989.
19. Scognamiglio R, Rahimtoola SH, Fasoli G, et al: Nifedipine in asymptomatic patients with severe aortic regurgitation and normal left ventricular function. *N Engl J Med* 331:689–694, 1994.
20. Evangelista A, Tornos P, Sambola A, et al: Long-term vasodilator therapy in patients with severe aortic regurgitation. *N Engl J Med* 353(13):1342–1349, 2005.
21. Sampat U, Varadarajan P, Turk R, et al: Effect of beta-blocker therapy on survival in patients with severe aortic regurgitation. *JACC* 54:452–457, 2009.
22. Elder DH, Wei L, Szwejkowski BR, et al: The impact of renin-angiotensin system blockade on heart failure outcomes and mortality in patients identified to have aortic regurgitation: a large population cohort study. *J Am Coll Cardiol* 58(20):2084–2091, 2011.
23. Chaliki HP, Mohty D, Avierinos JF, et al: Outcomes after aortic valve replacement in patients with severe aortic regurgitation and markedly reduced left ventricular function. *Circulation* 106(21):2687–2693, 2002.
24. Carabello BA: Mitral regurgitation: basic pathophysiologic principles. *Mod Concepts Cardiovasc Dis* 57:53–58, 1988.
25. Yoran C, Yellin EL, Becker RM, et al: Mechanism of reduction of mitral regurgitation with vasodilator therapy. *Am J Cardiol* 43:773–777, 1979.
26. Grigioni F, Enriquez-Sarano M, Ling LH, et al: Sudden death in mitral regurgitation due to flail leaflet. *J Am Coll Cardiol* 34:2078–2085, 1999.
27. Carabello BA: Sudden death in mitral regurgitation: why was I so surprised? *J Am Coll Cardiol* 34:2086–2087, 1999.
28. Nagatsu M, Ishihara K, Zile MR, et al: The effects of complete versus incomplete mitral valve repair in experimental mitral regurgitation. *J Thorac Cardiovasc Surg* 107(2):416–423, 1994.
29. Nagatsu M, Zile MR, Tsutsui H, et al: Native beta-adrenergic support for left ventricular dysfunction in experimental mitral regurgitation normalizes indexes of pump and contractile function. *Circulation* 89(2):818–826, 1994.
30. Mehta RH, Supiano MA, Oral H, et al: Relation of systemic sympathetic nervous system activation to echocardiographic left ventricular size and performance and its implications in patients with mitral regurgitation. *Am J Cardiol* 85(11):1193–1197, 2000.

31. Ling LH, Enrique-Sarano M, Seward JB, et al: Clinical outcome of mitral regurgitation due to flail leaflet. *N Engl J Med* 335:1417–1423, 1996.
32. Rosenhek R, Rader F, Klaar U, et al: Outcome of watchful waiting in asymptomatic severe mitral regurgitation. *Circulation* 113(18):2238–2244, 2006.
33. Urabe Y, Mann DL, Kent RL, et al: Cellular and ventricular contractile dysfunction in experimental canine mitral regurgitation. *Circ Res* 70(1):131–147, 1992.
34. Mulieri LA, Leavitt BJ, Kent RL, et al: Myocardial force-frequency defect in mitral regurgitation heart failure is reversed for forskolin. *Circulation* 88(6):2700–2704, 1993.
35. Carabello BA: The pathophysiology of mitral regurgitation. *J Heart Valve Dis* 9(5):600–608, 2000. Review.
36. Nagatamo Y, Carabello BA, Hamawaki M, et al: Translational mechanisms accelerate the rate of protein synthesis during canine pressure-overload hypertrophy. *Am J Physiol* 277(6 Pt 2):H2176–H2184, 1999.
37. Matsuo T, Carabello BA, Nagatamo Y, et al: Mechanisms of cardiac hypertrophy in canine volume overload. *Am J Physiol* 275(1 Pt 2):H65–H74, 1998.
38. Nakano K, Swindle MM, Spinale F, et al: Depressed contractile function due to canine mitral regurgitation improves after correction of the volume overload. *J Clinic Invest* 87(6):2077–2086, 1991.
39. Starling MR: Effects of valve surgery on left ventricular contractile function in patients with long-term mitral regurgitation. *Circulation* 92:811–818, 1995.
40. Tsutsui H, Spinale FG, Nagatsu M, et al: Effects of chronic beta-adrenergic blockade on the left ventricular and cardiocyte abnormalities of chronic canine mitral regurgitation. *J Clin Invest* 93:2639–2648, 1994.
41. Stewart RA, Raffel OC, Kerr AJ, et al: Pilot study to assess the influence of beta-blockade on mitral regurgitant volume and left ventricular work in degenerative mitral valve disease. *Circulation* 118(10):1041–1046, 2008.
42. Varadarajan P, Joshi N, Appel D, et al: Effect of beta-blocker therapy on survival in patients with severe mitral regurgitation and normal left ventricular ejection fraction. *Am J Cardiol* 102:611–615, 2008.
43. Ahmed MI, Aban I, Lloyd SG, et al: A randomized controlled phase IIb trial of β1-recepter blockade for chronic degenerative mitral regurgitation. *J Am Coll Cardiol* 60(9):833–838, 2012.
44. Tribouilloy CM, Enriquez-Sarano M, Schaff HV, et al: Impact of preoperative symptoms on survival after surgical correction of organic mitral regurgitation: rationale for optimizing surgical indications. *Circulation* 99(3):400–405, 1999.
45. Gillinov AM, Mihaljevic T, Blackstone EH, et al: Should patients with severe degenerative mitral regurgitation delay surgery until symptoms develop? *Ann Thorac Surg* 90(2):481–488, 2010.
46. Enriquez-Sarano M, Tajik AJ, Schaff HV, et al: Echocardiographic prediction of survival after surgical correction of organic mitral regurgitation. *Circulation* 90:830–837, 1994.
47. Matsumura T, Ohtaki F, Tanaka K, et al: Echocardiographic prediction of left ventricular dysfunction after mitral valve repair for mitral regurgitation as an indicator to decide the optimal timing of repair. *JACC* 42:458–463, 2003.
48. Tribouilloy C, Rusinaru D, Szymanski C, et al: Predicting left ventricular dysfunction after valve repair for mitral regurgitation due to leaflet prolapse: addictive value of left ventricular end-systolic dimension to ejection fraction. *Eur J Echocardiogr* 12(9):702–710, 2011.
49. Enriquez-Sarano M, Schaff HV, Orszulak TA, et al: Valve repair improves the outcome of surgery for mitral regurgitation: a multivariate analysis. *Circulation* 91:1022–1028, 1995.
50. Rozich JD, Carabello BA, Usher BW, et al: Mitral valve replacement with and without chordal preservation in patients with chronic mitral regurgitation: mechanisms for differences in postoperative ejection performance. *Circulation* 86:1718–1726, 1992.
51. Horskotte D, Schultz HD, Bircks W, et al: The effect of chordal preservation on late outcome after mitral valve replacement: a randomized study. *J Heart Valve Dis* 2:150–158, 1993.
52. David TE, Uden DE, Strauss HD: The importance of the mitral apparatus in left ventricular function after correction of mitral regurgitation. *Circulation* 68:1176–1182, 1983.
53. Bolling SF, Li S, O'Brien SM, et al: Predictors of mitral valve repair: clinical and surgeon factors. *Ann Thorac Surg* 90(6):1904–1911, discussion 1912, 2010.
54. St John Sutton MG, Plappert T, Abraham WT, et al: Effect of cardiac resynchronization therapy on left ventricular size and function in chronic heart failure. *Circulation* 107(15):1985–1990, 2003.
55. van Bommel RJ, Marsan NA, Delgado V, et al: Cardiac resynchronization therapy as a therapeutic option in patients with moderate-severe functional mitral regurgitation and high operative risk. *Circulation* 124(8):912–919, 2011.
56. Trichon BH, Fleker GM, Shaw LK, et al: Relation of frequency and severity of mitral regurgitation to survival among patients with left ventricular systolic dysfunction and heart failure. *Am J Cardiol* 91(5):538–543, 2003.
57. Rossi A, Dini FL, Faggiano P, et al: Independent prognostic value of functional mitral regurgitation in patients with heart failure. A quantitative analysis of 1256 patients with ischemic and non-ischemic dilated cardiomyopathy. *Heart* 97(20):1675–1680, 2011.
58. Bach DS, Bolling SF: Improvement following correction of secondary mitral regurgitation in end-stage cardiomyopathy with mitral annuloplasty. *Am J Cardiol* 78(8):966–969, 1996.
59. Wu AH, Aaronson KD, Bolling SF, et al: Impact of mitral valve annuloplasty on mortality risk in patients with mitral regurgitation and left ventricular systolic dysfunction. *J Am Coll Cardiol* 45(3):381–387, 2005.
60. Mihaljevic T, Lam BK, Rajeswaran J, et al: Impact of mitral valve annuloplasty combined with revascularization in patients with functional ischemic mitral regurgitation. *J Am Coll Cardiol* 49(22):2191–2201, 2007.
61. Fattouch K, Guccione F, Sampognaro S, et al: Rubolo G. Efficacy of adding mitral valve restrictive annuloplasty to coronary artery bypass grafting in patients with moderate ischemic mitral valve regurgitation: a randomized trial. *J Thorac Cardiovasc Surg* 138(2): 278–285, 2009.
62. Deja MA, Grayburn PA, Sun B, et al: Influence of mitral regurgitation repair on survival in the surgical treatment for ischemic heart failure trial. *Circulation* 125(21):2639–2648, 2012.
63. Pleger ST, Schulz-Schonhagen M, Geis N, et al: One year clinical efficacy and reverse cardiac remodeling in patients with severe mitral regurgitation and reduced ejection fraction after MitraClip implantation. *Eur J Heart Fail* 15:919–927, 2013.
64. Piazza N, Asgar A, Ibrahim R, et al: Transcatheter mitral and pulmonary valve therapy. *JACC* 53(20):1837–1851, 2009.
65. Roudaut R, Lafitte S, Roudaut MF, et al: Management of prosthetic heart valve obstruction: fibrinolysis versus surgery. Early results and long-term follow-up in a single-centre study of 263 cases. *Arch Cardiovasc Dis* 102(4):269–277, 2009.
66. Sasayama S, Ross J, Jr, Franklin D, et al: Adaptations of the left ventricle to chronic pressure overload. *Circ Res* 38:172–178, 1976.
67. Gunther S, Grossman W: Determinants of ventricular function in pressure-overload hypertrophy in man. *Circulation* 59(4):679–688, 1979.
68. Murakami T, Hess OM, Gage JE, et al: Diastolic filling dynamics in patients with aortic stenosis. *Circulation* 73:1162–1174, 1986.
69. Villari B, Campbell SE, Hess OM, et al: Influence of collagen network on left ventricular systolic and diastolic function in aortic valve disease. *J Am Coll Cardiol* 22:1477–1484, 1993.
70. Carabello BA, Green LH, Grossman W, et al: Hemodynamic determinants of prognosis of aortic valve replacement in critical aortic stenosis and advanced congestive heart failure. *Circulation* 62:42–48, 1980.
71. Huber D, Grimm J, Koch R, et al: Determinants of ejection performance in aortic stenosis. *Circulation* 64:126–134, 1981.
72. Carroll JD, Carroll EP, Feldman T, et al: Sex-associated differences in left ventricular function in aortic stenosis of the elderly. *Circulation* 86(4):1099–1107, 1992.
73. Kupari M, Turto H, Lommi J: Left ventricular hypertrophy in aortic valve stenosis: preventive or promotive of systolic dysfunction and heart failure? *Eur Heart J* 26:1790–1796, 2005.
74. Dumesnil JG, Pibarot P, Carabello B: Paradoxical low flow and/or low gradient severe aortic stenosis despite preserved left ventricular ejection fraction: implications for diagnosis and treatment. *Eur Heart J* 31:281–289, 2010.
75. Hachicha Z, Dumensnil JG, Bogaty P, et al: Paradoxical low-flow, low-gradient severe aortic stenosis despite preserved ejection fraction is associated with higher afterload and reduced survival. *Circulation* 115:2856–2864, 2007.
76. Clavel MA, Dumesnil JG, Capoulade R, et al: Outcome of patients with aortic stenosis, small valve area and low-flow, low-gradient despite preserved left ventricular ejection fraction. *J Am Coll Cardiol* 60:1259–1267, 2012.
77. Lorell BH, Carabello BA: Left ventricular hypertrophy: pathogenesis, detection, and prognosis. *Circulation* 102(4):470–479, 2000. Review.
78. Marcus ML, Doty DB, Hiratzka LF, et al: Decreased coronary reserve: a mechanism for angina pectoris in patients with aortic stenosis and normal coronary arteries. *N Engl J Med* 307:1362–1367, 1982.
79. Zile MR, Green GR, Schuyler GT, et al: Cardiocyte cytoskeleton in patients with left ventricular pressure overload hypertrophy. *J Am Coll Cardiol* 37(4):1080–1084, 2001.
80. Buermans HPJ, Redout EM, Schiel AE, et al: Micro-array analysis reveals pivotal divergent mRNA expression profiles early in the development of either compensated ventricular hypertrophy or heart failure. *Physiol Genomics* 21:314–323, 2005.
81. Connolly HM, Oh JK, Orszulak TA, et al: Aortic valve replacement for aortic stenosis with severe left ventricular dysfunction: prognostic indicators. *Circulation* 95:2395–2400, 1997.
82. Brogan WC, III, Grayburn PA, Lange RA, et al: Prognosis after valve replacement in patients with severe aortic stenosis and a low transvalvular pressure gradient. *J Am Coll Cardiol* 21:1657–1660, 1993.
83. Connolly HM, Oh JK, Schaff HV, et al: Severe aortic stenosis with low transvalvular gradient and severe left ventricular dysfunction: result of aortic valve replacement in 52 patients. *Circulation* 101:1940–1946, 2000.
84. Pereira JJ, Lauer MS, Bashier M, et al: Survival after aortic valve replacement for severe aortic stenosis with low transvalvular gradients and severe left ventricular dysfunction. *J Am Coll Cardiol* 39(8):1364–1365, 2002.
85. Monin JL, Quere JP, Monchi M, et al: Low-gradient aortic stenosis: operative risk stratification and predictors for long-term outcome: a multicenter study using dobutamine stress hemodynamics. *Circulation* 108(3):319–324, 2003.
86. Quere JP, Monin JL, Levy F, et al: Influence of preoperative left ventricular contractile reserve on postoperative ejection fraction in low-gradient aortic stenosis. *Circulation* 113(14):1738–1744, 2006.
87. Cannon JD, Zile MR, Crawford FA, et al: Aortic valve resistance as an adjunct to the Gorlin formula in assessing the severity of aortic stenosis in symptomatic patients. *J Am Coll Cardiol* 20:1517–1523, 1992.
88. DeFilippi Cr, Willett DL, Brickner ME, et al: Usefulness of dobutamine echocardiography in distinguishing severe from nonsevere valvular aortic stenosis in patients with depressed left ventricular function and low transvalvular gradients. *Am J Cardiol* 75:191–194, 1995.
89. Fougeres E, Tribouilloy C, Monchi M, et al: Outcomes of pseudo-severe aortic stenosis under conservative treatment. *Eur Heart J* 33(19):2426–2433, 2012.
90. Nishimura RA, Grantham JA, Connolly HM, et al: Low-output, low-gradient aortic stenosis in patients with depressed left ventricular systolic function: the clinical utility of the dobutamine challenge in the catheterization laboratory. *Circulation* 106:809–813, 2002.
91. Leon MB, Smith CR, Mack M, et al: Transcatheter aortic-valve implantation for aortic stenosis in patients who cannot undergo surgery. *N Engl J Med* 363:1597–1607, 2010.
92. Smith CR, Leon MB, Mack MJ, et al: Transcatheter versus surgical aortic-valve replacement in high-risk patients. *N Engl J Med* 364(23):2187–2198, 2011.
93. Clavel MA, Webb JG, Rodes-Cabau J, et al: Comparison between transcatheter and surgical prosthetic valve implantation in patients with severe aortic stenosis and reduced left ventricular ejection fraction. *Circulation* 122:1928–1936, 2010.
94. Gash AK, Carabello BA, Cepin D, et al: Left ventricular ejection performance and systolic muscle function in patients with mitral stenosis. *Circulation* 67(1):148–154, 1983.
95. Mohan JC, Khalilullah M, Arora R: Left ventricular intrinsic contractility in pure rheumatic mitral stenosis. *Am J Cardiol* 64:240, 1989.
96. Mahoney PD, Loh E, Blitz LR, et al: Hemodynamic effects of inhaled nitric oxide in women with mitral stenosis and pulmonary hypertension. *Am J Cardiol* 87(2):188–192, 2001.
97. Wroblewski E, James F, Spann JF, et al: Right ventricular performance in mitral stenosis. *Am J Cardiol* 47(1):51–55, 1981.
98. Stoll BC, Ashcom TL, Johns JP, et al: Effects of atenolol on rest and exercise hemodynamics in patients with mitral stenosis. *Am J Cardiol* 75:482–484, 1995.
99. Monmeneu Menadas JV, Marin Ortuno F, Reyes Gomis F, et al: Beta-blockade and exercise capacity in patients with mitral stenosis in sinus rhythm. *J Heart Valve Dis* 11:199–203, 2001.
100. Turi ZG, Reyes VP, Raju BS, et al: Percutaneous balloon versus surgical closed commissurotomy for mitral stenosis. A prospective, randomized trial. *Circulation* 83:1179–1185, 1991.
101. Reyes VP, Raju BS, Wynne J, et al: Percutaneous balloon valvuloplasty compared with open surgical commissurotomy for mitral stenosis. *NEJM* 331:961–967, 1994.
102. Ben Farhat M, Ayari M, Maatouk F, et al: Percutaneous balloon versus surgical closed and open mitral commissurotomy: seven-year follow-up results of a randomized trial. *Circulation* 97:245–250, 1998.
103. Messika-Zeitoun D, Thomson H, Bellamy M, et al: Medical and surgical outcome of tricuspid regurgitation caused by flail leaflets. *J Thorac Cardiovasc Surg* 128(2):296–302, 2004.
104. Ishibashi Y, Rembert JC, Carabello BA, et al: Normal myocardial function in severe right ventricular volume overload hypertrophy. *Am J Physiol Heart Circ Physiol* 280(1):H11–H16, 2001.

Heart Failure as a Consequence of Congenital Heart Disease

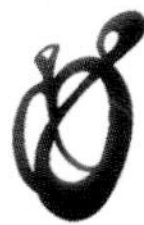

Eric V. Krieger and Anne Marie Valente

Adults with congenital heart disease (CHD) have multiple mechanisms placing them at risk for heart failure, leading one author to refer to congenital heart disease as "the original heart failure syndrome."[1] These mechanisms include chronic pressure and/or volume loading, inadequate myocardial preservation during prior surgeries, myocardial fibrosis, surgical injury to a coronary artery, and neurohormonal activation. The number of heart failure–related admissions for adult congenital heart disease (ACHD) patients has increased dramatically over the past decade,[2] and heart failure–related complications are the most common cause of death in these patients.[3] However, ACHD patients are commonly excluded from heart failure clinical trials, and there is little data to guide therapy in this growing population. This chapter will discuss the growing number of ACHD patients at risk for heart failure and the unique aspects of diagnostic testing and therapies in this group, and highlight several types of congenital heart disease posing the highest risk for development of heart failure.

EPIDEMIOLOGY

Due to tremendous advances in the diagnosis and management of CHD, there are now more adults than children alive with CHD and the incidence of CHD is approximately 4 per 1000 adults.[4] These advances have shifted mortality away from infants and toward adults living with CHD. The median age of death in patients with severe CHD has increased over 20 years since 1987.[5] The incidence of severe CHD has increased 85% in the adult population compared with a 22% increase in children, reflecting the increased survival in childhood. It is estimated that there are over 1 million adults living with CHD in the United States, with at least 15% being of severe complexity.[6]

There is also an increased recognition of heart failure–related complications in ACHD patients. However, the reported incidence of heart failure in ACHD patients is likely an underestimate. The reason for this is multifactorial, including challenges in making the diagnosis and gaps in care that exist for ACHD patients.[7] The prevalence of heart failure is highest in patients with complex anatomy, including single ventricle physiology, transposition of the great arteries (TGA), tetralogy of Fallot (TOF), and pulmonary hypertension (**Figure 25-1**).[8-10] Risk factors for the development of heart failure include high disease complexity, older age, more reoperations, and right ventricular dysfunction.[8]

Heart failure is the leading cause of death in ACHD patients, particularly those with complex anatomy (**Figure 25-2**).[3,9,10] In a cohort of 188 ACHD patients with either a systemic right ventricle (RV) or single ventricle, 15-year mortality for symptomatic patients was much greater than those without symptoms (47.1% versus 5%).[11] Zomer reported that ACHD patients admitted for heart failure had a fivefold higher risk of mortality than patients who were not hospitalized (HR = 5.3; 95% CI 4.2-6.9). One- and three-year mortality after the first heart failure admission was 24% and 35%, respectively.[12] Additionally, heart failure in ACHD patients is associated with increased morbidities and use of health care resources. In an analysis of the Nationwide Inpatient Sample (NIS), the number of heart failure–related admissions increased 82% from 1998-2005 in adults with CHD.[2] More recently, Rodriguez reported that heart failure accounted for 20% of the total ACHD admissions through a review of the 2007 NIS.[13] Heart failure–related hospitalizations were associated with a threefold increased risk of death compared with non–heart failure admissions.[13] Additionally, ACHD patients with pulmonary hypertension have a greater than 30% chance of developing heart failure.[14]

DIAGNOSIS

The mechanism of heart failure is heterogeneous in patients with CHD as discussed previously. Heart failure symptoms in ACHD patients may manifest as systolic and/or diastolic dysfunction of a morphologic left, right, or single ventricle. Other CHD patients may have normal ventricular function, but signs of end-organ dysfunction, such as the adult single ventricle patient with Fontan physiology and significant liver disease.

The diagnosis of heart failure in ACHD patients may be challenging. Patients with CHD, having lived their lives with cardiac disease, may not detect subtle changes in their exercise capacity. By the time they notice symptoms, the extent of ventricular dysfunction and valve disease may be severe and irreversible. Compared with patients with acquired heart disease, patients with CHD are more likely to overestimate their functional capacity and underreport heart failure symptoms.[15] Therefore, objective measures of ventricular function through imaging, exercise testing, and serum biomarkers can be very helpful in these patients. Exercise testing can be useful to uncover early signs of heart failure, even in patients who report that they are asymptomatic (**Figure 25-3**).[16] Patients with CHD and heart failure should be referred to a center with expertise in the care of these patients.[17]

Imaging

The imaging diagnosis of heart failure in ACHD patients can be challenging, and a multimodality approach is often used. The goals of diagnostic imaging in ACHD patients are to evaluate ventricular performance, identify anatomic and functional abnormalities, assess their severity, and provide information that informs clinical decisions. This includes identifying residual hemodynamic issues, such as valve dysfunction and shunts and evaluating for pulmonary hypertension.

Echocardiography

Echocardiography remains the first-line modality in CHD imaging; however, acoustic windows are often poor in older

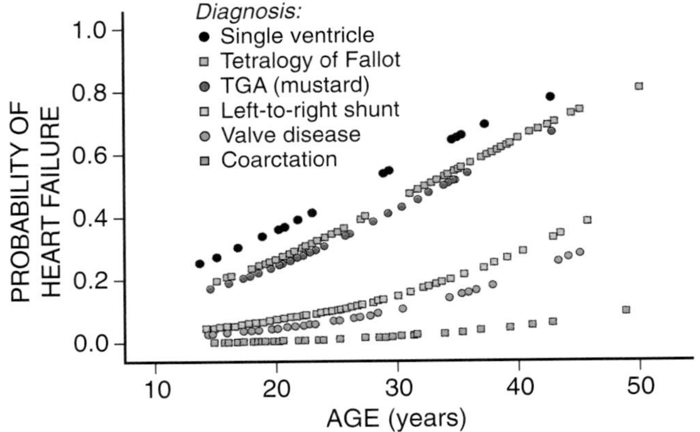

FIGURE 25-1 The probability of heart failure based on age and type of congenital heart defect. *Adapted from Norozi K, Wessel A, Alpers V, et al: Incidence and risk distribution of heart failure in adolescents and adults with congenital heart disease after cardiac surgery. Am J Cardiol 97:1238–1243, 2006.*

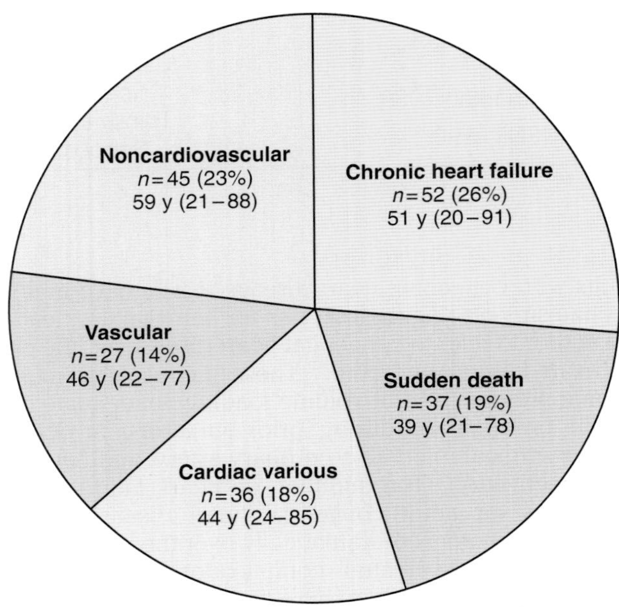

FIGURE 25-2 Modes of death in adult congenital heart patients. *Adapted from Verheugt CL, Uiterwaal CS, van der Velde ET, et al: Mortality in adult congenital heart disease. Eur Heart J 31:1220–1229, 2010.*

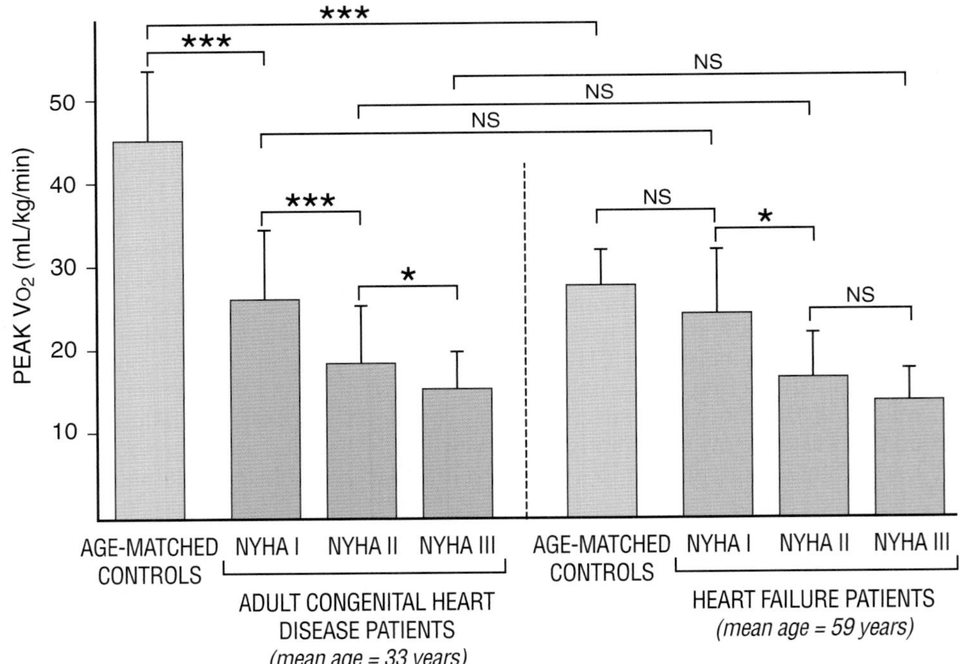

FIGURE 25-3 Peak oxygen consumption according to NYHA class for adult congenital heart patients, chronic heart failure patients and corresponding reference subjects. Bars and error markers represent mean and SD (*P <0.05, ***P <0.001). *Adapted from Diller GP, Dimopoulos K, Okonko D, et al: Exercise intolerance in adult congenital heart disease: comparative severity, correlates, and prognostic implication. Circulation 112:828–835, 2005.*

patients and those with multiple prior cardiac surgeries. It is often challenging to visualize certain parts of the right heart, which limits assessment of RV size and function.

Assessment of ventricular size and function is important in the ACHD patient. Left ventricular (LV) function is most often calculated as the ejection fraction (EF) based on the biplane Simpson or area-length method, both of which assume an ellipsoid shape of the ventricle. These methods are not applicable to the RV or single-ventricle patient because of the nonellipsoid shape of the ventricle. There are various echocardiographic techniques that can be used to evaluate RV function (see also Chapter 29). The RV fractional area change is defined as ([end-diastolic area – end-systolic area] / end-diastolic area). The lower reference value for normal RV systolic function using this method is 35%. This value correlates modestly with cardiac magnetic resonance (CMR) measurements in patients with CHD.[18] Three-dimensional echocardiography may provide a more accurate and reproducible quantification of RV volumes and function. However, it underestimates RV volumes and may overestimate EF, a discrepancy that may increase as the ventricle enlarges.[19] Over the past several years, several nongeometric echocardiographic parameters—such as the myocardial performance index, tissue Doppler imaging, and RV basal wall systolic excursion velocity—have been proposed for evaluation of RV performance in ACHD patients. However, the clinical utility of these parameters for ACHD patients with heart failure is unclear. Myocardial deformation imaging (strain and strain rate) is appealing in CHD patients as it may provide insights into mechanisms of both global and regional ventricular dysfunction.[20] The echocardiographic assessment of diastolic dysfunction in ACHD patients is even more challenging. Many factors contribute to the diastolic properties of ACHD patients, and the importance of diastolic dysfunction varies with the type of CHD.[21]

Cardiac Magnetic Resonance Imaging

The role of CMR is steadily increasing in the ACHD population. It is a particularly attractive imaging technique due to its excellent tissue border delineation, tissue characterization, and quantification of ventricular volumes and valvular regurgitation that allows for serial comparisons without the need for ionizing radiation.[22] CMR has become the gold standard for quantification of RV volumes and function. Phase-velocity imaging is used for assessment of cardiac output and valvular regurgitation. An additional strength of CMR is the ability to characterize myocardial tissue abnormalities. Specifically, late gadolinium enhancement suggestive of myocardial fibrosis has been associated with adverse clinical outcomes in patients with repaired TOF,[23] systemic RV,[24] and Fontan procedures.[25] Newer applications, which include quantification of the extracellular volume fraction using the modified look-locker inversion recovery sequence, may identify areas of more diffuse fibrosis. However, the clinical significance in ACHD patients is unknown.

Cardiopulmonary Exercise Testing

Cardiopulmonary exercise testing is a valuable tool in the assessment of ACHD patients at risk for heart failure. Objective testing is important in this population, because ACHD patients commonly overestimate their actual measured exercise capacity and are unaware of functional limitations.[15] Cardiopulmonary exercise testing is predictive of morbidity and mortality in CHD patients.[26] In a recent single-center experience of cardiopulmonary exercise testing in 1375 ACHD patients (age 33 ± 13 years), decreased peak oxygen consumption (V_{O_2}) and heart rate reserve were predictive of death over a median follow-up of 5.8 years. Additionally, an elevated VE/V_{CO_2} slope was associated with an increased risk of death in noncyanotic patients.[26] Diller reported the results of objective exercise testing in 335 ACHD patients and demonstrated that these patients, with a mean age of 33 years, had a similar distribution of heart failure symptoms and exercise capacity to a noncongenital heart failure population at a mean age of 59 years (see Figure 25-3).[16]

ACHD patients may have limited exercise capacity because of both cardiac and noncardiac causes. Ventricular dysfunction (both systolic and diastolic) and electromechanical dyssynchrony are increasingly recognized in ACHD patients. Residual hemodynamic lesions are common in ACHD patients, because almost no one who undergoes CHD surgery is "cured." Chronotropic incompetence is common in ACHD patients, often secondary to injury of the conduction system during surgery, intrinsic conduction abnormalities, or medications, and is associated with increased mortality.[27] Adults with CHD may have noncardiac limitations to exercise capacity. Restrictive lung disease is very common in those who underwent thoracotomies. Obstructive lung disease, diaphragmatic paralysis (due to phrenic nerve injury), liver dysfunction, skeletal muscle dysfunction, and hematologic derangements can also limit exercise capacity.

One of the challenges in interpreting the results and prognostic significance of cardiopulmonary exercise testing in ACHD patients is that the group is very heterogeneous. Recently, Kempny provided age and gender-specific reference values for peak V_{O_2} for groups of ACHD patients with various congenital heart conditions (**Figure 25-4**).[28] ACHD patients have elevations in the minute ventilation (VE) to carbon dioxide production (V_{CO_2}) slope and this finding is an independent predictor of mortality.[29] An elevated VE/V_{CO_2} slope may be seen in repaired TOF patients, when there is abnormal pulmonary blood flow distribution because of branch pulmonary artery stenosis.[30] Successful percutaneous interventions with relief of the stenosis result in improvement of the VE/V_{CO_2} slope.[31] However, an elevated VE/V_{CO_2} slope is not associated with increased mortality in single-ventricle patients who have undergone a Fontan procedure, where the elevation in the slope is a consequence of nonpulsatile pulmonary blood flow.[32] Additionally, Fontan patients commonly have a depressed oxygen pulse, even in the absence of ventricular dysfunction, indicating a failure of the Fontan to increase preload to the systemic ventricle during exercise.

Serum Biomarkers

ACHD patients with heart failure experience neurohormonal activation similar to those patients with heart failure from acquired heart disease. However, because of the diversity of CHD and the various mechanisms of heart failure in ACHD patients, there is not a consistent association of individual serum biomarkers to outcomes, which can be generalized across all ACHD patients. Even asymptomatic ACHD patients have significant neurohormonal activation, which

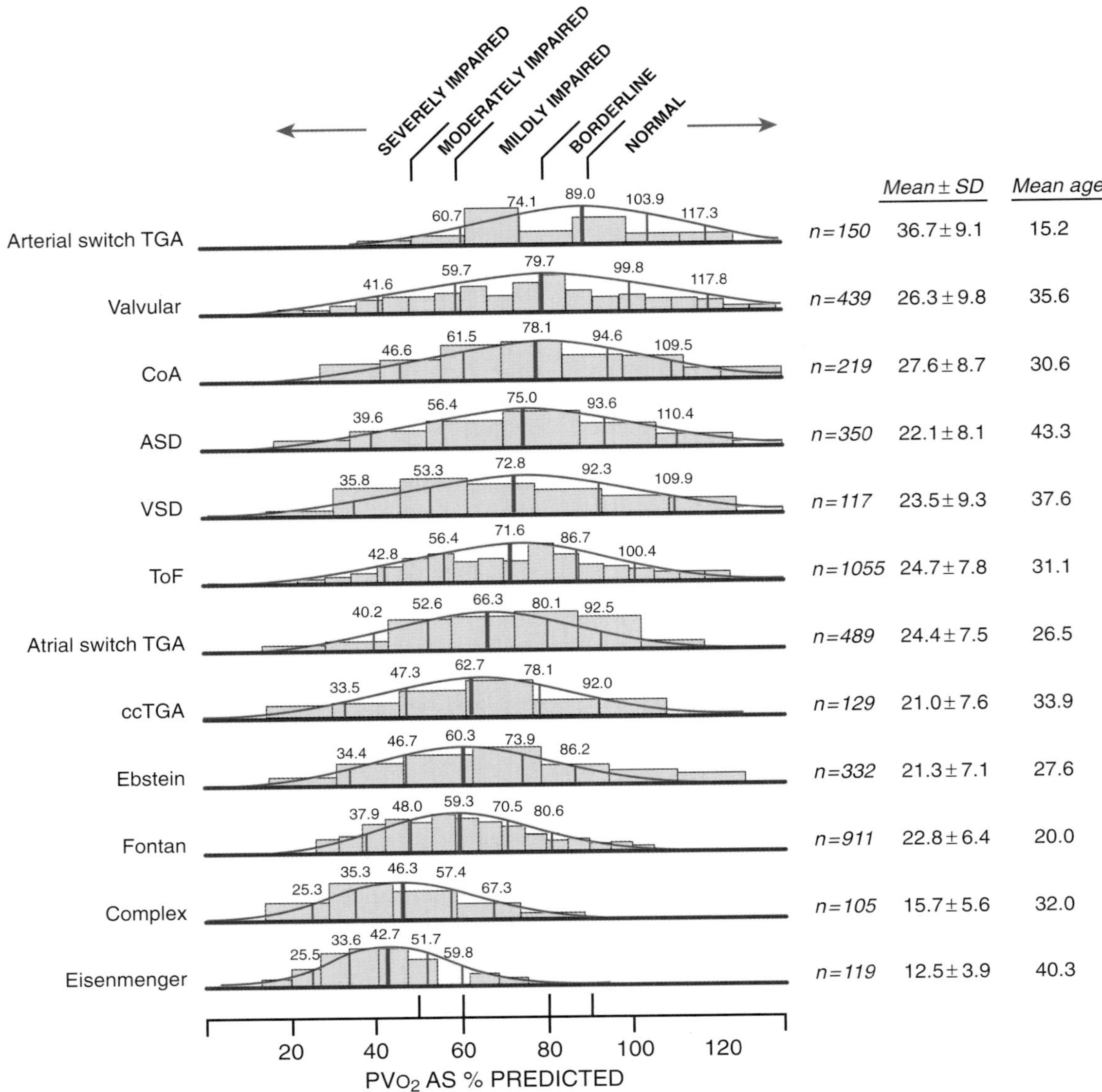

FIGURE 25-4 Peak oxygen uptake (peak VO_2) for various forms of congenital heart disease, expressed as a % of predicted value. The density lines above histograms and the numbers to the right of the graph relate to all patients with a given diagnosis. The numbers above the density lines indicate % peak VO_2 values for the 10th, 25th, 50th, 75th, and 90th percentile. *ASD,* Atrial septal defect; *ccTGA,* congenitally corrected TGA; *CoA,* coarctation of aorta; *complex,* complex congenital heart disease (including univentricular hearts); *Ebstein,* Ebstein anomaly; *Eisenmenger,* Eisenmenger syndrome; *Fontan,* patients after Fontan palliation; *TGA,* transposition of the great arteries; *TOF,* tetralogy of Fallot; *valvular,* mixed collective of patients with congenital valvular heart disease; *VSD,* ventricular septal defect. *From Kempny A, Dimopoulos K, Uebing A, et al: Reference values for exercise limitations among adults with congenital heart disease. Relation to activities of daily life—single centre experience and review of published data. Eur Heart J 33:1386–1396, 2012.*

demonstrates the occult nature of ventricular dysfunction in this group of patients.[33] Over the past decade, multiple investigators have reported results of abnormal biomarkers in ACHD patients that have been associated with mortality.[34,35] However, since natriuretic peptides are influenced by age, gender, and hypoxia, it is difficult to define normal levels for a diverse population of ACHD patients. In a recent investigation of 475 ACHD patients, Eindhoven reported that N-terminal-pro B-type natriuretic peptide (NT-proBNP) levels vary considerably by the type of underlying CHD, with the highest levels seen in patients with complex CHD, such as Fontan physiology and systemic RV.[36]

The utility of serum biomarkers in patients with Fontan physiology remains uncertain. In these patients, symptoms of heart failure may occur despite normal systolic ventricular function and unremarkable biomarker values. BNP values have not been shown to correlate with ventricular systolic dysfunction in this group of patients.[37,38] The data on BNP levels based on the morphology of the single ventricle (right, left, or mixed) are conflicting, with several studies documenting a higher BNP in patients with a single RV[39]; however, other studies have not confirmed this finding.[37,40]

TREATMENT

ACHD patients are commonly excluded from heart failure clinical trials and there is little data to guide therapy in this growing population. It may be tempting to simply extrapolate from established heart failure guidelines; however, this is dangerous due to the unique heterogeneous population of ACHD patients with heart failure. In ACHD patients, pulmonary venous hypertension may result from dysfunction of a systemic RV or single ventricle, with or without

TABLE 25-1 Selected Studies of Medical Therapy Trials in Adult Congenital Heart Patients

CHD GROUP	AUTHOR	YEAR	STUDY DESIGN	AGENT	N	DURATION (months)	ENDPOINTS	RESULTS
Tetralogy of Fallot								
	Norozi	2007	PDB-RCT	Bisoprolol	33	6	NT-proBNP, RVEF, LVEF	Negative
	Babu-Nararyan	2012	PDB-RCT	Ramipril	64	6	RVEF	Negative
Systemic RV								
	Dore	2005	PDB-COT	Losartan	29	3.5	Vo_{2max}, RVEF, NT-proBNP	Negative
	Giardini	2007	Prospective uncontrolled trial	Carvedilol	8	12	RVEF, LVEF, Vo_{2max}, exercise duration	Improvements in biventricular size and function
	Doughan	2007	Retrospective	Carvedilol or metoprolol	60	Retrospective	NYHA class, RV size	Positive
	Therrien	2008	PDB-RCT	Ramipril	17	12	RVEF, RVEDV	Negative
	van der Bom	2013	PDB-RCT	Valsartan	88	36	Primary: RVEF Secondary: RVEDV, Vo_{2max}, QOL	Negative except for small benefit on RVEDV
Fontan								
	Kouatli	1997	PDB-COT	Enalapril	18	2.5	Vo_{2max}, exercise duration	Negative
	Giardini	2008	PDB-RCT	Sildenafil	27	Single dose	Vo_{2max}, cardiac output, pulmonary blood flow	Positive
	Goldberg	2011	PDB-COT	Sildenafil	28	1.5	Primary: Vo_{2max} Secondary: VE/Vco_2 slope	Negative for primary outcome; positive for VE/Vco_2 slope
	Rhodes	2012	PDB-RCT	Iloprost	18	Single dose	Vo_{2max}, O_2 pulse	Positive

LVEF, Left ventricular ejection fraction; *NT-proBNP,* N-terminal-pro B-type natriuretic peptide; *PDB-COT,* prospective double-blind crossover trial; *PDB-RCT,* prospective double-blind randomized controlled trial; *QOL,* quality of life; *RVEDV,* right ventricular end-diastolic volume; *RVEF,* right ventricular ejection fraction.

systemic atrioventricular valve regurgitation. Conversely, central venous hypertension is very common in ACHD patients, often due to pulmonary ventricular systolic and diastolic dysfunction. Adults with Fontan physiology need to maintain higher central venous pressures because of the nonpulsatile flow to the pulmonary arteries. An additional cause of venous hypertension in ACHD patients is obstruction in surgical baffles or conduits. Therefore, the evaluation of new heart failure symptoms in an ACHD patient must be tailored to the patient's anatomy and surgical repair. It should include evaluation for residual shunts, baffle stenosis, valvular or conduit dysfunction, and collateral vessels, which may be amenable to interventions. All ACHD patients with new-onset heart failure should also be evaluated for pulmonary vascular disease. In a population-based study of more than 38,000 adults with CHD, Lowe reported a 6% incidence of pulmonary hypertension. Importantly, those subjects with pulmonary hypertension had a more than twofold higher risk of all-cause mortality and threefold higher risk of heart failure and arrhythmias compared with those without pulmonary hypertension.[14]

The treatment of heart failure in the ACHD patient must also address modifiable risk factors, such as hypertension, diabetes, and obesity.

Potential therapies for heart failure in ACHD patients include medical therapies, device therapies, and surgical interventions, such as mechanical assist devices and transplantation. The existing data for medical therapies in ACHD patients is limited, as no adequately powered clinical trials have been performed. Individual studies focused on medical therapies will be discussed in the lesion-specific section later and are listed in **Table 25-1**.

Cardiac Resynchronization Therapy and Implantable Defibrillators in Adult Congenital Heart Disease

In patients with chronic systolic heart failure and prolonged QRS duration, cardiac resynchronization therapy (CRT) improves symptoms, reduces hospitalizations, and reduces all-cause mortality.[41] However, there is comparatively little data on CRT in patients with CHD. There are various reasons why it may not be appropriate to apply standard CRT guidelines to ACHD patients. ACHD patients are considerably more heterogeneous than the population studied in the large resynchronization trials, so extrapolation is difficult. Patients with CHD are more likely to have predominantly right-sided heart disease, systemic RV, or single ventricle physiology, and the benefits of CRT are not well established in these groups. Additionally, due to shunts or variations in venous anatomy, patients with CHD are more likely to require epicardial pacing or defibrillation that increases the risk of implantation, reduces device longevity, and alters the risk-reward ratio of implanting a CRT device.

The three largest studies of CRT in CHD are retrospective uncontrolled case series that describe CRT response in 272 patients, 206 of whom had CHD (**Table 25-2**).[42-45] The patients were young (median age <18 years). The procedural complication rate ranged from 9% to 29% and included lead complications, pocket hematomas, blood loss, and, rarely, procedural mortality. Approximately half of devices were implanted with epicardial leads. As expected, patients who received CRT had a reduction in QRS width, with the greatest reduction in those being converted from single ventricular pacing. Overall rate of clinical response ranged from 32%

TABLE 25-2 Selected Studies of Cardiac Resynchronization Therapy Response in Pediatric and Congenital Heart Disease Patients

	CECCHIN ET AL	DUBIN ET AL	JANOUSEK ET AL
Year	2009	2005	2009
Number of patients	60	103	109
Median age (y)	15	13	17
Baseline data			
NYHA class I (%)	27	14	Median NYHA class 2.5
NYHA class II (%)	42	48	
NYHA class III-IV (%)	32	38	
Systemic ventricular EF (%)	36	26	27
Congenital heart disease (%)	77	71	80
Single ventricle (%)	22	7	4
Systemic RV (%)	12	17	33
QRS (ms)	149	166	160
Post-CRT data			
Change NYHA class	NR	NR	Decreased 1.5 grades
Systemic ventricular EF (%)	43	40	Median change +12
QRS (ms)	120	126	130
Improvement in EF or NYHA class (%)	87	76	72
Predictors of poor CRT response	Systemic RV	Higher baseline EF	Dilated cardiomyopathy, high baseline NYHA class

CRT, Cardiac resynchronization therapy; *EF*, ejection fraction; *NYHA*, New York Heart Association; *RV*, right ventricle.
Modified from van der Hulst AE, Delgado V, Blom NA, et al: Cardiac resynchronization therapy in paediatric and congenital heart disease patients. Eur Heart J *32:2236-2246, 2011.*

to 87% of treated patients and, depending on the study, the response was variably defined as improvement in systemic ventricular EF or improvement in New York Heart Association (NYHA) class.[43-45] Approximately one third of patients had a robust clinical response.[44] A few critically ill patients, who were dependent on intravenous inotropic support, could be weaned to oral therapy after CRT.[43]

Cardiac Resynchronization Therapy in Specific Populations

Tetralogy of Fallot

Patients with repaired TOF often have right bundle branch block because of RV dilation and myocardial fibrosis. QRS prolongation has been associated with adverse outcomes in this population.[46,47] For this reason some have speculated that CRT may be beneficial. However, in large CRT trials, patients with right bundle branch block have had disappointing results compared with those with left bundle branch block.[48] Right bundle branch block pattern is common in repaired TOF; therefore RV pacing with fusion of the spontaneous wave front is theoretically appealing. However, optimizing pacemaker settings is technically difficult and the negative impact of chronic RV pacing on LV systolic function needs to be considered. Additionally, as QRS prolongation in TOF is most often indicative of pathology in the RVOT rather than the body of the RV,[49] it is uncertain whether RV pacing can improve RV performance. Short-term hemodynamic studies have shown that CRT can improve right heart failure in patients with repaired TOF; however, there is very little long-term data on chronic CRT in this group.[50] In patients with TOF and LV dysfunction, CRT may be reasonable for conventional indications. However, the role of CRT in improving RV function in patients with right bundle branch block has not been established and is not routinely recommended.

Systemic Right Ventricle

Many patients with TGA have a morphologic RV, which functions as the systemic ventricle. These patients are predisposed to ventricular dysfunction and heart failure, as described elsewhere in this chapter. Approximately 40% of patients with a systemic RV have a wide QRS or echocardiographic features of dyssynchrony.[50-52] Up to 9% of patients with a systemic RV meet conventional indications for CRT (reduced EF, NYHA class ≥ 2, sinus rhythm, and QRS >120 msec).[51] Although it is possible that this population may benefit from CRT, robust data are lacking. Excluding individual case reports, there are fewer than 100 patients with systemic RV where the impact of CRT has been described in the literature. In a report of seven patients with systemic RV who underwent CRT, the results were encouraging: All patients had improved markers of dyssynchrony, improvement in NYHA class, and an improved exercise capacity.[53] Other studies have been less consistent. Approximately 20% of the patients in the studies by Janousek,[45] Cecchin,[44] and Dubin[43] had a systemic RV. Dubin found comparable improvement in those with systemic right and left ventricles. However, Janousek and Cecchin found that patients with systemic RV had less improvement compared with those with systemic LV. The authors speculate that the lack of improvement may be because of these patients' older age or that systemic atrioventricular (tricuspid) valve regurgitation did not improve after CRT. At this point the literature is conflicting and there is insufficient evidence to routinely recommend CRT for patients with systemic RV dysfunction; each case must be considered on an individual basis.

Single Ventricle

In patients with a functional single ventricle, the systemic ventricle can be either a morphologic left or right, depending on the initial cardiac anatomy. Patients with a Fontan operation who require ventricular pacing require an epicardial system to minimize the risk of stroke associated with thrombus formation on a lead in the systemic ventricle. Placement of multisite epicardial leads for CRT is also nonstandardized and optimal lead position is unknown, although an effort is made to place the CRT lead 180 degrees from the first pacing lead.[54]

In young children undergoing the Fontan operation, CRT acutely improves postoperative cardiac performance, as measured by echocardiographic markers of dyssynchrony and invasive hemodynamics.[55] Case reports have documented clinical improvement after multisite pacing in the failing Fontan circulation.[56] In the series by Janousek and Cecchin, most Fontan patients had improvement in NYHA class. Cecchin demonstrated on average a more than 10% improvement in EF after CRT.[44,45]

Transplantation and Mechanical Support

Myocardial dysfunction is common in patients with CHD and is a frequent cause of death in this population.[3,9,10] Therefore, for many patients with CHD, heart transplantation becomes the only potential treatment option. As with other forms of heart disease, transplantation is appropriate for patients with heart failure refractory to conventional medical therapy (see also Chapter 40).

Approximately 3% of adults who undergo heart transplantation have CHD, and the proportion is growing over time.[57,58] The most likely congenital diagnoses to result in transplantation include single-ventricle anatomy, TGA, and right ventricular outflow tract lesions. Most patients have had at least one prior corrective surgery.[59] Most, but not all,[59] studies have shown that transplanted patients with CHD have higher early mortality than patients without CHD.[60] The most frequent causes of early post-transplant mortality in patients with CHD are hemorrhage and acute graft failure.[61] Longer ischemic times are common in ACHD patients, likely as a result of technically difficult dissections, and are a risk factor for early postoperative death.[60] One-year mortality rates in the CHD population are approximately 20%.[62,63] Older recipient age, older donor age, longer ischemic times, and prior Fontan operation appear to be risk factors for early mortality.[59]

For patients with CHD who survive more than 3 months from the time of transplant, long-term survival is similar[58,64] to patients without CHD who receive heart transplantation, suggesting that the increased risk of mortality is related to peritransplant issues.[61] Outcomes for ACHD transplantation and risk factors for adverse outcomes are shown in **Table 25-3**.

Selecting appropriate congenital heart disease patients for cardiac transplantation is difficult. Risk models exist to predict the need for transplantation in acquired heart disease,[65] but these models are not validated in patients with ACHD. Therefore, it can be difficult to decide when it is appropriate to list a patient with CHD for transplantation. Poor exercise performance has been associated with poor outcomes in some, but not all congenital populations.[66,67] Appropriate timing for listing patients with Eisenmenger syndrome pose an additional challenge as these patients have improved survival compared with other patients with severe pulmonary arterial hypertension and require combined heart-lung transplantation, which carries a relatively poor prognosis.[68,69] In patients with Eisenmenger syndrome, it is appropriate to consider transplantation for patients with repeated hospitalizations, signs of refractory RV failure, arrhythmias, or worsening cyanosis.

Congenital patients often have complex postsurgical anatomy that can pose technical challenges at the time of transplantation. Systemic or pulmonary veins may need to be surgically redirected in patients with atrial situs inversus. Patients with TGA may require that additional lengths of great arteries be harvested at the time of donor organ procurement. Many patients with repaired CHD may have pulmonary vascular disease or distorted pulmonary artery anatomy because of prior shunts, branch pulmonary artery stenosis, or stents, which can increase RV afterload and predispose to early graft failure.

An additional barrier to transplantation in adult congenital patients is alloimmunization as a consequence of prior transfusions, homografts, or pregnancies. Patients with elevated preformed reactive antibodies have increased rejection and reduced post-transplant survival.[70] This can make it difficult to find a suitable donor organ. A panel of reactive antibodies should be checked early in the transplant evaluation to determine if the patient is appropriate for transplant listing and if a desensitization protocol is required. Most patients with CHD and end-stage heart failure who are considered for transplantation are never listed for transplantation because of high reactive antibodies, anatomic barriers, perceived surgical risk, or other reasons.[71]

Patients with CHD who are listed for transplant are more likely to be listed at a lower urgency status than patients with acquired heart disease; 64% of patients with CHD are listed as status 2, whereas only 44% of patients with acquired heart disease are listed as status 2. This discrepancy is in part because of the infrequent use of ventricular assist devices (which increase urgency status) in patients with CHD and end-stage heart failure. Therefore, listed patients with CHD have a longer time to transplantation and are less likely to receive a transplant once listed. Despite the lower listing priority, patients with CHD were more likely to experience cardiovascular death than patients with acquired heart disease.[72] The apparent penalty of transplant listing in patients with CHD could potentially be remedied by more judicious use of implantable defibrillators and ventricular assist devices in CHD patients[72] or by changing the urgency status upgrade given to patients with ventricular assist devices.[73]

Fontan patients undergoing transplantation require careful consideration. As discussed above, these patients are likely to have multiple prior palliative surgeries, complex anatomy, collateral vessels, and multiorgan dysfunction manifest by congestive hepatopathy, renal insufficiency, and coagulopathy.[74] They are also more likely to be cachectic and edematous. Fontan patients are therefore at increased risk of perioperative bleeding, postoperative hepato-renal syndrome, or serious infection. Fontan patients may also have in situ pulmonary artery thrombus, which can increase the risk of acute graft failure. Pulmonary vascular resistance is usually low in patients with Fontan physiology, but in the context of a failing Fontan it may be modestly elevated and can be difficult to calculate using standard techniques. Fontan patients appear to have increased post-transplant risk of death and higher risk of death from infection.[59,75]

Ventricular assist devices (VADs) (see also Chapter 42) have not gained widespread use in adult patients with CHD.[72] Most reports of VAD use in adult patients with CHD are limited to case reports or small case series of carefully selected patients. One larger series included six adult patients with a systemic RV and NYHA class IV symptoms. No patients required bilateral VAD placement. There were no operative deaths, and five patients survived more than 6 months, one was transplanted, and four patients survived more than 1 year.[76] In a second series of four adult CHD

TABLE 25-3 Outcomes of Heart Transplantation in Patients with Congenital Heart Disease

AUTHOR	YEAR	STUDY DESIGN	*N*	MEAN AGE (y)	1-YEAR SURVIVAL (%)	10-YEAR SURVIVAL (%)	PREDICTORS OF MORTALITY
Karamlou	2010	National database	575	28	76	52	Younger age, UNOS status I, ↑ ischemic time
Davies	2012	Single center, patients with prior Fontan	43	16	62	47	↑ operative bleeding, renal dysfunction
Davies	2012	Single center, patients *without* prior Fontan	129	14	≈80	≈50	NR
Irving	2010	Single center	38	34	68	53	Early era of surgery
Lamour	2009	Multicenter registry	488	12	≈80	≈55	Older age, Fontan, ↑ ischemic time, higher right atrial pressure higher PVR, CMV + donor
Patel	2009	UNOS database	689	>17	80	57	PVR >4 Woods units PRA >10%
Bernstein	2006	Multicenter, patients with prior Fontan	97	10	75	NR	NR
Jayakumar	2004	Multicenter, patients with Glenn or Fontan	35	16	72	62	NR
Chen	2004	Single center	106	15	≈77	≈55	Need for pulmonary artery reconstruction, ↑ PVR

CMV, Cytomegalovirus; *NR,* not reported; *PRA,* panel of reactive antibodies; *PVR,* pulmonary vascular resistance; *UNOS,* United Network for Organ Sharing.

patients who received VADs, 50% died in the first year.[71] There are numerous potential barriers to VAD use in patients with CHD. These include the higher frequency of right-sided heart failure in patients with CHD, a higher prevalence of pulmonary vascular disease, multiple prior chest surgeries, multiorgan dysfunction with coagulopathy, and renal dysfunction.

SPECIFIC CONDITIONS

Tetralogy of Fallot

TOF is the most common cyanotic CHD with an incidence of 0.3 to 0.5 per 1000 live births, accounting for 7% of CHD. It is characterized by deviation of the infundibular septum, creating a malalignment ventricular septal defect, aortic override, right ventricular outflow tract (RVOT) obstruction, and ventricular hypertrophy. Complete repair involves closure of the ventricular septal defect and relief of RVOT obstruction (**Figure 25-5**).

Despite excellent early surgical outcomes, multiple residual hemodynamic burdens can predispose to heart failure later in life. Often, pulmonary valve function is not preserved during repair, which leads to pulmonary valve regurgitation. Before the 1990s, surgery was most commonly performed through a large right ventriculotomy and a sizeable RVOT patch was used to relieve the obstruction. Free pulmonary valve regurgitation was considered to be an inevitable and acceptable tradeoff for complete relief of RVOT obstruction. The large transannular patch contributes to late pulmonary regurgitation[77] and predisposes to lower RV ejection fractions later in life.[78]

As a consequence of ongoing pulmonary regurgitation, many patients developed progressive RV dilation and systolic dysfunction.[79-81] Although free pulmonary regurgitation is initially well tolerated in childhood, changes in RV compliance and pulmonary artery capacitance as well as slower heart rates (allowing for more time in diastole) result in worsening regurgitation in adulthood. This often leads to RV dilation, functional tricuspid valve regurgitation, RV systolic dysfunction, and atrial and ventricular arrhythmias if left untreated.[80] RV function typically deteriorates and limits

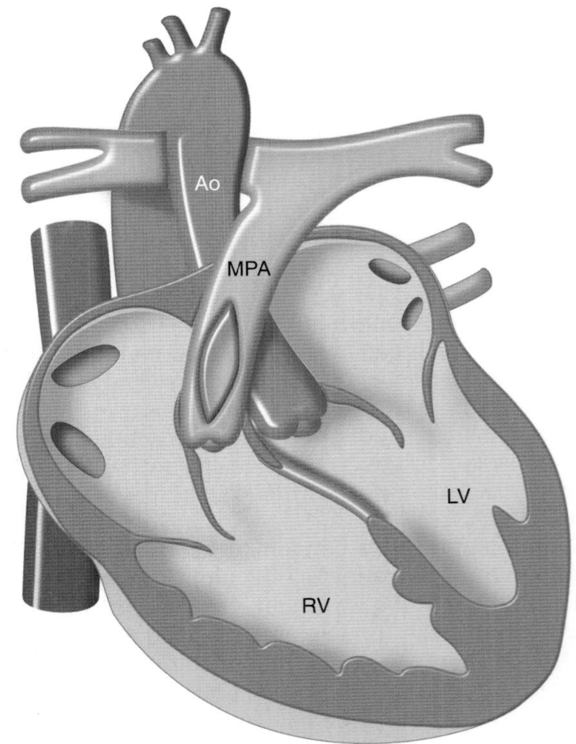

FIGURE 25-5 Diagrammatic representation of repaired tetralogy of Fallot. There is a patch across the right ventricular outflow tract and a patch closure of the ventricular septal defect. Of note, this diagram depicts a right-sided aortic arch, which may occur in conotruncal defects such as tetralogy of Fallot. *Ao,* Aorta; *LV,* left ventricle; *MPA,* main pulmonary artery; *RV,* right ventricle.

exercise tolerance,[80] and may cause overt right heart failure, usually in the third and fourth decades of life. Conversely, restrictive RV filling may limit adverse RV remodeling by limiting the amount of pulmonary regurgitation.[82]

Pulmonary valve replacement, if done before overt RV failure, leads to beneficial RV remodeling characterized by a reduction in end-diastolic volume and stabilization or improvement of RV EF.[83-85] However, not all authors have found an improvement in EF or exercise performance following surgery.[83,85-87] Earlier valve replacement may allow for greater improvement in function and exercise parameters.[79,88] The optimal timing for valve replacement remains controversial; the benefits of early pulmonary valve replacement in maximizing ventricular remodeling need to be weighed against the finite lifespan of prosthetic valves. Although optimal timing of pulmonary valve replacement in asymptomatic tetralogy patients remains controversial, various authors have demonstrated good short-term outcomes if surgery is done in the context of normal RV function, RV end-diastolic volumes less than 160 to 170 mL/m^2, and end-systolic volume less than 80 to 90 mL/m^2.[79,80,83,87-89] The role of medical therapy for patients with chronic pulmonary regurgitation is unknown; a small trial of ACE-inhibitors in patients with RV dilation and pulmonary regurgitation did not show a significant benefit, but larger trials are needed to further define the role of medical therapy in these patients.[90]

LV dysfunction is increasingly recognized in patients with TOF and appears to be an important determinant of outcome. Approximately 20% of adults with repaired TOF have LV systolic dysfunction.[88,91] Patients with LV dysfunction have more arrhythmias and worse outcomes than TOF patients with preserved LV systolic function.[91-93] The reason for LV dysfunction in patients with TOF is not fully understood, but it may be caused by interventricular interactions, chronic bundle branch block, aortic regurgitation, neonatal cyanosis, or LV volume overload from palliative shunts, or it may be a consequence of neurohormonal activation from RV failure.[33,91,94]

Systemic Right Ventricle

A systemic RV is one in which the morphologic RV delivers systemic output through the aorta (**Figure 25-6**). There is no standard definition for systemic RV dysfunction; therefore, its prevalence in ACHD patients is unknown and the response to medical therapies difficult to interpret. These patients are at high risk for sudden cardiac death and heart failure.[95] Additionally, much of the available literature concerning medical therapies in systemic RV patients includes both complete TGA (D-loop TGA) and physiologically corrected TGA (c-TGA; also called L-loop TGA, cc-TGA) patients. TGA and c-TGA patients may have very different responses to medical therapies. For example, TGA patients that have undergone an atrial switch procedure often have sinus node dysfunction, whereas c-TGA patients are at high risk for progressive atrioventricular block. Therefore, each group's responses to β-blockade may be quite different. The current ACHD guidelines recommend imaging every year or at least every other year to assess systemic RV function.[17]

Complete TGA (D-loop TGA) results from ventricular-arterial discordance such that the aorta connects to the RV pumping deoxygenated blood systemically. The pulmonary artery connects to the LV pumping oxygenated blood back to the lungs, which is a physiology incompatible with life without the presence of a shunt. In the 1960s to 1980s, the most common surgical procedure for this condition was the atrial switch procedure (Mustard or Senning operation), which directed deoxygenated blood via baffles to the LV and out the pulmonary artery and directed oxygenated blood to the RV and out the aorta. These procedures relieved the cyanosis, yet resulted in the RV ejecting to systemic pressure. RV dysfunction appears to be common following atrial switch, occurring in 8% to 61% of patients, depending on imaging modality used and length of follow-up.[96,97] The mechanisms for systemic RV dysfunction are incompletely understood but may include a suboptimal myofiber arrangement, myocardial ischemia from supply demand mismatch, and less robust conduction system. Additionally, these patients have rigid atrial baffles, which limit preload augmentation so that these patients may not be able to increase their ventricular stroke volume with exercise, resulting in abnormal atrioventricular coupling.[98]

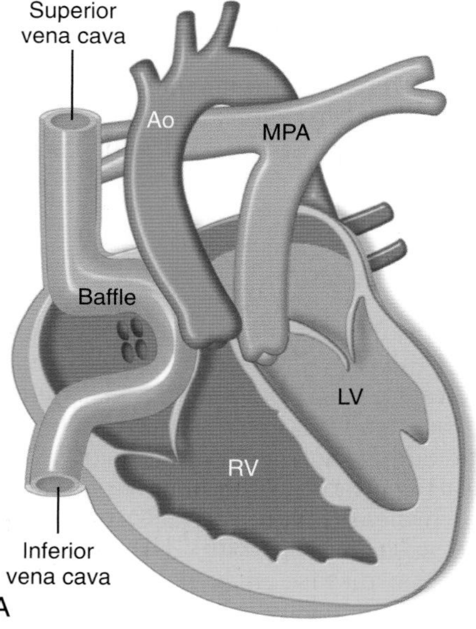

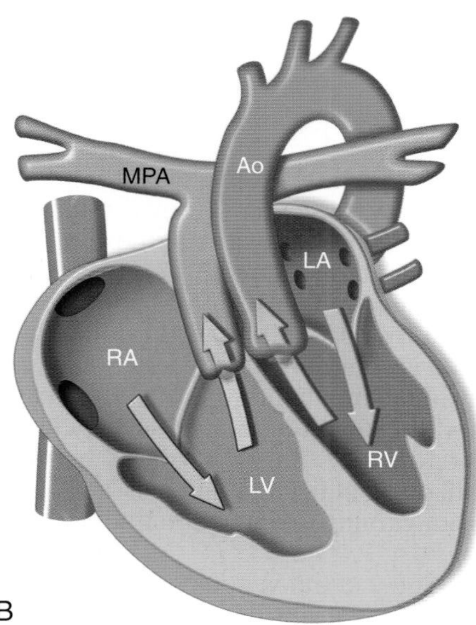

FIGURE 25-6 Diagrammatic representation of two types of systemic right ventricles. **A,** Complete transposition of the great arteries, status after an atrial switch (Mustard or Senning) procedure. **B,** Congenitally corrected transposition of the great arteries, with atrioventricular discordance and ventricular arterial discordance resulting in deoxygenated blood passing from the left ventricle to the pulmonary artery and oxygenated blood reaching the aorta through the systemic right ventricle. *Ao,* Aorta; *LA,* left atrium; *LV,* left ventricle; *MPA,* main pulmonary artery; *RA,* right atrium; *RV,* right ventricle. *Modified from Libby P: Essential atlas of cardiovascular disease, New York, 2009, Springer.*

Patients with c-TGA (L-loop TGA, cc-TGA) have atrioventricular discordance and ventricular arterial discordance such that deoxygenated blood passes through the LV and out the PA, whereas oxygenated blood passes to the systemic RV that pumps out the aorta; therefore, these patients are not cyanotic. However, most patients with c-TGA have associated cardiac anomalies, including VSD, pulmonary stenosis, or dysplastic tricuspid (systemic atrioventricular) valves. The prevalence of systemic RV dysfunction in this condition varies based on associated anomalies. In one large multicenter study of adults with c-TGA, systemic RV dysfunction and heart failure were higher with increasing age, the presence of significant associated cardiac lesions, history of arrhythmia, pacemaker implantation, and prior cardiac surgery.[99] Tricuspid (systemic atrioventricular) valve regurgitation contributes to systemic RV failure in c-TGA patients. Surgical replacement of the tricuspid valve should be considered before the RV EF falls below 40% and the pulmonary artery systolic pressure rises above 50 mm Hg.[100]

There have been several small case series examining the effectiveness of β-blockers in patients with a systemic RV, with a limited number of patients and follow-up and variable results (see Table 25-1).[101-103] The studies were all underpowered, making it difficult to draw definitive conclusions.

The data for use of agents to inhibit the renin-angiotensin-aldosterone system (RAAS) in patients with systemic RV are also limited (see Table 25-1). Therrien reported the results of a prospective, double-blind, randomized, placebo-controlled clinical trial of ramipril for 1 year in 17 adults with TGA who had undergone an atrial switch procedure and found no significant increase in the systemic RV EF.[104] Small trials of angiotensin receptor blockers have also showed conflicting results. Recently, van der Bom reported the results of a multicenter, double-blind, randomized controlled trial of valsartan compared with placebo in patients with a systemic RV. There was no significant treatment effect of valsartan on RV EF, exercise capacity, or quality of life during 3-year follow-up.[105] This study concluded that there is no evidence for the routine use of angiotensin receptor blockers in asymptomatic patients with a systemic RV.

Single Ventricle

Most patients with a single functional ventricle undergo the Fontan operation, whereby systemic venous return is diverted to the pulmonary arteries without the aid of a subpulmonic pumping chamber (**Figure 25-7**). This physiology requires chronic elevations in central venous pressure to maintain adequate blood flow through the pulmonary circulation. Heart failure is common after the Fontan operation and is more likely in older patients, those with conduction abnormalities, and those who had their surgery in an older era of Fontan operation.[106-108] Rather than being a single disease, the failing Fontan circulation is a diverse group of conditions with varying presentation and underlying pathophysiology.

In the Fontan circulation, central venous pressure drives blood through the lungs to the left heart. Therefore, any condition that elevates left atrial pressure or increases pulmonary vascular resistance has deleterious effects on Fontan hemodynamics and necessitates either a rise in central venous pressure, a drop in cardiac output, or the formation of decompressing systemic venous to pulmonary venous collaterals. Frequent culprit lesions that increase Fontan pressure include systolic dysfunction, restrictive ventricular physiology, pulmonary vein stenosis (particularly the left lower pulmonary vein), obstruction within the Fontan circuit (e.g., branch pulmonary artery stenosis), or pressure loss as a result of hemodynamic inefficiencies in the Fontan circuit.[109] These hemodynamic perturbations are poorly tolerated in Fontan circulation; therefore, pathway obstruction and valve dysfunction should be aggressively sought out and treated if found. In carefully selected patients, pulmonary artery vasodilators may be useful once mechanical issues have been addressed.[110,111]

Ventricular dysfunction is relatively common in patients with Fontan circulation, perhaps because of excessive afterload and resulting alterations in ventricular-vascular coupling.[112] In patients with systemic LV systolic dysfunction, conventional heart failure treatments with ACE inhibitors and β-blockers are used. Their utility in patients with a morphologic RV is not well established and is discussed in detail elsewhere in this chapter.

Many patients with Fontan circulation have clinical deterioration for reasons other than ventricular dysfunction or pathway obstruction. Atrial tachyarrhythmias, most commonly intra-atrial reentrant tachycardia or ectopic atrial tachycardia, are common in patients who had older style Fontan completion before the 1990s.[113] Atrial arrhythmias are poorly tolerated in Fontan circulation[114] and should be treated with cardioversion, antiarrhythmic medications, ablation, or surgical conversion to a modern extracardiac Fontan by a center with expertise in the management of arrhythmias in congenital heart disease.

Liver disease is common in Fontan patients due to a combination of high central venous pressure, reduced hepatic blood flow, and perioperative liver injury.[74] Liver dysfunction can manifest as radiologic evidence of fibrosis or as overt cirrhosis with ascites and varices. The presence of significant liver dysfunction carries poor prognosis[115] and should prompt a hemodynamic evaluation. Unfortunately, the presence of significant liver disease can be a barrier to heart transplantation in Fontan patients. Patients with cirrhosis are at risk for perioperative complications, such as hepatorenal syndrome, infection, and bleeding. There is no consensus on whether resolution of liver disease is expected after heart transplantation. Multidisciplinary care is needed from an adult CHD doctor, a transplant team, and a hepatologist.

SUMMARY

Heart failure is increasingly recognized in ACHD patients and heart failure–related complications are the most common cause of death in these patients.[3] The prevalence of heart failure is highest in patients with complex anatomy, including single-ventricle physiology, transposition of TGA, TOF, and those with pulmonary hypertension. The diagnosis of heart failure in ACHD patients may be challenging because patients with CHD, having lived their lives with cardiac disease, may not detect subtle changes in their exercise capacity and underreport their symptoms. By the time they notice symptoms, the extent of ventricular dysfunction and valve disease may be severe and irreversible. Objective measures of ventricular function through imaging, exercise testing, and serum biomarkers can be very helpful

CLASSIC FONTAN

A

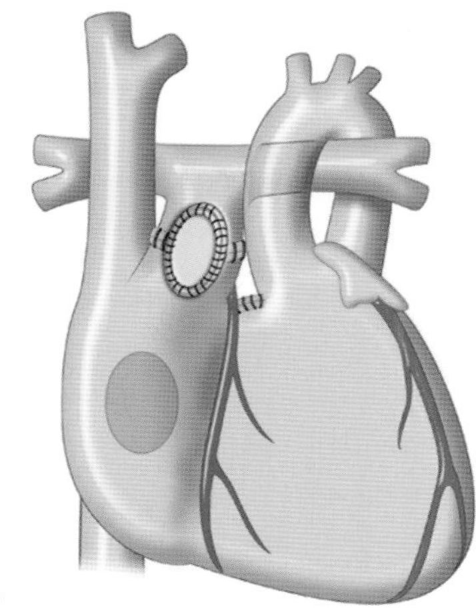

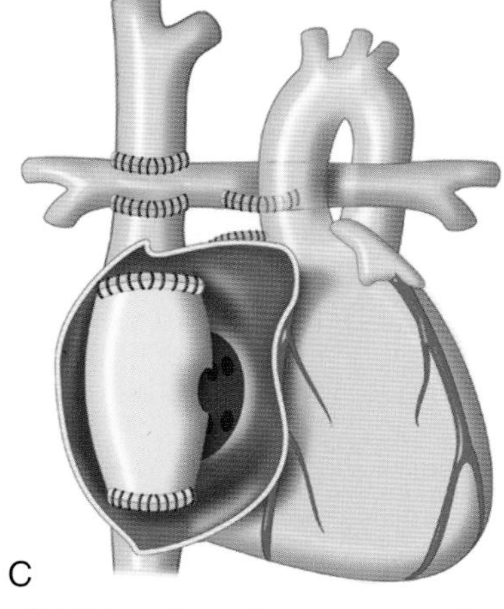

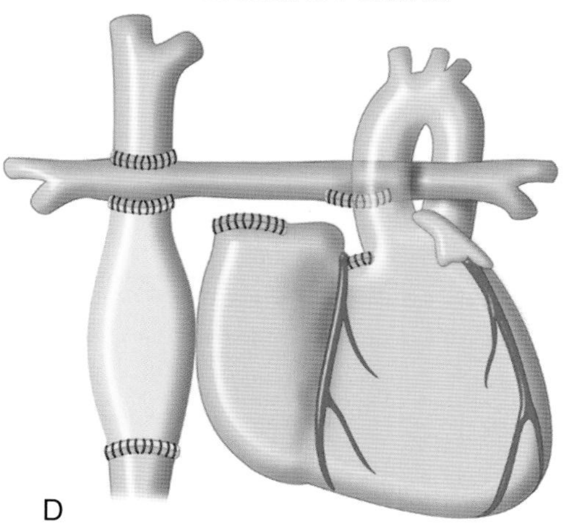

FIGURE 25-7 Diagrammatic representation of the various types of Fontan surgeries. **A,** The classic style Fontan, which consists of a conduit from the inferior vena cava to the left pulmonary artery and a classic right Glenn procedure (superior vena cava to the right pulmonary artery). **B,** The atriopulmonary connection has been largely abandoned because of dilation of the right atrium, predisposing to thrombosis and atrial arrhythmias. **C,** Lateral tunnel is widely used in part because of the ease of creating a fenestration in this type. **D,** Extracardiac conduits are often used because they do not create extensive atrial sutures and may be performed off bypass. *Modified from Libby P: Essential atlas of cardiovascular disease, New York, 2009, Springer.*

in these patients. The evaluation of heart failure symptoms in an ACHD patient must be tailored to the patient's anatomy and prior interventions and should include evaluation for residual shunts, baffle stenosis, valvular or conduit dysfunction, and collateral vessels, which may be amenable to interventions. Potential therapies for heart failure in ACHD patients include medical therapies, device therapies, and surgical interventions, such as mechanical assist devices and transplantation. However, guidelines for the management of acquired heart failure are often not applicable to the patient with CHD because of disease heterogeneity, unusual mechanisms of heart failure, and unique comorbidities in the ACHD patient. Multicenter trials are needed to better define the appropriate therapies for this growing group of patients, and a multidisciplinary team with expertise in ACHD and advanced heart failure is required to manage this challenging population.

References

1. Bolger AP, Coats AJ, Gatzoulis MA: Congenital heart disease: the original heart failure syndrome. *Eur Heart J* 24:970–976, 2003.
2. Opotowsky AR, Siddiqi OK, Webb GD: Trends in hospitalizations for adults with congenital heart disease in the U.S. *J Am Coll Cardiol* 54:460–467, 2009.
3. Verheugt CL, Uiterwaal CS, van der Velde ET, et al: Mortality in adult congenital heart disease. *Eur Heart J* 31:1220–1229, 2010.
4. O'Leary JM, Siddiqi OK, de Ferranti S, et al: The changing demographics of congenital heart disease hospitalizations in the United States, 1998 through 2010. *JAMA* 309:984–986, 2013.
5. Khairy P, Ionescu-Ittu R, Mackie AS, et al: Changing mortality in congenital heart disease. *J Am Coll Cardiol* 56:1149–1157, 2010.
6. Marelli AJ, Mackie AS, Ionescu-Ittu R, et al: Congenital heart disease in the general population: changing prevalence and age distribution. *Circulation* 115:163–172, 2007.
7. Gurvitz M, Valente AM, Broberg C, et al: Prevalence and predictors of gaps in care among adult congenital heart disease patients: HEART-ACHD (The Health, Education, and Access Research Trial). *J Am Coll Cardiol* 61:2180–2184, 2013.
8. Norozi K, Wessel A, Alpers V, et al: Incidence and risk distribution of heart failure in adolescents and adults with congenital heart disease after cardiac surgery. *Am J Cardiol* 97:1238–1243, 2006.
9. Oechslin EN, Harrison DA, Connelly MS, et al: Mode of death in adults with congenital heart disease. *Am J Cardiol* 86:1111–1116, 2000.
10. Nieminen HP, Jokinen EV, Sairanen HI: Causes of late deaths after pediatric cardiac surgery: a population-based study. *J Am Coll Cardiol* 50:1263–1271, 2007.
11. Piran S, Veldtman G, Siu S, et al: Heart failure and ventricular dysfunction in patients with single or systemic right ventricles. *Circulation* 105:1189–1194, 2002.
12. Zomer AC, Vaartjes I, van der Velde ET, et al: Heart failure admissions in adults with congenital heart disease; risk factors and prognosis. *Int J Cardiol* 168:2487–2493, 2013.
13. Rodriguez FH, 3rd, Moodie DS, Parekh DR, et al: Outcomes of heart failure-related hospitalization in adults with congenital heart disease in the United States. *Congenit Heart Dis* 8:513–519, 2013.
14. Lowe BS, Therrien J, Ionescu-Ittu R, et al: Diagnosis of pulmonary hypertension in the congenital heart disease adult population impact on outcomes. *J Am Coll Cardiol* 58:538–546, 2011.
15. Gratz A, Hess J, Hager A: Self-estimated physical functioning poorly predicts actual exercise capacity in adolescents and adults with congenital heart disease. *Eur Heart J* 30:497–504, 2009.

16. Diller GP, Dimopoulos K, Okonko D, et al: Exercise intolerance in adult congenital heart disease: comparative severity, correlates, and prognostic implication. *Circulation* 112:828–835, 2005.
17. Warnes CA, Williams RG, Bashore TM, et al: ACC/AHA 2008 guidelines for the management of adults with congenital heart disease: Executive summary: a report of the American College of Cardiology/American Heart Association task force on practice guidelines (writing committee to develop guidelines for the management of adults with congenital heart disease). *Circulation* 118:2395–2451, 2008.
18. Wang J, Prakasa K, Bomma C, et al: Comparison of novel echocardiographic parameters of right ventricular function with ejection fraction by cardiac magnetic resonance. *J Am Soc Echocardiogr* 20:1058–1064, 2007.
19. Crean AM, Maredia N, Ballard G, et al: 3D echo systematically underestimates right ventricular volumes compared to cardiovascular magnetic resonance in adult congenital heart disease patients with moderate or severe RV dilatation. *J Cardiovasc Magn Reson* 13:78, 2011.
20. Friedberg MK, Mertens L: Deformation imaging in selected congenital heart disease: is it evolving to clinical use? *J Am Soc Echocardiogr* 25:919–931, 2012.
21. Friedman KG, McElhinney DB, Rhodes J, et al: Left ventricular diastolic function in children and young adults with congenital aortic valve disease. *Am J Cardiol* 111:243–249, 2013.
22. Partington SL, Valente AM: Cardiac magnetic resonance in adults with congenital heart disease. *Methodist Debakey Cardiovasc J* 9:156–162, 2013.
23. Babu-Narayan SV, Kilner PJ, Li W, et al: Ventricular fibrosis suggested by cardiovascular magnetic resonance in adults with repaired tetralogy of Fallot and its relationship to adverse markers of clinical outcome. *Circulation* 113:405–413, 2006.
24. Babu-Narayan SV, Goktekin O, Moon JC, et al: Late gadolinium enhancement cardiovascular magnetic resonance of the systemic right ventricle in adults with previous atrial redirection surgery for transposition of the great arteries. *Circulation* 111:2091–2098, 2005.
25. Rathod RH, Prakash A, Powell AJ, et al: Myocardial fibrosis identified by cardiac magnetic resonance late gadolinium enhancement is associated with adverse ventricular mechanics and ventricular tachycardia late after fontan operation. *J Am Coll Cardiol* 55:1721–1728, 2010.
26. Inuzuka R, Diller GP, Borgia F, et al: Comprehensive use of cardiopulmonary exercise testing identifies adults with congenital heart disease at increased mortality risk in the medium term. *Circulation* 125:250–259, 2012.
27. Diller GP, Dimopoulos K, Okonko D, et al: Heart rate response during exercise predicts survival in adults with congenital heart disease. *J Am Coll Cardiol* 48:1250–1256, 2006.
28. Kempny A, Dimopoulos K, Uebing A, et al: Reference values for exercise limitations among adults with congenital heart disease. Relation to activities of daily life–single centre experience and review of published data. *Eur Heart J* 33:1386–1396, 2012.
29. Dimopoulos K, Okonko DO, Diller GP, et al: Abnormal ventilatory response to exercise in adults with congenital heart disease relates to cyanosis and predicts survival. *Circulation* 113:2796–2802, 2006.
30. Rhodes J, Dave A, Pulling MC, et al: Effect of pulmonary artery stenoses on the cardiopulmonary response to exercise following repair of tetralogy of Fallot. *Am J Cardiol* 81:1217–1219, 1998.
31. Sutton NJ, Peng L, Lock JE, et al: Effect of pulmonary artery angioplasty on exercise function after repair of tetralogy of Fallot. *Am Heart J* 155:182–186, 2008.
32. Fernandes SM, Alexander ME, Graham DA, et al: Exercise testing identifies patients at increased risk for morbidity and mortality following Fontan surgery. *Congenit Heart Dis* 6:294–303, 2011.
33. Bolger AP, Sharma R, Li W, et al: Neurohormonal activation and the chronic heart failure syndrome in adults with congenital heart disease. *Circulation* 106:92–99, 2002.
34. Giannakoulas G, Dimopoulos K, Bolger AP, et al: Usefulness of natriuretic peptide levels to predict mortality in adults with congenital heart disease. *Am J Cardiol* 105:869–873, 2010.
35. Koch AM, Zink S, Singer H, et al: B-type natriuretic peptide levels in patients with functionally univentricular hearts after total cavopulmonary connection. *Eur J Heart Fail* 10:60–62, 2008.
36. Eindhoven JA, van den Bosch AE, Ruys TP, et al: N-terminal pro-b-type natriuretic peptide and its relationship with cardiac function in adults with congenital heart disease. *J Am Coll Cardiol* 62:1203–1212, 2013.
37. Man BL, Cheung YF: Plasma brain natriuretic peptide and systemic ventricular function in asymptomatic patients late after the Fontan procedure. *Heart Vessels* 22:398–403, 2007.
38. Robbers-Visser D, Kapusta L, van Osch-Gevers L, et al: Clinical outcome 5 to 18 years after the Fontan operation performed on children younger than 5 years. *J Thorac Cardiovasc Surg* 138:89–95, 2009.
39. Lechner E, Schreier-Lechner EM, Hofer A, et al: Aminoterminal brain-type natriuretic peptide levels correlate with heart failure in patients with bidirectional Glenn anastomosis and with morbidity after the Fontan operation. *J Thorac Cardiovasc Surg* 138:560–564, 2009.
40. Lechner E, Gitter R, Mair R, et al: Aminoterminal brain natriuretic peptide levels in children and adolescents after Fontan operation correlate with congestive heart failure. *Pediatr Cardiol* 29:901–905, 2008.
41. Holzmeister J, Leclercq C: Implantable cardioverter defibrillators and cardiac resynchronisation therapy. *Lancet* 378:722–730, 2011.
42. van der Hulst AE, Delgado V, Blom NA, et al: Cardiac resynchronization therapy in paediatric and congenital heart disease patients. *Eur Heart J* 32:2236–2246, 2011.
43. Dubin AM, Janousek J, Rhee E, et al: Resynchronization therapy in pediatric and congenital heart disease patients: an international multicenter study. *J Am Coll Cardiol* 46:2277–2283, 2005.
44. Cecchin F, Frangini PA, Brown DW, et al: Cardiac resynchronization therapy (and multisite pacing) in pediatrics and congenital heart disease: five years experience in a single institution. *J Cardiovasc Electrophysiol* 20:58–65, 2009.
45. Janousek J, Gebauer RA, Abdul-Khaliq H, et al: Cardiac resynchronisation therapy in paediatric and congenital heart disease: differential effects in various anatomical and functional substrates. *Heart* 95:1165–1171, 2009.
46. Gatzoulis MA, Till JA, Somerville J, et al: Mechanoelectrical interaction in tetralogy of Fallot. QRS prolongation relates to right ventricular size and predicts malignant ventricular arrhythmias and sudden death. *Circulation* 92:231–237, 1995.
47. Gatzoulis MA, Balaji S, Webber SA, et al: Risk factors for arrhythmia and sudden cardiac death late after repair of tetralogy of Fallot: a multicentre study. *Lancet* 356:975–981, 2000.
48. Kaszala K, Ellenbogen KA: When right may not be right: right bundle-branch block and response to cardiac resynchronization therapy. *Circulation* 122:1999–2001, 2010.
49. Uebing A, Gibson DG, Babu-Narayan SV, et al: Right ventricular mechanics and QRS duration in patients with repaired tetralogy of Fallot: implications of infundibular disease. *Circulation* 116:1532–1539, 2007.
50. Thambo JB, Dos Santos P, Bordachar P: Cardiac resynchronization therapy in patients with congenital heart disease. *Arch Cardiovasc Dis* 104:410–416, 2011.
51. Diller GP, Okonko D, Uebing A, et al: Cardiac resynchronization therapy for adult congenital heart disease patients with a systemic right ventricle: analysis of feasibility and review of early experience. *Europace* 8:267–272, 2006.
52. Chow PC, Liang XC, Lam WW, et al: Mechanical right ventricular dyssynchrony in patients after atrial switch operation for transposition of the great arteries. *Am J Cardiol* 101:874–881, 2008.
53. Jauvert G, Rousseau-Paziaud J, Villain E, et al: Effects of cardiac resynchronization therapy on echocardiographic indices, functional capacity, and clinical outcomes of patients with a systemic right ventricle. *Europace* 11:184–190, 2009.
54. Silva JN, Ghosh S, Bowman TM, et al: Cardiac resynchronization therapy in pediatric congenital heart disease: insights from noninvasive electrocardiographic imaging. *Heart Rhythm* 6:1178–1185, 2009.
55. Bacha EA, Zimmerman FJ, Mor-Avi V, et al: Ventricular resynchronization by multisite pacing improves myocardial performance in the postoperative single-ventricle patient. *Ann Thorac Surg* 78:1678–1683, 2004.
56. Sojak V, Mazic U, Cesen M, et al: Cardiac resynchronization therapy for the failing Fontan patient. *Ann Thorac Surg* 85:2136–2138, 2008.
57. Taylor DO, Edwards LB, Aurora P, et al: Registry of the international society for heart and lung transplantation: twenty-fifth official adult heart transplant report–2008. *J Heart Lung Transplant* 27:943–956, 2008.
58. Patel ND, Weiss ES, Allen JG, et al: Heart transplantation for adults with congenital heart disease: analysis of the United Network for Organ Sharing database. *Ann Thorac Surg* 88:814–821, discussion 821–822, 2009.
59. Lamour JM, Kanter KR, Naftel DC, et al: The effect of age, diagnosis, and previous surgery in children and adults undergoing heart transplantation for congenital heart disease. *J Am Coll Cardiol* 54:160–165, 2009.
60. Karamlou T, Hirsch J, Welke K, et al: A United Network for Organ Sharing analysis of heart transplantation in adults with congenital heart disease: outcomes and factors associated with mortality and retransplantation. *J Thorac Cardiovasc Surg* 140:161–168, 2010.
61. Pigula FA, Gandhi SK, Ristich J, et al: Cardiopulmonary transplantation for congenital heart disease in the adult. *J Heart Lung Transplant* 20:297–303, 2001.
62. Chen JM, Davies RR, Mital SR, et al: Trends and outcomes in transplantation for complex congenital heart disease: 1984 to 2004. *Ann Thorac Surg* 78:1352–1361, discussion 1352–1361, 2004.
63. Lamour JM, Hsu DT, Quaegebeur JM, et al: Heart transplantation to a physiologic single lung in patients with congenital heart disease. *J Heart Lung Transplant* 23:948–953, 2004.
64. Hosseinpour AR, Cullen S, Tsang VT: Transplantation for adults with congenital heart disease. *Eur J Cardiothorac Surg* 30:508–514, 2006.
65. Levy WC, Mozaffarian D, Linker DT, et al: The Seattle heart failure model: prediction of survival in heart failure. *Circulation* 113:1424–1433, 2006.
66. Giardini A, Hager A, Lammers AE, et al: Ventilatory efficiency and aerobic capacity predict event-free survival in adults with atrial repair for complete transposition of the great arteries. *J Am Coll Cardiol* 53:1548–1555, 2009.
67. Diller GP, Giardini A, Dimopoulos K, et al: Predictors of morbidity and mortality in contemporary Fontan patients: results from a multicenter study including cardiopulmonary exercise testing in 321 patients. *Eur Heart J* 31:3073–3083, 2010.
68. Dimopoulos K, Inuzuka R, Goletto S, et al: Improved survival among patients with Eisenmenger syndrome receiving advanced therapy for pulmonary arterial hypertension. *Circulation* 121:20–25, 2010.
69. McGlothlin D, De Marco T: Transplantation in adults with congenital heart disease. *Prog Cardiovasc Dis* 53:312–323, 2011.
70. Nwakanma LU, Williams JA, Weiss ES, et al: Influence of pretransplant panel-reactive antibody on outcomes in 8,160 heart transplant recipients in recent era. *Ann Thorac Surg* 84:1556–1562, discussion 1562–1563, 2007.
71. Harper AR, Crossland DS, Perri G, et al: Is alternative cardiac surgery an option in adults with congenital heart disease referred for thoracic organ transplantation? *Eur J Cardiothorac Surg* 43:344–351, 2013.
72. Everitt MD, Donaldson AE, Stehlik J, et al: Would access to device therapies improve transplant outcomes for adults with congenital heart disease? Analysis of the United Network for Organ Sharing (UNOS). *J Heart Lung Transplant* 30:395–401, 2011.
73. Dardas T, Mokadam NA, Pagani F, et al: Transplant registrants with implanted left ventricular assist devices have insufficient risk to justify elective organ procurement and transplantation network status 1a time. *J Am Coll Cardiol* 60:36–43, 2012.
74. Wu FM, Ukomadu C, Odze RD, et al: Liver disease in the patient with Fontan circulation. *Congenit Heart Dis* 6:190–201, 2011.
75. Bernstein D, Naftel D, Chin C, et al: Outcome of listing for cardiac transplantation for failed Fontan: a multi-institutional study. *Circulation* 114:273–280, 2006.
76. Shah NR, Lam WW, Rodriguez FH, 3rd, et al: Clinical outcomes after ventricular assist device implantation in adults with complex congenital heart disease. *J Heart Lung Transplant* 32:615–620, 2013.
77. Davlouros PA, Kilner PJ, Hornung TS, et al: Right ventricular function in adults with repaired tetralogy of Fallot assessed with cardiovascular magnetic resonance imaging: detrimental role of right ventricular outflow aneurysms or akinesia and adverse right-to-left ventricular interaction. *J Am Coll Cardiol* 40:2044–2052, 2002.
78. Wald RM, Haber I, Wald R, et al: Effects of regional dysfunction and late gadolinium enhancement on global right ventricular function and exercise capacity in patients with repaired tetralogy of Fallot. *Circulation* 119:1370–1377, 2009.
79. Frigiola A, Redington AN, Cullen S, et al: Pulmonary regurgitation is an important determinant of right ventricular contractile dysfunction in patients with surgically repaired tetralogy of Fallot. *Circulation* 110:II153–II157, 2004.
80. Therrien J, Siu SC, McLaughlin PR, et al: Pulmonary valve replacement in adults late after repair of tetralogy of Fallot: are we operating too late? *J Am Coll Cardiol* 36:1670–1675, 2000.
81. Latus H, Binder W, Kerst G, et al: Right ventricular-pulmonary arterial coupling in patients after repair of tetralogy of Fallot. *J Thorac Cardiovasc Surg* 146:1366–1372, 2013.
82. Gatzoulis MA, Clark AL, Cullen S, et al: Right ventricular diastolic function 15 to 35 years after repair of tetralogy of Fallot. Restrictive physiology predicts superior exercise performance. *Circulation* 91:1775–1781, 1995.
83. Oosterhof T, van Straten A, Vliegen HW, et al: Preoperative thresholds for pulmonary valve replacement in patients with corrected tetralogy of Fallot using cardiovascular magnetic resonance. *Circulation* 116:545–551, 2007.
84. Vliegen HW, van Straten A, de Roos A, et al: Magnetic resonance imaging to assess the hmodynamic effects of pulmonary valve replacement in adults late after repair of tetralogy of Fallot. *Circulation* 106:1703–1707, 2002.
85. Buechel ER, Dave HH, Kellenberger CJ, et al: Remodelling of the right ventricle after early pulmonary valve replacement in children with repaired tetralogy of Fallot: assessment by cardiovascular magnetic resonance. *Eur Heart J* 26:2721–2727, 2005.
86. Vliegen HW, van Straten A, de Roos A, et al: Magnetic resonance imaging to assess the hemodynamic effects of pulmonary valve replacement in adults late after repair of tetralogy of Fallot. *Circulation* 106:1703–1707, 2002.
87. Therrien J, Provost Y, Merchant N, et al: Optimal timing for pulmonary valve replacement in adults after tetralogy of Fallot repair. *Am J Cardiol* 95:779–782, 2005.
88. Harrild DM, Berul CI, Cecchin F, et al: Pulmonary valve replacement in tetralogy of Fallot: impact on survival and ventricular tachycardia. *Circulation* 119:445–451, 2009.
89. Geva T, Gauvreau K, Powell AJ, et al: Randomized trial of pulmonary valve replacement with and without right ventricular remodeling surgery. *Circulation* 122:S201–S208, 2010.

90. Babu-Narayan SV, Uebing A, Davlouros PA, et al: Randomised trial of ramipril in repaired tetralogy of Fallot and pulmonary regurgitation: the appropriate study (ACE inhibitors for potential prevention of the deleterious effects of pulmonary regurgitation in adults with repaired tetralogy of Fallot). *Int J Cardiol* 154:299–305, 2012.
91. Broberg CS, Aboulhosn J, Mongeon FP, et al: Prevalence of left ventricular systolic dysfunction in adults with repaired tetralogy of Fallot. *Am J Cardiol* 107:1215–1220, 2011.
92. Khairy P, Aboulhosn J, Gurvitz MZ, et al: Arrhythmia burden in adults with surgically repaired tetralogy of Fallot: a multi-institutional study. *Circulation* 122:868–875, 2010.
93. Ghai A, Silversides C, Harris L, et al: Left ventricular dysfunction is a risk factor for sudden cardiac death in adults late after repair of tetralogy of Fallot. *J Am Coll Cardiol* 40:1675–1680, 2002.
94. Davlouros PA, Kilner PJ, Hornung TS, et al: Right ventricular function in adults with repaired tetralogy of Fallot assessed with cardiovascular magnetic resonance imaging: detrimental role of right ventricular outflow aneurysms or akinesia and adverse right-to-left ventricular interaction. *J Am Coll Cardiol* 40:2044–2052, 2002.
95. Kammeraad JA, van Deurzen CH, Sreeram N, et al: Predictors of sudden cardiac death after Mustard or Senning repair for transposition of the great arteries. *J Am Coll Cardiol* 44:1095–1102, 2004.
96. Kirjavainen M, Happonen JM, Louhimo I: Late results of Senning operation. *J Thorac Cardiovasc Surg* 117:488–495, 1999.
97. Hucin B, Voriskova M, Hruda J, et al: Late complications and quality of life after atrial correction of transposition of the great arteries in 12 to 18 year follow-up. *J Cardiovasc Surg (Torino)* 41:233–239, 2000.
98. Fratz S, Hager A, Busch R, et al: Patients after atrial switch operation for transposition of the great arteries cannot increase stroke volume under dobutamine stress as opposed to patients with congenitally corrected transposition. *Circ J* 72:1130–1135, 2008.
99. Graham TP, Jr, Bernard YD, Mellen BG, et al: Long-term outcome in congenitally corrected transposition of the great arteries: a multi-institutional study. *J Am Coll Cardiol* 36:255–261, 2000.
100. Mongeon FP, Connolly HM, Dearani JA, et al: Congenitally corrected transposition of the great arteries ventricular function at the time of systemic atrioventricular valve replacement predicts long-term ventricular function. *J Am Coll Cardiol* 57:2008–2017, 2011.
101. Lindenfeld J, Keller K, Campbell DN, et al: Improved systemic ventricular function after carvedilol administration in a patient with congenitally corrected transposition of the great arteries. *J Heart Lung Transplant* 22:198–201, 2003.
102. Doughan AR, McConnell ME, Book WM: Effect of beta blockers (carvedilol or metoprolol xl) in patients with transposition of great arteries and dysfunction of the systemic right ventricle. *Am J Cardiol* 99:704–706, 2007.
103. Josephson CB, Howlett JG, Jackson SD, et al: A case series of systemic right ventricular dysfunction post atrial switch for simple d-transposition of the great arteries: the impact of beta-blockade. *Can J Cardiol* 22:769–772, 2006.
104. Therrien J, Provost Y, Harrison J, et al: Effect of angiotensin receptor blockade on systemic right ventricular function and size: a small, randomized, placebo-controlled study. *Int J Cardiol* 129:187–192, 2008.
105. van der Bom T, Winter MM, Bouma BJ, et al: Effect of valsartan on systemic right ventricular function: a double-blind, randomized, placebo-controlled pilot trial. *Circulation* 127:322–330, 2013.
106. Gentles TL, Gauvreau K, Mayer JE, Jr, et al: Functional outcome after the Fontan operation: factors influencing late morbidity. *J Thorac Cardiovasc Surg* 114:392–403, discussion 404–405, 1997.
107. Gentles TL, Mayer JE, Jr, Gauvreau K, et al: Fontan operation in five hundred consecutive patients: factors influencing early and late outcome. *J Thorac Cardiovasc Surg* 114:376–391, 1997.
108. Khairy P, Fernandes SM, Mayer JE, Jr, et al: Long-term survival, modes of death, and predictors of mortality in patients with Fontan surgery. *Circulation* 117:85–92, 2008.
109. Deal BJ, Jacobs ML: Management of the failing Fontan circulation. *Heart* 98:1098–1104, 2012.
110. Goldberg DJ, French B, McBride MG, et al: Impact of oral sildenafil on exercise performance in children and young adults after the Fontan operation: a randomized, double-blind, placebo-controlled, crossover trial. *Circulation* 123:1185–1193, 2011.
111. Giardini A, Balducci A, Specchia S, et al: Effect of sildenafil on haemodynamic response to exercise and exercise capacity in Fontan patients. *Eur Heart J* 29:1681–1687, 2008.
112. Senzaki H, Masutani S, Ishido H, et al: Cardiac rest and reserve function in patients with Fontan circulation. *J Am Coll Cardiol* 47:2528–2535, 2006.
113. Nurnberg JH, Ovroutski S, Alexi-Meskishvili V, et al: New onset arrhythmias after the extracardiac conduit Fontan operation compared with the intraatrial lateral tunnel procedure: early and midterm results. *Ann Thorac Surg* 78:1979–1988, discussion 1988, 2004.
114. Ghai A, Harris L, Harrison DA, et al: Outcomes of late atrial tachyarrhythmias in adults after the Fontan operation. *J Am Coll Cardiol* 37:585–592, 2001.
115. Camposilvan S, Milanesi O, Stellin G, et al: Liver and cardiac function in the long term after Fontan operation. *Ann Thorac Surg* 86:177–182, 2008.

26 Heart Failure as a Consequence of Viral and Nonviral Myocarditis

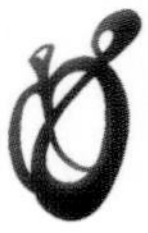

Dennis M. McNamara

In the attempt to diagnose heart disease more accurately, the term myocarditis is wisely being abandoned in large part; we must remember, nevertheless, that there does exist such a condition as myocarditis....

Paul Dudley White[1]

Dr. White's concerns about the "abandonment" of the term *myocarditis* were unfounded, and over half a century after his initial observations myocarditis remains an important pathologic term defining of diverse set of cardiac disorders involving primary myocardial inflammation. For his readership in the 1950s, the primary infectious causes of myocardial inflammation were rheumatic fever and diphtheroids, for which effective antibiotic therapies were later developed. In the present day, an ever-changing group of viral etiologies has proven much more difficult to eradicate. Acute myocardial inflammation plays a critical role in viral clearing, but in chronic pathologic states inflammation may play a role in the pathogenesis of nonischemic cardiomyopathy. However, while immune suppression plays an important role in very specific pathologic diagnostic subsets of myocarditis, for the vast majority of cases there is no proven benefit.

Although infectious causes remain important, the category of myocarditis includes a diverse set of disorders for which there is no discernible infectious cause, from transient myocardial dysfunction with allergic eosinophilic myocarditis to the progressive myocyte destruction that characterizes giant cell myocarditis (GCM). This chapter will discuss the pathogenesis of heart failure from viral and nonviral forms of myocarditis, the current practice of supportive heart failure treatment, the hope for future targeted therapeutics, and in the case of fulminant myocarditis, the role of mechanical therapy as a bridge to recovery. Despite decades of clinical and basic investigation since Paul Dudley White's initial observations,[1] the diagnosis and treatment of myocarditis remain extremely challenging.

HISTORY

The French pathologist Corvisart described "carditis" in 1806 as an important clinical syndrome, which most commonly was acute and fatal but could develop into more "chronic organic disease."[2] The term *carditis* was later refined to *myocarditis,* first introduced by Sobernheim in 1837,[3] to describe the myocardial inflammation presumed to be the cause of most nonvalvular cardiac dysfunction. By the latter part of the nineteenth century it was increasingly recognized that primary myocardial inflammation was responsible for only a small subset of nonvalvular cardiac dysfunction, because coronary disease and hypertensive heart disease were far more common causes. In contrast to the previous nondiscriminant use of the term, attempts at more accurate cardiac diagnosis of myocarditis in the twentieth century led to a mark diminishment in its recognition.

The emergence of endomyocardial biopsy (EMB) in the 1960s as a diagnostic tool[4] increased the ability of clinicians to delineate cellular inflammation of the myocardium, and led to the hope that this heterogeneous group of patients with primary cardiomyopathy could now be classified into histopathologic subsets with distinct therapies and outcomes. The Dallas criteria[5] were developed in 1986 by a group of leading cardiac pathologists to standardize the histologic definition of lymphocytic myocarditis, the most commonly observed form of cellular inflammation. They defined *borderline myocarditis* as mononuclear cell infiltrates without myocyte necrosis (**Figure 26-1**) and *myocarditis* as cellular infiltration with myocyte necrosis (**Figure 26-2**). Despite the wide acceptance of these histologic criteria for the pathologic assessment of myocarditis, significant variation in interpretation remained in the practical application.[6] A decade later, the World Health Organization task force defined inflammatory cardiomyopathy as "myocarditis in association with myocardial dysfunction. Myocarditis is an inflammatory disease of the myocardium and is diagnosed by established histologic, immunologic, and

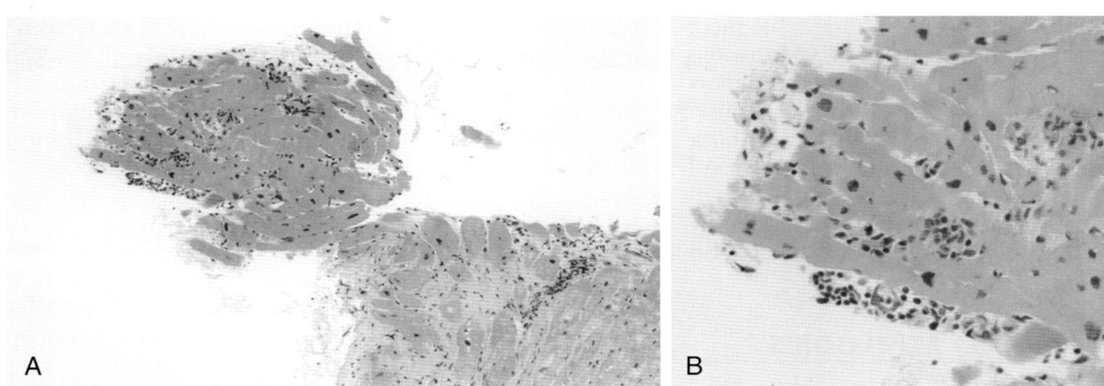

FIGURE 26-1 Histopathologic appearance of borderline myocarditis by Dallas criteria (lymphocytic infiltrates without myocyte necrosis) with routine staining with hematoxylin and eosin (H&E) under **A,** low power (100×) and **B,** high power (350×).

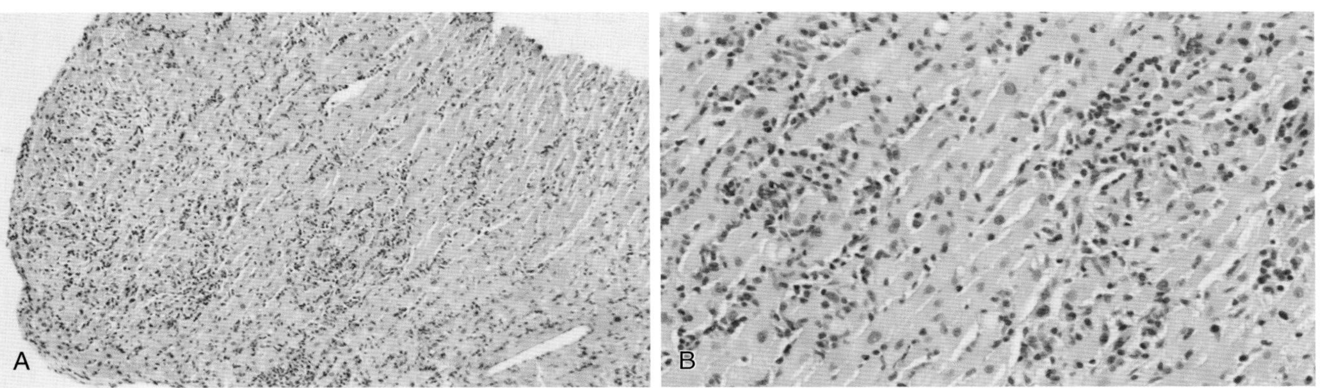

FIGURE 26-2 Histopathologic appearance of myocarditis by Dallas criteria (lymphocytic infiltrates with myocyte necrosis) with routine staining with hematoxylin and eosin under **A,** low power (100×) and **B,** high power (350×).

immunohistochemical criteria."[7] This task force expanded the definition by adding the quantitative criteria of diffuse mononuclear infiltrates with greater than 14 cells/mm^2, as well as immunohistochemical criteria for both detection of cellular infiltrates and expression of HLA class II molecules.

The observed histologic similarity of lymphocytic myocarditis to cardiac allograft rejection led to the hypothesis that a therapeutic strategy of immunosuppression would improve clinical outcomes. When the Myocarditis Treatment Trial demonstrated no benefit,[8] the absence of a histologically guided therapy led to a diminished role for endomyocardial biopsy, and native cardiac biopsy is not commonly performed in the United States. Efforts continue to improve the diagnostic utility of EMB with the addition of molecular diagnostics to detect viral nucleic acids and routine immunohistochemistry to improve the specificity, but this is only performed at selected centers.[9] The histologic and clinical diversity of myocarditis remains a challenge in terms of the development of targeted therapeutics.

VIRAL ETIOLOGIES

The most common infectious agents initiating myocarditis in North America are viral pathogens (**Table 26-1**), although the dominant viral species continues to evolve over time and differs across eras. Enteroviruses, in particular coxsackie B, were first described in clinical and serologic studies decades ago[10] and remain a major cause in infants and children.[11] In adults adenovirus, influenza A and B, and herpesviruses have also been implicated as important viral pathogens,[12-14] whereas hepatitis C has been implicated in Asia,[15] but less commonly reported in case series in the United States. Over the past decade influenza and erythroviruses, such as parvovirus B19,[16] emerged as two important pathogens associated with myocarditis. The changing viral milieu represents a considerable challenge for developing therapeutic efforts targeting specific viral pathogens. Effective viral therapies can diminish viral pathogenesis. For example, human immunodeficiency virus (HIV) infection has been associated with myocarditis and dilated cardiomyopathy[17]; however, the incidence of HIV-associated cardiomyopathy has been diminished with more aggressive antiviral therapies against HIV.[18]

TABLE 26-1 Viral Causes of Inflammatory Cardiomyopathy and Myocarditis

Parvovirus (Parvovirus B19)	Hepatitis B and C virus
Adenoviruses	Human immunodeficiency virus
Influenza A and B	Poliovirus
Enteroviruses (coxsackie A and B)	Variola virus (smallpox)
Herpesvirus (human herpesvirus-6)	Rubella virus
Varicella-zoster	Echovirus
Cytomegalovirus	Polio
Epstein-Barr virus	

In the developing world, bacterial pathogens remain important causes as the incidence of myocarditis as a complication of rheumatic fever and diphtheroids are much more prevalent.[19,20] In Central and South America, the most common infectious agent is the protozoa *Trypanosoma cruzi,* the causative agent for Chagas' disease, which is endemic in certain areas[21] and may affect 15 to 20 million people.[22] This disorder is not seen in North America without a travel history to endemic areas. In immunocompromised hosts other pathogens, such as toxoplasmosis[23] and aspergillus,[24] can cause myocardial inflammation but generally in the setting of a systemic infection and not as isolated myocarditis.

AUTOIMMUNE (NONVIRAL) ETIOLOGIES

There are several autoimmune forms of myocardial inflammation for which no infectious agent can be identified. For certain diagnoses, histopathology combined with the clinical setting can point toward targeted treatments. The demonstration of multinucleated giant cells in the myocardium in the setting of fulminant myocarditis suggests the diagnosis of GCM (**Figure 26-3**), a progressive and destructive form of myocarditis with a high mortality rate on conventional therapy[25] but responsive to immunosuppressive therapy.[26] Finding similar multinucleated granulomas in the myocardium, but with few other inflammatory cells in a more compensated patient, may suggest systemic sarcoidosis, a chronic disorder responsive to treatment with corticosteroids.[27]

Eosinophilic predominance of inflammatory cells in the myocardium of a subject with new myocardial dysfunction may suggest an allergic hypersensitivity myocarditis.[28-30] A number of pharmacologic agents, including tricyclic antidepressants, antipsychotics, and cephalosporin, have been implicated as triggering eosinophilic myocarditis. This disorder is rare and generally self-limited, because the myocardium will recover with removal of the triggering agent without immunosuppressive therapy. For persistent myocarditis in the setting of peripheral eosinophilia, a short course of corticosteroids can be considered. More chronic peripheral eosinophilia without a clear initiating agent should also result in consideration of a more serious systemic syndrome such as Churg-Strauss vasculitis[31] or hypereosinophilic syndrome (HES)[32] for which immunosuppressive therapy is generally indicated.

Myocarditis may also be a clinical feature of a number of systemic autoimmune disorders. Systemic lupus erythematosus (SLE),[33] dermatopolymyositis,[34] and rheumatoid arthritis[35] have also been associated with inflammatory myocarditis. In general, immunosuppressive therapy is directed toward the systemic autoimmune disorder and will result in recovery of myocardial function as well. Endomyocardial biopsy is rarely performed, except in cases where the systemic disorder is quiescent and the finding of myocardial inflammation may be the only indication for immunosuppressive therapy.

PATHOGENESIS IN MURINE MODELS

Much of what is known of the basic pathogenesis of viral myocarditis is derived from murine models of inoculation with the cardiotropic coxsackie group B virus[36] or encephalomyocarditis virus[37] into susceptible strains. The viral particles are taken up by myocytes via receptor-mediated endocytosis. Translation of viral proteins and replication of viral particles can result in cell lysis within 3 days (**Figure 26-4**) before the initiation of myocardial inflammation. Macrophage activation results in cytokine expression, including interferon-γ[38,39] and activation of natural killer cells,[40] both of which limit subsequent viral replication. Infiltrates of antigen-specific T lymphocytes including T-helper (CD4+) cells and cytotoxic T lymphocyte (CD8+) cells are seen within 7 days of the viral infection.[41] Recognition of viral peptides by cytotoxic T cells results in cellular toxicity of virally infected cells.[42] Up to 20% of infiltrating lymphocytes are B cells, and neutralizing antibodies are important in viral clearing although not in cytotoxicity.

Viral particles are no longer evident within 15 days of the initial inoculation, although inflammatory infiltrates may persist for 90 days.[43] Viral nucleic acid can be detected after 90 days in only a small percentage of virally infected mice; however, long-term ventricular dilation and remodeling may develop and are associated with myocardial fibrosis. Similar transient myocardial inflammation followed by ventricular dilation and fibrosis has been seen without viral infection in transgenic mice overexpressing TNF-α.[44] In addition, murine models using antimyosin antibodies also result in myocardial remodeling.[45] Such murine models point to the potential role of chronic myocardial inflammation, whether virally mediated or autoimmune, in the pathogenesis of nonischemic dilated cardiomyopathy.

CLINICAL PRESENTATION

Acute myocarditis will typically present with a variety of symptoms, including dyspnea, chest pain, palpitations, syncope, and near syncope, and when associated with left

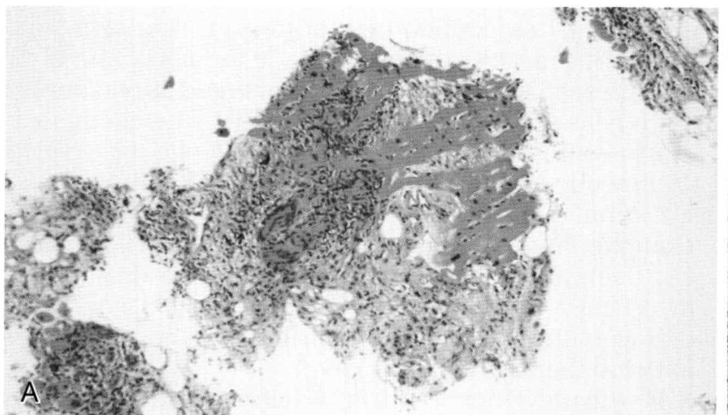

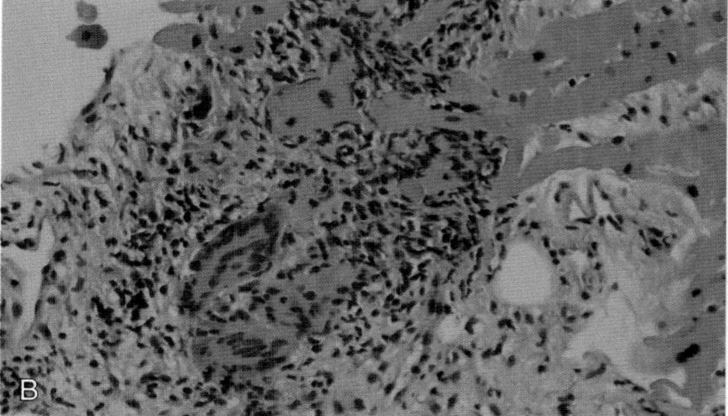

FIGURE 26-3 Histopathologic appearance of giant cell myocarditis (multinucleated giant cell) with routine staining with hematoxylin and eosin under **A,** low power (100×) and **B,** high power (350×).

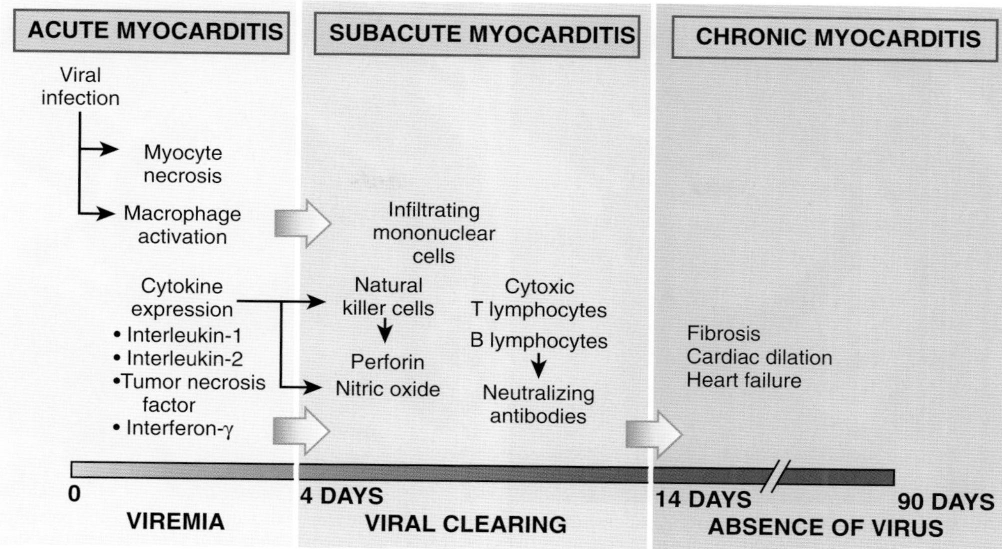

FIGURE 26-4 Timeline of progression in murine models from initial viral inoculation to acute myocarditis to subacute myocarditis to chronic myocarditis. *From Feldman AM, McNamara D: Myocarditis. N Engl J Med 343:1388–1398, 2000.*

ventricular dysfunction, most commonly presents with signs of heart failure.[46] A presentation with dyspnea or chest pain associated with electrocardiogram abnormalities[47] or an elevation of cardiac enzymes[48,49] may be the first sign of a possible myocarditis or myopericarditis. The cardiac examination may be fairly unremarkable or may reveal a pericardial rub. Tachycardia, relative hypotension, jugular venous distention, and peripheral edema may suggest more significant hemodynamic compromise. Chest examination may reveal congestion, and decreased breath sounds are suggestive of pleural effusions.

Electrocardiographic findings are generally diffuse and nonspecific. PR depression and global ST elevation may be seen in cases with an associated pericarditis. Low voltage may be evident, particularly subjects with an associated pericardial effusion. Heart block, ventricular tachycardia, or a new bundle branch block are all suggestive of a more fulminant disorder. Evaluation of biomarkers may reveal an elevation in cardiac troponin and brain natriuretic peptide. More fulminant myocarditis may be associated with elevated liver function tests and a compromise of renal function. Chest x-ray may be unremarkable or show evidence of heart failure and cardiomegaly.

CARDIAC IMAGING (see also Chapter 29)

Transthoracic echocardiography remains a critically important tool in the evaluation of myocarditis[50,51] and frequently provides the first evidence of ventricular impairment. Systolic dysfunction is generally global; however, it may be segmental and can mimic ischemic disease. Pericardial effusion may be present and provide supportive evidence of an inflammatory process. In severe myocarditis, the ventricular walls may be thickened due to edema; however, routine echocardiography is limited in terms of characterization of the myocardial tissue itself. The dimensions of the left ventricular diameter generally demonstrate minimal left ventricular (LV) enlargement and remodeling for an acute presentation, although remodeling may be more evident in more chronic insidious forms. The ease of the portable evaluation of ventricular function in the most critically ill patients greatly increases the importance of echocardiographic assessment in suspected fulminant myocarditis with hemodynamic compromise.

Cardiac magnetic resonance (CMR) imaging has had an increasing role in the diagnostic evaluation of myocarditis given its ability to characterize cardiac tissue and assess for inflammation[52,53] (**Figure 26-5**). The use of gadolinium on T1-weighted images allows for assessment of hyperemia and capillary leak with early enhancement, and more significant tissue injury and necrosis with late gadolinium enhancement (LGE). The anatomic distribution of gadolinium enhancement also assists in diagnosis, because an epicardial distribution of gadolinium enhancement is suggestive of myocarditis, whereas an endocardial predominance is more consistent with ischemic injury. The addition of T2-weighted images provides an assessment of myocardial water, and increased content is likely a marker of ongoing edema and inflammation.

The diagnostic criteria for myocarditis by CMR were established by a consensus panel, and the "Lake Louise" criteria were published in 2009.[54] These criteria noted that combining data from all three tissue markers, early and late gadolinium enhancement on T1-weighted images and myocardial edema by global and regional T2 relaxation times (**Table 26-2**), increased the utility of CMR and that myocardial inflammation could be predicted with a diagnostic accuracy of 78%. When only gadolinium enhancement on T1 images was used, CMR assessment would still yield an accuracy of 68%. Although CMR has greatly enhanced our ability to image the myocardium, the time required for data acquisition and the need to transport the patient to the imaging facility limit the ability of CMR to assess the most critically ill subjects. In addition, contrast imaging with gadolinium essential to the evaluation of myocardial inflammation cannot be performed in subjects with renal dysfunction.

ENDOMYOCARDIAL BIOPSY

Although the evaluation of myocardial histology by endomyocardial biopsy (EMB) remains the gold standard for the

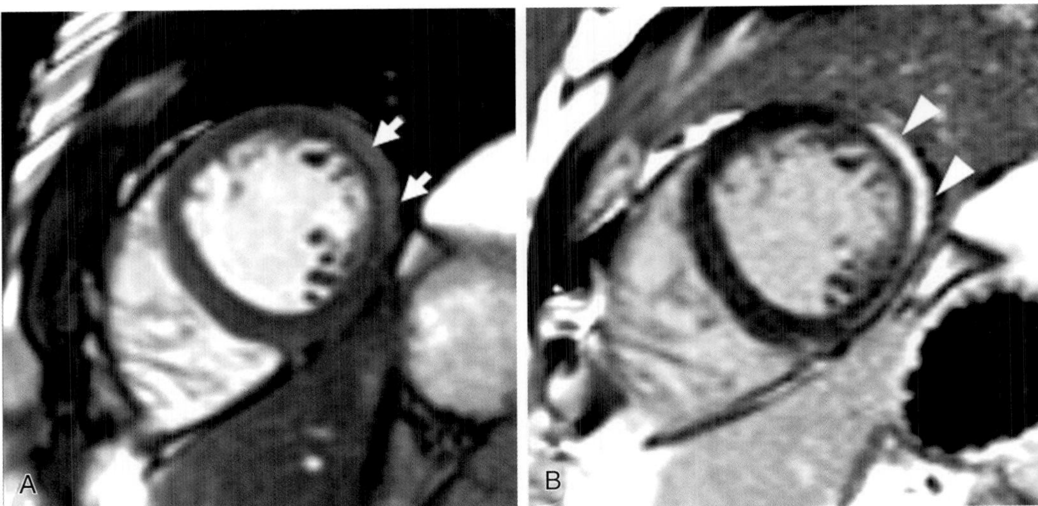

FIGURE 26-5 Cardiovascular magnetic resonance midventricular short-axis images from a 21-year-old man with acute myocarditis who presented with acute chest pain, peak troponin I of 15 ng/mL, and angiographically normal appearing coronary arteries. **A,** Myocardial edema *(white arrows)* in the epicardial portion of the inferolateral wall on T2-weighted images. **B,** Necrosis on late gadolinium enhancement images in the same region *(white arrowheads)* with uptake of contrast due to loss of cell membrane integrity (20 minutes following 0.2 mmol/kg of gadoteridol). *Courtesy of Timothy C. Wong, MD, MS, and Erik B. Schelbert, MD, MS.*

TABLE 26-2 Cardiac Magnetic Resonance Imaging (CMR) Criteria for Myocarditis (Lake Louise Consensus Criteria)*

In the clinical setting of suspected myocarditis, the CMR findings consistent with the diagnosis of myocardial inflammation (at least 2 of 3 criteria) are:

1. Regional or global myocardial increase in signal intensity in T2-weighted images
2. Increased global myocardial early gadolinium enhancement ratio between myocardium and skeletal muscle in gadolinium-enhanced T1-weighted images
3. At least one focal lesion with nonischemic regional distribution in inversion recovery-prepared gadolinium-enhanced T1-weighted images ("late gadolinium enhancement" or LGE)

CMR is consistent with myocyte injury and/or scar caused by myocardial inflammation, if:

- Criterion 3 is present.

Repeat CMR study between 1 and 2 weeks after the initial CMR study is recommended, if:

- None of the criteria is present, but the onset of symptoms has been very recent and there is strong clinical evidence for myocardial inflammation.
- One of the criteria is present.

The presence of left ventricular dysfunction or pericardial effusion provides additional, supportive evidence for myocarditis.

*Modified from Friedrich MG, Sechtem U, Schulz-Menger J, et al for the International Consensus Group on Cardiovascular Magnetic Resonance in Myocarditis: Cardiovascular magnetic resonance in myocarditis: a JACC White Paper. *J Am Coll Cardiol* 53:1475–1487, 2009.

TABLE 26-3 Major Indication for Endomyocardial Biopsy*

1. New-onset heart failure of less than 2 weeks' duration associated with a normal size or dilated left ventricle and hemodynamic compromise: recommendation class I, level of evidence B
2. New-onset heart failure of 2 weeks' to 3 months' duration associated with a dilated left ventricle and new ventricular arrhythmias, second- or third-degree heart block, or failure to respond to usual care within 2 to 3 weeks: recommendation class 1, level of evidence B
3. Heart failure of greater than 3 months' duration associated with a dilated left ventricle and new ventricular arrhythmias, second- or third-degree heart block, or failure to respond to usual care within 2 to 3 weeks: recommendation class IIa, level of evidence C
4. Heart failure associated with a DCM of any duration associated with suspected allergic reaction of eosinophilia: recommendation class IIa, level of evidence C

Class 1 recommendation, Condition for which there is evidence of general agreement that a given procedure is beneficial, useful, and effective; *Class IIa,* condition for which there is conflicting evidence but for which the weight of evidence/opinion is in favor of usefulness/efficacy; *DCM,* dilated cardiomyopathy; *level of evidence B,* limited number of randomized trials, nonrandomized studies, and registries; *level of evidence C,* primarily expert opinion.

*Modified from Cooper LT, Baughman KL, Feldman AM, et al: The role of endomyocardial biopsy in the management of cardiovascular disease: a scientific statement from the American Heart Association, the American College of Cardiology, and the European Society of Cardiology. *J Am Coll Cardiol* 50:1914–1931, 2007.

diagnosis of myocarditis, the diagnostic yield of biopsy remains low. In the large published biopsy series of over 2000 subjects screened for the myocarditis treatment trial with EMB, the prevalence of lymphocytic myocarditis (LM) was only 10%.[8] Myocardial histology generally does not affect treatment strategies, and although there are notable exceptions such as GCM, this is far less prevalent than LM and evident in no more than 2% of subjects who had biopsies[55] in published series. The current American Heart Association (AHA) and European Society of Cardiology guidelines[56] for the indication for EMB are driven by the need to detect histologic diagnoses, such as GCM, which change therapeutic recommendations. These guidelines give the strongest recommendation for endomyocardial biopsy in cases of acute fulminant myocarditis (acute myocarditis associated with hemodynamic compromise) and in acute myocarditis associated with ventricular tachycardia or heart block (**Table 26-3**). Although much interest exists in the enhancement of the diagnostic potential of EMB through the addition of molecular diagnostics, this remains an area of research at specialized centers and is not widely available, and the role of therapies guided by molecular diagnostics remains uncertain.

EMB does have defined risks, most notably the risk of cardiac perforation and tamponade, which can occur in up to 1% of subjects. These risks are diminished when performed by an experienced operator. Given that the risk of the procedure is increased by the inherent hemodynamic instability of suspected fulminant myocarditis, EMB in this scenario should be performed by an experienced operator at a tertiary center with the ability to provide mechanical support if required.

MEDICAL THERAPY

For myocarditis associated with left ventricular dysfunction, therapy remains supportive and similar to the medical therapy of more chronic forms of heart failure with reduced ejection fraction. Treatment with β-receptor antagonists and with either angiotensin-converting enzyme (ACE) inhibitors or angiotensin receptor antagonists remains the mainstay of therapy.[57] Digoxin should be avoided, as it has been shown to worsen injury in animal models.[58] Diuretics can be used for congestion and fluid overload, and generally should be used at the lowest dose required for symptomatic relief. For subjects with severe left ventricular dysfunction, anticoagulation should be considered and is definitively indicated for those subjects with evidence of left ventricular thrombus or those presenting with a thromboembolic event.

For subjects with suspected myocarditis and LV dysfunction, the management of potential arrhythmias should be tempered by the possibility of recovery. Even in those subjects with severe LV dysfunction, treatment with an implantable cardioverter defibrillator (ICD) should be deferred, given the potential for resolution.[59] An obvious exception to this general deferral of primary prevention ICDs is indicated for subjects presenting with "aborted sudden death" in which the placement of an ICD is required for secondary prevention. In subjects presenting with complex ventricular arrhythmias without sudden death, a temporary external defibrillator or life vest can be considered as an alternative to a more permanent device.

Systolic function recovers rapidly within weeks to months in many subjects with recent onset cardiomyopathy,[60] and the role of long-term therapy with ACE inhibitors and β-blockers in subjects who have recovered remains controversial. In subjects who have complete normalization of systolic function after a documented transient episode of myocarditis, medical therapy with ACE inhibitors and β-receptor antagonists can be gradually weaned off and discontinued with careful monitoring for subsequent declines in LVEF. Subjects with persistent abnormalities of either systolic function or remodeling (increased left ventricular diastolic diameter) should be continued on long-term heart failure therapy with either ACE inhibitors, β-receptor antagonists, or both. In subjects whose systolic function has completely recovered, abnormalities of diastolic function may persist for months[61] and may result in persistent symptoms of exertional dyspnea and fluid retention.

IMMUNOSUPPRESSIVE THERAPY

For subjects with heart failure and myocarditis, the role of immunosuppressive therapy remains controversial. While many anecdotal reports or small case series suggest benefit from immunosuppressive therapy, these must be viewed with caution given the high rate of spontaneous recovery for most subjects with suspected myocarditis. In several previous randomized trials, the role of immunosuppressive or immune modulatory therapy was evaluated in acute myocarditis or recent-onset nonischemic cardiomyopathy (with and without myocarditis) and failed to provide evidence of therapeutic benefit (**Table 26-4**).

The first randomized trial of immune suppression for inflammatory heart disease was a National Heart, Lung and Blood Institute–sponsored investigation of several months of oral prednisone for subjects with heart failure caused by dilated cardiomyopathy. The results demonstrated a modest but significant improvement in LV ejection fraction for subjects treated with steroid therapy with an "inflammatory" biopsy; however, the impact was modest, was not sustained after discontinuing treatment, and did not appear to warrant the side effects of therapy.[62] The Myocarditis Treatment Trial (MTT) evaluated treatment with prednisone and cyclosporine in subjects with biopsy-proven lymphocytic myocarditis. In the MTT, there was no benefit evident for immune suppression, because both the change in left ventricular function ejection fraction at 6 months and overall survival

TABLE 26-4 Randomized Trials of Immune Modulation or Immune Suppression in Myocarditis and Inflammatory Cardiomyopathy

REFERENCE	ENTRY CRITERIA	AGENT STUDIED	RANDOMIZED	OUTCOME MEASURES	RESULT
Parrillo et al[62]	Subjects with dilated cardiomyopathy divided into reactive versus nonreactive based on biopsy	Prednisone	102	Change in EF at 3 months	Modest benefit overall (4 EF units vs. 2 EF units with placebo); no benefit in nonreactive patients
Mason et al[8] (Myocarditis Treatment Trial)	Lymphocytic myocarditis	Prednisone and cyclosporine	111	Change in EF at 6 months	No significant effect (increase of 10 EF units vs. 7 EF units with placebo)
McNamara et al (IMAC Trial)[66]	History <6 months; subjects with recent onset with and without myocarditis	Immune globulin	62	Change in EF at 6 months	No treatment effect (increase of 14 EF units in both groups)
Wojnicz et al[69]	History >6 months; increased HLA expression on biopsy	Azathioprine and prednisone	84	LVEF after 3 months	Significant difference in LVEF (0.36 with immune suppression vs. 0.27 with placebo, $P<0.001$)
Frustaci et al[70] (TIMIC study)	History >6 months; lymphocytic myocarditis and viral negative	Azathioprine and prednisone	85	LVEF at 6 months	Significant difference in 6 months (0.46 with immune suppression vs. 0.21 with placebo, $P<0.001$)

during several years of follow-up were statistically no different in the treatment group receiving cyclosporine and prednisone from those receiving the placebo.[8]

Immune globulin was reported to be effective for the treatment of pediatric myocarditis in a large single-center series with historical controls.[63] This led to exploration of its use in adults and reports of efficacy in two case series with recent-onset nonischemic cardiomyopathy[64] and peripartum cardiomyopathy.[65] The Intervention in Myocarditis and Acute Cardiomyopathy (IMAC) trial evaluated the efficacy of therapy with intravenous immune globulin in adults in a multicenter placebo-controlled investigation and failed to demonstrate benefit.[66] There was a significant improvement in the mean LVEF overall with an increase of 14 EF units evident in subjects treated with immune globulin; however, this was identical to the mean improvement seen in those treated with the placebo (**Figure 26-6**). The MTT and IMAC investigations targeted very acute subjects, and in both spontaneous recovery in the placebo group limited the study power to determine the efficacy. However, there was no demonstrable treatment benefit in either investigation of immune modulation in acute inflammatory cardiomyopathy.

ACUTE VERSUS CHRONIC INFLAMMATORY CARDIOMYOPATHY

The inability to improve outcomes with immune suppression in acute myocarditis trials may reflect the fact that acute inflammation actually plays a beneficial role in viral clearing. Indeed, subjects with the histologically most severe form of lymphocytic myocarditis, so-called fulminant myocarditis, have better long-term outcomes than more subacute indolent forms.[67] In fulminant myocarditis, the clinical inflammation generally resolves rapidly and left ventricular systolic function recovers in parallel. This potential for full recovery with fulminant lymphocytic myocarditis with only supportive care supports the concept that inflammation itself in the acute setting is not necessarily pathologic, and indeed may be protective. Although inflammation may play a protective role during the acute phase, in later stages persistent chronic inflammation appears to play a more pathologic role. In a large study from Germany of subjects with primary dilated cardiomyopathy undergoing myocardial biopsy, those with evidence of persistent inflammation by cell markers and immunohistochemistry had poorer outcomes overall than those without myocardial inflammation.[68]

Two single-center studies from Europe evaluated immunosuppression in more chronic inflammatory heart disease and demonstrated the potential benefit for therapeutic intervention in this context (see Table 26-4). The first study from Poland performed EMB on 202 subjects with a nonischemic dilated cardiomyopathy of at least 6 months' duration, and performed immunohistochemical staining for expression of HLA antigens. The 84 subjects with strong expression of HLA antigens were defined as "inflammatory" and randomized to 3 months of treatment with either steroids plus azathioprine or a placebo, and followed for up to 2 years.[69] There was no difference in hospitalization-free survival; however, LVEF improved significantly by 3 months with immune suppression compared with placebo, and this improvement was maintained for the 2-year follow-up (**Figure 26-7**). In a second Italian study in chronic myocarditis, the TIMIC study,[70] 85 subjects with chronic heart failure (>6 months) and an EMB that demonstrated both active

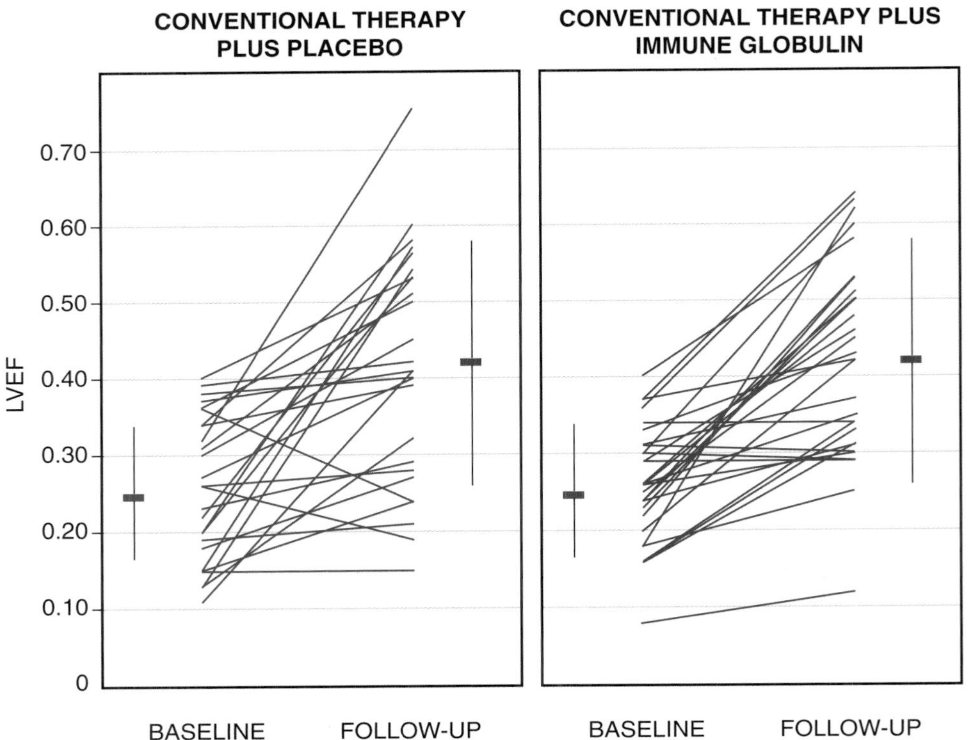

FIGURE 26-6 Left ventricular ejection fraction (LVEF) over time by treatment in the IMAC trial: LVEF by radionuclide scan at baseline and 12 months post randomization in patients randomized to placebo and immunoglobulin. Overall, LVEF improved significantly over time (12 months LVEF significantly higher than baseline, $P < 0.001$). However, no differences by treatment group were evident. *From McNamara DM, Holubkov R, Starling RC, et al for the IMAC investigators: A controlled trial of intravenous immune globulin for recent onset dilated cardiomyopathy. Circulation 103:2254–2259, 2001.*

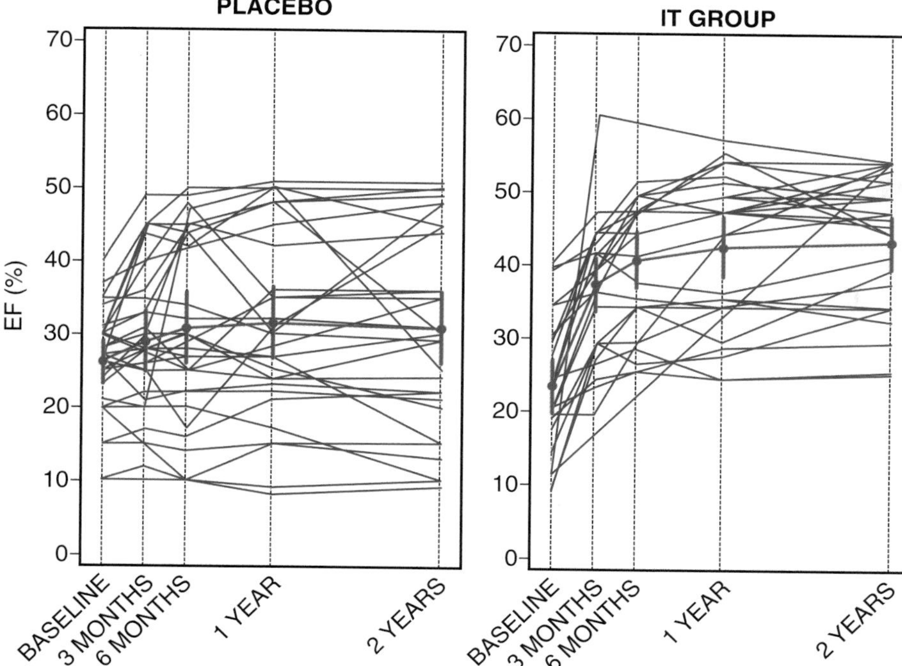

FIGURE 26-7 Serial left ventricular ejection fractions (EF) from 58 subjects (all with chronic cardiomyopathy but with increased HLA expression as evidence of pathologic inflammation on biopsy) receiving either placebo (n = 30) or immunosuppressive therapy (IT) with azathioprine and prednisone. Thickened line and bars delineate means and standard deviations. *From Wojnicz R, Nowalany-Kozielska E, Wojciechowska C, et al: Randomized, placebo-controlled study for immunosuppressive treatment of inflammatory dilated cardiomyopathy: two-year follow-up results. Circulation 104:39–45, 2001.*

lymphocytic myocarditis and no evidence of viral nucleic acids were randomized to azathioprine plus prednisone for 6 months versus a placebo. The primary endpoint was LVEF at 6 months, which improved almost 20 EF units in the treatment group and declined in the placebo group. These single-center investigations using a similar therapeutic strategy in two cohorts with chronic nonischemic cardiomyopathy support the hypothesis that immune suppression may be more beneficial in the chronic pathologic phase of myocardial inflammation.

Molecular diagnostics have been used over the past two decades to evaluate for the presence of viral nucleic acids in EMB specimens. Research of viral persistence has demonstrated that the specific species detected in cases of myocarditis and dilated cardiomyopathy continues to evolve over time, and represents a moving target in terms of therapeutic efforts to facilitate viral clearing. In several European investigations, these data have been used to triage subjects into therapeutic pathways. In the TIMIC trial, only patients with myocarditis who were "virus negative" were randomized to immune suppression. In subjects who were "viral positive" on EMB, small series have attempted to tailor therapy to the specific virus detected.[71,72] However, in the absence of controlled data, current European guidelines note the potential for antiviral therapy but do not advocate specific treatments.[73] The European Study of Epidemiology and Treatment of Cardiac Inflammatory Diseases (ESETCID) is a multicenter investigation initiated almost two decades ago to attempt to provide controlled data for the efficacy of molecular targeted therapeutic strategies. This placebo-controlled, multiple-arm therapeutic trial randomized viral-negative subjects into immune suppression with azathioprine and prednisone, enteroviral-positive patients to interferon-α, CMV-positive subjects to high-dose immune globulin, and adenoviral or parvo B19–positive subjects to intermediate-dose immune globulin.[74] Reports of the first 3000 subjects screened by EMB for this complicated randomization strategy found eligible subjects with myocarditis and reduced left ventricular ejection fraction in only 6%, and viral nucleic acid in only 11%.[75] The complexity of these molecular diagnostic strategies has limited the ability to validate these targeted strategies, and has prevented their widespread adoption outside of specialized centers.

MECHANICAL SUPPORT AND RECOVERY

In cases of fulminant myocarditis due to suspected viral myocarditis, mechanical support has been successfully used to provide hemodynamic support and allow full recovery (see also Chapter 42). Subjects with fulminant myocarditis often present with cardiogenic shock and associated multisystem failure. Such patients may require full cardiac support, which can be instituted using either temporary biventricular assist device (BiVAD) support or extracorporeal membrane oxygenation (ECMO). Even in such critically ill patients, mechanical support can allow successful cardiac rescue, with most subjects surviving to leave the hospital with normal cardiac function.[76]

The timetable for recovery from fulminant myocarditis can vary from weeks to months, and when support is anticipated for more than several weeks, a chronic long-term left ventricular assist device (LVAD) is required. Use of extracorporeal devices may allow simpler operative implantation and explanation, so the determination of recovery potential is of great assistance in planning specific LVAD support strategies. Factors predicting a greater likelihood of recovery include a short duration of symptoms before LVAD support and the absence of LV remodeling preimplant (i.e., a smaller LV end-diastolic diameter).[77] In a recent multicenter study of ventricular recovery on LVAD, 8 of 11 subjects with recent-onset cardiomyopathy with less than 4 months of symptoms at the time of LVAD implant were successfully recovered and explanted.[78] In this investigation myocardial histology at the time of implant was predictive of recovery, and cellular inflammation with either lymphocytic myocarditis or nonspecific inflammatory cells was seen in 75% of subjects who recovered. In contrast, only 25% of subjects with evidence of fibrosis at the time of implant recovered.

PEDIATRIC MYOCARDITIS

Pediatric myocarditis differs from that seen in adults as there is a greater likelihood of infectious viral causes, in part because the prevalence of the noninfectious causes is much lower in children. Children are more likely to have an inflammatory biopsy and have a greater probability of recovery.[79,80] The specific viral species involved have changed over time and closely mirror those seen in adults. While enteroviruses were once predominant, they were later surpassed first by adenoviruses[81] and more recently by erythroviruses, in particular parvovirus B19.[82] Notably, children have not been included in previous randomized trials of immune suppression or immune modulation. As a result, case series and anecdotal experience dictate practice, and children are much more likely to be treated with either steroids or immune globulin. Despite the absence of controlled data on the effectiveness of immune modulatory therapies in children, the use of these therapies has become common practice,[83] with immune globulin used in more than 70% of cases in a recent study of tertiary referral centers and prednisone used in 25% to 30%.[84]

PERIPARTUM CARDIOMYOPATHY (see also Chapter 19)

Peripartum cardiomyopathy (PPCM) is a form of nonischemic cardiomyopathy that occurs in women in the peripartum period. An autoimmune pathogenesis has been postulated,[85] likely triggered by fetal or placental antigens rather than viral, and PPCM generally presents at the precise time maternal cellular immunity is rebounding from the downregulation required for fetal tolerance. The frequency of lymphocytic myocarditis on endomyocardial biopsy varies widely in historical series of PPCM but appears similar to other forms of acute cardiomyopathy.[86] Therapy remains supportive and there is a high probability of ventricular recovery[87] during the first few months postpartum. Prolactin plays an important role in the resetting of maternal immunity, and inhibition of prolactin with the drug bromocriptine has been reported to improve recovery in women with PPCM in case reports[88] and a small randomized pilot in South Africa.[89] These reports are difficult to interpret given the high rate of spontaneous recovery, and a randomized trial is currently under way in Europe.

SUMMARY AND FUTURE THERAPEUTIC DIRECTIONS

Myocarditis from both viral and nonviral causes remains an important cause of myocardial dysfunction and heart failure. Current therapy for acute myocarditis with LV dysfunction remains the medical treatment for heart failure, and the role of immune suppression is limited to patients with GCM or those with a systemic autoimmune disorder. Although many subjects with acute myocarditis recover completely with no long-term sequelae, a percentage are left with chronic nonischemic cardiomyopathy and the clinical consequence of progressive heart failure.

The high spontaneous recovery rate on contemporary therapy complicates the ability to evaluate novel therapies designed to facilitate myocardial recovery. The ability to better decipher on presentation those subjects destined for recovery remains an active area of investigation, because this would allow future investigations of innovative therapies to focus on subjects predicted to have the poorest outcomes on conventional therapy. Analysis of transcriptional expression profiles on myocardial biopsies[90,91] appears to successfully predict subjects who will recover, and may one day be a useful adjunct to conventional histology and immunohistochemistry.

Single-center trials in chronic myocarditis have demonstrated great promise, and suggest that in this more pathologic form of myocardial inflammation, immune suppression may play a more important therapeutic role. These innovative investigations need to be replicated in larger multicenter trials to determine their therapeutic potential; however, the molecular diagnostic techniques used for evaluating myocardial biopsies in these investigations are not part of current practice. The ability to delineate subjects who had evidence of persistent chronic myocardial inflammation was a critical component for these investigations and an essential requirement for targeted immune suppression in the future. These future investigations will determine whether immune suppression has a significant role in the treatment of chronic myocardial inflammation.

References

1. Silverman ME: A view from the millennium: the practice of cardiology circa 1950 and thereafter. *J Am Coll Cardiol* 33:1141–1151, 1999.
2. O'Connell JB: The role of myocarditis in end-stage dilated cardiomyopathy. *Tex Heart Inst J* 14:268–275, 1987.
3. Waller BF, Slack JD, Orr CD, et al: "Flaming," "smoldering" and "burned out": the fireside saga of myocarditis. *JACC* 18:1627–1630, 1991.
4. Sakakibara S, Konno S: Endomyocardial biopsy. *Jpn Heart J* 3:537–543, 1962.
5. Aretz HT, Billingham ME, Edwards WD: Myocarditis, a histopathologic definition and classification. *Am J Cardiovasc Pathol* 1:3–14, 1987.
6. Shanes JG, Gahli J, Billingham ME, et al: Interobserver variability in the pathological interpretation of endomyocardial biopsy results. *Circulation* 75:401–405, 1987.
7. Richardson P, McKenna W, Bristow M: Report of the 1995 World Health Organization/International Society and Federation of Cardiology Task Force on the Definition and Classification of Cardiomyopathies. *Circulation* 93:841–842, 1996.
8. Mason JW, O'Connell JB, Herskowitz A, et al, for the Myocarditis Treatment Trial investigators: a clinical trial of immunosuppressive therapy for myocarditis. *N Engl J Med* 333:269–313, 1995.
9. Maisch B, Pankuweit S: Standard and etiology-directed evidence-based therapies in myocarditis: state of the art and future perspectives. *Heart Fail Rev* 18:761–795, 2013.
10. Fairly CK, Ryan M, Wall PG, et al: The organisms reported to cause infective myocarditis and pericarditis in England and Wales. *J Infect Dis* 32:223–225, 1996.
11. Bowles NE, Bowles KR, Towbin JA: Viral genomic detection and outcome in myocarditis. *Heart Fail Clin* 1:407–417, 2005.
12. Grumbach IM, Heim A, Pring-Akerblom P, et al: Adenoviruses and enteroviruses as pathogens in myocarditis and dilated cardiomyopathy. *Acta Cardiol* 54:83–88, 1999.
13. Mamas MA, Fraser D, Neyses L: Cardiovascular manifestations associated with influenza virus infection. *Int J Cardiol* 130:304–309, 2008.
14. Dennert R, Crijns HJ, Heymans S: Acute viral myocarditis. *Eur Heart J* 29:2073–2082, 2008.
15. Matsumori A: Hepatitis C virus infection. *Circ Res* 96:144–147, 2005.
16. Andréoletti L, Lévêque N, Boulagnon C, et al: Viral causes of human myocarditis. *Arch Cardiovasc Dis* 102:559–568, 2009.
17. Cohen IS, Anderson DW, Virmani R, et al: Congestive cardiomyopathy in association with the acquired immunodeficiency syndrome. *N Engl J Med* 315:628–630, 1986.
18. Ng B, Macpherson P, Haddad T, et al: Heart failure in HIV infection: focus on the role of atherosclerosis. *Curr Opin Cardiol* 29(2):174–179, 2014.
19. Lee JL, Naguwa SM, Cheema GS, et al: Acute rheumatic fever and its consequences: a persistent threat to developing nations in the 21st century. *Autoimmun Rev* 9:117–123, 2009.
20. Havaldar PV, Sankpal MN, Doddannavar RP: Diphtheritic myocarditis: clinical and laboratory parameters of prognosis and fatal outcome. *Ann Trop Paediatr* 20:209–215, 2000.
21. Dias JCP: Control of Chagas' disease in Brazil. *Parasitol Today* 3:336–339, 1987.
22. World Health Organization. Sixth program report: Chapter 6: Chagas' disease. Special Program for Research and Training in Tropical Diseases. Document TDR, PR-6, 83.6-CHA, YNDP, World Bank, WHO, 1983.
23. Montoya JG, Jordan R, Lingamneni S, et al: Toxoplasmic myocarditis and polymyositis in patients with acute acquired toxoplasmosis diagnosed during life. *Clin Infect Dis* 24:676–683, 1997.
24. Williams A: Aspergillus myocarditis. *Am J Pathol* 61:247–248, 1974.
25. Cooper LT, Berry GJ, Shabetai R, et al: Idiopathic giant-cell myocarditis—natural history and treatment. *N Engl J Med* 336:1860–1866, 1997.
26. Cooper LT, Jr, Hare JM, Tazelaar HD, et al: for the Giant Cell Myocarditis Treatment Trial Investigators. Usefulness of immunosuppression for giant cell myocarditis. *Am J Cardiol* 102:1535–1539, 2008.

27. Sadek MM, Yung D, Birnie DH, et al: Corticosteroid therapy for cardiac sarcoidosis: a systematic review. *Can J Cardiol* 29:1034–1041, 2013.
28. Aslan I, Fischer M, Laser KT, et al: Eosinophilic myocarditis in an adolescent: a case report and review of the literature. *Cardiol Young* 23:277–283, 2013.
29. Kounis NG, Zavras GM, Soufras GD, et al: Hypersensitivity myocarditis. *Ann Allergy* 62:71–74, 1989.
30. Galiuto L, Enriquez-Sarano M, Reeder GS, et al: Eosinophilic myocarditis manifesting as myocardial infarction: early diagnosis and successful treatment. *Mayo Clin Proc* 72:603–610, 1997.
31. Lim J, Sternberg A, Manghat N, et al: Hypereosinophilic syndrome masquerading as a myocardial infarction causing decompensated heart failure. *BMC Cardiovasc Disord* 13:75, 2013.
32. Shanks M, Ignaszewski AP, Chan SY, et al: Churg-Strauss syndrome with myocarditis manifesting as acute myocardial infarction with cardiogenic shock: case report and review of the literature. *Can J Cardiol* 19:1184–1188, 2003.
33. Mavrogeni S, Bratis K, Markussis V, et al: The diagnostic role of cardiac magnetic resonance imaging in detecting myocardial inflammation in systemic lupus erythematosus. Differentiation from viral myocarditis. *Lupus* 22:34–43, 2013.
34. Zhang L, Wang GC, Ma L, et al: Cardiac involvement in adult polymyositis or dermatomyositis: a systematic review. *Clin Cardiol* 35:686–691, 2012.
35. Mavrogeni S, Bratis K, Sfendouraki E, et al: Myopericarditis, as the first sign of rheumatoid arthritis relapse, evaluated by cardiac magnetic resonance. *Inflamm Allergy Drug Targets* 12:206–211, 2013.
36. Huber SA: Animal models: immunological aspects. In Banatvala JE, editor: *Viral infections of the heart*, London, 1993, Arnold, pp 82–109.
37. Matsumori A, Kawai C: An animal model of congestive (dilated) cardiomyopathy: dilatation and hypertrophy of the heart in the chronic stage in DBA/2 mice with myocarditis caused by encephalomyocarditis virus. *Circulation* 66:355–360, 1982.
38. Kawai C: From myocarditis to cardiomyopathy: mechanisms of inflammation and cell death. Learning from the past for the future. *Circulation* 99:1091–1100, 1999.
39. Feldman AM, McNamara D: Myocarditis. *N Engl J Med* 343:1388–1398, 2000.
40. Godeny EK, Gauntt CJ: Interferon and natural killer cell activity in coxsackie virus B3-induced myocarditis. *Eur Heart J* 8:433–435, 1987.
41. Liu CC, Young LHY, Young JDE: Mechanisms of disease: lymphocyte-mediated cytolysis and disease. *N Engl J Med* 335:1651–1659, 1996.
42. Seko Y, Tsuchimochi H, Nakamura T, et al: Expression of major histocompatibility complex class I antigen in murine ventricular myocytes infected with Coxsackie virus B3. *Circ Res* 69:360–367, 1990.
43. Kyu B, Matsumori A, Sato Y, et al: Cardiac persistence of cardioviral RNA detected by polymerase chain reaction in a murine model of dilated cardiomyopathy. *Circulation* 86:1605–1614, 1992.
44. Kubota T, McTiernan CF, Frye CS, et al: Dilated cardiomyopathy in transgenic mice with cardiac-specific overexpression of tumor necrosis factor-alpha. *Circ Res* 81:627–635, 1997.
45. Neumann DA, Lane JR, Wulff SM, et al: In vivo deposition of myosin-specific autoantibodies in the hearts of mice with experimental autoimmune myocarditis. *J Immunol* 148:3806–3813, 1992.
46. Dec GW, Palacios IF, Fallon JT, et al: Active myocarditis in the spectrum of acute dilated cardiomyopathies: clinical features, histologic correlates, and clinical outcome. *N Engl J Med* 312:885–890, 1985.
47. Heikkila J, Karjalainen J: Evaluation of mild acute infectious myocarditis. *Br Heart J* 7:381–391, 1982.
48. Smith SC, Ladenson JH, Mason JW, et al: Elevations of cardiac troponin I associated with myocarditis. Experimental and clinical correlates. *Circulation* 95:163–168, 1996.
49. Lauer B, Niederau C, Kuhl U, et al: Cardiac troponin T in patients with clinically suspected myocarditis. *J Am Coll Cardiol* 30:1354–1359, 1997.
50. Gibson DG: Value and limitations of echocardiography in the diagnosis of myocarditis. *Eur Heart J* 8:85–88, 1987.
51. Pinamonti B, Alberti E, Cigalotto A, et al: Echocardiographic findings in myocarditis. *Am J Cardiol* 62:285–291, 1988.
52. Abdel-Aty H, Boyé P, Zagrosek A, et al: Diagnostic performance of cardiovascular magnetic resonance in patients with suspected acute myocarditis. *J Am Coll Cardiol* 45:1815–1822, 2005.
53. Liu PP, Yan AT: Cardiovascular magnetic resonance for the diagnosis of acute myocarditis. *J Am Coll Cardiol* 45:1823–1825, 2005.
54. Friedrich MG, Sechtem U, Schulz-Menger J, et al: for the International Consensus Group on Cardiovascular Magnetic Resonance in Myocarditis. Cardiovascular magnetic resonance in myocarditis: a JACC White Paper. *J Am Coll Cardiol* 53:1475–1487, 2009.
55. Davidoff R, Palacios P, Southern J, et al: Giant cell versus lymphocytic myocarditis. A comparison of their clinical features and long term outcomes. *Circulation* 83:953–961, 1991.
56. Cooper LT, Baughman KL, Feldman AM, et al: The role of endomyocardial biopsy in the management of cardiovascular disease: a scientific statement from the American Heart Association, the American College of Cardiology, and the European Society of Cardiology. *J Am Coll Cardiol* 50:1914–1931, 2007.
57. Blauwet LA, Cooper LT: Myocarditis. *Prog Cardiovasc Dis* 52:274–288, 2010.
58. Matsumori A, Igata H, Ono K, et al: High doses of digitalis increase the myocardial production of proinflammatory cytokines and worsen myocardial injury in viral myocarditis: a possible mechanism of digitalis toxicity. *Jpn Circ J* 63:934–940, 1999.
59. Sheppard R, Mather PJ, Alexis JD, et al, for the IMAC Investigators: Implantable cardiac defibrillators and sudden death in recent onset non-ischemic cardiomyopathy: results from IMAC2. *J Card Fail* 18:675–681, 2012.
60. McNamara DM, Starling RC, Cooper LT, et al, for the IMAC Investigators: Clinical and demographic predictors of outcomes in recent onset dilated cardiomyopathy: results of the IMAC (Intervention in Myocarditis and Acute Cardiomyopathy)-2 study. *J Am Coll Cardiol* 58:1112–1118, 2011.
61. Semigran MJ, Thaik CM, Fifer MA, et al: Exercise capacity and systolic and diastolic ventricular function after recovery from acute dilated cardiomyopathy. *J Am Coll Cardiol* 24:462–470, 1994.
62. Parillo JE, Cunnion RE, Epstein SE, et al: A prospective, randomized, controlled trial of prednisone for dilated cardiomyopathy. *N Engl J Med* 321:1061–1068, 1989.
63. Drucker MA, Colan SD, Lewis AB, et al: Gammaglobulin treatment of acute myocarditis in the pediatric population. *Circulation* 89:252–257, 1994.
64. McNamara DM, Rosenblum WD, Janosko KM, et al: Intravenous immune globulin in the therapy of myocarditis and acute cardiomyopathy. *Circulation* 95:2476–2478, 1997.
65. Bozkurt B, Villanueva FS, Holubkov R, et al: Intravenous immune globulin in the therapy of peripartum cardiomyopathy. *J Am Coll Cardiol* 34:177–180, 1999.
66. McNamara DM, Holubkov R, Starling RC, et al, for the IMAC investigators: A controlled trial of intravenous immune globulin for recent onset dilated cardiomyopathy. *Circulation* 103:2254–2259, 2001.
67. McCarthy RE, Boehmer JP, Hruban RH, et al: Long-term outcome of fulminant myocarditis as compared with acute (nonfulminant) myocarditis. *N Engl J Med* 342:690–695, 2000.
68. Kindermann I, Kindermann M, Kandolf R, et al: Predictors of outcome in patients with suspected myocarditis. *Circulation* 118:639–648, 2008.
69. Wojnicz R, Nowalany-Kozielska E, Wojciechowska C, et al: Randomized, placebo-controlled study for immunosuppressive treatment of inflammatory dilated cardiomyopathy: two-year follow-up results. *Circulation* 104:39–45, 2001.
70. Frustaci A, Russo MA, Chimenti C: Randomized study on the efficacy of immunosuppressive therapy in patients with virus-negative inflammatory cardiomyopathy: the TIMIC study. *Eur Heart J* 30:1995–2002, 2009.
71. Daliento L, Calabrese F, Tona F, et al: Successful treatment of enterovirus-induced myocarditis with interferon-alpha. *J Heart Lung Transplant* 22:214–217, 2003.
72. Kuhl U, Pauschinger M, Schwimmbeck PL, et al: Interferon-beta treatment eliminates cardiotropic viruses and improves left ventricular function in patients with myocardial persistence of viral genomes and left ventricular dysfunction. *Circulation* 107:2793–2798, 2003.
73. Caforio AL, Pankuweit S, Arbustini E, et al: European Society of Cardiology Working Group on Myocardial and Pericardial Diseases. Current state of knowledge on aetiology, diagnosis, management, and therapy of myocarditis: a position statement of the European Society of Cardiology Working Group on Myocardial and Pericardial Diseases. *Eur Heart J* 34:2636–2648, 2013.
74. Maisch B, Hufnagel G, Schönian U, et al: The European Study of Epidemiology and Treatment of Cardiac Inflammatory Disease (ESETCID). *Eur Heart J* 16(Suppl O):173–175, 1995.
75. Hufnagel G, Pankuweit S, Richter A, et al: The European Study of Epidemiology and Treatment of Cardiac Inflammatory Diseases (ESETCID). First epidemiological results. *Herz* 25:279–285, 2000.
76. Mody KP, Takayama H, Landes E, et al: Acute mechanical circulatory support for fulminant myocarditis complicated by cardiogenic shock. *J Cardiovasc Transl Res* 7:156–164, 2014.
77. Simon MA, Kormos RL, Murali S, et al: Myocardial recovery using ventricular assist devices. Prevalence, clinical characteristics, and outcomes. *Circulation* 112(Suppl I):I-32–I-36, 2005.
78. Boehmer JP, Starling RC, Cooper LT, et al, for the IMAC Investigators: Left ventricular assist device support and myocardial recovery in recent onset cardiomyopathy. *J Card Fail* 18:755–761, 2012.
79. Kleinert S, Weintraub RG, Wilkinson JL, et al: Myocarditis in children with dilated cardiomyopathy: incidence and outcome after dual therapy immunosuppression. *J Heart Lung Transplant* 16:1248–1254, 1997.
80. Lee KJ, McCrindle BW, Bohn DJ, et al: Clinical outcomes of acute myocarditis in childhood. *Heart* 82:226–233, 1999.
81. Bowles NE, Ni J, Kearney DL, et al: Detection of viruses in myocardial tissues by polymerase chain reaction. Evidence of adenovirus as a common cause of myocarditis in children and adults. *J Am Coll Cardiol* 42:466–472, 2003.
82. Molina KM, Garcia X, Denfield SW, et al: Parvovirus B19 myocarditis causes significant morbidity and mortality in children. *Pediatr Cardiol* 34:390–397, 2013.
83. Canter CE, Simpson KP: Diagnosis and treatment of myocarditis in children in the current era. *Circulation* 129:115–128, 2014.
84. Ghelani SJ, Spaeder MC, Pastor W, et al: Demographics, trends, and outcomes in pediatric acute myocarditis in the United States, 2006 to 2011. *Circ Cardiovasc Qual Outcomes* 5:622–627, 2012.
85. Gleicher N, Elkayam U: Peripartum cardiomyopathy, an autoimmune manifestation of allograft rejection? *Autoimmun Rev* 8:384–387, 2009.
86. Pearson GD, Veille JC, Rahimtoola S, et al: Peripartum cardiomyopathy: National Heart, Lung, and Blood Institute and Office of Rare Diseases (National Institutes of Health) workshop recommendations and review. *JAMA* 283:1183–1188, 2000.
87. Haghikia A, Podewski E, Libhaber E, et al: Phenotyping and outcome on contemporary management in a German cohort of patients with peripartum cardiomyopathy. *Basic Res Cardiol* 108:366, 2013.
88. Hilfiker-Kleiner D, Meyer GP, Schieffer E, et al: Recovery from postpartum cardiomyopathy in 2 patients by blocking prolactin release with bromocriptine. *J Am Coll Cardiol* 50:2354–2355, 2007.
89. Sliwa K, Blauwet L, Tibazarwa K, et al: Evaluation of bromocriptine in the treatment of acute severe peripartum cardiomyopathy: a proof-of-concept pilot study. *Circulation* 121:1465–1473, 2010.
90. Heidecker B, Kittleson MM, Kasper EK, et al: Transcriptomic biomarkers for the accurate diagnosis of myocarditis. *Circulation* 123:1174–1184, 2011.
91. Ramani R, Vela D, Segura A, et al: A micro-ribonucleic acid signature associated with recovery from assist device support in 2 groups of patients with severe heart failure. *J Am Coll Cardiol* 58:2270–2278, 2011.

27 Heart Failure in the Developing World

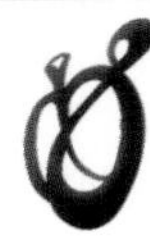

Karen Sliwa and Simon Stewart

IS ALL HEART FAILURE THE SAME AROUND THE GLOBE?

As a complex syndrome that had defied simple definitions, it is perhaps understandable that heart failure has been largely defined by epidemiologic studies undertaken in the developed world; most notably the Framingham Heart Study[1] (**see also Chapter 17**). In this respect, the central importance of underlying coronary artery disease and to a lesser extent hypertension, has remained pivotal to our evolving understanding of the syndrome. **Table 27-1** summarizes some of the key definitions that have shaped our collective perceptions of heart failure,[2] from a predominantly "systolic dysfunction" phenomenon to one that acknowledged neurohormonal activation and wider systemic responses to a "failing heart" and, more latterly, the concept of preserved systolic dysfunction.[3] Indeed, one can appreciate the fact that contemporary definitions of heart failure represent a "broad church" that accepts multiple pathways to the syndrome.

If one were to ask the question *"Is all heart failure the same around the globe?"* on the basis of contemporary guidelines, it is obvious that the answer could easily be "yes" on the basis of broad definitions. However, one cannot ignore the developed world–centric dominance of heart failure reports, nor the fact that most of the clinical trials of new pharmacologic agents and devices have gravitated toward predominantly younger men with an ischemic cause and impaired systolic function. This has been exacerbated by the general lack of evidence to support new therapeutic modalities for the treatment of those with preserved systolic function. Just as predominantly older women with heart failure have been underrepresented in clinical trials and popular perceptions of the syndrome in the developed world, there is little appreciation of the different pathways to the syndrome in the developing world, with potentially more women than men being affected and with much younger case presentations.

This chapter outlines the pattern of heart failure from a developing world perspective, outlining the differential pathways to the syndrome based on profound differences in risk profiles and socioeconomic factors. In presenting key data, it is important to acknowledge the challenge of presenting a global picture given the heterogeneous nature of different populations, the lack of standardized definitions and surveillance studies, in addition to the difficulty of prioritizing research in low-income settings.[4] Even if a coherent picture is not provided, it would be remiss not to remind readers of the enormity of the burden of heart failure in the developing world as it overcomes the traditional killers of malnutrition and infectious diseases and adopts the diseases of lifestyle that have fueled an epidemic of heart failure in the developed world.

GLOBAL BURDEN OF HEART FAILURE IN THE DEVELOPING WORLD

As indicated above, the pattern of heart failure is likely to vary across different regions of the world, based on different risk factor prevalence among the wide spectrum of ethnic groups influenced by socioeconomic factors. Differential coding of the syndrome, coupled with nuanced differences in defining cases, defies simple regional comparisons, particularly from a developed world perspective. For example, the current International Classification of Diseases (ICD) system classifies heart failure as an intermediate and not an underlying cause of death.[5] The recently published Global Burden of Disease (GBD) studies, undertaken in 1990 and 2000, reported the global death for 235 causes, including cardiovascular and circulatory diseases such as rheumatic heart disease, ischemic heart disease, cardiomyopathy, and others, but did not list heart failure as a cause of death.[6] However, heart failure was included as one of the nonfatal health outcomes and as a crucial parameter in the monitoring of population health. The GBD studies have been the only studies to quantify nonfatal health outcomes across an exhaustive set of disorders at the global and regional levels. Left-sided and right-sided symptomatic heart failure was one of the 289 impairments included in the GBD cause-sequelae list in many locations.[7] Worldwide an estimate of 37.7 million cases of prevalent heart failure was recorded in 2010, leading to 4.2 years lived with disability (YLDs). Heart failure was distributed across a number of causes (**Table 27-2**). More than two thirds (68.7%) of heart failure globally was attributable to four underlying causes: ischemic heart disease, chronic obstructive pulmonary disease, and hypertensive and rheumatic heart disease. Importantly, there were marked regional

TABLE 27-1 A Historical Perspective on Heart Failure Definitions

Wood, 1968	"A state in which the heart fails to maintain an adequate circulation for the needs of the body despite a satisfactory venous filling pressure."
Braunwald & Grossman, 1992	"A state in which an abnormality of cardiac function is responsible for the failure of the heart to pump blood at a rate commensurate with the requirements of the metabolizing tissues or, to do so only from an elevated filling pressure."
Packer, 1988	"A complex clinical syndrome characterized by abnormalities of left ventricular function and neurohormonal regulation which are accompanied by effort intolerance, fluid retention, and reduced longevity."
Poole-Wilson, 1987	"A clinical syndrome caused by an abnormality of the heart and recognized by a characteristic pattern of hemodynamic, renal, neural, and hormonal responses."
ACC/AHA Heart Failure Guidelines, 2005[95]	"Heart failure is a complex clinical syndrome that can result from any structural or functional cardiac disorder that impairs the ability of the ventricle to fill with or eject blood."
ESC Heart Failure Guidelines, 2005	"A syndrome in which the patients should have the following features: symptoms of heart failure, typically breathlessness or fatigue, either at rest or during exertion, or ankle swelling and objective evidence of cardiac dysfunction at rest."
ACC/AHA Heart Failure Guidelines, 2009 (Update)	Definition essentially unchanged, with reinforcement of the stages of heart failure (see legend below—note that the first two stages are not heart failure) and the central importance of the following statement: "The single most useful diagnostic test in the evaluation of patients with HF is the comprehensive two-dimensional echocardiogram coupled with Doppler flow studies to determine whether abnormalities of myocardium, heart valves, or pericardium are present and which chambers are involved. Three fundamental questions must be addressed: (1) Is the LV ejection fraction (EF) preserved or reduced? (2) Is the structure of the LV normal or abnormal? (3) Are there other structural abnormalities such as valvular, pericardial, or right ventricular abnormalities that could account for the clinical presentation?"
ESC Heart Failure Guidelines, 2012 (Update)[62]	"A syndrome in which patients have typical symptoms (e.g., breathlessness, ankle swelling, and fatigue) and signs (e.g., elevated jugular venous pressure, pulmonary crackles, and displaced apex beat) resulting from an abnormality of cardiac structure or function."

The AHA/ACC guidelines provide a map of the natural history of heart failure (from a developed world perspective) in respect to four distinct stages: **Stage A:** Those at risk for heart failure, but who have not yet developed structural heart changes (those with diabetes or coronary disease without prior infarct). **Stage B:** Individuals with structural heart disease (i.e., reduced ejection fraction, left ventricular hypertrophy, chamber enlargement); however, no symptoms of heart failure have ever developed. **Stage C:** Patients who have developed clinical heart failure. **Stage D:** Patients with refractory heart failure requiring advanced intervention (biventricular pacemakers, left ventricular assist device, or transplantation).

Data from Krum H, Jelinek MV, Stewart S, et al: 2011 update to National Heart Foundation of Australia and Cardiac Society of Australia and New Zealand Guidelines for the prevention, detection and management of chronic heart failure in Australia, 2006. Med J Aust 194:405–409, 2011.

TABLE 27-2 Global Years Lived with Disability (YLDs) for Heart Failure from a Comprehensive List of 289 Causes and Select Sequelae in 1990 and 2010 for All Ages, Both Sexes Combined, and per 100,000

	All Ages YLDs (thousands)			*YLDs (per 100,000)*		
CAUSE OF HEART FAILURE (HF)	**1990**	**2010**	**% Δ**	**1990**	**2010**	**% Δ**
Cardiovascular and circulatory diseases	14,373 (11,094-18,134)	21,985 (16,947-27,516)	53.0%	271 (209-342)	319 (246-399)	17.7%
Rheumatic heart disease (HD)	290 (191-412)	420 (278-592)	45.1%	5 (4-8)	6 (4-9)	11.6%
Ischemic HD	894 (609-1236)	1518 (1038-2128)	69.9%	17 (11-23)	22 (15-31)	30.8%
Hypertensive HD	292 (202-412)	460 (315-639)	57.4%	6 (4-8)	7 (5-9)	21.1%
HF due to cardiomyopathy and myocarditis	272 (183-378)	394 (269-551)	44.8%	5 (3-7)	6 (4-8)	11.4%
HF due to endocarditis	42 (28-59)	61 (42-87)	45.8%	1 (1-1)	1 (1-1)	12.2%
HF due to other circulatory diseases	183 (123-259)	268 (180-372)	46.3%	3 (2-5)	4 (3-5)	12.6%

Data from Vos T, Flaxman AD, Naghavi M, et al: Years lived with disability (YLDs) for 1160 sequelae of 289 diseases and injuries 1990-2010: a systematic analysis for the Global Burden of Disease Study 2010. Lancet 380:2163–2196, 2012.

differences, with hypertensive heart disease, rheumatic heart disease, cardiomyopathy, and myocarditis making a larger contribution in developing countries.

What Do We Know About the Variation of Risk Factor Prevalence?

A recently published systematic review on worldwide risk factors for heart failure by Khatibzadeh and colleagues[5] found 53 full-text surveys of heart failure patients eligible for inclusion and, after excluding 15 full text papers, sorted 38 studies by region, using them for a qualitative synthesis. Their analysis demonstrated that ischemic heart disease was a risk factor for heart failure in more than 50% of patients in Western high-income regions, as well as Eastern and Central European regions; 30% to 40% in East Asia, Asia Pacific high-income regions; and Latin American and Caribbean regions. In sub-Saharan Africa, ischemic heart disease contributed less than 10% to heart failure.

Hypertension substantially contributed to heart failure in all regions, with a 17% or more crude prevalence among all cases around the world. However, after age and gender adjustment, hypertension was distinctly more common in Eastern and Central Europe (35%, range 32.7%-37.3%) and sub-Saharan Africa (32.6%, range 29.6%-35.7%). Of the other two commonly reported antecedents, rheumatic heart disease was particularly prevalent in East Asia (34%) and sub-Saharan Africa (14%) cases. The heterogeneous group of cardiomyopathy, which can include numerous causes such as familial, peripartum, infectious, infiltrative, autoimmune, postmyocarditis, idiopathic, and many others, were reported with a particularly high prevalence in sub-Saharan Africa (age- and gender-adjusted prevalence 25.7%, range 22.8%-28.5%). Latin America and the Caribbean, as well as Asia Pacific high-income countries, had a prevalence of 19.8% (16.5%-23.4%) and 16.5% (12.8%-20.6%). The risk factors found in that systematic review was similar to other past reviews of international risk factors published in 1985[8] and 2001.[9] However, the review by Khatibzadeh used multiple risk factors, thus reflecting a more real-world scenario. The review has a number of limitations, because in many studies younger patients are not included, preclinical heart failure is usually not captured, and the duration of heart failure symptoms is rarely described.

What Do We Not Know?

As data from many regions of the world are scarce, there is a particular lack of data estimating urban/rural differences as well as change in contributing factors to heart failure over time. There is an overall underreporting on the specific factors contributing to the spectrum of cardiomyopathy because these investigations are costly and there is a shortage of diagnostic facilities, such as cardiac catheterization laboratories, access to magnetic resonance imaging, or cardiac biopsies in those areas where, in particular, infectious causes of cardiomyopathy occur. In general, right heart failure per se, or as a contributing factor to left-sided heart failure, is poorly documented and there is a paucity of detailed description of the subtypes of valvular heart disease, such as different types of rheumatic valve disease or function valve disease. Congenital heart disease, either operated or not operated, usually gets lumped in the category "other causes contributing to heart failure" and warrants further investigation. This is particularly important as the proportion of cases with operated congenital heart disease is increasing and congenital heart disease altogether is more commonly diagnosed.[10] Early heart failure needs to be diagnosed appropriately as it can be managed in multidisciplinary teams using pharmacologic or nonpharmacologic interventions.

PRIMARY CAUSE AND TYPE OF HEART FAILURE IN THE DEVELOPING WORLD

Heart failure in the developing world is mainly due to nonischemic causes, such as hypertensive heart disease, valvular heart disease as a result of rheumatic fever and its sequelae, and heart muscle disease caused by infectious or unknown agents. This includes region-specific cardiomyopathies, such as endomyocardial fibrosis (EMF) (Africa), Chagas disease (South America), and peripartum cardiomyopathy (PPCM), which has a particularly high prevalence in the black African population. Cardiac manifestations of HIV include forms of HIV cardiomyopathy,[11] which will be reviewed in the following sections. Reporting on the etiology and primary cause of heart failure was in the past only clinical-based and is only in the past 10 to 20 years supported by echocardiography. In addition, the focus is mainly on causes of heart failure due to systolic dysfunction. Reporting on heart failure with preserved systolic function, as commonly seen due to hypertensive heart disease or in addition to systolic heart failure, is rare from the developing world.[12,13] This needs to be addressed in future studies, because it is likely that the profile of heart failure will also change in those regions as a result of shifts in population demographics, prevalence of specific risk factors, and the influence of the evolution of and access to therapeutic options. In studies from the Western world, such as those by Owan and colleagues[14] reporting on 6076 patients with heart failure being discharged from the Mayo Clinic Hospitals in Olmsted County, Minnesota, an increase was shown in the prevalence of heart failure with preserved systolic function over a 15-year period. This is probably due to a number of factors, but is also likely due to the fact that the chance of survival after the diagnosis of heart failure has increased and overall management has improved.

SPECIFIC ASPECTS OF HEART FAILURE IN KEY REGIONS IN THE DEVELOPING WORLD

Sub-Saharan Africa

Cardiomyopathy and rheumatic heart disease have historically been considered to be the major causes of heart failure in sub-Saharan Africa, accounting for almost half of all cases presenting to hospitals in the period between 1957 and 2005.[15,16] They pose a great challenge even in the context of the increasing burden of other cardiovascular diseases, such as hypertensive heart disease, because they are difficult to diagnose in resource-poor environments as a result of the lack of specialized facilities and access to echocardiography. There is also a limit in effective interventions, such as medication, device therapy, valve replacement, and heart transplantation. There has been important new research on the epidemiology, pathogenesis, and prognosis of heart failure and cardiomyopathy in Africa in the past decade, as well as a few outcome studies.

Heart Failure Overall

Acute decompensated heart failure is the most common primary diagnosis for patients admitted to a hospital with heart disease in Africa.[17,18] Recent data from the Sub-Saharan Africa Survey of Heart Failure (THESUS-HF), the first and largest multicenter registry of acute heart failure in Africa to date, has characterized the causes and short-term outcomes in 1006 Africans with heart failure, from 12 tertiary cardiology centers in 9 countries in sub-Saharan Africa.[17] The diagnosis of heart failure in THESUS-HF was based on the presence of dyspnea associated with physical findings of congestive heart failure, necessitating admission to a hospital in a patient who was 12 years of age or older. Echocardiography was used in all patients included in the study. It is apparent from THESUS-HF that there are major differences between the epidemiology of acute decompensated heart failure in sub-Saharan Africa compared with North America and Europe (**Table 27-3**). One of the most striking features is the relative youth of the African patients affected by acute heart failure (mean age 52 years). In Western countries, acute decompensated heart failure is a disease of the elderly, with a mean age of 70 to 72 years.[19,20] Acute heart failure therefore strikes the generation of breadwinners and caregivers in African patients, thereby having major economic implications. The younger African patients with acute heart failure have a lower frequency of ischemic heart disease, hypertension, diabetes mellitus, atrial fibrillation, and renal insufficiency compared with elderly heart failure sufferers in developed countries. Compared with a summary of the causes of heart failure in sub-Saharan Africa, based on the case series published between 1957 and 2005,[15] THESUS-HF shows a changing trend in the epidemiology of acute heart failure in sub-Saharan Africa. There was a rise in the contribution of hypertension as a

TABLE 27-3 Features of Patients with Acute Decompensated Heart Failure in Registries in the ADHERE (United States), ADHERE-AP (Asia Pacific), EHFS II (Europe), and THESUS-HF (Sub-Saharan Africa) Registries

	ADHERE REGISTRY (n = 105,388)	ADHERE—AP (n = 10,171)	EHFS II REGISTRY (n = 3580)	THESUS-HF REGISTRY (n = 1006)
Male, %	48	57	61	49
Mean age, years	72	66	70	52
Hypertension	73	64	63	45
Coronary artery disease, %	57	50	54	7
Diabetes, %	44	45	33	11
Atrial fibrillation, %	31	24	39	18
Anemia, %	NA	NA	15	15
Renal insufficiency, %	30	NA	17	8

ADHERE, Acute Decompensated Heart Failure National Registry; *ADHERE-AP,* ADHERE Asia Pacific; *EHFS II,* EuroHeart Failure Survey II; *THESUS-HF,* The Sub-Saharan Africa Survey of Heart Failure.

cause of heart failure (from 23% to 45%), a reduction in the role of rheumatic heart disease (from 22% to 14%), and an apparent increase in recognition of ischemic heart disease as a cause of heart failure (from 2% to almost 8%). The high incidence of hypertension and relatively low rate of coronary artery disease have also been observed in other single-center studies, such as the Heart of Soweto Study, where less than 10% of cases of heart failure were attributed to coronary artery disease.[21]

A recent publication by Ojji et al[22] reported on carefully characterized, consecutively captured patients residing in Abuja/Nigeria (n = 1515), comparing them to 4626 patients from the Heart of Soweto project, South Africa,[18] showing that hypertension contributed to even 60% of all cases presented with heart failure (HF) in Abuja versus 33% in Soweto. In the Soweto Cohort, 66% had multiple risk factors versus only 12% in Abuja. On an age- and sex-adjusted basis, compared with the Soweto cohort, the Abuja cohort were more likely to present with a primary diagnosis of hypertension (adjusted odds ratio [OR] 2.10, 95% confidence interval [CI] 1.85-2.42) or hypertensive heart disease/failure (OR 2.48, 95% CI 2.18-2.83); P <0.001 for both. They were, however, far less likely to present with coronary artery disease (OR 0.04, 95% CI 0.02-0.11) and right heart failure (2.5% vs. 27%).

HF with systolic dysfunction appears to be the most common form in Africa.[23,24] However, most of the larger hospital- and community-based studies on HF were performed before the emphasis on HF with preserved ejection fraction. Data on treatment pattern are limited. In a registry in South Africa,[21] medication prescribed for patients presenting with systolic dysfunction (n = 417) was appropriately prescribed as loop diuretics (85%), ACE inhibitors (70%), β-blocker (64%), aldosterone inhibitors (60%), and digitalis (19%). In the same cohort study, 373 patients had heart failure with preserved ejection fraction and received therapy with diuretics (43%), β-blocker (25%), aldosterone antagonists (22%), and a calcium antagonist (18%). The THESUS study[17] showed an inappropriately high prescription of aspirin and digitalis. Data on compliance are limited but, if available, were comparable with other regions.[17,25]

Heart Failure Due to Hypertensive Heart Disease

The global impact of elevated blood pressure (BP)/hypertension is profound, being responsible for more deaths worldwide than any other risk factor, including tobacco use, obesity, and lipid disorders (see also Chapter 23).[7] Taking Africa as a whole, a systematic review by Ibrahim and Damasceno[26] estimate that the prevalence of hypertension (BP >160/95 mm Hg) in adults 55 years or older increased from 54% to 78% between 1998 and 2003. Based on the change in lifestyle (adopting Western lifestyles), the African Union estimates that 10 to 20 million people in sub-Saharan Africa may currently be having hypertension, providing a similar challenge to HIV/AIDS. As such, hypertension commonly manifests in Africa with stroke, chronic heart failure, and chronic kidney disease.[27] Hypertension in the black African population is considered to be a distinct biologic entity.[28] Not only do Africans develop more hypertension, but compared with other ethnic groups, hypertension in blacks is often more severe[29] and more resistant to treatment,[30] often leading to heart failure.

Studies on possible pathophysiologic mechanisms are not yet conclusive, particularly with respect to gender-based heterogeneity. However, observed gender-based differences in the underlying prevalence and characteristics of hypertension are often marked in black Africans. In the Heart of Soweto registry,[18,31,32] detailed information was captured on more than 6000 de novo presentations (5328 with confirmed heart disease) presenting to the cardiology unit of the Baragwanath Hospital, which services a community in profound epidemiologic transition. African women were the single biggest contributors to case presentations (2863 or 54%), with 575 (20%) presenting with a primary diagnosis of hypertension and a further 1196 (42%) with a secondary diagnosis of hypertension. Among the latter, hypertensive heart failure (682/1196 or 57%, mean age 60 ± 14 years) was the most common manifestation of hypertensive heart disease.[31] Interestingly the level of education and noncommunicable risk factors, such as family history of CVD, smoking, obesity, and type 2 diabetes, correlated with advance disease.

Historically, these data contrast with that collected in Nigeria in the 1960s and 1970s, showing a higher prevalence of hypertension in men than in women, at least up to the age of 40 years old when the prevalence equalized.[33,34] However, a more contemporary report from rural Nigeria showed that of 858 cases of hypertension, more than two thirds were female, suggesting a possible shift in epidemiology.[35]

Heart Failure Due to Cardiomyopathies

In adult Africans, cardiomyopathy accounts for 20% to 30% of cases and is a major cause of heart failure.[15,17] Dilated cardiomyopathy refers to a heterogeneous group of heart muscle diseases of diverse causes (see also Chapter 19). Presentation is usually with progressive heart failure.

Important causes in Africa include PPCM, endomyocardial fibrosis, HIV-related cardiomyopathies, genetic causes, and idiopathic cardiomyopathies.[36]

Data from studies in Europe and North America have for a long time indicated that as many as 20% to 50% of patients with dilated cardiomyopathy (DCM) may have familial disease,[37] but little is known about the frequency and clinical genetics of this disease in Africa (see also Chapter 22). Ntusi and coworkers found that familial DCM affected at least a quarter of African patients with DCM.[38] Patients presented at a young age (29 years old) compared with patients with idiopathic DCM (39 years old). Furthermore, this was associated with PPCM (7%) and followed an autosomal dominant pattern of inheritance in most families. This was the first study to report on the frequency and the probable mode of inheritance of familial DCM in patients who presented at a tertiary center in Cape Town. The recommendation for family screening for familial DCM in all cases of unexplained DCM, including patients with PPCM, to African patients with the disease[39] is supported by these findings.

Studies from South Africa have shown an association with HLA-DR1 and DRw10 antigens, as well as mitochondrial polymorphisms with idiopathic DCM.[40] Isolated left ventricular noncompaction (ILVNC)[41] is probably often unrecognized as a cause of heart failure and stroke.

The first population-based study of the epidemiologic features and early stages of EMF were reported by Mocumbi and coworkers.[42] In a random sample (1063 subjects) of all age groups from rural Mozambique, the prevalence of EMF (19.8% overall) was determined by transthoracic echocardiography. Patients 10 to 19 years old presented with the highest prevalence of EMF (28.1%), and EMF was higher in male compared to female subjects. Biventricular EMF was found to be the most common form (prevalence 55.5%), followed by right-sided EMF (prevalence 29.0%), with most affected patients displaying mild to moderate structural and functional echocardiographic abnormalities and only 48 being symptomatic with signs of heart failure (22.7%).

HIV/AIDS and its therapy can have effects on the cardiovascular system on several levels leading to heart failure (**Figure 27-1**).[43] Cardiomyopathy in HIV-seropositive patients is associated with a longer duration of HIV infection, low total lymphocyte count, low CD4 count, and high HIV-1 viral load.[11,44] A prospective study of 157 patients from Kinshasa showed that almost 50% of the patients developed a cardiac abnormality over a 7-year period.[45] A significant proportion of patients with HIV-associated cardiomyopathy are free of specific cardiac signs and symptoms. In the Heart of Soweto cohort, 24% of patients with HIV-associated cardiomyopathy had asymptomatic left ventricular dysfunction.[46] HIV-associated cardiomyopathy leads to rapid progression of death in patients who are not treated with antiretroviral therapy.[47] The majority of HIV-positive patients in Africa now have access to antiretroviral therapy, which can by itself have cardiac effects leading to heart failure, as recently reviewed by Thienemann and colleagues.[43]

PPCM is a relatively rare idiopathic disease associated with severe heart failure and occurs toward the end of pregnancy or in the months following delivery (see also Chapter 19).[48,49] Accurate data on the incidence of PPCM are unavailable as few population-based registries exist. Recent studies suggest a wide variation in the estimated incidences (**Table 27-4**). The reason for such a variation remains unclear and could possibly be linked to ethnic

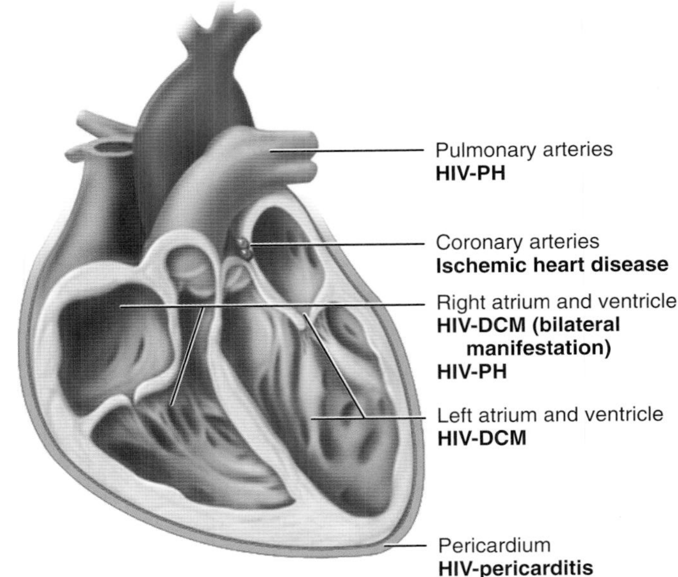

FIGURE 27-1 Effects of HIV on the heart.

and socioeconomic factors. Brar[50] found a large difference in the incidence among different ethnic groups in the United States, with 1:1421 in African Americans, 1:2675 in Asians, 1:4075 in Caucasians, and 1:9861 in Hispanics. Another study from the United States[51] found a 15-fold higher incidence of PPCM in African American women compared with non-African Americans. Interestingly, left ventricular recovery and survival rates of PPCM in African Americans are similar to those reported from Haiti and South Africa, and different from that of Caucasians diagnosed in the United States.[52] Socioeconomic factors may limit access to timely and advanced medical care. However, in the U.S. and South African studies, patients had a similar rate of optimal drug therapy, including ACE inhibitors and β-blockers, compared with the other ethnic groups.[52,53]

Novel molecular mechanisms of PPCM have been identified through research performed in the past 10 years. Studies using plasma from African patients with newly diagnosed PPCM have shown that elevated proinflammatory serum markers such as sFas/Apo1, C-reactive protein, interferon gamma, and interleukin-6 point to proinflammatory processes involved in the induction and the progression of PPCM and possibly impacting the prognosis.[54,55] Moreover, the findings of Hilfiker-Kleiner and colleagues point to possible involvement of a pathophysiologic circuit involving unbalanced oxidative stress and subsequent enhanced cleavage of the prolactin into an angiostatic and proapoptotic 16-kDa subfragment, leading to endothelial damage and ventricular dysfunction.[55] The significant role of endothelial damage is further supported by the significantly elevated endothelial microparticles found in acute PPCM, exhibiting apoptosis with impaired microcirculation.[56]

Hilfiker-Kleiner and coworkers went on to dissect the downstream effects of 16-kDa prolactin in PPCM. They discovered that 16-kDa prolactin, which is not signaling through the prolactin receptors, induces the expression of microRNA-146a (miR-146a) in endothelial cells.[57]

TABLE 27-4 Incidence of Peripartum Cardiomyopathy

AUTHOR	YEAR	COUNTRY	INCIDENCE	COHORT	DEFINITION OF PERIPARTUM CARDIOMYOPATHY	ECHOCARDIOGRAPHIC ASSESSMENT
Fett[96]	2002	Haiti	1 in 400 live births	Afro-Caribbean	1. CHF 1 month before to 5 months after delivery 2. No preexisting heart disease 3. No other cause identified for the CHF	EF <45%
Fett[97]	2005	Haiti	1 in 300 live births	Afro-Caribbean	1. CHF 1 month before to 5 months after delivery 2. No preexisting heart disease 3. No other cause identified for the CHF	EF <45%
Desai[98]	1995	South Africa	1 in 1000 live births	Black Africans	1. CHF 1 month before to 5 months after delivery 2. No preexisting heart disease 3. No other cause identified for the CHF	EF <45%
Mielniczuk[99]	2006	United States	1 in 2289 live births	50% nonwhite	1. CHF 1 month before to 5 months after delivery 2. No preexisting heart disease 3. No other cause identified for the CHF	Not defined
Chapa[100]	2005	United States	1 in 1149 live births	African American 80%	1. CHF 1 month before to 5 months after delivery 2. No preexisting heart disease 3. No other cause identified for the CHF	Not defined

Only studies using echocardiography have been included.
CHF, Congestive heart failure; *EF*, ejection fraction.

The angiogenic imbalance in PPCM as well as preeclampsia may not only depend on 16-kDA prolactin, but may rely on other factors such as soluble fms-like tyrosine kinase (sFlt-1).[58,59]

Bromocriptine, a prolactin-blocker, has recently emerged as a very promising therapeutic approach for the treatment of patients with PPCM,[60,61] based on the concept of enhanced cleavage of the nursing hormone prolactin into a deleterious, antiangiogenic, and proapoptotic form. A proof-of-concept pilot study with 20 African patients having PPCM showed that mortality was reduced and cardiac function improved in patients treated with bromocriptine, in contrast to patients receiving a placebo. That therapeutic option has been highlighted in the current European Society Guidelines on Cardiac Disease in Pregnancy[62] and received support from a recent study on a large cohort of German PPCM patients.[63]

Several prospective outcome studies in PPCM using contemporary diagnostic tools have been done in South Africa. A recent single-center study on 176 patients with PPCM in South Africa reports a poor outcome, defined as death, remaining in New York Heart Association (NYHA) functional class (FC) III-IV, or no improvement in ejection fraction greater than 35% in 26% of patients over 6 months on standard heart failure therapy, including ACE inhibitors and β-blockers. Left ventricular systolic dimension, lower body mass index, and low serum cholesterol at presentation were found to be predictors of poor outcome in African patients with PPCM. Advanced age and smaller left ventricular end-systolic dimensions appear to be independently associated with a higher incidence of left ventricular recovery.[53] A recent study from Nigeria by Karaye[64] reported, in addition to the low left ventricular ejection fraction (27.2 ± 9.4%), a frequent poor right ventricular function, as measured by echocardiographic tricuspid annular plane excursion, of less than 14 mm in more than 50% of the 55 patients studied.

Other forms of heart failure occurring commonly in Africa include heart failure associated with pericardial disease due to late recognition of and poorly managed rheumatic valvular disease and right heart failure. A recently published review on heart failure in sub-Saharan Africa summarized the recent literature of those conditions leading to heart failure.[13]

South America

Heart failure is the main cause of hospitalization based on available data from about 50% of the South American population.[12] With the Latin American countries undergoing marked epidemiologic changes with a marked increase in coronary artery disease due to an increasing prevalence of the traditional risk factors such as obesity, diabetes, hypertension, and aging population, coronary artery disease is now the main cause of congestive heart failure in the Latin Americans.[65] However, infectious diseases, such as Chagas disease and rheumatic heart disease—common causes of CHF in Latin America—still remain frequent in this region and contribute to the burden of disease.

A number of studies reported data on cause and outcome in patients with acute and chronic heart failure from South America versus other regions of the world. These are the Eplerenone Post-AMI Heart Failure Efficacy and Survival Study[66] and the EVEREST study,[67] comparing in particular North and South America. For example, the recently published data from the EVEREST study reported on the regional differences of the baseline demographics of patients with acute heart failure in regions such as North America (n = 1251), South America (n = 699), Western Europe (n = 564), and Eastern Europe (n = 1619). With a mean age of 62.2 years, the patients in South America were significantly younger compared with the other regions (P <0.001), with the same dominance of males (74.5%), but only half of the patients reporting were of white ethnicity (P <0.001). There were marked differences in the baseline characteristics with patients from South America having less coronary artery disease (39.9% versus 77.6%), less chronic obstructive pulmonary disease (5.7% versus 18.1%), less diabetes (29.9% versus 51.5%), and less frequent myocardial infarction (29.5% versus 55.6%) compared with patients in North America (for all P <0.001). There was therefore a significantly lower percentage of patients having had a coronary artery bypass graft (CABG) (13.3% in South America versus 41.4% in North America, P <0.001), and having had less frequently percutaneous coronary intervention (PCI) (12.3% versus 32.6%). There was also a difference in the use of medical therapy with patients in South America having a particularly high use of ACE inhibitors (93% versus 75%), higher use of aldosterone blockers (65% versus 35%), but a lower use of β-blockers (56% versus 78%). In general patients in South America were younger, had longer hospitalizations, and had lower PCI and CABG use, and there were some differences in event rates, risk factors, and therapeutic management. Some of the regional differences in drug use, cardiovascular interventions, and severity of the diseases appear to be related to economic factors.

Robust data on prevalence and outcome of heart failure in inpatients are also available from the Brazilian Ministry of Health (DATASUS).[12] Of the 743,763 hospitalizations due to cardiovascular disease in 2007, 39.4% were associated with HF. The mean period in the hospital was 5.8 days, with a mortality range from 6.5% to 6.9%.[12] Studies from Brazil (REMADHF),[68] Argentina (GESICA),[69] and Mexico[70] on outpatients reported high prevalences of ischemic cause, ranging from 22% to 47%, followed by hypertension and valvular disease. The RAMADHF and GESICA studies reported prevalence of Chagas disease as a cause of heart failure between 10% and 28%.

Chagas disease in Latin America remains common. Disease control programs have significantly reduced the number of infected individuals from approximately 16 to 18 million in the early 1990s to 10 to 12 million in the early 2000s.[71,72] Chagas disease is usually acquired during childhood as a result of *Trypanosoma cruzi* present in the feces of Reduviidae insects penetrating the skin or conjunctiva of people living in rural areas. The disease has an acute phase, presenting as a nonspecific febrile illness lasting several weeks, and is becoming clinically manifest in less than 1% of the infected subjects. Acute myocarditis leading to heart failure only occurs in 1 to 5 of every 10,000 infected people.[73] It commonly (>50%) has a significant pericardial effusion.[74]

Chronic Chagas cardiomyopathy evolves over several decades after infection. A recent review by Acquatella reported on the echocardiographic features in Chagas heart disease. More than half of the chronic Chagas cardiomyopathy subjects remain asymptomatic. Early Doppler abnormalities include prolongation of isovolumic contraction and relaxation times. Systolic function frequently is normal, but dysfunction can be provoked by stress testing. More than half of the symptomatic patients have left ventricular apical aneurysm and other contractile abnormalities. Other forms presenting with a generally dilated heart are indistinguishable from other cardiomyopathies. Patients presenting with heart failure in NYHA FC II and III commonly present with arrhythmias, an embolism, and sudden death. The heart is commonly dilated, and left ventricular (LV) systolic and diastolic parameters are usually abnormal.[75,76] Mitral and tricuspid valve regurgitation may be present. The estimated 10-year survival is 75% to 85%. Patients in NYHA FC IV have only a 50% chance of survival. Recent studies reported prognostic variables by echocardiography. Chagas-related electrocardiogram abnormalities, LV systolic and diastolic parameters, and LVEF were predictors of events. The prognosis of patients with Chagas heart disease is worse in comparison with other causes.[77] Heart transplantation is effective but is associated with reactivation of the *T. cruzi* infection.[78] Altogether the challenges of the management of Chagas disease need to be addressed and specific trials are necessary.

Asia and the Pacific Region

This large and heterogeneous region represents some of the most populous countries in the world; from well-known "giants" such as China (population 1.3 billion) to India (1.2 billion) to the often forgotten Indonesia (250 million). Any systematic review of the published literature, although revealing an increasing number of reports from the latter two countries, is characterized by a startling lack of data for midsize countries, such as Vietnam (population ≈90 million) and Malaysia (≈28 million), relative to those derived from smaller populations in Europe and North America. The difficulty of broadly characterizing the burden of heart failure in these countries is highlighted by the limited reports emanating from them. For example, Chong and colleagues[79] examined a total of 1435 medical admissions to a major hospital in Kuala Lumpur (the capital of Malaysia) over 4 weeks. They found that around 7% of these admissions were attributable (primary diagnosis of chronic heart failure) to coronary artery disease (50%) and hypertension (20%). However, considering the ethnic diversity of the Malaysian population (including the predominant Malay people plus significant portions of people from Chinese and Indian descent) with geographic differentials, their observation that associated causative factors varied according to ethnicity (e.g., markedly more diabetes in those of Indian descent) is notable. Although one might expect a less complex picture of heart failure in Vietnam (perhaps with northern versus southern differentials based on cultural and socioeconomic factors), there is a dearth of data to confirm this. Indeed, the most obvious report on heart failure represents the personal experiences of a visiting U.S. student with very little insight into the nature of the problem in that country.[80] Indeed, there are many such gaps in respect to describing heart failure in the largest (i.e., Indonesia) and smallest (the Pacific Islands) populations in the region.

Regional Comparisons

Given the paucity of data overall, it is fortunate that Atherton and colleagues[81] have reported on the ADHERE (Acute Decompensated Heart Failure National Registry) comprising 10,171 hospitalized cases of heart failure (principal diagnosis) captured via an electronic Web-based observational database during the period 2006 to 2008. Apart from those higher-income countries (including Australia, Hong Kong, Singapore, and Taiwan), a number of developing countries in the region were included—comprising Thailand (20% of clinical cases), Indonesia (17%), Malaysia (9%), and the Philippines (7%). **Figure 27-2** compares the median age of

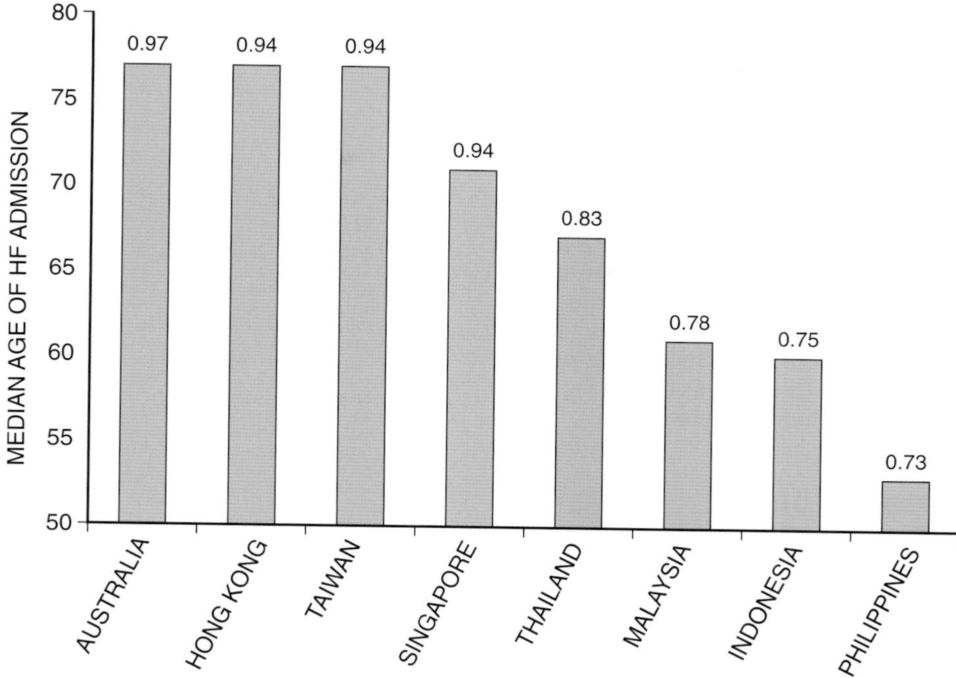

FIGURE 27-2 Median age of heart failure (HF) cases in ADHERE in countries of the Asia Pacific region, with the number above each bar representing the human development index (HDI). *Data from Atherton JJ, Hayward CS, Wan Ahmad WA, et al: Patient characteristics from a regional multicenter database of acute decompensated heart failure in Asia Pacific (ADHERE International-Asia Pacific) J Card Fail 18:82–88, 2012.*

heart failure cases for the developing countries with the developed countries included in the registry. Although not providing a perfect correlation, it is evident that in high-income countries in this region with associated high human development index scores, typical heart failure patients present with a median age older than 75 years and with profiles similar to those published in Europe via the EHS[20] and ADHERE data from North America.[19] Alternatively, as with other regions around the world such as sub-Saharan Africa, the median age of heart failure cases is markedly lower.

East Asia

In China alone it is estimated that just over 4 million individuals (only a million less than the United States but clearly at lower prevalence levels) currently have heart failure.[82] Guo and colleagues recently completed a systematic review of the literature relating to heart failure in East Asia.[83] This and other papers in a series seeking to provide a global picture of heart failure (see South Asia discussion later) provide the most contemporary and up-to-date picture of heart failure in developing countries (albeit mixed with summaries of developed countries in those regions). However, the same caveat in respect to lack of standardized data and enormous gaps in the literature (given the size of population) needs to be considered.

Using best available data (reports from China being a predominant feature), they concluded that the prevalence of heart failure in Malaysia was as high as 6.7% compared with 1.3% in China (with an associated incidence rate of 0.7-0.9 per 1000 per annum).[83] In comparison, the estimated prevalence of heart failure in the highly developed country of Singapore was estimated to be 4.5%.[84] As expected, profound socioeconomic dynamics continue to shape the underlying causes of an evolving burden of heart failure in the region. As such the reported presence of coronary artery disease in heart failure cases across the region ranged from as low as 25% to 47%.[83] In comparison, concurrent hypertension ranged from a low of 19% in Malaysia[85] to a high of 74% in the high-income country of Japan,[86] with markedly different figures in mainland China depending on the region (23%-47%).[87-89] Notably, concurrent cases of valvular disease varied across the region with fewer cases reported in East Asia; in most countries this figure ranged from 15% to 35%, but was only 4% in Malaysia.[83] Reports of heart failure associated with preserved systolic function and heart failure–related survival are few and far between, with almost all reports derived from high-income countries; perhaps not surprisingly given the high prevalence of hypertensive heart failure, Japanese reports dominate the former.

Indigenous Peoples

Any commentary on the burden of heart failure in this widely dispersed region is not complete without some consideration of indigenous populations living in countries otherwise designated as "developed." For example, New Zealand (population ≈4.5 million) has significant numbers of Pacific people who have similar health profiles to those living in the developed world. Data derived from these vulnerable populations share the same characteristics of relatively younger cases and more women affected with more diverse pathways to the syndrome.[90]

Carr and colleagues[91] undertook a retrospective, national analysis of mortality and morbidity data attributed to heart failure (data period 1988-1998) in Mäori and non-Mäori men and women aged 45 years or older. They found that heart failure–related case fatality was almost 9 times and 3.5 times, respectively, higher in Mäori men aged 45 to 64 years and older than 65 years, with similar patterns in women. A similar pattern (of markedly increased risk) was found in respect to the rate of heart failure admissions. More recent data from Sopoaga and colleagues[92] indicate that observed disparities remain high relative to the rest of the population, with Mäori people being six times more likely to be admitted to the hospital with cardiomyopathy and four to five times more likely to present with rheumatic heart disease. Across the Tasman Sea in Australia (population 20 million), McGrady[93] and colleagues undertook a population survey of heart failure in the isolated communities of Central Australia (≈15,000 Aboriginal people). Of 436 adults screened (mean 44 years and 64% women), a high proportion (relative to wider population estimates) were diagnosed with heart failure (5.3%) and asymptomatic left ventricular dysfunction (13%). The main drivers of heart failure were obesity (42%), hypertension (41%), and diabetes (40%), with the case prevalence of coronary artery disease the same as that of the relatively high figure for rheumatic heart disease (7%).

KEY CONSIDERATIONS FOR THE PREVENTION AND MANAGEMENT OF HEART FAILURE IN THE DEVELOPING WORLD

The epidemiology of heart failure in the different regions of the world remains poorly described. Therefore, geographically and ethnically diverse population studies including all ages and gender are urgently needed. Because much information is missing, it is not clear if the current guidelines developed by different societies apply in full, because they can only be based on the data that are currently available.

In Africa there is, at present, only a single outcome-based study on about 1000 patients admitted with acute heart failure.[17] This study has many limitations, because it was hospital-based, using selected centers that have access to echocardiography and a cardiologist. As highlighted above, future research on heart failure, not only in hospitals but also in the community, is urgently needed in several world regions. Prevalence studies are costly and are not receiving the necessary support. Multicountry case-control studies, such as the INTERCHF study, will help to get information on underlying risk factors. INTERCHF, a longitudinal case study, is under way in low- and middle-income countries in South America, Asia, and Africa and aims to recruit approximately 5000 heart failure patients from rural and urban areas, including inpatients and outpatients.

What Is Needed for a Global Heart Failure Prevention Strategy?

In many regions patients are dying of heart failure from preventable causes.[94] In some regions, for example, Brazil, Argentina, and South Africa, a large portion of the health care resources are spent on paying for high-complexity cardiac surgeries, and limited funds are allocated to prevention. Some regions have no specific prevention programs for rheumatic heart disease. Implementing what is known, tackling obesity, and preventing diabetes and subsequently hypertension and ischemic heart disease is probably the most important strategy worldwide. Early diagnosis of the risk factors via simple and affordable diagnostic tools could prevent communicable and emerging noncommunicable causes and lead to the use of already affordable pharmacologic therapy such as, in particular, ACE inhibitors and β-blockers.

References

1. D'Agostino RB, Russell MW, Huse DM, et al: Primary and subsequent coronary risk appraisal: new results from the Framingham study. *Am Heart J* 139:272281, 2000.
2. Krum H, Jelinek MV, Stewart S, et al: 2011 update to National Heart Foundation of Australia and Cardiac Society of Australia and New Zealand Guidelines for the prevention, detection and management of chronic heart failure in Australia, 2006. *Med J Aust* 194:405–409, 2011.
3. Chan MM, Lam CS: How do patients with heart failure with preserved ejection fraction die? *Eur J Heart Fail* 15:604–613, 2013.
4. Stewart S, Sliwa K: Preventing CVD in resource-poor areas: perspectives from the "real world." *Nat Rev Cardiol* 6:489–492, 2009.
5. Khatibzadeh S, Farzadfar F, Oliver J, et al: Worldwide risk factors for heart failure: a systematic review and pooled analysis. *Int J Cardiol* 168:1186–1194, 2013.
6. Lozano R, Naghavi M, Foreman K, et al: Global and regional mortality from 235 causes of death for 20 age groups in 1990 and 2010: a systematic analysis for the Global Burden of Disease Study 2010. *Lancet* 380:2095–2128, 2012.
7. Vos T, Flaxman AD, Naghavi M, et al: Years lived with disability (YLDs) for 1160 sequelae of 289 diseases and injuries 1990-2010: a systematic analysis for the Global Burden of Disease Study 2010. *Lancet* 380:2163–2196, 2012.
8. Killip T: Epidemiology of congestive heart failure. *Am J Cardiol* 56:2A–6A, 1985.
9. Mendez GF, Cowie MR: The epidemiological features of heart failure in developing countries: a review of the literature. *Int J Cardiol* 80:213–219, 2001.
10. van der Linde D, Konings EE, Slager MA, et al: Birth prevalence of congenital heart disease worldwide: a systematic review and meta-analysis. *J Am Coll Cardiol* 58:2241–2247, 2011.
11. Ntsekhe M, Mayosi BM: Cardiac manifestations of HIV infection: an African perspective. *Nat Clin Pract Cardiovasc Med* 6:120–127, 2009.
12. Bocchi EA: Heart failure in South America. *Curr Cardiol Rev* 9:147–156, 2013.
13. Bloomfield GS, Barasa FA, Doll JA, et al: Heart failure in sub-Saharan Africa. *Curr Cardiol Rev* 9:157–173, 2013.
14. Owan TE, Hodge DO, Herges RM, et al: Trends in prevalence and outcome of heart failure with preserved ejection fraction. *N Engl J Med* 355:251–259, 2006.
15. Mayosi BM: Contemporary trends in the epidemiology and management of cardiomyopathy and pericarditis in sub-Saharan Africa. *Heart* 93:1176–1183, 2007.
16. Sliwa K, Damasceno A, Mayosi BM: Epidemiology and etiology of cardiomyopathy in Africa. *Circulation* 112:3577–3583, 2005.
17. Damasceno A, Mayosi BM, Sani M, et al: The etiology, treatment, and outcome of acute heart failure in 1006 Africans from 9 countries: results of the Sub-Saharan Africa Survey of Heart Failure (THESUS-HF). *Arch Intern Med* 172:1386–1394, 2012.
18. Sliwa K, Wilkinson D, Hansen C, et al: Spectrum of heart disease and risk factors in a black urban population in South Africa (the Heart of Soweto Study): a cohort study. *Lancet* 371:915–922, 2008.
19. Adams KF, Jr, Fonarow GC, Emerman CL, et al: Characteristics and outcomes of patients hospitalized for heart failure in the United States: rationale, design, and preliminary observations from the first 100,000 cases in the Acute Decompensated Heart Failure National Registry (ADHERE). *Am Heart J* 149:209–216, 2005.
20. Nieminen MS, Brutsaert D, Dickstein K, et al: EuroHeart Failure Survey II (EHFS II): a survey on hospitalized acute heart failure patients: description of population. *Eur Heart J* 27:2725–2736, 2006.
21. Stewart S, Wilkinson D, Hansen C, et al: Predominance of heart failure in the Heart of Soweto Study cohort: emerging challenges for urban African communities. *Circulation* 118:2360–2367, 2008.
22. Ojji D, Stewart S, Ajayi S, et al: A predominance of hypertensive heart failure in the Abuja Heart Study cohort of urban Nigerians: a prospective clinical registry of 1515 de novo cases. *Eur J Heart Fail* 15:835–842, 2013.
23. Kingue S, Dzudie A, Menanga A, et al: [A new look at adult chronic heart failure in Africa in the age of the Doppler echocardiography: experience of the medicine department at Yaounde General Hospital]. *Ann Cardiol Angeiol (Paris)* 54:276–283, 2005.
24. Kengne AP, Dzudie A, Sobngwi E: Heart failure in sub-Saharan Africa: a literature review with emphasis on individuals with diabetes. *Vasc Health Risk Manag* 4:123–130, 2008.
25. Ruf V, Stewart S, Pretorius S, et al: Medication adherence, self-care behaviour and knowledge on heart failure in urban South Africa: the Heart of Soweto study. *Cardiovasc J Afr* 21:86–92, 2010.
26. Ibrahim MM, Damasceno A: Hypertension in developing countries. *Lancet* 380:611–619, 2012.
27. Opie LH: Controversies in cardiology. *Lancet* 367:13–14, 2006.
28. Drazner MH: The progression of hypertensive heart disease. *Circulation* 123:327–334, 2011.
29. Salako BL, Ogah OS, Adebiyi AA, et al: Unexpectedly high prevalence of target-organ damage in newly diagnosed Nigerians with hypertension. *Cardiovasc J Afr* 18:77–83, 2007.
30. Addo J, Smeeth L, Leon DA: Hypertension in sub-Saharan Africa: a systematic review. *Hypertension* 50:1012–1018, 2007.
31. Stewart S, Carrington M, Pretorius S, et al: Standing at the crossroads between new and historically prevalent heart disease: effects of migration and socio-economic factors in the Heart of Soweto cohort study. *Eur Heart J* 32:492–499, 2011.
32. Stewart S, Carrington MJ, Pretorius S, et al: Elevated risk factors but low burden of heart disease in urban African primary care patients: a fundamental role for primary prevention. *Int J Cardiol* 158:2005–2010, 2012.
33. Akinkugbe OO, Ojo AO: The systemic blood pressure in a rural Nigerian population. *Trop Geogr Med* 20:347–356, 1968.
34. Kramer H, Han C, Post W, et al: Racial/ethnic differences in hypertension and hypertension treatment and control in the multi-ethnic study of atherosclerosis (MESA). *Am J Hypertens* 17:963–970, 2004.
35. Ogah OS: Hypertension in Sub-Saharan African populations: the burden of hypertension in Nigeria. *Ethn Dis* 16:765, 2006.
36. Sliwa K, Mayosi BM: Recent advances in the epidemiology, pathogenesis and prognosis of acute heart failure and cardiomyopathy in Africa. *Heart* 99:1317–1322, 2013.
37. Watkins H, Ashrafian H, Redwood C: Inherited cardiomyopathies. *N Engl J Med* 364:1643–1656, 2011.
38. Ntusi NB, Badri M, Gumedze F, et al: Clinical characteristics and outcomes of familial and idiopathic dilated cardiomyopathy in Cape Town: a comparative study of 120 cases followed up over 14 years. *S Afr Med J* 101:399–404, 2011.
39. Hershberger RE, Siegfried JD: Update 2011: clinical and genetic issues in familial dilated cardiomyopathy. *J Am Coll Cardiol* 57:1641–1649, 2011.
40. Khogali SS, Mayosi BM, Beattie JM, et al: A common mitochondrial DNA variant associated with susceptibility to dilated cardiomyopathy in two different populations. *Lancet* 357:1265–1267, 2001.
41. Peters F, Khandheria BK, dos Santos C, et al: Isolated left ventricular noncompaction in sub-Saharan Africa: a clinical and echocardiographic perspective. *Circ Cardiovasc Imaging* 5:187–193, 2012.
42. Mocumbi AO, Ferreira MB, Sidi D, et al: A population study of endomyocardial fibrosis in a rural area of Mozambique. *N Engl J Med* 359:43–49, 2008.

43. Thienemann F, Sliwa K, Rockstroh JK: HIV and the heart: the impact of antiretroviral therapy: a global perspective. *Eur Heart J* 34:3538–3546, 2013.
44. Twagirumukiza M, Nkeramihigo E, Seminega B, et al: Prevalence of dilated cardiomyopathy in HIV-infected African patients not receiving HAART: a multicenter, observational, prospective, cohort study in Rwanda. *Curr HIV Res* 5:129–137, 2007.
45. Longo-Mbenza B, Bayekula M, Ngiyulu R, et al: Survey of rheumatic heart disease in school children of Kinshasa town. *Int J Cardiol* 63:287–294, 1998.
46. Sliwa K, Carrington MJ, Becker A, et al: Contribution of the human immunodeficiency virus/acquired immunodeficiency syndrome epidemic to de novo presentations of heart disease in the Heart of Soweto Study cohort. *Eur Heart J* 33:866–874, 2012.
47. Currie PF, Jacob AJ, Foreman AR, et al: Heart muscle disease related to HIV infection: prognostic implications. *BMJ* 309:1605–1607, 1994.
48. Sliwa K, Hilfiker-Kleiner D, Petrie M, et al: Current state of knowledge on aetiology, diagnosis, management, and therapy of peripartum cardiomyopathy: a position statement from the Heart Failure Association of the European Society of Cardiology Working Group on Peripartum Cardiomyopathy. *Eur Heart J* 12:767–778, 2010.
49. Sliwa K, Fett J, Elkayam U: Peripartum cardiomyopathy. *Lancet* 368:687–693, 2006.
50. Brar SS, Khan SS, Sandhu GK, et al: Incidence, mortality, and racial differences in peripartum cardiomyopathy. *Am J Cardiol* 100:302–304, 2007.
51. Gentry MB, Dias JK, Luis A, et al: African-American women have a higher risk for developing peripartum cardiomyopathy. *J Am Coll Cardiol* 55:654–659, 2010.
52. Modi KA, Illum S, Jariatul K, et al: Poor outcome of indigent patients with peripartum cardiomyopathy in the United States. *Am J Obstet Gynecol* 201:171 e1–171 e5, 2009.
53. Blauwet LA, Libhaber E, Forster O, et al: Predictors of outcome in 176 South African patients with peripartum cardiomyopathy. *Heart* 99:308–313, 2013.
54. Sliwa K, Forster O, Libhaber E, et al: Peripartum cardiomyopathy: inflammatory markers as predictors of outcome in 100 prospectively studied patients. *Eur Heart J* 27:441–446, 2006.
55. Hilfiker-Kleiner D, Kaminski K, Podewski E, et al: A cathepsin D-cleaved 16 kDa form of prolactin mediates postpartum cardiomyopathy. *Cell* 128:589–600, 2007.
56. Walenta K, Schwarz V, Schirmer SH, et al: Circulating microparticles as indicators of peripartum cardiomyopathy. *Eur Heart J* 33:1469–1479, 2012.
57. Halkein J, Tabruyn SP, Ricke-Hoch M, et al: MicroRNA-146a is a therapeutic target and biomarker for peripartum cardiomyopathy. *J Clin Invest* 123:2143–2154, 2013.
58. Patten IS, Rana S, Shahul S, et al: Cardiac angiogenic imbalance leads to peripartum cardiomyopathy. *Nature* 485:333–338, 2012.
59. Sliwa K, Mebaaza A: Possible joint pathways of early preeclampsia and congenital heart defects via angiogenic imbalance and potential evidence of cardio-placental syndrome. *Eur Heart J* In press, 2013.
60. Jahns BG, Stein W, Hilfiker-Kleiner D, et al: Peripartum cardiomyopathy—a new treatment option by inhibition of prolactin secretion. *Am J Obstet Gynecol* 199:e5–e6, 2008.
61. Sliwa K, Blauwet L, Tibazarwa K, et al: Evaluation of bromocriptine in the treatment of acute severe peripartum cardiomyopathy: a proof-of-concept pilot study. *Circulation* 121:1465–1473, 2010.
62. Regitz-Zagrosek V, Blomstrom Lundqvist C, Borghi C, et al: ESC Guidelines on the management of cardiovascular diseases during pregnancy: the Task Force on the Management of Cardiovascular Diseases during Pregnancy of the European Society of Cardiology (ESC). *Eur Heart J* 32:3147–3197, 2011.
63. Haghikia A, Podewski E, Libhaber E, et al: Phenotyping and outcome on contemporary management in a German cohort of patients with peripartum cardiomyopathy. *Basic Res Cardiol* 108:366, 2013.
64. Karaye KM: Right ventricular systolic function in peripartum and dilated cardiomyopathies. *Eur J Echocardiogr* 12:372–374, 2011.
65. Cubillos-Garzon LA, Casas JP, Morillo CA, et al: Congestive heart failure in Latin America: the next epidemic. *Am Heart J* 147:412–417, 2004.
66. Pitt B, Remme WJ, Zannad F, et al: Eplerenone, a selective aldosterone blocker in patients with left ventricular dysfunction after myocardial infarction. *N Engl J Med* 348:1309–1321, 2003.
67. Gheorghiade M, Pang PS, Ambrosy AP, et al: A comprehensive, longitudinal description of the in-hospital and post-discharge clinical, laboratory, and neurohormonal course of patients with heart failure who die or are re-hospitalized within 90 days: analysis from the EVEREST trial. *Heart Fail Rev* 17:485–509, 2012.
68. Bocchi EA, Cruz F, Guimaraes G, et al: Long-term prospective, randomized, controlled study using repetitive education at six-month intervals and monitoring for adherence in heart failure outpatients: the REMADHE trial. *Circ Heart Fail* 1:115–124, 2008.
69. Doval HC, Nul DR, Grancielli HO, et al: For Gruppo de Estudio de la Sobrevida en la Insuficiencia Cardiaca en Argentine (GESICA). Randomized trial of low-dose amiodarone in severe congestive heart failure. *Lancet* 344:493–498, 1994.
70. Mendez GF, Betancourt L, Galicia-Mora G: The impact of heart failure clinic in the improvement on quality of life of heart failure patients in Mexico. *Int J Cardiol* 115:242–243, 2007.
71. Acquatella H: Echocardiography in Chagas heart disease. *Circulation* 115:1124–1131, 2007.
72. Celermajer DS, Chow CK, Marijon E, et al: Cardiovascular disease in the developing world: prevalences, patterns, and the potential of early disease detection. *J Am Coll Cardiol* 60:1207–1216, 2012.
73. Rosenbaum MB: Chagasic myocardiopathy. *Prog Cardiovasc Dis* 7:199–225, 1964.
74. Parada H, Carrasco HA, Anez N, et al: Cardiac involvement is a constant finding in acute Chagas' disease: a clinical, parasitological and histopathological study. *Int J Cardiol* 60:49–54, 1997.
75. Carrasco HA, Barboza JS, Inglessis G, et al: Left ventricular cineangiography in Chagas' disease: detection of early myocardial damage. *Am Heart J* 104:595–602, 1982.
76. Espinosa R, Carrasco HA, Belandria F, et al: Life expectancy analysis in patients with Chagas' disease: prognosis after one decade (1973-1983). *Int J Cardiol* 8:45–56, 1985.
77. Issa VS, Amaral AF, Cruz FD, et al: Beta-blocker therapy and mortality of patients with Chagas cardiomyopathy: a subanalysis of the REMADHE prospective trial. *Circ Heart Fail* 3:82–88, 2010.
78. Campos KE, Volpato GT, Calderon IM, et al: Effect of obesity on rat reproduction and on the development of their adult offspring. *Braz J Med Biol Res* 41:122–125, 2008.
79. Chong PH, Boskovich A, Stevkovic N, et al: Statin-associated peripheral neuropathy: review of the literature. *Pharmacotherapy* 24:1194–1203, 2004.
80. Tong ST: Heart failure in Vietnam. *Fam Med* 44:656–657, 2012.
81. Atherton JJ, Hayward CS, Wan Ahmad WA, et al: Patient characteristics from a regional multicenter database of acute decompensated heart failure in Asia Pacific (ADHERE International-Asia Pacific). *J Card Fail* 18:82–88, 2012.
82. Cheng Z, Zhu K, Chen T, et al: Poor prognosis in chronic heart failure patients with reduced ejection fraction in China. *Congest Heart Fail* 18:165–172, 2012.
83. Guo Y, Lip GY, Banerjee A: Heart failure in East Asia. *Curr Cardiol Rev* 9:112–122, 2013.
84. Ng TP, Niti M: Trends and ethnic differences in hospital admissions and mortality for congestive heart failure in the elderly in Singapore, 1991 to 1998. *Heart* 89:865–870, 2003.
85. Chong AY, Rajaratnam R, Hussein NR, et al: Heart failure in a multiethnic population in Kuala Lumpur, Malaysia. *Eur J Heart Fail* 5:569–574, 2003.
86. Shiba N, Nochioka K, Miura M, et al: Trend of westernization of etiology and clinical characteristics of heart failure patients in Japan–first report from the CHART-2 study. *Circ J* 75:823–833, 2011.
87. Pei ZY, Zhao YS, Li JY, et al: [Fifteen-year evolving trends of etiology and prognosis in hospitalized patients with heart failure]. *Zhonghua Xin Xue Guan Bing Za Zhi* 39:434–439, 2011.
88. Yin Q, Zhao Y, Li J, et al: The coexistence of multiple cardiovascular diseases is an independent predictor of the 30-day mortality of hospitalized patients with congestive heart failure: a study in Beijing. *Clin Cardiol* 34:442–446, 2011.
89. Yu S, Cui H, Qin M, et al: Characteristics of in-hospital patients with chronic heart failure in Hubei province from 2000 to 2010. *Zhonghua Xin Xue Guan Bing Za Zhi* 39:549–552, 2011.
90. Riddell T: Heart failure hospitalisations and deaths in New Zealand: patterns by deprivation and ethnicity. *N Z Med J* 118:U1254, 2004.
91. Carr J, Robson B, Reid P, et al: Heart failure: ethnic disparities in morbidity and mortality in New Zealand. *N Z Med J* 115:15–17, 2002.
92. Sopoaga F, Buckingham K, Paul C: Causes of excess hospitalizations among Pacific peoples in New Zealand: implications for primary care. *J Prim Health Care* 2:105–110, 2010.
93. McGrady M, Krum H, Carrington MJ, et al: Heart failure, ventricular dysfunction and risk factor prevalence in Australian Aboriginal peoples: the Heart of the Heart Study. *Heart* 98:1562–1567, 2012.
94. Gersh BJ, Sliwa K, Mayosi BM, et al: Novel therapeutic concepts: the epidemic of cardiovascular disease in the developing world: global implications. *Eur Heart J* 31:642–648, 2010.
95. ACC/AHA 2005: Guideline update for the diagnosis and management of chronic heart failure in the adult. A report of the American College of Cardiology/American Heart Association Task Force on Practice Guidelines (Writing Committee to update the 2001 Guidelines for the Evaluation and Management of Heart Failure). *Circulation* 112:Published online September 13, 2005.
96. Fett JD, Carraway RD, Dowell DL, et al: Peripartum cardiomyopathy in the Hospital Albert Schweitzer District of Haiti. *Am J Obstet Gynecol* 186:1005–1010, 2002.
97. Fett JD, Christie LG, Carraway RD, et al: Unrecognized peripartum cardiomyopathy in Haitian women. *Int J Gynaecol Obstet* 90:161–166, 2005a.
98. Desai D, Moodley J, Naidoo D: Peripartum cardiomyopathy: experiences at King Edward VIII Hospital, Durban, South Africa and a review of the literature. *Trop Doct* 25:118–123, 1995.
99. Mielniczuk LM, Williams K, Davis DR, et al: Frequency of peripartum cardiomyopathy. *Am J Cardiol* 97:1765–1768, 2006.
100. Chapa JB, Heiberger HB, Weinert L, et al: Prognostic value of echocardiography in peripartum cardiomyopathy. *Obstet Gynecol* 105:1303–1308, 2005.

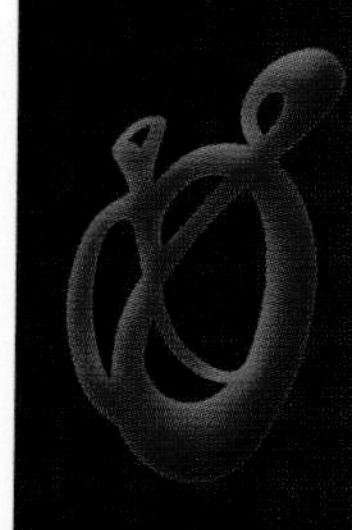

SECTION IV

CLINICAL ASSESSMENT OF HEART FAILURE

28 Clinical Evaluation of Heart Failure

W. H. Wilson Tang and Gary S. Francis

Heart failure is a clinical syndrome that presents in different stages with a wide spectrum of bedside presentations. Hence, the bedside evaluation of the patient with heart failure may vary, but is a critically important task. It calls for the use of clinical acumen and the proper use of laboratory resources in a very skillful manner. It also demands unrelenting vigilance to uncover precipitating factors and persistent counseling to ensure maximal effects in deterring disease progression. Heart failure is much like fever or anemia, and should not be considered as a "stand-alone" diagnosis, but be described with its associated cause (or causes), such as coronary artery disease, hypertension, valvular heart disease, and/or arrhythmia. Clearly, this evaluation will not be a one-time occurrence, but rather an ongoing process, and may evolve according to how the clinical course unfolds. Additional diagnostic information may be necessary to support the diagnosis and determine the precise mechanism of the symptoms, the severity of the problem, the natural history of the disorder, and the prognosis of an individual patient.

The clinical concept of heart failure has been largely historical and descriptive of volume overload (which may explain the common use of the term *congestive heart failure*). Today the availability of hemodynamic and imaging measures, quantification of the degree of cardiac insufficiency, and description of morphologic abnormalities are becoming increasingly important as part of the process of bedside clinical evaluation. With the recent adaptation of the staging system that extends beyond the presentation of signs and symptoms of heart failure, the evaluation process requires the integration of complex clinical and laboratory data. In particular, patients with "preclinical" heart failure can only be identified by careful imaging or other techniques that identify underlying structural abnormalities. Nevertheless, the recent departure from a purely symptomatic evaluation and management toward a process of disease progression allows for the opportunity to explore how to best evaluate patients afflicted by this condition.

This chapter provides a broad framework of clinical evaluation across the spectrum of heart failure to gain an appreciation of how the heart failure began, how the signs and symptoms are unfolding over time, and the pace whereby the signs and symptoms are occurring. Practical considerations of clinical evaluation of heart failure have been highlighted in the latest guideline recommendations.[1,2] Such information is critical when determining prognosis and devising precise management strategies, specific therapies, and interventions, including pharmacologic interdiction, percutaneous coronary intervention, surgery, or mechanical devices.

CLINICAL EVALUATION OF PRESENTING SYMPTOMS: THE MEDICAL HISTORY

One of the first principles of clinical evaluation of heart failure is to make the determination that the patient is indeed presenting with heart failure. Although this may sound obvious and self-fulfilling, presenting signs and symptoms of heart failure are often nonspecific. In fact, some patients can be labeled with a diagnosis of heart failure yet can be confounded by other noncardiac conditions. At the other end of the spectrum, there are patients without any signs and symptoms (or perhaps being overlooked) but overt cardiac dysfunction that remains undiagnosed. Despite these ambiguities, a series of questions should be addressed to every patient to understand the contributors and trajectory of disease progression: When did the symptoms start? Are the symptoms stable or are they getting worse? Are symptoms provoked or do they occur at rest? Are there accompanying symptoms (such as chest pain or calf claudication, palpitations, and dizziness)? How do the symptoms affect everyday activities? Illness narratives are particularly important, and sometimes patients may provide some clues as to how their conditions evolved, even though many of these questions may not yield immediate answers (and sometimes the answers may be sought from significant others or family members). Sometimes, several rounds of interviewing are necessary. It can be a time-consuming process and requires patience on the part of the person taking the history.

It is important to determine where the patient might be in the natural history of the disorder. Identification of risk factors for the development of heart failure is critically important in anticipating the eventuality of heart failure (so-called "stage A" heart failure in the latest heart failure guidelines; **Figure 28-1**).[3] Such risk factors include hypertension, coronary artery disease, previous myocardial infarction, diabetes mellitus, valvular heart disease, a positive family history of cardiomyopathy, or exposure to cardiotoxins (such as alcohol, anthracyclines, occupational exposures, ephedra-containing supplements, or illicit drugs). **Table 28-1** illustrates the prevalence and population-attributable risk of some of these risk factors, which are often substantial. In fact, several of these commonly available variables can be easily identified using a risk scoring system developed in an elderly cohort (HealthABC heart

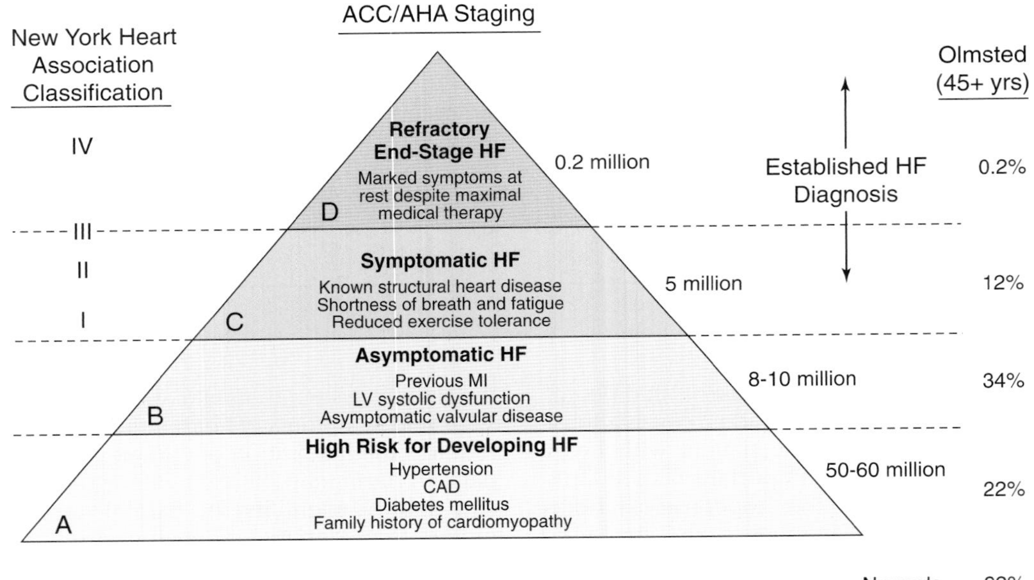

FIGURE 28-1 Heart failure staging and prevalence of stages in the Olmstead County Epidemiology Study. *CAD,* Coronary artery disease; *HF,* heart failure; *LV,* left ventricular; *MI,* myocardial infarction.[105] *Data on the right side of the figure are from Ammar KA, Jacobsen SJ, Mahoney DW, et al: Prevalence and prognostic significance of heart failure stages: application of the American College of Cardiology/American Heart Association heart failure staging criteria in the community. Circulation 115:1563–1570, 2007.*

TABLE 28-1 Prevalence and Population-Attributable Risk Factors for Developing Heart Failure

RISK FACTOR	AGE- AND RISK FACTOR–ADJUSTED HAZARD RATIO		% PREVALENCE	POPULATION-ATTRIBUTABLE RISK
Hypertension (BP ≥ 140/90 mm Hg)	Men	2.1	60	39
	Women	3.4	62	59
Myocardial infarction	Men	6.3	10	34
	Women	6.0	3	13
Angina	Men	1.4	11	5
	Women	1.7	9	5
Diabetes	Men	1.8	8	6
	Women	3.7	5	12
Left ventricular hypertrophy (EKG)	Men	2.2	4	4
	Women	2.9	3	5
Valvular heart disease	Men	2.5	5	7
	Women	2.1	8	8

BP, Blood pressure; *EKG,* electrocardiogram.

Age	
Years	**Points**
≤71	−1
72-75	0
76-78	1
≥79	2

Coronary artery disease	
Status	**Points**
No	0
Possible	2
Definite	5

LV hypertrophy	
Status	**Points**
No	0
Yes	2

Systolic blood pressure	
mm Hg	**Points**
≤90	−4
95-100	−3
105-115	−2
120-125	−1
130-140	0
145-150	1
155-165	2
170-175	3
180-190	4
195-200	5
>200	6

Heart rate	
bpm	**Points**
≤50	−2
55-60	−1
65-70	0
75-80	1
85-90	2
≥95	3

Smoking	
Status	**Points**
Never	0
Past	1
Current	4

Creatinine	
g/dL	**Points**
≤4.8	−3
4.5-4.7	−2
4.2-4.4	−1
3.9-4.1	0
3.6-3.8	1
3.3-3.5	2
≥3.2	3

Fasting glucose	
mg/dL	**Points**
≤80	−1
85-125	0
130-170	1
175-220	2
225-265	3
≥270	5

Creatinine	
mg/dL	**Points**
≤0.7	−2
0.8-0.9	−1
1.0-1.1	0
1.2-1.4	1
1.5-1.8	2
1.9-2.3	3
≥2.3	6

Key:
Systolic BP to nearest 5 mm Hg
Heart rate to nearest 5 bpm
Albumin to nearest 0.1 g/dL
Glucose to nearest 5 mg/dL
Creatinine to nearest 0.1 mg/dL

HF = Heart failure

Health ABC HF risk score	HF risk group	5-yr HF risk
≤2 points	Low	<5%
3-5 points	Average	5-10%
6-9 points	High	10-20%
≥10 points	Very high	>20%

FIGURE 28-2 HealthABC Heart Failure Risk Score. *BP,* Blood pressure; *HF,* heart failure; *LV,* left ventricular. *From Butler J, Kalogeropoulos A, Georgiopoulou V, et al: Incident heart failure prediction in the elderly: the health ABC heart failure score. Circ Heart Fail 1:125–133, 2008.*

failure risk score; **Figure 28-2**),[4] as well as in a younger population cohort (ARIC heart failure risk score, http://aricnews.net/HFCalcs/RiskCalcHFClinFac.html)[5] that may predict the risk of developing heart failure. Some of these risk factors may not be apparent, and it is not uncommon for a patient to trace back his or her past exposures or family histories to provide clues to possible underlying causes, particularly in those with nonischemic etiologies.

Even in the absence of symptoms, some patients may have structural and functional abnormalities of the heart and circulation that antedate the onset of symptoms (so-called "stage B" heart failure).[3] These structural abnormalities include left ventricular hypertrophy, asymptomatic left ventricular dysfunction, asymptomatic valvular dysfunction, or wall-motion abnormalities from prior myocardial infarction. The anticipation that heart failure will likely develop in these early stages in some patients is a strong incentive to institute preventive therapy or risk factor modification, as well as early use of neurohormonal antagonists, including angiotensin-converting enzyme (ACE) inhibitors, and in selected cases, β-adrenergic blockers and statin therapy.

Symptoms of heart failure may be well controlled with outpatient medical therapy ("stage C")[3] or may become refractory to conventional therapy ("stage D").[3] After establishing that symptoms may be caused by the syndrome of heart failure, ongoing review of the patient's clinical status is critical to the appropriate selection and monitoring of therapy. It is traditional to classify patients according to their extent of disability via the New York Heart Association (NYHA) functional classification (see Figure 28-1).[6] This classification system is notoriously subjective, yet it continues to be widely applied to patients with heart failure and reported in clinical trials as selection criteria or secondary outcome measures. Several other clinical scoring systems have been developed to define heart failure in population-based studies, but rarely are used at the bedside (**Table 28-2**).[7] We should point out an important distinction between Staging and Functional Classification assessment—the NYHA functional classification is based solely on clinical signs and symptoms and can improve or worsen, whereas heart failure staging can only advance forward. In other words, once a patient has reached stage C, even if he or she became asymptomatic with treatment (i.e., NYHA class I), he or she would not revert back to stage B because symptoms have already manifested themselves.

The pace at which heart failure develops and progresses can be highly variable, and sometimes it is difficult to

TABLE 28-2 Diagnostic Criteria for Heart Failure in Population-Based Studies

*Framingham Criteria**

MAJOR CRITERIA	MINOR CRITERIA	MAJOR OR MINOR CRITERIA
• Paroxysmal nocturnal dyspnea or orthopnea • Neck-vein distention • Rales • Cardiomegaly • Acute pulmonary edema • S_3 gallop • Increased venous pressure >6 cm H_2O • Circulation time >25 sec • Hepatojugular reflux	• Ankle edema, night cough, dyspnea on exertion • Hepatomegaly • Pleural effusion • Vital capacity decreased ⅓ from maximal capacity • Tachycardia (rate >120/min)	• Weight loss >4.5 kg in 5 days in response to treatment

Boston Criteria and NHANES Clinical Score†

CATEGORIES	CRITERIA	NHANES	BOSTON
History	Dyspnea		
	• At rest	1	4
	• On level ground	1	2
	• On climbing	2	1
	• Stop when walking at own pace or on level ground after 100 yards		
	Orthopnea		4
	Paroxysmal nocturnal dyspnea		3
Physical examination	Heart rate		
	• 91-110 beats/min	1	1
	• >110 beats/min	2	2
	Jugular venous pressure (>6 cm H_2O)		
	• Alone	1	2
	• Plus hepatomegaly or edema	2	3
	Rales/crackles		
	• Basilar crackles	1	1
	• More than basilar crackles	2	2
	Wheezing		3
	S_3 gallop		3
Chest radiography	Alveolar pulmonary edema		4
	Alveolar fluid plus pleural fluid	3	
	Interstitial pulmonary edema	2	3
	Interstitial edema plus pleural fluid	3	
	Bilateral pleural effusion		3
	Cardiothoracic ratio >0.5 (posteroanterior projection)		3
	Upper zone flow redistribution	1	2

*Diagnosis of heart failure: two major, or one major and two minor criteria are required.

†Diagnosis of heart failure: Boston criteria: definite (score 8-12 points), possible (score 5-7 points), unlikely (score ≤ 4 points). NHANES-1 criteria: diagnosis of heart failure if score ≥ 3 points.

NHANES, National Health and Nutrition Examination Survey.

From Rector TS, Cohn JN: Assessment of patient outcome with the Minnesota living with heart failure questionnaire: reliability and validity during a randomized, double-blind, placebo controlled trial of pimobendan. Am Heart J 124:1017, 1992.

distinguish stage C from stage D. The Interagency Registry for Mechanically Assisted Circulatory Support (INTERMACS) describes seven distinct profiles of disease severity in advanced heart failure (**Table 28-3**).[8] The timing and need for various diagnostic assessments will therefore depend on decisions regarding the appropriateness and timing of specialized interventions (such as revascularization or heart transplantation). In fact, the concept of "stage D heart failure" continues to evolve as more advanced therapeutics become available. For example, a young woman with decompensated heart failure as a result of acute inflammatory myocarditis may require full diagnostic workup and mechanical circulatory support to maximize the chances of recovery. Despite the clinical picture of cardiogenic shock, the designation of "stage D" in this case should be applied only when standard heart failure therapeutics have been exhausted without recovery. At the same time, the judgment of determining disease severity lies in the therapeutic options available, and often neglected is the preference of the patient to undergo diagnostic testing and various medical/surgical interventions. This is particularly important in patients with advanced heart failure where choices between improving the quality versus length of life can be highly variable.[9] For example, for an elderly patient who has long-standing rheumatic valve disease with stable symptoms of heart failure and has had repeatedly refused surgical therapy, routine clinical follow-up may be adequate if there are no interim changes in signs and symptoms.

When seeing a patient with new heart failure or decompensated heart failure, identification and correction of a *precipitating cause* is very important (**Table 28-4**). In some cases, this is obvious (such as dietary indiscretion), but in other cases it may be far more subtle. Unfortunately, such causes identified from clinical histories are often associative by nature, and therefore careful scrutiny should be given to the illness narrative. A prospective substudy of a large clinical trial demonstrated that the most common acute precipitants of heart failure exacerbations were noncompliance for salt restriction (22%), pulmonary infections (15%), or arrhythmias (13%). More alarming is the prevalence of iatrogenic causes of decompensation, such as use and misuse of antiarrhythmic agents (15%) or calcium channel blockers (13%), or inappropriate reductions in heart failure medications (10%).[10] Furthermore, different

TABLE 28-3 INTERMACS Profile

INTERMACS CLASS	DESCRIPTION	INOTROPIC SUPPORT	TIME FRAME TO INTERVENTION
1	Critical cardiogenic shock	Yes	Needed within hours
2	Progressive decline	Yes	Needed within days
3	Stable but inotrope dependent	Yes	Elective within weeks/months
4	Resting symptoms	No	Elective within weeks/months
5	Exertion intolerant	No	Variable, depending on condition
6	Exertion limited	No	Variable, depending on condition
7	Advanced NYHA III	No	Variable, depending on condition

Modifiers: A = Arrhythmia (any profile); FF = frequent flyer (profiles 3-6); TCS = temporary circulatory support (profiles 1-3 only).

TABLE 28-4 Factors That May Precipitate Worsening Heart Failure

Myocardial ischemia or infarction
Dietary sodium excess or excess fluid intake
Medication noncompliance
Iatrogenic volume overload
Uncontrolled hypertension
Arrhythmia
- Atrial fibrillation or flutter
- Ventricular tachyarrhythmias
- Bradyarrhythmias

Comorbidities
- Fever, infections/sepsis
- Thyroid dysfunction
- Anemia
- Renal insufficiency
- Nutritional deficiencies (such as thiamine deficiency)
- Pulmonary diseases (chronic obstructive pulmonary disease, pulmonary embolism, hypoxemia)

Inappropriate reduction of heart failure medications
Adverse drug effects
- Alcohol
- Overzealous administration of negative inotropic agents (such as β-blockers, calcium channel blockers, antiarrhythmic agents)
- Nonsteroidal anti-inflammatory drugs
- Fluid retention (e.g., thiazolidinediones)
- Corticosteroids

TABLE 28-5 Minnesota Living with Heart Failure Questionnaire

Did your heart failure prevent you from living as you wanted during the last month by:

1. Causing swelling in your ankles, legs, etc.?
2. Making you sit or lie down to rest during the day?
3. Making your walking about or climbing stairs difficult?
4. Making your working around the house or yard difficult?
5. Making your going places away from home difficult?
6. Making your sleeping well at night difficult?
7. Making your relating to or doing things with your friends and family difficult?
8. Making your working to earn a living difficult?
9. Making your recreational pastimes, sports, or hobbies difficult?
10. Making your sexual activities difficult?
11. Making you eat less of the foods you like?
12. Making you short of breath?
13. Making you tired, fatigued, or low on energy?
14. Making you stay in a hospital?
15. Costing you money for medical care?
16. Giving you side effects from medicine?
17. Making you feel you are a burden to your family or friends?
18. Making you feel a loss of self-control in your life?
19. Making you worry?
20. Making it difficult for you to concentrate or remember things?
21. Making you feel depressed?

precipitating factors may also have different implications. For example, heart failure decompensation due to ischemia or worsening renal function has poorer 60- to 90-day adverse outcomes than admissions to the hospital because of poor blood pressure control or arrhythmia (the latter being more likely to be reversible with appropriate treatment).[11]

Much effort has been made to develop objective assessment of health-related quality of life in heart failure (such as the Minnesota Living with Heart Failure questionnaire [**Table 28-5**][12] or the Kansas City Cardiomyopathy Questionnaire [**Table 28-6**]).[13] These disease-specific instruments have been developed with the goal of improving the measurement of health status and quality of life so as to compare within a specific population to gain insight into disease severity or to quantify their changes over time. Many of these have been used in substudies of clinical trials, and are now beginning to be incorporated into standardized registries as part of patient assessment tools and performance measures. Other objective measures of functional capacity, such as the six-minute walk test, have also been steadily adopted in the clinical setting, and assessment of frailty now plays a more important role in therapeutic decisions for more invasive interventions.

The cardinal symptoms of heart failure are dyspnea ("shortness of breath") and fatigue that occur either at rest and/or with exertion. Some patients may attribute their dyspnea to being "out of shape," or even "old age." Many patients may have lived with it for so long that they do not even notice the degree of slow but steady deterioration. At the other end of the spectrum, patients may present initially with severe acute pulmonary edema that can be rarely mistaken for any other condition. Most patients present somewhere between these two extremes, and the latest guideline updates have emphasized that the clinical presentation can be congestion, noncongestion, or asymptomatic. Like eliciting any medical history, many of the answers may only be apparent to the prepared mind, and most are from casual conversations regarding activities of daily living. A good example is when asking patients about their fluid status and dietary salt intake. Most people will claim that they have done everything in their efforts to reduce sodium intake. However, careful review of their dietary habits may indicate otherwise, or simply clear ignorance of salt-laden food intake. Probing into specifics often helps to better understand patients' condition and their immediate environment. Food diaries and nutritional consultations are often insightful and in some cases therapeutic. Patients may also be focused on any abnormal signs and symptoms that may be attributable to heart failure or its treatment side effects. Good rapport with patients and their families is vital in eliciting information regarding adherence to medical advice and reviewing abilities to provide appropriate self-care.

TABLE 28-6 Kansas City Cardiomyopathy Questionnaire

1. Please indicate how much you are limited by **heart failure** (shortness of breath or fatigue) in your ability to do the following activities *over the past 2 weeks* (extremely limited, quite a bit limited, moderately limited, slightly limited, not at all limited, or limited for other reasons or did not do the activity)?
   - Dress yourself
   - Showering/bathing
   - Walking 1 block on level ground
   - Doing yard work, housework, or carrying groceries
   - Climbing a flight of stairs without stopping
   - Hurrying or jogging (as if to catch a bus)
2. *Compared with 2 weeks ago,* have your symptoms of **heart failure** (shortness of breath, fatigue, or ankle swelling) changed? (much worse, slightly worse, not changed, slightly better, much better, I've had no symptoms over the past 2 weeks)
3. Over the *past 2 weeks,* how much have the following signs/symptoms bothered you? (extremely, quite a bit, moderately, slightly, not at all bothersome; no such signs/symptoms)
   - Swelling in your feet, ankles, or legs
   - Fatigue
   - Shortness of breath
4. Over the *past 2 weeks,* how many times did you have **swelling** in your feet, ankles, or legs when you woke up in the morning? (every morning, 3 or more times a week but not every day, 1-2 times/week, less than once a week, never over the past 2 weeks)
5. Over the *past 2 weeks,* on average, how many times has **fatigue** limited your ability to do what you want? (all the time, several times/day, at least once/day, 3 or more times/week but not every day, 1-2 times/week, less than once/week, never over past 2 weeks)
6. Over the *past 2 weeks,* on average, how many times have you been forced to sleep sitting up in a chair or with at least 3 pillows to prop you up because of **shortness of breath**? (every night, 3 or more times/week but not every day, 1-2 times/week, less than once/week, never over past 2 weeks)
7. **Heart failure** symptoms can worsen for a number of reasons. How sure are you that you know what to do, or whom to call, if your **heart failure** gets worse? (not at all sure, not very sure, somewhat sure, mostly sure, completely sure)
8. How well do you understand what things you are able to do to keep your **heart failure** symptoms from getting worse? (for example, weighing yourself, eating a low salt diet, etc.) (do not understand at all, do not understand very well, somewhat understand, mostly understand, completely understand)
9. Over the *past 2 weeks,* how much has your **heart failure** limited your enjoyment of life? (extremely, quite a bit, moderately, slightly, not limited)
10. If you had to spend the rest of your life with your **heart failure** the way it is *right now,* how would you feel about this? (not at all satisfied, mostly dissatisfied, somewhat satisfied, mostly satisfied, completely satisfied)
11. Over the *past 2 weeks,* how often have you felt discouraged or down in the dumps because of your **heart failure**? (all the time, most of the time, occasionally, rarely, never)
12. How much does your **heart failure** affect your lifestyle? Please indicate how your **heart failure** may have limited your participation in the following activities *over the past 2 weeks* (severely limited, limited quite a bit, moderately limited, slightly limited, did not limit at all, does not apply or did not do for other reasons)
    - Hobbies, recreational activities
    - Working or doing household chores
    - Visiting family or friends out of your home
    - Intimate relationships with loved ones

From Green CP, Porter CB, Bresnahan DR, et al: Development and evaluation of the Kansas City cardiomyopathy questionnaire: a new health status measure for heart failure. J Am Coll Cardiol 35:1245–1255, 2000.

Dyspnea

Dyspnea is the abnormal sensation of an uncomfortable awareness of breathing. When it occurs at rest or at a level of physical activity where it is not expected, it is abnormal. Dyspnea is a nonspecific symptom that occurs with a wide variety of cardiac, pulmonary, and chest wall disorders. It can also result from acute anxiety, acute coronary insufficiency, and anemia. Patients with heart failure may manifest a variety of types of dyspnea, including exertional dyspnea, orthopnea, paroxysmal nocturnal dyspnea, dyspnea at rest, and acute pulmonary edema with respiratory distress. An increase in respiratory rate (usually >16 breaths/min) usually accompanies dyspnea, and may signal the onset of acute decompensation of stable heart failure.

The mechanisms of dyspnea, fatigue, and exercise intolerance in patients with heart failure vary widely, and many are still not well understood because they are not simply due to increased pulmonary capillary wedge pressure and decreased cardiac output.[14-18] There is little correlation between pulmonary capillary wedge pressure and exertional dyspnea in individual patients with heart failure, unless frank pulmonary edema is present.[19] It is well known that auscultation of the lungs may be clear in a substantial proportion of patients with shortness of breath and heart failure.[20] The availability of implanted hemodynamic monitors has provided insights into dynamic changes in hemodynamics over time and with exertion.

All patients with heart failure should be carefully queried regarding the threshold of dyspnea onset during exercise. Specific examples of how and when the dyspnea occurs should be sought. The mechanism of dyspnea should be considered, particularly in relation to different types of daily activities. Difficulties with stairs or "air hunger" are particularly suspicious for underlying cardiac insufficiency. Shortness of breath may be due to concomitant pulmonary disease or respiratory muscle dysfunction.[21] Increased ventilatory drive or exercise hyperventilation is believed to be a common cause of dyspnea in patients with heart failure,[22-25] but the precise mechanism of dyspnea has remained elusive. The mechanism of increased ventilatory drive in patients with heart failure is multifactorial and incompletely understood, but may be due to increased peripheral chemosensitivity in the skeletal muscles and accumulation of lactic acid. Both of these may lead to exercise hyperpnea,[26,27] thus tiring the patient out at an earlier point in exercise. This concept is consistent with the so-called muscle hypothesis, which proposes that the real source of dyspnea in patients with heart failure begins in the skeletal muscles.[26,27] Exertional dyspnea can also occur when there is markedly elevated left ventricular filling pressure. Distinguishing these causes may require specific testing, including cardiopulmonary exercise testing and pulmonary function testing.

There are multiple, complex mechanisms operating in the production of exertional dyspnea in patients with heart failure, and no single mechanism is likely dominant. Nevertheless, the augmented ventilatory response to exercise in heart failure (such as increased breathing rate relative to the amount of exercise) correlates with hemodynamic alterations,[28] whereas peak VO_2 does not. The classic theory of increased exercise ventilatory response of heart failure embraces the concept that increases in carbon dioxide output relative to peak oxygen consumption lead to bicarbonate buffering and accumulation of lactic acid.[27] Lactic acid builds up at relatively low workloads in patients with heart failure and acts as an additional stimulus to breathing. It may also contribute to the sensation of dyspnea. In some patients there is also an increase in airway dead space because of reduced perfusion of ventilated lung tissue, leading to inefficient gas exchange. Despite this, arterial carbon dioxide concentration is driven to low levels during peak exercise in most patients with heart failure. The "muscle hypothesis" of exertional dyspnea would argue that peripheral (i.e., skeletal muscle) chemoreceptors have a higher gain for arterial oxygen and carbon dioxide concentrations in heart failure, leading to ergoreflex overactivation.[29] The overactivation of ergoreflexes increases both ventilatory drive and sympathetic nervous system activity through activation of a central mechanism. Physical training in patients with heart failure may reduce exaggerated ergoreflex activity and thereby improve the response to exercise.[30] Clearly, exertional dyspnea in patients with heart failure is complex, multifactorial, and not simply due to increased filling pressures. Reflex control mechanisms involving the heart, lungs, brain, and skeletal muscles and a buildup of lactic acid in the working muscles are likely involved, leading to an increased ventilatory response to exercise.

Fatigue

Similar to dyspnea, there are uncertainties regarding the mechanism of fatigue in patients with heart failure. There was a widely held assumption that cardiac fatigue is simply due to a low cardiac output, but in the past 10 to 15 years it has become clear that abnormalities of skeletal muscles, compensatory vascular and autonomic responses, and other noncardiac comorbidities such as anemia may contribute importantly to fatigue. Abnormalities of high-energy phosphates in the skeletal muscles of patients with heart failure are well documented,[31-35] even in the face of normal regional blood flow.[33] Muscle fatigue relates to abnormal phosphocreatinine depletion and/or acidosis in the working muscle. The anaerobic regeneration of adenosine triphosphate (ATP) is impaired in the skeletal muscles of patients with heart failure. There is also a shift in fiber distribution with increased percentage of the fast-twitch, glycolytic, easily fatigable type IIb fibers.[31] There are major alterations in skeletal muscle histology and biochemistry of patients with heart failure,[36] including the development of skeletal muscle atrophy.[37] Significant ultrastructural abnormalities are present,[38] leading to diminished oxidative capacity of working muscle.[39,40] Chronic fatigue begets further inactivity, leading to further deconditioning and a greater extent of disability. In the late stages of heart failure, a low cardiac output and anemia of chronic disease probably also contribute to fatigue. Like dyspnea, fatigue is multifactorial and may have important noncardiac mechanisms involving the skeletal muscles. Patients who are ambulatory with heart failure should be encouraged to stay physically active,[41,42] and participation in a structured exercise training program can improve exercise tolerance.[43-45]

Other Symptoms of Heart Failure

An occasional patient with heart failure will present with palpitations, light-headedness, or even frank syncope. In our experience, this is unusual and usually signifies underlying arrhythmia or outflow obstruction and less often in low output states. However, heart block, arrhythmias with circulatory collapse, or even atrial fibrillation or premature beats may be a presenting feature of heart failure, which is especially common in specific conditions, such as acute myocarditis, infiltrative cardiomyopathy (such as sarcoid or amyloid), Chagas disease, or some inherited cardiomyopathies. Right upper quadrant pain due to acute liver congestion or early satiety may be a presenting symptom. Abdominal fullness, particularly with meals, is often overlooked as indicative of worsening splanchnic congestion. Additional presenting symptoms might include nocturnal angina, weight loss (weight gain is more common), and cough (particularly at night). Usually there are other signs and symptoms of heart failure present. Sometimes patients may present with more subtle symptoms of heart failure, and are often mistakenly misdiagnosed with bronchitis (dry productive cough), asthma (wheezing due to cardiac asthma), or insomnia (Cheyne-Stokes respiration). Many endocrine abnormalities can be associated with heart failure, and may be treatable. It is not uncommon for asymptomatic people to be diagnosed with cardiomegaly on a routine chest x-ray, or have left bundle branch block or arrhythmia on an electrocardiogram—both of which are forerunners to the development of heart failure and cardiac dysfunction.

CLINICAL EVALUATION OF PRESENTING SIGNS: PHYSICAL EXAMINATION

A careful physical examination is always warranted in the evaluation of patients with heart failure. The purpose of the examination is to help determine the cause of heart failure and to assess the severity of the syndrome. Obtaining additional information about the hemodynamic profile and the response to therapy, and determination of the prognosis, are important additional goals of the physical examination.

General Inspection of the Patient

The diagnosis of heart failure is relatively straightforward by simple medical history and physical examination. It is not unusual for an experienced physician to sense the severity of the heart failure syndrome within the first few minutes of walking into the room, meeting the patient, and observing the patient carefully. Hospitalized patients often have labored or uncomfortable breathing. They may not be able to finish a sentence because of shortness of breath. Lying down may be difficult because of orthopnea, and sometimes patients may even describe sleeping in a recliner or chair. Altered respiratory signs such as coughing, undulating breathing patterns ("Cheyne-Stokes respiration"), and cyanosis are sometimes observed. Peripheral cyanosis is limited to exposed skin, and usually indicates inadequate perfusion or low cardiac output. They may feel cold and have slow capillary refill at their nail beds. In contrast, central cyanosis is uncommon but found predominantly in the tongue, uvula, and buccal mucosa, indicating intracardiac or intrapulmonary shunting. Some patients will demonstrate cachexia, a particularly poor prognostic sign. There may be severe peripheral edema and ascites that is obvious from simple inspection.

Examination of the arterial pulse is very important. The absence of pulses should be noted, as well as the character of the pulse. Pulsus alternans (a strong beat alternating with a weak beat), though unusual, is virtually diagnostic of severe advanced heart failure. Pulsus paradoxus (a substantial diminishment in the amplitude of the arterial pulse during inspiration) is found in pericardial tamponade. It is usually confirmed by measuring blood pressure carefully during the phases of inspiration and expiration. Pulsus paradoxus is also seen in an occasional patient with severe asthma, pulmonary embolism, pregnancy, marked obesity, and patients with superior vena cava syndrome. Patients with aortic stenosis may have diminished upstroke of the carotid pulse, whereas patients with severe, chronic aortic regurgitation manifest accentuated pulses and a series of findings related to a large stroke volume. Peripheral pulses may be absent in patients with coarctation of the aorta. Irregular rhythm is often detected by erratic peripheral pulses. Therefore, a thorough assessment of the pulses is always warranted.

Assessment of the Volume Status of the Patient

Volume status assessment is perhaps one of the most important skills needed for the care of the patient with heart failure. Pertinent features of the cardiac physical examination, such as jugular venous distention and tissue congestion, are especially important aspects in the accurate assessment of the patient with heart failure. It can be useful to dichotomize the signs of heart failure into those of volume overload and those of low cardiac output (**Figure 28-3**).[46] Signs of volume overload include increased jugular venous distention, prominent "v" waves, gallop heart rhythm (S_3), rales and pleural effusion, anasarca, ascites, and peripheral edema. Occasionally, specific organomegaly is present, including enlarged and sometimes tender liver, enlarged spleen (rare), and cardiomegaly. Recent analysis from the Evaluation Study of Congestive Heart Failure and Pulmonary Artery Catheterization Effectiveness (ESCAPE) trial observed that the presence of orthopnea and increased jugular venous distention may be useful to detect increased intracardiac filling pressures, whereas a global assessment of inadequate perfusion ("cold profile") may be useful to detect reduced cardiac index.[47]

Despite the historical use of the term *congestive heart failure,* it is not unusual to see patients with advanced heart failure who consistently demonstrate no evidence of volume overload.[20] For reasons that are unclear, such patients do not seem to retain significant amounts of salt and water, and are hence subject to overdiuresis, leading in some cases to "prerenal azotemia." Patients should be examined while lying down with their head tilted at 45 degrees. The physician should examine the patient from the patient's right side (Oslerian tradition). The most important assessment of volume status is careful examination of the jugular venous pressure. Unfortunately, this is somewhat of a lost art.[20,48,49] It is important to understand that jugular venous pressure often reflects left-sided and right-sided filling pressure, but that a substantial number of patients with heart failure have relatively normal intracardiac filling pressures and no distended neck veins. In patients with mild heart failure, the jugular venous pressure may be normal with the patient lying at 45 degrees, but rises to abnormal levels with compression to the right upper quadrant. This is referred to as *hepatojugular reflux.* To elicit this sign, the right upper quadrant should be compressed firmly, gradually, and continuously for 1 minute while the neck veins are being observed. The presence of hepatojugular reflux that very slowly dissipates on release of hand pressure is a sign that intracardiac filling pressures are abnormally increased.[50]

Despite the common lack of abdominal complaints, some patients do accumulate fluid in the form of ascites or visceral edema. Examination of the abdomen should be performed to determine the presence of ascites, hepatosplenomegaly, or pulsatile, tender liver. Splenomegaly is rare in heart failure. However, hepatomegaly is common, and acute congestion can lead to rather severe right upper quadrant tenderness that mimics cholecystitis. Occasionally, patients with acute decompensation and severe right upper quadrant pain may even go to the operating room where the diagnosis is found to be acute hepatic congestion. Liver transaminases are often elevated during acute passive congestion, and in severe right heart failure, clotting factors and total bilirubin may be increased. Recent recognition of raised intraabdominal pressures in

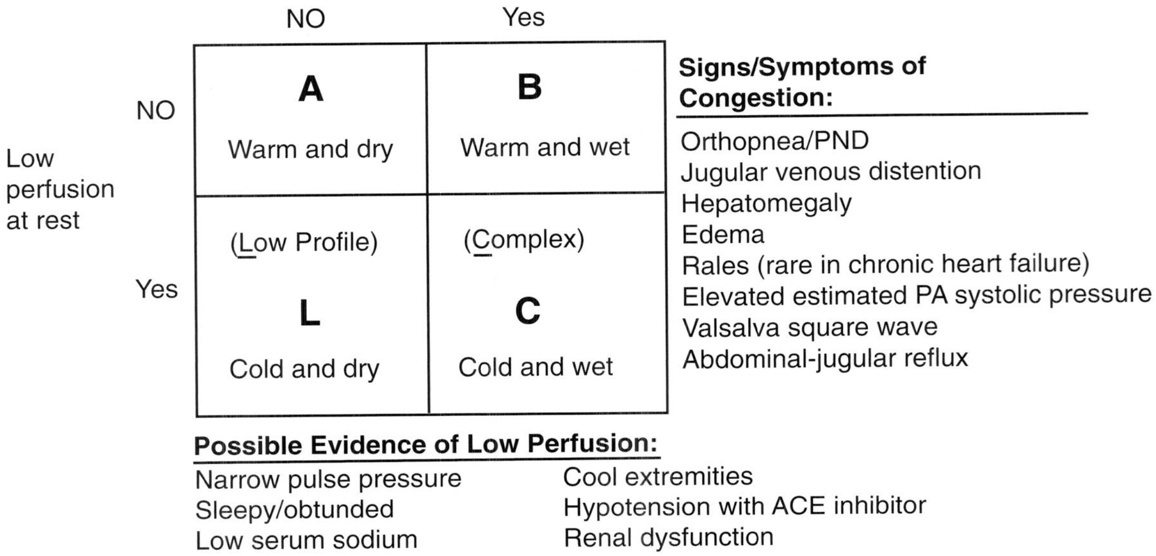

Low perfusion at rest		NO	Yes
	NO	**A** Warm and dry	**B** Warm and wet
	Yes	(Low Profile) **L** Cold and dry	(Complex) **C** Cold and wet

Signs/Symptoms of Congestion:
Orthopnea/PND
Jugular venous distention
Hepatomegaly
Edema
Rales (rare in chronic heart failure)
Elevated estimated PA systolic pressure
Valsalva square wave
Abdominal-jugular reflux

Possible Evidence of Low Perfusion:
Narrow pulse pressure
Sleepy/obtunded
Low serum sodium
Cool extremities
Hypotension with ACE inhibitor
Renal dysfunction

FIGURE 28-3 Heart failure profiles according to perfusion and congestion. *ACE,* Angiotensin-converting enzyme; *PA,* pulmonary artery; *PND,* paroxysmal nocturnal dyspnea. *From Nohria A, Lewis E, Stevenson LW: Medical management of advanced heart failure. JAMA 287:628–640, 2002.*

TABLE 28-7 Utility of Components of History and Physical Examination in Detecting Pulmonary Capillary Wedge Pressure >22 mm Hg

FINDING	SENSITIVITY	SPECIFICITY	Predictive Value POSITIVE	Predictive Value NEGATIVE	Likelihood Ratio POSITIVE	Likelihood Ratio NEGATIVE
Rales (≥⅓ lung field)	15	89	69	38	1.32	1.04
S_3	62	32	61	33	0.92	0.85
Ascites (≥ moderate)	21	92	81	40	2.44	1.15
Edema (≥2+)	41	66	67	40	1.20	1.11
Orthopnea (≥2 pillow)	86	25	66	51	1.15	1.80
Hepatomegaly (>4 fb)	15	93	78	39	2.13	1.09
Hepatojugular reflux	83	27	65	49	1.13	1.54
JVP ≥12 mm Hg	65	64	75	52	1.79	1.82
JVP <8 mm Hg	4.3	81	28	33	0.23	0.85

fb, Fingerbreadths; *JVP,* jugular venous pressure.
Modified from Drazner MH, Hellkamp AS, Leier CV, et al: Value of clinician assessment of hemodynamics in advanced heart failure: the escape trial. Circ Heart Fail 1:170–177, 2008.

congested patients with decompensated heart failure further illustrates the evidence and hemodynamic impact of abdominal congestion.[51]

There may be normal, hyperdynamic, or sustained precordial pulsations. Cardiomegaly tends to displace the point of maximal impulse, which is also sustained in cases of severe left ventricular hypertrophy. Physical examination of precordial pulsation, however, is inadequate to assess the degree of left ventricular dysfunction. In some patients, a third heart sound is audible and palpable at the apex. Patients with enlarged or hypertrophied right ventricles may have a sustained and prolonged left parasternal impulse extending throughout systole.

A third heart sound (or gallop rhythm) is most commonly present in patients with volume overload who have tachycardia and tachypnea. This may be absent in many patients with advanced heart failure, but the presence of a third heart sound can signify severe hemodynamic compromise.[52] The murmurs of mitral and tricuspid regurgitation are frequently present in patients with advanced heart failure, although severe regurgitation is frequently present in the absence of an audible murmur. The presence of jugular venous distention and a third heart sound predict a poor prognosis[53] and disease progression,[54] and should always be sought out and recorded.

Interestingly, signs of pulmonary congestion (such as rales, pulmonary edema, and elevated jugular venous pressure) are frequently absent, even in patients with raised pulmonary capillary wedge pressure[20] (**Table 28-7**). Patients with chronic, severe heart failure tend to have robust lymphatic drainage of the pulmonary interstitial spaces in a similar manner as those with long-standing mitral stenosis. The absence of rales does not exclude impending pulmonary edema, and direct hemodynamic measurements may sometimes be necessary. Instead, tachypnea (and in some extreme cases, hypoxia) is often associated with significant pulmonary congestion.

An increase in circulating volume is often associated with evidence of excessive adrenergic activity. This includes diaphoresis, tachycardia, pallor, and coldness of the extremities. The adrenergic nervous system is similarly activated during low cardiac output. Relief of congestion is always an important primary goal in the management of patients with chronic heart failure so that the identification of the volume-overloaded state is a critical step in the physical examination.[55]

Signs of Low Cardiac Output

Patients in a "low-output" state may present with a wide variety of clinical signs (from cool, dry skin, pallor, or peripheral cyanosis, to normal color, warmth, and appearance). In some cases, pulses may be diminished and blood pressure may be low with a narrow pulse pressure. Some patients will demonstrate virtually no signs of inadequate blood flow despite a low cardiac output. They may be alert and cognitively responsive despite extreme diminishment in cardiac index (i.e., less than 1.5 L/min/m^2). This probably relates to the body's remarkable ability to redistribute flow to vital organs (including the brain) in the face of very diminished cardiac output. This is in contrast with acute cardiogenic shock (e.g., acute myocardial infarction), where patients may develop cool skin, pallor, mental status changes or cognitive deficits, oliguria, peripheral cyanosis, and hypothermia. Pulsus alternans, if present, is virtually pathognomonic of a low-output state,[56] but is more often seen in the terminally ill patient. More commonly, compensatory tachycardia (especially in young patients) and low blood pressures in the setting of profound signs and symptoms of heart failure are concerning for low-output states. Apparently, clinical assessment of inadequate perfusion can be reasonably accurate.[47]

Signs of Cachexia

The importance of cachexia in patients with severe end-stage heart failure is currently the subject of intense research.[57,58] It is believed that unintentional weight loss and cachexia portend a very poor prognosis. Although the mechanism of cachexia is not entirely understood, it may be related to various cytokines, including tumor necrosis factor-α (TNF-α), that are known to be increased in patients with heart failure with poor prognosis.[59]

LABORATORY EVALUATION OF THE PATIENT WITH HEART FAILURE

As shown in **Table 28-8**, the diagnostic sensitivity and specificity of the clinical history and physical examination for diagnosing patients with heart failure is relatively poor. For this reason, laboratory testing has assumed a progressively greater role in establishing the diagnosis of heart failure, as will be discussed later.

Biochemical Evaluation: Biomarker Testing (see also Chapter 30)

It is recommended that patients with new-onset heart failure have a battery of routine laboratory tests when they are first diagnosed. This is also true of patients with chronic heart failure and acute decompensation, when there is a change in therapeutic intervention, or periodic monitoring for clinical stability. Often, a basic metabolic panel that includes electrolytes and renal markers is useful, sometimes with additional thyroid or liver function tests or markers of glycemic or lipid control.[60,61] Recognition of anemia in adverse heart failure prognosis has also prompted periodic evaluation of hemoglobin levels and iron profiles to better determine the presence of functional iron deficiency, but subsets of patients may have reversible abnormalities.[62]

TABLE 28-8 Sensitivity, Specificity, and Predictive Accuracy of Symptoms and Signs for Diagnosing Heart Failure

SYMPTOMS OR SIGNS	SENSITIVITY (%)	SPECIFICITY (%)	PREDICTIVE ACCURACY (%)
Exertional dyspnea	66	52	23
Orthopnea	21	81	2
Paroxysmal	33	76	26
History of edema	23	80	22
Resting heart rate	7	99	6
Rales	13	91	21
Third heart sound	31	95	61
Jugular venous distention	10	97	2
Edema (on examination)	10	93	3

From Harlan WR, Oberman A, Grimm R, et al: Chronic congestive heart failure in coronary artery disease: clinical criteria. Ann Intern Med 86:133–138, 1977.

Several cardiac biomarkers may provide incremental diagnostic and prognostic information, such as B-type natriuretic peptide (BNP) and cardiac troponin.[63] BNP and its aminoterminal fragment (NT-proBNP) in particular have provided important diagnostic utility for heart failure in the acute clinical setting (**Figure 28-4**). There are still ongoing clinical studies to determine the appropriateness of their uses to guide therapy, because clinical trials supporting the drugs and devices received their approval *before* broad adoption of biomarker testing. Testing for markers of inflammation (such as erythrocyte sedimentation rate, C-reactive protein, or other specific rheumatologic disease markers) can be helpful in some circumstances to unmask myocarditis or other inflammatory causes, but routine measurements are yet to be adopted.[63] Viral antibody titers have also been found to be low yield and are rarely indicated, because the appropriate treatment with positive viral antibody titers remains unclear at this point. Other commonly measured biomarkers indicate renal function (blood urea nitrogen, serum creatinine), electrolyte balance (sodium, potassium), oxidative process (uric acid), liver function (total bilirubin, aminotransferases, prothrombin time), and hematologic status (hemoglobin, red cell distribution width)—most of them being important prognostic indicators of disease severity.

Electrocardiographic Evaluation: Electrocardiography

Electrocardiographic evaluation remains a valuable and broadly available laboratory test in patients with heart failure. An electrocardiogram should be routinely performed and interrogated for evidence of underlying

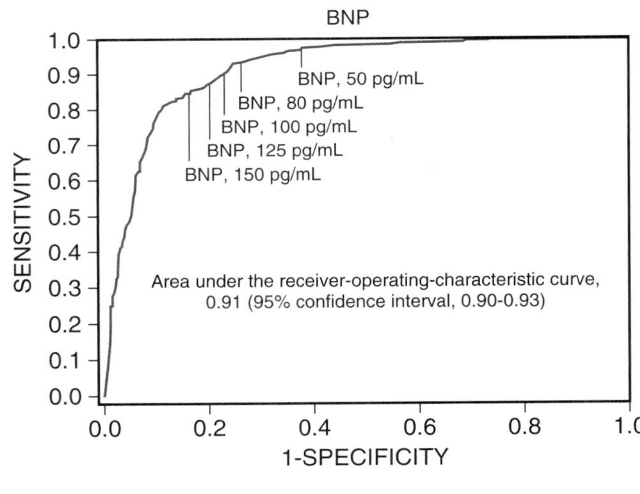

BNP pg/mL	Sensitivity	Specificity	PPV	NPV	Accuracy
	(95% confidence interval)				
50	97 (96-98)	62 (59-66)	71 (68-74)	96 (94-97)	79
80	93 (91-95)	74 (70-77)	77 (75-80)	92 (89-94)	83
100	90 (88-92)	76 (73-79)	79 (76-81)	89 (87-91)	83
125	87 (85-90)	79 (76-82)	80 (78-83)	87 (84-89)	83
150	85 (82-88)	83 (80-85)	83 (80-85)	85 (83-88)	84

Note: *PPV*, Positive predictive value; *NPV*, negative predictive value.

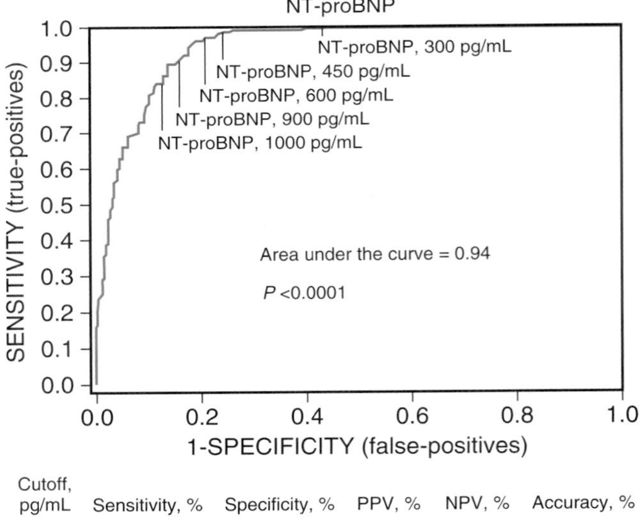

Cutoff, pg/mL	Sensitivity, %	Specificity, %	PPV, %	NPV, %	Accuracy, %
300	99	68	62	99	79
450	98	76	68	99	83
600	96	81	73	97	86
900	90	85	76	94	87
1000	87	86	78	91	87

Note: *PPV*, Positive predictive value; *NPV*, negative predictive value.

FIGURE 28-4 Receiver operator characteristic curves for diagnostic accuracies for B-type natriuretic peptide (BNP) and aminoterminal pro B-type natriuretic peptide (NT-proBNP). *Left from Maisel AS, Krishnaswamy P, Nowak RM, et al: Rapid measurement of b-type natriuretic peptide in the emergency diagnosis of heart failure. N Engl J Med 347:161–167, 2002; right from Januzzi JL, Jr., Camargo CA, Anwaruddin S, et al: The N-terminal pro-BNP investigation of dyspnea in the emergency department (PRIDE) study. Am J Cardiol 95:948–954, 2005.*

structural alterations (e.g., left ventricular hypertrophy, prior myocardial infarctions), rhythm abnormalities as a cause or consequence of heart failure decompensation (e.g., atrial fibrillation, frequent ectopic beats, or other sustained arrhythmias), or the presence of conduction abnormalities (such as bundle branch block or intraventricular conduction delays) that may lead to electrical dyssynchrony. Frequently, Holter monitoring or event monitoring can assist with the detection of such abnormalities.

The QT interval should be noted, as many therapies can further prolong the QT interval and provoke lethal arrhythmias. In patients who have undergone cardiac resynchronization therapy (CRT), acute changes in QRS complex or morphology may also signify underlying pacing or programming alterations (although such changes may or may not result in reversal of cardiac remodeling, nor are prerequisites for symptomatic improvement). The presence of ectopic beats, although benign in most cases, may also lead to cardiac insufficiency when the burden is high.

Morphologic Evaluation: Chest X-ray, Echocardiography, and Magnetic Resonance Imaging (see also Chapter 29)

It is our belief that the chest x-ray remains important in the assessment of patients with heart failure. Roentgenographic findings of pulmonary congestion may precede the presence of rales. Careful examination of the cardiac size and shape, as well as the pulmonary vasculature, remains part of routine evaluation of all patients with heart failure. In recipients of CRT implantation, posteroanterior and lateral views of chest x-rays may help determine inappropriate left ventricular lead positioning that may be contributory to persistent symptoms (**Figure 28-5**).

Echocardiographic evaluation remains an essential diagnostic tool for assessing cardiac structure and function. Although traditionally the focus has been on the left ventricular ejection fraction, the degree of underlying chamber dilation (or hypertrophy) can be overlooked. In fact, it is seldom recognized that the estimation of effective stroke volume (i.e., the ejection fraction relative to the left ventricular end-diastolic volume) is more appropriate in determining if the signs and symptoms can be explained by cardiac causes. Therefore, chamber size is an important indicator of compensatory progression of disease, and the propensity for long-term recovery. Other aspects of chamber dilation can lead to valvular regurgitation (from annular dilation) or mechanical dyssynchrony from prolonged interventricular and intraventricular conduction delays. Doppler estimates of right ventricular or pulmonary artery systolic pressure are helpful surrogates for pulmonary hypertension. Mitral, tricuspid, and pulmonary vein Doppler flow patterns can provide estimates of intracardiac pressures and diastolic staging, whereas tissue Doppler indices can characterize the myocardial abnormalities related to diastolic dysfunction and restrictive physiology. The clinical utility of mechanical dyssynchrony assessment is dwindling and is not routinely performed. Left atrial enlargement and left ventricular hypertrophy are common findings for heart failure with preserved ejection fraction, whereas the presence of left ventricular outflow tract obstruction (at rest or provoked by amyl nitrite) due to asymmetric septal hypertrophy and/or systolic anterior motion of the mitral leaflet may occur in the setting of hypertrophic cardiomyopathy. The presence of thrombus in the left ventricular and/or left atrium/left atrial appendage can be a reliable surrogate indicator of low cardiac output status and should warrant aggressive evaluation. Obviously, the presence of wall-motion abnormalities or abnormalities of cardiac structure and performance are hallmarks of stage B heart failure.

Magnetic resonance (MR) imaging has been shown to be of considerable use in the morphologic and functional assessment of the heart (see also Chapter 29). However, at present this technology is mainly used to gain additional information. Cardiac MR imaging requires acquisition of multiple oblique planes relative to the heart, similar to echocardiography. The imaging techniques are designed to render blood dark or bright and to depict various aspects of motion, flow, and perfusion (**Figure 28-6**). Different techniques have been used for assessing cardiac function with MR imaging. New MR sequences allow studying cardiac motion (myocardial tagging), blood flow velocity (phase contrast method), and myocardial scarring (late

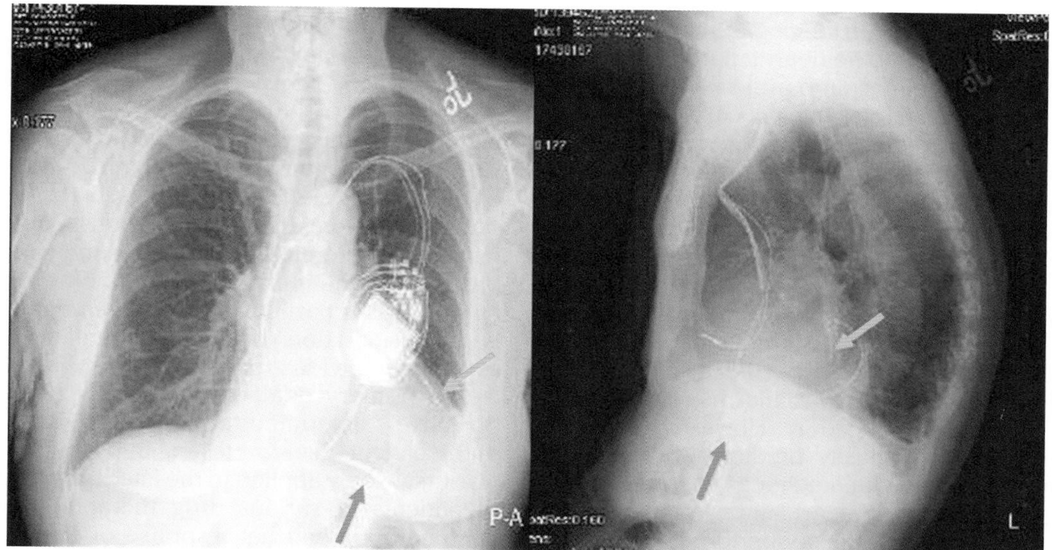

FIGURE 28-5 Appropriate lead placement *(arrows)* for cardiac resynchronization therapy by chest x-ray.

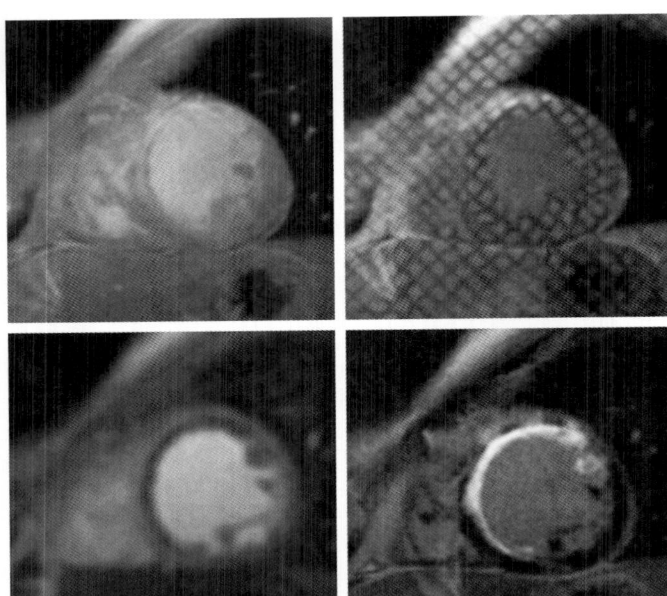

FIGURE 28-6 Cardiac magnetic resonance imaging (MRI) assessment of myocardial viability with cine imaging (cine), myocardial tagging imaging (TAG), TurboFlash perfusion imaging with gadolinium (Turbo+Gd), and delay-enhanced imaging with gadolinium (D-E+Gd).

enhancement technique), and specific patterns may indicate the presence of infiltrative diseases (such as amyloidosis, sarcoidosis, hemachromatosis) or myocarditis. In some cases, such findings from MRI may lead to more definitive tissue diagnosis and confirmation of the cause of cardiomyopathy.

Ischemic Evaluation: Myocardial Viability and Coronary Anatomy (see also Chapter 18)

Coronary artery disease is the cause of heart failure in about two thirds of patients with left ventricular systolic dysfunction, and up to one third of patients with nonischemic cardiomyopathy experience chest pain that mimics angina.[60,64] Studies have also pointed out that underdiagnosis or misdiagnosis of ischemic heart disease in the heart failure population is common if angiographic evaluation was not undertaken as part of the heart failure workup.[65,66]

Patients with systolic heart failure and severe coronary artery disease have by definition ischemic cardiomyopathy, and in some cases this reduction in myocardial function may be improved using percutaneous coronary intervention (PCI) or surgical revascularization. Most patients with heart failure should be considered as candidates for diagnostic coronary angiography to determine if there is significant coronary artery disease, especially in patients where revascularization is often very beneficial. Clearly this remains highly controversial, because the large majority of patients with a good clinical history and a low clinical suspicion based on lack of cardiovascular risk factors may not need such an invasive procedure. However, coronary artery disease may not be easily predicted by medical history, physical examination, and echocardiogram.[67] If the patient has angina pectoris and heart failure, an even more compelling argument can be made for performing diagnostic coronary angiography. On the other hand, if there is

TABLE 28-9 Weber Classification of Functional Impairment in Aerobic Capacity and Anaerobic Threshold as Measured during Incremental Exercise Testing

CLASS	DEGREE OF IMPAIRMENT	Vo_2 MAX (mL/min/kg)	ANAEROBIC THRESHOLD (mL/min/kg)
A	None to mild	>20	>14
B	Mild to moderate	16-20	11-14
C	Moderate to severe	10-16	8-11
D	Severe	6-10	5-8
E	Very severe	<6	≤4

severe coronary artery disease and reduced left ventricular function but minimal anginal symptoms, demonstration of myocardial viability may be of importance. It is also important to recognize that diagnostic evaluation for coronary artery disease only provides a snapshot at the time of evaluation, and clearly atherosclerotic diseases may progress over time, leading to progressive ischemia.

In the case of cardiac MR, assessment of myocardial viability has been considered important to detect ischemic but viable myocardium for potential therapeutic interventions. Recently, it has become apparent that myocardial viability assessment may not identify patients with a differential survival benefit from coronary artery bypass surgery.[68] In heart failure, where 60% to 70% of all patients suffer from coronary artery disease, these techniques can be helpful for therapeutic and prognostic stratification. Late enhancement MR imaging has become an important tool for determination of infarct size and scar burden in patients with myocardial infarction. The spatial and temporal relationship measured via differential uptake and release of contrast material in the viable versus scar tissue can provide the location as well as the extent of the scar. Nevertheless, widespread use of viability testing as a prerequisite for bypass surgery in patients with ischemic cardiomyopathy is now open to some questions.[68]

Functional Evaluation: Cardiopulmonary Exercise Testing

A fundamental requirement for many activities of daily living is the ability to perform aerobic work. Functional capacity is usually measured in metabolic equivalents (METs), where 1 MET represents 3.5 mL O_2/kg/min. Exercise testing is a valuable tool in the diagnosis and assessment of patients with heart failure[42] (**Table 28-9**). It has long been recognized that the simple history and physical examination, as well as various subjective functional classification systems, can be too nonspecific and relatively insensitive. Therefore, exercise testing can add substantial precision in the initial evaluation of the patient with heart failure. This is particularly true when heart transplantation is a consideration, or when quantitative information on assessing individual patient disability is necessary.

The primary goal of metabolic exercise testing is to objectively determine the functional status and prognosis of the patient. Exercise testing in patients with heart failure was first widely applied in the late 1970s to test the response of patients to various drug therapies.[17] Although it has become apparent that response of exercise to short-term drug therapy is not predictive of long-term drug efficacy,[69]

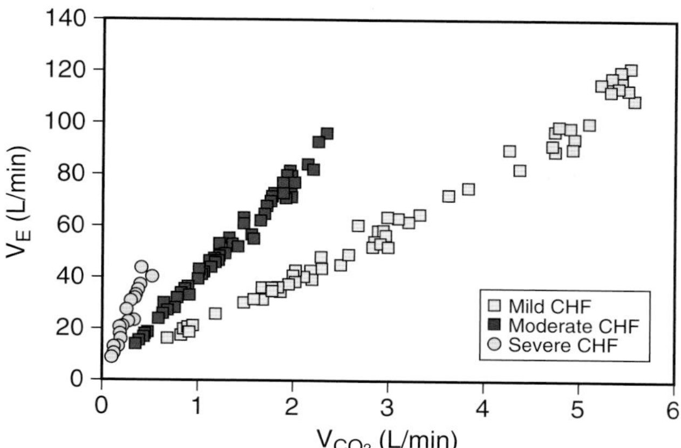

FIGURE 28-7 Plot of minute ventilation (V_E) versus the rate of carbon dioxide production (VCO_2) in patients with different degrees of severity of chronic heart failure (CHF). *From Coats AJ: Heart failure: what causes the symptoms of heart failure? Heart 86:574–578, 2001.*

useful information regarding how to gauge the degree of patient disability more precisely has emerged from these studies. Recent years have witnessed remarkable growth in the use of exercise testing to assess the severity of heart failure and to help to determine the prognosis of individual patients. In retrospect, it has become clear that measurements of the peak VO_2 and V_E/VCO_2 slopes are powerful predictors of the prognosis. Serial improvement in peak VO_2 in response to therapy or occurring spontaneously has also been demonstrated to have prognostic value.[70] However, the V_E/VCO_2 slope remains the strongest predictor of prognosis, better even than peak VO_2.[71] The usefulness of cardiac output estimation during standard metabolic exercise testing is under intense investigation.[72]

Metabolic exercise testing is of value in deciphering whether the heart or lungs are causing the dyspnea. Increased ventilation (V_E) with respect to carbon dioxide production is a hallmark finding of patients with heart failure[71,73] (**Figure 28-7**). The slope of the V_E/VCO_2 offers important prognostic information (particularly those >45), perhaps even more than peak ventilatory oxygen uptake (VO_2).[73,74] However, the increase in V_E/VCO_2 slope observed in patients with heart failure is nonspecific[75] and can also be abnormally steep in patients with primary lung disease.[76]

Assessment of functional capacity is typically performed on a motorized treadmill or stationary bicycle ergometer. The functional capacity can be estimated or measured directly by gas exchange methods (VO_2) from the highest work level achieved. Estimates of functional capacity such as exercise duration are less reliable than direct measurements of gas exchange. Peak VO_2 and anaerobic ventilatory threshold are highly reproducible and therefore recommended for evaluation of patients with heart failure.[42] The peak VO_2 is currently the standard used by most laboratories. However, there are well-known limitations of maximal exercise testing in the setting of heart failure.[77] Because patients generally have a reduced level of physical activity, peak VO_2 may not be a relevant indicator of everyday exercise activity. The six-minute walk or shuttle-walk tests, on the other hand, are simpler and do not require special equipment.[78,79] Simply assessing exercise duration can also provide important prognostic information. However, it is controversial whether these submaximal exercise tests are an accurate predictor of the prognosis,[80,81] because the results may depend on patient motivation and operator enthusiasm. The point of aerobic threshold is, however, insensitive to patient motivation. In this regard, submaximal exercise testing may be an ideal test of everyday activity capacity, but there is not uniform agreement on how to best perform it. A prime use of metabolic exercise testing is in the evaluation of patients for heart transplantation. A peak VO_2 of greater than 14 mL/kg/min is considered "too well" for transplant in many centers.[82] Because this was derived from a relatively aged population before the widespread use of β-adrenergic blockers, this criterion has posed some problems with younger individuals, in which extremely poor functional capacity is not below this cutoff range. The latest advanced heart failure guidelines have therefore refined the criteria to include an age- and gender-predicted comparison, and less than 50% of predicted normal is now often considered as being impaired to the point where heart transplant might be considered.[83]

Additional information from the exercise test includes assessment of the chronotropic response to exercise, which is indicative of abnormal parasympathetic activation, a well-described feature of heart failure.[84] Abnormal return of parasympathetic activity following exercise is also abnormal in many patients with heart failure (i.e., reduction in heart rate of 12 beats or less 1 minute following cessation of exercise).

Hemodynamic Evaluation: Cardiac Catheterization (see also Chapter 31)

There are individual circumstances when it may be prudent to consider invasive hemodynamic evaluation and monitoring as part of clinical evaluation of patients with heart failure. This was the predominant mode of quantifying disease during the development of neurohormonal antagonists. The main shift in practice occurred as a result of fading interests in using intravenous vasoactive therapies, as well as from increasing concerns regarding the lack of incremental long-term benefit (or even harm) using such strategies. Routine use of hemodynamic-guided therapy in advanced heart failure have been called to question with the equivocal results from the landmark Evaluation Study of Congestive Heart Failure and Pulmonary Artery Catheterization Effectiveness (ESCAPE) trial, which randomized 433 patients with advanced decompensated heart failure receiving acute management with or without pulmonary artery catheter-guided therapy. The 30-day mortalities were similar at 4.7% for the pulmonary artery catheter group and 5.0% for the clinically managed group. Also, rates of complications, adverse events, and clinical outcomes were not significantly different at 6 months.[85] Therefore, only patients who are doing poorly with severe congestion, ascites, anasarca, or obvious low-output signs and symptoms might be considered for hospitalization with hemodynamic monitoring. When constrictive physiology or restrictive cardiomyopathy is suspected, right-heart catheterization should also be considered. With improved imaging techniques, the role of right-heart catheterization is diminishing, although it is still useful as a confirmatory test in patients with complex or unusual forms of heart failure. Most right-heart catheterizations performed in patients with heart failure today are used to help guide therapy rather than to make a specific diagnosis.

With the broad adoption of implantable cardioverter-defibrillators and cardiac resynchronization therapy, there has been a dramatic rise in the number of chronic heart failure patients undergoing implantation of cardiac devices. Measurements that provide the necessary diagnostics in self-maintenance of the functionality of the devices and their electrode leads became notable physiologic assessment tools that allow clinicians to review an individual patient's clinical status. Not only different types of arrhythmic events and their corresponding treatments can be interrogated but also periodic trends in heart rate and patient activity, and in some cases measures of intrathoracic impedance, can be extrapolated. There have been consistent reports about their abilities to track with disease states, and may provide some prognostic insights into morbidity and mortality that may find its potential use as part of remote monitoring strategies in the care of these implanted devices.[86-88] However, the true clinical utility of these device diagnostics is still under question as clinical trials using these measures have yet to provide incremental benefits and in some reports actually presented with worse outcomes.[89]

Histologic Evaluation: Endomyocardial Biopsy

Over the years, it has become clear that there is a diminished role for diagnostic endomyocardial biopsy in patients with heart failure.[90] The early impetus for this nihilism stems from the results from the Myocarditis Treatment Trial, which implied a sense of futility regarding various treatment strategies for acute myocarditis[91] (see also Chapter 26). It is unclear if certain forms of cardiomyopathy and myocarditis can be managed better with the aid of diagnostic endomyocardial biopsy,[82] especially with some recent support for immunosuppression and immunoabsorption in the setting of chronic persistent myocarditis without viral persistence. If acute inflammatory myocarditis is suspected, endomyocardial biopsy should still be considered, especially with the current availability of newer molecular markers.[92] Selected patients may in fact respond to various immunosuppressant therapies, but success cannot be reliably predicted.[93]

Although the role of endomyocardial biopsy is diminishing in the evaluation of patients with heart failure, it is important that clinicians keep in mind that specific entities can only be diagnosed using this technique. Endomyocardial biopsy is a requirement for the diagnosis of acute myocarditis, because the clinical diagnosis of this entity is notoriously insensitive. The natural history and prognosis of some types of heart failure, including fulminant myocarditis, giant-cell myocarditis, sarcoidosis, and amyloid heart disease, are quite distinct and are variably responsive to different management strategies. For example, patients with amyloid heart disease are usually refractory to both conventional therapy and heart transplantation. Those with fulminant myocarditis may recover spontaneously following aggressive hemodynamic support.[94] Patients with giant-cell myocarditis often have a rapid downhill course, and may be suitable for immunosuppressive protocols or heart transplantation.[95] European data indicate the presence of a "viral cardiomyopathy" entity with persistent viral presence by polymerase chain reaction testing,[96] whereas those with no detectable viral genome tend to be more responsive to immunosuppressive therapies.[97] Therefore, the use of endomyocardial biopsy, though now more limited, clearly has a role when specific types of cardiomyopathy are suggested on clinical grounds, and the biopsy information may be quite helpful in planning therapy. **Table 28-10** outlines the 14 clinical scenarios where endomyocardial biopsy should be considered as recommended by a recently published consensus statement.[93]

TABLE 28-10 Fourteen Clinical Scenarios for Indications for Endomyocardial Biopsy

SCENARIO	RECOMMENDATION (STRENGTH/LEVEL)
New-onset heart failure of <2 weeks' duration associated with a normal-sized or dilated left ventricle and hemodynamic compromise.	I/B
New-onset heart failure of 2 weeks' to 3 months' duration associated with a dilated left ventricle and new ventricular arrhythmias, second- or third-degree heart block, or failure to respond to usual care within 1-2 weeks.	I/B
Heart failure of ≥3 months' duration associated with a dilated left ventricle and new ventricular arrhythmias, second- or third-degree heart block, or failure to respond to usual care within 1 to 2 weeks.	IIa/C
Heart failure associated with a dilated cardiomyopathy of any duration associated with suspected allergic reaction and/or eosinophilia.	IIa/C
Heart failure associated with suspected anthracycline cardiomyopathy.	IIa/C
Heart failure associated with unexplained restrictive cardiomyopathy.	IIa/C
Suspected cardiac tumors.	IIa/C
Unexplained cardiomyopathy in children.	IIa/C
New-onset heart failure of 2 weeks' to 3 months' duration associated with a dilated left ventricle, without new ventricular arrhythmias or second- or third-degree heart block, that responds to usual care within 1-2 weeks.	IIb/B
Heart failure of >3 months' duration associated with a dilated left ventricle, without new ventricular arrhythmias or second- or third-degree heart block, that responds to usual care within 1-2 weeks.	IIb/C
Heart failure associated with unexplained hypertrophic cardiomyopathy.	IIb/C
Suspected arrhythmogenic right ventricular dysplasia.	IIb/C
Unexplained ventricular arrhythmias.	IIb/C
Unexplained atrial fibrillation.	III/C

Modified from Cooper LT, Baughman KL, Feldman AM, et al: The role of endomyocardial biopsy in the management of cardiovascular disease: a scientific statement from the American Heart Association, the American College of Cardiology, and the European Society of Cardiology. Circulation 116:2216–2233, 2007.

Genetic Evaluation

Clinical genetic testing for monogenetic mutations of sarcomeric and metabolic genes in inherited cardiomyopathies has become a reality in recent years with the broad availability of commercial testing laboratories. Many of the inherited cardiomyopathies have been extensively reviewed in Chapter 22. There continue to be several important hurdles facing routine genetic testing. First, mapping specific gene mutations can be highly complex and some of the affected genes are large, which can translate into

TABLE 28-11 MAGGIC Risk Score for Prognosis in Heart Failure

RISK FACTOR	ADDITION TO RISK SCORE								RISK SCORE
Ejection fraction (%)	<20	20-24	25-29	30-34	35-39	40+			
	+7	+6	+5	+3	+2	0			
Extra for age (years)	<55	56-59	60-64	65-69	70-74	75-79	80+		
EF <30	0	+1	+2	+4	+6	+8	+10		
EF 30-39	0	+2	+4	+6	+8	+10	+13		
EF 40+	0	+3	+5	+7	+9	+12	+15		
Extra for systolic blood pressure (mm Hg)	<110	110-119	120-129	130-139	140-149	150+			
EF <30	+5	+4	+3	+2	+1	0			
EF 30-39	+3	+2	+1	+1	0	0			
EF 40+	+2	+1	+1	0	0	0			
BMI (kg/m^2)	<15	15-19	20-24	25-29	30+				
	+6	+5	+3	+2	0				
Creatinine (μmol/L)	<90	90-109	110-129	130-149	150-169	170-209	210-249	250+	
	0	+1	+2	+3	+4	+5	+6	+8	
NYHA class	1	2	3	4					
	0	+2	+6	+8					
Male				+1					
Current smoker				+1					
Diabetic				+3					
Diagnosis of COPD				+2					
First diagnosis of heart failure in the past 18 months				+2					
Not on β-blocker				+3					
Not on ACEI/ARB				+1					
							Total risk score =		

From Pocock SJ, Ariti CA, McMurray JJ, et al: Predicting survival in heart failure: a risk score based on 39,372 patients from 30 studies. Eur Heart J 34:1404–1413, 2012.

labor-intensive and expensive ventures. Second, despite the association between a family history of heart failure and underlying genetic predispositions, we only realize a small proportion of mutations that lead to inherited cardiomyopathies. This means that a negative test for unexplained cardiomyopathies cannot provide the confidence to rule out any underlying genetic mutations. Third, treatment options have yet to catch up with the availability of genetic information to help clinicians to tailor their management strategies. For now, the greatest impact of genetic testing remains identification of at-risk individuals for inherited cardiomyopathies who then require careful evaluation and close monitoring, particularly in the case of hypertrophic cardiomyopathy and arrhythmogenic right ventricular dysplasia.[98] Specific diseases, such as Fabry disease or transthyretin amyloidosis, also have genetic tests available for confirmatory purposes. Nevertheless, pharmacogenomic-guided therapy is still under intensive clinical investigation.

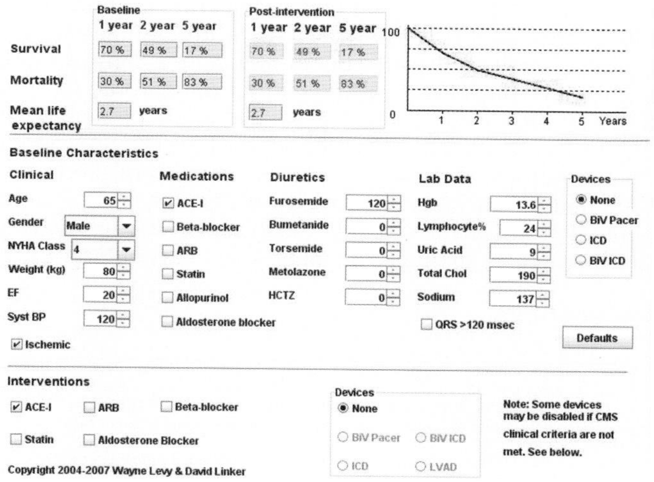

FIGURE 28-8 Seattle Heart Failure Model.

PROGNOSIS

Although the primary focus of clinical evaluation of heart failure is to establish the diagnosis of heart failure and to evaluate for treatable causes, the ability to determine an individual's short-term and long-term risk profile may provide insightful information to triage treatment approaches. This is particularly relevant when guideline-based therapies have already been instituted, and there is a need to establish meaningful expectations for patients and their care providers. Several "risk scores" have been developed over the past decades in both acute and chronic heart failure settings, and several have even been applied to clinical decision-making algorithms for advanced therapies (**Table 28-11**). Overall, readily-available variables needed for risk stratification include (1) measures of cardiac insufficiency (e.g., systolic blood pressure, symptom severity/functional impairment, or cardiac-specific biomarkers); (2) measures of end-organ dysfunction (e.g., kidney function, such as glomerular filtration or uremia); and (3) treatment requirements and responses (e.g., loop diuretic dosing needs, intolerance to neurohormonal antagonists). The Seattle Heart Failure Model has been commonly used for this purpose (www.seattleheartfailuremodel.org; **Figure 28-8**)[99] while a recent integer risk model (MAGGIC risk score) has also been proposed.[100] There is also the recent development of a mortality risk score (www.mortalityscore.org/heart_failure.php) and readmission risk score for heart failure (www.readmissionscore.org/heart_failure.php).[101] Abnormal levels of novel biomarkers that are clinically available, such as high-sensitivity cardiac troponins, ST2, and galectin-3, may also provide robust risk prediction (which will be discussed in Chapter 30).[102-104] However, translating such risk profiles into clinically meaningful actions remains a major challenge. Despite some endorsements of clinical practice guidelines and appropriate use statements, we still do not have a universally accepted algorithm to triage heart failure therapeutic approaches based on prognostic evaluation.

FUTURE DIRECTIONS

The present approach to clinical evaluation of heart failure still adheres to the traditional patient-doctor encounter, including the eliciting of medical history for suspicious symptoms, bedside examinations to detect clinical signs of congestion and perfusion, and the decision to undergo confirmatory or monitoring testing in search for therapeutic interventions. These require the patient's physical presence and may only capture the clinical picture as a snapshot. Simple longitudinal information such as daily weights, self-report health status, and vital signs have been widely used, but is often plagued with nonadherence, subjectivity, and selectivity in self-reporting. The next generation of clinical evaluation relies on the ability of technological advances to quantify disease severity both at the time of clinical encounter and at home. Some are already available as adjunctive parameters derived from interrogation of implantable devices, whereas others have linked to disease management and home care programs. Examples include arrhythmia detection and management, intracardiac impedance monitoring, and even detection of intracardiac filling pressures. External devices, both stand-alone and portable versions, are also becoming increasingly available to measure physiologic and electrocardiographic information that promises incremental values in the clinical evaluation of patients with heart failure. When the appropriate configurations and methodologies are established, such "ambulatory" insight can provide insight and clarity into the clinical profile, which could transform the way we evaluate (and ultimately manage) patients with heart failure.

References

1. Lindenfeld J, Albert NM, Boehmer JP, et al: HFSA 2010 comprehensive heart failure practice guideline. *J Card Fail* 16:e1–e194, 2010.
2. McMurray JJ, Adamopoulos S, Anker SD, et al: ESC guidelines for the diagnosis and treatment of acute and chronic heart failure 2012: the task force for the diagnosis and treatment of acute and chronic heart failure 2012 of the European Society of Cardiology. Developed in collaboration with the Heart Failure Association (HFA) of the ESC. *Eur Heart J* 33:1787–1847, 2012.
3. Hunt SA, Abraham WT, Chin MH, et al: 2009 focused update incorporated into the ACC/AHA 2005 guidelines for the diagnosis and management of heart failure in adults: a report of the American College of Cardiology Foundation/American Heart Association task force on practice guidelines: developed in collaboration with the International Society for Heart and Lung Transplantation. *Circulation* 119:e391–e479, 2009.
4. Butler J, Kalogeropoulos A, Georgiopoulou V, et al: Incident heart failure prediction in the elderly: the health ABC heart failure score. *Circ Heart Fail* 1:125–133, 2008.
5. Agarwal SK, Chambless LE, Ballantyne CM, et al: Prediction of incident heart failure in general practice: the Atherosclerosis Risk in Communities (ARIC) study. *Circ Heart Fail* 5:422–429, 2012.
6. Criteria committee of the New York Heart Association: *Nomenclature and criteria for diagnosis of diseases of the heart and great vessels*, ed 9, Boston, 1994, Little, Brown & Co.
7. Mosterd A, Deckers JW, Hoes AW, et al: Classification of heart failure in population based research: an assessment of six heart failure scores. *Eur J Epidemiol* 13:491–502, 1997.
8. Stevenson LW, Pagani FD, Young JB, et al: INTERMACS profiles of advanced heart failure: the current picture. *J Heart Lung Transplant* 28:535–541, 2009.
9. Lewis EF, Johnson PA, Johnson W, et al: Preferences for quality of life or survival expressed by patients with heart failure. *J Heart Lung Transplant* 20:1016–1024, 2001.
10. Tsuyuki RT, McKelvie RS, Arnold MO, et al: Acute precipitants of congestive heart failure exacerbations. *Arch Intern Med* 161:2337, 2001.
11. Fonarow GC, Abraham WT, Albert NM, et al: Factors identified as precipitating hospital admissions for heart failure and clinical outcomes: findings from OPTIMIZE-HF. *Arch Intern Med* 168:847–854, 2008.
12. Rector TS, Cohn JN: Assessment of patient outcome with the Minnesota Living with Heart Failure Questionnaire: reliability and validity during a randomized, double-blind, placebo controlled trial of pimobendan. *Am Heart J* 124:1017, 1992.
13. Green CP, Porter CB, Bresnahan DR, et al: Development and evaluation of the Kansas City Cardiomyopathy Questionnaire: a new health status measure for heart failure. *J Am Coll Cardiol* 35:1245–1255, 2000.
14. ACC/AHA guidelines for the management of patients with valvular heart disease. A report of the American College of Cardiology/American Heart Association. Task Force on Practice Guidelines (Committee on Management of Patients with Valvular Heart Disease). *J Am Coll Cardiol* 32:1486–1588, 1998.
15. Benge W, Litchfield RL, Marcus ML: Exercise capacity in patients with severe left ventricular dysfunction. *Circulation* 61:955–959, 1980.
16. Franciosa JA, Park M, Levine TB: Lack of correlation between exercise capacity and indexes of resting left ventricular performance in heart failure. *Am J Cardiol* 47:33–39, 1981.
17. Franciosa JA, Ziesche S, Wilen M: Functional capacity of patients with chronic left ventricular failure. Relationship of bicycle exercise performance to clinical and hemodynamic characterization. *Am J Med* 67:460–466, 1979.
18. Francis GS, Goldsmith SR, Cohn JN: Relationship of exercise capacity to resting left ventricular performance and basal plasma norepinephrine levels in patients with congestive heart failure. *Am Heart J* 104:725–731, 1982.
19. Fink LI, Wilson JR, Ferraro N: Exercise ventilation and pulmonary artery wedge pressure in chronic stable congestive heart failure. *Am J Cardiol* 57:249–253, 1986.
20. Stevenson LW, Perloff JK: The limited reliability of physical signs for estimating hemodynamics in chronic heart failure. *JAMA* 261:884–888, 1989.
21. Mancini DM, Henson D, LaManca J, et al: Respiratory muscle function and dyspnea in patients with chronic congestive heart failure. *Circulation* 86:909–918, 1992.
22. Clark AL, Poole-Wilson PA, Coats AJ: Exercise limitation in chronic heart failure: central role of the periphery. *J Am Coll Cardiol* 28:1092–1102, 1996.
23. MacGowan GA, Cecchetti A, Murali S: Ventilatory drive during exercise in congestive heart failure. *J Card Fail* 3:257–262, 1997.
24. Wasserman K: Dyspnea on exertion. Is it the heart or the lungs? *JAMA* 248:2039–2043, 1982.
25. Wilson JR, Mancini DM: Factors contributing to the exercise limitation of heart failure. *J Am Coll Cardiol* 22:93A–98A, 1993.
26. Chua TP, Clark AL, Amadi AA, et al: Relation between chemosensitivity and the ventilatory response to exercise in chronic heart failure. *J Am Coll Cardiol* 27:650–657, 1996.
27. Ponikowski P, Francis DP, Piepoli MF, et al: Enhanced ventilatory response to exercise in patients with chronic heart failure and preserved exercise tolerance: marker of abnormal cardiorespiratory reflex control and predictor of poor prognosis. *Circulation* 103:967–972, 2001.
28. Johnson RL, Jr: Gas exchange efficiency in congestive heart failure ii. *Circulation* 103:916–918, 2001.
29. Wasserman K: The peripheral circulation and lactic acid metabolism in heart, or cardiovascular, failure. *Circulation* 80:1084–1086, 1989.
30. Piepoli M, Clark AL, Volterrani M, et al: Contribution of muscle afferents to the hemodynamic, autonomic, and ventilatory responses to exercise in patients with chronic heart failure: effects of physical training. *Circulation* 93:940–952, 1996.
31. Mancini DM, Coyle E, Coggan A, et al: Contribution of intrinsic skeletal muscle changes to 31P NMR skeletal muscle metabolic abnormalities in patients with chronic heart failure. *Circulation* 80:1338–1346, 1989.
32. Mancini DM, Ferraro N, Tuchler M, et al: Detection of abnormal calf muscle metabolism in patients with heart failure using phosphorus-31 nuclear magnetic resonance. *Am J Cardiol* 62:1234–1240, 1988.
33. Massie B, Conway M, Yonge R, et al: Skeletal muscle metabolism in patients with congestive heart failure: relation to clinical severity and blood flow. *Circulation* 76:1009–1019, 1987.
34. Massie BM, Conway M, Yonge R, et al: 31P nuclear magnetic resonance evidence of abnormal skeletal muscle metabolism in patients with congestive heart failure. *Am J Cardiol* 60:309–315, 1987.
35. Wilson JR, Fink L, Maris J, et al: Evaluation of energy metabolism in skeletal muscle of patients with heart failure with gated phosphorus-31 nuclear magnetic resonance. *Circulation* 71:57–62, 1985.
36. Sullivan MJ, Green HJ, Cobb FR: Skeletal muscle biochemistry and histology in ambulatory patients with long-term heart failure. *Circulation* 81:518–527, 1990.
37. Mancini DM, Walter G, Reichek N, et al: Contribution of skeletal muscle atrophy to exercise intolerance and altered muscle metabolism in heart failure. *Circulation* 85:1364–1373, 1992.
38. Drexler H, Riede U, Munzel T, et al: Alterations of skeletal muscle in chronic heart failure. *Circulation* 85:1751–1759, 1992.
39. Schaefer S, Gober JR, Schwartz GG, et al: In vivo phosphorus-31 spectroscopic imaging in patients with global myocardial disease. *Am J Cardiol* 65:1154–1161, 1990.
40. Sullivan MJ, Green HJ, Cobb FR: Altered skeletal muscle metabolic response to exercise in chronic heart failure. Relation to skeletal muscle aerobic enzyme activity. *Circulation* 84:1597–1607, 1991.
41. Working Group on Cardiac Rehabilitation & Exercise Physiology and Working Group on Heart Failure of the European Society of Cardiology: Recommendations for exercise training in chronic heart failure patients. *Eur Heart J* 22:125–135, 2001.
42. Fleg JL, Pina IL, Balady GJ, et al: Assessment of functional capacity in clinical and research applications: an advisory from the Committee on Exercise, Rehabilitation, and Prevention, Council on Clinical Cardiology, American Heart Association. *Circulation* 102:1591–1597, 2000.
43. Minotti JR, Massie BM: Exercise training in heart failure patients. Does reversing the peripheral abnormalities protect the heart? *Circulation* 85:2323–2325, 1992.
44. Sullivan MJ, Higginbotham MB, Cobb FR: Exercise training in patients with chronic heart failure delays ventilatory anaerobic threshold and improves submaximal exercise performance. *Circulation* 79:324–329, 1989.
45. Sullivan MJ, Higginbotham MB, Cobb FR: Exercise training in patients with severe left ventricular dysfunction. Hemodynamic and metabolic effects. *Circulation* 78:506–515, 1988.
46. Nohria A, Lewis E, Stevenson LW: Medical management of advanced heart failure. *JAMA* 287:628–640, 2002.
47. Drazner MH, Hellkamp AS, Leier CV, et al: Value of clinician assessment of hemodynamics in advanced heart failure: the ESCAPE trial. *Circ Heart Fail* 1:170–177, 2008.
48. Economides E, Stevenson LW: The jugular veins: knowing enough to look. *Am Heart J* 136:6–9, 1998.
49. Perloff JK: The jugular venous pulse and third heart sound in patients with heart failure. *N Engl J Med* 345:612–614, 2001.
50. Wiese J: The abdominojugular reflux sign. *Am J Med* 109:59–61, 2000.
51. Mullens W, Abrahams Z, Skouri HN, et al: Elevated intra-abdominal pressure in acute decompensated heart failure: a potential contributor to worsening renal function? *J Am Coll Cardiol* 51:300–306, 2008.
52. Tribouilloy CM, Enriquez-Sarano M, Mohty D, et al: Pathophysiologic determinants of third heart sounds: a prospective clinical and doppler echocardiographic study. *Am J Med* 111:96–102, 2001.
53. Drazner MH, Rame JE, Stevenson LW, et al: Prognostic importance of elevated jugular venous pressure and a third heart sound in patients with heart failure. *N Engl J Med* 345:574–581, 2001.
54. Drazner MH, Rame JE, Dries DL: Third heart sound and elevated jugular venous pressure as markers of the subsequent development of heart failure in patients with asymptomatic left ventricular dysfunction. *Am J Med* 114:431–437, 2003.
55. Lucas C, Johnson W, Hamilton MA, et al: Freedom from congestion predicts good survival despite previous class IV symptoms of heart failure. *Am Heart J* 140:840–847, 2000.
56. Lee YC, Sutton FJ: Pulsus alternans in patients with congestive cardiomyopathy. *Circulation* 65:1533–1534, 1982.
57. Anker SD, Ponikowski P, Varney S, et al: Wasting as independent risk factor for mortality in chronic heart failure. *Lancet* 349:1050–1053, 1997.

58. Anker SD, Rauchhaus M: Insights into the pathogenesis of chronic heart failure: immune activation and cachexia. *Curr Opin Cardiol* 14:211–216, 1999.
59. Dunlay SM, Weston SA, Redfield MM, et al: Tumor necrosis factor-alpha and mortality in heart failure: a community study. *Circulation* 118:625–631, 2008.
60. Hunt SA, Abraham WT, Chin MH, et al: ACC/AHA 2005 guideline update for the diagnosis and management of chronic heart failure in the adult: a report of the American College of Cardiology/American Heart Association task force on practice guidelines (writing committee to update the 2001 guidelines for the evaluation and management of heart failure): developed in collaboration with the American College of Chest Physicians and the International Society for Heart and Lung Transplantation: endorsed by the Heart Rhythm Society. *Circulation* 112:e154–e235, 2005.
61. Heart Failure Society of America: Executive summary: HFSA 2006 comprehensive heart failure practice guideline. *J Card Fail* 12:10–38, 2006.
62. Tang WH, Tong W, Jain A, et al: Evaluation and long-term prognosis of new-onset, transient, and persistent anemia in ambulatory patients with chronic heart failure. *J Am Coll Cardiol* 51:569–576, 2008.
63. Tang WH, Francis GS, Morrow DA, et al: National Academy of Clinical Biochemistry Laboratory Medicine Practice Guidelines: clinical utilization of cardiac biomarker testing in heart failure. *Circulation* 116:e99–e109, 2007.
64. Gheorghiade M, Bonow RO: Chronic heart failure in the United States: a manifestation of coronary artery disease. *Circulation* 97:282–289, 1998.
65. Baba R, Tsuyuki K, Kimura Y, et al: Oxygen uptake efficiency slope as a useful measure of cardiorespiratory functional reserve in adult cardiac patients. *Eur J Appl Physiol Occup Physiol* 80:397–401, 1999.
66. Brookes CI, Hart P, Keogh BE, et al: Angiography and the aetiology of heart failure. *Postgrad Med J* 71:480–482, 1995.
67. Bortman G, Sellanes M, Odell DS, et al: Discrepancy between pre- and post-transplant diagnosis of end-stage dilated cardiomyopathy. *Am J Cardiol* 74:921–924, 1994.
68. Bonow RO, Maurer G, Lee KL, et al: Myocardial viability and survival in ischemic left ventricular dysfunction. *N Engl J Med* 364:1617–1625, 2011.
69. Smith RF, Johnson G, Ziesche S, et al: Functional capacity in heart failure. Comparison of methods for assessment and their relation to other indexes of heart failure. The V-HeFT VA cooperative studies group. *Circulation* 87:VI88–VI93, 1993.
70. Florea VG, Henein MY, Anker SD, et al: Prognostic value of changes over time in exercise capacity and echocardiographic measurements in patients with chronic heart failure. *Eur Heart J* 21:146–153, 2000.
71. Chua TP, Ponikowski P, Harrington D, et al: Clinical correlates and prognostic significance of the ventilatory response to exercise in chronic heart failure. *J Am Coll Cardiol* 29:1585–1590, 1997.
72. Lang CC, Agostoni P, Mancini DM: Prognostic significance and measurement of exercise-derived hemodynamic variables in patients with heart failure. *J Card Fail* 13:672–679, 2007.
73. Robbins M, Francis G, Pashkow FJ, et al: Ventilatory and heart rate responses to exercise: better predictors of heart failure mortality than peak oxygen consumption. *Circulation* 100:2411–2417, 1999.
74. Weber KT, Kinasewitz GT, Janicki JS, et al: Oxygen utilization and ventilation during exercise in patients with chronic cardiac failure. *Circulation* 65:1213–1223, 1982.
75. Russell SD, McNeer FR, Higginbotham MB: Exertional dyspnea in heart failure: a symptom unrelated to pulmonary function at rest or during exercise. Duke University Clinical Cardiology Studies (DUCCS) exercise group. *Am Heart J* 135:398–405, 1998.
76. Johnson RL, Jr: Gas exchange efficiency in congestive heart failure. *Circulation* 101:2774–2776, 2000.
77. Francis GS, Rector TS: Maximal exercise tolerance as a therapeutic end point in heart failure—are we relying on the right measure? *Am J Cardiol* 73:304–306, 1994.
78. Guyatt GH, Sullivan MJ, Thompson PJ, et al: The 6-minute walk: a new measure of exercise capacity in patients with chronic heart failure. *Can Med Assoc J* 132:919–923, 1985.
79. Morales FJ, Martinez A, Mendez M, et al: A shuttle walk test for assessment of functional capacity in chronic heart failure. *Am Heart J* 138:291–298, 1999.
80. Opasich C, Pinna GD, Mazza A, et al: Six-minute walking performance in patients with moderate-to-severe heart failure; is it a useful indicator in clinical practice? *Eur Heart J* 22:488–496, 2001.
81. Sharma R, Anker SD: The 6-minute walk test and prognosis in chronic heart failure—the available evidence. *Eur Heart J* 22:445–448, 2001.
82. Mancini DM, Eisen H, Kussmaul W, et al: Value of peak exercise oxygen consumption for optimal timing of cardiac transplantation in ambulatory patients with heart failure. *Circulation* 83:778–786, 1991.
83. Mehra MR, Kobashigawa J, Starling R, et al: Listing criteria for heart transplantation: International Society for Heart and Lung Transplantation guidelines for the care of cardiac transplant candidates—2006. *J Heart Lung Transplant* 25:1024–1042, 2006.
84. Lauer MS, Francis GS, Okin PM, et al: Impaired chronotropic response to exercise stress testing as a predictor of mortality. *JAMA* 281:524–529, 1999.
85. Binanay C, Califf RM, Hasselblad V, et al: Evaluation study of congestive heart failure and pulmonary artery catheterization effectiveness: the ESCAPE trial. *JAMA* 294:1625–1633, 2005.
86. Tang WH, Warman EN, Johnson JW, et al: Threshold crossing of device-based intrathoracic impedance trends identifies relatively increased mortality risk. *Eur Heart J* 33:2189–2196, 2012.
87. Cowie MR, Sarkar S, Koehler J, et al: Development and validation of an integrated diagnostic algorithm derived from parameters monitored in implantable devices for identifying patients at risk for heart failure hospitalization in an ambulatory setting. *Eur Heart J* 34:2472–2480, 2013.
88. Whellan DJ, Sarkar S, Koehler J, et al: Development of a method to risk stratify patients with heart failure for 30-day readmission using implantable device diagnostics. *Am J Cardiol* 111:79–84, 2013.
89. van Veldhuisen DJ, Braunschweig F, Conraads V, et al: Intrathoracic impedance monitoring, audible patient alerts, and outcome in patients with heart failure. *Circulation* 124:1719–1726, 2011.
90. Hrobon P, Kuntz KM, Hare JM: Should endomyocardial biopsy be performed for detection of myocarditis? A decision analytic approach. *J Heart Lung Transplant* 17:479–486, 1998.
91. Mason JW, O'Connell JB, Herskowitz A, et al: A clinical trial of immunosuppressive therapy for myocarditis. The Myocarditis Treatment Trial investigators. *N Engl J Med* 333:269–275, 1995.
92. Kawai C: From myocarditis to cardiomyopathy: mechanisms of inflammation and cell death: learning from the past for the future. *Circulation* 99:1091–1100, 1999.
93. Cooper LT, Baughman KL, Feldman AM, et al: The role of endomyocardial biopsy in the management of cardiovascular disease: a scientific statement from the American Heart Association, the American College of Cardiology, and the European Society of Cardiology. *Circulation* 116:2216–2233, 2007.
94. McCarthy RE, 3rd, Boehmer JP, Hruban RH, et al: Long-term outcome of fulminant myocarditis as compared with acute (nonfulminant) myocarditis. *N Engl J Med* 342:690–695, 2000.
95. Cooper LT, Jr, Berry GJ, Shabetai R: Idiopathic giant-cell myocarditis—natural history and treatment. Multicenter giant cell myocarditis study group investigators. *N Engl J Med* 336:1860–1866, 1997.
96. Basso C, Calabrese F, Angelini A, et al: Classification and histological, immunohistochemical, and molecular diagnosis of inflammatory myocardial disease. *Heart Fail Rev* 18:673–681, 2013.
97. Frustaci A, Russo MA, Chimenti C: Randomized study on the efficacy of immunosuppressive therapy in patients with virus-negative inflammatory cardiomyopathy: the TIMIC study. *Eur Heart J* 30:1995–2002, 2009.
98. Hershberger RE, Lindenfeld J, Mestroni L, et al: Genetic evaluation of cardiomyopathy—a Heart Failure Society of America practice guideline. *J Card Fail* 15:83–97, 2009.
99. Levy WC, Mozaffarian D, Linker DT, et al: The Seattle heart failure model: prediction of survival in heart failure. *Circulation* 113:1424–1433, 2006.
100. Pocock SJ, Ariti CA, McMurray JJ, et al: Predicting survival in heart failure: a risk score based on 39372 patients from 30 studies. *Eur Heart J* 34:1404–1413, 2012.
101. Keenan PS, Normand SL, Lin Z, et al: An administrative claims measure suitable for profiling hospital performance on the basis of 30-day all-cause readmission rates among patients with heart failure. *Circ Cardiovasc Qual Outcomes* 1:29–37, 2008.
102. Ky B, French B, McCloskey K, et al: High-sensitivity ST2 for prediction of adverse outcomes in chronic heart failure. *Circ Heart Fail* 4:180–187, 2011.
103. Nagarajan V, Hernandez AV, Tang WH: Prognostic value of cardiac troponin in chronic stable heart failure: a systematic review. *Heart* 98:1778–1786, 2012.
104. van der Velde AR, Gullestad L, Ueland T, et al: Prognostic value of changes in galectin-3 levels over time in patients with heart failure: data from CORONA and COACH. *Circ Heart Fail* 6:219–226, 2013.
105. Ammar KA, Jacobsen SJ, Mahoney DW, et al: Prevalence and prognostic significance of heart failure stages: application of the American College of Cardiology/American Heart Association heart failure staging criteria in the community. *Circulation* 115:1563–1570, 2007.

29 Cardiac Imaging in Heart Failure

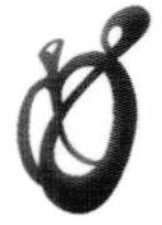

Martin St. John Sutton, Alan R. Morrison, Albert J. Sinusas, and Victor A. Ferrari

DEFINITION OF HEART FAILURE

Heart failure can be defined as an abnormality of cardiac structure or function that fails to deliver oxygen at a rate commensurate with the needs of the body tissues (systolic failure) or fails to receive blood at normal filling pressures (diastolic failure). The diagnosis of heart failure may be difficult to establish clinically, especially during its early stages, because the symptoms and physical signs are nonspecific, consisting of dyspnea, effort intolerance, fatigue, elevated jugular venous pressure, and lower extremity edema. As a result, cardiac imaging has assumed a pivotal role in the early diagnosis and optimal management of patients with heart failure from acquired and congenital heart disease.[1,2]

EPIDEMIOLOGY OF HEART FAILURE (see also Chapter 17)

Heart failure currently affects approximately 30 million people worldwide, 6 million of whom reside in the United States. There are an additional 650,000 new cases of heart failure diagnosed each year in the United States largely because of improved noninvasive cardiac imaging, typically transthoracic two-dimensional echocardiography (TTE).[3] The incidence of heart failure increases with advancing age, so that approximately 10% of all males and females older than 70 years of age have heart failure.[4] In addition, heart failure is the most frequent hospital discharge diagnosis in patients older than 65 years old. The health care cost for the diagnostic-related group (DRG) for heart failure at the present time exceeds $39 billion per year in the United States alone. Furthermore, based on the increase in life expectancy over the past three decades, it is predicted that by the year 2035 there will be approximately 70 million subjects in the United States older than 75 years of age, of whom 7 million (10%) will have heart failure. For this reason, heart failure has been targeted as a major health care initiative.

OBJECTIVES OF CARDIAC IMAGING IN HEART FAILURE

There are three major objectives of cardiac imaging. The primary objective of noninvasive and invasive cardiac imaging is to establish the definitive cardiac diagnosis *de novo*, or confirm the clinically suspected diagnosis with minimal risk to the patient. The secondary objective is to acquire reproducible high-quality, high-resolution images that enable accurate quantitative assessment of cardiac chamber size, architecture, and global and regional left ventricular (LV) function. The tertiary objective is to relate metrics of cardiac chamber size and function to early risk stratification and long-term clinical outcome.

The aim of this chapter is to discuss the optimal and appropriate use of the panoply of multimodal cardiovascular imaging techniques that are currently used routinely in patients with heart failure. We do not wish to compare and contrast the individual diagnostic strengths and weaknesses of each of the various imaging modalities in each clinical situation, but rather to describe the most efficacious contemporary use of imaging modalities for a range of specific causes of heart failure. Special attention is given to a number of different pathoetiologies of heart failure that include (1) systolic and diastolic heart failure; (2) valvular heart disease; (3) myocardial infarction, myocardial viability, and ventricular remodeling postinfarction; (4) detection of myocardial fibrosis; (5) selection of patients for device deployment; (6) genetically determined cardiomyopathy (DCM); and (7) right heart failure.

Choosing the cardiovascular imaging modality best suited to resolve the clinical differential diagnoses and to safely guide therapy can be challenging. This is because many of the cardiovascular symptoms in heart failure are nonspecific and correlate poorly with the degree of LV dysfunction.

COST OF IMAGING TESTS

Cardiac imaging is a frequent and costly component of cardiovascular health care. Thus when choosing a cardiovascular imaging modality, it is important to be cognizant of the cost of the desired diagnostic test and the next best alternative if the findings of the preferred test result are ambiguous, and to be fiscally responsible for its appropriate use as recommended by the American College of Cardiology Foundation/American Heart Association (ACCF/AHA) guidelines.[2] Adherence to the ACCF/AHA guidelines for the diagnosis and treatment of heart failure should curtail the inappropriate use of multimodal imaging, and also avoid the practice of defensive medicine that entails requesting multiple confirmatory imaging tests when the diagnosis has already been unequivocally established. The ultimate aim of cardiovascular imaging is to maximize diagnostic accuracy to improve patient care and clinical outcomes cost-effectively using evidence-based medicine to guide the appropriate use of the already limited health care system resources.[5]

HEART FAILURE WITH REDUCED EJECTION FRACTION VERSUS HEART FAILURE WITH PRESERVED EJECTION FRACTION

Between 35% and 50% of all patients with symptoms of heart failure have what was formerly called *diastolic heart failure,* now known as *heart failure with preserved ejection fraction* (HFpEF; see also Chapter 36). Patients with the new onset of heart failure and reduced LV ejection fraction (HFrEF/systolic heart failure) cannot always be reliably distinguished clinically from HFpEF patients. Lateral displacement of the LV apical impulse is the clinical clue to LV dilation that often cannot be appreciated in HFrEF due to an overweight condition, chronic lung disease, or a diffuse less forceful apical impulse. LV dilation can be easily confirmed by chest radiograph or TTE. LV dilation and decreased ejection fraction are crucial for the diagnosis of HFrEF. There is a preponderance of elderly women with systemic hypertension in HFpEF as compared with HFrEF.[6,7] More than two thirds of patients with HFrEF have an ischemic cause for their LV dysfunction (see also Chapter 18).[1] The diagnosis of HFpEF can strictly only be made by the combination of clinical demographics and computational image analysis that provides estimation of ejection fraction and assessment of the severity of LV diastolic dysfunction with TTE. HFpEF only recently has been acknowledged as a discrete pathophysiologic entity, because formerly it was considered to be a benign condition for which there is still no specific treatment. However, studies have demonstrated that HFpEF is a discrete entity with a significant annual morbidity, mortality, and readmission rate for acute exacerbations of heart failure.[8] Doppler echocardiographic imaging easily distinguishes HFpEF from HFrEF because in HFrEF there is obligatory LV dilation to maintain a normal stroke volume as LVEF declines.[9] In contrast, LV cavity size in HFpEF is normal or small and there is usually mild to moderate concentric hypertrophic remodeling (**Figure 29-1, A and B**) induced by concomitant HTN, with preserved LVEF (≥50%).

EVALUATION OF LEFT VENTRICULAR DIASTOLIC DYSFUNCTION

Diastolic dysfunction is the underlying pathophysiologic abnormality that typifies HFpEF.[10] Diastolic LV dysfunction includes abnormal transmitral peak E wave, peak A wave that ranges from delayed relaxation to irreversible restrictive physiology and severely elevated filling pressures (**Figure 29-2**; E/e′); reduced e′ myocardial velocities by tissue Doppler imaging (TDI) in the septum and lateral wall are consistent with delayed relaxation and an enlarged LA.[11,12] In addition, there is consistently abnormal pulmonary venous flow (see Figure 29-2). Diastolic ventricular function can also be assessed with nuclear techniques from ventricular volume curves in terms of LV peak filling rate, time to peak filling rate, and filling fractions. However, there is no single echo, Doppler, or nuclear parameter that is sufficiently robust to diagnose the presence of LV diastolic dysfunction.

The reason for distinguishing HFpEF from HFrEF patients is that they have different LV morphology, epidemiology, mechanisms of heart failure, and systolic and diastolic LV function, all of which are evident by two-dimensional (2-D) and three-dimensional (3-D) transthoracic echocardiographic imaging. Furthermore, patients with HFpEF have an absent or blunted response to traditional heart failure therapy, which includes β-adrenergic receptor blockers, angiotensin-converting enzyme inhibitors, angiotensin receptor blockers, and mineralocorticoid inhibitors.[13-15] Heart size in HFpEF remains stable, although LV hypertrophy may increase and diastolic dysfunction may worsen over time. In contrast, heart size in HFrEF is increased at the time of diagnosis and increases progressively thereafter (**Figure 29-3**). The prognosis of HFpEF is better than in HFrEF, although the rate of hospital readmission is similar for recurrent heart failure.

Echocardiographic changes in LV size, geometry, hypertrophy, and function have been reported prospectively in multiple studies of systolic heart failure/HFrEF for more

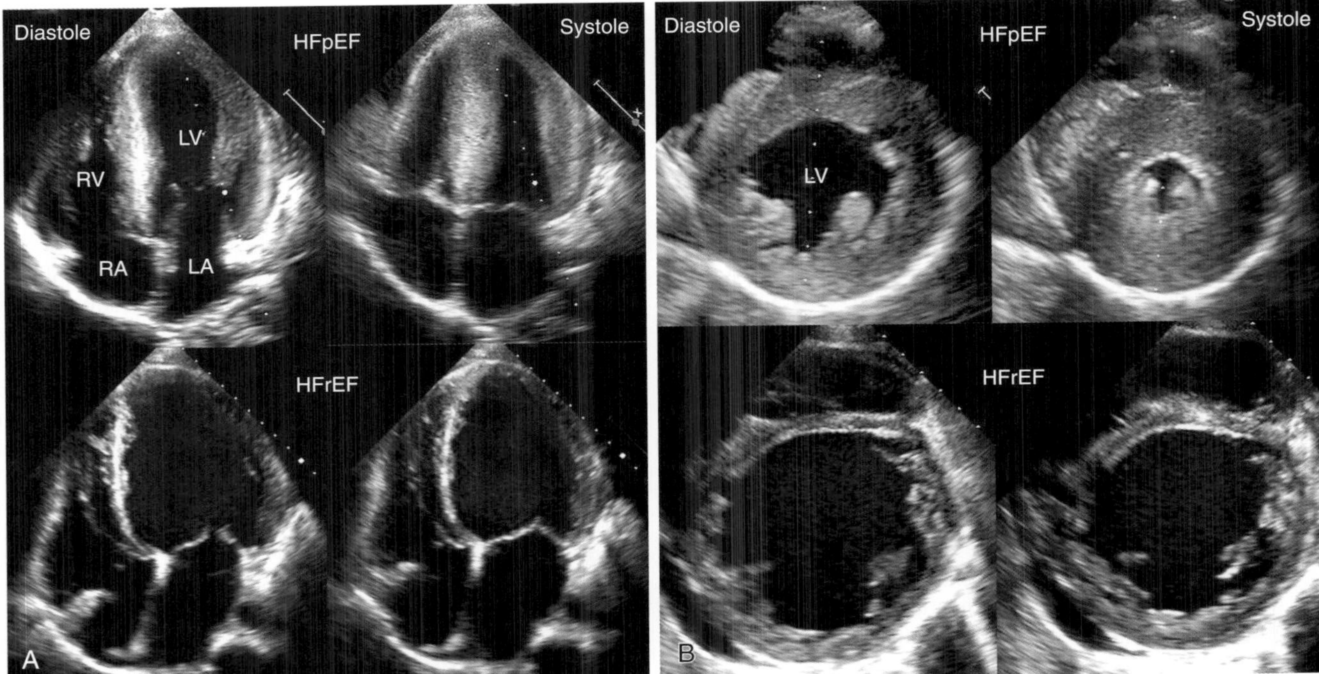

FIGURE 29-1 **A,** Transthoracic echocardiogram (TTE) of the apical four-chamber view at end-diastole *(top left)* and end-systole *(top right)* from a patient with HFpEF showing normal left ventricular (LV) cavity size and with an ejection fraction of 53%, moderate concentric LV hypertrophy, and an enlarged left atrium. The apical four-chamber view from a patient with HFrEF is seen at end-diastole *(bottom left)* and at end-systole *(bottom right).* In contrast to the patient in the top panels, the patient with HFrEF has a markedly enlarged LV with severely decreased function (EF of 20%), a distal septal scar from a remote myocardial infarction indicating an ischemic cause for the LV dysfunction, and an enlarged left atrium. **B,** TTE of the same two patients above showing images of the LV short-axis views at the level of the tips of the mitral valve leaflets at end-diastole *(top left)* and at end-systole *(top right)* with HFpEF *(top panels)* with marked concentric hypertrophy. The HFrEF patient shown at end-diastole *(bottom left)* and at end-systole *(bottom right)* has a much larger LV with poor function (EF 20%) and thinning of the septum.

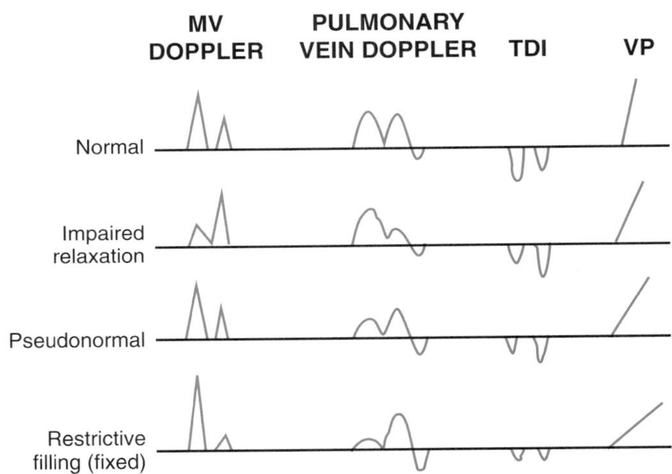

FIGURE 29-2 Doppler assessment of diastolic function: HFpEF is primarily a disorder of left ventricular diastolic function ranging from impaired myocardial relaxation to fixed restrictive filling manifested by abnormal transmitral blood flow velocities, pulmonary vein flow, tissue Doppler imaging, and a progressive decrease in propagation velocity. *MV,* Mitral valve; *TDI,* tissue Doppler imaging; *VP,* velocity of propagation.

than three decades. By comparison there is a paucity of Doppler echocardiographic information on HFpEF available for assessment of diastolic LV function over time, except for studies from the Framingham database.[7,16]

MULTIPLE MODALITY CARDIAC IMAGING

Cardiac diagnostic imaging techniques are used routinely in heart failure and range from simple assessment of overall heart size, cardiac silhouette, and the presence of pulmonary congestion by chest radiograph to real time 3-D Doppler echocardiographic reconstruction of the heart and great vessels, or cardiac magnetic resonance (CMR) perfusion showing delayed gadolinium enhancement due to myocardial fibrosis. Although computed tomography (CT) provides spectacular high-resolution cardiac imaging, the doses of ionizing radiation and of iodinated contrast agents precludes serial studies that are required in patients with heart failure undergoing LV remodeling.

Chest radiograph is obtained in all heart failure patients for detection of cardiomegaly, individual chamber and great vessel enlargement, pulmonary venous congestion, pericardial and pleural effusions that are frequent accompaniments of decompensated heart failure. Even minor hemodynamically irrelevant pericardial effusions in heart failure are associated with increased risk of cardiac mortality.[17]

Echocardiography is the imaging modality of choice in all causes of heart failure because it is portable, safe, and provides accurate quantitative information at the bedside that includes LV volumes, chamber architecture, regional and global systolic and diastolic function, valve function, and pulmonary artery systolic pressure, all of which correlate with clinical endpoints. In addition, Doppler measures of intracardiac blood flow velocities and myocardial velocities permit calculation of myocardial strain and torsion/rotation that enable complete assessment of global and regional myocardial mechanics. A great advantage of 2-D and 3-D echocardiography is that the information regarding myocardial mechanics is immediately available at the bedside, and furthermore it can be repeated without any negative impact on patient safety. However, misgivings

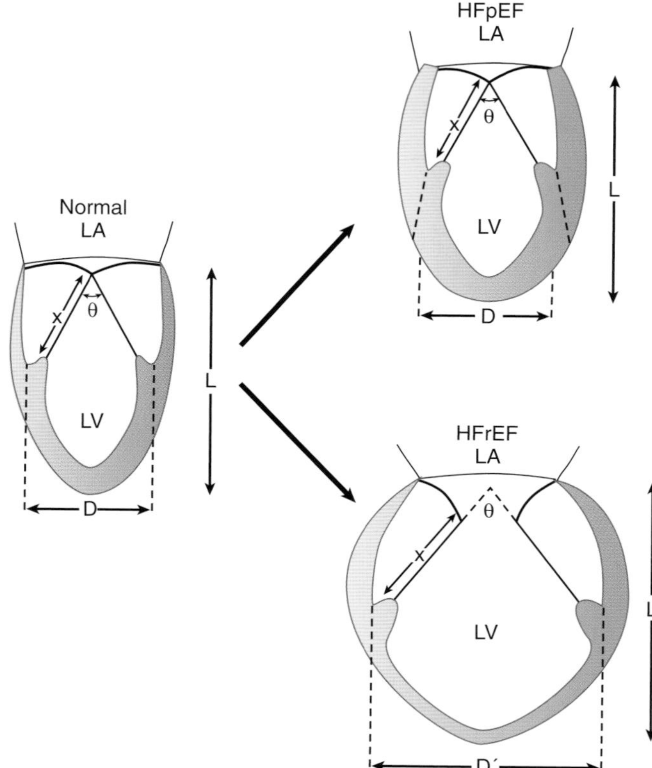

FIGURE 29-3 Remodeling-associated left ventricular (LV) geometry changes: Schema showing the cavity geometry in the normal heart *(left)*, a heart of a patient with HFpEF *(top right)* showing normal LV cavity dimensions and moderate LV hypertrophy consistent with concentric remodeling. The heart in the bottom right panel represents a heart with HFrEF that is typified by severe cavity dilation, distorted LV geometry, separation of the papillary muscles with an increase in the angle "ø" causing mal-coaptation of the mitral valve leaflets and mitral regurgitation.

have been expressed recently regarding the use of 2-D echocardiography to assess LV volumes, ejection fraction, and LV mass in serial studies because of the poor test and retest reproducibility and the magnitude of the standard deviations derived from a meta-analysis that involved a large number of studies.[18] However, these findings are discordant with a number of recent studies in which serial echoes were performed and consistently demonstrated important reproducible changes in LV size, mass, and function following intervention.[19-21]

Assessment of Left Ventricular Function by Echocardiography

M-mode echocardiography has been used for measurements of LV size, LV mass, LV loading conditions (end-systolic meridional and circumferential wall stress), and myocardial function (fractional and midwall shortening and velocity of circumferential fiber shortening peak Vcf). However, M-mode echo assessments of LV function are limited because it is assumed that there is uniform wall thickness and normal concentric wall motion. The majority (68%) of patients with HFrEF have coronary artery disease (CAD) and ischemic cardiomyopathy,[1] in which the hallmarks of CAD are LV wall motion abnormalities and variation in LV wall thickness. Thus M-mode echo measurements of LV size and function are not admissible in over two thirds of the HFrEF population. LV linear dimensions are still used in randomized clinical trials in hypertension that require serial measurements with or without an intervention as the primary outcome measure.

Two-dimensional Doppler echocardiography is the most frequently used and clinically most important diagnostic imaging modality in HFrEF and in HFpEF.[22] LV end-systolic, end-diastolic, and stroke volumes can be calculated from biplane orthogonal images of the left ventricle in the apical four-chamber and the apical two-chamber planes using the Simpson method of discs.[23] LV mass can also be estimated from measurements of end-diastolic wall thickness, LV cavity diameter/2, and LV length (5/6 short-axis area × length). The important fundamental relation between LV volume and mass can be examined. Estimates of LV volumes, LV mass, and ejection fraction by 2-D echo provide insight into the structural, geometric, and functional changes in the left ventricle as the heart remodels and the severity of heart failure progresses. Two-dimensional Doppler echocardiography has played a major role in elucidating our current understanding of the different natural histories and causative mechanisms involved in HFpEF and HFrEF.

In addition to TTE determination of LV volumes, mass (left ventricular hypertrophy [LVH] as increased relative wall thickness), LV shape, and ejection fraction have proved to be powerful predictors of clinical outcome in patients with heart failure.[24,25] LV stroke volume can be calculated from LV volumes (EDV − ESV = SV) by 2-D and 3-D TTE and also by Doppler measurement of intracardiac blood flow velocities in the LV outflow tract (LVOT). Blood volume flow in unit time can be assessed as the product of the time velocity integral (TVI) and the cross-sectional area (CSA) of the flow stream (TVI × CSA). When recorded from the LVOT, stroke volume correlates closely with stroke volume estimated from LV volumes. Recently, the LVOT has been shown to be elliptical rather than circular by transesophageal echocardiography (TEE), CMR, and CT, especially in the presence of LVH that protrudes into the LVOT in patients with hemodynamically important aortic stenosis and severe systemic hypertension. The influence of an abnormal LVOT cross-sectional shape can be minimized by planimetering the cross-section directly.[26]

Myocardial Strain and Strain Rate

Measurement of myocardial strain is a relatively new concept that describes global and regional ventricular systolic function using speckle-tracking echocardiography or magnetic resonance with myocardial tagging. Speckle tracking echocardiography depends upon the temporal and spatial tracking of naturally occurring intramyocardial reflectors of ultrasound (speckles) within the 2-D echocardiographic images of the LV walls. Displacement of these speckles is due to myocardial deformation[27] from which the myocardial strain is calculated. *Strain* is defined as the change in myocardial segment length (ΔL) divided by resting segment length (L_0): $S = \Delta L/L_0$. The insonating beam is directed parallel to the LV long axis. Myocardial strain is assessed in three planes—longitudinal, circumferential, and radial.

Longitudinal strain is calculated from the LV long-axis and radial and circumferential strains from LV short-axis images obtained at the LV midcavity level (**Figure 29-4**). Estimates of myocardial strains by speckle-tracking

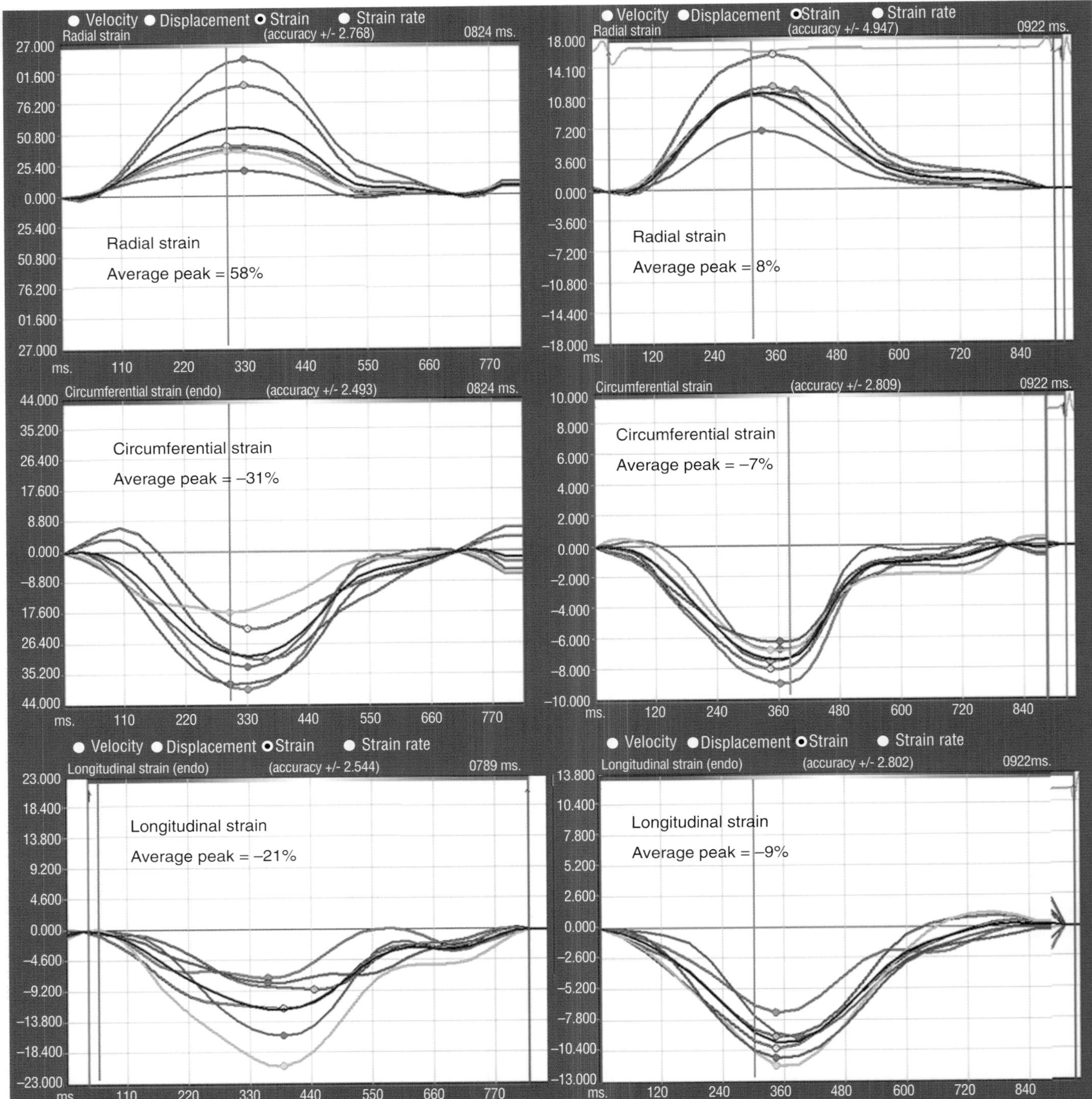

FIGURE 29-4 Left ventricular (LV) strain—normal versus cardiomyopathy: This six-panel figure shows radial strain in a normal subject with an average peak value of 58% *(top left)* and severely reduced average peak radial strain of 8% in a heart failure patient (*top right,* note difference in scale). Of note, there was no evidence for LV dyssynchrony in either subject or patient. In the middle and lower panels average peak circumferential strain and average peak longitudinal strain are shown with the normal in the left panels and the heart failure patient in the right panels. Note the major reduction in the average peak radial, circumferential, and longitudinal strains in heart failure without evidence for dyssynchrony.

echocardiography have been validated in humans by CMR with myocardial tagging and in animals by sonomicrometry.[27] Global systolic strains can be assessed in addition to simultaneous assessment of myocardial strains in each segment using the 16 or 17 segment model of the left ventricle. Myocardial strains can be recorded simultaneously from the interventricular septum and from the lateral LV wall in each of three myocardial segments (apical, mid, and proximal) from the apical four-chamber, two-chamber, and long-axis views (see Figure 29-4). Strain analysis can be quantified after acquisition of the echo images. Measurement of the time period from onset of QRS to peak strain for each myocardial segment provides insight as to the coordination of contraction and the degree of dyssynchrony. Strain can detect mild perturbations in LV function before any change is detectable in LV volumes or ejection fraction. Strain rate is the rate of change of strain, which has not always proved as robust or reproducible as measurement of deformation because of a number of confounding factors.

Three-dimensional echocardiography: Numerous studies have demonstrated the correlations between LV volumes, mass, and ejection fraction estimated by 2-D echocardiography and CMR. Still closer correlations have been demonstrated between real-time 3-D echocardiography and CMR with less variability about the mean.[28]

Real-time 3-D echocardiographic assessment of LV volumes, mass, and LVEF (**Figure 29-5**) correlates more closely to CMR than 2-D echo, with less variability than with 2-D.[29] However, the greater precision of measurement of LV mass and ejection fraction by CMR is the reason that CMR has become the standard of reference for quantification of LV mass and LV volumes.

A proportion of echocardiograms in heart failure patients is technically limited because endocardial definition is incomplete, resulting in poor image quality necessitating interpolation of extensive regions of the LV endocardium. This occurs especially in patients with emphysema or morbid obesity that may even preclude quantitative analysis. However, endocardial definition is improved with harmonic imaging and can be further enhanced with intravenous echo contrast so that a proportion of poor quality studies can be recovered for quantitative analysis.

Transesophageal echocardiography: When image quality is poor, switching to TEE or to an alternative imaging modality such as CMR for better image quality may be a better strategy. However, there is a tradeoff for the exquisite image quality attained by TEE, and that is that quantitation of LV volumes from biplane TEE images consistently underestimates volumes calculated by TTE. This occurs because of unavoidable foreshortening of the LV long axis in the apical imaging planes with TEE. This foreshortening results in underestimation of LV volumes, ejection fraction, and longitudinal strain.

TEE is not indicated in the routine assessment of patients with heart failure, except in special circumstances that include poor image quality, suspected vegetative endocarditis, and assessment of MR due to papillary muscle infarction and occasionally to measure left atrial size.

An additional important role performed by 2-D echocardiography is detection of LV cavity thrombus (**Figure 29-6**) adherent to severely hypokinetic or akinetic myocardial segments. Thrombus formation also occurs in the left atrial cavity and/or appendage, especially in patients with left atrial enlargement and atrial fibrillation. In patients with unexplained worsening symptoms, 2-D echocardiograms should be performed to rule out significant pericardial effusion, pleural effusion, or the onset of atrial fibrillation that is a common dysrhythmia in heart failure.

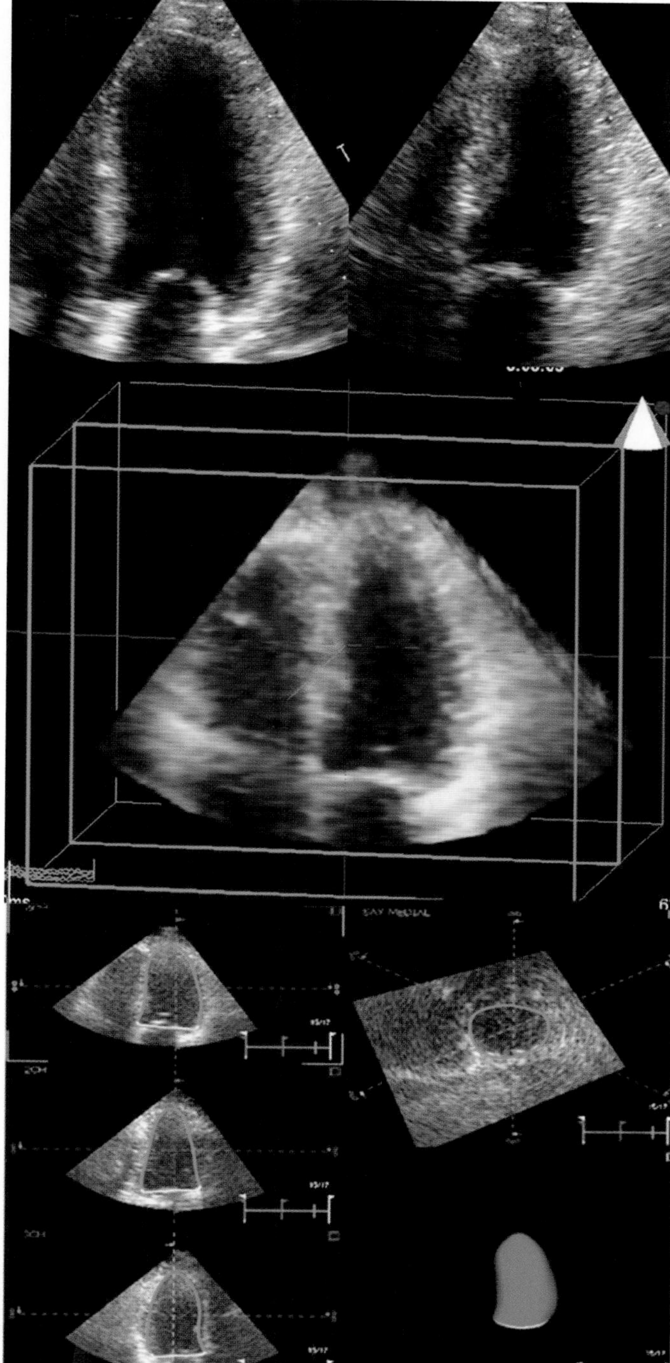

FIGURE 29-5 Three-dimensional (3-D) echocardiography: 3-D echocardiogram showing acquisition and processing of apical images of the LV from a normal subject. These 3-D echocardiograms allow for quantification of LV volumes and LV mass that compare favorably with those calculated from cardiac magnetic resonance (CMR) images. CMR has become the reference standard for quantitative analysis of LV geometry and function.

Radionuclide Single Photon Emission Computed Tomography and Positron Emission Tomography

Radionuclide and positron emission tomography (PET) provide unique information regarding ventricular volumes and function, myocardial perfusion, viability of noncontracting, hibernating myocardium and the likely benefit of revascularization and restoration of coronary flow by surgical or percutaneous interventions.

Radiotracer imaging: Single photon emission computed tomography (SPECT) and PET imaging have become standard approaches for quantitative physiologic imaging in patients with heart failure. Radiotracer techniques have been used to evaluate regional and global ventricular function and to detect myocardial ischemia, hibernation, infarction, and ventricular remodeling. Nuclear imaging techniques are also well suited for in vivo molecular imaging because of their high sensitivity, spatial resolution, and availability of new hybrid instrumentation and molecular

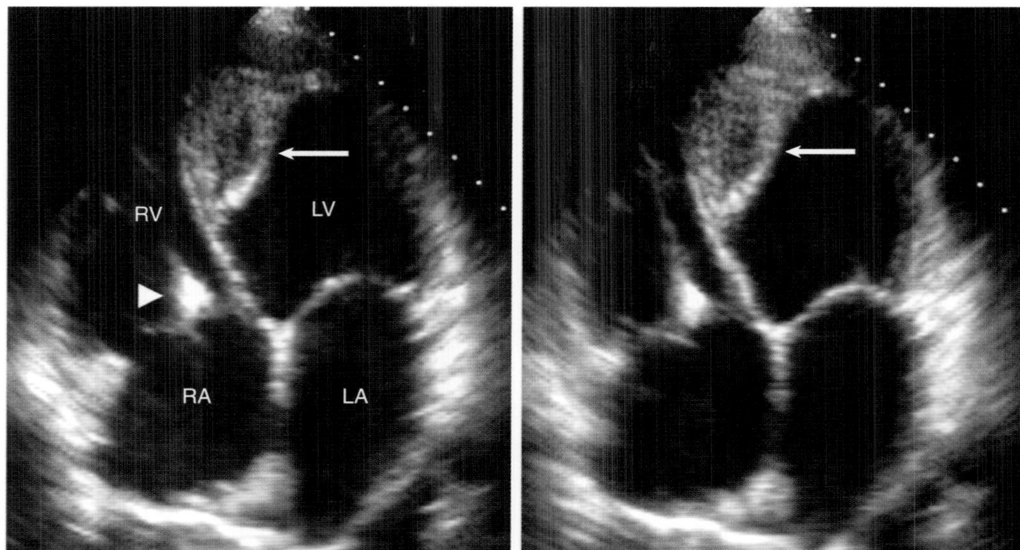

FIGURE 29-6 Left ventricular (LV) dysfunction with an apical thrombus: transthoracic echocardiogram showing an apical four-chamber view at end-diastole *(left)* and at end-systole *(right)* in a 60-year-old female who became acutely short of breath 2 weeks ago with easy fatigue, who previously walked to work 5 days per week. She did not seek medical help until she sustained a near syncopal episode. The LV is enlarged and there is severe hypokinesis of the mid-septum to the apex of the LV with a large adherent thrombus attached to the distal septum with liquefaction necrosis at the center *(arrows)*.

targeted probes.[30] Molecular imaging offers a novel approach for detecting molecular or cellular changes in vivo before development of any physiologic or anatomic changes. Recently dedicated hybrid imaging systems combining nuclear detector systems with high-resolution structural imaging modalities, such as x-ray computed tomography or magnetic resonance imaging, have been introduced into routine clinical practice. These hybrid systems provide important complementary anatomic, functional, and molecular information.

Assessment of right and left ventricular volumes and function: There are several radionuclide approaches to the assessment and management of patients with heart failure. The traditional radiotracer approaches included first-pass radionuclide angiocardiography and equilibrium radionuclide angiocardiography (ERNA) that employ imaging of ^{99m}Tc labeled red blood cells. The first-pass technique permits assessment of global right and left ventricular size and function, but is inadequate for evaluation of regional LV function, because only a single projection of the ventricle is obtained. To assess RV and LV functional reserve by the first-pass technique, separate injections of the radiotracer are made at rest and during peak exercise. The first-pass technique has been replaced by ERNA, which in turn has been superseded by gated SPECT blood pool angiography[31] and gated SPECT perfusion imaging.[32] Analysis of temporal changes in count density from four-dimensional (4-D) SPECT images provides an index of regional LV wall thickening.[33] New 3-D radiotracer-based imaging approaches offer a more comprehensive evaluation of regional and global LV function.[34] Serial equilibrium blood pool imaging can be performed at rest and during various levels of exercise or after pharmacologic perturbations to evaluate ventricular functional reserve. Gated SPECT perfusion imaging is primarily restricted to evaluation of resting function.

LV end-diastolic and end-systolic volumes can be evaluated serially using nuclear approaches in patients with heart failure and can be used to track LV remodeling and monitor therapy. Volumes from gated blood pool images are calculated based on radiotracer count density and are therefore relatively independent of alterations in regional geometry. Simple count-based techniques allow volume measurements to be made without the confounding technical issues of accurate measurement of attenuation.[35,36] These estimates of volumes can be improved by applying 3-D imaging techniques.

Assessment of diastolic function is also important in the evaluation of HFpEF and HFrEF in elderly patients with hypertension and/or CAD. Diastolic parameters such as filling rate, time to peak filling, and filling fractions can be readily assessed from the ventricular volume curve.[37] Such measurements should be routine in the assessment of heart failure in the presence of CAD.

Imaging autonomic dysfunction: Cardiac autonomic dysfunction is known to influence the risk of ventricular arrhythmia and sudden cardiac death in heart failure (see also Chapter 12). Alterations in presynaptic and postsynaptic cardiac sympathetic function can be assessed noninvasively using both SPECT and PET radiotracers.[38-40] The most widely used SPECT radiotracer for imaging of presynaptic function is ^{123}I-meta-iodobenzylguanidine (^{123}I-MIBG), which shares many cellular uptake and storage properties with norepinephrine. Many studies have demonstrated the clinical value of ^{123}I-MIBG imaging for both diagnostic and prognostic purposes in patients with heart failure. In patients with heart failure, ^{123}I-MIBG scans typically show a reduced heart-to-mediastinal uptake ratio (HMR), heterogeneous distribution within the myocardium, and increased ^{123}I-MIBG washout from the heart. HMR is a marker of specific sympathetic nerve terminal tracer retention and has prognostic value in heart failure.[41] The washout ratio of ^{123}I-MIBG predicts sudden cardiac death, independent of LVEF.[42] A large prospective study of ^{123}I-MIBG imaging demonstrated a significant relationship between the heart failure–related events and the HMR that was independent of LVEF and BNP.[43] This clinical study also showed an association between myocardial sympathetic neuronal dysfunction and risk for subsequent cardiac death. Moreover, the size

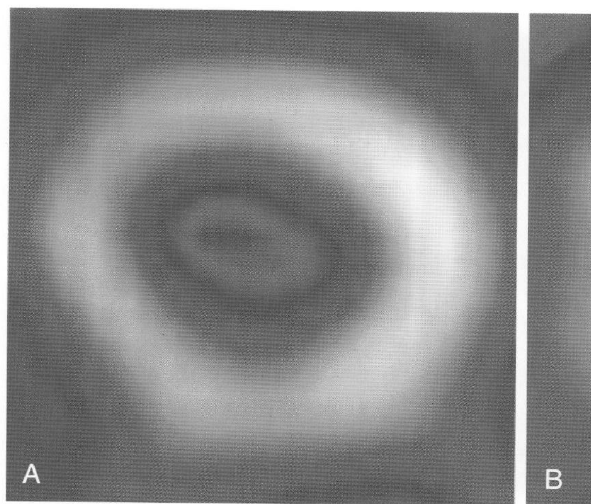

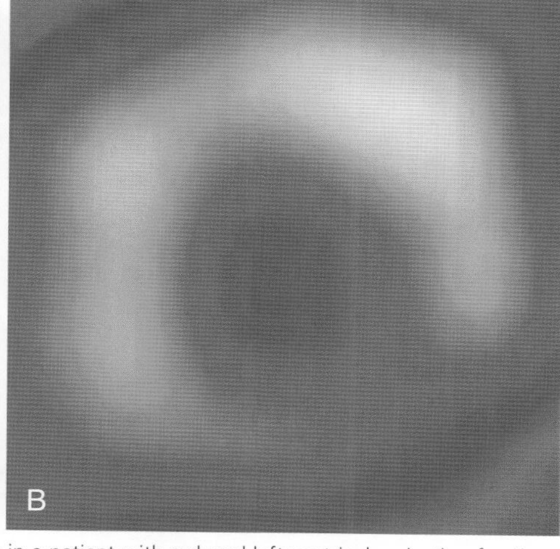

FIGURE 29-7 Resting myocardial perfusion and late ^{123}I MIBG myocardial imaging in a patient with reduced left ventricular ejection fraction: The patient demonstrates normal resting myocardial perfusion **(A)**, but abnormal regional ^{123}I meta-iodobenzylguanidine (^{123}I-MIBG) imaging **(B)**. A correlation has been demonstrated between the size of the ^{123}I-MIBG defect and the risk of ventricular arrhythmias. This relatively large area of abnormal sympathetic function accurately predicted this patient's appropriate implantable cardioverter-defibrillator therapy (antitachycardia pacing) after 18 months of follow-up. *Modified from Boogers MJ, Borleffs CJ, Henneman MM, et al: Cardiac sympathetic denervation assessed with 123-iodine metaiodobenzylguanidine imaging predicts ventricular arrhythmias in implantable cardioverter-defibrillator patients. J Am Coll Cardiol 55:2769–2777, 2010.*

of the MIBG defect on delayed SPECT imaging also predicts ventricular arrhythmias (**Figure 29-7**).

Presympathetic function can also be assessed by PET imaging with ^{11}C-meta-hydroxyephedrine (^{11}C-HED).[44] In nontransmural myocardial infarctions, the HED imaging defect can exceed perfusion defect, but it is not clear whether this is associated with higher ventricular arrhythmia risk. In patients with nonischemic cardiomyopathy, there is decreased HED uptake, and in a recent retrospective study, global HED uptake was an independent predictor of adverse outcomes in patients with New York Heart Association (NYHA) class II and III heart failure (**Figure 29-8**).[45] This PET sympathetic imaging approach is under evaluation in patients with CAD and depressed left ventricular function. A recently completed single-site prospective clinical study (PAREPET) showed that quantitative ^{11}C-HED PET imaging was one of the best predictors of sudden cardiac death (SCD).[46]

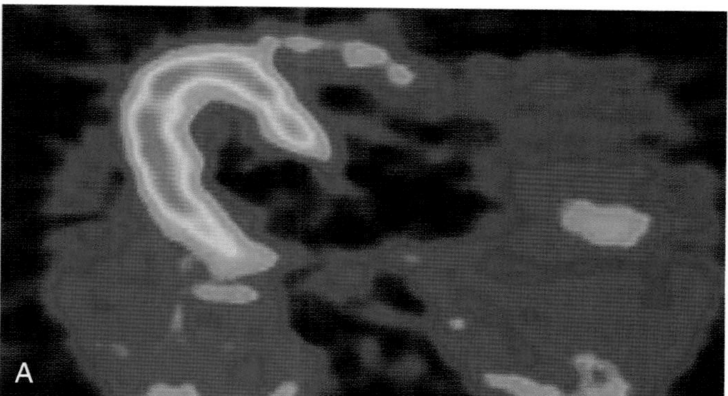

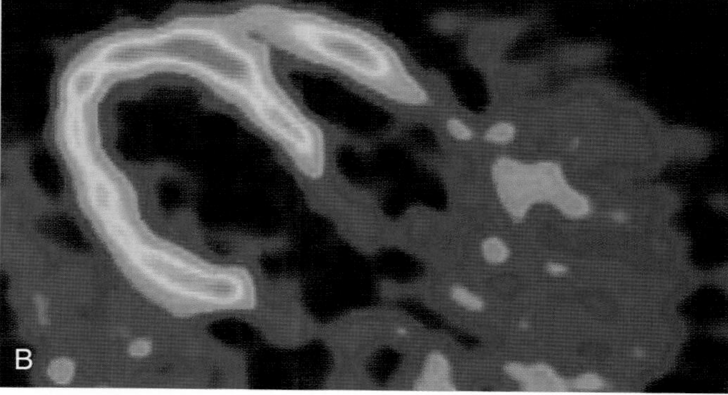

FIGURE 29-8 Myocardial ^{11}C-meta-hydroxyephedrine (^{11}C-HED) uptake in a healthy subject and a heart failure patient: The healthy subject **(A)** shows normal ^{11}C HED uptake, whereas the patient with dilated cardiomyopathy **(B)** demonstrates reduced ^{11}C HED uptake on quantitative evaluation. *Modified Pietila M, Malminiemi K, Ukkonen H, et al: Reduced myocardial carbon-11 hydroxyephedrine retention is associated with poor prognosis in chronic heart failure. Eur J Nucl Med 28:373–376, 2001.*

Computed Tomography

CT and CMR imaging both produce exquisite image quality with and without contrast enhancement and allow comprehensive quantitative assessment of LV and RV architecture and function, as well as delineation of the coronary artery anatomy. The disadvantage of CT is the exposure to both ionizing radiation and iodinated contrast agents. Recently, attempts have been made to minimize radiation exposure during CT and have had a modicum of success. However, serial evaluations of cardiac chamber volumes, mass, and function with CT, which are necessary in heart failure, are not recommended.

Cardiac Magnetic Resonance Imaging

The acquisition of such high-fidelity image quality is the reason that CMR has become the standard of reference for quantification of LV volumes, LVEF, and LV mass (**Figure 29-9A**). The accuracy and reproducibility of CMR makes it the ideal tool for serial assessment of ventricular size and function, and at the same time reduces the sample sizes necessary in clinical trials.[47,48] However, a substantial proportion of heart failure patients have implantable cardioverter-defibrillators (ICDs), permanent pacemakers, and there is an increasing number of cardiac resynchronization therapy (CRT) device implants in which CMR imaging is currently contraindicated. The numerical data generated

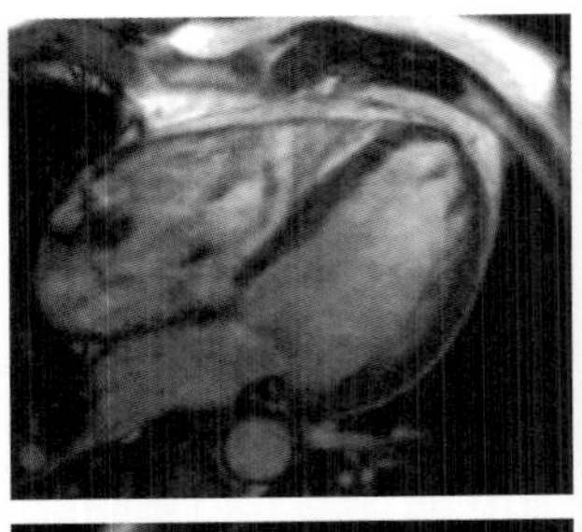
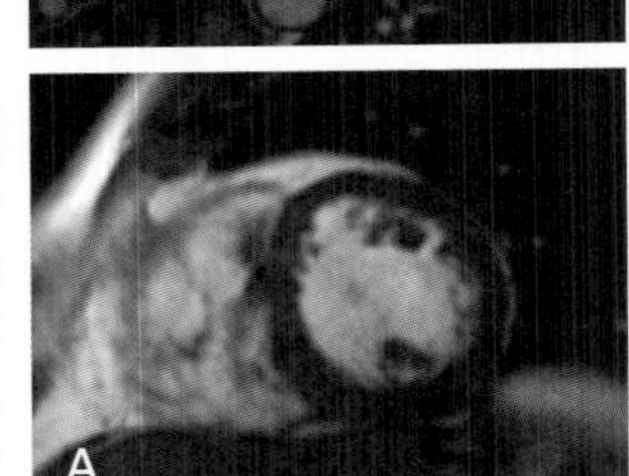

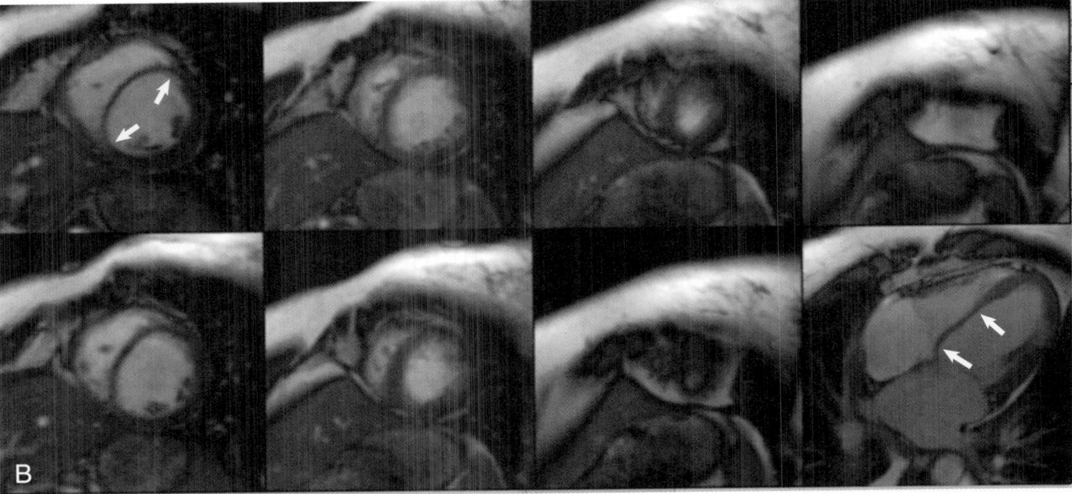

FIGURE 29-9 Short-axis and long-axis cardiac magnetic resonance images: Normal vs. heart failure: Representative single-slice short axis and four-chamber CMR images are shown in **(A)**. Note the excellent soft tissue contrast and depiction of intracardiac versus extracardiac structures. **B,** A series of end-diastolic short-axis images from base to apex is shown in a chronic heart failure patient following remote giant cell myocarditis, as well as a four-chamber view *(lower right)*. The more basal short-axis slices show thinning of the septum *(arrows)* from the base to the midventricle, which is confirmed by the four-chamber image *(lower right, arrows)*. Note detailed depiction of the right and left ventricular anatomy.

in healthy normal subjects and in acute and chronic heart failure by CMR are commonly used to risk stratify patients with heart failure. Serial imaging of the heart in patients with heart failure is frequently used to assess the rate of disease progression and the response to pharmacologic agents, devices, and surgical and cellular therapies. Serial evaluation of large patient cohorts has also been used to assess the efficacy of novel pharmacologic agents and device therapies for heart failure in large randomized clinical trials. Gadolinium-containing CMR contrast agents have been used safely in many millions of patients. A rare disorder known as *nephrogenic sclerosing fibrosis* was reported as a possible side effect following high-dose contrast use in patients with severe renal impairment (glomerular filtration rate <30 mL/min). The use of a cyclic chelate-based gadolinium agent has almost completely eliminated this problem. These agents continue to be used with caution in patients with renal failure because of the greater risks of iodinated contrast agents.

CMR avoids errors imposed by geometric assumptions during acquisition of 3-D stacked sets of contiguous cine slices, usually in the short-axis plane (see Figure 29-9B). End-diastolic and end-systolic volumes and mass for both ventricles are determined by planimetry of each slice and then summed for the entire ventricle. Measures of ventricular performance, including stroke volume, ejection fraction (EF), and cardiac output, may be accurately quantified using this methodology. Similarly, calculation of abnormal hemodynamic states resulting from coronary artery, valvular, and congenital heart disease, which cause left-sided or right-sided heart failure, may be performed routinely. The high quality of the data allows indexation to important variables such as body surface area, gender, and age. These data demonstrate that indexation is important for confident diagnosis of conditions in their early stages, for example, dilated or hypertrophic cardiomyopathy.[49] LV diastolic function can also be assessed by CMR. However, echocardiography is used routinely, is readily available, and has been the preferred imaging modality of choice in large randomized clinical trials.

VALVULAR HEART DISEASE AS A REMEDIAL CAUSE OF HEART FAILURE (see also Chapter 24)

Mitral Valve Regurgitation

Mitral regurgitation (MR) is more frequently associated with chronic HFrEF than with HFpEF, occurring in approximately 50% of patients, ranging in severity from mild to severe. MR is readily detected by Doppler because color flow velocity mapping is exquisitely sensitive even to trivial MR. The underlying mechanism of MR in HFrEF can be appreciated by 2-D and 3-D TTE imaging that demonstrates distortion of the geometry of the mitral subvalve apparatus and stretching of the mitral annulus, preventing adequate coaptation of the mitral valve leaflets caused by progressive LV cavity enlargement that results in MR (Figures 29-3 and **29-10**). Compared with HFrEF that undergoes eccentric remodeling, LV cavity size in HFpEF is not prone to dilation but instead undergoes concentric hypertrophic remodeling that only rarely results in severe MR.

Evaluation of the presence and severity of MR in heart failure is hemodynamically important because the excessive volume handling from MR increases LV loading conditions, causing further deterioration in LV function as predicted by the inverse relationship between load and ejection phase indices. This shows[50] that the greater the increase in LV load, the greater the reduction in LVEF. The corollary of this relationship provides the rationale for the chronic use of vasodilator therapy to reduce load and improve refractory heart failure. Another cause of MR that is also more frequent in HFrEF than HFpEF is due to recurrent episodes of myocardial ischemia triggered by worsening of regional myocardial blood flow that may cause severe sudden onset MR and flash pulmonary edema/acute heart failure. This can be documented by stress echo, radionuclide stress, or CMR perfusion studies.

The clinical question that often needs resolution when HFrEF and MR coexist is whether MR is the primary cause of the heart failure or whether the heart failure is the cause of the secondary MR. Since the majority of HFrEF cases has

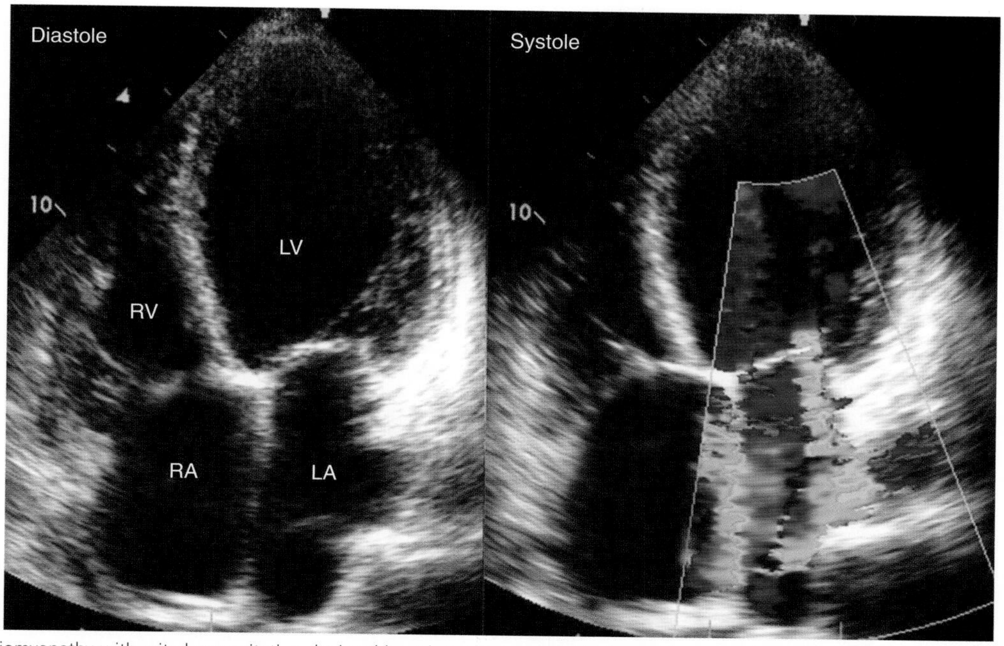

Diastole
10
LV
RV
RA
LA
Systole
10

FIGURE 29-10 Cardiomyopathy with mitral regurgitation depicted by echocardiography: A 2-D transthoracic echocardiogram in the apical four-chamber view from a patient with HFrEF at end-diastole *(left)* and in systole with color flow Doppler *(right)* shows moderately severe left ventricular enlargement and poor function *(left)*. In the right panel, color flow Doppler demonstrates two mitral regurgitant jets and moderately severe mitral regurgitation jet with proximal isovelocity surface area.

an ischemic cause, the development of MR is the result of postinfarction remodeling. When the MR is moderate to severe following remote myocardial infarction and the mitral valve leaflets and mitral annulus are intrinsically normal, it is more likely that the MR is secondary because of alteration of LV architecture by cavity dilation and remodeling that causes failure of the normal coaptation of the mitral leaflets in heart failure. In contrast, when the mitral valve leaflets are rheumatically thickened with commissural fusion or when the leaflets are myxomatous and degenerative, it is more than likely that the MR is primary and the heart failure is secondary to hemodynamically significant MR. The mitral valve can be imaged in exquisite detail by TTE and TEE such that there is little doubt as to its normality or abnormality. In a small minority of patients, it is not possible to determine which is the primary event. However, care should be taken to inspect the mitral valve leaflets, commissures, and subvalve tensor apparatus for undisclosed ruptured chordae tendineae from excessive traction. The hemodynamic severity of MR should be quantified noninvasively using proximal isovelocity surface area (PISA) and not by visual estimation alone.

When mitral regurgitation is severe, it may spuriously increase LVEF, causing delay in urgently needed surgical mitral valve repair or replacement. The presence of even trivial mitral regurgitation can be demonstrated by Doppler color flow velocity mapping. However, color flow mapping describes velocity distribution and not regurgitant volume flow. The severity of MR should be quantified by PISA, which relies upon the principle that blood flow velocity increases as it approaches a restrictive orifice, forming a series of hemispheric isovelocity shells. The finite orifice is the mitral regurgitant orifice, with the velocity shells forming on the ventricular side of the regurgitant orifice. The conservation of mass dictates that the flow rates at each of the hemispherical isovelocity shells are equal to the flow rates at the mitral regurgitant orifice. The flow rate can be calculated as the surface area of a hemisphere $2\pi r^2 \times$ aliasing velocity, where r = the radius of the hemisphere, which is the only Doppler parameter that needs to be measured. The severity of mitral regurgitation can be evaluated comprehensively by a number of echo parameters derived from PISA. These include the effective regurgitant orifice area = flow rate/peak mitral regurgitant jet velocity. The regurgitant volume = effective mitral regurgitant orifice area × the time velocity integral (TVI) of the mitral regurgitant jet. The regurgitant fraction = regurgitant volume/stroke volume.

Aortic Valve Disease as a Cause of Heart Failure

Aortic stenosis: Subjects with congenital aortic stenosis present in their late teens to early twenties with chest pain, syncope, or symptoms of heart failure for valvuloplasty or open-chest valve replacement. Adult-onset/acquired severe "senile" calcific aortic stenosis occurs from the sixth to ninth decades. Bicuspid valves require surgical intervention for valve replacement on average a decade earlier than stenotic trileaflet aortic valves. TTE is the diagnostic imaging modality of choice for aortic valve stenosis and enables precise assessment of the severity of aortic stenosis (AS) in terms of the aortic valve effective orifice area, and the peak and mean transaortic valve gradients and LV ejection fraction (**Figure 29-11**). A proportion of adults with severe or critical AS develop heart failure that is associated with a poor prognosis. If critical AS is not recognized and the left ventricle is allowed to dilate, the transaortic gradient falls as LV function deteriorates so that the aortic valve orifice area must be calculated by 2-D or 3-D echo. There is a growing appreciation for a proportion of symptomatic patients with severe AS, who have low transvalvular gradients as a result of LV systolic dysfunction and a low LV ejection fraction, known as low-flow AS.[51] It is important to identify these elderly

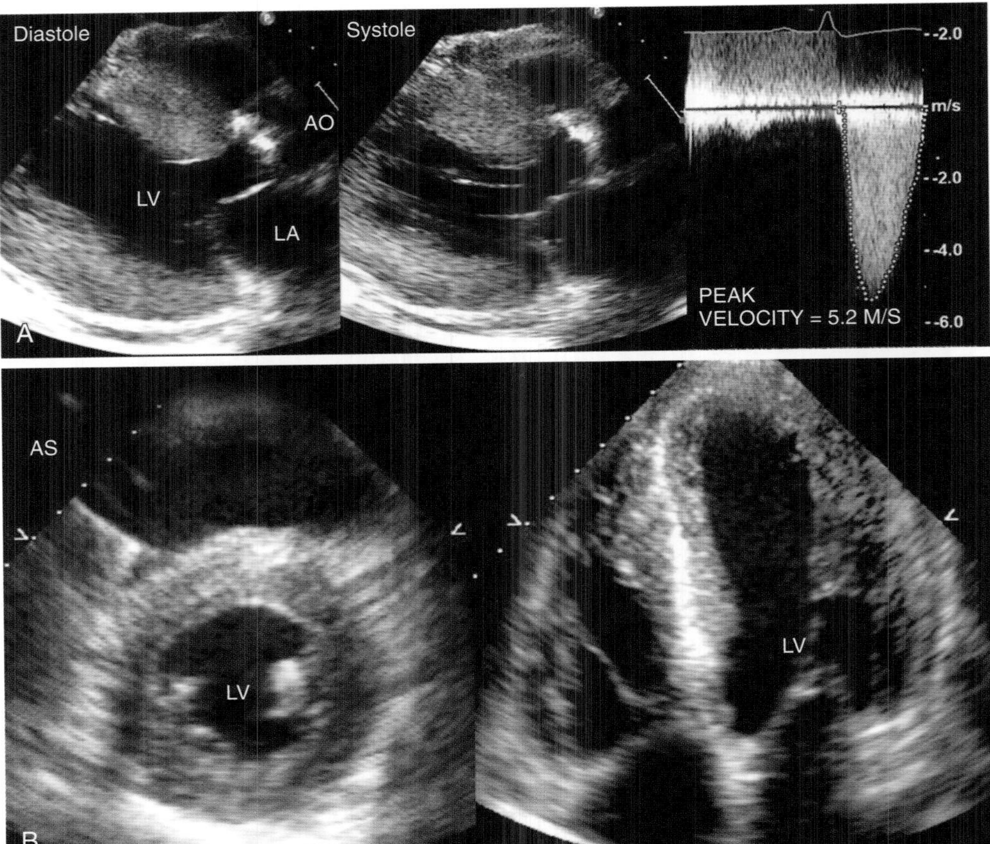

FIGURE 29-11 **A,** Aortic stenosis: Two-dimensional and Doppler evaluation: A left parasternal transthoracic echocardiogram (TTE) in an octogenarian with heart failure symptoms due to previously undiagnosed critical aortic stenosis showing top normal left ventricular (LV) size with severe LV hypertrophy *(left* and *middle)* and a heavily calcified immobile aortic valve with a transaortic peak systolic valve gradient of >100 mm Hg *(right)* by continuous-wave Doppler. The aortic valve area was 0.7 cm^2. **B,** LV remodeling in aortic stenosis: A TTE from a patient in the seventh decade with normal LV dimensions but with at least moderate concentric LV hypertrophy shown in the LV short-axis view *(left)* and the apical four-chamber view *(right)* with typical concentric remodeling.

patients because they do well clinically with transcutaneous intervention. Hemodynamically chronic decompensated calcific aortic stenosis is associated with LV dilation, and decreased LVEF must be differentiated from idiopathic dilated cardiomyopathy with concomitant age-related calcification of the aortic valve. This can be achieved with 2-D Doppler echo of the apical long-axis and the apical five-chamber view (see Figure 29-11). Two-dimensional, three-dimensional, or TEE are the imaging modalities of choice for diagnosis and quantification of the severity of AS. Bicuspid aortic valves (BAV) are associated with ascending aortic aneurysm formation, which is independent of the hydraulics across the aortic valve.[52,53] The extent and severity of the aortopathy should ideally be assessed by either CTA or CMR with contrast, and if the maximal dimension distal to the sinuses of Valsalva at the sinotubular junction is greater than 4.5 cm, surgical repair or endovascular stenting should be considered. The anatomy of the commissures can be determined best by 2-D, TEE, or 3-D echo. Once the diagnosis of hemodynamically significant aortic stenosis is established, management should follow the ACCF/AHA guidelines.[54] Ascending aortic aneurysms need to be carefully monitored by serial measurements of maximal diameter and growth rate that determine the timing of surgery or endovascular stenting. Dilation of the aortic root with effacement of the sinuses of Valsalva may disrupt the architecture of the aortic valve leaflets, resulting in secondary rather than primary aortic regurgitation.

Chronic aortic regurgitation (AR) has become a less common cause of congestive heart failure in the Western hemisphere because of the decline in incidence of rheumatic heart disease. The diagnosis of AR is easily made by documenting the regurgitant diastolic blood flow reversal in the LVOT flow by Doppler color flow velocity mapping that is extremely sensitive even to trivial AR. The cause of AR is either due to abnormalities of the aortic valve leaflets or to abnormalities of the aortic root geometry. The aortic valve is bicuspid in 1% of all live births and undergoes calcification, becoming either primarily stenotic or primarily regurgitant. Both lesions may be associated with ascending aortopathy that varies independently of the hemodynamic severity of the aortic valve pathology.[52,53] The valve leaflets may vary from rheumatic thickening with commissural fusion and calcification to floppy myxomatous leaflets that fail to coapt normally. The geometry of the aortic root may be altered by aneurysmal dilation or effacement of the sinuses of Valsalva, as occurs in Marfan syndrome, which exerts abnormal traction on the aortic valve leaflets preventing normal coaptation and resulting in secondary aortic regurgitation.

In heart failure due to chronic severe AR, the left ventricle is markedly dilated, with moderate to severe eccentric hypertrophy and initially preserved function that slowly but progressively deteriorates over time (**Figure 29-12**). Importantly, one third of patients with moderate to severe AR do not develop cardiovascular symptoms and only become

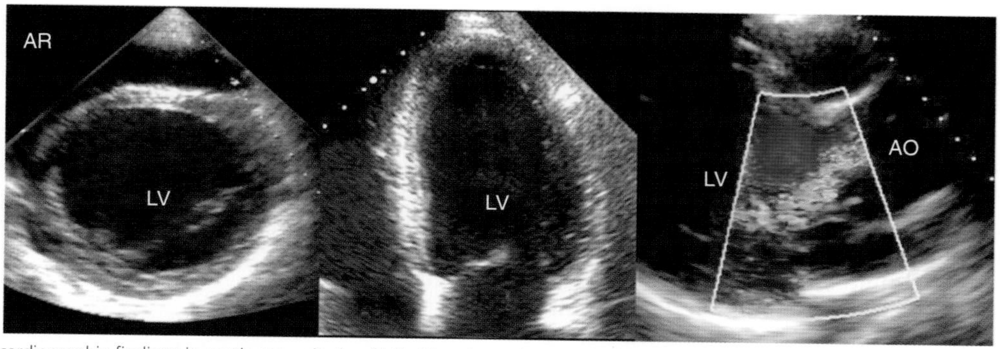

FIGURE 29-12 Echocardiographic findings in aortic regurgitation (AR): Chronic aortic regurgitation in a young female (age 39) who presented with fatigue and heart failure symptoms for almost 1 year. Left ventricular (LV) short-axis view *(left)* shows marked LV dilation but only mildly reduced contractile function *(middle)* consistent with eccentric LV remodeling and preserved systolic function and showing the appearance of an early diastolic color flow Doppler velocity signal of moderate aortic regurgitation *(right)*.

symptomatic late in the natural history of the disease when irreversible LV dysfunction develops; thus great reliance is placed upon Doppler echo findings. The severity of the AR can be accurately quantified by Doppler echo assessment of the deceleration rate of the regurgitant aortic jet, by the diameter of the vena contracta, regurgitant volume, regurgitant fraction and the effective regurgitant orifice area. Clinical decision making to recommend aortic valve replacement (AVR) is based largely on echo measurements of LV cavity size (end-systolic and end-diastolic dimensions) and ejection fraction (function; see Figure 29-12) together with onset of cardiac symptoms as recommended in the ACCF/AHA 2006 guidelines for the management of patients with valvular heart disease.[34] Thus TTE imaging provides all the requisite information regarding LV size, geometry, and hemodynamic assessment necessary to confidently advocate AVR to remove the regurgitant volume that is important in the appropriate management of patients with chronic AR and congestive heart failure.

Cardiac Magnetic Resonance Assessment of Valvular Heart Disease

CMR may be a useful alternative to echocardiography in patients with valvular disease with limited image quality, or those with conflicting or inconclusive results. Tissue characterization may help physicians to determine the cause and potential therapy of valvular heart disease, for example, in ischemic MR. Although regurgitant and stenotic jets are evident in cine images, a more complete valvular disease assessment requires quantitative evaluation of flow and flow velocity data that has been previously validated.[55,56]

The regurgitant volume and regurgitant fraction in MR may be measured by comparing the left ventricular stroke volume with systolic aortic flow. In AR, the regurgitant fraction is measured by integrating the diastolic flow across the aortic valve, and comparing it to the systolic forward flow (**Figure 29-13**). CMR can accurately quantify the effective cardiac output and provide an important objective parameter of heart failure related to low-output states.

In stenotic valvular disease, flow quantification can be used to identify increased transvalvular flow velocity and calculate pressure gradients.[57] By visualizing the stenotic orifice, CMR offers reliable aortic valve area quantification and avoids limitations related to oblique or turbulent jets and unreliable pressure gradients, particularly in low-output states.[2,58-60]

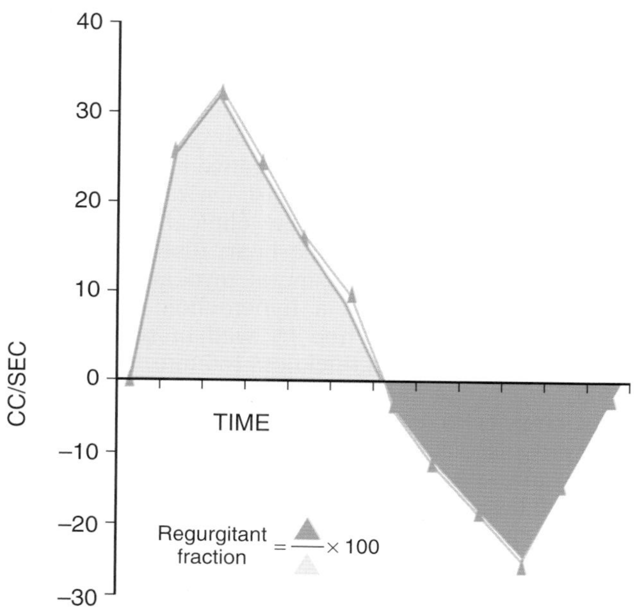

FIGURE 29-13 Cardiac magnetic resonance assessment of chronic aortic regurgitation: Forward *(gray curve)* and reverse *(yellow curve)* flow across the aortic valve is depicted in this graph. The forward stroke volume is calculated as the total blood flow across the valve in systole [Velocity-time integral via phase contrast images × blood vessel cross-sectional area = blood flow in cc/sec], whereas the regurgitant fraction is the integral of the reverse flow over time divided by the forward flow multiplied by 100. *Courtesy Mark Fogel, MD.*

MYOCARDIAL VIABILITY (see also Chapter 18)

HFrEF patients who have an ischemic cause may present with angina, shortness of breath, reduced exercise capacity, and a low LVEF because of the presence of noncontracting but viable myocardium. There are three noninvasive imaging methods commonly used for assessing myocardial viability: stress echocardiography, nuclear imaging, and CMR perfusion studies.

Stress Echocardiography

Viable noncontracting myocardium in heart failure can be detected by exercise and/or pharmacologic (low-dose dobutamine) stress echocardiography. The reason for identifying viable myocardium in selected heart failure patients is because restoration of myocardial perfusion targeted to the ischemic regions can potentially translate into increased regional and global (LVEF) function. There are three nonoverlapping phasic responses to dobutamine stress echocardiography. First, at low levels of stress there is recruitment of myocardial shortening that is lost as the level of stress (dobutamine dosage) increases, described as a "biphasic response." A second response to dobutamine stress echo is continued improvement in regional and global function known as a "contractile reserve." The third response to dobutamine stress echocardiography is no change or worsening global LV function, the so-called flat response. Technically limited image acquisition and image analysis due to lung disease, enhanced respiratory excursion, or abnormal body habitus (obesity) can usually be minimized by augmenting endocardial definition with intravenous echo contrast. The advantages of stress echocardiography for detecting viable noncontracting myocardium is that this method correlates with nuclear imaging, does not involve radiation exposure, is relatively inexpensive, and the results are available immediately. Patients with a biphasic response to stress benefit from revascularization more than those patients with contractile reserve. In contrast, those with a flat or negative response to stress usually do not benefit from revascularization and moreover are at high risk for adverse clinical cardiovascular outcomes. In chronic ischemic heart disease, there may be a history of remote transmural myocardial infarction that can be identified as a hyperechoic (highly echo reflective) region of the free LV wall or septum that is thinner than normal wall thickness (<6 mm) and does not contract or change in thickness with increasing workload during stress echo testing.

A prerequisite for diagnosis of viability and ischemic myocardium with noninvasive imaging tools is the acquisition of high-quality images at rest but especially during stress testing. CMR studies provide complete and continuous endocardial surfaces. By contrast, the 2-D and 3-D TTE images often need to be interpolated, although the need for major interpolation has diminished since the introduction of harmonic imaging and use of intravenous echo contrast for the express purpose of enhancing endocardial definition. Myocardial viability can also be detected by radionuclide angiography and CMR perfusion studies.

Nuclear Imaging: Evaluation of Ischemic Heart Disease

In the evaluation of patients with heart failure, it is important to rule out ischemic heart disease as the cause of the LV dysfunction. This can be accomplished by assessment of stress-induced changes in regional perfusion or function. Rest and stress myocardial perfusion imaging can be accomplished with either SPECT or PET perfusion imaging. Importantly, radionuclide myocardial perfusion imaging effectively visualizes regional changes in myocardial blood flow, a principal target of many therapies in patients with CAD. Rest and stress radiotracer studies continue to play a major role in the diagnosis of CAD, which is the major cause of heart failure. Thus stress/rest SPECT perfusion imaging can effectively separate ischemic from nonischemic cardiomyopathy.

The care of patients with acute myocardial infarction (MI) is directed at establishing early coronary reperfusion, because aborting ischemia may result in myocardial salvage. Myocardial salvage results in preservation of LV function, which is the most important predictor of long-term survival postinfarction. Radiotracer imaging has proved effective in estimation of infarct size and salvage of cardiomyocytes after MI. The radiotracer technique also provides a reliable estimation of residual LV function. There is a well-established relationship between survival and global RV and LV function in patients undergoing reperfusion with thrombolytic therapy or percutaneous coronary intervention (PCI).[61]

Radiotracer-Based Assessment of Myocardial Viability and Remodeling

Serial SPECT perfusion imaging can be used for the assessment of myocardial viability and salvage following reperfusion,[62-65] and later following PCI.[66,67] These indices of myocardial salvage derived from nuclear imaging are predictive of long-term outcome.

Nuclear imaging techniques have also been used specifically to predict LV remodeling. ^{201}Tl and ^{99m}Tc-labeled perfusion images have also been used to assess infarct size, and this radiotracer-based estimation of myocardial viability has correlated with subsequent LV remodeling. ^{99m}Tc-sestamibi imaging has been used to assess infarct size early post MI in patients, and these perfusion-based estimates of infarct size have correlated with LV volumes at 1 year.[68,69] Another study suggested that infarct severity on ^{99m}Tc-sestamibi imaging may be a better predictor of remodeling than infarct size alone.[69] Radionuclide assessment of viability was also shown to predict LV remodeling in a study of patients with ischemic cardiomyopathy.[70] In this study, viability was assessed with serial nitrate-enhanced ^{201}Tl and ^{99m}Tc-sestamibi imaging. Remodeling was prevented in patients with at least five viable segments who underwent revascularization at 21-month follow-up.[70] The direct relationship between the extent of ^{201}Tl defects and collagen content in severe ischemic cardiomyopathy was assessed in a study of hearts excised after cardiac transplantation. There was greater collagen content in segments with irreversible ^{201}Tl defects compared with segments with reversible defects or normal ^{201}Tl perfusion. Furthermore, noninfarcted segments in the cardiomyopathic hearts also had elevated collagen content compared with control hearts.[71]

Cardiac Magnetic Resonance Stress

CMR can also be used to predict post-revascularization recovery of LV function, using late gadolinium enhancement (LGE) and low-dose dobutamine stress testing. The degree of transmural LGE predicts regional functional recovery, and improvement in LVEF frequently occurs when there is hibernation of greater than 20% of the global LV myocardium. On a regional basis, LGE has an 80% positive predictive value for recovery in segments demonstrating no infarction, and a 90% negative predictive valve for no improvement in segments with greater than a 50% transmural scar.[72] Other work suggests that low-dose dobutamine stress CMR may be more sensitive for viability assessment, and additional clinical experience is accumulating. LGE demonstrates myocardium with nontransmural scar that is destined not to recover function despite revascularization (**Figure 29-14**). Failure of functional improvement may

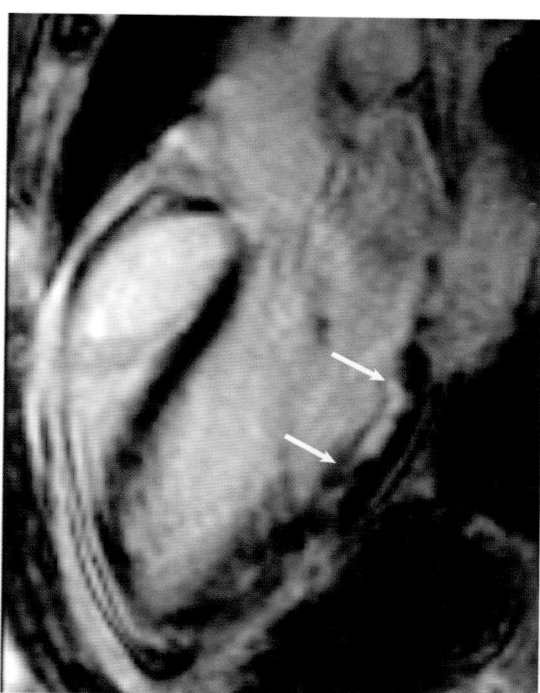

FIGURE 29-14 Cardiac magnetic resonance nontransmural scar: Note the nontransmural area of increased signal intensity (late gadolinium enhancement) at the basal inferolateral wall *(arrows)*, which represents nonviable myocardial tissue at the subendocardial level.

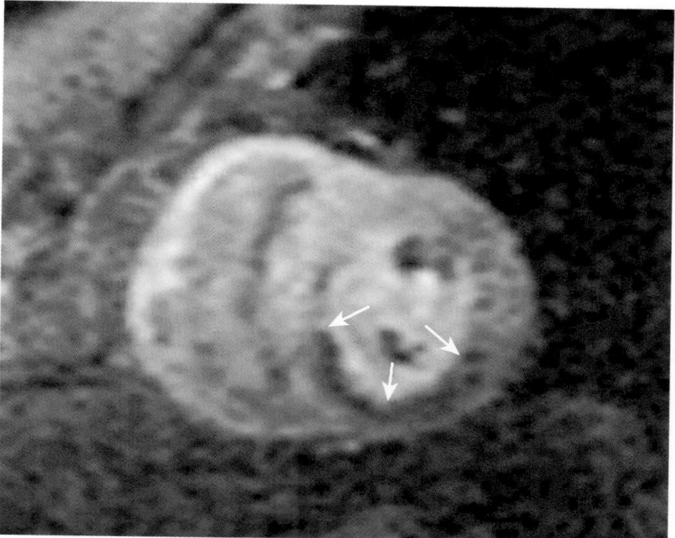

FIGURE 29-15 Nontransmural ischemia: The darker area in this image *(arrows)* represents hypoperfused (less contrast agent delivery) subendocardial tissue resulting from poststress perfusion imaging of a patient with an epicardial vessel stenosis of greater than 70%.

also be due to incomplete revascularization, persistent hibernation early post-revascularization, or abnormal wall mechanics that may be recruitable with dobutamine or exercise stress. CMR also predicts the response to β-blockers in heart failure patients, and demonstrates lower response rates in patients with larger myocardial infarctions.[73]

Detection of Myocardial Ischemia with Cardiac Magnetic Resonance

CMR may be used for ischemia assessment using either a first-pass stress myocardial perfusion strategy or dobutamine stress wall motion imaging as alternatives to myocardial perfusion SPECT and stress echocardiography, respectively. Dobutamine stress CMR (DSMR) is a technique that has been performed in a number of centers that have demonstrated its diagnostic accuracy and prognostic capability. DSMR studies may be used at low dose for viability, or at high dose (with or without atropine) for demonstrating supply/demand mismatch ischemia. Stress perfusion CMR has been proven accurate in multicenter studies, and has several advantages over conventional nuclear perfusion methods.[74] CMR does not suffer from the "roll-off" or plateau effect at high myocardial perfusion rates seen with SPECT, and the higher resolution CMR methods permit depiction of nontransmural ischemia that is easily detectable by visual inspection. Recent clinical trials, including the multicenter, multiple vendor, Magnetic Resonance Imaging for Myocardial Perfusion Assessment in Coronary Artery Disease Trial (MR-IMPACT) involving over 240 patients, have shown that perfusion CMR performs comparably or better than perfusion SPECT for detection of CAD.[75] Greater clinical utility will come from direct comparison between modalities, such as the recent Clinical Evaluation of MAgnetic Resonance imaging in Coronary heart disease (CE-MARC) trial, which performed a head-to-head comparison of adenosine stress perfusion CMR and adenosine stress ^{99}Tc tetrofosmin in 752 patients with angina and suspected CAD. The sensitivity and negative predictive value for CMR were greater than SPECT, whereas the specificity and positive predictive value were similar.[76]

The negative predictive value for cardiac events is excellent with a normal stress CMR, and cardiac risk increases corresponding to greater degrees of ischemia.[77] By adding myocardial tagging to stress CMR to measure myocardial strain, interobserver variability is reduced, accuracy may be improved, and new physiologic information may be obtained.[78-80] The addition of perfusion imaging to tagging provides a more complete characterization of the state of the myocardium, particularly at greater field strengths (i.e., 3T).[81] Clinical experience is increasing with CMR stress techniques, and protocols are being harmonized to minimize variability between interpreters and centers. Detection of nontransmural ischemia with stress DSMR perfusion techniques by abnormal wall motion will likely endorse these methods as valuable clinical tools (**Figure 29-15**).

Detection of Infarction with Cardiac Magnetic Resonance

LGE techniques have matured to the point where high-quality, reproducible detection of both nontransmural and transmural myocardial infarctions are achievable 10 minutes after intravenous injection of a gadolinium-containing contrast agent. The greater volume of distribution of the diseased tissue produces higher regional gadolinium concentration, which appears bright and readily identifiable on T1-weighted CMR pulse sequences. The LGE techniques depict both acute and chronic infarction, and focal as well as diffuse fibrosis, and are highly accurate and reproducible, as demonstrated by a recent large multicenter clinical trial.[82] LGE has advanced the assessment of myocardial infarctions because the technique shows greater sensitivity than SPECT perfusion and wall motion abnormality imaging techniques because of the vagaries of spatial resolution and endocardial detection, as well as other potential artifacts.[83] Studies focused on the prognostic impact of unrecognized infarctions have demonstrated additional incremental value over conventional risk measures in patients with clinically suspected CAD but no known previous infarction.[84] LGE has an important role in the assessment of heart failure patients in particular. In a series of 150 consecutive heart failure patients with an LVEF less than 50% and contemporaneous echo evaluation, CMR had a significant clinical impact in 65%—including a new diagnosis in 30%—predominantly related to detection of LGE.[85] LGE techniques also play an important role in heart failure related to infiltrative disorders. Diseases such as amyloidosis and sarcoidosis may be detected by their unique patterns on LGE imaging. Beyond LGE, CMR can detect and permit serial noninvasive evaluation of another important systemic disorder causing heart failure—hemochromatosis. Local myocardial iron concentration changes the signal properties such that greater tissue iron concentrations result in greater signal alterations. CMR thus becomes a tool to follow chelation or other therapies to optimally treat affected patients.

TRANSITION FROM MYOCARDIAL INFARCTION TO HEART FAILURE WITH REDUCED EJECTION FRACTION

More than two thirds of HFrEF patients have occlusive CAD or previous myocardial infarction, in whom ischemia may be ongoing, resulting in maladaptive changes not only in the surviving cardiomyocytes but also in the extracellular matrix. Heart failure is a progressive clinical syndrome with a poor prognosis that includes dyspnea, effort intolerance, and decreased exercise capacity. A proportion of patients in the advanced stages (level C/D or NYHA symptom class III/IV) have a seriously impaired quality of life that is punctuated by recurrent hospital admissions for acute exacerbations of heart failure requiring intravenous diuretics, inotropic agents, device therapy, and even heart transplantation. Myocardial infarction (MI) results in almost immediate cessation of myocardial contraction in the territory subtended by the occluded nutrient coronary artery. Echocardiographic imaging in acute MI shows a region of the LV wall that is akinetic or severely hypokinetic, with altered acoustic impedance that is spatially congruent with the infarct location and coronary artery perfusion defect at cardiac catheterization. The noncontracting infarct zone thins because of stretching by actively contracting myocardium contiguous and remote to the infarction zone, resulting in LV dilation and increased wall stress. Failure to normalize the increased wall stress is a trigger for progressive LV dilation and an adverse outcome. Disproportionate LV dilation causes an increase in load, which results in further deterioration in LV function. A number of factors are involved in the transition from the initial infarction to chronic HFrEF, which includes the initial infarct size, infarct location and transmurality, patency of the culprit infarct artery, activation of the neurohumoral RAAS and sympathetic nervous system, changes in the extracellular matrix (ECM), and local tropic factors. In this dynamic process of ventricular remodeling, a balance is sought between increased wall stress causing LV dilation and opposing restraining forces from the viscoelastic collagen scaffold formed by the ECM. When equilibrium between these opposing forces is not attained, progressive remodeling leads to further LV dilation, poor LV function, and the insidious onset of heart failure—a course that portends a poor prognosis. When equilibrium is achieved, myocardial repair begins with formation of a collagenous scar with a high enough tensile strength to prevent further infarct expansion and LV cavity dilation. Old MIs are common in HFrEF, accounting for the low LVEF. Old MIs are detectable by the highly echo reflective, thin (wall thickness <0.6 cm), noncontracting region of myocardium. The progressive structural and functional remodeling in HFrEF has been well characterized by 2-D TTE in a number of randomized clinical trials of chronic heart failure.[24,25,86-88] The changes in LV structure and function postinfarction described by serial TTE can be followed by serial CMR in HFrEF. Much less is known about the natural history of HFpEF except that the left ventricle usually does not dilate, LV hypertrophy may increase consistent with hypertrophic concentric remodeling, and diastolic dysfunction may worsen with time. Randomized controlled trials have shown that echocardiographically determined LV volumes, LV mass, LV shape, and ejection fraction are powerful predictors of clinical outcome.[24] Although LVEF is used for clinical decision making more than any other metric in the management of heart failure, it is not a measure of contractility and varies widely with changes in loading conditions. LV stroke volume is more robust and can be estimated from LV volumes and from Doppler velocity signals and diameters recorded from the LVOT. However, stroke volume in HFrEF has been shown by quantitative 2-D TTE to remain unchanged until LVEF falls to 20% or below, at which point the left ventricle can no longer modulate stroke volume by structural remodeling.[9,89] Increases in cardiac output are achieved either by increasing resting heart rate or by ejecting a smaller fraction of a larger end-diastolic volume. These two mechanisms work in concert to maintain cardiac output as ejection fraction falls.

Until the mid-1980s to the early 1990s, treatment of refractory heart failure was limited to digitalis, diuretics, vasodilators, cautious use of β-adrenergic receptor blockers, mitral valve surgery, or orthotopic heart transplantation. The introduction of ACE inhibitors (ACEi) and the angiotensin receptor blockers (ARBs) was followed by several large randomized controlled trials in which serial TTE imaging was used to assess their efficacy in reducing adverse events (see also Chapter 34).[25,86] Quantitative TTE demonstrated that angiotensin-converting enzyme inhibitors, ACEi, β-adrenergic receptor blockers, and aldosterone antagonists resulted in symptomatic benefit and improved clinical outcomes associated with structural and functional reverse remodeling mediated by attenuating neurohumoral activation.[87]

Follow-up of HFrEF patients revealed two major causes of death. In NYHA symptom class I-III patients, death was either due to pump failure or to SCD from life-threatening ventricular arrhythmias. Once these findings were confirmed in subsequent clinical studies patients were targeted for treatment with CRT in addition to the optimal drug therapy combined with ICD placement where indicated. A variety of imaging modalities including echo, nuclear, and CMR have since been employed in multiple prospective, randomized clinical trials in HFrEF testing the efficacy of novel pharmacologic agents, surgical interventions, and device placement over long-term follow-up. The control arms of these trials are useful data repositories that demonstrate changes in LV architecture and function and extent of LV remodeling over 5-year follow-up with serial quantitative analysis of echocardiographic images at 6 monthly intervals.[90] Studies involving large numbers of HFrEF patients of all NYHA symptom classes have shown the strong predictive value of the echocardiographic metrics for clinical outcomes.

As our understanding of the causative mechanisms of heart failure has improved, the number of treatment options for heart failure patients has diversified such that there are now specific therapies for selected patient populations. Cardiac imaging modalities have proved useful in identifying patients for consideration of orthotopic heart transplantation (see Chapter 40), ventricular assist device placement (see Chapter 42), CRT, internal cardiac defibrillator placement (see Chapter 35), and detection of hemodynamically severe mitral regurgitation requiring surgical repair or replacement (see Chapter 41).

Cardiac Magnetic Resonance Infarction

CMR provides much greater detail of infarcted myocardium and tissue that has experienced ischemia/reperfusion injury. In acute infarction, CMR can depict areas of microvascular obstruction—generally a subendocardial dark area on LGE—that identifies tissue with extremely long gadolinium inflow times. This abnormality is best detected 1 to 2 minutes after gadolinium contrast injection and is known as early gadolinium enhancement (EGE) imaging. Microvascular obstruction portends a poorer prognosis, more unfavorable remodeling, and is a negative prognostic indicator above and beyond LVEF.[91] Of note, microvascular obstruction is not seen in the chronic state because of infarct involution and collagen remodeling, and is present only in the first few weeks after infarction. EGE imaging is also more accurate than echocardiography for detection of LV thrombi, which are of low signal intensity in contrast to the brighter adjacent infarcted myocardium.

Other unique aspects of CMR include its ability to noninvasively depict areas of reversible ischemia, area at risk, and myocardial hemorrhage. A T2-weighted CMR pulse sequence is used to detect cellular edema, which distinguishes areas of recent ischemia/reperfusion injury from irreversibly injured tissue.[92] This method also allows for calculation of the area at risk following reperfusion of an acute infarction (the edematous area), whereas the salvaged myocardium corresponds to the difference between the infarcted territory (depicted by LGE), and the edematous area.[93] These changes can be seen for days or weeks after infarction or reperfusion, but SPECT methods have a narrow time window of only a few hours. T2* CMR may also detect intramyocardial hemorrhage related to acute infarction and the functional outcome of this process.[94]

CARDIAC RESYNCHRONIZATION THERAPY (see also Chapter 35)

CRT has been a significant advance in the treatment of patients with HFrEF. Enrollment criteria for randomized clinical CRT trials of patients with chronic refractory heart failure have been consistent and included a prolonged QRS duration greater than 120 ms, LV dilation (LVEDd >5.5 cm), and dysfunction (LVEF <35%) determined echocardiographically. Between 30% and 50% of HFrEF patients have a high degree of atrioventricular infra-Hisian conduction delay, most commonly with left bundle branch block (LBBB) morphology. There is a close relation between mortality and duration of the QRS, so that the longer the QRS duration, the higher the mortality.

LBBB occurs in approximately 70% of patients with idiopathic dilated cardiomyopathy. LBBB is associated with LV dyssynchrony that involves reversed septal motion and loss of coordinated systolic inward wall motion. There is also delay in the temporal acquisition of peak myocardial velocities in the 17-segment model of the left ventricle by Doppler echocardiography. LV dyssynchrony was initially regarded as being synonymous with prolonged QRS duration. A number of attempts were made using Doppler parameters to identify patients who responded and benefited before device deployment.[95] CRT was associated with symptomatic improvement because of LV reverse remodeling in approximately 65% to 70% of patients in all NYHA classes from I through IV heart failure.[88,96,97] The beneficial impact on mortality when CRT was combined with an ICD was greater than with CRT alone. HFrEF patients with nonischemic LV dysfunction experienced threefold greater reverse remodeling than patients with ischemic heart failure. This salutary impact of CRT on reverse remodeling is sustained for at least 5-year follow-up.[19,98]

Nuclear Imaging for Cardiac Resynchronization Therapy

Gated SPECT blood pool and perfusion imaging have recently been shown to be beneficial in the evaluation of resynchronization therapy in patients with end-stage heart failure.[99,100] The degree of intraventricular and interventricular dyssynchrony can be assessed by phase analysis. For gated SPECT blood pool imaging, the combination of a baseline LVEF greater than 15% with significant interventricular dyssynchrony were the best predictors for improvement in LV systolic function after 6 months of CRT.[101] Gated SPECT perfusion imaging is unique in allowing simultaneous assessment of the degree of LV dyssynchrony and site of latest activation along with the assessment of scar burden from perfusion imaging. Thus a single image acquisition provides a means for predicting CRT response in heart failure patients (**Figure 29-16**).

Cardiac Magnetic Resonance for Resynchronization Therapy

The disappointing response rate to CRT for patients with DCM (≈30% with LBBB/wide QRS) motivated a search for novel imaging indicators to identify potential responders. Studies have shown reduced response rates and poorer outcomes in patients with LV inferolateral scar.[102] Technical aspects of the procedure, such as avoiding areas of lateral wall scar during LV lead placement, have increased the response rate in small groups of patients.[103] However, the presence of midwall fibrosis appears to be an even stronger marker of potential responders to CRT. A recent study demonstrated a marked increase in both cardiovascular mortality and major adverse cardiac events, and a low rate of LV

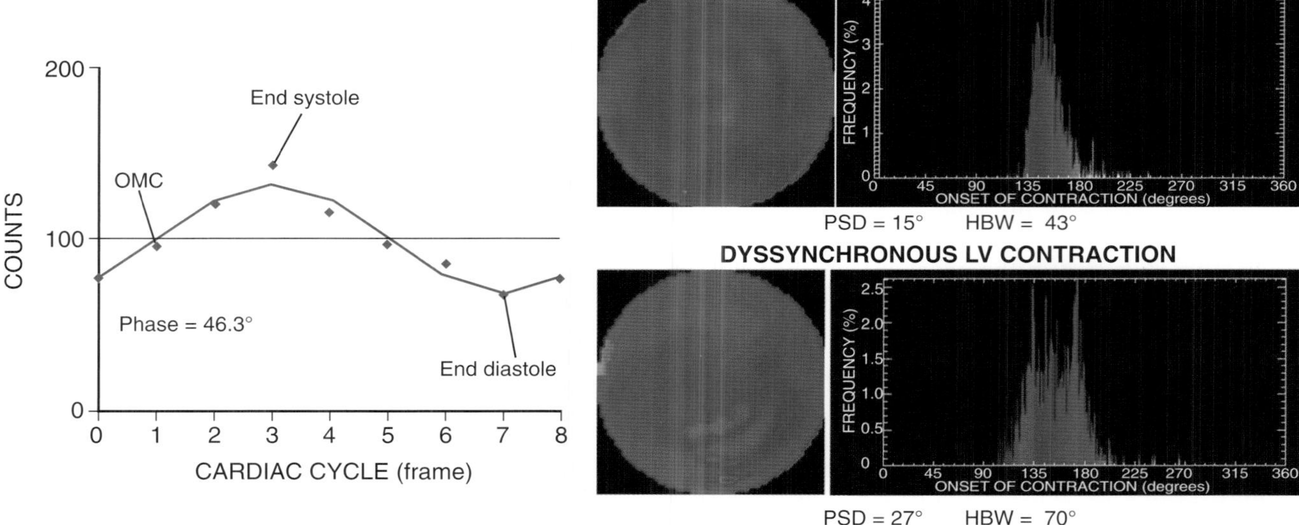

FIGURE 29-16 Single photon emission computed tomography approach to left ventricular (LV) dyssynchrony. The left panel shows the time-activity curve from a single myocardial segment. Based on the partial volume effect, this is essentially a thickening curve. The low fidelity curve based on 8-bin gating is converted to a continuous curve by Fourier transformation. For the purposes of comparing thickening among all myocardial segments, the point of inflection of the thickening curve on a horizontal line representing the average segmental counts during one cardiac cycle (onset of mechanical contraction [OMC]) is chosen as the reference point. The right panel shows the creation of a histogram and phase polar map of OMC from the approximately 600 myocardial segments acquired during a standard SPECT study. Top panel shows a narrow histogram and uniform phase polar map indicative of synchronous LV contraction. Bottom panel shows a wide histogram and nonuniform phase polar map indicative of dyssynchronous LV contraction. Automated measures of synchrony, which have been validated, are the phase standard deviation (PSD, standard deviation of the phase distribution) and the histogram bandwidth (HBW, the range of phases that encompasses 95% of the OMCs).

reverse remodeling (nonresponse rate) in those patients demonstrating midwall LGE.[104]

IDIOPATHIC DILATED CARDIOMYOPATHY

Idiopathic dilated cardiomyopathy (IDCM) accounts for approximately one quarter to one third of all patients presenting with HFrEF and one third of the prevalence of ischemic cardiomyopathy (**see Chapter 19**). Most patients with idiopathic DCM present with a slow and insidious progressive deterioration in exercise capacity. A minority of patients present with hemodynamic collapse due to sudden death from poorly tolerated and life-threatening ventricular arrhythmias. A proportion of DCM is genetically determined (**see Chapter 22**), occurring in multiple family members and varying severity of LV dysfunction and AV conduction abnormalities. Seventy percent of these DCM patients develop conduction delay that is typically of left bundle branch block morphology, with major prolongation of the QRS duration often becoming refractory to pharmacologic therapy. It is important to identify these patients because they are typically young with very low LVEF and respond especially well to resynchronization therapy. These patients are easy to diagnose by 2-D TTE that reveals massive LV cavity dilation, inadequate left ventricular hypertrophy, usually with severe dyssynchrony. Most of these patients with idiopathic DCM and especially those with LBBB respond favorably to CRT therapy. Moreover, there is a threefold greater reduction in LV volumes and more than a threefold greater increase in ejection fraction in idiopathic DCM than in patients with ischemic cardiomyopathy, indicating that more extensive reverse LV remodeling can be achieved in patients with nonischemic DCM.[88]

However, only two thirds of all heart failure patients respond to CRT, and attempts to preselect patients who respond to CRT using a number of Doppler echo parameters or clinical demographics by any imaging modality in the PROSPECT trial have not been successful.[95]

MISCELLANEOUS CAUSES OF HEART FAILURE

There are two additional causes of heart failure that both have a poor prognosis and yet should not be overlooked. These are (1) vegetative endocarditis and (2) partial rupture of an LV papillary muscle from ischemia. Both of these should be diagnosed unequivocally by 2-D TTE, 3-D TTE, or ideally TEE imaging. Vegetative endocarditis may destroy the mitral or aortic valve leaflets, resulting in severe MR or AR and causing myocardial abscess and congestive heart failure, especially when the definitive diagnosis and appropriate antibiotic therapy are delayed (**see also Chapter 24**). The diagnosis may be obscured because no organism is identified as a result of earlier administration of an inappropriately short course of antibiotics before the diagnosis of endocarditis was entertained. Severe MR or AR may also result when the causative micro-organism is especially virulent or resistant to the antibiotic therapy or when the vegetation is large and excessively mobile. Excessively mobile valve vegetation puts increased traction on the leaflets and mitral tensor apparatus, causing leaflet tears or avulsion of the valve and recurrent systemic embolization of septic vegetative material.

Diagnostic uncertainty regarding rupture of the chordae tendineae resulting in severe MR with flail or partially flail leaflets should be clarified by 3-D TTE or TEE (**Figure 29-17**) before surgical intervention. TEE provides essential information regarding the morphology of large vegetation prone to embolization and whether there is evidence of intramyocardial or valve ring abscess. These

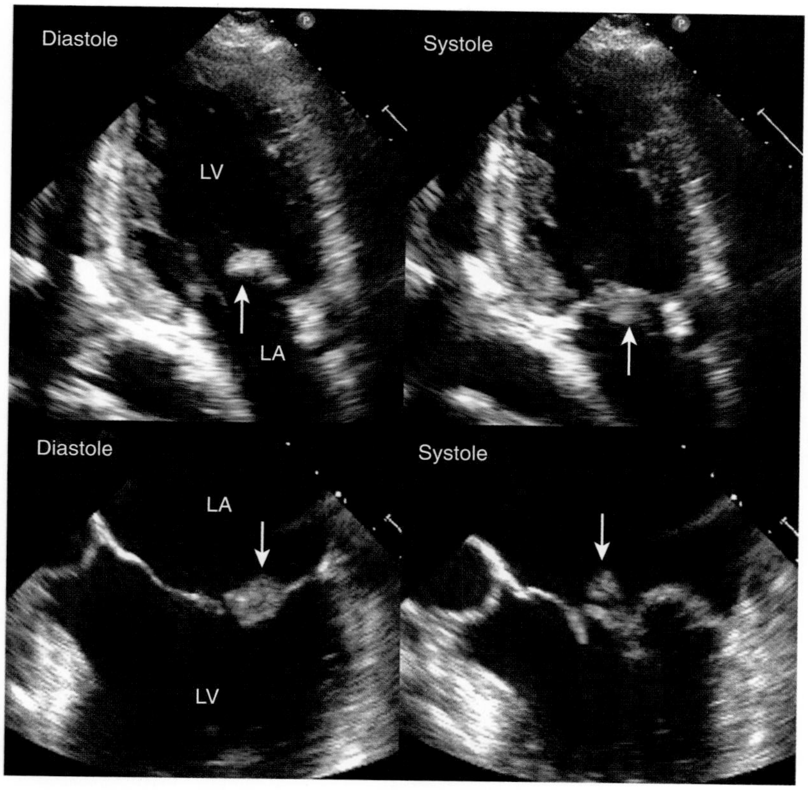

Diastole Systole LV LA Diastole Systole LA LV

FIGURE 29-17 Mitral valve vegetation by transesophageal echocardiography: transthoracic echocardiogram of the apical long-axis view showing mitral valve thickening that was mobile but was initially thought to be nonspecific in a 70-year-old male who developed spiking fevers, symptoms of heart failure, and increasingly severe mitral regurgitation with positive blood cultures. A TEE was performed that revealed a discrete vegetation on the mitral valve with ruptured chordae, allowing mild prolapse of the posterior valve leaflet and acute severe mitral regurgitation that worsened with stress.

echocardiographic findings impact directly on the timing of surgical intervention, the choice of the size, and the type of prosthesis.

Another valvular cause of acute hemodynamic instability is partial or complete rupture of a papillary muscle (inferior > anterior), causing severe MR. The increased mobility of the ruptured heads of a papillary muscle are often not well visualized by TTE or by contrast LV angiography. So when the diagnosis of ruptured papillary muscle is seriously entertained, urgent TEE should be performed as the imaging modality of choice. TEE lays out the anatomy and pathophysiology that facilitates complete diagnosis. Ischemic injury or rupture of a papillary muscle is more commonly associated with LV inferobasal than lateral hypokinesis.

ASSESSMENT OF RIGHT VENTRICULAR FUNCTION

The complex shape of the normal RV cannot be successfully modeled mathematically, and this poses difficulties in quantifying ventricular volumes and RV cavity function. Two-dimensional echo is limited to measurement of percent change of RV cavity areas at end diastole and end systole as indicators of RV size, while RV function is limited to percent change in LV area. The RV is important in heart failure because it is a strong and independent predictor of clinical outcome in HFrEF patients.[105] Quantification of RV volumes and ejection fraction with CTA or CMR imaging can be achieved with much greater precision than by Doppler echo. In addition, CMR can quantify the regurgitant fraction across both the pulmonary and tricuspid valves.

COMPLICATIONS OF HEART FAILURE

Detection of complications of heart failure is important and includes hemodynamic compromise caused by large pericardial and pleural effusions, onset of atrial fibrillation with rapid ventricular response, development of acute severe mitral regurgitation, and the increased stroke risk associated with intracardiac thrombus within the left heart chambers.[17] In idiopathic dilated and ischemic cardiomyopathies the combination of dilated chambers and decreased amplitude of left atrial and left ventricular wall motion results in low-velocity intracardiac blood flow, which predisposes to thrombus formation with the attendant risk of thrombus propagation to the systemic circulation, especially with the onset of atrial fibrillation, which is common in heart failure. The presence of left heart thrombus necessitates anticoagulation that has additional significant morbidity and mortality.

FUTURE DIRECTIONS IN CARDIAC IMAGING

Nuclear Imaging

Injury and inflammation: Myocardial injury and inflammation lead to disruption of cellular membranes and release of myosin heavy chain. Antimyosin, tenascin-C, and the LTB_4 receptor represent potential targets for assessing the severity of myocellular injury. ^{111}In-labeled antimyosin antibodies have been used to visualize myocardial damage in patients with heart failure caused by idiopathic and alcoholic cardiomyopathies. They have also been used to visualize myocyte damage in acute myocardial infarction.[106,107] It became apparent that noninvasive imaging of this extracellular exposure of myosin could provide early diagnostic,

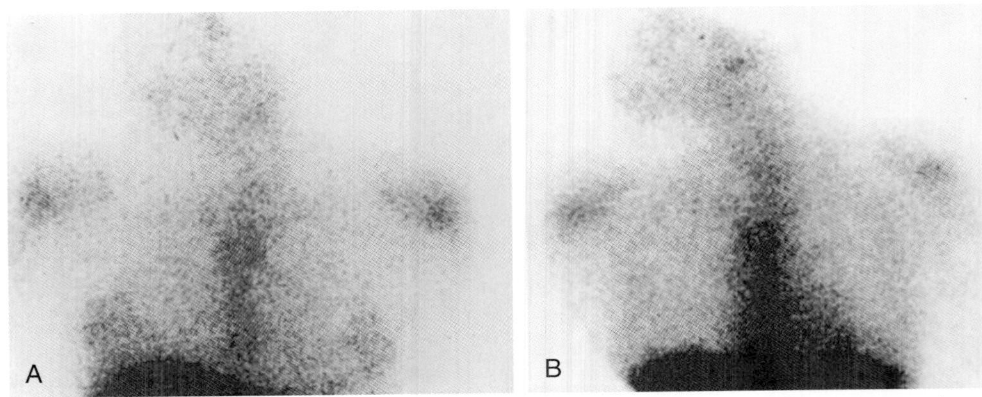

FIGURE 29-18 ^{111}In-antimyosin antibody uptake in myocarditis. **A,** No myocardial antimyosin uptake is seen in the left panel (heart to lung ratio [HLR] = 1.4) in a scan with normal findings. **B,** Moderate myocardial antimyosin uptake (HLR = 1.8) in a patient with active myocarditis. *Modified from Martin ME, Moya-Mur JL, Casanova M, et al: Role of noninvasive antimyosin imaging in infants and children with clinically suspected myocarditis. J Nucl Med 45:429–437, 2004.*

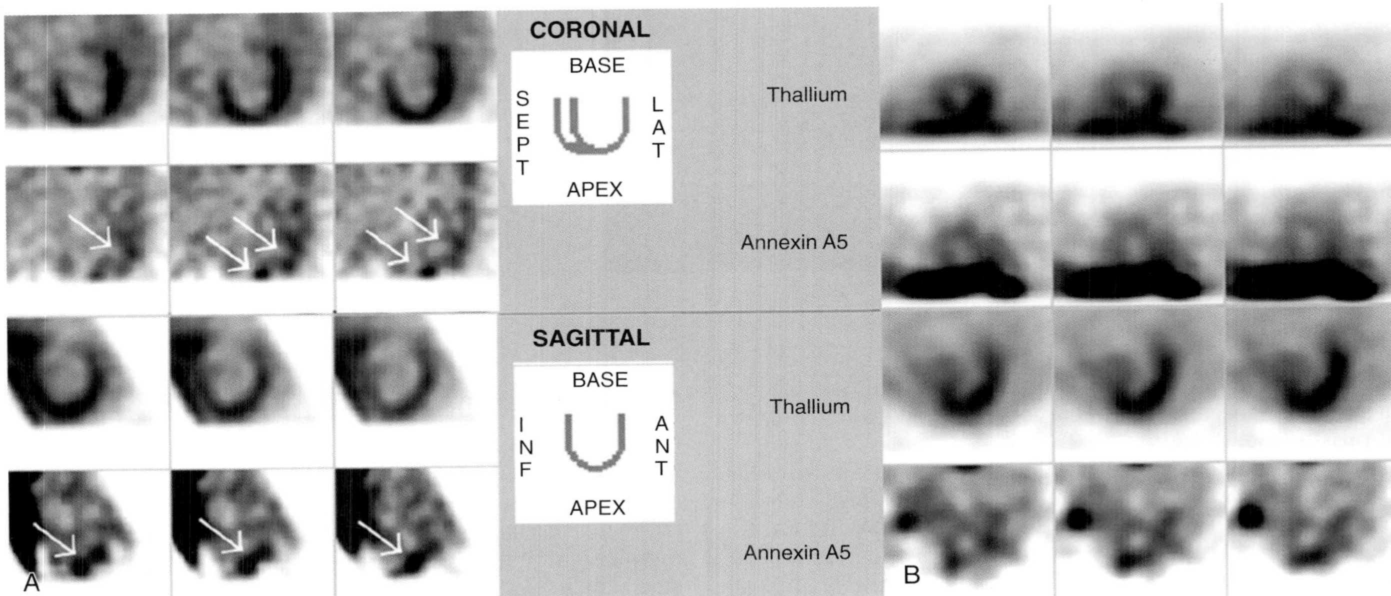

FIGURE 29-19 Dual isotope imaging with ^{201}Tl for left ventricular myocardial border detection and ^{99m}Tc-labeled annexin V in dilated cardiomyopathy (DCM). **A,** DCM patient with rapid deterioration of left ventricular function. There is apical and lateral wall focal uptake, and mild septal uptake. **B,** DCM patient with acute heart failure. There is global uptake of the tracer. *ANT,* Anterior; *INF,* inferior; *LAT,* lateral; *SEPT,* septal. *Modified from Kietselaer BL, Reutelingsperger CP, Boersma HH, et al: Noninvasive detection of programmed cell loss with 99mTc-labeled annexin A5 in heart failure. J Nucl Med 48:562–567, 2007.*

as well as longer term prognostic information[108,109] (**Figure 29-18**). Antimyosin antibody imaging has a high sensitivity (91%-100%) and high negative predictive value (93%-100%).[110]

Tenascin-C is a large extracellular matrix protein expressed in the heart during inflammation, wound healing, and remodeling.[111] Serum tenascin-C levels provide additional prognostic information to BNP in heart failure.[111,112] In-antitenascin-C monoclonal antibody fragments have also been used in a dual isotope SPECT imaging technique with ^{99m}Tc-MIBI to assess early inflammation in vivo during postinfarction remodeling.

Apoptosis and cell death: Apoptosis is the physiologic process of programmed cell death whereby organisms selectively target cells to be eliminated, whereas necrosis is a process of injury leading to cell death. Potential targets for the evaluation of myocellular apoptosis include annexin V and the critical apoptotic protease family of caspases. Pyrophosphate- and glucarate-based imaging allows for evaluation of necrotic cell death.

The cardiovascular pathologies of cardiomyopathy, heart failure, myocarditis, and myocardial infarction are associated with increased apoptosis. Apoptotic signaling pathways trigger the activation of caspases, cysteine proteases, and in particular the key effector caspase-3.[113] Caspase-3 disrupts the processes that regulate various subregions of the cell membrane, leading to increased phosphatidyl serine (PS) on the outer cell membrane.[114] Exposure of PS to the cell surface makes it an excellent target for imaging via the PS-binding protein annexin V.

^{99m}Tc-labeled annexin V was used to detect in vivo cell death in patients with myocardial infarction and who underwent percutaneous coronary intervention.[115] Revascularized patients had early ^{99m}Tc-labeled annexin V SPECT imaging and subsequent ^{99m}Tc-sestamibi-based perfusion imaging. Early regional retention of ^{99m}Tc-labeled annexin V correlated well with the perfusion defect. ^{99m}Tc labeled annexin V also appears to have predictive value in terms of deterioration of left ventricular function in patients with known cardiomyopathy (**Figure 29-19**).[116]

Heart transplant rejection is characterized by perivascular and interstitial mononuclear inflammatory infiltrates associated with myocyte apoptosis and necrosis. In a study of 18 patients undergoing apoptotic imaging within 1 year of cardiac transplantation, annexin V retention correlated with the severity of rejection.[117] Patients with a negative scan had a concomitant negative biopsy. The authors suggested that serial annexin V imaging for apoptotic cells could be used as a surrogate for detection of allograft rejection in place of serial biopsies in patients post heart transplant. As an alternative to visualizing apoptosis, several studies have demonstrated that certain agents allow visualization of ongoing myocardial necrosis as a mechanism of identifying acute infarction potentially even in the presence of prior myocardial infarction. ^{99m}Tc-glucarate enters necrotic cells by passive diffusion following breakdown of the sarcolemma and binds to exposed histones in cardiomyocyte nuclei, making it a useful an alternative to ^{99m}Tc-pyrophosphate.[118] Canine models for ischemia and infarction reveal a high affinity of ^{99m}Tc-glucarate for necrotic tissue versus ischemic but viable myocardium. Initial data in patients revealed that ^{99m}Tc-glucarate is able to diagnose myocardial infarction noninvasively in patients with chest pain, with a sensitivity that is dependent on time of presentation, specifically within the first 9 hours of symptom onset.[119]

Ventricular remodeling: Ventricular remodeling is a complex biologic process that involves angiogenesis, wound repair, and scarring. Several cell types modulate this adaptive remodeling process in ischemic and nonischemic cardiomyopathies. VEGF receptors, integrins, and matrix metalloproteinases are all potential new targets to modulate remodeling because of their association with neovascularization and turnover of the ECM.

VEGF receptors are potential targets for visualization of ventricular remodeling-associated angiogenesis. A PET tracer, ^{64}Cu-6DOTA-VEGF$_{121}$, was developed for this express purpose in patients with myocardial infarction.[120] The tracer is detectable by immunofluorescence microscopy in the infarct region and peaks with the changing levels of VEGFR expression in the tissue.

^{18}F-FHBG is a cardiac-specific reporter probe for use with micro-PET imaging in small animals. The reporter system was linked to VEGF to detect the impact of angiogenic therapy with an imaging-based approach.[121] Increased capillary density and small blood vessels were seen in the VEGF-treated myocardium before detectable increases in regional organ perfusion. These results provide evidence that a molecular reporter system can be developed in tandem with vasculogenic therapy.

During angiogenesis, there is upregulation of adhesion molecules, such as $\alpha_v\beta_3$ integrin. An ^{111}In-labeled quinolone (^{111}In-RP748) with high affinity and selectivity for $\alpha_v\beta_3$ integrin showed increased relative ^{111}In-RP748 uptake in acute myocardial infarcts, which persisted for at least 3 weeks post reperfusion (**Figure 29-20**).[122] The imaging of $\alpha_v\beta_3$ integrin by the PET imaging tracer, ^{18}F-Galakto-RGD, in a 35-year-old patient 2 weeks after a transmural myocardial infarction demonstrates the feasibility of using integrin-based imaging in human myocardial tissue (**Figure 29-21**).[123] A new biodegradable positron-emitting nanoprobe targeted at the $\alpha_v\beta_3$ integrin has been designed for noninvasive imaging of angiogenesis with a PET-based system[54] that promises an exciting future area of research.

Since collagen deposition and fibrosis in the failing heart are mediated by myofibroblasts, markers that indicate increased myofibroblast recruitment and activity are of interest. Myofibroblasts demonstrate an upregulation of integrins, leading to use of the ^{99m}Tc-labeled cy5.5-RGD peptide analogue, CRIP, to image upregulated $\alpha_v\beta_3$ integrins in a murine model of myocardial infarction.[124] A subgroup of animals was treated with either captopril or a combination of captopril and losartan to positively affect ventricular remodeling and visualize the effect on the CRIP-$\alpha_v\beta_3$ integrin signal. Ex vivo SPECT imaging of CRIP revealed lower signal intensity images in the treated hearts and correlated with smaller infarct size and increased LVEF, demonstrating the potential of integrin-targeted imaging in tracking response to therapy.

By radiolabeling molecules that target matrix metalloproteinases (MMPs), such as pharmacologic inhibitors

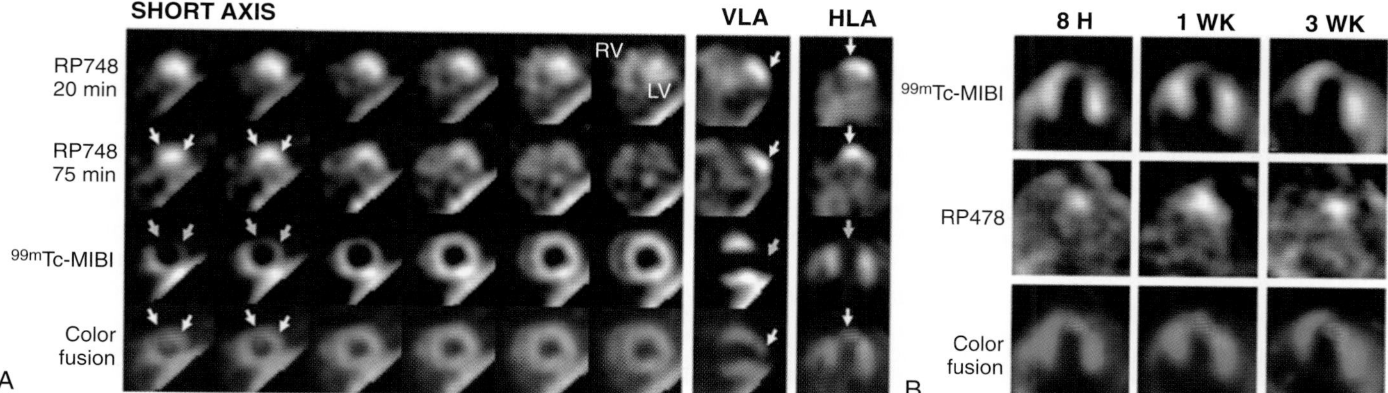

FIGURE 29-20 Angiogenesis demonstrated by in vivo ^{111}In-RP748 and ^{99m}Tc-sestamibi (^{99m}Tc-MIBI) images from dogs with chronic infarction. **A,** Serial in vivo canine ^{111}In-RP748 single photon emission computed tomography (SPECT) short-axis, vertical long-axis (VLA), and horizontal long-axis (HLA) images 3 weeks post-LAD infarction at 20 minutes and 75 minutes post injection. ^{111}In-RP748 SPECT images are shown registered with ^{99m}Tc-MIBI perfusion images *(third row).* The 75-minute ^{111}In-RP748 SPECT images were colored red and fused with MIBI images *(green)* to show localization of ^{111}In-RP748 activity within the heart *(color fusion, bottom row).* Right ventricular (RV) and left ventricular (LV) blood pool activity is seen at 20 minutes *(top row).* White arrows indicate region of increased ^{111}In-RP748 uptake in anterior wall. This corresponds to the anteroapical ^{99m}Tc-MIBI perfusion defect *(yellow arrows).* **B,** Sequential ^{99m}Tc-MIBI *(top row)* and ^{111}In-RP748 in vivo SPECT HLA images at 90 minutes post injection *(middle row)* from a dog at 8 hours, and 1 and 3 weeks post-LAD infarction. Increased myocardial ^{111}In-RP748 uptake is seen in the anteroapical wall at all three time points (although appears greatest 1 week postinfarction). Color fusion ^{99m}Tc-MIBI *(green)* and ^{111}In-RP748 *(red)* images *(bottom row)* demonstrate ^{111}In-RP748 uptake within ^{99m}Tc-MIBI perfusion defect. *Modified from Meoli DF, Sadeghi MM, Krassilnikova S, et al: Noninvasive imaging of myocardial angiogenesis following experimental myocardial infarction. J Clin Invest 113:1684–1691, 2004.*

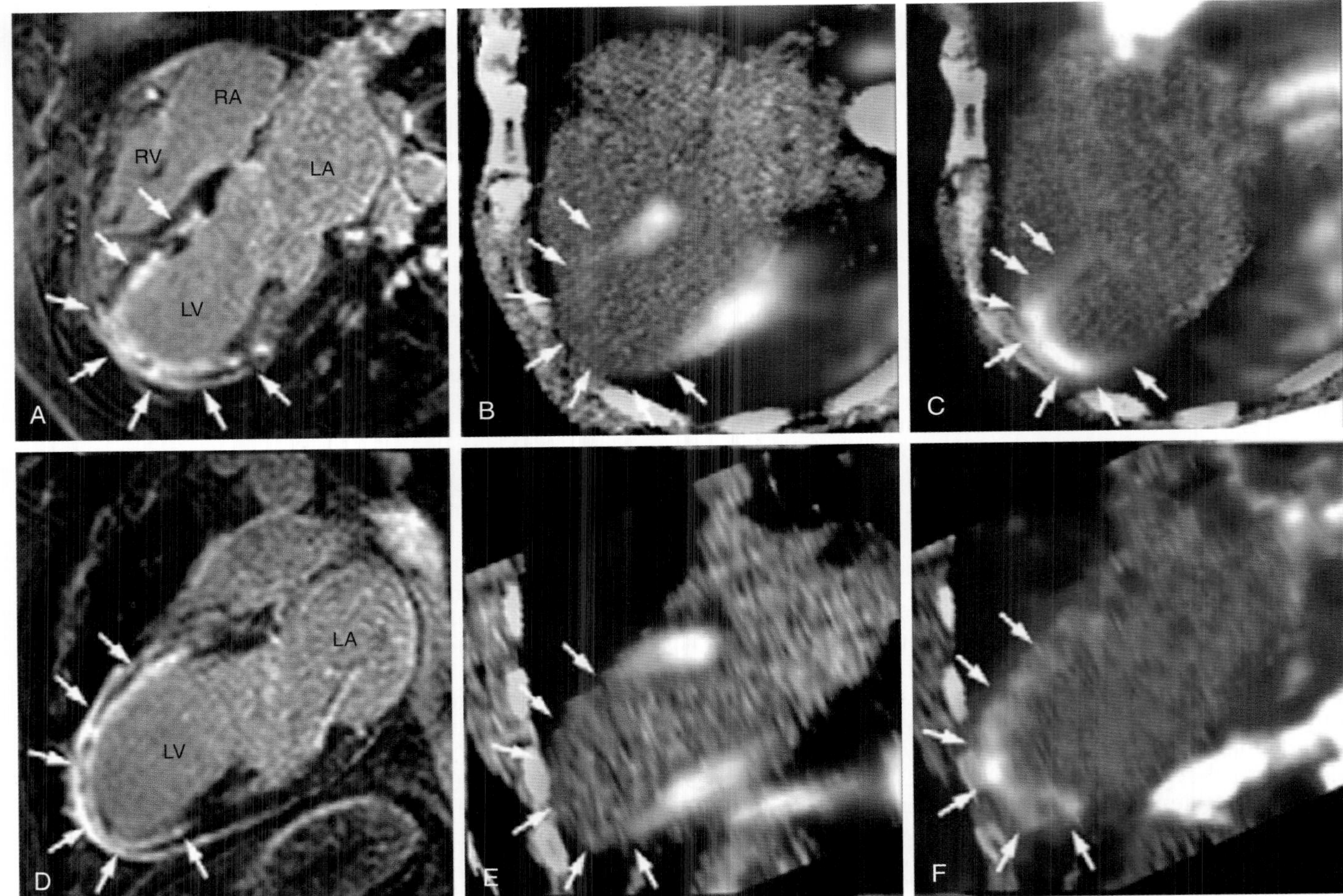

FIGURE 29-21 ^{18}F-Galakto-RGD positron emission tomography imaging. Cardiac magnetic resonance (CMR) image with extensive late gadolinium enhancement *(arrows)* from the anterior wall to the apical region in the four- **(A)** and two-chamber **(D)** views. **B** and **E,** Severely reduced myocardial blood flow shown using 13N-ammonia in similarly oriented images, corresponding to the regions of CMR delayed enhancement *(arrows).* **C** and **F,** Focal ^{18}F-RGD signal shown colocalized to the infarcted area. This signal likely reflects angiogenesis in the healing area *(arrows). Modified from Makowski MR, Ebersberger U, Nekolla S, et al: In vivo molecular imaging of angiogenesis, targeting alpha-v beta-3 integrin expression, in a patient after acute myocardial infarction. Eur Heart J 29:2201, 2008.*

that specifically bind to the catalytic domain, postinfarction MMP activation can be visualized in vivo (**Figure 29-22**).[125,126] Preclinical imaging studies were carried out using a ^{99m}Tc-labeled compound (^{99m}Tc-RP805) targeting MMP activation combined with hybrid SPECT/CT imaging. The hybrid method used a dual isotope imaging protocol with ^{99m}Tc-RP805 myocardial imaging and adjunctive ^{201}Tl perfusion imaging. These dual isotope imaging studies revealed significant MMP activation within the perfusion defect region, as well as lesser degrees of MMP activation in peri-infarct and remote areas of the heart. This suggests that MMP activation is taking place throughout the heart and supports the concept that molecules that target MMP activation may be used to evaluate ventricular remodeling.

Further imaging studies have been performed using ^{99m}Tc-labeled analog of RP782 (^{99m}Tc-RP805) and hybrid SPECT/CT imaging with a dual isotope protocol involving ^{99m}Tc-RP805 imaging and adjunctive ^{201}Tl-perfusion imaging. The dual isotope imaging studies showed MMP activation within the perfusion defect region, suggesting that MMP activation is taking place primarily within areas of injury and supports the concept that targeting MMP activation with imaging approaches might be used to evaluate ventricular remodeling.

Ischemic memory: Because ischemia leads to reduced fatty acid use and a transition to primarily glucose use, there is reduced 15-(*p*-[^{123}I]-iodophenyl)-3R,S-methyl pentadecanoic acid (BMIPP) uptake in ischemic tissue. Severe ischemia can lead to persistent suppression of fatty acid metabolism, so that loss of fatty acid metabolism can serve as a marker of myocardial "ischemic memory." Imaging of BMIPP acquired within 48 hours of the onset of chest pain demonstrated 74% sensitivity and 92% specificity for identifying coronary stenosis (**Figure 29-23**).[127] In heart failure, defects in myocardial BMIPP scintigraphy correlate with the severity of heart failure. Angiotensin II receptor blocker for 6 months improved BMIPP scintigraphy, suggesting that targeted metabolic imaging may serve as a useful tool in tracking therapeutic effectiveness.

Cardiac Magnetic Resonance

Four-dimensional flow for CRT optimization: Novel developments in pulse sequences have permitted visualization of intraventricular blood flow patterns. Using a noninvasive labeling technique that permits spatial tracking of regional flow, streamlines are formed that can follow 3-D blood flow over several heart cycles.[128] This 4-D (three dimensions over time) technique has been applied to large vessels (aorta),

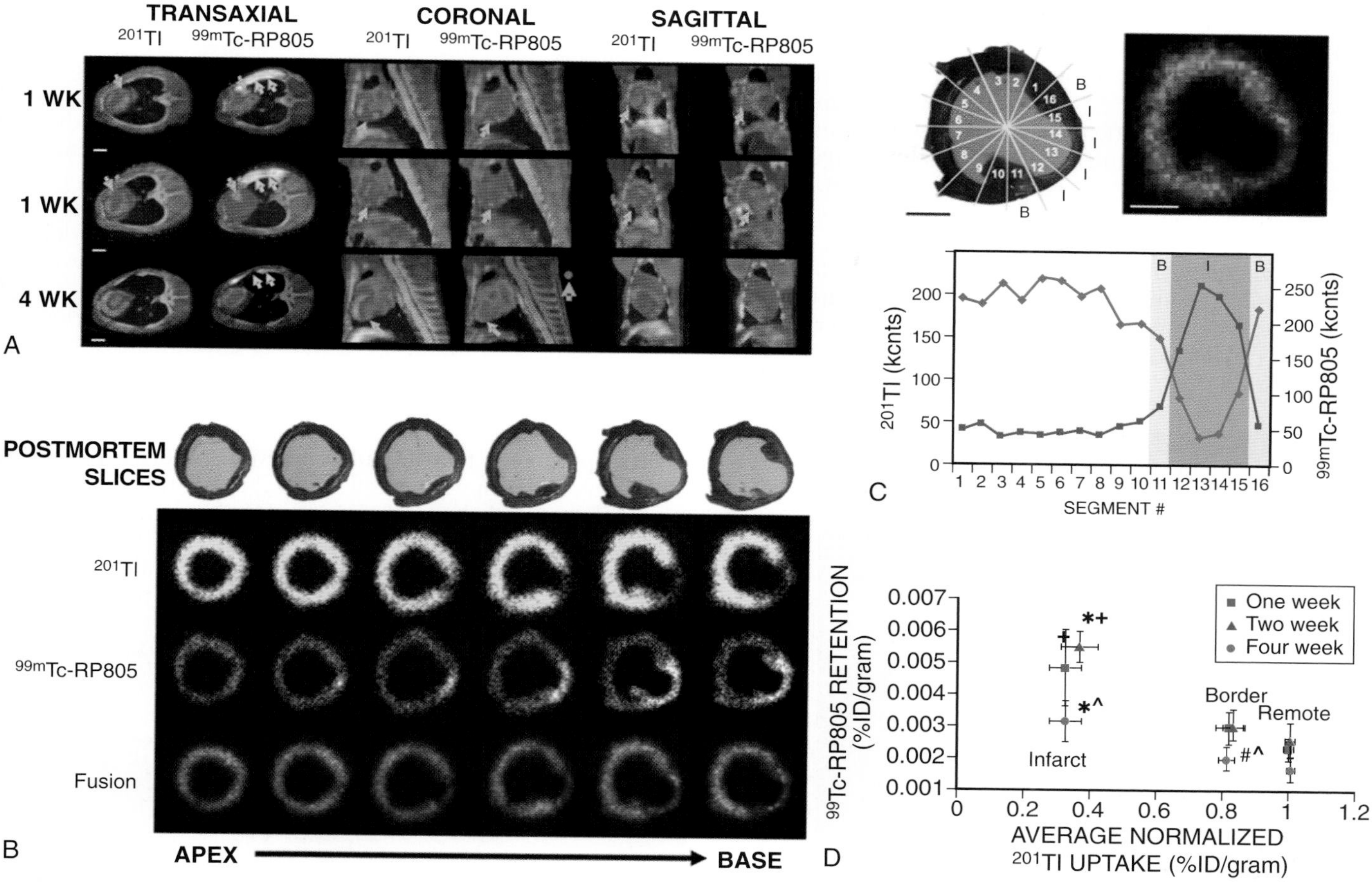

FIGURE 29-22 Dual-isotope in vivo single-photon emission computed tomography (SPECT)/CT imaging and ex vivo planar imaging of matrix metalloproteinase activation and perfusion. **A,** In vivo ^{201}Tl and ^{99m}Tc-RP805 SPECT/CT images of pig hearts at 1 week, 2 weeks, and 4 weeks after myocardial infarction (MI) are shown in transaxial, coronal, and sagittal views. Note the perfusion defect in the lateral wall and the time-dependent changes in the intensity of ^{99m}Tc-RP805 retention in the same regions *(green arrows)*. The yellow arrows point to ^{99m}Tc-RP805 activity in the surgical sternal wound. **B,** Postmortem short-axis myocardial slices filled with alginate are shown from a representative pig at 1 week post MI. Slices are oriented with the anterior wall on top. Below are the corresponding ex vivo short-axis ^{201}Tl perfusion images, ^{99m}Tc-RP805 images, and color-coded fused images (^{201}Tl, *green;* ^{99m}Tc-RP805, *red*). The infarct can be seen as a thinned fibrotic area in the lateral wall of the four most basal slices. The fused image clearly demonstrates maximal uptake of ^{99m}Tc-RP805 in the infarct region. **C,** Analysis of ^{201}Tl and ^{99m}Tc-RP805 radioactivity. Short-axis slice through the infarct region of a pig heart at 1 week after myocardial infarction, showing sections (numbered) used for determination of ^{201}Tl and ^{99m}Tc-RP805 uptake and corresponding ex vivo planar image of the same slice with circumferential count profiles of corresponding well-counting data. Increased ^{99m}Tc-RP805 activity in the region of diminished ^{201}Tl activity. **D,** Gamma well counting of ^{201}Tl and ^{99m}Tc-RP805 radioactivity. Correlation of the average relative myocardial ^{201}Tl activity and ^{99m}Tc-RP805 activity for infarct, border, and remote myocardial regions in pig hearts at 1, 2, and 4 weeks after MI as determined by gamma well counting. Notice that the relative ^{201}Tl perfusion deficit does not change over time, although there are dramatic time-dependent changes in ^{99m}Tc-RP805 activity. *P <0.05 versus remote. +P <0.05 versus border region, #P <0.05 versus 1 week post MI, ^P <0.05 versus 2 weeks post MI. *B,* Border region; *I,* infarct region. *Modified from Sahul ZH, Mukherjee R, Song J, et al: Targeted imaging of the spatial and temporal variation of matrix metalloproteinase activity in a porcine model of postinfarct remodeling: relationship to myocardial dysfunction. Circ Cardiovasc Imaging 4:381–391, 2011.*

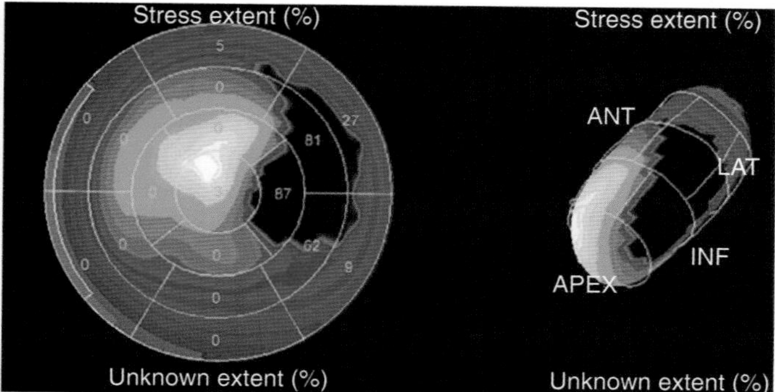

FIGURE 29-23 BMIPP SPECT imaging in a patient with suspected acute coronary syndrome. **A,** β-methyl-*p*-[^{123}I]-iodophenyl-pentadecanoic acid (BMIPP) single-photon emission computed tomography images demonstrating a large defect in the lateral wall. **B,** Corresponding coronary angiogram from the same patient demonstrating severe stenosis in the left circumflex coronary artery consistent with the vascular distribution of the BMIPP defect. *Modified from Kontos MC, Dilsizian V, Weiland F, et al: Iodofiltic acid I 123 (BMIPP) fatty acid imaging improves initial diagnosis in emergency department patients with suspected acute coronary syndromes: a multicenter trial. J Am Coll Cardiol 56:290, 2010.*

as well as the cardiac chambers, and allows assessment of slow flow areas, which are frequently adjacent to poorly contractile myocardium (**Figure 29-24**). Future CRT planning and optimization strategies may use these techniques to target areas for optimal lead placement. This may enable identification of patients who respond to CRT before device deployment to demonstrate efficacy and potentially improve response to CRT.

Creatine chemical exchange saturation transfer (CEST) imaging: The CEST technique is an MRI method that allows noninvasive detection of in vivo metabolites with exchangeable protons (such as glutamate and creatine) for use as endogenous biomarkers for disease detection and monitoring. Creatine is important in cellular bioenergetics in providing an energy balance in myocardial contraction, because ATP is generated from the conversion of phosphocreatine to creatine. Myocardial creatine may be imaged in high resolution by using the exchange of amine protons to bulk water, and the CEST technique affords two orders of magnitude greater sensitivity than conventional proton MR spectroscopy methods and allows more rapid data acquisition than other methods. Recent work has demonstrated the use of this technique in infarction and assessment of skeletal muscle energetics[129] (**Figure 29-25**). Future heart failure applications include effects of substrate changes on myocardial metabolism and energetics, testing of agents for myocardial preservation in ischemia/reperfusion injury, and assessment of skeletal muscle abnormalities in chronic congestive heart failure states.

Cardiac magnetic resonance assessment of myocardial fiber orientation: Changes in LV size and shape during the remodeling process result in altered fiber direction within the complex matrix of muscle sheets, bundles, and fibers that comprise the myocardial walls, and this leads to progressive ventricular distortion and dysfunction. Since the maximal myocardial force is generated along the axis of a fiber's direction, an improved understanding of the organization of myocardial architecture and fiber direction may aid in early disease detection and therapy. Recent studies have used MRI capabilities to detect fiber directions and map transmural myocardial architecture, even in the beating heart[130] (**Figure 29-26**). Understanding the mechanisms and constraints by which the heart remodels increases the likelihood of developing new and improved therapeutic strategies.

Cardiac magnetic resonance molecular imaging of apoptosis: A number of important signaling cascades resulting in programmed myocardial cell death have been identified and may be used to recognize cells or groups of cells that will not survive. Understanding mechanisms of cell death and the processes that modulate them may permit design of therapies for improving cell survival in heart failure and stress states such as ischemia/reperfusion injury. Most studies have used the ligand annexin V to bind to the cell surface of apoptotic cells, and many investigations have used radiotracers for detection of these cells. A recent MRI approach uses annexin-labeled nanoparticles, such as annexin-labeled cross-linked iron oxide [(CLIO)-Cy5.5] to

FIGURE 29-24 Four-dimensional (4-D) flow with CMR: pathline visualization of left ventricular flow patterns. Note the shorter red pathlines near the apex indicating slower blood flow, while the more basal yellow and green streamlines are longer and indicate more rapidly moving blood. *Courtesy Jonatan Eriksson, PhD, Carljohan Carlhäll, MD, Petter Dyverfeldt, PhD, Tino Ebbers, PhD, and Ann Bolger, MD.*

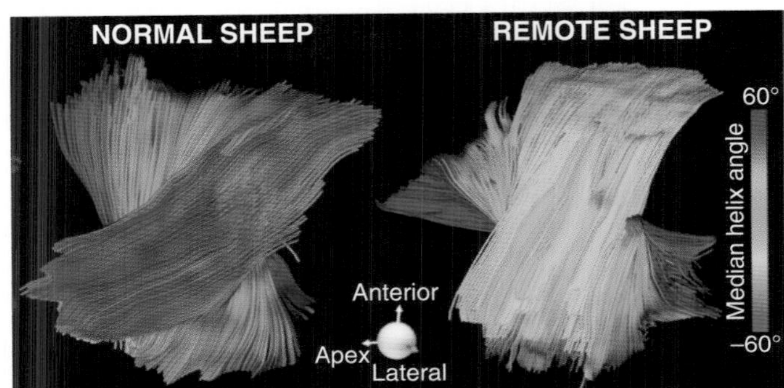

FIGURE 29-26 Noninvasive assessment of myocardial fiber orientation with cardiac magnetic resonance: These images identify the normal transmural fiber orientation pattern *(left)* and the altered fiber orientation pattern postinfarction on the right. The color pattern identifies both the layer (endocardial or epicardial) and direction of the fibers in that layer. Note the greater dispersion of fiber angles in the infarcted heart.

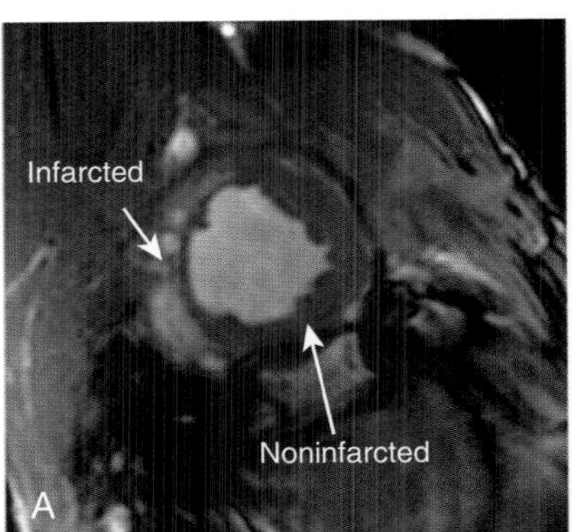

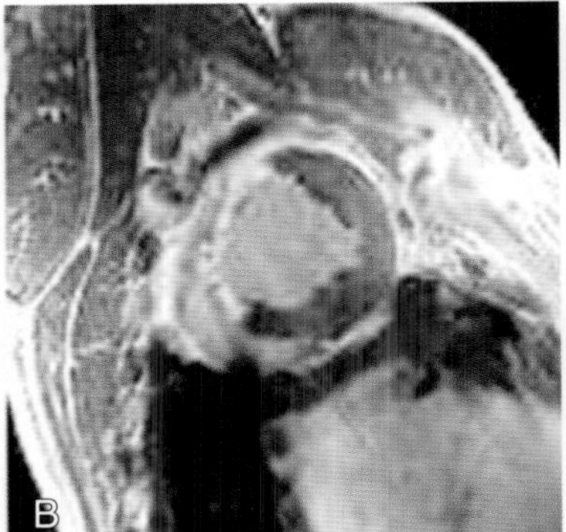

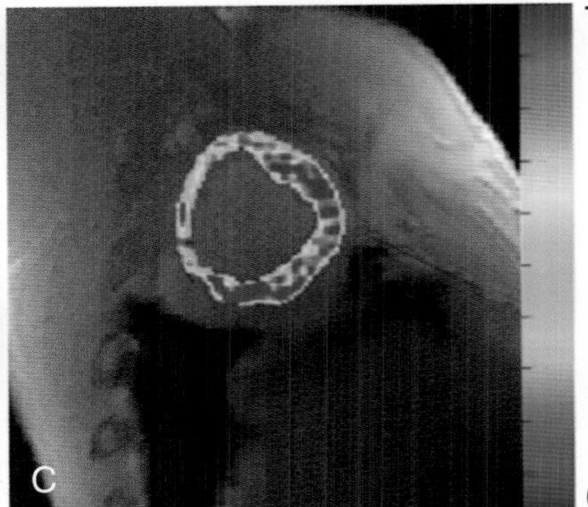

FIGURE 29-25 Creatine exchange saturation transfer (CrEST) imaging for direct imaging of high-energy phosphate metabolism: Left ventricular short-axis (3 Tesla) image at the midventricle in a chronic swine myocardial infarction model showing thinned areas (infarcted, *arrow*) and those of normal thickness (noninfarcted, *arrow*) **(A).** Late gadolinium enhancement images clearly depict the nonviable infarcted region *(bright/white tissue)* and noninfarcted tissue *(gray tissue)* **(B). C,** A CrEST pseudocolor map is shown of the same areas as in **B.** CrEST detects free creatine concentration in the tissue, and the mean CrEST contrast was 11.7% in the noninfarcted tissue and 6.4% in the infarcted territory. CrEST imaging provides two orders of magnitude greater sensitivity, significantly greater spatial resolution, and more rapid data acquisition than conventional proton magnetic resonance spectroscopy.

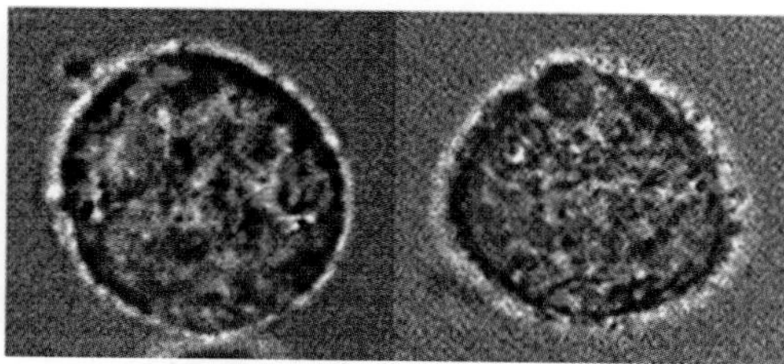

FIGURE 29-27 Cardiac magnetic resonance molecular imaging to assess myocyte apoptosis: Time lapse confocal microscopy shows the annexin cross-linked iron oxide nanoparticle bound predominantly to the apoptotic cell surface at less than 3 hours post incubation, but becomes internalized into the cells with more than 7 hours of exposure. Since the iron oxide is the component producing the signal in the annexin-bound nanoparticle complex, either location (surface or intracellular) will produce a contrast effect.

noninvasively image apoptotic cells in vivo. This agent not only permits detection of apoptotic cells, but has a cardioprotective effect by reducing cell death following injection[131] (**Figure 29-27**).

References

1. McMurray JJ, Adamopoulos S, Anker SD, et al: ESC guidelines for the diagnosis and treatment of acute and chronic heart failure 2012: the task force for the diagnosis and treatment of acute and chronic heart failure 2012 of the European Society of Cardiology. Developed in collaboration with the Heart Failure Association (HFA) of the ESC. *Eur Heart J* 33:1787–1847, 2012.
2. Yancy CW, Jessup M, Bozkurt B, et al: 2013 ACCF/AHA guideline for the management of heart failure: Executive summary: a report of the American College of Cardiology Foundation/American Heart Association task force on practice guidelines. *Circulation* 128:1810–1852, 2013.
3. Kirkpatrick JN, Vannan MA, Narula J, et al: Echocardiography in heart failure: applications, utility, and new horizons. *J Am Coll Cardiol* 50:381–396, 2007.
4. Mosterd A, Hoes AW: Clinical epidemiology of heart failure. *Heart* 93:1137–1146, 2007.
5. Taylor AJ, Cerqueira M, Hodgson JM, et al: ACCF/SCCT/ACR/AHA/ASE/ASNC/NASCI/SCAI/SCMR 2010 appropriate use criteria for cardiac computed tomography. A report of the American College of Cardiology Foundation appropriate use criteria task force, the Society of Cardiovascular Computed Tomography, the American College of Radiology, the American Heart Association, the American Society of Echocardiography, the American Society of Nuclear Cardiology, the North American Society for Cardiovascular Imaging, the Society for Cardiovascular Angiography and Interventions, and the Society for Cardiovascular Magnetic Resonance. *Circulation* 122:e525–e555, 2010.
6. Borlaug BA, Paulus WJ: Heart failure with preserved ejection fraction: pathophysiology, diagnosis, and treatment. *Eur Heart J* 32:670–679, 2011.
7. Brouwers FP, de Boer RA, van der Harst P, et al: Incidence and epidemiology of new onset heart failure with preserved vs. reduced ejection fraction in a community-based cohort: 11-year follow-up of PREVEND. *Eur Heart J* 34:1424–1431, 2013.
8. Pocock SJ, Ariti CA, McMurray JJ, et al: Predicting survival in heart failure: a risk score based on 39,372 patients from 30 studies. *Eur Heart J* 34:1404–1413, 2013.
9. Ky B, Plappert T, Kirkpatrick J, et al: Left ventricular remodeling in human heart failure: quantitative echocardiographic assessment of 1,794 patients. *Echocardiography* 29:758–765, 2012.
10. Zile MR, Baicu CF, Gaasch WH: Diastolic heart failure–abnormalities in active relaxation and passive stiffness of the left ventricle. *N Engl J Med* 350:1953–1959, 2004.
11. Paulus WJ, Tschope C, Sanderson JE, et al: How to diagnose diastolic heart failure: a consensus statement on the diagnosis of heart failure with normal left ventricular ejection fraction by the heart failure and echocardiography associations of the European Society of Cardiology. *Eur Heart J* 28:2539–2550, 2007.
12. Nagueh SF, Appleton CP, Gillebert TC, et al: Recommendations for the evaluation of left ventricular diastolic function by echocardiography. *Eur J Echocardiogr* 10:165–193, 2009.
13. Edelmann F, Wachter R, Schmidt AG, et al: Effect of spironolactone on diastolic function and exercise capacity in patients with heart failure with preserved ejection fraction: the aldo-DHF randomized controlled trial. *JAMA* 309:781–791, 2013.
14. Solomon SD, Zile M, Pieske B, et al: The angiotensin receptor neprilysin inhibitor LCZ696 in heart failure with preserved ejection fraction: a phase 2 double-blind randomised controlled trial. *Lancet* 380:1387–1395, 2012.
15. Massie BM, Carson PE, McMurray JJ, et al: Irbesartan in patients with heart failure and preserved ejection fraction. *N Engl J Med* 359:2456–2467, 2008.
16. Vasan RS, Benjamin EJ, Levy D: Prevalence, clinical features and prognosis of diastolic heart failure: an epidemiologic perspective. *J Am Coll Cardiol* 26:1565–1574, 1995.
17. Frohlich GM, Keller P, Schmid F, et al: Haemodynamically irrelevant pericardial effusion is associated with increased mortality in patients with chronic heart failure. *Eur Heart J* 34:1414–1423, 2013.
18. Thavendiranathan P, Grant AD, Negishi T, et al: Reproducibility of echocardiographic techniques for sequential assessment of left ventricular ejection fraction and volumes: application to patients undergoing cancer chemotherapy. *J Am Coll Cardiol* 61:77–84, 2013.
19. Linde C, Abraham WT, Gold MR, et al: Randomized trial of cardiac resynchronization in mildly symptomatic heart failure patients and in asymptomatic patients with left ventricular dysfunction and previous heart failure symptoms. *J Am Coll Cardiol* 52:1834–1843, 2008.
20. Tang AS, Wells GA, Talajic M, et al: Cardiac-resynchronization therapy for mild-to-moderate heart failure. *N Engl J Med* 363:2385–2395, 2010.
21. Curtis AB, Worley SJ, Adamson PB, et al: Biventricular pacing for atrioventricular block and systolic dysfunction. *N Engl J Med* 368:1585–1593, 2013.
22. Hunt SA, Abraham WT, Chin MH, et al: 2009 focused update incorporated into the ACC/AHA 2005 guidelines for the diagnosis and management of heart failure in adults. A report of the American College of Cardiology Foundation/American Heart Association task force on practice guidelines developed in collaboration with the International Society for Heart and Lung Transplantation. *J Am Coll Cardiol* 53:e1–e90, 2009.
23. Lang RM, Bierig M, Devereux RB, et al: Recommendations for chamber quantification. *Eur J Echocardiogr* 7:79–108, 2006.
24. St. John Sutton M, Pfeffer MA, Moye L, et al: Cardiovascular death and left ventricular remodeling two years after myocardial infarction: baseline predictors and impact of long-term use of captopril: information from the survival and ventricular enlargement (SAVE) trial. *Circulation* 96:3294–3299, 1997.
25. Effect of enalapril on survival in patients with reduced left ventricular ejection fractions and congestive heart failure. The SOLVD investigators. *N Engl J Med* 325:293–302, 1991.
26. Doddamani S, Bello R, Friedman MA, et al: Demonstration of left ventricular outflow tract eccentricity by real time 3D echocardiography: implications for the determination of aortic valve area. *Echocardiography* 24:860–866, 2007.
27. Amundsen BH, Helle-Valle T, Edvardsen T, et al: Noninvasive myocardial strain measurement by speckle tracking echocardiography: validation against sonomicrometry and tagged magnetic resonance imaging. *J Am Coll Cardiol* 47:789–793, 2006.
28. Lang RM, Badano LP, Tsang W, et al: EAE/ASE recommendations for image acquisition and display using three-dimensional echocardiography. *Eur Heart J Cardiovasc Imaging* 13:1–46, 2012.
29. Takeuchi M, Nishikage T, Mor-Avi V, et al: Measurement of left ventricular mass by real-time three-dimensional echocardiography: validation against magnetic resonance and comparison with two-dimensional and m-mode measurements. *J Am Soc Echocardiogr* 21:1001–1005, 2008.
30. Dobrucki LW, Sinusas AJ: PET and SPECT in cardiovascular molecular imaging. *Nat Rev Cardiol* 7:38–47, 2010.
31. Corbett JR, Jansen DE, Lewis SE, et al: Tomographic gated blood pool radionuclide ventriculography: analysis of wall motion and left ventricular volumes in patients with coronary artery disease. *J Am Coll Cardiol* 6:349–358, 1985.
32. Vallejo E, Dione DP, Sinusas AJ, et al: Assessment of left ventricular ejection fraction with quantitative gated SPECT: accuracy and correlation with first-pass radionuclide angiography. *J Nucl Cardiol* 7:461–470, 2000.
33. Shen MY, Liu YH, Sinusas AJ, et al: Quantification of regional myocardial wall thickening on electrocardiogram-gated SPECT imaging. *J Nucl Cardiol* 6:583–595, 1999.
34. Germano G, Kavanagh PB, Slomka PJ, et al: Quantitation in gated perfusion SPECT imaging: the Cedars-Sinai approach. *J Nucl Cardiol* 14:433–454, 2007.
35. Massardo T, Gal RA, Grenier RP, et al: Left ventricular volume calculation using a count-based ratio method applied to multigated radionuclide angiography. *J Nucl Med* 31:450–456, 1990.
36. Levy WC, Cerqueira MD, Matsuoka DT, et al: Four radionuclide methods for left ventricular volume determination: comparison of a manual and an automated technique. *J Nucl Med* 33:763–770, 1992.
37. Bonow RO: Radionuclide angiographic evaluation of left ventricular diastolic function. *Circulation* 84:I208–I215, 1991.
38. Carrio I, Cowie MR, Yamazaki J, et al: Cardiac sympathetic imaging with mIBG in heart failure. *JACC Cardiovasc Imaging* 3:92–100, 2010.
39. Link JM, Caldwell JH: Diagnostic and prognostic imaging of the cardiac sympathetic nervous system. *Nat Clin Pract Cardiovasc Med* 5(Suppl 2):S79–S86, 2008.
40. Henneman MM, Bengel FM, van der Wall EE, et al: Cardiac neuronal imaging: application in the evaluation of cardiac disease. *J Nucl Cardiol* 15:442–455, 2008.
41. Merlet P, Valette H, Dubois-Rande JL, et al: Prognostic value of cardiac metaiodobenzylguanidine imaging in patients with heart failure. *J Nucl Med* 33:471–477, 1992.
42. Tamaki S, Yamada T, Okuyama Y, et al: Cardiac iodine-123 metaiodobenzylguanidine imaging predicts sudden cardiac death independently of left ventricular ejection fraction in patients with chronic heart failure and left ventricular systolic dysfunction: results from a comparative study with signal-averaged electrocardiogram, heart rate variability, and QT dispersion. *J Am Coll Cardiol* 53:426–435, 2009.
43. Jacobson AF, Senior R, Cerqueira MD, et al: Myocardial iodine-123 meta-iodobenzylguanidine imaging and cardiac events in heart failure. Results of the prospective ADMIRE-HF (AdreView myocardial imaging for risk evaluation in heart failure) study. *J Am Coll Cardiol* 55:2212–2221, 2010.
44. Luisi AJ, Jr, Suzuki G, Dekemp R, et al: Regional 11C-hydroxyephedrine retention in hibernating myocardium: chronic inhomogeneity of sympathetic innervation in the absence of infarction. *J Nucl Med* 46:1368–1374, 2005.
45. Pietila M, Malminiemi K, Ukkonen H, et al: Reduced myocardial carbon-11 hydroxyephedrine retention is associated with poor prognosis in chronic heart failure. *Eur J Nucl Med* 28:373–376, 2001.
46. Fallavollita JA, Heavey BM, Luisi AJ, Jr, et al: Regional myocardial sympathetic denervation predicts the risk of sudden cardiac arrest in ischemic cardiomyopathy. *J Am Coll Cardiol* 63:141–149, 2014.
47. Grothues F, Smith GC, Moon JC, et al: Comparison of interstudy reproducibility of cardiovascular magnetic resonance with two-dimensional echocardiography in normal subjects and in patients with heart failure or left ventricular hypertrophy. *Am J Cardiol* 90:29–34, 2002.
48. Bellenger NG, Davies LC, Francis JM, et al: Reduction in sample size for studies of remodeling in heart failure by the use of cardiovascular magnetic resonance. *J Cardiovasc Magn Reson* 2:271–278, 2000.
49. Maceira AM, Prasad SK, Khan M, et al: Reference right ventricular systolic and diastolic function normalized to age, gender and body surface area from steady-state free precession cardiovascular magnetic resonance. *Eur Heart J* 27:2879–2888, 2006.
50. Dobrucki LW, Sinusas AJ: PET and SPECT in cardiovascular molecular imaging. *Nat Rev Cardiol* 7:38–47, 2010.

51. Herrmann HC, Pibarot P, Hueter I, et al: Predictors of mortality and outcomes of therapy in low-flow severe aortic stenosis: a placement of aortic transcatheter valves (PARTNER) trial analysis. *Circulation* 127:2316–2326, 2013.
52. Tzemos N, Therrien J, Yip J, et al: Outcomes in adults with bicuspid aortic valves. *JAMA* 300:1317–1325, 2008.
53. Keane MG, Wiegers SE, Plappert T, et al: Bicuspid aortic valves are associated with aortic dilatation out of proportion to coexistent valvular lesions. *Circulation* 102:III35–III39, 2000.
54. American College of Cardiology/American Heart Association Task Force on Practice Guidelines, Society of Cardiovascular Anesthesiologists, Society for Cardiovascular Angiography and Interventions, et al: ACC/AHA 2006 guidelines for the management of patients with valvular heart disease: a report of the American College of Cardiology/American Heart Association task force on practice guidelines (writing committee to revise the 1998 guidelines for the management of patients with valvular heart disease): developed in collaboration with the Society of Cardiovascular Anesthesiologists: endorsed by the Society for Cardiovascular Angiography and Interventions and the Society of Thoracic Surgeons. *Circulation* 114:e84–e231, 2006.
55. Higgins CB, Wagner S, Kondo C, et al: Evaluation of valvular heart disease with cine gradient echo magnetic resonance imaging. *Circulation* 84:1198–1207, 1991.
56. Globits S, Higgins CB: Assessment of valvular heart disease by magnetic resonance imaging. *Am Heart J* 129:369–381, 1995.
57. Caruthers SD, Lin SJ, Brown P, et al: Practical value of cardiac magnetic resonance imaging for clinical quantification of aortic valve stenosis: comparison with echocardiography. *Circulation* 108:2236–2243, 2003.
58. Friedrich MG, Schulz-Menger J, Poetsch T, et al: Quantification of valvular aortic stenosis by magnetic resonance imaging. *Am Heart J* 144:329–334, 2002.
59. John AS, Dill T, Brandt RR, et al: Magnetic resonance to assess the aortic valve area in aortic stenosis: how does it compare to current diagnostic standards? *J Am Coll Cardiol* 42:519–526, 2003.
60. Kupfahl C, Honold M, Meinhardt G, et al: Evaluation of aortic stenosis by cardiovascular magnetic resonance imaging: comparison with established routine clinical techniques. *Heart* 90:893–901, 2004.
61. Zaret BL, Wackers FJ, Terrin ML, et al: Assessment of global and regional left ventricular performance at rest and during exercise after thrombolytic therapy for acute myocardial infarction: results of the thrombolysis in myocardial infarction (TIMI) II study. *Am J Cardiol* 69:1–9, 1992.
62. Christian TF, Clements IP, Gibbons RJ: Noninvasive identification of myocardium at risk in patients with acute myocardial infarction and nondiagnostic electrocardiograms with technetium-99m-sestamibi. *Circulation* 83:1615–1620, 1991.
63. Pellikka PA, Behrenbeck T, Verani MS, et al: Serial changes in myocardial perfusion using tomographic technetium-99m-hexakis-2-methoxy-2-methylpropyl-isonitrile imaging following reperfusion therapy of myocardial infarction. *J Nucl Med* 31:1269–1275, 1990.
64. Gibbons RJ, Verani MS, Behrenbeck T, et al: Feasibility of tomographic 99mTc-hexakis-2-methoxy-2-methylpropyl-isonitrile imaging for the assessment of myocardial area at risk and the effect of treatment in acute myocardial infarction. *Circulation* 80:1277–1286, 1989.
65. Wackers FJ, Gibbons RJ, Verani MS, et al: Serial quantitative planar technetium-99m isonitrile imaging in acute myocardial infarction: efficacy for noninvasive assessment of thrombolytic therapy. *J Am Coll Cardiol* 14:861–873, 1989.
66. Gibbons RJ, Holmes DR, Reeder GS, et al: Immediate angioplasty compared with the administration of a thrombolytic agent followed by conservative treatment for myocardial infarction. The Mayo coronary care unit and catheterization laboratory groups. *N Engl J Med* 328:685–691, 1993.
67. O'Keefe JH, Jr, Grines CL, DeWood MA, et al: Factors influencing myocardial salvage with primary angioplasty. *J Nucl Cardiol* 2:35–41, 1995.
68. Christian TF, Behrenbeck T, Gersh BJ, et al: Relation of left ventricular volume and function over one year after acute myocardial infarction to infarct size determined by technetium-99m sestamibi. *Am J Cardiol* 68:21–26, 1991.
69. Lipiecki J, Cachin F, Durel N, et al: Influence of infarct-zone viability detected by rest Tc-99m sestamibi gated SPECT on left ventricular remodeling after acute myocardial infarction treated by percutaneous transluminal coronary angioplasty in the acute phase. *J Nucl Cardiol* 11:673–681, 2004.
70. Senior R, Kaul S, Raval U, et al: Impact of revascularization and myocardial viability determined by nitrate-enhanced Tc-99m sestamibi and Tl-201 imaging on mortality and functional outcome in ischemic cardiomyopathy. *J Nucl Cardiol* 9:454–462, 2002.
71. Shirani J, Lee J, Quigg R, et al: Relation of thallium uptake to morphologic features of chronic ischemic heart disease: evidence for myocardial remodeling in noninfarcted myocardium. *J Am Coll Cardiol* 38:84–90, 2001.
72. Kim RJ, Wu E, Rafael A, et al: The use of contrast-enhanced magnetic resonance imaging to identify reversible myocardial dysfunction. *N Engl J Med* 343:1445–1453, 2000.
73. Bello D, Shah DJ, Farah GM, et al: Gadolinium cardiovascular magnetic resonance predicts reversible myocardial dysfunction and remodeling in patients with heart failure undergoing beta-blocker therapy. *Circulation* 108:1945–1953, 2003.
74. Wolff SD, Schwitter J, Coulden R, et al: Myocardial first-pass perfusion magnetic resonance imaging: a multicenter dose-ranging study. *Circulation* 110:732–737, 2004.
75. Schwitter J, Wacker CM, van Rossum AC, et al: MR-IMPACT: comparison of perfusion-cardiac magnetic resonance with single-photon emission computed tomography for the detection of coronary artery disease in a multicentre, multivendor, randomized trial. *Eur Heart J* 29:480–489, 2008.
76. Greenwood JP, Maredia N, Younger JF, et al: Cardiovascular magnetic resonance and single-photon emission computed tomography for diagnosis of coronary heart disease (CE-MARC): a prospective trial. *Lancet* 379:453–460, 2012.
77. Dall'Armellina E, Morgan TM, Mandapaka S, et al: Prediction of cardiac events in patients with reduced left ventricular ejection fraction with dobutamine cardiovascular magnetic resonance assessment of wall motion score index. *J Am Coll Cardiol* 52:279–286, 2008.
78. Korosoglou G, Lossnitzer D, Schellberg D, et al: Strain-encoded cardiac MRI as an adjunct for dobutamine stress testing: incremental value to conventional wall motion analysis. *Circ Cardiovasc Imaging* 2:132–140, 2009.
79. Kuijpers D, Ho KY, van Dijkman PR, et al: Dobutamine cardiovascular magnetic resonance for the detection of myocardial ischemia with the use of myocardial tagging. *Circulation* 107:1592–1597, 2003.
80. Scott CH, Sutton MS, Gusani N, et al: Effect of dobutamine on regional left ventricular function measured by tagged magnetic resonance imaging in normal subjects. *Am J Cardiol* 83:412–417, 1999.
81. Thomas D, Strach K, Meyer C, et al: Combined myocardial stress perfusion imaging and myocardial stress tagging for detection of coronary artery disease at 3 tesla. *J Cardiovasc Magn Reson* 10:59, 2008.
82. Kim RJ, Albert TS, Wible JH, et al: Performance of delayed-enhancement magnetic resonance imaging with gadoversetamide contrast for the detection and assessment of myocardial infarction: an international, multicenter, double-blinded, randomized trial. *Circulation* 117:629–637, 2008.
83. Wagner A, Mahrholdt H, Holly TA, et al: Contrast-enhanced MRI and routine single photon emission computed tomography (SPECT) perfusion imaging for detection of subendocardial myocardial infarcts: an imaging study. *Lancet* 361:374–379, 2003.
84. Kwong RY, Chan AK, Brown KA, et al: Impact of unrecognized myocardial scar detected by cardiac magnetic resonance imaging on event-free survival in patients presenting with signs or symptoms of coronary artery disease. *Circulation* 113:2733–2743, 2006.
85. Abbasi SA, Ertel A, Shah RV, et al: Impact of cardiovascular magnetic resonance on management and clinical decision-making in heart failure patients. *J Cardiovasc Magn Reson* 15:89, 2013.
86. Effects of enalapril on mortality in severe congestive heart failure. Results of the Cooperative North Scandinavian Enalapril Survival study (CONSENSUS). The CONSENSUS Trial Study Group. *N Engl J Med* 316:1429–1435, 1987.
87. Pitt B, Zannad F, Remme WJ, et al: The effect of spironolactone on morbidity and mortality in patients with severe heart failure. Randomized aldactone evaluation study investigators. *N Engl J Med* 341:709–717, 1999.
88. Sutton MG, Plappert T, Hilpisch KE, et al: Sustained reverse left ventricular structural remodeling with cardiac resynchronization at one year is a function of etiology: quantitative doppler echocardiographic evidence from the Multicenter InSync Randomized Clinical Evaluation (MIRACLE). *Circulation* 113:266–272, 2006.
89. Gaasch WH, Delorey DE, St John Sutton MG, et al: Patterns of structural and functional remodeling of the left ventricle in chronic heart failure. *Am J Cardiol* 102:459–462, 2008.
90. Linde C, Gold MR, Abraham WT, et al: Long-term impact of cardiac resynchronization therapy in mild heart failure: 5-year results from the REsynchronization reVErses remodeling in systolic left vEntricular dysfunction (REVERSE) study. *Eur Heart J* 34:2592–2599, 2013.
91. Wu KC, Zerhouni EA, Judd RM, et al: Prognostic significance of microvascular obstruction by magnetic resonance imaging in patients with acute myocardial infarction. *Circulation* 97:765–772, 1998.
92. Abdel-Aty H, Zagrosek A, Schulz-Menger J, et al: Delayed enhancement and T2-weighted cardiovascular magnetic resonance imaging differentiate acute from chronic myocardial infarction. *Circulation* 109:2411–2416, 2004.
93. Abdel-Aty H, Cocker M, Meek C, et al: Edema as a very early marker for acute myocardial ischemia: a cardiovascular magnetic resonance study. *J Am Coll Cardiol* 53:1194–1201, 2009.
94. Kidambi A, Mather AN, Motwani M, et al: The effect of microvascular obstruction and intramyocardial hemorrhage on contractile recovery in reperfused myocardial infarction: insights from cardiovascular magnetic resonance. *J Cardiovasc Magn Reson* 15:58, 2013.
95. Chung ES, Leon AR, Tavazzi L, et al: Results of the predictors of response to CRT (PROSPECT) trial. *Circulation* 117:2608–2616, 2008.
96. Feldman AM, de Lissovoy G, Bristow MR, et al: Cost effectiveness of cardiac resynchronization therapy in the comparison of medical therapy, pacing, and defibrillation in heart failure (COMPANION) trial. *J Am Coll Cardiol* 46:2311–2321, 2005.
97. Ghio S, Freemantle N, Scelsi L, et al: Long-term left ventricular reverse remodelling with cardiac resynchronization therapy: results from the CARE-HF trial. *Eur J Heart Fail* 11:480–488, 2009.
98. Moss AJ, Hall WJ, Cannom DS, et al: Cardiac-resynchronization therapy for the prevention of heart-failure events. *N Engl J Med* 361:1329–1338, 2009.
99. Chen J, Boogers MJ, Bax JJ, et al: The use of nuclear imaging for cardiac resynchronization therapy. *Curr Cardiol Rep* 12:185–191, 2010.
100. Friehling M, Chen J, Saba S, et al: A prospective pilot study to evaluate the relationship between acute change in left ventricular synchrony after cardiac resynchronization therapy and patient outcome using a single-injection gated SPECT protocol. *Circ Cardiovasc Imaging* 4:532–539, 2011.
101. Toussaint JF, Lavergne T, Kerrou K, et al: Basal asynchrony and resynchronization with biventricular pacing predict long-term improvement of LV function in heart failure patients. *Pacing Clin Electrophysiol* 26:1815–1823, 2003.
102. Chalil S, Stegemann B, Muhyaldeen SA, et al: Effect of posterolateral left ventricular scar on mortality and morbidity following cardiac resynchronization therapy. *Pacing Clin Electrophysiol* 30:1201–1209, 2007.
103. Shetty AK, Duckett SG, Ginks MR, et al: Cardiac magnetic resonance-derived anatomy, scar, and dyssynchrony fused with fluoroscopy to guide LV lead placement in cardiac resynchronization therapy: a comparison with acute haemodynamic measures and echocardiographic reverse remodelling. *Eur Heart J Cardiovasc Imaging* 14:692–699, 2013.
104. Leyva F, Taylor RJ, Foley PW, et al: Left ventricular midwall fibrosis as a predictor of mortality and morbidity after cardiac resynchronization therapy in patients with nonischemic cardiomyopathy. *J Am Coll Cardiol* 60:1659–1667, 2012.
105. Kenchaiah S, Pfeffer MA, St John Sutton M, et al: Effect of antecedent systemic hypertension on subsequent left ventricular dilation after acute myocardial infarction (from the survival and ventricular enlargement trial). *Am J Cardiol* 94:1–8, 2004.
106. Johnson LL, Seldin DW, Becker LC, et al: Antimyosin imaging in acute transmural myocardial infarctions: results of a multicenter clinical trial. *J Am Coll Cardiol* 13:27–35, 1989.
107. Khaw BA, Gold HK, Yasuda T, et al: Scintigraphic quantification of myocardial necrosis in patients after intravenous injection of myosin-specific antibody. *Circulation* 74:501–508, 1986.
108. Dec GW, Palacios I, Yasuda T, et al: Antimyosin antibody cardiac imaging: its role in the diagnosis of myocarditis. *J Am Coll Cardiol* 16:97–104, 1990.
109. Martin ME, Moya-Mur JL, Casanova M, et al: Role of noninvasive antimyosin imaging in infants and children with clinically suspected myocarditis. *J Nucl Med* 45:429–437, 2004.
110. Narula J, Khaw BA, Dec GW, et al: Diagnostic accuracy of antimyosin scintigraphy in suspected myocarditis. *J Nucl Cardiol* 3:371–381, 1996.
111. Okamoto H, Imanaka-Yoshida K: Matricellular proteins: new molecular targets to prevent heart failure. *Cardiovasc Ther* 30:e198–e209, 2012.
112. Fujimoto N, Onishi K, Sato A, et al: Incremental prognostic values of serum tenascin-C levels with blood B-type natriuretic peptide testing at discharge in patients with dilated cardiomyopathy and decompensated heart failure. *J Card Fail* 15:898–905, 2009.
113. Tait JF: Imaging of apoptosis. *J Nucl Med* 49:1573–1576, 2008.
114. Martin SJ, Reutelingsperger CP, McGahon AJ, et al: Early redistribution of plasma membrane phosphatidylserine is a general feature of apoptosis regardless of the initiating stimulus: inhibition by overexpression of bcl-2 and abl. *J Exp Med* 182:1545–1556, 1995.
115. Hofstra L, Liem IH, Dumont EA, et al: Visualisation of cell death in vivo in patients with acute myocardial infarction. *Lancet* 356:209–212, 2000.
116. Kietselaer BL, Reutelingsperger CP, Boersma HH, et al: Noninvasive detection of programmed cell loss with 99mTc-labeled annexin A5 in heart failure. *J Nucl Med* 48:562–567, 2007.
117. Narula J, Petrov A, Pak KY, et al: Very early noninvasive detection of acute experimental nonreperfused myocardial infarction with 99mTc-labeled glucarate. *Circulation* 95:1577–1584, 1997.
118. Flotats A, Carrio I: Non-invasive in vivo imaging of myocardial apoptosis and necrosis. *Eur J Nucl Med Mol Imaging* 30:615–630, 2003.
119. Mariani G, Villa G, Rossettin PF, et al: Detection of acute myocardial infarction by 99mTc-labeled D-glucaric acid imaging in patients with acute chest pain. *J Nucl Med* 40:1832–1839, 1999.

120. Rodriguez-Porcel M, Cai W, Gheysens O, et al: Imaging of VEGF receptor in a rat myocardial infarction model using PET. *J Nucl Med* 49:667–673, 2008.
121. Wu JC, Chen IY, Wang Y, et al: Molecular imaging of the kinetics of vascular endothelial growth factor gene expression in ischemic myocardium. *Circulation* 110:685–691, 2004.
122. Kalinowski L, Dobrucki LW, Meoli DF, et al: Targeted imaging of hypoxia-induced integrin activation in myocardium early after infarction. *J Appl Physiol (1985)* 104:1504–1512, 2008.
123. Almutairi A, Rossin R, Shokeen M, et al: Biodegradable dendritic positron-emitting nanoprobes for the noninvasive imaging of angiogenesis. *Proc Natl Acad Sci U S A* 106:685–690, 2009.
124. van den Borne SW, Isobe S, Verjans JW, et al: Molecular imaging of interstitial alterations in remodeling myocardium after myocardial infarction. *J Am Coll Cardiol* 52:2017–2028, 2008.
125. Su H, Spinale FG, Dobrucki LW, et al: Noninvasive targeted imaging of matrix metalloproteinase activation in a murine model of postinfarction remodeling. *Circulation* 112:3157–3167, 2005.
126. Sahul ZH, Mukherjee R, Song J, et al: Targeted imaging of the spatial and temporal variation of matrix metalloproteinase activity in a porcine model of postinfarct remodeling: relationship to myocardial dysfunction. *Circ Cardiovasc Imaging* 4:381–391, 2011.
127. Kontos MC, Dilsizian V, Weiland F, et al: Iodofiltic acid I 123 (BMIPP) fatty acid imaging improves initial diagnosis in emergency department patients with suspected acute coronary syndromes: a multicenter trial. *J Am Coll Cardiol* 56:290–299, 2010.
128. Markl M, Kilner PJ, Ebbers T: Comprehensive 4D velocity mapping of the heart and great vessels by cardiovascular magnetic resonance. *J Cardiovasc Magn Reson* 13:7, 2011.
129. Cai K, Haris M, Singh A, et al: Magnetic resonance imaging of glutamate. *Nat Med* 18:302–306, 2012.
130. Mekkaoui C, Huang S, Chen HH, et al: Fiber architecture in remodeled myocardium revealed with a quantitative diffusion CMR tractography framework and histological validation. *J Cardiovasc Magn Reson* 14:70, 2012.
131. Chen HH, Yuan H, Josephson L, et al: Theranostic imaging of the kinases and proteases that modulate cell death and survival. *Theranostics* 2:148–155, 2012.

The Use of Biomarkers in the Evaluation of Patients with Heart Failure

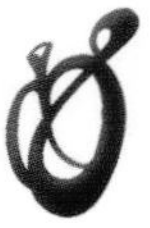

Hanna K. Gaggin and James L. Januzzi, Jr

The clinical syndrome of heart failure (HF) is characterized by the inability of cardiac output to meet the needs of the body, and can result from a multitude of cardiovascular disease processes. Accordingly, the underlying mechanisms in the development and progression of HF are complex, and involve an intricate interplay of cardiac strain and injury, tissue inflammation, neurohumoral activation, oxidative stress, and ventricular remodeling, all compounded by the impact of comorbidities, such as cardiorenal interactions and other medical conditions.

Traditionally, diagnostic evaluation of patients suspected of having HF has involved history, physical examination, and chest x-ray (see Chapter 28). However, the complex diagnosis of HF by clinical presentation alone may be challenging, because patients often have signs and symptoms that are vague and nonspecific. In fact, isolated findings from history or physical examination correlate poorly with objective methods of cardiac function, and clinical criteria that combine relevant findings perform poorly in accurately diagnosing HF (sensitivity 50%-73% and specificity 54%-78%). This challenge is associated with delays in definitive diagnosis and treatment, increased health care expenditures, and ultimately with poor prognosis. Although noninvasive and invasive diagnostic studies complement the initial history and physical examination in the evaluation of the HF patient, such methods, including echocardiography and right-heart catheterization, have limitations and the routine use of these methods is associated with significant cost and potential risk.

Given the complexity of HF biology—which includes processes that are not easily detectable with physical examination or imaging techniques—increased interest has been given to the use of biomarkers to supplement clinical judgment; many biomarkers are conveniently measured and easily interpretable and may support clinical evaluation, while at the same time reflecting important pathophysiologies involved in HF presence, severity, and prognosis.

BIOMARKERS IN HEART FAILURE: A HISTORICAL PERSPECTIVE

The early concept of biomarker testing in HF goes back decades, but among the earliest mentions of biomarker measurement in HF may be found in work by Braunwald and colleagues from the 1950s, where a crude version of a C-reactive protein (CRP) assay was first used to analyze serum from patients with advanced HF. In this context, elevated CRP concentrations were commonly present. Subsequent studies by this group examined measurement of norepinephrine in both blood and urine of patients with advanced HF; additionally, the detection of norepinephrine synthesis in the heart led to the visionary description of the heart as an endocrine organ,[1] hypothesizing clinical value from measurement of circulating substances produced by the myocardium.

In parallel, following very early electron microscopy studies in the 1950s revealing dense granules in the atrial myocardium quite comparable to those found in glandular tissue, pursuit of an atrial factor with endocrine, paracrine, and autocrine effects on the cardiovascular system followed. The pioneering work of Adolfo de Bold in 1981 led to the discovery of atrial natriuretic peptide (ANP). Following observations that the presence and density of atrial granules changed with intravascular volume, experiments were performed where intravenous injection of atrial myocardial extracts led to a rapid diuretic and natriuretic response in rats. Subsequent isolation and identification of the peptides responsible for this effect led to the first descriptions of the natriuretic peptide family.

The modern era of HF biomarker testing began in the early 2000s when large-scale clinical trials demonstrated the value of both B-type natriuretic peptide (BNP) and its amino-terminal propeptide counterpart (NT-proBNP).[2,3] These pivotal studies heralded the onset of the era of HF biomarkers. With more modern techniques of proteomics and mass spectroscopy becoming more widely available to stimulate biomarker discovery, a wave of studies pursuing other novel biomarkers followed.

BIOMARKERS: DEFINITION AND GUIDELINES FOR EVALUATION

Although biomarkers may be measured from multiple sources, most frequently, they are obtained from blood or urine samples; this chapter will focus on biomarkers derived from such sources. In general, a biomarker is typically a protein compound, quantifiable, easily available (at a reasonable cost and turnaround time), and indicative of the

TABLE 30-1 2013 ACC/AHA Heart Failure Guideline Recommendations for the Use of Biomarkers in Heart Failure

BIOMARKERS		CLASS OF RECOMMENDATION	LEVEL OF EVIDENCE
BNP or NT-proBNP	Diagnosis	I	A
	Prognosis	I	A
	Guided-therapy (chronic HF)	IIa	B
	Guided-therapy (acute HF)	IIb	C
Troponin T or I (Myocardial injury)	Prognosis	I	A
sST2, Galectin-3 (Myocardial fibrosis)	Prognosis	IIb	B for chronic A for acute

BNP, B-type natriuretic peptide; *HF,* heart failure; *sST2,* soluble ST2.
From Yancy CW, Jessup M, Bozkurt B, et al: 2013 ACCF/AHA guideline for the management of heart failure: a report of the American College of Cardiology Foundation/American Heart Association task force on practice guidelines. Circulation 128:e240–327, 2013.

biologic process underlying the disease, providing a special insight into the microcosms surrounding the disease.

As articulated by van Kimmenade and Januzzi,[4] measurement of a HF biomarker should be easily achieved through the use of assays with acceptable analytic precision and provide accurate results with well-defined biologic variation. The biomarker candidate should primarily reflect important processes involved in HF pathophysiology, and should not recapitulate clinical information already available at the bedside. The study of HF biomarkers should be appropriate to the clinical use being evaluated and design should be rigorous; new assays should be evaluated across a wide range of HF patients, and the statistical methods used to evaluate the biomarker (relative to clinical variables, as well as other biomarkers) should be contemporary and robust.

MAJOR SOCIETY GUIDELINES

Several major societies have set forth clinical practice guidelines for the diagnosis, prognosis, and treatment of HF, including the recent update by the American Heart Association/American College of Cardiology writing group on HF.[5] The use of BNP and NT-proBNP is now recommended in the routine evaluation of HF for the purposes of diagnosis and in determining prognosis. In point of fact, the recent ACC/AHA guideline update (**Table 30-1**) has given natriuretic peptide testing a class I (level of evidence A) for both diagnosis and prognosis of HF, while also upgrading the use of both natriuretic peptides for HF management to a class II recommendation. As will be discussed later, recent clinical practice guideline updates have considered the role of more novel biomarkers; troponin testing for risk assessment was given a class I (level of evidence A), whereas both soluble (s)ST2 and galectin-3 (biomarkers of myocardial fibrosis) were given a class II recommendation.

HEART FAILURE BIOMARKERS

A vast number of biomarkers in HF have been examined to date (examples are shown in **Table 30-2**). No single, standardized categorization of HF biomarkers exists, although several have been proposed. Braunwald suggested that markers may be considered in the following categories: (1) myocardial stretch, (2) myocyte injury, (3) extracellular matrix remodeling, (4) inflammation, (5) renal dysfunction, (6) neurohumoral activation, and (7) oxidative stress

TABLE 30-2 Biomarkers of Heart Failure

Myocardial Insult

• Myocyte stretch
  • BNP, NT-proBNP, MR-proANP
• Myocardial necrosis
  • Troponin T, troponin I, myosin light-chain kinase I, heart-type fatty-acid protein, CKMB
• Oxidative stress
  • Myeloperoxidase, uric acid, oxidized low-density lipoproteins, urinary biopyrrins, urinary and plasma isoprostanes, plasma malodialdehyde

Neurohormonal Activation

• Sympathetic nervous system
  • Norepinephrine, chromogranin A, MR-proADM
• Renin-angiotensin system
  • Renin, angiotensin II, aldosterone
• Arginine vasopressin system
  • Arginine vasopressin, copeptin
• Endothelins

Remodeling

• Inflammation
  • C-reactive protein, TNF-α, Fas, soluble TNF receptors, interleukins (1, 6, and 18), osteoprotegerin
• Hypertrophy/fibrosis
  • Soluble ST2, galectin-3
• Extracellular matrix remodeling
  • Collagen propeptides (PINP, PIIINP), matrix metalloproteinases (MMP-2, MMP-4, MMP-8), tissue inhibitors of MMP (TIMPS)
• Apoptosis
  • GDF-15
• Miscellaneous
  • MicroRNA, quiescin Q6, soluble fms-like tyrosine kinase-1 (also known as VEGFR-1)

Markers of Comorbidity

• Renal biomarkers
  • Renal function
    • Creatinine, BUN, eGFR, cystatin C, β trace protein
  • Renal injury markers
    • NGAL, KIM-1, NAG, liver-type fatty acid binding protein, IL-18
• Hematologic biomarkers
  • Hemoglobin, RDW
• Liver function tests
• Albumin
• Adiponectin

BNP, B-type natriuretic peptide; *BUN,* blood urea nitrogen; *CKMB,* creatine kinase-MB; *eGFR,* estimated glomerular filtration rate; *GDF,* growth differentiation factor; *MMP,* matrix metalloproteinases; *NAG, N*-acetyl β-(D)-glucosaminidase; *NGAL,* neutrophil-gelatinase–associated lipocalin; *RDW,* red blood cell distribution width; *TNF,* tumor necrosis factor

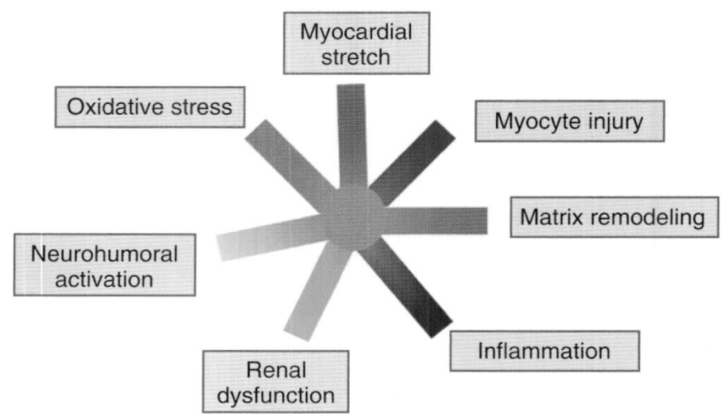

FIGURE 30-1 Schema for heart failure biomarker classification. *From Braunwald E: Heart failure. JACC Heart Failure 1:1–20, 2013.*

(**Figure 30-1**).[6] Clearly, significant overlaps among these various processes exist, which may allow further simplification of biomarker categories to (1) myocardial insult, (2) neurohormonal activation, (3) myocardial remodeling, and (4) markers of comorbidity.

Myocardial Insult

Various myocardial insults are among the initiating event in the cascade of changes that occur in HF. Within the context of myocardial insult are subcategories of biomarkers that reflect myocardial stretch, myocyte necrosis, and oxidative stress.

Myocardial Stretch

As noted, dense granules were noted in tissue derived from the atria of the heart by electron microscopy in the 1950s. Further, stretching of the canine left atrium was shown to increase urine output, and injection of atrial homogenates into rats caused diuresis and natriuresis. ANP was subsequently purified, sequenced, and reproduced. In the 1980s, a homologous peptide with similar biologic activity was discovered in porcine brain and named BNP. Soon other natriuretic peptides, sharing similar structural features, were discovered: urodilantin (a renally active isoform of ANP), C-type natriuretic peptide, and *Dendroaspis* natriuretic peptide, the latter found in snake venom. Although each of the natriuretic peptide family of markers is of potential use in the evaluation and management of the patient with HF, BNP and NT-proBNP are most studied, whereas ANP has been increasingly examined.[7]

BNP and NT-proBNP

Left ventricular (LV) wall stretch from increased pressure or volume is the most potent inducer of BNP gene transcription. One of the early products of the BNP gene is a 108-amino-acid peptide, $proBNP_{1-108}$, which is subsequently cleaved into the biologically active 32-amino-acid peptide, BNP, and a biologically inert 76-amino-acid peptide, NT-proBNP. Both BNP and NT-proBNP are released into the bloodstream within minutes of their synthesis. In addition, varying amounts of uncleaved $proBNP_{1-108}$ are released. Although the cause of this observation is not understood, it is now known that such concentrations of $proBNP_{1-108}$ are produced in increasing amounts in more advanced HF. Furthermore, the conventional assays for BNP or NT-proBNP measurement cross-react with circulating $proBNP_{1-108}$, which means that the overall measured natriuretic peptide value in patients evaluated clinically contains a mixture of cleaved and uncleaved peptide.

BNP binds to membrane-bound natriuretic peptide receptors (NPR) type A and B, activating intracellular cyclic guanosine monophosphate (cGMP) and beginning a cascade of events leading to natriuresis, diuresis, vasodilation, inhibition of renin and aldosterone, and inhibition of fibrosis. Besides being removed by receptor-mediated mechanisms (including by the NPR C receptor), BNP is also degraded by various enzymatic processes, including neutral endopeptidases, meprin-A, and dipeptidyl peptidase-IV. As well, BNP is cleared passively by numerous organs with high blood flows. Because of the multitude of means by which BNP is removed from circulation, the half-life of BNP is approximately 20 minutes. In contrast, NT-proBNP is only passively cleared by multiple organs including the kidneys.[8]

A major misconception about clearance of BNP and NT-proBNP relates to the degree of dependence on renal function for their removal from the circulation. Mechanistic studies actually suggest the degree of renal clearance to be identical for both BNP and NT-proBNP, with approximately 25% of both being cleared by renal mechanisms, down to an estimated glomerular filtration rate (eGFR) of less than 15 mL/min/1.73 m^2.[2,8]

Extensive studies have established BNP and NT-proBNP as the gold standard biomarkers for the diagnosis and prognostication of HF, and emerging data suggest value for their use in the management of patients with HF.

Diagnosis

In healthy adults, circulating concentrations of BNP are quite low and women tend to have slightly higher values than men (14 vs. 8 pg/mL), with similar findings observed with NT-proBNP.[9] Other conditions that affect concentrations of natriuretic peptides beyond cardiac structure and function include factors that may lead to higher values (advancing age, renal dysfunction), as well as those that may lead to lower than expected values (obesity). These factors are discussed below (**Tables 30-3** and **30-4**). In the context of pressure or volume overload states such as acutely decompensated HF (ADHF), BNP, or NT-proBNP concentrations typically dramatically increase.

When considering the interpretation of BNP or NT-proBNP, numerous data exist now to suggest that their concentrations hardly reflect a single physiology. Thus, although wall stress is a prime factor responsible for their release, a broad range of cardiac structural and functional abnormalities may trigger elevation in BNP or NT-proBNP (see Table 30-4). Appropriate interpretation of these natriuretic values in the context of each patient is crucial. **Table 30-5** details the recommended cutoff points for natriuretic peptide testing in HF.

BNP and NT-proBNP: ADHF Diagnosis

In 1586 patients presenting to the emergency department with acute dyspnea, the Breathing Not Properly Multinational Study[2] showed that patients diagnosed with ADHF had higher BNP levels compared with those without HF (mean 675 ± 450 vs. 110 ± 225 pg/mL, $P < 0.001$). Furthermore, an increasing concentration of BNP was associated with an increasing severity of HF as evidenced by New York Heart Association (NYHA) functional class ($P < 0.001$). In a multivariable logistic regression analysis, a BNP greater

TABLE 30-3 Factors Influencing the Clinical Interpretation of BNP or NT-proBNP Values

Factors Associated with Lower Than Expected BNP or NT-proBNP

- Obesity
- Flash pulmonary edema
- Heart failure causes upstream from left ventricle (e.g., acute mitral regurgitation, mitral stenosis)
- Cardiac tamponade
- Pericardial constriction

Factors Associated with Elevated BNP or NT-proBNP

Left ventricular dysfunction
- Hypertrophic heart muscle diseases
- Infiltrative myocardiopathies, such as amyloidosis
- Acute cardiomyopathies, such as apical ballooning syndrome
- Inflammatory, including myocarditis and chemotherapy
- Valvular heart disease

Previous heart failure
Arrhythmia
- Atrial fibrillation and flutter

Acute coronary syndromes
Cardiotoxic drugs
- Anthracyclines and related compounds

Significant pulmonary disease
- Acute respiratory distress syndrome, lung disease with right-sided heart failure, obstructive sleep apnea, pulmonary hypertension
- Pulmonary embolism

Advanced age
Renal dysfunction
Anemia
Critical illness
- Burns
- Stroke

High-output states
- Sepsis
- Cirrhosis
- Hyperthyroidism

BNP, B-type natriuretic peptide.

TABLE 30-4 Cardiac Abnormalities Associated with Increased Natriuretic Peptide Concentrations

Myocardial dysfunction	• Systolic dysfunction • Diastolic dysfunction • Fibrosis/scar • Hypertrophy • Infiltrative diseases
Valvular abnormalities	• Mitral stenosis, regurgitation • Aortic stenosis, regurgitation • Tricuspid regurgitation • Pulmonic stenosis
Cardiac chamber size	• Ventricular enlargement • Atrial enlargement
Filling pressures	• Atrial, ventricular • Pulmonary
Ischemic heart disease	• Coronary artery ischemia
Heart rhythm abnormalities	• Atrial fibrillation, flutter
Pericardial diseases	• Constriction, tamponade
Congenital abnormalities	• Shunts, stenotic lesions

than 100 pg/mL was the single most accurate predictor of the diagnosis of ADHF than any other single finding from history, physical examination, chest x-ray, or laboratory tests. A BNP cutoff value of 100 pg/mL had overall sensitivity of 90%, specificity of 76%, and accuracy of 85%, performing better than either the NHANES criteria (accuracy = 67%) or the Framingham criteria for the diagnosis of HF (accuracy = 73%). BNP added independent and additive information in the diagnosis of ADHF when added to the traditional evaluation of patients with HF. The performance of BNP in

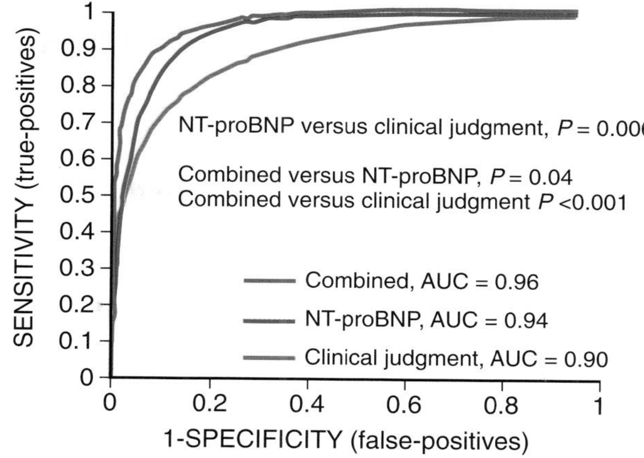

FIGURE 30-2 Comparison of NT-proBNP versus clinical judgment for the diagnosis of acutely decompensated heart failure. *From Januzzi JL, Jr, Camargo CA, Anwaruddin S, et al: The N-terminal Pro-BNP Investigation of Dyspnea in the Emergency Department (PRIDE) study. Am J Cardiol 95:948–954, 2005.*

the diagnosis of HF can be summarized by its receiver operating characteristic (ROC) curve area under the curve (AUC) of 0.91 (95% confidence interval [CI] = 0.90-0.93; P <0.001).

NT-proBNP has also been shown to be quite useful in the diagnosis of ADHF. In the ProBNP Investigation of Dyspnea in the Emergency Department (PRIDE) Study,[3] patients with ADHF had much higher NT-proBNP values compared with patients without HF (median 4054 [interquartile range 1675-10,028] vs. 131 [interquartile range 46-433] pg/mL, $P<0.001$); increasing NT-proBNP correlated well with increasing severity of HF ($P = 0.001$) and was the strongest predictor of ADHF diagnosis compared with any other single traditional finding. Despite the excellent diagnostic performance of NT-proBNP (AUC = 0.94) compared with clinical judgment alone (AUC = 0.90), the best approach in the evaluation of patients suspected of HF is a combination of both the NT-proBNP and clinical judgment (AUC = 0.96) as shown in **Figure 30-2**. Although an NT-proBNP cutoff value of 900 pg/mL provided identical performance to that reported for a BNP of 100 pg/mL in the Breathing Not Properly Multinational Study, the International Collaborative on NT-proBNP (ICON) investigators reported that age stratification of NT-proBNP reference limits (≥450, ≥900, and ≥1800 pg/mL for ages <50, 50-75, and >75 years old) improved performance even further.[10] Importantly, an NT-proBNP threshold value of less than 300 pg/mL was found to exclude ADHF with almost 100% negative predictive value.

Important insights from the Breathing Not Properly Multinational Study, PRIDE, and ICON include the fact that BNP and NT-proBNP were superior to radiographic standards for HF diagnosis, and both may also identify unsuspected HF in patients with underlying lung disease. Although renal function may impair the diagnostic performance of both BNP and NT-proBNP (as discussed below), with careful adjustment of reference limits, analyses suggest that both retain usefulness for evaluation of patients with acute dyspnea.[11,12]

As 50% of modern HF consists of patients with preserved left ventricular ejection fraction (LVEF), it is helpful to understand the performance of BNP and NT-proBNP in those with HF and preserved EF (HFpEF) versus those with HF and reduced EF (HFrEF). Abundant data indicate that natriuretic peptide concentrations are typically lower in

TABLE 30-5 Suggested Natriuretic Peptide Cut-Points in Heart Failure

	CUTOFF VALUE	SENSITIVITY	SPECIFICITY	POSITIVE PREDICTIVE VALUE	NEGATIVE PREDICTIVE VALUE
To Exclude Acutely Decompensated HF:					
BNP	<30-50 pg/mL	97%	*	*	96%
NT-proBNP	<300 pg/mL	99%	*	*	99%
MR-proANP	<57 pmol/L	98%	*	*	97%
To Identify Acutely Decompensated HF:					
Single Cutoff Point Strategy					
BNP	<100 pg/mL	90%	76%	79%	89%
NT-proBNP	<900 pg/mL	90%	85%	76%	94%
MR-proANP	<127 pmol/L	87%	79%	67%	93%
Multiple Cut-Point Strategy					
BNP, "gray zone" approach	<100 pg/mL to exclude	90%	73%	75%	90%
	100-400 pg/mL, "gray zone"	*	*	*	*
	>400 pg/mL, to rule in	63%	91%	86%	74%
NT-proBNP, "age-stratified" approach	<450 pg/mL for age <50 years <900 pg/mL for age 50-75 years <1800 pg/mL for age >75 years	90%	84%	88%	66%
MR-proANP, "age-stratified" approach	<104 pmol/L for age <65 years 214 pmol/L for age ≥65 years	82%	86%	75%	91%
Outpatient Application					
BNP	20 pg/mL (asymptomatic)	*	*	*	96%
	or 40 pg/mL (symptomatic)	*	*	*	
NT-proBNP, "age-stratified" approaches	<125 pg/mL for age <75 years	*	*	*	98%
	<450 pg/mL for age ≥75 years	*	*	*	91%
	or				
	<50 pg/mL for age <50 years	*	*	*	98%
	<75 pg/mL for age 50-75 years	*	*	*	98%
	<250 pg/mL for age >75 years	*	*	*	93%
MR-proANP	Unknown	Unknown	Unknown	Unknown	Unknown

*Not available.
BNP, B-type natriuretic peptide; *HF,* heart failure.

those with HFpEF; however, lower BNP or NT-proBNP concentrations are not pathognomonic for HFpEF by any means, and the same cutoff values for BNP and NT-proBNP are recommended for the diagnosis of HF in patients with HFpEF, as well as HFrEF, with the recognition that the sensitivity may be reduced in those with preserved LV function.[13,14] In this setting, values of BNP or NT-proBNP are rarely normal, but are more likely in a range between the "rule out" and "rule in" thresholds (the so-called gray zone; see later discussion).

Relative to the added value of natriuretic peptide testing when put together with standard clinical evaluation, the B-type natriuretic peptide for Acute Shortness of breath EvaLuation (BASEL),[15] the Improved Management of Patients With Congestive Heart Failure (IMPROVE-CHF),[16] and the NT-proBNP for EValuation of dyspneic patients in the Emergency Room and hospital (BNP4EVER)[17] studies all indicated an advantage to use of either BNP or NT-proBNP when added to clinical judgment. For example, in both BASEL and IMPROVE-CHF, the use of BNP and NT-proBNP, respectively, led to considerable cost savings, findings echoed by Siebert and colleagues in a report from the PRIDE study.[18] In BASEL, the use of BNP was associated with less use of intensive care unit admission, without excess hazard with such care. In the IMPROVE-CHF study, not only was NT-proBNP-supplemented evaluation superior diagnostically, but outcomes of patients in the NT-proBNP arm had better short-term outcomes as well.

When considering the appropriate application of BNP or NT-proBNP for diagnostic evaluation of ADHF, it is worth reviewing the circumstances where testing is most valuable. As shown by Green and colleagues,[19] indecision when evaluating patients with acute dyspnea occurs in approximately 30% of cases seen in the emergency department, and is associated with considerably higher short-term risk. Results by Steinhart and colleagues from the IMPROVE-CHF study lend important clarity regarding the importance of natriuretic peptide testing in this setting; although NT-proBNP correctly (and significantly) reclassified diagnoses in patients judged with confidence in this study, the value of the biomarker was considerably greater in those with uncertain diagnoses; these findings inform the current class I guideline recommendations for use of BNP or NT-proBNP for ADHF diagnosis.

BNP and NT-proBNP: Chronic HF Diagnosis

Not surprisingly, both BNP and NT-proBNP have been shown to be useful in the diagnosis of HF in the outpatient setting.[20] In contrast to the diagnostic application of BNP or NT-proBNP in the acute environment, however, both peptides have been mainly examined relative to their negative predictive value to exclude the diagnosis, rather than to confirm it. In this regard, the optimal reference limits for use in this setting are considerably lower than in patients with acute dyspnea (see Table 30-5). For NT-proBNP, the ICON-Primary Care group[21] showed that age stratification again improves diagnostic accuracy in this setting. If a patient is found to be above the BNP or NT-proBNP cutoffs, further diagnostic testing such as echocardiography is likely needed. Causes of falsely low BNP or NT-proBNP in the outpatient setting are comparable with those with acute dyspnea.

Another potential use of BNP or NT-proBNP in the nonacute setting is for the screening of at-risk patients for the presence of underlying structural heart disease. Although influenced by numerous cardiac correlates (see Table 30-4), a single measurement of BNP or NT-proBNP may be able to identify reduced LV function in asymptomatic individuals; in recognition of their dependence on diastolic indices, as well for their concentrations, both peptides appear to be useful in screening for diastolic ventricular dysfunction.[22]

Natriuretic Peptides: Caveats

Despite the promising information conveyed by BNP or NT-proBNP in the evaluation of HF patients, there are several important limitations that need to be considered in the interpretation of the results; several factors have been shown to alternately lead to higher than expected BNP or NT-proBNP values, as well as lower than expected values (see Table 30-3).

Beyond age, as discussed previously, a number of diagnoses have been associated with increased natriuretic peptide levels.[23] Many cardiac disorders characterized by structural heart disease in addition to HF are associated with elevated BNP or NT-proBNP concentrations, including apical ballooning syndrome, myocarditis, acute coronary artery disease, valvular heart disease (either stenotic or regurgitant), arrhythmias such as atrial fibrillation or flutter, and cardiotoxic drugs such as anthracycline chemotherapy. Many pulmonary disorders with resulting right ventricular strain are also associated with elevated natriuretic peptide levels, including pulmonary embolism, pulmonary hypertension, congenital heart disease, and sleep apnea. In these latter examples, the extent of increase in natriuretic peptide levels generally tends to be less than in ADHF. Some patients with acute stroke, severe anemia, and other critical illnesses such as bacterial sepsis, severe burns, and acute respiratory distress syndrome can have elevated BNP or NT-proBNP levels; exact mechanisms are less clear. Clinical judgment when interpreting natriuretic peptide concentrations is crucial. As with any diagnostic test, a differential diagnosis should be kept in mind when interpreting an elevated BNP or NT-proBNP value.

Although discussed previously, the importance of renal function in the interpretation of BNP or NT-proBNP deserves further detail. Patients with chronic kidney disease typically have higher BNP and NT-proBNP values. Mechanistically, this is due to both peptide accumulation, as well as increased release of BNP or NT-proBNP because of shared comorbidities such as hypertension, LV hypertrophy, and chronic volume overload. In patients with renal insufficiency (GFR <60 mL/min/1.73 m^2), a BNP cutoff of 200 pg/mL or NT-proBNP of 1200 pg/mL provides good diagnostic performance; alternatively, the age-stratified NT-proBNP cutoffs may be used with good accuracy and without adjustment.[11,12] Furthermore, both BNP and NT-proBNP are considerably prognostic in patients with chronic kidney disease, even in the absence of overt cardiovascular disease; NT-proBNP may even predict progression of renal dysfunction in population studies.

As mentioned above, BNP and NT-proBNP levels are lower in overweight and obese patients.[24,25] This phenomenon is hypothesized to be due to suppression of synthesis or release of natriuretic peptides in obese subjects. However, regardless of body-mass index (BMI), BNP or NT-proBNP concentrations are higher in patients with HF compared with patients without, and age-adjusted cutoff points retain usefulness for the diagnosis of acute HF. In the PRIDE study of acute dyspnea patients,[26] ROC analyses of NT-proBNP for diagnosis of acute HF had AUC of 0.94 for lean, 0.95 for overweight, and 0.94 for obese patients. An NT-proBNP value <300 pg/mL still had excellent diagnostic performance in ruling out acute HF across all BMI categories.

When a patient has a BNP or NT-proBNP between the optimized cutoff to exclude HF and the optimized cutoff to diagnose it, this is referred to as a *gray zone* result. van Kimmenade and colleagues reported that patients with a gray zone NT-proBNP in ICON were more likely to have ADHF when physical findings, such as elevated jugular venous pressure or pulmonary rales, were present.[27] Additionally, although complicating biomarker-based evaluation of the patient with suspected HF, gray zone values have prognostic meaning above that of patients with lower concentrations of BNP or NT-proBNP.

BNP and NT-proBNP: Prognosis

Concentrations of BNP or NT-proBNP are strong predictors of future clinical outcomes in a variety of populations spanning all stages of HF articulated by the American College of Cardiology/American Heart Association (ACC/AHA) guidelines: from patients without any cardiac dysfunction, but at high risk of developing HF in the future (stage A), through patients with asymptomatic LV dysfunction (stage B), to symptomatic HF (stage C) and advanced HF (stage D).

The largest body of data supporting the use of BNP and NT-proBNP is in patients with ADHF. The Acute Decompensated Heart Failure National Registry (ADHERE) registry[28] showed that higher admission BNP values were associated with increased in-hospital mortality among 48,629 patients admitted to the hospital with ADHF. Moreover, there was a linear relationship between increasing quartile of BNP and in-hospital mortality (**Figure 30-3**), even after adjusting for potential confounders such as age, gender, systolic blood pressure, pulse, renal function, sodium, and dyspnea in both HFpEF and HFrEF patients. In a similar manner, admission NT-proBNP concentrations were found to be strongly predictive of both short- and long-term clinical outcomes.[10,29] NT-proBNP values greater than 986 pg/mL predicted death

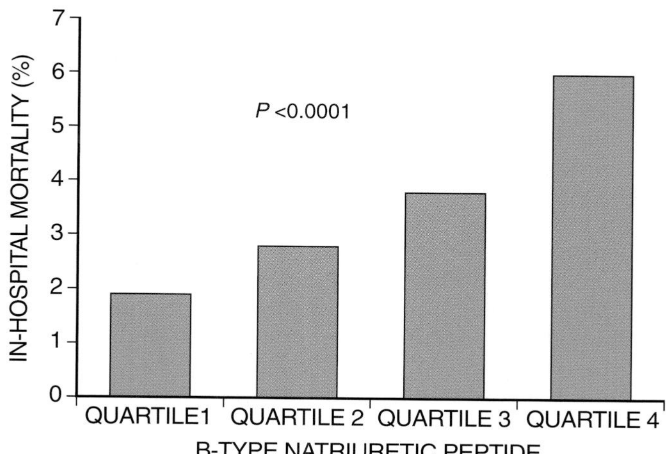

FIGURE 30-3 B-type natriuretic peptide and in-hospital mortality in 48,629 patients admitted to the hospital with acute decompensated heart failure. *Adapted from Fonarow GC, Peacock WF, Phillips CO, et al: Admission B-type natriuretic peptide levels and in-hospital mortality in acute decompensated heart failure. J Am Coll Cardiol 49:1943–1950, 2007.*

at 1 year (P<0.001, 79% sensitivity and 68% specificity), even after adjusting for relevant traditional factors. Some studies have examined the role of follow-up BNP or NT-proBNP measurement compared with admission. Indeed, discharge natriuretic peptides obtained after inpatient treatment for ADHF appeared to be even more predictive of future mortality and/or rehospitalization when compared with admission values.[30]

Serial assessment with BNP and NT-proBNP for prognosis has also been explored in those with chronic HF. For example, in a large population of ambulatory patients with chronic stable HF enrolled in the Valsartan Heart Failure Trial (Val-HeFT) study, NT-proBNP was measured at baseline and at 4 months; although baseline values were prognostically important, changes in NT-proBNP concentrations over 4 months and the relationship to all-cause mortality were more important in providing prognostic information.[31] Thus, in analogy to those patients with acute symptoms, serial assessment of BNP or NT-proBNP appears to provide incremental data regarding the likelihood of an adverse outcome. Recent data suggest that elevated values of NT-proBNP in chronic HF not only predict adverse outcome but also identify patients at highest risk for deleterious LV remodeling.[32]

An intriguing application that is yet well established is to use BNP or NT-proBNP to predict the onset of cardiovascular disease, including HF. In 3346 asymptomatic subjects without HF from the Framingham Offspring Study,[33] baseline elevated values of BNP or NT-proBNP strongly predicted future clinical outcomes, including all-cause mortality, first major cardiovascular event, HF, atrial fibrillation, and stroke or transient ischemia attack; most notably, BNP levels above 80th percentile (20.0 for men and 23.3 pg/mL for women) were associated with a 62% increase in the risk of death, a 76% increase in first cardiovascular event, and a 307% increase in the risk of HF (all P<0.05). Similar findings were seen with NT-proBNP, where values above 80th percentile (497 for men and 541 pg/mL for women) were associated with a 76% increase in the risk of death, a 52% increase in first cardiovascular event, and a 502% increase in the risk of HF (all P <0.05).

BNP and NT-proBNP: Management of HF

Coupled with their dynamic and prognostically meaningful behavior in the context of HF treatment is the interesting observation that natriuretic peptide concentrations appear to fall in the context of treatment with therapies shown to improve long-term mortality in HF, including β-blockers, angiotensin-converting enzyme inhibitors, angiotensin II receptor blockers, mineralocorticoid receptor antagonists, and cardiac resynchronization therapy.[34] Significant reduction in BNP or NT-proBNP concentrations typically occur within 2 to 4 weeks of successful therapy titration, allowing for a defined window for resampling and assessment for benefit of therapy. This concept of using BNP or NT-proBNP as a guide to HF care, with a goal of achieving excellent guideline-derived medical therapy plus natriuretic peptide suppression, was born. Since 2000, a number of trials have examined the use of natriuretic peptides in this manner.

Following the seminal pilot study by Troughton and colleagues from the Christchurch Cardioendocrine Group,[35] numerous studies have explored the topic of BNP- or NT-proBNP–guided HF care with mixed outcomes.[36] Nonetheless, meta-analyses combining findings from existing studies have shown a 20% to 30% mortality reduction associated with biomarker-guided HF management over standard HF care, raising the possibility of a personalized, biologically driven approach to HF management.[37] Lessons learned from the approach include that BNP- or NT-proBNP–guided care is typically well tolerated, and is associated with more application of guideline-derived medical therapies in the biomarker-guided arm. Further, experience would dictate that for natriuretic peptide–guided HF care to be successful, a low target value must be sought (BNP <100 pg/mL; NT-proBNP <1000 pg/mL), therapies must be titrated to lower the natriuretic peptide concentrations, and significant lowering of the biomarkers must occur. In those trials that had these three characteristics, substantial improvement in outcomes was observed.[35,38,39] Large, prospective, randomized multicenter trials are currently underway to better explore this topic.

Emerging Natriuretic Peptide Tests: MR-proANP

More attention has been given recently to ANP as a biomarker for HF. In parallel to the B-type peptides, circulating levels of ANP rapidly increase with cardiac stretch; unlike BNP, whose production is induced after myocyte stretch, ANP is premade and stored in the myocardium, predominantly in the atrium. Although discovered before BNP or NT-proBNP, the reliable detection of circulating ANP is challenging as its half-life is only 2 to 5 minutes, and attention shifted away from this class of peptide for a time. However, the immediate precursor protein, proANP, has a longer half-life and makes serum measurement possible. The development of a midregional propeptide assay for ANP (MR-proANP) assay has led to the examination of its use for HF applications. Table 30-5 details suggested cutoff points for MR-proANP for clinical use.

The role of MR-proANP in the diagnosis of ADHF was first examined in 1641 patients with acute dyspnea in the Biomarkers in the Acute Heart Failure (BACH) trial.[40] MR-proANP performed well in diagnosing ADHF, and was noninferior to BNP or NT-proBNP; a MR-proANP cutoff point of ≥120 pmol/L had a sensitivity of 97%, specificity of 60%, and accuracy of 74%, whereas BNP with a cutoff point of 100 pg/mL had a sensitivity of 96%, specificity of 62%, and accuracy of 73%. In the PRIDE study analysis of MR-proANP (cutoff value of 127 pmol/L),[41] NT-proBNP performed slightly better than MR-proANP in the diagnosis of ADHF (AUC of 0.94 for NT-proBNP vs. 0.90 for MR-proBNP, P = 0.001 for difference); however, MR-proANP was found to be an independent predictor of HF diagnosis even with NT-proBNP in a multivariable model (odds ratio = 4.34, 95% CI = 2.11-8.92, P <0.001) and when added to NT-proBNP measurement, correctly reclassified patients who had false-negative and false-positive results by NT-proBNP testing alone.

In the PRIDE study,[41] MR-proANP strongly and independently predicted 1- and 4-year mortality (adjusted hazard ratio [HR] = 2.99, P<0.001, and 3.12, P<0.001, respectively), and the addition of NT-proBNP to these models did not attenuate the predictive power of MR-proANP. Adding MR-proANP to base models containing NT-proBNP significantly improved the C-statistic at 1 and 4 years and reclassified mortality risk as a part of a multimarker strategy in determining prognosis.

In chronic HF, the Gruppo Italiano per lo Studio della Sopravvivenza nell'Insufficienza Cardiaca–Heart Failure

(GISSI-HF) study[42] examined the predictive power of MR-proANP in stable chronic HF patients. Investigators found that a MR-proANP of 278 pmol/L or more had the best prognostic accuracy for 4-year mortality among several novel and established biomarkers, including NT-proBNP, midregional proadrenomedullin (MR-proADM), C-terminal provasopressin (copeptin), and C-terminal proendothelin-1 (AUC of 0.74, 95% CI = 0.70-0.76). In addition, MR-proANP added independent prognostic information beyond NT-proBNP and relevant clinical characteristics in a reclassification analysis. Using the same biomarkers, only the change in MR-proANP over 3 months was found to be significant in predicting mortality.

Although initial data from the BACH study suggested that MR-proANP was less likely to be affected by covariates that reduce diagnostic accuracy of BNP or NT-proBNP (such as age, renal function, or obesity), subsequent data from other sources suggest that factors influencing BNP or NT-proBNP are quite likely to exert a similar effect on MR-proANP.[41] As an example, Richards and colleagues recently reported that atrial fibrillation reduced the diagnostic accuracy of MR-proANP for ADHF diagnosis just as much as it did BNP or NT-proBNP.[43]

Cardiac Necrosis

Cardiac Troponins

In the context of cardiomyocyte necrosis, disruption of normal cardiomyocyte membrane results in the inner contents of the damaged cells to be released into the extracellular space; a variety of cellular and structural proteins, such as troponin, creatine kinase, myoglobin, and cardiac fatty acid binding protein, are released into circulation and become detectable in peripheral blood. Of these, cardiac troponins have rapidly become the standard of care biomarker in diagnosing myocardial infarction (MI).[44] Cardiac troponin levels have also been found to be elevated in nonacute MI settings; one such setting is in HF.

The exact mechanism behind the release of troponins in HF is unclear, but may be related to either increased myocyte membrane permeability or necrosis. A variety of HF mechanisms are involved in the release of troponin: inflammation, neurohormonal activation, ventricular stretch, increased wall tension, supply-demand mismatch, cytotoxicity, cellular necrosis, apoptosis, or autophagy. Regardless, increased circulating levels of cardiac troponins in HF patients have been shown to be closely linked to future clinical outcomes. With the development and application of highly sensitive cardiac troponin (hsTn) assays that can accurately detect even minute concentrations, most patients with HF are found to have detectable levels of cardiac troponins with a substantial percentage demonstrating concentrations of the biomarker above the upper reference limit for a normal patient population, even in the absence of ischemic heart disease.

In the ADHERE registry,[45] 4240 patients (6.2%) out of 69,259 patients with ADHF had an elevated troponin, and in this context, higher in-hospital mortality (8.0% vs. 2.7%, $P<0.001$) was observed, with an adjusted odds ratio for death of 2.55 (95% CI = 2.24-2.89, $P<0.001$) compared with patients with a negative troponin measurement. Using a hsTnT assay, another group[46] found that 30.6% of patients with ADHF had elevated troponin values. In a multivariable model that included NT-proBNP and the interleukin receptor family member, sST2, hsTnT remained a significant and independent predictor of all-cause mortality with a HR of 1.16 (95% CI = 1.09-1.24, $P<0.001$). In a multimarker strategy, patients with all three biomarkers below their optimal cutoff point had the best survival (0% death) at a median follow-up of 739 days, whereas 53% of those with elevation of all three biomarkers died. In integrated discrimination analyses, the use of all three markers in a multimarker approach was the best model for mortality prediction. As might be expected, the use of highly sensitive assay was particularly helpful in determining the prognosis in patients with undetectable conventional TnT concentrations.

Although the prognostic ramification of an elevated troponin in patients with ADHF is clear, the therapeutic steps to follow with such an elevated value remain less well defined. Nonetheless, given the great importance of acute MI in the precipitation of ADHF, current position statements recommend the universal measurement of troponin in patients with acute symptoms to primarily diagnose or exclude an ischemic cause for the presentation.[44]

In chronic HF, cardiac troponin levels are also frequently increased (**Figure 30-4**), and in analogy to ADHF, such elevations are prognostically important. Using a conventional assay, only about 10% of patients had detectable TnT out of the 4035 stable chronic HF patients in the Val-HeFT study.[47] Not surprisingly, detectable troponin concentration was associated with an increased risk of death (HR 2.08, 95% CI = 1.72-2.52) and first hospitalization for HF (HR 1.55, 95% CI = 1.25-1.93) at 2 years in a model that adjusted for traditional risk factors. When hsTnT was measured in this same cohort, troponin was detectable in 92% of the cohort and predicted future adverse outcomes (HR 1.05, 95% CI = 1.04-1.07, $P<0.001$), as well as LV remodeling. Adding hsTnT to a baseline model including BNP and relevant clinical predictors significantly improved prognostic discrimination. Combining patients from both the Val-HeFT study and the GISSI-HF study, investigators looked at the role of serial hsTnT measurement in 5284 patients with chronic HF.[48] Increases in hsTnT over 3 to 4 months of follow-up strongly predicted all-cause mortality (adjusted HR 1.59, 95% CI = 1.39-1.82 and 1.88, 95% CI = 1.50-2.35 after adjustment for traditional risk factors, baseline hsTnT, and baseline NT-proBNP), but improvement in test performance was only modest over a single baseline measurement of hsTnT.

Concentrations of troponin—particularly when measured with a highly sensitive method—may be useful in predicting the onset of HF in apparently well individuals. For example, hsTnT measurement was found to be useful in predicting future development of HF in 4221 older, community dwelling adults; hsTnT >12.94 pg/mL was associated with HF incidence rate of 6.4 per 100 person-years (95% CI = 5.8-7.2) and an adjusted HR of 2.48 (95% CI = 2.04-3.00).[49] An elevated hsTnT was also predictive of future cardiovascular death (incidence rate of 4.8, 95% CI = 4.3-5.4 and adjusted HR 2.91, 95% CI = 0.9-1.2 compared with those with undetectable hsTnT). A repeat hsTnT measurement in 2 to 3 years showed that among patients with detectable hsTnT at baseline, greater than 50% change in hsTnT was associated with an even higher risk for HF (adjusted HR 1.61, 95% CI = 1.32-1.97) and cardiovascular death (adjusted HR 1.65, 95% CI = 1.35-2.03), whereas a decrease in hsTnT was associated with a lower risk for developing HF and having cardiovascular death. In a lower risk cohort from the Framingham Heart Study, Wang and colleagues similarly demonstrated the prognostic importance of hsTnI for predicting death and

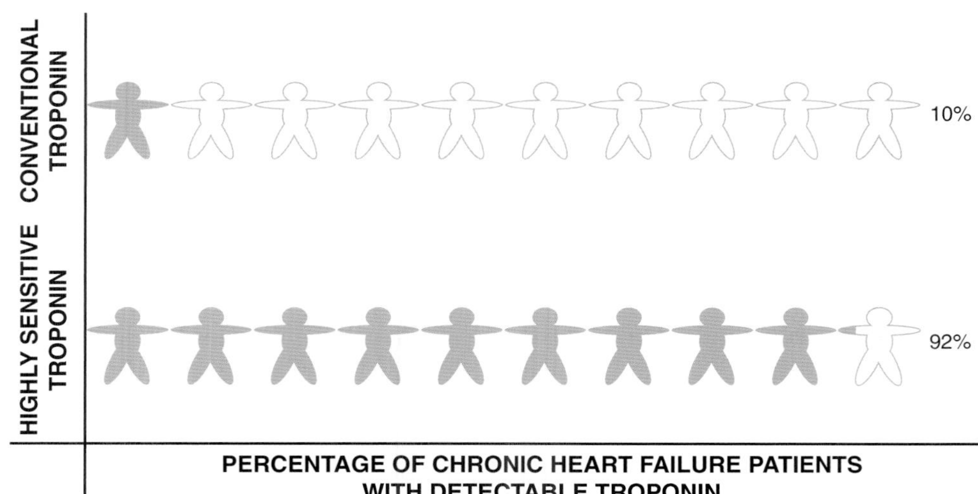

FIGURE 30-4 Percentage of patients with chronic heart failure with detectable troponin.

HF onset, even when extensively adjusted for relevant covariates, including other biomarkers.[50]

Oxidative Stress

As a consequence of normal aerobic metabolism, molecules called reactive oxygen species (ROS) are produced. ROS are involved in a variety of intracellular proteins and signaling pathways, including vital proteins involved in myocardial excitation-contraction coupling and myocyte growth. Under normal circumstances, ROS are scavenged and neutralized by antioxidants. However, in pathologic conditions such as HF, free radicals are present in relative excess to the antioxidants, creating a state of oxidative stress, which can exert direct toxic effect on myocardial structure and function.

An important biomarker of oxidative stress is myeloperoxidase (MPO), a 150-kDa protein. MPO is found in blood neutrophils, and through its activity produces hypochlorous acid, a potently oxidative cytotoxic compound. MPO appears to be prognostic in both acute and chronic settings; in acute settings, MPO may be additively prognostic to BNP for forecasting death by 1 year. In chronic HF, Tang and colleagues reported that MPO values were prognostic, even when adjusted for relevant covariates.[51]

Uric Acid

Xanthine oxidase is an important source of ROS, including superoxide anion and hydrogen peroxide. Serum uric acid has been shown to reflect the degree of xanthine oxidase activation in HF; in addition, uric acid may be a marker of cell death when other purines are degraded. When elevated, uric acid appears to predict HF onset; in 4912 unaffected participants from the Framingham Offspring Study, incident HF was about 6 times higher in patients with the highest quartile of serum uric acid level (≥6.3 mg/dL) compared with those at the lowest quartile (<3.4 mg/dL), with an adjusted HR of 2.1 (95% CI = 1.04-4.22).[52]

Beyond its link to incident HF, there is a strong association of serum uric acid with severity of the diagnosis with a particularly important role for prognostication. For example, among 112 patients with chronic HF, a uric acid level of 565 μmol/L or higher was strongly related to increased mortality at 1 year and was validated in a separate cohort of 182 patients with chronic HF (HR 7.14, 95% CI = 4.20-12.15, P<0.0001). In a multivariable Cox model containing relevant clinical, biochemical, and mechanical characteristics, uric acid remained independently predictive of clinical outcomes (P <0.0001), although to a lesser extent after adjustment. This association is less likely due to uric acid itself, but rather indicative of uric acid's role in xanthine oxidase activation; decreasing uric acid levels with a uricosuric agent, probenecid, did not improve endothelial function in HF, but inhibition of xanthine oxidase with allopurinol did.[53] Disappointingly, strategies to reduce ROS have not shown clinical benefit in HF outcomes in randomized controlled trials. In the Oxypurinol Therapy in Congestive Heart Failure (OPT-CHF) study,[54] oxipurinol, a xanthine oxidase inhibitor, reduced uric acid levels, but failed to show improvement in the composite primary endpoint that included hospitalization and cardiovascular death (**Table 30-6**).

TABLE 30-6 Composite Primary Endpoint* at 24 Weeks for Oxipurinol versus Placebo

	PLACEBO (n = 202)	OXYPURINOL (n = 203)	P-VALUE
Improved	91 (45.0%)	88 (43.3%)	0.42
Unchanged	72 (35.6%)	65 (32.0%)	
Worsened	39 (19.3%)	50 (24.6%)	

*Composite endpoint included cardiovascular death, hospitalization, emergency room or emergent clinic visit for worsening heart failure, administration of a new drug class for heart failure or intravenous diuretics for worsening heart failure, permanent withdrawal of study drug due to worsening heart failure, New York Heart Association functional class, or Patient Global Heart Failure Clinical Status.
From Hare JM, Mangal B, Brown J, et al: Impact of oxypurinol in patients with symptomatic heart failure. Results of the OPT-CHF study. J Am Coll Cardiol 51:2301–2309, 2008.

Neurohormonal Activation

Cardiac insults such as reduced LV function trigger production of biologically active proteins that attempt to maintain cardiac output. These proteins were originally termed *neurohormones* in reference to their production in neuroendocrine cells. These various proteins act to compensate for reduced myocardial function, resulting in increased retention of salt and water, peripheral arterial vasoconstriction, and increased contractility. These effects are responsible for raising blood pressure and improving perfusion of vital organs, and activation of inflammatory mediators responsible for cardiac repair and remodeling. However, overexpression and prolonged activation of the same proteins ultimately lead to deleterious long-term effects on the heart and the circulation, and end up contributing to progression of HF.

Sympathetic Nervous System

One of the first responses to cardiac and circulatory dysfunction is the activation of the sympathetic nervous system and inhibition of the parasympathetic tone, resulting in relative excess function of the adrenergic nervous system.

Norepinephrine

Activation of the sympathetic nervous system in HF results in an increased circulating concentration of the potent adrenergic neurotransmitter norepinephrine. Elevated norepinephrine results in increased heart rate and myocardial contraction, as well as peripheral vasoconstriction, but at the expense of an increased energy requirement. Early studies suggested that a single measurement of plasma norepinephrine in asymptomatic and symptomatic patients with HFrEF was independently predictive of future mortality in a multivariable analysis that included other relevant clinical and biochemical characteristics. However, in a more contemporary and comprehensive analysis of available novel and established biomarkers, as well as the Seattle Heart Failure Model, adding norepinephrine to the model did not improve prediction of mortality (HR 1.53, 95% CI = 0.87-2.67, $P = 0.14$).[55] Interestingly, in advanced HF patients, there is a paradoxical decline in myocardial concentration of norepinephrine as HF progresses. The mechanism behind this phenomenon of norepinephrine depletion is unclear, but may be related to decreased stimulation with prolonged adrenergic activation, deregulation of the synthesis of norepinephrine, or decreased reuptake of norepinephrine.

Chromogranin A

Chromogranin A (CgA) is a major component of chromaffin granules that are stored and released together in the adrenal glands with catecholamines, such as norepinephrine. CgA has also been found in the heart and colocalized to the atrial and ventricular myocardium with ANP and BNP. It has been shown that CgA is the precursor of several biologically active proteins, including vasostatin-1 and catestatin, and is intimately involved in the regulation of the adrenergic system activation. However, the exact mechanism and effect on the heart remain to be resolved. CgA levels are elevated in both acute and chronic HF syndromes and are directly related to severity of HF, although its ability to diagnose ADHF is poor. Nonetheless, in patients with ADHF, a CgA concentration greater than 6.6 nmol/L was independently predictive of mortality in a Cox proportional-hazards regression analysis with a risk ratio of 2.56 (95% CI = 1.33-4.95).[56] However, this relationship was not seen in a large study of 1233 patients with chronic HF; CgA was initially found to be predictive of all-cause mortality, but after adjusting for established risk factors in HF, this association was no longer significant.[57]

MR-proADM

Adrenomedullin is a potent vasodilator with cyclic adenosine monophosphate (AMP)–independent inotropic properties that was originally found to be produced by pheochromocytoma cells, arising from the adrenal medulla. Adrenomedullin levels are elevated in patients with chronic HF and in those with diastolic LV dysfunction and restrictive filling, and adrenomedullin concentrations increase with HF severity. However, adrenomedullin itself is biologically unstable and difficult to reliably measure; to address this, a novel assay measuring the midregion of a more stable prohormone, proadrenomedullin, was recently developed (MR-proADM). Much like its parent compound, MR-proADM is elevated in patients with HF and has been found to be a remarkably strong predictor of early mortality, adding value beyond BNP or NT-proBNP.[40,41]

In a study of chronic HF, MR-proADM was a strong and independent predictor of 18-month all-cause mortality (risk ratio 3.92, 95% CI = 1.76-8.7) and HF hospitalization (risk ratio 2.4, 95% CI = 1.3-4.5) even after a full adjustment for other biomarkers and clinical factors.[58] Notably, in this analysis from the Australia-New Zealand HF study, an interaction was found between carvedilol treatment and MR-proADM concentrations; in patients with above the median values of MR-proADM, treatment with carvedilol significantly reduced the risk of death or HF hospitalizations.

Determining short-term HF prognosis with MR-proADM appears promising, but more information is needed before routine clinical use can be recommended. In particular, a better understanding of the triggers for its release, the value of its serial measurement, and the approach from a therapy perspective for those patients with an elevated MR-proADM remain unclear.

Renin-Angiotensin-Aldosterone System

All of the components of the renin-angiotensin-aldosterone system can be measured in patients with HF; however, circulating concentrations of these hormones do not necessarily reflect the local tissue activities of these entities, and their measurement is complicated and costly. Plasma renin activity and aldosterone concentration are often normal in patients with chronic stable HF, despite evidence of increased local activity of angiotensin II and angiotensin-converting enzyme in the heart. In the setting of ADHF, circulating levels of renin, angiotensin II, and aldosterone appear to increase, but again, may not fully reflect the tissue activities of these entities.

Arginine Vasopressin

Sympathetic stimulation can also lead to increased release of arginine vasopressin (AVP), also known as vasopressin or antidiuretic hormone (ADH), from the posterior pituitary. AVP plays a central role in the regulation of free water clearance and plasma osmolality by increasing absorption of water from the collecting ducts of the kidneys. It also increases peripheral vasoconstriction and endothelin production, which further increases arterial blood pressure.

Circulating levels of AVP are elevated in patients with severe HF, but reliable measurement is quite challenging, similar to challenges posed by measurement of ANP or adrenomedullin. However, the c-terminal segment of the precursor of provasopressin, copeptin, is a reliable surrogate marker for AVP and has been shown to be a strong predictor of clinical outcomes in patients with HF. In the

Biomarkers in Acute Heart Failure (BACH) trial[59] of 557 patients with ADHF, elevated copeptin level at the highest quartile strongly predicted mortality (HR 3.85, $P < 0.001$). In the subgroup of patients with hyponatremia and elevated copeptin above the median value, the HR for mortality was even higher at 7.36 ($P < 0.001$). The predictive power of copeptin remained even after adjusting for NT-proBNP and traditional baseline characteristics. Although it is tempting to speculate that elevated concentrations of copeptin might identify those HF patients most likely to benefit from therapy with vasopressin receptor antagonists, this concept has yet to be comprehensively explored.

Endothelin

Endothelins are vasoconstrictive peptides that may play a role in the development and exacerbation of HF, as well as pulmonary hypertension. Big endothelin-1 is a 39-amino-acid propeptide that is cleaved into the biologically active endothelin-1; both have been shown to be elevated in patients with HF and to predict the presence of elevated pulmonary pressures, as well as mortality. In the Val-HeFT trial, concentrations of both big endothelin-1 and endothelin-1 were prognostic, even when adjusted for other relevant biomarkers and clinical factors. Although it is possible that measurement of endothelin-1 might be useful to predict benefits from drugs that oppose its biologic activity, such data are not yet available.

Myocardial Remodeling

Activation of the neurohormonal system does not fully explain the continued progression of HF in patients whose neurohormonal system appears to have stabilized. Ventricular remodeling is a deleterious process by which cellular and structural changes occur in the LV myocardium, resulting in dilation and reduced function; eventually, if unchecked, remodeling may result in worsening LVEF and progressively worse prognosis. Conversely, beneficial therapies for HF, such as ACE inhibitors or angiotensin II receptor blockers, β-blockers, mineralocorticoid inhibitors, or cardiac resynchronization therapy, may result in favorable "reverse" remodeling.

Several classes of biomarkers have been linked to myocardial remodeling; a theorized advantage of biomarker testing to predict remodeling is that such measurement might identify those patients with ongoing biologic changes likely to lead to deleterious remodeling before the structural changes of the LV have occurred. In this, directed therapy intervention might be more effective.

Inflammation

Several of the proteins involved in the inflammatory pathways are strongly recruited after myocardial insult and are thought to initiate the repair process. But when these proinflammatory cytokines, such as tumor necrosis factor (TNF) and interleukin (IL), are activated for a prolonged period of time, they also appear to contribute to the progression of adverse cardiac remodeling (**Figure 30-5**).[60] Cardiac remodeling involves not just the cardiomyocytes, but also nonmyocytes and the myocardial extracellular matrix. There is also a close connection between proinflammatory proteins and neurohormonal activation, and both processes often lead to further myocardial insult.

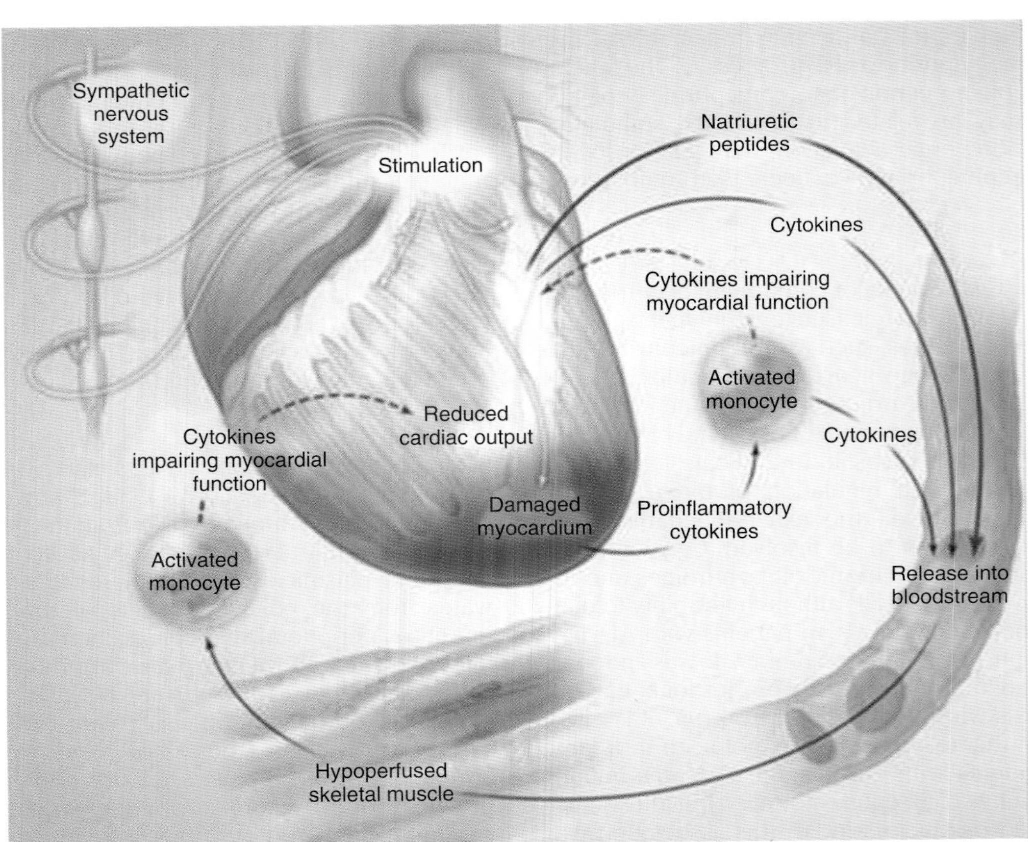

FIGURE 30-5 The role of inflammation in heart failure. *From Braunwald E: Biomarkers in heart failure. N Engl J Med 358:2148–2159, 2008.*

Abundant data have consistently linked inflammation, as assessed with various biomarkers with outcomes in HF.[61] Indeed, beyond CRP, elevated values for multiple members of the IL family (such as IL-1, IL-6, and IL-18), as well as TNF-α (and related compounds, such as Fas, a proapoptotic hormone linked to remodeling) are elevated in a prognostically meaningful fashion in patients with HF; whether these inflammatory biomarkers are byproduct markers or mediators of disease remains unclear. Nonetheless, compelling data suggest the importance of inflammation in prognosticating HF. For example, in the largest study to date, circulating levels of TNF, soluble TNF receptors, and IL-6 levels were obtained in patients with chronic HF and were found to be associated with increased risk of mortality, even after adjusting for all traditional risk factors and characteristics (all $P < 0.05$). Even in older patients without any cardiovascular disease, IL-6 and TNF-α, but not CRP, were significantly and independently associated with incident HF in a model that included traditional risk factors.[62]

In exploring a process as widespread and nonspecific as inflammation, it becomes very important to adjust for potential covariates that may influence the level of proinflammatory proteins. A further compounding problem with the measurement of inflammatory biomarkers is poor understanding of the triggers for their release, very little understanding of their biologic variability, and lack of relevant clinical tools for treating an elevated inflammatory biomarker concentration.

Hypertrophy/Fibrosis

Soluble ST2 (sST2)

ST2 was originally described in the context of inflammation, cell proliferation and autoimmune diseases involving T helper type 2 lymphocyte responses. Since then, ST2 is now known as a unique biomarker with pluripotent effects in vivo including a powerful role in cardiovascular disease. In the setting of mechanical cardiomyocyte and cardiac fibroblasts stretch, the ST2 gene is strongly induced and the resulting ST2 proteins are closely linked with cardiac remodeling and fibrosis in HF. In its interaction with IL-33, a protein with antifibrosis and antiremodeling effects, ST2 actively participates in inducible pathways in mitigating biomechanical stress.

The ST2 system includes a membrane-bound ligand receptor (ST2L) and the freely circulating sST2; both can bind with IL-33. When IL-33 binds to ST2L, it transduces favorable effects that mitigate ventricular remodeling in volume-overloaded states. On the other hand, excessive sST2 acts as a decoy receptor and IL-33 is no longer able to bind to ST2L, blocking the favorable effects from this ST2L. In experimental models, interruption of ST2L expression or infusion of high concentrations of sST2 leads to unchecked ventricular hypertrophy, fibrosis, remodeling, and higher risk for death (**Figure 30-6**).[63] These findings are recapitulated clinically, where elevated concentrations of sST2 have been closely associated with the phenotype of cardiac decompensation and remodeling, and very strongly linked

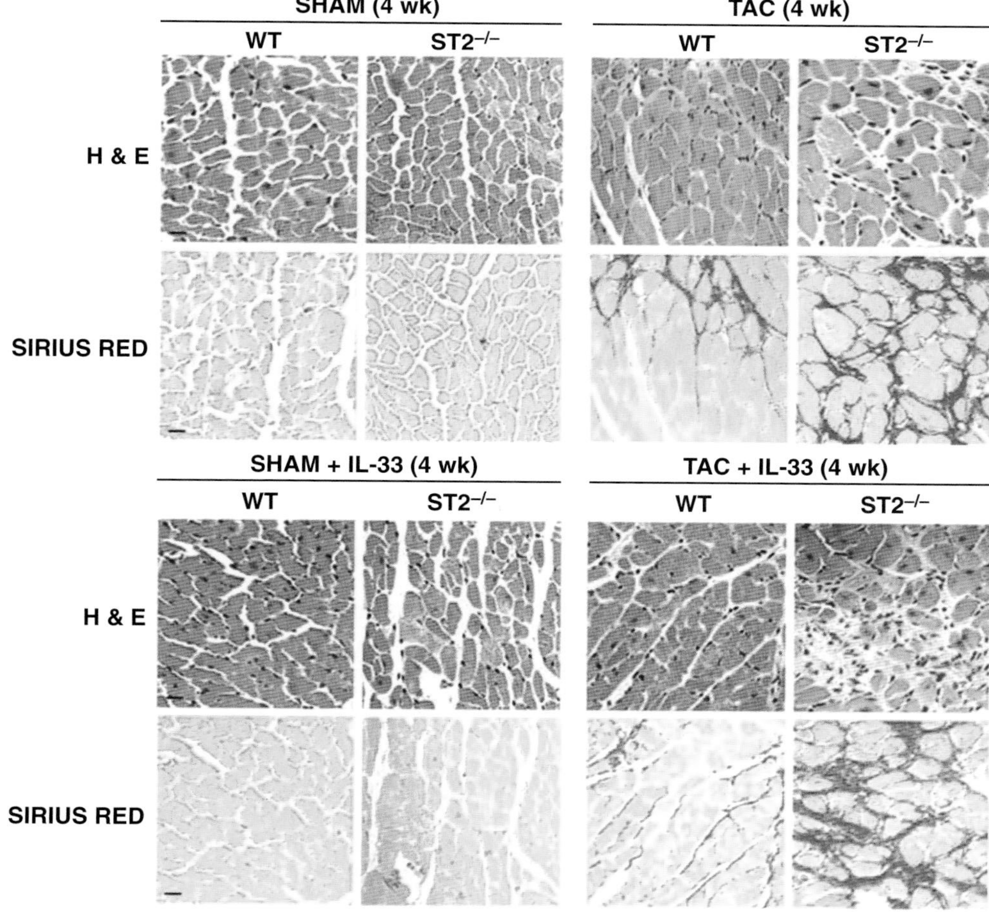

FIGURE 30-6 The importance of sST2 and IL-33 signaling in animal models of pressure overload. Substantial myocyte hypertrophy and fibrosis occurs in the setting of thoracic aortic constriction, a finding that is rescued by IL-33 infusion in wild-type, but not ST2, knockout animals. *H&E,* Hematoxylin and eosin stain; *IL,* interleukin; *SHAM,* sham-operated; *TAC,* thoracic aortic constriction; *WT,* wild type. *From Sanada S, Hakuno D, Higgins LJ, et al: Il-33 and ST2 comprise a critical biomechanically induced and cardioprotective signaling system. J Clin Invest 117:1538–1549, 2007.*

to adverse clinical outcomes in HF. An advantage of ST2 is that its concentration is not affected by age, renal function, or BMI, unlike natriuretic peptides.[64] sST2 testing for risk prediction in both acute and chronic HF recently received a class II recommendation in the recent ACC/AHA HF guidelines.

Studies show that sST2 is a consistently strong determinant of HF prognosis, adding independent information to the information already provided by natriuretic peptides and other biomarkers (**Figure 30-7**).[65] Increased circulating concentrations of sST2 are associated with HF severity as assessed by LVEF and NYHA functional class, and elevated sST2 concentrations predict mortality in ADHF patients in adjusted multivariable analysis, providing prognostic information superior to (and additive with) NT-proBNP (HR = 9.3, P = 0.003, AUC for 1-year mortality 0.80 P <0.001).[65] The prognostic information provided by sST2 was equivalent in those with HFrEF and HFpEF, and when measured serially in ADHF, sST2 provides incremental information beyond the baseline value; percent change in sST2 during treatment for ADHF is strongly predictive of 90-day mortality (AUC = 0.783, P <0.001), again superior to natriuretic peptides.[66] In a recent large-scale analysis of multiple biomarkers in a large, international analysis, sST2 values were among the strongest predictors of death by 30 days and 1 year, substantially reclassifying risk beyond clinical variables and other biochemical markers.[67]

In a chronic HF, similarly consistent data support measurement of sST2. For example, in a study of 1100 chronic HF patients,[68] those with elevated sST2 had a 3.2-fold risk increase in adverse outcomes (95% CI = 2.2-4.7, P <0.0001). In comparison with NT-proBNP, sST2 had similar prognostic ability, but again, the best strategy was to combine the information from both biomarkers. Adding sST2 and NT-proBNP to the Seattle Heart Failure Model improved reclassification.

Other applications of sST2 testing include prediction of incident HF and risk for death in those with acute MI; for example, in the Thrombolysis in Myocardial Infarction 36 trial, an elevated sST2 value at presentation identified patients at highest risk for incident HF by 30 days; similar data for death were also noted.[69] Concordant with these results, following acute MI, Weir and colleagues demonstrated concentrations of sST2 predict ventricular remodeling. In this same analysis, the benefits of mineralocorticoid receptor antagonism with eplerenone were explored. Only those patients with elevated sST2 concentrations showed protection from remodeling from eplerenone therapy, while those with low sST2 values did not.[70]

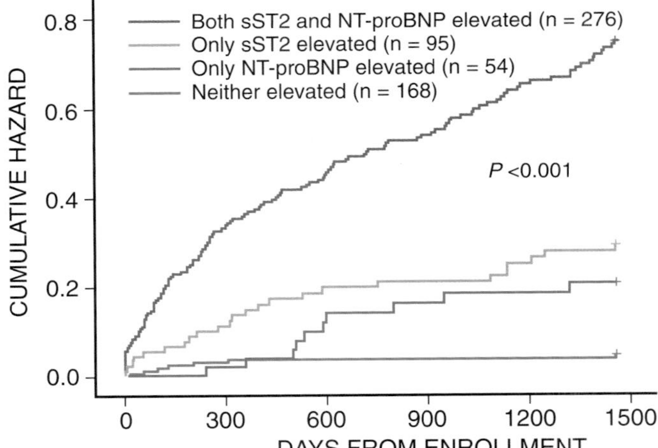

FIGURE 30-7 Additive value of sST2 to NT-proBNP in long-term heart failure prognosis (unpublished figure). *From Januzzi JL, Jr, Peacock WF, Maisel AS, et al: Measurement of the interleukin family member ST2 in patients with acute dyspnea: results from the pride (pro-brain natriuretic peptide investigation of dyspnea in the emergency department) study. J Am Coll Cardiol 50:607–613, 2007.*

Development of a highly sensitive sST2 assay with substantially improved analytic performance compared with earlier methods has allowed for testing in broader demographics and informing further value for sST2 testing. In a healthy cohort from the Framingham Heart Study,[50] sST2 concentrations were measureable in 100% of subjects, and when elevated, predicted onset of hypertension as well as incident HF, even after exhaustively adjusting for other novel and established biomarkers, as well as clinical variables.

Galectin-3

Galectin-3 is a member of the lectin family found in a wide variety of cells and tissues, including the heart. In the heart, it is closely involved in the initiation of the inflammatory cascade following cardiac insult and contributes to ventricular remodeling by the way of tissue repair, myofibroblast proliferation, and fibrogenesis. Soon after the galectin-3 gene was found to be induced in rat HF models, investigators demonstrated that instillation of galectin-3 in the pericardium resulted in considerable collagen deposition.[71] Consequently, galectin-3 genetic knockout mouse models were resistant to LV pressure and volume overload with a slower progression to LV dysfunction or HF.

In a cohort of patients with acute dyspnea,[72] circulating levels of galectin-3 were higher in patients with ADHF compared with those without (P <0.001) and were substantially prognostic for short-term hazard; since then, galectin-3 measurement has been shown to be predictive of clinical outcomes in patients with both acute and chronic HF syndromes.[72-74] Interestingly the ability of galectin-3 to predict adverse outcomes appeared to be better in patients with HFpEF compared with patients with HFrEF.[75] Recent data suggest that serial measurement of galectin-3 in chronic HF adds significantly to baseline values[76]; however, there are no known therapeutic interventions yet identified to respond to elevated galectin-3 values. On the other hand, lower galectin-3 values appear to predict benefit from both statin therapy as well as cardiac resynchronization therapy, suggesting that elevated values of galectin-3 identify a particularly malignant HF phenotype that may be resistant to conventional HF management. Similar to sST2, galectin-3 testing recently received a class II recommendation in the ACC/AHA HF guidelines for risk prediction in HF.

Extracellular Matrix Remodeling

An important component of the nonmyocardial tissue in the heart includes connective tissue and extracellular matrix (see also Chapter 4). Cardiac fibroblasts comprise greater than 90% of the nonmyocyte cells in the heart and are responsible for the secretion of the majority of extracellular matrix, such as collagens, laminin, and fibronectin. As such, fibroblasts are involved in fibrosis and scar formation in response to cardiac insult, neurohormonal activation, or remodeling itself; indeed histologically, one of the hallmarks of advanced HF is increased fibrosis as marked by increased collagen content. The N-terminal procollagens, such as type I amino-terminal (PINP) and procollagen type III amino-terminal (PIIINP), serve as markers of collagen turnover and elevated circulating concentrations of both have been detected in HF patients.[77] This finding is accompanied by loss of normal structural integrity of collagens and the resulting progressive LV enlargement, increased myocardial stiffness, and increased substrate for arrhythmias. The discovery of the matrix metalloproteinases (MMPs), a set of enzymes capable of breaking down collagens, and tissue inhibitors of matrix metalloproteinases (TIMPS) that regulate the activities of MMPs has provided further knowledge of matrix biology; increased MMP (coupled with TIMP) activities have been reported in LV myocardium of dilated cardiomyopathies and linked to adverse clinical outcomes.[78] In another study, a profile of extracellular matrix biomarkers that included MMP-2, MMP-4, PIIINP, and MMP-8 has been shown to be characteristic of HFpEF.[79]

Evaluation of therapeutic agents with close links to collagen synthesis and fibrosis, such as aldosterone antagonists, showed a reduction of PINP and PIIINP concentrations and improved outcomes in HF and may demonstrate how biomarkers can be leveraged to help guide therapy.[80]

MicroRNA (miRNA)

MiRNAs are small noncoding RNA molecules that are closely involved in the transcriptional and post-transcriptional regulation of gene expression. miRNAs were first described in both animal and human HF models by Van Rooij and colleagues.[81] Since then, promising data suggest that they play an important role in the pathogenesis of structural alternations of the failing heart through their ability to regulate the expression of genes that are closely involved in cardiac remodeling.

Because miRNAs are remarkably stable and disease-specific, several miRNAs have been demonstrated to be fairly accurate in the diagnosis of HF in small pilot studies; miR-423-5p was most strongly diagnostic of HF with AUC of 0.91 from healthy controls and 0.83 from acutely dyspneic patients and closely linked with HF severity including LVEF and NYHA.[82] One of the characteristics of an ideal biomarker is a change in the biomarker level with a change in clinical status, especially in response to therapy; levels of two of the identified miRNAs, miR-499-5p and miR-423-5p, changed in response to therapy that improved measures of cardiac remodeling and survival.[83] Again, the small number of subjects in the studies limits the wider implication of these results, and more research is needed to confirm these findings.

Apoptosis

Progressive loss of myocytes in HF contributes further to LV dysfunction and remodeling in a vicious cycle. The loss of myocyte can take several forms and apoptosis appears to play a prominent role in HF progression.

Growth Differentiation Factor (GDF)-15

GDF-15 is a protein that belongs to the transforming growth factor-β family, with a role in regulating response to injury in a broad array of tissues. In the heart, GDF-15 appears to participate in the modulation of myocardial strain, remodeling, and apoptosis. The gene for GDF-15 is robustly induced in cardiomyocytes after metabolic stress such as cardiac ischemia (nitric oxide–dependent) or increased cardiac tension such as HF; induction of GDF-15 expression in this setting occurs in an angiotensin II–dependent manner.[84]

Elevation of circulating GDF-15 levels is common in patients with chronic HF. Marked elevation in GDF-15 level is associated with worsening HF severity, but similar to many other HF biomarkers, the proposed usefulness of GDF-15 measurement in HF appears to be in its ability to independently forecast prognosis beyond the established natriuretic peptides. Increasing levels of GDF-15 in chronic HF was associated with increasing risk of adverse outcomes (risk of mortality of 10.0%, 9.4%, 33.4%, and 56.2% in increasing quartiles of GDF-15, $P < 0.001$). After adjusting for NT-proBNP and other traditional risk factors, GDF-15 was still predictive of mortality with an adjusted HR for a 1-unit increase in the natural log scale of 2.26 (95% CI = 1.52-3.37, $P < 0.001$).

In a study of 1734 patients from the Val-HeFT study,[85] a trial that randomized study participants to valsartan or a placebo in chronic HF patients, GDF-15 measurement was performed at baseline and after 12 months of study follow-up. In a comprehensive multivariable Cox regression model that included an exhaustive list of baseline characteristics, GDF-15 remained an independent predictor of all-cause mortality; however, its predictive power was minimal (HR = 1.007, 95% CI = 1.001-1.014, $P = 0.02$). Such results suggest that most of the prognosis can be explained by already available baseline characteristics. GDF-15 levels rose over time (145 ng/L in the placebo group vs. 173 ng/L in the valsartan group, $P = 0.94$) and such an increase was associated with increased risk of death and first morbid event even after adjustment for other baseline characteristics. Contrary to the theoretical link between GDF-15 and angiotensin II receptor, there was no significant interaction between clinical outcomes and valsartan treatment.

Quiescin Q6

The discovery of quiescin Q6 (also known as QSOX1) is another example of how the field of proteomics has impacted the discovery of biomarkers in HF. In patients with ADHF, liquid chromatography and mass spectrometry were used to provide a library of proteins that are present in the decompensated state. One of the best performing proteins in a small sample of patients was quiescin Q6, a protein closely linked to the formation of disulfide bridges; given the presence of a disulfide bond in the ubiquitous ring structure of natriuretic peptides, this is of note. Quiescin Q6 measurement identified patients with ADHF accurately (AUC 0.86, 95% CI = 0.79-0.92), and particularly was superior to BNP in discerning acute decompensation from chronic release.[86] In a larger cohort of 267 patients, this finding was validated with similar diagnostic accuracy independent of renal function. In particular, combining quiescin Q6 with BNP significantly improved its diagnostic performance by improving specificity.

Markers of Comorbidity

Renal Biomarkers

Renal Function Markers

Abnormal renal function is one of the most prognostically important comorbidities in patients with both acute and chronic HF syndromes. HF and abnormalities are so tightly intertwined that the term *cardiorenal syndrome* has been coined to describe this deleterious intersection (see also Chapter 14).

It is well established that standard measures of renal function, such as serum creatinine, eGFR, or blood urea nitrogen (BUN), are important predictors of outcome in patients with HF. For example, among those with ADHF in the ADHERE registry, both creatinine and BUN were independent predictors of hospital death; a classification and regression tree model containing both measures plus the presence of low blood pressure was useful to partition patients into various risk groups, with rates of death ranging from 2.1% to 21.9%.[87] Thus the value of renal function estimates to predict prognosis is additive (and frequently superior) to many risk factors in HF. Relative to other biomarkers, eGFR has been shown to be additive to natriuretic peptides for forecasting adverse outcome[8]; it has been postulated the definition of *cardiorenal syndrome* should be based on conjoined measurement of a cardiac biomarker such as NT-proBNP, plus a renal function marker such as eGFR.[88]

Beyond standard measures such as creatinine, newer methods to estimate renal function have been recently examined. Of these, cystatin C and β trace protein (BTP) appear most promising. Cystatin C is a 13-kDa protein produced at a constant rate by all nucleated cells that is filtered and then catabolized by tubular cells. BTP is a low-molecular-weight glycoprotein (between 23 and 29 kDa, depending on the degree of glycosylation) involved in prostaglandin metabolism. Compared to serum creatinine, both cystatin C and BTP provide consistently superior estimation of renal function, particularly in ranges of mild impairment of eGFR. As would be expected, both cystatin C and BTP are substantially prognostic in patients with HF, and were recently described to be superior to creatinine, eGFR, or BUN for this indication.[89] Considerably more data are needed before cystatin C or BTP would be considered ready for routine testing.

Renal Injury Markers

Rather than focusing on renal function, biomarkers that predict the presence of acute kidney injury (AKI) may be of particular value. This is because standard markers of renal function do not become abnormal until days after renal injury. Several early markers of renal injury have been discovered that appear to reflect the close interaction between the heart and the kidneys in cardiorenal dysfunction, whether from advanced HF and poor renal perfusion or because of excessive diuretic use and subsequent renal dysfunction.

Several biomarkers linked to AKI have been examined in patients with HF. Among these are neutrophil-gelatinase–associated lipocalin (NGAL), kidney injury molecule (KIM)-1, *N*-acetyl β-(D)-glucosaminidase (NAG), liver-type fatty acid binding protein, and IL-18.

NGAL is a siderophore protein involved in response to injury of epithelial cells, such as those in the kidneys. Concentrations of urine or serum NGAL have been suggested to be reflective of renal injury; notably, concentrations of NGAL are elevated in those with ADHF and prognosticate the onset of renal dysfunction in this setting.[90] However, the accuracy of NGAL to forecast imminent AKI was modest, with 68% sensitivity and 70% specificity (AUC 0.71, 95% CI = 0.58-0.84), and after adjustment for baseline renal function, the OR for AKI was 3.73 (95% CI = 1.26-11.01). Reflective of the poor prognosis in cardiorenal syndrome, patients with elevated NGAL had poor prognosis; NGAL greater than 167.5 ng/mL was associated with 2.7-fold increase in the risk of death and a 2.9-fold risk of death or hospitalization.[91] Similar findings were seen with urinary NGAL.

Despite generally favorable results, the role of NGAL remains uncertain, as conflicting evidence relative to its value exists. In a study of 1415 patients with HFrEF, the prognostic value of NGAL was less clear after adjusting for other traditional and biochemical factors, including NT-proBNP and eGFR.[92] Furthermore, NGAL may be nonspecific for renal injury due to its expression in a number of nonrenal tissues. It exists in more than one molecular form, and the relative advantage of plasma versus urine NGAL assays is not yet clear.

Fewer data exist for KIM-1 or NAG in HF. KIM-1 is a glycoprotein expressed in the proximal tubule. Urinary levels of KIM-1 have been shown to be an early indication of tubular injury in AKI. In patients with chronic HFrEF, urinary KIM-1 concentrations were reported to be higher than in those without HF (1460 vs. 56 pg/mL) and KIM-1 values correlated with LVEF and NYHA functional class.[93] NAG was originally described as a biomarker of AKI several years ago; it is a glycosidase found in renal tubular epithelia whose urinary concentrations are reasonably linked to acute tubular necrosis. Similar to KIM-1, concentrations of NAG correlate with LV function and HF severity in patients with chronic HF.[93] In 2130 patients from the GISSI-HF trial, NGAL, KIM-1, and NAG were independently associated with the combined endpoint of all-cause mortality and HF hospitalizations (NGAL, HR = 1.10, 95% CI = 1.00-1.20, $P = 0.04$; KIM-1, HR = 1.13, 95% CI = 1.02-1.24, $P = 0.02$; NAG, HR = 1.22, 95% CI = 1.10-1.36, $P < 0.001$); this association remained true even in patients with normal eGFR.

Hematologic Biomarkers

Abnormalities of hematologic indices are exceedingly common in patients with HF, and are of considerable prognostic importance. Anemia is caused by a multitude of abnormalities, including renal dysfunction, inflammation, and iron deficiency; it is typically defined as a serum hemoglobin less than 13 g/dL in men and less than 12 g/dL in women, and is associated with worse HF symptomatology and adverse outcomes in patients with both HFrEF and HFpEF, and it is additive to NT-proBNP for prognostication.[94] Unfortunately, treatment of anemia in HF does not appear to mitigate this risk.

Beyond hemoglobin, a curious association between red blood cell distribution width (RDW) and outcome in HF has been found. Felker and colleagues originally noted that for each increase in RDW in the Candesartan in HF: Assessment of Reduction in Mortality and Morbidity study, a 17% increase in risk for morbidity and mortality was observed.[95] In ADHF, RDW remained in adjusted models that included renal function and NT-proBNP, predicting death to 1 year from presentation.[96] Data from the Study of Anemia in a HF Population registry suggest the link between RDW and outcomes may be explained by inflammation and impaired iron mobilization.[97]

Liver Function Tests and Serum Albumin

Abnormalities of hepatic function, such as elevated aminotransferases, are common in patients with severe HF. This usually indicates significant congestion of the hepatic

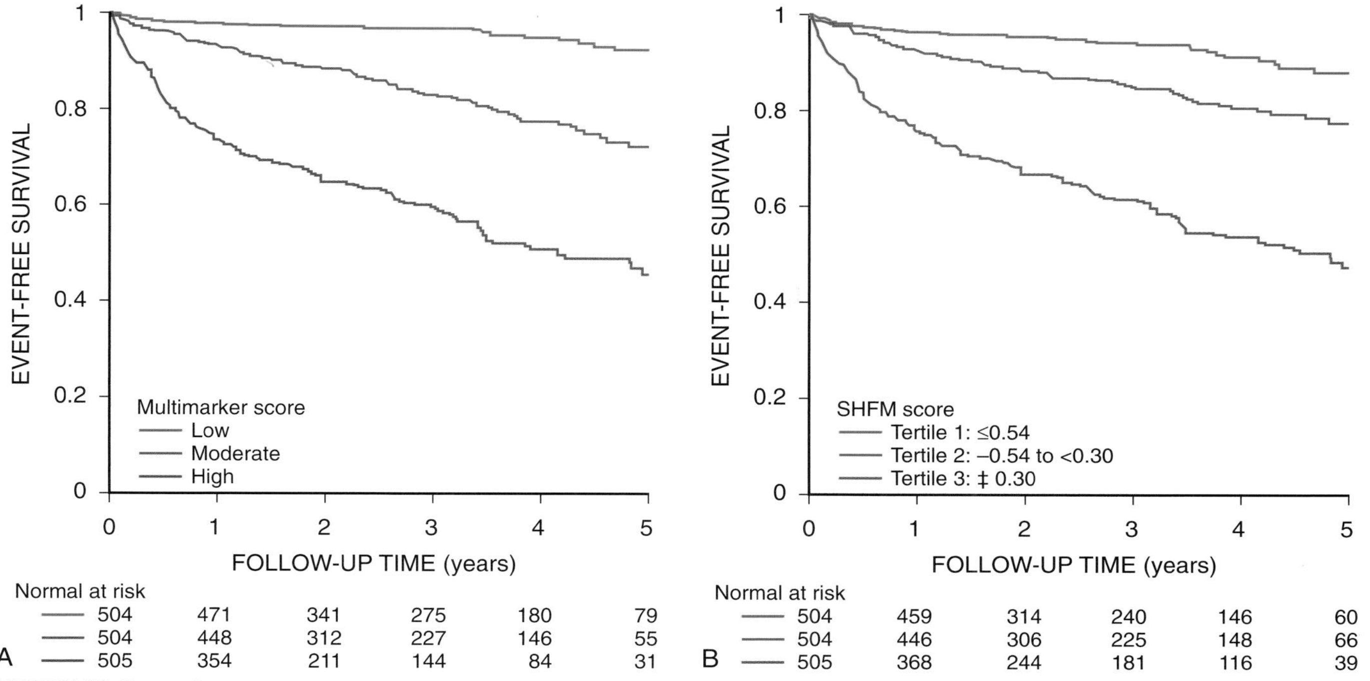

FIGURE 30-8 Event-free survival by multimarker score category **(A)** and tertiles of the Seattle Heart Failure Model (SHFM) score **(B)**. *From Ky B, French B, Levy WC, et al: Multiple biomarkers for risk prediction in chronic heart failure. Circ Heart Fail 5:183–190, 2012.*

venous system consequent to right heart congestion; however, low blood pressure may contribute. In a similar fashion, low serum albumin (e.g., <3.4 g/dL) is common in patients with HF, independent of BMI, possibly reflecting protein loss from enteral congestion due to right-sided HF. Both abnormal liver function tests and hypoalbuminemia in the context of HF are independently prognostic, even when considered in the context of natriuretic peptide measurement.

Adipokines

Adiponectin is a 244-amino-acid peptide involved in fatty acid metabolism, as well as glucose regulation. Concentrations of adiponectin are inversely related to body mass index, and may play a role in suppression of the metabolic disarray associated with obesity and metabolic syndrome. Elevated values of adiponectin have been reported in patients with cardiac cachexia, and may be prognostically meaningful.[25]

FUTURE DIRECTION: MULTIMARKER TESTING

With the rapid advancement in proteomic and genomic technologies and a growing fund of knowledge relative to the existing biomarkers currently available, the potential role of biomarkers in HF is likely to grow exponentially. Rather than focusing on the information provided by a single biomarker, it is likely that phenotyping patients using a mixture of biomarkers that provide "orthogonal" information will be of benefit. Such a multimarker strategy has potential to better personalize the care of patients with HF. As a proof-of-concept, Ky and colleagues examined a panel of biomarkers among 1513 patients with chronic HF (**Figure 30-8**), including BNP, CRP, MPO, soluble fms-like tyrosine kinase receptor-1, hsTnI, sST2, creatinine, and uric acid.[98] The score derived from this panel was independent (adjusted HR 6.80, 95% CI = 8.75-21.5), additive to the established clinical risk score from the Seattle Heart Failure Model with an improvement in the AUC of 0.803 from 0.756 ($P = 0.003$) and improved reclassification (net reclassification improvement of 25.2%, 95% CI = 14.2%-36.2%, $P<0.001$).

References

1. Braunwald E, Harrison DC, Chidsey CA: The heart as an endocrine organ. *Am J Med* 36:1–4, 1964.
2. Maisel AS, Krishnaswamy P, Nowak RM, et al: Rapid measurement of B-type natriuretic peptide in the emergency diagnosis of heart failure. *N Engl J Med* 347:161–167, 2002.
3. Januzzi JL, Jr, Camargo CA, Anwaruddin S, et al: The N-terminal pro-BNP investigation of dyspnea in the emergency department (pride) study. *Am J Cardiol* 95:948–954, 2005.
4. van Kimmenade RR, Januzzi JL, Jr: Emerging biomarkers in heart failure. *Clin Chem* 58:127–138, 2012.
5. Yancy CW, Jessup M, Bozkurt B, et al: 2013 ACCF/AHA guideline for the management of heart failure: a report of the American College of Cardiology Foundation/American Heart Association task force on practice guidelines. *Circulation* 128:e240–e327, 2013.
6. Braunwald E: Heart failure. *JACC Heart Fail* 1:1–20, 2013.
7. Januzzi JL, Jr: Natriuretic peptides as biomarkers in heart failure. *J Investig Med* 61:950–955, 2013.
8. van Kimmenade RR, Januzzi JL, Jr, Bakker JA, et al: Renal clearance of B-type natriuretic peptide and amino terminal pro-B-type natriuretic peptide: a mechanistic study in hypertensive subjects. *J Am Coll Cardiol* 53:884–890, 2009.
9. Wang TJ, Larson MG, Levy D, et al: Impact of age and sex on plasma natriuretic peptide levels in healthy adults. *Am J Cardiol* 90:254–258, 2002.
10. Januzzi JL, van Kimmenade R, Lainchbury J, et al: Nt-proBNP testing for diagnosis and short-term prognosis in acute destabilized heart failure: an international pooled analysis of 1256 patients: the international collaborative of NT-proBNP study. *Eur Heart J* 27:330–337, 2006.
11. McCullough PA, Duc P, Omland T, et al: B-type natriuretic peptide and renal function in the diagnosis of heart failure: an analysis from the Breathing Not Properly Multinational Study. *Am J Kidney Dis* 41:571–579, 2003.
12. Anwaruddin S, Lloyd-Jones DM, Baggish A, et al: Renal function, congestive heart failure, and amino-terminal pro-brain natriuretic peptide measurement: results from the ProBNP Investigation of Dyspnea in the Emergency Department (PRIDE) study. *J Am Coll Cardiol* 47:91–97, 2006.
13. Maisel AS, McCord J, Nowak RM, et al: Bedside B-type natriuretic peptide in the emergency diagnosis of heart failure with reduced or preserved ejection fraction. Results from the Breathing Not Properly Multinational Study. *J Am Coll Cardiol* 41:2010–2017, 2003.
14. O'Donoghue M, Chen A, Baggish AL, et al: The effects of ejection fraction on N-terminal proBNP and BNP levels in patients with acute CHF: analysis from the ProBNP Investigation of Dyspnea in the Emergency Department (PRIDE) study. *J Card Fail* 11:S9–S14, 2005.
15. Mueller C, Scholer A, Laule-Kilian K, et al: Use of B-type natriuretic peptide in the evaluation and management of acute dyspnea. *N Engl J Med* 350:647–654, 2004.
16. Moe GW, Howlett J, Januzzi JL, et al: N-terminal pro-B-type natriuretic peptide testing improves the management of patients with suspected acute heart failure: primary results of the Canadian prospective randomized multicenter improve-CHF study. *Circulation* 115:3103–3110, 2007.
17. Meisel SR, Januzzi JL, Medvedovski M, et al: Pre-admission NT-proBNP improves diagnostic yield and risk stratification—the NT-proBNP for evaluation of dyspnoeic patients in the emergency room and hospital (bnp4ever) study. *Eur Heart J Acute Cardiovasc Care* 1:99–108, 2012.

18. Siebert U, Januzzi JL, Jr, Beinfeld MT, et al: Cost-effectiveness of using N-terminal pro-brain natriuretic peptide to guide the diagnostic assessment and management of dyspneic patients in the emergency department. *Am J Cardiol* 98:800–805, 2006.
19. Green SM, Martinez-Rumayor A, Gregory SA, et al: Clinical uncertainty, diagnostic accuracy, and outcomes in emergency department patients presenting with dyspnea. *Arch Intern Med* 168:741–748, 2008.
20. Wright SP, Doughty RN, Pearl A, et al: Plasma amino-terminal pro-brain natriuretic peptide and accuracy of heart-failure diagnosis in primary care: a randomized, controlled trial. *J Am Coll Cardiol* 42:1793–1800, 2003.
21. Hildebrandt P, Collinson PO, Doughty RN, et al: Age-dependent values of N-terminal pro-B-type natriuretic peptide are superior to a single cut-point for ruling out suspected systolic dysfunction in primary care. *Eur Heart J* 31:1881–1889, 2010.
22. Suzuki T, Yamaoki K, Nakajima O, et al: Screening for cardiac dysfunction in asymptomatic patients by measuring B-type natriuretic peptide levels. *Jpn Heart J* 41:205–214, 2000.
23. Baggish AL, van Kimmenade RR, Januzzi JL, Jr: The differential diagnosis of an elevated amino-terminal pro-B-type natriuretic peptide level. *Am J Cardiol* 101:43–48, 2008.
24. Wang TJ, Larson MG, Levy D, et al: Impact of obesity on plasma natriuretic peptide levels. *Circulation* 109:594–600, 2004.
25. Kistorp C, Faber J, Galatius S, et al: Plasma adiponectin, body mass index, and mortality in patients with chronic heart failure. *Circulation* 112:1756–1762, 2005.
26. Bayes-Genis A, Lloyd-Jones DM, van Kimmenade RR, et al: Effect of body mass index on diagnostic and prognostic usefulness of amino-terminal pro-brain natriuretic peptide in patients with acute dyspnea. *Arch Intern Med* 167:400–407, 2007.
27. van Kimmenade RR, Pinto YM, Bayes-Genis A, et al: Usefulness of intermediate amino-terminal pro-brain natriuretic peptide concentrations for diagnosis and prognosis of acute heart failure. *Am J Cardiol* 98:386–390, 2006.
28. Fonarow GC, Peacock WF, Phillips CO, et al: Admission B-type natriuretic peptide levels and in-hospital mortality in acute decompensated heart failure. *J Am Coll Cardiol* 49:1943–1950, 2007.
29. Januzzi JL, Jr, Sakhuja R, O'Donoghue M, et al: Utility of amino-terminal pro-brain natriuretic peptide testing for prediction of 1-year mortality in patients with dyspnea treated in the emergency department. *Arch Intern Med* 166:315–320, 2006.
30. Kociol RD, Horton JR, Fonarow GC, et al: Admission, discharge, or change in B-type natriuretic peptide and long-term outcomes: data from Organized Program to Initiate Lifesaving Treatment in Hospitalized Patients with Heart Failure (OPTIMIZE-HF) linked to Medicare claims. *Circ Heart Fail* 4:628–636, 2011.
31. Masson S, Latini R, Anand IS, et al: Prognostic value of changes in n-terminal pro-brain natriuretic peptide in Val-HeFT (Valsartan Heart Failure trial). *J Am Coll Cardiol* 52:997–1003, 2008.
32. Weiner RB, Baggish AL, Chen-Tournoux A, et al: Improvement in structural and functional echocardiographic parameters during chronic heart failure therapy guided by natriuretic peptides: mechanistic insights from the ProBNP Outpatient Tailored Chronic Heart Failure (PROTECT) study. *Eur J Heart Fail* 15:342–351, 2013.
33. Wang TJ, Larson MG, Levy D, et al: Plasma natriuretic peptide levels and the risk of cardiovascular events and death. *N Engl J Med* 350:655–663, 2004.
34. Gaggin HK, Januzzi JL, Jr: Biomarkers and diagnostics in heart failure. *Biochim Biophys Acta* 1832:2442–2450, 2013.
35. Troughton RW, Frampton CM, Yandle TG, et al: Treatment of heart failure guided by plasma aminoterminal brain natriuretic peptide (n-BNP) concentrations. *Lancet* 355:1126–1130, 2000.
36. Kim HN, Januzzi JL, Jr: Biomarkers in the management of heart failure. *Curr Treat Options Cardiovasc Med* 12:519–531, 2010.
37. Felker GM, Hasselblad V, Hernandez AF, et al: Biomarker-guided therapy in chronic heart failure: a meta-analysis of randomized controlled trials. *Am Heart J* 158:422–430, 2009.
38. Jourdain P, Jondeau G, Funck F, et al: Plasma brain natriuretic peptide-guided therapy to improve outcome in heart failure: the Stars-BNP multicenter study. *J Am Coll Cardiol* 49:1733–1739, 2007.
39. Januzzi JL, Jr, Rehman SU, Mohammed AA, et al: Use of amino-terminal pro-b-type natriuretic peptide to guide outpatient therapy of patients with chronic left ventricular systolic dysfunction. *J Am Coll Cardiol* 58:1881–1889, 2011.
40. Maisel A, Mueller C, Nowak R, et al: Mid-region pro-hormone markers for diagnosis and prognosis in acute dyspnea: results from the BACH (Biomarkers in Acute Heart Failure) trial. *J Am Coll Cardiol* 55:2062–2076, 2010.
41. Shah RV, Truong QA, Gaggin HK, et al: Mid-regional pro-atrial natriuretic peptide and pro-adrenomedullin testing for the diagnostic and prognostic evaluation of patients with acute dyspnoea. *Eur Heart J* 33:2197–2205, 2012.
42. Masson S, Latini R, Carbonieri E, et al: The predictive value of stable precursor fragments of vasoactive peptides in patients with chronic heart failure: data from the GISSI-heart failure (GISSI-HF) trial. *Eur J Heart Fail* 12:338–347, 2010.
43. Richards M, Di Somma S, Mueller C, et al: Atrial fibrillation impairs the diagnostic performance of cardiac natriuretic peptides in dyspneic patients: results from the BACH study (Biomarkers in Acute Heart Failure). *JACC Heart Fail* 1:192–199, 2013.
44. Thygesen K, Alpert JS, Jaffe AS, et al: Third universal definition of myocardial infarction. *Circulation* 126:2020–2035, 2012.
45. Peacock WF, De Marco T, Fonarow GC, et al: Cardiac troponin and outcome in acute heart failure. *N Engl J Med* 358:2117–2126, 2008.
46. Xue Y, Clopton P, Peacock WF, et al: Serial changes in high-sensitive troponin I predict outcome in patients with decompensated heart failure. *Eur J Heart Fail* 13:37–42, 2011.
47. Latini R, Masson S, Anand IS, et al: Prognostic value of very low plasma concentrations of troponin T in patients with stable chronic heart failure. *Circulation* 116:1242–1249, 2007.
48. Masson S, Anand I, Favero C, et al: Serial measurement of cardiac troponin T using a highly sensitive assay in patients with chronic heart failure: data from 2 large randomized clinical trials. *Circulation* 125:280–288, 2012.
49. deFilippi CR, de Lemos JA, Christenson RH, et al: Association of serial measures of cardiac troponin T using a sensitive assay with incident heart failure and cardiovascular mortality in older adults. *JAMA* 304:2494–2502, 2010.
50. Wang TJ, Wollert KC, Larson MG, et al: Prognostic utility of novel biomarkers of cardiovascular stress: the Framingham Heart Study. *Circulation* 126:1596–1604, 2012.
51. Tang WHW, Brennan M-L, Philip K, et al: Plasma myeloperoxidase levels in patients with chronic heart failure. *Am J Cardiol* 98:796–799, 2006.
52. Krishnan E: Hyperuricemia and incident heart failure. *Circ Heart Fail* 2:556–562, 2009.
53. George J, Carr E, Davies J, et al: High-dose allopurinol improves endothelial function by profoundly reducing vascular oxidative stress and not by lowering uric acid. *Circulation* 114:2508–2516, 2006.
54. Hare JM, Mangal B, Brown J, et al: Impact of oxypurinol in patients with symptomatic heart failure. Results of the OPT-CHF study. *J Am Coll Cardiol* 51:2301–2309, 2008.
55. Cabassi A, Champlain JD, Maggiore U, et al: Prealbumin improves death risk prediction of BNP-added Seattle Heart Failure Model: results from a pilot study in elderly chronic heart failure patients. *Int J Cardiol* 168:3334–3339, 2013.
56. Dieplinger B, Gegenhuber A, Struck J, et al: Chromogranin a and c-terminal endothelin-1 precursor fragment add independent prognostic information to amino-terminal proBNP in patients with acute destabilized heart failure. *Clin Chim Acta* 400:91–96, 2009.
57. Rosjo H, Masson S, Latini R, et al: Prognostic value of chromogranin A in chronic heart failure: data from the GISSI-Heart Failure trial. *Eur J Heart Fail* 12:549–556, 2010.
58. Richards AM, Doughty R, Nicholls MG, et al: Plasma N-terminal pro-brain natriuretic peptide and adrenomedullin: prognostic utility and prediction of benefit from carvedilol in chronic ischemic left ventricular dysfunction. Australia-New Zealand heart failure group. *J Am Coll Cardiol* 37:1781–1787, 2001.
59. Maisel A, Xue Y, Shah K, et al: Increased 90-day mortality in patients with acute heart failure with elevated copeptin: secondary results from the Biomarkers in Acute Heart Failure (BACH) study. *Circ Heart Fail* 4:613–620, 2011.
60. Braunwald E: Biomarkers in heart failure. *N Engl J Med* 358:2148–2159, 2008.
61. Januzzi JL, Jr, Rehman S, Mueller T, et al: Importance of biomarkers for long-term mortality prediction in acutely dyspneic patients. *Clin Chem* 56:1814–1821, 2010.
62. Cesari M, Penninx BW, Newman AB, et al: Inflammatory markers and onset of cardiovascular events: results from the Health ABC study. *Circulation* 108:2317–2322, 2003.
63. Sanada S, Hakuno D, Higgins LJ, et al: Il-33 and ST2 comprise a critical biomechanically induced and cardioprotective signaling system. *J Clin Invest* 117:1538–1549, 2007.
64. Dieplinger B, Januzzi JL, Jr, Steinmair M, et al: Analytical and clinical evaluation of a novel high-sensitivity assay for measurement of soluble ST2 in human plasma–the presage ST2 assay. *Clin Chim Acta* 409:33–40, 2009.
65. Januzzi JL, Jr, Peacock WF, Maisel AS, et al: Measurement of the interleukin family member ST2 in patients with acute dyspnea: results from the PRIDE (Pro-brain Natriuretic Peptide Investigation of Dyspnea in the Emergency Department) study. *J Am Coll Cardiol* 50:607–613, 2007.
66. Boisot S, Beede J, Isakson S, et al: Serial sampling of ST2 predicts 90-day mortality following destabilized heart failure. *J Card Fail* 14:732–738, 2008.
67. Lassus J, Gayat E, Mueller C, et al: Incremental value of biomarkers to clinical variables for mortality prediction in acutely decompensated heart failure: the Multinational Observational Cohort on Acute Heart Failure (MOCA) study. *Int J Cardiol* 168:2186–2194, 2013.
68. Ky B, French B, McCloskey K, et al: High-sensitivity ST2 for prediction of adverse outcomes in chronic heart failure. *Circ Heart Fail* 4:180–187, 2011.
69. Kohli P, Bonaca MP, Kakkar R, et al: Role of ST2 in non-ST-elevation acute coronary syndrome in the MERLIN-TIMI 36 trial. *Clin Chem* 58:257–266, 2012.
70. Weir RA, Miller AM, Murphy GE, et al: Serum soluble ST2: a potential novel mediator in left ventricular and infarct remodeling after acute myocardial infarction. *J Am Coll Cardiol* 55:243–250, 2010.
71. Sharma UC, Pokharel S, van Brakel TJ, et al: Galectin-3 marks activated macrophages in failure-prone hypertrophied hearts and contributes to cardiac dysfunction. *Circulation* 110:3121–3128, 2004.
72. van Kimmenade RR, Januzzi JL, Jr, Ellinor PT, et al: Utility of amino-terminal pro-brain natriuretic peptide, galectin-3, and apelin for the evaluation of patients with acute heart failure. *J Am Coll Cardiol* 48:1217–1224, 2006.
73. Gullestad L, Ueland T, Kjekshus J, et al: Galectin-3 predicts response to statin therapy in the Controlled Rosuvastatin Multinational Trial in Heart Failure (CORONA). *Eur Heart J* 33:2290–2296, 2012.
74. Lok DJ, Van Der Meer P, de la Porte PW, et al: Prognostic value of galectin-3, a novel marker of fibrosis, in patients with chronic heart failure: data from the DEAL-HF study. *Clin Res Cardiol* 99:323–328, 2010.
75. de Boer RA, Lok DJ, Jaarsma T, et al: Predictive value of plasma galectin-3 levels in heart failure with reduced and preserved ejection fraction. *Ann Med* 43:60–68, 2011.
76. Motiwala SR, Szymonifka J, Belcher A, et al: Serial measurement of galectin-3 in patients with chronic heart failure: results from the proBNP Outpatient Tailored Chronic Heart Failure Therapy (PROTECT) study. *Eur J Heart Fail* 15:1157–1163, 2013.
77. Polyakova V, Loeffler I, Hein S, et al: Fibrosis in endstage human heart failure: severe changes in collagen metabolism and MMP/TIMP profiles. *Int J Cardiol* 151:18–33, 2011.
78. Jordan A, Roldan V, Garcia M, et al: Matrix metalloproteinase-1 and its inhibitor, timp-1, in systolic heart failure: relation to functional data and prognosis. *J Intern Med* 262:385–392, 2007.
79. Zile MR, Desantis SM, Baicu CF, et al: Plasma biomarkers that reflect determinants of matrix composition identify the presence of left ventricular hypertrophy and diastolic heart failure. *Circ Heart Fail* 4:246–256, 2011.
80. Iraqi W, Rossignol P, Angioi M, et al: Extracellular cardiac matrix biomarkers in patients with acute myocardial infarction complicated by left ventricular dysfunction and heart failure: insights from the Eplerenone Post-Acute Myocardial Infarction Heart Failure Efficacy and Survival study (EPHESUS) study. *Circulation* 119:2471–2479, 2009.
81. van Rooij E, Sutherland LB, Liu N, et al: A signature pattern of stress-responsive microRNAs that can evoke cardiac hypertrophy and heart failure. *Proc Natl Acad Sci U S A* 103:18255–18260, 2006.
82. Tijsen AJ, Creemers EE, Moerland PD, et al: Mir423-5p as a circulating biomarker for heart failure. *Circ Res* 106:1035–1039, 2010.
83. Montgomery RL, Hullinger TG, Semus HM, et al: Therapeutic inhibition of mir-208a improves cardiac function and survival during heart failure. *Circulation* 124:1537–1547, 2011.
84. Xu J, Kimball TR, Lorenz JN, et al: Gdf15/mic-1 functions as a protective and antihypertrophic factor released from the myocardium in association with SMAD protein activation. *Circ Res* 98:342–350, 2006.
85. Anand IS, Kempf T, Rector TS, et al: Serial measurement of growth-differentiation factor-15 in heart failure: relation to disease severity and prognosis in the Valsartan Heart Failure trial. *Circulation* 122:1387–1395, 2010.
86. Mebazaa A, Vanpoucke G, Thomas G, et al: Unbiased plasma proteomics for novel diagnostic biomarkers in cardiovascular disease: identification of quiescin q6 as a candidate biomarker of acutely decompensated heart failure. *Eur Heart J* 33:2317–2324, 2012.
87. Fonarow GC, Adams KF, Jr, Abraham WT, et al: Risk stratification for in-hospital mortality in acutely decompensated heart failure: classification and regression tree analysis. *JAMA* 293:572–580, 2005.
88. van Kimmenade RRJ, Pinto Y, Januzzi JL: When renal and cardiac insufficiencies intersect: Is there a role for natriuretic peptide testing in the "cardio-renal syndrome"? *Eur Heart J* 28:2960–2961, 2007.
89. Manzano-Fernández S, Januzzi JL, Jr, Boronat-Garcia M, et al: B-trace protein and cystatin c as predictors of long-term outcomes in patients with acute heart failure. *J Am Coll Cardiol* 57:849–858, 2011.
90. Macdonald S, Arendts G, Nagree Y, et al: Neutrophil gelatinase-associated lipocalin (NGAL) predicts renal injury in acute decompensated cardiac failure: a prospective observational study. *BMC Cardiovasc Disord* 12:8, 2012.
91. Alvelos M, Lourenco P, Dias C, et al: Prognostic value of neutrophil gelatinase-associated lipocalin in acute heart failure. *Int J Cardiol* 165:51–55, 2013.
92. Nymo SH, Ueland T, Askevold ET, et al: The association between neutrophil gelatinase-associated lipocalin and clinical outcome in chronic heart failure: results from CORONA*. *J Intern Med* 271:436–443, 2012.
93. Jungbauer CG, Birner C, Jung B, et al: Kidney injury molecule-1 and n-acetyl-beta-d-glucosaminidase in chronic heart failure: possible biomarkers of cardiorenal syndrome. *Eur J Heart Fail* 13:1104–1110, 2011.

94. Baggish AL, van Kimmenade R, Bayes-Genis A, et al: Hemoglobin and n-terminal pro-brain natriuretic peptide: independent and synergistic predictors of mortality in patients with acute heart failure results from the International Collaborative of NT-proBNP (ICON) study. *Clin Chim Acta* 381:145–150, 2007.
95. Felker GM, Allen LA, Pocock SJ, et al: Red cell distribution width as a novel prognostic marker in heart failure: data from the CHARM program and the Duke Databank. *J Am Coll Cardiol* 50:40–47, 2007.
96. van Kimmenade RR, Mohammed AA, Uthamalingam S, et al: Red blood cell distribution width and 1-year mortality in acute heart failure. *Eur J Heart Fail* 12:129–136, 2010.
97. Allen LA, Felker GM, Mehra MR, et al: Validation and potential mechanisms of red cell distribution width as a prognostic marker in heart failure. *J Card Fail* 16:230–238, 2010.
98. Ky B, French B, Levy WC, et al: Multiple biomarkers for risk prediction in chronic heart failure. *Circ Heart Fail* 5:183–190, 2012.

31 Hemodynamics in Heart Failure

John J. Ryan, Jose Nativi Nicolau, and James C. Fang

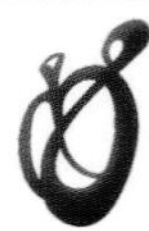

The first right-heart catheterization in humans was performed in 1929 by Dr. Werner Forssmann (on himself), who ultimately shared in the 1956 Nobel Prize in Medicine with Andre Cournand and Dickinson Richards for their work in cardiac catheterization. A right-heart catheter was further refined by the work of Drs. Bradley and Fife, and in 1969 Drs. Scheinman, Abbott, and Rapaport reported their use of a flow-directed right-heart catheter. Following their report of a bedside balloon flotation catheter by Drs. Swan and Ganz in the *New England Journal of Medicine* in 1970, right-heart catheterization became widespread both in the catheterization laboratory and in intensive care units for critically ill and unstable patients.[1] Despite advances in noninvasive hemodynamic assessment with echocardiography and cardiac magnetic resonance imaging (MRI), right- and left-heart catheterization (RHC, LHC) remains the gold standard for hemodynamic assessment in heart disease.[2] Today, the three predominant reasons to obtain invasive hemodynamics in heart failure are:

1. To resolve diagnostic uncertainty in patients with cryptic symptoms.
2. To assess the suitability for advanced therapies in chronic heart failure.
3. To investigate pulmonary hypertension.

TECHNICAL ISSUES

The technique for obtaining invasive hemodynamics is extensively and comprehensively discussed in other excellent sources (e.g., *Braunwald's Textbook of Cardiovascular Medicine*[3] and *Grossman's Cardiac Catheterization, Angiography, and Intervention*).[4] However, some specific technical points bear emphasis.

It is important to recognize that invasive hemodynamics are traditionally measured at rest, in the sedated state, and in a supine position. These limitations should be appreciated when invasive hemodynamics are used to reconcile cryptic symptoms, assess prognosis, or prepare patients for advanced therapies. However, most of our contemporary understanding of heart failure hemodynamics is derived from these resting, supine, and sedated studies. Exercise and upright hemodynamics can be obtained in the properly trained laboratory and are often necessary in certain clinical situations, but are not commonly performed on a routine basis in most clinical catheterization laboratories. The hemodynamic response to various physiologic and/or pharmacologic challenges should also be considered at the time of right-heart catheterization so as to maximize the information obtained during this invasive procedure. Finally, it should be appreciated that traditionally obtained hemodynamic measurements lack concomitant measurements of cardiac and/or intravascular volume so pressure is used as a surrogate for volume.

Pressure measurements in cardiac catheterization are recorded using fluid-filled catheters connected to strain-gauge pressure transducers using the principle of the Wheatstone bridge. Because of the need for pressure transmission to record a signal, a time delay is inherent and should be accounted for when assessing instantaneous pressure differences (e.g., gradients). Moreover, fluid-filled systems are influenced by various factors, including transducer height, patient position, catheter length, air bubbles, fluid frequency response/damping (e.g., catheter whip artifacts), and open connections.

These issues can be avoided by using micromanometer catheters that use high-fidelity pressure sensors at the point of measurement (Millar Instruments, Houston). Such systems can also be combined with special conductance catheters to provide simultaneous volume measurements but their use is confined to research laboratories. These systems provide more sophisticated measures of ventricular performance, such as contractility, diastolic function, and ventricular pressure-volume relationships.[5]

The impact of respiration on intracardiac pressures should be considered. The dynamic changes in intrathoracic pressures associated with respiration are usually modest (e.g., –1 to 5 mm Hg) but can be quite dramatic (e.g., severe obesity, obstructive pulmonary disease) and will have a significant influence on intracardiac pressures. However, it is common in both clinical practice and investigation that mean pressure measurements rather than respirophasic ranges are reported, which can lead to important misinterpretations. For example, the pulmonary capillary wedge pressure (PCWP) averaged over the duration of the respiratory cycle may underestimate the true end-expiratory left ventricular end-diastolic pressure (LVEDP) and lead to an erroneous diagnosis of World Health Organization (WHO) group 1 rather than group 2 or mixed pulmonary hypertension (PH).[6] It is optimal to manually measure end-expiratory pressures because the effects of negative intrathoracic pressures required for ventilation on intracardiac pressures are minimal at end expiration. A breath-hold can be useful if done at end expiration as long as a Valsalva maneuver does not ensue.

RHC is generally safe but its routine use in heart failure management should be tempered by complications associated with any invasive procedure. Serious complications, such as pneumothorax, pulmonary embolism, and pulmonary arterial rupture, however, are rare. In the ESCAPE trial, in-hospital adverse events were more common among patients in the RHC group compared with the clinical assessment group (22% vs. 11.5%; $P = 0.04$).[7] Adverse events due to the pulmonary artery catheter (PAC) occurred in 4% ($n = 9$) of the RHC group. The most common complication was access site bleeding. There were no hospital deaths attributed to the PAC. Adverse events included PAC-related infection, catheter knotting, pulmonary infarction and hemorrhage, and implantable cardioverter-defibrillator (ICD) shocks. Pulmonary arterial rupture and right bundle branch block (RBBB) with subsequent complete heart block in the setting of a baseline left bundle branch block (LBBB) did not occur. Pulmonary artery (PA) rupture is rare in clinical practice, but risk factors include severe PH, anticoagulation, mitral valve disease, and advanced age.[8,9]

HEMODYNAMIC WAVEFORMS

In clinical practice, it is difficult to measure LV volume throughout the cardiac cycle, rendering the use of pressure-volume (PV) loops for clinical care impractical. The difficulty in obtaining PV loops has resulted in a dependence on pressure versus time rather than pressure versus volume measurements to assess hemodynamic status and ventricular performance.

Each chamber has a distinct waveform and reflects cardiac filling and ventricular ejection. Personal inspection of specific cardiac chamber waveforms can often convey important hemodynamic information that is not appreciated by a single pressure measurement.

Right Atrium and Ventricle

The right atrial pressure (RAP) and waveform can provide simple yet important insight into a patient's overall hemodynamic status. During normal respiration, RAP decreases with inspiration to the same degree as the drop in intrapleural pressure (usually <5 mm Hg). Lack of an inspiratory fall, or even rise in RAP with inspiration (e.g., Kussmaul sign), is indicative of right ventricle (RV) diastolic dysfunction and often RV overload (**Figure 31-1**). Steep *y* descents are also indicative of RV diastolic dysfunction (**Figure 31-2**). The steep *y* descent results from the rapid inflow required to fill a stiff right ventricle in early diastole, particularly in the presence of an elevated RAP. Similarly, the "dip and plateau" appearance in the RV tracing indicates rapid, early diastolic filling and abrupt cessation of diastolic inflow as

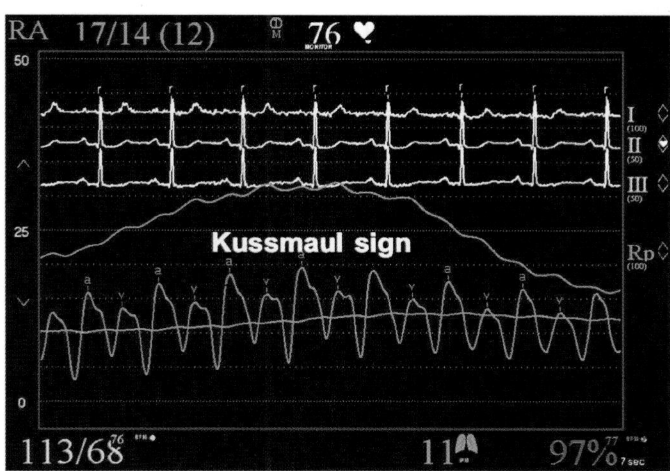

FIGURE 31-1 Right atrial pressure waveform. Kussmaul sign: increased right atrial pressure with inspiration. Waveform also demonstrates dynamic tricuspid regurgitation as a consequence of right ventricular enlargement and dysfunction with venous return.

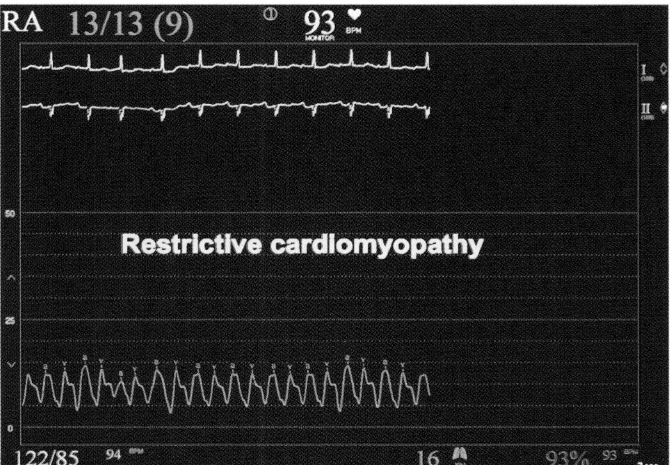

FIGURE 31-2 Right atrial pressure waveform. Restrictive cardiomyopathy: steep *x* and *y* descents. Appearance of the waveform conveys significant right ventricular dysfunction despite the minimal increase in right atrial pressure of 9 mm Hg.

the left and right ventricles reach the point of pericardial restraint. Such findings are commonly found in conditions associated with RV dysfunction, including advanced heart failure with reduced ejection fraction (HFrEF), restrictive cardiomyopathies, heart transplantation, and RV infarction. Prominent *v* wave is noted in severe tricuspid regurgitation (**Figure 31-3**).

The RV is a low-pressure chamber in normal individuals. A small systolic gradient between the RV systolic pressure (RVSP) and PA systolic pressure (PASP) facilitates forward flow in this low-pressure system. The RV waveform can be distinguished from the PA waveform by the rise in pressure during diastole in contrast to the fall in pressure in the PA tracing. The rise in the RVSP over time, dP/dt, can be used to estimate the PA diastolic pressure (ePAD) because the pulmonic valve opening will occur at the end of isovolumic contraction or maximum dP/dt (**Figure 31-4**). The ePAD will approximate the PCWP (e.g., within 2 to 3 mm Hg) as long as the pulmonary vascular resistance is normal. This strategy was used for the CHRONICLE device to provide a continuous estimate of the PCWP.[10]

Pulmonary Capillary Wedge Pressure

A common concern in RHC is whether a true PCWP has been obtained (**Figure 31-5**). Fluoroscopy and a visible change in the waveform is typically used to confirm the PCWP position. Loss of the pulmonary arterial waveform and a change to a "flattened" appearance with attenuated deflections usually signifies the PCWP. A prominent ***v*** wave can also be seen with a true PCWP but can be easily confused with the PASP. The ***v*** wave of PCWP occurs well after the T wave of the electrocardiogram (ECG), whereas the peak systolic wave of PASP occurs before or within the T wave. Difficulty in distinguishing between PCWP and PASP is particularly problematic in patients with prominent ***v*** waves (e.g., acute severe mitral regurgitation, ventricular septal defects, and severe diastolic dysfunction).

Hybrid tracings between PCWP and actual PAP result in an overestimation of PCWP and should be suspected when the PCWP exceeds the PAD pressure (**Figure 31-6**). Damping of the hemodynamic waveform should also be considered. Underdamping, which is often referred to as *ringing* or *whip* artifact, can lead to inaccurate pressure recordings and can be rectified by drawing a small amount of blood or contrast into the catheter to increase the viscosity of the fluid. In patients with severe right ventricular enlargement and dysfunction, caution must be used when it comes to interpreting an elevated PCWP or LVEDP. RV pressure overload from PAH can result in elevated LVEDP due to impaired relaxation of the LV secondary to RV enlargement, as well as pericardial restraint (see also later discussion). In this setting, LV diastolic dysfunction is a consequence and not independent of the primary abnormality (PAH).

If there is still uncertainty about the accuracy of the measured PCWP, it is best confirmed by other means. A common strategy is to use the O_2 saturation from a blood sample obtained from the PCWP position.[6] In the true PCWP position, the O_2 saturation from the PCWP blood sample should have an O_2 saturation comparable to systemic arterial saturation (in the absence of intracardiac shunts). Wedge position can also be confirmed by cautious injection of contrast to document true wedging of the balloon. LVEDP should be directly measured if uncertainty exists as to the accuracy of the PCWP as a surrogate for left ventricular filling. In circumstances where accurate assessment of left atrial pressure is critical, consideration should be given to directly measuring left atrial pressure across the atrial septum.

The PCWP waveform is similar to that seen in the left atrium with well-characterized *a* and *v* waves, in addition to *x* and *y* descent (*c* waves are less apparent in PCWP tracings). PCWP waveforms are also slightly damped and delayed compared with that seen in the left artery because of transmission of the pressures through the lung parenchyma. As noted above, in the absence of increased pulmonary vascular resistance, pulmonary artery diastolic pressure is similar to mean PCWP (e.g., within 2 to 3 mm Hg). If there is PH, the PA end-diastolic pressure will be markedly higher than PCWP.[11] Furthermore, when pulmonary vascular resistance is increased by pulmonary venous hypertension or mitral stenosis, PCWP may overestimate LVEDP.[12] PCWP may also underestimate LVEDP because PCWP is an intrathoracic pressure that is an indirect assessment of LVEDP and is not a direct measurement of LV filling pressure. In one study, PCWP was more than 5 mm Hg lower than LVEDP in about a third of cardiac patients.[13] Therefore, when it is critical to have a definitive

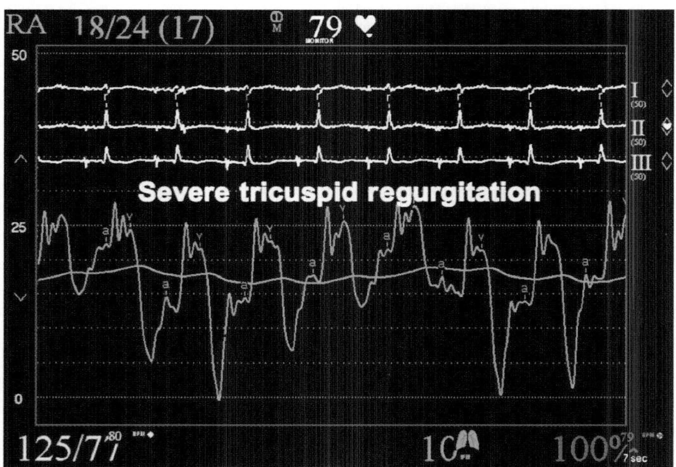

FIGURE 31-3 Right atrial pressure waveform. Severe tricuspid regurgitation: prominent *v* wave. Waveform appears ventricularized due to the organic disease of the tricuspid valve.

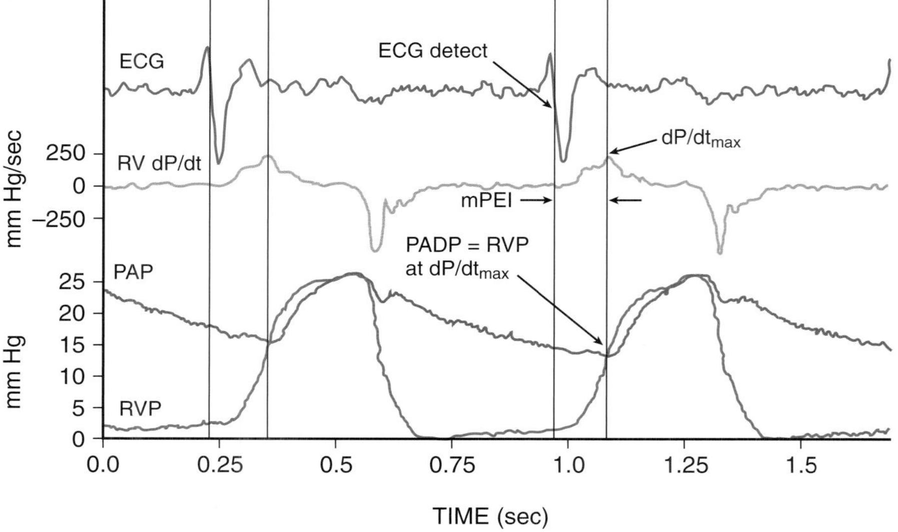

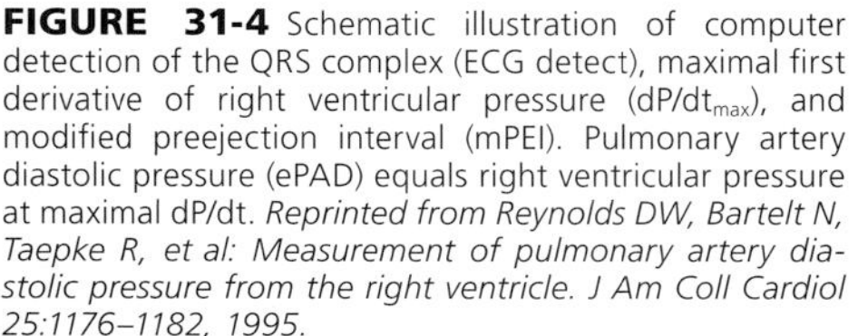
FIGURE 31-4 Schematic illustration of computer detection of the QRS complex (ECG detect), maximal first derivative of right ventricular pressure (dP/dt_{max}), and modified preejection interval (mPEI). Pulmonary artery diastolic pressure (ePAD) equals right ventricular pressure at maximal dP/dt. *Reprinted from Reynolds DW, Bartelt N, Taepke R, et al: Measurement of pulmonary artery diastolic pressure from the right ventricle. J Am Coll Cardiol 25:1176–1182, 1995.*

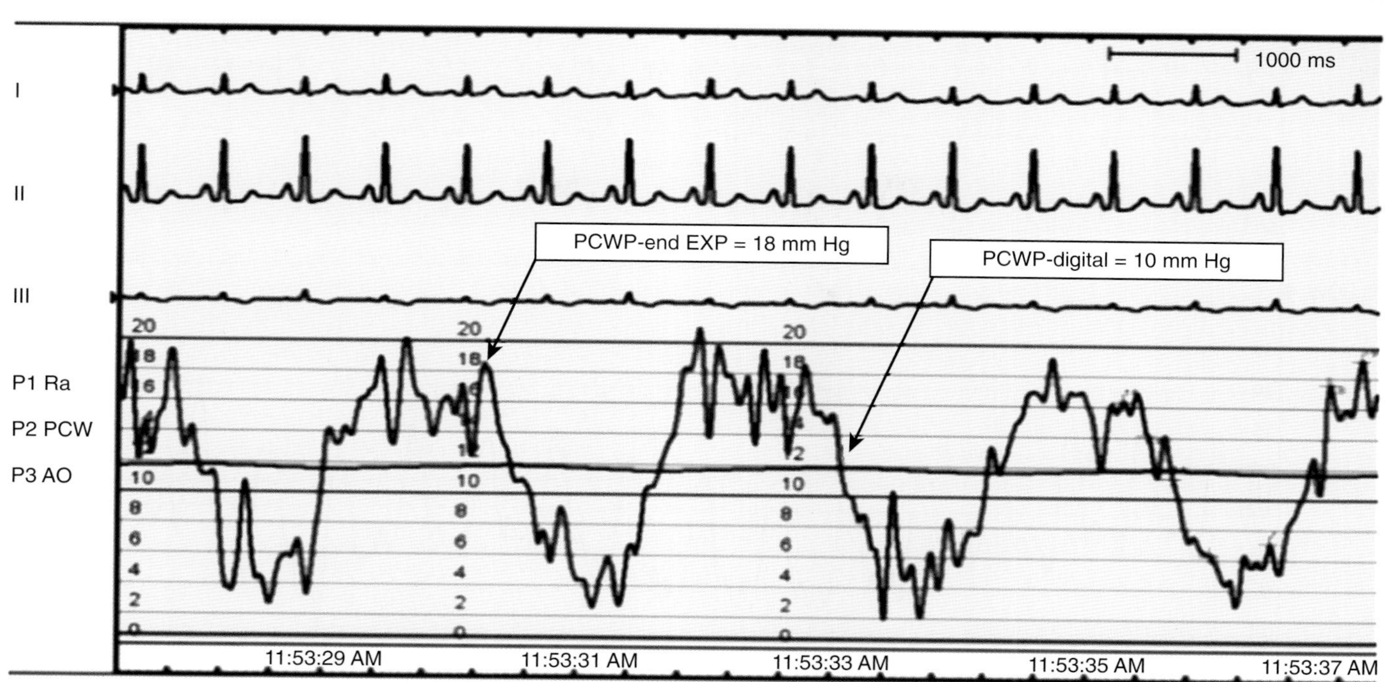

FIGURE 31-5 Errors in pulmonary capillary wedge pressure. Tracing illustrates the respirophasic waveforms with the digitized means. The difference between PCWP–end expiration versus PCWP-digital suggests misclassification of the type of pulmonary hypertension. *Reprinted from Ryan JJ, Rich JD, Thiruvoipati T, et al: Current practice for determining pulmonary capillary wedge pressure predisposes to serious errors in the classification of patients with pulmonary hypertension. Am Heart J 163:589–594, 2012.*

measure of LV filling pressure, direct measurement of LVEDP is necessary.

The height of the *v* wave should be reported separately from the mean PCWP, particularly when it exceeds the height of the *a* wave by >50%. The height of the *v* wave is determined by left atrial chamber compliance and distending blood volume. Although most commonly associated with acute severe mitral regurgitation (due to the sudden retrograde volume overwhelming the compliance of the left atrium), it is also characteristic of a large volume VSD and can be seen in severe left ventricular diastolic dysfunction.

Measuring Cardiac Output

The two most commonly used methods for measuring cardiac output (CO) are the thermodilution and the Fick methods. Both methods are limited by technical issues and physiologic assumptions. The indication-dilution technique is rarely used in contemporary clinical practice but forms the basis for the thermodilution method.

In the thermodilution method, a known volume of cold saline or dextrose is injected at a known temperature into the proximal port of the PAC. The subsequent change in temperature of this solution is measured by a thermistor at the distal end of the catheter. The change in temperature of the injectate allows measurement of the cardiac output. If the temperature does not change markedly and remains close to the temperature at which it was injected, this reflects a high cardiac output because there is insufficient time for the surrounding structures to transfer heat energy to the fluid. In contrast, if the cardiac output is low, there will be ample time to transfer heat energy from the blood to the injectate before it passes the thermistor at the distal end of the catheter. In this setting, the temperature of the injectate will change markedly and will be reflective of a decreased cardiac output. The cardiac output is calculated using an equation that incorporates a calibration factor plus the volume, the specific gravity, and the temperature of the injectate along with the temperature and specific gravity of the blood. The cardiac output is inversely related to the area under the thermodilution curve (e.g., change in temperature over time) with a larger area reflective of a lower cardiac output. Accuracy of the cardiac output measurement is improved by the greater the difference between the temperature of the injectate and the temperature of the blood. The thermodilution technique overestimates flow in patients with low-output states. Concern is frequently raised regarding the accuracy of thermodilution in patients with severe tricuspid regurgitation, but it remains remarkably useful even in this setting.

The Fick method is based upon the principle that O_2 consumption equals the product of the O_2 delivery rate (e.g., cardiac output) and O_2 extraction (e.g., the difference in O_2 content between the arterial and venous circulation). Thus cardiac output equals the ratio of O_2 consumption to O_2 extraction and is therefore directly proportional to O_2 consumption. Measurement of O_2 consumption requires specialized equipment (e.g., a metabolic cart) to measure the content of O_2 in expired air. Because most clinical laboratories lack the capacity to make this measurement, most clinical laboratories assume a uniform normalized O_2 consumption (e.g., 125 mL/min/m^2) for all patients. Corrections for metabolic state, age, and gender are generally not made, and errors in O_2 consumption can be as high as 50% because O_2 consumption varies widely between patients and clinical status. Such issues are compounded during exercise hemodynamics.[14] Errors in the Fick method can also occur if the mixed venous O_2 content is inaccurately measured because of contamination of the pulmonary arterial sample with blood from the pulmonary capillary wedge position or use of central venous samples rather than blood from the PA. Inaccurate assessment of hemoglobin content

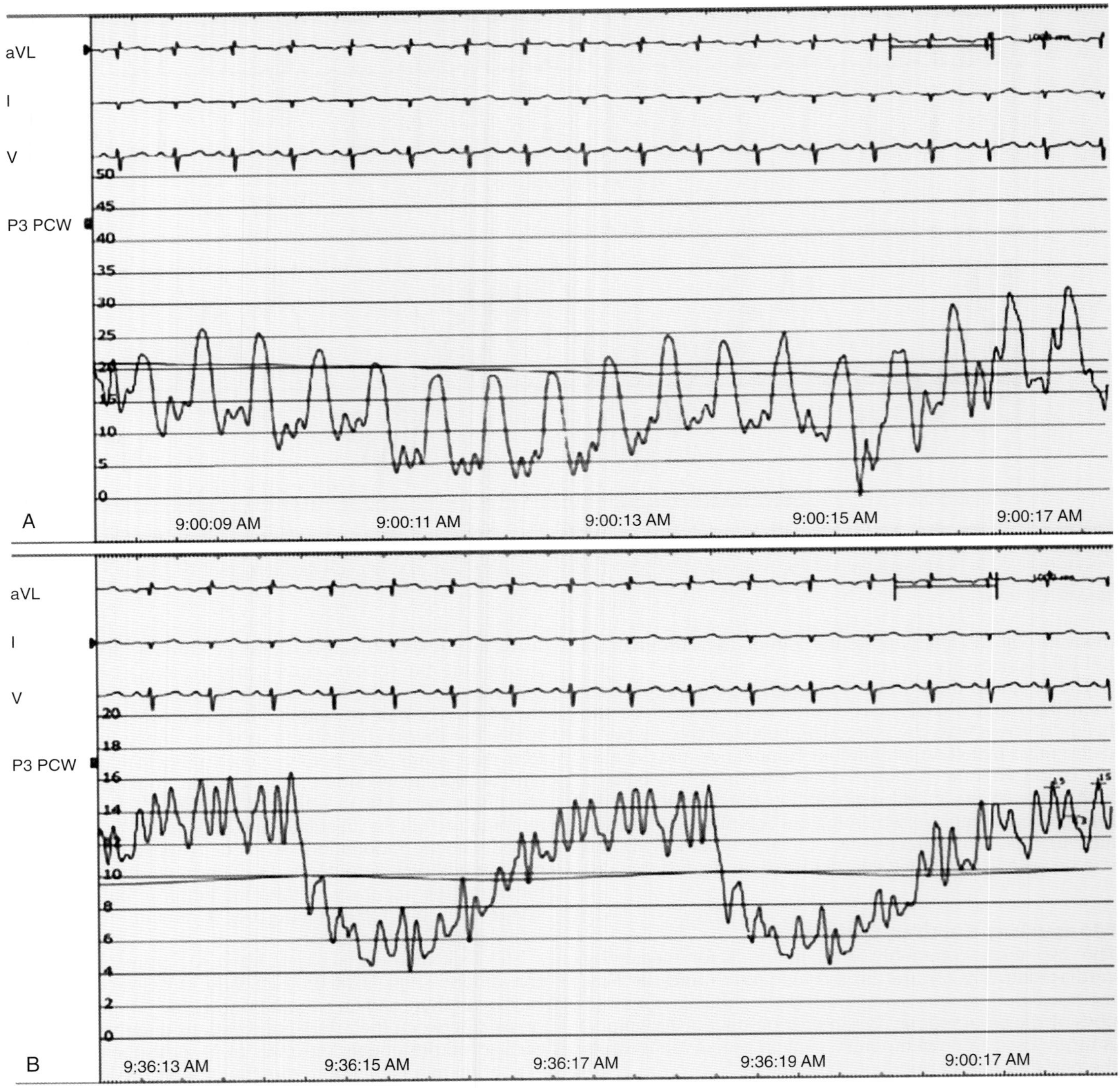

FIGURE 31-6 Errors in pulmonary capillary wedge pressure. **A,** Hybrid tracing of pulmonary artery pressure and wedge tracing overestimating wedge pressure. **B,** Actual pulmonary capillary wedge pressure tracing once the balloon is deflated and allowed to wedge in a smaller, more distal branch of the pulmonary artery. *Reprinted from Guillinta P, Peterson KL, Ben-Yehuda O: Cardiac catheterization techniques in pulmonary hypertension. Cardiol Clin 22:401–415, 2004.*

will also lead to measurement errors, and simultaneous measurement of hemoglobin concentration should be obtained if possible. If O_2 consumption is accurately measured, the Fick method is more accurate than thermodilution in patients with low cardiac output.

HEMODYNAMICS OF HEART FAILURE WITH REDUCED EJECTION FRACTION

The hemodynamic interaction between the left ventricle and the vascular system (e.g., ventricular-vascular coupling) for any degree of intrinsic myocardial contractility is best described with PV loops.[5] In a PV loop, load-independent contractility is characterized by the slope of the end-systolic pressure-volume relationship (ESPVR) curve, or end-systolic elastance (Ees), which is also influenced by chamber size. Vascular afterload is characterized by arterial stiffness or elastance (Ea) and determined from the negative slope of the line through the end-systolic and end-diastolic volumes (**Figure 31-7**); this measure integrates the resistive and pulsatile components of afterload.[15] Ejection fraction, systolic blood pressure, stroke volume, and stroke work can all

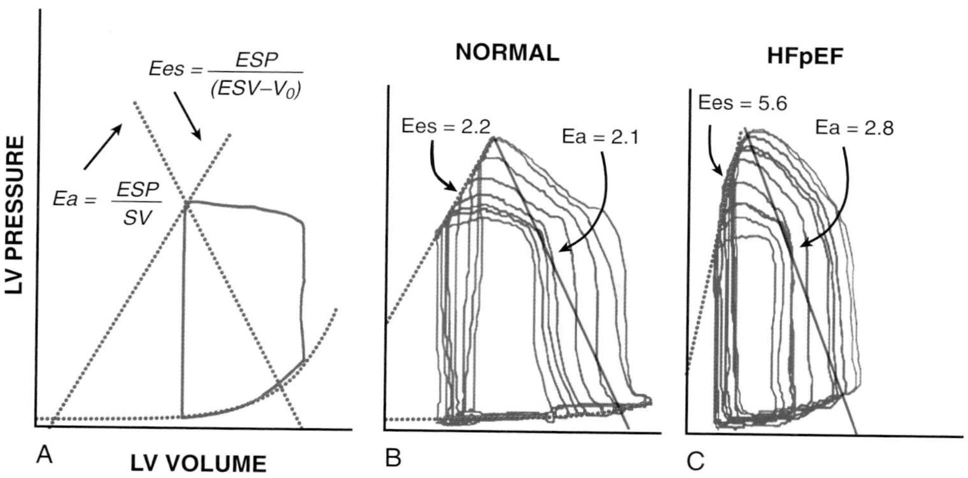

FIGURE 31-7 **A,** Left ventricular end-systolic elastance (Ees) is described by the slope and intercept of the end-systolic pressure-volume relationship; arterial elastance (Ea) is defined by the negative slope between the end-systolic pressure-volume point and end-diastolic volume. **B,** A normal adult has relatively low Ees and Ea, with a coupling ratio around unity, whereas older aged, hypertensive, and HFpEF subjects **(C)** display marked increases in ventricular and arterial elastance. *Reprinted from Borlaug BA, Kass DA: Ventricular-vascular interaction in heart failure. Cardiology Clin 29:447–459, 2011.*

be derived from end-diastolic volume (EDV) and these elastances.

The ratio of these two measurements represents ventricular-arterial coupling (Ea/Ees) and describes the "matching" of vascular load to myocardial function.[15-17] Experimental studies suggest an optimal Ea/Ees ratio is 0.6 to 1.2, which maximizes the efficient transfer of blood from the heart into the systemic circulation. In patients with HFrEF, this ratio is increased because ventricular elastance (Ees) is depressed from the underlying cardiomyopathy and arterial elastance (Ea) is increased from neurohormonal activation and vasoconstriction.[16] This afterload "mismatch" has prognostic implications independent of EF and can be a target for therapy (see later discussion). In a recent noninvasive multicenter study of HFrEF patients, an Ea/Ees ratio >2.34 was found an independent risk factor of all-cause mortality, cardiac transplantation, or VAD implantation (HR 2.1, 95% CI 1.3-3.3).[18]

It is important to note that systemic blood pressure and systemic vascular resistance do not adequately describe afterload in a pulsatile system. In clinical practice, the resistive load is described by the systemic vascular resistance (SVR) [(mean blood pressure – central venous pressure)/ cardiac output]; the pulsatile load is usually not described. The pulsatile load can be quantified by the total systemic arterial compliance (Ca) [stroke volume index/aortic pulse pressure]. Because the aorta provides the majority of this pulsatile load, central pulsatile load (or characteristic impedance, Zc = change in pressure/change in flow in early systole) better characterizes the work that must be overcome by the LV during ejection and is elevated in HFrEF.[19] Although not practical for routine clinical use, the effective arterial elastance (Ea = ESP/SV, where ESP = end systolic pressure, SV = stroke volume) combines the resistive and pulsatile components of LV afterload and best describes the impact of ventricular-vascular coupling to LV performance.

In HFrEF, vasodilation can dramatically improve stroke volume because the reduced contractile state is particularly afterload sensitive and characterized by an increased Ea/Ees ratio (e.g., afterload "mismatch"). Vasodilator therapy takes advantage of the inverse relationship between cardiac output and impedance. In HFrEF, the afterload-sensitive nature of the failing LV is reflected by the relatively flat end-systolic pressure-volume relationship (ESPVR) (i.e., shallow Ees). This flat ESPVR accounts for the marked improvement in stroke volume that occurs with vasodilator therapy without a significant drop in blood pressure (**Figure 31-8**).

HEMODYNAMICS FOR ASSESSMENT AND MANAGEMENT

A hemodynamically directed clinical assessment is prognostic. The 1-year risk of mortality or urgent transplantation increases with worsening hemodynamic status. With bedside evaluation of filling pressures and perfusion, the patient can be classified as profile A (warm and dry), B (warm and wet), C (cold and wet), and L (cold and dry). Congested patients (profile B) are at greater risk for death or transplant than those compensated (profile A) (HR 1.84, $P = 0.02$); the highest risk is associated with congestion and poor perfusion (profile C) (HR 2.48, $P = 0.03$).[20] Drazner and coworkers confirmed that a bedside clinical assessment (e.g., orthopnea, jugular venous distention, impression of inadequate perfusion) does parallel invasively obtained hemodynamics in a group of patients with advanced heart failure. Moreover, invasively obtained hemodynamics in this population did identify those at increased risk of morbidity and mortality.[21] The central venous pressure (CVP) is particularly useful because it is easy to obtain at the bedside or invasively. An elevated CVP is the hemodynamic abnormality most commonly associated with cardiorenal syndrome.[22] An increased RA/PCW ratio is also associated with more severe PH, RV dysfunction, and poor outcomes in advanced heart failure and with left ventricular assist device therapy (see Chapter 42).[23]

The hemodynamic profile can be used to guide therapy. Most patients with decompensated heart failure present congested but well perfused. Vasodilators and decongestion with diuretics or mechanical fluid removal are recommended for symptom relief, but this hemodynamic profile rarely requires invasively obtained hemodynamics to guide therapy. In contrast, selected patients with clinical evidence

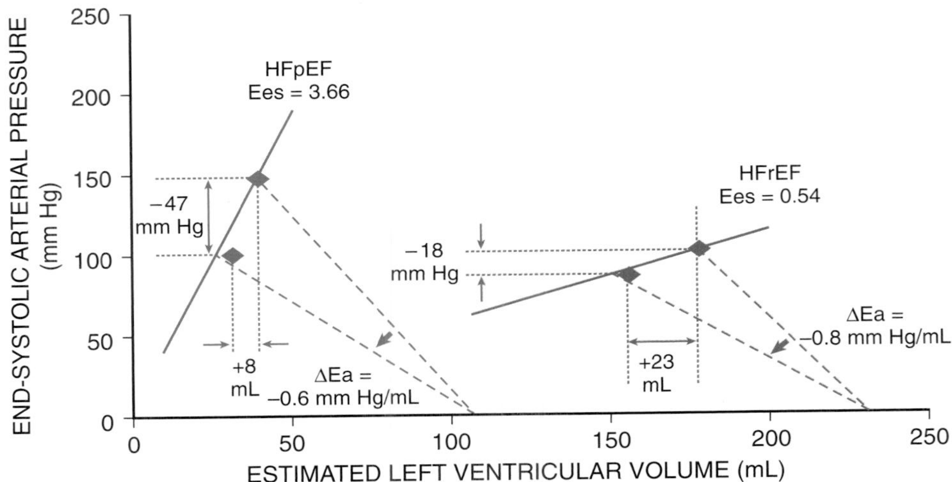

FIGURE 31-8 Differential effect of afterload reduction in HFpEF versus HFrEF. In HFpEF *(black)*, a reduction in afterload (Ea = −0.6 mm Hg/mL) with a vasodilator produces a large decrease in blood pressure (BP) (−47 mm Hg) but only a modest increase in stroke volume (+8 mL) because end-systolic elastance (Ees) is steep (3.66). In contrast, comparable vasodilation (Ea = −0.8 mm Hg/mL) produces only a modest decrease in BP (−18 mm Hg) but a large increase in stroke volume (+23 mL) because of the shallow Ees (0.54) in HFrEF *(red)*. *Reprinted from Schwartzenberg S, Redfield MM, From AM, et al: Effects of vasodilation in heart failure with preserved or reduced ejection fraction implications of distinct pathophysiologies on response to therapy. J Am Coll Cardiol 59:442–451, 2012.*

of inadequate perfusion (e.g., hypotension, end-organ dysfunction, lack of improvement with empiric therapy) may benefit from invasive hemodynamics to guide therapy. This approach can be particularly useful when there is hypotension, because the cause may be vasoplegic (e.g., low systemic vascular resistance) rather than due to poor perfusion (e.g., low cardiac index, high SVR). In this setting, if an inadequate cardiac output is confirmed (and hypovolemia is not present), subsequent therapy can be "tailored" to the total hemodynamic picture.[24,25] In the ESCAPE trial, the RA decreased from 14 ± 10 to 10 ± 7 mm Hg, PCW fell from 25 ± 9 to 17 ± 7 mm Hg, the CI rose from 1.9 ± 0.6 to 2.4 ± 0.7 L/min/m^2, and the SVR fell from 1500 ± 800 to 1100 ± 500 dynes/sec/cm^{-5} with tailored therapy.[7] Reasonable hemodynamic goals include a RA <10 mm Hg, PCWP <15 mm Hg, and an SVR <1200 dynes/sec/cm^{-5} to maximize the forward cardiac output while maintaining a mean BP >65-70 mm Hg or a systemic systolic blood pressure of at least 80 to 90 mm Hg. These goals are physiologically based; there is no randomized evidence to support these targets to improve symptoms or impact clinically important outcomes.

These hemodynamic goals are generally achieved with diuretic management and vasodilators. This approach is preferred over inotropic management when the cardiac index is low and SVR is elevated because of the increase in mortality associated with inotropic agents.[2] Often intravenous rather than oral vasodilators are elected to achieve rapid hemodynamic goals, which minimizes the duration of PA line placement. Sodium nitroprusside (SNP) is ideal in this regard because its effects are rapid in onset and it is rapidly cleared and is recommended in numerous guidelines.[2,24-26] Its balanced vasodilator effect is particularly useful when filling pressures are high, SVR is increased (e.g., >2000 dynes/sec/cm^{-5}), and the cardiac index is low. In a observational experience from the Cleveland Clinic, use of tailored therapy with SNP was associated with improved survival in patients presenting with a low cardiac index (1.6 ± 0.2 L/min/m^2) and elevated SVR (1846 ± 567 dynes/sec/cm^{-5}), without worsening renal function or the need for inotropic support.[25] Randomized experiences with SNP in chronic heart failure, however, are lacking. Nitroglycerin and nesiritide can also be used for "tailored" therapy.

An effective reduction in mitral regurgitation and an increase in forward stroke volume also occur with vasodilators because of a reduction in left ventricular volume and mitral annular orifice size.[27] In addition, relieving right-heart congestion leads to improved LV filling through reduction in the pericardial constraint imposed by an overdistended RV "crowding out" the LV.[28] In fact, almost half of the measured intraventricular diastolic pressure is a consequence of external forces from the pericardium and RV.[29,30] Diastolic ventricular interaction is most evident when RA pressure (an estimate of pericardial pressure) equals PCWP, effectively decreasing LV transmural pressure (e.g., LV preload).[31] "Release" of the pericardial constraint by decompressing the RV paradoxically increases LV transmural pressure, thereby optimizing LV preload (**Figure 31-9A-D**).

Hemodynamic profiles have changed over time. As a result of the routine use of aggressive oral vasodilators in chronic systolic heart failure, it is relatively uncommon to see patients with a low cardiac index and extremely elevated SVR. In advanced heart failure, a low cardiac index may be associated with an "abnormally" normal SVR (e.g., <1200 dynes/sec/cm^{-5}) or vasoplegic state. In this situation, inotropic support, with or without vasopressors, may be necessary in the acute setting. Unless there is another reason to explain the inappropriate vasoplegia (e.g., infection, adrenal insufficiency, etc.), this hemodynamic profile is difficult to treat, associated with poor outcomes, and should initiate a consideration of advanced therapies.

Despite the potential use of hemodynamics for "tailored" therapy, the *routine* use of invasive hemodynamics for the treatment of heart failure is not recommended. The 2013 ACCF/AHA guidelines for the management of heart failure observe that RHC and PA catheter is best reserved for situations where a particular therapeutic or clinical question is being addressed, such as inadequate clinical assessment and uncertain hemodynamics in patients with inadequate systemic perfusion and/or respiratory distress (**Table 31-1**).[2] The ESCAPE trial was a multicenter randomized

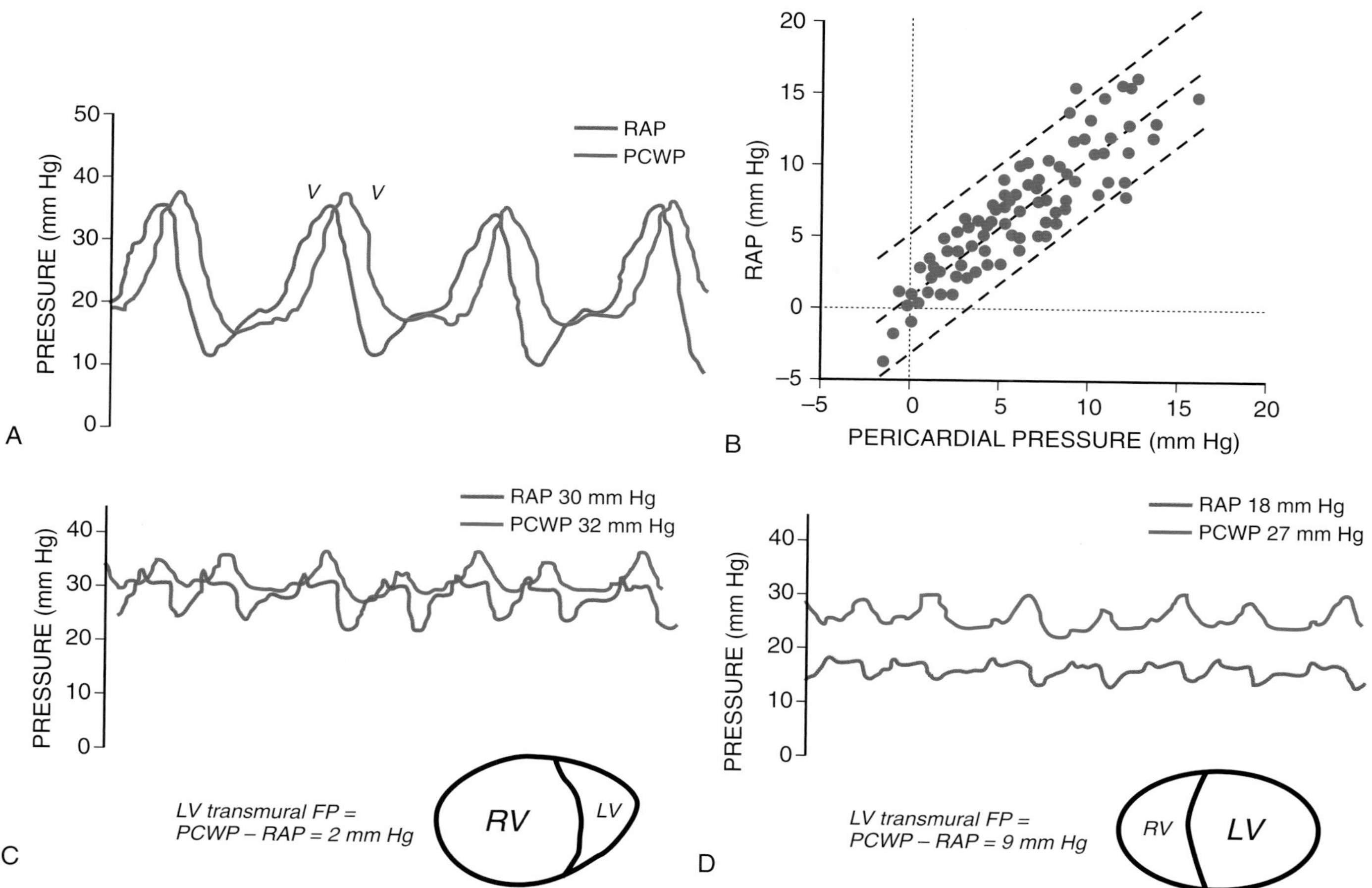

FIGURE 31-9 Ventricular interdependence in right heart failure from group 2 PH. **A,** Typical equalization in RAP and PCWP from enhanced interdependence in a patient with biventricular HF and severe functional tricuspid insufficiency. Note the prominent V wave in the PCWP that tracks closely with the RA V wave, even in the absence of significant mitral insufficiency. This is caused by pressure changes in the RA being transmitted to the LA across the interatrial septum. **B,** External pericardial pressure, which restrains left heart filling, can be estimated by RAP. Thus when RA pressure is elevated near PCWP, true LV preload volume may be reduced despite marked elevation in left PCWP, because transmural pressure is reduced. **C** and **D,** Unloading of right-heart congestion in this circumstance may enhance left-sided preload, even if PCWP drops, because transmural pressure increases. *FP,* Filling pressure; *HF,* heart failure; *LA,* left atrium; *LV,* left ventricle; *PCWP,* pulmonary capillary wedge pressure; *PH,* pulmonary hypertension; *RAP,* right atrial pressure; *RV,* right ventricle; *RA,* right atrium. *Reprinted from Guazzi M, Borlaug BA: Pulmonary hypertension due to left heart disease. Circulation 126:975–990, 2012.*

TABLE 31-1 Recommendations for Invasive Evaluation

RECOMMENDATIONS	COR	LOE
Monitoring with a pulmonary artery catheter should be performed in patients with respiratory distress or impaired systemic perfusion when clinical assessment is inadequate.	I	C
Invasive hemodynamic monitoring can be useful for carefully selected patients with acute HF with persistent symptoms and/or when hemodynamics are uncertain.	IIa	C
When ischemia may be contributing to HF, coronary arteriography is reasonable.	IIa	C
Endomyocardial biopsy can be useful in patients with HF when a specific diagnosis is suspected that would influence therapy.	IIa	C
Routine use of invasive hemodynamic monitoring is not recommended in normotensive patients with acute HF.	III: No benefit	B
Endomyocardial biopsy should not be performed in the routine evaluation of HF.	III: Harm	C

COR, Class of recommendation; *HF,* heart failure; *LOE,* level of evidence.
Adapted from Yancy CW, Jessup M, Bozkurt B, et al: 2013 ACCF/AHA guideline for the management of heart failure: a report of the American College of Cardiology Foundation/American Heart Association task force on practice guidelines. J Am Coll Cardiol 62:e147-239, 2013.

controlled trial of PA catheter–guided management in acute decompensated heart failure patients with a left ventricular ejection fraction (LVEF) <30%.[7] Compared with patients treated without a PA catheter, the use of invasive hemodynamics to guide therapy achieved no significant difference in mortality (10% vs. 9%, $P = 0.35$) or days hospitalized (8.7 vs. 8.3 days, $P = 0.67$). PA catheter–guided therapy was associated with more in-hospital adverse events as described previously. Use of PA catheter–guided therapy remains a reasonable approach in patients not responding to initial therapy or with deteriorating clinical status.

HEMODYNAMICS AND ADVANCED HEART FAILURE

Hemodynamic assessment in advanced heart failure is necessary to evaluate PH, RV function, and candidacy for advanced therapies. The primary hemodynamic

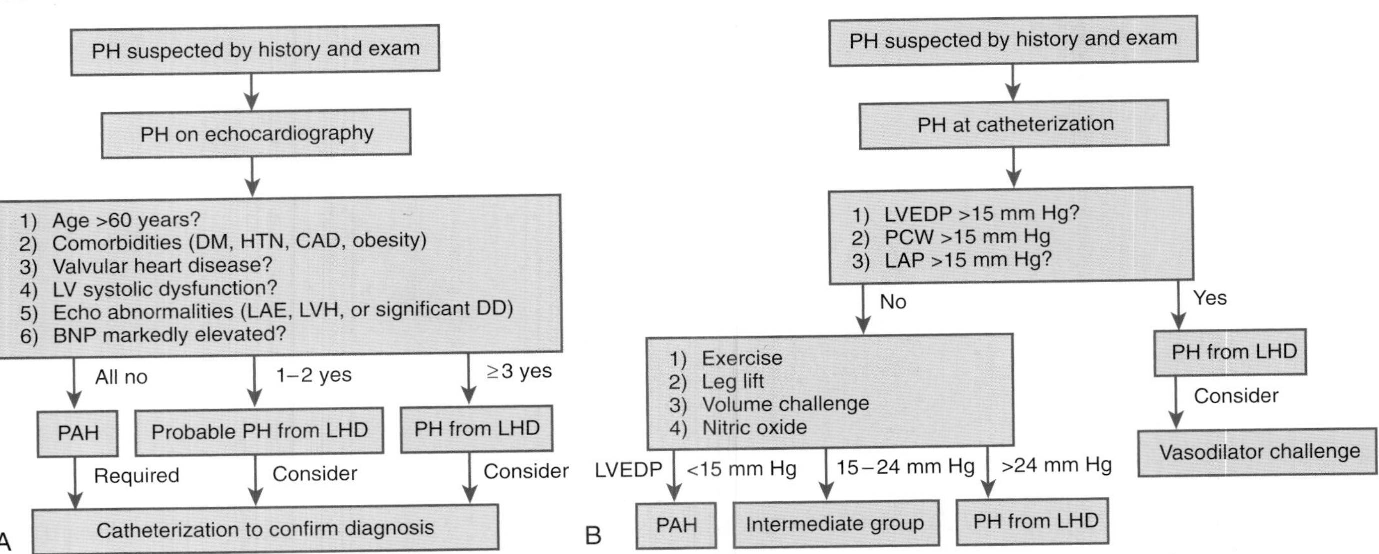

FIGURE 31-10 Echocardiographic **(A)** and hemodynamic **(B)** approach to pulmonary hypertension.

considerations when faced with PH and heart failure are to confirm its presence and severity, delineate cause, and assess reversibility (**Figure 31-10**). Excluding WHO Group 1 PH is crucial; it is defined by a mean PAP ≥25 mm Hg and a resting PCWP <15 mm Hg. Therefore, accurate measurement of PCWP is critical. If there is uncertainty regarding this measurement, LVEDP should be obtained directly. A fluid challenge or a selective pulmonary vasodilator (e.g., inhaled nitric oxide) can be used to selectively assess the LV filling pressure response to an increase in volume.[32] Hemodynamic assessment and treatment of WHO Group 1 PH is comprehensively reviewed in other excellent sources (**see also Chapter 39**).[33]

The PH of heart failure is defined by a mean PAP ≥25 mm Hg with resting PCWP ≥15 mm Hg (e.g., WHO Group 2 PH). In heart failure, the chronically elevated pressures of the left heart are passively transmitted back into the pulmonary circulation, leading to elevated pulmonary arterial pressures, variably referred to as *passive, postcapillary,* or *secondary* PH. PH is common in heart failure and is a marker of disease severity and is associated with increased mortality.[34,35] In a cohort of 337 patients with LVEF <30%, 62% had a mean PAP >20 mm Hg.[36] In a series from the Mayo Clinic, 75% of those presenting for resting RHC and LVEF ≤40% had a mean PAP ≥25 mm Hg and had a greater than twofold risk for mortality (HR 2.24; 95% CI 1.39-3.98; *P* <0.001). Although PH in heart failure has been defined by mean PAP, a PASP ≥35 mm Hg is a valid surrogate for a mean PAP ≥25 mm Hg.[37]

In heart failure, PH is commonly increased out of proportion to the predicted PH relative to the increase in left-heart filling pressure (e.g., "mixed" or reactive PH). It is defined by a mean PAP ≥25 mm Hg, PCWP ≥15 mm Hg, transpulmonary gradient (TPG) ≥12-15 mm Hg, and PVR ≥2.5-3.0 Wood units.[34] In this setting, this secondary pulmonary vasoreactivity is associated with greater diastolic dysfunction, mitral regurgitation, and RV dysfunction and may develop as an adaptive mechanism with anatomic remodeling.[38] In HFrEF, mixed PH is not easily predicted from clinical profiles but is associated with greater disease severity and increased mortality. In a study of 242 patients with HFrEF, 31% had passive PH (mPAP 38 ± 7 mm Hg, PVR 2.8 ± 1.9 WU, TPG 11 ± 6 mm Hg) and 13% had mixed PH (44 ± 8 mm Hg, PVR 4.2 ± 2.4 WU, TPG 14 ± 6 mm Hg).[39] However, there were no differences in RA (16 ± 7 vs. 16 ± 7 mm Hg), PCWP (28 ± 6 vs. 30 ± 6 mm Hg) or CI (2.2 ± 0.7 vs. 2.0 ± 0.8 L/min/m²), respectively. Importantly, mixed PH was an independent risk factor for mortality (HR 4.8) compared with passive PH (HR 2.8). In another experience of 463 HFrEF patients at the Mayo Clinic, more than half of patients with PH had mixed PH, which was associated with a greater risk for mortality when compared with passive PH (HR 1.55; 95% CI 1.11-2.20; *P* <0.001).[37] Due to its independent association with disease severity and mortality, PH and specifically mixed PH may be a novel target for therapy.

These clinical observations may be explained by the unique pathophysiology of PH in heart failure. Left-side diastolic dysfunction increases the RV afterload to a greater extent than the simple passive transmission of backpressure into the pulmonary circulation. In the pulmonary vasculature, arterial compliance is high and is evenly distributed across the lungs. The main pulmonary artery contributes relatively little to overall compliance and is minimally affected by age, which contrasts with the aorta, which accounts for more than 75% of the compliance of the systemic circulation.[40] There are also 10 times more vessels in the pulmonary bed than in the systemic circulation, and vascular resistance is 10-fold lower in the lung than in the systemic circulation. Therefore, the distal pulmonary vessels contribute to both vascular resistance and compliance. These circumstances lead to premature pulmonary arterial wave reflections, augmentation of the systolic PAP, and increases in the mean PAP. This combination of resistance and compliance in the same bed explains why elevations in PCWP result in both direct and indirect increases in mean PAP.

For a given left atrial pressure (LAP), the product of resistance and compliance has been shown to be constant and not significantly altered by PH.[40] Increases in LAP shift the resistance/compliance relationship to the left, such that compliance is lower at any given PVR (**Figure 31-11**). This increases the pulsatile component of RV afterload (e.g., impedance) relative to the resistive load, to which the normal RV is extremely sensitive. Therefore, RV hydraulic efficiency is compromised to a greater extent in patients with PH due to left-heart disease as a consequence of this

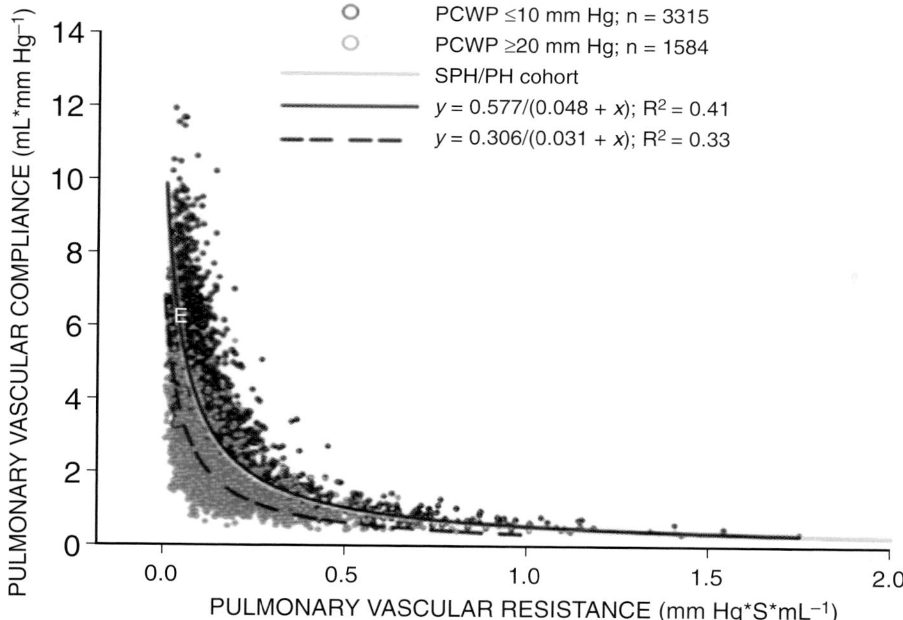

FIGURE 31-11 Inverse relationship between compliance and resistance in pulmonary circulation. Increased pulmonary capillary wedge pressure (PCWP) *(red)* moves this relationship to the left *(dotted line). Reprinted from Tedford RJ, Hassoun PM, Mathai SC, et al: Pulmonary capillary wedge pressure augments right ventricular pulsatile loading. Circulation 125:289–297, 2012.*

abnormal ventricular-vascular coupling and afterload mismatch. This impact on RV efficiency suggests increased pulmonary arterial compliance in heart failure could affect outcomes. Some have suggested that a PA compliance >2.0 mL/mm Hg is associated with increased mortality but there are few studies that have systematically addressed this parameter with partition values.

Heart Transplantation

An elevated PVR is an independent risk factor for RV failure and early mortality after heart transplantation (see also Chapter 40). Cardiac surgery alone may also exacerbate an elevated PVR through cardiopulmonary bypass, transfusions, and hypoxia. However, if PH is predominantly driven by an increase in PCWP and the PVR is reversible, successful transplantation is possible. The magnitude of PVR elevation does not appear to impact heart transplant outcomes as long as the PH is reversible.[41]

The ISHLT Cardiac Transplant Guidelines recommend assessment of pulmonary pressures and resistance in all transplant candidates.[42] A vasodilator challenge is advised when the PASP ≥50 mm Hg, TPG ≥15 mm Hg, or PVR ≥3 Wood units (or 240 dynes/sec/cm^{-5}). In the 1992 classic study at Stanford University, "reversible" PH was defined by a decrease in PVR to ≤2.5 Wood units without excessive hypotension (e.g., asymptomatic systolic BP ≥85 mm Hg) and was associated with a post-transplant mortality of 3.8%.[43] In that series, the inability to acutely achieve this goal (using SNP) suggested "fixed" PH and an unacceptable post-transplant mortality (e.g., 20%-40%). More contemporary experiences have confirmed those early observations. In 217 heart transplant patients from Germany, survival in the 22.6% patients with reversible PH with prostacyclin (PVR <2.5 Wood units; TPG <12 mm Hg) was comparable to patients without PH, despite more early right heart failure.[44] An upper limit to PVR for transplantation has not been established although most centers will not consider patients with fixed PVR >5 Wood units, PASP >60 mm Hg, or TPG >15-20 mm Hg without some chronic attempt to lower the PVR (e.g., chronic inotropes, IABP, VAD).[45] Regular surveillance RHC is also recommended since PH often gets worse with time, although this practice has little evidence base.

Several agents are available to assess pulmonary vasoreactivity (see previous discussion of SNP, **Table 31-2**). Bolus milrinone is useful because titration is not necessary and hypotension is uncommon. Fifty micrograms per kilogram over 10 minutes is well tolerated and produces its peak effect within minutes. The effects of inotropy and vasodilation produce a fall in PVR 30%, although there is usually minimal change in TPG. Selective pulmonary vasodilators (e.g., inhaled nitric oxide) can be used but can precipitate acute pulmonary edema if the diastolic compliance of the left ventricle is overwhelmed with the sudden increase in transpulmonary flow. If the resting PCWP is >20-25 mm Hg, milrinone, nitroprusside, or nitroglycerin are preferable for this reason. In contrast, sildenafil is well tolerated in chronic systolic heart failure when given acutely.[46]

Chronic lowering of LV filling pressures, whether by mechanical circulatory support or transplant, may ultimately reverse the PH and allow transplantation (see Chapters 40 and 42).[34] Retrospective studies have shown reduction in pulmonary pressures with prolonged mechanical circulatory support (MCS) in patients with HF and "fixed" PH.[47] Sildenafil has been used as an adjuvant in this setting to help lower the pulmonary pressures.[48]

Most post-transplant resting hemodynamics normalize within months following transplantation.[49] In 24 heart transplant recipients, the mean PAP fell from 38 ± 9 mm Hg to 19 ± 5 mm Hg, and the PVR fell from 2.5 ± 1.1 Wood units to 1.2 ± 0.4 Wood units 1 year after heart transplantation. However, there may be significant acute diastolic dysfunction of the left artery and LV, manifest by large *v* waves in the PCW tracing (in the absence of significant mitral regurgitation) in the immediate days to weeks after transplant. LV compliance improves but does not normalize; there is generally a rapid rise in LVEDP with exercise.[50] In some

TABLE 31-2 Selective Intravenous Pulmonary Vasodilators

AGENT	ROUTE	$T_{1/2}$	DOSE	INCREASE	mPAP	PVR	TPG	PCWP	SBP	SVR	CI	SIDE EFFECTS
Nitric oxide	Inhaled	15-30 s	10-40 ppm	10 ppm	Decrease	Decrease	Decrease	Increase	No effect	No change	Decrease	Increased LV pressure
Adenosine	Intravenous	5-10 s	50-150 µg/kg/min	50 µg/kg/min	Decrease	Decrease	Decrease	Possible increase	Decrease	No change	Increase	Chest pain, AV block
Epoprostenol	Intravenous	3 min	2-12 ng/kg/min	2 ng/kg/min	Decrease	Decrease	Decrease	Decrease	Decrease	Decrease	Increase	Headache, nausea
Nitroprusside	Intravenous	2 min	0.25 to 3 µg/kg/min	0.25 µg/kg/min	Decrease	Decrease	Decrease	Decrease	Decrease	Decrease	Increase	Flushing, hypotension
Milrinone	Intravenous	2.5 hr	50 µg/kg IV bolus	Maintenance: 0.375-0.75 µg/kg/minute	Decrease	Decrease	Decrease	Decrease	Decrease	Decrease	Increase	Atrial and ventricular arrhythmia

AV, Atrioventricular; *CI,* confidence interval; *IV,* intravenously; *LV,* left ventricular; *mPAP,* mean pulmonary artery pressure; *PCWP,* pulmonary capillary wedge pressure; *PVR,* pressure-volume relationship; *SBP,* systolic blood pressure; *SVR,* systemic vascular resistance; *TPG,* transpulmonary gradient.

Adapted from Fang JC, DeMarco T, Givertz MM, et al: World Health Organization pulmonary hypertension group 2: pulmonary hypertension due to left heart disease in the adult—a summary statement from the Pulmonary Hypertension Council of the International Society for Heart and Lung Transplantation. J Heart Lung Transplant 31:913–933, 2012.

instances, an increase in filling pressures and low index may be associated with severe cellular rejection, but rejection is generally hemodynamically silent.[51]

Left Ventricular Assist Devices

All patients who are evaluated for MCS should have invasive hemodynamics obtained to confirm the severity of heart failure, to measure pulmonary pressures and vascular resistance, and to assess RV function. Severe preimplant irreversible RV failure is a contraindication for LVAD implantation (see also Chapter 42). Physiologically, the LVAD depends on adequate left ventricular loading from the RV and therefore adequate RV function is required. In the case of bridging to transplant, consideration should be given to biventricular VADs or a total artificial heart if RV function is not adequate.

RV function may also suffer post implant because of the effects of cardiopulmonary bypass, transfusions, and ischemic injury on the RV and pulmonary vasculature during surgery. Postimplant RV failure is defined by (1) need for at least 14 days of continuous inotropic support or (2) the need for a right ventricular assist device (RVAD). The thresholds for these interventions are extremely variable among centers and clinicians and contribute to the wide range of postimplant RV failure rates from 4% to 40%.[52,53] Postimplant RV dysfunction is likely when there is a low mean PA pressure (with an elevated CVP), increased CVP or CVP/PCWP ratio, and a low right ventricular stroke work index (RVSWI). A low mean PAP with an elevated CVP suggests lack of RV preload recruitable stroke work and an RV that is not capable of generating enough PA pressure to overcome an elevated PVR. An elevated CVP, particularly in relation to the PCWP (e.g., CVP/PCWP ratio), suggests significant RV dysfunction; a CVP/PCWP ratio >0.63 is an independent risk factor for RV failure.[52]

A more load-independent measure of RV function is reflected in the RVSWI, which describes RV contractile performance for a given afterload/preload and is based upon the use of a PV loop. The right ventricular stroke work is calculated by multiplying stroke volume (indexed by body surface area [BSA)] and the pressure generated by the RV while ejecting that stroke volume (e.g., mean PAP – CVP).

$$
\begin{aligned}
\text{RVSWI} &= \text{Stroke volume index} \times (\text{mPAP} - \text{CVP}) \\
&\quad \times \text{conversion factor} \\
&= (\text{CO/HR})/\text{BSA} \times (\text{mPA} - \text{CVP}) \\
&\quad \times 0.0136\ \text{mm Hg/mL/m}^2
\end{aligned}
$$

In a single-center LVAD study, postimplant RV failure was rare if the RVSWI was >900 mm Hg/mL/m² (3%) but common when >600 mm Hg/mL/m² (29%-38%).[54] Risk scores have been proposed to determine the risk of RV failure after LVAD implantation and are dependent on specific hemodynamics, as well as other measures of RV function such as tricuspid annular plane systolic excursion (TAPSE), RVEF, tricuspid regurgitation, and RV size.[55] RV failure has continued to be an important clinical problem despite the almost universal adoption of continuous flow LVADs for durable support despite improvements in patient selection and postimplant management.

Continuous flow VADs are now the predominant devices used for durable long-term MCS. With the Heartmate II LVAD, blood is propelled forward from a low-pressure (e.g., LV) into a high-pressure (e.g., aorta) chamber under the influence of the Archimedes principle using a small impeller rotating between 6000 and 12,000 rpm. For this reason, continuous flow pumps are preload insensitive but afterload sensitive. Because the afterload is the distal pressure minus the proximal pressure, afterload varies continuously over the cardiac cycle, leading to variable flow over time. The variable flows can be quantified by the pulsatility index (PI = [max-min flow]/average flow). A palpable or Doppler-able pulse pressure >15-20 mm Hg generally signifies an aortic valve opening and is often desired to avoid the long-term complication of commissural fusion and aortic insufficiency. Pump speed is commonly adjusted to keep the interventricular septum midline and the aortic valve intermittently opening; the PCWP should generally be <15 mm Hg post implant if the LVAD cannula is adequately decompressing the LV.

THE HEMODYNAMICS OF HEART FAILURE WITH PRESERVED EJECTION FRACTION (HFpEF)

Initial studies in HFpEF were focused on the presence of diastolic dysfunction as the primary hemodynamic determinant of symptoms and pathophysiology. More recently, there is growing evidence for other pathophysiologic mechanisms to explain the dyspnea and exertional intolerance of these aged patients with multiple comorbidities.[56]

The hemodynamic characteristics of HFpEF can be characterized using a PV loop. Elegant studies by Kass and others have demonstrated that a steep ESPVR and noncompliant EDPVR combine to limit stroke volume.[57] Moreover, increased end-systolic stiffness (Ees) is associated with an increased effective arterial elastance (Ea). The hemodynamic consequences of a stiff ventricular-arterial system is a larger increase in blood pressure in response to increases in end-diastolic volume; similarly larger falls in blood pressure occur with modest decreases in end-diastolic volume.[58] However, the ventricular-arterial coupling (Ea/Ees) is comparable with age-matched asymptomatic and hypertensive subjects, although the absolute values for Ea and Ees are increased.[15] Stiffening of the aorta also leads to early wave reflection and an increased vascular load late into systole, prolonging relaxation and increased LVEDP.[59]

Some hemodynamic correlate of diastolic dysfunction is generally present and necessary for the diagnosis of HFpEF. In the European Society of Cardiology criteria for HFpEF, diastolic dysfunction should be documented, either invasively or noninvasively.[60] However, the hemodynamic nature of the diastolic dysfunction may not be uniform and may be associated with any of the four phases of diastole (isovolumic relaxation, early ventricular filling, diastasis, or atrial contraction). Moreover, diastolic dysfunction is not always associated with symptomatic heart failure.[61]

In clinical practice, the hemodynamic abnormality most commonly associated with HFpEF is an abnormally elevated filling pressure in the setting of a relatively normal LV volume, implying a steep end-diastolic pressure-volume relationship (EDPVR). In a study of predominantly middle-aged men with HFpEF, the end-diastolic pressure was higher (25 ± 6 vs. 8 ± 2 mm Hg, P <0.001) and the end-diastolic volume was lower (103 ± 22 mL vs. 115 ± 9 mL, P = 0.01), displacing the entire EDPVR upward and left.[61]

Patients with HFpEF also have higher stiffness constant compared with controls. Ventricular relaxation can also be quantified using the mono-exponential rate of isovolumic pressure decay (Tau) and is prolonged in HFpEF. Contractile reserve is blunted in HFpEF. Vasodilation (reduction in Ea and systemic vascular resistance index [SVRI]) is also impaired in HFpEF. These factors contribute to abnormal ventricular-arterial coupling responses (**Figure 31-12**).[62] However, these sophisticated measures of diastole are not obtained in clinical practice because of the complexity of making such measurements. Volume loading in the catheterization laboratory has been proposed to unmask diastolic dysfunction when resting PCWP <15-20 mm Hg and can be accomplished with bolus saline infusion or leg raising (see later discussion).

PH is also frequently noted in HFpEF. In fact, the most common cause of PH in the setting of a preserved ejection fraction is HFpEF. In a community-based echocardiographic study, 83% of the HFpEF population had a PASP >35 mm Hg and was also more severe than predicted from an estimate of the PCWP.[63]

HEMODYNAMIC CHALLENGES: EXERCISE AND VOLUME LOADING

In patients with cryptic exertional dyspnea or exertional intolerance and normal resting hemodynamics, invasive hemodynamics with exercise or volume challenge may uncover HFpEF or PH.[64]

Technical Considerations

Exercise hemodynamics are usually obtained in the supine position in most clinical catheterization laboratories; some academic laboratories have the technical expertise to perform upright studies and concomitant measurement of oxygen consumption (e.g., metabolic cart). Supine or upright bicycle ergometry is favored because of the ability to incrementally increase workload with a conventional activity. Upper extremity exercise with weights or straight leg raising for several minutes or until symptoms have been used by some investigators. However, published guidelines do not address how hemodynamic assessment should be performed during exercise nor what should be the goal of exercise. However, it is reasonable to (1) start at a low level of exercise, (2) titrate upward at fixed intervals until symptoms occur, and (3) measure hemodynamics at rest, peak exercise, and if possible, after each stage. During exercise, there can be dramatic fluctuations in intracardiac pressures secondary to wide swings in intrathoracic pressures, and measurements should be made at end expiration. Heart rate response should also be noted because chronotropic incompetence may be more relevant than the hemodynamic response as an explanation for exertional intolerance.

The normal response to exercise consists of increases in mean systemic and pulmonary arterial pressures, as well as heart rate and myocardial contractility.[64] Systemic vascular resistance decreases with exercise (despite the increase in mean arterial pressure); there is also a slight decrease in pulmonary vascular resistance with exercise. Oxygen consumption increases with exercise and is facilitated by an increase in cardiac output, as well as an increase in tissue oxygen extraction. An increase in PCWP is expected (e.g., preload recruitable stroke work) as venous return increases, but the magnitude should be modest (e.g., <20-25 mm Hg) and the rise in pressure gradual (see Figure 31-12). Eighty percent of the increase in PCWP during supine exercise occurs early and at low levels of exertion. There is some debate as to what constitutes a normal response of

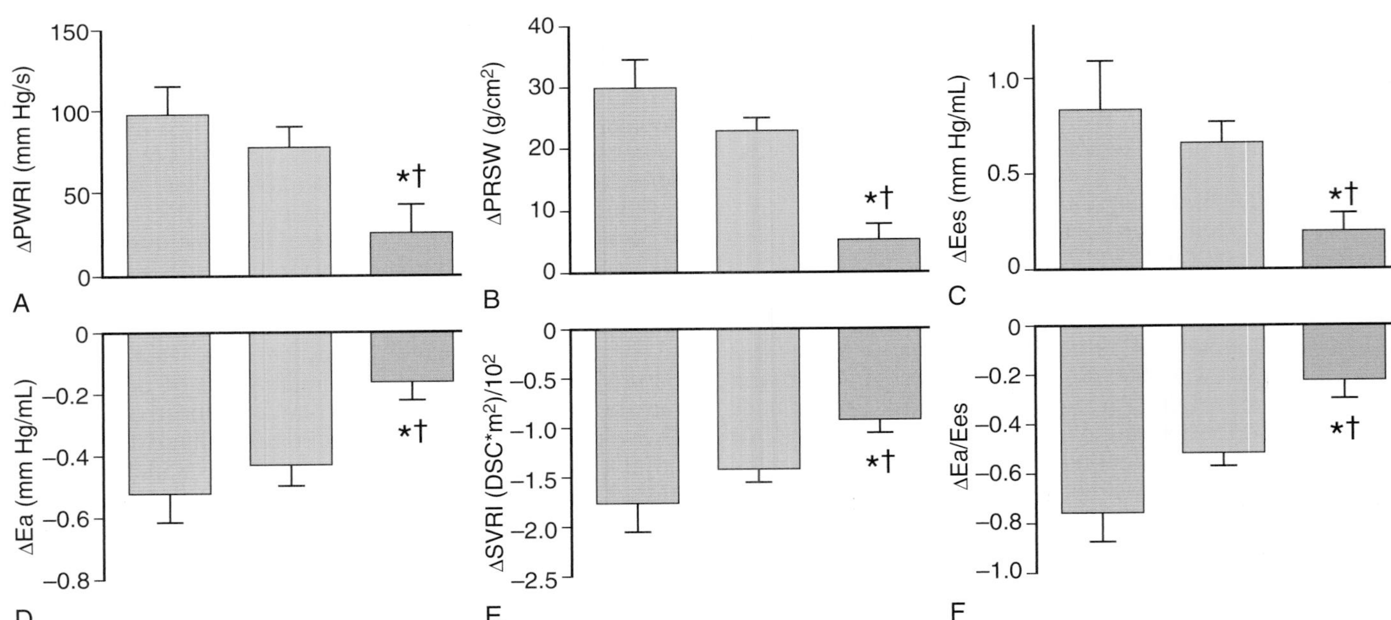

FIGURE 31-12 Contractile, vascular, and coupling reserve with low-level exercise (20 W). **A** to **C,** Compared with both control subjects *(blue bars)* and hypertensive subjects *(green bars)*, contractile reserve was blunted in heart failure with preserved ejection fraction (HFpEF) *(red bars)* at 20 W, evidenced by blunted increases in end-systolic elastance (Ees), preload recruitable stroke work (PRSW), and peak power index (PWRI). **D** and **E,** Vasodilation (reduction in arterial elastance [Ea] and systemic vascular resistance index [SVRI]) was also impaired in HFpEF. **F,** These deficits led to abnormal ventricular-arterial coupling responses in HFpEF subjects compared with controls and hypertensive subjects. *$P < 0.05$ versus hypertension; †$P < 0.05$ versus control. *Reprinted from Borlaug BA, Olson TP, Lam CS, et al: Global cardiovascular reserve dysfunction in heart failure with preserved ejection fraction. J Am Coll Cardiol 56:845–854, 2010.*

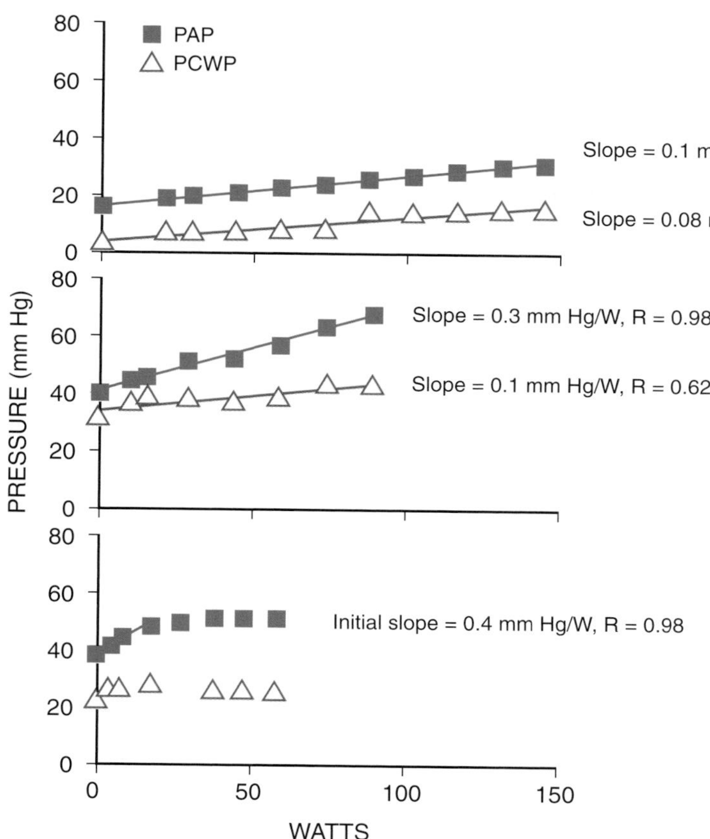

FIGURE 31-13 Representative patterns of pulmonary arterial pressure (PAP) and pulmonary capillary wedge pressure (PCWP) responses to exercise in controls *(top)*, patients with left ventricular systolic dysfunction (LVSD) with a linear PAP increment with exercise *(middle)*, and patients with LVSD with a PAP plateau pattern during exercise *(bottom)*. *Reprinted from Lewis GD, Murphy RM, Shah RV, et al: Pulmonary vascular response patterns during exercise in left ventricular systolic dysfunction predict exercise capacity and outcomes. Circ Heart Fail 4:276–285, 2011.*

intracardiac and pulmonary pressures to exercise. Previous definitions have relied on younger populations to define a normal response to exercise; a conservative definition is an exertional PCWP (at end-expiration) elevation of <25 mm Hg.[64]

LV diastolic compliance can also be assessed with a volume challenge. Volume loading can be accomplished by leg raising or the rapid infusion of saline. Leg raising provides 250-500 mL of blood volume into the chest within seconds. Infusion of warm isotonic saline can also be used but should be rapid (100-200 mL/min up to 1-2 L), and use of a pressurized bag is recommended. In healthy subjects, the PCWP increases from 10 ± 2 to 16 ± 3 mm Hg after 1 L and to 20 ± 3 mm Hg after 2 L. Older healthy women have a greater increase in PCW relative to infused volume (e.g., 16 ± 4 mm Hg/L/m^2, P <0.019) than men and younger women; there is also a greater increase in mean PAP relative to cardiac output in women compared with men, regardless of age. Selective volume loading of the LV can also be accomplished by administering selective pulmonary vasodilators (e.g., inhaled nitric oxide) if there is increased pulmonary vascular resistance and normal PCWP or LVEDP.

Specific Clinical Scenarios

In HFrEF, intracardiac pressures also rise but more rapidly and with a blunted cardiac output response. There is also a concomitant rapid rise in pulmonary pressures and transpulmonary gradient (**Figure 31-13**). In some HFrEF patients, the rise in PA pressures plateaus with exercise (**Figure 31-14**). The steep increase in PA pressures and the plateau pattern are associated with reduced peak VO_2, inability to augment RV stroke work, and increased mortality.[65]

In patients with LVEF >50%, exercise-induced HFpEF is defined as an increase in PCWP to >20-25 mm Hg with exercise and consistent with an inability to accommodate the venous return without an increase in left ventricular end-diastolic volume, limiting preload recruitable stroke work.[64] This response can also be elicited with leg raising or volume loading.[66] In HFpEF patients, rapid infusion of saline (100-200 mL/min, up to 1-2 L) results in a steeper increase in PCWP (25 ± 12 mm Hg/L/m^2) than healthy younger (12 ± 3 mm Hg/L/m^2) and older subjects (14 ± 5 mm Hg/L/m^2). An increase in PCWP >18 mm Hg suggests diastolic dysfunction,[67] although some investigators prefer more conservative values such as >25 mm Hg. In HFpEF, exercise testing also demonstrates a decrease in peak oxygen consumption because of reduced peak cardiac output secondary to blunted inotropic, chronotropic, and vasodilator reserve.

When the mean PAP exceeds 30 mm Hg in the setting of a PCWP <20 mm Hg during exercise, a diagnosis of exercise-induced PAH should be considered (**Figure 31-15**). In a study by Tolle and colleagues, 406 patients with dyspnea on exertion underwent upright cardiopulmonary exercise testing with hemodynamic monitoring. Exercise-related PAH was associated with a significant impairment in oxygen consumption (66.5 ± 16.3% of controls) and comparable to PAH.[68] However, the clinical relevance of exercise-induced PH in asymptomatic subjects is not clear. For example, elite athletes demonstrate a higher increase in mean PA pressure compared with healthy controls because of the marked increase in stroke volume with exercise.[69]

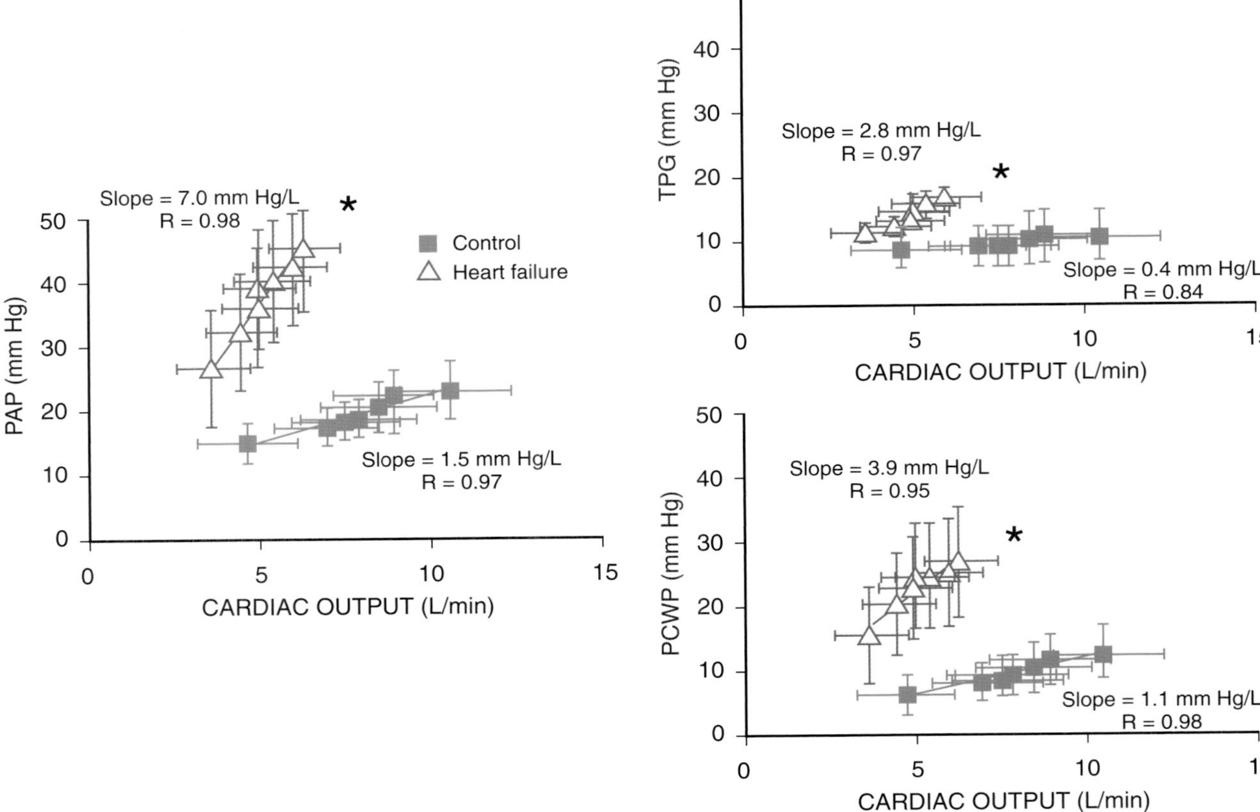

FIGURE 31-14 Mean pulmonary arterial pressures (PAP) relative to cardiac outputs during incremental exercise in patients with left ventricular systolic dysfunction (LVSD). Transpulmonary gradient (TPG) and pulmonary capillary wedge pressure (PCWP) responses to exercise relative to cardiac output in patients with LVSD. *$P < 0.005$ for the comparison of pressure changes in patients with LVSD with pressure changes in controls. *Reprinted from Lewis GD, Murphy RM, Shah RV, et al: Pulmonary vascular response patterns during exercise in left ventricular systolic dysfunction predict exercise capacity and outcomes. Circ Heart Fail 4:276–285, 2011.*

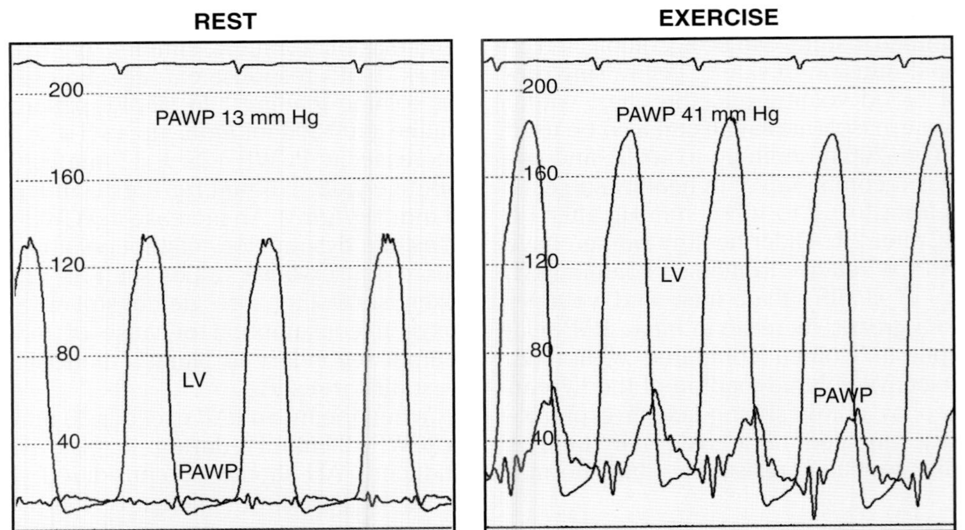

FIGURE 31-15 Effect of exercise in a patient with normal resting hemodynamics but significant exertional dyspnea and normal left ventricular ejection fraction. At a low level of supine bicycle exercise, there was a marked increase in pulmonary artery wedge pressure to 41 mm Hg with a large *v* wave. There was not significant mitral regurgitation by simultaneous echocardiography, indicating that these symptoms were from noncompliance of the left atrium and left ventricle. *Reprinted from Nishimura RA, Carabello BA: Hemodynamics in the cardiac catheterization laboratory of the 21st century. Circulation 125:2138–2150, 2012.*

IMPLANTABLE DEVICES

Technologic advances now permit the measurement of ambulatory hemodynamics with implantable monitors (see also Chapters 28 and 44). Current devices include RV leads that measure intrathoracic impedance and pressure, wireless pulmonary artery pressure monitors, and left atrial pressure sensors.[70] Such devices have provided valuable insights into the hemodynamic picture of ambulatory heart failure patients and the longitudinal changes in hemodynamics over time. For example, these devices have confirmed that a rise in LV filling pressure commonly occurs days before symptoms, changes in weight, or hospitalization occurs.[71]

However, the role of these invasive pressure sensors to guide therapy and ultimately prevent hospitalization has yet to be determined. The Chronicle device (Medtronic, Inc., Minneapolis) consists of a transvenous lead placed in the RV with a distal tip sensor that records intracardiac pressure. In the COMPASS trial, this device did not show a statistically significant decrease in heart failure hospitalization in NYHA III-IV heart failure patients, although the trial was underpowered for the HF hospitalization endpoint and target hemodynamics were not specified.[10] The CardioMEMS™ device is a radiofrequency-based wireless pressure sensor that is implanted into the branch pulmonary arteries, allowing transmission of PAP data. The accuracy of pressure measurement is comparable to that obtained through right-heart catheterization. In the randomized single-blind CHAMPION trial of 550 patients with NYHA III heart failure, clinicians were directed to use a medical algorithm to achieve protocol-specific hemodynamic targets: PASP 15-35 mm Hg, PAD 8-20 mm Hg, and mean PAP 10-25 mm Hg. With this study design, the CardioMEMS arm was associated with a 28% relative risk reduction (P = 0.0002) in HF hospitalization and a decrease in PA pressures over the 6-month study period.[71] However, the treatment effect may not be generalizable because the trial outcome was a result of the combination of the device and the elaborate clinical support system, which could be difficult to replicate in routine clinical practice. The LAPTOP-HF study will also assess the use of hemodynamic directed HF management with an implantable left atrial monitor to decrease HF hospitalization in NYHA III heart failure patients.[72]

References

1. Chatterjee K: The Swan-Ganz catheters: past, present, and future. A viewpoint. *Circulation* 119:147–152, 2009.
2. Yancy CW, Jessup M, Bozkurt B, et al: 2013 ACCF/AHA guideline for the management of heart failure: a report of the American College of Cardiology Foundation/American Heart Association task force on practice guidelines. *J Am Coll Cardiol* 2013.
3. Davidson C, Bonow R: Cardiac catheterization. In Libby P, Bonow R, Mann D, et al, editors: *Braunwald's heart disease: a textbook of cardiovascular medicine*, ed 8, Elsevier, 2008, Philadelphia, pp 439–462.
4. Baim D, Grossman W: Percutaneous approach, including transseptal and apical puncture. In Baim DS, Grossman W, editors: *Cardiac catheterization, angiography, and intervention*, ed 7, Philadelphia, 2006, Lea & Febiger, p 86.
5. Borlaug BA, Kass DA: Ventricular-vascular interaction in heart failure. *Heart Fail Clin* 4:23–36, 2008.
6. Ryan JJ, Rich JD, Thiruvoipati T, et al: Current practice for determining pulmonary capillary wedge pressure predisposes to serious errors in the classification of patients with pulmonary hypertension. *Am Heart J* 163:589–594, 2012.
7. Binanay C, Califf RM, Hasselblad V, et al: Evaluation study of congestive heart failure and pulmonary artery catheterization effectiveness: The escape trial. *JAMA* 294:1625–1633, 2005.
8. Kearney TJ, Shabot MM: Pulmonary artery rupture associated with the Swan-Ganz catheter. *Chest* 108:1349–1352, 1995.
9. Voyce S, Urbach D, Rippe J: Pulmonary artery catheters. In Rippe JM, Irwin RS, Alpert JS, et al, editors: *Intensive care medicine*, Boston, 1991, Little Brown, p 66.
10. Bourge RC, Abraham WT, Adamson PB, et al: Randomized controlled trial of an implantable continuous hemodynamic monitor in patients with advanced heart failure: the COMPASS-HF study. *J Am Coll Cardiol* 51:1073–1079, 2008.
11. Gerges C, Gerges M, Lang MB, et al: Diastolic pulmonary vascular pressure gradient: a predictor of prognosis in "out-of-proportion" pulmonary hypertension. *Chest* 143:758–766, 2013.
12. Hildick-Smith DJ, Walsh JT, Shapiro LM: Pulmonary capillary wedge pressure in mitral stenosis accurately reflects mean left atrial pressure but overestimates transmitral gradient. *Am J Cardiol* 85:512–515, A511, 2000.
13. Flores ED, Lange RA, Hillis LD: Relation of mean pulmonary arterial wedge pressure and left ventricular end-diastolic pressure. *Am J Cardiol* 66:1532–1533, 1990.
14. Fakler U, Pauli C, Hennig M, et al: Assumed oxygen consumption frequently results in large errors in the determination of cardiac output. *J Thorac Cardiovasc Surg* 130:272–276, 2005.
15. Borlaug BA, Kass DA: Ventricular-vascular interaction in heart failure. *Cardiol Clin* 29:447–459, 2011.
16. Asanoi H, Sasayama S, Kameyama T: Ventriculoarterial coupling in normal and failing heart in humans. *Circ Res* 65:483–493, 1989.
17. Kass DA, Kelly RP: Ventriculo-arterial coupling: concepts, assumptions, and applications. *Ann Biomed Eng* 20:41–62, 1992.
18. Ky B, French B, Khan AM, et al: Ventricular-arterial coupling, remodeling, and prognosis in chronic heart failure. *J Am Coll Cardiol* 2013.
19. Mitchell GF, Tardif JC, Arnold JM, et al: Pulsatile hemodynamics in congestive heart failure. *Hypertension* 38:1433–1439, 2001.
20. Nohria A, Tsang SW, Fang JC, et al: Clinical assessment identifies hemodynamic profiles that predict outcomes in patients admitted with heart failure. *J Am Coll Cardiol* 41:1797–1804, 2003.
21. Drazner MH, Hellkamp AS, Leier CV, et al: Value of clinician assessment of hemodynamics in advanced heart failure: the ESCAPE trial. *Circ Heart Fail* 1:170–177, 2008.
22. Nohria A, Hasselblad V, Stebbins A, et al: Cardiorenal interactions: insights from the ESCAPE trial. *J Am Coll Cardiol* 51:1268–1274, 2008.
23. Drazner MH, Velez-Martinez M, Ayers CR, et al: Relationship of right- to left-sided ventricular filling pressures in advanced heart failure: insights from the ESCAPE trial. *Circ Heart Fail* 6:264–270, 2013.
24. Stevenson LW, Tillisch JH: Maintenance of cardiac output with normal filling pressures in patients with dilated heart failure. *Circulation* 74:1303–1308, 1986.
25. Mullens W, Abrahams Z, Francis GS, et al: Sodium nitroprusside for advanced low-output heart failure. *J Am Coll Cardiol* 52:200–207, 2008.
26. Guiha NH, Cohn JN, Mikulic E, et al: Treatment of refractory heart failure with infusion of nitroprusside. *N Engl J Med* 291:587–592, 1974.
27. Rosario LB, Stevenson LW, Solomon SD, et al: The mechanism of decrease in dynamic mitral regurgitation during heart failure treatment: importance of reduction in the regurgitant orifice size. *J Am Coll Cardiol* 32:1819–1824, 1998.
28. Atherton JJ, Moore TD, Lele SS, et al: Diastolic ventricular interaction in chronic heart failure. *Lancet* 349:1720–1724, 1997.
29. Dauterman K, Pak PH, Maughan WL, et al: Contribution of external forces to left ventricular diastolic pressure. Implications for the clinical use of the Starling law. *Ann Intern Med* 122:737–742, 1995.
30. Frenneaux M, Williams L: Ventricular-arterial and ventricular-ventricular interactions and their relevance to diastolic filling. *Prog Cardiovasc Dis* 49:252–262, 2007.
31. Tyberg JV, Taichman GC, Smith ER, et al: The relationship between pericardial pressure and right atrial pressure: an intraoperative study. *Circulation* 73:428–432, 1986.
32. Hemnes AR, Forfia PR, Champion HC: Assessment of pulmonary vasculature and right heart by invasive haemodynamics and echocardiography. *Int J Clin Pract Suppl* 4-19, 2009.
33. McLaughlin VV, Archer SL, Badesch DB, et al: ACCF/AHA 2009 expert consensus document on pulmonary hypertension: a report of the American College of Cardiology Foundation task force on expert consensus documents and the American Heart Association developed in collaboration with the American College of Chest Physicians; American Thoracic Society, Inc.; and the Pulmonary Hypertension Association. *J Am Coll Cardiol* 53:1573–1619, 2009.
34. Fang JC, DeMarco T, Givertz MM, et al: World Health Organization pulmonary hypertension group 2: pulmonary hypertension due to left heart disease in the adult—a summary statement from the Pulmonary Hypertension Council of the International Society for Heart and Lung Transplantation. *J Heart Lung Transplant* 31:913–933, 2012.
35. Guazzi M, Borlaug BA: Pulmonary hypertension due to left heart disease. *Circulation* 126:975–990, 2012.
36. Ghio S, Gavazzi A, Campana C, et al: Independent and additive prognostic value of right ventricular systolic function and pulmonary artery pressure in patients with chronic heart failure. *J Am Coll Cardiol* 37:183–188, 2001.
37. Miller W, Grill D, Borlaug B: Clinical features, hemodynamics, and outcomes of pulmonary hypertension due to chronic heart failure with reduced ejection fraction. *JACC Heart Fail* 1:290–299, 2013.
38. Delgado JF, Conde E, Sanchez V, et al: Pulmonary vascular remodeling in pulmonary hypertension due to chronic heart failure. *Eur J Heart Fail* 7:1011–1016, 2005.
39. Aronson D, Eitan A, Dragu R, et al: Relationship between reactive pulmonary hypertension and mortality in patients with acute decompensated heart failure. *Circ Heart Fail* 4:644–650, 2011.
40. Tedford RJ, Hassoun PM, Mathai SC, et al: Pulmonary capillary wedge pressure augments right ventricular pulsatile loading. *Circulation* 125:289–297, 2012.
41. Drakos SG, Kfoury AG, Gilbert EM, et al: Effect of reversible pulmonary hypertension on outcomes after heart transplantation. *J Heart Lung Transplant* 26:319–323, 2007.
42. Jessup M, Banner N, Brozena S, et al: Optimal pharmacologic and non-pharmacologic management of cardiac transplant candidates: approaches to be considered prior to transplant evaluation: International Society for Heart and Lung Transplantation guidelines for the care of cardiac transplant candidates—2006. *J Heart Lung Transplant* 25:1003–1023, 2006.
43. Costard-Jackle A, Fowler MB: Influence of preoperative pulmonary artery pressure on mortality after heart transplantation: testing of potential reversibility of pulmonary hypertension with nitroprusside is useful in defining a high risk group. *J Am Coll Cardiol* 19:48–54, 1992.
44. Klotz S, Wenzelburger F, Stypmann J, et al: Reversible pulmonary hypertension in heart transplant candidates: to transplant or not to transplant. *Ann Thorac Surg* 82:1770–1773, 2006.
45. Mehra MR, Kobashigawa J, Starling R, et al: Listing criteria for heart transplantation: International Society for Heart and Lung Transplantation guidelines for the care of cardiac transplant candidates—2006. *J Heart Lung Transplant* 25:1024–1042, 2006.
46. Lewis GD, Shah R, Shahzad K, et al: Sildenafil improves exercise capacity and quality of life in patients with systolic heart failure and secondary pulmonary hypertension. *Circulation* 116:1555–1562, 2007.
47. Nair PK, Kormos RL, Teuteberg JJ, et al: Pulsatile left ventricular assist device support as a bridge to decision in patients with end-stage heart failure complicated by pulmonary hypertension. *J Heart Lung Transplant* 29:201–208, 2010.
48. Tedford RJ, Hemnes AR, Russell SD, et al: Pde5a inhibitor treatment of persistent pulmonary hypertension after mechanical circulatory support. *Circ Heart Fail* 1:213–219, 2008.
49. Bhatia SJ, Kirshenbaum JM, Shemin RJ, et al: Time course of resolution of pulmonary hypertension and right ventricular remodeling after orthotopic cardiac transplantation. *Circulation* 76:819–826, 1987.
50. Stinson EB, Griepp RB, Schroeder JS, et al: Hemodynamic observations one and two years after cardiac transplantation in man. *Circulation* 45:1183–1194, 1972.
51. Bolling SF, Putnam JB, Jr, Abrams GD, et al: Hemodynamics versus biopsy findings during cardiac transplant rejection. *Ann Thorac Surg* 51:52–55, 1991.

52. Kormos RL, Teuteberg JJ, Pagani FD, et al: Right ventricular failure in patients with the Heartmate II continuous-flow left ventricular assist device: incidence, risk factors, and effect on outcomes. *J Thorac Cardiovasc Surg* 139:1316–1324, 2010.
53. Slaughter MS, Rogers JG, Milano CA, et al: Advanced heart failure treated with continuous-flow left ventricular assist device. *N Engl J Med* 361:2241–2251, 2009.
54. Schenk S, McCarthy PM, Blackstone EH, et al: Duration of inotropic support after left ventricular assist device implantation: risk factors and impact on outcome. *J Thorac Cardiovasc Surg* 131:447–454, 2006.
55. Drakos SG, Janicki L, Horne BD, et al: Risk factors predictive of right ventricular failure after left ventricular assist device implantation. *Am J Cardiol* 105:1030–1035, 2010.
56. Borlaug BA, Paulus WJ: Heart failure with preserved ejection fraction: pathophysiology, diagnosis, and treatment. *Eur Heart J* 32:670–679, 2011.
57. Kass DA, Yamazaki T, Burkhoff D, et al: Determination of left ventricular end-systolic pressure-volume relationships by the conductance (volume) catheter technique. *Circulation* 73:586–595, 1986.
58. Chen CH, Nakayama M, Nevo E, et al: Coupled systolic-ventricular and vascular stiffening with age: implications for pressure regulation and cardiac reserve in the elderly. *J Am Coll Cardiol* 32:1221–1227, 1998.
59. Borlaug BA, Melenovsky V, Redfield MM, et al: Impact of arterial load and loading sequence on left ventricular tissue velocities in humans. *J Am Coll Cardiol* 50:1570–1577, 2007.
60. McMurray JJ, Adamopoulos S, Anker SD, et al: ESC guidelines for the diagnosis and treatment of acute and chronic heart failure 2012: the Task Force for the Diagnosis and Treatment of Acute and Chronic Heart Failure 2012 of the European Society of Cardiology. Developed in collaboration with the Heart Failure Association (HFA) of the ESC. *Eur Heart J* 33:1787–1847, 2012.
61. Zile MR, Baicu CF, Gaasch WH: Diastolic heart failure—abnormalities in active relaxation and passive stiffness of the left ventricle. *N Engl J Med* 350:1953–1959, 2004.
62. Borlaug BA, Olson TP, Lam CS, et al: Global cardiovascular reserve dysfunction in heart failure with preserved ejection fraction. *J Am Coll Cardiol* 56:845–854, 2010.
63. Lam CS, Roger VL, Rodeheffer RJ, et al: Pulmonary hypertension in heart failure with preserved ejection fraction: a community-based study. *J Am Coll Cardiol* 53:1119–1126, 2009.
64. Maron BA, Cockrill BA, Waxman AB, et al: The invasive cardiopulmonary exercise test. *Circulation* 127:1157–1164, 2013.
65. Lewis GD, Murphy RM, Shah RV, et al: Pulmonary vascular response patterns during exercise in left ventricular systolic dysfunction predict exercise capacity and outcomes. *Circ Heart Fail* 4:276–285, 2011.
66. Borlaug BA, Nishimura RA, Sorajja P, et al: Exercise hemodynamics enhance diagnosis of early heart failure with preserved ejection fraction. *Circ Heart Fail* 3:588–595, 2010.
67. Hoeper MM, Barbera JA, Channick RN, et al: Diagnosis, assessment, and treatment of non-pulmonary arterial hypertension pulmonary hypertension. *J Am Coll Cardiol* 54:S85–S96, 2009.
68. Tolle JJ, Waxman AB, Van Horn TL, et al: Exercise-induced pulmonary arterial hypertension. *Circulation* 118:2183–2189, 2008.
69. Reeves J, Dempsey J, Grover R: Pulmonary circulation during exercise. In Weir EK, Reeves JT, editors: *Pulmonary vascular physiology and physiopathology*, New York, 1989, Marcel Dekker, pp 107–133. Chapter 104.
70. Abraham WT: Disease management: remote monitoring in heart failure patients with implantable defibrillators, resynchronization devices, and haemodynamic monitors. *Europace* 15(Suppl 1):i40–i46, 2013.
71. Abraham WT, Adamson PB, Bourge RC, et al: Wireless pulmonary artery haemodynamic monitoring in chronic heart failure: a randomised controlled trial. *Lancet* 377:658–666, 2011.
72. St. Jude Medical: Left atrial pressure monitoring to optimize heart failure therapy (LAPTOP-HF) (website). http://clinicaltrials.Gov/show/nct01121107.

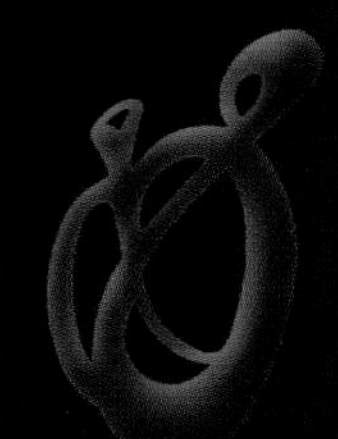

SECTION V

THERAPY FOR HEART FAILURE

32 Disease Prevention in Heart Failure

Viorel G. Florea and Jay N. Cohn

Medicine is not only a science; it is also an art. It does not consist of compounding pills and plasters; it deals with the very processes of life, which must be understood before they may be guided.

Paracelsus

Prevention of heart failure is an urgent public health need with national and global implications. Despite recent advances in the therapy of cardiovascular disorders, heart failure remains a challenging disease with a high prevalence (**Figure 32-1**) and a dismal long-term prognosis.[1] Although survival after a diagnosis of heart failure has improved during the past several decades,[2-4] the incidence of heart failure has not declined[4] and remains high in both genders (**Figure 32-2**). The "aging of the population" and improved survival and "salvage" of patients with acute myocardial infarction are believed to be some factors contributing to the growing burden of heart failure (see also Chapter 17). Projections show that by 2030, the prevalence of heart failure will increase 25% from 2013 estimates.[5] It becomes evident that the heart failure burden will not be eliminated by an improvement in the survival of patients who are already affected with the disease; instead, a drastic reduction in the incidence of heart failure is required to prevent an increase in the heart failure burden. It is therefore important that we develop a population-level strategy to prevent the lifetime risk of heart failure that applies to the large number of "at-risk" individuals. Such a strategy would complement our current approaches that are aimed at intensive management of patients with manifest heart failure (**Figure 32-3**).

Given the sizeable public health burden posed by heart failure and limited health care resources, it is critical to identify the primary "drivers" of this problem. In 2001, a new approach to the classification of heart failure was adopted by the American College of Cardiology/American Heart Association, which included stage A patients who have no structural disorder of the heart or heart failure symptoms but have risk factors that clearly predispose them toward the development of heart failure.[6] It is estimated that 74 million people in the United States are living with risk factors for heart failure (i.e., are in stage A of heart failure).[7] The new classification scheme adds a useful dimension to our understanding of heart failure, recognizing that there are established risk factors and structural prerequisites for the development of heart failure and that therapeutic interventions performed even before the appearance of left ventricular dysfunction or symptoms can prevent the development of heart failure. In 2008, the American Heart Association published a scientific statement on heart failure prevention.[8] The progression of heart failure mandates that an all-out effort be made to prevent its development in the first place, and the best time to intervene would be before or at pre–heart failure stage A.

A number of risk factors have been identified that may lead to heart failure. These exert their adverse effects through functional and structural influence on the left ventricle, characterized as ventricular remodeling and defined as progressive ventricular hypertrophy, enlargement, and

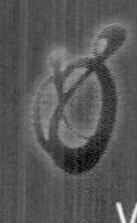

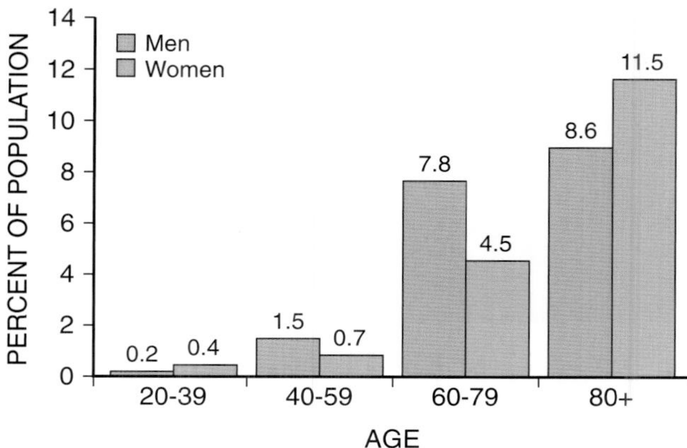

FIGURE 32-1 Prevalence of heart failure by sex and age (National Health and Nutrition Examination Survey: 2007-2010). Source: National Center for Health Statistics and National Heart, Lung, and Blood Institute. *From Go AS, Mozaffarian D, Roger VL, et al: Heart disease and stroke statistics—2013 update: a report from the American Heart Association. Circulation 127:e6–e245, 2013.*

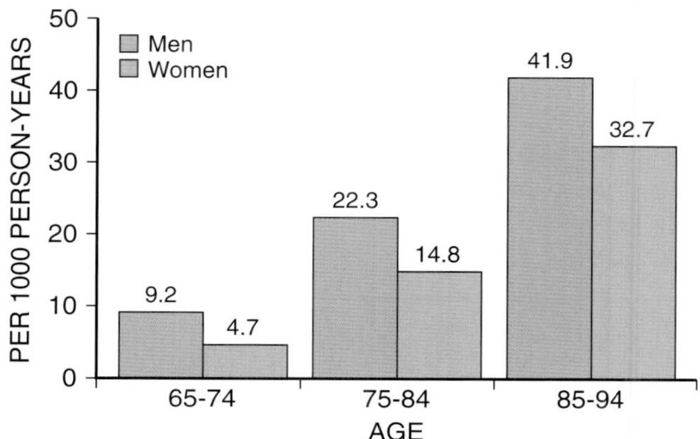

FIGURE 32-2 Incidence of heart failure (heart failure based on physician review of medical records and strict diagnostic criteria) by age and sex (Framingham Heart Study: 1980-2003). Source: National Heart, Lung, and Blood Institute. *From Go AS, Mozaffarian D, Roger VL, et al: Heart disease and stroke statistics—2013 update: a report from the American Heart Association. Circulation 127:e6–e245, 2013.*

cavity distortion over time.[9,10] These risk factors include hypertension, diabetes mellitus, atherosclerotic disease, metabolic syndrome, obesity, chronic obstructive pulmonary disease, and the use of many therapeutic and recreational agents that can exert important cardiotoxic effects. Hypertension and myocardial infarction together account for approximately three fourths of the population-attributable risk of heart failure,[11] and both are, by and large, preventable with currently known and available strategies. The burden of heart failure risk factors, comorbid conditions, and their treatment on incident heart failure is examined in this chapter. As the primary mechanisms of the development of heart failure may be cardiac (structural remodeling, decreased compliance, impaired contractility) or peripheral (fluid retention, vascular remodeling), this discussion is an attempt to characterize the specific mechanisms of the effect of the comorbid conditions and their treatment on the development of heart failure.

DIASTOLIC AND SYSTOLIC HEART FAILURE

Although the existence of diastolic as distinguished from systolic heart failure was recognized more than 70 years ago,[12] the mechanisms that ultimately produce these two phenotypes of chronic heart failure remain, presently, largely unknown.[13] Furthermore, whereas in systolic heart failure diastolic dysfunction is common,[14] in diastolic heart failure left ventricular systolic performance, function, and contractility in general remain normal.[15] The myocardium and left ventricle of most patients with heart failure have, in fact, many similarities and are abnormal, regardless of ejection fraction. The myocardium in patients with ischemic cardiomyopathy or hypertensive heart disease is similarly characterized by increased left ventricular mass, myocyte hypertrophy, and increased interstitial collagen (see also Chapters 2 and 4).[16,17] Hypertrophic myocardium in these and other conditions have similar abnormalities of calcium handling and similar functional abnormalities of contraction and relaxation,[18] regardless of ejection fraction.

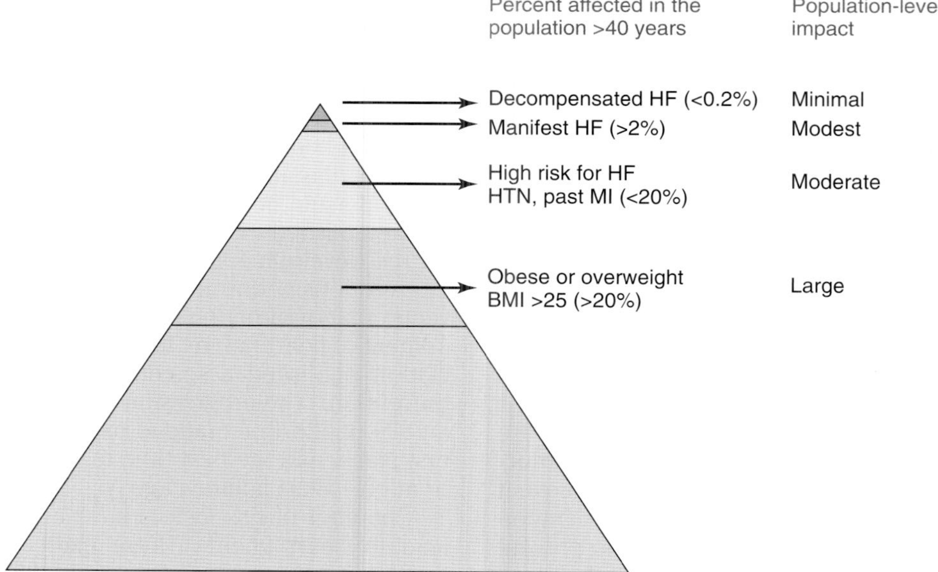

FIGURE 32-3 The pyramid of heart failure in the population and the potential effect of a range of preventive and treatment strategies in lowering age-specific mortality rates. *BMI,* Body mass index; *HF,* heart failure; *HTN,* hypertension; *MI,* myocardial infarction. *From Young J, Narula J: Preface: prevention should take center stage. Cardiol Clin 25:xi–xiii, 2007; data from Yusuf S, Pitt B: A lifetime of prevention: the case of heart failure. Circulation 106:2997–2998, 2002.*

Myocardium from patients with dilated cardiomyopathy and from those with hypertrophic cardiomyopathy shows similar delay in diastolic cytosolic calcium reuptake, associated with delayed relaxation.[18]

Although there has been some recent challenge in classifying systolic and diastolic heart failure,[19] the key element differentiating the two types of heart failure is in the presence or absence of ventricular dilation and remodeling (see Chapter 11).[9] Presence of risk factors such as hypertension or diabetes leads to myocyte apoptosis and necrosis.[20] The resultant fibrosis forms the basis of impaired ventricular relaxation and reduced ventricular compliance.[21] When this process is slow and chronic, the ventricle maintains its size and shape (does not remodel) and therefore preserves its ejection fraction.[22] In acute insults to the ventricle, such as in myocardial infarction, alterations in the topography of both the infarcted and noninfarcted regions of the ventricle may lead to progressive ventricular enlargement.[23] The decrease in global left ventricular ejection fraction results largely from ventricular dilation and remodeling (**Figure 32-4**).[24]

The distinctive features of remodeling in diastolic heart failure and systolic heart failure are illustrated in **Figure 32-5**.[25,26] In systolic heart failure, the left ventricular cavity size is increased; the ventricular shape and geometry is altered, with a greater increase in transverse than in long axis; the wall stress is increased; and the ejection fraction is reduced. The mass is increased, but the mass/cavity ratio remains unchanged or is decreased. In diastolic heart failure, the cavity size remains unchanged or may even decrease. There is usually an increase in wall thickness and mass; however, the mass/cavity ratio is substantially increased, the end-diastolic wall stress is increased, systolic wall stress remains normal, and the ejection fraction remains normal or may even be higher than normal.[15,25]

Ejection fraction provides no information regarding functional capacity.[27] Rather, in patients with normal ejection fraction[28] and in those with low ejection fraction,[29] functional status is linked in part to the ventricular capacity for diastolic distention and preload recruitment during exertion. Konstam and colleagues[29] have observed that among

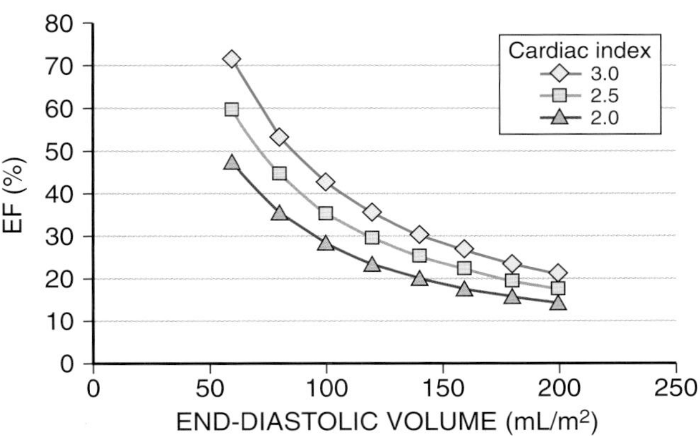

FIGURE 32-4 Relationship between left ventricular end-diastolic volume and ejection fraction (EF) at three levels of cardiac index, and a constant heart rate of 70 beats/min. For patients with chronic heart failure, a low EF relates little about contractility or left ventricular load, but mostly identifies a patient whose left ventricle has remodeled with dilation. *From Konstam MA: "Systolic and diastolic dysfunction" in heart failure? Time for a new paradigm. J Card Fail 9:1–3, 2003.*

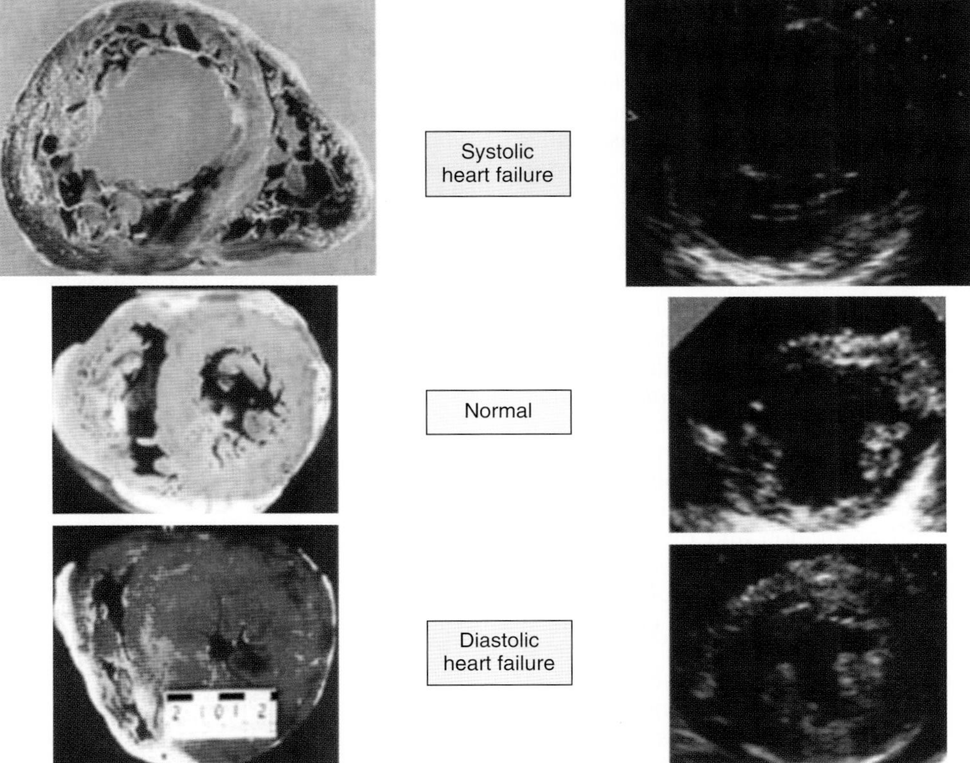

FIGURE 32-5 Ventricular remodeling in systolic and diastolic heart failure. *Left,* Autopsy samples; *right,* cross-sectional two-dimensional echocardiographic views of systolic *(top)* and diastolic *(bottom)* heart failure, in comparison with normal heart function *(middle).* In systolic heart failure, the left ventricular cavity is markedly dilated, and wall thickness is not increased. In diastolic heart failure, the cavity size is normal or decreased, and wall thickness is markedly increased. *From Chatterjee K, Massie B: Systolic and diastolic heart failure: differences and similarities. J Card Fail 13:569–576, 2007.*

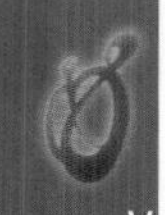

patients with low ejection fraction, diastolic distention during exercise, with associated stroke volume augmentation, distinguishes asymptomatic patients from those with symptoms of heart failure. Therefore, both patients with heart failure and low ejection fraction and those with heart failure and more normal ejection fraction have myocardium and a left ventricle that function abnormally during both systole and diastole. Ejection fraction in patients with chronic heart failure, rather than signifying distinct pathophysiology, principally distinguishes the pattern of hypertrophic left ventricular remodeling: hypertrophic cavity dilation versus hypertrophic concentric thickening without cavity dilation.

DISTINGUISHING FLUID RETENTION FROM ABNORMALITIES IN VENTRICULAR PERFORMANCE

The clinical syndrome of heart failure usually results from both impaired left ventricular performance and congestion secondary to sodium and fluid retention. Consequently, heart failure may develop as a result of the effects of disease or drugs either on left ventricular performance or on renal sodium excretion.

HEALTHY LIFESTYLE TO PREVENT HEART FAILURE

Among 20,900 male physicians in the Physicians Health Study, healthy lifestyle habits (normal body weight, not smoking, regular exercise, moderate alcohol intake, consumption of breakfast cereals, and consumption of fruits and vegetables) were individually and jointly associated with a lower lifetime risk of heart failure, with the highest risk in men adhering to none of the six lifestyle factors and the lowest risk in men adhering to four or more desirable factors.[30] Moderate physical activity is associated with a lower long-term incidence of heart failure, preventing cardiac injury and neurohormonal activation.[31] Prevention of heart failure should therefore start with healthy lifestyle education. The American Heart Association created in 2010 a new set of national goals for cardiovascular health promotion and disease reduction.[32] Specifically, the American Heart Association committed itself to achieving the following central organizational goals: *"By 2020, to improve the cardiovascular health of all Americans by 20% while reducing deaths from cardiovascular diseases and stroke by 20%."*[32] These goals will require new strategic directions for the American Heart Association in its research, clinical, public health, and advocacy programs for cardiovascular health promotion and disease prevention in the next decade and beyond. These goals introduce the concept of *ideal cardiovascular health,* which is defined by the absence of clinically manifest cardiovascular disease together with the simultaneous presence of optimal levels of seven health metrics, including four health behaviors (nonsmoking, body mass index <25 kg/m^2, physical activity at goal levels, and pursuit of a diet consistent with current guideline recommendations) and three ideal health factors (untreated total cholesterol <200 mg/dL, untreated blood pressure <120/<80 mm Hg, and fasting blood glucose <100 mg/dL).[32]

HYPERTENSION AND HEART FAILURE

Considerable evidence from experimental and clinical studies and epidemiologic investigations indicate the critical role of hypertension in the pathogenesis of heart failure (see Chapter 23). Elevated levels of diastolic and especially systolic blood pressure are major risk factors for the development of heart failure.[33,34] The lifetime risk of heart failure for people with blood pressure >160/90 mm Hg is double that of those with blood pressure <140/90 mm Hg.[1] Also, hypertension is frequently accompanied by metabolic risk factors and obesity, which themselves increase the risk of heart failure. On the basis of the 44-year follow-up of the Framingham Heart Study, 75% of heart failure cases have antecedent hypertension.[11] The population-attributable risk for heart failure associated with hypertension is 39% in men and 59% in women.[33] Because 1 in 3 adults in the United States has high blood pressure,[1] strategies to control blood pressure are an integral part of any effort to prevent heart failure.

Both acute and chronic hypertension has been linked to the risk of heart failure. Sudden elevation of blood pressure (such as in hypertensive emergencies) can lead to acute left ventricular strain and acute heart failure,[35] and is a common precipitating cause for decompensation in a patient with chronic heart failure.[36] Progression from chronic hypertension to structural ventricular changes, and then to asymptomatic diastolic and systolic ventricular dysfunction is well established by natural history investigations from longitudinal epidemiologic cohort studies, such as the Framingham Heart Study.[33]

Elevated blood pressure places greater hemodynamic burden on the myocardium and leads to left ventricular hypertrophy[37,38] (**Figure 32-6**). Left ventricular hypertrophy is associated with increased myocardial stiffness and decreased compliance, initially during exercise and subsequently at rest.[39-41] The initial concentric hypertrophy (thick wall, normal chamber volume, and high mass-to-volume ratio), per the Laplace law, helps keep wall tension normal despite high intraventricular pressure (**Figure 32-7**). Because systolic stress (afterload) is a major determinant of ejection performance, normalization of systolic stress helps maintain a normal stroke volume despite the need to generate high levels of systolic pressure.[42]

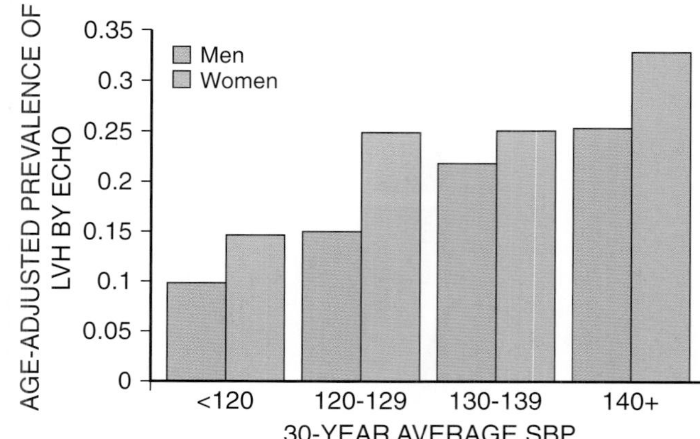

FIGURE 32-6 Prevalence of left ventricular hypertrophy (LVH), demonstrated by echocardiography (ECHO), as a function of 30-year average systolic blood pressure (SBP). *From Lauer MS, Anderson KM, Levy D: Influence of contemporary versus 30-year blood pressure levels on left ventricular mass and geometry: the Framingham Heart Study. J Am Coll Cardiol 18:1287–1294, 1991.*

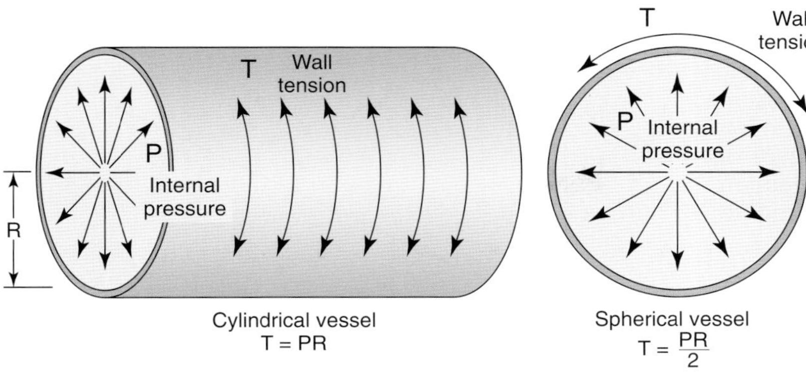

FIGURE 32-7 Laplace law. The larger the vessel radius (R) is, the higher the wall tension (T) must be to withstand a given internal fluid pressure (P). For a given vessel radius and internal pressure, a spherical vessel has half the wall tension of a cylindrical vessel.

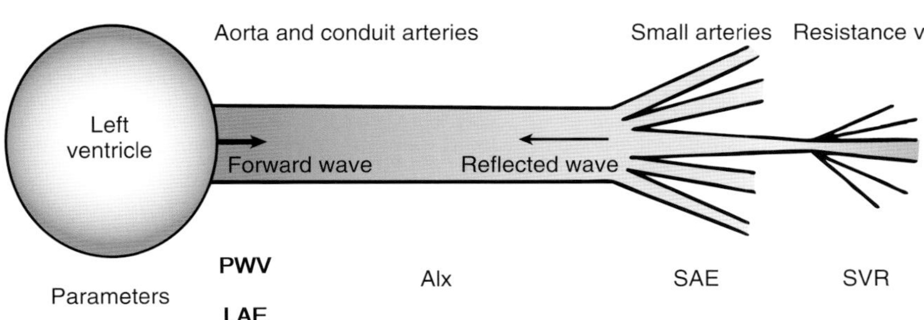

FIGURE 32-8 The different parameters of arterial stiffness/elasticity and the information they provide along the arterial system. *AIx,* Augmentation index; *LAE,* large artery elasticity; *PWV,* pulse wave velocity; *SAE,* small artery elasticity; *SVR,* systemic vascular resistance. *From Duprez DA: Arterial stiffness/elasticity in the contribution to progression of heart failure. Heart Fail Clin 8:135–141, 2012.*

Because the impedance load facing the left ventricle is dependent on pressure at all pressure levels, the benefit of lowering this vascular load may be demonstrated in all patients with left ventricular dysfunction, regardless of the absolute pressure level. Furthermore, changes in brachial artery pressure may not serve as an adequate guide to reductions in impedance load on the left ventricle. Constriction and stiffening of small arteries at branch points and in the microcirculation augment reflected waves that may impose a late systolic aortic pressure load on left ventricular emptying that is not detectable in the arm (**Figure 32-8**).[43] Therapy that relaxes these small arteries may therefore exert a greater benefit than is apparent from standard blood pressure measurement. In addition, however, some of the benefits of antihypertensive therapy on the development of heart failure may be mediated by nonpressure mechanisms. Improved endothelial function may favorably affect coronary perfusion, and some drugs may inhibit structural changes in the left ventricle independent of pressure reduction.

Aggressive blood pressure control is the most effective approach to reduce the incidence of heart failure in a hypertensive population.[44] A number of clinical trials demonstrate the benefit of treating hypertension in the prevention of heart failure.[45-49] Primary prevention trials demonstrate up to a 50% reduction in the incidence of heart failure in patients with hypertension who are treated with blood pressure–lowering agents.[50,51] Hypertension in the Very Elderly trial showed a 64% relative risk reduction in heart failure with the diuretic indapamide with or without the angiotensin-converting enzyme (ACE) inhibitor perindopril (**Figure 32-9**).[52]

Inhibition of the renin-angiotensin system with ACE inhibitors or angiotensin receptor blockers (ARBs) appears to exert a greater benefit on left ventricular hypertrophy and remodeling than would be predicted from their pressure-lowering effect. Their effectiveness in reducing morbid events in nonhypertensive patients with atherosclerotic disease may involve pressure-independent as well as pressure-dependent mechanisms.[53,54]

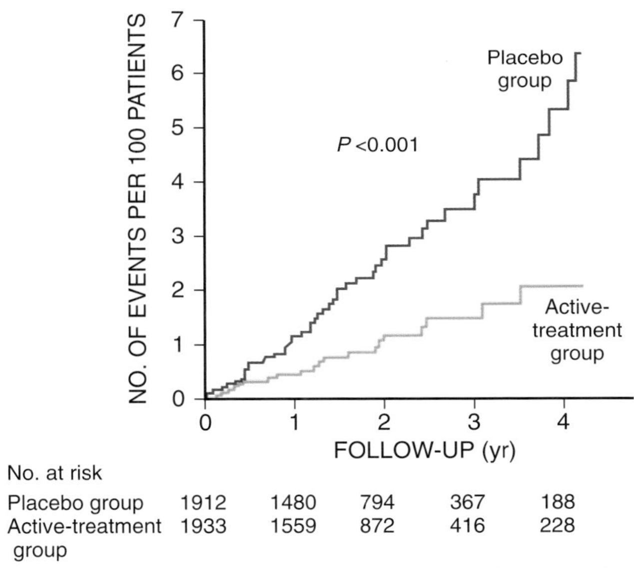

FIGURE 32-9 Kaplan-Meier estimates of the rate of heart failure according to study group in the Hypertension in the Very Elderly trial. For subjects receiving active treatment, in comparison with those receiving a placebo, the unadjusted hazard ratio was 0.36 (95% confidence interval, 0.22 to 0.58). *From Beckett NS, Peters R, Fletcher AE, et al: Treatment of hypertension in patients 80 years of age or older. N Engl J Med 358:1887–1898, 2008.*

β-blockers are also effective in preventing heart failure in hypertensive patients, in part through pressure reduction and in part through inhibition of structural remodeling of the left ventricle. Diuretic therapy also is effective in preventing heart failure, not only through blood pressure reduction but also by intravascular volume contraction, reducing the risk of congestion. Diuretics are not known to directly affect remodeling. Calcium antagonists, especially amlodipine, contribute to prevention of heart failure by their powerful vascular effects that reduce blood pressure and diminish reflected waves. These drugs probably do not directly inhibit left ventricular remodeling. The failure of α-blockers to prevent heart failure or to slow its progression is consistent with the lack of effectiveness of these drugs to inhibit structural cardiac remodeling.

DIABETES MELLITUS AND HEART FAILURE (see also Chapter 45)

The number of patients with diabetes mellitus continues to rise in industrial societies, owing mainly to changes in lifestyle (excessive calorie and fat intake and decreased physical activity).

On the basis of data from the National Health and Nutrition Examination Survey 2007-2010, an estimated 19.7 million Americans 20 years of age or older have physician-diagnosed diabetes mellitus.[1] An additional 8.2 million adults have undiagnosed diabetes mellitus, and approximately 87.3 million adults have prediabetes (e.g., fasting blood glucose of 100 to <126 mg/dL).[1] The prevalence of diagnosed diabetes mellitus in adults 65 years of age or older was 26.9% in 2010.[1] Since 1990, the prevalence of those diagnosed with diabetes increased 61%.[55] A total of 1.9 million new cases of diabetes mellitus (type 1 or type 2) were diagnosed in the United States in adults 20 years of age or older in 2010.[1] Data from Framingham Heart Study indicate a doubling in the incidence of diabetes over the past 30 years, most dramatically during the 1990s. Type 2 diabetes accounts for 90% to 95% of all diagnosed cases of diabetes in adults.[1] Most of the increase in absolute incidence of diabetes occurred in individuals with a body mass index (BMI) of 30 kg/m^2 or more.[56] Worldwide, the prevalence of diabetes for all age groups was estimated to be 2.8% in 2000 and is projected to be 4.4% in 2030.[57]

Diabetes and insulin resistance are important risk factors for the development of heart failure.[58] The presence of clinical diabetes mellitus markedly increases the likelihood of heart failure in patients without structural heart disease[59] and adversely affects the outcomes of patients with established heart failure.[60,61] In a study of patients with type 2 diabetes mellitus older than 50 years of age who had urinary albumin >20 mg/L, 4% of patients developed heart failure over the study period, of whom 36% died.[62] The Framingham Heart Study showed that the prevalence of heart failure was twice as high in diabetic men and five times as high in diabetic women aged between 45 and 74 years old when compared with age-matched controls.[63] Over the age of 65 years, the association became even stronger, with a fourfold higher prevalence in diabetic males and an eightfold higher prevalence in diabetic females.[63] A study of the predictors of heart failure among women with coronary disease found that diabetes was the strongest risk factor.[64] Diabetic women with elevated body mass index or depressed creatinine clearance were at highest risk. Diabetics with fasting glucose >300 mg/dL had a threefold adjusted risk of developing heart failure, compared with diabetics with controlled fasting blood sugar levels.[64]

The occurrence of heart failure represents a major and adverse prognostic turn in a diabetic patient's life. Heart failure is the most common admission diagnosis for the diabetic patient, and more than one third of type 2 diabetic patients die of heart failure.[63,65-67] Of patients requiring hospitalization for heart failure in the United States, 44% have diabetes, a percentage that seems to be increasing with time.[68] In a community-based cohort of 665 subjects with heart failure in Olmsted County, Minnesota, the 5-year survival was 46% for those with heart failure alone but only 37% for those with heart failure and diabetes mellitus.[69]

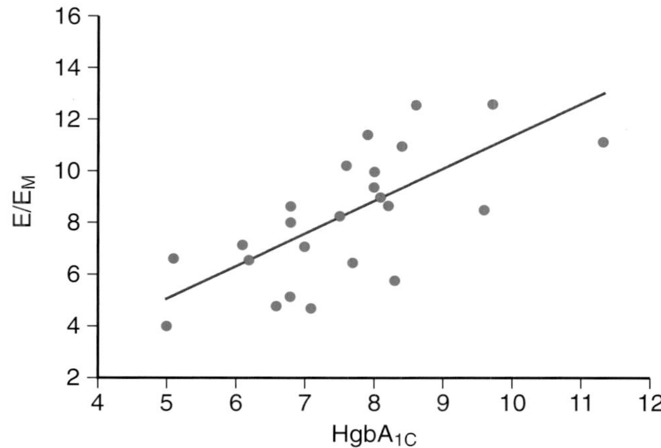

FIGURE 32-10 Relationship between glycosylated hemoglobin ($HgbA_{1c}$) and left ventricular diastolic function in patients with type 1 diabetes and without overt heart failure ($r = 0.68$, $P < 0.0002$). E/Em = relation of peak early diastolic transmitral flow (E) to myocardial relaxation velocity during early diastole (Em). *From Shishehbor MH, Hoogwerf BJ, Schoenhagen P, et al: Relation of hemoglobin A_{1c} to left ventricular relaxation in patients with type 1 diabetes mellitus and without overt heart disease. Am J Cardiol 91:1514–1517, 2003.*

The basic reason for the increased prevalence of heart failure in the diabetic patient is the presence of a distinct diabetic cardiomyopathy that is structurally characterized by cardiomyocyte hypertrophy, microangiopathy, endothelial dysfunction, and myocardial fibrosis.[20,70] At the cellular level, diabetic cardiomyopathy is associated with defects in subcellular organelles and downregulation of catecholamine receptors due to chronically elevated catecholamine levels.[71,72] Also, in animal models with the onset of hyperglycemia, changes in myocardial calcium transportation and alterations in contractile proteins occur, both of which lead to systolic and diastolic dysfunction that worsens as the collagen content of the myocardium increases.[71,73,74] Doppler imaging studies have been used to provide load-independent assessments of cardiac relaxation. These studies not only have confirmed evidence of diastolic dysfunction in asymptomatic patients with diabetes but also have shown a direct relationship between the extent of diastolic dysfunction and glycemic control (**Figure 32-10**).[75] Although diastolic dysfunction is the hallmark of diabetic cardiomyopathy, concomitant subtle systolic dysfunction is present even at earlier stages of the disease.[65]

Although neither the Diabetes Control and Complications Trial (DCCT) in type 1 diabetes nor the UK Prospective Diabetes Study (UKPDS) in type 2 diabetes showed a reduction in cardiovascular events with intensive glycemic control,[76,77] a prospective, observational component of UKPDS revealed a continuous relationship between glycemic exposure and the development of heart failure with no threshold of risk, such that for each 1% absolute reduction in glycosylated hemoglobin (HbA_{1c}), there was

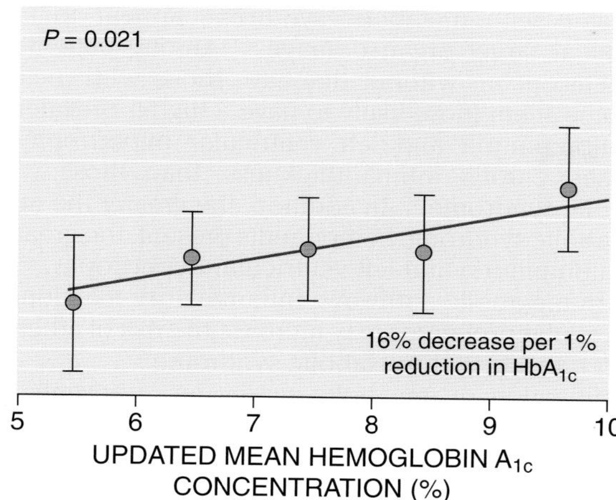

FIGURE 32-11 Relative risk of heart failure in relation to glycosylated hemoglobin ($HgbA_{1c}$) in the U.K. Prospective Diabetes Study. *From Stratton IM, Adler AI, Neil HA, et al: Association of glycaemia with macrovascular and microvascular complications of type 2 diabetes (UKPDS 35): prospective observational study. BMJ 321:405–412, 2000.*

an associated 16% decrease in the risk for heart failure (**Figure 32-11**).[78] Similar findings were also reported recently in a large cohort study from the United States.[79] The Atherosclerosis Risk in Communities (ARIC) study demonstrated that chronic hyperglycemia before the development of diabetes contributes to development of heart failure.[80] Glucose levels predict hospitalizations for congestive heart failure with a 10% increase in the risk of heart failure hospitalization for each 18-mg/dL (1-mmol) increase in fasting glucose level.[81]

Attaining optimal glycemic control should be a goal in both the prevention and treatment of heart failure in patients with diabetes. The Action to Control Cardiovascular Risk in Diabetes (ACCORD) study indicated a previously unrecognized harm of intensive glucose lowering in patients with type 2 diabetes[82]; however, these results were not confirmed in the Action in Diabetes and Vascular Disease: Preterax and Diamicron Modified Release Controlled Evaluation (ADVANCE) trial,[83] and should not be interpreted as diminishing the importance of glycemic control.[84] The choice of oral hypoglycemic agent that may be used is restricted. For example, metformin is contraindicated in the presence of either heart failure or renal impairment, and precautions also apply to the use of the thiazolidinediones.[85,86] In addition to treating hyperglycemia, controlling all other cardiovascular and metabolic risks and preventing complications in patients with diabetes is of utmost importance. ACE inhibitors or ARBs can prevent the development of end-organ disease and the occurrence of clinical events in diabetic patients, even in those who do not have hypertension.[53,87] Long-term treatment with several ACE inhibitors or ARBs has been shown to decrease the risk of renal disease in diabetic patients,[88,89] and prolonged therapy with the ACE inhibitor ramipril has been shown to lower the likelihood of heart failure, myocardial infarction, and cardiovascular death.[53] Likewise, the use of ARBs in patients with diabetes mellitus and hypertension or left ventricular hypertrophy has been shown to reduce the incidence of first hospitalization for heart failure, in addition to having other beneficial effects on renal function.[90-92]

ATHEROSCLEROTIC DISEASE AND HEART FAILURE

Patients with known atherosclerotic disease (e.g., of the coronary, cerebral, or peripheral blood vessels) are at increased risk of developing heart failure (see Chapter 18). The role of coronary artery disease and myocardial infarction as major antecedents of heart failure has been well established.[93,94]

Myocardial infarction is an important risk factor for heart failure, increasing risk twofold to threefold.[59,95,96] Myocardial infarction stimulates cardiac remodeling.[23,97] The percentage of people with a first myocardial infarction who will have heart failure in 5 years is 8% of men and 18% of women at 45 to 64 years of age, and 20% of men and 23% of women at 65 years of age or older.[1] Even in heart failure patients classified clinically as "nonischemic cardiomyopathy," up to a fourth may have evidence of coronary artery disease at autopsy.[98] Indeed, patients with "nonischemic cardiomyopathy" may develop clinical ischemic events, an observation that suggests that coronary disease may not be just an "innocent bystander" in these patients.[99] In addition to epicardial disease, microvascular coronary disease is also both widespread and often underrecognized.[100] The presence of underlying coronary artery disease contributes to the morbidity and mortality of patients with heart failure.[101] Clinically silent coronary atherosclerosis is highly prevalent in the general population, including children and young adults.[102,103] These data suggest that coronary atherosclerotic disease (epicardial or microvascular, clinically overt or silent) can lead to acute or chronic ischemia, thereby predisposing to left ventricular dysfunction and symptomatic heart failure.

The risk of coronary artery disease and myocardial infarction can be reduced by modification of risk factors.[50,51] Hydroxymethylglutaryl-coenzyme A reductase inhibitors (statins) reduce cardiovascular events in patients with myocardial infarction and the occurrence of heart failure in patients with coronary heart disease.[104-107] Uncertainty, however, remains regarding the role of statins in patients with established heart failure. Although observational studies and small clinical investigations have suggested that statins may be beneficial in patients with ischemic and nonischemic heart failure,[108-111] the first prospective randomized clinical outcome trial with statins focused specifically on patients with heart failure. The Controlled Rosuvastatin in Multinational Trial in Heart Failure (CORONA) showed no significant differences in the primary composite endpoint of death from cardiovascular causes, nonfatal myocardial infarction, or nonfatal stroke.[112]

ACE inhibitors reduce incidence of heart failure by 23% among patients who have coronary artery disease and normal systolic function and by 37% among patients who have reduced left ventricular systolic function.[50] In one large-scale trial, long-term treatment with an ACE inhibitor decreased the risk of the primary endpoint of cardiovascular death, myocardial infarction, and stroke in patients with high-risk established vascular disease who were without evidence of heart failure or reduced left ventricular ejection fraction.[53] Among patients with stable coronary artery disease and no heart failure, ACE inhibitor therapy significantly reduced the incidence of death, myocardial infarction, or cardiac arrest.[113] β-blockers,[114] aldosterone antagonists,[115] and angiotensin II receptor antagonists[116] reduce mortality and the need for hospitalization for heart failure in patients with myocardial infarction and left ventricular systolic dysfunction but without overt heart failure.[117,118]

METABOLIC SYNDROME AND HEART FAILURE

Metabolic syndrome refers to a cluster of risk factors for cardiovascular disease and type 2 diabetes mellitus. Although several different definitions for metabolic syndrome have been proposed, the International Diabetes Federation and others recently proposed a harmonized definition for metabolic syndrome.[119] By this definition, metabolic syndrome is diagnosed when three or more of the following five risk factors are present: (1) fasting plasma glucose of 100 mg/dL or more or undergoing drug treatment for elevated glucose, (2) HDL cholesterol <40 mg/dL in men or <50 mg/dL in women or undergoing drug treatment for reduced HDL cholesterol, (3) triglycerides of 150 mg/dL or more or undergoing drug treatment for elevated triglycerides, (4) waist circumference 102 cm or more in men or 88 cm or more in women, and (5) blood pressure 130 mm Hg or more systolic or 85 mm Hg or more diastolic or undergoing drug treatment for hypertension.

Approximately 34% of adults 20 years of age or older met the criteria for metabolic syndrome.[120] The prevalence of metabolic syndrome ranges from 6.7% among people 20 to 29 years of age to 43.5% for people 60 to 69 years of age and 42.0% for those 70 years of age or older.[121,122] The age-adjusted prevalence of metabolic syndrome was 35.1% for men and 32.6% for women.[1]

Although the designation of metabolic syndrome as a unique pathophysiologic condition and as a predictor of disease has recently been questioned,[123] most clinicians and researchers have long maintained that certain metabolic risk factors are prone to cluster, and that this clustering increases the risk of diabetes,[124] atrial fibrillation,[125] heart failure,[126] and overall cardiovascular morbidity and mortality.[127] According to the National Health and Nutrition Examination Survey (NHANES) data, people who did not have metabolic syndrome had the lowest risk for cardiovascular events, those with metabolic syndrome had an intermediate level of risk, and those with diabetes mellitus had the highest level of risk (**Figure 32-12**).[128]

Mechanisms underlying elevated cardiovascular risk associated with metabolic syndrome appear to involve subclinical target organ damage.[129] Among patients with hypertension but without diabetes, those with metabolic syndrome seem more likely to have a higher prevalence of microalbuminuria and left ventricular hypertrophy, and increased carotid intima thickness, than those without metabolic syndrome.[129] In addition, the greater the number of metabolic syndrome components present, the greater the microalbuminuria and left ventricular hypertrophy.[129] Alterations in metabolic pathways, inflammatory reactions, and other cellular processes may increase the risk of atherosclerosis in patients with metabolic syndrome.

Identification of metabolic syndrome represents a call to action for the health care provider and patient to address the underlying lifestyle-related risk factors, including abdominal obesity, physical inactivity, and atherogenic diet, as well as clinical management to address the characteristic atherogenic dyslipidemia, elevated blood pressure, elevated glucose, and prothrombotic state that are common to people with metabolic syndrome. A multidisciplinary team of health care professionals is desirable to adequately address these multiple issues in patients with the metabolic syndrome.

OBESITY AND HEART FAILURE

Obesity continues to be a leading public health concern in the United States.[130,131] Overall, 68% of adults in the United States are overweight or obese (73% of men and 64% of women).[1] The trend toward increasing obesity in this country is alarming.[132] Between 1980 and 2002, obesity prevalence doubled in adults aged 20 years or older and overweight prevalence tripled in children and adolescents aged 6 to 19 years.[133,134]

Obesity has been consistently associated with left ventricular hypertrophy and dilation,[135-138] which are known precursors of heart failure.[139,140] In the Framingham Heart Study population, overweight and lesser degrees of obesity were associated with an increased risk of heart failure (**Figure 32-13**).[141] Extreme obesity has also been associated with heart failure.[142] Excess body weight was found to be a strong predictor of mortality[143-145] and associated with a significant increase in the risk of stroke.[146] There are several plausible mechanisms for the association between obesity and heart

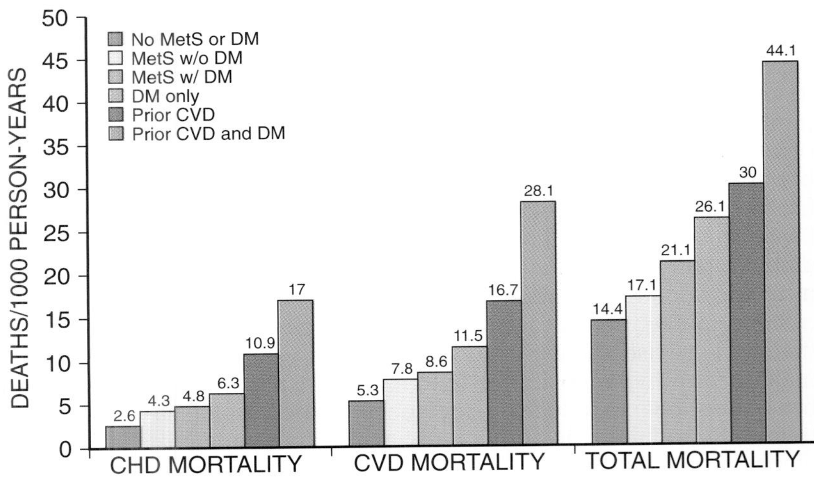

FIGURE 32-12 Mortality rates among adults in the United States, 30 to 75 years of age, with metabolic syndrome (MetS), with and without diabetes mellitus (DM) and preexisting cardiovascular disease (CVD). *CHD*, Coronary heart disease; *w/*, with; *w/o*, without. *From Malik S, Wong ND, Franklin SS, et al: Impact of the metabolic syndrome on mortality from coronary heart disease, cardiovascular disease, and all causes in United States adults. Circulation 110:1245–1250, 2004.*

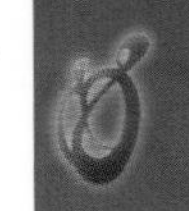

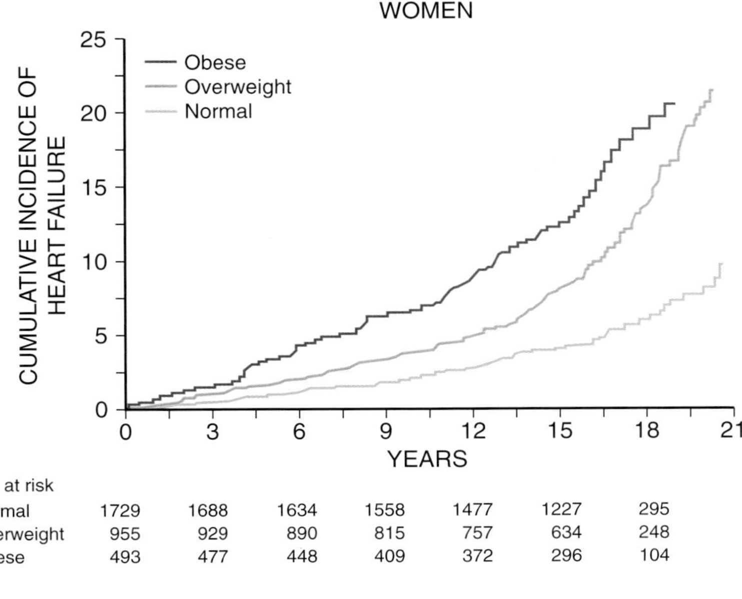

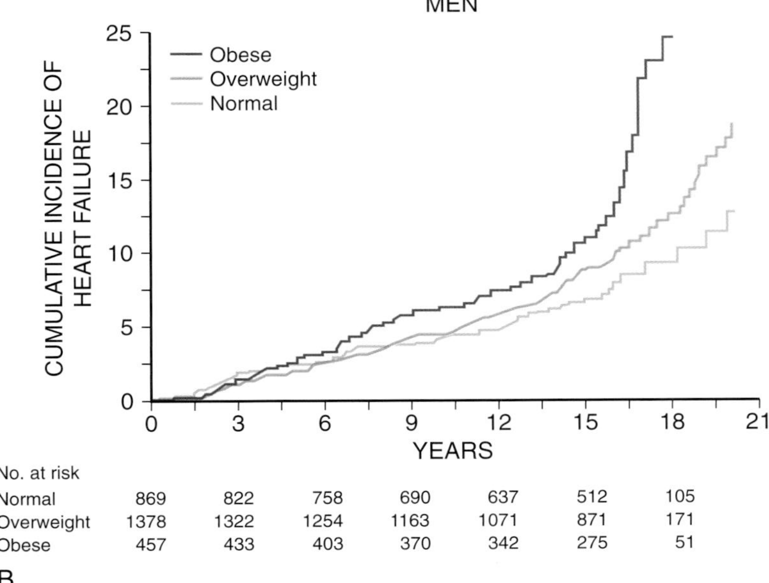

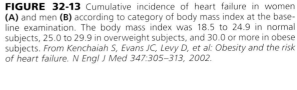

FIGURE 32-13 Cumulative incidence of heart failure in women **(A)** and men **(B)** according to category of body mass index at the baseline examination. The body mass index was 18.5 to 24.9 in normal subjects, 25.0 to 29.9 in overweight subjects, and 30.0 or more in obese subjects. *From Kenchaiah S, Evans JC, Levy D, et al: Obesity and the risk of heart failure. N Engl J Med 347:305–313, 2002.*

failure. Increased body mass index (BMI) is a risk factor for hypertension,[147] diabetes mellitus,[147,148] and dyslipidemia,[132] all of which augment the risk of myocardial infarction,[149,150] an important antecedent of heart failure.[34,59,95,151] In addition, hypertension and diabetes mellitus independently increase the risk of heart failure.[33,34,59,95,151] Elevated body mass index is associated with altered left ventricular remodeling,[135-139] possibly owing to increased hemodynamic load,[152,153] neurohormonal activation,[154] and increased oxidative stress.[154,155] Adipose tissue acts as an endocrine organ, secreting hormones and other substances that create a proinflammatory state and promote formation of atherosclerotic plaques.[156]

Despite the known strong association between overweight/obesity and cardiovascular risk factors and the development of cardiovascular diseases, numerous studies, including in heart failure, have demonstrated an "obesity paradox," in that obese patients with established cardiovascular diseases appear to have a more favorable clinical prognosis in heart failure, hypertension, coronary heart disease, and atrial fibrillation than do their leaner counterparts with the same cardiovascular diseases.[157,158] In the Atrial Fibrillation Follow-up Investigation of Rhythm Management (AFFIRM) study, a multicenter trial of atrial fibrillation, obese patients had lower all-cause mortality (HR = 0.77, $P = 0.01$) than normal-weight patients after multivariable adjustment over a 3-year follow-up period.[159] The reasons for the obesity paradox remain unclear. Because heart failure is a catabolic state, obese patients may have more metabolic reserve, and there is no doubt that cachexia is associated with adverse prognosis in heart failure.[160,161] Various cytokines and neuroendocrine profiles of obese patients may be protective.[158,160,161] Adipose tissue is known to produce soluble tumor necrosis factor-α receptors, which could have a protective effect in obese patients with both acute and chronic heart failure by neutralizing the adverse biologic effects of tumor necrosis factor-α.[162] In addition, higher circulating lipoproteins in obese patients may bind and detoxify lipopolysaccharides that play a role in stimulating the release of inflammatory cytokines, all of which may serve to protect obese heart failure patients.[158,163]

While weight reduction clearly has beneficial effects on cardiac structure and function and efforts to promote optimal body weight are likely to have an impact on a number of risk factors for heart failure and other cardiovascular diseases, only limited data are available to base current recommendations for intentional weight loss in patients with established heart failure.[157] Although the "weight" of evidence supports intentional weight reduction in heart failure, especially for those with more significant obesity,[157] better clinical studies are needed to define optimal body composition in patients with heart failure.

IDENTIFYING PATIENTS WITH EARLY HEART FAILURE FOR PREVENTIVE THERAPY

Several clinical tools have been studied for detecting patients with early heart failure in whom appropriate preventive and therapeutic interventions can be instituted. These include risk prediction scores, circulating biomarkers, and imaging techniques for detecting alterations in myocardial structure and function.

Use of Risk Scores for Prediction of Incident Heart Failure

Two epidemiology studies have developed heart failure risk prediction scores that generally have only a moderate discriminative value for identifying whether or not an individual will develop overt heart failure. The original Framingham Heart Study (FHS) heart failure prediction score was developed in the late 1990s in individuals with hypertension, coronary heart disease, or valve disease and used simple clinical data available from the medical record. This risk score identified patients with incremental risk of future heart failure.[151] The Health Aging and Body Composition (ABC) study enrolled 3075 well-functioning community-dwelling elderly persons aged 70 to 79 years and derived a risk score predictive of incident heart failure at 5 years.[164] The ABC risk score was superior to the FHS score but still provided only moderate discrimination for incident heart failure. The ABC heart failure model was externally validated in the Cardiovascular Health Study (CHS).[165] The ABC study and CHS define the numbers of older individuals without prevalent heart failure who have low (<5%), average (5%-10%), high (10%-20%), and very high (>20%) risk of overt heart failure over 5 years and thus provide insight into the number of persons who would be suitable for an intervention to prevent incident heart failure. Findings in the ABC study and CHS indicate that approximately 40% of older individuals have a risk of more than 5% of heart failure over 5 years and that approximately 75% of heart failure events occur in these individuals. Thus intervening with a heart failure prevention strategy in those at a risk of more than 5% of developing heart failure would limit the application of the intervention to 40% of the older population and offer the potential to affect 75% of future heart failure events. Intervening in those at more than 10% risk of developing heart failure would limit the application of the intervention to 20% of the older population and offer the potential to affect 50% of future heart failure events.

Use of Biomarkers for Screening and Prevention of Heart Failure

Biomarkers encompass an expanding array of biochemical variables, the levels of which may reflect various aspects of the pathophysiology of heart failure (see also Chapter 30). Putative biomarkers can be broadly classified into (a) biomarkers of neurohormonal activation, (b) myocyte injury, (c) extracellular matrix remodeling, (d) inflammation, (e) oxidative stress, and (f) newer biomarkers whose pathophysiologic associations are less well defined (**Table 32-1**).[166]

Most of the early studies of natriuretic peptides have focused on the role of B-type natriuretic peptide (BNP) or *N*-terminal pro-B-type natriuretic peptide (NT-proBNP) testing among patients presenting with signs and symptoms of heart failure ("stage C and D heart failure"). The diagnostic and prognostic utility of plasma natriuretic peptide levels in the overt heart failure setting has prompted interest in evaluation of these biomarkers as screening tools for patients with risk factors for heart failure and asymptomatic left ventricular dysfunction ("stage A and B heart failure").

Luchner A and colleagues[167] evaluated BNP as a marker of left ventricular dysfunction and hypertrophy in a population-based sample of middle-aged subjects and showed that compared with subjects with normal left ventricular function and mass, subjects with left ventricular dysfunction or hypertrophy had increased BNP levels. Recent data from Olmsted County, Minnesota, showed that in stage A and B heart failure, plasma NT-proBNP values

TABLE 32-1 Putative Biomarkers in Heart Failure

Neurohormonal activation	B-type natriuretic peptide (BNP)
	NT-proBNP
	Atrial natriuretic peptide (ANP)
	Norepinephrine
	Endothelin
	Adrenomedullin
	Urocortin
	Apelin
	Plasma renin activity (PRA)
	Angiotensin II
	Aldosterone
	Arginine vasopressin (AVP)
Myocyte injury	Cardiac troponin I (TnI)
	Cardiac troponin T (TnT)
	Heart-type fatty acid-binding protein (H-FABP)
	Myosin light chain-1 (MLC-1)
Extracellular matrix remodeling	Matrix metalloproteinases (MMPs)
	Tissue inhibitors of metalloproteinases (TIMPs)
Inflammation	C-reactive protein (CRP)
	Tumor necrosis factor-α (TNF-α)
	Interleukins 1, 6, and 18 (IL-1, IL-6, IL-18)
	Adhesion molecules
	ST2
Oxidative stress	Myeloperoxidase (MPO)
	Urinary biopyrrins
	Urinary and plasma isoprostanes
	8-epi prostaglandin-F-a
	Reduced glutathione/oxidized glutathione ratio
	Plasma malondialdehyde
New biomarkers	Osteoprotegerin
	Galectin-3
	Chromogranin A
	Adipokines
	Adiponectin
	Leptin
	Resistin
	Growth differentiation factor 15 (GDF-15)

From Florea VG, Anand IS: Biomarkers. Heart Fail Clin 8:207–224, 2012.

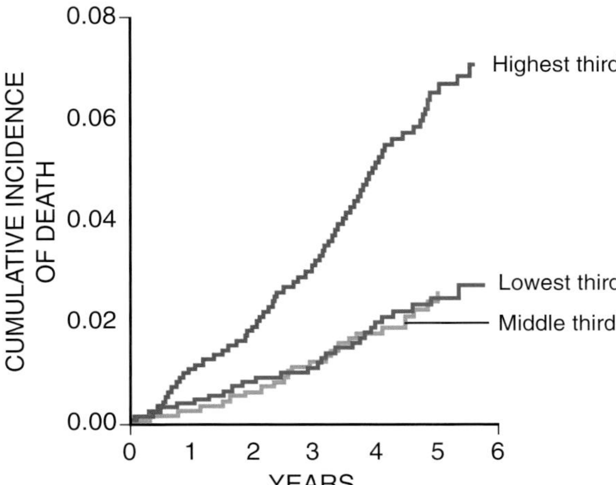

No. at risk							
Lowest third	1191	1188	1160	1051	959	697	331
Middle third	1073	1070	1053	959	882	673	369
A Highest third	1082	1073	1047	945	865	666	361

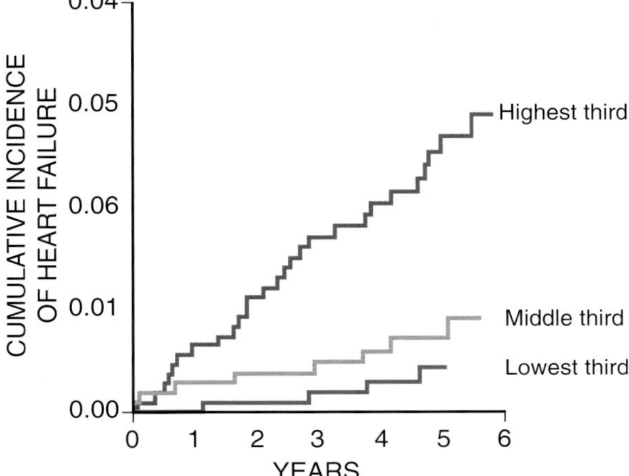

No. at risk							
Lowest third	1191	1188	1160	1050	957	695	331
Middle third	1073	1068	1050	957	878	670	368
B Highest third	1082	1068	1038	932	850	653	355

FIGURE 32-14 Cumulative incidence of death **(A)** and heart failure **(B)**, according to the plasma B-type natriuretic peptide level at baseline. *From Wang T, Larson M, Levy D, et al: Plasma natriuretic peptide levels and the risk of cardiovascular events and death. N Engl J Med 350:655–663, 2004.*

greater than age-/sex-specific 80th percentiles were associated with increased risk of death, heart failure, cerebrovascular accident, and myocardial infarction even after adjustment for clinical risk factors and structural cardiac abnormalities.[168] Higher NT-proBNP levels have also been associated with the greater likelihood of detecting incident heart failure in a population with stable coronary artery disease.[169] Recent investigations from the Framingham Heart Study reported that plasma natriuretic peptide levels predicted the risk of death and first cardiovascular event including heart failure, atrial fibrillation, and stroke or transient ischemic attack (**Figure 32-14**).[170]

Both the Framingham Heart Study and the Health Aging and Body Composition study have explored the ability of several biomarkers to enhance clinical scores for heart failure risk assessment. In the FHS, BNP and the urinary albumin to creatinine ratio (but not C-reactive protein, plasminogen activator inhibitor 1, homocysteine, or aldosterone to renin ratio) increased the discrimination of a clinical heart failure prediction score modestly.[171] In the ABC study, the additive value of inflammatory markers (interleukin-6, tumor necrosis factor-α, and C-reactive protein) to the ABC clinical risk score was assessed. Interleukin-6 provided modest but statistically significant additive discrimination and improved the risk stratification.[172] These studies suggest that heart failure risk stratification can be improved by biomarkers that might be useful if a prevention strategy was targeting those with increased heart failure risk.

The Dallas Heart Study included a cardiac magnetic resonance (CMR) examination in 2339 participants aged 30 to 65 years old and found that 12.5% of participants met the definition of stage B heart failure defined as the presence of left ventricular hypertrophy, reduced ejection fraction, or prior myocardial infarction.[173] They then examined the ability of the ABC heart failure risk score, BNP, NT-proBNP, and the combination of BNP or NT-proBNP and clinical risk score to detect stage B heart failure. The combination of a high clinical risk score and an elevated BNP or NT-proBNP had the best predictive characteristics for identifying stage B heart failure, but positive predictive values were quite low and indicate that 70% of imaging studies obtained in response to screening would not identify left ventricular hypertrophy or systolic dysfunction.[173]

The Olmsted County Heart Study examined the potential utility of plasma BNP as a stand-alone screening intervention to detect asymptomatic left ventricular systolic dysfunction in the general population.[174] The predictive characteristics of BNP for detection of ejection fraction of 40% or less were better than for detection of ejection fraction of 50% or less, but even focusing on detection of EF of 40% or less, the burden of imaging and yield on imaging would preclude a biomarker-only strategy from becoming widely accepted because most follow-up study results would be negative. A similar analysis with NT-proBNP in the same cohort was largely identical.[175] Similar findings were found in the Framingham Heart Study.[176] Although other investigators postulate that natriuretic peptides could be cost-effective,[177] the low prevalence of systolic dysfunction provides a very high bar for using natriuretic peptides as screening biomarkers. As a result, most guidelines currently do not support routine blood natriuretic peptide testing for screening large asymptomatic patient populations for left ventricular systolic dysfunction.[178]

Use of Imaging for Evaluation of Newly Suspected or Potential Heart Failure

In patients with signs and symptoms that raise suspicion of heart failure, assessment of left ventricular systolic and diastolic function is important and can be performed with a variety of imaging techniques (**see also Chapter 29**). The same holds true for patients who are at risk for heart failure, such as patients after acute myocardial infarction, those with hypertension and left ventricular hypertrophy, those who are exposed to potentially cardiotoxic chemotherapeutic agents,[179] and first-degree relatives of those with an inherited cardiomyopathy. The main objectives of imaging for heart failure evaluation revolve primarily around understanding both cardiac structure and function, and secondarily in determining the underlying cause, so that proven therapies may be targeted to appropriate patients.

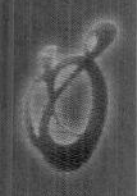

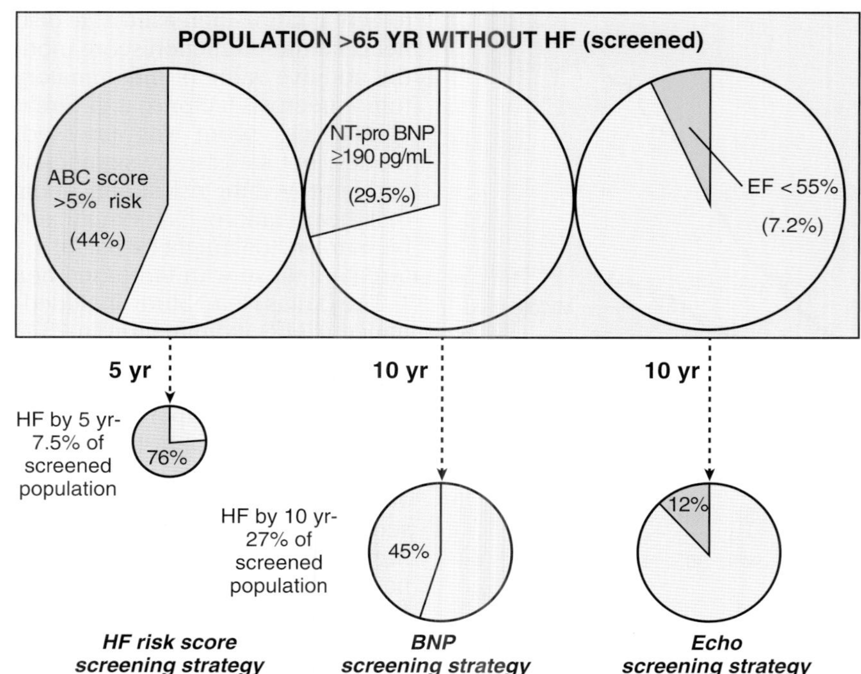

FIGURE 32-15 The ABC Heart Failure risk score, *N*-terminal pro-B-type natriuretic peptide (NT-proBNP) levels, and echocardiography-based screening in the Cardiovascular Health Study cohort. The percentage of the cohort with a positive screening result, the percentage of the cohort who went on to develop incident heart failure, and the percentage of the patients who developed heart failure who would have been identified by the screening intervention are shown (please see text for details). *BNP*, B-type natriuretic peptide; *EF*, ejection fraction; *HF*, heart failure. *From Redfield MM: Strategies to screen for stage B as a heart failure prevention intervention. Heart Fail Clin 8:285–296, 2012.*

Although a complete history and physical examination are the first steps in evaluating the cause of newly suspected heart failure, or factors predisposing to heart failure, identification of structural abnormalities leading to heart failure generally requires imaging of the cardiac chambers and great vessels.[180,181] Imaging may be used in new-onset heart failure to determine whether abnormalities of the myocardium, valves, or pericardium are present, which chambers are involved, and whether secondary pulmonary arterial hypertension is present. Imaging is also often very useful in such patients for early prognostication. For example, left ventricular ejection fraction after myocardial infarction remains a strong predictor of risk, with lower ejection fraction associated with worse outcome.[182]

Although the prevalence of asymptomatic left ventricular systolic dysfunction in the general adult population (3%-6%) may be too low to advocate use of traditional imaging techniques as a primary screening modality, population studies have identified subsets with sufficient prevalence of systolic dysfunction (elderly men with prevalent cardiovascular disease in whom the prevalence of asymptomatic left ventricular ejection fraction of 50% or less was 17%) that may warrant a primary imaging strategy.[183]

There are many diagnostic procedures used to evaluate patients with newly suspected or potential heart failure (see Chapter 28). Resting electrocardiogram or chest x-rays are part of the routine data collected with general history and physical examinations when appropriate. More advanced procedures include both rest and stress tests for echocardiography, radionuclide imaging (including radionuclide ventriculography [RNV], single photon emission computed tomography [SPECT], positron emission tomography [PET], and cardiovascular magnetic resonance [CMR]). Additionally, imaging of cardiac structures and coronary angiography with cardiac computer tomography and invasive cardiac catheterization may be considered. The use of these procedures should prudently take into account their possible technical capabilities, safety, and cost-effectiveness, according to the recently published appropriate use criteria.[184]

Figure 32-15 shows the utility of the ABC Heart Failure risk score, *N*-terminal pro-B-type natriuretic peptide (NT-proBNP) levels, and echocardiography in detecting incident heart failure in the Cardiovascular Health Study population.[183] The percentage of the cohort with a positive screening result, the percentage of the cohort who went on to develop incident heart failure, and the percentage of the patients who developed heart failure who would have been identified by the screening intervention are shown. The ABC Heart Failure risk score indicated higher (>5%) risk of heart failure at 5 years in 44% of the cohort and identified 76% of those who developed heart failure by 5 years. As the score was validated to predict 5-year risk of heart failure, only data on 5-year heart failure incidence were reported. An abnormal NT-proBNP level was present in 29.5% of the cohort and identified 45% of those who developed heart failure within 10 years. The baseline (screening) echocardiography identified reduced left ventricular ejection fraction in 7.2% of the population, but a low ejection fraction on screening identified only 12% of those who developed heart failure within 10 years.

FUTURE DIRECTIONS

Thus far, research aimed at preventing heart failure in high-risk individuals has been relatively modest in comparison with the extensive efforts at discovering new treatments for patients after heart failure has developed. Because preventive efforts are likely to be applicable to much larger numbers of individuals, such efforts could lead to greater population-level benefits. It is therefore important that we develop a strategy of prevention of heart failure that applies to the large number of "at-risk" individuals. Such a strategy would complement our current approaches that are aimed at intensive management of patients with manifest heart failure. Implementation of our current knowledge of both prevention and treatment of hypertension, obesity, and atherosclerotic vascular disease has the potential to have a large impact on the incidence and mortality from heart failure.

The ability to identify noninvasively early abnormalities of cardiovascular function and structure has led to the concept that it would be preferable to screen for and treat abnormalities that lead to all cardiovascular morbid events, not only heart failure. Because heart failure is a manifestation of chronic progression of these functional and structural defects, and some of these same abnormalities may lead to myocardial infarction, stroke, renal failure, peripheral vascular disease, and other morbid cardiovascular events, efforts to reduce the prevalence of all these events would appear to be more cost-effective than focusing specifically on heart failure.[185] One approach to this effort is the disease score for detection of early cardiovascular disease developed by Cohn and colleagues.[186] This method of performing 10 noninvasive tests of vascular and cardiac health has led to a scoring system that has been remarkably sensitive and specific in predicting future morbid events, including heart failure.[187] This testing array includes an ultrasound examination of the left ventricle, an electrocardiogram, and a plasma NT-proBNP level among the 10 tests. Thus it includes what may be viewed as the optimal approach to identifying early cardiac disease, as well as seven additional tests of vascular health.

Screening to identify candidates for aggressive preventive pharmacotherapy has not yet become an accepted standard approach to disease prevention. Nonetheless, the growing cost of advanced cardiovascular disease care will eventually demand that more effort be expended on prevention. Risk factor control will be part of that strategy, but pharmacologic interference with disease progression for those with early disease must become a priority.

References

1. Go AS, Mozaffarian D, Roger VL, et al: Heart disease and stroke statistics—2013 update: a report from the American Heart Association. *Circulation* 127:e6–e245, 2013.
2. Chen J, Normand SL, Wang Y, et al: National and regional trends in heart failure hospitalization and mortality rates for Medicare beneficiaries, 1998-2008. *JAMA* 306:1669–1678, 2011.
3. Levy D, Kenchaiah S, Larson MG, et al: Long-term trends in the incidence of and survival with heart failure. *N Engl J Med* 347:1397–1402, 2002.
4. Roger VL, Weston SA, Redfield MM, et al: Trends in heart failure incidence and survival in a community-based population. *JAMA* 292:344–350, 2004.
5. Heidenreich PA, Trogdon JG, Khavjou OA, et al: Forecasting the future of cardiovascular disease in the United States: a policy statement from the American Heart Association. *Circulation* 123:933–944, 2011.
6. Hunt SA, Baker DW, Chin MH, et al: ACC/AHA guidelines for the evaluation and management of chronic heart failure in the adult: executive summary a report of the American College of Cardiology/American Heart Association task force on practice guidelines (committee to revise the 1995 guidelines for the evaluation and management of heart failure): Developed in collaboration with the International Society for Heart and Lung Transplantation; Endorsed by the Heart Failure Society of America. *Circulation* 104:2996–3007, 2001.
7. Velagaleti RS, Vasan RS: Heart failure in the twenty-first century: is it a coronary artery disease or hypertension problem? *Cardiol Clin* 25:487–495, 2007.
8. Schocken DD, Benjamin EJ, Fonarow GC, et al: Prevention of heart failure: a scientific statement from the American Heart Association Councils on Epidemiology and Prevention, Clinical Cardiology, Cardiovascular Nursing, and High Blood Pressure Research; Quality of care and outcomes research interdisciplinary working group; and functional genomics and translational biology interdisciplinary working group. *Circulation* 117:2544–2565, 2008.
9. Cohn JN, Ferrari R, Sharpe N: Cardiac remodeling—concepts and clinical implications: a consensus paper from an international forum on cardiac remodeling. Behalf of an International Forum on Cardiac Remodeling. *J Am Coll Cardiol* 35:569–582, 2000.
10. Florea VG, Mareyev VY, Samko AN, et al: Left ventricular remodelling: common process in patients with different primary myocardial disorders. *Int J Cardiol* 68:281–287, 1999.
11. Lloyd-Jones DM, Larson MG, Leip EP, et al: Lifetime risk for developing congestive heart failure: the Framingham Heart Study. *Circulation* 106:3068–3072, 2002.
12. Fishberg AM: *Heart failure*, Philadelphia, 1937, Lea & Febiger.
13. Chatterjee K, Massie B: Systolic and diastolic heart failure: differences and similarities. *J Card Fail* 13:569–576, 2007.
14. Bursi F, Weston SA, Redfield MM, et al: Systolic and diastolic heart failure in the community. *JAMA* 296:2209–2216, 2006.
15. Baicu CF, Zile MR, Aurigemma GP, et al: Left ventricular systolic performance, function, and contractility in patients with diastolic heart failure. *Circulation* 111:2306–2312, 2005.
16. Huysman JA, Vliegen HW, Van der Laarse A, et al: Changes in nonmyocyte tissue composition associated with pressure overload of hypertrophic human hearts. *Pathol Res Pract* 184:577–581, 1989.
17. Pearlman ES, Weber KT, Janicki JS, et al: Muscle fiber orientation and connective tissue content in the hypertrophied human heart. *Lab Invest* 46:158–164, 1982.
18. Gwathmey JK, Copelas L, MacKinnon R, et al: Abnormal intracellular calcium handling in myocardium from patients with end-stage heart failure. *Circ Res* 61:70–76, 1987.
19. Florea VG: Classifying systolic and diastolic heart failure. *JAMA* 297:1058–1059, author reply 1059, 2007.
20. Factor SM, Minase T, Sonnenblick EH: Clinical and morphological features of human hypertensive-diabetic cardiomyopathy. *Am Heart J* 99:446–458, 1980.
21. Weber KT, Brilla CG, Janicki JS: Myocardial fibrosis: functional significance and regulatory factors. *Cardiovasc Res* 27:341–348, 1993.
22. Lauer MS, Anderson KM, Levy D: Influence of contemporary versus 30-year blood pressure levels on left ventricular mass and geometry: the Framingham Heart Study. *J Am Coll Cardiol* 18:1287–1294, 1991.
23. Pfeffer MA, Braunwald E: Ventricular remodeling after myocardial infarction. Experimental observations and clinical implications. *Circulation* 81:1161–1172, 1990.
24. Cohn JN: Critical review of heart failure: the role of left ventricular remodeling in the therapeutic response. *Clin Cardiol* 18:IV4–IV12, 1995.
25. Aurigemma GP, Zile MR, Gaasch WH: Contractile behavior of the left ventricle in diastolic heart failure: with emphasis on regional systolic function. *Circulation* 113:296–304, 2006.
26. Konstam MA: "Systolic and diastolic dysfunction" in heart failure? Time for a new paradigm. *J Card Fail* 9:1–3, 2003.
27. Baker BJ, Wilen MM, Boyd CM, et al: Relation of right ventricular ejection fraction to exercise capacity in chronic left ventricular failure. *Am J Cardiol* 54:596–599, 1984.
28. Kitzman DW, Higginbotham MB, Cobb FR, et al: Exercise intolerance in patients with heart failure and preserved left ventricular systolic function: failure of the Frank-Starling mechanism. *J Am Coll Cardiol* 17:1065–1072, 1991.
29. Konstam MA, Kronenberg MW, Udelson JE, et al: Effectiveness of preload reserve as a determinant of clinical status in patients with left ventricular systolic dysfunction. The SOLVD investigators. *Am J Cardiol* 69:1591–1595, 1992.
30. Djousse L, Driver JA, Gaziano JM: Relation between modifiable lifestyle factors and lifetime risk of heart failure. *JAMA* 302:394–400, 2009.
31. deFilippi CR, de Lemos JA, Tkaczuk AT, et al: Physical activity, change in biomarkers of myocardial stress and injury, and subsequent heart failure risk in older adults. *J Am Coll Cardiol* 60:2539–2547, 2012.
32. Lloyd-Jones DM, Hong Y, Labarthe D, et al: Defining and setting national goals for cardiovascular health promotion and disease reduction: the American Heart Association's strategic impact goal through 2020 and beyond. *Circulation* 121:586–613, 2010.
33. Levy D, Larson MG, Vasan RS, et al: The progression from hypertension to congestive heart failure. *JAMA* 275:1557–1562, 1996.
34. Wilhelmsen L, Rosengren A, Eriksson H, et al: Heart failure in the general population of men—morbidity, risk factors and prognosis. *J Intern Med* 249:253–261, 2001.
35. Gandhi SK, Powers JC, Nomeir AM, et al: The pathogenesis of acute pulmonary edema associated with hypertension. *N Engl J Med* 344:17–22, 2001.
36. Gheorghiade M, Zannad F, Sopko G, et al: Acute heart failure syndromes: current state and framework for future research. *Circulation* 112:3958–3968, 2005.
37. Kannel WB, Gordon T, Offutt D: Left ventricular hypertrophy by electrocardiogram. Prevalence, incidence, and mortality in the Framingham study. *Ann Intern Med* 71:89–105, 1969.
38. Urbina EM, Gidding SS, Bao W, et al: Effect of body size, ponderosity, and blood pressure on left ventricular growth in children and young adults in the Bogalusa Heart Study. *Circulation* 91:2400–2406, 1995.
39. Devereux RB: Left ventricular diastolic dysfunction: early diastolic relaxation and late diastolic compliance. *J Am Coll Cardiol* 13:337–339, 1989.
40. Inouye I, Massie B, Loge D, et al: Abnormal left ventricular filling: an early finding in mild to moderate systemic hypertension. *Am J Cardiol* 53:120–126, 1984.
41. Smith VE, Schulman P, Karimeddini MK, et al: Rapid ventricular filling in left ventricular hypertrophy: II. Pathologic hypertrophy. *J Am Coll Cardiol* 5:869–874, 1985.
42. Gunther S, Grossman W: Determinants of ventricular function in pressure-overload hypertrophy in man. *Circulation* 59:679–688, 1979.
43. Duprez DA: Arterial stiffness/elasticity in the contribution to progression of heart failure. *Heart Fail Clin* 8:135–141, 2012.
44. Chobanian AV, Bakris GL, Black HR, et al: Seventh report of the Joint National Committee on Prevention, Detection, Evaluation, and Treatment of High Blood Pressure. *Hypertension* 42:1206–1252, 2003.
45. Effects of treatment on morbidity in hypertension. II. Results in patients with diastolic blood pressure averaging 90 through 114 mm Hg. *JAMA* 213:1143–1152, 1970.
46. Izzo JL, Jr, Gradman AH: Mechanisms and management of hypertensive heart disease: from left ventricular hypertrophy to heart failure. *Med Clin North Am* 88:1257–1271, 2004.
47. Kostis JB, Davis BR, Cutler J, et al: Prevention of heart failure by antihypertensive drug treatment in older persons with isolated systolic hypertension. SHEP Cooperative Research Group. *JAMA* 278:212–216, 1997.
48. Dahlof B, Lindholm LH, Hansson L, et al: Morbidity and mortality in the Swedish Trial in Old Patients with Hypertension (STOP-Hypertension). *Lancet* 338:1281–1285, 1991.
49. Moser M, Hebert PR: Prevention of disease progression, left ventricular hypertrophy and congestive heart failure in hypertension treatment trials. *J Am Coll Cardiol* 27:1214–1218, 1996.
50. Baker DW: Prevention of heart failure. *J Card Fail* 8:333–346, 2002.
51. Vasan RS, Levy D: The role of hypertension in the pathogenesis of heart failure. A clinical mechanistic overview. *Arch Intern Med* 156:1789–1796, 1996.
52. Beckett NS, Peters R, Fletcher AE, et al: Treatment of hypertension in patients 80 years of age or older. *N Engl J Med* 358:1887–1898, 2008.
53. Yusuf S, Sleight P, Pogue J, et al: Effects of an angiotensin-converting-enzyme inhibitor, ramipril, on cardiovascular events in high-risk patients. The Heart Outcomes Prevention Evaluation Study Investigators. *N Engl J Med* 342:145–153, 2000.
54. Yusuf S, Teo KK, Pogue J, et al: Telmisartan, ramipril, or both in patients at high risk for vascular events. *N Engl J Med* 358:1547–1559, 2008.
55. Mokdad AH, Ford ES, Bowman BA, et al: Prevalence of obesity, diabetes, and obesity-related health risk factors, 2001. *JAMA* 289:76–79, 2003.
56. Fox CS, Pencina MJ, Meigs JB, et al: Trends in the incidence of type 2 diabetes mellitus from the 1970s to the 1990s: the Framingham Heart Study. *Circulation* 113:2914–2918, 2006.

57. Wild S, Roglic G, Green A, et al: Global prevalence of diabetes: estimates for the year 2000 and projections for 2030. *Diabetes Care* 27:1047–1053, 2004.
58. Taegtmeyer H, McNulty P, Young ME: Adaptation and maladaptation of the heart in diabetes: Part I: general concepts. *Circulation* 105:1727–1733, 2002.
59. He J, Ogden LG, Bazzano LA, et al: Risk factors for congestive heart failure in US men and women: NHANES I epidemiologic follow-up study. *Arch Intern Med* 161:996–1002, 2001.
60. Krumholz HM, Chen YT, Wang Y, et al: Predictors of readmission among elderly survivors of admission with heart failure. *Am Heart J* 139:72–77, 2000.
61. Shindler DM, Kostis JB, Yusuf S, et al: Diabetes mellitus, a predictor of morbidity and mortality in the Studies of Left Ventricular Dysfunction (SOLVD) Trials and Registry. *Am J Cardiol* 77:1017–1020, 1996.
62. Vaur L, Gueret P, Lievre M, et al: Development of congestive heart failure in type 2 diabetic patients with microalbuminuria or proteinuria: observations from the DIABHYCAR (type 2 DIABetes, Hypertension, CArdiovascular Events and Ramipril) study. *Diabetes Care* 26:855–860, 2003.
63. Kannel WB, McGee DL: Diabetes and cardiovascular disease. The Framingham study. *JAMA* 241:2035–2038, 1979.
64. Bibbins-Domingo K, Lin F, Vittinghoff E, et al: Predictors of heart failure among women with coronary disease. *Circulation* 110:1424–1430, 2004.
65. Bell DS: Heart failure in the diabetic patient. *Cardiol Clin* 25:523–538, 2007.
66. Cook CB, Tsui C, Ziemer DC, et al: Common reasons for hospitalization among adult patients with diabetes. *Endocr Pract* 12:363–370, 2006.
67. Reis SE, Holubkov R, Edmundowicz D, et al: Treatment of patients admitted to the hospital with congestive heart failure: specialty-related disparities in practice patterns and outcomes. *J Am Coll Cardiol* 30:733–738, 1997.
68. Adams KF, Jr, Fonarow GC, Emerman CL, et al: Characteristics and outcomes of patients hospitalized for heart failure in the United States: rationale, design, and preliminary observations from the first 100,000 cases in the Acute Decompensated Heart Failure National Registry (ADHERE). *Am Heart J* 149:209–216, 2005.
69. From AM, Leibson CL, Bursi F, et al: Diabetes in heart failure: prevalence and impact on outcome in the population. *Am J Med* 119:591–599, 2006.
70. Fang ZY, Prins JB, Marwick TH: Diabetic cardiomyopathy: evidence, mechanisms, and therapeutic implications. *Endocr Rev* 25:543–567, 2004.
71. Ganguly PK, Pierce GN, Dhalla KS, et al: Defective sarcoplasmic reticular calcium transport in diabetic cardiomyopathy. *Am J Physiol* 244:E528–E535, 1983.
72. Huggett RJ, Scott EM, Gilbey SG, et al: Impact of type 2 diabetes mellitus on sympathetic neural mechanisms in hypertension. *Circulation* 108:3097–3101, 2003.
73. Giacomelli F, Wiener J: Primary myocardial disease in the diabetic mouse. An ultrastructural study. *Lab Invest* 40:460–473, 1979.
74. Poirier P, Bogaty P, Garneau C, et al: Diastolic dysfunction in normotensive men with well-controlled type 2 diabetes: importance of maneuvers in echocardiographic screening for preclinical diabetic cardiomyopathy. *Diabetes Care* 24:5–10, 2001.
75. Shishehbor MH, Hoogwerf BJ, Schoenhagen P, et al: Relation of hemoglobin A1c to left ventricular relaxation in patients with type 1 diabetes mellitus and without overt heart disease. *Am J Cardiol* 91:1514–1517, 2003.
76. The effect of intensive treatment of diabetes on the development and progression of long-term complications in insulin-dependent diabetes mellitus. The Diabetes Control and Complications Trial Research Group. *N Engl J Med* 329:977–986, 1993.
77. Intensive blood-glucose control with sulphonylureas or insulin compared with conventional treatment and risk of complications in patients with type 2 diabetes (UKPDS 33). UK Prospective Diabetes Study (UKPDS) Group. *Lancet* 352:837–853, 1998.
78. Stratton IM, Adler AI, Neil HA, et al: Association of glycaemia with macrovascular and microvascular complications of type 2 diabetes (UKPDS 35): prospective observational study. *BMJ* 321:405–412, 2000.
79. Iribarren C, Karter AJ, Go AS, et al: Glycemic control and heart failure among adult patients with diabetes. *Circulation* 103:2668–2673, 2001.
80. Matsushita K, Blecker S, Pazin-Filho A, et al: The association of hemoglobin a1c with incident heart failure among people without diabetes: the Atherosclerosis Risk in Communities study. *Diabetes* 59:2020–2026, 2010.
81. Held C, Gerstein HC, Yusuf S, et al: Glucose levels predict hospitalization for congestive heart failure in patients at high cardiovascular risk. *Circulation* 115:1371–1375, 2007.
82. Gerstein HC, Miller ME, Byington RP, et al: Effects of intensive glucose lowering in type 2 diabetes. *N Engl J Med* 358:2545–2559, 2008.
83. Patel A, MacMahon S, Chalmers J, et al: Intensive blood glucose control and vascular outcomes in patients with type 2 diabetes. *N Engl J Med* 358:2560–2572, 2008.
84. Dluhy RG, McMahon GT: Intensive glycemic control in the ACCORD and ADVANCE trials. *N Engl J Med* 358:2630–2633, 2008.
85. Gilbert RE, Connelly K, Kelly DJ, et al: Heart failure and nephropathy: catastrophic and interrelated complications of diabetes. *Clin J Am Soc Nephrol* 1:193–208, 2006.
86. Lipscombe LL, Gomes T, Levesque LE, et al: Thiazolidinediones and cardiovascular outcomes in older patients with diabetes. *JAMA* 298:2634–2643, 2007.
87. Effects of ramipril on cardiovascular and microvascular outcomes in people with diabetes mellitus: results of the HOPE study and MICRO-HOPE substudy. Heart Outcomes Prevention Evaluation Study Investigators. *Lancet* 355:253–259, 2000.
88. Kasiske BL, Kalil RS, Ma JZ, et al: Effect of antihypertensive therapy on the kidney in patients with diabetes: a meta-regression analysis. *Ann Intern Med* 118:129–138, 1993.
89. Lewis EJ, Hunsicker LG, Bain RP, et al: The effect of angiotensin-converting-enzyme inhibition on diabetic nephropathy. The Collaborative Study Group. *N Engl J Med* 329:1456–1462, 1993.
90. Berl T, Hunsicker LG, Lewis JB, et al: Cardiovascular outcomes in the Irbesartan Diabetic Nephropathy Trial of patients with type 2 diabetes and overt nephropathy. *Ann Intern Med* 138:542–549, 2003.
91. Brenner BM, Cooper ME, de Zeeuw D, et al: Effects of losartan on renal and cardiovascular outcomes in patients with type 2 diabetes and nephropathy. *N Engl J Med* 345:861–869, 2001.
92. Zanella MT, Ribeiro AB: The role of angiotensin II antagonism in type 2 diabetes mellitus: a review of renoprotection studies. *Clin Ther* 24:1019–1034, 2002.
93. Bourassa MG, Gurne O, Bangdiwala SI, et al: Natural history and patterns of current practice in heart failure. The Studies of Left Ventricular Dysfunction (SOLVD) Investigators. *J Am Coll Cardiol* 22:14A–19A, 1993.
94. Kenchaiah S, Narula J, Vasan RS: Risk factors for heart failure. *Med Clin North Am* 88:1145–1172, 2004.
95. Chen YT, Vaccarino V, Williams CS, et al: Risk factors for heart failure in the elderly: a prospective community-based study. *Am J Med* 106:605–612, 1999.
96. Gottdiener JS, Arnold AM, Aurigemma GP, et al: Predictors of congestive heart failure in the elderly: the Cardiovascular Health Study. *J Am Coll Cardiol* 35:1628–1637, 2000.
97. Pfeffer MA: Left ventricular remodeling after acute myocardial infarction. *Annu Rev Med* 46:455–466, 1995.
98. Repetto A, Dal Bello B, Pasotti M, et al: Coronary atherosclerosis in end-stage idiopathic dilated cardiomyopathy: an innocent bystander? *Eur Heart J* 26:1519–1527, 2005.
99. Hedrich O, Jacob M, Hauptman PJ: Progression of coronary artery disease in non-ischemic dilated cardiomyopathy. *Coron Artery Dis* 15:291–297, 2004.
100. Mohri M, Takeshita A: Coronary microvascular disease in humans. *Jpn Heart J* 40:97–108, 1999.
101. Bart BA, Shaw LK, McCants CB, Jr, et al: Clinical determinants of mortality in patients with angiographically diagnosed ischemic or nonischemic cardiomyopathy. *J Am Coll Cardiol* 30:1002–1008, 1997.
102. Kavey RE, Daniels SR, Lauer RM, et al: American Heart Association guidelines for primary prevention of atherosclerotic cardiovascular disease beginning in childhood. *Circulation* 107:1562–1566, 2003.
103. Tuzcu EM, Kapadia SR, Tutar E, et al: High prevalence of coronary atherosclerosis in asymptomatic teenagers and young adults: evidence from intravascular ultrasound. *Circulation* 103:2705–2710, 2001.
104. Randomised trial of cholesterol lowering in 4444 patients with coronary heart disease: the Scandinavian Simvastatin Survival Study (4S). *Lancet* 344:1383–1389, 1994.
105. Prevention of cardiovascular events and death with pravastatin in patients with coronary heart disease and a broad range of initial cholesterol levels. The Long-Term Intervention with Pravastatin in Ischaemic Disease (LIPID) Study Group. *N Engl J Med* 339:1349–1357, 1998.
106. Kjekshus J, Pedersen TR, Olsson AG, et al: The effects of simvastatin on the incidence of heart failure in patients with coronary heart disease. *J Card Fail* 3:249–254, 1997.
107. Lewis SJ, Moye LA, Sacks FM, et al: Effect of pravastatin on cardiovascular events in older patients with myocardial infarction and cholesterol levels in the average range. Results of the Cholesterol and Recurrent Events (CARE) trial. *Ann Intern Med* 129:681–689, 1998.
108. Go AS, Lee WY, Yang J, et al: Statin therapy and risks for death and hospitalization in chronic heart failure. *JAMA* 296:2105–2111, 2006.
109. Horwich TB, MacLellan WR, Fonarow GC: Statin therapy is associated with improved survival in ischemic and non-ischemic heart failure. *J Am Coll Cardiol* 43:642–648, 2004.
110. Ramasubbu K, Estep J, White DL, et al: Experimental and clinical basis for the use of statins in patients with ischemic and nonischemic cardiomyopathy. *J Am Coll Cardiol* 51:415–426, 2008.
111. Sola S, Mir MQ, Lerakis S, et al: Atorvastatin improves left ventricular systolic function and serum markers of inflammation in nonischemic heart failure. *J Am Coll Cardiol* 47:332–337, 2006.
112. Kjekshus J, Apetrei E, Barrios V, et al: Rosuvastatin in older patients with systolic heart failure. *N Engl J Med* 357:2248–2261, 2007.
113. Fox KM: Efficacy of perindopril in reduction of cardiovascular events among patients with stable coronary artery disease: randomised, double-blind, placebo-controlled, multicentre trial (the EUROPA study). *Lancet* 362:782–788, 2003.
114. Dargie HJ: Effect of carvedilol on outcome after myocardial infarction in patients with left-ventricular dysfunction: the CAPRICORN randomised trial. *Lancet* 357:1385–1390, 2001.
115. Pitt B, Remme W, Zannad F, et al: Eplerenone, a selective aldosterone blocker, in patients with left ventricular dysfunction after myocardial infarction. *N Engl J Med* 348:1309–1321, 2003.
116. Pfeffer MA, McMurray JJ, Velazquez EJ, et al: Valsartan, captopril, or both in myocardial infarction complicated by heart failure, left ventricular dysfunction, or both. *N Engl J Med* 349:1893–1906, 2003.
117. Ambrosioni E, Borghi C, Magnani B: The effect of the angiotensin-converting-enzyme inhibitor zofenopril on mortality and morbidity after anterior myocardial infarction. The Survival of Myocardial Infarction Long-Term Evaluation (SMILE) Study Investigators. *N Engl J Med* 332:80–85, 1995.
118. Pfeffer MA, Braunwald E, Moye LA, et al: Effect of captopril on mortality and morbidity in patients with left ventricular dysfunction after myocardial infarction. Results of the survival and ventricular enlargement trial. The SAVE Investigators. *N Engl J Med* 327:669–677, 1992.
119. Alberti KG, Eckel RH, Grundy SM, et al: Harmonizing the metabolic syndrome: a joint interim statement of the International Diabetes Federation Task Force on Epidemiology and Prevention; National Heart, Lung, and Blood Institute; American Heart Association; World Heart Federation; International Atherosclerosis Society; and International Association for the Study of Obesity. *Circulation* 120:1640–1645, 2009.
120. Ervin RB: Prevalence of metabolic syndrome among adults 20 years of age and over, by sex, age, race and ethnicity, and body mass index: United States, 2003-2006. *Natl Health Stat Report* 1–7, 2009.
121. Ford ES, Giles WH, Dietz WH: Prevalence of the metabolic syndrome among US adults: findings from the third National Health and Nutrition Examination Survey. *JAMA* 287:356–359, 2002.
122. Kereiakes DJ, Willerson JT: Metabolic syndrome epidemic. *Circulation* 108:1552–1553, 2003.
123. Kahn R, Buse J, Ferrannini E, et al: The metabolic syndrome: time for a critical appraisal: joint statement from the American Diabetes Association and the European Association for the Study of Diabetes. *Diabetes Care* 28:2289–2304, 2005.
124. Grundy SM, Brewer HB, Jr, Cleeman JI, et al: Definition of metabolic syndrome: report of the National Heart, Lung, and Blood Institute/American Heart Association conference on scientific issues related to definition. *Circulation* 109:433–438, 2004.
125. Chamberlain AM, Agarwal SK, Ambrose M, et al: Metabolic syndrome and incidence of atrial fibrillation among blacks and whites in the Atherosclerosis Risk in Communities (ARIC) Study. *Am Heart J* 159:850–856, 2010.
126. Horwich TB, Fonarow GC: Glucose, obesity, metabolic syndrome, and diabetes relevance to incidence of heart failure. *J Am Coll Cardiol* 55:283–293, 2010.
127. Lakka HM, Laaksonen DE, Lakka TA, et al: The metabolic syndrome and total and cardiovascular disease mortality in middle-aged men. *JAMA* 288:2709–2716, 2002.
128. Malik S, Wong ND, Franklin SS, et al: Impact of the metabolic syndrome on mortality from coronary heart disease, cardiovascular disease, and all causes in United States adults. *Circulation* 110:1245–1250, 2004.
129. Leoncini G, Ratto E, Viazzi F, et al: Metabolic syndrome is associated with early signs of organ damage in nondiabetic, hypertensive patients. *J Intern Med* 257:454–460, 2005.
130. Overweight, obesity, and health risk. National Task Force on the Prevention and Treatment of Obesity. *Arch Intern Med* 160:898–904, 2000.
131. Flegal KM, Graubard BI, Williamson DF, et al: Excess deaths associated with underweight, overweight, and obesity. *JAMA* 293:1861–1867, 2005.
132. Clinical Guidelines on the Identification, Evaluation, and Treatment of Overweight and Obesity in Adults—The Evidence Report. National Institutes of Health. *Obes Res* 6(Suppl 2):51S–209S, 1998.
133. Hedley AA, Ogden CL, Johnson CL, et al: Prevalence of overweight and obesity among US children, adolescents, and adults, 1999-2002. *JAMA* 291:2847–2850, 2004.
134. Ogden CL, Carroll MD, Curtin LR, et al: Prevalence of overweight and obesity in the United States, 1999-2004. *JAMA* 295:1549–1555, 2006.
135. Alpert MA, Lambert CR, Terry BE, et al: Influence of left ventricular mass on left ventricular diastolic filling in normotensive morbid obesity. *Am Heart J* 130:1068–1073, 1995.
136. Hammond IW, Devereux RB, Alderman MH, et al: Relation of blood pressure and body build to left ventricular mass in normotensive and hypertensive employed adults. *J Am Coll Cardiol* 12:996–1004, 1988.
137. Lauer MS, Anderson KM, Kannel WB, et al: The impact of obesity on left ventricular mass and geometry. The Framingham Heart Study. *JAMA* 266:231–236, 1991.

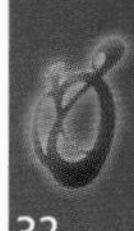

138. Messerli FH, Sundgaard-Riise K, Reisin ED, et al: Dimorphic cardiac adaptation to obesity and arterial hypertension. *Ann Intern Med* 99:757–761, 1983.
139. Gardin JM, McClelland R, Kitzman D, et al: M-mode echocardiographic predictors of six- to seven-year incidence of coronary heart disease, stroke, congestive heart failure, and mortality in an elderly cohort (the Cardiovascular Health Study). *Am J Cardiol* 87:1051–1057, 2001.
140. Vasan RS, Larson MG, Benjamin EJ, et al: Left ventricular dilatation and the risk of congestive heart failure in people without myocardial infarction. *N Engl J Med* 336:1350–1355, 1997.
141. Kenchaiah S, Evans JC, Levy D, et al: Obesity and the risk of heart failure. *N Engl J Med* 347:305–313, 2002.
142. Alpert MA: Obesity cardiomyopathy: pathophysiology and evolution of the clinical syndrome. *Am J Med Sci* 321:225–236, 2001.
143. Adams KF, Schatzkin A, Harris TB, et al: Overweight, obesity, and mortality in a large prospective cohort of persons 50 to 71 years old. *N Engl J Med* 355:763–778, 2006.
144. Hu FB, Willett WC, Li T, et al: Adiposity as compared with physical activity in predicting mortality among women. *N Engl J Med* 351:2694–2703, 2004.
145. McGee DL: Body mass index and mortality: a meta-analysis based on person-level data from twenty-six observational studies. *Ann Epidemiol* 15:87–97, 2005.
146. Hu G, Tuomilehto J, Silventoinen K, et al: Body mass index, waist circumference, and waist-hip ratio on the risk of total and type-specific stroke. *Arch Intern Med* 167:1420–1427, 2007.
147. Stamler J: Epidemiologic findings on body mass and blood pressure in adults. *Ann Epidemiol* 1:347–362, 1991.
148. Chan JM, Rimm EB, Colditz GA, et al: Obesity, fat distribution, and weight gain as risk factors for clinical diabetes in men. *Diabetes Care* 17:961–969, 1994.
149. Kannel WB, McGee DL: Diabetes and glucose tolerance as risk factors for cardiovascular disease: the Framingham study. *Diabetes Care* 2:120–126, 1979.
150. Manson JE, Colditz GA, Stampfer MJ, et al: A prospective study of obesity and risk of coronary heart disease in women. *N Engl J Med* 322:882–889, 1990.
151. Kannel WB, D'Agostino RB, Silbershatz H, et al: Profile for estimating risk of heart failure. *Arch Intern Med* 159:1197–1204, 1999.
152. Alexander JK, Dennis EW, Smith WG, et al: Blood volume, cardiac output, and distribution of systemic blood flow in extreme obesity. *Cardiovasc Res Cent Bull* 1:39–44, 1962.
153. Messerli FH, Sundgaard-Riise K, Reisin E, et al: Disparate cardiovascular effects of obesity and arterial hypertension. *Am J Med* 74:808–812, 1983.
154. Engeli S, Sharma AM: The renin-angiotensin system and natriuretic peptides in obesity-associated hypertension. *J Mol Med* 79:21–29, 2001.
155. Vincent HK, Powers SK, Stewart DJ, et al: Obesity is associated with increased myocardial oxidative stress. *Int J Obes Relat Metab Disord* 23:67–74, 1999.
156. Lau DC, Dhillon B, Yan H, et al: Adipokines: molecular links between obesity and atherosclerosis. *Am J Physiol Heart Circ Physiol* 288:H2031–H2041, 2005.
157. Lavie CJ, Alpert MA, Arena R, et al: Impact of obesity and the obesity paradox on prevalence and prognosis in heart failure. *J Am Coll Cardiol HF* 1:93–102, 2013.
158. Lavie CJ, Milani RV, Ventura HO: Obesity and cardiovascular disease: risk factor, paradox, and impact of weight loss. *J Am Coll Cardiol* 53:1925–1932, 2009.
159. Badheka AO, Rathod A, Kizilbash MA, et al: Influence of obesity on outcomes in atrial fibrillation: yet another obesity paradox. *Am J Med* 123:646–651, 2010.
160. Anker SD, Negassa A, Coats AJ, et al: Prognostic importance of weight loss in chronic heart failure and the effect of treatment with angiotensin-converting-enzyme inhibitors: an observational study. *Lancet* 361:1077–1083, 2003.
161. Kalantar-Zadeh K, Block G, Horwich T, et al: Reverse epidemiology of conventional cardiovascular risk factors in patients with chronic heart failure. *J Am Coll Cardiol* 43:1439–1444, 2004.
162. Mohamed-Ali V, Goodrick S, Bulmer K, et al: Production of soluble tumor necrosis factor receptors by human subcutaneous adipose tissue in vivo. *Am J Physiol* 277:E971–E975, 1999.
163. Rauchhaus M, Coats AJ, Anker SD: The endotoxin-lipoprotein hypothesis. *Lancet* 356:930–933, 2000.
164. Butler J, Kalogeropoulos A, Georgiopoulou V, et al: Incident heart failure prediction in the elderly: the health ABC heart failure score. *Circ Heart Fail* 1:125–133, 2008.
165. Kalogeropoulos A, Psaty BM, Vasan RS, et al: Validation of the health ABC heart failure model for incident heart failure risk prediction: the Cardiovascular Health Study. *Circ Heart Fail* 3:495–502, 2010.
166. Florea VG, Anand IS: Biomarkers. *Heart Fail Clin* 8:207–224, 2012.
167. Luchner A, Burnett JC, Jr, Jougasaki M, et al: Evaluation of brain natriuretic peptide as marker of left ventricular dysfunction and hypertrophy in the population. *J Hypertens* 18:1121–1128, 2000.
168. McKie PM, Cataliotti A, Lahr BD, et al: The prognostic value of N-terminal pro-B-type natriuretic peptide for death and cardiovascular events in healthy normal and stage A/B heart failure subjects. *J Am Coll Cardiol* 55:2140–2147, 2010.
169. Bibbins-Domingo K, Gupta R, Na B, et al: N-terminal fragment of the prohormone brain-type natriuretic peptide (NT-proBNP), cardiovascular events, and mortality in patients with stable coronary heart disease. *JAMA* 297:169–176, 2007.
170. Wang TJ, Larson MG, Levy D, et al: Plasma natriuretic peptide levels and the risk of cardiovascular events and death. *N Engl J Med* 350:655–663, 2004.
171. Velagaleti RS, Gona P, Larson MG, et al: Multimarker approach for the prediction of heart failure incidence in the community. *Circulation* 122:1700–1706, 2010.
172. Kalogeropoulos A, Georgiopoulou V, Psaty BM, et al: Inflammatory markers and incident heart failure risk in older adults: the Health ABC (Health, Aging, and Body Composition) study. *J Am Coll Cardiol* 55:2129–2137, 2010.
173. Gupta S, Rohatgi A, Ayers CR, et al: Risk scores versus natriuretic peptides for identifying prevalent stage B heart failure. *Am Heart J* 161:923–930, e922, 2011.
174. Redfield MM, Rodeheffer RJ, Jacobsen SJ, et al: Plasma brain natriuretic peptide to detect preclinical ventricular systolic or diastolic dysfunction: a community-based study. *Circulation* 109:3176–3181, 2004.
175. Costello-Boerrigter LC, Boerrigter G, Redfield MM, et al: Amino-terminal pro-B-type natriuretic peptide and B-type natriuretic peptide in the general community: determinants and detection of left ventricular dysfunction. *J Am Coll Cardiol* 47:345–353, 2006.
176. Vasan RS, Benjamin EJ, Larson MG, et al: Plasma natriuretic peptides for community screening for left ventricular hypertrophy and systolic dysfunction: the Framingham Heart Study. *JAMA* 288:1252–1259, 2002.
177. Heidenreich PA, Gubens MA, Fonarow GC, et al: Cost-effectiveness of screening with B-type natriuretic peptide to identify patients with reduced left ventricular ejection fraction. *J Am Coll Cardiol* 43:1019–1026, 2004.
178. Tang WH, Francis GS, Morrow DA, et al: National Academy of Clinical Biochemistry Laboratory Medicine practice guidelines: clinical utilization of cardiac biomarker testing in heart failure. *Circulation* 116:e99–e109, 2007.
179. Sawaya H, Sebag IA, Plana JC, et al: Assessment of echocardiography and biomarkers for the extended prediction of cardiotoxicity in patients treated with anthracyclines, taxanes, and trastuzumab. *Circ Cardiovasc Imaging* 5:596–603, 2012.
180. Fonseca C, Morais H, Mota T, et al: The diagnosis of heart failure in primary care: value of symptoms and signs. *Eur J Heart Fail* 6:795–800, 2004.
181. Hunt SA, Abraham WT, Chin MH, et al: 2009 Focused update incorporated into the ACC/AHA 2005 Guidelines for the Diagnosis and Management of Heart Failure in Adults: a report of the American College of Cardiology Foundation/American Heart Association Task Force on Practice Guidelines Developed in Collaboration With the International Society for Heart and Lung Transplantation. *J Am Coll Cardiol* 53:e1–e90, 2009.
182. Solomon SD, Anavekar N, Skali H, et al: Influence of ejection fraction on cardiovascular outcomes in a broad spectrum of heart failure patients. *Circulation* 112:3738–3744, 2005.
183. Redfield MM: Strategies to screen for stage B as a heart failure prevention intervention. *Heart Fail Clin* 8:285–296, 2012.
184. Patel MR, White RD, Abbara S, et al: 2013 ACCF/ACR/ASE/ASNC/SCCT/SCMR Appropriate Utilization of Cardiovascular Imaging in Heart Failure: a joint report of the American College of Radiology Appropriateness Criteria Committee and the American College of Cardiology Foundation Appropriate Use Criteria Task Force. *J Am Coll Cardiol* 61:2207–2231, 2013.
185. Cohn JN: Preventing heart failure: a critique of strategies. *J Card Fail* 19:211–213, 2013.
186. Cohn JN, Hoke L, Whitwam W, et al: Screening for early detection of cardiovascular disease in asymptomatic individuals. *Am Heart J* 146:679–685, 2003.
187. Duprez DA, Florea N, Zhong W, et al: Vascular and cardiac functional and structural screening to identify risk of future morbid events: preliminary observations. *J Am Soc Hypertens* 5:401–409, 2011.

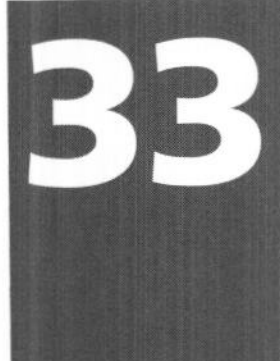

Management of Acute Decompensated Heart Failure

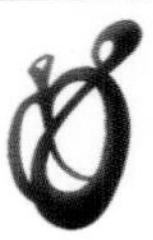

Lynne Warner Stevenson

Heart failure is the primary diagnosis for more than 1 million hospitalizations yearly, and approximately 2 million more include heart failure as a secondary diagnosis, particularly with pulmonary or renal disease (**see also Chapter 17**).[1] Heart failure hospitalizations can be divided about evenly between those for heart failure with reduced ejection fraction (HFrEF) and those for heart failure with "preserved" ejection fraction (HFpEF)[2] (**Figure 33-1**), which in turn is divided between those in which left ventricular ejection fraction (LVEF) is 40% to 55% and those in which LVEF exceeds 55%[3] (**Table 33-1**). In contrast to patients in trial populations, the average patient admitted with heart failure in the community is 75 years old, with a high burden of comorbid conditions that strongly influence medical therapy and prognosis.

Most admissions are for exacerbation of chronic heart failure,[4,5] which will be the focus of this chapter. New diagnoses of heart failure resulting from acute myocardial infarction, acute valvular regurgitation, or hypertensive emergencies require specific therapy directed to those conditions. Acute heart failure occasionally results from fulminant myocarditis (**see Chapter 26**), which necessitates rapid institution of life-saving therapies for cardiogenic shock with good potential for ultimate recovery.[6] Although the term *acute decompensated heart failure* (ADHF) and the frequently rapid evolution of symptoms imply sudden decompensation, insights from home monitoring indicate that most episodes of decompensation follow a gradual increase of intracardiac filling pressures for both HFrEF and HFpEF. Although the evidence base for chronic therapy exists only for HFrEF, the initial assessment and therapy for most patients with decompensation of chronic heart failure are guided by similar principles regardless of the ejection fraction.

COMPONENTS OF THE 5-POINT ASSESSMENT

For patients admitted with heart failure, the initial assessment should include consideration of the cause and potential factors contributing to decompensation (**Table 33-2**). For patients with known coronary artery disease, active ischemia should always be considered (**see also Chapter 18**). Other common exacerbating factors are tachyarrhythmias, thyroid disease, anemia, infections, and chronic pulmonary disease (**Figure 33-2**). Although pulmonary emboli can certainly occur and exacerbate heart failure,[7] careful clinical consideration should minimize the use of computed tomography (CT) scanning during decompensation, where dye has higher likelihood of worsening renal function than of identifying significant pulmonary emboli. Adherence to the outpatient regimen can be challenged by inadequate support structure, lack of patient-appropriate education about heart failure, limited literacy and numeracy skills, and other factors.

Within minutes of arrival, a bedside clinical assessment should be performed to identify the profile of fluid status and perfusion that will guide initial therapy.[5,8,9] Because chronic circulatory adaptations can mask evidence of decompensation, the severity and urgency may be underappreciated during initial triage in urgent care settings.[10] Comorbidities can trigger, mimic, or mask heart failure decompensation, and can also complicate the hemodynamic assessment, such as with pulmonary disease or sepsis.

After initial stabilization, causative factors can be reviewed in more detail. Interventions related to longer-term treatment for rhythms and embolic risks can be considered. Disease-modifying therapies with neurohormonal antagonists and other guideline-based therapies should be redesigned as appropriate. Some patients may be candidates for catheter-based or surgical interventions to treat structural heart disease. A small minority of patients may be eligible for therapies that exchange diseases and change lives with cardiac transplantation or mechanical circulatory devices. For most other patients, however, repeated hospitalizations with heart failure should trigger review of the disease trajectory and the goals of care after discharge.

Initial Profiles

The central hemodynamic components of decompensated heart failure are the elevation of filling pressures ("wet")

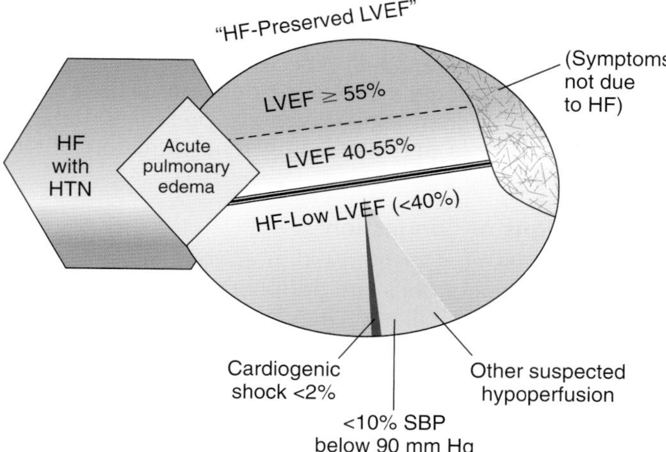

FIGURE 33-1 Estimation of typical proportions of patients accounting for hospitalizations for heart failure (HF) in the community. Approximately half of such hospitalizations are for heart failure with left ventricular ejection fraction (LVEF) exceeding 40%. Patients with acute pulmonary edema frequently have uncontrolled hypertension (HTN). Only a small fraction of patients present in cardiogenic shock. Clinical hypoperfusion at hospital admission may be present in up to 25% of patients with low ejection fraction in large tertiary centers, but this proportion is much smaller in community hospitals. *SBP,* Systolic blood pressure. *Data from large registries (Acute Decompensated Heart Failure Registry [ADHERE][1-3]).*

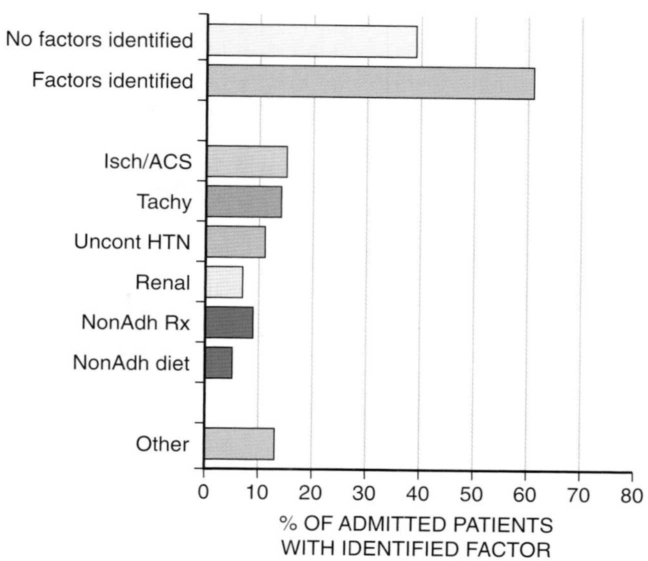

FIGURE 33-2 Bar graph showing factors identified as leading to hospitalization in patients with previously known diagnosis of heart failure. The data reported in 48,612 patients from the OPTIMIZE-HF database are represented.[7] Two or more factors were identified in 19% of patients. *ACS,* Acute coronary syndrome; *Isch,* ischemia; *NonAdh,* nonadherence; *Tachy,* tachycardia; *Uncont HTN,* uncontrolled hypertension.

TABLE 33-1 Typical Community Hospitalizations for Heart Failure Classified by LVEF

CHARACTERISTIC	LVEF <0.40	LVEF 0.40-0.55	LVEF ≥0.55
Age	70	74	74
% Women	40	54	69
% African American	22	17	17
% With coronary artery disease	59	61	48
% With hypertension	69	76	78
Systolic blood pressure (average; mm Hg)	139	150	152
% Diabetes mellitus	40	48	44
% With atrial fibrillation	29	33	32
% With COPD	27	32	34
% With renal insufficiency	26	31	27

COPD, Chronic obstructive pulmonary disease; *LVEF,* left ventricular ejection fraction.
Data from publications describing the Acute Decompensated Heart Failure National Registry (ADHERE) database.[2,3]

TABLE 33-2 5-Point Assessment at Heart Failure Admission

I. Cause and contributing factors
 Primary diagnosis
 Potential exacerbating medical factors
 Adherence challenges
II. Profiles
 2 × 2 hemodynamic profiles of filling pressures and perfusion
  Consider acute coronary syndrome
  Triage for cardiogenic shock and urgent support
  Reverse acute pulmonary edema
 Baseline function before decompensation
III. Noncardiac comorbidities
 As triggers of decompensation
 As confounders for assessment
 As causes of other limiting symptoms
 As obstacles to effective therapy
 General frailty
IV. Beats and clots
 Atrial and ventricular tachyarrhythmias
 ICD/CRT device function if in place
 If low EF without device, indications/contraindications
 Presence or need of chronic anticoagulation
V. The road ahead
 Prospect for decongestion
 Potential for major intervention
  Optimization of guideline-driven medical therapy
  Structural disease amenable to catheter-based or surgical intervention
  General eligibility for durable circulatory support or cardiac transplantation
 Alignment with long-term goals of care

CRT, Cardiac resynchronization therapy; *EF,* ejection fraction; *ICD,* implantable cardioverter-defibrillator.

and the reduction of cardiac output ("cold," although often not reflected in skin temperature). These two hemodynamic perturbations do not necessarily occur together, as shown in **Figure 33-3**.[9] Initial triage should identify the emergency situations of cardiogenic shock with severe perturbations of both filling pressures and hypoperfusion, acute pulmonary edema often in the setting of acute myocardial infarction or severe hypertension, and other acute ischemic syndrome presentations (see Chapter 17). Whether the left ventricular ejection fraction is low or "preserved," the most common profile of decompensation is "warm and wet" (profile B), with congestion and adequate perfusion.

Symptoms of Congestion

The most helpful symptom is orthopnea, which indicates elevated pulmonary venous pressures until proven otherwise (such as in a patient with severe emphysema or obesity), and is specifically associated with pulmonary capillary wedge pressures over 30 mm Hg.[10,11] Immediate dyspnea on light exertion (IDLE), such as dressing or walking from room to room, usually indicates high left-sided filling pressures. Dyspnea and fatigue with more strenuous exertion are typical even in compensated heart failure, but rarely lead to hospitalization. Shortness of breath or discomfort from "head fullness" during tasks requiring bending, such as putting on shoes, has recently been termed *bendopnea* by Drazner and associated with elevation of both right- and left-sided filling pressures.

Most patients describe a combination of symptoms at hospital admission for decompensation, with dyspnea the most common. When asked to specify their "worst" symptom at the time of admission with low ejection fraction heart failure, about half of patients in the ESCAPE trial indicated dyspnea and a third indicated fatigue, which was associated with slightly less symptomatic improvement after therapy (**Figure 33-4**). The remaining patients who cited either abdominal symptoms or edema as their worst symptom had higher jugular venous pressures initially, with more diuresis and worsening renal function before discharge.[12]

TWO-MINUTE ASSESSMENT OF HEMODYNAMIC PROFILE

Low perfusion at rest?	Congestion at rest? NO	Congestion at rest? YES
NO	*Warm & dry* A	*Warm & wet* B
YES	*Cold & dry* L	*Cold & wet* C

Evidence for congestion
- Orthopnea
- Elevated jugular venous pressure
- Bendopnea
- Rales (rarely)
- New S3
- Hepatomegaly
- Ascites
- Edema (more common in older patients)
- Valsalva square wave

Evidence for low perfusion
- Narrow auscultated pulse pressure
- Cool extremities
- May be sleepy, obtunded
- Suspect from ACEI/ARB hypotension
- Progressive oliguria

FIGURE 33-3 Hemodynamic profiles of patients hospitalized for heart failure. Most patients can be classified as having one of these four profiles in a 2-minute bedside assessment, although in practice some patients may qualify for both profile B and profile C. This classification helps guide consideration of initial therapy and prognosis.[9] The clinical criteria for congestion *(columns)* concern dryness or wetness; the clinical evidence for perfusion *(rows)* concerns coldness or warmth. For the "cold and dry" category, the label "L" is used instead of "D" to avoid the implication that heart failure invariably progresses. Many patients never develop a profile "L," which can stand for "heart failure light," because it is without congestion. *ACEI,* Angiotensin-converting enzyme inhibitor; *ARB,* angiotensin receptor blocker.

Physical Signs of Congestion

Physical assessment of congestion is complicated by the frequent absence of rales and peripheral edema in patients with chronic heart failure.[11] Jugular venous pressure provides the most visible and reliable index of elevated filling pressures on physical examination[11] (**Table 33-3**). Although this assesses only the right-sided filling pressures, jugular venous pressure elevation is nonetheless the best clinical sign of elevated left-sided pressures. Right- and left-sided pressure elevations in chronic heart failure are concordant in about 75% of cases if thresholds of right atrial pressure greater than 10 mm Hg and pulmonary capillary wedge pressure greater than 22 mm Hg are used.[13,14] Hepatomegaly suggests high right-sided pressures. Increased radiation of the pulmonary second sound (P2) away from the left sternal border suggests high pulmonary artery pressure, which often reflects left-sided filling pressures unless there is intrinsic pulmonary hypertension. Serial changes in the intensity of a third heart sound or regurgitant murmur can indicate changes in right- or left-sided filling pressures. The Valsalva maneuver square-wave response can help identify elevated filling pressures, particularly when cardiac and pulmonary causes of dyspnea coexist.[15] The abdominojugular reflex is a sensitive measure that can be positive in patients with only mild elevation in venous volume or tone.[16] Elevated natriuretic peptide levels are chronically elevated in most patients with a previous diagnosis of heart failure (see also Chapter 30); therefore, the finding of a high level may not indicate the presence or severity of worsening congestion.[17] Other clues for elevated filling pressures can be present in

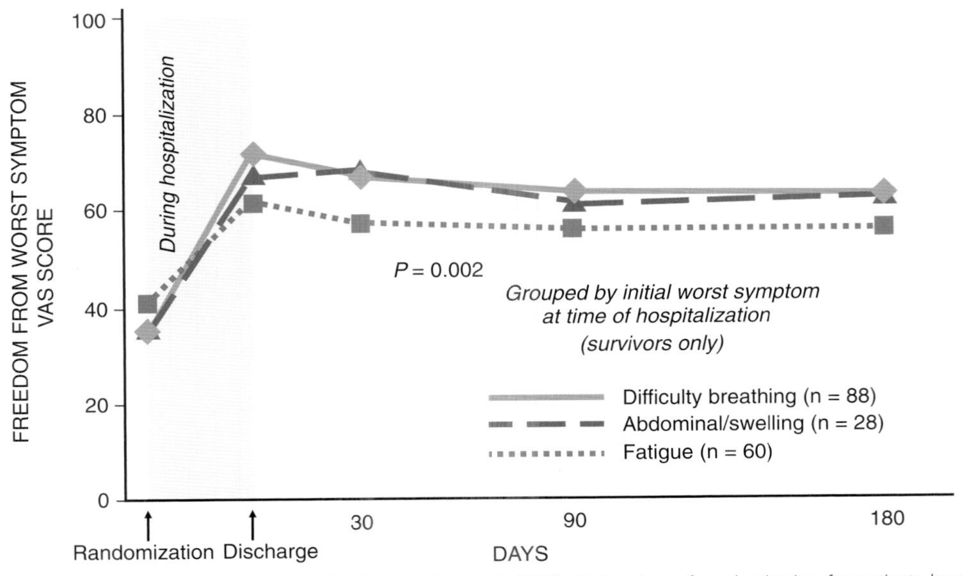

FIGURE 33-4 The time course of symptomatic improvement by visual analog scale (VAS). At the time of randomization for patients hospitalized with at least one symptom and one sign of congestion, patients selected their worst symptom from difficulty breathing, fatigue, abdominal discomfort, or body swelling; subsequent assessment by each patient was of that same worst symptom. Graph includes only patients for whom there is a complete set of scores at all time points: Difficulty breathing, $n = 88$; fatigue, $n = 60$; abdominal discomfort or body swelling, $n = 28$ (abdominal/swelling). Symptoms improved during hospitalization and declined slightly after discharge but remained improved at 6 months, with significantly less improvement when the worst symptom was fatigue ($P = 0.002$). *Data from the ESCAPE trial; Kato M, Stevenson LW, Palardy M, et al: The worst symptom as defined by patients during heart failure hospitalization: implications for response to therapy. J Card Fail 18:524–533, 2012.*

TABLE 33-3 Detection of Elevated Left-Sided Filling Pressures during Hospitalization with Low Ejection Fraction Heart Failure

FINDING	SENSITIVITY FOR PCW >22 MM HG	SPECIFICITY FOR PCW >22 MM HG
Orthopnea	86%	25%
Rales more than basilar	15%	89%
Third heart sound	62%	32%
Right-Sided Signs		
Estimated JVP >12 cm	65%	64%
Edema >2+	41%	66%
Hepatomegaly >4 cm	15%	93%
Abdominojugular reflex	83%	27%
Measured RAP >10 mm Hg	76%	83%
Echocardiographic Assessment		
Pulmonary artery systolic pressure >60 mm Hg	47%	96%
Tricuspid regurgitation > moderate	78%	70%
Mitral regurgitation > moderate	78%	43%

JVP, Jugular venous pressure; *RAP,* right atrial pressure; *PCW,* pulmonary capillary wedge pressure.
Modified from Drazner MH, Hellkamp AS, Leier CV, et al: Value of clinician assessment of hemodynamics in advanced heart failure. The ESCAPE trial. Circ Heart Fail 1:170–177, 2008; and Drazner MH, Hamilton MA, Fonarow G, et al: Relationship between right and left-sided filling pressures in 1000 patients with advanced heart failure. J Heart Lung Transplant 18:1126–1132, 1999.

echocardiographic findings of moderate or severe mitral or tricuspid regurgitation or pulmonary hypertension in the absence of other causes.[13] Echocardiography with handheld devices to interrogate mitral inflow patterns, pulmonary artery pressure, and hepatic veins may help to assess volume status in the absence of skilled physical examination (see also Chapter 29).[18]

Careful attention to the pattern of respiration can support or challenge the diagnosis of dyspnea related to elevated intracardiac filling pressures. Orthopnea may sometimes be observed as an increase in respiratory rate because the head of the bed is lowered, even in patients who deny supine dyspnea. The dyspnea of congestion usually causes relatively rapid and shallow breathing, while accessory muscle use and an emphasis on exhalation are more consistent with pulmonary disease. Regular deep excursion breathing may be caused by metabolic acidosis or hepatic encephalopathy. Periodic breathing without frank apnea is common in late-stage heart failure while awake, as well as while asleep (see also Chapter 45).[19] During the tachypneic phase of periodic breathing, characterized by large and rapid respiratory excursions, patients often perceive respiratory distress, which may be mistreated as attacks of panic or anxiety when the contrasting hypopneic periods are overlooked.

Blood Pressure and Perfusion

Bedside estimation of hypoperfusion is less reliable than for congestion, even for the skilled examiner.[11] Significant reduction of cardiac output may be missed in a patient with chronic low cardiac output who appears oriented. Accurate assessment of blood pressure is crucial, and requires a skilled examiner listening to each beat. This is particularly important when an irregular rhythm of atrial fibrillation or frequent premature beats lead to wide variability and overestimation of average systolic blood pressure from an automated machine. In patients compensated on optimal heart failure therapy, systolic blood pressure is often below 100 mm Hg but rarely below 85 mm Hg, except right after taking oral medications. Conversely, critically low perfusion can exist at higher systolic blood pressure, in which case the pulse pressure is surprisingly narrow, sometimes less than 10 mm Hg. The proportional pulse pressure (systolic minus diastolic divided by systolic blood pressure) can be more informative than the systolic blood pressure alone. Normally at least 30%, when the pulse pressure is less than 25%, the cardiac index is often below 2.2 L/min/m^2.[10] Auscultation is useful also to detect pulsus alternans, attributed to regular alternation in the release and reuptake of calcium during sequential beats, which should raise concern about more unstable hemodynamic status than is otherwise apparent. Palpation of the brachial pulse is usually sensitive enough to detect variations of 10 mm Hg or more between alternate beats.

Temperature of the extremities relates to perfusion. Warm hands and feet provide reassurance regarding adequate perfusion, but are frequently cool in normal patients with high sympathetic tone due to anxiety. However, adequate systemic blood flow usually maintains warm calves and forearms, except in a very cold room. Fluctuating mentation, often attributed to depression or sleep deprivation, may instead be a key sign of low cardiac output. Typical is the patient who is oriented and appropriate but appears to be nodding in and out of sleep during the initial history. Patients who describe a history of hypotension or dizziness with even low doses of ACE inhibitors or β-blockers may be suspected of having low baseline perfusion that is further undermined by inhibition of compensatory reflex systems. Some patients fall into an intermediate "lukewarm" group in which perfusion status may be ambiguous. This is particularly true for patients with prominent right ventricular dysfunction and worsening renal function.

PRINCIPLES OF THERAPY GUIDED BY PROFILES

For most patients admitted with heart failure, symptoms and physical examination findings provide sufficient information to guide initial therapy (see Figure 33-3).[9,11] Invasive hemodynamic monitoring is not often indicated at the time of admission for either diagnosis or therapy. For patients who appear to be profile A (warm and dry), without clinical evidence of elevated filling pressures or hypoperfusion on clinical examination, the diagnosis of heart failure may not adequately explain the presenting symptoms, which could be caused by other conditions, such as pulmonary or hepatic disease, or by transient events, such as ischemia or arrhythmias. Up to half of rehospitalizations in patients with chronic heart failure are for diagnoses other than heart failure.[20]

Profile B: Wet and Warm

The most common profile is the "warm and wet" (profile B[1,21]), accounting for about 90% of community hospitalizations and most of those in referral centers for advanced heart failure therapies. This is almost always the profile in

HFpEF unless due to hypertrophic or restrictive physiology with small ventricular volumes. Even in HFrEF in which cardiac output may be lower than normal, the congestion profile with adequate perfusion describes most typical decompensation events, some of which may be treated at home or in short-stay outpatient units. The initial goal is the relief of congestion with reduction of filling pressures ("get to dry"). Although heart failure was once considered primarily a condition of low cardiac output, therapies designed to stimulate contractility and cardiac output have to date been deleterious, leading to increased arrhythmias and ischemia and an apparent acceleration of progressive disease, often compared with "whipping a tired horse." Although cardiac output frequently improves with better loading conditions, increase of cardiac output is not a *primary* target of acute therapy unless organ perfusion is critically compromised, or when systemic or renal hypoperfusion prevents effective diuresis.

Elevated filling pressures can result from elevated intravascular volume, systemic vasoconstriction (venous or arterial or both), severe intrinsic diastolic dysfunction, and combinations of the above. Most patients presenting with profile B have at least some component of total-body fluid overload that necessitates net fluid removal, with an average of about 4 kg during a hospitalization. For the occasional "wet and warm" exacerbations in which vasoconstriction dominates, as in settings of severe hypertension with incipient pulmonary edema, intravenous vasodilators are the first line of therapy (see Use of Specific Intravenous Agents during Hospitalization, later), although adding a dose of intravenous diuretics may accelerate initial relief. Positive-pressure ventilation may also help avert the need for urgent intubation in patients with upright tachypnea and hypoxia. However, most profile B decompensation can be managed with a stepwise approach to achieve effective diuresis to target filling pressures.

What Is the Target Level of Left Ventricular Filling Pressures?

In patients with heart failure caused by chronic dilated cardiomyopathy, filling pressures can often be lowered to levels below 18 mm Hg despite initial elevation over 30 mm Hg at admission.[22-25] This contrasts with the requirement for higher filling pressures with acutely decreased compliance that has been described during acute myocardial infarction.[26] Most dilated hearts operate far beyond the level of filling at which stroke volume depends on increments in filling pressures. In fact, as high filling pressures are reduced in chronic dilated heart failure, cardiac output usually increases (**Figure 33-5**).[22,27]

The improvement in cardiac output with diuresis may reflect multiple factors, including an increase in contractility from decreased myocardial oxygen consumption and improved gradient for myocardial perfusion, improvement in ejection related to decreased systemic vascular resistance, and redistribution of mitral regurgitant volumes to supplement forward flow. Although all these may contribute, the most easily measured change is that of decreased mitral regurgitation caused by a reduction in the effective mitral regurgitant orifice, which in turn results from small reductions in left ventricular distention.[24,28,29] Both the landmark original study of nitroprusside[30] and later studies with tailored therapy have confirmed the central role of changes in mitral regurgitant flow.[29] The mitral regurgitant fraction

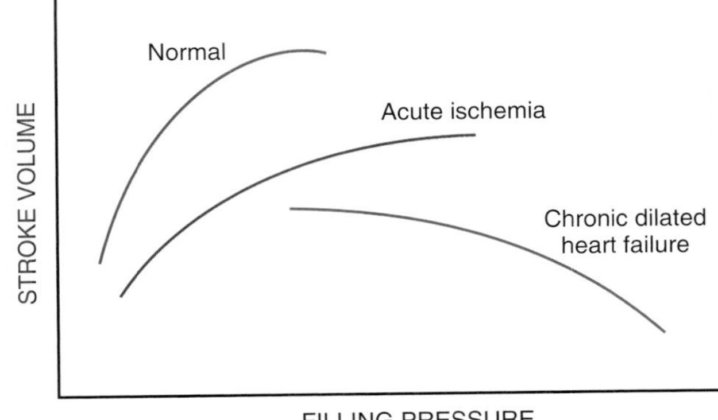

FIGURE 33-5 Curves demonstrating relationship of filling pressures to stroke volume. In the acutely ischemic ventricle, compliance is decreased with little change in volume, and the curve is shifted to the right, as described by Russell and colleagues.[106] In the chronically dilated ventricle, the "Starling curve" is actually reversed in that reduction of markedly elevated filling pressures leads to higher stroke volume.[22]

during therapy may decrease from 0.50 to less than 0.20,[23] which appears to account for most of the improvement in measured cardiac output with vasodilators. Similar considerations affect tricuspid regurgitation and right ventricular stroke volume.

Reduction of pulmonary capillary wedge pressures has long been observed, and more recently demonstrated directly to reduce the symptoms of congestion that lead to most hospitalizations for heart failure.[31] Although immediate symptomatic improvement often occurs when filling pressures are still severely elevated, therapy should continue until optimal filling pressures have been reached. Many patients perceive early relief from the most oppressive symptoms and do not appreciate that symptoms could be improved further until afterward. Target filling pressures measured invasively are generally described as goals of 15 to 18 mm Hg for pulmonary capillary wedge pressure and less than 8 mm Hg for right atrial pressure for patients with low ejection fraction. Results achieved with invasive hemodynamic monitoring approach these goals (**Table 33-4**).

Even in the absence of apparent symptoms, elevated filling pressures have a deleterious impact on disease progression. High pulmonary capillary wedge pressures are linked to greater activation of the renin-angiotensin and sympathetic nervous systems.[32,33] Chronic elevation of left-sided filling pressures contributes to valvular regurgitation, pulmonary hypertension, and eventually to right ventricular dysfunction, all of which lead to disease progression and worse outcomes. Whether near-normal filling pressures are measured invasively, assessed clinically from absence of signs and symptoms of congestion, or reflected by echocardiographic assessment, the ability to achieve them and maintain them over time[34-38] is associated with better survival and fewer rehospitalizations. It is not known to what extent current outcomes could be improved by more intensive reduction and prevention of recurrent congestion during chronic outpatient disease management. However, data from investigational chronic home monitoring devices indicates that maintenance of a daily median pulmonary artery diastolic pressure of 18 mm Hg or less is associated with the lowest risk for recurrent heart failure events.

Current data are insufficient to define the usual filling pressure target for patients with heart failure and preserved ejection fraction. Like patients with heart failure and low ejection fraction, patients with heart failure and preserved ejection fraction retain fluid to a level substantially higher than needed for cardiac output, although fluid retention is commonly aggravated by intrinsic renal impairment.[39] In addition, the development of symptomatic pulmonary congestion in patients hospitalized with HF and preserved left ventricular ejection may be accelerated by lower oncotic pressure because of inadequate nutrition. The heterogeneity of myocardial disease and degrees of hypertrophy may dictate more heterogeneity in the optimal fluid levels for these patients. Similar to HFrEF, chronic studies suggest that the optimal filling pressure for HFpEF is in the range of 18 mm Hg, but the window between too high and too low may be narrower in this population.[40]

Getting to Dry

Intravenous diuretic therapy is the major intervention that relieves congestion. As most patients admitted with decompensated heart failure are already receiving chronic oral diuretic therapy, their total daily dose guides the choice of an initial inpatient dose. For furosemide, this is commonly the outpatient total oral daily dose given as an intravenous bolus (usually 3-4 times more potent) to be repeated at least every 12 hours, or more often. In the DOSE study, the largest randomized study of acute diuretics done to date, a higher initial dose of 2.5 times the total daily dose in the loop diuretic dosing trial achieved about 30% more net fluid loss and greater relief of dyspnea in the first 3 days.[41] The higher diuresis was associated with slightly more frequent increase in creatinine during hospitalization but no difference after discharge. Continuous loop diuretic infusions are frequently employed in patients on high-dose diuretic therapy, particularly those with hypotension, hypokalemia, or renal dysfunction. However, in the same DOSE trial, continuous infusion of the same daily dose did not show any overall benefit compared with bolus administration.

After escalation to high doses of intravenous loop diuretics two or more times daily, the next step generally includes addition of metolazone or a thiazide if net diuresis is not at least 1 to 2 L daily. As the next step, the aggressive diuretic protocol developed for patients with worsening renal function during decompensation in the CARRESS trial included the addition of low doses (usually about 2 μg/kg/min) of dobutamine or dopamine.[42]

The general clinical goals for "getting to dry" in profile B patients are resolution of edema and orthopnea, and reduction of jugular venous pressure to 8 cm or less. Patients should be able to ambulate with upright systolic blood pressure of at least 80 mm Hg and without postural symptoms. Net diuresis during the first day is often 1.5 to 2 L, but may be up to 3 L or more daily in patients with large visible volume reservoirs of anasarca ("tree-trunk legs"). In general, diuretic therapy should be continued intravenously until the desired fluid balance has been achieved. The length of time required depends on the efficacy of the diuretic regimen and the degree of initial volume overload. The median diuresis in most trials of acute decompensated heart failure is between 4 and 5 kg (**Figure 33-6**). Some patients with massive anasarca may require more than 2 weeks of diuresis to achieve necessary loss of 20 to 30 kg of fluid.

Evidence is accumulating that some acute contraction of intravascular volume as indicated by a rising creatinine may now be a marker for effective intervention, with subsequent gradual reequilibration.[43] The detection of an increased hematocrit during hospital diuresis has been associated with improved outcome after discharge.[44] This association has been shown in trial populations carefully screened for clear evidence of intravascular fluid overload at admission, usually requiring at least one definitive sign and one resting symptom of congestion. Beyond the qualitative association, it is not clear how any marker of dilution/concentration could be used to guide therapy

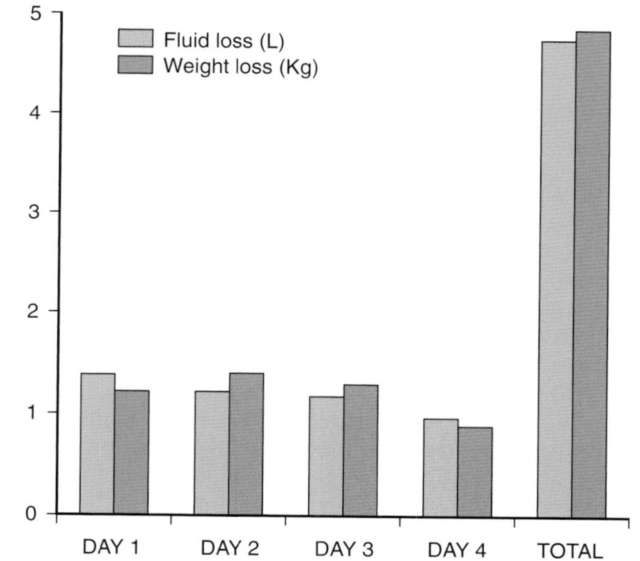

FIGURE 33-6 Bar graph demonstrating median daily diuresis and measured weight loss during hospitalization in the DOSE trial of diuretics in acute decompensated heart failure.[41]

TABLE 33-4 Responses to Therapy Tailored with Pulmonary Artery Catheter to Relieve Congestion

MEASUREMENT	BASELINE	ON REVISED ORAL THERAPY	CHANGE AFTER THERAPY
Right atrial pressure (mm Hg)	14 ± 10	7 ± 4	
Pulmonary capillary wedge pressure (mm Hg)	25 ± 9	17 ± 7	
Cardiac index (L/min/m^2)	1.9 ± 0.6	2.4 ± 0.7	
Systemic vascular resistance (dynes/sec/cm^{-5})	1500 ± 800	1100 ± 500	
Systolic blood pressure	106 ± 17	102 ± 15	
Weight			−4 kg
Creatinine			0.0 mg/dL
Mitral regurgitation area (echocardiographic)			−2 cm^2 (−20%)
Global symptoms			
Visual Analog Scale (0-100)			−25
Preference for survival (time trade-off tool)			+6.2 months

Data from ESCAPE Investigators and Coordinators: Evaluation study of congestive heart failure and pulmonary artery catheterization. JAMA 294:1625–1633, 2005.

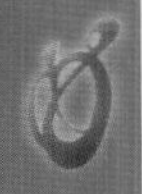

TABLE 33-5 Indications for Invasive Hemodynamic Monitoring with Pulmonary Artery Catheter

Class I. Acute Circulatory Compromise
Should be performed to guide therapy in patients who have respiratory distress of clinical evidence of impaired perfusion in whom the adequacy or excess of intracardiac filling pressures cannot be determined from clinical assessment.
Class IIa. Diagnostic Uncertainty or Need for Escalating Therapies
Can be useful for carefully selected patients with acute heart failure who have persistent symptoms despite empiric adjustment of standard therapies, and a. Whose fluid status, perfusion, or systemic or pulmonary vascular resistances are uncertain* b. Whose systolic pressure remains low or is associated with symptoms, despite initial therapy c. Whose renal function is worsening with therapy d. Who require parenteral vasoactive agents e. Who may need consideration for mechanical circulatory support or transplantation
Class III
Routine use is not recommended in normotensive patients with acute decompensated heart failure and congestion with symptomatic response to diuretics and vasodilators.

*Uncertainty regarding the level of left-sided filling pressures is particularly common in the setting of concomitant noncardiac conditions, such as chronic pulmonary disease or sepsis.

From Yancy CW, Jessup M, Bozkurt B, et al: 2013 ACCF/AHA guideline for the management of heart failure: a report of the American College of Cardiology Foundation/American Heart Association Task Force on practice guidelines. Circulation 128(16):e240–327, 2013.

without more precise quantitation of the amount of excess fluid at admission.

Difficulty with Decongestion

In some patients who appear to have uncomplicated congestion, escalating diuretic therapy fails to relieve signs and symptoms of congestion as anticipated. Symptoms that persist unabated despite ongoing daily weight loss may reflect slow resolution of a large peripheral volume reservoir of peripheral edema and/or ascites that must be mobilized before detectable decrease in intravascular volume, jugular venous pressure, and symptoms. On the other hand, large negative net fluid balance by intake/output measurements that do not translate to weight loss usually reflect high unrecorded oral intake by patients over their fluid restriction (commonly set at 2 L of oral intake during heart failure hospitalization). This can include omission of water consumed while at the lavatory or walking around the wards, or disregard for the high fluid content of fruits.

When patients are not responding as anticipated to diuretic therapy, the hemodynamic profile should be reassessed. Failure to relieve symptoms despite empiric adjustment of therapy is one of the indications for invasive hemodynamic assessment (**Table 33-5**). The most common limitation to effective decongestion is renal dysfunction. Multiple factors can lead to worsening renal function during a hospitalization for heart failure, including contrast agents, kidney stones, and urinary retention. Although these should be systematically considered, worsening renal function during diuretic therapy often does not have an obvious single cause or treatment.

Cardiorenal Limitation to Diuresis

Baseline Renal Dysfunction. There is increasing recognition of the relationship between renal function and outcomes in heart failure even when renal dysfunction and heart failure are both mild.[45] Patients admitted with creatinine greater than 2.75 mg/dL or BUN over 43 mg/dL have worse outcomes during hospitalization.[46] Chronically elevated right atrial pressures, often with substantial tricuspid regurgitation, are increasingly implicated in the renal dysfunction seen with both HFpEF and HFrEF.[47] Some studies have demonstrated the added contribution of elevated intraperitoneal pressures to renal dysfunction, sometimes improving after paracentesis of tense ascitic fluid.[48] Interestingly, patients admitted with renal dysfunction are almost as likely to have improvement as deterioration in renal function.

Changing Renal Function during Diuresis. Patients with renal dysfunction at admission are at higher risk for worsening renal function during diuresis. In the past, worsening renal function during an admission for heart failure decompensation was often attributed incorrectly to reduction in cardiac output from excessive diuresis. However, serial hemodynamic monitoring has shown that worsening renal function in this setting usually occurs without a decline in cardiac output and is most likely in the patients with persistently high right atrial pressures.[47,49]

The original descriptions of worsening renal function during heart failure hospitalization indicated that about 25% of patients would develop a creatinine increase of 0.3 mg/dL or more, with worse outcomes after discharge.[50] Similarly poor outcomes were seen when the BUN (blood urea nitrogen) levels increase substantially even with minimal increase in creatinine. However, the adverse prognostic impact of worsening renal function seems to have diminished in recent trials of strategies for ADHF, possibly due to greater attention to renal function. Small increases in serum creatinine during major diuresis have recently been associated with improved long-term outcomes in patients, presumably reflecting more effective decongestion.[43] In these studies, the creatinine generally returns to baseline early after discharge.

Right-Left Mismatch

Although most patients have concordant elevations of right- and left-sided filling pressures, right-left mismatch may be present in one of every four to five patients hospitalized with heart failure.[51] If the right-sided pressure elevation is disproportionately high, diuresis guided by jugular venous pressure may lead to inadequate left-sided filling, such as in patients with intrinsic pulmonary hypertension. Patients with disproportionate elevation of left-sided filling pressures without jugular venous distention may have congestive symptoms incorrectly attributed to noncardiac disease. This may be suspected when elevated pulmonary artery pressures are detected on echocardiography in the presence of normal hepatic vein motion, but often requires invasive measurement to verify. Results of prior right-heart catheterization should be diligently retrieved as they may provide sufficient indication of the patient's underlying right-left relationship to obviate the need for new hemodynamic measurement.

High or Low Systemic Vascular Resistance

Diuresis can exacerbate renal dysfunction without symptom relief when elevated filling pressures result more from very high systemic vascular resistance with fluid redistribution rather than from fluid overload. This is easy to recognize and treat when blood pressure is high in profile B patients. In other patients, it can be suspected on the basis of a very narrow pulse pressure. However, when both blood pressure and cardiac output are low, severe vasoconstriction is difficult to confirm or treat without direct hemodynamic monitoring.

Some patients have persistent hypotension with diuretic or vasodilator therapy despite apparently adequate cardiac output, as judged by reasonable pulse pressure and warm extremities. Such patients occasionally have marked intrinsic vasodilation unrelated to pharmacotherapy. Their systemic vascular resistances can be too low to support perfusion if further lowered by neurohormonal antagonists or other vasodilators. The most common cause is the autonomic neuropathy of amyloid infiltration. However, circulating vasodilator substances have been implicated in severe intrinsic liver disease. This may be suspected in patients in whom the degree of ascites is disproportionate to the other evidence of heart failure. Patients particularly at risk may be those with long-standing cirrhosis caused by alcohol or other toxins, hepatitis or, in some cases, cardiac cirrhosis after many years of right-sided heart failure from valvular disease, restrictive disease, or congenital heart disease.

"Lukewarm"

As the clinical assessment for hypoperfusion is less reliable than that for congestion,[11] patients with unrecognized or borderline low cardiac output may lack adequate perfusion to support blood pressure and renal function; this situation is sometimes referred to as an intermediate "wet and lukewarm" profile, which may lead to treatment as for profile C. The possibility should also be considered that perfusion has become compromised since admission, by ongoing myocardial injury, infection, or negative inotropy from new therapies, such as amiodarone or uptitration of β-blockers.

Adjunctive Agents during Diuresis—Profile B

Use of adjunctive intravenous therapies beyond diuretics has not been demonstrated to improve long-term outcomes in any randomized trials of acute decompensated heart failure. It is important to note, however, that trials are limited to those patients for whom the clinicians had equipoise and did *not* perceive a strong rationale for any adjunctive therapies. Multiple uncontrolled experiences confirm the worse early and late outcomes of patients who received infusions of approved intravenous inotropic agents to facilitate diuresis in the absence of clinical hypoperfusion.[52] The randomized study with milrinone[53] revealed increased arrhythmias and trends toward more ischemic events in hospital and more adverse events in the 60 days after discharge; this last effect was more evident in the patients with underlying coronary artery disease. Although sometimes considered for therapy of hypotension, milrinone actually caused more hypotension than placebo. Inotropic infusions may increase low levels of troponin leakage during hospitalization for heart failure, particularly in patients with underlying coronary artery disease.[54] The calcium-sensitizing agents, such as levosimendan, demonstrated no clinically significant benefit in either symptoms or outcomes.[55] Infusions of nitroglycerin and the synthetic B-type natriuretic peptide nesiritide at doses with significant hemodynamic effect were both associated with early symptomatic improvement but have not been proved to affect overall outcomes either positively or negatively during hospitalization or after discharge.[56] Both can cause hypotension, particularly when used in patients for whom circulating volume overload has been overestimated. Nesiritide has occasionally been implicated in the worsening of renal function, usually in association with hypotension.[57] The recent ASCEND-HF trial of nesiritide infusion in over 7000 patients confirmed a modest improvement in self-reported dyspnea in the first 24 hours during nesiritide treatment, which had no impact on death or rehospitalization.[58] Endothelin antagonists have not improved symptom relief or outcomes after discharge.[59] Therapy with vasopressin antagonists is effective in increasing serum sodium levels in the setting of hyponatremia, usually with some enhancement of diuresis and acceleration of relief of dyspnea.[60] However, initial benefits for fluid balance have not been not sustained during longer follow-up, in part because of increased thirst and water consumption.

Trials focused specifically on patients with renal dysfunction and congestion have not yet demonstrated any adjunctive therapy to be beneficial in this more compromised population. The strategy of bedside ultrafiltration yielded equivalent volume diuresis but was associated with more procedural complexity and slightly more frequent creatinine elevation than an aggressive regimen of escalating diuretic therapy.[42] The adenosine A1 antagonist rolofylline showed promising initial results for renal function that were not seen in the subsequent PROTECT trial.

Interest has risen in using nesiritide or dopamine in low doses anticipated to act primarily on the kidney ("renal-dose"). Evaluation of these adjunctive strategies was the focus of the NHLBI-sponsored ROSE trial.[61] In patients admitted with clinical congestion and estimated glomerular filtration rate between 15 and 60 mL/min, there was no significant impact overall of either therapy on diuresis or renal function during hospitalization. Prespecified analysis of patients according to ejection fraction showed an unfavorable trend in patients with preserved ejection fraction. There was a trend toward benefit in patients with reduced ejection fraction and with initial systolic blood pressure less than 120 mm Hg.

New agents in ongoing clinical trials of hospitalized heart failure populations include the cardiac myosin activator omecamtiv mecarbil, the endogenous pregnancy peptide active relaxin, and the synthetic natriuretic peptide ularitide.

Profile C: Wet and Cold

Fewer than 3% of patients present with true cardiogenic shock, in which organ function is jeopardized, and lactate is accumulating[1,4] (see Figure 33-1). These patients are classified as Circulatory Support (INTERMACS) profile 1 (precipitous deterioration despite rapidly escalating therapy "crash and burn") or profile 2 (failing on inotropes).[62] After ruling out correctable lesions, these patients require rapid intervention and decisions regarding mechanical circulatory support (see Chapter 42) or realistic revision of the goals of care (see Chapter 47).

Most profile C patients with recognized hypoperfusion and congestion do not require emergency intervention, but expeditious attention to improving perfusion and relieving congestion.[21] Effective stabilization generally requires more than 48 hours of hospitalization to optimize therapy except when goals of care have been revised to support care in the home until death. Although reduction of filling pressures alone can lead to increased cardiac output through decrease of mitral regurgitation discussed above for profile B,[22] it is often not possible to establish effective diuresis until perfusion is adequate. The conceptual approach to the cold and wet profile is summarized by "Patients need to warm up to dry out."

Intravenous Vasodilators or Inotropic Agents?

The initial choice of adjunctive agents for hypoperfusion depends on the assessment of systemic vascular resistance. When systemic vascular resistance is very high, the intravenous vasodilators can simultaneously increase cardiac output and decrease filling pressures.[63] In addition, the hemodynamic benefit achieved with intravenous vasodilators can often be translated into equivalent effects with oral vasodilators. Hemodynamic profiles of decompensated heart failure as described from the 1980s and early 1990s were frequently characterized by severe vasoconstriction, for which titration of vasodilator therapy was key to the reduction of elevated filling pressures.[13] This is uncommon now in patients who have been maintained chronically on neurohormonal antagonist therapy. In the presentation of profile C now, patients with severe vasoconstriction are usually those whose disease has progressed in the absence of chronic renin-angiotensin system inhibition (either not prescribed or not taken as prescribed). For hypoperfusion in the face of vasoconstriction, both direct vasodilators and inotropic therapy with vasodilator effects will increase cardiac output, but inotropic therapy can increase myocardial oxygen demands, ischemia, and arrhythmias. In addition to precipitating clinical ischemic events, these agents may cause silent myocardial injury, as reflected in low-level troponin release that may worsen long-term outcomes after discharge.[53,54] Multiple observational studies support long-term deleterious effects of brief infusions of inotropic agents in the hospital,[52] but it is not possible to separate this from the increased acuity of illness likely to trigger their use.

For most patients with critically low perfusion in the current era who do not have severe vasoconstriction, increased contractility may be necessary to allow effective diuresis. The simplest way to increase contractility is to decrease the dose of β-blocker therapy. If this has already been done, or the initial dose is very low, empiric addition of low-dose intravenous inotropic therapy is reasonable. However, serious consideration should always be given to the possibility of subsequent inability to wean inotropic therapy for discharge. When review of the journey suggests end-stage disease without other options, it may be more appropriate to focus on other ways to palliate symptoms, perhaps with plans for hospice (see also Chapter 47).

Dosages of inotropic therapy should be as low as possible to minimize the deleterious effect of increased calcium loading and increased myocardial energy requirements and to minimize the risk of atrial fibrillation and ventricular tachyarrhythmias. Therapy should be continued until the desired goals of initial stabilization and volume reduction are achieved, but weaning should begin quickly thereafter. Specific agents and weaning of inotropic therapy are discussed below.

Profile L: Dry and Cold

Patients rarely present for hospitalization with true profile L (cold and dry)[9]; therefore, a patient with apparent profile L should be carefully evaluated for occult elevation of filling pressures indicative of profile C instead. In the unusual event that they have documented low filling pressures (pulmonary capillary wedge pressure <12 mm Hg, or right atrial pressure <5 mm Hg), a cautious trial of oral fluid repletion may be considered. Oral replacement while holding diuretics is better tolerated than is intravenous fluid supplementation, which tends to leak into the lungs. Unless postural hypotension is present, fluid supplementation does not often improve chronic clinical status in this population and may lead to congestive symptoms.

Patients with pulmonary capillary wedge pressures of approximately 16 mm Hg with normal right atrial pressures generally look surprisingly comfortable at rest even if the cardiac output is quite low. Intravenous inotropic therapy provides only temporary effects and may be followed by clinical deterioration after discontinuation. Cardiac resynchronization may be very useful in patients with appropriately long QRS and left bundle branch block pattern (see Chapter 35). The goals of further therapy depend on the clinical situation, but the main limitation of exercise and cardiac reserve is hard to address with oral medications. Further vasodilation may increase resting cardiac output, but it frequently causes symptomatic hypotension, particularly upon standing. In patients with stable renal function, the addition of digoxin is reasonable. Cautious initiation or uptitration of therapy with β-blocking agents may lead to later improvement in systolic function and cardiac output, particularly if resting heart rate is high. Any uptitration of β-blocking agents should proceed very slowly with care in patients with suspected or proven low cardiac output.

Use of Invasive Hemodynamic Monitoring

Right-heart catheterization is recommended for those situations where a specific clinical or therapeutic question needs to be addressed as summarized in Table 33-5 (see also Chapter 31). Invasive monitoring with a pulmonary artery catheter should be performed in patients with known or suspected cardiogenic shock to guide use of multiple vasopressors and consideration of urgent mechanical circulatory support (see Chapter 42).

Hemodynamic Diagnosis

Direct hemodynamic monitoring is occasionally necessary to clarify hemodynamic status before initiating therapy for decompensated heart failure, although skilled clinical assessment is adequate to place most patients into one of the four profiles of fluid status and perfusion for initiation of therapy. In the Evaluation Study of Congestive Heart Failure and Pulmonary Artery Catheterization Effectiveness (ESCAPE) study, clinical assessment was very reliable for elevated filling pressures but only modestly accurate for adequacy of cardiac output.[11] In patients in whom assessment yields limited or ambiguous findings, hemodynamic measurements may help define the appropriate first targets of filling pressures and perfusion. Diagnosis and therapy can also be informed by elective hemodynamic measurement for ambulatory patients when symptoms exceed clinical evidence of hemodynamic abnormalities, sometimes in conjunction with exercise testing. Hemodynamic measurement may clarify the contribution of heart failure to decompensation in the setting of other concomitant diagnoses. These may be cardiac conditions such as aortic valve disease, or noncardiac conditions, of which the most common one confounding assessment is chronic pulmonary disease, present in about a third of patients hospitalized with heart failure.

Hemodynamic Monitoring while Tailoring Therapy

One of the first routine uses of pulmonary artery catheterization in heart failure was to determine pulmonary pressures and reversibility of pulmonary hypertension during evaluation for cardiac transplantation in patients with advanced heart failure and low ejection fraction. When pulmonary vascular resistance was high in the setting of high left-sided filling pressures, the catheters were often left in place to determine reversibility of pulmonary hypertension during reduction of left ventricular filling pressures with diuretics and vasodilators. Because severe vasoconstriction was commonly present in the era before chronic renin-angiotensin system inhibition became standard, vasodilation with nitroprusside or nitroglycerin was frequently necessary in combination with and occasionally instead of diuretic therapy to achieve near-normal filling pressures. Use of rapid-acting intravenous vasodilators facilitates more rapid and definitive testing of the vasodilator strategy, particularly in someone with marginal blood pressure, than is possible with titration of oral vasodilators. Oral vasodilators can then be substituted to maintain the lower filling pressures and vascular resistances as patients are weaned from the intravenous vasodilators.[63,64] After major improvement in symptoms and intermediate-term outcomes were noted, this strategy of tailored therapy was employed for many patients admitted with advanced heart failure at specialized centers.[65]

The knowledge gained from physiology and therapeutic responses during hemodynamic monitoring has helped refine serial goals as clinically assessed. Therapy guided by clinical assessment was compared with therapy guided additionally with a pulmonary artery catheter in the ESCAPE trial (see Table 33-4) during hospitalization for decompensation of advanced heart failure. Evidence of right-sided congestion, based on jugular venous pressure and edema, was alleviated similarly in both groups; in patients with the pulmonary artery catheter, renal function was better and mitral regurgitation was lower at the time of hospital discharge, perhaps in relation to the ability to better assess and lower left-sided filling directly.[14,29] Symptomatic improvement was better at 1 month for the patients who underwent catheter-guided therapy, but there were no differences between the patient groups by 6 months, during which fluid retention recurred in both.[37]

Contemporary Hemodynamic Monitoring

The need for invasive monitoring to guide initial treatment is thus unusual except in the setting of life-threatening cardiogenic shock. Baseline vasoconstriction is less common now in subacute decompensation of chronic heart failure given the background of chronic renin-angiotensin system inhibition. Current "tailoring" is thus not often directed to vasoconstriction, but to volume overload, which can usually be tracked by expert clinical assessment during simple diuretic therapy, or sometimes tailored to reduce secondary pulmonary hypertension, which still requires invasive measurement to determine responsiveness.

In patients initially managed by clinical assessment, hemodynamic monitoring should still be considered if patients fail to respond to or deteriorate during usual therapy. This may lead to detection of right-left mismatch of filling pressures or unusually high or low systemic vascular resistance. Hemodynamic monitoring is strongly recommended to help optimize filling pressures and systemic vascular resistance on oral agents to facilitate weaning of inotropic infusions in patients who appear to be dependent on them. The value of hemodynamic information is less clear in patients who develop the cardiorenal syndrome during diuresis, in which the hemodynamic values obtained are often as anticipated from clinical assessment.

Hemodynamic parameters related to filling pressures are robust predictors of functional outcomes, rehospitalization, and survival. High pulmonary capillary wedge pressure, right atrial pressure, and pulmonary artery systolic and mean pressures all predict rehospitalization and death on a continuum, without a sharp threshold, and predict better when measured after therapy has been optimized. Indices of cardiac output offer little prediction in patients with advanced heart failure.[25,37] Invasive hemodynamic monitoring is *not* indicated purely to stratify risk in this population, for which there are many noninvasive prognostic parameters. Repeated right-sided heart catheterization should not be necessary during long-term management, except when the clinical situation worsens in the setting of new events, such as myocardial infarction or pulmonary emboli. However, it should again be emphasized that the right-left relationship should be carefully noted from previously available invasive hemodynamic measurement, including not only cardiac catheterization but also perioperative pulmonary artery catheter measurement.

Other markers that can correlate with elevated filling pressures include echocardiographic mitral valve flow patterns (Chapter 29) and natriuretic peptides (Chapter 30). Both of these can be useful for diagnosis of heart failure and for prognosis both at admission and discharge. However, they have not been demonstrated useful in titration of therapy during hospitalization. Several approaches to measuring thoracic impedance have been shown to correlate directionally with developed intrathoracic fluid but none has been sufficiently reliable to guide diagnosis and therapy of decompensation in individual patients.[66] Further refinements of handheld echocardiographic measurements may offer useful information, particularly when serial information is available for individual patients.

USE OF SPECIFIC INTRAVENOUS AGENTS DURING HOSPITALIZATION

Diuretics, intravenous vasodilators, and intravenous inotropic agents are the major medications used during acute management of decompensated heart failure. Use of diuretics in patients with ADHF is described earlier in the chapter (see Getting to Dry, earlier).

Intravenous Vasodilators

After diuretics, intravenous vasodilators are the most useful medications for the acute relief of congestive symptoms of heart failure. They reduce filling pressures and symptoms immediately. Cardiac output often increases as vasodilation and diuresis occur, primarily as a result of decreased mitral regurgitation, as discussed previously. These agents do not usually increase heart rate or exacerbate arrhythmias unless titrated to excessive levels of vasodilation and severe hypotension. Renal function can worsen if systemic hypotension develops.

Nitroprusside

Nitroprusside was the first vasodilator shown to improve cardiac output in heart failure.[30] It has dramatic efficacy in therapy for severe hypertension, in which systemic vascular resistance is also severely elevated. Although useful for hypertensive crises, nitroprusside is rarely associated with serious hypotension when titrated carefully in heart failure. Nitroprusside in heart failure has traditionally been monitored invasively through pulmonary artery catheters.[67] Noninvasive blood pressure monitoring with an automated cuff usually obviates the need for an indwelling arterial catheter as well. The rapidity of onset and offset, with a half-life of approximately 2 minutes, can facilitate early establishment of optimal vasodilation in a patient with severe vasoconstriction, and then allow efficient weaning onto an oral vasodilator regimen that is adjusted for equivalent hemodynamic effects. Nitroprusside is generally initiated at 10 μg/min and increased by 10 to 20 μg every 10 to 20 minutes as tolerated.[63,65] Doses may be measured in absolute doses or calculated per kilogram, starting at about 0.15 μg/kg/min but rarely exceeding 4 μg/kg (**Table 33-6**). The primary hemodynamic goal is reduction of the pulmonary capillary wedge pressure to 16 mm Hg without lowering systolic blood pressure below 80 mm Hg. The systemic vascular resistance is used to guide the relative emphasis on vasodilation versus diuresis. Although cardiac output is not the primary target, it often improves with treatment of these loading conditions because of the reduction of mitral and tricuspid regurgitation. Individual response varies markedly; 30 to 100 μg/min is effective in some patients, whereas others require over 200 μg/min to overcome severe vasoconstriction.

TABLE 33-6 Common Intravenous Vasoactive Agents for Heart Failure

AGENT	INITIAL DOSE	EFFECTIVE DOSE RANGE
Vasodilators		
Nitroglycerin	20 μg/min	40-400 μg/min*
Nitroprusside	10 μg/min	30-350 μg/min* Usually <4 μg/kg/min
Nesiritide	With or without 1- to 2-μg/kg bolus	0.005-0.03 μg/kg/min
Inotropic Agents†		
Dobutamine	1-2 μg/kg/min	2-10 μg/kg/min for inotropy and vasodilation
Dopamine		
To augment diuresis	2 μg/kg/min	2-4 μg/kg/min for vasodilation and inotropy
To treat hypotension	4-5 μg/kg/min	5-15 μg/kg/min for inotropy and vasoconstriction
Milrinone	50- to 75-μg/kg bolus may be administered over 10 min	0.10-0.75 μg/kg/min for vasodilation and inotropy

*Customarily titrated to effect, using absolute doses rather than per kilogram.
†These inotropic agents also cause vasodilation. The more potent inotropic agents epinephrine and norepinephrine and the pressor agent vasopressin are rarely used for chronic decompensated heart failure but are discussed in the Use of Specific Intravenous Agents during Hospitalization section.

The major side effects of nitroprusside in this setting are from the cyanide, which is most likely to accumulate in patients in whom hepatic perfusion is severely reduced as a result of low cardiac output or in whom hepatic function is decreased as a result of elevated right-sided pressures or previous underlying liver disease. Cyanide toxicity is most likely to develop in patients receiving more than 250 μg/min for more than 48 hours. These symptoms are predominantly gastrointestinal and central nervous system manifestations, often manifested by nausea and "feeling weird." Cyanide level results are rarely available in time to be useful; suspected toxicity is treated by decreasing or discontinuing the nitroprusside infusion, and additional therapy is almost never required in this setting. Less important during short-term nitroprusside administration is the thiocyanate metabolite, which can accumulate over days during more chronic use, particularly when renal function is impaired. Although it is the most effective intravenous vasodilator available, decreasing familiarity with nitroprusside has unfortunately limited its use in heart failure to specialized centers.

Nitroglycerin

Regardless of the route of administration, nitroglycerin is one of the safest and most versatile agents in acute therapy for decompensated heart failure. Nitroglycerin infusion is most commonly used for treatment of acute ischemic syndromes or heart failure in which acute ischemia is suspected. However, nitrates are very effective arterial vasodilators in the setting of vasoconstriction, although they are commonly misclassified as venodilators.[68-70] Dose responses for both nitroglycerin and nitroprusside are markedly variable between individuals, but treatment of vasoconstriction requires higher doses of nitroglycerin than of nitroprusside. Dosing is generally begun at 20 μg/min of nitroglycerin, increased in 20-μg increments to the hemodynamic goals described previously. The most common side effect of intravenous or oral nitrates is headache, which, if mild, can be treated with analgesics and often resolves during continued therapy.[56] As with all vasodilating agents, blood pressure often decreases, and it may decrease precipitously if filling pressures were incorrectly assessed to be elevated. A dramatic but rare reaction is a prolonged episode of profound hypotension with bradycardia, usually when initial filling pressures are normal or low.

Nesiritide

Nesiritide is a recombinant form of the endogenous B-type natriuretic peptide secreted primarily from the left ventricle in response to wall stress. Like nitroprusside and nitroglycerin, nesiritide acts to increase cyclic guanosine monophosphate. Nesiritide lowers filling pressures and improves symptoms during therapy for decompensated heart failure.[71] Although both nesiritide and nitroglycerin are systemic vasodilators, nesiritide is used more often than nitroglycerin for pulmonary vasodilation. As with nitroglycerin, blood pressure must be monitored closely during nesiritide therapy because hypotension can occur. Because nesiritide has a longer half-life (18 minutes), hypotension can last longer than with intravenous nitroglycerin, but it is usually well tolerated in the supine position. Inappropriate bradycardia occasionally accompanies hypotension. Headache is less common with nesiritide than nitroglycerin. Both agents have been shown to be effective for decreasing filling pressures and relieving symptoms early during heart failure hospitalization.[56]

Nesiritide has not been associated with major diuresis when used alone, but appears to potentiate the effect of concomitant diuretics, so that the total diuretic dose required may be reduced. Controversy regarding potential deleterious effects of nesiritide has been noteworthy.[57] Although it was considered at one time to be renal-sparing, in standard doses it does not appear to improve renal function and may in fact worsen it if hypotension develops. Nesiritide is sometimes used specifically to decrease pulmonary vascular resistance in patients with heart failure, particularly after cardiac surgery. The recent large trial in acute decompensation (ASCEND) showed neither benefit nor adverse impact on outcomes, and confirmed a previous modest trend toward early symptom relief.[58] The more recent ROSE trial examined the use of lower-dose nesiritide (0.005 μg/kg/min) with the intent of isolated renal effects, and found no significant impact on diuresis or renal function during hospitalization.[61] There was more hypotension with nesiritide, suggesting that even this dose has systemic hemodynamic effects. There was a trend for worse outcome in patients with preserved ejection fraction, with suggestion of benefit for some patients with reduced ejection fraction and initial systolic blood pressure below 120 mm Hg.

Weaning from Intravenous Vasodilator Agents

Once patients are considered to have reached optimal circulatory status, they are weaned from intravenous agents as oral agents are adjusted.[64,65] It is important to recognize that the current intravenous vasodilators cause both arterial and venous dilation. As patients are weaned from these agents, filling pressures frequently rise again as venous capacitance decreases, necessitating either further diuresis or effective substitution with oral vasodilators. When oral agents are adjusted according to clinical assessment, the jugular venous pressure, supine blood pressure, and upright blood pressure guide dosing. Nitrates and hydralazine in combination or individually offer the most direct transition from intravenous to chronic oral vasodilation. For patients who have required tailoring with intravenous vasodilators for stabilization, angiotensin-converting enzyme inhibitors often need to be supplemented with oral nitrates to achieve comparable oral vasodilation.[72]

Intravenous Inotropic Agents

The perception that intravenous inotropic agents are easy to use has led to their frequent initiation at the time of hospitalization for heart failure in the absence of any specific indications for inotropic support. These agents are associated with more tachyarrhythmias and ischemic events than seen with infusions of placebo or vasodilators.[53] In addition, the presence of inotropic infusions complicates the redesign of oral therapy for discharge; the efficacy of diuretics and tolerability of neurohormonal antagonist doses may be artificially boosted by lingering effects of inotropic stimulation. This may increase the likelihood of early rehospitalization. The use of current inotropic agents, therefore, should be limited to those cases where recommended therapies have failed to relieve congestion or establish adequate perfusion.

Specific Inotropic Agents

Dobutamine

The most commonly used inotropic agent during hospitalization for heart failure is dobutamine, an agent that stimulates β-adrenergic receptors with little effect on α-adrenergic receptors, so that contractility is increased with peripheral and pulmonary vasodilation. Dobutamine was introduced as an alternative to dopamine, one that produces less tachycardia and does not affect dopaminergic receptors. Early uncontrolled studies demonstrated increased cardiac output with decreased filling pressures. Myocardial stores of adenosine triphosphate were shown to be improved after a brief period of dobutamine therapy, and sometimes symptomatic benefit persisted.[73] Much of this early reported benefit has been attributed to the potentiation of diuresis when fewer options were available for enhancement of diuretic therapy.

Heart rate is consistently increased during dobutamine therapy, particularly in patients with atrial fibrillation. Atrial and ventricular tachyarrhythmias and symptoms of ischemia are increased during dobutamine therapy for decompensated heart failure. A comparison of dobutamine with nesiritide revealed increased premature ventricular contractions, episodes of nonsustained ventricular tachycardia, and signs that fulfilled criteria for the diagnosis of proarrhythmia.[74]

When dobutamine therapy is considered warranted despite these risks, the lowest dosage possible should be used for the desired effect. Enhancement of diuresis and improvement of renal function can be observed at doses of 1 to 2 μg/kg/min (see Table 33-6). Treatment for symptomatic hypotension usually necessitates higher doses. Patients receiving chronic maintenance infusions generally exhibit tachyphylaxis and require increasing dosages over time. There may be little benefit from increasing the dosage to more than 10 μg/kg/min, however, and other therapy should be added or substituted as the dosage approaches 15 μg/kg/min in an acute setting. An exception may be in patients with hypotension during chronic therapy with β-adrenergic antagonists. Dobutamine is often adequate for improving cardiac output in this setting, but dosages higher than usual may be required.[75]

On occasion, patients taking dobutamine for prolonged periods of many weeks may develop an eosinophilic hypersensitivity manifested in an elevated circulating eosinophil count and sometime in urine eosinophil levels as well. This can take the form of a skin rash, but of greater importance, eosinophilic myocarditis has been found in the explanted hearts of about 15% of patients receiving chronic infusions before cardiac transplantation.

Dopamine

Dopamine stimulates β-receptors, α-receptors, and dopaminergic receptors that cause vasodilation in the renal and peripheral vasculature. At dosages of 3 μg/kg/min or less, dopamine is predominantly vasodilatory. The dopaminergic receptors are overwhelmed by α-adrenergic stimulation when dopamine doses reach 5 μg/kg/min, or when other vasoconstricting pressors are given. Dopamine also causes release of norepinephrine from nerve terminals, which

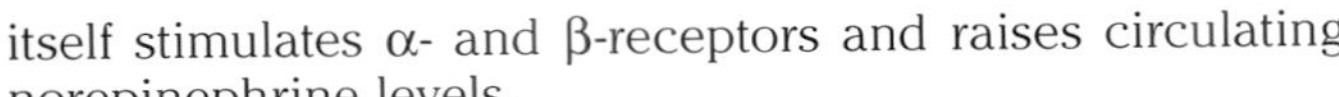

itself stimulates α- and β-receptors and raises circulating norepinephrine levels.

In response to observed effects on dopaminergic receptors in animal models and restrictions placed on "cardiac infusions" outside intensive care units, the concept of "renal-dose dopamine" at 1 to 3 μg/kg/min has been popularized. For patients with renal dysfunction and normal circulation, it is controversial whether this therapy enhances renal function specifically. In patients with heart failure, any dose of dopamine can have central hemodynamic effects to increase cardiac output and decrease systemic vascular resistance, and has been associated with tachyarrhythmias and ischemic episodes. The effect of low-dose dopamine (2 μg/kg/min) to enhance diuresis has recently been examined in the randomized ROSE trial as described previously.

Dopamine is a reasonable choice when inotropic therapy is indicated in rapidly evolving situations where blood pressure support may require dose escalation, particularly when the systemic vascular resistance and cardiac output are not known. When blood pressure support is the initial trigger for inotropic therapy, dopamine should be started at a dosage of 3 to 5 μg/kg/min. Similarly, when patients are weaned from the use of dopamine as a pressor agent, it may be necessary to discontinue it once a dosage of 2 to 3 μg/kg/min is reached, because gradual weaning through lower doses may in fact cause vasodilation and hypotension. There is little evidence to support the addition of dopamine to dobutamine for enhanced renal function for patients with heart failure, and it would be expected to increase the risk of arrhythmias and ischemia.

Milrinone

Milrinone, and other agents with phosphodiesterase inhibition, lead to increased levels of cyclic adenosine monophosphate by inhibiting its breakdown, rather than by increasing its production through stimulation of β-receptors. These agents then may act synergistically with β-adrenergic agents to achieve a further increase in cardiac output than either agent alone. They may also be more effective than β-adrenergic receptor stimulation for increasing cardiac output when excess β-blocking agents have been given. Phosphodiesterase inhibition increases contractility and causes vasodilation. The relative effects on cardiac output and systemic vascular resistance vary markedly, so that some patients exhibit predominant vasodilation. This can cause significant hypotension, unlike dobutamine, which rarely causes hypotension except in unappreciated vasodilatory states such as sepsis. In a trial of patients hospitalized with heart failure and an average baseline blood pressure of 120 mm Hg, 10% of the patients randomized to milrinone developed clinically significant hypotension, a higher percentage than with a placebo.[53] When hypotension is considered the indication for use of an intravenous inotropic agent, milrinone is rarely an appropriate choice.

Milrinone has been associated with slightly less elevation in heart rate than have dobutamine and dopamine.[76] Like the other intravenous inotropic agents, however, milrinone increases the frequency of atrial and ventricular tachyarrhythmias and ischemic events. A trial of a 48-hour infusion of milrinone during heart failure hospitalization increased adverse events of atrial and ventricular tachyarrhythmias, cardiac arrest, and myocardial infarction.[53]

The use of milrinone for short-term stabilization is complicated by its prolonged half-life. Unlike the pharmacologic half-lives of dopamine and dobutamine, which are in minutes, the elimination half-life of milrinone is about 2.5 hours, and the physiologic half-life is closer to 6 hours. Although bolus therapy was originally recommended, milrinone is frequently used without a bolus to avoid rapid initial effects, at doses as low as 0.01 μg/kg/min. The drug is then titrated to the desired hemodynamic effect, in increments of the lowest doses possible, up to a maximum of 0.75 μg/kg/min. Because the drug is excreted renally, dosage adjustment is recommended. In the setting of renal dysfunction, effects accumulate and persist over a longer period of time. When milrinone is discontinued after several days, the physiologic half-life often seems to exceed 12 or even 18 hours. As a result, patients are frequently assumed to have tolerated milrinone weaning only to deteriorate hours after transfer out of the intensive care unit or discharge home. It is thus particularly important to follow patients weaned from milrinone for at least 48 hours to ensure adequate fluid balance and blood pressure on oral therapy before discharge.

Patients awaiting cardiac transplantation may be supported with extended infusions of milrinone either alone or in combination with dobutamine.[77] Patients requiring inotropic infusions are moving earlier to mechanical support devices as bridges to transplantation, where possible (see also Chapters 40 and 42). Although intermittent outpatient inotropic infusions were occasionally administered in the past, this practice is not supported by evidence.

Epinephrine and Norepinephrine

Epinephrine and norepinephrine are full β-receptor agonists, in contrast to dopamine and dobutamine. Significant additional inotropic and blood pressure support can be provided by these agents for short-term life-saving intervention over a span of minutes to hours before definitive therapy. Although norepinephrine is commonly confused with phenylephrine (Neo-Synephrine, a pure peripheral α-vasoconstrictor), both norepinephrine and epinephrine stimulate type 1 β-adrenergic receptors and α-adrenergic receptors, which increase contractility, heart rate, and peripheral vascular resistance, while promoting cardiac arrhythmias and ischemia. Kidney failure, hepatic failure, and gangrene can result from use of these agents, which should not be administered except in true emergency situations. Compared with norepinephrine, epinephrine has more affinity for type 2 β-receptors, and thus is slightly less likely to cause tissue necrosis from intense vasoconstriction, although both are profound vasoconstrictors appropriate only for therapy of life-threatening shock.

When fatal hypotension is imminent, epinephrine or norepinephrine is used at a starting dose of 1 μg/min, less often expressed as per-kilogram dosing. Before this point, injection of 0.25 mg of epinephrine from the code cart may provide several minutes of stabilization during which to make more definitive plans for circulatory support or the orchestration of the end of life. To maintain survival for brief periods until definitive therapy, boluses of calcium can also be helpful, particularly in the presence of conditions that may acutely lower serum calcium, such as transfusion, dialysis, or cardiopulmonary bypass. Contractility increases rapidly with increased circulating calcium concentration.[78] Intravenous calcium administration is highly arrhythmogenic and may exacerbate ongoing myocardial necrosis.

Vasopressin is used increasingly to potentiate the effects of catecholamines in patients who remain severely hypotensive on catecholamines. This experience is derived from early postoperative management after heart transplantation or insertion of mechanical support devices.[79,80] Some patients with life-threatening hypotension develop profound vasoplegia during cardiac surgery, with low systemic vascular resistance states of the systemic inflammatory response syndrome. Vasopressin has been used for periods of hours to days, in doses of 0.05 to over 0.1 U/min. At these doses, patients already receiving norepinephrine frequently have further 30 mm Hg increases in systolic blood pressure.[79,80] As a potent vasoconstricting hormone itself, vasopressin can contribute to ischemic injury and necrosis of organs and limbs during use of other vasoconstricting agents.

Weaning of Intravenous Inotropic Therapy

Inotropic therapy has been regarded as the "until" therapy, which should not be started without careful consideration of a predefined endpoint.[81] It may be used *until* the underlying hemodynamic profile and need for emergency support are determined. It may be used *until* diuresis is effective in patients with conditions refractory to escalating diuretic therapy. It may be used *until* kidney, lung, or liver function has improved to establish eligibility for cardiac transplantation or for operative intervention. It may be used *until* recovery from a superimposed insult such as pneumonia, pulmonary embolus, myocardial infarction, or surgery. Much of the experience with prolonged infusions has derived from patients waiting *until* an appropriate heart can be found for cardiac transplantation. More recently, experience with implantable ventricular assist devices suggests that ambulatory patients with class IV symptoms at home may have better postoperative outcomes following a period of stabilization on intravenous inotropic therapy *until* elective device implantation. For patients in whom transplantation and mechanical support are not options, inotropic therapy initiated with the intent of brief support may be difficult to wean without symptomatic deterioration. Often, inotropic therapy can be weaned slowly and successfully with careful tailoring onto oral therapy to optimize filling pressures and systemic vascular resistance during invasive hemodynamic monitoring.[63,82] This may necessitate discontinuation of β-adrenergic antagonists and ACE inhibitors to avoid their negative inotropic effects in severely compromised patients. In patients with adequate renal function, the addition of digoxin may be particularly useful at this time. The use of nitrates and the addition of hydralazine may be particularly effective in restoring compensation with oral vasodilators after prolonged inotropic infusion.[82]

However, sometimes inotropic therapy initiated for temporary support cannot be weaned without symptomatic deterioration. Many of these patients are those in whom right ventricular failure has become prominent and the cardiorenal syndrome is manifest. Collaboration with palliative care services may be necessary to decide with families whether weaning should proceed after preparing for possible death in hospital or whether the short-term goals for the patient and family can better be met during continuous inotropic therapy (see also Chapter 47). Continuous intravenous inotropic infusions have been recognized as palliative care *until* death for some of these patients. This therapy has been associated with frequent complications from indwelling catheters and with sepsis.[73] Escalating doses are usually required, and survival expectancy is less than 50% during the next 3 to 6 months. Patients should not be discharged on home inotropic therapy unless they demonstrate initial clinical stability and reasonable function with this regimen to justify the cost and inconvenience to the patient and family. Although in rare cases patients may stabilize to allow later weaning of intravenous therapy, patients should understand that long-term stability is unlikely and that discontinuation of inotropic therapy may become necessary, particularly for some hospice programs. Palliative inotropic therapy is not an indication for an implantable cardioverter-defibrillator in end-stage heart failure, and deactivation should be discussed with patients who already have a device. For many patients, the last part of their journey with heart failure is smoother and more comfortable if they are not tethered to a catheter and pump for continuous infusion.

CONTINUING THE JOURNEY

Serial evaluation and adjustments in therapy usually lead to resolution of the acute decompensation that led to the hospitalization for heart failure. Primary and exacerbating causes of heart failure will have been explored and addressed if possible. After initial stabilization or attempted stabilization, the previous history and current state will be incorporated into a view of the next part of the journey. This will include considerations of both the severity of heart disease and the severity and contribution of comorbidities to survival and quality of life. For those few patients with advanced heart failure and reduced ejection fraction who are still eligible for cardiac transplantation or mechanical circulatory support, subsequent care is directed toward ensuring the best outcomes with those therapies. For some patients there may be investigational therapies that could be considered, although at the present time these are more numerous for patients with mild to moderate disease without recent decompensation. For most patients with heart failure, regardless of the ejection fraction, the focus is on reevaluation of the goals of care and redesign of their chronic medical regimen in light of both the cardiac condition and the common comorbidities.[83]

Aligning Goals of Care

Mapping the journey is crucial for aligning medications with the goals of care (see also Chapter 47). For a patient with advanced disease who was just weaned with difficulty from intravenous inotropic therapy, the prognosis for extended good quality survival is poor. These patients may not tolerate reinitiation of neurohormonal antagonists that undermine the reflex systems necessary to maintain tenuous perfusion. Although this is well-known for β-blockers, the potential for ACEI, ARB, and spironolactone to decrease blood pressure and perfusion is less appreciated. The renin-angiotensin system potentiates effects of endogenous catecholamines, such that its inhibition may decrease effective inotropic state and cause hypotension, which is further aggravated by the bradykinin that accumulates when the angiotensin-converting enzyme is inhibited. There is no demonstrated benefit of neurohormonal antagonists in these patients, who would have been excluded from the definitive studies that form the basis of evidence for recommended therapies, and in whom remodeling has already progressed to a state unlikely to be reversed. Even if not receiving intravenous inotropic therapy, there are other patients in whom a history of frequent heart failure hospitalizations, progressive renal dysfunction, or other trends indicate a very limited prognosis. When the goals of care are to maximize mobility, relieve symptoms, and maintain social exchange toward the end of life, thoughtful review is warranted regarding medications for which benefits may have been outlived when those medications undermine marginal blood pressure and renal function or otherwise detract from energy desired for meaningful interaction.

Transition to Oral Diuretics—All EF

Although one of the most critical factors in stability in the early days after discharge, how to establish the home diuretic regimen is one of the questions un-informed by any basis of evidence.[84] Consideration includes the previous home diuretic dose and the intensity of diuretics required in hospital. Lower doses are required to maintain stability after diuresis than were required to achieve net fluid loss. However, bed rest enhances diuretic efficacy, which is reduced when patients return to a more ambulatory routine. In addition, patients often consume more sodium and fluid at home than when restricted in the hospital. It is crucial to adjust oral diuretics in the hospital to achieve at least even fluid balance. Discharge preparation should include instructions on how to measure and act on daily weights after discharge, and the identification of a "first response plan" for the diuretic change to be initiated if the weight increases above target (see also Chapter 44). This first response plan should be recorded for the patient and shared with all providers involved in the outpatient setting. Too often the first call responder, not knowing what diuretic change to suggest, decides to wait for another day or another provider before action is taken. Similarly, although additional potassium supplementation may still be required according to a "sliding scale," discontinuation of intravenous diuretics should trigger reinstitution of a regular oral potassium replacement schedule. If an aldosterone antagonist is to be started or increased before discharge, it ideally should be early enough so that its effect is present before the decision regarding maintenance potassium doses for discharge.[85] Maintenance of excessive replacement once net diuresis has stopped, particularly in the presence of aldosterone antagonists, is a common cause of life-threatening hyperkalemia in and out of the hospital.

Redesign of Oral Regimen—HF Low EF (see also Chapter 34)

Neurohormonal Antagonist Therapy

For patients with low ejection fraction, there are multiple other components of the medical regimen in addition to the diuretic plan as discussed previously. Most patients will have been admitted as profile B, for which there has been no need for intravenous inotropic therapy to support perfusion during diuresis. Most patients will already have been on neurohormonal antagonist therapy, for which discharge doses should be carefully reviewed in relation to the doses on admission. Some patients may have needed decreases in the dose of ACEI/ARB or β-blockers initially because of concerns regarding low blood pressure or renal function. On the other hand, major correction of volume status may decrease tolerability of vasodilating drugs that were less potent in the volume-loaded state. ACEI/ARB and other vasodilators can be increased in small increments before discharge as allowed by blood pressure and renal function. Changes in general should be made at least 48 hours before discharge, and the medication records should be carefully reviewed to ensure that doses are not being held for low blood pressure or heart rate. The aldosterone antagonists can decrease blood pressure and renal function, as well as cause hyperkalemia. Whether initiated primarily for neurohormonal effects, potentiation of diuresis, or reduction of potassium supplementation, they should be started several days before discharge. All patients should be checked for postural hypotension before the day of discharge to allow further changes if necessary to avoid symptoms that may undermine adherence to the regimen at home.

Initiation of β-adrenergic blocking agents is not recommended during hospitalization for heart failure decompensation when hypoperfusion[5] has been prominent or intravenous inotropic therapy has been used. However, most patients admitted in profile B can undergo cautious initiation of β-blocker therapy in the hospital once fluid status has been stabilized, if blood pressure has not been low.[86] β-Blocker therapy initially causes elevation of filling pressures and reduction of cardiac output; therefore, patients should have sufficient hemodynamic margin to tolerate this challenge. When successful, initiation in the hospital has been associated with a higher adherence and higher maintenance dose of β-blocker after discharge.[86] However, after the first one or two uptitrations, establishment of the appropriate target doses of β-blockers should proceed gradually in the outpatient setting.

Other Therapies

Hydralazine-Nitrates. Addition of the hydralazine-nitrate combination to the ACE inhibitor/angiotensin receptor blocker (ARB) regimens should be considered when class III or IV symptoms persist in African American patients for whom substantial improvement in both function and survival was demonstrated in the African American Heart Failure Trial (A-HeFT) (see also Chapter 34).[87] Although there have been no definitive randomized trials, addition of nitrates to ACE inhibitor/ARB regimens in other patient populations has commonly been implicated in symptomatic improvement,[70] particularly for exertional dyspnea or exertional chest pain in nonischemic, as well as ischemic cardiomyopathy.

Depending on the referral population, up to 30% of patients with advanced heart failure may not be able to tolerate ACE inhibitors because of hypotension or severe renal dysfunction.[88] In these patients, the usual regimen is hydralazine, 25 to 150 mg three to four times daily, and oral isosorbide dinitrate, 10 to 80 mg three times daily. Although ACE inhibitors were shown to be superior in patients with class II heart failure, the Veterans Administration Cooperative Vasodilator–Heart Failure Trial II (V-HeFT II) demonstrated equivalent rates of survival with enalapril and with hydralazine and nitrates in class III and class IV heart failure.[89] Most experience has been with the short-acting nitrate, although longer acting oral nitrates have also been used. When hydralazine is not tolerated, vasodilation can also be achieved with high doses of oral nitrates alone. There is currently no accepted regimen for patients who cannot tolerate ACE inhibitors, hydralazine, or nitrates.

Digoxin. There is wide variability regarding the use of digoxin in heart failure. The most convincing data on digoxin confirm increased risk of deterioration in the weeks after withdrawal of digoxin. As digoxin has been shown to decrease hospitalization,[90] it is reasonable to consider the initiation of digoxin in hospitalized patients with stable renal function for whom the likelihood of digoxin toxicity is low.

Implantable Pacing and Defibrillation Devices. Cardiac resynchronization therapy is indicated in selected ambulatory patients who have had severe symptoms but have stabilized on an oral medical regimen (see also Chapter 35).[91] Good clinical responses are most likely in patients with baseline QRS duration of 150 msec or more, and left bundle branch block.[41] Even when electrocardiographic criteria are met, outcomes have been poor in patients who have required intravenous inotropic therapy. Depending on the overall likelihood of clinical response and the patients' preferences regarding mode of death and inappropriate shocks, cardiac resynchronization devices without defibrillation capability may often be appropriate.[92]

Implantable devices for defibrillation as primary prevention are indicated only in patients who have a reasonable expectation of survival, with good functional status, for more than 1 year. Implantation of cardioverter-defibrillators for primary prevention of sudden death is contraindicated in patients with class IV symptoms of heart failure, except in ambulatory patients with a high likelihood of benefit from resynchronization therapy.[93] Among large community populations, the rate of mortality within 1 year of the first hospitalization for heart failure is 20% to 35%, and over 40% after rehospitalization.[94] In patients with heart failure burden indicated by more than two previous heart failure hospitalizations or hospital stay at least a week before implantation, 3-year survival is less than 50% even with an implantable cardioverter-defibrillator (ICD).[95]

For patients recognized to have a declining course with anticipated survival of less than a year, it is appropriate to review the option of deactivation of defibrillation from an ICD already in place. Many patients who decline initially will later request device inactivation. Although most heart failure patients, with or without ICDs, die from progression to refractory hemodynamic compromise or from other chronic conditions, most have not previously discussed inactivation of ICDs.

Redesign of Regimen for HF with Preserved EF (see also Chapter 36)

No medications have been shown to modify the course of heart failure with preserved ejection fraction beyond treatment of fluid retention and hypertension. Other therapies should be prescribed as indicated for coronary artery disease, diabetes, and other comorbidities. In view of differences in mean age, renal function, and fall risk, the effects and interactions of medicines to cause excessive lowering of blood pressure should be closely reviewed. Evidence of fluid retention should be carefully sought in patients taking drugs that can exacerbate peripheral edema attributed to local vascular factors, such as the glitazones, calcium channel blockers, and gabapentin. Many older patients who eat alone or otherwise have poor appetite can benefit from nutritional supplements to ensure adequate caloric intake and maintenance of serum oncotic pressure.

TABLE 33-7 Discharge Criteria for Hospitalization with Heart Failure

Clinical Status Goals
Achievement of optimal volume status Definition of acceptable blood pressure range Walking without dyspnea or dizziness
Ideal Stability Goals
• ≥48 hours off intravenous inotropic agents, if used • 24 hours without changes in oral regimen for heart failure (no doses held for hypotension or other symptoms) • Even fluid balance on oral diuretics • Renal function stable or improving
Discharge Regimen
• Estimated diuretic dose, with first response plan for escalation if needed • Potassium replacement • ACE inhibitor/ARB or documented contraindication (Level I) • β-Blocker or documented contraindication (Level I) • Anticoagulation for atrial fibrillation unless contraindicated (Level I)
Patient/Family Education About Heart Failure (Level I)
• Sodium restriction, fluid limitation if indicated • Medication schedule, effects and side effects • Exercise prescription
Monitoring and Management
• Monitoring of weight • Recognition of sentinel symptom • Instructions regarding when and whom to call • Scheduled call to patient within 3 days (Level IIa) • Clinic appointment within 7 to 14 days (Level IIa) • Information hand-off to monitoring physician • Multidisciplinary HF disease management for high-risk patients (Level I) • Use of risk prediction tools and/or biomarkers to identify patients at higher risk for postdischarge events (Level IIa)

ACE, Angiotensin-converting enzyme; *ARB*, angiotensin receptor blocker.

Transitions to Home

Achieving Goals for Discharge

As discussed previously, the patient course should be reviewed early and often during hospitalization to set reasonable expectations before and after discharge (**Table 33-7**). For most patients, stabilization before discharge has been possible on oral regimens of guideline-driven medical therapies. Stability includes fluid balance, blood pressure, and renal function that have not worsened for at least 24 hours on the oral regimen planned for home, without doses held. As a general rule, patients should be free of orthopnea, dyspnea on minimal exertion such as washing and walking on the ward, and without peripheral edema, ascites, or significant pleural effusions related to elevated cardiac filling pressures. The goal for jugular venous pressure is 8 cm or less above the right atrium, except in the presence of high right-left mismatch, limiting renal function, or chronic nonadherence to the regimen of medications and dietary restrictions. Hospital dosing should be modified to schedules that are feasible for patients at home, such as timing a second diuretic dose for midafternoon rather than evening. At least 48 hours of monitoring on the oral regimen is needed before discharge for patients who have received intravenous inotropic agents, which can mask the inadequacy or intolerability of the discharge regimen. Failure to meet criteria for discharge contributes to increased rates of rehospitalization.[95] For patients in whom stability goals cannot be achieved and for whom there are no definitive therapies, it is appropriate to shift the

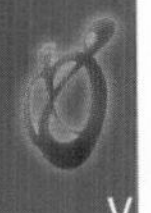

direction of the regimen toward palliation and in some cases hospice-supported care.

Patient Education

Patient education should take place during the entire hospitalization, with specific focus on fundamental heart failure physiology such as fluid retention, which many patients do not recognize as integral to their heart problem. They need specific information regarding their salt and fluid intake, medication schedules, and a flexible diuretic regimen, including a first response plan for increased diuretic triggered by weight gain or other signals identified specifically as sentinel for an individual patient, such as orthopnea, edema, or right upper quadrant discomfort.[97-99] Participation in the ritual of daily weights and diuretic dosing during hospitalization reinforces the concepts of fluid balance. Both patients and family members should hear specific instructions regarding desirable and allowable activity levels. It is often useful to assure families that even if a patient "does too much," the likely outcome is only the need to rest, not further injury to the heart. Although hospitalization is considered a true "teachable moment," too often the discharge information is rushed as the patients are packing their belongings. In addition to information about what they should not do, patients need positive information on the activities they can pursue, reinforcing that they should "Keep dry, keep active, and keep doing what you enjoy."

Connection through the Transition

As separation increases between inpatient and outpatient care and those who provide it, seamless transitions demand more effort and collaboration (see also Chapter 44). Medication reconciliation for patient and care providers should detail all additions, subtractions, and dose changes between the time of admission and discharge. A follow-up call within the first 3 days is recommended to elicit early symptoms of recurrent decompensation or medication side effects, as well as discrepancies and problems with prescriptions at local pharmacies. Patients should leave the hospital with a written appointment reminder for follow-up within 7 to 14 days in person, or occasionally by video-assist technology in remote areas. All patients need also to go home with information regarding how to contact a member of their care team at any hour. The first response diuretic plan should be known to patient and family and all members of the care team likely to connect with the patient during this transition. Many of these elements of the discharge process are amenable to process improvement systems, which are recommended to improve outcomes during and after the transition to home.

Heart Failure Readmissions

Risk for Readmissions

Between 30% and 50% of patients discharged with a diagnosis of heart failure are rehospitalized within the next 3 to 6 months.[1] Risk factors for readmission are similar to those for hospitalization for heart failure in general. The BUN level, BNP level, and systolic blood pressures have been strong predictors of in-hospital mortality and also contribute to risk of heart failure–related events after discharge.[46,100] The ESCAPE risk score was designed specifically from information at *discharge* to determine risk for death or readmission within 6 months, and it includes two thresholds of BNP and BUN levels (500 and 1300 pg/mL for BNP, 40 and 90 mg/dL for BUN), diuretic dose greater than 240 mg of furosemide or greater than 120 mg of torsemide, serum sodium level (<130 mEq/L), inability to tolerate β-blocker therapy, 6-minute walk distance <300 feet), need for cardiopulmonary resuscitation or intubation during hospitalization, and age older than 70 years.[101] Multidisciplinary heart failure disease management programs are recommended for patients at high risk for readmission.

Three-Phase Terrain of Readmissions

The First Month. When admissions are tracked between the first discharge and death, three periods can be distinguished[102,103] (**Figure 33-7**). Within 30 days of discharge, 20% to 25% of patients are readmitted.[104] This early peak

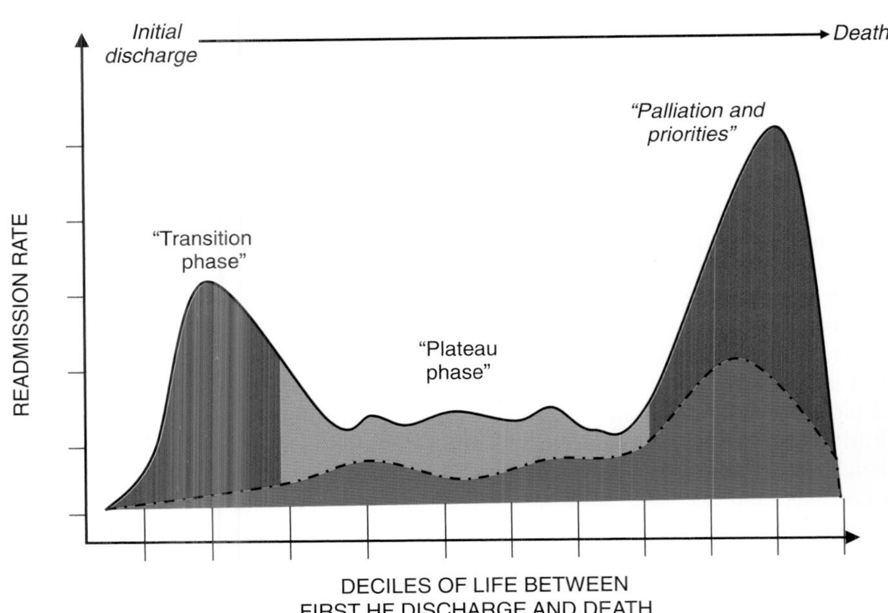

FIGURE 33-7 Three-phase terrain of rehospitalizations during the patient journey with heart failure (HF). The initial peak reflects the transitions into outpatient HF management. The plateau reflects a period of relative stability during which many hospitalizations may be averted by early detection of increasing filling pressures. The last peak represents progression to end-stage disease. The green color is a theoretical depiction of a proportion of hospitalizations that may be indicated for major reevaluation and revision of care. *Adapted from Desai AS, Stevenson LW: Rehospitalization for heart failure: predict or prevent? Circulation 126:501–506, 2012, with incorporation of data from Russo MJ, Gelijns AC, Stevenson LW, et al: The cost of medical management in advanced heart failure during the final two years of life. J Card Fail 14:651–658, 2008; and Chun S, Tu JV, Wijeysundera HC, et al: Lifetime analysis of hospitalizations and survival of patients newly admitted with heart failure. Circ Heart Fail 5:414–421, 2012.*

may be most sensitive to gaps in the transition processes between inpatient and outpatient. During this month, initial adjustments in the discharge regimen may be made, education should be reinforced, and identified deficits in the home environment have been addressed if possible. Reevaluation at the 1-month point provides a key opportunity for further refinement of prognosis and plans.[38,105] Patients demonstrating persistent or recurrent evidence of congestion are likely to suffer declining functional capacity and quality of life, and are at more than twice the risk for death or readmission than are those who remain free of congestion.[105]

The Plateau Period. The rate of admissions is lower during the plateau period, which for most patients is the longest of the three periods of life remaining after discharge from the first heart failure hospitalization. Whether ejection fraction is preserved or reduced, rehospitalizations after initial stabilization are preceded by a gradual increase in right- and left-sided filling pressures over at least 2 weeks.[39] These increases occur many days before recognized symptom deterioration, which occurs late and may appear to be sudden. Taking daily weights fails to identify most of these gradual changes in the chronic outpatient setting, where changing balance of caloric intake and expenditure also alters weight without fluid changes. Home pressure monitoring systems have just been approved with the hope that early detection of these changes will allow early response and the opportunity for additional response if necessary to avert decompensation.

The Last Hill. After the transition month following hospital discharge, the highest rate of rehospitalization is experienced later, during the weeks before death. Although brief improvement may occur during therapy with diuresis and possibly with temporary intravenous inotropic support, typically the goals of decongestion and stabilization can no longer be met during hospitalization, and patients return soon after discharge. This period of major distress with refractory congestion has lengthened dramatically compared with 30 years ago, when most patients died at home in their sleep, often prematurely and tragically before the end stage of disease. The decrease in sudden death was already apparent after the advances of chronic neurohormonal antagonist therapy, preceding the further impact of implantable defibrillators. We have successfully prolonged the good quality phase of life with heart failure, and have also prolonged the passage of death with heart failure. Our new responsibilities to guide our patients also through this phase of the journey are discussed in Chapter 47.

The Medical Village

The heavy burden of heart failure hospitalizations can be reduced but not eliminated with more attention to specialized heart failure management. As half of rehospitalizations after heart failure result from non–heart failure comorbidities, we also need better integration with primary care management teams as the "medical home," which will be facilitated by better linking of electronic medical records. In addition to better detection of early decompensation, we need to design more facilities devoted to acute outpatient intervention, in some cases offering a "day camp" for repeated visits. In the face of the widening mismatch between the large heart failure population and the small advanced heart disease physician work force, the health care system will evolve to support reimbursement and focused specialization in heart failure training for midlevel health professionals. The heart failure teams will recognize further obligation to refine triage of high-technology options to be offered responsibly to patients most likely to benefit, while finding the fortitude and palliative care support to guide other patients through the end of the journey with their original hearts.[83] As patients, care teams, and medical institutions recognize their shared responsibility for managing heart failure in the population, it will increasingly "take a village" to sustain patients beyond hospitalization to enjoy meaningful lives in their communities.

References

1. Gheorghiade M, Pang PS: Acute heart failure syndromes. *J Am Coll Cardiol* 53:557–573, 2009.
2. Yancy CW, Lopatin M, Stevenson LW, et al: Clinical presentation, management, and in-hospital outcomes of patients admitted with acute decompensated heart failure with preserved systolic function: a report from the Acute Decompensated Heart Failure National Registry (ADHERE) Database. *J Am Coll Cardiol* 47:76–84, 2006.
3. Sweitzer NK, Lopatin M, Yancy CW, et al: Comparison of clinical features and outcomes of patients hospitalized with heart failure and normal ejection fraction (> or =55%) versus those with mildly reduced (40% to 55%) and moderately to severely reduced (<40%) fractions. *Am J Cardiol* 101:1151–1156, 2008.
4. Dickstein K, Cohen-Solal A, Filippatos G, et al: ESC Guidelines for the diagnosis and treatment of acute and chronic heart failure 2008: the Task Force for the Diagnosis and Treatment of Acute and Chronic Heart Failure 2008 of the European Society of Cardiology. Developed in collaboration with the Heart Failure Association of the ESC (HFA) and endorsed by the European Society of Intensive Care Medicine (ESICM). *Eur Heart J* 29:2388–2442, 2008.
5. Jessup M, Abraham WT, Casey DE, et al: 2009 focused update: ACCF/AHA Guidelines for the Diagnosis and Management of Heart Failure in Adults: a report of the American College of Cardiology Foundation/American Heart Association Task Force on Practice Guidelines: developed in collaboration with the International Society for Heart and Lung Transplantation. *Circulation* 119:1977–2016, 2009.
6. McCarthy RE, 3rd, Boehmer JP, Hruban RH, et al: Long-term outcome of fulminant myocarditis as compared with acute (nonfulminant) myocarditis. *N Engl J Med* 342:690–695, 2000.
7. Fonarow GC, Abraham WT, Albert NM, et al: Factors identified as precipitating hospital admissions for heart failure and clinical outcomes: findings from OPTIMIZE-HF. *Arch Intern Med* 168:847–854, 2008.
8. Acker MA, Pagani FD, Stough WG, et al: Statement regarding the pre and post market assessment of durable, implantable ventricular assist devices in the United States: executive summary. *Circ Heart Fail* 6:145–150, 2013.
9. Nohria A, Tsang SW, Fang JC, et al: Clinical assessment identifies hemodynamic profiles that predict outcomes in patients admitted with heart failure. *J Am Coll Cardiol* 41:1797–1804, 2003.
10. Stevenson LW, Perloff JK: The limited reliability of physical signs for estimating hemodynamics in chronic heart failure. *JAMA* 261:884–888, 1989.
11. Drazner MH, Hellkamp AS, Leier CV, et al: Value of clinician assessment of hemodynamics in advanced heart failure. The ESCAPE trial. *Circ Heart Fail* 1:170–177, 2008.
12. Kato M, Stevenson LW, Palardy M, et al: The worst symptom as defined by patients during heart failure hospitalization: implications for response to therapy. *J Card Fail* 18:524–533, 2012.
13. Drazner MH, Hamilton MA, Fonarow G, et al: Relationship between right and left-sided filling pressures in 1000 patients with advanced heart failure. *J Heart Lung Transplant* 18:1126–1132, 1999.
14. Campbell P, Drazner MH, Kato M, et al: Right-left mismatch in the ESCAPE population: discordance between right and left-sided filling pressures before and after therapy. *J Card Fail* 15:S28, 2009.
15. Zema MJ, Restivo B, Sos T, et al: Left ventricular dysfunction–bedside Valsalva manoeuvre. *Br Heart J* 44:560–569, 1980.
16. Butman SM, Ewy GA, Standen JR, et al: Bedside cardiovascular examination in patients with severe chronic heart failure: importance of rest or inducible jugular venous distension. *J Am Coll Cardiol* 22:968–974, 1993.
17. Maisel AS, McCord J, Nowak RM, et al: Bedside B-type natriuretic peptide in the emergency diagnosis of heart failure with reduced or preserved ejection fraction. Results from the Breathing Not Properly Multinational Study. *J Am Coll Cardiol* 41:2010–2017, 2003.
18. Nguyen VT, Ho JE, Ho CY, et al: Handheld echocardiography offers rapid assessment of clinical volume status. *Am Heart J* 156:537–542, 2008.
19. Sobh JF, Lucas C, Stevenson LW, et al: Altered cardiorespiratory control in patients with severe congestive heart failure: a transfer function analysis approach. *Comput Cardiol* 1-4, 1996.
20. Setoguchi S, Nohria A, Rassen JA, et al: Maximum potential benefit of implantable defibrillators in preventing sudden death after hospital admission because of heart failure. *Can Med Assoc J* 180:611–616, 2009.
21. Nohria A, Lewis E, Stevenson LW: Medical management of advanced heart failure. *JAMA* 287:628–640, 2002.
22. Stevenson LW, Tillisch JH: Maintenance of cardiac output with normal filling pressures in patients with dilated heart failure. *Circulation* 74:1303–1308, 1986.
23. Stevenson LW, Brunken RC, Belil D, et al: Afterload reduction with vasodilators and diuretics decreases mitral regurgitation during upright exercise in advanced heart failure [see comments]. *J Am Coll Cardiol* 15:174–180, 1990.
24. Rosario LB, Stevenson LW, Solomon SD, et al: The mechanism of decrease in dynamic mitral regurgitation during heart failure treatment: importance of reduction in the regurgitant orifice size. *J Am Coll Cardiol* 32:1819–1824, 1998.
25. Stevenson LW, Tillisch JH, Hamilton M, et al: Importance of hemodynamic response to therapy in predicting survival with ejection fraction less than or equal to 20% secondary to ischemic or nonischemic dilated cardiomyopathy. *Am J Cardiol* 66:1348–1354, 1990.
26. Rackley CE, Russell RO, Jr: Left ventricular function in acute and chronic coronary artery disease. *Annu Rev Med* 26:105–120, 1975.
27. Wilson JR, Reichek N, Dunkman WB, et al: Effect of diuresis on the performance of the failing left ventricle in man. *Am J Med* 70:234–239, 1981.
28. Stevenson L, Bellil D, Grover-McKay M, et al: Effects of afterload reduction (diuretics and vasodilators) on left ventricular volume and mitral regurgitation in severe congestive heart failure secondary to ischemic or idiopathic dilated cardiomyopathy. *Am J Cardiol* 60:654–658, 1987.
29. Palardy M, Stevenson LW, Tasissa G, et al: Reduction in mitral regurgitation during therapy guided by measured filling pressures in the ESCAPE trial. *Circ Heart Fail* 2:181–188, 2009.

30. Guiha NH, Cohn JN, Mikulic E, et al: Treatment of refractory heart failure with infusion of nitroprusside. *N Engl J Med* 291:587–592, 1974.
31. Solomonica A, Burger AJ, Aronson D: Hemodynamic determinants of dyspnea improvement in acute decompensated heart failure. *Circ Heart Fail* 6:53–60, 2013.
32. Kaye DM, Lambert GW, Lefkovits J, et al: Neurochemical evidence of cardiac sympathetic activation and increased central nervous system norepinephrine turnover in severe congestive heart failure. *J Am Coll Cardiol* 23:570–578, 1994.
33. Johnson W, Omland T, Collins CM, et al: Neurohormonal activation rapidly decreases after intravenous vasodilator and diuretic therapy for class IV heart failure. *Circulation* 98:I–780 (abstr), 1998.
34. Morley D, Brozena SC: Assessing risk by hemodynamic profile in patients awaiting cardiac transplantation. *Am J Cardiol* 73:379–383, 1994.
35. Aaronson KD, Schwartz JS, Chen TM, et al: Development and prospective validation of a clinical index to predict survival in ambulatory patients referred for cardiac transplant evaluation. *Circulation* 95:2660–2667, 1997.
36. Lucas CJW, Flavell C, Fonarow G, et al: Freedom from congestion at one month predicts good two-year survival after hospitalization for class IV heart failure. *Circulation* 94(Suppl I):I–193, 1996.
37. ESCAPE Investigators and Coordinators: Evaluation Study of Congestive Heart Failure and Pulmonary Artery Catheterization. *JAMA* 294:1625–1633, 2005.
38. Rogers JG, Nohria A, Hellkamp A, et al: Warm-dry clinical profiles at 1 month after HF hospitalization can be used for triage in advanced heart failure (abstract). *J Am Coll Cardiol* 49:2007.
39. Zile MR, Bennett TD, St John Sutton M, et al: Transition from chronic compensated to acute decompensated heart failure: pathophysiological insights obtained from continuous monitoring of intracardiac pressures. *Circulation* 118:1433–1441, 2008.
40. Stevenson LW, Zile M, Bennett TD, et al: Chronic ambulatory intracardiac pressures and future heart failure events. *Circ Heart Fail* 3:580–587, 2010.
41. Felker GM, Lee KL, Bull DA, et al: Diuretic strategies in patients with acute decompensated heart failure. *N Engl J Med* 364:797–805, 2011.
42. Bart BA, Goldsmith SR, Lee KL, et al: Ultrafiltration in decompensated heart failure with cardiorenal syndrome. *N Engl J Med* 367:2296–2304, 2012.
43. Testani JM, Chen J, McCauley BD, et al: Potential effects of aggressive decongestion during the treatment of decompensated heart failure on renal function and survival. *Circulation* 122:265–272, 2010.
44. Testani JM, Brisco MA, Chen J, et al: Timing of hemoconcentration during treatment of acute decompensated heart failure and subsequent survival: importance of sustained decongestion. *J Am Coll Cardiol* 62:516–524, 2013.
45. Dries DL, Exner DV, Domanski MJ, et al: The prognostic implications of renal insufficiency in asymptomatic and symptomatic patients with left ventricular systolic dysfunction. *J Am Coll Cardiol* 35:681–689, 2000.
46. Fonarow GC, Adams KF, Jr, Abraham WT, et al: Risk stratification for in-hospital mortality in acutely decompensated heart failure: classification and regression tree analysis. *JAMA* 293:572–580, 2005.
47. Mullens W, Abrahams Z, Francis GS, et al: Importance of venous congestion for worsening of renal function in advanced decompensated heart failure. *J Am Coll Cardiol* 53:589–596, 2009.
48. Mullens W, Abrahams Z, Skouri HN, et al: Elevated intra-abdominal pressure in acute decompensated heart failure: a potential contributor to worsening renal function? *J Am Coll Cardiol* 51:300–306, 2008.
49. Weinfeld MS, Chertow GM, Stevenson LW: Aggravated renal dysfunction during intensive therapy for advanced chronic heart failure. *Am Heart J* 138:285–290, 1999.
50. Forman DE, Butler J, Wang Y, et al: Incidence, predictors at admission, and impact of worsening renal function among patients hospitalized with heart failure. *J Am Coll Cardiol* 43:61–67, 2004.
51. Campbell P, Drazner MH, Kato M, et al: Mismatch of right- and left-sided filling pressures in chronic heart failure. *J Card Fail* 17:561–568, 2011.
52. Elkayam U, Tasissa G, Binanay C, et al: Use and impact of inotropes and vasodilator therapy in hospitalized patients with severe heart failure. *Am Heart J* 153:98–104, 2007.
53. O'Connor CM: OPTIME in CHF trial. *Eur Heart J* 5:9–12, 2003.
54. Beohar N, Erdogan AK, Lee DC, et al: Acute heart failure syndromes and coronary perfusion. *J Am Coll Cardiol* 52:13–16, 2008.
55. Mebazaa A, Nieminen MS, Packer M, et al: Levosimendan vs dobutamine for patients with acute decompensated heart failure: the SURVIVE Randomized Trial. *JAMA* 297:1883–1891, 2007.
56. VMAC Investigators: Intravenous nesiritide vs nitroglycerin for treatment of decompensated congestive heart failure: a randomized controlled trial. *JAMA* 287:1531–1540, 2002.
57. Sackner-Bernstein JD, Skopicki HA, Aaronson KD: Risk of worsening renal function with nesiritide in patients with acutely decompensated heart failure. *Circulation* 111:1487–1491, 2005.
58. Dandamudi S, Chen HH: The ASCEND-HF trial: an acute study of clinical effectiveness of nesiritide and decompensated heart failure. *Expert Rev Cardiovasc Ther* 10:557–563, 2012.
59. McMurray JJ, Teerlink JR, Cotter G, et al: Effects of tezosentan on symptoms and clinical outcomes in patients with acute heart failure: the VERITAS randomized controlled trials. *JAMA* 298:2009–2019, 2007.
60. Pang PS, Konstam MA, Krasa HB, et al: Effects of tolvaptan on dyspnoea relief from the EVEREST trials. *Eur Heart J* 30:2233–2240, 2009.
61. Chen HH, Anstrom KJ, Givertz MM, et al: Low-dose dopamine or low-dose nesiritide in acute heart failure with renal dysfunction: the ROSE acute heart failure randomized trial. *JAMA* 310(23):2533–2543, 2013.
62. Stevenson LW, Pagani FD, Young JB, et al: INTERMACS profiles of advanced heart failure: the current picture. *J Heart Lung Transplant* 28:535–541, 2009.
63. Stevenson LW, Dracup KA, Tillisch JH: Efficacy of medical therapy tailored for severe congestive heart failure in patients transferred for urgent cardiac transplantation. *Am J Cardiol* 63:461–464, 1989.
64. Kovick RB, Tillisch JH, Berens SC, et al: Vasodilator therapy for chronic left ventricular failure. *Circulation* 53:322–328, 1976.
65. Steimle AE, Stevenson LW, Chelimsky-Fallick C, et al: Sustained hemodynamic efficacy of therapy tailored to reduce filling pressures in survivors with advanced heart failure. *Circulation* 96:1165–1172, 1997.
66. Kamath SA, Drazner MH, Tasissa G, et al: Correlation of impedance cardiography with invasive hemodynamic measurements in patients with advanced heart failure: the BioImpedance CardioGraphy (BIG) substudy of the Evaluation Study of Congestive Heart Failure and Pulmonary Artery Catheterization Effectiveness (ESCAPE) Trial. *Am Heart J* 158:217–223, 2009.
67. Pierpont GL, Cohn JN, Franciosa JA: Combined oral hydralazine-nitrate therapy in left ventricular failure. Hemodynamic equivalency to sodium nitroprusside. *Chest* 73:8–13, 1978.
68. Massie B, Chatterjee K, Werner J, et al: Hemodynamic advantage of combined administration of hydralazine orally and nitrates nonparenterally in the vasodilator therapy of chronic heart failure. *Am J Cardiol* 40:794–801, 1977.
69. Cohn JN: Nitrates are effective in the treatment of chronic congestive heart failure: the protagonist's view. *Am J Cardiol* 66:444–446, 1990.
70. Elkayam U: Nitrates in the treatment of congestive heart failure. *Am J Cardiol* 77:41C–51C, 1996.
71. Colucci WS, Elkayam U, Horton DP, et al: Intravenous nesiritide, a natriuretic peptide, in the treatment of decompensated congestive heart failure. Nesiritide Study Group. *N Engl J Med* 343:246–253, 2000.
72. Fonarow GC, Chelimsky-Fallick C, Stevenson LW, et al: Effect of direct vasodilation with hydralazine versus angiotensin- converting enzyme inhibition with captopril on mortality in advanced heart failure: the Hy-C trial. *J Am Coll Cardiol* 19:842–850, 1992.
73. Unverferth DA, Blanford M, Kates RE, et al: Tolerance to dobutamine after a 72 hour continuous infusion. *Am J Med* 69:262–266, 1980.
74. Silver MA, Horton DP, Ghali JK, et al: Effect of nesiritide versus dobutamine on short-term outcomes in the treatment of patients with acutely decompensated heart failure. *J Am Coll Cardiol* 39:798–803, 2002.
75. Tsvetkova TFD, Abraham WT, Kelly P, et al: Comparative hemodynamic effects of milrinone and dobutamine in heart failure patients treated chronically with carvedilol. *J Card Fail* 4(Suppl 1):36, 1998.
76. Biddle TL, Benotti JR, Creager MA, et al: Comparison of intravenous milrinone and dobutamine for congestive heart failure secondary to either ischemic or dilated cardiomyopathy. *Am J Cardiol* 59:1345–1350, 1987.
77. Miller LW: Outpatient dobutamine for refractory congestive heart failure: advantages, techniques, and results. *J Heart Lung Transplant* 10:482–487, 1991.
78. Lang RM, Fellner SK, Neumann A, et al: Left ventricular contractility varies directly with blood ionized calcium. *Ann Intern Med* 108:524–529, 1988.
79. Argenziano M, Choudhri AF, Oz MC, et al: A prospective randomized trial of arginine vasopressin in the treatment of vasodilatory shock after left ventricular assist device placement. *Circulation* 96:II-286-90, 1997.
80. Morales DL, Gregg D, Helman DN, et al: Arginine vasopressin in the treatment of 50 patients with postcardiotomy vasodilatory shock. *Ann Thorac Surg* 69:102–106, 2000.
81. Stevenson LW: Clinical use of inotropic therapy for heart failure: looking backward or forward? Part II: chronic inotropic therapy. *Circulation* 108:492–497, 2003.
82. Binkley PF, Starling RC, Hammer DF, et al: Usefulness of hydralazine to withdraw from dobutamine in severe congestive heart failure. *Am J Cardiol* 68:1103–1106, 1991.
83. Allen LA, Stevenson LW, Grady KL, et al: Decision making in advanced heart failure: a scientific statement from the American Heart Association. *Circulation* 125:1928–1952, 2012.
84. Shah MR, Stevenson LW: Searching for evidence: refractory questions in advanced heart failure. *J Card Fail* 10:210–218, 2004.
85. Masoudi FA, Gross CP, Wang Y, et al: Adoption of spironolactone therapy for older patients with heart failure and left ventricular systolic dysfunction in the United States, 1998-2001. *Circulation* 112:39–47, 2005.
86. Gattis WA, O'Connor CM: Predischarge initiation of carvedilol in patients hospitalized for decompensated heart failure. *Am J Cardiol* 93:74B–76B, 2004.
87. Taylor AL, Ziesche S, Yancy C, et al: Combination of isosorbide dinitrate and hydralazine in blacks with heart failure. *N Engl J Med* 351:2049–2057, 2004.
88. Kittleson M, Hurwitz S, Shah MR, et al: Development of circulatory-renal limitations to angiotensin-converting enzyme inhibitors identifies patients with severe heart failure and early mortality. *J Am Coll Cardiol* 41:2029–2035, 2003.
89. Cohn JN, Johnson G, Ziesche S, et al: A comparison of enalapril with hydralazine-isosorbide dinitrate in the treatment of chronic congestive heart failure. *N Engl J Med* 325:303–310, 1991.
90. Digitalis Investigation Group: The effect of digoxin on mortality and morbidity in patients with heart failure. *N Engl J Med* 336:525–533, 1997.
91. Bristow MR, Saxon LA, Boehmer J, et al: Cardiac-resynchronization therapy with or without an implantable defibrillator in advanced chronic heart failure. *N Engl J Med* 350:2140–2150, 2004.
92. Cleland JG, Daubert JC, Erdmann E, et al: The effect of cardiac resynchronization on morbidity and mortality in heart failure. *N Engl J Med* 352:1539–1549, 2005.
93. Epstein AE, Dimarco JP, Ellenbogen KA, et al: ACC/AHA/HRS 2008 Guidelines for device-based therapy of cardiac rhythm abnormalities. *Heart Rhythm* 5:e1–e62, 2008.
94. Setoguchi S, Stevenson LW, Schneeweiss S: Repeated hospitalizations predict mortality in the community population with heart failure. *Am Heart J* 154:260–266, 2007.
95. Chen CY, Stevenson LW, Stewart GC, et al: Impact of baseline heart failure burden on post-implantable cardioverter-defibrillator mortality among medicare beneficiaries. *J Am Coll Cardiol* 61:2142–2150, 2013.
96. Ashton CM, Kuykendall DH, Johnson ML, et al: The association between the quality of inpatient care and early readmission. *Ann Intern Med* 122:415–421, 1995.
97. Albert NM: Improving medication adherence in chronic cardiovascular disease. *Crit Care Nurse* 28:54–64, quiz 5, 2008.
98. Albert NM, Buchsbaum R, Li J: Randomized study of the effect of video education on heart failure healthcare utilization, symptoms, and self-care behaviors. *Patient Educ Couns* 69:129–139, 2007.
99. Koelling TM, Johnson ML, Cody RJ, et al: Discharge education improves clinical outcomes in patients with chronic heart failure. *Circulation* 111:179–185, 2005.
100. Mebazaa A, Gheorghiade M, Pina IL, et al: Practical recommendations for prehospital and early in-hospital management of patients presenting with acute heart failure syndromes. *Crit Care Med* 36:S129–S139, 2008.
101. O'Connor CM, Hasselblad V, Mehta RH, et al: Triage after hospitalization with advanced heart failure: the ESCAPE (Evaluation Study of Congestive Heart Failure and Pulmonary Artery Catheterization Effectiveness) risk model and discharge score. *J Am Coll Cardiol* 55:872–878, 2010.
102. Desai AS, Stevenson LW: Rehospitalization for heart failure: predict or prevent? *Circulation* 126:501–506, 2012.
103. Chun S, Tu JV, Wijeysundera HC, et al: Lifetime analysis of hospitalizations and survival of patients newly admitted with heart failure. *Circ Heart Fail* 5:414–421, 2012.
104. Hummel SL, Pauli NP, Krumholz HM, et al: Thirty-day outcomes in Medicare patients with heart failure at heart transplant centers. *Circ Heart Fail* 3:244–252, 2010.
105. Lucas C, Johnson W, Hamilton MA, et al: Freedom from congestion predicts good survival despite previous class IV symptoms of heart failure. *Am Heart J* 140:840–847, 2000.
106. Russell RO, Jr, Rackley CE, Pombo J, et al: Effects of increasing left ventricular filling. Pressure in patients with acute myocardial infarction. *J Clin Invest* 49:1539–1550, 1970.

GUIDELINES

The Hospitalized Patient with Heart Failure*

Below we review the most recent heart failure guidelines regarding the patient hospitalized with acute heart failure, those released by the American College of Cardiology/American Heart Association (ACC/AHA) in 2013 (Table 33G-1). These new guidelines expand the 2009 ACC/AHA guidelines with several new class I recommendations. These include the use of BNP or NT-proBNP and/or troponin for establishing prognosis in AHF, more detailed recommendations about the appropriate use of diuretics, and more comprehensive and detailed recommendations about transitions of care from the hospital to the ambulatory setting. Although the 2013 ACC/AHA guidelines are in general agreement with the 2012 European Society of Cardiology (ESC) Heart Failure guidelines in most areas, there are some distinct areas of emphasis. These differing emphases can be seen in part in the use of the terms *hospitalized patient with HF* (in the ACC/AHA guidelines) compared to *acute heart failure* (in the ESC Guidelines). The ESC Guidelines focus in significantly more detail on specific issues of acute therapy, specifically to distinguish particular sets of more detailed recommendations in AHF patients based on phenotype (e.g., AHF with pulmonary congestion without shock, AHF with ACS, ACS with atrial fibrillation, etc.). Parenteral vasodilators receive a stronger of recommendation (IIA) in the ESC guidelines compared with the new ACC/AHA guidelines (IIB). In contrast, the new ACC/AHA guidelines provide more detailed recommendations about transitions and follow-up after discharge from the hospital.

*From Felker GM, Teerlink JR: Guidelines: management of heart failure with reduced ejection fraction. In Mann DL, Zipes DP, Libby P, et al, editors: *Braunwald's heart disease: a textbook of cardiovascular medicine*, ed 10, Philadelphia, 2015, Saunders.

TABLE 33G-1 ACC/AHA Recommendations for the Hospitalized Patient

CLASS	INDICATION	LEVEL OF EVIDENCE
Biomarkers		
I	Measurement of BNP or NT-proBNP is useful to support clinical judgment for the diagnosis of acutely decompensated HF, especially in the setting of uncertainty for the diagnosis.	A
I	Measurement of BNP or NT-proBNP and/or cardiac troponin is useful for establishing prognosis or disease severity in acutely decompensated HF.	A
IIB	The usefulness of BNP- or NT-proBNP–guided therapy for acutely decompensated HF is not well established.	C
IIB	Measurement of other clinically available tests such as biomarkers of myocardial injury or fibrosis may be considered for additive risk stratification in patients with acutely decompensated HF.	A
Precipitating Causes of AHF		
I	ACS precipitating acute HF decompensation should be promptly identified by ECG and serum biomarkers, including cardiac troponin testing, and treated optimally as appropriate to the overall condition and prognosis of the patient.	C
I	Common precipitating factors for acute HF should be considered during initial evaluation, as recognition of these conditions is critical to guide appropriate therapy.	C
Invasive Evaluation		
I	Invasive hemodynamic monitoring with a pulmonary artery catheter should be performed to guide therapy in patients who have respiratory distress or clinical evidence of impaired perfusion in whom the adequacy or excess of intracardiac filling pressures cannot be determined from clinical assessment.	C
IIA	Invasive hemodynamic monitoring can be useful for carefully selected patients with acute HF who have persistent symptoms despite empiric adjustment of standard therapies and: a. Whose fluid status, perfusion, or systemic or pulmonary vascular resistance is uncertain; b. Whose systolic pressure remains low, or is associated with symptoms, despite initial therapy; c. Whose renal function is worsening with therapy; d. Who require parenteral vasoactive agents; or e. Who may need consideration for MCS or transplantation	C
III	Routine use of invasive hemodynamic monitoring is not recommended in normotensive patients with acute decompensated HF and congestion with symptomatic response to diuretics and vasodilators.	B
Maintenance of GDMT During Hospitalization		
I	In patients with HFrEF experiencing a symptomatic exacerbation of HF requiring hospitalization during chronic maintenance treatment with GDMT, it is recommended that GDMT be continued in the absence of hemodynamic instability or contraindications.	B
I	Initiation of β-blocker therapy is recommended after optimization of volume status and successful discontinuation of intravenous diuretics, vasodilators, and inotropic agents. β-blocker therapy should be initiated at a low dose and only in stable patients. Caution should be used when initiating β-blockers in patients who have required inotropes during their hospital course.	B
Diuretics		
I	Patients with HF admitted with evidence of significant fluid overload should be promptly treated with intravenous loop diuretics to reduce morbidity.	B
I	If patients are already receiving loop diuretic therapy, the initial intravenous dose should equal or exceed their chronic oral daily dose and should be given as either intermittent boluses or continuous infusion. Urine output and signs and symptoms of congestion should be serially assessed, and the diuretic dose should be adjusted accordingly to relieve symptoms, reduce volume excess, and avoid hypotension.	B

Continued

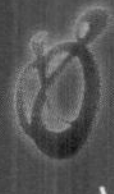

TABLE 33G-1 ACC/AHA Recommendations for the Hospitalized Patient—cont'd

CLASS	INDICATION	LEVEL OF EVIDENCE
I	The effect of HF treatment should be monitored with careful measurement of fluid intake and output, vital signs, body weight that is determined at the same time each day, and clinical signs and symptoms of systemic perfusion and congestion. Daily serum electrolytes, urea nitrogen, and creatinine concentrations should be measured during the use of intravenous diuretics or active titration of HF medications.	C
IIA	When diuresis is inadequate to relieve symptoms, it is reasonable to intensify the diuretic regimen using either: a. Higher doses of intravenous loop diuretics b. Addition of a second (e.g., thiazide) diuretic	B
IIB	Low-dose dopamine infusion may be considered in addition to loop diuretic therapy to improve diuresis and better preserve renal function and renal blood flow.	B
Venous Thromboembolism Prophylaxis		
I	A patient admitted to the hospital with decompensated HF should receive venous thromboembolism prophylaxis with an anticoagulant medication if the risk-benefit ratio is favorable.	B
Ultrafiltration		
IIB	Ultrafiltration may be considered for patients with obvious volume overload to alleviate congestive symptoms and fluid weight.	B
IIB	Ultrafiltration may be considered for patients with refractory congestion not responding to medical therapy.	C
Parenteral Therapy		
IIB	If symptomatic hypotension is absent, intravenous nitroglycerin, nitroprusside, or nesiritide may be considered an adjuvant to diuretic therapy for relief of dyspnea in patients admitted with acutely decompensated HF.	A
Inotropic Support and Mechanical Circulatory Support (MCS)		
I	Until definitive therapy (e.g., coronary revascularization, MCS, heart transplantation) or resolution of the acute precipitating problem, patients with cardiogenic shock should receive temporary intravenous inotropic support to maintain systemic perfusion and preserve end-organ performance.	C
IIA	Nondurable MCS is reasonable as a "bridge to recovery" or "bridge to decision" for carefully selected patients with HF and acute profound disease.	B
IIB	Short-term, continuous intravenous inotropic support may be reasonable in those hospitalized patients presenting with documented severe systolic dysfunction who present with low blood pressure and significantly depressed cardiac output to maintain systemic perfusion and preserve end-organ performance.	B
III	Use of parenteral inotropic agents in hospitalized patients without documented severe systolic dysfunction, low blood pressure, or impaired perfusion, and evidence of significantly depressed cardiac output, with or without congestion, is potentially harmful.	B
Arginine Vasopressin Antagonists		
IIB	In patients hospitalized with volume overload, including HF, who have persistent severe hyponatremia and are at risk for or having active cognitive symptoms despite water restriction and maximization of GDMT, vasopressin antagonists may be considered in the short term to improve serum sodium concentration in hypervolemic, hyponatremic states with either a V2 receptor selective or a nonselective vasopressin antagonist.	B
Transitions of Care		
I	The use of performance improvement systems and/or evidence-based systems of care is recommended in the hospital and early postdischarge outpatient setting to identify appropriate HF patients for GDMT, provide clinicians with useful reminders to advance GDMT, and assess the clinical response.	B
I	Throughout the hospitalization as appropriate, before hospital discharge, at the first postdischarge visit, and in subsequent follow-up visits, the following should be addressed: a. Initiation of GDMT if not done or contraindicated; b. Causes of HF, barriers to care, and limitations in support; c. Assessment of volume status and blood pressure with adjustment of HF therapy; d. Optimization of chronic oral HF therapy; e. Renal function and electrolytes; f. Management of comorbid conditions; g. HF education, self-care, emergency plans, and adherence; h. Palliative or hospice care	B
I	Multidisciplinary HF disease-management programs are recommended for patients at high risk for hospital readmission, to facilitate the implementation of GDMT, to address different barriers to behavioral change, and to reduce the risk of subsequent rehospitalization for HF.	B
IIA	Scheduling an early follow-up visit (within 7 to 14 days) and early telephone follow-up (within 3 days) of hospital discharge is reasonable.	B
IIA	Use of clinical risk-prediction tools and/or biomarkers to identify patients at higher risk for postdischarge clinical events is reasonable.	B

34 Contemporary Medical Therapy for Heart Failure Patients with Reduced Ejection Fraction

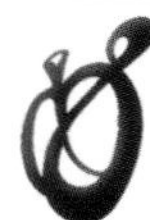

Robert J. Mentz, Douglas L. Mann, and G. Michael Felker

Heart failure (HF) is a complex clinical syndrome that represents a final common pathway for many types of cardiovascular disease. Multiple overlapping frameworks for classifying heart failure exist (**see also Chapters 17 and 28**). HF can be viewed as continuum that is comprised of four interrelated stages as defined by the American College of Cardiology and the American Heart Association (ACC/AHA) Guidelines (**Figure 34-1**).[1] Stage A patients represent the largest group, defined as patients who are at high risk for developing HF, but who do not yet have evidence of structural heart disease or symptoms of HF (e.g., patients with diabetes or hypertension; **see also Chapter 32**). Stage B includes patients who have structural heart disease, but without symptoms of HF (e.g., patients with a previous myocardial infarction (MI), left ventricular hypertrophy, or asymptomatic left ventricular [LV] dysfunction). Stage C includes patients who have structural heart disease and have developed symptoms of HF. Stage D includes patients with refractory HF requiring special interventions (e.g., patients who may be candidates for left ventricular assist devices or cardiac transplantation; **see also Chapters 40 and 42**).

Epidemiologically, a large (and growing) proportion of patients with symptomatic heart failure have normal or near normal ejection fraction, so-called heart failure with preserved ejection fraction or HFpEF. This clinical entity, for which highly effective therapies have yet to be developed, is covered in detail in **Chapter 36**. Similarly, acute decompensated heart failure leading to hospitalization is a major public health problem and is covered in detail in **Chapter 33**. In the current chapter, we will focus on contemporary medical therapy for patients with symptomatic heart failure and reduced ejection fraction (HFrEF), with a focus on both the biologic rationale and the clinical evidence supporting contemporary treatment. Notably, few areas in medicine have seen as much progress in the development of effective new therapies over recent decades as has the treatment of HFrEF, with multiple classes of agents and devices (which are covered separately in **Chapter 35**) having demonstrated major improvements in morbidity and mortality over this period (**Figure 34-2**).

GOALS OF THERAPY IN HFrEF

The main goals of treatment in heart failure are to reduce symptoms, improve quality of life and functional capacity, prolong survival, and prevent disease progression. Although different therapies may impact these goals to varying degrees, the contemporary medical therapy for HFrEF has made a significant impact on each of these outcomes, as detailed later.

General Measures

Diet and Fluid Restriction

Dietary restriction of sodium (2-3 g daily) is commonly recommended in all patients with symptomatic heart failure, based on the rationale that sodium and fluid retention are a central aspect of heart failure pathophysiology. Although the recommendation for sodium restriction has been a long-standing cornerstone of heart failure management, the body of evidence on which these recommendations are based is relatively scant, and the level of evidence for fluid restriction in recent guidelines is based primarily on expert opinion only (class IIa recommendation, level of evidence C).[1] Indeed, some studies have suggested that sodium restriction may actually worsen the neurohormonal profile and may lead to worsened outcomes.[2] Strict fluid restriction is generally unnecessary in most patients unless the patient is hyponatremic (<130 mEq/L), which may develop because of activation of the renin-angiotensin system, excessive secretion of arginine vasopressin (AVP), or loss of salt in excess of water from prior diuretic use. Fluid restriction (<2 L day) should be considered in hyponatremic patients or for those patients whose fluid retention is difficult to control despite high doses of diuretics and sodium restriction.

Activity

Regular physical activity or exercise training is recommended for heart failure patients (class I, level of evidence A) by the current ACC-AHA guidelines.[1] This recommendation is based on studies and meta-analyses suggesting that

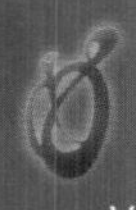

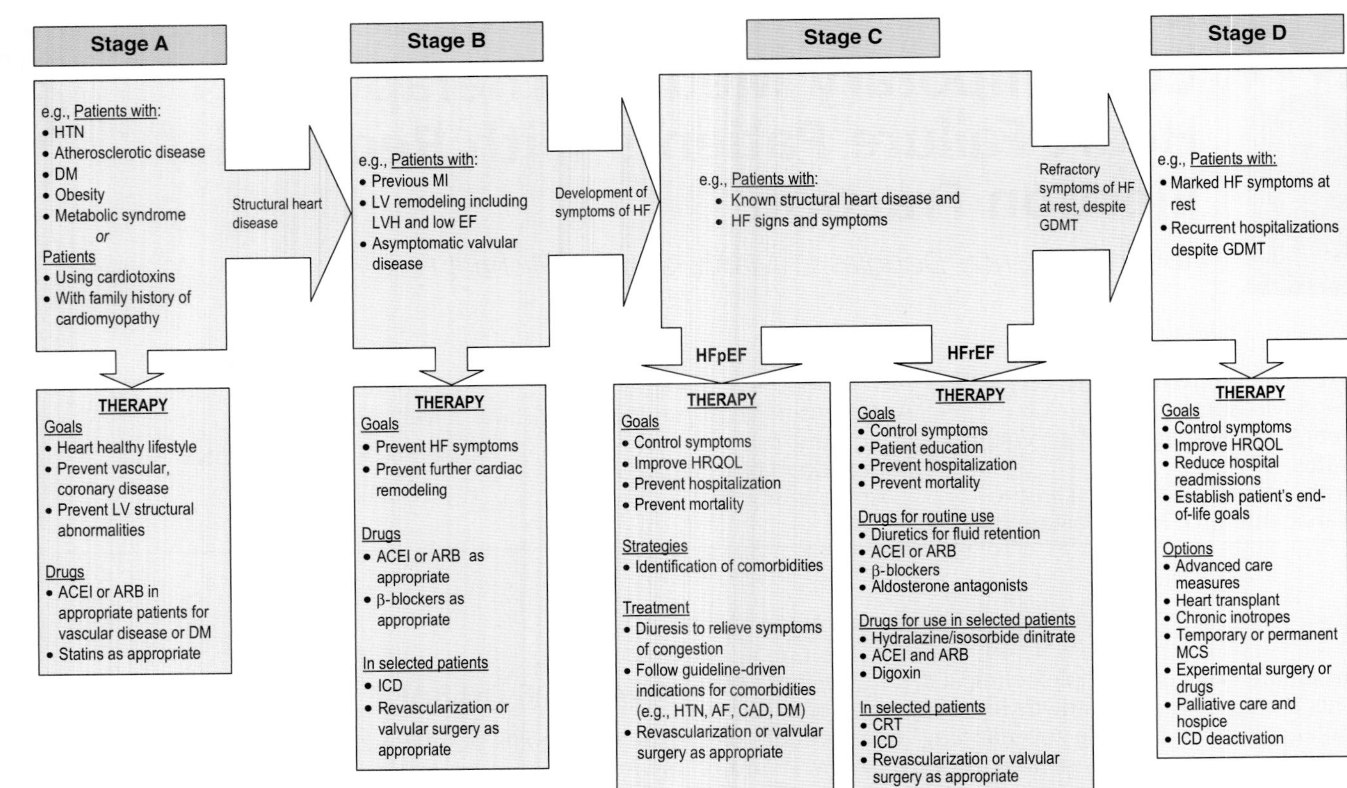

FIGURE 34-1 AHA-ACC stages of heart failure. *ACEI,* Angiotensin-converting enzyme inhibitor; *AF,* atrial fibrillation; *ARB,* angiotensin receptor blocker; *CAD,* coronary artery disease; *CRT,* cardiac resynchronization therapy; *DM,* diabetes mellitus; *EF,* ejection fraction; *GDMT,* guideline-directed medical therapy; *HF,* heart failure; *HRQOL,* health-related quality of life; *HTN,* hypertension; *ICD,* implantable cardioverter-defibrillator; *LV(H),* left ventricular hypertrophy; *MCS,* mechanical circulatory support; *MI,* myocardial infarction. *Modified from Hunt SA, Abraham WT, Chin MH, et al: 2009 focused update incorporated into the ACC/AHA 2005 guidelines for the diagnosis and management of heart failure in adults: a report of the American College of Cardiology Foundation/American Heart Association task force on practice guidelines: developed in collaboration with the International Society for Heart and Lung Transplantation. Circulation 119:e391–e479, 2009; and Yancy CW, Jessup M, Bozkurt B, et al: 2013 ACCF/AHA guideline for the management of heart failure: a report of the American College of Cardiology Foundation/American Heart Association task force on practice guidelines. Circulation 128:e240–327, 2013.*

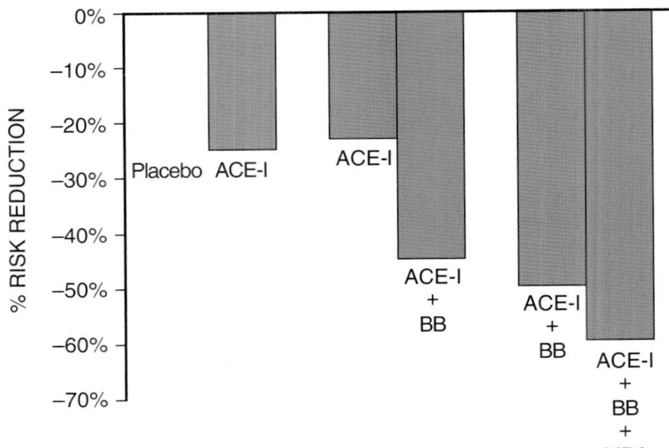

FIGURE 34-2 Mortality improvements for contemporary HFrEF medications. *ACEI,* Angiotensin-converting enzyme inhibitor; *BB,* β-blocker; *MRA,* mineralocorticoid receptor antagonist.

exercise training improves functional capacity, quality of life, and clinical outcomes in patients with heart failure. Unlike many lifestyle interventions, exercise training has been rigorously studied in a large randomized outcomes trial. The HF-ACTION trial (A Controlled Trial Investigating Outcomes of Exercise Training) was a large multicenter randomized controlled study of exercise training that enrolled patients with an ejection fraction (EF) of 35% or less and NYHA class II-IV symptoms with a primary endpoint of all-cause mortality and all-cause hospitalization.[3] In this study, structured exercise training demonstrated a modest improvement in all-cause mortality and hospitalizations after adjustment for other variables, as well as improvements in functional capacity and quality of life (**Figure 34-3**). Notably, in the HF-ACTION study there was no evidence that exercise training in heart failure was unsafe, even in patients with relatively severe heart failure symptoms.

Therapies to Avoid

Several common classes of medications may exacerbate symptoms of heart failure and potentially lead to disease progression, and thus should be avoided in patients with heart failure. Nonsteroidal anti-inflammatory drugs (NSAIDs) inhibit the synthesis of prostaglandins and lead to sodium and fluid retention, and may lead to worsening heart failure. Thiazolidinediones are a class of antidiabetic agents that may lead to fluid retention and have been shown to increase the rate of heart failure events in previous clinical trials. Calcium channel blockers, which are frequently used for the management of hypertension and angina, have negative inotropic properties that may worsen heart failure and should generally not be used in patients with heart failure. The dihydropyridine calcium channel blockers (e.g., amlodipine) have been studied in HF, and although

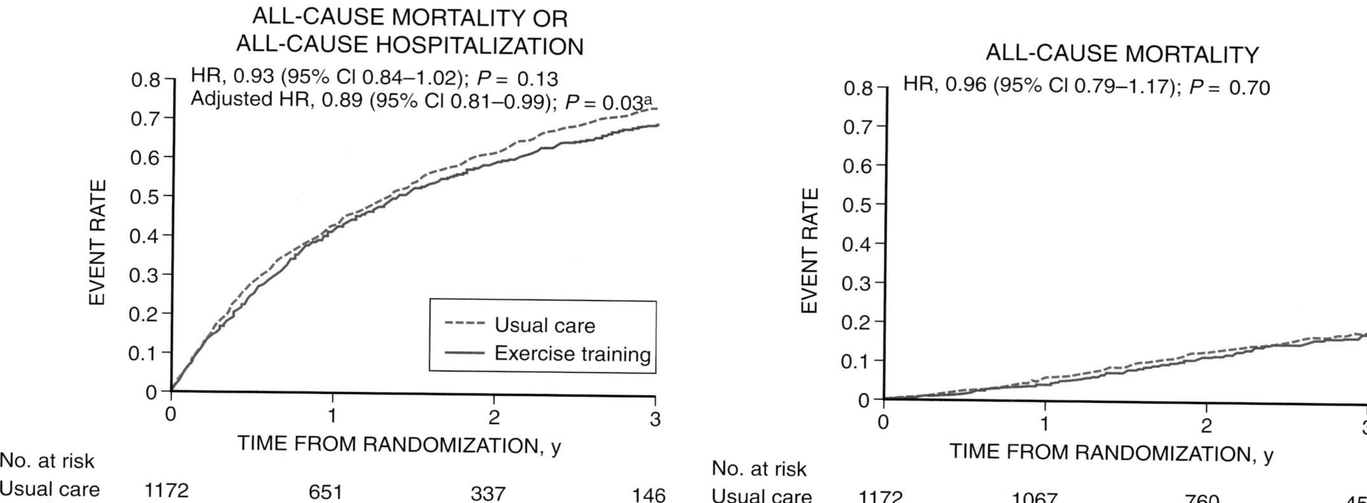

FIGURE 34-3 Time to all-cause mortality or all-cause hospitalization and to all-cause mortality with structured exercise training compared with usual care in the HF-ACTION trial. *CI*, Confidence interval; *HR*, hazard ratio. [a]Adjusted for key prognostic factors. *Reproduced from O'Connor CM, Whellan DJ, Lee KL, et al: Efficacy and safety of exercise training in patients with chronic heart failure: HF-ACTION randomized controlled trial. JAMA 301:1439–1450, 2009.*

not efficacious as a heart failure therapy, appear to be safe in heart failure patients if needed for management of hypertension or angina.[4,5] The use of dietary supplements should generally be avoided in the management of symptomatic HF because of the lack of proven benefit and the potential for significant interactions with proven HF therapeutics.

Diuretics and Management of Volume Status

Many of the cardinal clinical manifestations of HF result from excessive salt and water retention that leads to an inappropriate volume expansion of the vascular and extravascular space. Most patients with symptomatic chronic heart failure therefore require diuretic therapy to maintain appropriate volume status and to control symptoms related to fluid retention.

A number of classification schemes have been proposed for diuretics on the basis of their mechanism of action and their anatomic locus of action within the nephron. The most common classification for diuretics employs an admixture of chemical (e.g., "thiazide" diuretic), site of action (e.g., "loop" diuretics), or clinical outcomes (e.g., "potassium-sparing" diuretics). Classes of diuretics and their mechanisms of action are shown in **Figure 34-4**.

Loop Diuretics

The loop diuretics are the primary form of diuretic used in patients with heart failure. These agents increase sodium excretion by up to 20% to 25% of the filtered load of sodium, enhance free water clearance, and maintain their efficacy unless renal function is severely impaired. The agents in this class, which include furosemide, bumetanide, and torsemide, act by reversibly inhibiting the Na^+-K^+-$2Cl^-$ symporter (cotransporter) on the apical membrane of epithelial cells in the thick ascending loop of Henle (see Figure 34-4), resulting in decreased urine sodium and chloride reabsorption with natriuresis and diuresis. The increase in delivery of Na^+ and water to the distal nephron segments also markedly enhances K^+ excretion, particularly in the presence of elevated aldosterone levels. Loop diuretics have a sigmoidal-shaped dose response relationship (**Figure 34-5**).[6] Importantly, in both heart failure and renal insufficiency, the dose response for loop diuretics curve shifts downward and to the right, thereby necessitating a higher dose to achieve the same effect.

Because furosemide, bumetanide, and torsemide are bound extensively to plasma proteins, delivery of these drugs to the tubule by filtration is limited. However, these drugs are secreted efficiently by the organic acid transport system in the proximal tubule and thereby gain access to their binding sites on the Na^+-K^+-$2Cl^-$ symporter in the luminal membrane of the ascending limb. Thus the efficacy of loop diuretics is dependent upon sufficient renal plasma blood flow and proximal tubular secretion to deliver these agents to their site of action. Although these drugs have similar mechanisms of action, they differ in terms of bioavailability and pharmacokinetics in ways that may have important clinical implications (**Table 34-1**).[7]

Thiazides and Thiazide-Like Diuretics

Thiazide-type diuretics inhibit the Na/Cl cotransporter in the distal tubule, thus blocking sodium resorption[8] (see Figure 34-4). Commonly used drugs in this class include hydrochlorothiazide, chlorthalidone, chlorothiazide, and metolazone (which is not technically a thiazide but has similar properties). Thiazides have been shown to be a potentially powerful adjunct to loop diuretics (so-called sequential nephron blockade), especially in patients demonstrating a substantial degree of diuretic resistance and/or with significant renal dysfunction. The potential benefits imparted by the addition of a thiazide-type diuretic must be balanced against the potential risks, specifically the risk of resulting electrolyte and metabolic abnormalities. Hypokalemia in particular is a frequent consequence of the sequential nephron blockade that results from combining a thiazide-type diuretic with a loop diuretic. Other electrolyte abnormalities, such as hyponatremia and hypomagnesemia, are also common and may be severe. Use of these agents as an adjunct to loop diuretics in the outpatient setting should generally be done with caution and only with frequent monitoring.

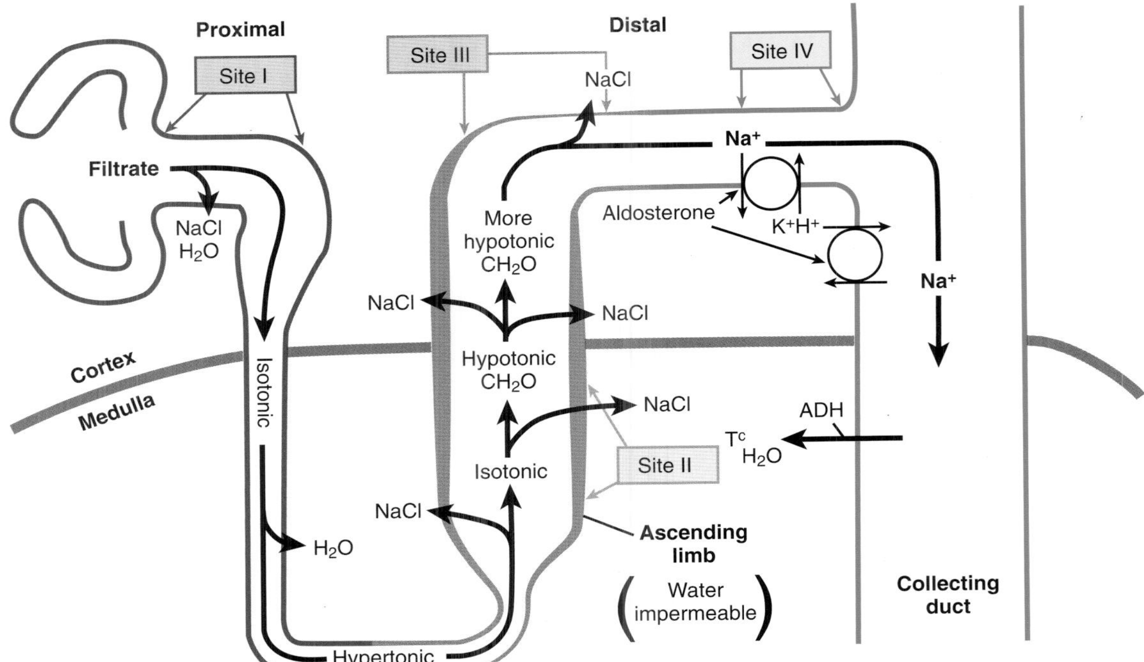

FIGURE 34-4 Classes of diuretics and their mechanisms of actions. *MRA,* Mineralocorticoid receptor antagonist. *Modified from Wile D: Diuretics: a review. Ann Clin Biochem 49:419–431, 2012.*

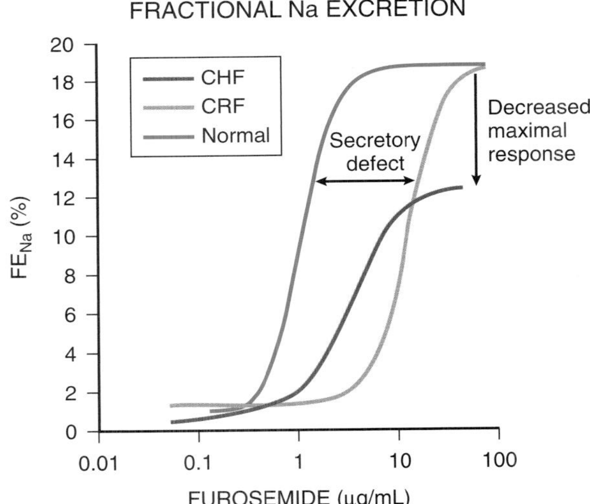

FIGURE 34-5 Dose response curves of loop diuretics in chronic heart failure (CHF) and chronic renal failure (CRF) patients compared with normal controls. In heart failure patients, higher doses are required to achieve a given diuretic effect and the maximal effect is blunted. *Reproduced from Ellison DH: Diuretic therapy and resistance in congestive heart failure. Cardiology 96:132–143, 2001.*

Mineralocorticoid Receptor Antagonists and Potassium Sparing Diuretics

Mineralocorticoid receptor antagonists (MRAs), such as spironolactone and eplerenone, are weak diuretics at commonly used doses, but are generally used in HF patients as neurohormonal antagonists rather than for their diuretic properties (as described in detail later). High doses of MRAs (e.g., doses of spironolactone of 100 mg/day or more) may induce substantial diuresis, and can be used as a therapy for refractory diuretic resistance, although careful monitoring of potassium and renal function is required.[9] Potassium sparing diuretics such as triamterene are mild diuretics, but are typically not effective in HF patients and are seldom used clinically in this population.

Vasopressin Antagonists

Increased circulating levels of the pituitary hormone AVP contribute to the increased systemic vascular resistance and positive water balance in HF patients. The cellular effects of AVP are mediated by interactions with three types of receptors: V_{1a}, V_{1b}, and V_2. Selective V_{1a} antagonists block the vasoconstricting effects of AVP in peripheral vascular smooth muscle cells, whereas V_2 selective receptor antagonists inhibit recruitment of aquaporin water channels into the apical membranes of collecting duct epithelial cells, thereby reducing the ability of the collecting duct to resorb water. The AVP antagonists or "vaptans" were developed to selectively block the V_2 receptor (tolvaptan) or nonselectively block both the V_{1a}/V_2 receptors (conivaptan). These agents are not diuretics per se but have been termed *aquaretics* because they lead to exertion of free water rather than natriuresis. Long-term therapy with the V_2 selective vasopressin antagonist tolvaptan did not improve mortality but appears to be safe when given chronically after a heart failure hospitalization.[10] There was some evidence to suggest that tolvaptan improved short-term symptoms of dyspnea, a concept currently undergoing further study.[11] The two currently FDA-approved vasopressin antagonists (conivaptan and tolvaptan) are not specifically approved for HF, but are approved for the treatment of hyponatremia in patients with HF.

TABLE 34-1 Pharmacokinetics of the Loop Diuretics

PROPERTY	FUROSEMIDE	BUMETANIDE	TORSEMIDE
Relative IV potency	40 mg	1 mg	20 mg
Bioavailability (%)	10-100 (average = 50)	80-100	80-100
PO to IV conversion	2:1	1:1	1:1
Initial outpatient PO dose (mg)	20-40	0.5-1	5-10
Maintenance outpatient PO dose (mg)	40-240	1-5	10-20
Maximum daily IV dose (mg)	400-600	10	200
Onset (min)			
Oral	30-60	30-60	30-60
Intravenous	5	2-3	10
Peak serum concentration after PO administration (h)	1	1-2	1
Affected by food	Yes	Yes	No
Metabolism	50% renal conjugation	50% hepatic	80% hepatic
Half-life (h)			
Normal	1.5-2	1	3-4
Renal dysfunction	2.8	1.6	4-5
Hepatic dysfunction	2.5	2.3	8
Heart failure	2.7	1.3	6
Average duration of effect (h)	6-8	4-6	6-8

From Felker GM, Mentz RJ: Diuretics and ultrafiltration in acute decompensated heart failure. J Am Coll Cardiol 59:2145–2153, 2012.

Practical Issues in the Use of Diuretics in Heart Failure

Patients with evidence of volume overload or a history of fluid retention should be treated with a diuretic to relieve their symptoms. In patients who have moderate to severe HF symptoms and/or renal insufficiency, a loop diuretic is generally required. Diuretics should generally be titrated as needed to relieve signs and symptoms of fluid overload. One commonly used method for finding the appropriate dose is to double the dose until the desired effect is achieved or the maximal dose of diuretic is reached. Patients with chronic heart failure can be instructed on parameters for self-adjustment of diuretics based on daily weights and symptoms (see also Chapter 44). Although furosemide is the most commonly used loop diuretic, bumetanide or torsemide may be preferable in selected patients because of their increased bioavailability (see Table 34-1). Changing to torsemide in particular may induce diuresis in patients seemingly refractory to oral furosemide. With the exception of torsemide, the commonly used loop diuretics are short acting (<3 hours). For this reason, loop diuretics usually are more effective when given at least twice daily to minimize periods where the concentration in the tubular fluid declines below a therapeutic level, which may produce postdiuretic sodium retention or "rebound."[6] Infrequent dosing may therefore lead to sodium retention that exceeds natriuresis, especially if dietary sodium intake is not restricted.

Risks of Diuretic Use

Observational studies have shown associations between loop diuretics, especially at higher doses, and adverse clinical outcomes in patients with heart failure.[12] These observations are confounded by the fact that patients receiving higher doses of diuretics tend to have greater disease severity or comorbidity, making it difficult to determine whether higher doses of diuretics are simply a marker for greater heart failure severity or are actually causing harm in HF patients. Postulated mechanisms for worse outcomes with loop diuretics include stimulation of the RAAS and sympathetic nervous system, electrolyte disturbances, and deterioration of renal function. Although randomized data on the use of diuretics in HF are limited, the largest randomized study to date of diuretics in patients with acute decompensated heart failure (the DOSE study) did not suggest that higher doses of diuretics were associated with significant harm (see also Chapter 33).[13]

Patients with HF who are receiving diuretics should be monitored for complications of diuretics on a regular basis. The major complications of diuretic use include electrolyte and metabolic disturbances, volume depletion, and worsening azotemia. The interval for reassessment should be individualized based on severity of illness and underlying renal function; the use of concomitant medications such as angiotensin-converting enzyme inhibitors (ACEIs), angiotensin receptor blockers (ARBs), and MRAs; the past history of electrolyte imbalances; and/or need for more aggressive diuresis.

Diuretic use can lead to potassium depletion, which can predispose the patient to significant cardiac arrhythmias and sudden death.[14] Renal potassium losses from diuretic use can be also exacerbated by the increase in circulating levels of aldosterone observed in patients with advanced HF, as well by the marked increases in distal nephron Na^+ delivery that follow use of either loop or distal nephron diuretics. Serum potassium levels should generally be maintained between 4.0 and 5.0 mEq/L. Hypokalemia can be prevented by increasing the dietary intake of KCL, although most patients on significant doses of loop diuretics will require oral potassium supplementation. Diuretics may be associated with multiple other metabolic and electrolyte disturbances, including hyponatremia, hypomagnesemia, metabolic alkalosis, hyperglycemia, hyperlipidemia, and hyperuricemia.

Diuretic Resistance and Management

One inherent limitation of diuretics is that they achieve water loss via excretion of solute at the expense of glomerular filtration, which in turn activates a set of homeostatic mechanisms that ultimately limit their effectiveness. The term *diuretic resistance* typically defines a clinical scenario with progressively diminished responsiveness to diuretics despite persistent signs and/or symptoms of volume excess. One common cause of diuretic resistance is the so-called braking phenomenon to the effect of loop

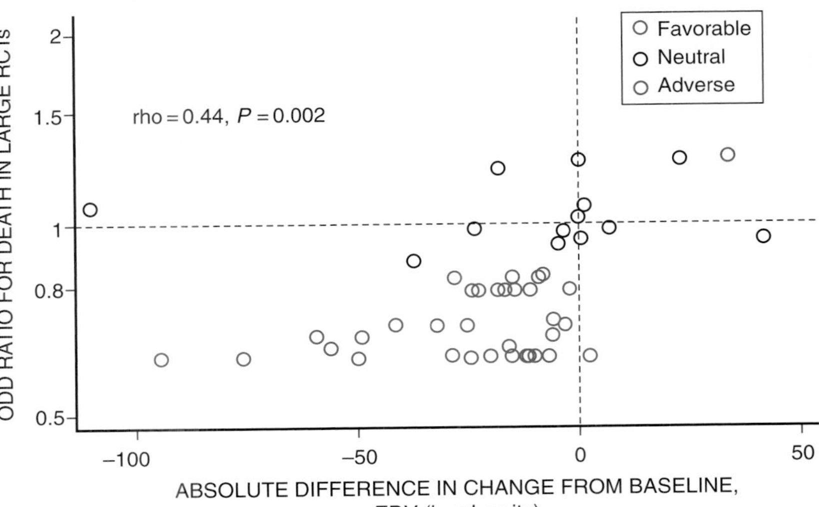

FIGURE 34-6 Relationship between drug effect on ventricular remodeling and mortality in randomized trials. Quantitative relationship between drug effects on end-diastolic volume and mortality: each data point represents a placebo-corrected change in EDV from an individual remodeling trial plotted against the mortality odds ratio (OR) for the specific therapy. Interventions were classified as favorable *(blue circles)* if the upper limit of the 95% confidence interval (CI) of the OR for death from the mortality trials was less than 1, neutral *(black circles)* if the 95% CI crossed 1, and adverse *(red circles)* if the lower limit of the 95% CI was greater than 1. There were significant correlations between short-term therapeutic effects on EDV and longer-term therapeutic effect on mortality. *EDV,* End-diastolic volume; *RCTs,* randomized clinical trials. *Reproduced from Kramer DG, Trikalinos TA, Kent DM, et al: Quantitative evaluation of drug or device effects on ventricular remodeling as predictors of therapeutic effects on mortality in patients with heart failure and reduced ejection fraction: a meta-analytic approach. J Am Coll Cardiol 56:392–406, 2010.*

diuretics—this results from hemodynamic changes at the glomerulus mediated by the RAAS and sympathetic nervous system[15] and adaptive changes in the distal nephron.[16] Additionally, as mentioned above, most loop diuretics, with the exception of torsemide, are short-acting drugs. Accordingly, after a period of natriuresis, the diuretic concentration in plasma and tubular fluid declines below the diuretic threshold. In this situation, renal Na^+ reabsorption is no longer inhibited and a period of antinatriuresis or postdiuretic NaCl retention ensues. If dietary NaCl intake is moderate to excessive, postdiuretic NaCl retention may overcome the initial natriuresis in patients with excessive activation of the adrenergic nervous system and renin-angiotensin system. Other potential contributors to apparent diuretic resistance include changes in cardiac or renal function or patient noncompliance with their diuretic regimen or diet. Concurrent use of drugs that adversely affect renal function, such as NSAIDs and COX-2 inhibitors, may contribute to diuretic resistance.

Management of patients with progressive resistance to diuretics requires careful consideration of potential causes (see also Chapter 33). Increasing doses of diuretics to ensure that therapeutic concentrations are achieved in the tubule is the typical initial step. Another common method for treating the diuretic-resistant patient is to administer two classes of diuretic concurrently ("sequential nephron blockade"). Most commonly, this involves adding a thiazide-like diuretic to a loop diuretic. Many clinicians choose metolazone because its half-life is longer than that of some other distal collecting tubule diuretics, and because it has been reported to remain effective even when the glomerular filtration rate is low. As noted above, careful monitoring of fluid status, renal function, and electrolytes is critical with this approach, as sequential nephron blockade can be associated with dramatic fluid shifts and electrolyte disturbances.

Neurohormonal Antagonists in the Management of Heart Failure

Maladaptive chronic activation of the renin-angiotensin-aldosterone axis and sympathetic nervous system is central to modern understanding of the pathophysiology of heart failure (see Chapters 5 and 6). The clinical development of drugs that antagonize these axes has been the most fundamental and important development in the management of chronic HF, establishing for the first time the ability of medical therapy to change the natural history of the disease process. In this regard, inhibitors of the renin-angiotensin-aldosterone system (ACEIs, ARB, and MRAs) and β-blockers have emerged as cornerstones of modern HF therapy for patients with HFrEF (see Figure 34-2). The ability of therapies to effectively intervene on ventricular remodeling has been consistently shown to be the most reliable surrogate for predicting subsequent efficacy in improving clinical outcomes (**Figure 34-6**). These classes of agents, often collectively referred to as *neurohormonal antagonists,* have been shown to arrest, prevent, and even (particularly for β-blockers) potentially reverse the process of progressive ventricular remodeling that is associated with disease progression in heart failure (**Figure 34-7**). As will be described in detail later, these agents have a large evidence base definitively establishing their efficacy in improving morbidity and mortality in patients with chronic heart failure and reduced EF, which are summarized in current ACC/AHA guidelines as "guideline-directed medical therapy," or GDMT (see Figure 34-1).

ACE Inhibitors and ARBs

Rationale/Pathophysiologic Basis for Use

Activation of the renin-angiotensin-aldosterone system (RAAS) plays a key role in the pathophysiology of the development and progression of HF. The fundamental biology of this complex neurohormonal axis as it relates to HF is covered in Chapter 5. The RAAS may be inhibited at many levels: renin inhibition, inhibition of the conversion of angiotensin I to angiotensin II, antagonism of one or more angiotensin II receptors, and blockade of the primary target of aldosterone, the mineralocorticoid receptor.

ACE Inhibitors

Angiotensin-converting enzyme (ACE) inhibitors were the first agents clinically available for inhibiting the RAAS and continue to be the most widely used in clinical practice. ACE inhibitors interfere with the renin-angiotensin system by inhibiting the enzyme that is responsible for the conversion of angiotensin I to angiotensin II. These agents act by

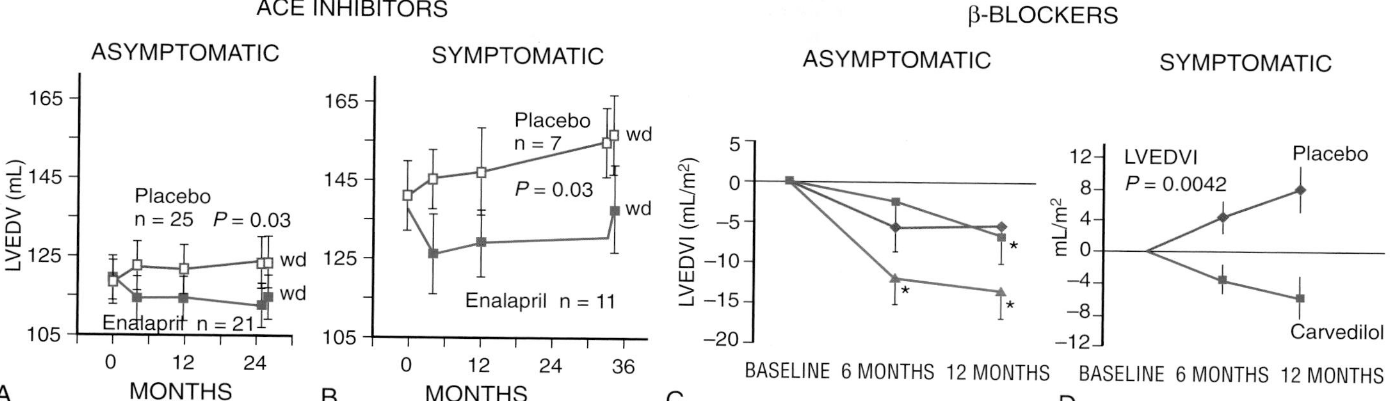

FIGURE 34-7 The effect of angiotensin-converting enzyme (ACE) inhibitors and β-blockers on ventricular remodeling. **A** and **B**, Left ventricular end-diastolic volumes (LVEDV) (mean ± SE) in enalapril and placebo patients within the prevention trial and the previously reported treatment trial who had measurements made at all five time points. Measurements are at baseline, 4 months, 1 year, and at study end (mean of 25 months and 33 months for prevention trial and treatment trial patients, respectively). The final data point on each graph is after withdrawal (wd) of study drug for a minimum of 5 days. *P* values shown are for comparison of placebo and enalapril groups by repeated-measures analysis applied to all time points. Baseline volumes were significantly higher in treatment trial patients ($P < 0.005$). In the prevention trial and the treatment trial, placebo-treated patients manifested progressive increases in ventricular volumes, whereas enalapril-treated patients showed an early and sustained reduction in LV volumes. Treatment difference between the placebo and enalapril groups was significantly greater within the treatment trial than within the prevention trial ($P < 0.02$ at 1 year). **C**, Effect of metoprolol succinate on LV volumes. Shown are the least square mean changes (SE) in LVEDVI (B) compared with baseline for patients receiving metoprolol succinate 200 mg *(triangles)*, 50 mg *(squares)*, or placebo *(diamonds)*. $^*P < 0.05$ versus baseline. **D**, Changes in left ventricular end-diastolic volume index (LVEDVI) from baseline (BL) to 6 months (6M) and 12 months (12M). Data are presented as mean value ± SE. *P* values comparing carvedilol and placebo are for repeated measures multivariate analysis of variance (MANOVA) over 12 months of treatment. ***A** and **B**, Reproduced from Konstam MA, Kronenberg MW, Rousseau MF, et al: Effects of the angiotensin converting enzyme inhibitor enalapril on the long-term progression of left ventricular dilatation in patients with asymptomatic systolic dysfunction. SOLVD (Studies of Left Ventricular Dysfunction) Investigators. Circulation 88:2277–2283, 1993. **C**, Reproduced from Colucci WS, Kolias TJ, Adams KF, et al: Metoprolol reverses left ventricular remodeling in patients with asymptomatic systolic dysfunction: the REversal of VEntricular Remodeling with Toprol-XL (REVERT) trial. Circulation 116:49–56, 2007. **D**, Reproduced from Doughty RN, Whalley GA, Gamble G, et al: Left ventricular remodeling with carvedilol in patients with congestive heart failure due to ischemic heart disease. Australia-New Zealand Heart Failure Research Collaborative Group. J Am Coll Cardiol 29:1060–1066,1997.*

inhibiting one of several proteases responsible for cleaving angiotensin I to form angiotensin II. However, alternative enzymatic pathways have become recognized as playing a major role in angiotensin II production in humans.[17] For example, in the failing human heart, angiotensin II formation is only partially inhibited by an ACE inhibitor but almost completely blocked by an inhibitor of chymase, another protease that catalyzes the formation of angiotensin II from angiotensin I.[18] Accordingly, ACE inhibitor therapy achieves only partial inhibition of angiotensin II production.

To the extent that ACE inhibitors reduce production of angiotensin II, effects attributable to angiotensin II are diminished regardless of which receptor mediates the particular effect (i.e., both AT_1 and AT_2 receptors). ACE not only cleaves angiotensin I to form angiotensin II, but also is the principal protease that degrades bradykinin; thus ACE inhibition leads to increased levels of bradykinin within the circulation and at the tissue level.[19] The hemodynamic effects of ACE inhibitors may be mediated in part through increases in regional bradykinin levels. Bradykinin stimulates endothelial release of nitric oxide and vasodilator prostaglandins,[20,21] contributing to the vasodilator effects of ACE inhibitors. In some animal models of myocardial injury or pressure overload, the beneficial effects of ACE inhibitors mitigating cardiomyocyte hypertrophy and fibroblast hyperplasia within the myocardium are blocked by a bradykinin antagonist.[22-24] Thus, reduction of bradykinin metabolism, resulting in potentiation of local bradykinin levels, potentially contributes to the therapeutic benefit of ACE inhibitors.

ARBs

Although ACE inhibitors and ARBs both inhibit RAAS, they do so by different mechanisms. ARBs block the effects of angiotensin II on the angiotensin type 1 receptor, the receptor subtype that is responsible for virtually all the adverse biologic effects relevant to angiotensin II on cardiac remodeling. In contrast to ACE inhibitors, effects of angiotensin II receptor antagonists limit the responses specifically mediated by that receptor. Because most of the clinically relevant effects of angiotensin II appear to be mediated through the AT_1 receptor, AT_1 receptor antagonists mirror the actions anticipated through the blockade of angiotensin II production. However, loss of feedback inhibition results in increased angiotensin II levels after administration of an AT_1 receptor antagonist, which leads to overstimulation of alternative angiotensin II receptors. The unopposed activation of non-AT_1 receptors may mediate some of the clinically relevant effects attributable to AT_1 receptor blockade. For example, stimulation of the AT_2 receptor may be responsible for the antiproliferative and antifibrotic effects of AT_1 antagonists[25] within the cardiovascular system. Unopposed activation of the AT_2 receptor may, however, also promote apoptosis.[26]

Effects on Hemodynamics

The primary acute hemodynamic effect of both ACE inhibitors and ARBs is vasodilation. In the early investigations of ACE inhibitors, captopril, enalapril, and lisinopril all produced dose-dependent decreases in right atrial pressure, pulmonary capillary wedge pressure, and systemic vascular resistance, with a resultant increase in cardiac index.[27-29] In studies in which follow-up hemodynamic measurements were obtained, these hemodynamic benefits of ACE inhibitor therapy were shown to be sustained.[27,29] In addition, inhibition of neurohormonal activation over time is evident from decreases in heart rates and plasma catecholamine levels at rest and with exercise.[29,30] Similarly, ARBs such as losartan and irbesartan produce dose-dependent decreases in right atrial pressure, pulmonary capillary wedge pressure, and systemic vascular resistance in association with increased cardiac index, which are sustained over time in the absence of tachyphylaxis.[31-33] These hemodynamic effects of ARBs occur without increases in heart rate or neurohormonal activation. Beneficial hemodynamic and clinical effects of irbesartan were reported by Havranek and colleagues in patients already taking ACE inhibitors.[32] Likewise, the administration of valsartan (160 mg) to patients with HF who were already taking ACE inhibitors produced acute and sustained hemodynamic benefits, accompanied by a reduction in aldosterone levels and by a trend for reduction in plasma norepinephrine levels.[34]

In summary, these data indicate that ACE inhibitors and ARBs produce similar hemodynamic benefits in patients with heart failure and LV systolic dysfunction. The addition of ARBs to ACE inhibitor therapy also produces significant and sustained hemodynamic benefits, which are consistent with results of clinical studies demonstrating that angiotensin II levels remain elevated in patients receiving ACE inhibitor therapy.[35,36]

Effects on Ventricular Structure

In addition to a wealth of experimental evidence supporting the important role of the RAAS in the pathophysiologic processes of ventricular remodeling (see Chapter 11), clinical evidence also supports this premise. Because of the large number of trials demonstrating consistent benefits of ACE inhibitors in rates of mortality and morbidity, these agents have become a mainstay of therapy for patients with LV systolic dysfunction. Sharpe and associates demonstrated that captopril initiated within 48 hours after Q wave myocardial infarction reduced the increase in LV end-diastolic volume after only 3 months of therapy.[37] Similarly, in the multicenter Survival and Ventricular Enlargement (SAVE) trial, captopril improved survival among patients after myocardial infarction with reduced LVEF (<40%) and mitigated the degree of LV chamber dilation after the first year of therapy.[38] Konstam and associates demonstrated that ACE inhibitors prevent progressive LV remodeling in patients with LV systolic dysfunction with or without symptoms of heart failure[39,40] (see Figure 34-7). In a substudy of the Studies of Left Ventricular Dysfunction (SOLVD) trial, the placebo recipients exhibited LV dilation over the span of this study (1 year), whereas the enalapril recipients exhibited the opposite, which was consistent with a decrease in LV chamber size for a given LV pressure. This study demonstrated clinically that ACE inhibition prevents, and perhaps reverses, the extent of ventricular remodeling in patients with LV systolic dysfunction.

The precise effect of AT_1 receptor antagonists on ventricular remodeling is not as well studied. In the Evaluation of Losartan In The Elderly (ELITE) radionuclide substudy, researchers compared the effect of losartan, an AT_1 antagonist, with that of the ACE inhibitor captopril on LV remodeling in elderly patients with HF and systolic dysfunction (EF <40%).[41] After 48 weeks of therapy, captopril and losartan demonstrated statistically equivalent effects in reducing LV end-diastolic and end-systolic volumes, although there was a trend toward a greater beneficial effect of captopril in this study. McKelvie and coworkers compared the effects of the AT_1 antagonist candesartan with those of the ACE inhibitor enalapril and the effects of their combination on LV remodeling as part of the Randomized Evaluation Strategies for Left Ventricular Dysfunction (RESOLVD) pilot study.[42] With combination therapy, they observed a significant reduction in LV end-systolic volume at 43 weeks in comparison with enalapril treatment alone; this finding suggested that the combination of an ACE inhibitor and ARB in the clinical setting may have additive benefits. Whether these effects were secondary to beneficial changes in myocardial structure or were related purely to afterload reduction is unknown. Perhaps the largest study of whether combination therapy with an ACE inhibitor and ARB produces greater reduction in LV remodeling has been the Valsartan in Acute Myocardial Infarction Trial (VALIANT), in which investigators examined the effect of valsartan alone, captopril alone, and their combination in patients after an acute myocardial infarction complicated by heart failure, LV dysfunction, or both.[43] Although the patient population in this trial differed from that in heart failure trials (after myocardial infarction, mean LVEF among the groups was 39%), the degree of LV remodeling (increase in LV end-diastolic volume and change in LVEF) was similar among all three groups of patients.[44] The results of the VALIANT substudy do not support the view that combination therapy in patients with HF or LV dysfunction after myocardial infarction exerts a greater effect in limiting LV remodeling than either class of agent alone.

Effects on Functional Capacity and Symptoms

ACE Inhibitors

Reduced functional capacity in patients with HF caused by systolic dysfunction results from a variety of cardiac and noncardiac factors. ACE inhibitors have variably been shown to improve exercise capacity in patients with HF and systolic dysfunction, presumably through their sustained hemodynamic benefits, as described previously. However, the improvement in exercise capacity noted with ACE inhibitors is often modest in clinical trials. The lack of more dramatic improvements in exercise capacity in clinical trials may result in part from improved survival among patients with advanced HF being treated with ACE inhibitors. For example, in the Vasodilators in Heart Failure Treatment (V-HeFT) II trial, in which ACE inhibition was compared with the combination of hydralazine and isosorbide dinitrate, subjects receiving the latter regimen had a more pronounced improvement in exercise capacity as judged by peak exercise oxygen consumption.[45] However, the survival rate among patients treated with the ACE inhibitor was better than that among subjects taking hydralazine and isosorbide, which raised the question of whether more differentially better survival among patients treated with enalapril may have diluted any improvements in exercise capacity.[46]

A number of studies have demonstrated that ACE inhibitors improve exercise time and ameliorate symptoms of HF. The benefits of ACE inhibitors in the management of HF symptoms have long been recognized. In the early 1980s, captopril treatment was shown to improve exercise time by 25% and to reduce HF symptoms and NYHA class in patients with severe HF treated with digoxin and diuretics.[47] Similar improvements in exercise capacity and HF symptoms were noted with the ACE inhibitors enalapril, lisinopril, and quinapril.[27,28,48] Taken together, these clinical data demonstrate that ACE inhibitors favorably influence symptoms of HF and exercise capacity in patients with LV systolic dysfunction.

ARBs

ARBs also improve exercise capacity and symptoms in patients with HF. Losartan has been shown to improve symptoms of HF after 12 weeks of therapy in patients with reduced LVEF (<45%).[33] In a comparative trial with the ACE inhibitor enalapril, losartan-treated patients demonstrated similar exercise capacity and symptoms of HF after 12 weeks of treatment.[49] Vescovo and associates evaluated exercise capacity in small groups of patients, one treated with enalapril and the other with losartan.[50] Both groups demonstrated similar improvements in exercise capacity, as demonstrated by peak oxygen consumption. Interestingly, Vescovo and associates also compared the myosin profiles in skeletal muscle and demonstrated a myosin heavy chain shift toward slow, fatigue-resistant isoforms, which suggested that improvement in exercise capacity by these agents may be in part related to noncardiac factors.

Riegger and colleagues studied the effects of various doses of the ARB candesartan (4, 8, and 16 mg) in patients with HF and LV systolic dysfunction.[51] In this study, ACE inhibitors were withdrawn 2 weeks before the placebo run-in period. With all three doses of candesartan, patients demonstrated improved score of heart failure symptoms and improved exercise capacity in comparison with placebo-treated patients. Researchers in the RESOLVD pilot study compared candesartan alone, enalapril alone, and their combination over a 43-week period.[42] Each agent resulted in similar improvements in exercise capacity and quality of life. Thus, available studies suggest that ARBs produce improvements in exercise capacity and HF symptoms that are similar to those produced by ACE inhibitors, either historically or in a direct, individual manner.

Effects on Morbidity and Mortality

Although the hemodynamic and clinical effects of ACE inhibitors are notably similar to those of ARBs, these two classes of agents should not be considered interchangeable, inasmuch as they possess both overlapping and distinct effects. Clinical evidence for the benefit of ACE inhibitors exceeds that for ARBs, a finding that is strongly influenced by the earlier development of ACE inhibitors. Results of clinical trials, both early and more recent, have helped determine whether and under what circumstances these agents can be used interchangeably or in combination.

ACE Inhibitors

ACE inhibitors were the first class of agents shown to significantly alter the natural history of HF, as demonstrated by a reduction in the frequency of death and of other morbid events. Most of these data have been accumulated from patients with reduced LVEF, and clinicians have therefore recognized the necessity for measuring ventricular systolic function and prescribing ACE inhibitors to patients with reduced EF (e.g., ≤35%) as standards of care for patients with HF. **Table 34-2** lists the key trials demonstrating benefit of ACE inhibitors in this population. These trials recruited a broad variety of patients, including women and the elderly, as well as patients with a wide range of causes and severity of LV dysfunction.

The consistency of data from the Studies on Left Ventricular Dysfunction (SOLVD) Prevention Study,[52] Survival and Ventricular Enlargement (SAVE),[53] and Trandolapril Cardiac Evaluation (TRACE)[54] has shown that asymptomatic patients with LV dysfunction (stage B) have less remodeling and a reduced risk of progressing to symptomatic heart failure when treated with ACE inhibitors. ACE inhibitors have also consistently shown benefit for patients with symptomatic LV dysfunction (stage C). All significant placebo-controlled ACE inhibitors in HFrEF patients have demonstrated a reduction in mortality. Further, the absolute benefit is greatest in patients with the most severe HF. Indeed, the patients with NYHA class IV HF in the Cooperative North Scandinavian Enalapril Survival Study (CONSENSUS I)[55] had a much larger effect size than the SOLVD Treatment Trial,[56] which in turn had a larger effect size than the SOLVD Prevention Trial.[52] Although only three placebo-controlled mortality trials have been conducted in patients with chronic HF, the aggregate data suggest that ACE inhibitors reduce mortality in direct relation to the degree of

TABLE 34-2 Key Randomized Trials of ACE Inhibitors and ARBs in Heart Failure

TRIAL NAME	AGENT	NYHA CLASS	NO. OF SUBJECTS ENROLLED	12-MONTH PLACEBO MORTALITY (%)	12-MONTH EFFECT SIZE (%)	*P* VALUE 12 MONTHS (FULL F/U)
ACEIs						
HF						
CONSENSUS-1	Enalapril	IV	253	52	↓31	0.01 (0.0003)
SOLVD-Rx	Enalapril	I-III	2569	15	↓21	0.02 (0.004)
SOLVD-Asx	Enalapril	I, II	4228	5	0	0.82 (0.30)
Post-MI						
SAVE	Captopril	—	2231	12	↓18	0.11 (0.02)
AIRE	Ramipril	—	1986	20	↓22	0.01 (0.002)
TRACE	Trandolapril	—	1749	26	↓16	0.046 (0.001)
ARBs						
HF						
VAL-HeFT	Valsartan	II-IV	5010	9	0	NS (0.80)
CHARM-Alternative	Candesartan	II-IV	2028	NS	NS	NS (0.02)
CHARM-Added	Candesartan	II-IV	2547	NS	NS	NS (0.11)
HEAAL	Losartan	II-IV	3846	NS	NS	NS (0.24)

ACE, Angiotensin-converting enzyme; *ACEI,* angiotensin-converting enzyme inhibitor; *ARB,* angiotensin receptor blocker; *HF,* heart failure; *MI,* myocardial infarction; *NYHA,* New York Heart Association.

severity of chronic HF. A pooled analysis of placebo-controlled trials of ACE inhibitors suggested a 23% reduction in mortality and a 35% reduction in the combined endpoint of death or HF hospitalization compared with a placebo (**Figure 34-8**).[57] The V-HeFT-II trial provided evidence that ACE inhibitors improve the natural history of HF through mechanisms other than vasodilation, inasmuch as subjects treated with enalapril had significantly lower mortality than subjects treated with the vasodilatory combination of hydralazine plus isosorbide dinitrate (which does not directly inhibit neurohormonal systems).[58] Although enalapril is the only ACE inhibitor that has been used in placebo-controlled mortality trials in chronic HF, multiple ACE inhibitors have proven to be roughly equally effective when administered in oral form within the first week of the ischemic event in myocardial infarction trials, supporting the general notion that the ACE inhibitor effect is a class effect in HF. In a direct randomized comparison study of high dose (≈35 mg of lisinopril) compared with low dose (≈5 mg of lisinopril), the ATLAS study suggested that mortality was similar, although higher doses were associated with lower rates of HF hospitalization.[59]

Importantly, it should be emphasized that patients with a low blood pressure (<90 mm Hg systolic) or impaired renal function (serum creatinine greater than 2.5 mg per mL) were not recruited and/or represent a small proportion of patients who participated in these trials. Thus the efficacy of these agents for these patient populations is less well established.[60]

Mechanisms Underlying These Effects

The original hypothesis behind investigation of ACE inhibitors in patients with HF was that these agents would reduce the progression of clinical HF through vasodilation. As noted above, direct comparison between ACE inhibitors and other vasodilatory regimens (e.g., nitrates and hydralazine in the V-HeFT studies) support the concept that ACE inhibitors alter the natural history of HF via mechanisms distinct from their hemodynamic effects, including direct effects on the cellular mechanisms responsible for progressive changes in the myocyte and the interstitium. Beyond an effect on clinical events linked to progressive HF, both the SOLVD and SAVE studies demonstrated significant reductions in the incidence of myocardial infarction, which potentially contributed to the overall influence of ACE inhibitors on mortality. Furthermore, within the SOLVD population, enalapril caused a significant reduction in number of patients hospitalized for unstable angina. These findings provided, for the first time, evidence for an influence of ACE inhibitors on the pathogenesis of acute coronary syndromes, an influence potentially mediated by effects on the arterial wall, on the balance between thrombosis and thrombolysis, or on both.

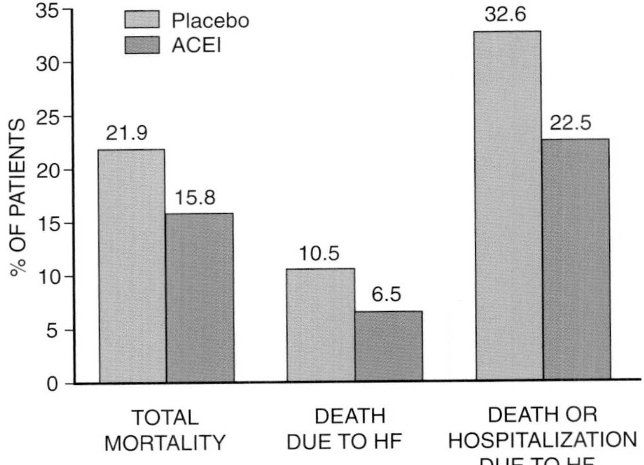

FIGURE 34-8 Outcomes with ACE inhibitors compared with placebo in a pooled analysis of placebo-controlled trials in heart failure patients. *From Garg R, Yusuf S: Overview of randomized trials of angiotensin-converting enzyme inhibitors on mortality and morbidity in patients with heart failure. Collaborative Group on ACE Inhibitor Trials. JAMA 273:1450–1456, 1995.*

ARBs

In symptomatic HF patients who were intolerant of ACE inhibitors, the aggregate clinical data suggest that ARBs are roughly as effective as ACE inhibitors in reducing HF morbidity and mortality. Candesartan significantly reduced all-cause mortality, cardiovascular death, or hospitalization in ACE-intolerant patients in the Candesartan Heart Failure: Assessment of Reduction in Mortality and Morbidity (CHARM-Alternative) trial.[61] Similar findings were shown with valsartan in the small subgroup of patients not receiving an ACE inhibitor in the Valsartan Heart Failure Trial (Val-HeFT)[62] (**Figure 34-9**). A direct comparison of ACE inhibitors and ARBs was assessed in the Losartan Heart Failure Survival Study (ELITE-II), which showed that losartan was not associated with improved survival in elderly HF patients when compared with captopril, but was significantly better tolerated.[63] Two trials have evaluated ARBs compared to ACE inhibition in postmyocardial infarction patients who developed LV dysfunction or signs of HF. The direct comparison of losartan with captopril indicated that losartan was not as effective as captopril on all-cause mortality, whereas valsartan was shown to be noninferior to captopril on all-cause mortality in the Valsartan in Acute Myocardial Infarction Trial (VALIANT).[43] The combination of captopril and valsartan produced no further reduction in mortality in VALIANT, although the number of adverse events increased. When given in addition to ACE inhibitors in general cohorts of patients with symptomatic HF, the effects of ARBs were shown to have a modest beneficial effect in the CHARM-Added trial.[64] However, the addition of valsartan to ACE inhibitors had no beneficial effect on mortality in Val-HeFT, although the combined endpoint mortality and morbidity was significantly (13.2%) lower with valsartan than with the placebo because of a reduction in the number of patients hospitalized for HF.[65] The question of high-dose versus low-dose angiotensin receptor antagonism on clinical outcomes was evaluated in the Heart Failure Endpoint Evaluation of Angiotensin II Antagonist Losartan (HEAAL) trial.[66] This study showed that the use of a high-dose losartan was not associated with a significant reduction in the primary endpoint of all-cause death or admission for HF (hazard ratio [HR] 0.94, 95% confidence interval [CI] 0.84-1.04, $P = 0.24$) when compared with low-dose losartan, but was associated with a significant reduction in HF admissions (HR 0.94, 95% CI 0.84-1.04, $P = 0.24$), suggesting that uptitration of ARBs may confer clinical benefit.

Although one meta-analysis suggests that ARBs and ACEIs have similar effects on all-cause mortality and heart failure hospitalizations,[67] and although ARBs may be considered as initial therapy rather than ACE inhibitors

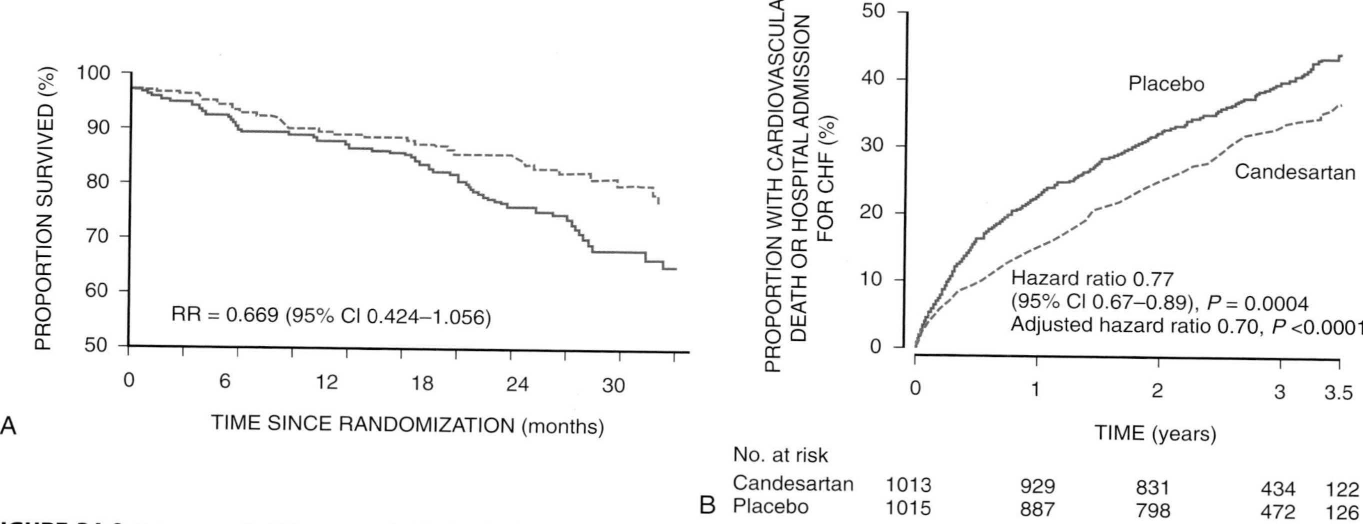

FIGURE 34-9 Outcomes with ARBs compared with the placebo in heart failure. **A,** Kaplan-Meier curves for mortality in the valsartan *(dotted line)* and placebo *(solid line)* groups (n = 185 and 181, respectively) without angiotensin-converting enzyme (ACE) inhibitor background therapy (P = 0.017 by log-rank test) in the Valsartan Heart Failure Trial (Val-HeFT). **B,** Kaplan-Meier cumulative event curves for the primary outcome (all-cause mortality, cardiovascular death, or hospitalization) in the Candesartan Heart Failure: Assessment of Reduction in Mortality and Morbidity trial (CHARM-Alternative) in ACE-intolerant patients. ***A,*** *Reproduced from Maggioni AP, Anand I, Gottlieb SO, et al: Effects of valsartan on morbidity and mortality in patients with heart failure not receiving angiotensin-converting enzyme inhibitors. J Am Coll Cardiol 40:1414–1421, 2002;* ***B,*** *Reproduced from Granger CB, McMurray JJ, Yusuf S, et al: Effects of candesartan in patients with chronic heart failure and reduced left-ventricular systolic function intolerant to angiotensin-converting-enzyme inhibitors: the CHARM-Alternative trial. Lancet 362:772–776, 2003.*

following myocardial infarction, the general consensus is that ACE inhibitors remain first-line therapy for the treatment of HF, whereas ARBs are recommended for ACE inhibitor-intolerant patients. Combination therapy can be considered in persistently symptomatic patients, although the risk of side effects is higher (see later discussion), particularly in patients also treated with MRAs (the triple combination of ACE inhibitors, ARBs, and MRAs is specifically discouraged (class III recommendation for harm) in current guidelines.[1]

Side Effects, Complications, and Drug Interactions

ACE Inhibitors

Most of the adverse effects of ACE inhibitors are related to suppression of the renin-angiotensin system. The decreases in blood pressure and mild azotemia are often seen during the initiation of therapy are, in general, well tolerated and do not require a decrease in the dose of the ACE inhibitor. However, if hypotension is accompanied by dizziness or if the renal dysfunction becomes severe, it may be necessary to decrease the dose of the diuretic if significant fluid retention is not present, or alternatively, decrease the dose of the ACE inhibitor if significant fluid retention is present. Hyperkalemia may also become problematic if the patient is receiving potassium supplements or a potassium-sparing diuretic. Potassium retention that is not responsive to these measures may require a reduction in the dose of ACE inhibitor or (rarely) discontinuation. The side effects of ACE inhibitors that are related to kinin potentiation include a nonproductive cough (10%-15% of patients) and angioedema (1% of patients). In patients who cannot tolerate ACE inhibitors because of cough or angioedema, ARBs are the next recommended line of therapy. Patients intolerant to ACE inhibitors because of hyperkalemia or renal insufficiency are likely to experience the same side effects with ARBs. The combination of hydralazine and an oral nitrate should be considered for these latter patients (see later discussion).

Early clinical evidence suggested that aspirin use may prevent or limit the hemodynamic and survival benefits of ACE inhibitors. Importantly, contemporary studies derived from registry data and population-based cohorts have refuted these earlier concerns related to a potential aspirin and ACE inhibitor interaction. In multiple recent systematic reviews of ACE inhibitor trials, improvement in clinical outcomes continued to be evident in patients receiving aspirin at baseline, although the magnitude of the benefit tended to be lower.[68,69]

ARBs

ARBs are well tolerated and highly efficacious in patients who are intolerant of ACE inhibitors because of cough, skin rash, and angioedema and should therefore be used in symptomatic and asymptomatic patients with an EF less than 40% who are ACE inhibitor-intolerant for reasons other than hyperkalemia or renal insufficiency. Both ACE inhibitors and ARBs have similar effects on blood pressure, renal function, and potassium. Therefore, the problems of symptomatic hypotension, azotemia, and hyperkalemia will be similar for both of these agents. Although less frequent than with ACE inhibitors, angioedema has also been reported in some patients who receive ARBs. In patients who are intolerant to ACE inhibitors and ARBs, the combined use of hydralazine and isosorbide dinitrate may be considered as a therapeutic option in such patients.

Practical Tips

ACE Inhibitors

Starting and target doses for commonly used ACE inhibitors and ARBs are shown in **Table 34-3**. Because fluid retention can attenuate the effects of ACE inhibitors, it is preferable to optimize the dose of diuretic first before starting the ACE inhibitor. However, it may be necessary to reduce the dose of diuretic during the initiation of an ACE inhibitor to prevent symptomatic hypotension. ACE inhibitors should be initiated in low doses, followed by increments in dose if lower

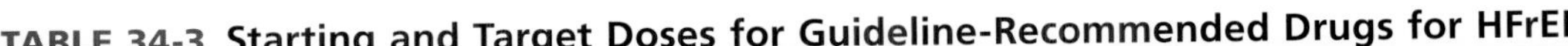

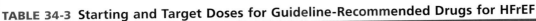

TABLE 34-3 Starting and Target Doses for Guideline-Recommended Drugs for HFrEF

DRUG	INITIAL DAILY DOSE(S)	MAXIMUM DOSE(S)	MEAN DOSES ACHIEVED IN CLINICAL TRIALS
ACE Inhibitors			
Captopril	6.25 mg 3 times	50 mg 3 times	122.7 mg/day
Enalapril	2.5 mg twice	10-20 mg twice	16.6 mg/day
Fosinopril	5-10 mg once	40 mg once	N/A
Lisinopril	2.5-5 mg once	20-40 mg once	32.5-35.0 mg/day
Perindopril	2 mg once	8-16 mg once	N/A
Quinapril	5 mg twice	20 mg twice	N/A
Ramipril	1.25-2.5 mg once	10 mg once	N/A
Trandolapril	1 mg once	4 mg once	N/A
ARBs			
Candesartan	4-8 mg once	32 mg once	24 mg/day
Losartan	25-50 mg once	50-150 mg once	129 mg/day
Valsartan	20-40 mg twice	160 mg twice	254 mg/day
Aldosterone Antagonists			
Spironolactone	12.5-25.0 mg once	25 mg once or twice	26 mg/day
Eplerenone	25 mg once	50 mg once	42.6 mg/day
β-Blockers			
Bisoprolol	1.25 mg once	10 mg once	8.6 mg/day
Carvedilol	3.125 mg twice	50 mg twice	37 mg/day
Carvedilol CR	10 mg once	80 mg once	N/A
Metoprolol succinate extended release (metoprolol CR/XL)	12.5-25 mg once	200 mg once	159 mg/day
Hydralazine and Isosorbide Dinitrate			
Fixed-dose combination	37.5 mg hydralazine/20 mg isosorbide dinitrate 3 times daily	75 mg hydralazine/40 mg isosorbide dinitrate 3 times daily	≈175 mg hydralazine/90 mg isosorbide dinitrate daily
Hydralazine and isosorbide dinitrate	Hydralazine: 25 to 50 mg, 3 or 4 times daily and isosorbide dinitrate: 20-30 mg 3 or 4 times daily	Hydralazine: 300 mg daily in divided doses and isosorbide dinitrate: 120 mg daily in divided doses	N/A

ACE, Angiotensin-converting enzyme; *ARB,* angiotensin receptor blocker; *HFrEF,* heart failure with reduced ejection fraction; *N/A,* not applicable.
From Yancy CW, Jessup M, Bozkurt B, et al: 2013 ACCF/AHA guideline for the management of heart failure: a report of the American College of Cardiology Foundation/American Heart Association task force on practice guidelines. Circulation 128:e240–e327, 2013.

doses have been well tolerated. Titration is generally achieved by doubling doses every 3 to 5 days. The dose of ACEI should be increased until the doses used are similar to those that have been shown to be effective in clinical trials or to the maximally tolerated dose. Higher doses are more effective than lower doses in preventing hospitalization based on the ATLAS trial.[59] For stable patients, it is acceptable to add therapy with β-blocking agents before full target doses of ACE inhibitors are reached. Blood pressure (including postural changes), renal function, and potassium should be evaluated within 1 to 2 weeks after initiation of ACE inhibitors, especially in patients with preexisting azotemia, hypotension, hyponatremia, diabetes mellitus, or in those taking potassium supplements. Abrupt withdrawal of treatment with an ACE inhibitor may lead to clinical deterioration and should therefore be avoided in the absence of life-threatening complications (e.g., angioedema, hyperkalemia).

ARBs

Multiple ARBs that are approved for the treatment of hypertension are now available to clinicians. Three of these, losartan, valsartan, and candesartan, have been extensively evaluated in the setting of HF. ARBs should be initiated with the starting doses shown in Table 34-2, which can be uptitrated every 3 to 5 days by doubling the dose of ARB. As with ACE inhibitors, blood pressure, renal function, and potassium should be reassessed within 1 to 2 weeks after initiation and followed closely after changes in dose.

Angiotensin–Neprilysin Inhibition

Neprilysin is a neutral endopeptidase (NEP) that degrades several peptides in the neurohormonal axis, including natriuretic peptides, bradykinin, and adrenomedullin. NEP inhibition increases levels of these vasoactive peptides and counters adverse vasoconstriction, sodium retention, and ventricular remodeling. Neprilysin inhibition was combined with ACE inhibition in the medication omapatrilat. Data in HF animal models demonstrated that combined ACE and NEP inhibition with omapatrilat was more effective than ACE inhibition alone in preventing adverse changes in LV geometry.[69a] In the Omapatrilat Versus Enalapril Randomized Trial of Utility in Reducing Events (OVERTURE) conducted in 5770 chronic HF patients, omapatrilat reduced cardiovascular death or hospitalization (HR 0.91, 95% CI 0.84-0.99, $P = 0.024$), but there was no difference between the therapies for the primary endpoint of death or HF hospitalization ($P = 0.187$).[69b] However, studies with omapatrilat in patients with hypertension demonstrated an increased risk for serious angioedema[69c] and the compound was not developed further.

LCZ696, which consists of the ARB valsartan and the NEP inhibitor sacubitril, was developed to minimize the risk of angioedema. This medication class is referred to as an angiotensin receptor–neprilysin inhibitor or ARNI. In the phase 2 study, Prospective comparison of ARNI with ARB on Management Of heart failUre with preserved ejectioN fracTion (PARAMOUNT) ($N = 301$), LCZ696 led to greater reductions in N-terminal pro-B-type natriuretic peptide

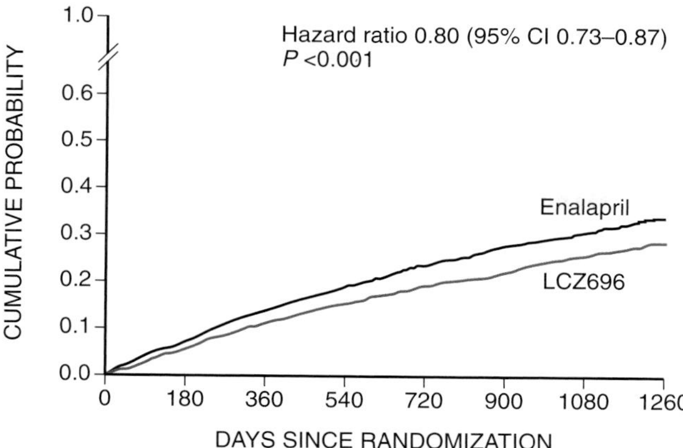

No. at risk								
LCZ696	4187	3922	3663	3018	2257	1544	896	249
Enalapril	4212	3883	3579	2922	2123	1488	853	236

FIGURE 34-10 Kaplan-Meier curve for the primary composite endpoint (death from cardiovascular causes or first hospitalization for heart failure), according to Study Group. *Reproduced with permission from McMurray JJ, Packer M, Desai AS, et al, for the PARADIGM-HF Investigators and Committees: Angiotensin-neprilysin inhibition versus enalapril in heart failure. N Engl J Med 371:993–1004, 2014.*

(NT-proBNP) than valsartan at 12 weeks and was well tolerated.[69d]

The effect of LCZ696 on morbidity and mortality in HFrEF was evaluated in the Prospective Comparison of ARNI with ACEI to Determine Impact on Global Mortality and Morbidity in Heart Failure (PARADIGM-HF) trial.[69e] PARADIGM-HF was a double-blind randomized controlled trial of enalapril versus LCZ696 in 8442 patients with NYHA class II-IV symptoms and an LVEF ≤ 40% with a primary endpoint of cardiovascular death or HF hospitalization. The trial was stopped early by the Data Safety Monitoring Board with a median follow-up of 27 months given the overwhelming evidence for a clinical important benefit of LCZ696 on cardiovascular mortality. There was a 20% relative reduction in the primary endpoint with LCZ696 compared with enalapril (**Figure 34-10**). The benefits with LCZ696 were consistent across study endpoints including all-cause mortality (HR 0.84, 95% CI 0.76-0.93, $P<0.001$), cardiovascular mortality (HR 0.80, 95% CI 0.71-0.89, $P<0.001$), and HF hospitalization (HR 0.79, 95% CI 0.71-0.89, $P<0.001$). Patients receiving LCZ696 had more symptomatic hypotension and nonserious angioedema, but less renal impairment, hyperkalemia, and cough than the enalapril group. The findings of this large clinical trial provide strong support for using LCZ696 instead of ACE inhibitors in the treatment of chronic HF.

β-Blockers

Rationale/Pathophysiologic Basis for Use

A detailed description of the role of the adrenergic system in HF is included in Chapter 6. Early studies demonstrating that the failing heart was subjected to too much adrenergic stimulation provided the rationale for β-blocker therapy. In 1966, investigators at the National Institutes of Health found that biopsy samples from failing human hearts were depleted of the adrenergic neurotransmitter norepinephrine[70] and that plasma norepinephrine or urinary catecholamine metabolites were elevated in patients with HF.[71] To address the question of whether adrenergic activity and β-adrenergic signaling were increased or decreased in the failing human heart, end-stage failing hearts from cardiac transplant recipients were compared with nonfailing unused organ donor hearts; in failing hearts, β-receptor density and signaling were found to be markedly reduced, which was interpreted as evidence both of exposure to increased adrenergic activity and of a mechanism responsible for compromised myocardial reserve.[72] A short time later, it was proved—first by direct coronary sinus norepinephrine measurements[73] and then by isotope dilution techniques to measure norepinephrine spillover[74]—that adrenergic activity is increased in the failing human heart.

Because of their acute negative inotropic effects resulting from interruption of adrenergic support of the failing heart, these agents were initially considered to be contraindicated in patients with heart failure. However, β-blocking agents also prevent the adverse biologic effects of chronically elevated adrenergic signaling in the failing heart, which is the basis for their salutary therapeutic effects. β-blockers competitively antagonize one or more adrenergic receptors (α_1, β_1, and β_2). Although there are a number of potential benefits to blocking all three receptors, most of the deleterious effects of sympathetic activation are mediated by the β_1-adrenergic receptor. Indeed, demonstration of the beneficial effects of β-blocking agents on cardiac function and outcomes is the final proof of the hypothesis that chronic adrenergic activation is a major determinant of the progressive clinical course of HF. In addition, detailed functional, structural, and gene expression analyses have demonstrated that with β-blocker treatment, the dysfunctional, remodeled left or right ventricle can improve in HF patients.

When given in concert with ACE inhibitors, β-blockers reverse the process of LV remodeling, improve patient symptoms, prevent hospitalization, and prolong life (see Figures 34-2 and 34-7). Indeed, the effects of β-blockade on remodeling and clinical events are probably the most dramatic of any single intervention in HF. Therefore, β-blockers are routinely indicated for all patients with symptomatic or asymptomatic HF and LVEF less than 40%.

Effects on Ventricular Structure

Multiple studies have consistently shown the beneficial effects of chronic β-blocker therapy on LV function and structure (see Figure 34-7).[75,76] Long-term benefits include an increase in LVEF, a decrease in LV volumes and in mitral regurgitation (when present), and a reversion of the left ventricle to a more elliptical shape. Improvement in load-independent indices of myocardial contractility has also been shown, which demonstrates that the improvement is related to changes in the intrinsic properties of the myocardium. LV diastolic function and right ventricular function are also improved by long-term β-blocker therapy. Although RAAS inhibitors have also been shown to impact LV remodeling, the effects of β-blocker therapy are generally more dramatic and include "normalization" or near normalization of ventricular structure and LV function in a minority of patients.

The functional effects of β-blocker therapy on the failing heart are biphasic.[77,78] Administration of β-blockers may be associated with an early, short-term deterioration in cardiac function, which is consistent with the negative inotropic effects of adrenergic drive withdrawal and is enhanced in the failing heart because of its dependence on adrenergic support. Carefully performed studies with serial echocardiography have shown a decrease from baseline in LVEF in the first few days of treatment, followed by return to baseline values after 1 month.[77,79] An increase in LVEF from

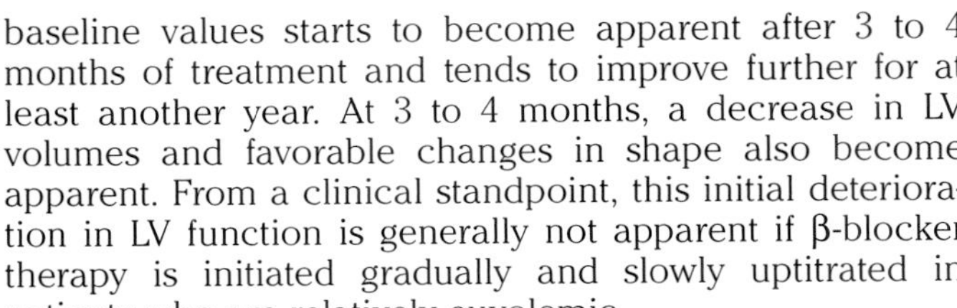

baseline values starts to become apparent after 3 to 4 months of treatment and tends to improve further for at least another year. At 3 to 4 months, a decrease in LV volumes and favorable changes in shape also become apparent. From a clinical standpoint, this initial deterioration in LV function is generally not apparent if β-blocker therapy is initiated gradually and slowly uptitrated in patients who are relatively euvolemic.

Predictors of changes in parameters of LV function have been identified and are rather consistent across multiple studies. Predictors of an improvement in LVEF include a nonischemic cause of HF, higher blood pressure at baseline, the administration of a higher β-blocker dose, and higher baseline heart rates.[80-83] Patients with a nonischemic cause generally show a greater contractile reserve. Higher heart rate at baseline and the administration of a higher, rather than lower, β-blocker dosage are related to the level of adrenergic drive and the degree of β-blockade, respectively. A higher blood pressure at baseline is a rather accurate index of contractile reserve in left ventricles with systolic dysfunction. Accordingly, the demonstration of contractile reserve by dobutamine echocardiography is an excellent predictor of a favorable response to β-blocker therapy.[84,85] In patients with HF of ischemic origin, a direct relation exists between the number of LV segments showing myocardial hibernation and change in LVEF after β-blocking treatment.[86] The basis of all these observations is the fact that the magnitude of the improvement in LV function after chronic β-blockade is directly related to the amount of viable myocardium present at baseline.

Changes in LV function are related to subsequent prognosis.[80,81,87] Patients with the greatest increase in LVEF and reduction in volumes have an excellent long-term prognosis. A post hoc analysis of the Cardiac Insufficiency BIsoprolol Study (CIBIS) confirmed these findings.[88] Patients who showed an improvement in LV fractional shortening after 5 months of treatment had a survival advantage over other patients.

Effects on Functional Capacity/Symptoms

The impairment of exercise capacity in patients with HF is related both to myocardial dysfunction and to the abnormalities in β-adrenergic receptor signal transduction that result in reduced cardiac sensitivity to sympathetic stimulation.[89,90] β-Blocker therapy improves myocardial function and, on that basis, would be expected to improve exercise performance. However, if β-adrenergic receptors are blocked by higher doses of β-blocking agents or are not upregulated by therapy, then exercise tolerance may not improve. This is because the failing heart is dependent on increasing heart rate for improving exercise capacity, more so than is the nonfailing heart. Thus despite the improvement in cardiac function and stroke volume, both at rest and during exercise, the β-blocker–related reduced chronotropic response to exercise may prevent cardiac output to rise sufficiently during exercise to allow an improvement in exercise capacity.[79,91] A direct correlation between change from baseline in maximal exercise capacity and change from baseline in peak exercise heart rate after β-blocker therapy has been observed in multiple-dose studies[92] and in comparisons of multiple β-blockers.[93]

In general, β_1-selective β-blocking agents, such as metoprolol, which at lower doses do not block myocardial β_2-adrenergic receptors and upregulate myocardial β_1-receptors, slightly improve maximal exercise capacity.[94,95] In contrast, agents such as carvedilol and bucindolol—which may not alter myocardial β_1-adrenergic receptor density, have slower offset kinetics from β_1-adrenergic receptors, and also block β_2-adrenergic receptors—may not allow an increase in peak exercise cardiac output and heart rate sufficient to improve exercise capacity and peak VO_2.[91,96,97] On the basis of results of a few single-center studies, it was initially thought that β-blockers might be able to improve submaximal exercise.[91,96] However, multicenter trials failed to show any change also in submaximal exercise capacity.[98-100]

In contrast to direct measurements of exercise capacity, most controlled studies have shown a significant improvement in symptoms and functional class in patients with HF treated with β-blockers. The results obtained are consistent in single-center[91,96,97] and in multicenter trials.[87,94,98,99] According to a meta-analysis by Lechat and associates,[88] patients treated with a β-blocker were 32% more likely to experience an improvement and 30% less likely to experience a worsening in NYHA class. Direct assessment of HF symptoms, as well as global clinical assessment (a quality-of-life measurement) by either the patient or the physician, has been similarly sensitive, showing an improvement in clinical status.[94,98,99] The interpretation of the functional capacity and symptom outcomes of these studies is that β-blockade does not worsen exercise capacity, and the improvement in cardiac function is associated, albeit indirectly, with an improvement in symptoms and quality-of-life measures.

Effects on Morbidity and Mortality

There are three β-blockers that have been shown to be effective in reducing the risk of death in patients with chronic HF: bisoprolol and sustained-release metoprolol succinate both competitively block the β_1 receptor, and carvedilol competitively blocks the α_1, β_1, and β_2 receptors. A summary of the major outcome trials of β-blockers is provided in **Table 34-4**.

The first placebo-controlled multicenter trial with a β-blocking agent was the Metoprolol in Dilated Cardiomyopathy (MDC) trial,[94] which used the shorter acting tartrate preparation at a target dose of 50 mg three times a day in symptomatic HF patients with idiopathic dilated cardiomyopathy. Metoprolol tartrate at an average dose of 108 mg/day reduced the prevalence of the primary endpoint of death or need for cardiac transplantation by 34%, which did not quite reach statistical significance ($P = 0.058$). The benefit was due entirely to a reduction by metoprolol in the morbidity component of the primary endpoint, with no favorable trends in the mortality component of the primary endpoint.

A more efficacious formulation of metoprolol was subsequently developed, metoprolol (succinate) CR/XL, which has a better pharmacologic profile than metoprolol tartrate because of its controlled-release profile and longer half-life. In the Metoprolol CR/XL Randomized Intervention Trial in Congestive Heart Failure (MERIT-HF), metoprolol CR/XL provided a significant relative risk reduction in mortality of 34% in subjects with mild to moderate HF and moderate to severe systolic dysfunction when compared with the placebo group.[101] Importantly, metoprolol CR/XL reduced mortality from both sudden death and progressive pump failure. Further, mortality was reduced across most demographic groups, including older versus younger subjects,

TABLE 34-4 Key Randomized Placebo-Controlled Trials of β-Blockers in Heart Failure

TRIAL NAME	AGENT	NYHA CLASS	NO. OF SUBJECTS ENROLLED	12-MONTH CONTROL MORTALITY (%)	12-MONTH EFFECT SIZE (%)	*P* VALUE 12 MONTHS (FULL F/U)
Heart Failure						
CIBIS-I	Bisoprolol	III, IV	641	21	↓20	NS (0.22)
U.S. Carvedilol	Carvedilol	II, III	1094	8	↓66	NS (<0.001)
ANZ Carvedilol	Carvedilol	I-III	415	NS	NS	NS (>0.1)
CIBIS-II	Bisoprolol	III, IV	2647	12	↓34	NS (0.001)
MERIT-HF	Metoprolol CR	II-IV	3991	10	↓35	NS (0.006)
BEST	Bucindolol	III, IV	2708	23	↓10	NS (0.16)
COPERNICUS	Carvedilol	Severe	2289	28	↓38	NS (0.0001)
Post-MI						
CAPRICORN	Carvedilol	I	1959		↓23	NS (0.03)
BEAT	Bucindolol	I	343	NS	↓12	NS (0.06)

MI, Myocardial infarction; *NS*, not specified; *NYHA*, New York Heart Association.

nonischemic versus ischemic causes, and lower versus higher ejection fractions.

Bisoprolol is a second-generation β_1 receptor-selective blocking agent with approximately 120-fold higher affinity for human β_1 versus β_2 receptors. The first trial performed with bisoprolol was the Cardiac Insufficiency Bisoprolol Study I (CIBIS-I) trial,[102] which examined the effects of bisoprolol on mortality in subjects with symptomatic ischemic or nonischemic cardiomyopathy. CIBIS-I showed a nonsignificant 20% risk reduction for mortality at 2 years' follow-up (P = 0.22). Because the sample size for CIBIS-I was based on an unrealistically high expected event rate in the control group, a follow-up trial with more conservative effect size estimates and sample size calculations was conducted. In CIBIS-II, bisoprolol reduced all-cause mortality by 32% (11.8% vs. 17.3%, P = 0.002), sudden cardiac death by 45% (3.6% vs. 6.4%, P = 0.001), HF hospitalizations by 30% (11.9% bisoprolol vs. 17.6% placebo, P <0.001), and all-cause hospitalizations by 15% (33.6% vs. 39.6%, P = 0.002).[103] The CIBIS-III trial addressed the important question of whether an initial treatment strategy using the β-blocker bisoprolol was noninferior to a treatment strategy of using an ACE inhibitor (enalapril) first, among patients with newly diagnosed mild to moderate HF.[104] The two strategies were compared in a blinded manner with regard to the combined primary endpoint of all-cause mortality or hospitalization, as well as with regard to each of the components of the primary endpoint individually. Although the per-protocol primary endpoint analysis of death or rehospitalization did not meet the prespecified criteria for noninferiority, the intent-to-treat analysis showed that bisoprolol was noninferior to enalapril (HR 0.94, 95% CI 0.77-1.16, P = 0.019 for noninferiority). Although CIBIS-III did not provide clear-cut evidence to justify starting with a β-blocker first, the overall safety profile of the two strategies was similar. Current guidelines continue to recommend starting with an ACE inhibitor first, followed by the subsequent addition of a β-blocker.

Of the three β-blockers that are approved for the treatment of HF, carvedilol has been studied most extensively. The phase III U.S. Trials Program, composed of four individual trials managed by a single Steering and Data and Safety Monitoring Committee, was stopped prematurely because of a highly significant 65% reduction in mortality by carvedilol that was observed across all four trials (P <0.0001). This was followed by a second study, the Australia-New Zealand Heart failure Research Collaborative Group Carvedilol Trial (ANZ-Carvedilol), which showed there was a significant improvement in LVEF (P <0.0001) and a significant (P = 0.0015) reduction in LV end-diastolic volume index in the carvedilol treated group at 12 months, as well a significant relative risk reduction of 26% in the clinical composite of death or hospitalization for the carvedilol group at 19 months.[105] Rates of hospitalization were also significantly lower for patients treated with carvedilol (48%) compared with the placebo (58%). The Carvedilol Prospective Randomized Cumulative Survival (COPERNICUS) study extended these benefits to patients with more advanced HF.[106] In COPERNICUS, patients with advanced HF symptoms had to be clinically euvolemic and have an LVEF less than 25%. When compared with placebo, carvedilol reduced the mortality risk at 12 months by 38% and the relative risk of death or HF hospitalization by 31%. Carvedilol has also been evaluated in a postmyocardial infarction trial in which patients had to exhibit LV dysfunction. The Carvedilol Post-Infarct Survival Controlled Evaluation (CAPRICORN) trial was a randomized, placebo-controlled trial designed to test the long-term efficacy of carvedilol on morbidity and mortality in patients with LV dysfunction after myocardial infarction who were already treated with ACE inhibitors.[107] Although carvedilol did not reduce the prespecified primary endpoint of mortality plus cardiovascular hospitalization, it did significantly reduce total mortality by 23% (P = 0.03), cardiovascular mortality by 25% (P <0.05), and nonfatal myocardial infarction by 41% (P = 0.014). Finally, in the Carvedilol or Metoprolol European Trial (COMET) carvedilol (target dose, 25 mg twice daily) was compared with immediate-release metoprolol tartrate (target dose, 50 mg twice daily) with respect to the primary endpoint of all-cause mortality.[108] In COMET, carvedilol was associated with a significant 33% reduction in all-cause mortality when compared with metoprolol tartrate (33.9% vs. 39.5%, HR 0.83, 95% CI 0.74-0.93, P = 0.0017) (**Figure 34-11**). Based on the results of the COMET trial, short-acting metoprolol tartrate is not recommended for use in the treatment of HF. The results of the COMET trial emphasize the importance of using doses and formulations of β-blockers that have been shown to be effective in clinical trials. There have been no head-to-head trials to ascertain whether the survival benefits of carvedilol are greater than those of metoprolol (succinate) CR/XL when both drugs are used at the appropriate target doses.

Not all studies with β-blockers have been universally successful, suggesting that the effects of β-blockers should not necessarily be viewed broadly as a class effect. Indeed early studies with the first generation of nonspecific β_1 and β_2 receptors without ancillary vasodilating properties (e.g., propranolol) resulted in significant worsening of HF and death. The Beta-blocker Evaluation of Survival Trial (BEST) evaluated the third-generation β-blocking agent bucindolol, which is a completely nonselective β_1 and β_2 blocker with some α_1-receptor blockade properties.[109] Although the BEST trial showed that there was a nonsignificant ($P = 0.10$) 10% reduction in total mortality in the bucindolol-treated group, there was a statistically significant 19% reduction in mortality in white patients ($P = 0.01$). The differential response of bucindolol in white patients has been suggested to be secondary to a polymorphism (Arginine 389) in the β_1-adrenergic receptor that is more prevalent in white patients[110] (see also Chapter 6). Nebivolol is a selective β_1 receptor antagonist with ancillary vasodilatory properties that are mediated, at least in part, by nitric oxide. In the Study of Effects of Nebivolol Intervention on Outcomes and Rehospitalization in Seniors with Heart Failure (SENIORS), nebivolol significantly reduced the composite outcome of death or cardiovascular hospitalizations (HR 0.86, 95% CI 0.74-0.99, $P < 0.04$), which was the primary endpoint of the trial, but did not reduce mortality.[111] Although approximately 35% of the patients in SENIORS had an LVEF greater than 35%, more than half of these patients had an EF ranging from 35% to 50% and thus would not be considered as HFpEF patients. Nebivolol is not currently FDA approved for the treatment of HF.

Side Effects

The adverse effects of β-blockers are generally related to the predictable complications that arise from interfering with the adrenergic nervous system. These reactions generally occur within several days of initiating therapy, and are generally responsive to adjusting concomitant medications as described above. The problem of fluid retention is discussed later. Treatment with a β-blocker can be accompanied by feelings of general fatigue or weakness. In most cases, the increased fatigue spontaneously resolves within several weeks or months; however, in some patients, it may be severe enough to limit the dose of β-blocker or require the withdrawal or reduction of treatment. Therapy with β-blockers can lead to bradycardia and/or exacerbate heart block. Moreover, β-blockers (particularly those that block the α_1 receptor) can lead to vasodilatory side effects. Accordingly, the dose of β-blockers should be decreased if the heart rate decreases to less than 50 beats/min and/or second- or third-degree heart block develops, or symptomatic hypotension develops. Continuation of β-blocker treatment during an episode of acute HF decompensation has been shown to be safe in randomized trials.[112] β-blockers are not recommended for patients with asthma with active bronchospasm.

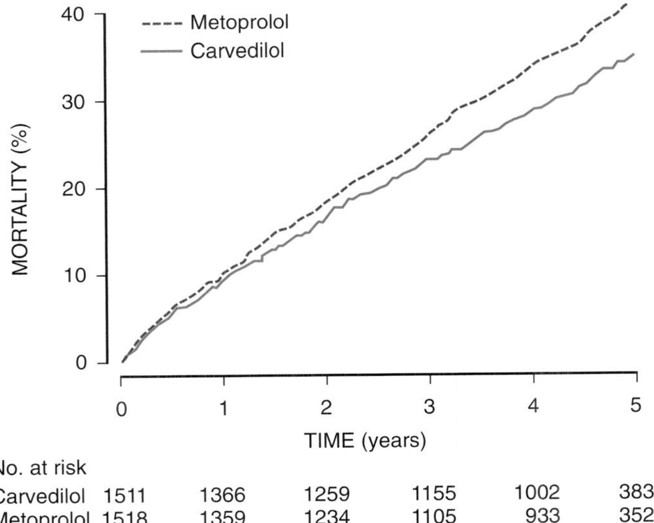

FIGURE 34-11 All-cause mortality in the Carvedilol or Metoprolol European Trial (COMET) with carvedilol compared with immediate-release metoprolol tartrate. *Reproduced from Poole-Wilson PA, Swedberg K, Cleland JG, et al: Comparison of carvedilol and metoprolol on clinical outcomes in patients with chronic heart failure in the Carvedilol Or Metoprolol European Trial (COMET): randomised controlled trial. Lancet 362:7–13, 2003.*

Practical Tips

Analogous to the use of ACE inhibitors, β-blockers should be initiated in low doses (see Table 34-3), followed by gradual increments in the dose if lower doses have been well tolerated. The dose of β-blocker should be increased until the doses used are similar to those that have been reported to be effective in clinical trials (see Table 34-3). Furthermore, in patients taking a low dose of an ACE inhibitor, the addition of a β-blocker appears to produce a greater improvement in symptoms and reduction in the risk of death than an increase in the dose of the ACE inhibitor, although this question has never been specifically subjected to randomized trials. However, unlike ACE inhibitors, which may be uptitrated relatively rapidly, the dose titration of β-blockers should proceed no sooner than 2-week intervals, because the initiation and/or increased dosing of these agents may lead to worsening fluid retention because of the abrupt withdrawal of adrenergic support to the heart and the circulation. Therefore, it is important to optimize the dose of diuretic before starting therapy with β-blockers. If worsening fluid retention does occur, it is likely to occur within 3 to 5 days of initiating therapy and will be manifest as an increase in body weight and/or symptoms of worsening HF. The increased fluid retention can usually be managed by increasing the dose of diuretics. Patients need not be taking high doses of ACE inhibitors before being considered for treatment with a β-blocker, because most patients enrolled in the β-blocker trials were not taking high doses of ACE inhibitors.

Randomized trial data from the IMPACT HF study show that β-blockers can be safely started before discharge even in patients hospitalized for HF, provided that the patients are stable and do not require intravenous HF therapy.[113] Contrary to initial concerns, the aggregate results of clinical trials suggest that β-blocker therapy is well tolerated by the great majority of HF patients (>85%), including patients with comorbid conditions, such as diabetes mellitus, chronic obstructive lung disease, and peripheral vascular disease. Nonetheless, there are a subset of patients (10%-15%) who remain intolerant to β-blockers because of worsening fluid retention or symptomatic hypotension and a minority who are intolerant because of reactive airway disease.

Mineralocorticoid Receptor Antagonists

Rationale/Pathophysiologic Basis for Use

Effects of RAAS activation are also mediated through aldosterone, the secretion of which is partially under the control of angiotensin II stimulation of the AT_1 receptor.[114] Even in

TABLE 34-5 Key Randomized Controlled Trials of Mineralocorticoid Antagonists in Heart Failure

TRIAL NAME	AGENT	NYHA CLASS	NO. OF SUBJECTS ENROLLED	12-MONTH PLACEBO MORTALITY (%)	12-MONTH EFFECT SIZE (%)	*P* VALUE 12 MONTHS (FULL F/U)
Heart Failure						
RALES	Spironolactone	III, IV	1663	24	↓25	NS (<0.001)
EMPHASIS	Eplerenone	II	2737	9	NS	NS (<0.01)
Post-MI						
EPHESUS	Eplerenone	I	6632	12	↓15	NS (0.005)

MI, Myocardial infarction; *NS,* not specified; *NYHA,* New York Heart Association.

presence of angiotensin II inhibition, increases in aldosterone persist in the circulation (endocrine effects) and at tissue levels (autocrine and paracrine effects).[35,115] Clinical studies have shown a "breakthrough" of aldosterone levels after prolonged treatment with an ARB or an ACE inhibitor in chronic HF.[42] Furthermore, the mineralocorticoid receptor can be activated by other factors, independent of aldosterone. For example, glucocorticoids bind to and activate the mineralocorticoid receptor in the presence of an increased oxidative state.[116] Aside from its effect on renal sodium-potassium exchange, the mineralocorticoid receptor mediates a wide array of effects across the cardiovascular system. There is substantial experimental evidence that mineralocorticoid receptor activation contributes to several adverse myocardial effects, such as increased myocardial fibrosis, inflammation, myocyte hypertrophy, and apoptosis.[116-124] Clinical observations that mineralocorticoid receptor blockade reduces vascular events such as acute coronary syndromes[125] have generated interest in exploring the biologic processes of vascular mineralocorticoid receptor action. Jaffe and associates reported that mineralocorticoid receptors are expressed in blood vessels and regulate gene transcription in vascular smooth muscle cells.[126,127] Using a gene-chip microarray approach, they observed an increase in the expression of collagen subtypes and of factors known to promote vascular calcification and inflammation. They also reported the intriguing finding that angiotensin II promoted mineralocorticoid receptor–specific effects in the absence of aldosterone.[126] Thus indirect mineralocorticoid receptor activation probably contributes importantly to RAAS-induced pathologic effects throughout the cardiovascular and renal systems.

The fact that the mineralocorticoid receptor may be activated by aldosterone and alternative stimuli, and the multifaceted means through which such activation may accelerate the advance of cardiovascular disease, represents a rationale for exploring the benefits of mineralocorticoid receptor antagonists, on top of ACE inhibitors or ARBs.

Effects on Ventricular Structure/Hemodynamics

Findings related to effects of mineralocorticoid receptor inhibition on cardiac remodeling in HF have been mixed. Some studies have suggested a benefit. For example, Hayashi and colleagues demonstrated that administration of the MRA spironolactone prevents postinfarct left ventricular remodeling associated with suppression of a marker of myocardial collagen synthesis.[128] Kasama and colleagues also showed that spironolactone has positive effects on cardiac sympathetic nerve activity and left ventricular remodeling in patients with dilated cardiomyopathy.[129] In contrast, Udelson and colleagues found no remodeling effect with the selective MRA eplerenone when added to an ACE inhibitor and β-blocker during 9 months of randomized, controlled treatment in patients with NYHA class II to class III HF and reduced LVEF.[130] It is possible that the reduction in mortality observed with mineralocorticoid receptor blockers in selected populations with heart failure is at least partly mediated by vascular effects or other pleiotropic effects, as opposed to myocardial effects. Although the mechanism for the beneficial effect of spironolactone has not been fully elucidated, prevention of extracellular matrix remodeling and prevention of hypokalemia are plausible mechanisms.

Effects on Morbidity and Mortality

Three landmark studies demonstrated reduced mortality when patients with HF and reduced LVEF were treated with an MRA (**Table 34-5**). The first evidence that MRAs could produce a major clinical benefit in HF was demonstrated by the Randomized Aldactone Evaluation Study (RALES) trial, which evaluated spironolactone (25 mg per day initially, titrated to 50 mg/day for signs of worsening HF) versus a placebo in NYHA class III or IV HF patients with an LVEF less than 35%, who were being treated with an ACE inhibitor, a loop diuretic, and in most cases digoxin.[131] Spironolactone led to a 30% reduction in total mortality when compared with the placebo ($P = 0.001$). The frequency of hospitalization for worsening HF was also 35% lower in the spironolactone group than in the placebo group.

The Eplerenone in Mild Patients Hospitalization and Survival Study in Heart Failure (EMPHASIS-HF) trial, which was performed in patients with NYHA class II HF with an EF less than 30% (or 35% if the QRS width was >130 msec), demonstrated that eplerenone (titrated to 50 mg/day) led to a significant 27% decrease in cardiovascular death or HF hospitalization (HR 0.63, 95% CI 0.54-0.74, $P < 0.001$).[132] There were also significant decreases in all-cause death (24%), cardiovascular death (24%), all-cause hospitalization (23%), and HF hospitalizations (43%). Importantly, the effect of eplerenone was consistent across all prespecified subgroups. In contrast to the RALES trial, which was conducted before the widespread adoption of β-blockers, the background therapy for EMPHASIS-HF included ACE inhibitors or ARBs and β-blockers.

The findings in RALES and EMPHASIS-HF are consistent with findings in randomized clinical trials in patients with acute myocardial infarction and LV dysfunction. The Eplerenone Post-Acute Myocardial Infarction Heart Failure Efficacy and Survival Study (EPHESUS) evaluated the effect of eplerenone (titrated to a maximum of 50 mg per day) on morbidity and mortality among patients with acute myocardial infarction complicated by LV dysfunction and HF.[133] Treatment with eplerenone led to 15% decrease in all-cause death in the EPHESUS trial (RR 0.85, 95 CI 0.75-0.96, P = 0.008). Based on the results of the RALES and EMPHASIS-HF trials, MRAs are currently recommend for all patients with persistent NYHA class II–IV symptoms and an EF <35%, despite treatment with an ACE inhibitor (or an ARB if an ACE inhibitor is not tolerated) and a β-blocker.

Side Effects

The major problem with the use of MRAs is the development of life-threatening hyperkalemia, which is more prone to occur in patients who are receiving potassium supplements or who have underlying renal insufficiency. Aldosterone antagonists are not recommended when the serum creatinine is greater than 2.5 mg/dL (or creatinine clearance is <30 mL/min) or the serum potassium is greater than 5.5 mmol/L. The development of worsening renal function should lead to consideration regarding stopping aldosterone antagonists because of the potential risk of hyperkalemia. Although the rate of significant hyperkalemia is relatively modest in clinical trials (≈2%-3%), outcomes data suggest that it is potentially much higher in clinical practice with less intensive monitoring of potassium.[134] Painful gynecomastia may develop in 10% to 15% of patients who use spironolactone, in which case eplerenone may be substituted.

Practical Tips

The administration of an MRA is recommended for patients with NYHA class II to IV HF who have ejection fraction less than 35% and who are receiving standard therapy, including diuretics, ACEIs, and β-blockers. Spironolactone should be initiated at a dose of 12.5 to 25 mg daily, and uptitrated to 25 to 50 mg daily, whereas eplerenone should be initiated at doses of 25 mg/day and increased to 50 mg daily. As noted previously, potassium supplementation is generally stopped after the initiation of aldosterone antagonists, and patients should be counseled to avoid high potassium-containing foods. Potassium levels and renal function should be rechecked within 3 days and again at 1 week after initiation of an aldosterone antagonist. Subsequent monitoring should be dictated by the general clinical stability of renal function and fluid status but should occur at least monthly for the first 6 months.

Hydralazine and Nitrates

Therapy with the combination of hydralazine and isosorbide dinitrate (H-ISDN) has been shown to reduce all-cause mortality and morbidity in African Americans. There are two placebo-controlled (V-HeFT-I and A-HeFT) randomized trials and one active-controlled (V-HeFT-II) randomized trial with H-ISDN.

The biology of nitrate therapy in heart failure is complex (**Figure 34-12**), and is complicated by issues such as nitrate tolerance and variations in nitrate dosing.[135] Studies have demonstrated several mechanisms for nitrate tolerance, which occur within several days of initiating therapy.[136,137] In brief, chronic nitrate therapy increases vascular oxidative stress via production of superoxide from mitochondrial sources, as well as vascular smooth muscle and endothelium. The resulting reactive oxygen species (ROS) inhibit the bioactivation of administered nitrate into nitric oxide (NO). This "quenching of NO" by ROS reduces dilator metabolites.

To combat these mechanisms, radical scavengers and substances, which reduce oxidative stress indirectly, are able to relieve tolerance and endothelial dysfunction.[137] For example, hydralazine is an efficient ROS scavenger, which prevents the development of nitrate tolerance when given concomitantly with nitrates. Additional agents postulated to limit or reverse nitrate tolerance include ACE inhibitors, ARBs, β-blockers, statins, folic acid, and vitamin C.[138,139]

The Veterans Administration Cooperative Study on Vasodilator Therapy of Heart Failure (V-HeFT-I) investigated 642 male patients with chronic HF treated with digoxin and diuretics. Patients were randomized to H-ISDN, prazosin, or a placebo.[58] Published in 1986, no study patients were treated with β-blockers or ACE inhibitors. H-ISDN increased exercise capacity and LVEF compared with placebo. Treatment with H-ISDN produced a 28% reduction in mortality compared with the placebo. The benefit of H-ISDN was particularly prominent in younger patients with a lower EF. H-ISDN did not reduce hospitalizations.

In V-HeFT-II, 804 men, mainly with NYHA class II or III symptoms, were randomized to enalapril or H-ISDN (300 mg/160 mg), added to a diuretic and digoxin.[45] No patients were treated with a β-blocker. Enalapril produced more favorable effects on survival. There was a trend in the H-ISDN group toward an increase in all-cause mortality during the overall period of follow-up (mean 2.5 years): relative increase in risk was 28%. However, H-ISDN increased peak oxygen consumption and resulted in a greater increase in LVEF compared with enalapril.

A post hoc retrospective analysis of these vasodilator trials demonstrated particular efficacy of H-ISDN in the African American cohort.[140] Thus a subsequent trial of H-ISDN was conducted that was limited to patients self-described as African American, the African-American Heart Failure Trial (AHEFT).[141] In A-HeFT, 1050 African American men and women with NYHA class III or IV HF symptoms were randomized to a placebo or a fixed-dose combination H-ISDN. The initial dose of treatment was 37.5 mg hydralazine/20 mg ISDN three times daily, increasing to a target of 75 mg/40 mg three times daily. Published in 2004, study patients received medical management similar to contemporary guideline recommendations: ACE inhibitor (70%), ARB (17%), β-blocker (74%), and spironolactone (39%). The trial was discontinued prematurely after a median follow-up of 10 months because of a significant reduction in mortality with H-ISDN (**Figure 34-13**). H-ISDN also reduced the risk of HF hospitalization and improved quality of life. Despite these impressive results, uptake of this therapy in African American patients has been modest, with data suggesting that fewer than 10% of eligible patients are treated with this therapy.[142] Many potential factors may contribute to the underutilization of this therapy. The inclusion criteria of only self-identified African American patients has led to some uncertainty, given that this is as much a social construct as a specific genetic population. Additionally, the relatively small RCT that was terminated early, the complexity of the regimen (as well as uncertainty about the suitability of substitution of inexpensive forms of the generic drugs), and access to care issues are all potential contributors for low prescription rates for this form of treatment.

Side Effects

The most common adverse effects with H-ISDN in the landmark trials were headache, dizziness/hypotension, and

Nitroglycerin
Pseudotolerance
Tolerance
Aldehyde dehydrogenase
↑ Norepinephrine
↓ GPT-cyclo-hydrolase
Impaired NTG bioactivation in mitochondria
Vasodilation
↑ Arginine vasopressin
Tetrahydro-biopterin
Uncoupling
Dihydrobiopterin
Peroxynitrite
O_2^-
↑ Phospho-diesterases
Nitric oxide synthase
Soluble guanylate cyclase
cGMP
GMP
↑ Renin activity
NO^-
Peroxynitrite
Prostacyclin synthase
↓ Prostacyclin
↑ Angiotensin II
Protein kinase C
NADPH oxidase
O_2^-
Endothelin-1
Protein kinase C
Vasoconstriction
↑ Aldosterone
Endothelial dysfunction
Smooth muscle dysfunction
↑ Sodium and water retention
Vascular dysfunction
Intravascular expansion

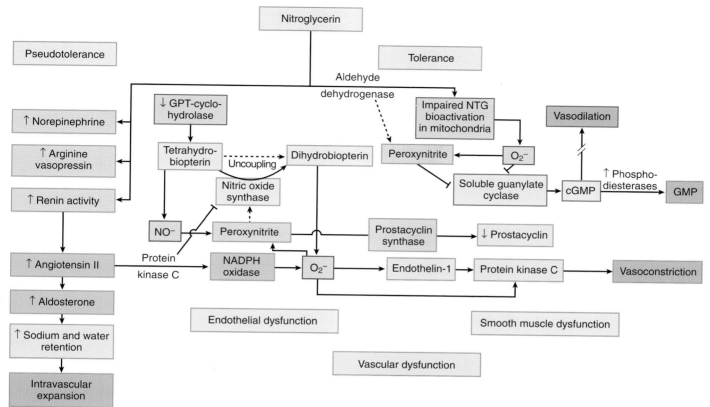

FIGURE 34-12 The biology of nitrate therapy in heart failure. Nitrate use leads to neurohormonal activation, which results in intravascular expansion through increased sodium and water retention *(Pseudo-tolerance)*. Later during therapy, changes in endothelial and smooth muscle cells function, resulting in vascular dysfunction *(Tolerance)*. These changes include (i) Activation of NADPH oxidase by angiotensin II through protein kinase C, which in turn results in superoxide (O_2^-) production. Superoxide results in vasoconstriction through endothelin-1 and protein kinase C. (ii) Protein kinase C directly inhibits nitric oxide synthase. (iii) Reduced expression of GTP-cyclohydrolase and peroxynitrite-induced oxidation of tetrahydrobiopterin causes limited tetrahydrobiopterin availability, which in turn causes uncoupling of endothelial nitric oxide synthase resulting in superoxide production and nitric oxide anions (NO^-). Nitric oxide anions through peroxynitrite cause inhibition of prostacyclin synthase, resulting in reduced prostacyclin levels. (iv) Impaired bioactivation of nitroglycerin (NTG) caused by inhibition of aldehyde dehydrogenase results in O_2^- production, which in turn inhibits smooth muscle soluble guanylate cyclase both directly and through peroxynitrite. (v) Cyclic-guanosine monophosphate (cGMP) vasodilatory properties are diminished secondary to cGMP inactivation by phosphodiesterases and low cGMP production because of the inhibition of soluble guanylate cyclase. *Reproduced from Gupta D, Georgiopoulou VV, Kalogeropoulos AP, et al: Nitrate therapy for heart failure: benefits and strategies to overcome tolerance. JACC Heart Fail 1:183–191, 2013.*

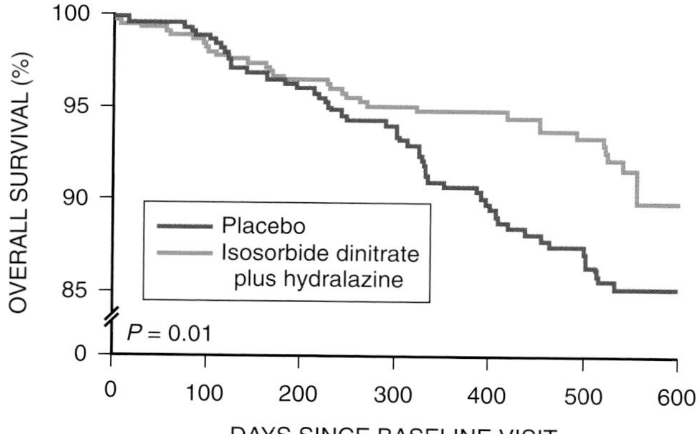

FIGURE 34-13 Kaplan-Meier estimates of overall survival with isosorbide dinitrate plus hydralazine compared with placebo in the African-American Heart Failure Trial (AHEFT). *Reproduced from Taylor AL, Ziesche S, Yancy C, et al: Combination of isosorbide dinitrate and hydralazine in blacks with heart failure. N Engl J Med 351:2049–2057, 2004.*

nausea. Arthralgia leading to discontinuation or reduction in dose of H-ISDN occurred in 5% to 10% of patients in V-HeFT I and II. A lupus-like syndrome has also been rarely reported, but a sustained increase in antinuclear antibody occurs in 2% to 3% of patients.

Practical Tips

H-ISDN should not be used in patients who have no prior use of ACE inhibitors/ARBs or β-blockers and should not be substituted for ACE inhibitors/ARBs in patients who are tolerating therapy without difficulty. Adherence to this combination has generally been poor because of the number of daily doses and tablets required, and the side effect profile including headache and dizziness. However, the benefit of these drugs can be substantial in specific patient populations who have been studied in randomized trials. Therefore, slower titration of the drugs should be performed to enhance tolerance of the therapy. If the fixed-dose combination is available, the initial dose should be one tablet containing 37.5 mg of hydralazine hydrochloride and 20 mg of isosorbide dinitrate three times daily. The dose can be increased to two tablets three times daily for a total daily dose of 225 mg of hydralazine hydrochloride and 120 mg of isosorbide dinitrate. When the two drugs are used separately, both pills should be administered at least three times daily. Initial low doses of the drugs given separately may be progressively increased to a goal similar to that achieved in the fixed-dose combination trial.

Ivabradine

Ivabradine is a heart rate–lowering agent that acts by selectively blocking the cardiac pacemaker *If* ("*f*unny") current

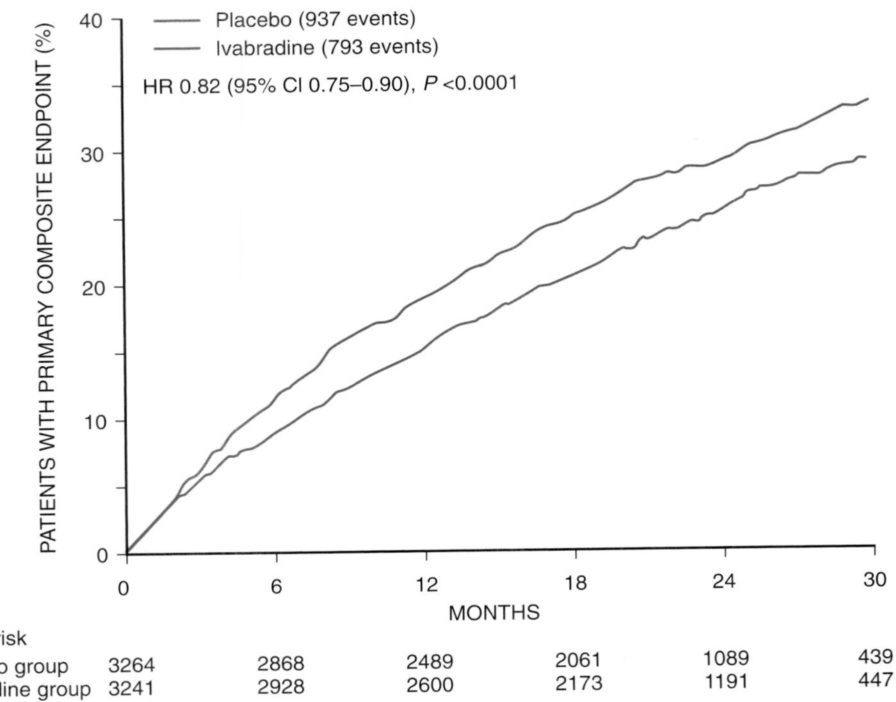

FIGURE 34-14 Kaplan-Meier cumulative event curves for the primary composite endpoint of cardiovascular death or hospital admission for worsening heart failure in the Systolic Heart failure treatment with the If inhibitor Ivabradine Trial (SHIFT). *Reproduced from Swedberg K, Komajda M, Böhm M, et al: Ivabradine and outcomes in chronic heart failure (SHIFT): a randomised placebo-controlled study. Lancet 376:875–885, 2010.*

that controls the spontaneous diastolic depolarization of the sinoatrial node. Ivabradine blocks I_f channels in a concentration-dependent manner by entering the channel pore from the intracellular side, and thus can only block the channel when it is open. The magnitude of I_f inhibition is directly related to the frequency of channel opening and would therefore be expected to be most effective at higher heart rates. Initially developed and approved as an antianginal agent in Europe, ivabradine was also shown to improve outcomes in the Systolic Heart failure treatment with the If inhibitor Ivabradine Trial (SHIFT), which enrolled symptomatic patients with an LVEF of 35% or less who were in sinus rhythm with a heart rate of 70 beats/min or more and on standard medical therapy for HF (including β-blockers).[143] SHIFT showed that ivabradine (uptitrated to a maximal dosage of 7.5 mg twice daily) reduced the primary composite outcome of cardiovascular death or HF hospitalization by 18% (HR 0.82, 95% CI 0.75-0.90, $P<0.0001$ (**Figure 34-14**). The composite endpoint was driven primarily by reducing hospital admissions for worsening HF (HR 0.74, CI 0.66-0.83, $P<0.0001$), insofar as there was no decrease in cardiovascular deaths (HR 0.91, 95% CI 0.80-1.03, $P=0.13$) or all-cause deaths. Given that ivabradine lowered heart rate by approximately 10 beats/min and that only 26% of the patients in the trial were on optimal doses of β-blockers, it is possible that titrating β-blockers to recommended disease may have reduced the HF hospitalizations to a similar degree. Additional safety evidence for ivabradine comes from the morbidity-mortality evaluation of the I_f inhibitor ivabradine in patients with coronary disease and left ventricular dysfunction (BEAUTIFUL) trial, in which over 10,000 patients with coronary heart disease and an EF less than 40% were randomized to treatment with ivabradine 7.5 mg twice daily.[144] Although this trial did not meet its primary endpoint of reducing cardiovascular death, myocardial infarction, or HF hospitalization, it was well tolerated in this patient population. Ivabradine use has been incorporated into European heart failure guidelines, but is not yet available in the United States.[145]

FUTURE DIRECTIONS

The progressive development of neurohormonal antagonists for chronic HF with systolic dysfunction has been one of the major success stories of modern cardiology. However, some have questioned whether the field has reached the ceiling benefits that can be provided by progressive neurohormonal blockade.[146] Notably, attempts to intervene on another major pathophysiologic mechanism associated with heart failure progression, such as inflammation and oxidative stress, have not been successful[147,148] (**see also Chapters 7 and 8**). Moving forward, therapeutic development for chronic HF is increasingly focused on novel approaches covered elsewhere in this textbook, including modulation of myocardial metabolism (**see Chapter 16**), device therapies (**see Chapter 35**), cellular and gene-based therapies (**see Chapter 38**), and mechanical circulatory support (**see Chapter 42**). In addition to ongoing development of new treatments, broad-based implementation of currently proven therapies remains a major unmet public health issue (**Chapter 46**).

References

1. Yancy CW, Jessup M, Bozkurt B, et al: 2013 ACCF/AHA guideline for the management of heart failure: a report of the American College of Cardiology Foundation/American Heart Association Task Force on Practice Guidelines. *Circulation* 128:e240–e327, 2013.
2. Paterna S, Fasullo S, Parrinello G, et al: Short-term effects of hypertonic saline solution in acute heart failure and long-term effects of a moderate sodium restriction in patients with compensated heart failure with New York Heart Association class III (Class C) (SMAC-HF Study). *Am J Med Sci* 342:27–37, 2011.
3. O'Connor CM, Whellan DJ, Lee KL, et al: Efficacy and safety of exercise training in patients with chronic heart failure: HF-ACTION randomized controlled trial. *JAMA* 301:1439–1450, 2009.
4. Packer M, Carson P, Elkayam U, et al: Effect of amlodipine on the survival of patients with severe chronic heart failure due to a nonischemic cardiomyopathy results of the PRAISE-2 study (Prospective Randomized Amlodipine Survival Evaluation 2). *JACC Heart Fail* 1:308–314, 2013.
5. Packer M, O'Connor CM, Ghali JK, et al: Effect of amlodipine on morbidity and mortality in severe chronic heart failure. *N Engl J Med* 335:1107–1114, 1996.
6. Ellison DH: Diuretic therapy and resistance in congestive heart failure. *Cardiology* 96:132–143, 2001.

7. Felker GM, Mentz RJ: Diuretics and ultrafiltration in acute decompensated heart failure. *J Am Coll Cardiol* 59:2145–2153, 2012.
8. Jentzer JC, DeWald TA, Hernandez AF: Combination of loop diuretics with thiazide-type diuretics in heart failure. *J Am Coll Cardiol* 56:1527–1534, 2010.
9. Bansal S, Lindenfeld J, Schrier RW: Sodium retention in heart failure and cirrhosis: potential role of natriuretic doses of mineralocorticoid antagonist? *Circ Heart Fail* 2:370–376, 2009.
10. Konstam MA, Gheorghiade M, Burnett JC, Jr, et al: Effects of oral tolvaptan in patients hospitalized for worsening heart failure: the EVEREST Outcome Trial. *JAMA* 297:1319–1331, 2007.
11. Pang PS, Konstam MA, Krasa HB, et al: Effects of tolvaptan on dyspnoea relief from the EVEREST trials. *Eur Heart J* 30:2233–2240, 2009.
12. Felker GM, O'Connor CM, Braunwald E, for the Heart Failure Clinical Research Network Investigators: Loop diuretics in acute decompensated heart failure: Necessary? Evil? A necessary evil? *Circ Heart Fail* 2:56–62, 2009.
13. Felker GM, Lee KL, Bull DA, et al: Diuretic strategies in patients with acute decompensated heart failure. *N Engl J Med* 364:797–805, 2011.
14. Cooper HA, Dries DL, Davis CE, et al: Diuretics and risk of arrhythmic death in patients with left ventricular dysfunction. *Circulation* 100:1311–1315, 1999.
15. Loon NR, Wilcox CS, Unwin RJ: Mechanism of impaired natriuretic response to furosemide during prolonged therapy. *Kidney Int* 36:682–689, 1989.
16. Kaissling B, Bachmann S, Kriz W: Structural adaptation of the distal convoluted tubule to prolonged furosemide treatment. *Am J Physiol* 248:F374–F381, 1985.
17. Urata H, Healy B, Stewart RW, et al: Angiotensin II-forming pathways in normal and failing human hearts. *Circ Res* 66:883–890, 1990.
18. Urata H, Boehm KD, Philip A, et al: Cellular localization and regional distribution of an angiotensin II-forming chymase in the heart. *J Clin Invest* 91:1269–1281, 1993.
19. Linz W, Wiemer G, Gohlke P, et al: Contribution of kinins to the cardiovascular actions of angiotensin-converting enzyme inhibitors. *Pharmacol Rev* 47:25–49, 1995.
20. Mombouli J-V, Vanhoutte PM: Endothelial dysfunction: from physiology to therapy. *J Mol Cell Cardiol* 31:61–74, 1999.
21. Yamasaki S, Sawada S, Komatsu S, et al: Effects of bradykinin on prostaglandin I2 synthesis in human vascular endothelial cells. *Hypertension* 36:201–207, 2000.
22. McDonald KM, Mock J, D'Aloia A, et al: Bradykinin antagonism inhibits the antigrowth effect of converting enzyme inhibition in the dog myocardium after discrete transmural myocardial necrosis. *Circulation* 91:2043–2048, 1995.
23. Wollert KC, Studer R, Doerfer K, et al: Differential effects of kinins on cardiomyocyte hypertrophy and interstitial collagen matrix in the surviving myocardium after myocardial infarction in the rat. *Circulation* 95:1910–1917, 1997.
24. Linz W, Schölkens BA: A specific B2-bradykinin receptor antagonist HOE 140 abolishes the antihypertrophic effect of ramipril. *Br J Pharmacol* 105:771–772, 1992.
25. Matsubara H: Pathophysiological role of angiotensin II type 2 receptor in cardiovascular and renal diseases. *Circ Res* 83:1182–1191, 1998.
26. Yamada T, Horiuchi M, Dzau VJ: Angiotensin II type 2 receptor mediates programmed cell death. *PNAS* 93:156–160, 1996.
27. Levine TB, Olivari MT, Garberg V, et al: Hemodynamic and clinical response to enalapril, a long-acting converting-enzyme inhibitor, in patients with congestive heart failure. *Circulation* 69:548–553, 1984.
28. Uretsky BF, Shaver JA, Liang C-S, et al: Modulation of hemodynamic effects with a converting enzyme inhibitor: acute hemodynamic dose-response relationship of a new angiotensin converting enzyme inhibitor, lisinopril, with observations on long-term clinical, functional, and biochemical responses. *Am Heart J* 116:480–488, 1988.
29. Patten RD, Kronenberg MW, Benedict CR, et al: Acute and long-term effects of the angiotensin-converting enzyme inhibitor, enalapril, on adrenergic activity and sensitivity during exercise in patients with left ventricular systolic dysfunction. *Am Heart J* 134:37–43, 1997.
30. Benedict CR, Johnstone DE, Weiner DH, et al: Relation of neurohumoral activation to clinical variables and degree of ventricular dysfunction: a report from the registry of studies of left ventricular dysfunction. *J Am Coll Cardiol* 23:1410–1420, 1994.
31. Gottlieb SS, Dickstein K, Fleck E, et al: Hemodynamic and neurohormonal effects of the angiotensin II antagonist losartan in patients with congestive heart failure. *Circulation* 88:1602–1609, 1993.
32. Havranek EP, Thomas I, Smith WB, et al: Dose-related beneficial long-term hemodynamic and clinical efficacy of irbesartan in heart failure. *J Am Coll Cardiol* 33:1174–1181, 1999.
33. Crozier I, Ikram H, Awan N, et al: Losartan in heart failure: hemodynamic effects and tolerability. *Circulation* 91:691–697, 1995.
34. Baruch L, Anand I, Cohen IS, et al: Augmented short- and long-term hemodynamic and hormonal effects of an angiotensin receptor blocker added to angiotensin converting enzyme inhibitor therapy in patients with heart failure. *Circulation* 99:2658–2664, 1999.
35. MacFadyen RJ, Lee AF, Morton JJ, et al: How often are angiotensin II and aldosterone concentrations raised during chronic ACE inhibitor treatment in cardiac failure? *Heart* 82:57–61, 1999.
36. Roig E, Perez-Villa F, Morales M, et al: Clinical implications of increased plasma angiotensin II despite ACE inhibitor therapy in patients with congestive heart failure. *Eur Heart J* 21:53–57, 2000.
37. Sharpe N, Smith H, Murphy J, et al: Early prevention of left ventricular dysfunction after myocardial infarction with angiotensin-converting-enzyme inhibition. *Lancet* 337:872–876, 1991.
38. St John Sutton M, Pfeffer MA, Plappert T, et al: Quantitative two-dimensional echocardiographic measurements are major predictors of adverse cardiovascular events after acute myocardial infarction. The protective effects of captopril. *Circulation* 89:68–75, 1994.
39. Konstam MA, Rousseau MF, Kronenberg MW, et al: Effects of the angiotensin converting enzyme inhibitor enalapril on the long-term progression of left ventricular dysfunction in patients with heart failure. SOLVD Investigators. *Circulation* 86:431–438, 1992.
40. Konstam MA, Kronenberg MW, Rousseau MF, et al: Effects of the angiotensin converting enzyme inhibitor enalapril on the long-term progression of left ventricular dilatation in patients with asymptomatic systolic dysfunction. SOLVD (Studies of Left Ventricular Dysfunction) Investigators. *Circulation* 88:2277–2283, 1993.
41. Konstam MA, Patten RD, Thomas I, et al: Effects of losartan and captopril on left ventricular volumes in elderly patients with heart failure: results of the ELITE ventricular function substudy. *Am Heart J* 139:1081–1087, 2000.
42. McKelvie RS, Yusuf S, Pericak D, et al: Comparison of candesartan, enalapril, and their combination in congestive heart failure: randomized evaluation of strategies for left ventricular dysfunction (resolvd) pilot study: the resolvd pilot study investigators. *Circulation* 100:1056–1064, 1999.
43. Pfeffer MA, McMurray JJV, Velazquez EJ, et al: Valsartan, captopril, or both in myocardial infarction complicated by heart failure, left ventricular dysfunction, or both. *N Engl J Med* 349:1893–1906, 2003.
44. Solomon SD, Skali H, Anavekar NS, et al: Changes in ventricular size and function in patients treated with valsartan, captopril, or both after myocardial infarction. *Circulation* 111:3411–3419, 2005.
45. Cohn JN, Johnson G, Ziesche S, et al: A comparison of enalapril with hydralazine-isosorbide dinitrate in the treatment of chronic congestive heart failure. *N Engl J Med* 325:303–310, 1991.
46. Ziesche S, Cobb FR, Cohn JN, et al: Hydralazine and isosorbide dinitrate combination improves exercise tolerance in heart failure. Results from V-HeFT I and V-HeFT II. The V-HeFT VA Cooperative Studies Group. *Circulation* 87:VI56–VI64, 1993.
47. A placebo-controlled trial of captopril in refractory chronic congestive heart failure. *J Am Coll Cardiol* 2:755–763, 1983.
48. Riegger GA: Effects of quinapril on exercise tolerance in patients with mild to moderate heart failure. *Eur Heart J* 12:705–711, 1991.
49. Lang RM, Elkayam U, Yellen LG, et al: Comparative effects of losartan and enalapril on exercise capacity and clinical status in patients with heart failure. *J Am Coll Cardiol* 30:983–991, 1997.
50. Vescovo G, Dalla Libera L, Serafini F, et al: Improved exercise tolerance after losartan and enalapril in heart failure: correlation with changes in skeletal muscle myosin heavy chain composition. *Circulation* 98:1742–1749, 1998.
51. Riegger GAJ, Bouzo H, Petr P, et al: Improvement in exercise tolerance and symptoms of congestive heart failure during treatment with candesartan cilexetil. *Circulation* 100:2224–2230, 1999.
52. Effect of enalapril on mortality and the development of heart failure in asymptomatic patients with reduced left ventricular ejection fractions. The SOLVD Investigattors. *N Engl J Med* 327:685–691, 1992.
53. Pfeffer MA, Braunwald E, Moye LA, et al: Effect of captopril on mortality and morbidity in patients with left ventricular dysfunction after myocardial infarction. Results of the survival and ventricular enlargement trial. The SAVE Investigators. *N Engl J Med* 327:669–677, 1992.
54. Kober L, Torp-Pedersen C, Carlsen JE, et al: A clinical trial of the angiotensin-converting-enzyme inhibitor trandolapril in patients with left ventricular dysfunction after myocardial infarction. Trandolapril Cardiac Evaluation (TRACE) Study Group. *N Engl J Med* 333:1670–1676, 1995.
55. Effects of enalapril on mortality in severe congestive heart failure. *NEJM* 316:1429–1435, 1987.
56. Effect of enalapril on survival in patients with reduced left ventricular ejection fractions and congestive heart failure. *NEJM* 325:293–302, 1991.
57. Garg R, Yusuf S: Overview of randomized trials of angiotensin-converting enzyme inhibitors on mortality and morbidity in patients with heart failure. *J Am Med Assoc* 273:1450–1456, 1995.
58. Cohn JN, Archibald DG, Ziesche S, et al: Effect of vasodilator therapy on mortality in chronic congestive heart failure. Results of a Veterans Administration Cooperative Study. *N Engl J Med* 314:1547–1552, 1986.
59. Packer M, Poole-Wilson PA, Armstrong PW, et al: Comparative effects of low and high doses of the angiotensin-converting enzyme inhibitor, lisinopril, on morbidity and mortality in chronic heart failure. ATLAS Study Group. *Circulation* 100:2312–2318, 1999.
60. Damman K, Tang WH, Felker GM, et al: Current evidence on treatment of patients with chronic systolic heart failure and renal insufficiency: practical considerations from published data. *J Am Coll Cardiol* 63:853–871, 2014.
61. Granger CB, McMurray JJV, Yusuf S, et al: Effects of candesartan in patients with chronic heart failure and reduced left-ventricular systolic function intolerant to angiotensin-converting-enzyme inhibitors: the CHARM-Alternative trial. *Lancet* 362:772–776, 2003.
62. Maggioni AP, Anand I, Gottlieb SO, et al: Effects of valsartan on morbidity and mortality in patients with heart failure not receiving angiotensin-converting enzyme inhibitors. *J Am Coll Cardiol* 40:1414–1421, 2002.
63. Pitt B, Poole-Wilson PA, Segal R, et al: Effect of losartan compared with captopril on mortality in patients with symptomatic heart failure: randomised trial—the Losartan Heart Failure Survival Study ELITE II. *Lancet* 355:1582–1587, 2000.
64. McMurray JJV, Ostergren J, Swedberg K, et al: Effects of candesartan in patients with chronic heart failure and reduced left-ventricular systolic function taking angiotensin-converting-enzyme inhibitors: the CHARM-Added trial. *Lancet* 362:767–771, 2003.
65. Cohn JN, Tognoni G, Valsartan Heart Failure Trial Investigators: A randomized trial of the angiotensin-receptor blocker valsartan in chronic heart failure. *N Engl J Med* 345:1667–1675, 2001.
66. Konstam MA, Neaton JD, Dickstein K, et al: Effects of high-dose versus low-dose losartan on clinical outcomes in patients with heart failure (HEAAL study): a randomised, double-blind trial. *Lancet* 374:1840–1848, 2009.
67. Lee VC, Rhew DC, Dylan M, et al: Meta-analysis: angiotensin-receptor blockers in chronic heart failure and high-risk acute myocardial infarction. *Ann Intern Med* 141:693–704, 2004.
68. Latini R, Tognoni G, Maggioni AP, et al: Clinical effects of early angiotensin-converting enzyme inhibitor treatment for acute myocardial infarction are similar in the presence and absence of aspirin: systematic overview of individual data from 96,712 randomized patients. Angiotensin-converting Enzyme Inhibitor Myocardial Infarction Collaborative Group. *J Am Coll Cardiol* 35:1801–1807, 2000.
69. Teo KK, Yusuf S, Pfeffer M, et al: Effects of long-term treatment with angiotensin-converting-enzyme inhibitors in the presence or absence of aspirin: a systematic review. *Lancet* 360:1037–1043, 2002.

69a. Trippodo NC, Fox M, Monticello TM, et al: Vasopeptidase inhibition with omapatrilat improves cardiac geometry and survival in cardiomyopathic hamsters more than does ACE inhibition with captopril. *J Cardiovasc Pharmacol* 34:782–790, 1999.

69b. Packer M, Califf RM, Konstam MA, et al: Comparison of omapatrilat and enalapril in patients with chronic heart failure: the Omapatrilat Versus Enalapril Randomized Trial of Utility in Reducing Events (OVERTURE). *Circulation* 106:920–926, 2002.

69c. Kostis JB, Packer M, Black HR, et al: Omapatrilat and enalapril in patients with hypertension: the Omapatrilat Cardiovascular Treatment vs. Enalapril (OCTAVE) trial. *Am J Hypertens* 17:103–111, 2004.

69d. Solomon SD, Zile M, Pieske B, et al: The angiotensin receptor neprilysin inhibitor LCZ696 in heart failure with preserved ejection fraction: a phase 2 double-blind randomised controlled trial. *Lancet* 380:1387–1395, 2012.

69e. McMurray JJ, Packer M, Desai AS, et al, for the PARADIGM-HF Investigators and Committees: Angiotensin-neprilysin inhibition versus enalapril in heart failure. *N Engl J Med* 371:993–1004, 2014.

70. Chidsey CA, Sonnenblick EH, Morrow AG, et al: Norepinephrine stores and contractile force of papillary muscle from the failing human heart. *Circulation* 33:43–51, 1966.
71. Chidsey CA, Braunwald E, Morrow AG: Catecholamine excretion and cardiac stores of norepinephrine in congestive heart failure. *Am J Med* 39:442–451, 1965.
72. Bristow MR, Ginsburg R, Minobe W, et al: Decreased catecholamine sensitivity and β-adrenergic-receptor density in failing human hearts. *NEJM* 307:205–211, 1982.
73. Swedberg K, Viquerat C, Rouleau JL, et al: Comparison of myocardial catecholamine balance in chronic congestive heart failure and in angina pectoris without failure. *Am J Cardiol* 54:783–786, 1984.
74. Hasking GJ, Esler MD, Jennings GL, et al: Norepinephrine spillover to plasma in patients with congestive heart failure: evidence of increased overall and cardiorenal sympathetic nervous activity. *Circulation* 73:615–621, 1986.
75. Doughty RN, Whalley GA, Gamble G, et al: Left ventricular remodeling with carvedilol in patients with congestive heart failure due to ischemic heart disease. Australia-New Zealand Heart Failure Research Collaborative Group. *J Am Coll Cardiol* 29:1060–1066, 1997.
76. Colucci WS, Kolias TJ, Adams KF, et al: Metoprolol reverses left ventricular remodeling in patients with asymptomatic systolic dysfunction: the REversal of VEntricular Remodeling with Toprol-XL (REVERT) trial. *Circulation* 116:49–56, 2007.

77. Hall SA, Cigarroa CG, Marcoux L, et al: Time course of improvement in left ventricular function, mass and geometry in patients with congestive heart failure treated with beta-adrenergic blockade. *J Am Coll Cardiol* 25:1154–1161, 1995.
78. Waagstein F, Caidahl K, Wallentin I, et al: Long-term beta-blockade in dilated cardiomyopathy. Effects of short- and long-term metoprolol treatment followed by withdrawal and readministration of metoprolol. *Circulation* 80:551–563, 1989.
79. Metra M, Nodari S, D'Aloia A, et al: A rationale for the use of β-blockers as standard treatment for heart failure. *Am Heart J* 139:511–521, 2000.
80. Metra M, Nodari S, Parrinello G, et al: Marked improvement in left ventricular ejection fraction during long-term β-blockade in patients with chronic heart failure: clinical correlates and prognostic significance. *Am Heart J* 145:292–299, 2003.
81. de Groote P, Delour P, Mouquet F, et al: The effects of β-blockers in patients with stable chronic heart failure. Predictors of left ventricular ejection fraction improvement and impact on prognosis. *Am Heart J* 154:589–595, 2007.
82. Schleman KA, Lindenfeld JA, Lowes BD, et al: Predicting response to carvedilol for the treatment of heart failure: a multivariate retrospective analysis. *J Card Fail* 7:4–12, 2001.
83. Di Lenarda A, Gregori D, Sinagra G, et al: Metoprolol in dilated cardiomyopathy: Is it possible to identify factors predictive of improvement? *J Card Fail* 2:87–102, 1996.
84. Eichhorn EJ, Grayburn PA, Mayer SA, et al: myocardial contractile reserve by dobutamine stress echocardiography predicts improvement in ejection fraction with β-blockade in patients with heart failure: the β-Blocker Evaluation of Survival Trial (BEST). *Circulation* 108:2336–2341, 2003.
85. Seghatol FF, Shah DJ, Diluzio S, et al: Relation between contractile reserve and improvement in left ventricular function with beta-blocker therapy in patients with heart failure secondary to ischemic or idiopathic dilated cardiomyopathy. *Am J Cardiol* 93:854–859, 2004.
86. Cleland JGF, Pennell DJ, Ray SG, et al: Myocardial viability as a determinant of the ejection fraction response to carvedilol in patients with heart failure (CHRISTMAS trial): randomised controlled trial. *Lancet* 362:14–21, 2003.
87. Bristow MR, Gilbert EM, Abraham WT, et al: Carvedilol produces dose-related improvements in left ventricular function and survival in subjects with chronic heart failure. *Circulation* 94:2807–2816, 1996.
88. Lechat P, Escolano S, Golmard JL, et al: Prognostic value of bisoprolol-induced hemodynamic effects in heart failure during the Cardiac Insufficiency BIsoprolol Study (CIBIS). *Circulation* 96:2197–2205, 1997.
89. Bristow MR: β-adrenergic receptor blockade in chronic heart failure. *Circulation* 101:558–569, 2000.
90. White M, Yanowitz F, Gilbert EM, et al: Role of beta-adrenergic receptor downregulation in the peak exercise response in patients with heart failure due to idiopathic dilated cardiomyopathy. *Am J Cardiol* 76:1271–1276, 1995.
91. Metra M, Nardi M, Giubbini R, et al: Effects of short- and long-term carvedilol administration on rest and exercise hemodynamic variables, exercise capacity and clinical conditions in patients with idiopathic dilated cardiomyopathy. *J Am Coll Cardiol* 24:1678–1687, 1994.
92. Bristow MR, Roden RL, Lowes BD, et al: The role of third-generation beta-blocking agents in chronic heart failure. *Clin Cardiol* 21:I3–I13, 1998.
93. Metra M, Nodari S, D'Aloia A, et al: Effects of neurohormonal antagonism on symptoms and quality-of-life in heart failure. *Eur Heart J* 19(Suppl B):B25–B35, 1998.
94. Waagstein F, Hjalmarson A, Swedberg K, et al: Beneficial effects of metoprolol in idiopathic dilated cardiomyopathy. *Lancet* 342:1441–1446, 1993.
95. Heilbrunn SM, Shah P, Bristow MR, et al: Increased beta-receptor density and improved hemodynamic response to catecholamine stimulation during long-term metoprolol therapy in heart failure from dilated cardiomyopathy. *Circulation* 79:483–490, 1989.
96. Krum H, Sackner-Bernstein JD, Goldsmith RL, et al: Double-blind, placebo-controlled study of the long-term efficacy of carvedilol in patients with severe chronic heart failure. *Circulation* 92:1499–1506, 1995.
97. Olsen SL, Gilbert EM, Renlund DG, et al: Carvedilol improves left ventricular function and symptoms in chronic heart failure: a double-blind randomized study. *J Am Coll Cardiol* 25:1225–1231, 1995.
98. Packer M, Colucci WS, Sackner-Bernstein JD, et al: Double-blind, placebo-controlled study of the effects of carvedilol in patients with moderate to severe heart failure: the PRECISE Trial. *Circulation* 94:2793–2799, 1996.
99. Colucci WS, Packer M, Bristow MR, et al: Carvedilol inhibits clinical progression in patients with mild symptoms of heart failure. *Circulation* 94:2800–2806, 1996.
100. Abdulla J, Køber L, Christensen E, et al: Effect of beta-blocker therapy on functional status in patients with heart failure—a meta-analysis. *Eur J Heart Fail* 8:522–531, 2006.
101. Group M-HS: Effect of metoprolol CR/XL in chronic heart failure: Metoprolol CR/XL Randomised Intervention Trial in Congestive Heart Failure (MERIT-HF). *Lancet* 353:2001–2007, 1999.
102. A randomized trial of beta-blockade in heart failure. The Cardiac Insufficiency Bisoprolol Study (CIBIS). CIBIS Investigators and Committees. *Circulation* 90:1765–1773, 1994.
103. The CIII: the Cardiac Insufficiency Bisoprolol Study II (CIBIS-II): a randomised trial. *Lancet* 353:9–13, 1999.
104. Willenheimer R, van Veldhuisen DJ, Silke B, et al: Effect on survival and hospitalization of initiating treatment for chronic heart failure with bisoprolol followed by enalapril, as compared with the opposite sequence. Results of the randomized Cardiac Insufficiency Bisoprolol Study (CIBIS) III. *Circulation* 112:2426–2435, 2005.
105. Randomised, placebo-controlled trial of carvedilol in patients with congestive heart failure due to ischaemic heart disease. Australia/New Zealand Heart Failure Research Collaborative Group. *Lancet* 349:375–380, 1997.
106. Packer M, Coats AJ, Fowler MB, et al: Effect of carvedilol on survival in severe chronic heart failure. *N Engl J Med* 344:1651–1658, 2001.
107. Dargie HJ: Effect of carvedilol on outcome after myocardial infarction in patients with left-ventricular dysfunction: the CAPRICORN randomised trial. *Lancet* 357:1385–1390, 2001.
108. Poole-Wilson PA, Swedberg K, Cleland JGF, et al: Comparison of carvedilol and metoprolol on clinical outcomes in patients with chronic heart failure in the Carvedilol Or Metoprolol, European Trial (COMET): randomised controlled trial. *Lancet* 362:7–13, 2003.
109. Beta-Blocker Evaluation of Survival Trial Investigators: A trial of the beta-blocker bucindolol in patients with advanced heart failure. *N Engl J Med* 344:1659–1667, 2001.
110. Liggett SB, Mialet-Perez J, Thaneemit-Chen S, et al: A polymorphism within a conserved beta(1)-adrenergic receptor motif alters cardiac function and beta-blocker response in human heart failure. *Proc Natl Acad Sci U S A* 103:11288–11293, 2006.
111. Flather MD, Shibata MC, Coats AJ, et al: Randomized trial to determine the effect of nebivolol on mortality and cardiovascular hospital admission in elderly patients with heart failure (SENIORS). *Eur Heart J* 26:215–225, 2005.
112. Jondeau G, Neuder Y, Eicher J-C, et al: B-CONVINCED: Beta-blocker CONtinuation Vs. INterruption in patients with Congestive heart failure hospitalizED for a decompensation episode. *Eur Heart J* 30:2186–2192, 2009.
113. Gattis WA, O'Connor CM, Gallup DS, et al: Predischarge initiation of carvedilol in patients hospitalized for decompensated heart failure: results of the Initiation Management Predischarge: Process for Assessment of Carvedilol Therapy in Heart Failure (IMPACT-HF) trial. *J Am Coll Cardiol* 43:1534–1541, 2004.
114. Mulrow PJ: Angiotensin II and aldosterone regulation. *Regul Pept* 80:27–32, 1999.
115. Biollaz J, Brunner HR, Gavras I, et al: Antihypertensive therapy with MK 421: angiotensin II–renin relationships to evaluate efficacy of converting enzyme blockade. *J Cardiovasc Pharmacol* 4:966–972, 1982.
116. Young MJ, Lam EY, Rickard AJ: Mineralocorticoid receptor activation and cardiac fibrosis. *Clin Sci (Lond)* 112:467–475, 2007.
117. Delyani JA, Robinson EL, Rudolph AE: Effect of a selective aldosterone receptor antagonist in myocardial infarction. *Am J Physiol Heart Circ Physiol* 281:H647–H654, 2001.
118. Suzuki G, Morita H, Mishima T, et al: Effects of long-term monotherapy with eplerenone, a novel aldosterone blocker, on progression of left ventricular dysfunction and remodeling in dogs with heart failure. *Circulation* 106:2967–2972, 2002.
119. Silvestre J-S, Heymes C, Oubénaïssa A, et al: Activation of cardiac aldosterone production in rat myocardial infarction: effect of angiotensin II receptor blockade and role in cardiac fibrosis. *Circulation* 99:2694–2701, 1999.
120. Weber K, Brilla CG, Campbell SE, et al: Myocardial fibrosis: role of angiotensin II and aldosterone. In Grobecker H, Heusch G, Strauer BE, editors: *Angiotensin and the heart*, Darmstadt, 1993, Steinkopff, pp 107–124.
121. Weber KT: Aldosterone and spironolactone in heart failure. *NEJM* 341:753–755, 1999.
122. Zhao W, Ahokas RA, Weber KT, et al: ANG II-induced cardiac molecular and cellular events: Role of aldosterone. *Am J Physiol Heart Circ Physiol* 291:H336–H343, 2006.
123. Rude MK, Duhaney T-AS, Kuster GM, et al: Aldosterone stimulates matrix metalloproteinases and reactive oxygen species in adult rat ventricular cardiomyocytes. *Hypertension* 46:555–561, 2005.
124. Mano A, Tatsumi T, Shiraishi J, et al: Aldosterone directly induces myocyte apoptosis through calcineurin-dependent pathways. *Circulation* 110:317–323, 2004.
125. Pitt B, Zannad F, Remme WJ, et al: The effect of spironolactone on morbidity and mortality in patients with severe heart failure. *N Engl J Med* 341:709–717, 1999.
126. Jaffe IZ, Mendelsohn ME: Angiotensin II and aldosterone regulate gene transcription via functional mineralocortocoid receptors in human coronary artery smooth muscle cells. *Circ Res* 96:643–650, 2005.
127. Jaffe IZ, Tintut Y, Newfell BG, et al: Mineralocorticoid receptor activation promotes vascular cell calcification. *Arterioscler Thromb Vasc Biol* 27:799–805, 2007.
128. Hayashi M, Tsutamoto T, Wada A, et al: Immediate administration of mineralocorticoid receptor antagonist spironolactone prevents post-infarct left ventricular remodeling associated with suppression of a marker of myocardial collagen synthesis in patients with first anterior acute myocardial infarction. *Circulation* 107:2559–2565, 2003.
129. Kasama S, Toyama T, Kumakura H, et al: Effect of spironolactone on cardiac sympathetic nerve activity and left ventricular remodeling in patients with dilated cardiomyopathy. *J Am Coll Cardiol* 41:574–581, 2003.
130. Udelson JE, Feldman AM, Greenberg B, et al: Randomized, double-blind, multicenter, placebo-controlled study evaluating the effect of aldosterone antagonism with eplerenone on ventricular remodeling in patients with mild-to-moderate heart failure and left ventricular systolic dysfunction. *Circulation* 3:347–353, 2010.
131. Pitt B, Zannad F, Remme WJ, et al: The effect of spironolactone on morbidity and mortality in patients with severe heart failure. Randomized Aldactone Evaluation Study Investigators. *N Engl J Med* 341:709–717, 1999.
132. Zannad F, McMurray JJ, Krum H, et al: Eplerenone in patients with systolic heart failure and mild symptoms. *N Engl J Med* 364:11–21, 2011.
133. Pitt B, Remme W, Zannad F, et al: Eplerenone, a selective aldosterone blocker, in patients with left ventricular dysfunction after myocardial infarction. *N Engl J Med* 348:1309–1321, 2003.
134. Juurlink DN, Mamdani MM, Lee DS, et al: Rates of hyperkalemia after publication of the Randomized Aldactone Evaluation Study. *N Engl J Med* 351:543–551, 2004.
135. Gupta D, Georgiopoulou VV, Kalogeropoulos AP, et al: Nitrate therapy for heart failure benefits and strategies to overcome tolerance. *JACC Heart Fail* 1:183–191, 2013.
136. Daiber A, Mulsch A, Hink U, et al: The oxidative stress concept of nitrate tolerance and the antioxidant properties of hydralazine. *Am J Cardiol* 96:25i–36i, 2005.
137. Munzel T, Daiber A, Mulsch A: Explaining the phenomenon of nitrate tolerance. *Circ Res* 97:618–628, 2005.
138. Horowitz JD: Amelioration of nitrate tolerance: matching strategies with mechanisms. *J Am Coll Cardiol* 41:2001–2003, 2003.
139. Liuni A, Luca MC, Di Stolfo G, et al: Coadministration of atorvastatin prevents nitroglycerin-induced endothelial dysfunction and nitrate tolerance in healthy humans. *J Am Coll Cardiol* 57:93–98, 2011.
140. Carson P, Ziesche S, Johnson G, et al: Racial differences in response to therapy for heart failure: analysis of the vasodilator-heart failure trials. Vasodilator-Heart Failure Trial Study Group. *J Card Fail* 5:178–187, 1999.
141. Taylor AL, Ziesche S, Yancy C, et al: Combination of isosorbide dinitrate and hydralazine in blacks with heart failure. *N Engl J Med* 351:2049–2057, 2004.
142. Cole RT, Kalogeropoulos AP, Georgiopoulou VV, et al: Hydralazine and isosorbide dinitrate in heart failure: historical perspective, mechanisms, and future directions. *Circulation* 123:2414–2422, 2011.
143. Swedberg K, Komajda M, Bohm M, et al: Ivabradine and outcomes in chronic heart failure (SHIFT): a randomised placebo-controlled study. *Lancet* 376:875–885, 2010.
144. Fox K, Komajda M, Ford I, et al: Effect of ivabradine in patients with left-ventricular systolic dysfunction: a pooled analysis of individual patient data from the BEAUTIFUL and SHIFT trials. *Eur Heart J* 34:2263–2270, 2013.
145. McMurray JJ, Adamopoulos S, Anker SD, et al: ESC Guidelines for the diagnosis and treatment of acute and chronic heart failure 2012: the Task Force for the Diagnosis and Treatment of Acute and Chronic Heart Failure 2012 of the European Society of Cardiology. Developed in collaboration with the Heart Failure Association (HFA) of the ESC. *Eur Heart J* 33:1787–1847, 2012.
146. Mehra MR, Uber PA, Francis GS: Heart failure therapy at a crossroad: are there limits to the neurohormonal model? *J Am Coll Cardiol* 41:1606–1610, 2003.
147. Mann DL: Inflammatory mediators and the failing heart: past, present, and the foreseeable future. *Circ Res* 91:988–998, 2002.
148. Hare JM, Mangal B, Brown J, et al: Impact of oxypurinol in patients with symptomatic heart failure. Results of the OPT-CHF study. *J Am Coll Cardiol* 51:2301–2309, 2008.

GUIDELINES

Management of Heart Failure with a Reduced Ejection Fraction*

A joint task force of the American College of Cardiology and the American Heart Association (ACC/AHA) published updated guidelines for the evaluation and management of heart failure (HF) in 2013.[1] These guidelines replaced previous sets of recommendations issued by the ACC/AHA in 2005[2] and updated in 2009.[3] New guidelines from the Heart Failure Society were published in 2010,[4] which superseded guidelines published in 2006.[4] The European Society of Cardiology (ESC) guidelines for the diagnosis and treatment of chronic heart failure were published in 2012,[5] which superseded guidelines published in 2008.[6]

As reviewed in **Chapter 34**, the ACC/AHA guidelines classify patients according to four stages: stage A—patients at high risk for developing heart failure but without structural disorders of the heart; stage B—patients with a structural disorder of the heart but no symptoms of heart failure; stage C—patients with past or current symptoms of heart failure associated with underlying structural heart disease; and stage D—patients with end-stage disease who require specialized treatment strategies, such as mechanical circulatory support, continuous inotropic infusions, cardiac transplantation, or hospice care. The guidelines are organized into recommendations for each stage (see Figure 34-1). As with other ACC/AHA guidelines, these recommendations classify interventions into one of three classes as follows, including two levels of the intermediate group:

Class I: Procedure/Treatment **SHOULD** be performed/administered (Benefit >>> Risk)

Class IIa: Additional studies with focused objectives needed. **IT IS REASONABLE** to perform procedure/administer treatment (Benefit >>> Risk)

Class IIb: Additional studies with broad objectives needed; additional registry data would be helpful. Procedure/administer treatment **MAY BE CONSIDERED** (Benefit ≥ Risk).

Class III: No Benefit (not helpful and of no proven benefit) or class III Harm (excessive cost without benefit or harmful)

The ACC/AHA guidelines also adopt a convention for rating levels of evidence on which recommendations have been based. Level A recommendations are derived from data from multiple populations with data from multiple randomized clinical trials and/or meta-analyses; level B recommendations are derived from data from limited populations with data from a single randomized clinical trial or nonrandomized studies; and level C recommendations are based on very limited populations or the consensus opinion of experts or case studies. The guidelines emphasize that the strength of evidence does not necessarily reflect the strength of a recommendation. A treatment may be controversial despite having been evaluated in controlled clinical trials; conversely, a strong recommendation may be supported only by historical data or by no data at all. New for the current set of guidelines is the introduction of the term *guideline-directed medical therapy (GDMT)*, which represents optimal medical therapy as defined by the ACC/AHA guideline-recommended therapies (primarily class I).

*Modified from Mann DL: Guidelines: management of heart failure with reduced ejection fraction. In Mann DL, Zipes DP, Libby P, et al, editors: *Braunwald's heart disease: a textbook of cardiovascular medicine,* ed 10, Philadelphia, 2015, Saunders.

INITIAL PATIENT EVALUATION

The ACC/AHA guidelines state that a complete history and physical examination should be the first step in the evaluation of patients with heart failure (**Table 34G-1**). This evaluation may provide insight into the cause of the patient's heart failure and the presence or absence of structural cardiovascular abnormalities. Other issues to be addressed include presence or absence of history of diabetes, rheumatic fever, chest radiation, exposure to cardiotoxic drugs, and use or abuse of alcohol, illicit drugs, or alternative therapies. The patient's functional and volume status should also be evaluated to assess prognosis and guide management. New recommendations include a three-generational family history for patients with dilated cardiomyopathy (DCM) and the use of validated multivariable risk models for assessing subsequent mortality risk.

The guidelines recommend that the initial evaluation should include a complete blood count, urinalysis, serum electrolytes (including calcium and magnesium), blood urea nitrogen, serum creatinine, glucose, fasting lipid profile, liver function tests, and thyroid-stimulating hormone, and that serial monitoring of electrolytes should be performed when indicated. The guidelines also recommend a chest radiograph; a 12-lead electrocardiogram; two-dimensional echocardiography with Doppler to assess left ventricular function and detect underlying myocardial, valvular, or pericardial disease. Echocardiography was considered a more valuable initial test than radionuclide ventriculography or magnetic resonance imaging. Screening for hemochromatosis, amyloidosis, the human immunodeficiency virus, sleep-disturbed breathing, connective tissue diseases, or pheochromocytoma is also a reasonable step in selected patients.

The updated ACC/AHA and European Society of Cardiology guidelines both reflect recent research on biomarkers, including B-type natriuretic peptide (BNP) and N-terminal pro-B-type natriuretic peptide (NT-proBNP). The 2013 ACC/AHA guidelines give a class I (level of evidence A) recommendation for the measurement of BNP or NT-proBNP in ambulatory patients with dyspnea to support clinical decision making regarding the diagnosis of HF, especially in the setting of clinical uncertainty and measurement of BNP or NT-proBNP, which is useful for establishing a prognosis or disease severity in chronic HF.

Screening for and assessment of coronary artery disease in patients with heart failure are given less weight in the 2013 ACC/AHA guidelines than in previous guidelines. When ischemia may be contributing to HF, the guidelines indicate that coronary arteriography is reasonable for patients eligible for revascularization (class IIa, level of evidence C). The guidelines also support noninvasive imaging to detect myocardial ischemia and viability in patients presenting with de novo HF who have known coronary artery disease (CAD) and no angina, unless the patient is not

TABLE 34G-1 ACC/AHA Guidelines for Initial and Serial Evaluation of Heart Failure

CLASS	INDICATION: HISTORY, PHYSICAL EXAM, AND RISK SCORING	LEVEL OF EVIDENCE
I	A thorough history and physical examination should be obtained/performed in patients presenting with HF to identify cardiac and noncardiac disorders or behaviors that might cause or accelerate the development or progression of HF.	C
	In patients with idiopathic DCM, a three-generational family history should be obtained to aid in establishing the diagnosis of familial DCM.	C
	Volume status and vital signs should be assessed at each patient encounter. This includes serial assessment of weight, as well as estimates of jugular venous pressure and the presence of peripheral edema or orthopnea.	B
IIa	Validated multivariable risk scores can be useful to estimate subsequent risk of mortality in ambulatory or hospitalized patients with HF.	C
Indication: Diagnostic Tests and Biomarkers		
I	Initial laboratory evaluation of patients presenting with HF should include complete blood count, urinalysis, serum electrolytes (including calcium and magnesium), blood urea nitrogen, serum creatinine, glucose, fasting lipid profile, liver function tests, and thyroid-stimulating hormone.	C
	Serial monitoring, when indicated, should include serum electrolytes and renal function.	C
	A 12-lead ECG should be performed initially on all patients presenting with HF.	C
	In ambulatory patients with dyspnea, measurement of BNP or N-terminal pro-B-type natriuretic peptide (NT-proBNP) is useful to support clinical decision making regarding the diagnosis of HF, especially in the setting of clinical uncertainty, and measurement of BNP or NT-proBNP is useful for establishing prognosis or disease severity in chronic HF.	A
IIa	Screening for hemochromatosis or HIV is reasonable in selected patients who present with HF.	C
	Diagnostic tests for rheumatologic diseases, amyloidosis, or pheochromocytoma are reasonable in patients presenting with HF in whom there is a clinical suspicion of these diseases.	C
	BNP- or NT-proBNP–guided HF therapy can be useful to achieve optimal dosing of GDMT in select clinically euvolemic patients followed in a well-structured HF disease management program.	B
IIb	The usefulness of serial measurement of BNP or NT-proBNP to reduce hospitalization or mortality in patients with HF is not well established. The measurement of other clinically available tests such as biomarkers of myocardial injury or fibrosis may be considered for additive risk stratification in patients with chronic HF.	B
Indication: Noninvasive Cardiac Imaging		
I	Patients with suspected or new-onset HF, or those presenting with acute decompensated HF, should undergo a chest x-ray to assess heart size and pulmonary congestion and to detect alternative cardiac, pulmonary, and other diseases that may cause or contribute to the patient's symptoms.	C
	A two-dimensional echocardiogram with Doppler should be performed during initial evaluation of patients presenting with HF to assess ventricular function, size, wall thickness, wall motion, and valve function.	C
	Repeat measurement of EF and measurement of the severity of structural remodeling are useful to provide information in patients with HF who have had a significant change in clinical status; who have experienced or recovered from a clinical event; or who have received treatment, including GDMT, that might have had a significant effect on cardiac function; or who may be candidates for device therapy.	C
IIa	Noninvasive imaging to detect myocardial ischemia and viability is reasonable in patients presenting with de novo HF who have known CAD and no angina unless the patient is not eligible for revascularization of any kind.	C
	Viability assessment is reasonable in select situations when planning revascularization in HF patients with CAD.	B
	Radionuclide ventriculography or magnetic resonance imaging can be useful to assess LVEF and volume when echocardiography is inadequate.	C
	Magnetic resonance imaging is reasonable when assessing myocardial infiltrative processes or scar burden.	B
III: No Benefit	Routine repeat measurement of LV function assessment in the absence of clinical status change or treatment interventions should not be performed.	B
Indication: Invasive Evaluation		
I	Invasive hemodynamic monitoring with a pulmonary artery catheter should be performed to guide therapy in patients who have respiratory distress or clinical evidence of impaired perfusion in whom the adequacy or excess of intracardiac filling pressures cannot be determined from clinical assessment.	C
IIa	Invasive hemodynamic monitoring can be useful for carefully selected patients with acute HF who have persistent symptoms despite empiric adjustment of standard therapies and (a) whose fluid status, perfusion, or systemic or pulmonary vascular resistance is uncertain; (b) whose systolic pressure remains low, or is associated with symptoms, despite initial therapy; (c) whose renal function is worsening with therapy; (d) who require parenteral vasoactive agents; or (e) who may need consideration for mechanical circulatory support or transplantation.	C
	When ischemia may be contributing to HF, coronary arteriography is reasonable for patients eligible for revascularization.	C
	Endomyocardial biopsy can be useful in patients presenting with HF when a specific diagnosis is suspected that would influence therapy.	C
III (no benefit)	Routine use of invasive hemodynamic monitoring is not recommended in normotensive patients with acute decompensated HF and congestion with symptomatic response to diuretics and vasodilators.	B
III (harm)	Endomyocardial biopsy should not be performed in the routine evaluation of patients with HF.	C

ACC, American College of Cardiology; *AHA,* American Heart Association; *BNP,* B-type natriuretic peptide; *CAD,* coronary artery disease; *DCM,* dilated cardiomyopathy, *GDMT,* guideline-directed medical therapy.

eligible for revascularization of any kind, as well as viability testing in select patients when planning revascularization (class IIa, level of evidence B-C). Although the guidelines support the use of endomyocardial in patients presenting with HF when a diagnosis that would influence therapy is suspected (class IIb, level of evidence C), the routine use of endomyocardial biopsy is not recommended (class III: Harm). The guidelines do not support serial measurement of left ventricular (LV) function in the absence of change in clinical status. The updated ACC/AHA guidelines now give a class I (level of evidence C) recommendation for the use of invasive hemodynamic monitoring with a pulmonary artery catheter to guide therapy in patients who have respiratory distress or clinical evidence of impaired perfusion in whom the adequacy or excess of intracardiac filling pressures cannot be determined from clinical assessment (see Chapter 33G for discussion of guidelines for hospitalized patients).

TREATMENT OF PATIENTS AT HIGH RISK OF DEVELOPING HEART FAILURE (STAGE A)

The 2013 ACC/AHA guidelines for stage A patients (**Table 34G-2**) are simplified from previous guidelines and continue to provide strong recommendations (class I) for treating hypertension and lipid disorders in accordance with contemporary guidelines to lower the risk of HF. The guidelines also suggest that other conditions that may lead to or contribute to HF, such as obesity, diabetes mellitus, tobacco use, and known cardiotoxic agents, should be controlled or avoided.

TREATMENT OF PATIENTS WITH LEFT VENTRICULAR DYSFUNCTION WHO HAVE NOT DEVELOPED SYMPTOMS (STAGE B)

The goal of therapy in stage B HF is to reduce the risk of further damage to the heart and to minimize the rate of progression of LV dysfunction (**Table 34G-3**). In the absence of contraindications, β-blockers and angiotensin-converting enzyme (ACE) inhibitors (or angiotensin receptor blockers [ARBs] in those intolerant of ACE inhibitors) are recommended for all patients with histories of myocardial infarction, regardless of ejection fraction, and for all patients with diminished ejection fraction, regardless of history of myocardial infarction (class I, level of evidence A-C). In contrast, the guidelines discourage use of calcium channel blockers with negative inotropic action in this population. The guidelines also support the use of an ICD (class IIb, level of evidence B) in patients with asymptomatic ischemic cardiomyopathy who have had a recent (>40 days) myocardial infarction with and EF of 30% or less, who are on appropriate medical therapy, and who have a reasonable expectation of life greater than 1 year.

TABLE 34G-2 ACC/AHA Guidelines for Treating Patients at High Risk of Developing Heart Failure (Stage A)

CLASS	INDICATION	LEVEL OF EVIDENCE
I	Hypertension and lipid disorders should be controlled in accordance with contemporary guidelines to lower the risk of HF.	A
	Other conditions that may lead to or contribute to HF, such as obesity, diabetes mellitus, tobacco use, and known cardiotoxic agents, should be controlled or avoided.	C

ACC, American College of Cardiology; *AHA*, American Heart Association.

TREATMENT OF PATIENTS WITH LEFT VENTRICULAR DYSFUNCTION AND CURRENT OR PRIOR SYMPTOMS (STAGE C)

Application of the same measures recommended for preventing or minimizing progression of left ventricular dysfunction for stage A and B patients is supported for stage C patients who have current or prior symptoms attributable to left ventricular dysfunction (**Table 34G-4**). Physical activity and cardiac rehabilitation are recommended for stage C patients. The updated guidelines also reflect the results of the recent HF-ACTION trial, in which exercise training did not have a favorable impact on all-cause mortality or heart failure hospitalization. Maximal exercise testing with or without measurement of respiratory gas exchange to facilitate an appropriate exercise program, which was a class IIa indication in 2009, is not recommended in the 2013 ACC/AHA guidelines, although it is still recommended in the 2012 ESC guidelines.

The 2013 ACC/AHA updated guidelines support the use of β-blockers (bisoprolol, carvedilol, and sustained-release metoprolol succinate) and ACE inhibitors (ARBs for patients who cannot tolerate ACE inhibitors) for all stage C patients, in the absence of contraindications, and use of diuretics for patients with fluid overload. Based on the results of the Eplerenone in Mild Patients Hospitalization and Survival Study in Heart Failure (EMPHASIS-HF [see Chapter 34]), aldosterone antagonists are now recommended for all NYHA class II-IV heart failure patients with an EF of 35% or less to reduce morbidity and mortality, unless contraindicated (class I, level of evidence A). As with the 2009 guidelines, the use of hydralazine and isosorbide remains a class I indication for self-identified African Americans who remain symptomatic in NYHA class III-IV HF despite optimal therapy. The combination of hydralazine and isosorbide is recommended in patients who are intolerant of an ACE inhibitor or an ARB. Digitalis remains a reasonable approach to decrease hospitalizations in symptomatic patients. Based on the results of the WARCEF (Warfarin vs. Aspirin in Reduced Cardiac Ejection Fraction [see Chapter 34]), anticoagulation is not recommended in patients with chronic HF without atrial fibrillation, a prior embolic event, or a cardioembolic source (class III: No Benefit). However, anticoagulation continues to be recommended for patients with chronic HF and permanent/persistent/paroxysmal atrial fibrillation who have an additional risk factor for cardioembolic stroke (class I, level of evidence B). The guidelines explicitly discourage the routine use of a combination of an ACE inhibitor, ARB, and aldosterone antagonist: calcium channel blockers, long-term infusion of positive inotropic drugs (except as palliation in patients with end-stage disease; **Table 34G-5**), use of nutritional supplements, statins as adjunctive therapy for HF, and hormonal

TABLE 34G-3 ACC/AHA Guidelines for Treatment of Asymptomatic Left Ventricular Systolic Dysfunction (Stage B)

CLASS	INDICATION	LEVEL OF EVIDENCE
I	In all patients with a recent or remote history of MI or ACS and reduced EF, ACE inhibitors should be used to prevent symptomatic HF and reduce mortality. In patients intolerant of ACE inhibitors, ARBs are appropriate unless contraindicated.	A
	In all patients with a recent or remote history of MI or ACS and reduced EF, evidence-based β-blockers should be used to reduce mortality β-blockade and ACE inhibition in all patients with a recent or remote history of MI regardless of ejection fraction or presence of heart failure.	B
	In all patients with a recent or remote history of MI or ACS, statins should be used to prevent symptomatic HF and cardiovascular events.	A
	Blood pressure should be controlled in accordance with clinical practice guidelines for hypertension to prevent symptomatic HF.	A
	ACE inhibitors should be used in all patients with a reduced EF to prevent symptomatic HF.	A
	β-blockers should be used in all patients with a reduced EF to prevent symptomatic HF.	C
IIa	To prevent sudden death, placement of an ICD is reasonable in patients with asymptomatic ischemic cardiomyopathy who are at least 40 days post-MI, have an LVEF of 30% or less, are on appropriate medical therapy, and have reasonable expectation of survival with a good functional status for more than 1 year.	B
III: Harm	Nondihydropyridine calcium channel blockers with negative inotropic effects may be harmful in asymptomatic patients with low LVEF and no symptoms of HF after MI.	B

ACC, American College of Cardiology; *ACE,* angiotensin-converting inhibitor; *ACS,* acute coronary syndrome; *AHA,* American Heart Association; *ARB,* angiotensin receptor blocker; *MI,* myocardial infarction.

TABLE 34G-4 ACC/AHA Guidelines for Treatment of Symptomatic Left Ventricular Systolic Dysfunction (Stage C)

CLASS	INDICATION	LEVEL OF EVIDENCE
Nonpharmacologic Interventions		
I	Patients with HF should receive specific education to facilitate HF self-care.	B
	Exercise training (or regular physical activity) is recommended as safe and effective for patients with HF who are able to participate to improve functional status.	A
IIa	Cardiac rehabilitation can be useful in clinically stable patients with HF to improve functional capacity, exercise duration, HRQOL, and mortality.	B
	Sodium restriction is reasonable for patients with symptomatic HF to reduce congestive symptoms.	C
	Continuous positive airway pressure (CPAP) can be beneficial to increase LVEF and improve functional status in patients with HF and sleep apnea.	B
Pharmacologic Interventions		
I	Measures listed as class I recommendations for patients in stages A and B are recommended where appropriate.	A, B, C
	GDMT should be the mainstay of pharmacologic therapy for HFrEF.	A
Diuretics		
I	Diuretics are recommended in patients with HFrEF who have evidence of fluid retention, unless contraindicated, to improve symptoms.	C
ACE/ARBs		
I	ACE inhibitors are recommended in patients with HFrEF and current or prior symptoms, unless contraindicated, to reduce morbidity and mortality.	A
	ARBs are recommended in patients with HFrEF with current or prior symptoms who are ACE inhibitor intolerant, unless contraindicated, to reduce morbidity and mortality.	A
IIa	ARBs are reasonable to reduce morbidity and mortality as alternatives to ACE inhibitors as first-line therapy for patients with HFrEF, especially for patients already taking ARBs for other indications, unless contraindicated.	A
IIb	Addition of an ARB may be considered in persistently symptomatic patients with HFrEF who are already being treated with an ACE inhibitor and a β-blocker in whom an aldosterone antagonist is not indicated or tolerated.	A
III: Harm	Routinely combining an ACE inhibitor, an ARB, and an aldosterone antagonist.	C
β-Blockers		
I	Use of one of the three β-blockers proven to reduce mortality (i.e., bisoprolol, carvedilol, and sustained-release metoprolol succinate) is recommended for all patients with current or prior symptoms of HFrEF, unless contraindicated, to reduce morbidity and mortality.	A
Aldosterone Receptor Antagonists		
I	Aldosterone receptor antagonists (or mineralocorticoid receptor antagonists) are recommended in patients with NYHA class II-IV and who have LVEF ≤ 35%, unless contraindicated, to reduce morbidity and mortality.	A

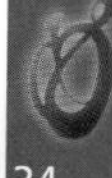

TABLE 34G-4 ACC/AHA Guidelines for Treatment of Symptomatic Left Ventricular Systolic Dysfunction (Stage C)—cont'd

CLASS	INDICATION	LEVEL OF EVIDENCE
I	Aldosterone receptor antagonists are recommended to reduce morbidity and mortality following an acute MI in patients who have LVEF ≤ 40% who develop symptoms of HF or who have a history of diabetes mellitus, unless contraindicated.	B
III: Harm	Inappropriate use of aldosterone receptor antagonists is potentially harmful because of life-threatening hyperkalemia or renal insufficiency when serum creatinine is more than 2.5 mg/dL in men or more than 2.0 mg/dL in women (or estimated glomerular filtration rate <30 mL/min/1.73 m^2), and/or potassium more than 5.0 mEq/L.	B
Hydralazine and Isosorbide Dinitrate		
I	The combination of hydralazine and isosorbide dinitrate is recommended to reduce morbidity and mortality for patients self-described as African Americans with NYHA class III–IV HFrEF receiving optimal therapy with ACE inhibitors and β-blockers, unless contraindicated.	A
IIa	A combination of hydralazine and isosorbide dinitrate can be useful to reduce morbidity or mortality in patients with current or prior symptomatic HFrEF who cannot be given an ACE inhibitor or ARB because of drug intolerance, hypotension, or renal insufficiency, unless contraindicated.	B
Digoxin		
IIa	Digoxin can be beneficial in patients with HFrEF, unless contraindicated, to decrease hospitalizations for HF.	B
Anticoagulation		
I	Patients with chronic HF with permanent/persistent/paroxysmal AF and an additional risk factor for cardioembolic stroke (history of hypertension, diabetes mellitus, previous stroke or transient ischemic attack, or ≥75 years of age) should receive chronic anticoagulant therapy.	A
I	The selection of an anticoagulant agent (warfarin, dabigatran, apixaban, or rivaroxaban) for permanent/persistent/paroxysmal AF should be individualized on the basis of risk factors, cost, tolerability, patient preference, potential for drug interactions, and other clinical characteristics, including time in the international normalized ratio therapeutic range if the patient has been taking warfarin.	C
IIa	Chronic anticoagulation is reasonable for patients with chronic HF who have permanent/persistent/paroxysmal AF but are without an additional risk factor for cardioembolic stroke.	B
III: No Benefit	Anticoagulation is not recommended in patients with chronic HFrEF without AF, a prior thromboembolic event, or a cardioembolic source.	B
Statins		
III: No Benefit	Statins are not beneficial as adjunctive therapy when prescribed solely for HF.	A
Omega-3 Fatty Acids		
IIa	Omega-3 polyunsaturated fatty acid (PUFA) supplementation is reasonable to use as adjunctive therapy in patients with NYHA class II-IV symptoms and HFrEF or HFpEF, unless contraindicated, to reduce mortality and cardiovascular hospitalizations.	B
Drugs of Unproven Value or That May Cause Harm		
III: No Benefit	Nutritional supplements as treatment for HF are not recommended in patients with current or prior symptoms of HFrEF.	B
	Hormonal therapies other than to correct deficiencies are not recommended for patients with current or prior symptoms of HFrEF.	C
III: Harm	Drugs known to adversely affect the clinical status of patients with current or prior symptoms of HFrEF are potentially harmful and should be avoided or withdrawn whenever possible (e.g., most antiarrhythmic drugs, most calcium channel blocking drugs (except amlodipine), NSAIDs, or thiazolidinediones).	B
	Long-term use of infused positive inotropic drugs is potentially harmful for patients with HFrEF, except as palliation for patients with end-stage disease who cannot be stabilized with standard medical treatment (see recommendations for stage D).	C
Calcium Channel Blockers		
III: No Benefit	Calcium channel blocking drugs are not recommended as routine therapy for patients with HFrEF.	A

ACC, American College of Cardiology; *ACE,* angiotensin-converting inhibitor; *AHA,* American Heart Association; *ARB,* angiotensin receptor blocker; *HFpEF,* heart failure with a preserved ejection fraction; *HFrEF,* heart failure with a reduced ejection fraction.

TABLE 34G-5 ACC/AHA Guidelines for Treatment of Patients with End-Stage Heart Failure (Stage D)

CLASS	INDICATION	LEVEL OF EVIDENCE
Nonpharmacologic Interventions		
IIa	Fluid restriction (1.5 to 2 L/day) is reasonable in stage D, especially in patients with hyponatremia.	B
Inotropic Support		
I	Until definitive therapy (e.g., coronary revascularization, MCS, heart transplantation) or resolution of the acute precipitating problem, patients with cardiogenic shock should receive temporary intravenous inotropic support to maintain systemic perfusion and preserve end-organ performance.	C
IIa	Continuous intravenous inotropic support is reasonable as "bridge therapy" in patients with stage D refractory to GDMT and device therapy who are eligible for and awaiting MCS or cardiac transplantation.	B
IIb	Short-term, continuous intravenous inotropic support may be reasonable in those hospitalized patients presenting with documented severe systolic dysfunction who present with low blood pressure and significantly depressed cardiac output to maintain systemic perfusion and preserve end-organ performance.	B
	Long-term, continuous intravenous inotropic support may be considered as palliative therapy for symptom control in select patients with stage D despite optimal GDMT and device therapy who are not eligible for either MCS or cardiac transplantation.	B
III: Harm	Long-term use of either continuous or intermittent intravenous parenteral positive inotropic agents, in the absence of specific indications or for reasons other than palliative care, is potentially harmful in the patient with HF.	B
	Use of parenteral inotropic agents in hospitalized patients without documented severe systolic dysfunction, low blood pressure, or impaired perfusion, and evidence of significantly depressed cardiac output, with or without congestion, is potentially harmful.	B
Mechanical Circulatory Support (MCS)		
IIa	MCS is beneficial in carefully selected patients with stage D HFrEF in whom definitive management (e.g., cardiac transplantation) or cardiac recovery is anticipated or planned.	B
	Nondurable MCS, including the use of percutaneous and extracorporeal ventricular assist devices (VADs), is reasonable as a "bridge to recovery" or "bridge to decision" for carefully selected patients with HFrEF with acute, profound hemodynamic compromise.	B
	Durable MCS is reasonable to prolong survival for carefully selected patients with stage D HFrEF.	B
Cardiac Transplantation		
I	Evaluation for cardiac transplantation is indicated for carefully selected patients with stage D HF despite GDMT, device, and surgical management.	C

ACC, American College of Cardiology; *AHA*, American Heart Association; *GDMT*, guideline-directed medical therapy; *HFrEF*, heart failure with a reduced ejection fraction; *MCS*, mechanical circulatory support.

therapies other than those needed to replete deficiencies. The recommendations regarding the use of implantable cardiac defibrillators (ICDs) and cardiac resynchronization (CRT) are reviewed in **Chapter 35 and 35G**.

TREATMENT OF PATIENTS WITH REFRACTORY END-STAGE HEART FAILURE (STAGE D)

The 2009 ACCF/AHA HF guidelines define stage D as "patients with truly refractory HF who might be eligible for specialized, advanced treatment strategies, such as mechanical circulatory support (MCS), procedures to facilitate fluid removal, continuous inotropic infusions, or cardiac transplantation or other innovative or experimental surgical procedures, or for end-of-life care, such as hospice." The guidelines provide clear indications for the use of inotropic agents and mechanical circulatory support in stage D patients (see Table 34G-5). The guidelines endorse the use of continuous intravenous inotropic support until definitive therapy can be performed (e.g., MCS, heart transplantation), and/or to maintain systemic perfusion and preserve end-organ performance until the acute precipitating problem is resolved (class I, level of evidence C). The guidelines also support inotropic support as "bridge therapy" to GDMT and/or device therapy (class IIa, level of evidence B), as well as short-term continuous intravenous inotropic support in hospitalized patients with documented severe systolic dysfunction who present with low blood pressure and significantly depressed cardiac output, to maintain systemic perfusion and preserve end-organ performance, or as palliative therapy for symptom control (class IIb, level of evidence B). The guidelines regard long-term use of either continuous or intermittent intravenous parenteral positive inotropic agents, in the absence of specific indications or for reasons other than palliative care, as potentially harmful (class III: Harm, level of evidence B).

The 2013 ACC/AHA guidelines provide qualified support for MCS in carefully selected patients with stage D heart failure with a reduced ejection fraction (HFrEF) for whom definitive management (e.g., cardiac transplantation) or cardiac recovery is anticipated or planned, and also indicate that percutaneous and extracorporeal ventricular assist devices (VADs) are reasonable as a "bridge to recovery" or "bridge to decision" for carefully selected patients with HFrEF with acute profound hemodynamic compromise (class IIb, level of evidence B). The guidelines also provide qualified support for the use of durable VADs to prolong survival in carefully selected patients with stage D HFrEF. As in previous guidelines, cardiac transplantation remains a class I indication (level of evidence C) for carefully selected patients with stage D HFrEF despite GDMT, device, and surgical management.

COMORBIDITIES IN HEART FAILURE PATIENTS

The 2013 ACC/AHA practice guidelines recognize the importance of comorbidities in heart failure, including hypertension, anemia, diabetes, arthritis, chronic kidney disease, and depression. However, the guidelines did not generate specific recommendations, given the status of current evidence.

THE HOSPITALIZED PATIENT

The updated 2010 Heart Failure Society of America (HFSA), 2012 ESC, and 2013 ACC/AHA guidelines included specific recommendations regarding the hospitalized patient and are reviewed in Chapter 33G (Table 33G-1).

HEART FAILURE WITH A PRESERVED EJECTION FRACTION

The updated 2010 HFSA, 2012 ESC, and 2013 ACC/AHA guidelines included specific recommendations regarding management of patients with heart failure with a preserved ejection fraction and are reviewed in Chapter 36G (Table 36G-1).

SURGICAL/PERCUTANEOUS/ TRANSCATHETER INTERVENTIONAL TREATEMENTS OF HEART FAILURE

The 2013 ACC/AHA guidelines reviewed surgical therapies and percutaneous interventions that are commonly integrated in the management of heart failure patients, including coronary revascularization (e.g., CABG, angioplasty, stenting); aortic valve replacement, mitral valve replacement, and LV surgical reconstruction (**Table 34G-6**). The revised guidelines recommend coronary artery revascularization via CABG or percutaneous intervention for patients on GDMT with angina and suitable coronary anatomy, especially for a left main stenosis (>50%) or left main equivalent disease (class I, level of evidence C). CABG was also recommended to improve survival in mild to moderate LV dysfunction (EF 35% to 50%) and significant (≥70% diameter stenosis) multivessel CAD or proximal left anterior descending coronary artery stenosis when viable myocardium is present, as well as to improve morbidity and cardiovascular mortality for patients with severe LV dysfunction (EF <35%), HF, and significant CAD (class IIa, level of evidence B). Qualified support was provided for a survival benefit for CABG (class IIb, level of evidence B) in patients with ischemic heart disease with severe LV systolic dysfunction (EF <35%) and operable coronary anatomy irrespective of whether viable myocardium was present. The new guidelines provide a class IIa (level of evidence B) recommendation for surgical aortic valve replacement in patients with a predicted surgical mortality of less than 10% and a class IIa (level of evidence B) recommendation for transcatheter aortic valve replacement in inoperable patients with critical aortic valve disease. The guidelines offer qualified support for transcatheter mitral valve repair or mitral valve surgery for functional mitral insufficiency and recommend that this approach should be considered after careful candidate selection and in addition to GDMT (class IIb, level of evidence B). A similar level of qualified support was given for surgical reverse remodeling or LV aneurysmectomy for intractable heart failure and ventricular arrhythmias.

COORDINATING CARE FOR PATIENTS WITH CHRONIC HEART FAILURE

The guidelines recognize that systems of care designed to support patients with HF and other cardiac diseases can produce significant improvement in outcomes, but indicate that the quality of evidence is mixed for specific components of HF clinical management interventions, such as

TABLE 34G-6 ACC/AHA Guidelines for Surgical/Percutaneous/Transcatheter Interventional Treatments of Heart Failure

CLASS	INDICATION	LEVEL OF EVIDENCE
I	Coronary artery revascularization via CABG or percutaneous intervention is indicated for patients (HFpEF and HFrEF) on GDMT with angina and suitable coronary anatomy, especially for a left main stenosis (>50%) or left main equivalent disease.	C
IIa	CABG to improve survival is reasonable in patients with mild to moderate LV systolic dysfunction (EF 35% to 50%) and significant (≥70% diameter stenosis) multivessel CAD or proximal left anterior descending coronary artery stenosis when viable myocardium is present in the region of intended revascularization.	B
	CABG or medical therapy is reasonable to improve morbidity and cardiovascular mortality for patients with severe LV dysfunction (EF <35%), HF, and significant CAD.	B
	Surgical aortic valve replacement is reasonable for patients with critical aortic stenosis and a predicted surgical mortality of no greater than 10%.	B
	Transcatheter aortic valve replacement after careful candidate consideration is reasonable for patients with critical aortic stenosis who are deemed inoperable.	B
IIb	CABG may be considered with the intent of improving survival in patients with ischemic heart disease with severe LV systolic dysfunction (EF <35%) and operable coronary anatomy whether or not viable myocardium is present.	B
	Transcatheter mitral valve repair or mitral valve surgery for functional mitral insufficiency is of uncertain benefit and should only be considered after careful candidate selection and with a background of GDMT.	B
	Surgical reverse remodeling or LV aneurysmectomy may be considered in carefully selected patients with HFrEF for specific indications, including intractable HF and ventricular arrhythmias.	B

ACC, American College of Cardiology; *AHA,* American Heart Association; *CABG,* coronary artery bypass grafting; *CAD,* coronary artery disease; *GDMT,* guideline-directed medical therapy; *HFpEF,* heart failure with a preserved ejection fraction; *HFrEF,* heart failure with a reduced ejection fraction.

TABLE 34G-7 Coordinating Care for Patients with Chronic Heart Failure

CLASS	INDICATION	LEVEL OF EVIDENCE
I	Effective systems of care coordination with special attention to care transitions should be deployed for every patient with chronic HF that facilitate and ensure effective care that is designed to achieve GDMT and prevent hospitalization.	B
	Every patient with HF should have a clear, detailed, and evidence-based plan of care that ensures the achievement of GDMT goals, effective management of comorbid conditions, timely follow-up with the health care team, appropriate dietary and physical activities, and compliance with Secondary Prevention Guidelines for cardiovascular disease. This plan of care should be updated regularly and made readily available to all members of each patient's health care team.	C
	Palliative and supportive care is effective for patients with symptomatic advanced HF to improve quality of life.	B

ACC, American College of Cardiology; *AHA,* American Heart Association; *GDMT,* guideline-directed medical therapy; *IV,* intravenous; *NYHA,* New York Heart Association.

home-based care, disease management, and remote telemonitoring programs. Hence, the guidelines recommend that interventions should focus on improving adherence to GDMT (**Table 34G-7**). The updated guidelines advocate patient education and involvement of patients with HF and their families, especially during transitions of care, to ensure effective care that is designed to achieve GDMT and prevent hospitalizations (class I, level of evidence B). The guidelines also recommend that every patient with HF should have a clear, detailed, and evidence-based plan of care that ensures the achievement of GDMT goals, effective management of comorbid conditions, timely follow-up with the health care team, appropriate dietary and physical activities, and compliance with secondary prevention guidelines for cardiovascular disease (class I, level of evidence C). The guidelines recommend that the HF and palliative care teams are best suited to help patients and families decide when end-of-life care (including hospice) is appropriate (class I, level of evidence C). The core elements of comprehensive palliative care for HF include expert symptom assessment and management, including symptom control, psychosocial distress, health-related quality of life, preferences about end-of-life care, caregiver support, and assurance of access to evidence-based disease-modifying interventions.

REFERENCES

1. Yancy CW, Jessup M, Bozkurt B, et al: 2013 ACCF/AHA guideline for the management of heart failure: a report of the American College of Cardiology Foundation/American Heart Association Task Force on Practice Guidelines. *Circulation* 2013.
2. Hunt SA, Abraham WT, Chin MH, et al: ACC/AHA 2005 guideline update for the diagnosis and management of chronic heart failure in the adult: a report of the American College of Cardiology/American Heart Association Task Force on Practice Guidelines (Writing Committee to Update the 2001 Guidelines for the Evaluation and Management of Heart Failure): developed in collaboration with the American College of Chest Physicians and the International Society for Heart and Lung Transplantation: endorsed by the Heart Rhythm Society. *Circulation* 112:e154–e235, 2005.
3. Jessup M, Abraham WT, Casey DE, et al: 2009 focused update: ACCF/AHA guidelines for the diagnosis and management of heart failure in adults: a report of the American College of Cardiology Foundation/American Heart Association Task Force on Practice Guidelines: developed in collaboration with the International Society for Heart and Lung Transplantation. *Circulation* 119:1977–2016, 2009.
4. Heart Failure Society of America: HFSA 2006 comprehensive heart failure practice guideline. *J Card Fail* 12:e1–e2, 2006.
5. McMurray JJ, Adamopoulos S, Anker SD, et al: ESC guidelines for the diagnosis and treatment of acute and chronic heart failure 2012: the Task Force for the Diagnosis and Treatment of Acute and Chronic Heart Failure 2012 of the European Society of Cardiology. Developed in collaboration with the Heart Failure Association (HFA) of the ESC. *Eur Heart J* 2012.
6. Dickstein K, Cohen-Solal A, Filippatos G, et al: ESC guidelines for the diagnosis and treatment of acute and chronic heart failure 2008: the Task Force for the Diagnosis and Treatment of Acute and Chronic Heart Failure 2008 of the European Society of Cardiology. Developed in collaboration with the Heart Failure Association of the ESC (HFA) and endorsed by the European Society of Intensive Care Medicine (ESICM). *Eur Heart J* 10:933–989, 2008.

Management of Arrhythmias and Device Therapy in Heart Failure

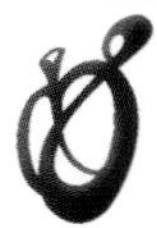

Christopher P. Porterfield and John P. DiMarco

Arrhythmias are common in heart failure patients. This chapter will discuss the diagnosis and therapy of arrhythmias in patients with heart failure.

ATRIAL FIBRILLATION

Atrial fibrillation (AF) is the most common sustained cardiac arrhythmia. Its prevalence increases with age and with both systolic and diastolic heart failure.[1-4] It has been reported that up to 25% of patients with chronic heart failure will have permanent atrial fibrillation.[5,7-9] Atrial fibrillation is one of the strongest predictors for the development of heart failure. In the Framingham Heart Study, the development of AF was responsible for worsening heart failure symptoms and was seen as the second greatest reason for hospitalization, second to acute heart failure exacerbation.[5] AF is also associated with significant morbidity and mortality, due primarily to the increased risk of thromboembolic events and adverse hemodynamic effects that may result in new onset or worsening heart failure, decreased exercise tolerance, as well as impaired quality of life.[6]

Epidemiology

In the Framingham Heart Study, 2326 men and 2866 women were followed for 2 years, and the risk of developing permanent AF was 8.5% for men and 13.7% for women. Paroxysmal AF was seen in 8.2% of men and 20.4% of women. In those without prior or concurrent congestive heart failure or myocardial infarction, the lifetime risks for atrial fibrillation were approximately 16%.[10] In diastolic heart failure, approximately 25% to 30% of patients have evidence of atrial fibrillation.[11] The prevalence increases with the severity of diastolic heart failure, reaching up to 40% in advanced stages.[12] Sustained high ventricular rates during atrial arrhythmias may result in a tachycardia-induced cardiomyopathy that in the absence of any other myopathic process may be completely reversible. However, in patients who develop AF in the setting of established heart failure atrial fibrosis with deleterious electrical remodeling is the primary cause for the arrhythmia.

Pathophysiology

The clinical manifestations of atrial fibrillation relate to the loss of atrial systolic function and an irregular, ventricular response whose rate is typically determined by the conduction and refractory properties of the atrioventricular (AV) node. Left atrial systole contributes up to 25% of the cardiac output, and this fraction may increase to 50% in left ventricular failure.[13-14] The loss of atrial systolic function results in impaired hemodynamic function of the heart. Atrial fibrillation causes a fall in cardiac stroke volume of about 10% in normal subjects, with a greater decrease seen at fast ventricular rates. This loss becomes more important clinically with increasing age and progressive impairment of left ventricular systolic or diastolic function, because atrial systole makes a greater contribution toward the overall stroke volume in these conditions. In addition to the loss of AV synchrony, the irregular and often inappropriate ventricular rates seen in atrial fibrillation result in suboptimal ventricular filling. These may further compromise cardiac output, an effect particularly seen in patients with mitral stenosis or diastolic dysfunction. Cardioversion of atrial fibrillation with poorly controlled ventricular rates usually improves left ventricular ejection fraction and exercise capacity, but the improvement occurs gradually after the procedure.[13]

Loss of atrial systolic function results in stasis within the left atrium, leading to intra-atrial thrombus formation and an increased risk of stroke and thromboembolism. During episodes of atrial fibrillation, echocardiography can detect spontaneous echo contrast as a result of the formation of erythrocyte aggregations and thrombus in the atria. Stasis within the left atrium has been related to hemostatic abnormalities that are suggestive of a hypercoagulable state and that involve coagulation factors and abnormal endothelial and platelet function. These abnormalities of hemostasis have been related to changes in inflammatory indices and growth factors.[14-15] The hypercoagulable state is often exaggerated in low flow states such as left ventricular dysfunction.[15] Hypercoagulability is altered by antithrombotic therapy and gradually by cardioversion of atrial fibrillation to sinus rhythm. Prothrombotic indices in atrial fibrillation have been shown to be prognostically relevant, being predictive of stroke and vascular events, and can be used to refine clinical stroke risk stratification.[16-17] Atrial natriuretic peptide levels are also increased in patients who have atrial fibrillation, which contributes to hemoconcentration and an increased risk for thrombus formation.

Prolonged atrial fibrillation with rapid ventricular rates produces functional, ultra-structural, and microscopic changes within the myocardium that may result in progressive left ventricular dilation and reduction of left ventricular systolic function; this is referred to as *tachycardia-induced cardiomyopathy.* In a patient who has chronic heart failure and is in sinus rhythm, increased intracardiac pressures may lead to atrial stretch and dilation, predisposing to both the development and the recurrence of atrial fibrillation. Several potential electrophysiologic mechanisms may be responsible for atrial fibrillation.[4,18] One postulated mechanism is multiple wavelet reentry, in which wavefronts continuously sweep through the atria in a random fashion. The multiple wavelet hypothesis requires that a minimum number of wavefronts and enough atrial tissue to permit their simultaneous propagation exist. An alternate hypothesis is that there are only one or two primary reentrant circuits or rotors that are constantly forming and disappearing, but the cycle lengths in these circuits are too short to allow the rest of the atria to follow in an organized fashion, resulting in fibrillatory conduction.[18] It has been shown clinically that atrial fibrillation may be produced by rapid tachycardias from either focal sources, commonly found in musculature of the pulmonary veins, or stable reentrant circuits that drive the remaining atrial tissue until degeneration to atrial fibrillation occurs.[18,19] The pulmonary veins, which include muscular sleeves that may be electrically active, and the posterior left atrial wall are considered to be the critical structures involved in the pathogenesis of atrial fibrillation.[19]

Clinical Presentation

The classification of atrial fibrillation focuses on temporal pattern after onset. Paroxysmal AF is a recurrence of AF that terminates spontaneously in 7 days or less. Persistent AF is recurrent AF that lasts longer than 7 days. Patients who undergo cardioversion within 48 hours of onset are described as paroxysmal and persistent if done after 48 hours. Longstanding persistent AF is continuous AF that has lasted longer than 1 year. Permanent AF is when the patient remains in longstanding persistent AF and there is no plan for rhythm control.[20]

Among patients who have recurrent forms of atrial fibrillation, this temporally based clinical classification can assist management strategies, particular in relation to considering rhythm control or rate control. In paroxysmal atrial fibrillation, the episodes are generally self-terminating, and thus the goals of therapy are the prevention of paroxysms and the long-term maintenance of sinus rhythm. In sustained atrial fibrillation, the therapeutic goal is either cardioversion to sinus rhythm or heart rate control. Antithrombotic therapy for moderate or high-risk patients is an important component of both strategies.

The differentiation between these clinical categories is dependent on the history given by the patient, electrocardiogram (ECG) documentation of the episode, and the duration of the most recent previous episode of AF. Although this classification is helpful, there is considerable variability, both between patients and in the same patient, in the temporal pattern of atrial fibrillation episodes, and approaches to therapy must be individualized, especially in relation to symptoms. Furthermore, paroxysmal atrial fibrillation may become permanent (8% at 1 year, 18% at 4 years), especially with increasing age.[21] The EURO Heart Survey showed that hypertension, age older than 75 years, previous transient ischemic attack or stroke, chronic obstructive pulmonary disease, and heart failure were independent predictors of AF progression.[21] These investigators used these factors to develop the HATCH score, which predicts the probability of progression of AF. With an increasing HATCH score, the percentage of patients in whom AF progressed to persistent forms was significantly higher. Fifty percent of the patients with a HATCH score more than 5 progressed to persistent AF compared with only 6% of the patients with a HATCH score of 0.[21,22]

Diagnosis

The investigation of a patient with atrial fibrillation requires a careful clinical history (including a past medical history) with emphasis on certain clinical features. The history should cover whether the symptoms are sustained or intermittent and whether any complications (such as heart failure, stroke, or thromboembolism) are present. Other useful data include the date of the first episode, information about acute precipitating factors or chronic conditions linked to atrial fibrillation, how symptoms are relieved, the typical duration of episodes and the typical interval between them, the duration of the current or most recent episode, and current and past drug treatment.

At the initial consultation, basic blood tests, including full blood count, biochemistry (renal function, electrolytes), and thyroid function tests, are taken. A full blood count is useful to exclude anemia because anticoagulation may be considered. Serum urea and electrolytes are relevant for consideration of drug therapy (e.g., the dose of digoxin would be reduced in renal impairment). The risk of atrial fibrillation is increased by clinical and subclinical hyperthyroidism, and thus the serum thyroid stimulating hormone level should be measured in all patients who have atrial fibrillation, even if there are no symptoms suggestive of thyrotoxicosis.

The arrhythmia should be documented, ideally with a standard 12-lead ECG. The characteristic ECG findings in atrial fibrillation include rapid baseline oscillations or fibrillatory waves that vary in size, shape, and timing; the absence of discrete P waves; and an irregularly irregular ventricular rate.

The ECG may also provide a clue to the electrophysiologic features that may have caused atrial fibrillation (e.g., a previous myocardial infarction, left ventricular hypertrophy, or preexcitation). Often, patients present with previous symptoms suggestive of atrial fibrillation but are in sinus rhythm at the time of their evaluation. If symptoms occur on a daily basis, a 24-hour ambulatory ECG should provide the diagnosis. If symptoms occur less frequently, a patient-activated event recorder or an implanted loop recorder would be more likely to provide a diagnosis.

An echocardiogram provides important information for the initial evaluation of most patients with atrial fibrillation.[4,23] Either transthoracic echocardiography or transesophageal echocardiography (TEE), or a combination of the two, may be appropriate. The initial goal of the echocardiographic evaluation should be to establish the presence or absence of structural heart disease, including valvular abnormalities, congenital anomalies, chamber dimensions, pericardial thickening or effusions, and ventricular function.

Left atrial size is an important predictor of outcome in patients with atrial fibrillation because the presence of significant left atrial enlargement has been shown to reduce the chances of successful cardioversion and long-term maintenance of sinus rhythm in most series. Left atrial enlargement may also increase the risk of stroke, owing to a greater potential for stasis in the dilated chamber.[4]

Although transthoracic echocardiography is acceptable for assessing chamber size, detection of thrombi or the assessment of left atrial appendage anatomy and function requires the TEE approach. Using TEE, up to 27% of patients with atrial fibrillation of more than 3 days' duration may have detectable thrombi. A prethrombotic finding, spontaneous echo contrast (SEC, also called "smoke"), is due to erythrocyte aggregation in the low-flow state and is even more commonly seen. Other TEE indices of high stroke risk include the presence of left atrial thrombus, low left atrial appendage velocities, dense SEC, and complex aortic plaque in the descending aorta.[23]

Invasive electrophysiologic studies have only a limited role in the routine evaluation of patients with atrial fibrillation unless catheter ablation is planned. Electrophysiologic studies of atrial fibrillation should be reserved for the following situations: when another arrhythmia (e.g., atrial flutter or atrial or supraventricular tachycardia) is thought to be the cause of the atrial fibrillation; when other electrophysiologic abnormalities or symptoms (e.g., preexcitation, sinus node dysfunction, syncope) require clarification or therapy; or when catheter ablation is planned.

Management of Acute Episodes of Atrial Fibrillation

Successful management of acute episodes of atrial fibrillation requires attention to several issues, including rate control, pharmacologic or electrical conversion, and protection against thromboembolic events. When patients present with new onset or a recurrent episodes of atrial fibrillation, the initial step should be to assess their symptoms and hemodynamic status. Rarely, the patient will be so severely compromised that urgent electrical cardioversion will be required despite a high risk for early recurrence. In most patients, however, the first step for stabilization should be to lower the ventricular rate. In an intensive care unit or other monitored setting, intravenous β-blockers are usually the first choice in patients with heart failure and systolic dysfunction. Intravenous digoxin may be a useful adjunct but its onset of action is delayed and its inability to lower rate is lessened during periods of high sympathetic tone. The non-dihydropyridine calcium channel blockers, diltiazem and verapamil, are effective alternatives in patients with preserved systolic function but must be used with caution, if at all, in patients with known systolic dysfunction. Intravenous amiodarone can play a dual role since it will both slow ventricular rates and may eventually cardiovert the rhythm. The heart rate target during attempts at rate control will depend on the patient's condition. In a resting, minimally symptomatic patient, one tries to approximate what the average rate would be in sinus rhythm (i.e., 60 to 100 beats/min). During periods of stress, however, this degree of rate control may not be achievable and rates up to 110 to 120 beats/min are usually adequate to control symptoms.

Once the patient's rate had been controlled, a decision about possible cardioversion should be made. Anticoagulation issues that will affect this decision will be discussed later. Most patients with new onset atrial fibrillation will be candidates for at least one attempt at cardioversion. Elective direct-current cardioversion without addition of an antiarrhythmic drug is an appropriate strategy for patients with recent onset AF in whom the risk of recurrence is thought to be only moderate or low. After cardioversion, the patient can be followed off antiarrhythmic drugs until a recurrence has been documented. AV nodal blocking agents are often continued at least during the early period after cardioversion. Although intravenous ibutilide and vernakalant (not currently available in the United States) are effective for conversion of recent onset AF, neither of these agents is advisable in patients with systolic heart failure or left ventricular hypertrophy. Intravenous or oral loading with amiodarone or oral loading with dofetilide is the best approach for pharmacologic cardioversion if long-term therapy is planned in the heart failure patient.[24]

Chemical or electrical cardioversion of AF of more than 2 days' duration is associated with a significant risk (2%-8%) of stroke or systemic thromboembolism in all patients with nonvalvular AF not on anticoagulants.[25] A prudent approach is to start anticoagulation in patients without contraindications scheduled for cardioversion if the cardioversion is to be delayed or if the duration of the episode is uncertain. For episodes of greater than 48 hours' duration, two anticoagulation strategies are acceptable. If early cardioversion is planned, the patient should undergo a transesophageal echocardiogram to exclude the presence of left atrial appendage thrombus. If no thrombus is visualized, anticoagulation is continued and cardioversion may be performed. The alternate strategy is to delay cardioversion until the patient has been adequately anticoagulated for at least 3 weeks. Although warfarin with an international normalized ratio (INR) between 2.0 and 3.0 has long been the anticoagulation standard, preliminary data suggest that a similar duration of anticoagulation with dabigatran, rivaroxaban, and apixaban would be similarly effective. The TEE-guided and delayed treatment approaches were compared in the

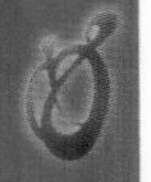

TABLE 35-1 Rate Control Agents for Primary Rate Control Strategy

DRUG CLASS	SPECIFIC DRUG	LOADING DOSE	MAINTENANCE DOSE	ADVERSE EFFECTS
β-Blockers	Bisoprolol	2.5-20 mg PO daily	Same	Bronchospasm, sinus bradycardia, AV block, exercise intolerance, hypotension, fatigue, depression
	Carvedilol	3.125-25 mg PO bid or sustained release 10-80 mg PO daily	Same	
	Metoprolol	2.5-5 mg IV or 25-100 mg PO bid or ER 25-200 mg PO daily	Same as PO dose	
	Nebivolol	5-40 mg PO daily	Same	
Calcium channel blockers	Diltiazem*	0.25 mg/kg IV bolus followed by 5-15 mg/hr infusion	120-480 mg ER PO daily	Sinus bradycardia, heart failure, AV block, hypotension, digoxin interaction (verapamil), peripheral edema
	Verapamil*	0.075-0.15 mg/kg IV bolus or 120-480 mg ER PO daily		
Other	Digoxin†	0.25 mg IV q4-6 hours (max 1 mg)	0.125-0.25 mg PO daily	Bradycardia, AV block, ventricular ectopy

*Use only in heart failure with preserved ejection fraction.
†Best used in conjunction with β-blocker for rate control.
AV, Atrioventricular.
From Fuster V, Ryden LE, Cannom DS, et al: ACC/AHA/ESC 2006 guidelines for the management of patients with atrial fibrillation: a report of the American College of Cardiology/American Heart Association task force on practice guidelines and the European Society of Cardiology committee for practice guidelines (Writing committee to revise the 2001 guidelines for the management of patients with atrial fibrillation). J Am Coll Cardiol 48:e149–246, 2006.

ACUTE trial. Both approaches were associated with a low rate of thromboembolic events after cardioversion and similar probabilities for sinus rhythm maintenance and bleeding.[26,27]

Chronic Management of Atrial Fibrillation

Patients with recurrent forms of atrial fibrillation will require a treatment program that provides rate control, an assessment of the benefits and feasibility of restoring and maintaining sinus rhythm, and mitigation of the risks for stroke and systemic embolism.

Rate Control versus Rhythm Control

The first question that must be addressed in patients with recurrent atrial fibrillation is whether a rate control or a rhythm control strategy is most appropriate. Factors that should be considered include the temporal pattern (paroxysmal versus persistent) of the arrhythmia, the frequency of episodes, the severity of symptoms, patient factors, and the probabilities for maintaining sinus rhythm or effectively controlling ventricular rates.

Although a rhythm control strategy would seem intuitively to be superior to a rate control strategy, a series of randomized trials have been unable to demonstrate this with pharmacologically based therapies. The two most relevant trials for heart failure patients were the AFFIRM trial and the AF-CHF trial.[28,29] AFFIRM randomized 4060 patients, 23% of whom had heart failure, between rate control and rhythm control strategies. No difference in total mortality or stroke was seen between the two strategies, with a slight trend favoring rate control. Patients in whom sinus rhythm was maintained during the study had improved outcomes but this likely represents a "healthy responder" phenomenon. A second trial, AF-CHF, compared rate control and rhythm control strategies in patients required to have heart failure and depressed left ventricular systolic function. There was no significant difference between the two strategies in the three primary endpoints, mortality, stroke, and heart failure hospitalizations. In addition, even when patients were grouped into those with high and low prevalence of sinus rhythm during the course of the study, no benefit on these outcomes could be demonstrated. However, it must be remembered that entry into all of the rate control versus rhythm control strategy trials required that the patient be a candidate for both approaches. Highly symptomatic patients therefore were unlikely to be randomized. Therefore, most clinicians recommend that heart failure patients with persistent symptoms related to their atrial fibrillation should have at least an initial attempt to restore and maintain sinus rhythm with rate control a fallback approach if rhythm control is unsuccessful or poorly tolerated.

Rate Control

The optimal range for ventricular rates during atrial fibrillation is still controversial. In AF-CHF the heart rate goals were 80 beats/min or less at rest and 110 beats/min or less during a 6-minute walk test. Similar heart rate targets were used in AFFIRM. In RACE II, a trial specifically designed to assess strict and lenient rate control, however, no adverse effects were seen with a more lenient heart rate target. RACE II, however, included very few patients with a history of heart failure.[30]

Options for rate control are shown in **Table 35-1**. β-blockers should be first-line therapy for rate control in patients with AF and heart failure. In addition to controlling rates in AF, several β-blockers have been shown to reduce mortality in heart failure patients in general. Nondihydropyridine calcium channel blockers, verapamil and diltiazem, may be used in patients with heart failure and preserved systolic function, but their negative inotropic actions make them contraindicated in patients with a depressed ejection fraction. Digoxin remains a potentially useful adjunct to β-blockers for rate control but must be used with caution due to its narrow therapeutic range.

For patients with permanent AF in whom rate cannot be controlled and for those with drug refractory highly symptomatic recurrent episodes, AV junctional ablation can be an effective strategy. The potentially deleterious effects of RV apical pacing must be considered. In some patients, poor rate control alone may be responsible for the low ejection fraction, and these patients may be managed with just RV pacing. If LV function is depressed even when the patient is in sinus rhythm, biventricular pacing for cardiac resynchronization will be the method of choice.

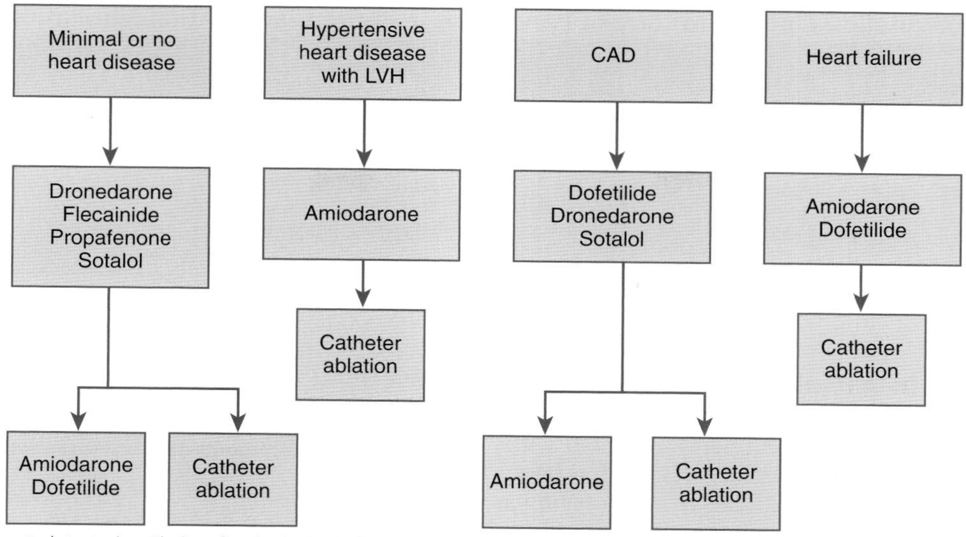

FIGURE 35-1 Rhythm control strategies. Choice of antiarrhythmic drug therapy based on comorbidities. *CAD*, Coronary artery disease; *LVH*, left ventricular hypertrophy. *From Camm AJ, Lip GYH, De Caterina R, et al: 2012 focused update of the ESC guidelines for the management of atrial fibrillation. Eur Heart J 33:2719–2747, 2012.*

Pharmacologic Rhythm Control

As shown in **Figure 35-1**, pharmacologic treatment options for maintaining sinus rhythm in patients with heart failure are limited. With the possible exception of disopyramide in patients with hypertrophic cardiomyopathy, class IA agents are not useful due to the high prevalence of side effects. Flecainide and propafenone are contraindicated in patients with heart failure. Dronedarone is similarly contraindicated in heart failure patients based on the data from the ANDROMEDA and PALLAS trials, both of which showed increased mortality with dronedarone therapy in patients with heart failure. Drug selection in patients with left ventricular hypertrophy is also limited by the risk for QT prolongation and *torsades de pointes* with class III agents like sotalol. These observations frequently leave only dofetilide (not currently marketed in the European Union) and amiodarone as treatment options for heart failure patients. Dofetilide is a relatively pure I_{Kr} blocker that is effective for both converting AF episodes and for maintaining sinus rhythm. In the Diamond-HF trial, dofetilide did not increase overall mortality and improved outcomes in the subgroup with AF but careful attention to dose and effects on the QTc during therapy is required. Heart failure patients with unstable renal function would not be good candidates for dofetilide. Amiodarone, therefore, frequently remains the only reasonable choice for sinus rhythm maintenance in patients with heart failure. Amiodarone was the drug most frequently used in both AFFIRM and AF-CHF. The estimated probability of maintaining sinus rhythm with selective use of electrical cardioversion in patients on amiodarone is 60% to 80% at 2 to 3 years but decreases over time. Amiodarone has many side effects, however, and should be used at the lowest effective chronic dose, usually 200 mg daily.

A number of agents and interventions that do not have classic antiarrhythmic effects are also likely to be important to the overall management of AF in heart failure. Angiotensin-converting enzyme (ACE) inhibitors, angiotensin receptor blockers (ARBs), β-adrenergic blockers, and aldosterone antagonists may be useful in this regard because they may both delay the onset of AF initially and act synergistically with more traditional antiarrhythmic drugs long-term. Sleep apnea is another risk factor for AF that should also be treated when present.[32]

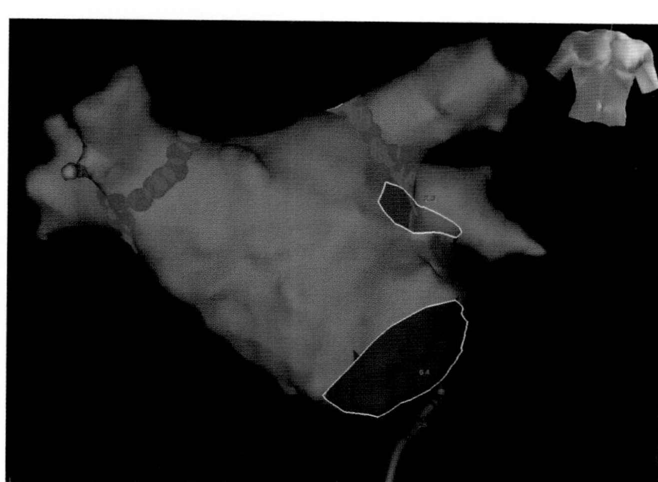

FIGURE 35-2 Atrial fibrillation ablation. An anteroposterior view of the left atrium demonstrating radiofrequency ablation lesions around the pulmonary veins.

Atrial Fibrillation Ablation in Heart Failure

Atrial fibrillation ablation may be technically challenging in patients with congestive heart failure. The basic technique of pulmonary vein antral isolation alone is rarely successful due to left atrial enlargement, chronic left atrial hypertension, and diffuse atrial scarring (**Figure 35-2**). Additional linear lesions, both left and right atrial, and lesions targeting atrial electrograms that are fractionated are often placed with a modest increase in efficacy. Nevertheless, even though only intermediate success rate should be anticipated, catheter or surgical ablation may be a useful option in selected patients.[24] Catheter ablation should probably be attempted before AV junctional ablation in younger patients without AV block because the latter procedure is irreversible and creates a situation of life-long pacemaker dependency.

TABLE 35-2 Anticoagulation Options for Stroke Prevention in Patients with Atrial Fibrillation[31,32]

DRUG	MECHANISM OF ACTION	DOSE	RENAL DOSE ADJUSTMENT	HALF-LIFE	ELIMINATION
Warfarin	Vitamin K antagonist	Variable INR 2-3	N/A	35-45 hr	Hepatic CYP450
Dabigatran	Direct thrombin inhibitor	150 mg bid	75 mg bid if CrCl 15-30	12-17 hr	80% renal 20% hepatic
Apixaban	Factor Xa direct inhibitor	5 mg bid	2.5 mg bid if CrCl 15-30	8-15 hr	75% hepatic 25% renal
Rivaroxaban	Factor Xa direct inhibitor	20 mg daily	15 mg daily if CrCl 15-50	5-9 hr	66% hepatic 33% renal

INR, International normalized ratio.

Anticoagulation in Atrial Fibrillation and Atrial Flutter

Non-rheumatic atrial fibrillation has been associated with a fivefold increase in the risk of ischemic stroke. It has been estimated that 15% of all ischemic strokes occur in patients with atrial fibrillation. Patients with stroke and atrial fibrillation are at higher risk for recurrent stroke and more severe stroke leading to greater disability and loss of independence. Stroke in patients with AF are 1.5 to 3.0 times more likely to be fatal than those in patients in sinus rhythm. Balanced against the increased risk for stroke and systemic embolism in patients with AF is the risk of bleeding associated with long-term anticoagulant therapy. For each patient, these risks must be carefully weighed to achieve optimal outcomes. Several new anticoagulation options are now available in addition to warfarin (see later discussion and **Table 35-2**).

Several scoring systems for stroke risk in patients with AF have been proposed. Although all the proposals have limitations, they remain clinically useful. In North America and Europe, the CHADS2 and CHA2DS2-VASc schemes are used most commonly. Heart failure is a risk factor in both these scoring systems so virtually all patients with heart failure and AF are candidates for chronic anticoagulation. In the absence of contraindications, oral anticoagulation is recommended for patients with CHADS2 or CHADSVASc (**Table 35-3**) scores of 2 or greater and should be considered for scores of 1. Bleeding risk is also a critical factor in decisions about long-term anticoagulation and scoring systems to predict risk have also been described. An example, the HAS-BLED score, is shown in **Table 35-4**.[32,33]

Warfarin has long been the primary oral anticoagulant for patients with atrial fibrillation. In a series of randomized trials in patients with nonvalvular AF, warfarin was shown to decrease stroke rate by approximately two thirds. Similar effects were seen in patients with both paroxysmal and permanent AF. The target INR should be 2.0 to 3.0, with increased rates of stroke clearly seen below an INR of 1.7 and increased bleeding when INR values were over 4.0. Recently, new oral anticoagulants have been introduced. Dabigatran, a direct thrombin inhibitor, and two factor 10a inhibitors, rivaroxaban and apixaban, have been shown to be noninferior to warfarin in large randomized clinical trials in nonvalvular AF.[32,33]

TABLE 35-3 Stroke Risk Scores

CHADS2 RISK	SCORE	CHA_2DS_2-VASc RISK	SCORE
CHF	1	CHF (or LVEF ≤ 40%)	1
Hypertension	1	Hypertension	1
Age >75	1	Age ≥ 75	2
Diabetes	1	Diabetes	1
Stroke or TIA	2	Stroke or TIA	2
		Vascular disease	1
		Age 65 to 74	1
		Female	1
Maximum	6	Maximum	10

Stroke risk scores estimate the stroke risk based on comorbid conditions to help determine appropriate anticoagulation for patients with atrial fibrillation.

CHF, Congestive heart failure; *LVEF*, left ventricular ejection fraction; *TIA*, transient ischemic attack.

From Camm, AJ, Lip GYH, De Caterina R, et al: 2012 focused update of the ESC guidelines for the management of atrial fibrillation. Eur Heart J 33:2719–2747, 2012.

TABLE 35-4 HAS-BLED Scores

HAS-BLED RISK	SCORE
Hypertension	1
Abnormal renal and/or liver function (1 point each)	1 or 2
Stroke or TIA	1
Bleeding	1
Labile INR	1
Elderly (Age >65)	1
Drugs and/or alcohol use (1 point each)	1 or 2
Maximum	9

HAS-BLED scores estimate bleeding risk in patients to be placed on systemic anticoagulation.

INR, International normalized ratio; *TIA*, transient ischemic attack.

From Camm, AJ, Lip GYH, De Caterina R, et al; 2012 focused update of the ESC guidelines for the management of atrial fibrillation. Eur Heart J 33:2719–2747, 2012.

Prognosis

Atrial fibrillation may adversely influence prognosis both by increasing the risk of thromboembolic events and by aggravating or directly causing heart failure or ischemia. Proarrhythmic responses to drug therapy or bleeding from anticoagulants may also contribute to an increase in mortality in patients who have atrial fibrillation. In the Framingham study, atrial fibrillation was associated with an odds ratio (OR) for death of 1.5 (95% CI 1.2-1.8) among men and 1.9 (95% CI 1.5-2.2) among women after adjustment for multiple clinical parameters.[5] The greatest absolute impact of atrial fibrillation on prognosis is seen when it occurs in patients who have advanced heart disease or other comorbid diseases.[6] In patients who do not have significant heart disease, atrial fibrillation has lesser effects on survival. As strategies for appropriate anticoagulation, effective rate control and heart failure management continue to evolve; it may be that the magnitude of the independent effect of atrial fibrillation will be lessened in the future. Atrial fibrillation is the most common sustained arrhythmia in adult populations.[5] Although atrial fibrillation itself is usually not life threatening, it leads to significant patient morbidity and economic costs, and contributes to stroke and heart failure.

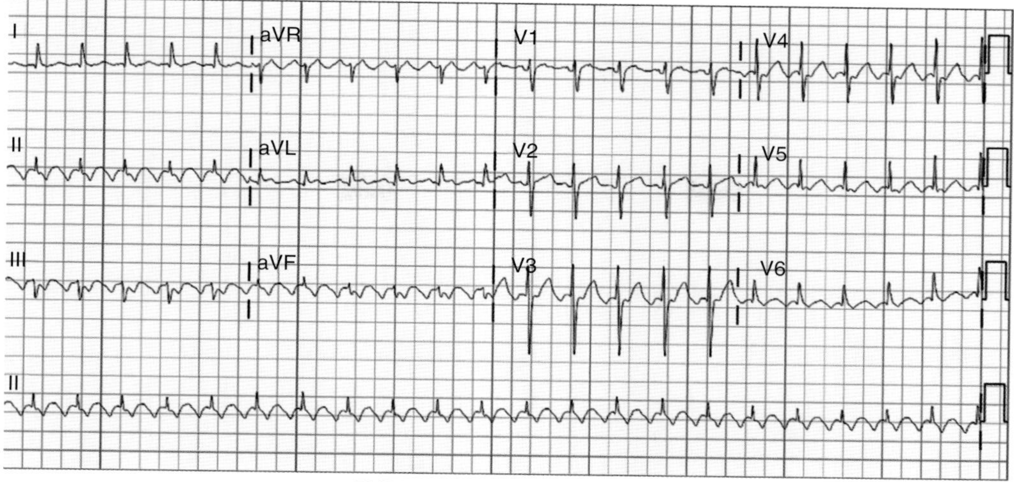

FIGURE 35-3 Typical atrial flutter.

Clinical decisions in patients who have atrial fibrillation are often difficult, and no uniformly effective therapies are available. In some patients, ventricular rate control and anticoagulation may be preferable to aggressive attempts to maintain sinus rhythm with repeat cardioversions and antiarrhythmic drug therapy. Newer strategies, such as less toxic antiarrhythmic agents, catheter ablation, improved surgical approaches, and new oral anticoagulants, offer promise for the future, but their efficacy and optimal uses still need to be demonstrated.

ATRIAL FLUTTER

Atrial flutter is defined as a rapid, regular atrial rhythm, with an atrial rate of 240 to 350 beats/min. Atrial flutter has an electrophysiologic mechanism different from atrial fibrillation but is often caused by the same factors and has a similar overall management strategy. When atrial flutter and atrial fibrillation are documented in the same patient, both will require treatment.

Epidemiology

Using the Marshfield Epidemiological Study Area, Granada and colleagues demonstrated an overall incidence of 88/100,000 person-years. Atrial flutter was found to be 2.5 times more common in men and 3.5 times more common in heart failure patients.[34] The highest rates of atrial flutter are seen post open heart surgery, with a 10% incidence in the first week.[35] This type of atrial flutter may resolve within weeks of the operation and not recur.

Pathophysiology and Diagnosis

The most common electrophysiologic mechanism for atrial flutter is a single macro-reentrant circuit located in the atrium. The rhythm is regular and ranges from 240 to 350 beats/min.[35] The ventricular rate that presents with atrial flutter depends on the atrioventricular nodal conduction and refractoriness. Atrioventricular conduction is often 2 : 1 or 4 : 1, but may be variable. In 2 : 1 atrial flutter, the ventricular rate is often close to 150 beats/min. Atrial flutter is often classified as either typical or atypical. In typical flutter, the atrial impulse travels in a counterclockwise fashion up the right atrial septum, across and down the right atrial free wall, and then along the tricuspid isthmus. The activation sequence results in the classic findings of "sawtooth" flutter waves in the inferior ECG leads and an upright flutter wave in lead V1 (**Figure 35-3**). Reverse typical flutter is when the atrial impulse travels in the opposite direction, also known as "clockwise" flutter (**Figure 35-4**). Other macro-reentrant atrial tachycardias are also possible and are frequently seen after cardiac surgery that involves atrial incisions or after ablation procedures for atrial fibrillation (scar-related atrial tachycardias) (**Figure 35-5**).[35]

The electrocardiogram is helpful in diagnosis of atrial flutter. In typical atrial flutter, the flutter waves are seen in the inferior leads II, III, and aVF as well as in lead V1 (see Figure 35-3). Flutter waves should have the same axis and cycle length often resembling a sawtooth pattern. Typical flutter can be identified with negative flutter waves in the inferior leads and positive flutter waves in V1. If atrial flutter is suspected but is difficult to identify, vagal maneuvers or other measures to block the AV node can be used to reveal flutter waves.[35]

Management

In acute atrial flutter, hemodynamic stability is the first important concern. Patients with left ventricular dysfunction are often unable to compensate for sudden increases in ventricular rates. Rate control can be attempted with intravenous calcium channel blockers or β-blockers, but is often difficult to maintain because there is little concealed conduction in the AV node during flutter. If patients are clinically unstable, direct current cardioversion is often the fastest option to restore hemodynamic stability. If the patient has an intracardiac device with pacing capabilities, rapid atrial pacing can be used for termination. Bipolar atrial pacing via the ramp or burst pacing algorithm can be performed starting at 10 beats/min faster than the atrial rate of the flutter cycle length. Pacing is often performed for at least 10 to 30 seconds until the flutter wave axis in lead II becomes positive. The stimulus strength often needed is greater than 10 mA and several attempts may be required to terminate.[35]

Before termination of atrial flutter, one must assess the stroke risk associated with return of normal sinus rhythm.

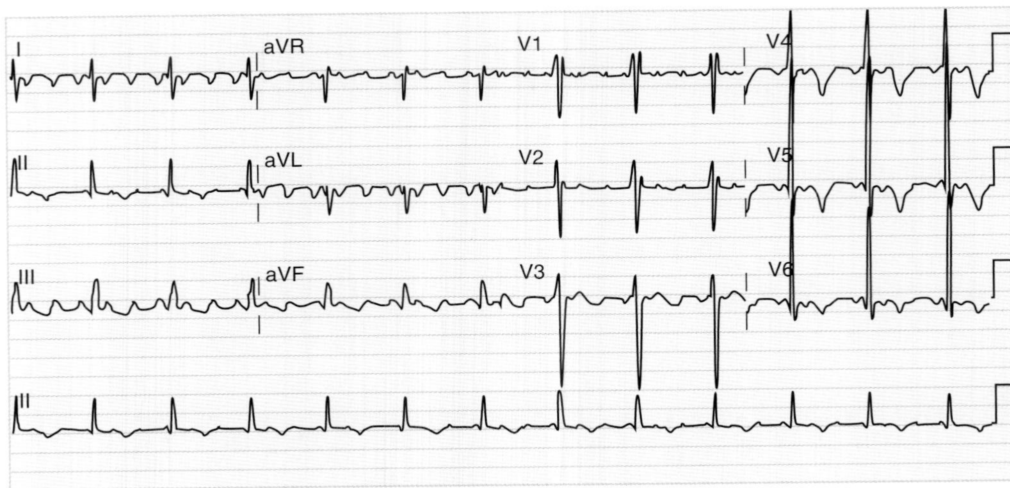

FIGURE 35-4 Atypical atrial flutter.

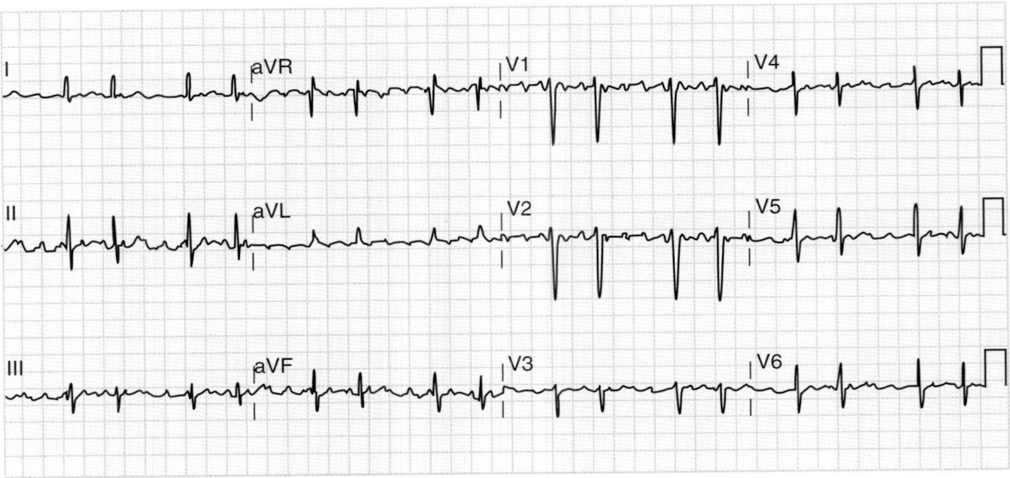

FIGURE 35-5 Scar-related atrial tachycardia.

Anticoagulation guidelines for cardioversion of atrial flutter are similar to those for cardioversion of atrial fibrillation. If the patient has been anticoagulated for the duration of the arrhythmia, the stroke risk is low. If the patient has been in sustained atrial flutter for less than 48 hours, the risk for thromboembolism is also considered low.

Similar to atrial fibrillation, amiodarone and dofetilide are the only drug options for patients with left ventricular dysfunction. Both have limited success in conversion of patients from atrial flutter to normal sinus rhythm. They may play a role in maintenance of sinus rhythm after electrical cardioversion, especially in patients with recurrence or patients with concomitant atrial fibrillation.

Radiofrequency catheter ablation of atrial flutter has become a safe and effective treatment option for most patients. If the reentrant circuit incorporates the cavotricuspid isthmus, then creating a linear lesion on the isthmus from the tricuspid annulus to the inferior vena cava will terminate the rhythm. Left atrial flutter or scar lesion–related flutter often require detailed mapping before radiofrequency ablation. Due to the high acute success rates of catheter ablation and the side effects of antiarrhythmic medications, radiofrequency ablation is first-line therapy for appropriate patients. Patients with previously documented atrial fibrillation will usually continue to have atrial fibrillation after a successful ablation for isthmus-dependent flutter and should be managed appropriately. Rate control is often more effective if the patient no longer has atrial flutter. Even if a patient has no history of prior AF, the likelihood of developing AF after a flutter ablation is at least 50% after 3 years.[36]

VENTRICULAR ARRHYTHMIAS

Ventricular arrhythmias are common in heart failure patients. Almost half of all patients with heart failure will die suddenly, mostly from ventricular arrhythmias. Implantable cardioverter-defibrillator (ICD) therapy is the main option for both primary and secondary prevention of sustained ventricular tachycardia (VT) and sudden death, but drug therapy and ablation are frequently important adjuncts.[37]

There is no one mechanism that causes ventricular arrhythmias in patients with heart failure. Instead, multiple elements contribute to the arrhythmogenesis, including increased sympathetic tone, ischemia, myocardial scar, conduction delay, increased diastolic calcium levels, early and delayed afterdepolarizations, electrolyte abnormalities,

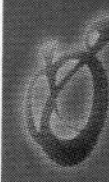

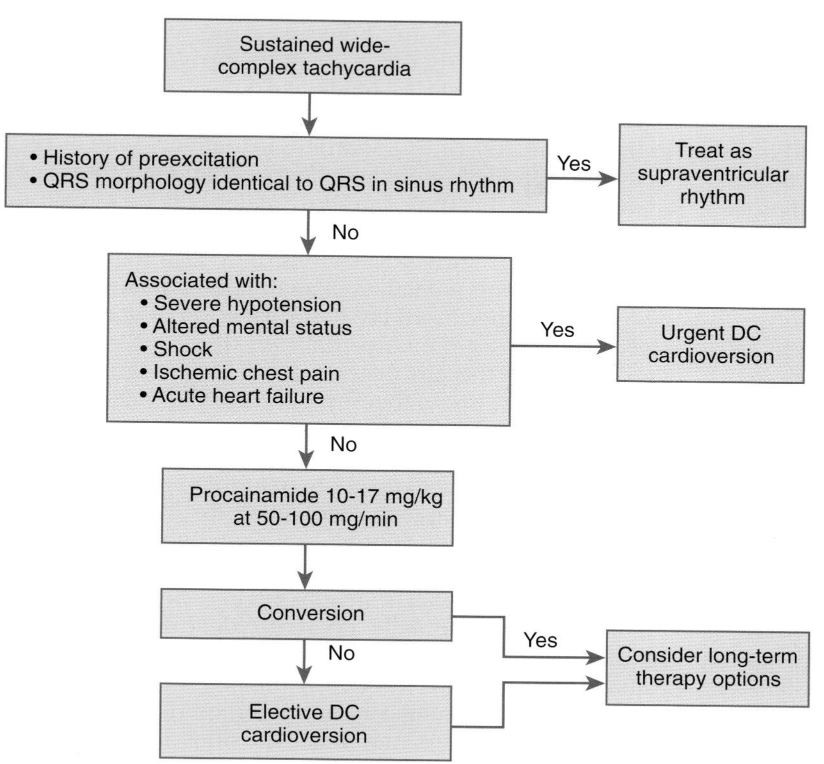

FIGURE 35-6 Wide-complex tachycardia management. *DC,* Direct-current.

and drugs. Common drugs that potentiate VT are antiarrhythmics, phosphodiesterase inhibitors, sympathomimetic drugs, and digoxin.[38]

Acute Episodes of Sustained Monomorphic Ventricular Tachycardia

The goal of acute therapy for sustained VT is to restore rapidly a stable rhythm with a physiologically appropriate rate and thereby prevent organ damage or further hemodynamic deterioration. Patients with severe hypotension, chest pain, or evidence for hypoperfusion of critical organs should be considered hemodynamically unstable and direct current cardioversion is usually the most expeditious method for terminating the arrhythmia. In many patients, however, the tachycardia is not immediately life threatening and the patient is conscious and not in severe distress. In such patients, pharmacologic cardioversion is the procedure of choice.[37,39]

Pharmacologic conversion of sustained monomorphic VT episodes has not been studied in large controlled randomized trials. Observational and limited controlled trial data, however, indicate that intravenous procainamide is the most effective agent.[40-42] Because procainamide-induced conversion is related to peak plasma drug concentrations, conversion is more likely with faster infusion rates (50-100 mg/min up to 15-17 mg/kg). These infusion rates, however, may cause hypotension and QT prolongation so blood pressure and the ECG must be frequently monitored throughout the infusion. Typically, the VT cycle length will lengthen and the slower rate will partially mitigate the vasodilating and negative inotropic effects of the drug. If the cycle length fails to lengthen, the ECG morphology changes, or the patient develops symptomatic hypotension, the infusion should be immediately stopped and electrical cardioversion considered.

Intravenous lidocaine and β-adrenergic blocking agents have very limited efficacy for terminating episodes of sustained VT in patients with heart failure. Verapamil and diltiazem are contraindicated in wide-complex tachycardias of unknown mechanism in patients with structural heart disease.[37,39] Rarely, if there is a strong possibility that the wide-complex tachycardia is supraventricular in origin, adenosine may be used. In most supraventricular arrhythmias, adenosine will either terminate the tachycardia or provide diagnostic information if AV block occurs. Intravenous amiodarone may be useful to treat recurrent episodes or if incessant monomorphic VT is seen (**Figure 35-6**).

Nonsustained Ventricular Tachycardia

Nonsustained VT is commonly detected during ECG monitoring in heart failure patients with both ischemic and nonischemic cardiomyopathies.[43] The frequency and complexity of ventricular ectopy are likely to increase during periods of worsening heart failure. A number of trials have tested the hypothesis that antiarrhythmic drug therapy either empirically administered or when guided by arrhythmia suppression during serial ambulatory ECG monitoring would improve survival and prevent sudden death. The drug most carefully evaluated has been amiodarone. In 1997, the Amiodarone Trials Meta-analysis Investigators reviewed 13 randomized controlled trials comparing amiodarone to placebo in patients with either recent myocardial infractions or congestive heart failure.[44] They estimated that prophylactic amiodarone would reduce arrhythmic/sudden death by 29% and total mortality by 13%. The studies included in this meta-analysis were completed before modern therapy for heart failure, including aggressive revascularization, renin-angiotensin system, β-adrenergic blockade, and aldosterone antagonism, was widely practiced. In the Sudden Cardiac Death-Heart Failure Trial

(SCD-HeFT), which was completed in 2004, empiric amiodarone had no advantage over a placebo in patients with New York Heart Association (NYHA) class II symptoms and actually increased mortality in patients with class III symptoms. A more recent meta-analysis of 15 randomized trials showed that prophylactic amiodarone had no overall benefit regarding mortality.[45] In most situations, asymptomatic ventricular ectopy should be considered a risk factor for future events and not as a target for therapy. However, in patients with very high frequency monomorphic premature ventricular contractions (PVCs) and VT, mapping and ablation of the site of origin may improve function and eliminate symptoms.

Sudden Cardiac Death in Patients with Heart Failure

The risk of sudden cardiac death (SCD) in heart failure patients is a major contributor to morbidity and mortality in this population. The annual incidence varies according to observational data, but ranges from 200,000 to 460,000. In the Metoprolol CR/XL Randomized Intervention Trial in Congestive Heart Failure (MERIT-HF), 64% of patients in NYHA class II who died had SCD compared with 59% of patients in class III and 33% of patients in class IV. The reasons for the elevated risk of SCD in heart failure patients are unknown but multiple theories have arisen. These include subendocardial ischemia, left ventricular hypertrophy, myocardial stretch, increased sympathetic tone, and aberrant baroreceptor response increasing ventricular arrhythmias, electrolyte abnormality, and coronary artery emboli. In the Assessment of Treatment with Lisinopril and Survival (ATLAS) trial, Uretsky and associates looked at 3164 patients with moderate to severe systolic heart failure. There were a total of 1382 deaths (43.7%) during the follow-up period of 36 to 60 months. Autopsy was performed in 188 patients and acute coronary causes were found in 54% of those with SCD.

Pharmacologic Therapy for Chronic Management of Ventricular Tachycardia

Although ICD therapy has evolved into the primary therapeutic modality to prevent death from ventricular arrhythmias, frequent ICD shocks are painful and may cause significant psychological distress. Therefore, concomitant antiarrhythmic drugs are often prescribed in an effort to reduce shock frequency.

Amiodarone and sotalol are the drugs most commonly used as adjuncts to ICD therapy in patients with structural heart disease and heart failure.[46-48] Pacifico and associates randomized 302 patients with prior sustained arrhythmias and secondary prevention ICDs to either sotalol (160-320 mg daily) or a placebo.[46] Sotalol resulted in a 48% reduction of the primary endpoint of death from any cause or delivery of first shock for any cause. Overall shock frequency was significantly reduced to 1.43 ± 3.53 shocks per year in the sotalol group from 3.89 ± 10.65 shocks per year in the placebo group. In the Optimal Pharmacological Therapy in Cardioverter Defibrillator Patients Trial (OPTIC), β-adrenergic blockade only, sotalol, and amiodarone plus β-blockade were compared.[47] Sotalol and, to a greater degree, amiodarone plus β-blockade significantly decreased the frequency of shocks, both appropriate and inappropriate. There are, however, more recent data that suggest that antiarrhythmic drug therapy to prevent ICD shocks may not always be beneficial. Kowey and colleagues reported a phase II dose-ranging study of celivarone, a non-iodinated analog of amiodarone, in patients with ICDs.[49] Celivarone had no significant effect on ICD shock frequency or mortality in this trial. The study included a small calibrator group treated with amiodarone. Although the amiodarone group had fewer ICD shocks, they also had a higher mortality. Patients with class III heart failure on amiodarone also had a higher mortality than placebo patients in SCD-HeFT. Until more definitive data on the value of adjunct antiarrhythmic therapy become available, it seems reasonable to restrict such therapy to only ICD patients with frequent, symptomatic episodes of atrial or ventricular arrhythmias.

In addition to the known extracardiac side effects of antiarrhythmic drugs, the potential for drug-ICD interactions must be considered. Antiarrhythmic drugs with sodium channel blocking properties may increase the defibrillation threshold. Pure class III agents are unlikely to do so and may actually decrease defibrillation energy requirements. Pacing thresholds may rarely be affected. Antiarrhythmic drugs frequently prolong VT cycle lengths and may require changes in programmed detection zones. Antiarrhythmic drugs may result in sinus bradycardia or worsen AV conduction, increasing the need for atrial and/or ventricular pacing.[50,51]

Catheter Ablation of Ventricular Tachycardia

Catheter ablation works best when a single structure or site not required for normal function but critical for the arrhythmia can be identified and safely ablated. Success rates with catheter ablation for some arrhythmias (e.g., supraventricular tachycardias mediated by accessory pathways or dual AV nodal pathways) are so high that catheter ablation has largely supplanted drug therapy in patients with these arrhythmias. Unfortunately, the results of catheter ablation for ventricular arrhythmias in patients with heart failure are much less favorable, but catheter ablation remains an important option for many patients.

The most common indication for catheter ablation in patients with heart failure is sustained monomorphic VT. Unless the tachycardia is quite slow, most patients will have an ICD for primary therapy and catheter ablation will be used to decrease the need for frequent ICD therapies. Catheter ablation may be used in these patients either alone or with concomitant antiarrhythmic drug therapy. Catheter ablation may be guided in several ways. If the VT is well tolerated, the arrhythmia is induced at electrophysiologic study with programmed ventricular stimulation and critical portions of the VT circuit defined by activation sequence and entrainment mapping. A three-dimensional electroanatomic mapping system is usually used to help guide catheter positioning. If circulatory support is used during the procedure, even rapidly organized tachycardias can usually be mapped and ablated in this fashion. An alternate technique uses voltage mapping to define areas of myocardial scarring and then places linear ablation lesions around the border zone of the scar. Pace mapping to match a known QRS morphology helps guide the region to be isolated. Most VT ablation is done using an endocardial approach, but

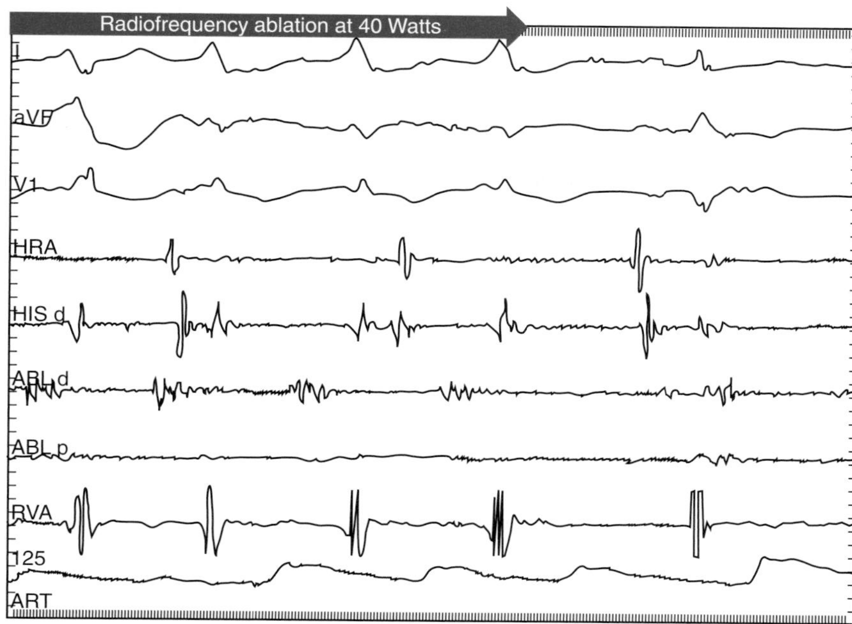

FIGURE 35-7 Ventricular tachycardia (VT) ablation intracardiac electrogram. Note the diastolic potential that changes to a systolic potential during ablation and termination of VT.

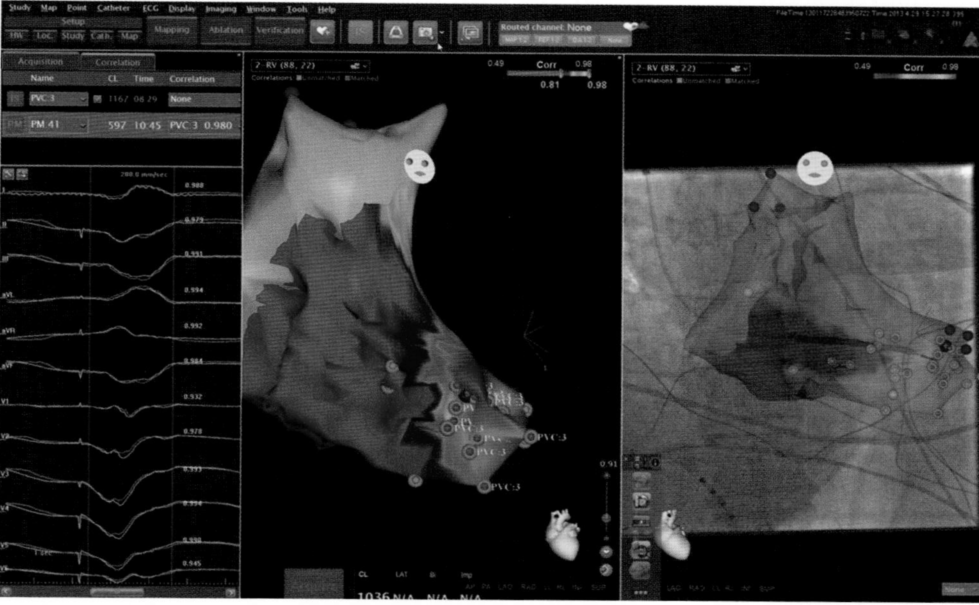

FIGURE 35-8 Ventricular tachycardia (VT) ablation activation map using Biosense Webster's CartoUnivu and PASO to determine location and optimal ablation sight of this right ventricular apical VT near the implantable cardioverter-defibrillator lead tip.

recent observations suggest that epicardial ablation may be required, particularly for patients with nonischemic forms of cardiomyopathy. Unfortunately many patients will have either multiple VT circuits at the time of their initial ablation attempt or will manifest new VTs during long-term follow-up, and the overall success rate for complete elimination of VT may be only 40% to 60%.[52] Despite this, decreasing the frequency of required ICD therapies may be an important part of patient management (**Figures 35-7 and 35-8**).

The second most common indication for VT ablation in patients with heart failure is when frequent PVCs by themselves compromise ventricular function and result in a tachycardia-induced cardiomyopathy. This is usually seen with extremely high-density PVCs in patients without other forms of heart disease, with a threshold for onset at about 10,000 PVCs per day. If the PVC morphology is stable, the site of origin can usually be mapped and identified by activation mapping, confirmed with pace mapping, and ablated with local RF energy delivery. For patients without disease that causes myocardial scarring, this type of PVC ablation may be curative and their left ventricular ejection fraction may return to normal.[53]

Finally, several groups have reported success in eliminating recurrent episodes of ventricular fibrillation (VF) by targeting a PVC focus whose firing triggers recurrent episodes. For this to be effective, the patient should have multiple VF episodes triggered by a PVC with a single morphology.

Risks of catheter ablation for VT are considerably higher than those for most other arrhythmias. In patients with peripheral vascular disease, vascular complications at access sites or inability to access the left ventricle may be problems. Valve or coronary artery damage, embolic events, cardiac perforations, bleeding, and hemodynamic

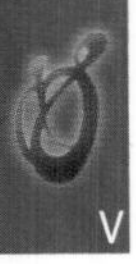

compromise from the mapping procedure are also potential complications.[52]

Device Therapy

Implantable Cardioverter-Defibrillator

The first clinical use of a totally implanted defibrillator was reported in 1980.[54] In the ensuing years, the ICD has developed into the most important therapy for preventing sudden death and treating sustained ventricular tachyarrhythmias. In the United States over 130,000 ICDs are implanted annually with over three fourths of the implants used for primary prevention of sudden cardiac death in patients with systolic heart failure.[55-57]

An ICD has two essential components: an ICD generator and a lead system for sensing, pacing, and shock delivery. The initial ICD generator was a bulky (230-g) device that required an abdominal implant and used epicardial leads and patches. Over time, advances in technology have allowed the devices to become smaller and permitted the use of transvenous or subcutaneous lead systems. The ICD generator contains sensing circuits, memory storage, capacitors, voltage enhancers, a battery, a telemetry module, and a control microprocessor. The initial implanted defibrillator detected only VF using a probability density function analysis of the sensed ventricular electrogram. It was soon recognized that organized VT also needed to be a target of ICD therapy and sensed ventricular rate is now the basic measure used to detect arrhythmias. Current ICDs have programming options that include pacing for bradycardia, resynchronization therapy, biphasic defibrillation, anti-tachycardia pacing, advanced arrhythmia discrimination in slower zones, and remote monitoring.

After implant, the ICD is programmed with one or more VT and/or VF detection zones. In slower zones, discrimination algorithms may be used to identify supraventricular arrhythmias so that therapy may be withheld. Episodes of a tachycardia in a VT zone are often treated with several bursts of anti-tachycardia pacing (ATP) first followed by a shock, if necessary. In a VF zone, a single burst of ATP during high-voltage charging is often used before shock delivery. Electrograms from each episode are stored and may be retrieved for subsequent analysis.

The ICD has been shown repeatedly to be effective for preventing sudden cardiac death in a number of randomized clinical trials (**Table 35-5**).[58-67] These trials are usually referred to as either secondary prevention trials in which patients had previously experienced a prior episode of cardiac arrest, VF, or VT, or primary prevention trials in which patients were studied who had high risk for sudden death but without known prior episodes.

The three most important secondary prevention ICD trials were the Antiarrhythmics Versus Implantable Defibrillators (AVID) Study, the Canadian Implantable Defibrillator Study (CIDS), and the Cardiac Arrest Study-Hamburg (CASH).[59-61] In AVID, 1016 cardiac arrest and unstable VT survivors were randomly assigned to either drug therapy (amiodarone or infrequently sotalol) or an ICD. Other indicated therapies were permitted, including β-adrenergic blockers, renin-angiotensin system inhibitors, and revascularization. The primary endpoint, total mortality, was decreased by 39%, 27%, and 31% at 1, 2, and 3-year time points, respectively. In CIDS, 696 patients with cardiac arrest, sustained VT, or syncope with induced VT were randomized between an ICD and amiodarone. ICD therapy resulted in a 19.7% lower mortality at the 2-year follow-up point. CASH included only cardiac arrest survivors ($N = 346$) and randomized them to either an ICD or drug therapy (amiodarone, metoprolol, or propafenone). The propafenone arm was terminated early because of excess mortality. At the 2-year time point, the mortality rate was 37% lower in the ICD group than in the combined amiodarone and metoprolol group.

TABLE 35-5 Primary and Secondary ICD Prevention Trials

TRIAL	RANDOMIZATION	YEAR	PATIENTS	ENTRY CRITERIA	MORTALITY RISK REDUCTION WITH ICD
Primary Prevention ICD Trials					
MADIT[62]	ICD vs. medical therapy	1996	196	NYHA I-II with prior MI and LVEF ≤ 35% with inducible VT	0.46 ($P = 0.009$)
CABG-PATCH[64]	Epicardial ICD vs. no ICD	1997	900	LVEF ≤ 35% with abnormal SAECG and CABG	1.07 ($P = 0.64$)
MADIT II[63]	ICD vs. no ICD	2002	1232	NYHA class I-III with LVEF ≤ 30% post MI	0.69 ($P = 0.016$)
DINAMIT[66]	ICD or no ICD (<40 days after MI)	2004	674	Up to 40 days post MI with LVEF ≤ 35%	1.08 ($P = 0.78$)
DEFINITE[65]	ICD vs. no ICD	2004	458	Nonischemic heart failure patients, LVEF <36% with >10 PVCs/hr or NSVT	0.65 ($P = 0.08$)
SCD-HeFT[58]	ICD vs. amiodarone vs. placebo	2005	2521	NYHA II-III and LVEF ≤ 35%; ischemic or nonischemic	0.77 ($P = 0.007$)
IRIS[67]	Randomized to ICD vs. no ICD	2009	898	Up to 31 days post MI with LVEF ≤ 40%, NSVT or HR >90	1.04 ($P = 0.78$)
Secondary Prevention ICD Trials					
AVID[59]	ICD vs. amiodarone	1997	1016	VF arrest or VT and syncope with EF ≤ 40%	0. 73 ($P <0.02$)
CIDS[60]	Amiodarone vs. ICD	2000	696	VF/VT arrest or syncope	0. 70 ($P = 0.142$)
CASH[61]	ICD vs. amiodarone vs. metoprolol	2000	346	VT/VF arrest	0.61 ($P = 0.2$)

CABG, Coronary artery bypass graft; *EF*, ejection fraction; *HR*, hazard ratio; *ICD*, implantable cardioverter-defibrillator; *LVEF*, left ventricular ejection fraction; *MI*, myocardial infarction; *NSVT*, nonsustained ventricular tachycardia; *NYHA*, New York Heart Association; *PVC*, premature ventricular contraction; *SAECG*, single-averaged electrocardiography; *VF*, ventricular fibrillation; *VT*, ventricular tachycardia.

Even in localities with skilled and efficient emergency medical care; most out-of-hospital cardiac arrest victims will not survive. Limiting ICD therapy to cardiac arrest survivors would therefore miss a large proportion of sudden death victims. A number of ICD trials have been completed that demonstrated conclusively that ICD therapy is also often effective for primary prevention of sudden death in patients with both ischemic and nonischemic cardiomyopathies. The two most important primary prevention trials were the Multicenter Automatic Defibrillator Implantation Trial II (MADIT II) and the Sudden Cardiac Death—Heart Failure Trial (SCD-HeFT).[58,63] In MADIT II, patients had ischemic heart disease with prior myocardial infarction and a left ventricular ejection fraction less than 0.30. ICD therapy compared with investigator-selected standard medical therapy resulted in a hazard ratio of 0.69. SCD-HeFT included patients with both ischemic and nonischemic cardiomyopathy, class II or class III heart failure symptoms, and a left ventricular ejection fraction less than 35%. Patients were randomized to an ICD, amiodarone, or placebo. Overall, ICD therapy resulted in a hazard ratio of 0.77, with the benefits seen in the subgroup having class II heart failure.

Not all primary prevention ICD trials have been positive. The Coronary Artery Bypass Graft-Patch Trial (CABG-Patch) randomized low ejection fraction in patients undergoing surgical coronary revascularization to either no therapy or an epicardial ICD system.[64] Mortality was slightly higher in the ICD group. Two studies have looked at ICD therapy for primary prevention in high-risk patients early after myocardial infarction. In both the Defibrillator in Acute Myocardial Infarction Trial (DINAMIT) and the Immediate Risk Stratification Improves Survival (IRIS) study, no overall benefit was seen.[66,67] In these two studies, a decrease in arrhythmic deaths in the ICD group was balanced by a corresponding increase in nonarrhythmic mortality. Based on these results, the Center for Medicare Services issued a National Coverage Decision related to ICD therapy in 2005.[68] Appropriate use criteria for ICD implantation and cardiac resynchronization covering over 500 clinical scenarios were published in 2013.[69]

ICD therapy has evolved during a period in which pharmacologic management of patients with heart failure has improved dramatically. As a result, survival rates in heart failure patients during medical therapy are now much better than they were when the first ICD trials were reported. For this reason, there has been considerable interest in defining the "optimal" candidate for a primary prevention ICD. In an analysis of data from MADIT II, the authors identified five factors that influenced ICD benefit. These five factors were NYHA function class III, atrial fibrillation, QRS duration greater than 120 msec, age older than 70 years, and BUN greater than 26 mg/dL. Patients with no risk factors had no benefit from ICD therapy and benefit attenuated in patients with three or more risk factors. Patients with one or two risk factors had the greatest change in benefit.[70] In an analysis of the national Medicare ICD registry data, Bilchick and colleagues identified seven predictors of mortality after ICD implantation.[71] These included age older than 75, class III heart failure, chronic lung disease, chronic kidney disease, atrial fibrillation, ejection fraction less than 0.20, and diabetes. Points were assigned to each risk factor and nomograms relating survival to total point score were calculated. It must be remembered, however, that cardiac resynchronization has independent positive effects on mortality in addition to simply symptoms of heart failure.[72] In the United States, over 40% of current primary prevention ICD recipients now receive a cardiac resynchronization device.

Implantable Cardioverter-Defibrillator Follow-up and Complications

All patients who received an ICD should have both periodic routine follow-up and urgent follow-up if problems arise.[73] With current ICD models, most follow-up device interrogations can be performed remotely, but virtually all ICD patients should still be seen in person by their cardiologist or electrophysiologist at least once or twice annually.[74]

At each device interrogation, the programmed parameter for bradycardia and tachycardia detection and therapy should be confirmed; expected device longevity can be estimated based on battery voltage, device parameters, and therapy history. Sensing and capture thresholds and pacing impedance values for each active lead should be measured. All devices also include event logs and store electrograms from specified arrhythmic events. These electrograms should be examined to make sure that tachycardia identification is accurate and therapy effective (**Figure 35-9**). Pocket erosions and lead and pocket infections remain common clinical problems. Patients should be instructed to call if they note any change in their pocket or if they have unexplained bloodstream infections. At each clinic visit, the pocket should be carefully examined for signs of infection or inflammation. Pain in a chronic ICD pocket should always arouse suspicion for a chronic low-grade infection.

The most common in-hospital complications after ICD insertion are lead dislodgment or perforation, pocket hematoma, pneumothorax, arrhythmias, and if a left ventricular lead is attempted, coronary sinus dissection.[75,76] Early complications are related to the experience and training of the operator, the type of device selected, and certain patient characteristics. Early ICD implants using epicardial patch systems that required a thoracotomy were associated with significant mortality (2%-8%), but with transvenous systems, early mortality is much lower and usually caused by recurrent arrhythmias. Procedural complications are more frequent with ICD generator changes, particularly if a new lead is added.[77]

Complications after hospital discharge are also unfortunately common during ICD therapy. The most frequent device-related adverse events are inappropriate shocks, infections, lead or device malfunction, and pacing- or lead-related hemodynamic effects. Psychological well-being may also be affected in patients with multiple shocks, either inappropriate or appropriate. Infections related to ICDs are a growing problem.[77-79] Superficial incisional infections that do not invade the pocket may be seen early after implant and can often be managed with antibiotics and good wound care. Late infections, either direct infection of the pocket or secondary infection of the leads from a remote site, are much more serious. Complete removal of the device and leads and antibiotic therapy are required to control the infection. Patients with evidence for associated valvular endocarditis will need a prolonged course of therapy.

A number of events can result in the delivery of inappropriate shocks in ICD recipients. Atrial tachyarrhythmias and antiarrhythmic drugs are the most common causes;

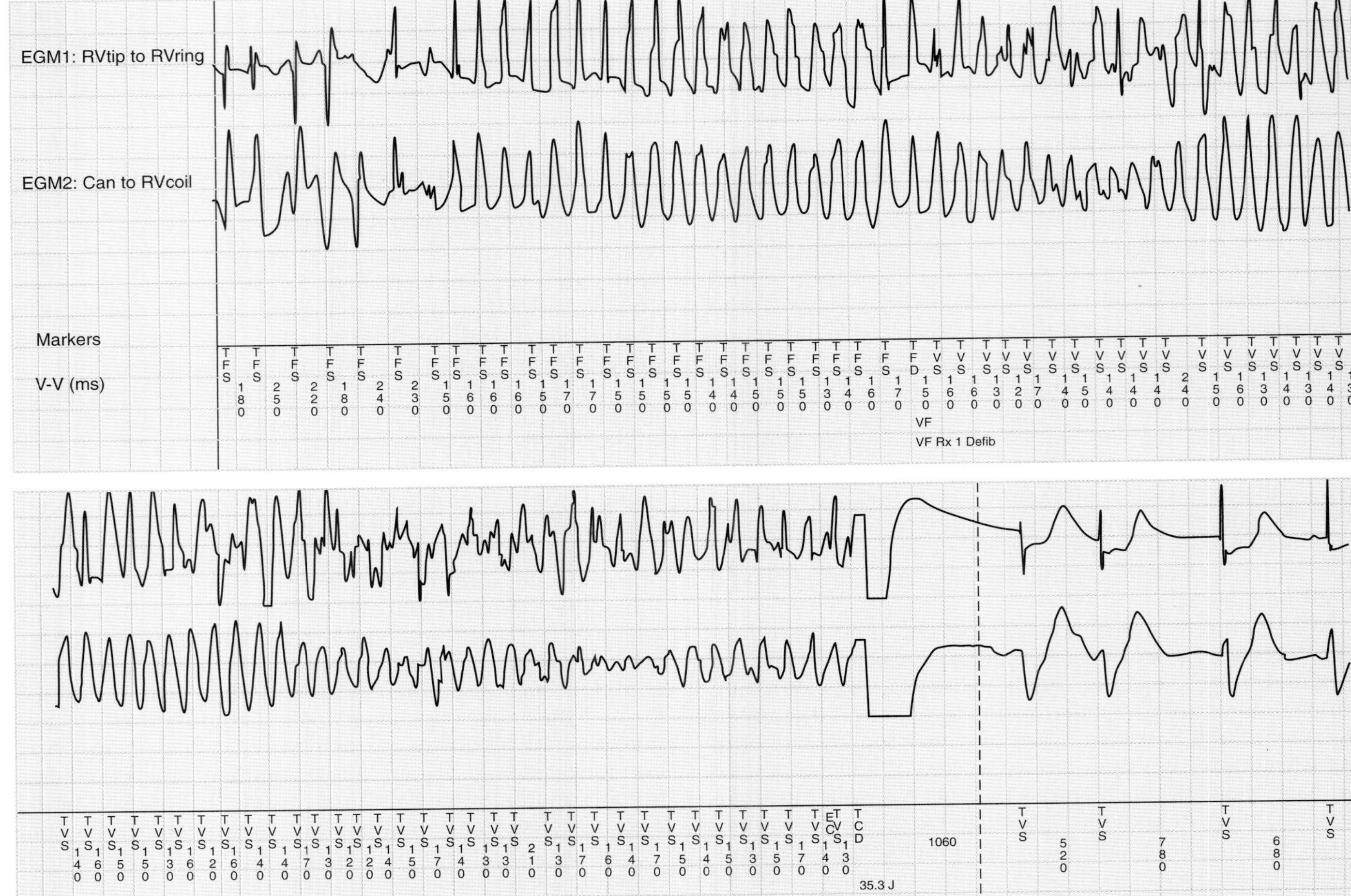

FIGURE 35-9 Implantable cardioverter-defibrillator stored electrogram showing termination of an episode of ventricular fibrillation.

β-adrenergic blocking agents and electrogram discrimination algorithms are the most common approaches for prevention. Lead or device malfunctions leading to oversensing are also frequently encountered. Some ICD leads have experienced a higher than expected fracture rate. Newer ICD models have incorporated automatic checks of lead integrity to prevent inappropriate shocks because of lead fractures, but these are not always effective. Recent studies have shown increasing detection rates and times help reduce inappropriate shocks without compromising efficacy.[80-81]

Congestive heart failure may be caused by lead-induced tricuspid valve dysfunction and by dyssynchrony caused by inappropriate right ventricular apical pacing. Loss of left ventricular lead capture during cardiac resynchronization therapy (CRT) is another common cause of ICD-related heart failure worsening.

Anxiety, depression, and post-traumatic stress disorder may be seen in ICD recipients. Rare or single shocks are well tolerated by most, but frequent shocks consistently will result in emotional distress and a reduced quality of life.[82]

Cardiac Resynchronization Therapy

Abnormalities of atrioventricular and intraventricular conduction are common in patients with heart failure and mortality increases in patients with longer QRS durations. A prolonged AV interval delays ventricular systole leading to diastolic mitral regurgitation and prevents optimal ventricular preload in patients with heart failure. Intraventricular conduction delays, particularly those that delay left ventricular activation, result in a dyssynchronous and inefficient pattern of contraction characterized by papillary muscle dysfunction, reduced stroke volumes, and adverse LV remodeling. Insertion of a cardiac resynchronization pacing device allows optimization of the AV interval and coordinates contraction between ventricles and within the left ventricle. Favorable effects include an improved LV ejection fraction, decreased functional mitral regurgitation, better septal contraction, and decreased LV end-diastolic and end-systolic volumes.

It has been well established in multiple clinical trials that CRT improves exercise parameters and quality of life measures and decreases heart failure hospitalizations and mortality in patients with low ejection fraction class II-III heart failure symptoms and wide QRS complex.[83] In a summary of clinical trials included in the 2013 European Society of Cardiology Guidelines on Cardiac Pacing and Cardiac Resynchronization Therapy, a 22% reduction in mortality and a 35% reduction in heart failure hospitalizations with CRT alone are described.[84] Addition of defibrillation capability to the device further improved outcomes in appropriately selected patients in the COMPANION Trial.[85]

Most of the early trials of CRT required a QRS duration of greater than 120 or 130 msec for entry, but the majority of patients had left bundle branch block (LBBB) and the efficacy of CRT in patients with non–left bundle intraventricular conduction defects (IVCDs) is not as well established. MADIT-CRT looked at QRS morphology on 1817 patients' 12-lead ECGs and divided them into LBBB and non-LBBB. There were 1281, or 70%, of patients with LBBB and 536, or 30%, non-LBBB patients. There was significant reduction in left ventricular volumes and an increase in ejection fraction with CRT-defibrillator (CRT-D) in LBBB compared with non-LBBB patients. The rates of VT, VF, or death were decreased significantly in CRT-D patients with LBBB compared with non-LBBB patients. They concluded that patients with NYHA class I or II and left ventricular ejection fraction of 30% or less and LBBB have a significant reduction in heart failure progression and risk of ventricular arrhythmias.[86]

Further analysis of MADIT-CRT showed that patients with LBBB morphology and QRS duration of 150 msec or greater were associated with the greatest reduction in heart failure events and mortality. They also found that women obtained greater reductions in death or heart failure and all-cause mortality with CRT-D therapy compared to men.[87] These observation are incorporated in updated guidelines for CRT therapy that were released in 2012 by the American College of Cardiology and in 2013 by the European Society of Cardiology.[84,88]

Studies demonstrating the efficacy of CRT are summarized in **Table 35-6**. Current indications for CRT include patients with a wide QRS of greater than 120 msec. However, patients with LBBB morphology and QRS duration of 150 msec or greater have a higher rate of responding to left ventricular pacing. Patients with indications for ICD therapy should be implanted with CRT-D therapy. CRT-pacemaker (CRT-P) has been suggested in patients with reduced life expectancy or in patients with reduced left ventricular ejection fraction (LVEF) and dependence for ventricular pacing.

Coronary Sinus or Left Ventricular Epicardial Lead Placement

For most patients that qualify for CRT at time of pacemaker or ICD implant, the coronary sinus is cannulated with a long sheath. A venogram is then often performed to identify the coronary sinus branches. The most desirable location is typically on the left lateral wall, the site with the greatest delay in activation in LBBB. Anterior or apical vein locations for pacing have been found to be less likely to result in improved ventricular function and may be detrimental. Once the lead is in an acceptable location, impedance, sensing, and threshold measurements are made. It is important to test for phrenic nerve capture, as the nerve is often close to this location. If phrenic nerve capture is obtained, the lead often needs to be moved. If there are no suitable options for coronary sinus pacing or it is not possible to cannulate the coronary sinus, an epicardial surgical procedure can be performed using a left lateral thoracotomy. The epicardial lead is then tunneled to the device site and connected.

Response to Cardiac Resynchronization Therapy

The definition of CRT response is poorly defined but is often thought of as a change in echocardiographic findings and clinical symptoms. Echocardiographic response is typically assessed by quantifying the change in LVEF or left ventricular end-systolic volume (LVESV) 3 to 6 months after CRT implantation. Clinical response is assessed with the increase in the distance walked in 6 minutes or improvement in NYHA functional class 3 to 6 months after CRT implantation. Studies have defined response to CRT as a combination of several clinical measures or as a combination of both clinical and echocardiographic measures.

In the Multicenter InSync Randomized Clinical Evaluation (MIRACLE) trial, there was a 67% improvement in the group randomized to CRT using a clinical composite score

TABLE 35-6 Selected Cardiac Resynchronization Therapy Trials

TRIAL	RANDOMIZATION	YEAR	PATIENTS	ENTRY CRITERIA	CRT OUTCOMES
MIRACLE[89]	CRT vs. OMT, 6 mo	2002	453	NYHA class III-IV and LVEF ≤ 35% with QRS ≥ 130	Improved NYHA class, LVEF, QoL, and 6MWD; reduced LVEDD and MR
MIRACLE-ICD[92]	CRT-D vs. ICD, 6 mo	2003	369	NYHA class III-IV and LVEF ≤ 35% with QRS ≥ 130	Improved, NYHA class, QoL, and peak Vo_2
CONTAK-CD[93]	CRT-D vs. ICD, 6 mo	2003	490	NYHA class II-IV with LVEF ≤ 35% and QRS ≥ 120	Improved 6MWD, NYHA class, QoL, and LVEF with reduced LV volume
COMPANION[94]	OMT vs. CRT-P or vs. CRT-D, 15 mo	2004	1520	NYHA class III-IV with LVEF ≤ 35% and QRS ≥ 120	Reduced all-cause mortality and hospitalization
CARE-HF[72]	OMT vs. CRT-P, 29.4 mo	2005	813	NYHA class III-IV with LVEF ≤ 35% and QRS ≥ 120	Reduced all-cause mortality and hospitalization; improved NYHA class and QoL
REVERSE[95]	CRT-ON vs. CRT-OFF, 12 mo	2008	610	NYHA class I-II with LVEF ≤ 40% and QRS ≥ 120	CRT did not reduce all-cause mortality but reduced LVESV index and hospitalization*
MADIT-CRT[87]	CRT-D vs. ICD, 12 mo	2009	1820	NYHA class I-II with LVEF ≤ 30% and QRS ≥ 130	34% reduction in the risk of death or heart failure events*
RAfT[96]	CRT-D vs. ICD, 40 mo	2010	1798	NYHA class II-III with LVEF ≤ 30% and QRS ≥ 120	Reduced all-cause mortality and hospitalization

*Benefits largely in NYHA class II.

6MWD, Six-minute walk distance; *CRT-D,* cardiac resynchronization therapy defibrillator; *CRT-P,* cardiac resynchronization therapy pacemaker; *GDMT;* guideline-directed medical therapy; *ICD,* implantable cardioverter-defibrillator; *LVEDD,* left ventricular end-diastolic dimension; *LVEF,* left ventricular ejection fraction; *LVESV,* left ventricular end-systolic volume; *MR,* mitral regurgitation; *NYHA,* New York Heart Association; *OMT,* optimal medical therapy; *QoL,* quality of life.

to determine which patients were improved, unchanged, or worsened.[89] Intriguingly, a more recent Frequent Optimization Study Using the QuickOpt Method (FREEDOM) trial, designed to assess strategies for atrioventricular (AV) and interventricular (VV) interval optimization, reported a 67.5% improvement after CRT using the same clinical composite score.[90] Despite advances in knowledge and experience with CRT, the proportion of patients considered clinical nonresponders has remained at roughly 30%.

In nonresponders, first the electrocardiogram can be checked with and without pacing to confirm left ventricular pacing. If the underlying QRS is narrower than the paced QRS, pacing may not benefit. Next the device should be interrogated to ensure optimal pacing with greater than 90% biventricular pacing. If the percentage of biventricular pacing is less than 90%, the reason should be determined and corrected. Most frequently, this is due to atrial or ventricular arrhythmia. Next the lead position should be confirmed on posteroanterior and lateral chest x-ray. It is generally recommended to implant the LV lead in a basal to midlateral or posterolateral branch of the coronary sinus, if there is an eligible vein. Lead reposition can be changed if there are options for a more suitable vein position. Echocardiographic assessment immediately after the device implantation or during the follow-up procedures provides further information on the reasons for response and nonresponse to CRT. The transmitral filling profile improves acutely in most patients with the initiation of CRT. If it remains below 40% to 45% of the corresponding cycle length, changing the AV-delay of the device programming can optimize it. The SMART AV trial showed that patients with normal AV-delay did not derive benefit from echo-guided or device-guided AV-optimization compared with the empiric settings; however, patients with prolonged AV-conduction were not included in this prospective, randomized study.[91] The presence or even worsening of intraventricular dyssynchrony is a common problem in CRT nonresponders. VV-optimization is a useful tool to correct intraventricular dyssynchrony by device programming. Optimal VV-delay settings are highly variable in CRT patients, and therefore echocardiography-guided VV-optimization is recommended.

Arrhythmias Associated with Left Ventricular Assist Device Therapy (see Chapter 43)

Left ventricular assist devices (LVADs) have become more common in the treatment of advanced heart failure patients. With the advancement of these mechanical circulatory support systems, they can be used not only for a bridge to heart transplant but also for destination therapy.[97,98]

Atrial arrhythmias are common in patients with LVADs. Atrial fibrillation is the most common atrial arrhythmia in patients with LVADs. Treatment for this is the same as in any patient with heart failure. β-blockers are the preferred treatment, namely metoprolol tartrate, because carvedilol may cause a significant drop in blood pressure. Calcium channel blockers should be avoided, because they are contraindicated in most heart failure patients due to the negative inotropic response. Catheter ablation in this population may be difficult and has not been studied in a prospective trial. All patients with LVADs are typically anticoagulated; thus the risk of thromboembolism because of atrial fibrillation is low.[99]

Ventricular arrhythmias are common in patients with end-stage heart failure. The substrate causing these arrhythmias does not change with the placement of an LVAD; thus the risk of developing ventricular arrhythmias is unchanged. There is a theoretical reduction of VT as the left ventricular end-diastolic pressure is lowered, thereby decreasing the risk of ventricular arrhythmias. However, with the addition of an inflow cannula inserted into the left ventricle, the risk of developing ventricular arrhythmias greatly increases. This occurs when the left ventricle is underfilled, especially when the inflow cannula touches any of the endocardial structures, most commonly the septal wall. This occurs any time the patient loses intracardiac volume, as with diuresis, significant blood loss, or increased LVAD speed, resulting in overpumping and collapse of the ventricle. Treatment involves resolving the underlying issue by turning the LVAD speed down, replacing blood loss, or reducing diuretics. Drug therapy includes β-blockers, amiodarone, or dofetilide. Mexiletine can be added if breakthrough occurs.[100]

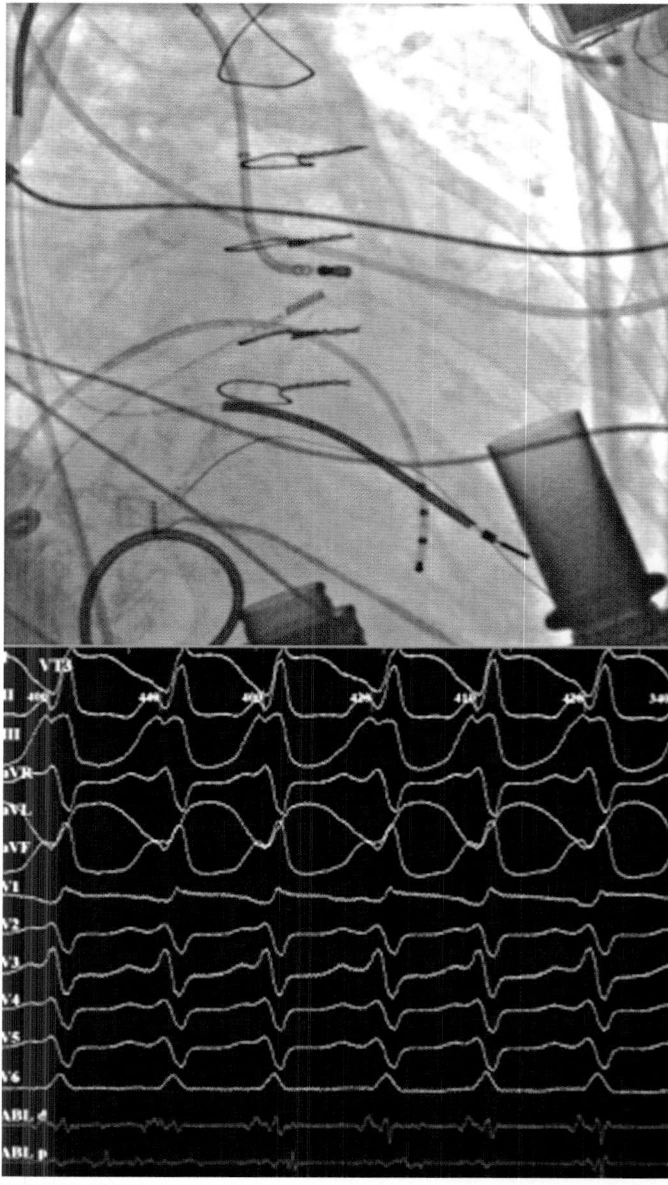

FIGURE 35-10 Ventricular tachycardia ablation in a patient with a left ventricular assist device. Notice the early ventricular signals on the intracardiac electrograms from the ablation catheter.

Limited data suggest that ranolazine may reduce ventricular arrhythmia burden in antiarrhythmic drug refractory cases.[101] Catheter ablation has been performed on patients with drug refractory ventricular arrhythmias. Ablation should be a secondary treatment because it is more difficult due to the presence of an inflow cannula as well as increased blood flow (**Figure 35-10**).[102]

Arrhythmia Management after Heart Transplantation

Improved outcomes after heart transplantation have led to a median survival time exceeding 10 years. The fact that patients live longer has led to increased occurrence of arrhythmias.

Sinus node ischemia, graft ischemia, drug effects, and sympathetic denervation all predispose patients to postsurgical bradycardia. Temporary pacing is often established via epicardial wires to keep ventricular rates greater than 90 beats/min. Permanent pacemaker implantation is reserved for symptomatic bradycardia or sinus node dysfunction.[103]

Atrial arrhythmias range in incidence from 0.3% to 24% for atrial fibrillation and 2.8% to 30% for atrial flutter after heart transplantation. Atrial fibrillation is the most common, especially early after surgery. Atrial flutter and other atrial tachycardias are more common later in the course after transplant. Interestingly, atrial fibrillation within 2 weeks has been associated with rejection, and atrial flutter after 3 weeks is the most common arrhythmia associated with rejection. Management of these arrhythmias is similar to other patients; however, prolonged antiarrhythmic drug therapy is not usually indicated.[103]

Nonsustained VT is somewhat common in the early postoperative period. This will typically become less frequent after transplant. If VT occurs late after heart transplant, severe cardiac allograft vasculopathy should be suspected. These patients may need antiarrhythmic therapy and should be considered for ICD placement. Up to 25% of patients with ventricular arrhythmias may have sudden cardiac death, and this is the most common cause of death after heart transplantation.[103]

References

1. Benjamin EJ, Wolf PA, D'Agostino RB, et al: Impact of atrial fibrillation on the risk of death. *Circulation* 98:946–952, 1998.
2. Lip GYH, Golding DJ, Nazir M, et al: A survey of atrial fibrillation in general practice: the West Birmingham Atrial Fibrillation Project. *Br J Gen Pract* 47:285–289, 1997.
3. Psaty BM, Manolio TA, Kuller LH, et al: Incidence of and risk factors for atrial fibrillation in older adults. *Circulation* 96:2555–2561, 1997.
4. Fuster V, Ryden LE, Cannom DS, et al: ACC/AHA/ESC 2006 guidelines for the management of patients with atrial fibrillation: a report of the American College of Cardiology/American Heart Association Task Force on Practice Guidelines and the European Society of Cardiology Committee for Practice Guidelines (Writing Committee to Revise the 2001 Guidelines for the Management of Patients with Atrial Fibrillation). *J Am Coll Cardiol* 48:e149–e246, 2006.
5. Benjamin EJ, Levy D, Vaziri SM, et al: Independent risk factors for atrial fibrillation in a population-based cohort: the Framingham Heart Study. *JAMA* 271(11):840–844, 1994.
6. Thrall G, Lane D, Carroll D, et al: Quality of life in patients with atrial fibrillation: a systematic review. *Am J Med* 119(5):448:e1–448:e19, 2006.
7. De Ferrari GM, Klersy C, Ferrero P, et al: Atrial fibrillation in heart failure patients: prevalence in daily practice and effect on the severity of symptoms. Data from the ALPA study registry. *Eur J Heart Fail* 9:502, 2007.
8. Cha YM, Redfield M, Shen WK, et al: Atrial fibrillation and ventricular dysfunction: a vicious electromechanical cycle. *Circulation* 109:2839, 2004.
9. Olivotto I, Cecchi F, Casey SA, et al: Impact of atrial fibrillation on the clinical course of hypertrophic cardiomyopathy. *Circulation* 104:2517, 2001.
10. Lloyd-Jones DM, Wang TJ, Leip EP, et al: Lifetime risk for development of atrial fibrillation: the Framingham Heart Study. *Circulation* 110:1042–1046, 2004.
11. Chen HH, Lainchbury JG, Senni M, et al: Diastolic heart failure in the community: clinical profile, natural history, therapy, and impact of proposed diagnostic criteria. *J Card Fail* 8:279–287, 2002.
12. Middlekauff HR, Stevenson WG, Stevenson LW: Prognostic significance of atrial fibrillation in advanced heart failure. A study of 390 patients. *Circulation* 84:40–48, 1991.
13. Ruo B, Capra AM, Jensvold NG, et al: Racial variation in the prevalence of atrial fibrillation among patients with heart failure. *J Am Coll Cardiol* 43(3):429–435, 2004.
14. Choudhury A, Lip GY: Atrial fibrillation and the hypercoagulable state: from basic science to clinical practice. *Pathophysiol Haemost Thromb* 33:282–289, 2003.
15. Boos CJ, Anderson RA, Lip GY: Is atrial fibrillation an inflammatory disorder? *Eur Heart J* 27:136–149, 2006.
16. Lip GY, Tse HF: Management of atrial fibrillation. *Lancet* 370(9587):604–618, 2007.
17. Lip GY, Lane D, Van Walraven C, et al: Additive role of plasma von Willebrand factor levels to clinical factors for risk stratification of patients with atrial fibrillation. *Stroke* 37:2294–2300, 2006.
18. Jalife J, Berenfield O, Mansour M: Mother rotors and fibrillatory conduction: a mechanism for atrial fibrillation. *Cardiovasc Res* 54:204–216, 2002.
19. Allessie MA, Boyden PA, Camm AJ, et al: Pathophysiology and prevention of atrial fibrillation. *Circulation* 103:769–777, 2001.
20. Calkins H, Kuck KH, Cappato R, et al: 2012 HRS/EHRA/ECAS expert consensus statement on catheter and surgical ablation of atrial fibrillation. *Heart Rhythm* 9(4):632–696, 2012.
21. Nieuwlaat R, Capucci A, Camm AJ, et al: Atrial fibrillation management: a prospective survey in ESC member countries: the Euro Heart Survey on Atrial Fibrillation. *Eur Heart J* 26:2422–2434, 2005.
22. De Vos CB, Pisters R, Nieuwlaat R, et al: Progression from paroxysmal to persistent atrial fibrillation. *J Am Coll Cardiol* 55(8):725–731, 2010.
23. The Stroke Prevention in Atrial Fibrillation Investigators Committee on Echocardiography: Transesophageal echocardiographic correlates of thromboembolism in high-risk patients with nonvalvular atrial fibrillation. *Ann Intern Med* 128:639–647, 1998.
24. Park KL, Anter E: Atrial fibrillation and heart failure: a review of the intersection of two cardiac epidemics. *J of Atrial Fibrillation* 6(1):1–12, 2013.
25. Heart Disease and stroke statistics—2007 update: a report from the American Heart Association Statistics Committee and Stroke Statistics Subcommittee. *Circulation* 115:e69–e171, 2007.
26. Asher CR, Klein AL: The ACUTE trial. Transesophageal echocardiography to guide electrical cardioversion in atrial fibrillation. Assessment of cardioversion using transesophageal echocardiography. *Cleve Clin J Med* 69(9):713–718, 2002.
27. Hart RG, Pearce LA, Rothbart RM, et al: Stroke with intermittent atrial fibrillation: incidence and predictors during aspirin therapy. Stroke Prevention in Atrial Fibrillation Investigators. *J Am Coll Cardiol* 35:183–187, 2000.
28. Wyse DG, Waldo AL, DiMarco JP, et al: A comparison of rate control and rhythm control in patients with atrial fibrillation. *N Engl J Med* 347:1825–1833, 2002.
29. Roy D, Talajic M, Nattel S, et al: Rhythm control versus rate control for atrial fibrillation and heart failure (AF-CHF). *N Engl J Med* 358:2667–2677, 2008.
30. Van Gelder IC, Hessel HF, Crijns HJGM, et al: Lenient versus strict rate control in patients with atrial fibrillation. *N Engl J Med* 362(15):1363–1373, 2010.
31. Singer DE, Albers GW, Dalen JE, et al: Antithrombotic therapy in atrial fibrillation: the Seventh ACCP Conference on Antithrombotic and Thrombolytic Therapy. *Chest* 126(3 Suppl):429S–456S, 2004.
32. Camm AJ, Lip GYH, De Caterina R, et al: 2012 focused update of the ESC guidelines for the management of atrial fibrillation. *Eur Heart J* 33:2719–2747, 2012.
33. Olesen JB, Fauchier L, Lane DA, et al: Risk factors for stroke and thromboembolism in relation to age among patients with atrial fibrillation: the Loire Valley Atrial Fibrillation Project. *Chest* 141:147–153, 2012.
34. Granada J, Uribe W, Chyou P, et al: Incidence and predictors of atrial flutter in the general population. *J Am Coll Cardiol* 36(7):2242–2246, 2000.
35. Waldo AL: Atrial flutter: from mechanism to treatment. In Camm AJ, editor: *Clinical approaches to tachyarrhythmias*, Armonk, NY, 2001, Futura Publishing, pp 1–56.
36. Perez FJ, Schubert CM, Parvez B, et al: Long-term outcomes after catheter ablation of cavo-tricuspid isthmus dependent atrial flutter: a meta-analysis. *Circ Arrhythm Electrophysiol* 2:393–401, 2009.
37. Zipes DP, Camm AJ, Borggrefe M, et al for the American College of Cardiology/American Heart Association Task Force, European Society of Cardiology Committee for Practice Guidelines, European Heart Rhythm Associates, Heart Rhythm Society: ACC/AHA/ESC 2006 guidelines for management of patients with ventricular arrhythmias and the prevention of sudden cardiac death. *Circulation* 114:e385–e484, 2006.
38. Jin H, Lyon AR, Akar FG: Arrhythmia mechanisms in the failing heart. *Pacing Clin Electrophysiol* 31:1048, 2008.
39. Neumar RW, Otto CW, Link MS, et al: Part 8: adult advanced cardiovascular life support: 2010 American Heart Association Guidelines for Cardiopulmonary Resuscitation and Emergency Cardiovascular Care. *Circulation* 122(18 Suppl 3):S729–S767, 2010.
40. Gorgels AP, van den Dool A, Hofs A, et al: Comparison of procainamide and lidocaine in terminating sustained monomorphic ventricular tachycardia. *Am J Cardiol* 78:43–46, 1996.
41. Marill KA, deSouza IS, Nishijima DK, et al: Amiodarone is poorly effective for the acute termination of ventricular tachycardia. *Ann Emerg Med* 47(3):217–224, 2006.
42. Marill KA, deSouza IS, Nishijima DK, et al: Amiodarone or procainamide for the termination of sustained stable ventricular tachycardia: an historical multicenter comparison. *Acad Emerg Med* 17(3):297–306, 2010.
43. Katritsis DG, Zareba W, Camm AJ: Nonsustained ventricular tachycardia. *J Am Coll Cardiol* 60:1993–2004, 2012.
44. Amiodarone Trials Meta-Analysis Investigators: Effect of prophylactic amiodarone on mortality after acute myocardial infarction and in congestive heart failure: meta-analysis of individual data from 6500 patients in randomised trials. *Lancet* 350(9089):1417–1424, 1997.
45. Piccini JP, Berger JS, O'Connor CM: Amiodarone for the prevention of sudden cardiac death: a meta-analysis of randomized controlled trials. *Eur Heart J* 30(10):1245–1253, 2009.
46. Pacifico A, Hohnloser SH, Williams JH, et al: Prevention of implantable-defibrillator shocks by treatment with sotalol. d,l-Sotalol Implantable Cardioverter-Defibrillator Study Group. *N Engl J Med* 340(24):1855–1862, 1999.
47. Connolly SJ, Dorian P, Roberts RS, et al: Comparison of beta-blockers, amiodarone plus beta-blockers, or sotalol for prevention of shocks from implantable cardioverter defibrillators: the OPTIC Study: a randomized trial. *JAMA* 295:165–171, 2006.
48. Ferreira-González I, Dos-Subira L, Guyatt G: Adjunctive antiarrhythmic drug therapy in patients with implantable cardioverter defibrillators: a systematic review. *Eur Heart J* 28:469–477, 2007.
49. Kowey PR, Crijns HJ, Aliot EM, et al: Efficacy and safety of celivarone, with amiodarone as calibrator, in patients with an implantable cardioverter-defibrillator for prevention of implantable cardioverter-defibrillator interventions or death: the ALPHEE study. *Circulation* 124(24):2649–2660, 2011.
50. Bollmann A, Husser D, Cannom DS: Antiarrhythmic drugs in patients with implantable cardioverter-defibrillators. *Am J Cardiovasc Drugs* 5(6):371, 2005.
51. Beadle R, Williams L, Lim HS: Drug-implantable cardioverter-defibrillator interactions. *Expert Rev Cardiovasc Ther* 8(9):1267–1273, 2010.
52. Stevenson WG, Soejima K: Catheter ablation for ventricular tachycardia. *Circulation* 115:2750–2760, 2007.
53. Lakkireddy D, Di Biase L, Ryschon K, et al, Radiofrequency ablation of premature ventricular ectopy improves the efficacy of cardiac resynchronization therapy in nonresponders. *J Am Coll Cardiol* 60(16):1531–1539, 2012.
54. Mirowski M, Reid PR, Mower MM, et al: Termination of malignant ventricular arrhythmias with an implantable automatic defibrillator in human beings. *N Engl J Med* 303:322–324, 1980.

55. Hammill SC, Kremers MS, Stevenson LW, et al: Review of the registry's fourth year, incorporating lead data and pediatric ICD procedures, and use as a national performance measure. *Heart Rhythm* 7(9):1340–1345, 2010.
56. DiMarco JP: Implantable cardioverter-defibrillators. *N Engl J Med* 349(19):1836–1847, 2003.
57. Epstein AE, DiMarco JP, Ellenbogen KE, et al: ACC/AHA/HRS 2008 Guidelines for Device-Based Therapy of Cardiac Rhythm Abnormalities: executive summary a report of the American College of Cardiology/American Heart Association Task Force on Practice Guidelines (Writing Committee to Revise the ACC/AHA/ NASPE 2002 Guideline Update for Implantation of Cardiac Pacemakers and Antiarrhythmia Devices). *Heart Rhythm* 5:934–955, 2008.
58. Bardy GH, Lee KL, Mark DB, et al, for the Sudden Cardiac Death in Heart Failure Trial (SCD-HeFT) Investigators: Amiodarone or an implantable cardioverter-defibrillator for congestive heart failure. *N Engl J Med* 352:225–237, 2005.
59. The Antiarrhythmics Versus Implantable Defibrillators (AVID) Investigators: A comparison of antiarrhythmic drug therapy with implantable defibrillators in patients resuscitated from near fatal ventricular arrhythmias. *N Engl J Med* 337:1576–1583, 1997.
60. Connolly SJ, Gent M, Roberts RS, et al: Canadian Implantable Defibrillator Study (CIDS): a randomized trial of the implantable cardioverter defibrillator against amiodarone. *Circulation* 101:1297–1302, 2000.
61. Kuck KH, Cappato R, Siebels J, et al: Randomized comparison of antiarrhythmic drug therapy with implantable defibrillators in patients resuscitated from cardiac arrest: the cardiac arrest study Hamburg (CASH). *Circulation* 102:748–754, 2000.
62. Moss AJ, Hall JW, Cannom DS, et al: Multicenter Automatic Defibrillator Implantation Trial Investigators. Improved survival with an implantable defibrillator in patients with coronary disease at high risk for ventricular arrhythmia. *N Engl J Med* 335:1933–1940, 1996.
63. Moss AJ, Zareba W, Hall WJ, et al: Prophylactic implantation of a defibrillator in patients with myocardial infarction and reduced ejection fraction. *N Engl J Med* 346:877–883, 2002.
64. Bigger JT, Jr: Prophylactic use of implanted cardiac defibrillators in patients at high risk for ventricular arrhythmias after coronary-artery bypass graft surgery. *N Engl J Med* 337:1569–1575, 1997.
65. Kadish A, Dyer A, Daubert JP, et al: Prophylactic defibrillator implantation in patients with non-ischemic dilated cardiomyopathy. *N Engl J Med* 350:2151–2158, 2004.
66. Hohnloser SH, Kuck KH, Dorian P, et al: Prophylactic use of an implantable cardioverter–defibrillator after acute myocardial infarction. *N Engl J Med* 351:2481–2488, 2004.
67. Steinbeck G, Andersen D, Seidi K, et al: Defibrillator implantation early after myocardial infarction. *N Engl J Med* 361:1427–1436, 2009.
68. Center for Medicare Services: Implantable automatic defibrillators, http://www.cms.gov/transmittals/downloads/R29NCD.pdf.
69. Russo AM, Stainback RF, Bailey SR, et al: ACCF/HRS/AGS/AHA/ASE/HFSA/SCAI/SCCT/SCMR 2013 appropriate use criteria for implantable cardioverter-defibrillators and cardiac resynchronization therapy. *J Am Coll Cardiol* 61:1318–1368, 2013.
70. Goldenberg I, Vyas AK, Hall WJ, et al: Risk stratification for primary implantation of a cardioverter-defibrillator in patients with ischemic left ventricular dysfunction. *J Am Coll Cardiol* 51:288–296, 2008.
71. Bilchick KC, Stukenborg GJ, Kamath S, et al: Prediction of mortality in clinical practice for Medicare patients undergoing defibrillator implantation for primary prevention of sudden cardiac death. *J Am Coll Cardiol* 60:1647–1655, 2012.
72. Cleland JG, Daubert JC, Erdmann E, et al for the CARE-HF Study Investigators: The effect of cardiac resynchronization on morbidity and mortality in heart failure. *N Engl J Med* 352:1539–1549, 2005.
73. Chugh SS, Wood MA: ICD follow up and troubleshooting. In Ellenbogen K, Wood M, editors: *Cardiac pacing and ICDs*, Oxford, 2008, Blackwell, pp 463–497.
74. Varma N, Epstein AE, Irimpen A, et al: Efficacy and safety of automatic remote monitoring for implantable cardioverter-defibrillator follow-up. The Lumos-T Safely Reduces Routine Office Device Follow-Up (TRUST) Trial. *Circulation* 122:325–332, 2010.
75. Freeman JV, Wang Y, Curtis JP, et al: The relation between hospital procedure volume and complications of cardioverter-defibrillator implantation from the implantable cardioverter-defibrillator registry. *J Am Coll Cardiol* 56(14):1133–1139, 2010.
76. Van Rees JB, de Bie MK, Thijssen J, et al: Implantation-related complications of implantable cardioverter-defibrillators and cardiac resynchronization therapy devices: a systematic review of randomized clinical trials. *J Am Coll Cardiol* 58(10):995–1000, 2011.
77. Poole JE, Gleva MJ, Mela T, et al: Complication rates associated with pacemaker or implantable cardioverter-defibrillator generator replacements and upgrade procedures: results from the REPLACE registry. *Circulation* 122(16):1553–1561, 2010.
78. Baddour LM, Cha YM, Wilson WR: Clinical practice. Infections of cardiovascular implantable electronic devices. *N Engl J Med* 367(9):842–849, 2012.
79. Baddour LM, Epstein AE, Erickson CC, et al, American Heart Association Rheumatic Fever, Endocarditis, and Kawasaki Disease Committee; Council on Cardiovascular Disease in Young; Council on Cardiovascular Surgery and Anesthesia; Council on Cardiovascular Nursing; Council on Clinical Cardiology; Interdisciplinary Council on Quality of Care; American Heart Association: Update on cardiovascular implantable electronic device infections and their management: a scientific statement from the American Heart Association. *Circulation* 121:458–477, 2010.
80. Moss A, Schuger C, Beck CA, et al: Reduction in inappropriate therapy and mortality through ICD programming (MADIT-RIT). *N Engl J Med* 367:2275–2283, 2012.
81. Wilkoff BL, Williamson BD, Stern RS, et al: Strategic programming of detection and therapy parameters in implantable cardioverter-defibrillators reduces shocks in primary prevention patients: results from the PREPARE (Primary Prevention Parameters Evaluation) study. *J Am Coll Cardiol* 52(7):541–550, 2008.
82. Sears S, Conti J: Understanding implantable cardioverter defibrillator shocks and storms: medical and psychosocial considerations for research and clinical care. *Clin Cardiol* 26(3):107–111, 2003.
83. Moss AJ, Hall WJ, Cannom DS, et al: Cardiac-resynchronization therapy for the prevention of heart failure events. *N Engl J Med* 361:1329–1338, 2009.
84. Brignole M, Auricchio A, Baron-Esquivias G, et al: 2013 ESC Guidelines on cardiac pacing and cardiac resynchronization therapy. *Eur Heart J* 34:2281–2329, 2013.
85. Bristow MR, Saxon LA, Boehmer J, et al: Cardiac-resynchronization therapy with or without an implantable defibrillator in advanced chronic heart failure. *N Engl J Med* 350:2140–2150, 2004.
86. Zareba W, Klein H, Cygankiewicz I, et al: Effectiveness of cardiac resynchronization therapy by QRS morphology in the multicenter automatic defibrillator implantation trial-cardiac resynchronization therapy (MADIT-CRT). *Circulation* 123:1061–1072, 2011.
87. Moss AJ, Hall WJ, Cannom DS, et al: Cardiac-resynchronization therapy for the prevention of heart-failure events. *N Engl J Med* 361:1329–1338, 2009.
88. Tracy CM, Epstein AE, Darbar D, et al: 2012 ACCF/AHA/HRS focused update of the 2008 guidelines for device-based therapy of cardiac rhythm abnormalities. *J Am Coll Cardiol* 60(14):1297–1313, 2012.
89. Abraham WT, Fisher WG, Smith AL, et al: Cardiac resynchronization in chronic heart failure. *N Engl J Med* 246:1845–1853, 2002.
90. Abraham WT, Gras D, Yu CM, et al: Rational and design of a randomized clinical trial to assess the safety and efficacy of frequent optimization of cardiac resynchronization therapy: the frequent optimization study using the QuickOpt method (FREEDOM) trial. *Am Heart J* 159(6):944–948, 2010.
91. Ellenbogen KA, Gold MR, Meyer TE, et al: Primary results from the SmartDelay determined AV optimization: a comparison to other AV delay methods used in cardiac resynchronization therapy (SMART-AV) trial. *Circulation* 122:2660–2668, 2010.
92. Young JB, Abraham WT, Smith AL, et al: Combined cardiac resynchronization and implantable cardioversion defibrillation in advanced chronic heart failure: the MIRACLE ICD Trial. *JAMA* 289:2685–2694, 2003.
93. Higgins SL, Hummel JD, Niazi IK, et al: Cardiac resynchronization therapy for the treatment of heart failure in patients with intraventricular conduction delay and malignant ventricular tachyarrhythmias. *J Am Coll Cardiol* 42:1454–1459, 2003.
94. Bristow MR, Saxon LA, Boehmer J, et al: Cardiac-resynchronization therapy with or without an implantable defibrillator in advanced chronic heart failure. *N Engl J Med* 350:2140–2150, 2004.
95. Linde C, Abraham WT, Gold MR, et al: Randomized trial of cardiac resynchronization in mildly symptomatic heart failure patients and in asymptomatic patients with left ventricular dysfunction and previous heart failure symptoms. *J Am Coll Cardiol* 52:1834–1843, 2008.
96. Tang AS, Wells GA, Talajic M, et al: Cardiac-resynchronization therapy for mild-to-moderate heart failure. *N Engl J Med* 363:2385–2395, 2010.
97. Boyle A, Ascheim D, Russo M, et al: Clinical outcomes for continuous-flow left ventricular assist device patients stratified by preoperative INTERMACS classification. *J Heart Lung Transplant* 30:402–407, 2011.
98. Starling R, Naka Y, Boyle A, et al: Results of the post-U.S. Food and Drug Administration approval study with a continuous flow left ventricular assist device as a bridge to heart transplantation. *J Am Coll Cardiol* 57:1890–1898, 2011.
99. Maisel W, Stevenson L: Atrial fibrillation in heart failure: epidemiology, pathophysiology, and rationale for therapy. *Am J Cardiol* 91(Suppl):2D–8D, 2003.
100. Anderson M, Videbaek R, Boesgaard S, et al: Incidence of ventricular arrhythmias in patients on long-term support with a continuous-flow assist device (HeartMate II). *J Heart Lung Transplant* 28:733–735, 2009.
101. Bunch TJ, Mahapatra S, Murdock D, et al: Ranolazine reduces ventricular tachycardia burden and ICD shocks in patients with drug-refractory ICD shocks. *Pacing Clin Electrophysiol* 34(12):1600–1606, 2011.
102. Dandamudi G, Ghumman W, Das M, et al: Endocardial catheter ablation of ventricular tachycardia in patients with ventricular assist devices. *Heart Rhythm* 4:1165–1169, 2007.
103. Thajudeen A, Stecker EC, Shehata M, et al: Arrhythmias after heart transplantation: mechanisms and management. *J Am Heart Assoc* 112:1–8, 2012.

GUIDELINES

Cardiac Resynchronization Therapy and Implantable Cardioverter-Defibrillators for Heart Failure with a Reduced Ejection Fraction*

In 2012 the ACC/AHA/HRS updated the 2008 guidelines for device-based therapy of cardiac rhythm abnormalities.[1] These revised guidelines were incorporated into the 2013 American College of Cardiology Foundation and American Heart Association (ACCF/AHA) heart failure guidelines.[2] The revised guidelines (**Table 35G-1**) include a comprehensive revision of CRT indications based on all available studies through 2013. The guidelines expand the indications for CRT to some NYHA class II and very selected class I patients, limit CRT indications by QRS morphology and QRS duration, and attempt to harmonize indications across NYHA classes when possible. The most certain indications are for those patients who have LVEF less than or equal to 35%, sinus rhythm, LBBB with a QRS duration greater than or equal to 150 msec, and NYHA class II, III, or ambulatory IV symptoms on optimal medical treatment.

Patients with reduced LVEF are at increased risk for ventricular tachyarrhythmias leading to sudden cardiac death.

*From Abraham WT: Guidelines: cardiac resynchronization therapy and implantable cardioverter-defibrillators for heart failure with a reduced ejection fraction. In Mann DL, Zipes DP, Libby P, et al, editors: *Braunwald's heart disease: a textbook of cardiovascular medicine*, ed 10, Philadelphia, 2015, Saunders.

TABLE 35G-1 ACCF/AHA Guidelines for Cardiac Resynchronization

CLASS	INDICATION	LEVEL OF EVIDENCE
I	CRT is indicated for patients who have LVEF of 35% or less, sinus rhythm, left bundle branch block (LBBB) with a QRS duration of 150 ms or greater, and NYHA class II, III, or ambulatory IV symptoms on GDMT.	Level of Evidence A for NYHA class III/I, Level of Evidence: B for NYHA class II
IIa	CRT can be useful for patients who have LVEF of 35% or less, sinus rhythm, a non-LBBB pattern with a QRS duration of 150 ms or greater, and NYHA class III/ambulatory class IV symptoms on GDMT.	A
	CRT can be useful for patients who have LVEF of 35% or less, sinus rhythm, LBBB with a QRS duration of 120 to 149 ms, and NYHA class II, III, or ambulatory IV symptoms on GDMT.	B
	CRT can be useful in patients with AF and LVEF of 35% or less on GDMT if (a) the patient requires ventricular pacing or otherwise meets CRT criteria and (b) atrioventricular nodal ablation or pharmacologic rate control will allow near 100% ventricular pacing with CRT.	B
	CRT can be useful for patients on GDMT who have LVEF of 35% or less, and are undergoing placement of a new or replacement device with anticipated requirement for significant (>40%) ventricular pacing.	C
IIb	CRT may be considered for patients who have LVEF of 35% or less, sinus rhythm, a non-LBBB pattern with QRS duration of 120 to 149 ms, and NYHA class III/ambulatory class IV on GDMT.	B
	CRT may be considered for patients who have LVEF of 35% or less, sinus rhythm, a non-LBBB pattern with a QRS duration of 150 ms or greater, and NYHA class II symptoms on GDMT.	B
	CRT may be considered for patients who have LVEF of 30% or less, ischemic etiology of HF, sinus rhythm, LBBB with a QRS duration of 150 ms or greater, and NYHA class I symptoms on GDMT.	C
III: No Benefit	CRT is not recommended for patients with NYHA class I or II symptoms and non-LBBB pattern with QRS duration less than 150 ms.	
	CRT is not indicated for patients whose comorbidities and/or frailty limit survival with good functional capacity to less than 1 year.	

ACCF, American College of Cardiology Foundation; *AHA,* American Heart Association; *CRT,* Cardiac resynchronization therapy; *GDMT,* guideline-directed medical therapy; *LBBB,* left bundle branch block; *LVEF,* left ventricular ejection fraction; *NYHA,* New York Heart Association.

TABLE 35G-2 ACCF/AHA Guidelines for Indications for Implantable Cardioverter-Defibrillators

CLASS	INDICATION	LEVEL OF EVIDENCE
I	ICD therapy is recommended for primary prevention of SCD in selected patients with HFrEF at least 40 days post MI with LVEF <35% and NYHA class II or III symptoms on chronic GDMT, who are expected to live >1 year.	A
I	ICD therapy is recommended for primary prevention of SCD in selected patients with HFrEF at least 40 days post MI with LVEF <30% and NYHA class I symptoms while receiving GDMT, who are expected to live >1 year.	B
IIa	To prevent sudden death, placement of an ICD is reasonable in patients with asymptomatic ischemic cardiomyopathy who are at least 40 days post MI, have an LVEF of 30% or less, are on appropriate medical therapy, and have reasonable expectation of survival with a good functional status for more than 1 year.	B
IIb	ICD therapy to prevent SCD in patients with nonischemic cardiomyopathy who are at least 40 days post MI, have an LVEF <35%, with NYHA functional class II or III symptoms while undergoing chronic optimal medical therapy, and who have reasonable expectation of survival for more than 1 year with good functional status.	B
	The usefulness of implantation of an ICD is of uncertain benefit to prolong meaningful survival in patients with a high risk of nonsudden death as predicted by frequent hospitalizations, advanced frailty, or comorbidities such as systemic malignancy or severe renal dysfunction.	B

ACCF, American College of Cardiology Foundation; *AHA,* American Heart Association; *GDMT,* guideline-directed medical therapy; *HFrEF,* heart failure with a reduced ejection fraction; *ICD,* implantable cardioverter-defibrillator; *LVEF,* left ventricular ejection fraction; *MI,* myocardial infarction; *NYHA,* New York Heart Association; *SCD,* sudden cardiac death.

Patients who have had sustained ventricular tachycardia, ventricular fibrillation, unexplained syncope, or cardiac arrest are at the highest risk for recurrence. Indications for ICD therapy as secondary prevention of sudden cardiac death are also discussed in the 2013 ACCF/AHA guidelines for heart failure (**Table 35G-2**),[2] as well as the ACCF/AHA/HRS device-based therapy guidelines.[3]

REFERENCES

1. Tracy CM, Epstein AE, Darbar D, et al: 2012 ACCF/AHA/HRS focused update of the 2008 guidelines for device-based therapy of cardiac rhythm abnormalities: a report of the American College of Cardiology Foundation/American Heart Association task force on practice guidelines and the Heart Rhythm Society [corrected]. *Circulation* 126:1784–1800, 2012.
2. Yancy CW, Jessup M, Bozkurt B, et al: 2013 ACCF/AHA Guideline for the Management of Heart Failure: a report of the American College of Cardiology Foundation/American Heart Association task force on practice guidelines. *Circulation* 128:e240–327, 2013.
3. Epstein AE, DiMarco JP, Ellenbogen KA, et al: ACC/AHA/HRS 2008 Guidelines for device-based therapy of cardiac rhythm abnormalities: a report of the American College of Cardiology/American Heart Association task force on practice guidelines (Writing committee to revise the ACC/AHA/NASPE 2002 guideline update for implantation of cardiac pacemakers and antiarrhythmia devices) developed in collaboration with the American Association for Thoracic Surgery and Society of Thoracic Surgeons. *J Am Coll Cardiol* 51:e1–e62, 2008.

36 Treatment of Heart Failure with Preserved Ejection Fraction

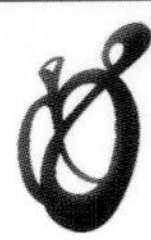

Anita Deswal and Sukhdeep S. Basra

Over the past two decades, it has become increasingly apparent that approximately 50% of patients with heart failure (HF) have a normal or almost normal ejection fraction (see also Chapter 17), referred to variably as *diastolic heart failure* or *heart failure with preserved ejection fraction* (HFpEF).[1-4] The prevalence of this condition will likely keep increasing as the prevalence of the elderly with comorbid conditions such as hypertension, diabetes, obesity, and renal disease increases.[5-7] Although the rates of mortality and morbidity associated with HFpEF and compared with HF with reduced ejection fraction (systolic HF) have varied, there is consensus that HFpEF is a condition associated with substantial morbidity and mortality and the frequency of clinical events increases markedly once a patient is hospitalized for HF.[1,7] However, until recently, most randomized clinical trials for HF underrepresented this population. A recent study examining secular trends in HF within Olmstead County found that survival improved significantly over time among patients with systolic HF (likely related to use of evidence-driven therapies), but no such trend toward improvement was noted for patients with HFpEF.[7] Therefore, there exists an urgent need to develop effective treatment strategies for the management of patients with this condition.

DEVELOPMENT OF TREATMENT STRATEGIES BASED ON THE PATHOPHYSIOLOGY OF HEART FAILURE WITH PRESERVED EJECTION FRACTION

The development of treatment strategies for HFpEF is based on our evolving understanding of the pathophysiology of this condition (reviewed in detail in Chapter 10). HFpEF commonly afflicts elderly patients with comorbidities of hypertension, left ventricular (LV) hypertrophy, diabetes mellitus, myocardial ischemia, and obesity. Of these risk factors, hypertension and subsequent LV hypertrophy are the most prevalent and highly associated with HFpEF. Less commonly, HFpEF may occur as a result of restrictive and infiltrative cardiomyopathies and transplant rejection.[8] In the presence of the conditions listed previously, clinical symptoms and signs of HF are commonly precipitated by concomitant anemia, pulmonary disease, renal insufficiency, and atrial fibrillation. In patients with HFpEF, in the absence of significant valvular or pericardial disease, diastolic dysfunction consisting of abnormalities of LV relaxation and increased LV stiffness have long been thought to be the central pathophysiologic abnormality contributing to the development of HF.[9,10] This has led to the term *diastolic heart failure* to describe this condition. Even though mechanistic studies demonstrate that abnormalities of diastolic function are invariably present in HFpEF, there is some disagreement concerning the relative contribution of diastolic dysfunction in clinical HF in an elderly comorbid population in whom there is a high prevalence of diastolic dysfunction even in the absence of clinical HF. However, it is likely that these elderly patients frequently experience clinical decompensation when the precipitants listed previously occur in the presence of the underlying substrate of diastolic dysfunction. Decompensated HF would be unlikely when the same precipitants occur in patients without underlying diastolic dysfunction. Factors other than diastolic dysfunction that have also been suggested as contributors to the development of HFpEF include increased vascular and LV systolic stiffness, volume overload secondary to renal disease with abnormal renal sodium handling, atrial dysfunction, neurohumoral (specifically renin-angiotensin-aldosterone system) activation, reduced vasodilator reserve, and chronotropic incompetence during exercise.[11-13] Aging is associated with a reduction in the elastic properties of the heart and vasculature associated with an increase in systolic blood pressure. This likely contributes to the much higher prevalence of HFpEF in the elderly. In addition, the comorbidities described earlier are more frequently prevalent in the elderly, contributing further to the increasing prevalence of this condition with increasing age.

The following sections in this chapter will provide an overview of therapeutic modalities that may be effective in patients with HFpEF based either on symptomatic benefit or on targeting pathophysiologic mechanisms. The clinical approach to management of these patients with HFpEF will then be summarized based on current evidence and consensus opinion.

TREATMENT OF VOLUME OVERLOAD AND CONGESTION

Although diuretics may not alter the pathophysiologic processes responsible for HFpEF, they do reduce ventricular filling pressures and are therefore very useful in providing symptomatic benefit in patients presenting with pulmonary vascular congestion and peripheral edema. It should be noted that some patients that fit the classic profile of "diastolic heart failure" with significant left hypertrophy and small LV volumes may exhibit a fall in cardiac output with rapid diuresis, resulting in hypotension and prerenal azotemia. This results from the fact that these patients have a very steep LV diastolic pressure-volume curve such that a small change in diastolic volume causes a large change in pressure and cardiac output.[14] Interestingly, although such caution may be particularly applicable to the subgroup of patients having HFpEF with significant left hypertrophy and small LV volumes, recent analyses demonstrated that the overall incidence of worsening renal function with diuresis was found to be similar in patients with HFpEF compared with HF with reduced LV ejection fraction (LVEF) in a substudy[15] of the DOSE (Diuretic Optimization Strategies Evaluation) trial, which compared diuretic dosing strategies in HF patients with both reduced and preserved LVEF.[16] Diuretics may also benefit patients based on other potential pathogenic mechanisms. First, it is known that the right ventricle forms the external pressure for approximately one third of the surface area of the left ventricle.[8,17] Therefore, elevation of right-heart diastolic pressures can constrain the filling of the left ventricle. In some patients, reduction of right-sided diastolic pressures by diuretics may unload the interventricular septum, improving LV distensibility,[18] and may therefore be associated with a reduction in pulmonary venous pressures while maintaining LV filling and cardiac output. More recently, Maurer and colleagues have demonstrated that in a subgroup of patients with hypertensive HFpEF, the LV end-diastolic pressure-volume relationship may be shifted rightward with somewhat increased end-diastolic volumes (in contrast to the classic paradigm of diastolic HF with a leftward- and upward-shifted end-diastolic pressure volume relationship and smaller LV volume).[13] This may be a result of a volume overload state contributed to by extracardiac factors such as renal dysfunction with abnormal renal sodium handling, obesity, and anemia. This could also represent a group of patients that would also respond more favorably to diuretic therapy. Lastly, low dose diuretics, especially thiazide diuretics, are useful in the treatment of hypertension, a key pathophysiologic factor in HFpEF.[19,20] Some patients with HFpEF and severe volume overload may also be candidates for ultrafiltration (discussed in Chapter 33).

Therapy with nitrates may also provide symptomatic benefit in patients with HFpEF with pulmonary vascular congestion. Nitrates are primarily venodilators with some arterial vasodilating action. They may benefit patients with HFpEF by reducing preload, thus leading to a reduction in ventricular filling pressures and pulmonary congestion. In acute decompensated HF, they can be used intravenously and may improve symptoms by reducing filling pressures, as well as by controlling systemic hypertension. Theoretically, by releasing nitric oxide, nitrates may improve the diastolic distensibility of the ventricle.[21] Again, as with diuretics, caution is required when nitrates are used in patients without hypertension or with severe diastolic dysfunction, with monitoring for a significant reduction in cardiac output and blood pressure as a result of preload reduction.

TREATMENT OF HYPERTENSION (see also Chapter 23)

Of the various risk factors for the development of HFpEF, hypertension and subsequent LV hypertrophy are the most prevalent and highly associated with the condition. The significant contribution of hypertensive heart disease to the development of diastolic dysfunction and HFpEF (reviewed in Hoit and Walsh[22]) implies that treating hypertension should be beneficial not only for the treatment but also for the prevention of HFpEF. Also, the increased afterload imposed by significant arterial hypertension reduces LV relaxation and filling rates.[23] Stiffening of the aorta and the left ventricle, as occurs in elderly patients with HFpEF, increases the tightness of the coupling of arterial systolic and left atrial pressures, with an increase in systolic arterial pressure resulting in elevation of left atrial pressures.[11,24] Controlling systolic hypertension could allow the left ventricle to eject to a smaller end-systolic volume, thus allowing the ventricle to operate with a smaller diastolic volume and reduced left atrial pressure. Lowering the systolic pressure allows the left ventricle to relax more rapidly, enhancing early filling.[25] In addition, concentrically hypertrophied hearts demonstrate increased passive stiffness and impaired relaxation independent of hemodynamic loads, and have limited coronary vascular reserve that can contribute to myocardial ischemia even in the absence of epicardial coronary artery disease. Adequate control of hypertension should benefit patients with HFpEF by favorably altering loading conditions in the short term, and in the long term, by leading to regression of LV hypertrophy. Although there may be some additional benefits of using one class of drugs versus others,[19] the most important goal is achieving an adequate reduction in blood pressure. Several trials evaluating reduction of blood pressure using angiotensin-converting enzyme (ACE) inhibitors or angiotensin receptor blockers (ARBs) compared with other agents have suggested that ultimately blood pressure control rather than the specific class of antihypertensive agents used may be the major determinant of regression of hypertrophy and improvement in diastolic function.[20,26,27] Moreover, trials have definitively demonstrated approximately 50% reduction in the incidence of HF in patients treated for hypertension, especially in the elderly population.[28,29]

Drugs such as β-blockers and calcium channel blockers that reduce blood pressure and heart rate and thus indirectly improve diastolic function as well as increase diastolic filling time may be beneficial in patients with HFpEF. On the other hand, the direct myocardial effects of slowing the relaxation rate of the ventricle and the negative inotropic actions of these drugs may be detrimental with respect to diastolic function.[8] In addition, a recent study demonstrated that during exercise, patients with HFpEF achieved less of an increase in heart rate (inadequate chronotropic response) and thus cardiac output despite a similar rise in end-diastolic volume, stroke volume, and contractility compared with matched subjects with hypertensive cardiac hypertrophy.[12] These data suggest possible deleterious effects of heart rate–reducing drugs, such as β-blockers and certain calcium channel blockers, in patients in whom reduced exercise capacity may partly result from reduced chronotropic reserve.

Over the years, a number of small studies evaluating calcium channel blockers, β-blockers, ACE inhibitors, and ARBs have variably suggested modest benefit in exercise capacity, New York Heart Association (NYHA) class, quality of life, and diastolic function in patients with HFpEF. However, until recently, none of the studies performed were large or randomized multicenter trials and thus definitive evidence of benefit on longer term outcomes was not available.

RENIN-ANGIOTENSIN-ALDOSTERONE BLOCKADE

Angiotensin-Converting Enzyme Inhibitors and Angiotensin Receptor Blockers

As in systolic HF, preclinical and clinical evidence suggest that the activation of the renin-angiotensin-aldosterone system (RAAS) is a contributing factor in the development of HFpEF, principally through the trophic effects of angiotensin II on the vasculature and myocardium, but perhaps also through myocardial fibrosis mediated by aldosterone (see also Chapter 10).[30,31] In addition, angiotensin II slows LV relaxation resulting in elevation of LV diastolic pressure.[32] Therefore, agents such as ACE inhibitors and ARBs, with their antihypertensive and angiotensin II-attenuating effects, were attractive options in the treatment of HFpEF. Furthermore, clinical trials have shown ACE inhibitors and ARBs to be effective in improving cardiovascular outcomes in populations with diabetes, coronary artery disease, vascular disease, and hypertension[33,34]; comorbidities that are frequently present in and contribute to the development of HFpEF.

On the basis of a strong theoretical rationale for RAAS blockade in patients with HFpEF, three large randomized clinical trials were designed specifically to evaluate ACE inhibitors and ARBs in patients with HFpEF. These include the Candesartan in Heart failure Assessment of Reduction in Mortality and morbidity-Preserved (CHARM-Preserved) Trial, the Perindopril in Elderly People with Chronic Heart Failure (PEP-CHF) trial,[35,36] and the Irbesartan in heart failure with PRESERVED ejection fraction (I-PRESERVE) trial.[37] The characteristics of the patient populations evaluated in these trials are summarized in **Table 36-1**.

Of the 3023 patients enrolled in the CHARM-Preserved trial, almost 20% were on ACE inhibitors and 56% on β-blockers at the time of randomization to candesartan or a placebo. After a median follow-up of approximately 37 months, the primary endpoint (cardiovascular death or HF hospitalization) occurred in 22% of the candesartan and 24% of the placebo group (hazard ratio [HR] 0.89, 95% confidence interval [CI] 0.77-1.03, P = 0.118; covariate-adjusted HR 0.86, 95% CI 0.74-1.00, P = 0.051) (**Figure 36-1**). The difference, which was of borderline statistical significance only for the adjusted hazard ratios, was driven mostly by a difference in HF hospitalizations between the candesartan- and placebo-treated groups (HR 0.85, 95% CI 0.72, 1.01, P = 0.072) with almost identical cardiovascular mortality rates between the two groups (**Figure 36-2**). In addition, the total number of HF hospitalizations was noted to be significantly lower in the candesartan group. Of note, at 6 months into the trial, the blood pressure was significantly more reduced in the candesartan group (6.9 mm Hg systolic and 2.9 mm Hg diastolic) compared with the placebo group (P <0.0001). It is therefore difficult to tease out whether the modest 15% relative reduction in HF hospitalizations with candesartan compared with a placebo in patients with HFpEF was mostly a result of blood pressure reduction versus any other more specific angiotensin-blocking effects of candesartan, and whether any other drugs causing similar blood pressure reduction would have led to similar effects. The lack of a greater benefit from the use of the ARB in CHARM-Preserved may also have been contributed to by the fact that ACE inhibitors were allowed for patients in the trial, with 20% of patients being on ACE inhibitors even at the beginning of the trial, and the relatively lower than expected annual event rates of the primary composite outcome of 9.1% in the placebo group.

The PEP-CHF trial of perindopril in HFpEF was conducted in a more elderly patient population compared with the CHARM-Preserved trial (see Table 36-1). However, the results of the study were neutral with respect to the primary outcome (composite of all-cause mortality and unplanned HF-related hospitalization), and demonstrated only a trend toward modest benefit in other endpoints.[36] As compared with the CHARM-Preserved trial, the PEP-CHF study enrolled only 850 patients with HFpEF, who in addition to having relatively preserved LVEF also had objective evidence of diastolic dysfunction at enrollment. The mean follow-up of 26 months was shorter than the CHARM-Preserved trial. The event rate was much lower than expected and despite much longer follow-up than originally intended, only 46% of the expected events occurred, giving the study only 25% power to show a difference in the primary endpoint. Furthermore, a large number of patients stopped their assigned treatment after 1 year, and most of them started taking open label ACE inhibitors (discontinuation rate of 38% at 18 months, ≈36% of patients on open-label ACE inhibitor treatment by the end of the study). Over the total duration of follow-up, perindopril was not associated with an improvement in the primary composite endpoint of death or HF hospitalization (HR 0.92, 95% CI 0.70-1.21, P = 0.55; **Figure 36-3A**). If, however, analysis was confined to 1 year of follow-up, at which point most patients were still taking the assigned medication, perindopril was associated with a statistically borderline significant 31%

TABLE 36-1 Study Characteristics of Some Multicenter Clinical Trials Evaluating Morbidity and Mortality in HFpEF

	CHARM-PRESERVED[35]	PEP-CHF[36]	I-PRESERVE[37]	TOP-CAT[40,106]	JAPANESE DIASTOLIC HEART FAILURE TRIAL[47]
HF trial population	N = 3023 LVEF >40% NYHA class II-IV NYHA III/IV: 39% Mean age: 67 years >75 years: 23% Male: 60%	N = 850 LVEF >40% NYHA class I-IV NYHA III/IV: 24% Mean age: 75 years ≥70 years: 100% Male: 45% Diastolic dysfunction	N = 4128 LVEF ≥ 45% NYHA class II-IV NYHA III/IV: 79% Mean age: 72 years ≥60 years: 100% Male 40% HF hospitalization or substrate for HF	N = 3445 LVEF ≥ 45% NYHA class II-IV NYHA III/IV: 34% Mean age: 69 years Male: 48% HF hospitalization or BNP ≥ 100 pg/mL or NT-proBNP ≥ 360 pg/mL	N = 245 LVEF >40% NYHA class I-IV NYHA III/IV: 11% Mean age: 72 years Male: 58%
Major exclusion criteria	Significant hypotension Creatinine >3 mg/dL Serum K >5.5 mEq/L	Systolic BP <100 mm Hg Creatinine >2.3 mg/dL Serum K >5.4 mEq/L	Systolic BP <100 or >160 mm Hg Creatinine >2.5 mg/dL	GFR <30 mL/min/1.73 m² or Creatinine ≥ 2.5 mg/dL Serum K ≥ 5.0 mEq/L Uncontrolled hypertension	Significant hypotension Creatinine >3 mg/dL Serum K >5.5 mEq/L Heart rate <50/min
Use of ACE inhibitors/ARBs at baseline	ACE inhibitor use allowed	No concomitant ACE inhibitor/ARB	ACE inhibitors allowed in one third of patients when indicated for diabetes or vascular disease	ACE inhibitor/ARB allowed	ACE inhibitor/ARB use allowed
Protocol	*Candesartan vs. placebo, uptitrated to target 32 mg/day Median follow-up: 36.6 months	*Perindopril vs. placebo, uptitrated to target 4 mg/day Median follow-up: 25.2 months	*Irbesartan vs. placebo, uptitrated to target 300 mg/day Mean follow-up: 49.5 months	*Spironolactone vs. placebo uptitrated to target 45 mg/day Mean follow-up: 3.3 years	Randomized, open label carvedilol vs. placebo uptitrated to target 20 mg twice daily Median follow-up: 3.2 years
Primary endpoint	Composite of CV mortality or HF hospitalization	Composite of all-cause mortality or HF hospitalization	Composite of all-cause mortality or CV hospitalization	Composite of CV mortality, aborted cardiac arrest, or HF hospitalization	Composite of CV mortality or HF hospitalization

ACE, Angiotensin-converting enzyme; *ARB,* angiotensin receptor blocker; *BNP,* B-type natriuretic peptide; *BP,* blood pressure; *CV,* cardiovascular; *GFR,* glomerular filtration rate; *HF,* heart failure; *HFpEF,* heart failure with preserved ejection fraction; *LVEF,* left ventricular ejection fraction; *NYHA,* New York Heart Association.
*Randomized, double-blind trial.

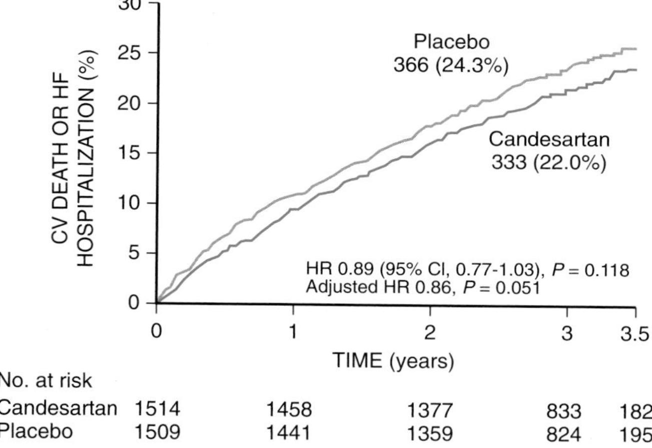

FIGURE 36-1 Kaplan-Meier curves for time to first occurrence of the primary endpoint in patients with heart failure with preserved ejection fraction in the CHARM-Preserved Trial. *CV,* Cardiovascular; *HF,* heart failure. *From Yusuf S, Pfeffer MA, Swedberg K, et al: Effects of candesartan in patients with chronic heart failure and preserved left-ventricular ejection fraction: the CHARM-Preserved Trial. Lancet. 362:777–781, 2003.*

relative reduction in the primary endpoint (HR 0.69, 95% CI 0.47-1.01, $P = 0.055$). Similarly, although perindopril was not associated with a benefit in HF hospitalization over the entire duration of the trial (see Figure 36-3B), at 1 year of follow-up, the perindopril group had a lower rate of HF hospitalizations (HR 0.63, 95% CI 0.41-0.97, $P = 0.03$). Thus, although perindopril did not have a beneficial effect on the overall primary outcome, there was a suggestion of reduction in HF hospitalizations at 1 year when patients were on assigned treatment.[36] In addition, significant improvements were observed compared with the placebo group in some other secondary endpoints, including the proportion of patients in NYHA functional class I and change in six-minute-walk distance at 1 year. Similar to the observation in the CHARM-preserved trial, the active arm of perindopril had a significantly greater reduction in systolic blood pressure (mean difference = 3 mm Hg, $P = 0.03$) compared with the placebo arm. Furthermore, it was noted that patients with a higher baseline blood pressure appeared to have a greater benefit with perindopril. Therefore, similar to the CHARM-preserved trial, it is not possible to rule out a significant contribution of the blood pressure–lowering effect of the ACE inhibitor as opposed to other RAAS-blocking actions of perindopril toward the observed short-term beneficial effect on HF hospitalizations. Also, both trials illustrate the encountered difficulty of lower event rates of patients enrolled in clinical trials compared with those seen in the general population. The switch over to open label ACE inhibitors illustrates the many existing indications for the use of ACE inhibitors or ARBs in patients with vascular disease, diabetes, and hypertension, the same group of comorbidities that are frequently encountered in patients with HFpEF, thus potentially limiting the opportunities to add ACE inhibitors or ARBs specifically for HFpEF.

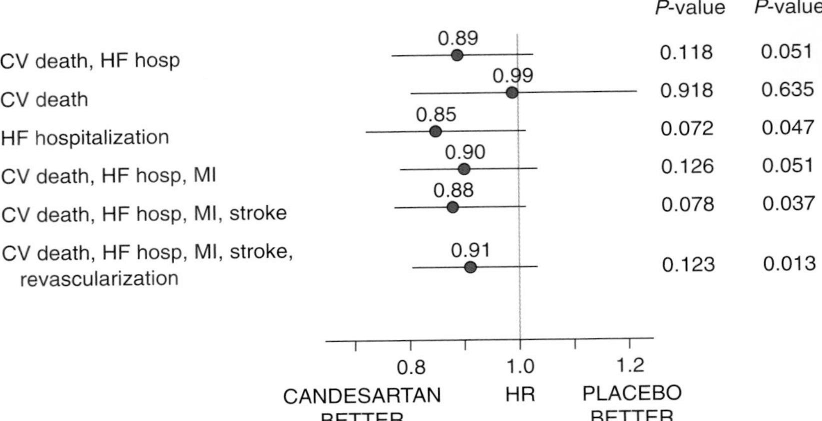

FIGURE 36-2 Hazard ratios and 95% confidence intervals for candesartan vs. placebo for selected secondary endpoints in the CHARM-Preserved Trial. *CV*, Cardiovascular; *HF*, heart failure; *MI*, myocardial infarction. *From Yusuf S, Pfeffer MA, Swedberg K, et al: Effects of candesartan in patients with chronic heart failure and preserved left-ventricular ejection fraction: the CHARM-Preserved Trial. Lancet. 362:777–781, 2003.*

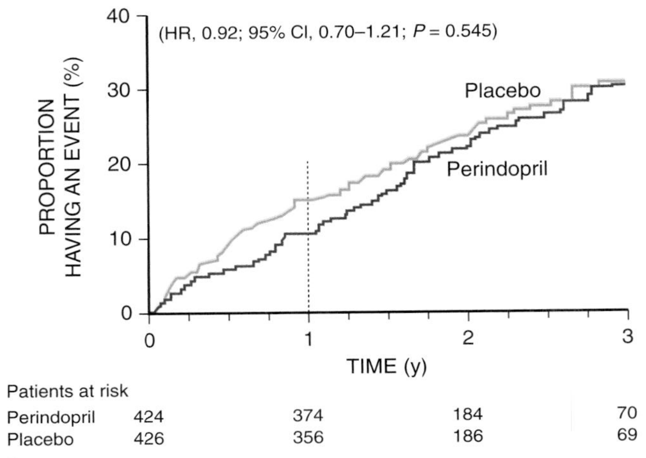

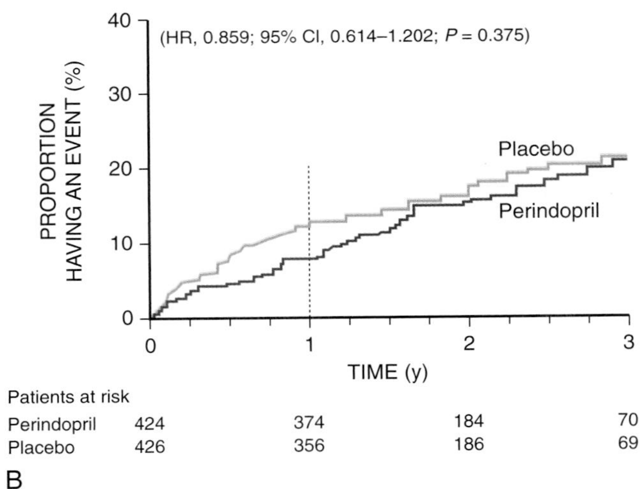

FIGURE 36-3 Effect of perindopril on clinical outcomes. **A,** Kaplan-Meier curves showing time to first occurrence of the primary endpoint, all-cause mortality or unplanned heart failure–related hospitalization. The dotted line points out the occurrence of the endpoint at 1 year of follow-up. **B,** Kaplan-Meier curves showing time to first occurrence of the prespecified secondary endpoint of unplanned heart failure–related hospitalization. The dotted line points out the occurrence of the endpoint at 1 year of follow-up. *From Cleland JG, Tendera M, Adamus J, et al: The perindopril in elderly people with chronic heart failure (PEP-CHF) study. Eur Heart J 27:2338–2345, 2006.*

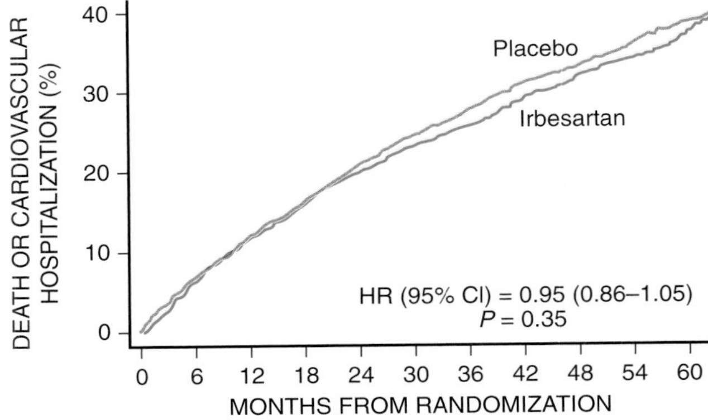

FIGURE 36-4 Kaplan-Meier curves for time to first occurrence of the primary endpoint in the I-PRESERVE trial. *From Massie BM, Carson PE, McMurray JJ, et al: Irbesartan in patients with heart failure and preserved ejection fraction. N Engl J Med 359:2456–2467, 2008.*

The largest trial, I-PRESERVE, enrolled 4128 patients with HFpEF (see Table 36-1).[37] The patients were randomly assigned to the ARB, irbesartan, or placebo. During a mean follow-up of 49.5 months, there was no significant difference in the occurrence of the primary outcome (death from any cause or hospitalization for a cardiovascular cause, i.e., HF, myocardial infarction, unstable angina, arrhythmia, or stroke) between irbesartan and the placebo (HR 0.95; 95% CI 0.86-1.05; $P = 0.35$; **Figure 36-4**). Overall rates of death were also similar (HR 1.00; 95% CI 0.88-1.14; $P = 0.98$) as were rates of cardiovascular hospitalization, HF hospitalization, and other secondary outcomes. Although, compared with the CHARM-preserved trial, the I-PRESERVE trial studied a greater number of patients, with slightly better preserved EF (≥45% vs. >40% in CHARM-Preserved), greater specificity of the substrate for HFpEF, and with a greater proportion of older patients and women (i.e., a study cohort more representative of the "real world" HFpEF population), this trial did not provide any evidence for overall benefit of ARBs on cardiovascular outcomes in HFpEF patients.

Thus apart from the modest signal of 15% relative reduction in HF hospitalizations with candesartan compared with a placebo in HFpEF patients observed in the

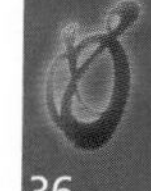

CHARM-Preserved trial and a possible benefit on HF hospitalizations and functional class at an intermediate time point in PEP-CHF (in the absence of benefit over the entire duration of follow-up), neither ACE inhibitors nor ARBs have been proven to have a convincing beneficial effect on clinical outcomes in HFpEF.

Aldosterone Receptor Antagonists

Mineralocorticoid receptor activation by aldosterone contributes to the pathophysiology of HF through several mechanisms, including sodium retention, potassium loss, endothelial dysfunction, vascular inflammation, fibrosis, and hypertrophy. It remains unclear whether aldosterone antagonists have more success in improving clinical outcomes in patients with HFpEF than ACE inhibitors and ARBs. Smaller trials suggested benefit on diastolic function without improvement in functional capacity in this group of patients. The recently published Aldo-DHF trial was a prospective, randomized, double-blind, placebo-controlled trial evaluating the effect of spironolactone on diastolic function and exercise capacity in 422 patients with HFpEF (**Table 36-2**).[38] At the end of 12 months of treatment, compared with a placebo, spironolactone use resulted in improvement in echocardiographic parameters of diastolic dysfunction (mitral annular E/e′ adjusted mean difference between the placebo and spironolactone −1.5; 95% CI −2.0 to −0.9, P <0.001), neuroendocrine activation (NT-proBNP geometric ratio 0.86, 95% CI 0.75-0.99, P = 0.03), and induced reverse remodeling (decline in LV mass index; difference −6 g/m^2, 95% CI −10 to −1 g/m^2; P = 0.009), but did not improve HF symptoms or quality of life and slightly reduced the 6-minute walking distance with no effect on hospitalizations. There was associated mild increase in serum potassium (P <0.001) and reduction in the glomerular filtration rate (P <0.001). The lack of clinical improvement despite improvement in echocardiographic and laboratory parameters may have been caused by the relatively younger and healthier patient cohort (86% NYHA class II, ≈50% on diuretics and baseline median NT-proBNP 158 ng/mL), a low event rate, and shorter follow-up. Similarly, another smaller study, the Randomized Aldosterone Antagonism in Heart Failure with Preserved Ejection Fraction (RAAM-PEF) trial, evaluated the effects of the more selective aldosterone receptor blocker, eplerenone, compared with a placebo on a 6-minute walk distance, diastolic function, and markers of collagen turnover after 6 months of treatment. The use of eplerenone was associated with improvement in diastolic dysfunction (E/e′, $P \le 0.01$) and reduced collagen turnover but no change in 6-minute walk distance (P = 0.91) as compared with a placebo.[39] The results of the large multicenter trial, the Treatment of Preserved Cardiac function heart failure with an Aldosterone Antagonist (TOPCAT), became available recently. This randomized, double-blind, placebo-controlled trial evaluated the effects of spironolactone on morbidity and mortality in 3445 patients with HFpEF (LVEF >45%; see Table 36-1). The primary endpoint of cardiovascular death, HF hospitalization, or resuscitated cardiac arrest was similar between the spironolactone and the placebo arms (18.6% vs. 20.4%, HR 0.89, 95% CI 0.77-1.04, P = 0.14; **Figure 36-5A**). Individual components, including CV mortality and aborted cardiac arrest, were similar between the two arms. However, HF hospitalizations were lower (12.0% vs. 14.2%, P = 0.042; see Figure 36-5B); all-hospitalizations were similar (P = 0.25). Hyperkalemia (18.7% vs. 9.1%, P<0.001) and renal failure, defined as serum creatinine ≥ 2 times the baseline value and above the upper limit of the normal range, were both significantly higher in the spironolactone arm. The results of the TOPCAT trial indicate that spironolactone is not overall superior to a

TABLE 36-2 Study Characteristics of Selected Recent Multicenter Clinical Trials in HFpEF with Non–Morbidity-Mortality Endpoints

	RELAX[70]	ALDO-DHF[38]	PARAMOUNT[45]	RHEOS DIASTOLIC HEART FAILURE TRIAL[70]
HF trial population	N = 190 NYHA class II-IV LVEF ≥ 50% BNP >200 pg/mL or NT-BNP >400 pg/mL Abnormal peak Vo_2 Median age: 69 years Male 52%	N = 422 NYHA class II-III LVEF ≥ 50% Diastolic dysfunction Mean age: 67 years Male 48%	N = 301 NYHA class II-III LVEF >45% NT-proBNP >400 pg/mL Mean age: 71 years Male 47%	N = 60 LVEF ≥ 45% Elevated BNP/NT-proBNP Bilateral carotid bifurcations below the level of the mandible Results awaited
Some exclusion criteria	GFR <20 mL/min/1.73 m^2 On nitrates or alpha antagonists Morbid obesity ACE inhibitor/ARB allowed	Significant CAD Potassium ≥ 5.1 mmol/L eGFR <30 mL/min/1.73 m^2 Concomitant therapy with potassium-sparing diuretics ACE inhibitor/ARB allowed	Potassium >5.2 mEq/L eGFR <30 mL/min/1.73 m^2 ACE inhibitor/ARB stopped at enrollment	History of suspected baroreflex failure or autonomic neuropathy ACE inhibitor/ARB allowed
Protocol: All double-blind, randomized	Sildenafil vs. placebo Target dose 60 mg, thrice daily Duration: 24 weeks	Spironolactone (25 mg daily) vs. placebo Duration: 12 months	LCZ696 (target 200 mg twice daily) vs. valsartan (target 160 mg twice daily) Duration: 12 weeks main; 24 weeks extension	Rheos Baroreflex Activation system implanted in all patients with device either on or off for 6 months
Primary endpoint	Exercise tolerance: Peak oxygen consumption	Coprimary: peak oxygen consumption and diastolic function (E/E′)	Change in NT-proBNP from baseline to 12 weeks	Left ventricular mass index

ACE, Angiotensin-converting enzyme; *ARB*, angiotensin receptor blocker; *BNP*, B-type natriuretic peptide; *CAD*, coronary artery disease; *eGFR*, estimated glomerular filtration rate; *HF*, heart failure; *HFpEF*, heart failure with preserved ejection fraction; *LVEF*, left ventricular ejection fraction; *NYHA*, New York Heart Association.

placebo in improving CV outcomes in patients with HFpEF. Most of these patients were already on an ACEI/ARB. There was also a significantly higher rate of hyperkalemia and renal failure in patients treated with spironolactone. The reduction in HF hospitalizations with spironolactone is encouraging but this finding will need to be confirmed and should be approached with caution because all-cause hospitalizations were similar between the placebo and spironolactone arms. An interesting post hoc analysis revealed a disparity in outcomes between the centers in North and South America and those in Eastern Europe. In the United States, Canada, Brazil, and Argentina, where the rate of the primary composite outcome was 31.8% in the placebo group, spironolactone had a significant benefit (HR 0.82, 95% CI 0.69-0.98). However, in Russia and the Republic of Georgia, where the primary outcome occurred in only 8.4% of patients taking the placebo, spironolactone did not have any effect (HR 1.10, 95% CI 0.79-1.51). Whether this could suggest that spironolactone may be useful in higher-risk patients is up for debate.[40]

Angiotensin Receptor Neprilysin Inhibitor

Natriuretic peptides have been associated with potent natriuresis, vasodilation, and inhibition of the renin-angiotensin-aldosterone system and may have antifibrotic and antisympathetic effects.[41,42] Neprilysin (neutral endopeptidase 24-11) inhibition leads to increased circulating levels of natriuretic peptides by preventing their breakdown with consequent cardiac, vascular, and renal protective effects. In addition, the augmentation of active natriuretic peptides increases generation of myocardial cGMP, which improves myocardial relaxation and decreases hypertrophy. However, neprilysin inhibition also prevents breakdown of vasoconstrictors like angiotensin II, thus diminishing the beneficial effects of neprilysin inhibition. Concomitant inhibition of the renin-angiotensin-aldosterone system, along with neprilysin inhibition, helps overcome this limitation and is the basis of dual-acting vasopeptidase inhibitors. Previous studies showed promising effects of a combination drug with neutral endopeptidase and an ACE inhibitor (omapatrilat) for treatment of patients with hypertension and HF.[43] However, further development of this agent was stopped due to increased occurrence of angioedema, likely from increased bradykinin levels from neprilysin and ACE inhibition. Angiotensin receptor blockers are associated with a lower incidence of angioedema as compared with ACE inhibitors and were substituted for ACE inhibitors in the development of a new dual vasopeptidase inhibitor, LCZ696 (combination of ARB, valsartan, and neprilysin inhibitor, AHU377), with higher antihypertensive potency as compared with valsartan and similar tolerability.[44] The use of LCZ696 in patients with HFpEF was recently evaluated in a phase 2 double-blind, randomized, parallel group trial, the Prospective comparison of the Angiotensin Receptor Neprilysin Inhibitor (ARNI) with ARB on Management Of heart failUre with preserved ejectioN fracTion (PARAMOUNT) trial.[45] The trial evaluated 301 patients with NYHA class II-III HFpEF (LVEF ≥ 45%) and NT-proBNP ≥ 400 pg/mL; randomized patients to LCZ696 titrated to 200 mg twice daily or valsartan titrated to 160 mg twice daily and treated for 36 weeks (see Table 36-2). The primary endpoint, a decrease in NT-proBNP from baseline to 12 weeks, was significantly greater in the LCZ696 group compared with the valsartan group (ratio of change LCZ696/valsartan at 0.77, 95% CI 0.64-0.92, $P = 0.005$; **Figure 36-6**). Although, NT-proBNP remained significantly reduced at 36 weeks compared with baseline, the difference between the two treatment groups was no longer statistically significant ($P = 0.2$). However, left atrial volume ($P = 0.003$) and left atrial dimension ($P = 0.034$) were significantly reduced and NYHA class improved at 36 weeks in patients in the LCZ696 group. No other echocardiographic parameters (including measures of diastolic function) differed between the treatment groups. The effect of LCZ696 on NT-proBNP appeared greater in subgroups of patients with systolic blood pressure higher than 140 mm Hg and in diabetic patients. LCZ696 was well tolerated overall and its side effect profile was similar to that of valsartan. Although the positive results of the study on biomarkers and surrogate endpoints are encouraging, only the larger planned phase III trial will determine the effects of LCZ696 on clinical outcomes.

β-BLOCKADE

A smaller trial, the Swedish Doppler-echocardiographic study (SWEDIC), examined the effect of the β-blocker carvedilol on diastolic function in patients with HFpEF

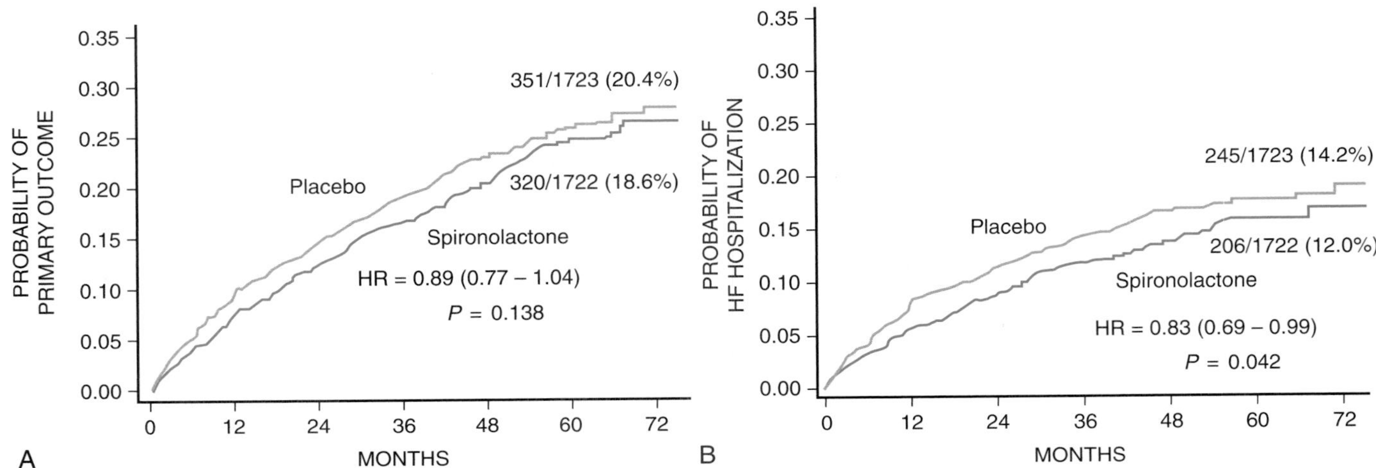

FIGURE 36-5 Kaplan-Meier curves of time to first occurrence of the primary endpoint of cardiovascular death, heart failure hospitalization, or resuscitated cardiac arrest **(A)** and of HF hospitalization **(B)** in the TOPCAT trial. *From Pitt B, Pfeffer MA, Assmann SF, et al: TOPCAT Investigators. Spironolactone for heart failure with preserved ejection fraction. N Engl J Med 370(15):1383–1392, 2014.*

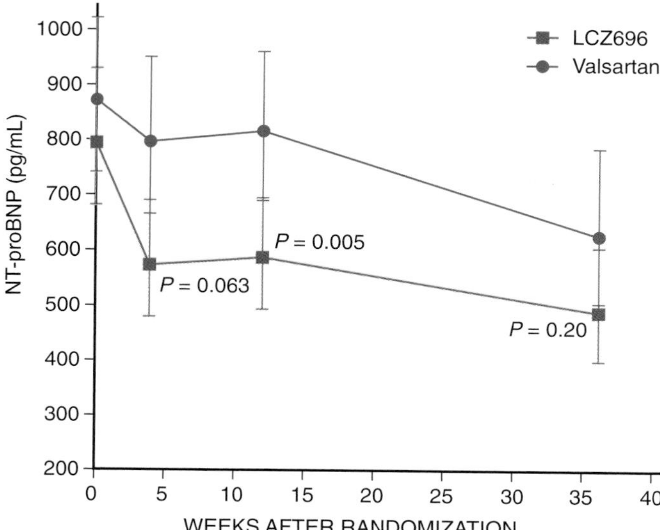

FIGURE 36-6 PARAMOUNT trial: NT-proBNP at 4, 12, and 36 weeks in the LCZ696 and valsartan groups. *Modified from Solomon SD, Zile M, Pieske B, et al: The angiotensin receptor neprilysin inhibitor LCZ696 in heart failure with preserved ejection fraction: a phase 2 double-blind randomised controlled trial. Lancet 380:1387–1395, 2012.*

(LVEF >45%) who also met conventional Doppler criteria for diastolic dysfunction.[46] In the 95 patients that completed the 6-month study, there were no significant differences between the carvedilol and placebo-treated patients for the primary endpoint, a composite evaluating either improved, unchanged, or worsened diastolic function, or for clinical endpoints. Of note, at baseline, most patients had only mild diastolic dysfunction and had NYHA class I or II functional status, making improvement in these parameters less likely.

The Japanese Diastolic Heart Failure Study (J-DHF) trial was a multicenter, randomized, placebo-controlled, open, blinded-endpoint trial, which evaluated the effects of carvedilol in 245 patients with HFpEF (LVEF >40%) during a median follow-up of 3.2 years.[47] There was no difference in the primary composite outcome of cardiovascular death or HF hospitalization or in the secondary composite outcome of cardiovascular death or any cardiovascular hospitalization. Although the overall results did not demonstrate a benefit of carvedilol on clinical outcomes in HFpEF, it should be pointed out that only 245 of the planned 800 patients were enrolled, resulting in the trial being underpowered and attesting to the difficulties in enrolling patients into clinical trials of HFpEF. Also, 78% of the patients in the trial did not reach the target dose of 20 mg/day, with the median prescribed dose being 7.5 mg/day. In a post hoc analysis, the investigators observed that in patients prescribed carvedilol more than 7.5 mg/day, the composite secondary outcome of cardiovascular death and unplanned hospitalization for any cardiovascular causes was significantly lower than in the controls (HR 0.54, 95% CI 0.30-0.96; $P = 0.04$), although it was comparable with controls in patients treated with carvedilol ≤ 7.5 mg/day.[48] It is not known if patients that could be titrated to higher doses were a healthier subset and thus had better outcomes compared with all controls analyzed as one group or whether the lack of use of higher doses of carvedilol in the study population contributed to the neutral results of the overall trial. Furthermore, it is difficult to interpret the significance of the observed trend toward lower BNP levels at 2 years after randomization in the carvedilol compared with the placebo group (164.9 ± 199.5 vs. 222.7 ± 288.7, respectively, $P = 0.11$) in view of the overall neutral results of this underpowered trial.

Another multicenter trial evaluated the effects of nebivolol in elderly patients with HF, irrespective of LV ejection fraction (LVEF). Nebivolol is a β_1 selective blocker that also has vasodilating properties and improves endothelial dysfunction via its effects on the endothelial nitric oxide synthase and its antioxidative properties.[49] In the Study of the Effects of Nebivolol Intervention on Outcomes and Rehospitalizations in Seniors with heart failure (SENIORS), 2128 patients aged ≥ 70 years with history of HF were randomized to receive nebivolol or the placebo.[50] Of these, 35% of patients had LVEF greater than 35%. In the overall study, nebivolol was associated with a modest 14% reduction in the primary composite endpoint of death or cardiovascular hospitalization (HR 0.84, 95% CI 0.74-0.99), contributed to by a reduction in both mortality and cardiovascular hospitalization. A similar magnitude of reduction was noted in the subgroup with LVEF greater than 35%; however, it did not reach statistical significance, possibly as a result of fewer patients in the subgroup (HR 0.82, 95% CI 0.63-1.05). Although labeled as patients with preserved ejection fraction or HFpEF, this subgroup of patients with EF greater than 35% clearly consisted of a heterogeneous patient population with both preserved and reduced LVEF. The proportion of patients with truly preserved LVEF (≥50%) was small (<15% of all patients in the trial). Therefore, although the overall trial suggests a modest cardiovascular benefit of the β-blocker, nebivolol, in elderly patients with HF, the results did not convincingly demonstrate a benefit in elderly patients with HFpEF.

Another smaller trial, the Effects of the Long-term Administration of Nebivolol on the clinical symptoms, exercise capacity, and LV function of patients with Diastolic Dysfunction: (ELANDD) study evaluated 116 patients with NYHA class II-III symptoms, LVEF greater than 45%, and echocardiographic signs of LV diastolic dysfunction. The patients were randomized to 6 months of treatment with nebivolol or a placebo. There was no difference in 6-minute walk distance or peak oxygen consumption between the two groups. The resting and peak blood pressure decreased in patients on nebivolol; there was a significant interaction between change in peak exercise heart rate and peak oxygen consumption ($r = 0.391$, $P = 0.003$), and it was postulated that the negative chronotropic effect of the β-blocker may have contributed to the neutral results of the study.[51]

In summary, these trials of the β-blockers carvedilol and nebivolol, although limited by sample size, have not demonstrated definitive benefits, or harm, on exercise and functional capacity, on diastolic dysfunction, or on clinical outcomes in patients with HFpEF.

SELECTIVE PHOSPHODIESTERASE TYPE 5 INHIBITION

Selective inhibitors of phosphodiesterase-5 (PDE5) are known to enhance nitric oxide-mediated vasodilation by inhibiting degradation of cyclic GMP, a key intracellular second messenger (see also Chapters 1, 2, and 13).[52] Whereas inhibitors of the cyclic AMP-specific phosphodiesterase-3 or PDE3 (including inotropic agents, such as milrinone and enoximone) augment intracellular

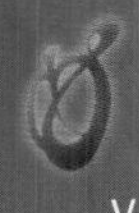

levels of cyclic AMP and increase mortality in patients with HF (see Chapter 33),[53] selective inhibitors of PDE-5 such as sildenafil are highly selective for human PDE5, do not increase cyclic AMP, and lack inotropic effects. Therefore, they are thought to not share the toxicity associated with PDE3 inhibition.

Several experimental observations suggest that sildenafil may be beneficial in the treatment of patients with HFpEF. In mice exposed to sustained pressure overload, chronic PDE5A inhibition led to attenuation of cardiac and myocyte hypertrophy and interstitial fibrosis, and improved cardiac functioning.[54] Sildenafil treatment applied to well-established hypertrophic cardiac disease in mice also prevented further cardiac and myocyte dysfunction, as well as progressive remodeling.[55] The investigators demonstrated that PDE-5 is upregulated in the heart in response to pressure overload and that the effects of PDE-5 inhibition are not mediated by an effect on blood pressure. In addition, PDE-5 inhibition has been associated with improvement in flow-mediated vasodilation in patients with systolic HF and an improvement in large artery stiffness in hypertensive men.[56,57] Beneficial effects on pulmonary vasculature with reduction in pulmonary pressures, as well as reduction in right ventricular hypertrophy, have been demonstrated with patients with pulmonary hypertension.[58] Furthermore, PDE-5 inhibition may restore renal responsiveness to natriuretic peptides in several states of abnormal sodium handling including HF.[59] The fact that PDE-5 is upregulated in cardiovascular disease states such as HF, with resultant greater susceptibility to PDE-5 inhibition in these disease states along with the previously summarized potential beneficial effects on LV hypertrophy, endothelial function, arterial stiffness, pulmonary hypertension, and renal responsiveness to natriuretic peptides, makes selective PDE-5 inhibition an attractive therapeutic target in the treatment of patients with HFpEF.

This hypothesis was tested in the PhosphodiesteRasE-5 Inhibition to improve cLinical status And eXercise Capacity in Diastolic Heart Failure (RELAX) trial. This study was a multicenter, double-blind, placebo-controlled, randomized clinical trial of 216 stable outpatients with HFpEF (LVEF ≥ 50%), elevated N-terminal brain-type natriuretic peptide or elevated invasively measured filling pressures, and reduced exercise capacity (see Table 36-2). Patients were randomized to a placebo or sildenafil 20 mg thrice daily for 12 weeks followed by 60 mg thrice daily for the next 12 weeks. The primary outcome—a change in peak oxygen consumption after 24 weeks of therapy and secondary endpoints, including change in 6-minute walk distance and a composite clinical status score—was not significantly different between the two groups at 24 weeks. Additionally, no differences were noted in Doppler assessed LV diastolic function parameters or in the pulmonary arterial systolic pressures between the two treatment groups. Serious adverse events occurred in 22% of sildenafil patients and 16% of placebo patients. Unexpectedly, there was modest but statistically significant worsening of renal function observed in patients treated with sildenafil, which was associated with concordant increases in NT-proBNP, uric acid, and endothelin-1, suggesting that the decline in renal function was physiologically significant. There were more (not statistically significant) patients who withdrew consent, died, or were too ill to perform the cardiopulmonary exercise test in the sildenafil treatment group, potentially accentuating the lack of benefit observed, particularly if those who withdrew did so due to adverse effects or poor clinical status.[60] The lack of clinical benefit in the RELAX study was in contrast to a smaller prior study of sildenafil in HFpEF ($n = 44$), which had demonstrated significant reductions in pulmonary artery and right heart pressures, right ventricular function, and some benefits for left heart diastolic pressures and diastolic function.[61] No exercise testing was performed in that study. Importantly, compared with the RELAX trial, HFpEF patients in that study had fewer comorbidities and significantly higher blood pressure, LV mass, pulmonary arterial hypertension, profound right ventricular systolic dysfunction, and right ventricular failure. Thus it can be hypothesized that the primary therapeutic effects of PDE-5 inhibitors in HF involve the drugs' ability to dilate the pulmonary vascular bed, enhance right ventricular contractility, and reduce ventricular interdependence, and that pulmonary arterial hypertension and right ventricular failure must be significant to observe clinical benefit in HFpEF.

DIGOXIN

Digoxin is one of the oldest drugs that has been used in the management of HF, but has been historically thought to be contraindicated in HFpEF. Theoretical considerations suggest potential benefit, as well as harm from digoxin, in this group of patients. For example, digoxin may improve the active energy-dependent myocardial early diastolic function, and may improve the neurohormonal profile in patients with HFpEF.[62] However, it may produce an increase in systolic energy demands, adding to a relative calcium overload in diastole, especially during periods of hemodynamic stress or ischemia and thus contribute to diastolic dysfunction.[14] The Digitalis Investigators Group (DIG) investigated the effects of digoxin on morbidity and mortality in HF patients in normal sinus rhythm, most of whom had systolic HF.[63] However, the trial population also included a small group of patients with HFpEF (EF >45%). In a post hoc analysis, among the 988 patients with chronic HFpEF, digoxin had no significant effect on the composite primary endpoint of HF mortality or HF hospitalizations (hazard 0.82, 95% CI 0.63-1.07, $P = 0.14$).[64] Similarly, there was no benefit of digoxin on the composite of cardiovascular mortality or HF hospitalization. Although the use of digoxin was associated with a trend toward a reduction in hospitalizations for worsening HF (HR 0.79, 95% CI 0.99-1.91, $P = 0.09$), it was also associated with a trend toward an increase in hospitalizations for unstable angina (HR 1.37, 95% CI, 0.99-1.91, $P = 0.06$). Thus, digoxin was not associated with any overall reduction in cardiovascular hospitalizations. This post hoc analysis would suggest that digoxin should not be recommended as treatment for all patients with HFpEF except, if required, as an agent for rate control in patients with concomitant atrial fibrillation. As noted previously, the DIG trial only enrolled patients in sinus rhythm.

OTHER TARGETS FOR MEDICAL THERAPY

Endothelin Antagonists

Experimental studies suggested that selective antagonists of endothelin type A (ETA) could exert beneficial effects in diastolic HF through attenuation of the progression of LV hypertrophy and fibrosis with resultant improvement in diastolic function.[65] In addition, in patients with moderate to severe HF, acute ETA receptor blockade with sitaxsentan caused selective pulmonary vasodilation. Therefore, sitaxsentan was thought to be of potential value in the treatment of patients with pulmonary hypertension secondary to chronic HF. Based on these considerations, a small trial with the selective endothelin (ETA) antagonist, sitaxsentan, was performed in patients with HFpEF. Although preliminary results suggested that patients treated with sitaxsentan had a significant increase in treadmill exercise time (90 seconds) compared with the placebo (37 seconds, $P = 0.03$) without other differences in diastolic parameters or functional status,[66] further work with sitaxsentan is not possible because the agent was withdrawn from clinical use because of the potential for significant liver toxicity.

Advanced Glycation End Products Cross-Link Breakers

Increased LV and arterial stiffness, which may be involved in the pathophysiology of HFpEF (see Chapter 10), especially in elderly subjects,[11,67] is at least partially contributed to by nonenzymatic cross-links that develop between advanced glycation end products (AGE) on long-lived proteins, such as collagen and elastin. Alagebrium chloride (ALT-711) nonenzymatically breaks AGE cross-links and has been shown to improve LV distensibility and arterial compliance in elderly subjects with systolic hypertension.[68] A small open-label study that evaluated the use of alagebrium in elderly patients with stable HFpEF[69] found that alagebrium was associated with a reduction of LV mass, improved tissue Doppler indices of diastolic function (e′), and improved quality of life. However, there was no change in blood pressure, pulse pressure, peak oxygen consumption, or aortic distensibility. Although a number of trials with this agent in HF including HFpEF were initiated, the studies were terminated without completion.[70]

Anti-inflammatory Agents

Enhanced inflammation is associated with worsening outcomes in HF patients, and may play a direct role in disease progression (see Chapter 7). Interleukin-1β (IL-1β) is a proinflammatory cytokine that is chronically elevated in HF and has been associated with adverse ventricular-vascular remodeling, pressure overload-induced cardiac hypertrophy, negative inotropy, as well as reduced β-adrenergic receptor responsiveness.[71] Anakinra, an IL-1 receptor antagonist used to treat rheumatoid arthritis, was recently evaluated in seven patients with HF with reduced LVEF and elevated inflammatory markers, and was associated with an 84% reduction in hsCRP ($P = 0.016$) as well as an improvement in peak oxygen consumption ($\dot{V}O_2$).[72] Anakinra is currently being evaluated in a pilot study in patients with HFpEF (NCT01542502).[70]

Lusitropic Agents

Ranolazine is an anti-ischemic drug, which inhibits the late sodium current in cardiac myocytes. In patients with HF, the late sodium current is increased,[73] leading to increased sodium accumulation, which reverses the direction of the Na^+/Ca^{2+}-exchanger, contributing to a Ca^{2+} overload in the cell. By inhibiting the late Na^+ current (INa), ranolazine is expected to prevent (or reduce) sodium accumulation in the myocyte, thus improving calcium extrusion through the Na^+/Ca^{2+}-exchanger and thereby improve relaxation of the myocardium.[74] Data from in vitro, ex vivo, and animal studies indicate that ranolazine improved diastolic function of the myocardium.[75] The RAnoLazIne for the Treatment of Diastolic Heart Failure (RALI-DHF) was a prospective, single-center, randomized, double-blind, placebo-controlled study of ranolazine compared with placebo in patients with HFpEF. Patients with LVEF greater than 45%, echo E/e′ greater than 15, NT-proBNP greater than 220 pg/mL, LVEDP greater than 18 mm Hg, and time constant of relaxation tau greater than 50 ms were randomized to receive an infusion of ranolazine for 24 hours followed by 1000 mg twice daily for 14 days ($n = 12$) or placebo ($n = 8$). There was a significant decline in LVEDP ($P = 0.04$) as well as PCWP ($P = 0.04$) 30 minutes after infusion of ranolazine but not with placebo.[76] Mean pulmonary artery pressure showed a trend toward a decrease in the ranolazine group that was significant under pacing conditions at 120 beats/min ($P = 0.02$), but not for the placebo group. These changes occurred without changes in LV end-systolic pressure or systemic or pulmonary resistance but in the presence of a small but significant decrease in cardiac output ($P = 0.04$). Relaxation parameters were unaltered. Echocardiographically, the E/e′ ratio did not significantly change after 22 hours. After 14 days of treatment, no significant changes were observed in echocardiographic or cardiopulmonary exercise test parameters without significant changes in NT-proBNP levels. The clinical significance of the results of this small short-term study with ranolazine improving some hemodynamic measures but without any improvement in relaxation parameters remains uncertain at this time.

POTENTIAL DEVICE-BASED THERAPY

Treatment of Obstructive Sleep Apnea

Obstructive sleep apnea (OSA) has been detected in 11% to 37% of patients with HF with systolic dysfunction,[77,78] but in a small study, sleep-disordered breathing was reported in greater than 50% of patients with HFpEF, with most patients having OSA (see also Chapter 12).[79] Patients with HFpEF and sleep-disordered breathing had worse diastolic dysfunction compared with patients without sleep-disordered breathing. Unlike systolic HF, where a number of studies have shown an increased prevalence of central sleep apnea, HFpEF may be more often associated with OSA. Several theoretical mechanisms are postulated for the contribution of OSA toward the development of diastolic dysfunction and HF.[80] The most direct mechanism may be through longstanding OSA causing hypertension, a major risk factor for the development and progression of HFpEF. LV hypertrophy may be more closely linked to hypertension during sleep than during wakefulness.[81] Thus the higher nocturnal blood pressure in hypertensive patients with OSA may place such individuals at greater risk in the long term for LV hypertrophy and HF. In patients with HF, the coexistence of OSA may also be associated with higher sympathetic nerve activity and higher systolic blood pressure during wakefulness, despite more intense antihypertensive therapy.[82] Responses to cytokines, catecholamines, endothelin, and other growth factors produced in OSA may also contribute to ventricular hypertrophy independently of hypertension. In addition, nocturnal oxygen desaturation is an independent predictor of impaired ventricular relaxation.[83] Long-term exposure to markedly subatmospheric pressure during OSA could also promote hypertrophy and diastolic dysfunction. Furthermore, a leftward shift of the interventricular septum due to overdistention of the right ventricle during OSAs may limit LV filling and thus decrease cardiac output. Some of these cardiovascular changes may be reversible with effective continuous positive airway pressure (CPAP) treatment.[80]

At this time, little evidence is available regarding the benefit of CPAP on patients with HFpEF. In a small group of patients with OSA, but without hypertension, diabetes, and other factors that could contribute to diastolic dysfunction, 12 weeks of CPAP was reported to attenuate abnormalities in diastolic function.[84] Adaptive servo ventilation, a novel method of noninvasive positive airway pressure that continuously monitors breathing patterns and provides real time adjusted airway support for patients with sleep-disordered breathing, was evaluated in another small study of HFpEF patients with moderate to severe sleep-disordered breathing (apnea-hypopnea index >15/hr; 18 patients, 18 controls). After 6 months, patients treated with adaptive servo-ventilation had improvement in diastolic function, BNP, and NYHA class, and during a longer follow-up period (mean 543 days), the treated patients had lower cardiac event rates (death and rehospitalization for worsening HF; $P < 0.01$) as compared with controls.[85] Larger clinical outcome studies are, however, needed to examine the clinical benefit of CPAP in patients with HFpEF.

Pacemakers

Patients with HFpEF also have chronotropic incompetence in response to exercise that may contribute to significant limitation of their physical activity. Borlaug and colleagues showed that at matched low-level workload as well as at peak workload, patients with HFpEF had less of an increase in heart rate and cardiac output and less systemic vasodilation than control subjects despite a similar rise in end-diastolic volume, stroke volume, and contractility.[12] Although these findings first question the conventional wisdom of using β-blockers, which are negative chronotropic agents, in HFpEF patients, especially the elderly, they also provide a potential target for treatment of HFpEF. One such trial to evaluate the effect of atrial rate-responsive pacing on exercise capacity and quality of life in patients with HFpEF, the Restoration of Chronotropic Competence in Heart Failure Patients With Normal Ejection Fraction (RESET) trial, was terminated because of difficulties with patient enrollment, and future trials evaluating this therapy are awaited (NCT00670111).[70]

Device-Based Treatment of Resistant Hypertension

Several patients with HFpEF have uncontrolled hypertension that is resistant to a combination of multiple antihypertensive agents (see also Chapter 23). The importance of the carotid sinus baroreceptors in modulating autonomic tone and regulating blood pressure has long been recognized (baroreflex mechanism). It is also well established that the arterial baroreflex buffers short-term fluctuations in blood pressure. Although its role in long-term blood pressure control has been debated, studies suggest that the baroreflex system is important in chronic hypertension and that renal sympathoinhibition with a resultant increase in natriuresis may be one of the mechanisms by which the baroreflex participates in long-term blood pressure control. Animal and human studies have demonstrated a safe and effective lowering of blood pressure with chronic electrical stimulation of the carotid sinus. The postulated mechanism is that activation of the baroreceptors is interpreted by the brain as elevation in blood pressure with resultant activation of the cardiac parasympathetic tone along with diminished sympathetic outflow to the heart, kidneys, and peripheral vasculature.[86,87] The most recent studies have been performed with the Rheos System (CVRx, Inc.). The system consists of an implantable pulse generator, the energy from which is conducted through leads to the left and right carotid sinus resulting in carotid sinus stimulation (**Figure 36-7**). Based on initial studies suggesting significant benefit in blood pressure reduction, the blood pressure–lowering efficacy and safety of this device were investigated in a multicenter randomized clinical trial (phase III Rheos Pivotal Trial) among 265 patients with resistant hypertension.[88] After device implantation, one set of subjects started active baroreflex therapy (BAT) 1 month later (group 1), whereas the second group (group 2) was randomized to a delayed treatment limb with the device activated after 6 months. There were five primary outcomes prespecified: acute efficacy, sustained efficacy, procedural safety, BAT safety, and device safety. Overall the results were mixed. The trial successfully met three of the five outcomes in that the sustained efficacy endpoint fulfilled an objective performance criterion of maintaining at least half the initial 6-month reduction in systolic blood pressure out to 12 months and the BAT safety endpoint and the device safety endpoints were met. Although the acute response endpoint was not met, the overall trial was encouraging in that those patients who did demonstrate a reduction in blood pressure initially were able to maintain it at 12 months. There was no "tachyphylaxis" or resetting of the baroreflex system to overcome the benefits seen. The implication is that while the blood pressure reductions demonstrated with BAT require some duration of therapy to exhibit the full effect, presumptively related to a need to reset the neurovascular tone, the reduction was durable in nature. However, there were also some concerning treatment-induced adverse events related to lead placement including transient (4.4%) or permanent nerve injury (4.8%), along with a 4.8% surgical complication rate and procedure safety yielded an event-free rate of 74.8%. Future studies are planned that may employ improved technology (device miniaturization) along with less invasive implantation procedures and predominantly unilateral carotid stimulation (which was shown to be successful for inducing blood pressure lowering among 75% of subjects in the pivot trial). Also, a phase II randomized, placebo-controlled study with this system has been completed to examine the safety and efficacy of baroreceptor activation on LV mass in 60 patients with HFpEF and the results are awaited (see Table 36-2).[70] Of note, a different approach using catheter-based renal sympathetic denervation also has been recently reported to show similar significant and sustained improvement in blood pressure in patients with resistant hypertension.[89] It is likely that a sustained improvement of blood pressure in

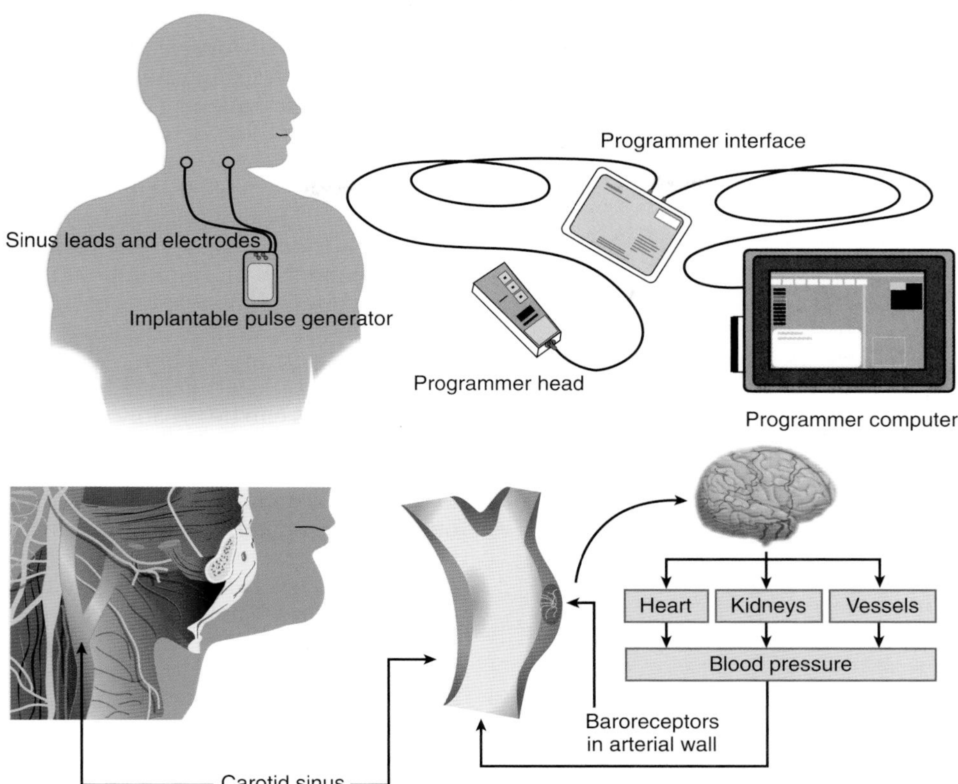

FIGURE 36-7 Representation of Rheos system (CVRx) of carotid baroreceptor stimulation. *Modified from Krum H, Schlaich M, Sobotka P, et al: Novel procedure- and device-based strategies in the management of systemic hypertension. Eur Heart J 32:537–544, 2011.*

patients with HFpEF and resistant hypertension will translate into improvement in cardiovascular outcomes.

Targeting Diastolic Suction

Another mechanism being targeted is a proposed abnormality of early diastolic suction of the left ventricle in patients with diastolic HF. The elastic recoil of the ventricle during early diastole contributes significantly to an early diastolic pressure gradient from the left atrium to the LV apex and allows the left ventricle to actively "suck" blood from the left atrium during early diastole, thus contributing to early LV filling.[90,91] Diastolic suction allows the LV to decrease its pressure despite its filling during early diastole. A major determinant of diastolic suction is the potential energy stored as myocytes are compressed and the elastic elements in the LV wall are compressed and twisted during systole. This energy is released as the elastic elements recoil during relaxation. With diastolic dysfunction (slowed relaxation and reduced elastic recoil), this diastolic suction is reduced and LV early filling is likely impaired. A series of passive diastolic assist devices (CorAssist Cardiovascular Limited) are being developed and studied.[92] The initial device, ImCardia, is attached to the epimyocardial surface of the left ventricle. The design is based on the principle of restoring normal balance of myocardial dynamic energy by the transfer of energy from preserved systole to underfunctioning diastole in a stiff ventricle. Potential energy produced by the left ventricle during systole is stored in the device—essentially being loaded like a spring—and is released during diastole, providing a recoiling force to restore the myocardium to its resting length. After initial feasibility and proof of concept studies in animals, initial small studies are under way in human subjects.[93,94]

EXERCISE TRAINING IN HFpEF

Exercise intolerance is often one of the debilitating symptoms in patients with HFpEF (see also Chapter 15). A meta-analysis of five studies evaluated the benefit of exercise training in patients with HFpEF. Three randomized controlled trials, one non-randomized controlled trial and one pre-post study were included (total n = 228).[95-100] The combined duration of exercise programs and follow-up ranged from 12 to 24 weeks. Exercise was found to be safe with no deaths, hospital admissions, or serious adverse events observed during or immediately following exercise training. In four trials that used peak oxygen uptake as an endpoint, compared with control, the change in exercise capacity was higher with exercise training (between-group mean difference: 3.0 mL/kg/min, 95% CI 2.4-2.6). In the four studies using the Minnesota Living with Heart Failure questionnaire, there was evidence of a larger gain in health-related quality of life with exercise training (7.3 units, 95% CI 3.3-11.4). The largest study showed some evidence of improvement in the echocardiographic E/e′ ratio with exercise training, but this was not confirmed in the other studies. In another recently reported trial, the Prospective Aerobic Reconditioning Intervention Study (PARIS), a total of 63 HFpEF patients (mean age 70) were randomized to 16 weeks of exercise training or to attention control.[101] In the exercise training group, after 16 weeks peak oxygen consumption improved significantly compared with controls, without a significant change in

TABLE 36-3 Exercise Regimens Used in Clinical Trials in HFpEF

STUDY	EXERCISE REGIMEN USED
Edelman et al[96]	Supervised center-based, 24-week aerobic (cycling): Weeks 1-4: 2 sessions/week, 20-40 min/session, 50%-60% peak V_{O_2}; Weeks 5-12: 3 sessions/ week, 20-40 min/session, 70% peak V_{O_2} plus resistance training
Gary et al[99]	Self-monitored community-based, 12-week aerobic (walking) exercise: 3 sessions/week, 30-40 min/ session, 40%-70% THR
Kitzman et al[97]	Supervised center-based, 16-week aerobic (cycling) exercise: 3 sessions/week, 1 hr/session, 40%-70% HRR
Kitzman et al[101]	Supervised: 3 sessions/week, 1 hr/session for 16 weeks Aerobic (track and cycle ergometry) and isolated arm ergometry; 40%-70% HRR
Korzeniowska-Kubacka et al[98]	Supervised center-based, 18-week aerobic (cycling and gymnastics) exercise: 3 sessions/week, 40 min/session, 80% maximum HR
Smart et al[100]	Supervised center-based, 16-week aerobic (cycling) exercise: 3 sessions/week, 1 hr/session, 60%-70% peak V_{O_2} plus resistance training weeks 8-16

HR, Heart rate; *HRR,* heart rate reserve; *THR,* target heart rate.

endothelial function or arterial stiffness. In another small randomized trial of 26 patients with HFpEF (median age 73 years), inspiratory muscle training for 12 weeks was associated with significant improvement in maximal inspiratory pressure, peak V_{O_2}, exercise oxygen uptake at anaerobic threshold, ventilatory efficiency, 6-minute walk distance, and quality of life as compared with the control group. No changes on diastolic function parameters or biomarker levels were observed between both groups.[102] The findings of these two trials, as well as other mechanistic studies, suggest that improvement in peripheral mechanisms, such as enhanced skeletal muscle perfusion and/or oxygen use, rather than central cardiovascular mechanisms may be responsible for the exercise-mediated increase in peak V_{O_2} in older HFpEF patients.[103] The training programs used in these trials are described in **Table 36-3**. Although data for improvement in clinical outcomes with exercise training in HFpEF is not available, the results of the described studies are promising if the improvement in exercise capacity as well as quality of life can be demonstrated in larger multicenter trials and sustained over longer periods of time.

CURRENT RECOMMENDATIONS FOR THE MANAGEMENT OF PATIENTS WITH HFpEF

The clinical diagnosis of HFpEF depends on the presence of clinical symptoms and signs of HF with preserved LVEF (≥45% or 50%) measured by any cardiac imaging technique. The presence of diastolic abnormalities, evidence of elevated LV filling pressures and left atrial enlargement, as well as substrate for diastolic dysfunction (i.e., LV hypertrophy) on echocardiography may provide supportive evidence. Although considered rudimentary, the clinical confirmation of the diagnosis of HF is key, especially in ruling out other causes of symptoms such as lung disease and obesity. Several conditions need to be considered in the differential diagnosis before treating for the prototypic "diastolic heart failure" or HFpEF. The algorithm suggested in the Heart Failure Society of America Heart Failure Practice Guidelines provides a useful guiding framework for the initial workup of these patients (**Figure 36-8**).[104] Conditions that require specific intervention need to be identified, such as valvular heart disease, coronary artery disease, pericardial disease, isolated right HF due to primary pulmonary conditions, or contributing systemic conditions such as anemia and thyrotoxicosis. Once these conditions are ruled out or treated, patients with HFpEF should be managed based on the general recommendations provided by the most recent 2013 American College of Cardiology Foundation and American Heart Association (ACCF/AHA) Guideline for the Management of Heart Failure (**Table 36G-1**).[105] Treatment considerations can be broadly grouped under the following categories: treatment of volume overload; aggressive control of hypertension; treatment of factors contributing to decompensation, most commonly atrial fibrillation; uncontrolled hypertension, ischemia, anemia, and infections; and therapies based on associated cardiovascular diagnoses or risk factors. Of note in the practice guidelines, most recommendations (other than the treatment of hypertension and possible consideration of ARBs to reduce hospitalization) are based on consensus opinion of experts rather than on definitive clinical trial data. In addition, the general principles of treatment of HF can be applied to patients with HFpEF in regard to fluid and salt restriction and avoidance of potentially harmful drugs, such as nonsteroidal anti-inflammatory agents and thiazolidinediones. In contrast to patients with HF with reduced ejection fraction, nondihydropyridine calcium channel blockers with potential negative inotropic effects such as diltiazem and verapamil could be considered to treat hypertension and angina, and to control the rate in atrial fibrillation, in patients with HFpEF.

SUMMARY AND FUTURE DIRECTIONS

The recognition of the high prevalence of HFpEF, with its associated substantial morbidity and mortality, has initiated a quest for effective therapy for the condition. Unlike in systolic HF, where RAAS blockers have been proven to have definite beneficial effects on mortality and morbidity, none of the clinical trials to date with ACE inhibitors or ARBs has demonstrated definitive benefit in clinical outcomes in patients with HFpEF. A number of novel therapies that are being currently tested for HFpEF are targeting alternate pathophysiologic mechanisms. At present, recommended therapy is aimed at relief of symptoms, control of hypertension, and management of other contributory comorbidities. Although RAAS blockers and β-blockers are not routinely recommended at present specifically for the treatment of HFpEF, their use will remain important for proven indications for other comorbid conditions that frequently coexist. We may need to reconsider traditional endpoints such as mortality for the efficacy evaluation of therapies in patients with HFpEF, a highly comorbid population with many competing risks for mortality, and we need to consider whether hospitalization and exercise capacity are more meaningful endpoints in this patient population. In addition, because of the heterogeneity of patients with HFpEF, it may be difficult to prove a "one-size-fits-all" therapeutic agent and there may be a need to study relevant interventions in more homogeneous subgroups of patients.

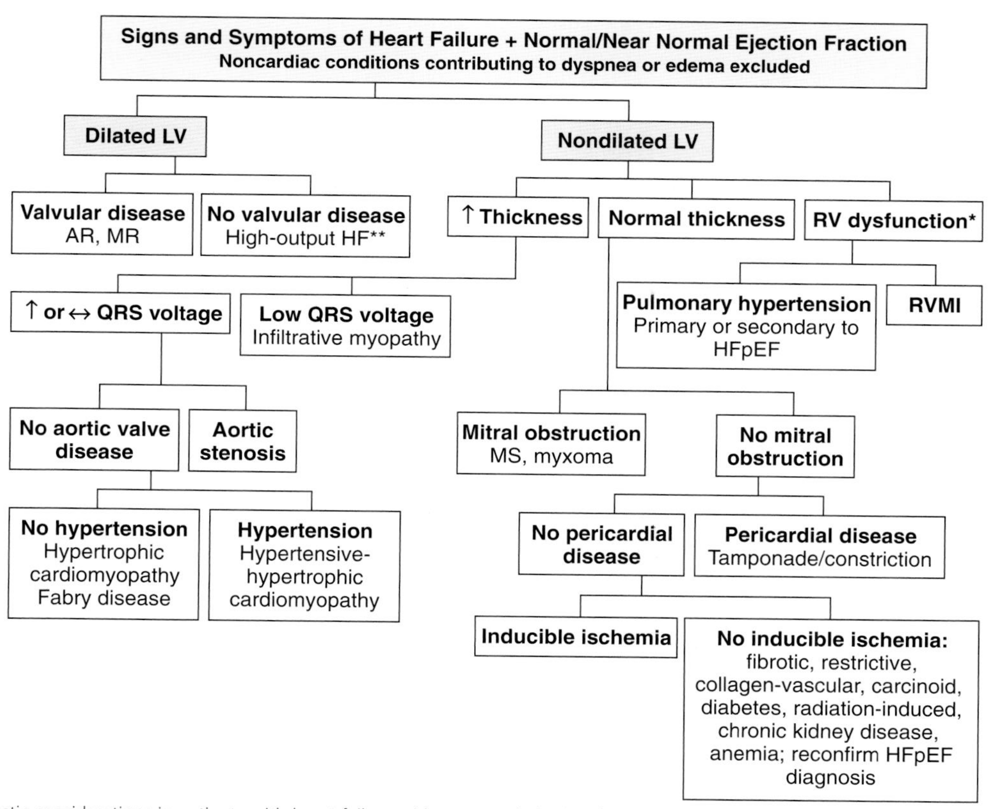

FIGURE 36-8 Diagnostic considerations in patients with heart failure with preserved ejection fraction. *Some patients with right ventricular dysfunction have LV dysfunction due to ventricular interaction. **E.g., anemia, thyrotoxicosis, arteriovenous fistulae. *AR,* Aortic regurgitation; *HF,* heart failure; *HFpEF,* heart failure with preserved ejection fraction; *LV,* left ventricle; *MR,* mitral regurgitation; *MS,* mitral stenosis; *RV,* right ventricl; *RVMI,* right ventricular myocardial infarction. *Adapted from Adams KF, Lindenfeld J, Arnold JMO, et al: Executive summary: HFSA 2006 comprehensive heart failure practice guideline. J Card Fail 12:10–38, 2006.*

References

1. Hogg K, Swedberg K, McMurray J: Heart failure with preserved left ventricular systolic function; epidemiology, clinical characteristics, and prognosis. *J Am Coll Cardiol* 43:317–327, 2004.
2. Kitzman DW, Gardin JM, Gottdiener JS, et al: Importance of heart failure with preserved systolic function in patients ≥65 years of age. *Am J Cardiol* 87:413–419, 2001.
3. Cleland JG, Swedberg K, Follath F, et al: The EuroHeart Failure survey programme—a survey on the quality of care among patients with heart failure in Europe. Part 1: patient characteristics and diagnosis. *Eur Heart J* 24:442–463, 2003.
4. Fonarow GC: The Acute Decompensated Heart Failure National Registry (ADHERE): opportunities to improve care of patients hospitalized with acute decompensated heart failure. *Rev Cardiovasc Med* 4(Suppl 7):S21–S30, 2003.
5. Cohen-Solal A, Desnos M, Delahaye F, et al: A national survey of heart failure in French hospitals. The Myocardiopathy and Heart Failure Working Group of the French Society of Cardiology, the National College of General Hospital Cardiologists and the French Geriatrics Society. *Eur Heart J* 21:763–769, 2000.
6. Zile MR: Heart failure with preserved ejection fraction: is this diastolic heart failure? *J Am Coll Cardiol* 41:1519–1522, 2003.
7. Owan TE, Hodge DO, Herges RM, et al: Trends in prevalence and outcome of heart failure with preserved ejection fraction. *N Engl J Med* 355:251–259, 2006.
8. Little WC, Brucks S: Therapy for diastolic heart failure. *Prog Cardiovasc Dis* 47:380–388, 2005.
9. Zile MR, Baicu CF, Gaasch WH: Diastolic heart failure—abnormalities in active relaxation and passive stiffness of the left ventricle. *N Engl J Med* 350:1953–1959, 2004.
10. Zile MR, Gaasch WH, Carroll JD, et al: Heart failure with a normal ejection fraction: is measurement of diastolic function necessary to make the diagnosis of diastolic heart failure? *Circulation* 104:779–782, 2001.
11. Kawaguchi M, Hay I, Fetics B, et al: Combined ventricular systolic and arterial stiffening in patients with heart failure and preserved ejection fraction: implications for systolic and diastolic reserve limitations. *Circulation* 107:714–720, 2003.
12. Borlaug BA, Melenovsky V, Russell SD, et al: Impaired chronotropic and vasodilator reserves limit exercise capacity in patients with heart failure and a preserved ejection fraction. *Circulation* 114:2138–2147, 2006.
13. Maurer MS, King DL, El Khoury RL, et al: Left heart failure with a normal ejection fraction: identification of different pathophysiologic mechanisms. *J Card Fail* 11:177–187, 2005.
14. Zile MR, Brutsaert DL: New concepts in diastolic dysfunction and diastolic heart failure: Part II: causal mechanisms and treatment. *Circulation* 105:1503–1508, 2002.
15. Deswal A, Bozkurt B, Pritchett A, et al: Worsening renal function in hospitalized heart failure patients with preserved vs. reduced ejection fraction. *Circulation* 122:A11035, 2010.
16. Felker GM, Lee KL, Bull DA, et al: Diuretic strategies in patients with acute decompensated heart failure. *N Engl J Med* 364:797–805, 2011.
17. Little WC, Badke FR, O'Rourke RA: Effect of right ventricular pressure on the end-diastolic left ventricular pressure-volume relationship before and after chronic right ventricular pressure overload in dogs without pericardia. *Circ Res* 54:719–730, 1984.
18. Dauterman K, Pak PH, Maughan WL, et al: Contribution of external forces to left ventricular diastolic pressure: implications for the clinical use of the Starling law. *Ann Intern Med* 122:737–742, 1995.
19. The ALLHAT Officers and Coordinators for the ALLHAT Collaborative Research Group: Major outcomes in high-risk hypertensive patients randomized to angiotensin-converting enzyme inhibitor or calcium channel blocker vs diuretic: the Antihypertensive and Lipid-Lowering Treatment to Prevent Heart Attack Trial (ALLHAT). *JAMA* 288:2981–2997, 2002.
20. Kostis JB, Davis BR, Cutler J, et al: Prevention of heart failure by antihypertensive drug treatment in older persons with isolated systolic hypertension. *JAMA* 278:212–216, 1997.
21. Matter CM, Mandinov L, Kaufmann PA, et al: Effect of NO donors on LV diastolic function in patients with severe pressure-overload hypertrophy. *Circulation* 99:2396–2401, 1999.
22. Hoit BD, Walsh RA: In Gaasch WH, LeWinter MM, editors: *Left ventricular diastolic dysfunction and heart failure,* Philadelphia, 1994, Lea & Febiger, pp 354–372.
23. Leite-Moreira AF, Correia-Pinto J: Load as an acute determinant of end-diastolic pressure-volume relation. *Am J Physiol Heart Circ Physiol* 280:H51–H59, 2001.
24. Hundley WG, Kitzman DW, Morgan TM, et al: Cardiac cycle-dependent changes in aortic area and distensibility are reduced in older patients with isolated diastolic heart failure and correlate with exercise intolerance. *J Am Coll Cardiol* 38:796–802, 2001.
25. Little WC, Ohno M, Kitzman DW, et al: Determination of left ventricular chamber stiffness from the time for deceleration of early left ventricular filling. *Circulation* 92:1933–1939, 1995.
26. Devereux RB, Palmieri V, Sharpe N, et al: Effects of once-daily angiotensin-converting enzyme inhibition and calcium channel blockade-based antihypertensive treatment regimens on left ventricular hypertrophy and diastolic filling in hypertension: the prospective randomized enalapril study evaluating regression of ventricular enlargement (preserve). *trial. Circulation* 104:1248–1254, 2001.
27. Solomon SD, Janardhanan R, Verma A, et al: Effect of angiotensin receptor blockade and antihypertensive drugs on diastolic function in patients with hypertension and diastolic dysfunction: a randomised trial. *Lancet* 369:2079–2087, 2007.
28. Moser M, Hebert PR: Prevention of disease progression, left ventricular hypertrophy and congestive heart failure in hypertension treatment trials. *J Am Coll Cardiol* 27:1214–1218, 1996.
29. Beckett NS, Peters R, Fletcher AE, et al: Treatment of hypertension in patients 80 years of age or older. *N Engl J Med* 358:1887–1898, 2008.
30. Yamamoto K, Masuyama T, Sakata Y, et al: Roles of renin-angiotensin and endothelin systems in development of diastolic heart failure in hypertensive hearts. *Cardiovasc Res* 47:274–283, 2000.
31. Martos R, Baugh J, Ledwidge M, et al: Diastolic heart failure: evidence of increased myocardial collagen turnover linked to diastolic dysfunction. *Circulation* 115:888–895, 2007.
32. Cheng CP, Ukai T, Onishi K, et al: The role of ANG II and endothelin-1 in exercise-induced diastolic dysfunction in heart failure. *Am J Physiol Heart Circ Physiol* 280:H1853–H1860, 2001.
33. Yusuf S, Sleight P, Pogue J, et al: Effects of an angiotensin-converting-enzyme inhibitor, ramipril, on cardiovascular events in high-risk patients. The Heart Outcomes Prevention Evaluation Study Investigators. *N Engl J Med* 342:145–153, 2000.
34. Dagenais GR, Pogue J, Fox K, et al: Angiotensin-converting-enzyme inhibitors in stable vascular disease without left ventricular systolic dysfunction or heart failure: a combined analysis of three trials. *Lancet* 368:581–588, 2006.
35. Yusuf S, Pfeffer MA, Swedberg K, et al: Effects of candesartan in patients with chronic heart failure and preserved left-ventricular ejection fraction: the CHARM-Preserved Trial. *Lancet* 362:777–781, 2003.

36. Cleland JGF, Tendera M, Adamus J, et al: The perindopril in elderly people with chronic heart failure (PEP-CHF) study. *Eur Heart J* 27:2338–2345, 2006.
37. Massie BM, Carson PE, McMurray JJ, et al: Irbesartan in patients with heart failure and preserved ejection fraction. *N Engl J Med* 359:2456–2467, 2008.
38. Edelmann F, Wachter R, Schmidt AG, et al: Effect of spironolactone on diastolic function and exercise capacity in patients with heart failure with preserved ejection fraction: the Aldo-DHF randomized controlled trial. *JAMA* 309:781–791, 2013.
39. Deswal A, Richardson P, Bozkurt B, et al: Results of the Randomized Aldosterone Antagonism in Heart Failure with Preserved Ejection Fraction trial (RAAM-PEF). *J Card Fail* 17:634–642, 2011.
40. Pitt B, Pfeffer MA, Assmann SF, et al: TOPCAT Investigators. Spironolactone for heart failure with preserved ejection fraction. *N Engl J Med* 370(15):1383–1392, 2014.
41. Gardner DG, Chen S, Glenn DJ, et al: Molecular biology of the natriuretic peptide system: implications for physiology and hypertension. *Hypertension* 49:419–426, 2007.
42. Potter LR, Abbey-Hosch S, Dickey DM: Natriuretic peptides, their receptors, and cyclic guanosine monophosphate-dependent signaling functions. *Endocr Rev* 27:47–72, 2006.
43. Kostis JB, Packer M, Black HR, et al: Omapatrilat and enalapril in patients with hypertension: the Omapatrilat Cardiovascular Treatment vs. Enalapril (OCTAVE) trial. *Am J Hypertens* 17:103–111, 2004.
44. Ruilope LM, Dukat A, Bohm M, et al: Blood-pressure reduction with LCZ696, a novel dual-acting inhibitor of the angiotensin II receptor and neprilysin: a randomised, double-blind, placebo-controlled, active comparator study. *Lancet* 375:1255–1266, 2010.
45. Solomon SD, Zile M, Pieske B, et al: The angiotensin receptor neprilysin inhibitor LCZ696 in heart failure with preserved ejection fraction: a phase 2 double-blind randomised controlled trial. *Lancet* 380:1387–1395, 2012.
46. Bergstrom A, Andersson B, Edner M, et al: Effect of carvedilol on diastolic function in patients with diastolic heart failure and preserved systolic function. Results of the Swedish Doppler-echocardiographic study (SWEDIC). *Eur J Heart Fail* 6:453–461, 2004.
47. Hori M, Kitabatake A, Tsutsui H, et al: Rationale and design of a randomized trial to assess the effects of beta-blocker in diastolic heart failure; Japanese Diastolic Heart Failure Study (J-DHF). *J Card Fail* 11:542–547, 2005.
48. Yamamoto K, Origasa H, Hori M: Effects of carvedilol on heart failure with preserved ejection fraction: the Japanese Diastolic Heart Failure Study (J-DHF). *Eur J Heart Fail* 15:110–118, 2013.
49. Kamp O, Metra M, Bugatti S, et al: Nebivolol. *Drugs* 70:41–56, 2010.
50. Flather MD, Shibata MC, Coats AJ, et al: Randomized trial to determine the effect of nebivolol on mortality and cardiovascular hospital admission in elderly patients with heart failure (SENIORS). *Eur Heart J* 26:215–225, 2005.
51. Conraads VM, Metra M, Kamp O, et al: Effects of the long-term administration of nebivolol on the clinical symptoms, exercise capacity, and left ventricular function of patients with diastolic dysfunction: results of the ELANDD study. *Eur J Heart Fail* 14:219–225, 2012.
52. Semigran MJ: Type 5 phosphodiesterase inhibition: the focus shifts to the heart. *Circulation* 112:2589–2591, 2005.
53. Nony P, Boissel JP, Lievre M, et al: Evaluation of the effect of phosphodiesterase inhibitors on mortality in chronic heart failure patients. A meta-analysis. *Eur J Clin Pharmacol* 46:191–196, 1994.
54. Takimoto E, Champion HC, Li M, et al: Chronic inhibition of cyclic GMP phosphodiesterase 5A prevents and reverses cardiac hypertrophy. *Nat Med* 11:214–222, 2005.
55. Nagayama T, Hsu S, Zhang M, et al: Sildenafil stops progressive chamber, cellular, and molecular remodeling and improves calcium handling and function in hearts with pre-existing advanced hypertrophy caused by pressure overload. *J Am Coll Cardiol* 53:207–215, 2009.
56. Katz SD, Balidemaj K, Homma S, et al: Acute type 5 phosphodiesterase inhibition with sildenafil enhances flow-mediated vasodilation in patients with chronic heart failure. *J Am Coll Cardiol* 36:845–851, 2000.
57. Mahmud A, Hennessy M, Feely J: Effect of sildenafil on blood pressure and arterial wave reflection in treated hypertensive men. *J Hum Hypertens* 15:707–713, 2001.
58. Ghofrani HA, Osterloh IH, Grimminger F: Sildenafil: from angina to erectile dysfunction to pulmonary hypertension and beyond. *Nat Rev Drug Discov* 5:689–702, 2006.
59. Chen HH, Huntley BK, Schirger JA, et al: Maximizing the renal cyclic 3′-5(-guanosine monophosphate system with type V phosphodiesterase inhibition and exogenous natriuretic peptide: a novel strategy to improve renal function in experimental overt heart failure. *J Am Soc Nephrol* 17:2742–2747, 2006.
60. Redfield MM, Chen HH, Borlaug BA, et al: Effect of phosphodiesterase-5 inhibition on exercise capacity and clinical status in heart failure with preserved ejection fraction: a randomized clinical trial. *JAMA* 309:1268–1277, 2013.
61. Guazzi M, Vicenzi M, Arena R, et al: PDE5 inhibition with sildenafil improves left ventricular diastolic function, cardiac geometry, and clinical status in patients with stable systolic heart failure: results of a 1-year, prospective, randomized, placebo-controlled study. *Circ Heart Fail* 4:8–17, 2011.
62. Massie BM, Abdalla I: Heart failure in patients with preserved left ventricular systolic function: do digitalis glycosides have a role? *Prog Cardiovasc Dis* 40:357–369, 1998.
63. Digitalis Investigation Group: The effect of digoxin on mortality and morbidity in patients with heart failure. *N Engl J Med* 336:525–533, 1997.
64. Ahmed A, Rich MW, Fleg JL, et al: Effects of digoxin on morbidity and mortality in diastolic heart failure: the ancillary digitalis investigation group trial. *Circulation* 114:397–403, 2006.
65. Yamamoto K, Masuyama T, Sakata Y, et al: Prevention of diastolic heart failure by endothelin type A receptor antagonist through inhibition of ventricular structural remodeling in hypertensive heart. *J Hypertens* 20:753–761, 2002.
66. Zile MR, Barst RJ, Bourge R, et al: Phase 2 randomized, double-blind, placebo-controlled exploratory efficacy study of sitaxsentan sodium to improve impaired exercise tolerance in subjects with diastolic heart failure. *J Card Fail* 15:S63, 2009.
67. Zile MR, Brutsaert DL: New concepts in diastolic dysfunction and diastolic heart failure: Part I: diagnosis, prognosis, and measurements of diastolic function. *Circulation* 105:1387–1393, 2002.
68. Kass DA, Shapiro EP, Kawaguchi M, et al: Improved arterial compliance by a novel advanced glycation end-product crosslink breaker. *Circulation* 104:1464–1470, 2001.
69. Little WC, Zile MR, Kitzman DW, et al: The effect of alagebrium chloride (ALT-711), a novel glucose cross-link breaker, in the treatment of elderly patients with diastolic heart failure. *J Card Fail* 11:191–195, 2005.
70. U.S. NIH clinical trials website. www.clinicaltrials.gov. 2013.
71. Bujak M, Frangogiannis NG: The role of IL-1 in the pathogenesis of heart disease. *Arch Immunol Ther Exp (Warsz)* 57:165–176, 2009.
72. Van Tassell BW, Arena RA, Toldo S, et al: Enhanced interleukin-1 activity contributes to exercise intolerance in patients with systolic heart failure. *PLoS ONE* 7:e33438, 2012.
73. Valdivia CR, Chu WW, Pu J, et al: Increased late sodium current in myocytes from a canine heart failure model and from failing human heart. *J Mol Cell Cardiol* 38:475–483, 2005.
74. Hasenfuss G, Maier LS: Mechanism of action of the new anti-ischemia drug ranolazine. *Clin Res Cardiol* 97:222–226, 2008.
75. Sossalla S, Wagner S, Rasenack EC, et al: Ranolazine improves diastolic dysfunction in isolated myocardium from failing human hearts—role of late sodium current and intracellular ion accumulation. *J Mol Cell Cardiol* 45:32–43, 2008.
76. Maier LS, Layug B, Karwatowska-Prokopczuk E, et al: RAnoLazIne for the treatment of diastolic heart failure in patients with preserved ejection fraction: the RALI-DHF proof-of-concept study. *JACC: Heart Fail* 1:115–122, 2013.
77. Javaheri S, Parker TJ, Liming JD, et al: Sleep apnea in 81 ambulatory male patients with stable heart failure: types and their prevalences, consequences, and presentations. *Circulation* 97:2154–2159, 1998.
78. Lanfranchi PA, Somers VK, Braghiroli A, et al: Central sleep apnea in left ventricular dysfunction: prevalence and implications for arrhythmic risk. *Circulation* 107:727–732, 2003.
79. Chan J, Sanderson J, Chan W, et al: Prevalence of sleep-disordered breathing in diastolic heart failure. *Chest* 111:1488–1493, 1997.
80. Somers VK, White DP, Amin R, et al: Sleep apnea and cardiovascular disease: an American Heart Association/American College of Cardiology Foundation Scientific Statement From the American Heart Association Council for High Blood Pressure Research Professional Education Committee, Council on Clinical Cardiology, Stroke Council, and Council on Cardiovascular Nursing In Collaboration With the National Heart, Lung, and Blood Institute National Center on Sleep Disorders Research (National Institutes of Health). *J Am Coll Cardiol* 52:686–717, 2008.
81. Verdecchia P, Schillaci G, Guerrieri M, et al: Circadian blood pressure changes and left ventricular hypertrophy in essential hypertension. *Circulation* 81:528–536, 1990.
82. Spaak J, Egri ZJ, Kubo T, et al: Muscle sympathetic nerve activity during wakefulness in heart failure patients with and without sleep apnea. *Hypertension* 46:1327–1332, 2005.
83. Fung JW, Li TS, Choy DK, et al: Severe obstructive sleep apnea is associated with left ventricular diastolic dysfunction. *Chest* 121:422–429, 2002.
84. Arias MA, Garcia-Rio F, Onso-Fernandez A, et al: Obstructive sleep apnea syndrome affects left ventricular diastolic function: effects of nasal continuous positive airway pressure in men. *Circulation* 112:375–383, 2005.
85. Yoshihisa A, Suzuki S, Yamaki T, et al: Impact of adaptive servo-ventilation on cardiovascular function and prognosis in heart failure patients with preserved left ventricular ejection fraction and sleep-disordered breathing. *Eur J Heart Fail* 15:543–550, 2013.
86. Filippone JD, Bisognano JD: Baroreflex stimulation in the treatment of hypertension. *Curr Opin Nephrol Hypertens* 16:403–408, 2007.
87. Krum H, Schlaich M, Sobotka P, et al: Novel procedure- and device-based strategies in the management of systemic hypertension. *Eur Heart J* 32:537–544, 2011.
88. Bisognano JD, Bakris G, Nadim MK, et al: Baroreflex activation therapy lowers blood pressure in patients with resistant hypertension: results from the double-blind, randomized, placebo-controlled rheos pivotal trial. *J Am Coll Cardiol* 58:765–773, 2011.
89. Krum H, Schlaich M, Whitbourn R, et al: Catheter-based renal sympathetic denervation for resistant hypertension: a multicentre safety and proof-of-principle cohort study. *Lancet* 373:1275–1281, 2009.
90. Cheng CP, Freeman GL, Santamore WP, et al: Effect of loading conditions, contractile state, and heart rate on early diastolic left ventricular filling in conscious dogs. *Circ Res* 66:814–823, 1990.
91. Little WC: Diastolic dysfunction beyond distensibility: adverse effects of ventricular dilatation. *Circulation* 112:2888–2890, 2005.
92. Feld Y, Dubi S, Reisner Y, et al: Future strategies for the treatment of diastolic heart failure. *Acute Card Care* 8:13–20, 2006.
93. Little WC, Schwammenthal E, Dubi S, et al: Safety of new device-based approach for treating diastolic heart failure. *J Card Fail* 13:S120, 2007.
94. Elami A, Sherman A, Lak L, et al: Efficacy assessment of a new device-based approach for treating diastolic heart failure. *J Card Fail* 14(Suppl 6S):46, 2008.
95. Taylor RS, Davies EJ, Dalal HM, et al: Effects of exercise training for heart failure with preserved ejection fraction: a systematic review and meta-analysis of comparative studies. *Int J Cardiol* 162:6–13, 2012.
96. Edelmann F, Gelbrich G, Düngen HD, et al: Exercise training improves exercise capacity and diastolic function in patients with heart failure with preserved ejection fraction: results of the Ex-DHF (Exercise training in Diastolic Heart Failure) Pilot Study. *J Am Coll Cardiol* 58:1780–1791, 2011.
97. Kitzman DW, Brubaker PH, Morgan TM, et al: Exercise training in older patients with heart failure and preserved ejection fraction: a randomized, controlled, single-blind trial. *Circ Heart Fail* 3:659–667, 2010.
98. Korzeniowska-Kubacka I, Bilinska M, Michalak E, et al: Influence of exercise training on left ventricular diastolic function and its relationship to exercise capacity in patients after myocardial infarction. *Cardiol J* 17:136–142, 2010.
99. Gary R, Lee SY: Physical function and quality of life in older women with diastolic heart failure: effects of a progressive walking program on sleep patterns. *Prog Cardiovasc Nurs* 22:72–80, 2007.
100. Smart N, Haluska B, Jeffriess L, et al: Exercise training in systolic and diastolic dysfunction: effects on cardiac function, functional capacity, and quality of life. *Am Heart J* 153:530–536, 2007.
101. Kitzman DW, Brubaker PH, Herrington DM, et al: Effect of endurance exercise training on endothelial function and arterial stiffness in older patients with heart failure and preserved ejection fraction: a randomized, controlled, single-blind trial. *J Am Coll Cardiol* 62:584–592, 2013.
102. Palau P, Dominguez E, Nunez E, et al: Effects of inspiratory muscle training in patients with heart failure with preserved ejection fraction. *Eur J Prev Cardiol* 21:1465–1473, 2014.
103. Kitzman DW, Haykowsky MJ: Invited editorial commentary for American Heart Journal mechanisms of exercise training in heart failure with preserved ejection fraction: central disappointment and peripheral promise. *Am Heart J* 164:807–809, 2012.
104. Lindenfeld J, Albert NM, Boehmer JP, et al: HFSA 2010 comprehensive heart failure practice guideline. *J Card Fail* 16:e1–e194, 2010.
105. Yancy CW, Jessup M, Bozkurt B, et al: 2013 ACCF/AHA guideline for the management of heart failure: a report of the American College of Cardiology Foundation/American Heart Association Task Force on Practice Guidelines. *J Am Coll Cardiol* 62:e147–e239, 2013.
106. Shah SJ, Heitner JF, Sweitzer NK, et al: Baseline characteristics of patients in the treatment of preserved cardiac function heart failure with an aldosterone antagonist trial. *Circ Heart Fail* 6:184–192, 2013.

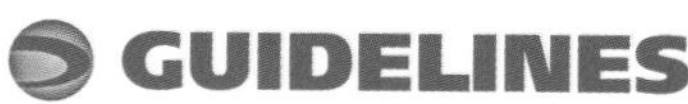

Treatment of Heart Failure with Preserved Ejection Fraction

TABLE 36G-1 Guideline Recommendations for the Treatment of Patients with HFpEF

RECOMMENDATIONS	CLASS OF RECOMMENDATION	LEVEL OF EVIDENCE
Systolic and diastolic blood pressure should be controlled according to published guidelines.	I	B
Diuretics should be used for relief of symptoms due to volume overload.	I	C
Coronary revascularization for patients with CAD in whom angina or demonstrable myocardial ischemia is present despite medical therapy.	IIa	C
Management of atrial fibrillation according to published guidelines in patients with HFpEF is reasonable to improve symptomatic HF.	IIa	C
Use of β-blockers, ACE inhibitors, and ARBs for hypertension in patients with HFpEF.	IIa	C
ARBs might be considered to decrease hospitalizations for patients with HFpEF.	IIb	B
Nutritional supplementation is not recommended in HFpEF.	III	C

Recommendations in the table are from the 2013 ACCF/AHA Guideline for the Management of Heart Failure.[1]

Strength of recommendations: Class I: Recommendation that treatment is useful or effective; Class IIa: Recommendation in favor of treatment being useful or effective; Class IIb: Greater conflicting evidence from multiple randomized trials or meta-analyses.

Level of Evidence: A: Data derived from multiple randomized clinical trials or meta-analyses; B: Data derived from a single randomized clinical trial or nonrandomized studies; C: Only consensus opinion of experts, case studies, or standard of care.

ACE, Angiotensin-converting enzyme; *ARB,* angiotensin receptor blocker; *CAD,* coronary artery disease; *HFpEF,* heart failure with preserved ejection fraction.

REFERENCE

1. Yancy CW, Jessup M, Bozkurt B, et al: 2013 ACCF/AHA guideline for the management of heart failure: a report of the American College of Cardiology Foundation/American Heart Association Task Force on Practice Guidelines. *J Am Coll Cardiol* 62:e147–e239, 2013.

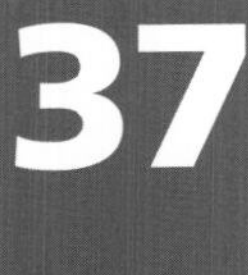

Management of Heart Failure in Special Populations: Older Patients, Women, and Racial/Ethnic Minority Groups

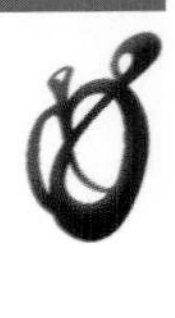

Susan M. Joseph, Angela L. Brown, Mathew S. Maurer, and Michael W. Rich

Although heart failure (HF) affects all segments of the population, older patients, women, and racial and ethnic minority groups have been markedly underrepresented in most major HF trials. This chapter provides a brief summary of the epidemiology, clinical features, and management of HF in these large and important subgroups of the HF population.

HEART FAILURE IN OLDER PATIENTS

Epidemiology

Heart failure (HF) is principally a disorder of older adults with prevalence and incidence rates that increase progressively with age. Of the greater than 6 million adults with HF in the United States, 50% are at least 75 years of age and prevalence among those over the age of 80 years is greater than 11% (see also Chapter 17). The disparity between genders seen in younger adults is abolished at advanced age with a slightly higher prevalence in women than men.[1] The prevalence and incidence of HF are similar in older whites and African-Americans.

In addition to age, risk factors for the development of HF in the older population include male gender, ischemic heart disease, systolic hypertension, widened pulse pressure, diabetes,[2] chronic lung disease, renal dysfunction, atrial fibrillation, left ventricular hypertrophy,[2] and obesity.[3] Of these risk factors, systolic hypertension has the greatest population attributable risk (see Chapter 23), especially among women, for the development of HF. HF has a profound impact on quality of life in older adults and is an independent risk factor for cessation of driving[4] and loss of functional capacity as evidenced by a decline in activities of daily living (ADLs) and independent ADLs (IADLs).[5]

Incident heart failure in older adult patients is predominantly characterized by the phenotype of HF with normal or preserved left ventricular (LV) systolic function (HFpEF)[6] (see also Chapter 36). More than 50% of older HF patients have HFpEF and the proportion increases with age.[7-10] There is also a female preponderance in HFpEF. Women with HFpEF are more likely than men to be older, obese, and to have chronic kidney disease and hypertension, but less likely to have an ischemic cause, atrial fibrillation, or chronic obstructive pulmonary disease.[11] Thus the profile of the typical older person with HF contrasts with that of middle-aged patients enrolled in HF trials (**Table 37-1**).

Prognosis

Older age is an independent predictor of reduced survival in patients with HF. In addition, common age-associated comorbidities, such as anemia, chronic kidney disease, and cognitive impairment, contribute to increased mortality after adjusting for age, gender, and race.[12]

Although the overall hospitalization rate for HF has declined from 1998 to 2008,[13] hospitalization for HFpEF is increasing relative to HF with reduced ejection fraction (HFrEF).[14] Among Medicare beneficiaries, HF is associated with the highest 30-day readmission rate.[15] Among older patients discharged with HF, most 30-day readmissions are for conditions other than HF, suggesting that interventional strategies will need to be patient-centered rather than HF-specific.[16] Despite major advances in HF therapy over the past two to three decades, overall mortality rates among patients with HFpEF have not declined (see also Chapter 36).[8] In the Framingham Heart Study, the annual mortality rate for HFpEF was 8.9% (i.e., about twofold higher than age-matched controls), but only half that reported for HFrEF

TABLE 37-1 Heart Failure in Older Adults

CHARACTERISTIC	OLDER ADULTS	MIDDLE AGED
Prevalence	≈10%	<1%
Incidence (per 1000)	>10	2-3
Gender	Predominantly women	Predominantly men
Etiology	Hypertension	Coronary artery disease
LV systolic function	Normal or preserved	Impaired
Comorbidities	Multiple	Few

LV, Left ventricular.

(19.6%).[17] However, among patients hospitalized for HF, mortality is similar in HFpEF and HFrEF.

Data from community-dwelling elderly subjects with HF suggest that the cause of death differs between patients with HFpEF versus HFrEF. Among patients with HFpEF, noncardiovascular conditions were the leading cause of death (49%), whereas coronary heart disease accounted for the greatest proportion (43%) in patients with HFrEF.

Pathophysiology

The pathophysiology of HF differs in older compared with younger adults because of age-related declines in cardiovascular reserve.[18,19] As a result, mild to moderate stressors that would be well tolerated in younger patients can precipitate acute HF in older adults. Age-related changes in other organ systems can also impair the ability of older adults to compensate for HF and can alter the response to pharmacologic therapy. The superimposition of normal aging changes implies that at equivalent levels of pathophysiology, the clinical severity of HF is more advanced in older patients (i.e., higher New York Heart Association [NYHA] functional class).

Diagnosis and Clinical Features

Elderly HF patients have chronic exercise intolerance, reduced quality of life, frequent hospitalizations, and high health care costs. Importantly, morbidity is *similar* in patients with either HFrEF or HFpEF. Notably, exercise intolerance in older HFpEF patients is as severe as in those with HFrEF, and impairments in quality of life are comparable.[20]

The diagnosis of HF is challenging in older adults who are more likely to have other conditions that mimic the symptoms and signs of HF. A reliable history may be more difficult to obtain because of cognitive dysfunction or sensory impairment, making corroborating history from a family member or caregiver very helpful. Atypical presentations are more common in older adults in whom HF may manifest as somnolence, confusion, disorientation, weakness, fatigue, gastrointestinal disturbances, or failure to thrive. Older adults may fail to perceive a gradual but progressive decline in exercise tolerance, and physicians often attribute this to advancing age or other conditions, thereby limiting early identification of HF. Care must be taken to exclude other potential causes for the signs and symptoms of HF (**Table 37-2**). Serial assessments of functional capacity using standard tests (e.g., 6-minute walk distance and gait speed)[21,22] and evaluation of ADLs and IADLs[23] can be helpful adjuncts in quantifying and monitoring functional

TABLE 37-2 Challenges to the Diagnosis of Heart Failure in Older Adults

CHALLENGE	EXAMPLE
Atypical symptoms	Malaise, confusion, irritability, anorexia, sleep disturbance, decreased activity, abdominal complaints
Alternative explanations for symptoms and signs	Fluid retention: drugs (NSAIDs), venous insufficiency Dyspnea: chronic lung disease, anemia, pneumonia Fatigue: anemia, hypothyroidism, obesity, deconditioning, depression Lower extremity edema: calcium channel blockers, venous insufficiency
Minimize symptoms	"I just can't get around, I'm 87."
Fewer exertional symptoms	Osteoarthritis, sarcopenia, loss of balance, poor vision

NSAIDs, Nonsteroidal anti-inflammatory drugs.

capacity. Both chest radiography and echocardiography have lower specificity for diagnosing HF in the elderly, thus contributing to diagnostic uncertainty.[24]

Natriuretic peptide assays aid in diagnosing HF, assessing disease severity, and evaluating response to treatment (see also Chapter 30). Natriuretic peptide levels increase mildly with aging, are higher in women than in men, and are affected by renal function, anemia and obesity; thus the specificity of the assays is reduced in older patients.[25]

Amyloidosis (see also Chapter 20)

Senile cardiac amyloidosis is a disorder that typically afflicts older adult males with an average age at clinical diagnosis of 70 to 75 years.[26] In this form of amyloidosis, deposition of insoluble protein fibrils impairs cardiac tissue structure and function. Amyloid infiltration results in a restrictive cardiomyopathy, atrial arrhythmias, heart failure, and advanced conduction disease. These disorders are more common than previously thought,[26] and the diagnosis of transthyretin (TTR) cardiac amyloidosis has become easier in recent years with advances in cardiac imaging and more widespread use of genetic analysis. Current therapy includes supportive medical care, avoidance of potentially toxic agents (including digoxin and calcium channel blockers, which can promote high degree heart block), and rarely organ transplantation. However, novel approaches that target the underlying biologic mechanisms of this disorder are under development. These therapies aim to stabilize the TTR tetramer,[27] thereby preventing the precursor protein from forming the amyloid fibrils that are deposited in the heart and nerves, or silencing TTR using siRNA or oligonucleotides.[28,29]

Cognitive Dysfunction

Cognitive dysfunction is highly prevalent in older patients with HF, ranging from 25% to 80%,[30] which is almost double the prevalence in age-matched cohorts.[31] Conservative estimates suggest that at least 25% to 30% of older adults with HF have some degree of cognitive dysfunction.[32] Cognitive impairment independently predicts mortality in patients with HF, and the magnitude of effect is similar to traditional measures, such as ejection fraction or systolic blood pressure.[32] Patients with HF are also at significantly increased

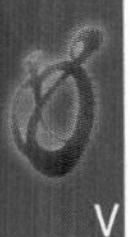

risk for dementia.[33] Because of the variable manifestations of cognitive dysfunction in patients with HF, particularly in the early stages, periodic cognitive screening is recommended.

Given the chronic nature of HF and the importance of self-care in management (i.e., adherence to a complex and ever-changing medical regimen, the need to follow dietary restrictions, monitoring of symptoms, engaging in exercise or physical therapy, and keeping follow-up appointments with multiple providers), altered cognitive function can significantly contribute to adverse outcomes, including recurrent hospitalizations and mortality.[32,34-36] Unfortunately, despite the negative impact of cognitive dysfunction on outcomes, these deficits often go unrecognized.[37] Accordingly, implementation of strategies to improve recognition of cognitive impairment and tailoring treatment to individuals with cognitive dysfunction may enhance patient care and outcomes.[38]

Identification of cognitive impairment in older adults with HF should prompt interventions to maximize adherence to self-management programs and minimize the hazards of complex medical regimens. As the risk for adverse drug effects increases exponentially with the number of drugs prescribed, all unnecessary (and perhaps even some indicated) medications should be discontinued. Basic principles of transitional care dictate that early clinical follow-up is essential in this vulnerable subset of patients. Clear written instructions and communication of medication changes to individuals assisting frail older adults with HF is mandatory. If mobility limits an older adult's ability to attend an office visit, then an early postdischarge home health visit by trained allied health professionals should be scheduled to reduce unplanned readmissions or death.

Treatment

Goals of therapy in older HF patients include relief of symptoms, improvement in functional capacity and quality of life, reduction in hospital admissions, and improved survival. In older patients, preservation of independence and maintenance of a satisfactory quality of life may be more important than survival.[39] Optimal management requires a systematic approach comprising (1) accurate diagnosis, (2) search for reversible or treatable causes, (3) judicious use of medications, (4) management of risk factors, (5) patient and caregiver education, (6) enhancement of self-management skills, (7) coordination of care across disciplines, and (8) close follow-up. Given these complexities, a team approach to treating heart failure in older patients is critical (**Table 37-3**). Several studies have confirmed the efficacy of a multidisciplinary approach to care in reducing hospitalizations, improving quality of life, reducing total costs, and, in one study, increasing survival (see also Chapter 44). Many of these studies included older patients who are ideal candidates for multidisciplinary care. One randomized trial involving patients aged 70 and older with either HFpEF or HFrEF demonstrated a 56% reduction in 90-day HF rehospitalizations.[40] Other important strategies in HF disease management include (1) smoking cessation, (2) moderation in alcohol use, (3) administration of pneumococcal and influenza vaccinations, (4) control of polypharmacy and over-the-counter medications, (5) consideration of cardiac rehabilitation, and (6) palliative care and end-of-life planning.

TABLE 37-3 Multidisciplinary Team for Older Adults with Heart Failure

POTENTIAL CONSULTANTS	ROLES
Geriatrician	Provides comprehensive evaluation and management strategy for all medical, social, and psychological issues
Palliative care consultation	Provides evaluation and management strategy to address palliative care needs including but not limited to pain, dyspnea, depression, and end of life issues
Nurse practitioner	Provides ongoing patient and family education, disease management
Medical subspecialists	Assist in managing comorbid conditions including renal insufficiency, arthritis, chronic lung disease, etc.
Psychiatrist	Evaluate for and treat comorbid psychiatric conditions, including depression, delirium, and dementia
Pharmacist	Systematically evaluate for medication appropriateness, proper dosing, and drug-drug interactions
Physical therapist	Assess home safety, evaluate rehabilitation potential, and develop individualized physical therapy program
Occupational therapist	Evaluate home and determine safety of environment, provide alternative approaches to perform activities
Nutritionist	Evaluate current dietary intake, modify diet to limit salt intake, manage caloric content, and develop appropriate diets for patients with comorbid conditions, including obesity, diabetes, and chronic renal disease
Social worker	Evaluate psychosocial situation, assist in family counseling, ensure optimal use of health care services, and engage in long-term care planning

Pharmacologic Interventions for HFrEF (see also Chapter 34)

Although clinical trials have demonstrated the beneficial effects of ACE inhibitors in patients with HFrEF, older patients have been underrepresented and there have been no specific trials evaluating outcomes in the elderly. However, a meta-analysis of published trials with stratification by age (<55 years, 55-64 years, 65-74 years, ≥75 years) demonstrated no heterogeneity in treatment effects by age for the combined outcomes of death or myocardial infarction (MI) and death or readmission for HF, suggesting a consistent benefit even among those over the age of 75 years.[41,42] The use of ACE inhibitors in older patients may be complicated by preexisting renal dysfunction, renal artery stenosis, orthostatic hypotension, and increased susceptibility to side effects because of concomitant therapy with NSAIDs or other medications.

Angiotensin-receptor blockers (ARBs) are a reasonable alternative to ACE inhibitors in chronic HF, but since many older adults have low serum sodium, diabetes mellitus, or impaired renal function, combination therapy with an ACE inhibitor and ARB is not recommended because of increased risk for adverse events without clear benefit.

Several large randomized trials have shown that long-term β-blockade is beneficial in patients with HFrEF. Patients up to age 80 have been included in these trials, and subgroup analyses indicate that β-blockers are as effective in older as in younger adults. Older patients often have relative contraindications to β-blockers, such as bradycardia, heart block, bronchospastic lung disease, or severe

TABLE 37-4 Clinical Trials in Heart Failure with Preserved Ejection Fraction

TRIAL	MEAN AGE	DRUG	EF	RESULTS
DIG Study	63	Digoxin	>45	No reduction in composite of death or HF hospitalization (HR 0.82; 95% CI 0.63-1.07)
CHARM-P	67	Candesartan	>40	No mortality benefit (HR 0.89; 95% CI 0.77-1.03; $P = 0.118$); ↓ 3-yr hospitalizations ($P = 0.017$)
SWEDIC	67	Carvedilol	>45	No significant change in composite diastolic LV function; ↑ E/A ($P \le 0.05$)
PEP-CHF	75	Perindopril	≥40	No mortality benefit was seen over 2.1 yr (HR 0.92; 95% CI 0.70-1.21, $P = 0.545$), ↓ 1-yr hospitalizations (HR 0.628; 95% CI 0.408-0.966; $P = 0.033$)
SENIORS	76	Nebivolol	≥35	No reduction in composite all-cause mortality or CV hospitalizations (HR (0.81; 95% CI 0.63-1.04; $P = 0.720$)
I-PRESERVE	72	Irbesartan	≥40	No reduction over 49.5 months of follow-up in composite all-cause mortality or CV hospitalizations (HR 0.95; 95% CI 0.86-1.05; $P = 0.35$)
RAAM-PEF	70	Eplerenone	≥50	No improvement ($P = 0.91$) in 6MWD
ELAND	66	Nebivolol	>45	No improvement ($P = 0.094$) in 6MWD
TOPCAT	69	Spironolactone	≥45	No reduction in composite CV mortality, aborted cardiac arrest, or HF admission (HR 0.89, 95% CI 0.77-1.04, $P = 0.14$); HF admissions reduced (HR 0.83, 95% CI 0.69-0.99, $P = 0.04$)
RELAX	69	Sildenafil	<50	No improvement in exercise capacity or clincal status

6MWD, Six-minute walk distance; *CI*, confidence interval; *CV*, cardiovascular; *EF*, ejection fraction; *HF*, heart failure; *HR*, hazard ratio; *LV*, left ventricular.

peripheral arterial disease. Nonetheless, indications for β-blockers are similar in older and younger patients with HFrEF, although initiation and dose titration should be more cautious.

The DIG study demonstrated similar effects of digoxin in younger and older patients, but toxicity was more common in older adults. The volume of distribution and renal clearance of digoxin decline with age, so that lower doses (e.g., 0.125 mg daily or less) are needed to achieve a therapeutic effect in older adults.

In the Randomized Aldactone Evaluation Study (RALES), subgroup analysis showed similar mortality benefits in patients ≥ 67 years of age (relative risk 0.68) compared with those less than 67 years of age (relative risk 0.74). Because the incidence of serious hyperkalemia is more common in older adults prescribed spironolactone in usual care settings, close monitoring is warranted for side effects including renal impairment and hyperkalemia.

Pharmacologic Interventions for HFpEF

Pharmacologic therapies for HFpEF have been reviewed in detail in Chapter 36. As shown in **Table 37-4**, although some of these agents exhibited favorable effects on surrogate or secondary outcomes, all of the trials were negative for the primary endpoint, and none of the drugs have been shown to reduce mortality. In the PEP-CHF trial, perindopril improved symptoms and exercise capacity and reduced hospitalizations for HF in the first year, but did not reduce long-term morbidity or mortality.[43] β-adrenergic antagonists reduce blood pressure, promote regression of ventricular hypertrophy, and increase the ischemic threshold, all of which may have theoretical importance in HFpEF, but these agents have not been shown to improve outcomes in older adults with HFpEF. Similarly, in the DIG Ancillary Trial, digoxin had no effect on mortality or hospitalizations in HFpEF patients.[44] In the Aldo-DHF trial, spironolactone induced reverse remodeling, reduced neuroendocrine activation, and improved diastolic function, but there was no improvement in HF symptoms or quality of life, peak oxygen consumption did not change significantly, and 6-minute walking distance was slightly reduced compared with a placebo.[45] In the TOPCAT trial, spironolactone did not reduce the primary composite endpoint of cardiovascular mortality, aborted cardiac arrest, or HF hospitalization, but HF hospitalizations were reduced by 17%. Finally, the RELAX trial evaluating phosphodiesterase-5 inhibition in a heterogeneous population of older adults with HFpEF failed to demonstrate any clinical benefit.[46]

Although extracardiac comorbidities are common in older adults with HF and have been suggested as potential therapeutic targets,[47] recent trials of erythropoiesis-stimulating agents for treating anemia in subjects with HFrEF[48] and HFpEF[49] have not demonstrated efficacy.

Biomarker-Guided Therapy (see also Chapter 30)

Given the high prevalence of chronic HF in older adults, coupled with the fact that HF is associated with the highest rate of 30-day readmissions of all chronic conditions,[15] there has been significant interest in the use of biomarkers to guide therapy. The TIME-CHF investigators[50] demonstrated that HF therapy guided by N-terminal BNP did not improve overall clinical outcomes or quality of life compared with symptom-guided treatment in a cohort of older adults. A meta-analysis of 12 randomized studies[51] demonstrated that the use of cardiac peptides to guide pharmacologic therapy significantly reduced mortality and HF hospitalizations in patients with chronic HF. However, there was a strong interaction with age, such that outcomes were significantly improved by natriuretic peptide-guided therapy in younger patients (≤75 years; odds ratio [OR] 0.45, 95% confidence interval [CI] 0.21 to 0.97, $P = 0.043$), but not in older patients (>75 years; OR 0.80, 95% CI 0.42 to 1.51, $P = 0.493$).

Nonpharmacologic Interventions

Although pharmacologic interventions for HFpEF in older adults have been disappointing, nonpharmacologic approaches, including diet and exercise, are emerging as promising areas of investigation. Indeed, an exercise training study demonstrated improved peak oxygen consumption mediated primarily to be an increase in peak arterial-venous oxygen difference. This suggests that peripheral mechanisms (i.e., improved microvascular and/or skeletal muscle function) contribute to improved exercise capacity after exercise training in HFpEF.[52] Dietary interventions are also

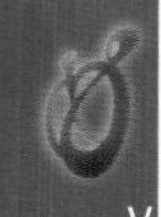

understudied in older adults, especially those with HFpEF. In animal studies, salt sensitivity is associated with a low renin state accompanied by renal dysfunction, hypertension, and obesity. In a small study in patients with HFpEF, the DASH/sodium restriction diet reduced systolic blood pressure, arterial stiffness, and oxidative stress and improved submaximal exercise tolerance,[53] suggesting that additional investigation of dietary interventions is warranted.

HEART FAILURE IN WOMEN

Epidemiology (see also Chapter 17)

More than 40% of HF patients are women, and among the elderly the prevalence of heart failure is greater in women than in men.[54,55] Women with HF are twice as likely to have HFpEF compared with men,[56,57] and women with HFrEF tend to have a higher left ventricular ejection fraction (LVEF) than men.[56,57] In the Atherosclerosis Risk in Communities Study, white women had the lowest age-adjusted rate of developing HF at 3.4 per 1000 person-years, as compared with white men (6.0), black women (8.1), and black men (9.1).[58] In Olmstead County, Minnesota, the incidence of HF increased 8% in women and 3% in men from 1979 to 2000,[59] whereas the Framingham investigators reported an increase in HF incidence for both women and men from 1980 to 1999.[60] During both time periods, age-adjusted 5-year mortality rates declined for both sexes.[17,59] Although age-adjusted HF incidence is higher in men than in women, men also have shorter survival.[59,60] However, the female survival advantage is limited to patients with nonischemic HF.[60]

Clinical Features

In the SOLVD database, women with chronic HF and impaired LV systolic function were more likely than men to have dependent edema, jugular venous distention, and an S_3 gallop.[61] However, women (n = 54,674) in the ADHERE registry for acute decompensated HF (impaired and preserved systolic function) did not differ from men (n = 50,713) with respect to the frequency of HF symptoms and signs.[56]

Comorbidities differ between men and women. Compared with men, women with HF are more likely to have hypertension, whereas men are more likely to have coronary artery disease (CAD) and a history of smoking. In the A-HeFT trial,[62] African American women had lower hemoglobin and more diabetes but less renal insufficiency than men. Thyroid disease is more frequent in women with acute decompensated HF, whereas chronic obstructive lung disease, peripheral vascular disease, and renal insufficiency are more common in men.[56,57] Pregnancy-related cardiomyopathy, a condition unique to women, is discussed in more detail in Chapter 19.

Data regarding sex differences for biomarkers of HF are scarce. A recent study demonstrated that levels of biomarkers related to inflammation, including C-reactive protein and interleukin 6, were significantly lower in women than in men. In this study, mortality was also lower in women compared with men, independent of differences in clinical characteristics.[63]

Women with HF tend to have lower quality of life than men, with greater impairment in functional capacity,[64] more HF hospitalizations,[55,56,64] and more depression.[65] Although women are more likely than men to have HFpEF, two large observational studies showed similar mortality rates for patients with HFpEF or HFrEF.[8,66]

Ischemic Heart Failure in Women (see also Chapter 18)

Women develop ischemic heart disease at an older age than men. Although coronary artery disease (CAD) is a less common cause of HF in women than in men, the presence of CAD is a more potent risk factor for HF than hypertension in both sexes.[67] Diabetes mellitus is common in both men and women with HF,[56] and it is a strong risk factor for the development of HF in women with CAD.[68]

Therapy in Women

Although women have been included in clinical trials in greater numbers than minorities, they have still been significantly underrepresented. Thus evidence-based treatment guidelines for HF therapy provide similar recommendations for men and women.[69] Although some studies have shown that women hospitalized with HF receive HF medications at similar rates as men,[70-72] others have reported that women receive less evidence-based therapies or are less likely to reach target doses of medications.[73] Notably, the Get With the Guidelines HF Registry demonstrated that women and men were treated equally with respect to most guideline-recommended HF therapies and that use of ACE inhibitors and β-blockers approached 90% in both genders.[74]

Angiotensin-Converting Enzyme Inhibitors

A meta-analysis of 30 ACE inhibitor studies that included a total of 1587 women with HF demonstrated trends toward improvement in survival (13.4% vs. 20.1%) and in the combined endpoint of survival and hospitalization (20.2% vs. 29.5%) among women randomized to ACE inhibitors[75] (**Table 37-5** and **Figure 37-1**).[76]

TABLE 37-5 Effect of ACE Inhibitors on Mortality by Sex

STUDY NAME	MALE *N*	FEMALE *N*	RR MALE (95% CI)	RR FEMALE (95% CI)
CONSENSUS	179	74	0.61 (0.44-0.85)	1.14 (0.68-1.90)
SAVE	1841	390	0.80 (0.68-0.95)	0.99 (0.67-1.47)
SMILE	1128	428	0.61 (0.39-0.96)	0.74 (0.47-1.18)
SOLVD-Prevention	3752	476	0.90 (0.77-1.05)	1.15 (0.74-1.78)
SOLVD-Treatment	2065	504	0.89 (0.80-0.99)	0.86 (0.67-1.09)
TRACE	1248	501	0.79 (0.68-0.91)	0.90 (0.74-1.11)
Random effects pooled estimate	*10,213*	*2373*	*0.82 (0.74-0.90)*	*0.92 (0.81-1.04)*

RR, Relative risk.

From Shekelle PG, Rich MW, Morton SC, et al: Efficacy of angiotensin-converting enzyme inhibitors and beta-blockers in the management of left ventricular systolic dysfunction according to race, gender, and diabetic status. J Am Coll Cardiol 41:1529–1538, 2003.

Angiotensin Receptor Blockers

Sex-specific data for ARBs are limited. Pooled data from the CHARM-Alternative and the CHARM-Added trials that included 1188 women with NYHA functional class II-IV HF and LVEF ≤ 40% showed that candesartan reduced the combined endpoint of cardiovascular death or HF hospitalization in women.[77] In the CHARM-Overall population, reduction in the combined endpoint was similar for men and women (**Figure 37-2**).[77]

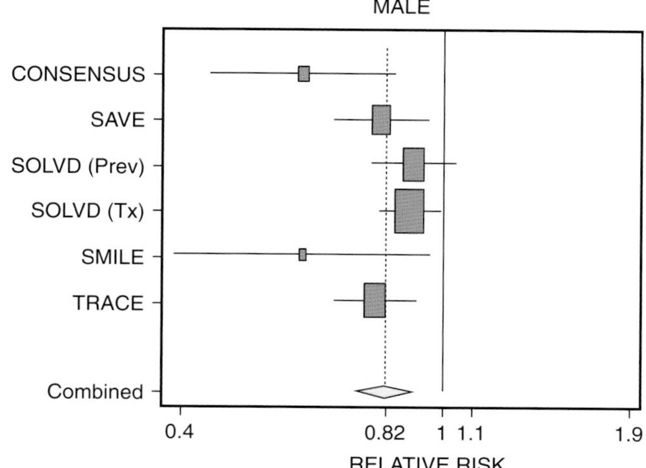

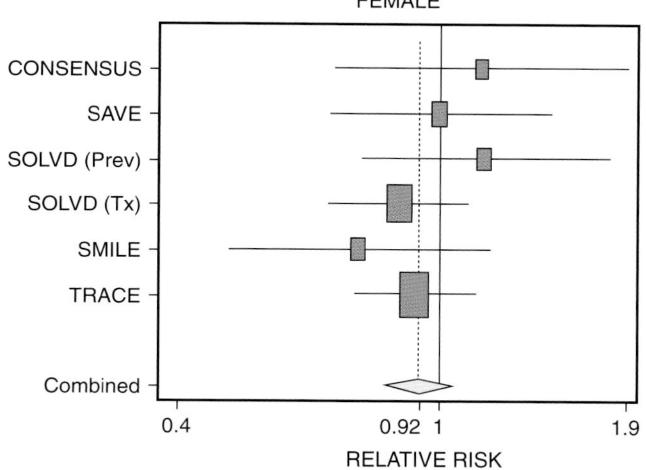

FIGURE 37-1 Effect of angiotensin-converting enzyme inhibitors and β-blockers in the management of left ventricular systolic dysfunction according to race, gender, and diabetic status. *From Shekelle PG, Rich MW, Morton SC, et al: Efficacy of angiotensin-converting enzyme inhibitors and beta-blockers in the management of left ventricular systolic dysfunction according to race, gender, and diabetic status. J Am Coll Cardiol 41:1529–1538, 2003.*

β-Blockers

As with ACE-Is and ARBs, meta-analyses of β-blocker trials suggest that these agents are equally beneficial in women and men with HF (**Table 37-6**).

Aldosterone Antagonists

Subgroup analysis of the RALES trial with spironolactone and the EPHESUS trial with eplerenone revealed similar mortality benefits for men and women with systolic HF.[78,79]

Hydralazine/Isosorbide Dinitrate

The early Veterans Administration HF trials using the combination of hydralazine/isosorbide dinitrate were limited to men.[80,81] In the African American Heart Failure Trial, combination hydralazine/isosorbide dinitrate was added to ACE inhibitor/ARB and β-blocker therapy in 1050 self-identified African Americans with NYHA functional class III-IV HF (420 women). Survival benefits were noted for both women (HR 0.33, 95% CI 0.16-0.71, $P = 0.003$) and men (HR 0.79, 95% CI 0.46-1.35, $P = 0.385$) with no significant treatment interaction by sex.[62]

Digoxin

In a post hoc subgroup analysis of the Digitalis Investigation Group (DIG) trial, women with HF and impaired systolic function (LVEF <45%) were reported to have increased mortality when treated with digoxin compared with a placebo (adjusted HR 1.23, 95% CI 1.02-1.47), whereas in men digoxin had no effect on mortality (adjusted HR 0.93, 95% CI 0.85-1.02).[82,83] However, subsequent analysis of the DIG trial data showed that digoxin at serum concentrations of 0.5 to 0.9 ng/mL was safe and effective for both women and men.[84]

Cardiac Resynchronization Therapy (CRT) (see also Chapter 35)

Although few studies have reported sex-specific data, there is some evidence that women may derive greater benefit from CRT compared with men. In the MADIT-CRT trial, which randomized 1367 men and 453 women with an LVEF ≤ 30% and NYHA class II HF to CRT plus implantable cardioverter-defibrillator (ICD) versus ICD alone, CRT was associated with better outcomes and greater degree of reverse remodeling in women compared with men.[85] In the Comparison of Medical Therapy, Pacing, and Defibrillation in Heart Failure (COMPANION) study, which included 299

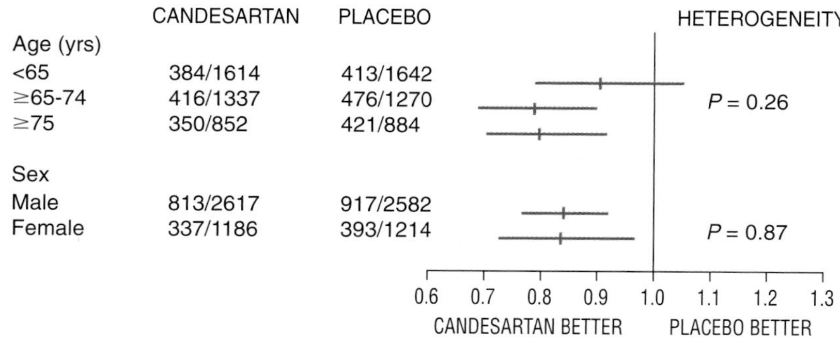

FIGURE 37-2 Effects of candesartan on cardiovascular death or heart failure hospitalizations in the CHARM study. *From Pfeffer MA, Swedberg K, Granger CB, et al: Effects of candesartan on mortality and morbidity in patients with chronic heart failure: the CHARM-Overall programme. Lancet 362:759–766, 2003.*

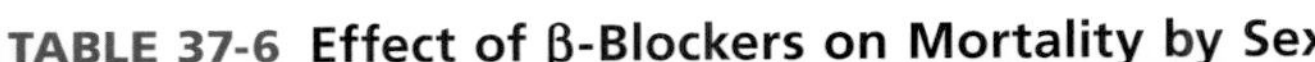

TABLE 37-6 Effect of β-Blockers on Mortality by Sex

STUDY NAME	MALE N	FEMALE N	RR MALE (95% CI)	RR FEMALE (95% CI)
CIBIS-II	2132	515	0.71 (0.58-0.87)	0.52 (0.30-0.89)
COOPERNICUS	1822	465	0.68 (0.54-0.86)	0.63 (0.39-1.04)
MERIT-HF	3093	898	0.63 (0.50-0.78)	0.93 (0.58-1.49)
U.S. carvedilol HF	838	256	0.44 (0.24-0.82)	0.32 (0.11-0.93)
Random effects pooled estimate	7885	2134	0.66 (0.59-0.75)	0.63 (0.44-0.91)

CI, Confidence interval; *RR*, relative risk.
From Shekelle PG, Rich MW, Morton SC, et al: Efficacy of angiotensin-converting enzyme inhibitors and beta-blockers in the management of left ventricular systolic dysfunction according to race, gender, and diabetic status. J Am Coll Cardiol 41:1529–1538, 2003.

STUDY NAME	HAZARD RATIO	(95% CI)	NO. OF WOMEN	P VALUE
MUSTT	1.64	(0.92–2.92)	68	0.09
MADIT II	0.57	(0.28–1.18)	192	0.12
DINAMIT	1.00	(0.49–2.04)	160	>0.99
DEFINITE	1.14	(0.50–2.64)	132	0.76
SCD-HeFT	0.90	(0.56–1.43)	382	0.66
Combined	**1.01**	**(0.76–1.33)**	**934**	**0.95**

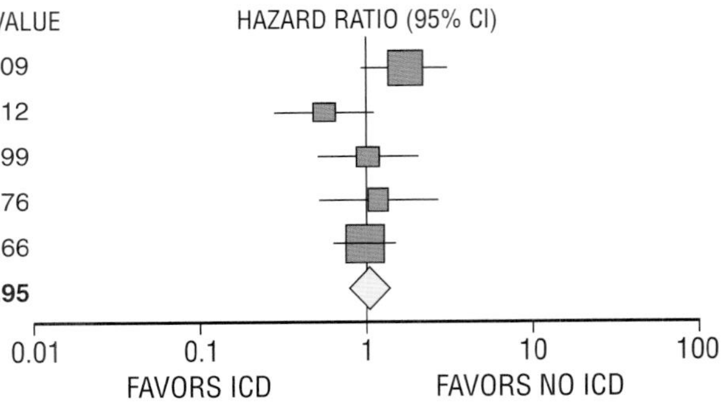

FIGURE 37-3 Effectiveness of implantable cardioverter-defibrillators for the primary prevention of sudden cardiac death in women with advanced heart failure: a meta-analysis of randomized controlled trials. *DEFINITE,* Defibrillators in Non-Ischemic Cardiomyopathy Treatment Evaluation; *DINAMIT,* Defibrillator In Acute Myocardial Infarction Trial; *MADIT,* Multicenter Automatic Defibrillator Implantation Trial; *MUSTT,* Multicenter Unsustained Tachycardia Trial; *SCD-HeFT,* Sudden Cardiac Death in Heart Failure Trial. *From Ghanbari H, Dalloul G, Hasan R, et al: Effectiveness of implantable cardioverter-defibrillators for the primary prevention of sudden cardiac death in women with advanced heart failure: a meta-analysis of randomized controlled trials. Arch Intern Med 169:1500–1506, 2009.*

women, women receiving CRT had a significant reduction in the combined endpoint of total mortality or hospitalization for any cause compared with women randomized to medical therapy, and there was no interaction by sex.[86]

Implantable Cardioverter Defibrillator

Guideline recommendations for ICD implantation to prevent sudden death are based on many multicenter studies, but women have been underrepresented and few studies have provided adequate sex-specific data.[86,87] The limited analyses available for women do not clearly demonstrate a mortality benefit.[84,86-88] In the SCD-HeFT trial, which included 382 women with NYHA class II-III HF and LVEF ≤ 35% (ischemic and nonischemic cardiomyopathy), ICD therapy did not reduce mortality in women (HR 0.96, 95% CI 0.58-1.61); however, the trial was not powered to detect sex differences. In the MADIT-II study, which included 119 women with ischemic cardiomyopathy and LVEF ≤ 30%, there was a nonsignificant trend toward lower mortality in women receiving an ICD (adjusted HR 0.57, $P = 0.132$), suggesting that women with ischemic cardiomyopathy may benefit.[89] A meta-analysis of ICD therapy in women found no overall benefit (**Figure 37-3**).[88] Due to the low inclusion of women in clinical trials and the lower use of ICDs in women, current data are insufficient to support differential use of ICDs by sex.

Left Ventricular Assist Devices (see also Chapter 42)

Implantable LV assist devices (LVADs) are being used more frequently for the treatment of end-stage refractory HF.[90] Although there are no sex differences in the surgical techniques for implanting LVADs, small women have limited LVAD options because the devices require a minimum body size to fit properly. In studies of first-generation pulsatile-flow LVADs, enrollment of women was less than 10%, primarily because the devices were too large to fit most women.[91] Current U.S. Food and Drug Administration (FDA)-approved continuous-flow devices, including the HeartMate II and the HeartWare, are smaller and more women have been enrolled in clinical trials with similar survival rates compared with men.[92] However, women tend to have more hemorrhagic strokes and fewer device-related infections relative to men.[92]

Heart Transplantation (see also Chapter 40)

Based on data from the International Society of Heart and Lung Transplantation registry, women received 23.7% of the 17,868 heart transplants performed from 2006 to June 2011,[93] representing significant increases from 22.3% and 19.3% in the prior 5- and 10-year periods. Overall survival rates are now similar in women and men, although female recipients of a male donor heart may be at higher risk of 1-year mortality than male recipients from a male donor.[93] Reasons for lower rates of transplantation in women are not clear, but may be partially explained by higher levels of reactive antibodies in parous women, making it more challenging to find a suitable donor. Women also tend to be older, possibly decreasing candidacy for transplantation.[94]

HEART FAILURE IN RACIAL/ETHNIC MINORITY GROUPS

Despite advances in therapy, racial and ethnic disparities persist in HF prevalence and outcomes. The complex interaction of genetics, social factors, environment, and lifestyle may affect pathophysiologic and therapeutic observations seen in these racial and ethnic populations, which exhibit considerable heterogeneity.[95,96] Because these groups are underrepresented in clinical trials, specific recommendations are derived from extrapolated data or post hoc analyses that lack statistical power and methodologic rigor.[97]

Prevalence

The prevalence of HF by sex and race/ethnicity is shown in **Table 37-7**.[98] African Americans have a disproportionately high prevalence of HF compared with the general population and other racial groups. The prevalence for Mexican Americans is less than that of non-Hispanic men and women.[98] Annual rates of new HF events per 1000 population by age, sex, and race are shown in **Table 37-8**.[98] The prevalence of HF in minority populations is projected to increase substantially over the next 20 years, reflecting demographic shifts in the U.S. population (**Figure 37-4**).[99-101]

In the Multi-Ethnic Study of Atherosclerosis, which included 6814 participants (38.5% white, 27.8% African American, 21.9% Hispanic, and 11.2% Chinese American),[102] the 5-year risk for HF by race/ethnicity was highest in African Americans, followed by Hispanics, non-Hispanic whites, and Chinese Americans (**Figure 37-5**).

TABLE 37-7 Heart Failure Prevalence by Sex and Race/Ethnicity

POPULATION GROUP	PREVALENCE, 2010 AGE ≥ 20 YR
Both sexes, *n* (%)	5,100,000 (2.1)
Males, *n* (%)	2,700,000 (2.5)
Females, *n* (%)	2,400,000 (1.8)
NH white males, %	2.2
NH white females, %	1.7
NH black males, %	4.1
NH black females, %	3.0
Mexican American males, %	1.9
Mexican American females, %	1.1

NH, non-Hispanic.
From Go AS, Mozaffarian D, Roger VL, et al: Heart disease and stroke statistics—2013 update: a report from the American Heart Association. Circulation 127:e6–e245, 2013.

Clinical Features

HF in African Americans occurs at an earlier age and is more frequently associated with hypertension and diabetes

TABLE 37-8 Annual Rates of New Heart Failure Events by Age, Sex, and Race (per 1000 individuals)

	WHITE MALES	WHITE FEMALES	BLACK MALES	BLACK FEMALES
Age 65-74	15.2	8.2	16.9	14.2
Age 75-84	31.7	19.8	25.5	25.5
Age ≥ 85	65.2	45.6	50.6	44.0

From Go AS, Mozaffarian D, Roger VL, et al: Heart disease and stroke statistics—2013 update: a report from the American Heart Association. Circulation 127:e6–e245, 2013.

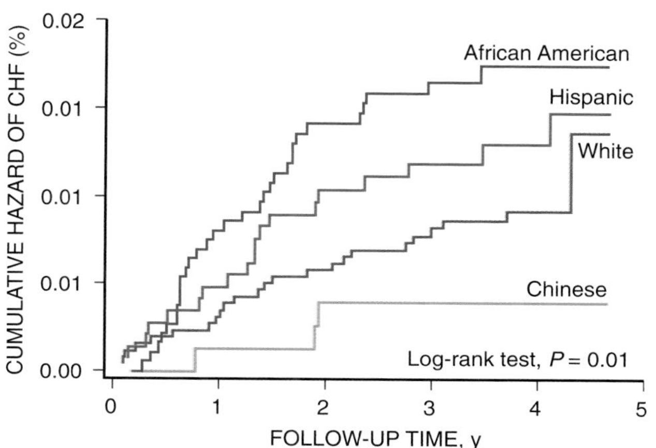

FIGURE 37-5 Cumulative hazards ratio for the development of heart failure by racial/ethnic group in the MESA (Multi-Ethnic Study of Atherosclerosis) study. *CHF*, Congestive heart failure. *From Bahrami H, Kronmal R, Bluemke DA, et al: Difference in the incidence of congestive heart failure by ethnicity: the multi-ethnic study of atherosclerosis. Arch Intern Med 168:2138–2145, 2008.*

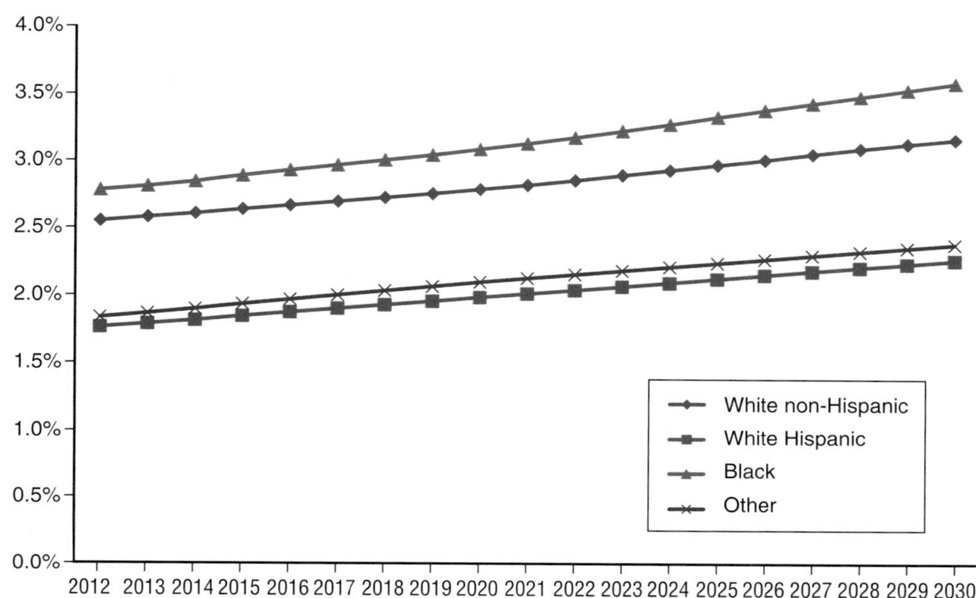

FIGURE 37-4 Projected U.S. prevalence of heart failure from 2012 to 2030 for different races. *From Heidenreich PA, Albert NM, Allen LA, et al: Forecasting the impact of heart failure in the United States: a policy statement from the American Heart Association. Circ Heart Fail 6:606–619, 2013.*

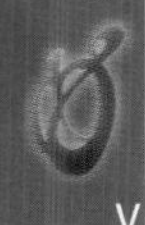

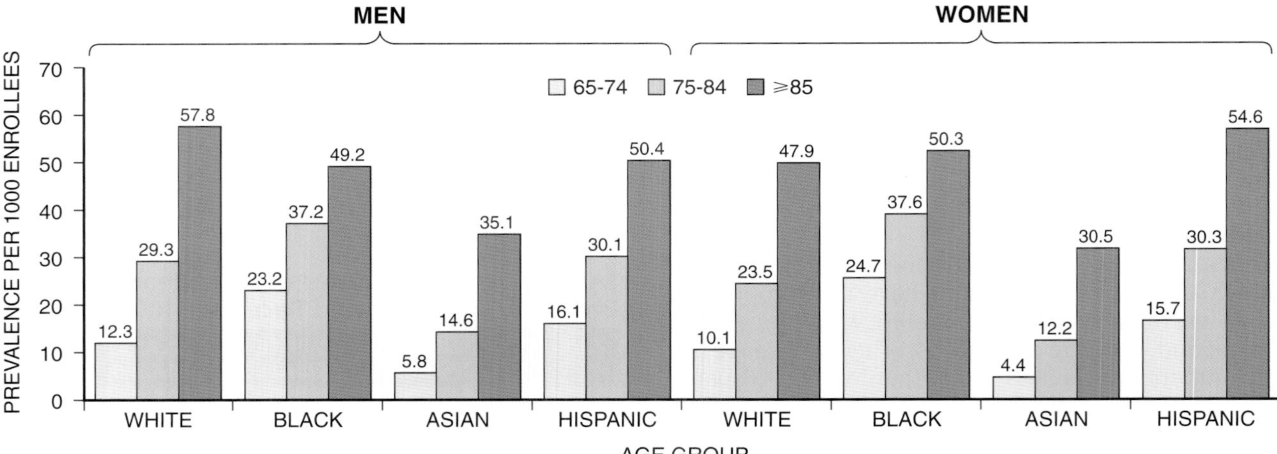

FIGURE 37-6 Age-specific prevalence of hospitalization with a first-listed diagnosis of heart failure among Medicare enrollees aged 65 years or older by sex and race/ethnicity. *Modified from Brown D, Haldeman G, Croft J, et al: Racial or ethnic differences in hospitalization for heart failure among elderly adults: Medicare, 1990-2000. Am Heart J 150:448–454, 2005.*

than with ischemic heart disease.[103-108] Hispanics with HF are younger than other racial groups and have higher rates of diabetes and renal disease. Rates of ischemic cardiomyopathy are intermediate between non-Hispanic and African American populations.[109]

HF data for Asian populations are limited. A review of Asian populations residing in Canada found that South Asian patients with HF tend to be younger and are more likely to have diabetes and lower body mass index.[110] In the Strong Heart Study, an observational study of American Indians with high prevalence of diabetes, obesity, and metabolic syndrome, the incidence of HF was 6.4 per 1000 person-years during 11 years of follow-up. Higher levels of C-reactive protein and fibrinogen were associated with increased risk.[111]

Observed racial differences in morbidity from HF may be related to differences in comorbid conditions (e.g., hypertension, diabetes, renal disease), effectiveness of treatment, socioeconomic factors (access to insurance and specialty care), lifestyle, and health care–seeking behaviors (time between symptom onset and presentation for care).[102,105,109,112] Data from Medicare enrollees showed that compared with white Americans, HF hospitalization was 50% more likely for African Americans and 20% more likely for Hispanics, but 50% less likely for Asian patients.[113] African Americans and Hispanics with HF have higher hospitalization and readmission rates compared with whites (**Figure 37-6**).[109,114-119] Length of stay is highest among non-Hispanic whites, intermediate among Hispanics, and shortest in African Americans.[109]

Mortality data for African Americans with HF is conflicting,[117,119-121] in part due to differences in study period, methodology (registries, observational databases, administrative databases, or randomized clinical trials), pathophysiology (HFpEF vs. HFrEF), and patient age.

Data from a meta-analysis of studies reporting mortality by race after hospitalization for HF showed that mortality in African Americans was 32% lower during short-term follow-up and 16% lower during long-term follow-up compared with white patients.[122] Hispanics have also been reported to have lower in-hospital and short-term mortality compared with whites.[109] Mechanisms for differences in outcomes by race/ethnicity are poorly understood.

Pathophysiology

Evolving data suggest that African Americans may have altered nitric oxide–dependent vascular function and less responsiveness to renin-angiotensin system inhibition.[123] African Americans have lower norepinephrine levels, a trend toward lower plasma renin activity, and reduced nitric oxide availability compared with other racial groups.[124,125] This imbalance may contribute to adverse ventricular remodeling (**see Chapter 11**).[123]

Certain genetic markers have been shown to exist in linkage disequilibrium in African American populations. African Americans who are homozygous for polymorphisms in genes encoding for both β_1-adrenergic receptors and α_2-adrenergic receptors are at 10-fold greater risk for HF.[126] Overexpression of transforming growth factor β_1 may imply worse prognosis,[127,128] and overexpression of other polymorphisms (e.g., endothelial nitric oxide synthase (eNOS), aldosterone synthase, and the G protein 825-T allele) may influence HF risk.[129] Although the study of gene variants represents an expanding area for research, caution must be employed when considering race as a surrogate for disease expression or response to therapy.[97]

Although HFpEF is more prevalent in African Americans, data on prognosis are limited.[130] In a middle-aged African American cohort of the Atherosclerosis Risk in Communities study, HFpEF was the most common form of HF and was associated with better prognosis compared with HFrEF.[130]

Racial Differences in Response to Drug Treatment

The efficacy of pharmacologic treatment in minority populations is controversial because there have been few clinical trials in HF that have prespecified subgroup analysis by race/ethnicity or have included sufficient numbers of subjects for meaningful statistical analysis. Retrospective analyses suggest differences between African American and white populations in response to HF pharmacotherapy, but few data exist for Hispanics and Asians.

ACE Inhibitors

Pooled data from the Studies of Left Ventricular Dysfunction (SOLVD) prevention and treatment trials found that

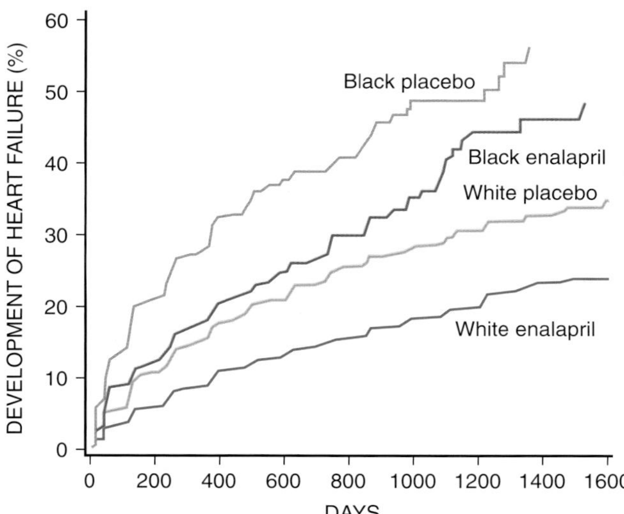

FIGURE 37-7 Effect of angiotensin-converting enzyme inhibition on the prevention of development of symptomatic heart failure in black and white patients with asymptomatic left ventricular dysfunction. *Adapted from Dries D, Strong M, Cooper R, et al: Efficacy of angiotensin-converting enzyme inhibition in reducing progression from asymptomatic left ventricular dysfunction to symptomatic heart failure in black and white patients. J Am Coll Cardiol 40:311–317, 2002.*

enalapril therapy was associated with similar reductions in mortality in African American and white patients, although overall mortality and mortality due to pump failure, stroke, and pulmonary embolism were all higher in African Americans.[131,132] Enalapril was also associated with a significant reduction in the risk of hospitalization for HF among white patients but not among African American patients. African Americans assigned to receive enalapril experienced a 44% increased risk of HF hospitalization (7.9 more admissions per 100 person-years of follow-up) compared with white patients assigned to enalapril.[132] In whites treated with enalapril, significant reductions in both systolic (5 ± 17.1 mm/Hg) and diastolic blood pressure (3.6 ± 10.6 mm/Hg) were observed, whereas no reduction in blood pressure was seen in African Americans. In a post hoc analysis of the SOLVD prevention study,[133] enalapril delayed the progression from asymptomatic LV dysfunction to symptomatic HF in both African American and white subjects. However, despite the comparable relative reduction in risk for the development of symptomatic HF, differences in baseline risk were such that African Americans randomized to enalapril were at higher risk than whites randomized to placebo for progression to clinical HF. Furthermore, this difference persisted after adjusting for potential confounders, including LVEF, NYHA class, serum sodium, and cause of LV dysfunction (**Figure 37-7**).[133]

β-Blockers

Although β-blockers are of proven benefit in HFrEF,[134] enrollment of African Americans in clinical trials has been limited.[135-137] Post hoc analyses show trends toward beneficial effects in African Americans for carvedilol and metoprolol, but hazard ratios failed to reach statistical significance due to low sample size.

In the Beta-blocker Evaluation of Survival Trial (BEST), the only trial prospectively stratified by African American or white race, bucindolol significantly reduced the risk of death or hospitalization among white patients but was associated with a nonsignificant increase in the risk of serious clinical events in African Americans (**Figure 37-8**).[76]

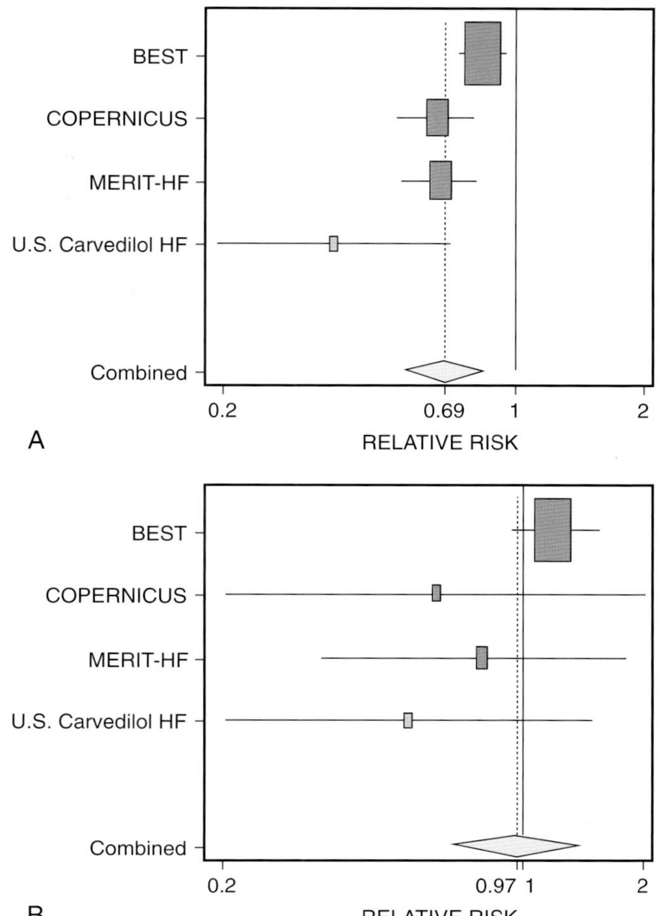

FIGURE 37-8 Effect of β-blocking agents in black and white patients. **A,** Effects of β-blocking agents in white patients. **B,** Effects of β-blocking agents in black patients. *Adapted from Shekelle PG, Rich MW, Morton SC, et al: Efficacy of angiotensin-converting enzyme inhibitors and beta-blockers in the management of left ventricular systolic dysfunction according to race, gender, and diabetic status: a meta-analysis of major clinical trials. J Am Coll Cardiol 41:1529–1538, 2003.*

Hydralazine/Isosorbide Dinitrate

Retrospective analyses of the Vasodilator HF Trials (V-HeFT I and II),[138,139] which included 28% to 30% African Americans, suggested racial differences in response to treatment.[124] In V-HeFT I,[124] which compared the combination of hydralazine/isosorbide dinitrate to prazosin or a placebo, a mortality benefit was observed in African American but not in white patients treated with hydralazine and isosorbide dinitrate. In the V-HeFT II trial, which compared enalapril with hydralazine/isosorbide dinitrate, a survival advantage of enalapril was observed only in white patients; in African Americans, mortality was similar in those randomized to enalapril or hydralazine/isosorbide dinitrate. The African-American Heart Failure Trial (A-HeFT) tested the hypothesis that the addition of isosorbide dinitrate and hydralazine to background neurohormonal blockade would improve HF outcomes in African American patients with low ejection fractions and advanced symptoms.[108] Compared with a placebo, hydralazine and isosorbide dinitrate significantly reduced mortality by 43% and the rate of first hospitalization by 33% in self-identified African American men and women (**Figure 37-9**).[108,109,113] The impact of this therapy in other populations requires further testing.

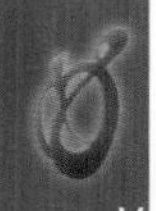

Angiotensin Receptor Blockers, Aldosterone Antagonists, Digoxin

Clinical trials of other pharmacotherapeutic agents included small numbers of racial/ethnic minorities and do not permit conclusions regarding treatment by race.

ICDs and CRT

Minorities have also been underrepresented in trials testing the utility of ICDs[89,140] and CRT,[141] as well as in registries tracking use of these devices.[142] The Sudden Cardiac Death in HF Trial (SCD-HeFT) enrolled 23% minorities and compared conventional therapy alone to conventional therapy plus amiodarone or an ICD.[143] Benefits of ICD therapy were similar in African Americans and whites.[144] However, examination of the National Cardiovascular Data Registry for racial/ethnic differences in CRT-D use revealed that CRT-eligible black and Hispanic patients were less likely to receive CRT-D than eligible white patients.[145] Conversely, white patients were more likely to receive CRT-D outside of established guidelines.[145]

Heart Transplantation

Retrospective analysis of data from the Organ Procurement and Transplantation database revealed that the overall risk of death or retransplantation within 6 months was similar in all racial groups. However, long-term survival was lower in black and Hispanic patients compared with whites, suggesting that further investigation and targeted interventions may be warranted for these racial/ethnic groups.[146]

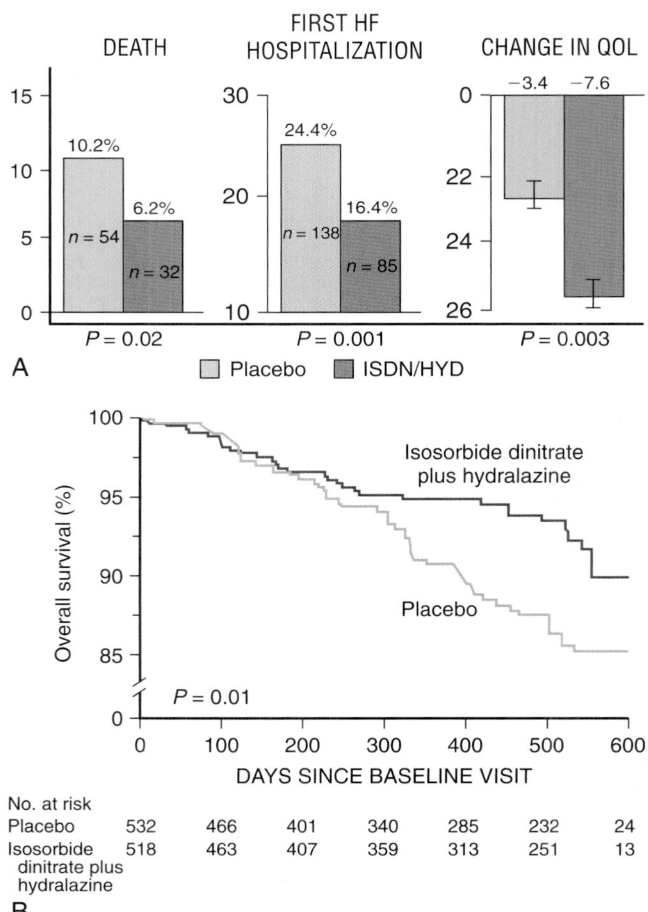

FIGURE 37-9 Clinical outcomes in the A-HeFT trial. **A,** Components of composite score in A-HeFT. **B,** Effect of fixed dose hydralazine isosorbide on mortality in A-HeFT. *HF,* Heart failure; *ISDN/HYD,* isosorbide dinitrate/hydralazine; *QoL,* quality of life. *Modified from Taylor AL, Ziesche S, Yancy C, et al: Combination of isosorbide dinitrate and hydralazine in blacks with heart failure. N Engl J Med 351:2049–2057, 2004.*

SUMMARY

Heart failure in older patients, women, and racial/ethnic minority groups is often associated with distinct differences in prevalence, pathophysiology, clinical features, and response to treatment relative to HF in younger white men (i.e., the demographic group with highest enrollment in most clinical trials). Additional studies are needed to define optimal strategies for prevention and treatment of HF in these populations.

References

1. Roger VL, Go AS, Lloyd-Jones DM, et al: Heart disease and stroke statistics—2012 update: a report from the American Heart Association. *Circulation* 125:e2–e220, 2012.
2. Roy B, Pawar PP, Desai RV, et al: A propensity-matched study of the association of diabetes mellitus with incident heart failure and mortality among community-dwelling older adults. *Am J Cardiol* 108:1747–1753, 2011.
3. Nicklas BJ, Cesari M, Penninx BW, et al: Abdominal obesity is an independent risk factor for chronic heart failure in older people. *J Am Geriatr Soc* 54:413–420, 2006.
4. Sims RV, Mujib M, McGwin G, Jr, et al: Heart failure is a risk factor for incident driving cessation among community-dwelling older adults: findings from a prospective population study. *J Card Fail* 17:1035–1040, 2011.
5. Tinetti ME, McAvay G, Chang SS, et al: Effect of chronic disease-related symptoms and impairments on universal health outcomes in older adults. *J Am Geriatr Soc* 59:1618–1627, 2011.
6. Gurwitz JH, Magid DJ, Smith DH, et al: Contemporary prevalence and correlates of incident heart failure with preserved ejection fraction. *Am J Med* 126:393–400, 2013.
7. Kitzman DW, Gardin JM, Gottdiener JS, et al: Importance of heart failure with preserved systolic function in patients > or = 65 years of age. CHS Research Group. Cardiovascular Health Study. *Am J Cardiol* 87:413–419, 2001.
8. Owan TE, Hodge DO, Herges RM, et al: Trends in prevalence and outcome of heart failure with preserved ejection fraction. *N Engl J Med* 355(3):251–259, 2006.
9. Ho JE, Lyass A, Lee DS, et al: Predictors of new-onset heart failure: differences in preserved versus reduced ejection fraction. *Circ Heart Fail* 6:279–286, 2013.
10. Devereux RB, Roman MJ, Liu JE, et al: Congestive heart failure despite normal left ventricular systolic function in a population-based sample: the Strong Heart Study. *Am J Cardiol* 86:1090–1096, 2000.
11. Lam CS, Carson PE, Anand IS, et al: Sex differences in clinical characteristics and outcomes in elderly patients with heart failure and preserved ejection fraction: the Irbesartan in Heart Failure with Preserved Ejection Fraction (I-PRESERVE) trial. *Circ Heart Fail* 5:571–578, 2012.
12. Ahluwalia SC, Gross CP, Chaudhry SI, et al: Impact of comorbidity on mortality among older persons with advanced heart failure. *J Gen Intern Med* 27:513–519, 2012.
13. Chen J, Normand SL, Wang Y, et al: National and regional trends in heart failure hospitalization and mortality rates for Medicare beneficiaries, 1998–2008. *JAMA* 306:1669–1678, 2011.
14. Steinberg BA, Zhao X, Heidenreich PA, et al: Trends in patients hospitalized with heart failure and preserved left ventricular ejection fraction: prevalence, therapies, and outcomes. *Circulation* 126:65–75, 2012.
15. Jencks SF, Williams MV, Coleman EA: Rehospitalizations among patients in the Medicare fee-for-service program. *N Engl J Med* 360:1418–1428, 2009.
16. Dharmarajan K, Hsieh AF, Lin Z, et al: Diagnoses and timing of 30-day readmissions after hospitalization for heart failure, acute myocardial infarction, or pneumonia. *JAMA* 309:355–363, 2013.
17. Levy D, Kenchaiah S, Larson MG, et al: Long-term trends in the incidence of and survival with heart failure. *N Engl J Med* 347:1397–1402, 2002.
18. Lakatta EG, Levy D: Arterial and cardiac aging: major shareholders in cardiovascular disease enterprises: Part II: the aging heart in health: links to heart disease. *Circulation* 107:346–354, 2003.
19. Lakatta EG, Levy D: Arterial and cardiac aging: major shareholders in cardiovascular disease enterprises: Part I: aging arteries: a "set up" for vascular disease. *Circulation* 107:139–146, 2003.
20. Kitzman DW, Little WC, Brubaker PH, et al: Pathophysiological characterization of isolated diastolic heart failure in comparison to systolic heart failure. *JAMA* 288:2144–2150, 2002.
21. Newman AB, Simonsick EM, Naydeck BL, et al: Association of long-distance corridor walk performance with mortality, cardiovascular disease, mobility limitation, and disability. *JAMA* 295:2018–2026, 2006.
22. Studenski S, Perera S, Patel K, et al: Gait speed and survival in older adults. *JAMA* 305:50–58, 2011.
23. Katz S, Ford AB, Moskowitz RW, et al: Studies of illness in the aged. The index of ADL: A standardized measure of biological and psychosocial function. *JAMA* 185:914–919, 1963.
24. Le Jemtel TH, Padeletti M, Jelic S: Diagnostic and therapeutic challenges in patients with coexistent chronic obstructive pulmonary disease and chronic heart failure. *J Am Coll Cardiol* 49:171–180, 2007.
25. Maisel AS, Clopton P, Krishnaswamy P, et al: Impact of age, race, and sex on the ability of B-type natriuretic peptide to aid in the emergency diagnosis of heart failure: results from the Breathing Not Properly (BNP) multinational study. *Am Heart J* 147:1078–1084, 2004.
26. Dharmarajan K, Maurer MS: Transthyretin cardiac amyloidoses in older North Americans. *J Am Geriatr Soc* 60:765–774, 2012.
27. Bulawa CE, Connelly S, Devit M, et al: Tafamidis, a potent and selective transthyretin kinetic stabilizer that inhibits the amyloid cascade. *Proc Natl Acad Sci U S A* 109:9629–9634, 2012.
28. Benson MD, Pandey S, Witchell D, et al: Antisense oligonucleotide therapy for TTR amyloidosis. *Amyloid* 18(Suppl 1):60, 2011.
29. Coelho T, Adams D, Silva A, et al: Safety and efficacy of RNAi therapy for transthyretin amyloidosis. *N Engl J Med* 369:819–829, 2013.
30. Vogels RL, Scheltens P, Schroeder-Tanka JM, et al: Cognitive impairment in heart failure: a systematic review of the literature. *Eur J Heart Fail* 9:440–449, 2007.
31. Pressler SJ: Cognitive functioning and chronic heart failure: a review of the literature (2002–July 2007). *J Cardiovasc Nurs* 23:239–249, 2008.

32. Pressler SJ, Kim J, Riley P, et al: Memory dysfunction, psychomotor slowing, and decreased executive function predict mortality in patients with heart failure and low ejection fraction. *J Card Fail* 16:750–760, 2010.
33. Gure TR, Blaum CS, Giordani B, et al: Prevalence of cognitive impairment in older adults with heart failure. *J Am Geriatr Soc* 60:1724–1729, 2012.
34. Cameron J, Worrall-Carter L, Page K, et al: Does cognitive impairment predict poor self-care in patients with heart failure? *Eur J Heart Fail* 12:508–515, 2010.
35. Riegel B, Moelter ST, Ratcliffe SJ, et al: Excessive daytime sleepiness is associated with poor medication adherence in adults with heart failure. *J Card Fail* 17:340–348, 2011.
36. Kindermann I, Fischer D, Karbach J, et al: Cognitive function in patients with decompensated heart failure: the Cognitive Impairment in Heart Failure (CogImpair-HF) study. *Eur J Heart Fail* 14:404–413, 2012.
37. Dodson JA, Truong TT, Towle VR, et al: Cognitive impairment in older adults with heart failure: prevalence, documentation, and impact on outcomes. *Am J Med* 126:120–126, 2013.
38. Green P, Maurer MS: Geriatric assessment of older adults with heart failure: an essential tool in planning of care. *Am J Med* 126:93–94, 2013.
39. Brunner-La Rocca HP, Rickenbacher P, Muzzarelli S, et al: End-of-life preferences of elderly patients with chronic heart failure. *Eur Heart J* 33:752–759, 2012.
40. Rich MW, Beckham V, Wittenberg C, et al: A multidisciplinary intervention to prevent the readmission of elderly patients with congestive heart failure. *N Engl J Med* 333:1190–1195, 1995.
41. Garg R, Yusuf S: Overview of randomized trials of angiotensin-converting enzyme inhibitors on mortality and morbidity in patients with heart failure. Collaborative Group on ACE Inhibitor Trials. *JAMA* 273:1450–1456, 1995.
42. Flather MD, Yusuf S, Kober L, et al: Long-term ACE-inhibitor therapy in patients with heart failure or left-ventricular dysfunction: a systematic overview of data from individual patients. ACE-Inhibitor Myocardial Infarction Collaborative Group. *Lancet* 355:1575–1581, 2000.
43. Cleland JG, Tendera M, Adamus J, et al: Perindopril for elderly people with chronic heart failure: the PEP-CHF study. The PEP investigators. *Eur J Heart Fail* 1:211–217, 1999.
44. Ahmed A, Rich MW, Fleg JL, et al: Effects of digoxin on morbidity and mortality in diastolic heart failure: the ancillary digitalis investigation group trial. *Circulation* 114:397–403, 2006.
45. Edelmann F, Wachter R, Schmidt AG, et al: Effect of spironolactone on diastolic function and exercise capacity in patients with heart failure with preserved ejection fraction: the Aldo-DHF randomized controlled trial. *JAMA* 309:781–791, 2013.
46. Redfield MM, Chen HH, Borlaug BA, et al: Effect of phosphodiesterase-5 inhibition on exercise capacity and clinical status in heart failure with preserved ejection fraction: a randomized clinical trial. *JAMA* 309:1268–1277, 2013.
47. Shah SJ, Gheorghiade M: Heart failure with preserved ejection fraction: treat now by treating comorbidities. *JAMA* 300:431–433, 2008.
48. Swedberg K, Young JB, Anand IS, et al: Treatment of anemia with darbepoetin alfa in systolic heart failure. *N Engl J Med* 368:1210–1219, 2013.
49. Maurer MS, Teruya S, Chakraborty B, et al: Treating anemia in older adults with heart failure with a preserved ejection fraction with epoetin alfa: single-blind randomized clinical trial of safety and efficacy. *Circ Heart Fail* 6:254–263, 2013.
50. Pfisterer M, Buser P, Rickli H, et al: BNP-guided vs symptom-guided heart failure therapy: the Trial of Intensified vs Standard Medical Therapy in Elderly Patients With Congestive Heart Failure (TIME-CHF) randomized trial. *JAMA* 301:383–392, 2009.
51. Savarese G, Trimarco B, Dellegrottaglie S, et al: Natriuretic peptide-guided therapy in chronic heart failure: a meta-analysis of 2,686 patients in 12 randomized trials. *PLoS ONE* 8:e58287, 2013.
52. Haykowsky MJ, Brubaker PH, Stewart KP, et al: Effect of endurance training on the determinants of peak exercise oxygen consumption in elderly patients with stable compensated heart failure and preserved ejection fraction. *J Am Coll Cardiol* 60:120–128, 2012.
53. Hummel SL, Seymour EM, Brook RD, et al: Low-sodium dietary approaches to stop hypertension diet reduces blood pressure, arterial stiffness, and oxidative stress in hypertensive heart failure with preserved ejection fraction. *Hypertension* 60:1200–1206, 2012.
54. Kimmelstiel CD, Konstam MA: Heart failure in women. *Cardiology* 86(4):304–309, 1995.
55. Rosamond W, Flegal K, Furie K, et al: Heart disease and stroke statistics—2008 update: a report from the American Heart Association Statistics Committee and Stroke Statistics Subcommittee. *Circulation* 117(4):e25–e146, 2008.
56. Galvao M, Kalman J, DeMarco T, et al: Gender differences in in-hospital management and outcomes in patients with decompensated heart failure: analysis from the Acute Decompensated Heart Failure National Registry (ADHERE). *J Card Fail* 12(2):100–107, 2006.
57. Nieminen MS, Harjola VP, Hochadel M, et al: Gender related differences in patients presenting with acute heart failure. Results from EuroHeart Failure Survey II. *Eur J Heart Fail* 10(2):140–148, 2008.
58. Loehr LR, Rosamond WD, Chang PP, et al: Heart failure incidence and survival (from the atherosclerosis risk in communities study). *Am J Cardiol* 101:1016–1022, 2008.
59. Roger VL, Weston SA, Redfield MM, et al: Trends in heart failure incidence and survival in a community based population. *JAMA* 292:344–350, 2004.
60. Adams FK, Dunlap SH, Sueta CA, et al: Relation between gender, etiology and survival in patients with symptomatic heart failure. *J Am Coll Cardiol* 28(7):1781–1788, 1996.
61. Johnstone D, Limacher M, Rousseau M, et al: Clinical characteristics of patients in studies of left ventricular dysfunction (SOLVD). *Am J Cardiol* 70(9):894–900, 1992.
62. Taylor AL, Lindenfeld J, Ziesche S, et al: Outcomes by gender in the African-American Heart Failure Trial. *J Am Coll Cardiol* 48(11):2263–2267, 2006.
63. Meyer S, van der Meer P, van Deursen VM, et al: Neurohormonal and clinical sex differences in heart failure. *Eur Heart J* 34:2538–2547, 2013.
64. Deswal A, Bozkurt B: Comparison of morbidity in women versus men with heart failure and preserved ejection fraction. *Am J Cardiol* 97:1228–1231, 2006.
65. Gottlieb SS, Khatta M, Friedmann E, et al: The influence of age, gender, and race on the prevalence of depression in heart failure patients. *J Am Coll Cardiol* 43(9):1542–1549, 2004.
66. Bhatia RS, Tu JV, Lee DS, et al: Outcome of heart failure with preserved ejection fraction in a population-based study. *N Engl J Med* 355(3):260–269, 2006.
67. He J, Ogden LG, Bazzano LA, et al: Risk factors for congestive heart failure in US men and women: NHANES I epidemiologic follow-up study. *Arch Intern Med* 161(7):996–1002, 2001.
68. Bibbins-Domingo K, Lin F, Vittinghoff E, et al: Predictors of heart failure among women with coronary disease. *Circulation* 110(11):1424–1430, 2004.
69. Heart Failure Society of America: Executive summary: HFSA 2006 Comprehensive Heart Failure Practice Guideline. *J Card Fail* 12(1):10–38, 2006. Review.
70. Yancy CW, Fonarow GC, Albert NM, et al: Influence of patient age and sex on delivery of guideline-recommended heart failure care in the outpatient cardiology practice setting: findings from IMPROVE HF. *Am Heart J* 157(4):754–62.e2, 2009.
71. Forman DE, Cannon CP, Hernandez AF, et al: Influence of age on the management of heart failure: findings from Get With the Guidelines-Heart Failure (GWTG-HF). *Am Heart J* 157(6):1010–1017, 2009.
72. Fonarow GC, Abraham WT, Albert NM, et al: Age- and gender-related differences in quality of care and outcomes of patients hospitalized with heart failure (from OPTIMIZE-HF). *Am J Cardiol* 104(1):107–115, 2009.
73. McSweeney J, Pettey C, Lefler LL, et al: Disparities in heart failure and other cardiovascular diseases among women. *Womens Health (Lond Engl)* 8(4):473–485, 2012.
74. Shah B, Hernandez AF, Liang L, et al: Hospital variation and characteristics of implantable cardioverter-defibrillator use in patients with heart failure: data from the GWTG-HF (Get With The Guidelines-Heart Failure) registry. *J Am Coll Cardiol* 53(5):416–422, 2009.
75. Garg R, Yusuf S: Overview of randomized trials of angiotensin-converting enzyme inhibitors on mortality and morbidity in patients with heart failure. Collaborative Group on ACE Inhibitor Trials. *JAMA* 273(18):1450–1456. Erratum in: *JAMA* 274(6):462, 1995.
76. Shekelle PG, Rich MW, Morton SC, et al: Efficacy of angiotensin-converting enzyme inhibitors and beta-blockers in the management of left ventricular systolic dysfunction according to race, gender, and diabetic status. *J Am Coll Cardiol* 41:1529–1538, 2003.
77. O'Meara E, Clayton T, McEntegart MB, et al: Sex differences in clinical characteristics and prognosis in a broad spectrum of patients with heart failure: results of the Candesartan in Heart failure: Assessment of Reduction in Mortality and morbidity (CHARM) program. *Circulation* 115(24):3111–3120, 2007.
78. Pitt B, Remme W, Zannad F, et al for the Eplerenone Post-Acute Myocardial Infarction Heart Failure Efficacy and Survival Study Investigators: Eplerenone, a selective aldosterone blocker, in patients with left ventricular dysfunction after myocardial infarction. *N Engl J Med* 348:1309–1321, 2003.
79. Pitt B, Zannad F, Remme WJ, et al, for the Randomized Aldactone Evaluation Study Investigators: The effect of spironolactone on morbidity and mortality in patients with severe heart failure. *N Engl J Med* 341:709–717, 1999.
80. Cohn JN, Archibald DG, Ziesche S, et al: Effect of vasodilator therapy on mortality in chronic congestive heart failure: results of a Veterans Administration Cooperative Study. *N Engl J Med* 314:1547–1552, 1986.
81. Cohn JN, Johnson G, Ziesche S, et al: A comparison of enalapril with hydralazine-isosorbide dinitrate in the treatment of chronic congestive heart failure. *N Engl J Med* 325:303–310, 1991.
82. Digitalis Investigation Group: The effect of digoxin on mortality and morbidity in patients with heart failure. *N Engl J Med* 336:525–533, 1997.
83. Rathore SS, Wang Y, Krumholz HM: Sex-based differences in the effect of digoxin for the treatment of heart failure. *N Engl J Med* 347(18):1403–1411, 2002.
84. Adams KF, Jr, Patterson JH, Gattis WA, et al: Relationship of serum digoxin concentration to mortality and morbidity in women in the digitalis investigation group trial: a retrospective analysis. *J Am Coll Cardiol* 46(3):497–504, 2005.
85. Arshad A, Moss AJ, Foster E, et al: Cardiac resynchronization therapy is more effective in women than in men: the MADIT-CRT (Multicenter Automatic Defibrillator Implantation Trial with Cardiac Resynchronization Therapy) trial. *J Am Coll Cardiol* 57(7):813–820, 2011.
86. Bristow MR, Saxon LA, Boehmer J, et al: Cardiac-resynchronization therapy with or without an implantable defibrillator in advanced chronic heart failure. *N Engl J Med* 350(21):2140–2150, 2004.
87. Bardy GH, Lee KL, Mark DB, et al: Amiodarone or an implantable cardioverter-defibrillator for congestive heart failure. *N Engl J Med* 352(3):225–237, 2005. Erratum in: *N Engl J Med* 352(20):2146, 2005.
88. Ghanbari H, Dalloul G, Hasan R, et al: Effectiveness of implantable cardioverter-defibrillators for the primary prevention of sudden cardiac death in women with advanced heart failure: a meta-analysis of randomized controlled trials. *Arch Intern Med* 169(16):1500–1506, 2009.
89. Moss AJ, Zareba W, Hall J, et al, for the Multicenter Automatic Defibrillator Implantation Trial II Investigators. *N Engl J Med* 346:877–883, 2002.
90. Miller LW, Pagani FD, Russell SD, et al: Use of a continuous-flow device in patients awaiting heart transplantation. *N Engl J Med* 357(9):885–896, 2007.
91. Rose EA, Gelijns AC, Moskowitz AJ, et al: Long-term use of a left ventricular assist device for end-stage heart failure. *N Engl J Med* 345(20):1435–1443, 2001.
92. Bogaev RC, Pamboukian SV, Moore SA, et al: Comparison of outcomes in women versus men using a continuous-flow left ventricular assist device as a bridge to transplantation. *J Heart Lung Transplant* 30(5):515–522, 2011.
93. Stehlik J, Edwards LB, Kucheryavaya AY, et al: The Registry of the International Society for Heart and Lung Transplantation: 29th official adult heart transplant report—2012. *J Heart Lung Transplant* 31(10):1052–1064, 2012.
94. Shin JJ, Hamad E, Murthy S, et al: Heart failure in women. *Clin Cardiol* 35(3):172–177, 2012.
95. Taylor AL, Wright JT, Jr: Should ethnicity serve as the basis for clinical trial design? Importance of Race/Ethnicity in Clinical Trials: Lessons from the African-American Heart Failure Trial (A-HeFT), the African-American Study of Kidney Disease and Hypertension (African Americans), and the Antihypertensive and Lipid-Lowering Treatment to Prevent Heart Attack Trial (ALLHAT). *Circulation* 112(23):3654–3660, 2005.
96. Hunt SA, Abraham WT, Chin MH, et al: 2009 Focuses update incorporated into the ACC/AHA 2005 guidelines for the diagnosis and management of heart failure in adults: a report of the American College of Cardiology Foundation/American Heart Association Task Force on Practice Guidelines. *Circulation* 119:e391–e479, 2009.
97. Mitchell JE, Ferdinand KC, Watson KE, et al: Treatment of heart failure in African Americans—a call to action. *J Natl Med Assoc* 103:86–98, 2011.
98. Go AS, Mozaffarian D, Roger VI, et al on behalf of the American Heart Association Statistics Committee and Stroke Statistics Subcommittee: Heart disease and stroke statistics—2013 Update: a report from the American Heart Association. *Circulation* 127:e6–e245, 2013.
99. Heidenreich PA, Albert NM, Allen LA, et al, on behalf of the American Heart Association Advocacy Coordinating Committee, Council of Arteriosclerosis, Thrombosis, and Vascular Biology, Council of Cardiovascular Radiology and Intervention, Council of Clinical Cardiology, Council of Epidemiology and Prevention, and Stroke Council: Forecasting the impact of heart failure in the United States: a policy statement from the American Heart Association. *Circ Heart Fail* 6:606–619, 2013.
100. U.S. Census Bureau: Facts for features: Hispanic Heritage Month 2012. http://www.census.gov/newsroom.releases.archives/facts_for_features_special_editions/cb12_ff19.html.
101. Qian F, Ling F, Deedwania P, et al: Care and outcomes of Asian-American acute myocardial infarction patients: findings from the American Heart Association Get with the Guidelines—coronary artery disease program. *Circ Cardiovasc Qual Outcomes* 5:126–133, 2012.
102. Bahrami H, Kronmal R, Bluemke DA, et al: Difference in the incidence of congestive heart failure by ethnicity: the multi-ethnic study of atherosclerosis. *Arch Intern Med* 168(19):2138–2145, 2008.
103. Yancy C: Heart failure in African Americans: a cardiovascular enigma. *J Card Fail* 6(3):183–186, 2000.
104. Yancy C: Heart failure in African Americans: pathophysiology and treatment. *J Card Fail* 9(5):S210–S215, 2003.
105. Philbin E, Weil H, Francis C, et al: Observations from a biracial angiographic cohort. *J Card Fail* 6(3):187–193, 2000.
106. Afzal A, Ananthasubramaniam K, Sharma N, et al: Racial differences in patients with heart failure. *Clin Cardiol* 22:791–794, 1999.
107. Mathew J, Davidson S, Narra L, et al: Etiology and characteristics of congestive heart failure in blacks. *Am J Card* 78:1447–1450, 1996.
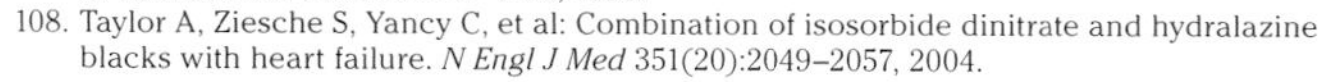
108. Taylor A, Ziesche S, Yancy C, et al: Combination of isosorbide dinitrate and hydralazine in blacks with heart failure. *N Engl J Med* 351(20):2049–2057, 2004.

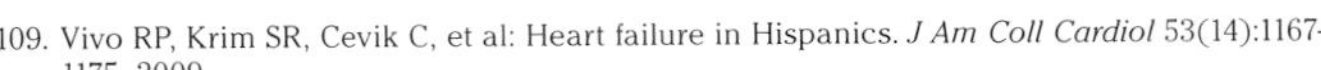

109. Vivo RP, Krim SR, Cevik C, et al: Heart failure in Hispanics. *J Am Coll Cardiol* 53(14):1167–1175, 2009.
110. Moe GW, Tu J: Heart failure in ethnic minorities. *Curr Opin Cardiol* 25(2):124–130, 2010.
111. Barac A, Wang H, Shara NM, et al: Inflammation, metabolic risk factors, and incident heart failure in American Indians: the Strong Heart Study. *J Clin Hypertens* 14(1):13–19, 2012.
112. Ghali J: Race, ethnicity, and heart failure. *J Card Fail* 8(6):387–389, 2002.
113. Brown D, Haldeman G, Croft J, et al: Racial or ethnic differences in hospitalization for heart failure among elderly adults: Medicare, 1990-2000. *Am Heart J* 150(3):448–454, 2005.
114. Vaccarino V, Gahbauer E, Kasl SV, et al: Differences between African Americans and whites in the outcome of heart failure: evidence for a greater functional decline in African Americans. *Am Heart J* 143(6):1058–1067, 2002.
115. Lafata JE, Pladevall M, Divine G, et al: Are there race/ethnicity differences in outpatient congestive heart failure management, hospital use, and morality among an insured population? *Med Care* 42(7):680–689, 2004.
116. Deswal A, Petersen NJ, Urbauer DL, et al: Racial variations in quality of care and outcomes in an ambulatory heart failure cohort. *Am Heart J* 152(2):348–354, 2006.
117. Rathore S, Foody J, Wang Y, et al: Race, quality of care, and outcomes of elderly patients hospitalized with heart failure. *JAMA* 289(19):2517–2524, 2003.
118. Philbin EF, Di Salvo TG: Influence of race and gender on care process, resource use, and hospital based outcomes in congestive heart failure. *Am J Cardiol* 82(1):76–81, 1998.
119. Mathew J, Wittes J, McSherry F, et al and the Digitalis Investigation Group: Racial differences in outcome and treatment effect in congestive heart failure. *Am Heart J* 150(5):968–976, 2005.
120. Agoston I, Cameron C, Yao D, et al: Comparison of outcomes in white versus black patients hospitalized with heart failure and preserved ejection fraction. *Am J Card* 94:1003–1007, 2004.
121. Singh H, Gordon H, Deswal A: Variation by race in factors contributing to heart failure hospitalizations. *J Card Fail* 11(1):23–29, 2005.
122. Gordon HS, Nowlin PR, Maynard D, et al: Mortality after hospitalization for heart failure in blacks compared to whites. *Am J Cardiol* 105:694–700, 2010.
123. Franciosa JA, Ferdinand KC, Yancy CW: Treatment of heart failure in African Americans: a consensus statement. *Congestive Heart Failure* 16(1):27–38, 2010.
124. Carson P, Ziesche S, Johnson G, et al: Racial differences in response to therapy for heart failure: analysis of the vasodilator-heart failure trials. Vasodilator-Heart Failure Trial Study Group. *J Card Fail* 5(3):178–187, 1999.
125. Kalinowski L, Dobrucki IT, Malinski T: Race-specific differences in endothelial function: predisposition of African Americans to vascular disease. *Circulation* 109:2511–2517, 2004.
126. Small KM, Wagoner LE, Levin AM, et al: Synergistic polymorphisms of beta 1- and alpha 2c- adrenergic receptors and the risk of congestive heart failure. *N Engl J Med* 347:1135–1142, 2002.
127. Cucoranu I, Clempus R, Dikalova A, et al: NAD(P)H oxidase 4 mediates transforming growth factor-beta 1-induced differentiation of cardiac fibroblasts into myofibroblasts. *Circ Res* 97:900–907, 2005.
128. Suthanthiran M, Li B, Song JO, et al: Transforming growth factor-beta 1 hyperexpression in African-American hypertensives: a novel mediator of hypertension and/or target organ damage. *Proc Natl Acad Sci U S A* 97:3479–3484, 2000.
129. Yancy CW: Heart failure in African Americans. *Am J Cardiol* 96:3i–12i, 2005.
130. Gupta DK, Shah AM, Castagno D, et al: Heart failure with preserved ejection fraction in African Americans. *J Am Coll Cardiol Heart Fail* 1:156–163, 2013.
131. Exner D, Dries D, Domanski M, et al: Lesser response to angiotensin-converting-enzyme inhibitor therapy in black as compared with white patients with left ventricular dysfunction. *N Engl J Med* 344(18):1351–1357, 2001.
132. Dries D, Exner D, Gersh B, et al: Racial differences in the outcome of left ventricular dysfunction. *N Engl J Med* 340(8):609–616, 1999.
133. Dries D, Strong M, Cooper R, et al: Efficacy of angiotensin-converting enzyme inhibition in reducing progression from asymptomatic left ventricular dysfunction to symptomatic heart failure in black and white patients. *J Am Coll Card* 40(2):311–317, 2002.
134. Packer M, Coats AJS, Fowler MB, et al: Effect of carvedilol on survival in severe chronic heart failure. *N Engl J Med* 344:1651–1658, 2001.
135. Goldstein S, Deedwania P, Gottlieb S, et al, for the MERIT-Heart Failure Study Group. Metoprolol CR/XL in black patients with heart failure. *Am J Card* 92:478–480, 2003.
136. Yancy C, Fowler M, Colucci W, et al: Race and the response to adrenergic blockade with carvedilol in patients with chronic heart failure. *N Engl J Med* 344(18):1358–1365, 2001.
137. Eichhorn E, Domanski M, Krause-Steinrauf H, et al: A trial of the beta-blocker bucindolol in patients with advanced chronic heart failure. *N Engl J Med* 344(22):1659–1667, 2001.
138. Cohn JN, Archibald DG, Ziesche S, et al: Effect of vasodilator therapy on mortality in chronic congestive heart failure: results of a Veterans Administration Cooperative Study. *N Engl J Med* 314:1547–1552, 1986.
139. Cohn JN, Johnson G, Ziesche S, et al: A comparison of enalapril with hydralazine-isosorbide dinitrate in the treatment of chronic congestive heart failure. *N Engl J Med* 325:303–310, 1991.
140. Hernandez AF, Fonarrow GC, Liang L, et al: Sex and racial differences in the use of implantable cardioverter-defibrillators among patients hospitalized with heart failure. *JAMA* 298: 1525–1532, 2007.
141. Cleland JGF, Daubert JC, Erdmann E, et al, for the Cardiac Resynchronization—Heart Failure (CARE-Heart Failure) Study Investigators: The effect of cardiac resynchronization on morbidity and mortality in heart failure. *N Engl J Med* 352:1539–1549, 2005.
142. Hernandez AF, Yancy C, Fonarrow GC, et al: A gender and racial gap in implantable cardioverter defibrillator use among hospitalized heart failure patients: data from the American Heart Association's Get with the Guidelines Heart Failure (GWTG-Heart Failure) Program. *J Am Coll Card* 49(9):830–833, 2007.
143. Mehra MR, Yancy CW, Albert NM, et al: Evidence of clinical practice heterogeneity in the use of implantable cardioverter-defibrillators in heart failure and post myocardial infarction left ventricular dysfunction. Findings from IMPROVE-HF. *Heart Rhythm* 6:1727–1734, 2009.
144. Mitchell Je, Hellkamp AS, Mark DB, et al: Outcome in African Americans and other minorities in the Sudden Cardiac Death in Heart Failure Trial (SCD-HeFT). *Am Heart J* 155:501–506, 2008.
145. Farmer SA, Kirkpatrick JN, Heidenreich PA, et al: Ethnic and racial disparities in cardiac resynchronization therapy. *Heart Rhythm* 6:325–331, 2009.
146. Singh TP, Almond CA, Givertz MM, et al: Improved survival in heart transplant recipients in the United States. *Circ Heart Fail* 4(2):153–160, 2011.

38 Stem Cell–Based and Gene Therapies in Heart Failure

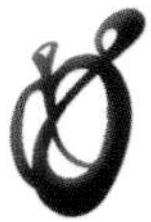

John Mignone and W. Robb MacLellan

Acute myocardial infarction (MI) remains a leading cause of mortality and morbidity despite significant advances in reperfusion strategies and pharmacologic management. The lost myocardium is ultimately replaced by scar tissue, leading to progressive left ventricular (LV) remodeling and dysfunction in many patients (see Chapters 11 and 18). This scar forms because the capacity of the adult heart for regeneration is extremely limited, and there are few, if any options, to reverse or repair damage after a myocardial infarction (MI). Although pharmacologic approaches have been responsible for significant reductions in heart failure mortality, attempts to make further gains by adding additional agents have largely been unsuccessful. Additionally, currently used pharmacologic therapies slow the progress of the remodeling but do not address the underlying cause, namely critical loss of contractile myocardium in the infarcted area. Although heart transplantation is an option when pharmacologic therapies fail, it is severely limited because the need exceeds organ availability 10-fold, and the long-term effects of rejection and side effects of immunosuppression have limited its durability (median survival post transplant is 9 years). Several new biologic therapies and strategies for the treatment of heart failure have emerged in recent years, which will be reviewed in this chapter. Two main approaches will be reviewed here, including cardiac cell therapy and gene therapy, which hold great promise for changing our current approach to heart failure treatment.

CARDIAC CELL THERAPY

Cardiac cell therapy has now been in clinical use for over 10 years. First proposed in the 1990s, cell replacement therapy was an attempt by investigators to address the limited availability of donor organs for cardiac transplantation. Instead of replacing the whole heart, investigators endeavored to restore cardiac function after MI by transplanting cells directly into and around the infarct zone. For lack of a better alternative, the first cell type tested was skeletal muscle cells.[1,2] Although initially thought to transdifferentiate into cardiac muscle, it is now known that these cells do not persist in the heart to any significant degree.[3] Furthermore, studies demonstrated the lack of electrical coupling of these cells to host myocardium and an increase in ventricular arrhythmias. After human studies of autologous skeletal myoblast transplantation in patients with heart failure did not improve regional or global LV function or result in a reduction of adverse cardiac events, this approach has been abandoned.[4] The field of cardiac cell therapy has moved entirely to adult cell types as the primary source of cells after a landmark, but controversial, paper in 2001. Despite questions as to the reproducibility of these findings,[5,6] cell therapy with bone marrow–derived cells was translated into human subjects almost immediately.[7,8] The cell types currently under evaluation in clinical and preclinical studies will be reviewed along with the biology of cell therapy and results of recent clinical trials.

Cell Types Used for Cardiac Cell Therapy

Adult and Endogenous Stem Cells

Adult stem cells used for cardiac cell therapy can be grouped into four categories: (1) circulating or mobilized cells, which are at least in part derived from the bone marrow; (2) bone marrow–derived stem or progenitor cells (BMC); (3) mesenchymal stem cell–like cells from various sources, such as adipose tissue; and (4) endogenous cardiac stem cells (**Figure 38-1**). Most studies have focused on the first two cell types because of a report in 2001 in which circulating cells were harvested and reinjected into the heart after treatment with cytokines commonly used to mobilize hematopoietic stem cells.[9] In mouse studies, the mobilized circulating cells were isolated based on the expression of the cytokine receptor c-kit, which had traditionally been thought to mark hematopoietic stem cells. When these mobilized c-kit+ cells were injected into infarcted heart tissue, a robust repair process was observed with replacement of 60% of the infarcted left ventricle wall and dramatic improvement in survival and LV function.[9] However, this experiment has been difficult to reproduce and lacked direct evidence that the transplanted cells were the same cells that became the new cardiomyocytes.[5,6] Several laboratories attempted to reproduce this study and trace the transplanted c-kit–positive bone marrow stem cells after injection into the myocardium. These studies did not demonstrate any significant conversion of c-kit expressing bone marrow cell conversion into cardiomyocytes or any significant capacity of these cells to restore heart function.[5,6] Other circulating blood-derived progenitors have also been tested, primarily for their potential to stimulate vasculogenesis. Endothelial progenitor cells (EPCs), which express hematopoietic markers, such as CD133+ or CD34+,

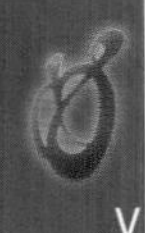

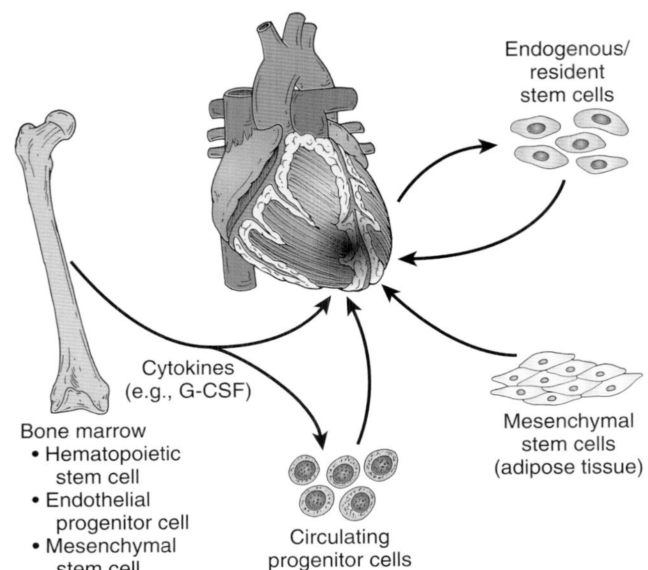

FIGURE 38-1 Adult cell types used for cardiac cell therapy. Schematic diagram outlining the sources of adult cells types that have been used for cardiac cell therapy. Each of these cell types has now been used in clinical trials. *G-CSF,* Granulocyte-colony stimulating factor.

and endothelial markers for vascular endothelial growth factor receptor 2 (KDR or flk-1), can form new blood vessels and enhance neovascularization after ischemia.[10,11] Whether these cells form new vessels by differentiating into endothelial cells or preferentially act as proangiogenic cells inducing neovascularization remains unclear. Regardless, several of these circulating cell types have made their way into the clinics and are currently being tested for clinical efficacy.

Bone marrow, the presumed source of the c-kit+ and other circulating progenitor cells, has been used extensively in preclinical and clinical trials.[12] Unfractionated bone marrow is a heterogeneous mix of cells, including hematopoietic stem cells, fibroblasts, endothelial cells, endothelial progenitor cells, and mesenchymal stem cells (MSCs) or stromal cells. Although the exact regenerative capability of each of these cell types is strongly debated, positive preclinical studies have resulted in numerous phase I clinical trials. However, to date, there is no direct evidence that any bone marrow cell can differentiate into a mature cardiomyocyte (without genetic reprogramming), so any regenerative effects are most likely indirect.

Several endogenous or resident cardiac stem cell/progenitors have now been described.[13] The best characterized of these is again a population of c-kit expressing cells but found within the myocardium with the potential to differentiate into all three cardiovascular cell types—cardiac myocytes, and endothelial and smooth muscle cells. These cardiac c-kit cells could be isolated and transplanted into recipient animals, reconstituting the infarcted ventricular wall and reducing infarct size.[14] Recently, a clinical trial isolating c-kit+ cells from left atrial appendage at the time of bypass surgery were isolated and reinjected into infarcted tissue (SCIPIO trial).[15] Although c-kit+ cells in the heart have garnered a significant amount of attention, it is not the only cell type that has been promoted as a potential source for cardiogenic stem cells. Other markers of hematologic stem cells have been promoted in mice as a potential source for resident cardiac stem cells, including the SCA-1 (Ly6A)[16] and the ABC transporter[17] (side population cells that efflux

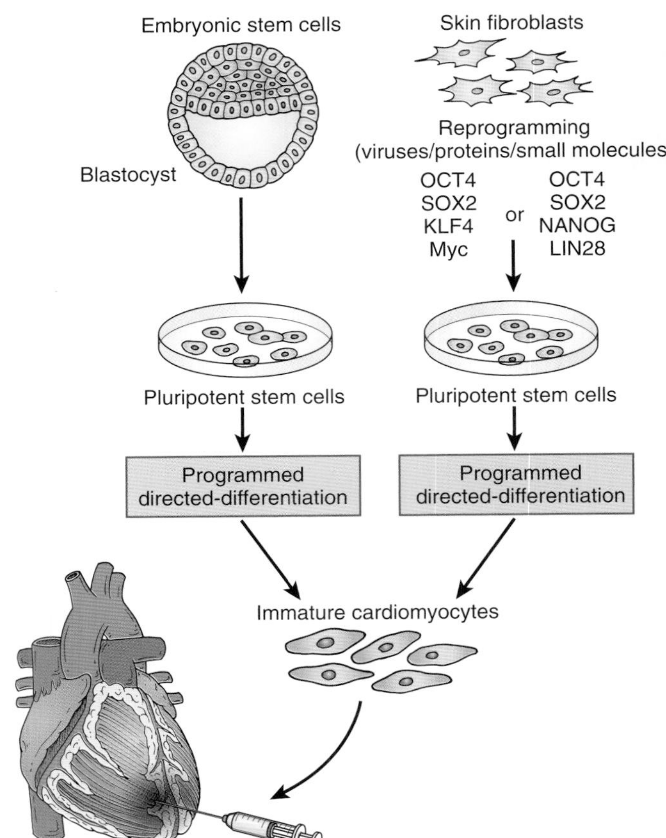

FIGURE 38-2 Use of pluripotent stem cells for cardiac repair. Embryonic stem cells are generated from the inner cell mass of blastocysts. They have the capacity to differentiate into cells of all three germ lines, including cardiac myocytes. Somatic cells such as skin fibroblasts can be reprogrammed to a pluripotent state with a cocktail of reprogramming factors.

Hoechst dye on flow cytometry). Unfortunately, there is no human orthologue for SCA-1, so translation of these results to humans is problematic. Finally, a cardiac progenitor cell has been reported to exist in cardiospheres, although its identity remains unknown.[18,19] These cardiospheres are three-dimensional clusters of cells formed from the cellular outgrowth of cardiac tissue explants.[20,21] Cardiospheres are a heterogeneous mix of nonmyocyte cells, which includes mesenchymal stem cells, smooth muscle cells, endothelial cells, cardiac fibroblasts, and presumably a cardiac progenitor cell. In preclinical studies, cardiosphere-derived cells improve LV function when transplanted into infarcted myocardium.[22]

Pluripotent Stem Cells

Embryonic Stem Cells

Human embryonic stem cells (ESC), first isolated in 1998,[23] are isolated from the inner cell mass of the blastocyst in the early stages of embryogenesis (**Figure 38-2**). These cells retain the potential to differentiate into any cell type if given the appropriate growth factors.[24,25] Initially, there was a belief that the heart milieu itself could provide either critical cell-cell interactions or growth factors to direct ESC to a cardiac phenotype and integrate into surrounding myocardium. This notion was quickly dispelled as injected ESC into mouse myocardium formed large teratomas rather than mature cardiomyocytes.[26,27] These studies also demonstrated that ESCs are not "immune-privileged" and therefore are quickly rejected by recipient animals unless these animals are properly immune-suppressed. Human ESC can be transplanted and survive in normal rodent hearts[28] and electrically couple with existing cardiomyocytes in porcine models.[29] When transplanted into recipient rodent models of MI, there was a reproducible improvement of 20% to 40% in fractional shortening of the mouse myocardium,[30,31] or ejection fraction (EF). These cells can grow and divide within the recipient heart, as well as form gap junctions and become electrically coupled to the host myocardium. In postinfarct models, not only have these cells proven to improve function but have also demonstrated reduced rates of ventricular arrhythmia either spontaneously or with attempted induction through electrical stimulation.[32] Although exciting, there has been at least some discussion that these improvements are not long lasting, and by 12 weeks the improvement in function is not statistically different from that in the control animals.[33] Although holding great promise, in contrast to adult cell types, there has been very limited application of ESC-derived cells in clinical trials, with studies limited to spinal cord injury and macular degeneration.[34] There have been no trials of ESC-derived cells in the heart, although one trial involving the transplantation of human ESC-derived CD15+ Isl-1+ progenitors in severe heart failure has been approved in France (www.clinicaltrials.gov).

Induced Pluripotent Stem Cells

Although the mature somatic cells contain all the genetic information of that first totipotent zygote, throughout development, a series of genetic modifications occur inhibiting a cell's ability to revert back to an earlier state. In 1996, the sheep, Dolly, was cloned by a method of transferring the nucleus from a somatic cell (in her case the mammary gland) to an unfertilized egg,[35] thus proving in the correct setting a cell can be converted to any other cell type. This discovery led to a flurry of excitement regarding methods of rewiring cells to an embryonic state. In 2007 a landmark paper demonstrated that a cocktail of four genes *(c-Myc, Oct3/4, SOX2,* and *Klf4)* known to maintain a pluripotent state in stem cells were expressed in mouse fibroblasts using retroviruses. A percentage of these fibroblasts converted into cells with embryonic stem cell capability. These cells were called *induced pluripotent stem cells* (iPSCs) (see Figure 38-2).[36] Since these initial discoveries, many papers have emerged demonstrating novel methods for achieving similar results using fewer genes,[37,38] addition of small molecule protein inhibitors,[38] hypoxic growth conditions,[39] or culture in mildly acidic media.[40] There has been success with the generation of cardiomyocytes from mouse or human iPSCs, which appear to function indistinguishably from cardiomyocytes derived from ESCs.[41] Transplantation of iPSC-derived cardiac myocytes improved LV function after MI in animal models.[42] In this model, iPSC treatment restored postischemic contractile performance, ventricular wall thickness, and electric stability while achieving in situ regeneration of cardiac, smooth muscle, and endothelial tissue. An added benefit with iPSCs is that they can be derived from the same patient they are intended to treat, thus by definition being an HLA match for the patient and obviating any need for immunosuppression. Although exciting, extending these results into humans would require derivation of clonal lineage committed cardiac cells or very efficient purification protocols to minimize any teratoma potential. Furthermore, the epigenetic profiles of different iPSC lines are quite varied, whether due to different donor cell types or the reprogramming methods used to generate the cells, which affects the differentiation potential of these iPSCs[43,44] and influence the oncogenic risk. Human iPSC generation by reprogramming of differentiated human somatic cells into a pluripotent state may someday eliminate the need for controversial human ESC and provide a mechanism to generate customized, patient-specific pluripotent cells for cardiac regenerative therapies and cardiovascular tissue engineering, but much work remains to be done.

Mechanisms of Action of Cardiac Cell Therapy

Early reports suggested that adult cell types, particularly the MSC from bone marrow, could differentiate into cardiovascular lineages including smooth muscle cells, endothelial cells, and cardiac myocytes. They did not differentiate spontaneously but required co-culture with existing cardiac myocytes,[45] or priming with demethylating agents[46] or cardiopoietic cytokines.[47] Thus when translating these cells in vivo investigators initially believed that the benefits of these BMCs would arise from their ability to form cardiomyocytes by transdifferentiation. A major limitation of the adult cardiac stem cell field is the inability to get full differentiation from putative stem/progenitor cells in vitro or in vivo. In fact, although expression of cardiac genes and proteins is demonstrated frequently, the levels, relative to authentic cardiac myocytes, and their ability to form sarcomeres and display calcium transients are rarely quantified.[48-50] In vivo engraftment studies have often demonstrated low-level retention of cells that, while expressing sarcomeric proteins, do not morphologically appear to resemble adult cardiac myocytes.[51] There is now general agreement that significant transdifferentiation of the injected BMC to cardiomyocytes is very limited, if it occurs at all. Identification of subsets of adult stem cells with a higher capacity to differentiate into cardiac myocytes and strategies to enhance cardiac differentiation are areas of intense research interest and at least one clinical trial has attempted to use bone marrow–derived MSCs pretreated with a cocktail of cytokines thought to cardiogenically orient them.[52] It has been suggested the resident cardiac stem cells have a greater cardiogenic differentiation potential, but whether this underlies their beneficial effects remains to be determined. The concept that new myogenesis cannot explain the benefits of most cell therapy is further supported by studies showing that cell transplantation clearly demonstrates a benefit but is not associated with significant engraftment.[53] In fact, there is a poor correlation between engraftment and functional benefit.[53] Thus the only stem cell type currently available with a robust ability to differentiate into mature cardiac myocytes remains pluripotent stem cells.

The reasons for the paradox between engraftment and benefit are unknown, although a number of alternative explanations have been proposed (**Figure 38-3**). One explanation for the regenerative effect of cardiac cell therapy is the possibility that injected cells activate endogenous repair mechanisms. Using genetic tracking mouse models, it was initially reported that new myocytes were being formed from a nonmyocyte, progenitor pool after MI,[54] which was enhanced by cell therapy.[55] However, in response to criticisms regarding the model used, investigators

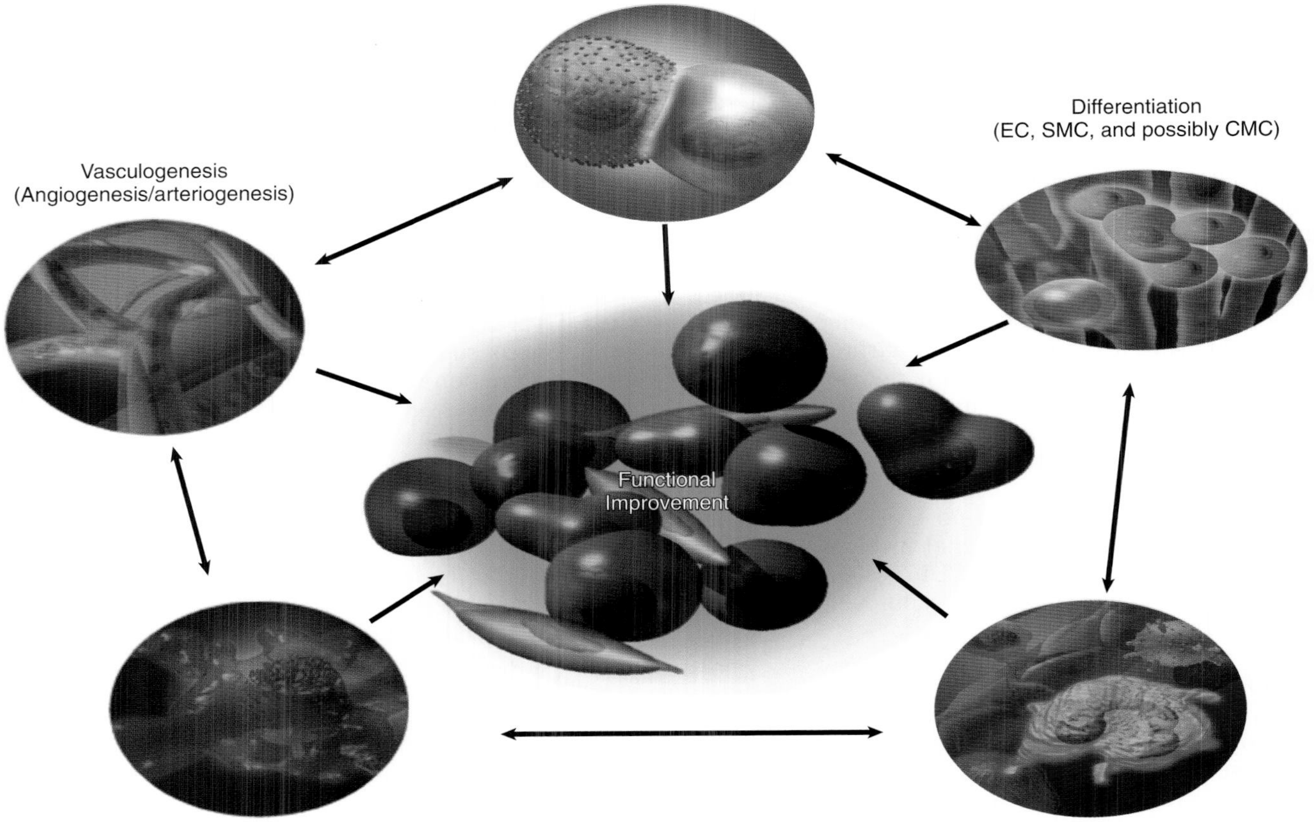

FIGURE 38-3 Mechanisms of benefit of cardiac cell therapy. The proposed mechanisms of action of transplanted cells in cardiac cell therapy are depicted. Direct cardiac myocyte transdifferentiation likely has a minor role in the beneficial effects in contrast to multiple paracrine effects, including neovascularization, activation of endogenous repair mechanisms, modulation of inflammation, and reducing apoptosis. *CMC,* Cardiac myocyte; *EC,* endothelial cells; *SMC,* smooth muscle cell.

developed a pulse-chase approach with stable isotope labeling and multi-isotope imaging mass spectrometry. This demonstrated that the genesis of cardiomyocytes occurs at a low rate (<1%) predominantly by the division of preexisting cardiomyocytes during normal aging, a process that increases adjacent to areas of myocardial injury.[56] This is consistent with recent studies using human heart samples that demonstrated that at the age of 25, approximately 1% of the cardiomyocytes per year are being regenerated; by the age of 75, the number falls to 0.45% per year.[57] It is not clear how these discrepancies will ultimately be resolved, but heavy isotope labeling is feasible in human patients, which will hopefully bring clarity to these issues.[58]

In addition to regenerative properties of stem cells, several other mechanisms have been proposed to explain their beneficial effects, including enhanced neovascularization, modulation of inflammation and scar formation, and cytoprotection (see Figure 38-3). Stem cells secrete paracrine factors, which could beneficially impact the repair process by preventing apoptosis and cardiac remodeling.[59] These paracrine factors can alter the development of fibrosis development during scar formation and/or modulate inflammatory processes.[60,61] Numerous animal studies support the ability of transplanted cells to increase capillary density and improved blood flow after ischemic injury. Augmenting blood flow to ischemic or hibernating myocardium can improve contractile function and prevent further damage. Neovascularization can be mediated by the physical incorporation of progenitor cells into new capillaries[10] or by perivascular accumulation of cells. Incorporated progenitor cells of most if not all types may release growth factors that promote angiogenesis by acting on mature endothelial cells.[62] When the cells expressing vascular markers were removed from BMCs, it resulted in an abrogation of the BMC-induced improved contractile recovery after MI.[63] Interestingly, transplanted cells can also stimulate the recruitment of proangiogenic monocytes.[64] Importantly, this proangiogenic effect persisted well beyond the survival of transplanted cells, potentially providing an explanation for lasting benefits in the absence of transplanted cells.

Clinical Trials of Cardiac Cell Therapy

Currently, there are over 75 trials of cardiac cell therapy listed on the Clinical Trials website (www.clinicaltrials.gov) using various adult progenitor cells at different stages of evaluation, but BMCs account for most of the trials performed thus far. Bone marrow is easily and safely aspirated even from patients who recently suffered an MI. Most human studies used the entire mononuclear cell fraction from bone marrow without further purification or ex vivo expansion in patients after an MI. There is a much more limited experience with cell therapy in heart failure patients.

TABLE 38-1 Randomized Cell Therapy Trials in Patients with Acute Myocardial Infarction and Ischemic Cardiomyopathy

		Number of Subjects					*Outcome*	
STUDY	**DESIGN**	**T**	**C**	**CELL TYPE**	**CELL NUMBER (×10^6)**	**TIME OF CELL DELIVERY (AFTER AMI)**	**IMPROVED**	**NO CHANGE**
Wollert et al, 2004 (BOOST)[87]	Open, controlled	30	30	BMCs	2460	6 ± 1 days	Global LVEF	LVEDV
Schachinger et al, 2006 (REPAIR-AMI)[88]	Placebo-controlled	95	92	BMCs	236	3-6 days	Global LVEF	LVEDV
Janssens et al, 2006 (Leuven-AMI)[89]	Placebo-controlled	32	34	BMCs	476	1 day	Regional contractility	Global LVEF LVEDV
Lunde et al, 2006 (ASTAMI)[90]	Open, controlled	47	50	Lymphocytic BMCs	54-130	6 ± 1 days	—	Global LVEF LVEDV
Huikuri et al, 2008 (FINCELL)[91]	Placebo-controlled	39	38	BMCs	402	≈3 days	Global LVEF	LVESV, LVEDV
Tendera et al, 2009 (REGENT)[92]	Open, controlled	97	20	BMCs vs. CD34+/CXCR4+ BMCs	178	3-12 days	Global LVEF	LVESV, LVEDV
Assmus et al, 2006 (TOPCARE-CHD)[93]	Open, controlled	35	23	BMCs	205	81 ± 72 months	Global LVEF	LVEDV
Menasche et al, 2008 (MAGIC)[4]	Placebo-controlled	67	30	Skeletal myoblasts	400 or 800	>4 weeks	LVEDV, LVESV	Regional contractility Global LVEF
Meluzin et al, 2008[94]	Parallel RCT	20	20	BMCs	10-100	7 days	LVEF LVESV	Perfusion defect, LVEDV
Lipiec et al, 2008[95]	Open, controlled	26	10	BMCs	NR (mBMC from 100 mL BM)	4-11 days	LV MPI	LVEF, LVEDV, LVESV
Cao et al, 2009[96]	Parallel RCT	41	45	BMCs	500	7 days	LVEF, LVEDV, LVESV	Perfusion defect
Grajek et al, 2010[97]	Parallel RCT	31	14	BMCs	410	4-5 days		
Roncalli et al, 2010 (BONAMI)[98]	Parallel RCT	52	49	BMCs	100	9 days		
Chen et al, 2004[99]	Parallel RCT	34	35	BMCs	8000-10,000	19 days		
Li et al, 2007[100]	Parallel RCT	35	35	BMCs	72.5	6 days		
Traverse et al, 2010[101]	Parallel RCT	30	10	BMCs	100	5		
Wohrle et al, 2010[102]	Parallel RCT	29	13	BMCs	381	6		
Hirsch et al, 2011 (HEBE)[103]	Parallel RCT	69	65	BMCs	2460	6 ± 1 days	Global LVEF	LVEDV
Traverse et al, 2011 (LateTIME Trial)	Parallel RCT	58	29	BMCs	236	3-6 days	Global LVEF	LVEDV
Chen et al, 2006[104]	Parallel RCT	24	24		476	1 day	Regional contractility	Global LVEF LVEDV
Yao et al, 2009[105]	Parallel RCT	15	15	BMCs	54-130	6 ± 1 days	—	Global LVEF LVEDV
Van Ramshort et al, 2009[106]	Parallel RCT	25	25		402	≈3 days	Global LVEF	LVESV, LVEDV
Perin et al, 2011 (FOCUS-HF)[107]	Parallel RCT	20	10		178	3-12 days	Global LVEF	LVESV, LVEDV
Hu et al, 2011[108]	Parallel RCT	31	29		205	81 ± 72 months	Global LVEF	LVEDV
Perin et al, 2012 (FOCUS-CCTRN)[109]	Parallel RCT	61	31		400 or 800	>4 weeks	LVEDV, LVESV	Regional contractility Global LVEF
Strauer et al, 2010 (STAR-heart)[110]	Parallel RCT	191	200		10-100	7 days	LVEF LVESV	Perfusion defect, LVEDV

AMI, Acute myocardial infarction; *BMC,* bone marrow cell; *C,* control; *LVEDV,* left ventricular end-diastolic volume; *LVEF,* left ventricular ejection fraction; *LVESV,* left ventricular end-systolic volume; *MPI,* myocardial perfusion index; *RCT,* randomized controlled study; *T,* treatment.

Also, a few trials have isolated specific endothelial progenitor cell subpopulations from bone marrow (CD133+ cells) or blood-derived cells.[11,65,66]

The results of clinical trials published to date using BMCs post-MI and ischemic cardiomyopathy are summarized in **Table 38-1** and have been reviewed by several recent publications.[12,67] Infusion of autologous BMC appears to be safe and well tolerated in patients with ischemic heart disease. Although large phase III trials that are adequately powered to determine the benefits of cell therapy are still lacking, a meta-analysis was recently released regarding the published trials involving over 2000 patients.[12] Overall, BMC therapy was associated with a significant increase in left ventricular ejection fraction (LVEF) of 2.8% and a significant decrease in perfusion defect size by 3.8% when compared with conventional therapy. The effect of BMC therapy was similar whether the cells were administered via intracoronary or intramyocardial routes and was not influenced by baseline EF or perfusion defect size. Although the magnitude of benefit of contractile function was similar in patients with heart failure, it did not reach statistical significance. Another recent meta-analysis focused solely on those patients receiving BMC for chronic ischemic cardiomyopathy. Cell therapy improved LVEF at 6 months

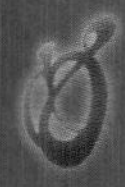

Study or Subgroup	BMC Mean	BMC SD	BMC Total	Control Mean	Control SD	Control Total	Weight	Mean Difference IV, Random, 95% CI
Ang IC 2008	−0.5	1.81	20	0.7	1.96	21	10.2%	−1.20 (−2.35, −0.05)
Ang IM arm 2008	4.3	1.58	21	0.7	1.96	21	10.3%	3.60 (2.52, 4.68)
Assmus 2006	2.9	3.6	28	−1.2	3	23	9.8%	4.10 (2.29, 5.91)
FOCUS-CCTRN trial	1.4	5.2	54	−1.3	5.1	28	9.3%	2.70 (0.36, 5.04)
FOCUS-HF 2011	3	2.66	20	3	3.34	10	9.3%	0.00 (−2.38, 2.38)
Hendrix et al 2006	6.1	8.6	10	3.6	9.1	10	4.2%	2.50 (−5.26, 10.26)
Hu et al 2011	10.62	11.98	31	5.69	6.87	29	6.6%	4.93 (0.03, 9.83)
Patel AN et al 2005	16.6	1.287	10	6.5	1.33	10	10.2%	10.10 (8.95, 11.25)
Pokushalov et al 2010	5	0.95	53	−0.6	0.978	46	10.5%	5.60 (5.22, 5.98)
Stamm et al 2007	9.7	2.31	20	3.4	3.07	20	9.9%	6.30 (4.62, 7.98)
Zhao et al 2008	13.25	2.6	16	3.93	3.1	18	9.7%	9.32 (7.40, 11.24)
Total (95% CI)			**283**			**236**	**100.0%**	**4.48 (2.43, 6.53)**

Heterogeneity: $Tau^2 = 10.33$; $Chi^2 = 244.99$, df = 10 (P <0.00001); $I^2 = 96\%$
Test for overall effect: Z = 4.28 (P <0.0001)

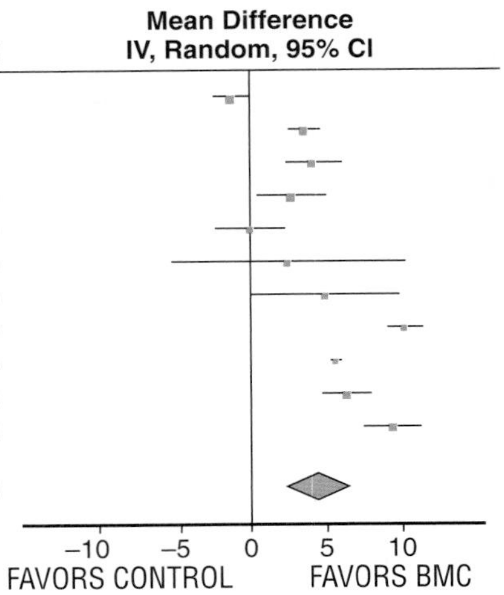

Mean Difference IV, Random, 95% CI: −10 −5 0 5 10; FAVORS CONTROL FAVORS BMC

A

Study or Subgroup	BMC Mean	BMC SD	BMC Total	Control Mean	Control SD	Control Total	Weight	Mean Difference IV, Random, 95% CI
Ang IC 2008	9.9	14.64	21	17.9	15.2	21	19.5%	−8.00 (−17.03, 1.03)
Ang IM arm 2008	−19.3	14.82	21	17.9	15.2	21	19.5%	−37.20 (−46.28, −28.12)
FOCUS-HF 2011	−18.9	13.07	20	−9.9	15.4	10	18.6%	−9.00 (−20.13, 2.13)
Pokushalov et al 2010	−27	6.71	55	7	8.5	54	21.5%	−34.00 (−36.88, −31.12)
Stamm et al 2007	−19.1	7.865	22	−5.5	9.58	21	20.9%	−13.60 (−18.85, −8.35)
Total (95% CI)			**139**			**127**	**100.0%**	**−20.64 (−33.21, −8.07)**

Heterogeneity: $Tau^2 = 189.39$; $Chi^2 = 79.41$, df = 4 (P <0.00001); $I^2 = 95\%$
Test for overall effect: Z = 3.22 (P = 0.001)

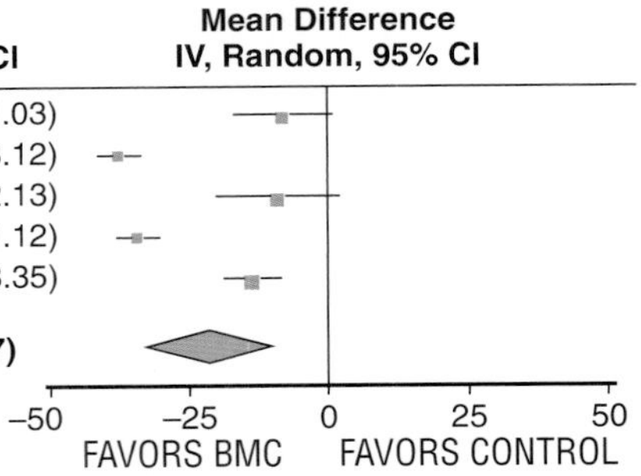

Mean Difference IV, Random, 95% CI: −50 −25 0 25 50; FAVORS BMC FAVORS CONTROL

B

Study or Subgroup	BMC Mean	BMC SD	BMC Total	Control Mean	Control SD	Control Total	Weight	Mean Difference IV, Random, 95% CI
Ang IC 2008	8.3	14.64	21	27	14.92	21	20.2%	−18.70 (−27.64, −9.76)
Ang IM arm 2008	−16.8	14.48	21	27	14.92	21	20.2%	−43.10 (−51.99, −34.21)
FOCUS-HF 2011	−9.3	14.91	20	−12.2	16.8	10	18.9%	2.90 (−9.39, 15.19)
Patel AN et al 2005	−22	12.31	10	−5	10.06	10	19.9%	−17.00 (−26.85, −7.15)
Stamm et al 2007	−11.1	11.28	20	−4.4	11.06	20	20.8%	−6.70 (−13.62, 0.22)
Total (95% CI)			**92**			**82**	**100.0%**	**−16.71 (−31.36, −2.06)**

Heterogeneity: $Tau^2 = 255.97$; $Chi^2 = 51.80$, df = 4 (P <0.00001); $I^2 = 92\%$
Test for overall effect: Z = 2.24 (P = 0.03)

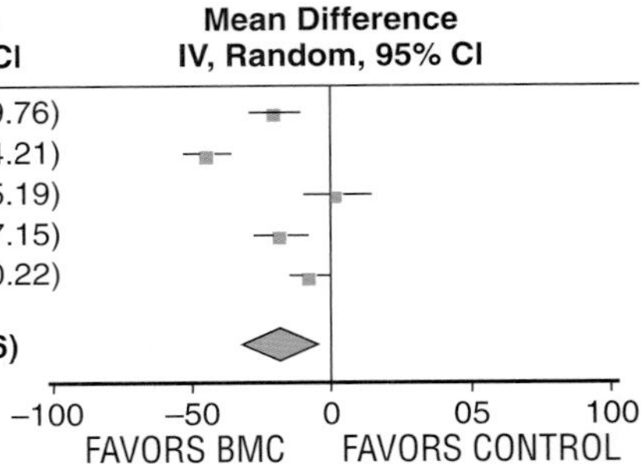

Mean Difference IV, Random, 95% CI: −100 −50 0 05 100; FAVORS BMC FAVORS CONTROL

C

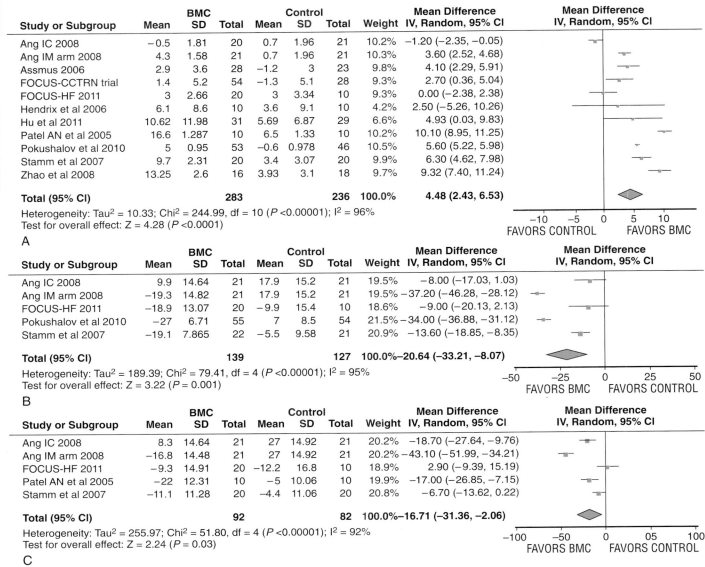

FIGURE 38-4 Benefits of bone marrow cell therapy in ischemic cardiomyopathy. Forest plot of weighted difference in mean (95% CI) improvements in **(A)** the LVEF, **(B)** LV end-systolic volume, and **(C)** LV end-diastolic volume. *BMC,* Bone marrow stem cell therapy; *FOCUS-CCTRN,* First Mononuclear Cells Injected in the United States conducted by the Cardiovascular Cell Therapy Research Network; *FOCUS-HF,* First Mononuclear Cells Injected in the United States in Ischemic Heart Failure; *IV,* inverse variance. *From Kandala J, et al: Meta-analysis of stem cell therapy in chronic ischemic cardiomyopathy. Am J Cardiol 112:217–225, 2013.*

by 4.48% and reduced LV end-systolic and end-diastolic volumes (**Figure 38-4**).[67] Interestingly, there was a greater improvement in the LVEF with intramyocardial injection compared with intracoronary infusion, which may suggest intramyocardial injection may be superior to intracoronary infusion in patients with LV systolic dysfunction. Although bone marrow cell therapy remains a promising approach acutely after ischemic injury or chronically in patients with ischemic cardiomyopathy, the absolute changes in EF or perfusion defects are relatively small and within the error margin of the imaging techniques used. Thus the final assessment of the benefits of this therapy must await larger randomized trials, some of which are currently under way.

It should be noted that while the results with BMC transplantation are encouraging, numerous questions remain unanswered. Although the meta-analysis suggests a positive effect on LV function, most of the studies were small and results of multimodality imaging sometimes discordant, even in the same study. Further, there remains no consensus on the most effective way to prepare cells, optimal dosing or delivery, and timing of administration. There is also concern that LVEF, although used as the primary endpoint in most studies, may not be the best endpoint. Cell therapies may have a disproportionately greater impact on clinical outcomes, such as functional status or quality of life relative to the increase in EF. The REPAIR-AMI trial suggested a potential benefit to clinical endpoints with BMC treatment despite its limited sample size. The incidence of the cumulative endpoint deaths, MIs, and rehospitalizations for HF was significantly lower in the BMC-treated patients compared with a placebo after 1-year follow-up.[68] Consistent with this, the meta-analysis of BMC therapy in patients with chronic ischemic cardiomyopathy demonstrated improvements in NYHA class and Minnesota Living With Heart Failure Questionnaire (MLHFQ) score.[67] Finally, durability of the effects of cell transplantation has

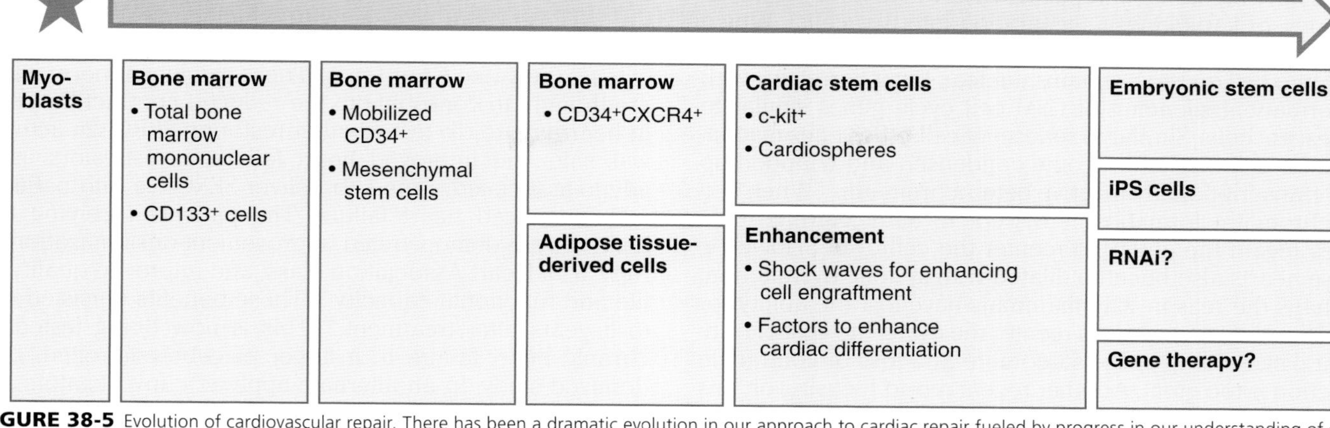

FIGURE 38-5 Evolution of cardiovascular repair. There has been a dramatic evolution in our approach to cardiac repair fueled by progress in our understanding of stem cells. The relative role of newer approaches, including pluripotent stem cells and gene therapy, remain to be determined.

been questioned[69]; however, long-term follow-up is limited and additional studies will need to be done to confirm this.

The first phase I trials using autologous, resident cardiac cells, SCIPIO,[15] and CADUCEUS[70] studies have now been reported. The SCIPIO trial randomized 33 patients with LV dysfunction (EF <40%) undergoing coronary artery bypass graft surgery to intracoronary injection of c-kit+, lineage-negative autologous cardiac stem cells, or usual care. At 4 months, CSC therapy demonstrated an increase in LVEF from a baseline of 29.0 ± 1.7% to 36.0 ± 2.5%.[15] This improvement was sustained at 1 year, improving an additional 8.1%.[71] Additionally, scar size was reduced 44.8% and viable LV tissue mass by 31.5 g at 1 year. CADUCEUS randomized 31 patients with ischemic cardiomyopathy to intracoronary administration of autologous CDCs approximately 2 months after an MI. There was no significant difference in LVEF or volumes between groups; however, compared with the control group, CDC-treated patients showed an increase in viable myocardium and reductions in scar mass at the 6-month time point. CDC-treated patients also demonstrated improvements in functional capacity but no improvement in quality of life. Although exciting, these results need to be viewed with caution as the numbers of patients were small and a significant number of patients did not receive follow-up magnetic resonance imaging, which could affect the LV parameters. Clinical trials with larger numbers of patients and longer follow-up are necessary to establish efficacy of endogenous cardiac cells in ischemic cardiomyopathy. Which cell type will ultimately triumph as the preferred cell for cardiac cell therapy is unknown at this point, but clearly there has been a rapid progress in our understanding and application of this promising therapy (**Figure 38-5**).

GENE THERAPIES IN HEART FAILURE

Gene Therapy Targeting Regeneration

Attempts to reactivate cardiomyocyte proliferation after injury have proven remarkably difficult. Early studies using overexpression of viral oncogene induced cardiac myocyte death.[72,73] More recently investigators have used adenoviral gene transfer targeted delivery of cyclin A2 into failing hearts and have demonstrated improvements in hemodynamic function and ventricular wall thickness. Whether this represents true cardiac regeneration and whether it can be translated to humans remains to be determined. In an alternative approach investigators injected DNA plasmids, which overexpress stromal cell-derived factor-1 (SDF-1), a cytokine implicated in stem cell homing.[74] This resulted in improvements in functional class and quality of life. There were no safety concerns but the promising efficacy of SDF-1 therapy should be interpreted with caution as there was no control group.

Interestingly, the progress in the reprogramming field has prompted researchers to determine if fibroblasts can be directly transformed into differentiated cells. A combination of three transcription factors was used to convert exocrine pancreatic cells to endocrine cells or neurons.[75] In 2010, a trio of transcription factors (Gata4, Mefc2, and Tbx5) were identified after screening a pool of 14 candidate genes involved in cardiomyocyte development that when infected into mouse fibroblasts could induce 20% of cells to become cardiomyocytes,[76] with the first signs of cardiomyocyte-specific protein expression after only 3 days. The robustness of the conversion to cardiomyocytes should only get better as scientists further dissect the pathways involved in the conversion of fibroblasts to cardiomyocytes. Infecting the postinfarct heart with these transcription factors[77] or combining them with HAND2[78] resulted in 4% to 35% of the cardiomyocytes in the region bordering the infarct zone being derived from the infected fibroblasts with almost a 50% reduction in scar area and improved LV function. Obviously, if these findings prove reproducible, it could obviate the need for cell therapy entirely, avoiding the concerns for rejection or infection. However, these studies are in their infancy, and it is likely as the field matures that issues will also arise from this approach. Retroviral infection of fibroblasts has many caveats when considering human applications, namely concern for infection frequency, random genomic insertion sites, tissue-specific infection, and inflammatory reaction. Furthermore, although the results are indeed exciting, the frequency of fibroblast-derived cardiomyocytes in the infarct border region was small; however, there was surprisingly significant improvement in heart function and decreased scar size. Further studies will dissect the conclusions of these papers' determining mechanism and exact the contribution of the infected cells to the improved function. These papers set a fascinating baseline from which further research will with hope only improve.

Clearly, in disease states, some mammalian cardiomyocytes have an ability to replicate DNA but to not advance to the step of karyokinesis (separation into two cells). Why a mature mammalian cardiac myocyte loses its ability to undergo cell division remains unclear, but it correlates with a permanent silencing of G2M cell cycle genes similar to senescent cells. Similar to senescent cells, the genes responsible for cell division become condensed and wrapped up into transcriptionally inactive heterochromatin.[79] When heterochromatin formation is disrupted, adult cardiac myocytes regain the ability to reenter the cell cycle. However, these hearts also became dilated with systolic dysfunction, perhaps the reason why mammals have lost the ability for adult cardiac myocytes to reenter the cycle; the cost of transient disassembly of the sarcomere and loss of contractile function is too great. Another recent report focusing on this perinatal period from day 3 to day 7, when the cardiomyocytes lose their ability to divide, demonstrated that a protein named Meis1 (myeloid ecotropic viral integration site 1 homolog), a protein involved in developmental regulation of hematopoietic cells but also upregulated in myocardium in the early postnatal period, may also repress the ability for cardiomyocytes to undergo replication. When Meis1 protein levels were reduced, a 10-fold increase in proliferation of cardiomyocytes could be seen within 1 week.[80]

MicroRNAs (miRNAs) regulate many regulatory pathways in cardiac development; thus it is not surprising that a number have been identified as regulating cardiac myocyte proliferation and as potential therapeutics. To identify miRNAs that might promote cardiac myocyte proliferation, investigators performed a high-throughput screen using a whole genome miRNA library in neonatal cardiomyocytes. Of the 875 miRNA mimics examined, 40 induced cell cycle progression including miR-590-3p and miR-199a-3p, which were selected for further studies of adult heart regeneration.[81] Overexpression of miR-590-3p and miR-199a-3p in neonatal mice increased cardiomyocyte, but not cardiac fibroblast, proliferation as well as reducing scar formation and improving cardiac function post MI.[81] Although the definitive targets of these miRNAs are unknown, it does suggest that they could be used as therapeutic reagents to promote myocardial regeneration following cardiac injury. Using a different approach based on developmental expression, miR-195 (a member of the miR-15 family) was identified as the most highly upregulated miRNA during the perinatal period. Knockdown of the miR-15 family in neonatal mice was associated with an increased number of mitotic cardiomyocytes,[82] extending the regenerative window and improving LV function after myocardial infaction.[83]

Although we have believed for decades that cardiomyocytes permanently exit the cell cycle after birth, effectively preventing a regenerative response, new data suggest the cardiac myocytes can be coaxed back into the cell cycle and create more new cardiomyocytes. There are now molecular targets that can be exploited for this purpose; however, this therapy is not without risks. Cardiac myocyte dedifferentiation could induce heart failure if cardiac myocyte cell cycle reentry is associated with reduced contractile function.[79]

Gene Therapy Targeting Contractility

The development of heart failure is associated with a series of modifications in the molecular regulation of cardiac contractility and particularly calcium handling. Classically, this includes a downregulation of sarcoplasmic reticulum Ca^{2+}-ATPase (SERCA2a) activity, which controls movement of calcium ions into the sarcoplasmic reticulum from the cytosol (see also Chapter 2). These calcium abnormalities are thought to contribute to the reduced contractility seen in heart failure. To test whether restoring SERCA2a activity was safe and improved heart failure, investigators used adeno-associated virus 1 to deliver SERCA2a into patients with advanced heart failure. The patients receiving the highest dose demonstrated improvement or stabilization in New York Heart Association class, and improved quality of life and functional capacity.[84] These benefits persisted out to 3 years after treatment.[85] This is now being tested in chronic heart failure in a larger placebo-controlled, randomized study. In an alternate approach, investigators are attempting to improve cardiac contractility using adenoviral-mediated gene transfer of human adenylyl cyclase type 6 (AC6).[86] This ongoing phase I trial will test safety and whether this agent may be of benefit in heart failure patients.

References

1. Murry CE, Wiseman RW, Schwartz SM, et al: Skeletal myoblast transplantation for repair of myocardial necrosis. *J Clin Invest* 98(11):2512–2523, 1996.
2. Taylor DA, Silvestry SC, Bishop SP, et al: Delivery of primary autologous skeletal myoblasts into rabbit heart by coronary infusion: a potential approach to myocardial repair. *Proc Assoc Am Physicians* 109(3):245–253, 1997.
3. Dib N, McCarthy P, Campbell A, et al: Feasibility and safety of autologous myoblast transplantation in patients with ischemic cardiomyopathy. *Cell Transplant* 14(1):11–19, 2005.
4. Menasche P, Alfieri O, Janssens S, et al: The Myoblast Autologous Grafting in Ischemic Cardiomyopathy (MAGIC) trial: first randomized placebo-controlled study of myoblast transplantation. *Circulation* 117(9):1189–1200, 2008.
5. Murry CE, Soonpaa MH, Reinecke H, et al: Haematopoietic stem cells do not transdifferentiate into cardiac myocytes in myocardial infarcts. *Nature* 428(6983):664–668, 2004.
6. Balsam LB, Wagers AJ, Christensen JL, et al: Haematopoietic stem cells adopt mature haematopoietic fates in ischaemic myocardium. *Nature* 428(6983):668–673, 2004.
7. Assmus B, Schachinger V, Teupe C, et al: Transplantation of Progenitor Cells and Regeneration Enhancement in Acute Myocardial Infarction (TOPCARE-AMI). *Circulation* 106(24):3009–3017, 2002.
8. Strauer BE, Brehm M, Zeus T, et al: Repair of infarcted myocardium by autologous intracoronary mononuclear bone marrow cell transplantation in humans. *Circulation* 106(15):1913–1918, 2002.
9. Orlic D, Kajstura J, Chimenti S, et al: Bone marrow cells regenerate infarcted myocardium. *Nature* 410(6829):701–705, 2001.
10. Kawamoto A, Tkebuchava T, Yamaguchi J, et al: Intramyocardial transplantation of autologous endothelial progenitor cells for therapeutic neovascularization of myocardial ischemia. *Circulation* 107(3):461–468, 2003.
11. Erbs S, Linke A, Schuler G, et al: Intracoronary administration of circulating blood-derived progenitor cells after recanalization of chronic coronary artery occlusion improves endothelial function. *Circ Res* 98(5):e48, 2006.
12. Sadat K, Ather S, Aljaroudi W, et al: The effect of bone marrow mononuclear stem cell therapy on left ventricular function and myocardial perfusion. *J Nucl Cardiol* 21:351–367, 2014.
13. Epstein JA, Parmacek MS: Recent advances in cardiac development with therapeutic implications for adult cardiovascular disease. *Circulation* 112(4):592–597, 2005.
14. Beltrami AP, Barlucchi L, Torella D, et al: Adult cardiac stem cells are multipotent and support myocardial regeneration. *Cell* 114(6):763–776, 2003.
15. Bolli R, Chugh AR, D'Amario D, et al: Cardiac stem cells in patients with ischaemic cardiomyopathy (SCIPIO): initial results of a randomised phase 1 trial. *Lancet* 378(9806):1847–1857, 2011.
16. Oh H, Bradfute SB, Gallardo TD, et al: Cardiac progenitor cells from adult myocardium: homing, differentiation, and fusion after infarction. *Proc Natl Acad Sci U S A* 100(21):12313–12318, 2003.
17. Pfister O, Oikonomopoulos A, Sereti KI, et al: Role of the ATP-binding cassette transporter Abcg2 in the phenotype and function of cardiac side population cells. *Circ Res* 103(8):825–835, 2008.
18. Masuda S, Montserrat N, Okamura D, et al: Cardiosphere-derived cells for heart regeneration. *Lancet* 379(9835):2425–2426, 2012.
19. Smith RR, Barile L, Cho HC, et al: Regenerative potential of cardiosphere-derived cells expanded from percutaneous endomyocardial biopsy specimens. *Circulation* 115(7):896–908, 2007.
20. Messina E, De AL, Frati G, et al: Isolation and expansion of adult cardiac stem cells from human and murine heart. *Circ Res* 95(9):911–921, 2004.
21. Davis DR, Zhang Y, Smith RR, et al: Validation of the cardiosphere method to culture cardiac progenitor cells from myocardial tissue. *PLoS ONE* 4(9):e7195, 2009.
22. Lee ST, White AJ, Matsushita S, et al: Intramyocardial injection of autologous cardiospheres or cardiosphere-derived cells preserves function and minimizes adverse ventricular remodeling in pigs with heart failure post-myocardial infarction. *J Am Coll Cardiol* 57(4):455–465, 2011.
23. Thomson JA, Itskovitz-Eldor J, Shapiro SS, et al: Embryonic stem cell lines derived from human blastocysts. *Science* 282(5391):1145–1147, 1998.
24. Ladd AN, Yatskievych TA, Antin PB: Regulation of avian cardiac myogenesis by activin/TGFbeta and bone morphogenetic proteins. *Dev Biol* 204(2):407–419, 1998.
25. Sugi Y, Lough J: Activin-A and FGF-2 mimic the inductive effects of anterior endoderm on terminal cardiac myogenesis in vitro. *Dev Biol* 168(2):567–574, 1995.
26. Nussbaum J, Minami E, Laflamme MA, et al: Transplantation of undifferentiated murine embryonic stem cells in the heart: teratoma formation and immune response. *FASEB J* 21(7):1345–1357, 2007.

27. Swijnenburg RJ, Tanaka M, Vogel H, et al: Embryonic stem cell immunogenicity increases upon differentiation after transplantation into ischemic myocardium. *Circulation* 112(9 Suppl):I166–I172, 2005.
28. Laflamme MA, Gold J, Xu C, et al: Formation of human myocardium in the rat heart from human embryonic stem cells. *Am J Pathol* 167(3):663–671, 2005.
29. Kehat I, Khimovich L, Caspi O, et al: Electromechanical integration of cardiomyocytes derived from human embryonic stem cells. *Nat Biotechnol* 22(10):1282–1289, 2004.
30. Laflamme MA, Chen KY, Naumova AV, et al: Cardiomyocytes derived from human embryonic stem cells in pro-survival factors enhance function of infarcted rat hearts. *Nat Biotechnol* 25(9):1015–1024, 2007.
31. Caspi O, Huber I, Kehat I, et al: Transplantation of human embryonic stem cell-derived cardiomyocytes improves myocardial performance in infarcted rat hearts. *J Am Coll Cardiol* 50(19):1884–1893, 2007.
32. Shiba Y, Fernandes S, Zhu WZ, et al: Human ES-cell-derived cardiomyocytes electrically couple and suppress arrhythmias in injured hearts. *Nature* 489(7415):322–325, 2012.
33. van Laake LW, Passier R, Monshouwer-Kloots J, et al: Monitoring of cell therapy and assessment of cardiac function using magnetic resonance imaging in a mouse model of myocardial infarction. *Nat Protoc* 2(10):2551–2567, 2007.
34. Schwartz SD, Hubschman JP, Heilwell G, et al: Embryonic stem cell trials for macular degeneration: a preliminary report. *Lancet* 379(9817):713–720, 2012.
35. Wilmut I, Schnieke AE, McWhir J, et al: Viable offspring derived from fetal and adult mammalian cells. *Nature* 385(6619):810–813, 1997.
36. Takahashi K, Yamanaka S: Induction of pluripotent stem cells from mouse embryonic and adult fibroblast cultures by defined factors. *Cell* 126(4):663–676, 2006.
37. Nakagawa M, Koyanagi M, Tanabe K, et al: Generation of induced pluripotent stem cells without Myc from mouse and human fibroblasts. *Nat Biotechnol* 26(1):101–106, 2008.
38. Huangfu D, Maehr R, Guo W, et al: Induction of pluripotent stem cells by defined factors is greatly improved by small-molecule compounds. *Nat Biotechnol* 26(7):795–797, 2008.
39. Yoshida Y, Takahashi K, Okita K, et al: Hypoxia enhances the generation of induced pluripotent stem cells. *Cell Stem Cell* 5(3):237–241, 2009.
40. Obokata H, Wakayama T, Sasai Y, et al: Stimulus-triggered fate conversion of somatic cells into pluripotency. *Nature* 505(7485):641–647, 2014.
41. Schenke-Layland K, Rhodes KE, Angelis E, et al: Reprogrammed mouse fibroblasts differentiate into cells of the cardiovascular and hematopoietic lineages. *Stem Cells* 26(6):1537–1546, 2008.
42. Nelson TJ, Martinez-Fernandez A, Yamada S, et al: Repair of acute myocardial infarction by human stemness factors induced pluripotent stem cells. *Circulation* 120(5):408–416, 2009.
43. Cahan P, Daley GQ: Origins and implications of pluripotent stem cell variability and heterogeneity. *Nat Rev Mol Cell Biol* 14(6):357–368, 2013.
44. Ghosh Z, Wilson KD, Wu Y, et al: Persistent donor cell gene expression among human induced pluripotent stem cells contributes to differences with human embryonic stem cells. *PLoS ONE* 5(2):e8975, 2010.
45. Condorelli G, Borello U, De AL, et al: Cardiomyocytes induce endothelial cells to transdifferentiate into cardiac muscle: implications for myocardium regeneration. *Proc Natl Acad Sci U S A* 98(19):10733–10738, 2001.
46. Makino S, Fukuda K, Miyoshi S, et al: Cardiomyocytes can be generated from marrow stromal cells in vitro. *J Clin Invest* 103:697–705, 1999.
47. Behfar A, Yamada S, Crespo-Diaz R, et al: Guided cardiopoiesis enhances therapeutic benefit of bone marrow human mesenchymal stem cells in chronic myocardial infarction. *J Am Coll Cardiol* 56(9):721–734, 2010.
48. Barile L, Messina E, Giacomello A, et al: Endogenous cardiac stem cells. *Prog Cardiovasc Dis* 50(1):31–48, 2007.
49. Bearzi C, Rota M, Hosoda T, et al: Human cardiac stem cells. *Proc Natl Acad Sci U S A* 104(35):14068–14073, 2007.
50. He JQ, Vu DM, Hunt G, et al: Human cardiac stem cells isolated from atrial appendages stably express c-kit. *PLoS ONE* 6(11):e27719, 2011.
51. Li TS, Cheng K, Lee ST, et al: Cardiospheres recapitulate a niche-like microenvironment rich in stemness and cell-matrix interactions, rationalizing their enhanced functional potency for myocardial repair. *Stem Cells* 28(11):2088–2098, 2010.
52. Bartunek J, Behfar A, Dolatabadi D, et al: Cardiopoietic stem cell therapy in heart failure: the C-CURE (Cardiopoietic stem Cell therapy in heart failURE) multicenter randomized trial with lineage-specified biologics. *J Am Coll Cardiol* 61(23):2329–2338, 2013.
53. Tang XL, Rokosh G, Sanganalmath SK, et al: Intracoronary administration of cardiac progenitor cells alleviates left ventricular dysfunction in rats with a 30-day-old infarction. *Circulation* 121(2):293–305, 2010.
54. Hsieh PC, Segers VF, Davis ME, et al: Evidence from a genetic fate-mapping study that stem cells refresh adult mammalian cardiomyocytes after injury. *Nat Med* 13(8):970–974, 2007.
55. Loffredo FS, Steinhauser ML, Gannon J, et al: Bone marrow-derived cell therapy stimulates endogenous cardiomyocyte progenitors and promotes cardiac repair. *Cell Stem Cell* 8(4):389–398, 2011.
56. Senyo SE, Steinhauser ML, Pizzimenti CL, et al: Mammalian heart renewal by pre-existing cardiomyocytes. *Nature* 493(7432):433–436, 2013.
57. Bergmann O, Bhardwaj RD, Bernard S, et al: Evidence for cardiomyocyte renewal in humans. *Science* 324(5923):98–102, 2009.
58. Busch R, Neese RA, Awada M, et al: Measurement of cell proliferation by heavy water labeling. *Nat Protoc* 2(12):3045–3057, 2007.
59. Anderson CD, Heydarkhan-Hagvall S, Schenke-Layland K, et al: The role of cytoprotective cytokines in cardiac ischemia/reperfusion injury. *J Surg Res* 148(2):164–171, 2008.
60. Ma S, Xie N, Li W, et al: Immunobiology of mesenchymal stem cells. *Cell Death Differ* 21(2):216–225, 2014.
61. El-Jawhari JJ, El-Sherbiny YM, Jones EA, et al: Mesenchymal stem cells, autoimmunity and rheumatoid arthritis. *QJM* 107:505–514, 2014.
62. Urbich C, Aicher A, Heeschen C, et al: Soluble factors released by endothelial progenitor cells promote migration of endothelial cells and cardiac resident progenitor cells. *J Mol Cell Cardiol* 39(5):733–742, 2005.
63. Yoon CH, Koyanagi M, Iekushi K, et al: Mechanism of improved cardiac function after bone marrow mononuclear cell therapy: role of cardiovascular lineage commitment. *Circulation* 121(18):2001–2011, 2010.
64. Ryu JC, Davidson BP, Xie A, et al: Molecular imaging of the paracrine proangiogenic effects of progenitor cell therapy in limb ischemia. *Circulation* 127(6):710–719, 2013.
65. Assmus B, Schachinger V, Teupe C, et al: Transplantation of Progenitor Cells and Regeneration Enhancement in Acute Myocardial Infarction (TOPCARE-AMI). *Circulation* 106(24):3009–3017, 2002.
66. Losordo DW, Schatz RA, White CJ, et al: Intramyocardial transplantation of autologous CD34+ stem cells for intractable angina: a phase I/IIa double-blind, randomized controlled trial. *Circulation* 115(25):3165–3172, 2007.
67. Kandala J, Upadhyay GA, Pokushalov E, et al: Meta-analysis of stem cell therapy in chronic ischemic cardiomyopathy. *Am J Cardiol* 112(2):217–225, 2013.
68. Schachinger V, Erbs S, Elsasser A, et al: Intracoronary bone marrow-derived progenitor cells in acute myocardial infarction. *N Engl J Med* 355(12):1210–1221, 2006.
69. Meyer GP, Wollert KC, Lotz J, et al: Intracoronary bone marrow cell transfer after myocardial infarction: 5-year follow-up from the randomized-controlled BOOST trial. *Eur Heart J* 30(24):2978–2984, 2009.
70. Makkar RR, Smith RR, Cheng K, et al: Intracoronary cardiosphere-derived cells for heart regeneration after myocardial infarction (CADUCEUS): a prospective, randomised phase 1 trial. *Lancet* 379(9819):895–904, 2012.
71. Chugh AR, Beache GM, Loughran JH, et al: Administration of cardiac stem cells in patients with ischemic cardiomyopathy: the SCIPIO trial: surgical aspects and interim analysis of myocardial function and viability by magnetic resonance. *Circulation* 126(11 Suppl 1):S54–S64, 2012.
72. Kirshenbaum LA, Schneider MD: Adenovirus E1A represses cardiac gene transcription and reactivates DNA synthesis in ventricular myocytes, via alternative pocket protein- and p300-binding domains. *J Biol Chem* 270:7791–7794, 1995.
73. Kirshenbaum LA, Chakraborty S, Schneider MD: Human E2F-1 reactivates cell cycle progression in ventricular myocytes and represses cardiac gene transcription. *Dev Biol* 179:402–411, 1996.
74. Penn MS, Mendelsohn FO, Schaer GL, et al: An open-label dose escalation study to evaluate the safety of administration of nonviral stromal cell-derived factor-1 plasmid to treat symptomatic ischemic heart failure. *Circ Res* 112(5):816–825, 2013.
75. Zhou Q, Brown J, Kanarek A, et al: In vivo reprogramming of adult pancreatic exocrine cells to beta-cells. *Nature* 455(7213):627–632, 2008.
76. Ieda M, Fu JD, Delgado-Olguin P, et al: Direct reprogramming of fibroblasts into functional cardiomyocytes by defined factors. *Cell* 142(3):375–386, 2010.
77. Qian L, Berry EC, Fu JD, et al: Reprogramming of mouse fibroblasts into cardiomyocyte-like cells in vitro. *Nat Protoc* 8(6):1204–1215, 2013.
78. Song K, Nam YJ, Luo X, et al: Heart repair by reprogramming non-myocytes with cardiac transcription factors. *Nature* 485(7400):599–604, 2012.
79. Sdek P, Zhao P, Wang Y, et al: Rb and p130 control cell cycle gene silencing to maintain the postmitotic phenotype in cardiac myocytes. *J Cell Biol* 194(3):407–423, 2011.
80. Mahmoud AI, Kocabas F, Muralidhar SA, et al: Meis1 regulates postnatal cardiomyocyte cell cycle arrest. *Nature* 497(7448):249–253, 2013.
81. Eulalio A, Mano M, Dal FM, et al: Functional screening identifies miRNAs inducing cardiac regeneration. *Nature* 492(7429):376–381, 2012.
82. Porrello ER, Johnson BA, Aurora AB, et al: MiR-15 family regulates postnatal mitotic arrest of cardiomyocytes. *Circ Res* 109(6):670–679, 2011.
83. Porrello ER, Mahmoud AI, Simpson E, et al: Regulation of neonatal and adult mammalian heart regeneration by the miR-15 family. *Proc Natl Acad Sci U S A* 110(1):187–192, 2013.
84. Jessup M, Greenberg B, Mancini D, et al: Calcium Upregulation by Percutaneous Administration of Gene Therapy in Cardiac Disease (CUPID): a phase 2 trial of intracoronary gene therapy of sarcoplasmic reticulum Ca2+-ATPase in patients with advanced heart failure. *Circulation* 124(3):304–313, 2011.
85. Zsebo K, Yaroshinsky A, Rudy JJ, et al: Long-term effects of AAV1/SERCA2a gene transfer in patients with severe heart failure: analysis of recurrent cardiovascular events and mortality. *Circ Res* 114(1):101–108, 2014.
86. Phan HM, Gao MH, Lai NC, et al: New signaling pathways associated with increased cardiac adenylyl cyclase 6 expression: implications for possible congestive heart failure therapy. *Trends Cardiovasc Med* 17(7):215–221, 2007.
87. Wollert KC, Meyer GP, Lotz J, et al: Intracoronary autologous bone-marrow cell transfer after myocardial infarction: the BOOST randomised controlled clinical trial. *Lancet* 364(9429):141–148, 2004.
88. Schachinger V, Erbs S, Elsasser A, et al: Intracoronary bone marrow-derived progenitor cells in acute myocardial infarction. *N Engl J Med* 355(12):1210–1221, 2006.
89. Janssens S, Dubois C, Bogaert J, et al: Autologous bone marrow-derived stem-cell transfer in patients with ST-segment elevation myocardial infarction: double-blind, randomised controlled trial. *Lancet* 367(9505):113–121, 2006.
90. Lunde K, Solheim S, Aakhus S, et al: Intracoronary injection of mononuclear bone marrow cells in acute myocardial infarction. *N Engl J Med* 355(12):1199–1209, 2006.
91. Huikuri HV, Kervinen K, Niemela M, et al: Effects of intracoronary injection of mononuclear bone marrow cells on left ventricular function, arrhythmia risk profile, and restenosis after thrombolytic therapy of acute myocardial infarction. *Eur Heart J* 29(22):2723–2732, 2008.
92. Tendera M, Wojakowski W, Ruzyllo W, et al: Intracoronary infusion of bone marrow-derived selected CD34+CXCR4+ cells and non-selected mononuclear cells in patients with acute STEMI and reduced left ventricular ejection fraction: results of randomized, multicentre Myocardial Regeneration by Intracoronary Infusion of Selected Population of Stem Cells in Acute Myocardial Infarction (REGENT) Trial. *Eur Heart J* 30(11):1313–1321, 2009.
93. Assmus B, Honold J, Schachinger V, et al: Transcoronary transplantation of progenitor cells after myocardial infarction. *N Engl J Med* 355(12):1222–1232, 2006.
94. Brocheriou V, Hagege AA, Oubenaissa A, et al: Cardiac functional improvement by a human Bcl-2 transgene in a mouse model of ischemia/reperfusion injury. *J Gene Med* 2(5):326–333, 2000.
95. Lipiec P, Krzeminska-Pakula M, Plewka M, et al: Impact of intracoronary injection of mononuclear bone marrow cells in acute myocardial infarction on left ventricular perfusion and function: a 6-month follow-up gated 99mTc-MIBI single-photon emission computed tomography study. *Eur J Nucl Med Mol Imaging* 36(4):587–593, 2009.
96. Cao F, Sun D, Li C, et al: Long-term myocardial functional improvement after autologous bone marrow mononuclear cells transplantation in patients with ST-segment elevation myocardial infarction: 4 years follow-up. *Eur Heart J* 30(16):1986–1994, 2009.
97. Grajek S, Popiel M, Gil L, et al: Influence of bone marrow stem cells on left ventricle perfusion and ejection fraction in patients with acute myocardial infarction of anterior wall: randomized clinical trial: impact of bone marrow stem cell intracoronary infusion on improvement of microcirculation. *Eur Heart J* 31(6):691–702, 2010.
98. Roncalli J, Mouquet F, Piot C, et al: Intracoronary autologous mononucleated bone marrow cell infusion for acute myocardial infarction: results of the randomized multicenter BONAMI trial. *Eur Heart J* 32(14):1748–1757, 2011.
99. Chen SL, Fang WW, Ye F, et al: Effect on left ventricular function of intracoronary transplantation of autologous bone marrow mesenchymal stem cell in patients with acute myocardial infarction. *Am J Cardiol* 94(1):92–95, 2004.
100. Li ZQ, Zhang M, Jing YZ, et al: The clinical study of autologous peripheral blood stem cell transplantation by intracoronary infusion in patients with acute myocardial infarction (AMI). *Int J Cardiol* 115(1):52–56, 2007.
101. Traverse JH, McKenna DH, Harvey K, et al: Results of a phase 1, randomized, double-blind, placebo-controlled trial of bone marrow mononuclear stem cell administration in patients following ST-elevation myocardial infarction. *Am Heart J* 160(3):428–434, 2010.
102. Wohrle J, Merkle N, Mailander V, et al: Results of intracoronary stem cell therapy after acute myocardial infarction. *Am J Cardiol* 105(6):804–812, 2010.
103. Hirsch A, Nijveldt R, van der Vleuten PA, et al: Intracoronary infusion of mononuclear cells from bone marrow or peripheral blood compared with standard therapy in patients after acute myocardial infarction treated by primary percutaneous coronary intervention: results of the randomized controlled HEBE trial. *Eur Heart J* 32(14):1736–1747, 2011.

104. Chen S, Liu Z, Tian N, et al: Intracoronary transplantation of autologous bone marrow mesenchymal stem cells for ischemic cardiomyopathy due to isolated chronic occluded left anterior descending artery. *J Invasive Cardiol* 18(11):552–556, 2006.
105. Yao K, Huang R, Sun A, et al: Repeated autologous bone marrow mononuclear cell therapy in patients with large myocardial infarction. *Eur J Heart Fail* 11(7):691–698, 2009.
106. van RJ, Bax JJ, Beeres SL, et al: Intramyocardial bone marrow cell injection for chronic myocardial ischemia: a randomized controlled trial. *JAMA* 301(19):1997–2004, 2009.
107. Perin EC, Silva GV, Henry TD, et al: A randomized study of transendocardial injection of autologous bone marrow mononuclear cells and cell function analysis in ischemic heart failure (FOCUS-HF). *Am Heart J* 161(6):1078–1087, 2011.
108. Hu S, Liu S, Zheng Z, et al: Isolated coronary artery bypass graft combined with bone marrow mononuclear cells delivered through a graft vessel for patients with previous myocardial infarction and chronic heart failure: a single-center, randomized, double-blind, placebo-controlled clinical trial. *J Am Coll Cardiol* 57(24):2409–2415, 2011.
109. Perin EC, Willerson JT, Pepine CJ, et al: Effect of transendocardial delivery of autologous bone marrow mononuclear cells on functional capacity, left ventricular function, and perfusion in chronic heart failure: the FOCUS-CCTRN trial. *JAMA* 307(16):1717–1726, 2012.
110. Strauer BE, Yousef M, Schannwell CM: The acute and long-term effects of intracoronary Stem cell Transplantation in 191 patients with chronic heARt failure: the STAR-heart study. *Eur J Heart Fail* 12(7):721–729, 2010.

Pulmonary Hypertension

Shannon M. Dunlay, Garvan C. Kane, and Margaret M. Redfield

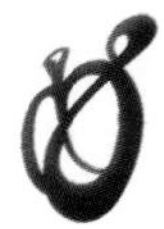

PULMONARY HYPERTENSION: DEFINITION AND CLASSIFICATION

Pulmonary hypertension (PH) is a hemodynamic finding and is considered to be present when the mean pulmonary artery pressure (mPAP) is 25 mm Hg or more (**Table 39-1**). PH is *suspected* based on clinical features or when echocardiography reveals an elevation in Doppler-derived estimates of PAPs and/or unexplained right ventricular enlargement or dysfunction. When the clinical situation and/or Doppler findings raise the suspicion of PH, a right-heart catheterization must be performed to confirm the presence of PH and determine the specific hemodynamic perturbation causing the elevation of mPAP. Pulmonary venous hypertension (PVH), pulmonary arterial hypertension (PAH), increased cardiac output, or some combination of these patterns (see Table 39-1) may cause PH. Finally, the underlying disease process or processes leading to PH must be defined.

A wide range of diseases can cause PH. The outdated separation of PH into primary and secondary causes has been replaced by a classification where PH is apportioned to five broad groups according to the specific hemodynamic abnormalities and underlying disease processes (**Table 39-2**). In general, the five PH groups identify common pathophysiology and treatment response and thus provide a context in which to structure the diagnostic evaluation.

The prevalence of PH and the contribution of each PH group to the global burden of PH have not been well defined and will vary according to practice setting and adequacy of diagnostic evaluation. An observational cohort study of an echocardiographic laboratory serving a region of Australia confirmed the predominance of group 2 PH among patients with elevated right ventricular systolic pressure (RVSP) at echocardiography (**Figure 39-1**),[1] many of whom have clear left-heart abnormalities.

CLINICAL FEATURES RAISING THE SUSPICION OF PULMONARY HYPERTENSION

The symptoms of PH are nonspecific and influenced by the hemodynamic type and underlying disease, but PH should be suspected in patients complaining of dyspnea, fatigue, exercise intolerance, chest pain, syncope, or edema. The physical examination may reveal evidence of PH, as well as clues to the cause of PH (**Table 39-3**).

Enlargement of the central pulmonary arteries with peripheral pruning of the pulmonary vasculature may be present on a chest radiograph (CXR) in patients with PAH. In the case of concomitant right ventricular failure, right ventricular enlargement (decrease in retrosternal space) and right atrial enlargement (enlarged right-heart border) may also be seen (**Figure 39-2**). Findings on electrocardiography (ECG) include signs of right ventricular hypertrophy, such as right-axis deviation, tall R wave in V_1, inverted T waves and ST depression in lead V_1 to V_3, and tall p waves in lead II because of right atrial enlargement.

DIAGNOSTIC EVALUATION OF PULMONARY HYPERTENSION

In general, evidence of PH is discovered when echocardiography is obtained during the evaluation of known or

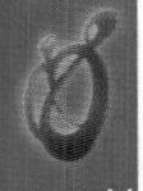

TABLE 39-1 Hemodynamic Parameters Defining Types of Pulmonary Hypertension

	TRUE NORMAL	PAH	PVH	MIXED	HIGH OUTPUT STATE
Established Parameters					
Mean PAP (mPAP, mm Hg)	<15	>25	>25	>25	>25
Systolic PAP (PASP, mm Hg)	<25	>35-40	>35-40	>35-40	>35-40
Mean PCWP (mm Hg)	<12	<15	≥15	≥15	variable
PVR ([mPAP-PCWP]/CO, Wood units)	<2	>3	≤3	>3	<3
Cardiac index (L/min/m²)	>2.5	variable	variable	variable	>5
Emerging Parameters					
Mean TPG (mPAP-PCWP, mm Hg)	<7	>12	≤12	>12	<12
Diastolic TPG (PADP-PCWP, mm Hg)	<5	≥7	<7	≥7	<7
Reactivity Testing in Group 1 PAH	Appropriate agents Inhaled NO, IV adenosine, IV prostacyclin			Positive response ↓mPAP ≥ 10 mm Hg *and* to <40 mm Hg without ↓ in CO	

CO, Cardiac output; *IV,* intravenously; *NO,* nitric oxide; *PAH,* pulmonary arterial hypertension; *PAP,* pulmonary artery pressure; *PCWP,* pulmonary capillary wedge pressure; *PVH,* pulmonary venous hypertension; *PVR,* pulmonary vascular resistance; *TPG,* transpulmonary gradient.

TABLE 39-2 Classification of Pulmonary Hypertension

Group 1 PH: Pulmonary Arterial Hypertension
Idiopathic (IPAH)
Familial (FPAH)
Associated With (APAH)
Collagen vascular disease
Congenital systemic-to-pulmonary shunts
Portal hypertension
Human immunodeficiency virus infection
Drugs and toxins
Other (thyroid disorders, glycogen storage disease, Gaucher disease, hereditary hemorrhagic telangiectasia, hemoglobinopathies, chronic myeloproliferative disorders, splenectomy)
Associated with substantial venous or capillary involvement
Pulmonary veno-occlusive disease
Pulmonary capillary hemangiomatosis
Persistent pulmonary hypertension of the newborn
Group 2 PH: PH (PVH or Mixed) Due to Left Heart Disease
Left-sided atrial or ventricular heart disease
Left-sided valvular heart disease
Group 3 PH: PH (PAH) Associated with Lung Disease or Hypoxemia
Chronic obstructive pulmonary disease
Interstitial lung disease
Sleep-disordered breathing
Alveolar hypoventilation disorders
Long-term exposure to high altitude
Developmental abnormalities
Group 4 PH: PAH Due to Chronic Thromboembolic Disease
Thromboembolic obstruction of proximal pulmonary arteries
Thromboembolic obstruction of distal pulmonary arteries
Nonthrombotic pulmonary embolism (tumor, parasites, fat)
Group 5 PH: Miscellaneous Rare Causes of PAH
Sarcoidosis, histiocytosis X, lymphangiomatosis, compression of pulmonary vessels

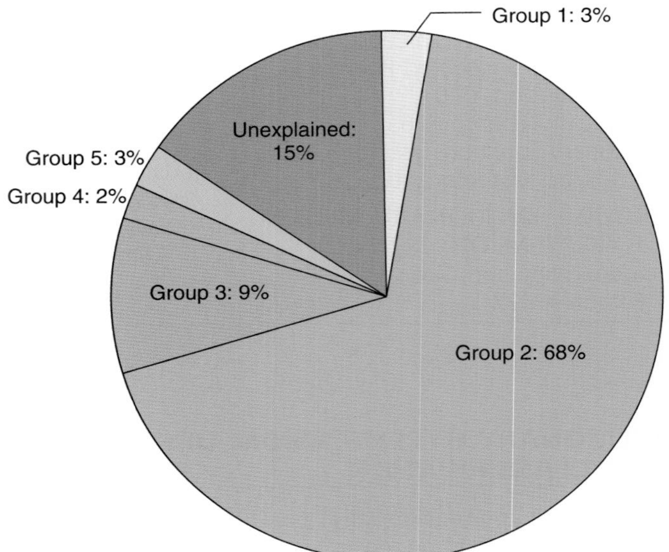

FIGURE 39-1 Distribution of the underlying cause of pulmonary hypertension. The proportion of patients with pulmonary hypertension (PH) classified as group 1 (pulmonary arterial hypertension), group 2 (PH due to left-sided disease), group 3 (PH due to lung disease), group 4 (PH due to chronic thromboembolic disease), group 5 (PH due to rare miscellaneous causes) or unexplained among an Australian cohort are shown. *From Strange G, Playford D, Stewart S, et al: Pulmonary hypertension: prevalence and mortality in the Armadale echocardiography cohort. Heart 98:1805–1811, 2012.*

suspected left heart or lung disease (group 2 and 3 PH). If the severity of PH at Doppler echocardiography is consistent with the severity of left-heart or lung disease, PH is usually attributed to the underlying process without further evaluation. However, if the severity of PH appears out of proportion to the severity of left-heart or lung disease or if PH is found in the absence of an obvious underlying cause, a rigorous evaluation should be performed to characterize the severity of PH and ascertain the cause. Guidelines recommend a comprehensive evaluation when the Doppler-estimated RVSP exceeds 40 to 50 mm Hg in the absence of a clear cause,[2] particularly in the setting of right-heart structural and functional abnormalities and in patient cohorts at an elevated risk of PAH (e.g., scleroderma, chronic liver disease, HIV infection).

Even in the setting of an obvious cause, the potential for a second process contributing to PH should be entertained so as to address concomitant and potentially treatable causes of PH. Left heart or pulmonary disease are risk factors for thromboembolic disease (group 4 PH), and patients with pulmonary disease may have unrecognized left heart disease (and vice versa). Understanding the degree of PH expected in patients with left-heart or pulmonary disease is required to appreciate when PH, is "out of proportion" and suggestive of additional processes.

The accepted diagnostic evaluation of PH is shown in **Table 39-4** and focuses on pivotal tests warranted in the evaluation of patients with PH in whom the cause is not obvious from the history, physical examination, CXR, and ECG. When pivotal tests are positive, contingent tests are

TABLE 39-3 Physical Examination in Pulmonary Hypertension

FINDING	IMPLICATIONS	FINDING	ETIOLOGIC INSIGHTS
Inspection		Clubbing	Congenital HD, PVOD
↑ JVP	RV failure	Central cyanosis	Hypoxia; R→L shunt
↑ A wave	Early RV failure	Sclerodactyly	Collagen vascular disease
V wave	Tricuspid regurgitation	Telangiectasia	
Ascites	RV failure	Rash	
Edema	RV failure	Raynaud	
Palpation		Varicose veins	Thromboembolic disease
Right parasternal lift	RV enlargement	Stasis pigment/ulcer	
Hepatomegaly	RV failure	Splenomegaly	Portopulmonary PH
Pulsatile liver	Tricuspid regurgitation	Spider angioma	
Auscultation		Palmer erythema	
↑ S_2P	Elevated PAP	Icterus	
Early systolic click	Elevated PAP	Caput medusa	
Holosystolic murmur RSB	Tricuspid regurgitation	Velcro rales	Interstitial lung disease
Inspiratory accentuation	Tricuspid regurgitation	Left sided murmur	Left heart disease
Diastolic murmur ULSB	Pulmonic regurgitation	Apical S_3 or S_4	
S_3 or S_4 RSB	RV failure	Laterally displaced apex	

JVP, Jugular venous pressure; *PAP,* pulmonary artery pressure; *PH,* pulmonary hypertension; *PVOD,* pulmonary veno-occlusive disease; *RSB,* right sternal border; *RV,* right ventricular; *S_2P,* pulmonic component of the second heart sound; *ULSB,* upper left sternal border.

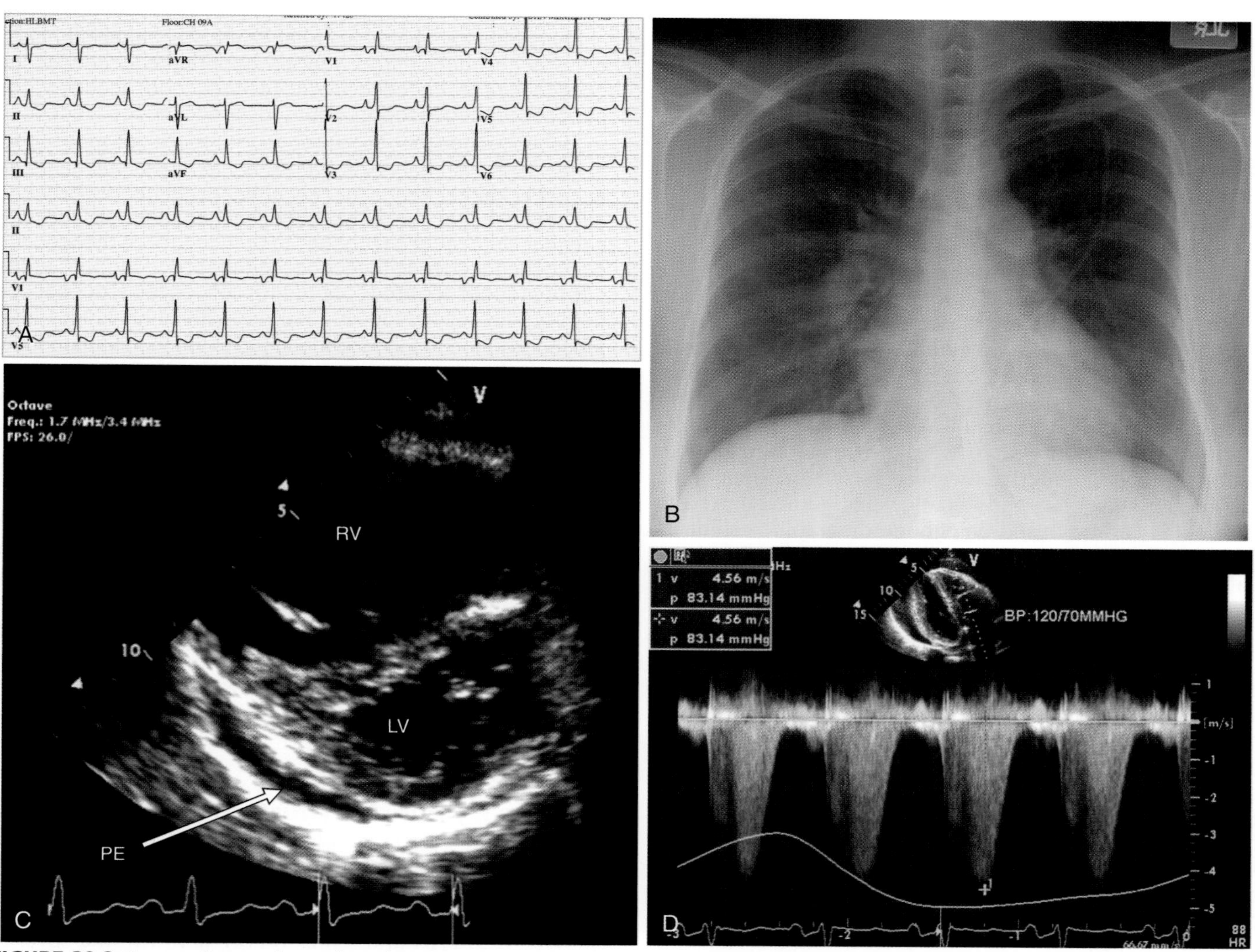

FIGURE 39-2 Electrocardiogram, chest radiograph, and echocardiographic findings in patients with pulmonary arterial hypertension. **A,** Typical ECG findings include right-axis deviation, right atrial enlargement, and right ventricular hypertrophy. **B,** Enlargement of the central pulmonary arteries with peripheral pruning of the pulmonary vasculature and evidence of right-sided chamber enlargement may be seen on chest radiograph. **C,** Right ventricular (RV) enlargement, flattening of the intraventricular septum resulting in a D-shaped left ventricle (LV) may be seen on echocardiography. A pericardial effusion (PE) may be present. **D,** The peak tricuspid regurgitation velocity can be used to estimate the right ventricular systolic pressure (elevated at >4 m/s).

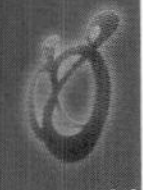

TABLE 39-4 Diagnostic Evaluation of Pulmonary Hypertension

PIVOTAL TESTS	CONTINGENT TESTING	TO ASSESS...
History and physical examination, CXR, and electrocardiogram		Suspect PH
Transthoracic echo	Transesophageal echo (select cases)	Doppler estimated PASP RV size and function Presence of left heart disease Congenital abnormalities
Ventilation/perfusion scan	Pulmonary angiography, CT angiography, coagulopathy evaluation	Chronic thromboembolic disease Low probability: no further testing Intermediate or high probability: CT or invasive pulmonary angiography
Overnight oximetry	Polysomnography	Sleep-disordered breathing–related PH
Pulmonary function testing	Arterial blood gas, chest CT	Lung disease–related PH
HIV	Infectious disease evaluation	HIV-related PH
Antinuclear antibody	Other CTD serologies, rheumatology evaluation	Connective tissue disease–related PH
Liver function tests	Liver ultrasound; echo shunt study	Portopulmonary hypertension
6-Minute Walk Test; BNP or NT-proBNP, CPXT		Prognosis and baseline to assess therapeutic response
Right-heart catheterization		Presence, severity, and type of PH (see Table 39-1) Exclude intracardiac shunt PAH—assess vasodilator response to guide therapy

BNP, B-type natriuretic peptide; *CPXT,* cardiopulmonary exercise test; *CT,* computed tomography; *CTD,* connective tissue disease; *CXR,* chest x-ray; *HIV,* human immunodeficiency virus; *NT-proBNP,* amino terminal BNP; *PAH,* pulmonary arterial hypertension; *PASP,* pulmonary artery systolic pressure; *PH,* pulmonary hypertension; *RV,* right ventricle.

obtained. The order and extent of the evaluation will be influenced by clinical suspicion, but echocardiography should be performed in all patients.

Echocardiographic Evaluation of Known or Suspected Pulmonary Hypertension

Echocardiography is a central test in the clinical evaluation of known or suspected PH (see also Chapter 29). The echocardiogram should address three key features. The first is an assessment of pulmonary hemodynamics. With close attention to technical details, the echocardiogram may provide reasonably accurate estimates of systolic, mean, and diastolic PAPs based on the Doppler velocity profiles of the peak tricuspid regurgitation (TR) and pulmonary valve regurgitation signals (see Figure 39-2). This information is integrated with a two-dimensional and Doppler estimation of right atrial pressure based on imaging of the inferior vena cava and hepatic veins. Although a suspicion of PH can be based on echocardiographic estimates, the diagnosis *cannot be established* without right-heart catheterization.

The second key feature in an echo evaluation of a PH patient is the evaluation of a host of variables that help define the severity of disease. These relate to quantitative assessment of right-sided enlargement and dysfunction.[3] With regard to right ventricular contractility, a key feature to note is that in contrast to the left ventricle the predominant direction of contractility is in the longitudinal plane with the base of the right ventricle moving down toward the apex. Hence measures of longitudinal contractility such as the tricuspid annular plane systolic excursion (TAPSE), the peak systolic velocity of the tricuspid annulus by tissue Doppler, and longitudinal systolic strain best reflect right ventricular performance and prognosis.[4,5] Other findings that indicate more severe disease include the presence of a "D-shaped" left ventricle, a delayed relaxation mitral inflow pattern, a high estimated right atrial pressure, more tricuspid valve regurgitation, and right-sided chamber enlargement.

The presence of a pericardial effusion, common in PAH, reflects chronic central venous hypertension and/or the presence of connective tissue disease, both features that indicate an increased mortality risk in PAH.[6,7]

The third important focus of an echocardiographic study in a patient with PH is the separation of a precapillary from a postcapillary form of PH. Indeed, many features of advanced left-heart disease, such as significant left-sided valvular stenosis or regurgitation or myocardial disease, are easily characterized by echocardiography. Although echocardiographic features, including left atrial size may be helpful, the separation of a patient with heart failure with preserved ejection fraction (HFpEF) and advanced right-heart dysfunction from a patient with a restricted pulmonary vascular mechanism of PH can be challenging solely on the basis of echo.

Laboratory Testing

All patients should have a complete blood cell count with platelet count and liver function tests. Antinuclear antibody titer is used to screen for connective tissue disease. Although 40% of patients with idiopathic PAH have positive but low antinuclear antibody (ANA) titers (≥1 : 80 dilutions), patients with a substantially elevated ANA or suspicious clinical findings require further serologic assessment and rheumatology consultation. Human immunodeficiency virus (HIV) serology should be considered.

Pulmonary Function Testing

Pulmonary function testing (PFT) is used to diagnose and quantify the underlying airway or parenchymal lung disease and should be performed in all patients with PH. The diffusing capacity for carbon monoxide (DLCO) is reduced in patients with PAH and tends to correlate with the severity of the disease. A patient with PAH would be expected to have normal spirometry and lung volumes. In all forms of PAH, desaturation during exercise is primarily related to the inability of the right ventricle to augment cardiac output, resulting in further depression of mixed venous oxygen saturation. Overnight oximetry can screen for clinically significant sleep apnea or hypopnea during sleep. In the evaluation of patients with PH, an assessment of sleep-disordered breathing is recommended.

Right-Heart Catheterization

Right-heart catheterization is *mandatory* to confirm the diagnosis of PH and should be completed on all patients before initiating therapy (see also Chapter 31). Cardiac output, pulmonary vascular resistance, PA pressure, and pulmonary artery wedge pressure (PAWP) should all be determined. Intracardiac shunting should also be excluded.

GROUP 1: PULMONARY ARTERIAL HYPERTENSION

PAH describes a group of various pulmonary hypertensive diseases that have similar histopathology, clinical presentations, and in whom approaches to therapy are similar. These include idiopathic and heritable causes and PH related to a number of associated conditions, including connective tissue diseases, systemic-to-pulmonary shunts, chronic liver disease, HIV infection, exposure to certain drugs or dietary products, and persistent PH of the newborn. In addition, pulmonary veno-occlusive disease and pulmonary capillary hemangiomatosis are included in the category of PAH, because they also are characterized by arteriopathy and by similar risk factors and possibly genetic substrates.

Epidemiology and Clinical Features

Idiopathic PAH

Idiopathic PAH, previously referred to as *primary pulmonary hypertension,* is a rare disease with an annual incidence of 1 to 2 cases per million and occurs more commonly in women than men. The average age at diagnosis is in the fourth decade.

Heritable PAH

Heritable causes of PAH include either a family history of PAH or a de novo mutation that imparts a heritable risk. These include alterations in genes from the transforming growth factor-β family, including bone morphogenetic protein receptor type 2 (BMPR2) and activin-like kinase 1 (ALK1).[8,9] ALK-1 mutations are most commonly found in patients with hereditary hemorrhagic telangiectasia and PAH. BMPR2 mutations are present in 20% of PAH cases, but have a lifetime penetrance of only 10% to 20%.[9] Testing for BMPR2 mutations is available and should be considered in patients with idiopathic PAH, particularly in those with a family history of PAH and to relatives of patients with heritable PAH, but should be preceded by genetic counseling.

Pulmonary Arterial Hypertension–Associated Conditions

Connective Tissue Disease

PAH can occur in conjunction with all forms of connective tissue diseases but occurs most commonly in systemic sclerosis (typically limited scleroderma), occurring in approximately 12% of cases.[10] As such, routine screening for PAH with symptom assessment, PFT (evaluating for abnormalities in diffusion capacity), and echocardiography every 1 to 2 years should be considered in patients with systemic sclerosis. Patients with PAH associated with connective tissue diseases often have a less robust response to PAH-specific medications and a poorer prognosis than those with idiopathic PAH.[11] All patients with unexplained PAH should have clinical and autoantibody testing for connective tissue disease.

Systemic-Pulmonary Shunts

PAH is a known complication of congenital heart disease, frequently associated with systemic to pulmonary shunts (see also Chapter 25). Initially systemic-pulmonary shunts lead to a period of high pulmonary flow but low pulmonary resistance. However, over time the high vascular shear stress related to elevated blood flow induces endothelial damage and progressive irreversible pulmonary vascular remodeling. The term *Eisenmenger syndrome* refers to the irreversible state of PAH mediated through arterial shunts causing pulmonary vasculopathy and ultimately resulting in a right-to-left or bidirectional shunt. The likelihood of PAH developing usually depends on the site and severity of the defect with ventricular septal defects causing PAH more commonly than atrial septal defects or a patent ductus arteriosus. Rarely, PAH may develop even after the defect is corrected.

The early diagnosis of lesions and appropriate timing of corrective surgery are critical to the prevention of PAH with congenital heart disease. Although multifactorial, persistent exposure to increased blood flow can result in progressive endothelial dysfunction, vasoconstriction, and vascular remodeling in the pulmonary circulation, which is not always reversible. Some patients will have residual elevation in pulmonary vascular resistance and PAH even following repair if irreversible changes have occurred in the pulmonary circulation.[12] PAH may also be seen in other forms of left-right shunts, including large peripheral arteriovenous malformations and even iatrogenic A-V fistulae placed for dialysis.

Compared with a patient who has idiopathic PAH, a patient with Eisenmenger syndrome and a comparable degree of PH has a greater probability of longer survival.[13]

Drugs and Toxins

Drugs and toxins have been implicated in the pathogenesis of some cases of PAH, including the use of central nervous system stimulants and appetite suppressants. In the 1960s, the anorexigen aminorex was first reported to be associated with PAH, and withdrawn from the market in 1972. In the 1980s and 1990s, fenfluramine and dexfenfluramine were reported to be associated with a marked increase in the risk of PAH if used for more than 3 months. The fenfluramines act by stimulating serotonin release; serotonin is a potent pulmonary vasoconstrictor and smooth muscle mitogen.[14] Central nervous system stimulants, such as amphetamine and methamphetamine, may also cause PAH.[15]

Chronic Liver Disease

A patient with advanced liver disease has a greatly increased risk of PH, and although often asymptomatic, it requires

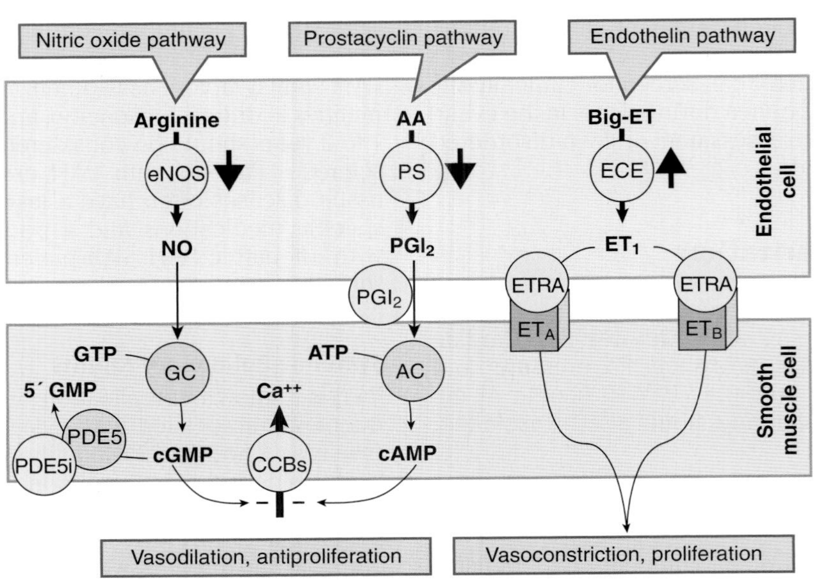

FIGURE 39-3 Disturbed mechanistic pathways in patients with pulmonary arterial hypertension (PAH). The three mechanistic pathways known to be disturbed in patients with PAH are shown. The short, thick black arrows depict aberrations observed in these pathways in patients with PAH. The points at which drug treatment affects these mechanistic pathways are shown in blue circles. *Left,* The nitric oxide (NO) pathway. Nitric oxide is created in endothelial cells by type III (i.e., endothelial) NO synthase (eNOS), which in pulmonary arterial smooth muscle cells (PASMCs) induces guanylate cyclase (GC) to convert guanylate triphosphate (GTP) to cyclic guanylate monophosphate (cGMP). Cyclic GMP is a second messenger that constitutively maintains PASMC relaxation and inhibition of PASMC proliferation by ultimately reducing inward flux of calcium ions (Ca^{++}). Cyclic GMP is removed by the PDE5 enzyme to yield the inactive product 5′GMP. Patients with PAH have reduced expression and activity of eNOS. *Middle,* The prostacyclin pathway. The production of prostaglandin I2 (PGI2 [i.e., prostacyclin]) is catalyzed by prostacyclin synthase (PS) in endothelial cells. In PASMCs, PGI2 stimulates adenylate cyclase (AC), thus increasing production of cyclic adenosine monophosphate (cAMP) from adenosine triphosphate (ATP). Cyclic AMP is a second messenger that constitutively maintains PASMC relaxation and inhibition of PASMC proliferation. Patients with PAH have reduced expression and activity of PS. *Right,* The endothelin (ET) pathway. Big- (i.e., pro-) ET is converted in endothelial cells to ET1 (a 21–amino acid peptide) by endothelin-converting enzyme (ECE). ET1 binds to PASMC ETA and ETB receptors, ultimately leading to PASMC contraction, proliferation, and hypertrophy. Patients with PAH have increased expression and activity of ECE. *AA,* Arachidonic acid; *CCB,* calcium channel blocker; *ETRA,* endothelin receptor antagonist; *PDE5i,* phosphodiesterase 5 inhibitor. *From McGoon MD, Kane GC: Pulmonary hypertension: diagnosis and management. Mayo Clin Proceed 84:191–207, 2009.*

consideration because patients undergoing liver transplantation with PH are at high mortality risk.[16] Patients with portopulmonary hypertension have a spectrum of hemodynamics but frequently have a hyperdynamic circulation with high cardiac output.

Pulmonary Veno-occlusive Disease and Pulmonary Capillary Hemangiomatosis

These are rare causes of PAH. Pathologically, pulmonary veno-occlusive disease is characterized by extensive occlusion of the pulmonary veins by fibrous tissue. In pulmonary capillary hemangiomatosis, there is proliferation of benign thin-walled capillary vessels in the lung parenchyma. They should be suspected when patients present with severe precapillary PH and evidence of pulmonary edema, often triggered by pulmonary vascular targeted therapies. Typically the PAWP is normal or low. Lung biopsy is required to confirm the diagnosis; however, often the procedural risk is prohibitive. Prognosis is poor, and there is a variable response to therapy. Lung transplantation is the only successful management strategy.

Pathophysiology of Group 1 Pulmonary Arterial Hypertension

In PAH, there is a disruption in the balance of vasodilators and vasoconstrictors, smooth muscle mitogens, growth inhibitors, and prothrombotic and anticoagulant compounds (**Figure 39-3**). As such, it is characterized by vasoconstriction, smooth muscle cell proliferation, and thrombosis.

Prostacyclin and thromboxane A2 are arachidonic acid metabolites. Prostacyclin is a potent vasodilator that inhibits platelet activation, and has been shown to be deficient in PAH. Conversely, thromboxane A2 is prothrombotic, and is found in elevated levels in PAH.[17] Nitric oxide is a known vasodilator and inhibitor of smooth muscle proliferation and platelet activation. It is produced by the family of nitric oxide synthase enzymes, which are reduced in the endothelium in PAH.[18] Endothelin-1 is a potent vasoconstrictor and inhibits pulmonary artery smooth muscle cell proliferation. Plasma levels of endothelin-1 are high in PAH,[19] and its clearance is reduced. Additional vascular substances, including serotonin, vasoactive intestinal peptide, and vascular endothelial growth factor, have altered homeostasis in PAH.[20]

Prognosis in Group 1 Pulmonary Arterial Hypertension

In patients with untreated PAH, the median survival is 2.8 years, with 1-, 3-, and 5-year survival of 68%, 48%, and 34%, respectively.[21] Patients with connective tissue disease and HIV tend to have a worse prognosis, whereas patients with congenital heart disease have more favorable outcomes. Additional markers of adverse prognosis are shown in **Figure 39-4**. Prognosis is best determined in patients with PAH by integration of cause and functional class with clinical, echocardiographic, and hemodynamic factors.[22,23] A number of integrative prognostic scores are now available to aid the PH physician in this assessment.[24,25]

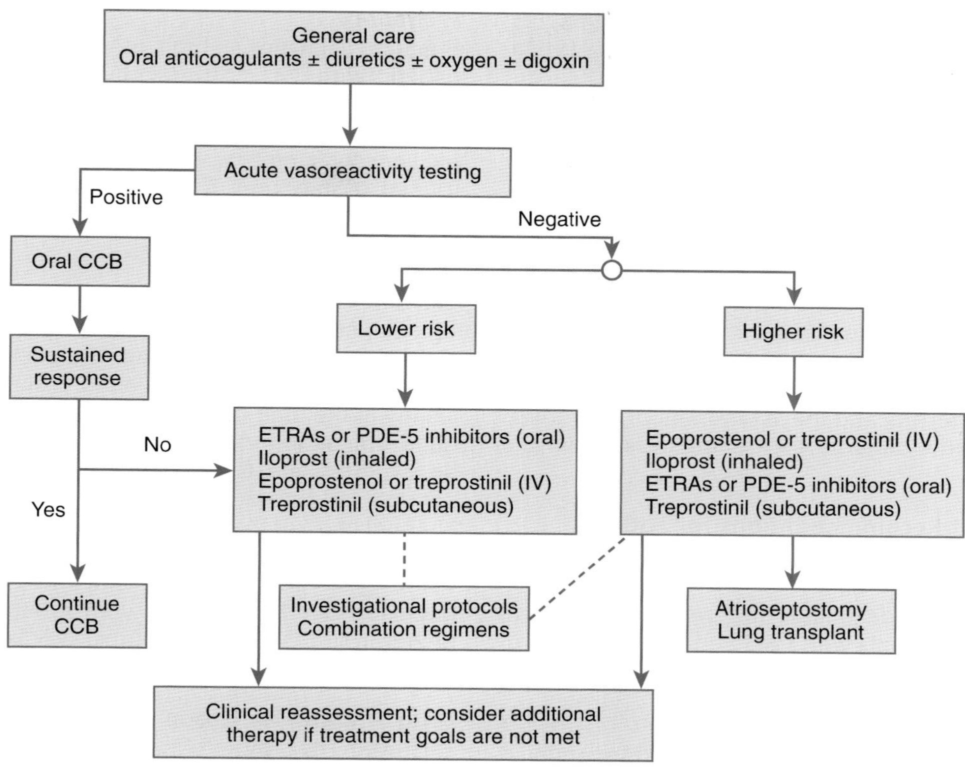

DETERMINANTS OF RISK	LOWER RISK	HIGHER RISK
Clinical evidence of RV failure	No	Yes
Progression	Gradual	Rapid
WHO class	II, III	IV
6-min walk distance	Longer (>400 m)	Shorter (<300 m)
Brain natriuetic peptide level	Minimally elevated	Very elevated
Echocardiographic findings	Minimal RV dysfunction	Percardial effusion: substantial RV dysfunction
Hemodynamics	Normal/near normal right arterial pressure and cardiac index	High right arterial pressure, low cardiac index

FIGURE 39-4 Algorithm for the pharmacologic management of pulmonary arterial hypertension. Assessment of risk for each patient includes clinical variables as outlined in the table below the algorithm. Patients deemed to be at highest risk on the basis of clinical assessment should be considered for early intravenous (IV) therapy. Those at lower risk are candidates for oral therapy. Patients should be followed up closely, and their response to therapy should be assessed within several months. If treatment goals are not met, addition of a second agent may be warranted. *CCB,* Calcium channel blocker; *ETRA,* endothelin receptor antagonist; *PDE-5,* phosphodiesterase 5; *RV,* right ventricular; *WHO,* World Health Organization. *Reused with permission from McGoon MD, Kane GC: Pulmonary hypertension: diagnosis and management. Mayo Clin Proceed 84:191–207, 2009.*

Clinical Assessment

Clinical evidence of right ventricular failure and rapidly progressive symptoms is associated with adverse prognosis in PAH. In particular, syncope, as a sign of poor cardiac output, is an independent predictor of mortality in PAH. The World Health Organization (WHO) functional class categorizes a patient based on his or her symptoms and functionality (class I, no limitation in physical activity; class II, slight limitation in physical activity; class III, no symptoms at rest but marked limitation in physical activity; class IV, symptoms with any physical activity and possibly at rest). Although somewhat controversial,[26] most studies demonstrate that the 6-minute walk test is a good indicator of prognosis and response to therapy; distances greater than 500 meters are associated with good prognosis, and less than 300 meters should trigger a change in therapy.

Biomarkers (see also Chapter 30)

Although several biomarkers have been assessed for their use in determining prognosis in PAH, the most widely tested is B-type natriuretic peptide (BNP) and its amino-terminal fragment (NT-proBNP). Elevated BNP and NT-proBNP levels reflect right ventricular dysfunction and are associated with increased mortality risk.[27,28]

Hemodynamics

Hemodynamic variables that reflect the degree of right ventricular decompensation or integrative parameters of function and load provide critically important prognostic information. These include measures of right atrial pressure, cardiac output, pulmonary resistance, and compliance. Vasoreactivity testing in group 1 PAH is routinely performed (see Table 39-1). A positive response to acute administration of a pulmonary vasodilator occurs in less than 10% of patients but identifies a cohort who may respond to calcium channel antagonists and who have a better prognosis. As described previously, echocardiography provides important noninvasive hemodynamic information but also measures of right-sided enlargement and right ventricular dysfunction that reflect disease severity.

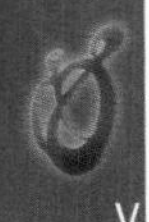

Computed tomography and magnetic resonance imaging of the right ventricle also provide useful measures of right ventricular enlargement and cardiac output.

Management of Group 1 Pulmonary Arterial Hypertension

Management of PAH includes general lifestyle modifications applicable to patients with all forms of PH, as well as pulmonary vascular targeted medications, adjuvant therapies, and advanced therapies. Treatment of associated conditions (connective tissue disease, HIV, etc.) is also important to slow progression but is not discussed here.

Choice of initial therapies for PAH is contingent on the results of reactivity testing and the assessment of prognosis. A recommended flow diagram for treatment is shown in Figure 39-4.

General Treatment Recommendations for Patients with Pulmonary Hypertension

Heart Failure Management

Salt restriction (<2.4 g/day) may be needed to avoid volume overload in patients with PAH and right ventricular dysfunction.

Exercise

Low-level aerobic exercise, as tolerated, is recommended.[2] Heavy exertion and isometric exercise should be avoided in advanced cases of PH, because they may trigger syncope. Cardiopulmonary rehabilitation programs should be considered in the overall PH management program and are usually beneficial.

Oxygen Therapy

Hypoxemia is a potent pulmonary vasoconstrictor and can contribute to the development or progression of PH. Supplemental oxygen should be used to maintain an oxygen saturation of more than 90% if possible at all times, although considerable shunting may preclude achieving this goal. In patients with obstructive sleep apnea and PH, treatment of obstructive sleep apnea with positive airway pressure therapy should be provided, with the expectation that pulmonary pressures will decrease, although they may not normalize, particularly when PH is more severe.

Pregnancy

Pregnancy carries a high associated mortality (30%) in patients with PAH.[29] Several physiologic changes contribute to the potential deterioration during pregnancy, including an increase in hypercoagulability, blood volume, and oxygen consumption, which can contribute to right ventricular dysfunction. As such, pregnancy is not advised in patients with PAH and non–estrogen-based contraceptive programs are recommended.

Calcium Channel Blockers

Calcium channel blockers have no role in the management of PAH, except in the setting of a subset of patients (less than 10%) with a significant acute response to vasodilatory testing at the time of right-heart catheterization. Nifedipine, diltiazem, or amlodipine can be used, but verapamil should be avoided due to its negative inotropic effects. If the patients fail to reach functional class I or II with calcium channel blocker therapy, then alternative PH-specific medications should be prescribed. Although improved systemic blood pressure control by calcium channel blockers is often indicated in patients with group 2 PH, there is no proven role for calcium channel blockers to lower pulmonary pressures in other PH settings and may be of harm.

Drug Therapy for Group 1 PAH: Vascular Targeted Therapy

Therapy for PAH has rapidly evolved in the past 15 years from the use of unselected vasodilating drugs to the use of therapies, which more effectively target pulmonary dilation and vascular remodeling with an impact on mortality in many PH patients and morbidity in most. The vascular-targeted therapies are outlined in **Table 39-5** and summarized here.

Phosphodiesterase-5 Inhibitors

The phosphodiesterase-5 (PDE-5) inhibitors, sildenafil, tadalafil, and vardenafil, have been shown to be efficacious therapies for patients with PAH. They are selective inhibitors of PDE-5 that degrade cyclic guanosine monophosphate (cGMP), which is found in high concentrations in the pulmonary arteries and corpora cavernosum.[30] Normally, endothelium-derived nitric oxide stimulates intracellular guanylate cyclase resulting in increased levels of cGMP,

TABLE 39-5 Vascular Targeted Therapies for Pulmonary Hypertension

MEDICATION	ROUTE	DOSAGE	SIDE EFFECTS	MONITORING
Calcium Channel Blockers			Hypotension, peripheral edema	
Amlodipine	PO	2.5-10 mg/day		
Diltiazem	PO	120-480 mg/day		
Nifedipine	PO	120-240 mg/day		
PDE-5 Inhibitors			Headache, hypotension, visual disturbances	
Sildenafil	PO	20-40 mg three times daily		
Tadalafil	PO	40 mg/day		
Endothelin Receptor Antagonists			Hepatotoxicity, peripheral edema	Monthly AST/ALT monitoring with bosentan
Bosentan	PO	62.5-125 mg twice daily		
Ambrisentan	PO	5-10 mg/day		
Prostanoids			Jaw pain, diarrhea, arthralgias, headache	
Epoprostenol	IV	1-20 ng/kg/min		
Treprostinil	IV, SC	Initial dose 0.625-1.25 ng/kg/min	Pain, erythema at SC site with treprostinil	
	INH	6-18 μg 4 times/day		
Iloprost	INH	2.5-5 μg 6 times/day	Cough	

ALT, Alanine aminotransferase; *AST,* aspartate aminotransferase; *PDE-5,* phosphodiesterase-5.

which then act to mediate smooth muscle relaxation. PDE-5 inhibitors prevent the breakdown of cGMP, thus prolonging its effects.

Sildenafil and tadalafil have been shown to improve exercise capacity and pulmonary hemodynamics in PAH.[31,32,33] These oral therapies are generally well tolerated with most notable adverse effects of headache, nasal congestion, epistaxis, and gastroesophageal reflux. Rare adverse effects of acute visual or auditory loss have been reported. The effects of PDE-5 inhibitors on mortality in PAH are unclear.

Endothelin Receptor Antagonists

Endothelin-1 is a potent vasoconstrictor and smooth muscle mitogen and is overexpressed in several forms of pulmonary vascular disease. Endothelin receptor antagonists emerged in the 1990s as important therapies in PAH. Bosentan is a nonselective endothelin-receptor antagonist, whereas ambrisentan selectively inhibits the type A endothelin-1 receptor.

Bosentan is U.S. Food and Drug Administration approved for use in WHO functional class II through IV PAH patients based on its proven efficacy in several randomized controlled trials.[34-36] In the BREATHE trial, bosentan improved 6-minute walk distance, Borg dyspnea index, and time to clinical worsening compared with a placebo in patients with WHO class III or IV PAH.[34] Bosentan also improved 6-minute walk distance and mean pulmonary vascular resistance in patients with WHO functional class II PAH.[36] Bosentan has been demonstrated to improve survival compared with model-predicted estimates.[37] Ambrisentan improves exercise capacity in PAH.

Hepatotoxicity is a primary complication with use of endothelin receptor antagonists. Bosentan requires monthly monitoring of liver function tests; ambrisentan no longer requires regular laboratory monitoring.

Prostacyclin Analogs

Prostanoids available to treat PAH include epoprostenol (intravenous, IV), treprostinil (IV, subcutaneous, inhaled) and iloprost (inhaled). This class of medications is expensive, associated with numerous side effects, and often reserved for patients with more advanced stages of disease. Epoprostenol has been best studied, and is first-line therapy for patients with severe PAH. It improves functional class, hemodynamics, and survival. In a randomized, multicenter trial of 81 patients, epoprostenol was associated with improved quality of life, a reduction in mPAP, and an improvement in 6-minute walk distance compared with placebo.[38] Survival at 1, 2, 3, and 5 years is improved with epoprostenol compared with historical PAH controls and equation-predicted survival.[39,40] Therapy is complicated, requiring a central venous catheter for a continuous IV infusion through a portable pump. The half-life is very short (5-6 minutes) and hence interruption of therapy may result in life-threatening rebound PH. Treprostinil can be administered subcutaneously, as a continuous IV infusion, or in lower doses via inhalation. Iloprost can be delivered by adapted aerosol device. Common dose-dependent adverse effects include jaw, diarrhea, nausea, an erythematous rash, and musculoskeletal pains, predominantly involving the legs and feet.

Choice and Order of Therapy

The choice of therapy is best determined by an experienced PH care team and the patient, based on a host of factors including disease severity, economic, individual capabilities, and family support. In principle, patients with advanced disease at presentation should be considered for parenteral prostanoid therapy with other therapies considered in milder forms of disease or as second-line agents. Indeed as there are multiple biologic pathways involved in the pathogenesis of PAH, there is a strong rationale to use combination medical therapy in its treatment. Studies continue to emerge demonstrating the safety and efficacy of combination therapy in PAH.[41-43] PAH is a very expensive disease, both in terms of the high patient morbidity and mortality but also the diagnostic and serial evaluation and the cost of pulmonary vascular-targeted therapies.

Drug Therapy for Group 1 PAH: Adjuvant Therapy

Anticoagulation

PAH is a prothrombotic state due to an imbalance of the homeostasis of prothrombotic and antithrombotic factors. PAH patients are also at risk for intrapulmonary thrombosis due to sluggish blood flow in the pulmonary circulation and endothelial dysfunction. Given this predisposition, it is generally recommended that patients with PAH have systemic anticoagulation with warfarin.[2]

Management of Right-Heart Failure

Diuretics are used to manage volume overload in patients with right-heart failure; if hospitalized, IV diuretics may be indicated. Digoxin is prescribed in some circumstances because it increases cardiac output in patients with right-heart failure and PAH.[44] However, there are no long-term clinical data to support its use. Inotropes can be used in patients as a bridge to heart-lung transplantation or as palliative therapy in some settings. Treatment with β-blockers is not recommended due to their potential negative inotropic and pulmonary vasoconstrictive effects. Angiotensin receptor blockers and angiotensin-converting enzyme inhibitors may contribute to systemic hypotension and have no current role in the treatment of PAH patients.

Atrial Septostomy

Atrial septostomy is considered in highly specialized centers in selected patients with severe PAH and right ventricular dysfunction. The creation of a right-to-left shunt allows improved left-sided filling and cardiac output at the expense of systemic oxygen desaturation. Careful selection is required as in the presence of very advanced disease (e.g., with severe elevations of right atrial pressure or poor baseline systemic oxygen saturations) periprocedural mortality can be high.[45] There is a carefully selected role as a bridge to transplant or as a palliative procedure when surgical options are not feasible.

Lung Transplantation

Transplantation remains an option in patients with PAH but is generally reserved for patients with progressive disease despite advanced medical therapies.[46] The optimal type of transplant is challenging. Heart-lung transplant is hampered by a shortage of available organs, although it has the advantages of requiring only one airway anastomosis yielding a very low rate of vascular complications and generally the best hemodynamic outcomes. Patients should be considered for heart-lung transplant if their degree of right ventricular dysfunction is felt to be irreversible, with resolution of the PH with lung transplant alone. Single lung transplant

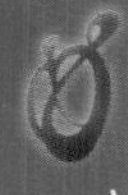

is easier than bilateral lung transplant to perform and requires less operative, ischemic, and cardiopulmonary bypass time, but there is the potential for ventilation-perfusion (V/Q) mismatch and reperfusion injury. Bilateral lung transplant may produce better hemodynamics, less V/Q mismatch, fewer early complications, better immediate overall lung function, and possibly improved long-term survival, but the operation is longer and more difficult to perform.[47]

GROUP 2: PULMONARY HYPERTENSION WITH LEFT-SIDED DISEASE

Patients with left-sided heart disease have PH due to a combination of PVH, pulmonary artery vasoconstriction, and pulmonary vascular remodeling. When the transpulmonary gradient and pulmonary vascular resistance (PVR) are normal, the PH is passive and a result of elevation in PAWP. This is most common in the early stages of heart failure, and may respond to measures to reduce the PAWP, such as diuretics and afterload reduction. When the PVR and transpulmonary gradient are elevated, this indicates reactive or mixed PH, and suggests that both pulmonary vascular changes and PVH are contributing to the PH. The potential reversibility of reactive PH can be tested during a hemodynamic catheterization by administering a vasodilator challenge and calculating the change in PVR. In the case of reversible reactive PH, lowering of the PAWP with heart failure therapies will result in return of the pulmonary vascular resistance to normal. If the pulmonary vascular resistance cannot be reduced to normal with correction of the PAWP, then the reactive PH is fixed but may respond to dramatic sustained unloading with inotropic therapy or left ventricular assist device (LVAD).[48] The reversibility of reactive PH in patients with left-sided heart failure is an important consideration in evaluating patients for heart transplantation.

PH may arise as a result of disease of the left-sided heart valves, left ventricular systolic dysfunction, left ventricular diastolic dysfunction, or left atrium.

Pulmonary Hypertension Due to Left-Sided Valvular Heart Disease (see also Chapter 24)

Mitral valve disease results in elevated left atrial pressure, and, as a result, elevation in pulmonary pressures, both due to passive backward transmission of the elevated left atrial pressure and reactive pulmonary artery changes. Mitral stenosis results in an obstruction in blood flow from the left atrium to the left ventricle, and accordingly, left atrial pressures must rise so that blood flow may continue. The development of PH plays an important role in the recommended timing of intervention in mitral stenosis, as surgical mortality is higher once PH has developed.[49] Mitral regurgitation can lead to PH through volume overload to the left atrium causing passive PVH, which, if longstanding, can trigger vasoconstriction and remodeling in the pulmonary arterial circulation. In mitral regurgitation due to degenerative disease, the development of PH (pulmonary artery systolic pressure ≥ 50 mm Hg) is common (present in 23% of cases) and increases the risk of all-cause and perioperative death.[50] In asymptomatic moderate or severe mitral regurgitation, exercise-induced PH (pulmonary artery systolic pressure ≥ 60 mm Hg) is present in 46% of patients, is associated with reduced 2-year symptom-free survival,[51] and represents an important indication for surgery. Aortic stenosis can contribute to PH by promoting left ventricular hypertrophy and diastolic dysfunction, which triggers elevation in left atrial pressures and PVH. Aortic regurgitation can rarely contribute to PH through elevation in left ventricular end-diastolic pressure.

Pulmonary Hypertension in Heart Failure with Preserved or Reduced Ejection Fraction

Both systolic and diastolic dysfunction of the left ventricle can result in elevation in left ventricular end-diastolic pressure (LVEDP), left atrial pressure, and pulmonary venous pressure, and can thus result in PH. The degree of PH in heart failure is thought to be proportional to the duration and intensity of exposure to PVH, which occurs independent of left ventricular ejection fraction (EF).[52] In heart failure with reduced EF (HFrEF, EF <50%), the prevalence of PH varies depending on the study population and definition used. In one study performed in 377 consecutive patients with heart failure and EF less than 35%, the prevalence of a mPAP greater than 20 mm Hg was 62% and was highly correlated with PAWP.[53] Diastolic dysfunction can also result in PH. Ventricular systolic and diastolic stiffness increases with age even in the absence of clinical heart failure, particularly in females.[54] Both diastolic dysfunction prevalence[55] and pulmonary artery pressures[56] increase with age. In HFpEF (EF ≥ 50%), PH is also quite common. In an Olmsted County community study of patients with HFpEF, the median estimated RVSP by echocardiography was 48 mm Hg, and 83% of patients had an RVSP ≥ 35 mm Hg.[57] Elevation in pulmonary artery pressures is associated with adverse prognosis in both HFpEF and HFrEF.[53,57,58]

The recognition that heart failure can occur in patients with preserved EF and that PH is as common in HFpEF as in HFrEF has complicated the assessment of PH as elderly patients with dyspnea frequently undergo echocardiography and may be found to have normal EF and elevated estimated RVSP. An approach to such patients has been suggested (**Figure 39-5**).[59]

Pulmonary Hypertension Due to Left Atrial Disease

Reduced left atrial compliance is common in both HFpEF and HFrEF and is manifest by large "V" waves in the pulmonary capillary wedge pressure (PCWP) tracing in the absence of mitral regurgitation. However, isolated or predominant left atrial pathology ("stiff left atrial syndrome" or "left atrial hypertension") can occur following left atrial radiofrequency ablation or surgical MAZE procedure performed for atrial arrhythmias. These patients may present with dyspnea on exertion, elevated pulmonary artery pressures, and large "v" waves on pulmonary capillary wedge pressure tracings that accentuate with volume load.[60] Although little is known about this entity, because it is associated with extensive left atrial scar formation, it is difficult to treat.

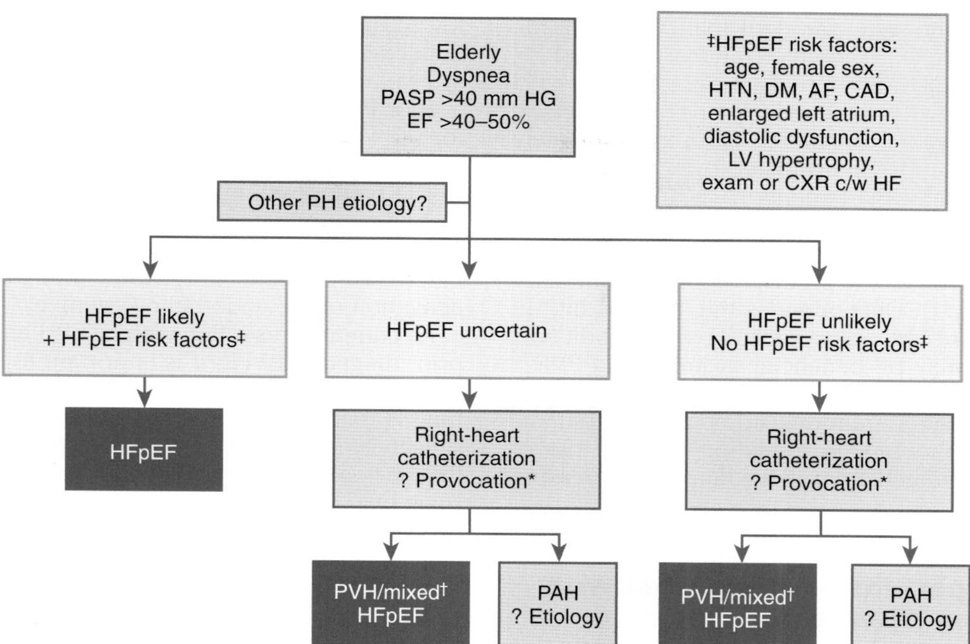

FIGURE 39-5 Algorithm to evaluate elderly patients with dyspnea, normal ejection fraction, and unexplained pulmonary hypertension (PH) at echocardiography. Decision to proceed to right-heart catheterization is driven by the severity of PH and the clinical evidence suggesting the presence of HFpEF. In many cases, the diagnosis of HFpEF can be made on the basis of clinical features and risk factors for HFpEF. In patients in whom the diagnosis of HFpEF is not evident, right-heart catheterization should be considered. If resting hemodynamics does not clarify diagnosis, provocative measures* should be considered and may include normal pulmonary capillary wedge pressure (PCWP) but HFpEF strongly suspected—exercise or volume expansion; elevated PCWP and pulmonary vascular resistance (mixed PH)—systemic vasodilator (nipride) particularly if systemic blood pressure is elevated; and PAH—pulmonary vasodilator to assess responsiveness and potential for treatment with calcium channel blocker. †See Table 39-1. ‡HFpEF risk factors: age, female sex, HTN, DM, AF, CAD, enlarged left atrium, diastolic dysfunction, LV hypertrophy, exam or CXR c/w HF. *AF,* Atrial fibrillation; *CAD,* coronary artery disease; *CXR,* chest radiograph; *DM,* diabetes mellitus; *EF,* ejection fraction; *HF,* heart failure; *HTN,* hypertension; *LV,* left ventricular; *PAH,* pulmonary artery hypertension; *PASP,* pulmonary artery systolic pressure; *PVH,* pulmonary venous hypertension. *Modified from Hoeper MM, Barbera JA, Channick RN, et al: Diagnosis assessment and treatment of non-pulmonary arterial hypertension pulmonary hypertension. J Am Coll Cardiol 54:S85–96, 2009.*

Treatment

In PH due to left heart disease, treatment of the underlying left heart disease is the mainstay of therapy. In valvular heart disease, surgical repair of the valvular abnormality, if indicated, may resolve the PH. In HFrEF, the use of evidence-based medications, such as angiotensin-converting enzyme inhibitors, angiotensin receptor blockers, β-blockers, aldosterone antagonists, and diuretics may result in improvement in afterload reduction, reverse remodeling, and improvement in ventricular mechanics and function that will lower LVEDP and PAWP and thus may reduce pulmonary artery pressures. Control of systemic hypertension and volume optimization are also advocated in HFpEF, though no therapies have been demonstrated to improve outcomes. However, if pulmonary artery pressures remain elevated despite hemodynamic optimization and normalization of the PAWP, there are no guidelines for use of PH-specific therapies in either HFpEF or HFrEF. Despite promising results in animal models and small single-center studies using the endothelin receptor antagonist bosentan, trials have not consistently shown efficacy.[61] There has been recent interest in using PDE-5 inhibitors to treat patients with left ventricular dysfunction, particularly HFpEF. A small single-center study demonstrated improvement in hemodynamics and left ventricular diastolic function with sildenafil.[62] However, the RELAX (Phosphodiesterase-5 Inhibition to Improve Clinical Status and Exercise Capacity in HFpEF) multicenter randomized controlled trial found no change in exercise capacity or clinical status after 24 weeks of sildenafil compared with a placebo.[63]

GROUP 3: PULMONARY HYPERTENSION ASSOCIATED WITH LUNG DISEASES AND/OR HYPOXEMIA

The respiratory diseases most commonly associated with PH are chronic obstructive pulmonary disease (COPD), interstitial lung disease, and sleep-disordered breathing. PH associated with advanced respiratory diseases is common but usually mild. An mPAP between 25 and 35 mm Hg is often seen in advanced disease and is associated with a worse prognosis. An mPAP greater than 35 mm Hg in the setting of advanced lung disease denotes a very high risk and such patients should be evaluated in a specialized center with consideration given toward transplantation. In milder forms of disease (e.g., forced expiratory volume in 1 second, FEV1, greater than 60% predicted and a forced vital capacity, FVC, greater than 70%), PH is uncommon and alternate mechanisms should be considered. Regardless of the mechanism, attention should be given to aggressively treating hypoxia.

Pulmonary Hypertension Associated with Chronic Obstructive Pulmonary Disease

COPD is a common lung disorder characterized by chronic obstruction of air inflow that is usually progressive and inhibits normal breathing. Chronic hypoxic vasoconstriction of the pulmonary arteries can lead to changes in the pulmonary vasculature, including intimal hyperplasia and smooth muscle hypertrophy. The exact prevalence of PH in

COPD is unclear. Among a cohort of COPD patients followed with serial right-heart catheterizations, none had PH at baseline, though 25% developed mild to moderate PH over time, which appeared to be associated with worsening hypoxemia.[64] In patients with severe COPD, approximately two thirds had elevated RVSP estimated by echocardiography.[65] Although most COPD patients have mild PH, there appears to be a group of patients who have severe PH out of proportion to their pulmonary mechanics, suggesting this group may have a genetic predisposition to pulmonary vascular disease, and COPD provides the "second hit." In addition to standard therapies such as bronchodilators for COPD, oxygen may be beneficial in improving PVR.[66] Although there has been interest in using PH-specific medications in this population, randomized controlled trial evidence is lacking. Pulmonary vasodilation runs the risk of perfusing poorly ventilated areas of the lung and increasing V/Q mismatch.

Pulmonary Hypertension Associated with Interstitial Lung Disease

Interstitial lung disease (also known as diffuse parenchymal lung disease) is a group of clinical disorders affecting the interstitium. Although the prevalence of PH has varied widely depending on the patient population and method of measurement, studies that have used right-heart catheterization and defined PH as a mean pulmonary artery pressure of ≥ 25 mm Hg have demonstrated a prevalence from 8.1% in a cohort with interstitial lung disease[67] to 73.8% in those with sarcoidosis who are listed for lung transplantation.[68] Therapy for PH in interstitial lung disease consists of treatment of the underlying disease and oxygen. There are insufficient data to assess the efficacy of the use of pulmonary vasodilators in this setting.

Pulmonary Hypertension and Sleep-Disordered Breathing (see also Chapter 45)

Sleep-disordered breathing can be categorized as obstructive sleep apnea (OSA), where there is cessation of air flow because of mechanical obstruction, or central sleep apnea (CSA), where there is absence of respiratory effort and air flow. OSA is highly prevalent and associated with obesity, whereas CSA is most often associated with heart failure. Repetitive apneic events lead to frequent recurring hypoxemia and hypercapnea, sympathetic-mediated vasoconstriction,[69] and abrupt changes in intrathoracic pressure, venous return, and cardiac output.[70] Sleep apnea can contribute to the development of PH, though the degree of PH tends to be mild.[71] Patients with sleep apnea and PH should be evaluated at a sleep center and treated with positive airway pressure therapy.

GROUP 4: PULMONARY HYPERTENSION DUE TO THROMBOTIC AND/OR EMBOLIC DISEASE

Chronic thromboembolic pulmonary hypertension (CTEPH) is defined by PH caused by emboli in the pulmonary arterial system. It is characterized by intra-arterial thrombus organization that fibroses and leads to intraluminal obliteration. The inciting event is thought to be a single or multiple recurrent pulmonary emboli (PE), followed by progressive vascular remodeling. The cumulative incidence of CTEPH following a clinical PE approaches 4% at 2 years.[72] Risk factors for CTEPH included younger age, a prior PE, a large perfusion defect, and idiopathic cause for PE.[72] However, up to 63% of patients diagnosed with CTEPH never have a history of clinically diagnosed PE.[73]

The pathophysiology of CTEPH is not entirely explained by pulmonary arterial obliteration but rather secondary downstream vascular remodeling because of molecular mechanisms similar to PAH, including inflammation[74] and activation of the endothelin system.[75]

As patients presenting with CTEPH and PH may have no prior diagnosis of PE, it is important to screen for chronic thromboembolic disease. Ventilation-perfusion lung scanning is recommended for screening because it has a high sensitivity (90%-100%) for the detection of CTEPH, meaning that a negative or very low probability result essentially rules out CTEPH. A segmental perfusion defect visualized on ventilation-perfusion scanning should be evaluated for definitive assessment with pulmonary angiography. PE-protocol CT scans have a significantly lower sensitivity for CTEPH and should not be used for screening.

With the identification of CTEPH, the patient should be referred to a specialized center for consideration of surgical pulmonary endarterectomy because outcome can be dramatically improved by resection of the fibrotic intraluminal material.[76] All patients should receive life-long anticoagulation with warfarin to achieve an INR goal of 2.0 to 3.0. The goal of anticoagulation is to reduce the risk of further thromboembolic events. Selective use of pulmonary vascular targeted therapies may play a role but only in those patients whose disease is too distal for a surgical approach or the minority of patients who have persistent PH postoperatively.

References

1. Strange G, Playford D, Stewart S, et al: Pulmonary hypertension: prevalence and mortality in the Armadale echocardiography cohort. *Heart* 98:1805–1811, 2011.
2. McLaughlin VV, Archer SL, Badesch DB, et al: ACCF/AHA 2009 expert consensus document on pulmonary hypertension: a report of the American College of Cardiology Foundation Task Force on Expert Consensus Documents and the American Heart Association developed in collaboration with the American College of Chest Physicians; American Thoracic Society, Inc.; and the Pulmonary Hypertension Association. *J Am Coll Cardiol* 53:1573–1619, 2009.
3. Rudski LG, Lai WW, Afilalo J, et al: Guidelines for the echocardiographic assessment of the right heart in adults: a report from the American Society of Echocardiography endorsed by the European Association of Echocardiography, a registered branch of the European Society of Cardiology, and the Canadian Society of Echocardiography. *J Am Soc Echocardiogr* 23:685–713, 2010.
4. Ghio S, Klersy C, Magrini G, et al: Prognostic relevance of the echocardiographic assessment of right ventricular function in patients with idiopathic pulmonary arterial hypertension. *Int J Cardiol* 140:272–278, 2010.
5. Sachdev A, Villarraga HR, Frantz RP, et al: Right ventricular strain for prediction of survival in patients with pulmonary arterial hypertension. *Chest* 139:1299–1309, 2011.
6. Forfia PR, Vachiery JL: Echocardiography in pulmonary arterial hypertension. *Am J Cardiol* 110:16S–24S, 2012.
7. Raymond RJ, Hinderliter AL, Willis PW, et al: Echocardiographic predictors of adverse outcomes in primary pulmonary hypertension. *J Am Coll Cardiol* 39:1214–1219, 2002.
8. Deng Z, Morse JH, Slager SL, et al: Familial primary pulmonary hypertension (gene PPH1) is caused by mutations in the bone morphogenetic protein receptor-II gene. *Am J Hum Genet* 67:737–744, 2000.
9. Machado RD, Eickelberg O, Elliott CG, et al: Genetics and genomics of pulmonary arterial hypertension. *J Am Coll Cardiol* 54:S32–S42, 2009.
10. Mukerjee D, St George D, Coleiro B, et al: Prevalence and outcome in systemic sclerosis associated pulmonary arterial hypertension: application of a registry approach. *Ann Rheum Dis* 62:1088–1093, 2003.
11. Fisher MR, Mathai SC, Champion HC, et al: Clinical differences between idiopathic and scleroderma-related pulmonary hypertension. *Arthritis Rheum* 54:3043–3050, 2006.
12. Diller GP, Gatzoulis MA: Pulmonary vascular disease in adults with congenital heart disease. *Circulation* 115:1039–1050, 2007.
13. Hopkins WE, Ochoa LL, Richardson GW, et al: Comparison of the hemodynamics and survival of adults with severe primary pulmonary hypertension or Eisenmenger syndrome. *J Heart Lung Transplant* 15:100–105, 1996.
14. Fishman AP: Aminorex to fen/phen: an epidemic foretold. *Circulation* 99:156–161, 1999.
15. Chin KM, Channick RN, Rubin LJ: Is methamphetamine use associated with idiopathic pulmonary arterial hypertension? *Chest* 130:1657–1663, 2006.
16. Krowka MJ, Plevak DJ, Findlay JY, et al: Pulmonary hemodynamics and perioperative cardiopulmonary-related mortality in patients with portopulmonary hypertension undergoing liver transplantation. *Liver Transpl* 6:443–450, 2000.

17. Christman BW, McPherson CD, Newman JH, et al: An imbalance between the excretion of thromboxane and prostacyclin metabolites in pulmonary hypertension. *N Engl J Med* 327:70–75, 1992.
18. Giaid A, Saleh D: Reduced expression of endothelial nitric oxide synthase in the lungs of patients with pulmonary hypertension. *N Engl J Med* 333:214–221, 1995.
19. Rubens C, Ewert R, Halank M, et al: Big endothelin-1 and endothelin-1 plasma levels are correlated with the severity of primary pulmonary hypertension. *Chest* 1562–1569, 2001.
20. Farber HW, Loscalzo J: Pulmonary arterial hypertension. *N Engl J Med* 1655–1665, 2004.
21. D'Alonzo GE, Barst RJ, Ayres SM, et al: Survival in patients with primary pulmonary hypertension. Results from a national prospective registry. *Ann Intern Med* 115:343–349, 1991.
22. Kane GC, Maradit-Kremers H, Slusser JP, et al: Integration of clinical and hemodynamic parameters in the prediction of long-term survival in patients with pulmonary arterial hypertension. *Chest* 139:1285–1293, 2011.
23. Humbert M, Montani D, Souza R: Predicting survival in pulmonary arterial hypertension: time to combine markers. *Chest* 139:1263–1264, 2011.
24. Benza RL, Miller DP, Gomberg-Maitland M, et al: Predicting survival in pulmonary arterial hypertension: insights from the Registry to Evaluate Early and Long-Term Pulmonary Arterial Hypertension Disease Management (REVEAL). *Circulation* 122:164–172, 2010.
25. Benza RL, Gomberg-Maitland M, Miller DP, et al: The REVEAL Registry risk score calculator in patients newly diagnosed with pulmonary arterial hypertension. *Chest* 141:354–362, 2012.
26. Farber HW: Validation of the 6-minute walk in patients with pulmonary arterial hypertension: trying to fit a square PEG into a round hole? *Circulation* 126:258–260, 2012.
27. Nagaya N, Nishikimi T, Uematsu M, et al: Plasma brain natriuretic peptide as a prognostic indicator in patients with primary pulmonary hypertension. *Circulation* 102:865–870, 2000.
28. Fijalkowska A, Kurzyna M, Torbicki A, et al: Serum N-terminal brain natriuretic peptide as a prognostic parameter in patients with pulmonary hypertension. *Chest* 129:1313–1321, 2006.
29. Weiss BM, Zemp L, Seifert B, et al: Outcome of pulmonary vascular disease in pregnancy: a systematic overview from 1978 through 1996. *J Am Coll Cardiol* 31:1650–1657, 1998.
30. Rabe KF, Tenor H, Dent G, et al: Identification of PDE isozymes in human pulmonary artery and effect of selective PDE inhibitors. *Am J Physiol* 266:L536–L543, 1994.
31. Galie N, Ghofrani HA, Torbicki A, et al: Sildenafil citrate therapy for pulmonary arterial hypertension. *N Engl J Med* 353:2148–2157, 2005.
32. Rubin LJ, Badesch DB, Fleming TR, et al: Long-term treatment with sildenafil citrate in pulmonary arterial hypertension: the SUPER-2 study. *Chest* 140:1274–1283, 2011.
33. Galie N, Brundage BH, Ghofrani HA, et al: Tadalafil therapy for pulmonary arterial hypertension. *Circulation* 119:2894–2903, 2009.
34. Rubin LJ, Badesch DB, Barst RJ, et al: Bosentan therapy for pulmonary arterial hypertension. *N Engl J Med* 346:896–903, 2002.
35. Channick RN, Simonneau G, Sitbon O, et al: Effects of the dual endothelin-receptor antagonist bosentan in patients with pulmonary hypertension: a randomised placebo-controlled study. *Lancet* 358:1119–1123, 2001.
36. Galie N, Rubin L, Hoeper M, et al: Treatment of patients with mildly symptomatic pulmonary arterial hypertension with bosentan (EARLY study): a double-blind, randomised controlled trial. *Lancet* 371:2093–2100, 2008.
37. McLaughlin VV: Survival in patients with pulmonary arterial hypertension treated with first-line bosentan. *Eur J Clin Invest* 36(Suppl 3):10–15, 2006.
38. Barst RJ, Rubin LJ, Long WA, et al: A comparison of continuous intravenous epoprostenol (prostacyclin) with conventional therapy for primary pulmonary hypertension. *N Engl J Med* 334:296–301, 1996.
39. McLaughlin VV, Shillington A, Rich S: Survival in primary pulmonary hypertension: the impact of epoprostenol therapy. *Circulation* 106:1477–1482, 2002.
40. Sitbon O, Humbert M, Nunes H, et al: Long-term intravenous epoprostenol infusion in primary pulmonary hypertension: prognostic factors and survival. *J Am Coll Cardiol* 40:780–788, 2002.
41. Gruenig E, Michelakis E, Vachiery JL, et al: Acute hemodynamic effects of single-dose sildenafil when added to established bosentan therapy in patients with pulmonary arterial hypertension: results of the COMPASS-1 study. *J Clin Pharmacol* 49:1343–1352, 2009.
42. Humbert M, Barst RJ, Robbins IM, et al: Combination of bosentan with epoprostenol in pulmonary arterial hypertension: BREATHE-2. *Eur Respir J* 24:353–359, 2004.
43. Simonneau G, Rubin LJ, Galie N, et al: Addition of sildenafil to long-term intravenous epoprostenol therapy in patients with pulmonary arterial hypertension: a randomized trial. *Ann Intern Med* 149:521–530, 2008.
44. Rich S, Seidlitz M, Dodin E, et al: The short-term effects of digoxin in patients with right ventricular dysfunction from pulmonary hypertension. *Chest* 114:787–792, 1998.
45. Kurzyna M, Dabrowski M, Bielecki D, et al: Atrial septostomy in treatment of end-stage right heart failure in patients with pulmonary hypertension. *Chest* 131:977–983, 2007.
46. Orens JB, Estenne M, Arcasoy S, et al: International guidelines for the selection of lung transplant candidates: 2006 update–a consensus report from the Pulmonary Scientific Council of the International Society for Heart and Lung Transplantation. *J Heart Lung Transplant* 25:745–755, 2006.
47. Conte JV, Borja MJ, Patel CB, et al: Lung transplantation for primary and secondary pulmonary hypertension. *Ann Thorac Surg* 1673–1679, 2001.
48. Zimpfer D, Zrunek P, Roethy W, et al: Left ventricular assist devices decrease fixed pulmonary hypertension in cardiac transplant candidates. *J Thorac Cardiovasc Surg* 133:689–695, 2007.
49. Vincens JJ, Temizer D, Post JR, et al: Long-term outcome of cardiac surgery in patients with mitral stenosis and severe pulmonary hypertension. *Circulation* 92:II137–II142, 1995.
50. Barbieri A, Bursi F, Grigioni F, et al: Prognostic and therapeutic implications of pulmonary hypertension complicating degenerative mitral regurgitation due to flail leaflet: a multicenter long-term international study. *Eur Heart J* 32:751–759, 2011.
51. Magne J, Lancellotti P, Pierard LA: Exercise pulmonary hypertension in asymptomatic degenerative mitral regurgitation. *Circulation* 122:33–41, 2010.
52. Georgiopoulou VV, Kalogeropoulos AP, Borlaug BA, et al: Left ventricular dysfunction with pulmonary hypertension: part 1: epidemiology, pathophysiology, and definitions. *Circ Heart Fail* 6:344–354, 2013.
53. Ghio S, Gavazzi A, Campana C, et al: Independent and additive prognostic value of right ventricular systolic function and pulmonary artery pressure in patients with chronic heart failure. *J Am Coll Cardiol* 37:183–188, 2001.
54. Redfield MM, Jacobsen SJ, Borlaug BA, et al: Age- and gender-related ventricular-vascular stiffening: a community-based study. *Circulation* 112:2254–2262, 2005.
55. Redfield MM, Jacobsen SJ, Burnett JC, Jr, et al: Burden of systolic and diastolic ventricular dysfunction in the community: appreciating the scope of the heart failure epidemic. *JAMA* 289:194–202, 2003.
56. Lam CS, Borlaug BA, Kane GC, et al: Age-associated increases in pulmonary artery systolic pressure in the general population. *Circulation* 119:2663–2670, 2009.
57. Lam CS, Roger VL, Rodeheffer RJ, et al: Pulmonary hypertension in heart failure with preserved ejection fraction: a community-based study. *J Am Coll Cardiol* 53:1119–1126, 2009.
58. Bursi F, McNallan SM, Redfield MM, et al: Pulmonary pressures and death in heart failure: a community study. *J Am Coll Cardiol* 59:222–231, 2012.
59. Hoeper MM, Barbera JA, Channick RN, et al: Diagnosis, assessment, and treatment of non-pulmonary arterial hypertension pulmonary hypertension. *J Am Coll Cardiol* 54:S85–S96, 2009.
60. Shoemaker MB, Hemnes AR, Robbins IM, et al: Left atrial hypertension after repeated catheter ablations for atrial fibrillation. *J Am Coll Cardiol* 57(19):1918–1919, 2011.
61. Kalra PR, Moon JC, Coats AJ: Do results of the ENABLE (Endothelin Antagonist Bosentan for Lowering Cardiac Events in Heart Failure) study spell the end for non-selective endothelin antagonism in heart failure? *Int J Cardiol* 85:195–197, 2002.
62. Guazzi M, Vicenzi M, Arena R, et al: Pulmonary hypertension in heart failure with preserved ejection fraction: a target of phosphodiesterase-5 inhibition in a 1-year study. *Circulation* 124:164–174, 2011.
63. Redfield MM, Chen HH, Borlaug BA, et al: Effect of phosphodiesterase-5 inhibition on exercise capacity and clinical status in heart failure with preserved ejection fraction: a randomized clinical trial. *JAMA* 309:1268–1277, 2013.
64. Kessler R, Faller M, Weitzenblum E, et al: "Natural history" of pulmonary hypertension in a series of 131 patients with chronic obstructive lung disease. *Am J Respir Crit Care Med* 164:219–224, 2001.
65. Scharf SM, Iqbal M, Keller C, et al: Hemodynamic characterization of patients with severe emphysema. *Am J Respir Crit Care Med* 166:314–322, 2002.
66. Timms RM, Khaja FU, Williams GW: Hemodynamic response to oxygen therapy in chronic obstructive pulmonary disease. *Ann Intern Med* 102:29–36, 1985.
67. Hamada K, Nagai S, Tanaka S, et al: Significance of pulmonary arterial pressure and diffusion capacity of the lung as prognosticator in patients with idiopathic pulmonary fibrosis. *Chest* 131:650–656, 2007.
68. Shorr AF, Helman DL, Davies DB, et al: Pulmonary hypertension in advanced sarcoidosis: epidemiology and clinical characteristics. *Eur Respir J* 25:783–788, 2005.
69. Somers VK, Dyken ME, Clary MP, et al: Sympathetic neural mechanisms in obstructive sleep apnea. *J Clin Invest* 96:1897–1904, 1995.
70. Shamsuzzaman AS, Gersh BJ, Somers VK: Obstructive sleep apnea: implications for cardiac and vascular disease. *JAMA* 290:1906–1914, 2003.
71. Atwood CW, Jr, McCrory D, Garcia JG, et al: Pulmonary artery hypertension and sleep-disordered breathing: ACCP evidence-based clinical practice guidelines. *Chest* 126:S72–S77, 2004.
72. Pengo V, Lensing AW, Prins MH, et al: Incidence of chronic thromboembolic pulmonary hypertension after pulmonary embolism. *N Engl J Med* 350:2257–2264, 2004.
73. Lang IM: Chronic thromboembolic pulmonary hypertension–not so rare after all. *N Engl J Med* 350:2236–2238, 2004.
74. Kimura H, Okada O, Tanabe N, et al: Plasma monocyte chemoattractant protein-1 and pulmonary vascular resistance in chronic thromboembolic pulmonary hypertension. *Am J Respir Crit Care Med* 164:319–324, 2001.
75. Bauer M, Wilkens H, Langer F, et al: Selective upregulation of endothelin B receptor gene expression in severe pulmonary hypertension. *Circulation* 105:1034–1036, 2002.
76. Klepetko W, Mayer E, Sandoval J, et al: Interventional and surgical modalities of treatment for pulmonary arterial hypertension. *J Am Coll Cardiol* 43:73S–80S, 2004.

40 Cardiac Transplantation

Mariell Jessup and Pavan Atluri

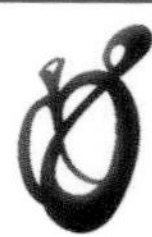

Cardiac transplantation is the treatment of choice for eligible patients with refractory heart failure. Nevertheless, the survival benefit of cardiac transplantation in advanced heart failure, as compared with conventional treatment, has never been tested in a prospective randomized trial. Shumway and colleagues developed surgical techniques for the procedure as early as 1966, and Barnard performed the first clinical human cardiac transplant in 1967.[1] By the time a review panel was convened in the 1980s, the U.S. Health Care Financing Administration (HCFA) concluded that heart transplantation was no longer experimental. Accordingly, in 1986, HCFA issued proposed regulations for reimbursement of Medicare-eligible patients undergoing heart transplant in centers that met HCFA-specified standards of experience and performance.

Many advances have occurred in the management of cardiac transplant recipients since the mid-1980s, including new immunosuppression modalities, therapies for chronic rejection, and improved operative and cardiac preservation techniques. This is reflected by the enhanced survival over the same time period. Three-year survival from 1975 to 1981, before the routine use of cyclosporine, was 40%, compared with 70% in the era from 1982 to 1994, representing the early use of cyclosporine.[2] The number of heart transplants worldwide has declined somewhat from the peak of approximately 4500 per year in 1994, perhaps as a reflection of better medical and device therapies for heart failure and a better understanding of prognostic indicators.[3] Nonetheless, identification of potential organ donors cannot meet the demand created by growing heart transplant waiting lists. As a result, other modalities for the treatment of Stage D heart failure have been created and are being assessed in clinical trials.[4] The approval of continuous flow left ventricular assist devices (LVAD) for destination therapy has provided alternative treatment options for patients who may not be considered candidates for heart transplant (see Chapter 42).[5] More recently, many patients referred for heart transplant have usually failed one, if not more, of alternative therapeutic options,[6] and are becoming progressively older and more ill, with increasing medical comorbidities. Similarly, there has been an expansion in the selection criteria for donors to increase the number of organs available.[7] As a result of these changes, the patients selected for heart transplantation are increasingly those with more acute disease, and, simultaneously, the available organs have been of poorer quality.[1,7]

PATIENT POPULATION

Which Patient Needs to Be Considered for Transplant?

The purpose of performing a heart transplant for an individual patient is to both prolong life and to improve the overall quality of life. The heart failure community has yet to agree on a single prognostic algorithm that will allow clinicians to accurately predict impending morbidity or mortality of an individual patient, although multiple scoring systems have been developed to help with this critical analysis.[8-11] It is important for referring physicians to understand the potential benefits a cardiac transplantation might confer on a recipient, as well as comorbidities that might predict an unsatisfactory outcome. An individualized risk-benefit assessment is ultimately the focus of deliberations by transplant committees in making decisions about process.

Evaluation of the Potential Recipient

Figure 40-1 outlines the questions that must be answered to evaluate a potential patient for cardiac transplantation. Patients estimated to have less than a 1-year life expectancy are the usual candidates. Typically, patients for consideration either have (1) cardiogenic shock requiring mechanical support or high-dose inotropic or vasopressor drugs (in which case the irreversibility of their course is usually clear); (2) chronic progressive, refractory, or Stage D heart failure symptoms despite optimal therapy[12]; (3) recurrent life-threatening arrhythmias despite maximal interventions, including implanted defibrillators; or, rarely, (4) refractory

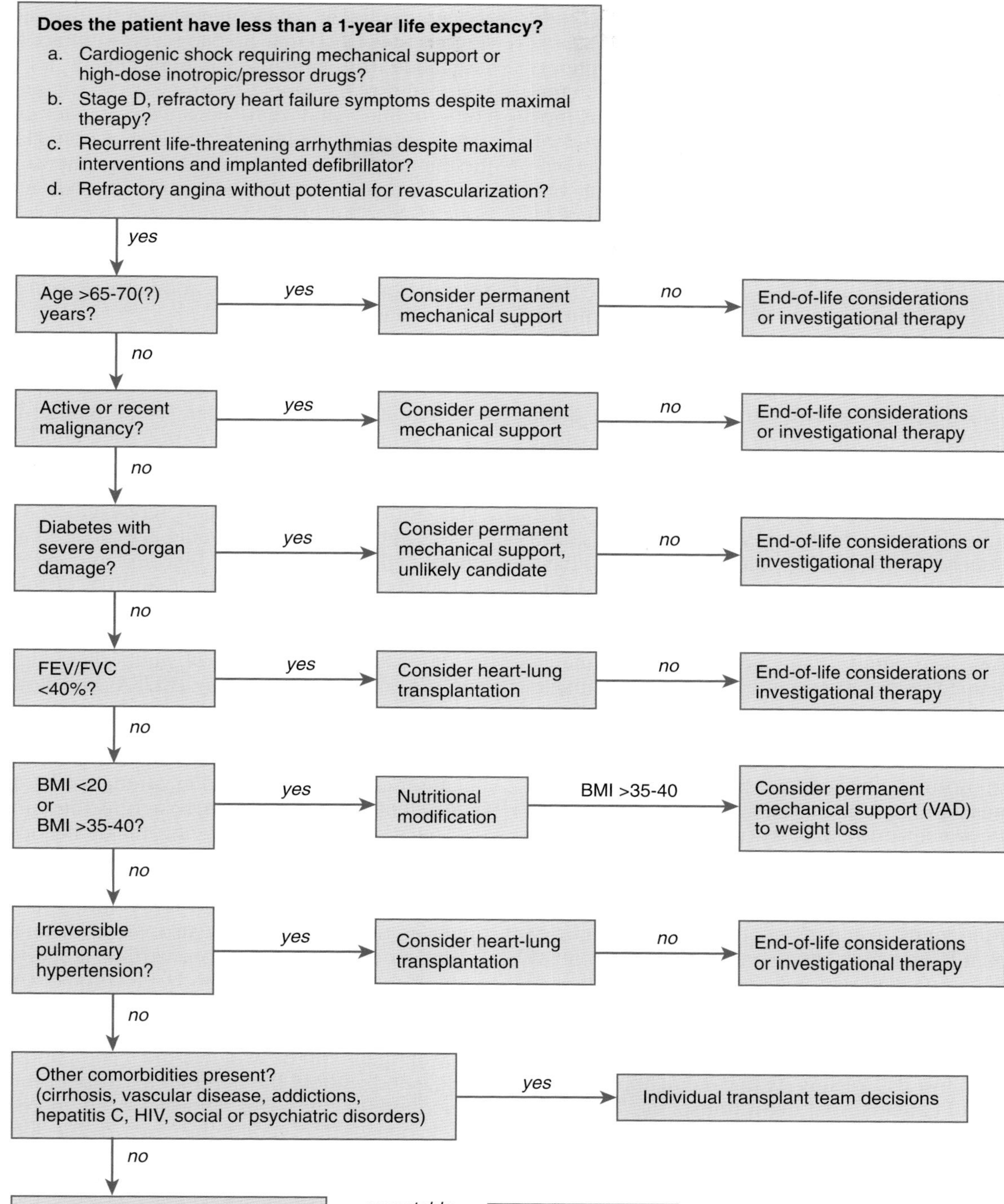

FIGURE 40-1 Evaluation of the potential heart transplant recipient. *BMI,* Body mass index; *FEV/FVC,* forced expiratory flow/forced vital capacity.

angina without potential for revascularization.[4] As continuous flow mechanical assist device experience grows, more and more patients are being "bridged" to transplant with an LVAD to provide hemodynamic stability while awaiting heart transplant (see Chapter 42). Moreover, as the number of patients with congenital heart disease are surviving to an older age, adult patients with repaired congenital heart disease are developing progressive heart failure and are being increasingly considered for heart transplant (see Chapter 25).[13] Optimal outcomes can be achieved in this complex patient population, with appropriate selection criteria.[14]

Several models have been proposed to assist in the risk stratification of patients with heart failure using both invasive and noninvasive methods.[8,9] The most potent predictor of outcome in ambulatory patients with heart failure is a symptom-limited metabolic stress test to calculate peak oxygen consumption, or peak $\dot{V}O_2$.[15] A peak $\dot{V}O_2$ of less than 12 mL/kg/min indicates a poor prognosis, with a survival that is less than that of a transplant.[16] Ideally, this information is organized in a score that also considers other important prognostic information, such as blood pressure, biologic assays such as BNP (blood natriuretic peptide), renal function, and frequency of hospitalization.[17,18] Nonambulatory patients who require continuous intravenous inotropic support that cannot be weaned or require mechanical support to maintain adequate cardiac index are more obviously at risk for a poor outcome without transplant, but often manifest signs and symptoms of end-organ failure of the pulmonary, hepatic, and renal systems that may signal an ominous prognosis even with a transplant procedure.

Each patient must then undergo an extensive medical and psychosocial evaluation by the transplant team to exclude contraindications for transplant, to further efforts at prognosis and the urgency of transplant, and to determine immunologic status. There are a number of relative contraindications to heart transplant; one of the most debated and variable among centers is the upper age limit for consideration. In general, patients older than 65 years of age are ineligible, and are more often approached for high-risk reparative surgery, permanent cardiac assist devices, or investigational therapies, such as cell transplantation, or to receive hearts from an alternate list of less than optimal donors.[19] However, a recent heart transplant guideline indicated the maximum age for eligibility could be as old as 70 years of age, so that individual centers must determine their own age cutoff.[20,21] An active or recent malignancy and diabetes with severe end-organ damage limit life expectancy following transplant, and are common reasons to exclude potential recipients. Significant lung disease complicates postoperative management and precludes the possibility of normal physical functioning; extremes of weight, as measured by body mass index (BMI), have also been shown to worsen post-transplant prognosis.[4] Advanced heart failure patients with renal dysfunction are generally excluded from heart transplant because abnormal renal function increases morbidity post transplantation. Thus it is important to clearly distinguish patients with potentially reversible renal failure from those patients in whom renal dysfunction is associated with advanced, irreversible end-stage renal disease. Many transplant centers have chosen to perform combined heart-kidney transplant procedures in selected patients.[22,23] Similarly, advanced liver disease results in prohibitive risk for surgery in general, thus excluding this subset of patients from heart transplant. There are a select few centers that have performed combined heart and liver transplants in patients with heart failure and concomitant hepatic failure. Very good long-term results have been achieved with combined transplants that are comparable to isolated heart or liver transplant.[24] Moreover, it appears that the hepatic transplant may be protective for rejection of the cardiac allograft.[25]

Pulmonary arterial hypertension, with a pulmonary vascular resistance of greater than 6 Wood units that cannot be reduced by medical therapy, or after the placement of a VAD, is considered an absolute contraindication for cardiac transplant. In the setting of fixed pulmonary hypertension, the donor right ventricle will often fail, leading to a high rate of early postoperative mortality.[26] In patients with moderate pulmonary arterial hypertension, it is important to select a suitable donor heart with good right ventricular function and suitable size. For those patients with irreversible pulmonary pressures, some centers may consider individual patients for a combined heart-lung transplant procedure. Recent data suggest that the implant of a continuous flow LVAD may help to reverse pulmonary vascular resistance, thus making a patient eligible for subsequent heart transplant (see Chapter 42).[27-29] There are other comorbidities that may negatively impact a transplant team's decision to further consider a potential recipient, including hepatitis C or cirrhosis, peripheral or cerebral vascular disease, advanced neuropathy, HIV status, addictions to alcohol or illicit drugs, and social or psychiatric disorders. Importantly, appropriate counseling of the patient excluded from heart transplant should include end-of-life preparation and discussions about possible investigational approaches.[30]

An increasingly sophisticated immunologic evaluation is done on each patient to determine ABO blood type and antibody screen, a panel reactive antibody (PRA) level and human leukocyte antigen (HLA) typing. Traditionally ("gold standard" method) the presence and levels of anti-HLA antibodies were determined by cytotoxic testing in which the recipient's serum was incubated with lymphocytes from 30 to 60 individuals representing a wide range of HLA antigens. The PRA value is expressed as a percentage of cell panel members that undergo cytolysis, and is considered positive if greater than 10% of the wells (cell panel members) undergo cytolysis. The PRA test can identify the presence of circulating anti-HLA antibodies but not the specificity or strength of antibodies. More recently, enzyme-linked immunoassay (ELISA) and flow cytometry have become the more commonly used means to determine PRA, because they are more sensitive than the cytotoxic test.[31] These more recent techniques allow quantification of the relative binding strength and specificity of preexistent antibodies. Assays such as the Luminex assay use beads coated with specific major histocompatibility complex (MHC) class I and II antigens to allow detection of these specific HLA antibodies. The most common cause of sensitization or elevated PRA levels is pregnancy; however, sensitization can also occur with transfusions (blood or platelets), infection, cardiac surgery, homograft material, prior transplantation, or insertion of a VAD. Virtual crossmatch is performed for all patients with an elevated PRA. By using virtual crossmatch, prospective donors with these antigens can be avoided and a compatible donor can be selected without the need for a prospective crossmatch (described below). This allows for an increased donor match outside the geographic area of the local OPO.[32,33] Virtual crossmatch utilizes specific MHC/HLA antibodies that are identified by PRA testing to avoid donors with the respective antigens.

There are a select group of patients with variable antibody titers on repeat testing (i.e., highly sensitized, recent VAD implant, recent transfusions) who must undergo a prospective crossmatch at the time of the identification of a prospective donor. This involves testing the recipient's serum with donor cells, in the presence of complement, to see if cytotoxicity occurs. The cell destruction predicts an unacceptably increased potential for either hyperacute, acute, or more chronic, recurrent rejections. Patients with high circulating levels of pre-formed antibodies, or highly sensitized patients, often have to wait long periods of time before a suitable donor can be found. Unfortunately, prospective crossmatch can only be performed within a single geographic region and hence further limits the pool of available donor hearts for recipients requiring the testing.

Managing the Sensitized Patient

Increasingly, patients who are being considered for heart transplant are found to be sensitized before listing. This can be attributed to an increase in the utilization of VADs as a bridge to transplant, a larger incidence of prior transfusion or previous cardiac surgery (e.g., mitral valve, coronary revascularization), and a greater number of patients with congenital heart disease under consideration for transplant. Unfortunately, the management of these highly sensitized patients can be quite challenging. A high circulating antibody titer can substantially reduce the available donor pool for an individual patient, markedly increasing waiting time and mortality while awaiting transplant.

Several desensitization strategies have been investigated, with varied anecdotal reports of subsequent successful transplant. Unfortunately, once these patients are transplanted they face a higher rate of rejection and likely diminished long-term survival. Two desensitization protocols have been described for managing these patients: (1) high-dose IVIG with or without rituximab, and (2) low-dose IVIG combined with plasmapheresis.[34-36] Antibody monitoring assays are utilized to determine the pre- and post-transplant treatments required to reduce HLA antibody titers and minimize rejection. Even with these protocols, patients can remain with high levels of antibodies. For this challenging subset, bortezomib (26s proteasome inhibitor that decreases antibody production) or eculizumab (monoclonal antibody that prevents the activation of C5 complex), among others, are being investigated.[37] Bortezomib in multidrug therapy, as well in combination with plasmapheresis as desensitization therapy, are currently being investigated in clinical trials.

The Management of the Patient Waiting for Cardiac Transplant

In the United States, solid organ transplantation is regulated, audited and facilitated by the government. The United Network of Organ Sharing (UNOS) is the national organization that maintains organ transplant waiting lists and allocates identified donor organs; UNOS is organized by regions throughout the country, integrated closely with local organ procurement organizations (OPOs). Donor hearts are assigned to recipients according to a priority status that is standardized nationally. The priority status is based on the recipient's medical urgency level, blood type, body size, and duration of time at a particular status level. Patients awaiting heart transplant are assigned a risk status according to the level of medical support they require. Patients who can be maintained safely and successfully outside the hospital are the lowest priority, status II. Intermediate priority is given to those patients requiring hospitalization and some continuous inotropic support or who require ongoing ventricular assist device (VAD) therapy, status 1B. The highest priority, status 1A, is given to patients requiring high-dose, continuous, inotropic infusions or mechanical support, such as intra-aortic balloon counterpulsation (IABP), ventilator, or VAD therapy. Such critically ill patients must be located in an intensive care unit and be undergoing continuous hemodynamic monitoring with Swan-Ganz catheters. Patients waiting for transplant with VADs as a bridge to transplant are given an automatic 30-day status 1A listing, with the timing at the discretion of the site. Thereafter, if the function of the VAD is normal, the patient reverts to a status 1B. Those patients with VADs that have complications (bleeding, infection, mechanical complications) are given an indefinite status 1A listing. Donor hearts are offered geographically using the location of the donor, and sequentially to patients with the highest priority and the appropriate blood type. In the past several years this process has been facilitated by a computerized system that requires transplant teams to have online access at all times. Nevertheless, speed and timing are critical aspects of optimal donor allocation, as potential donors often exist in an unstable hemodynamic environment that may impact on the viability of the donor heart, as well as other suitable organs. In addition, transport of donor hearts is generally limited by an ischemic time of approximately 4 hours once harvest of the organ has occurred.

Pretransplantation waiting times in the 11 UNOS donor regions vary considerably, and the challenges to individual transplant teams to manage waiting recipients similarly varies throughout the United States. The ability of potential recipients to be listed for and receive an organ transplant is influenced by a number of different factors, including candidate gender, size and blood group, presensitization antibody status, source of health insurance or lack thereof, type of cardiac disease, proximity to a transplant center, and even the number of other transplant centers in the region. This information and many other parameters of the U.S. transplant program are available to the public on a variety of websites, including the official UNOS link (http://optn.transplant.hrsa.gov/), where site-specific data may also be compared by city, region, or nationally. In the past 10 years, there have been an increasing number of heart transplant patients who are being listed and transplanted as status 1A or 1B, as compared with the less urgent status of years past.[38] This most likely represents the increasing use of VADs as a method to bridge the desperately ill patient to transplant, rather than watching similar patients succumb as was done a decade ago. Mechanical support devices often allow patients to be successfully managed as an outpatient while awaiting transplant, but the implantation of the device qualifies the recipient to at least a status 1B. A considerable debate about the outcome of these so-called bridged patients as compared with patients who are transplanted without a prior VAD has developed, with strong arguments on either side.[39] Nevertheless, the available data from the Organ Procurement and Transplantation Network (OPTN) and the Scientific Registry of Transplant Recipients (SRTR) website (www.ustransplant.org) suggest that overall survival is no different for patients transplanted without a VAD as status 1A, 1B, or status II, illustrated in **Figure 40-2**.

Patients waiting for transplant must be regularly reevaluated for the possibility of worsening status, obligating a change in priority, the development of a new comorbidity that would preclude transplant, or significant clinical improvement that would warrant a reconsideration of the listing. Each year a percentage of patients are removed from the waiting list because of marked clinical improvement, despite the great care in patient selection.[40]

THE CARDIAC TRANSPLANT PROCEDURE

The Cardiac Donor

In light of an increasing organ demand, efficacious donor management and meticulous selection are crucial in maintaining excellent transplant outcomes. Organ procurement representatives have become highly skilled in the rapid but thorough evaluation of potential donors, often screening for multiple organ harvests from a single donor. Obviously, any medical history about the donor is critical to obtain, including any relevant cardiovascular disorders before brain death. All donors are screened for communicable diseases, including viral disorders such as hepatitis and HIV. Unlike the restriction of risky individuals from blood bank donation, donors with behavioral risk factors are not barred from contributing to the organ supply. Accordingly, there has been an increased debate about the risk associated with transplant and how much of the donor-associated risk should be conveyed to the potential recipient.[41] Specific information that is relevant for the assessment of cardiac donor suitability also includes the presence or absence of thoracic trauma, donor hemodynamic stability, pressor and inotropic requirements, duration of cardiac arrest, the need for cardiopulmonary resuscitation, and number of hypotensive episodes and the method by which hypotension was managed. The use of echocardiography as a screening method to evaluate potential donors is invaluable. Some potential donors undergo hemodynamic deterioration caused by brain death, which requires inotropic or pressor infusions and substantial fluid administration with subsequent derangements in electrolytes and hemoglobin concentration. The resultant cardiovascular instability leads to suboptimal use of some donor hearts and has compounded the problem of donor shortage. To increase the donor yield, recommendations have been published to improve the evaluation and successful use of potential cardiac donors.[7,42]

The acceptable cold ischemia time (the time from harvest to recipient implantation) for cardiac transplantation is approximately 4 hours. Prolonged ischemic time has been shown to be a significant risk factor for mortality after cardiac transplantation, especially when coupled with other risk factors, such as older donor age. In the first two decades of heart transplant, the upper limit of donor age was 35 years, but older donors are now used frequently, with an age up to 60 years considered safe by most centers.[43] It has become quite standard to perform cardiac catheterization on the older donor to further clarify the integrity of the coronary circulation. The final decision to accept a heart for transplantation is made at the time of harvesting, after direct examination of the heart for myocardial infarction, trauma, coronary calcification, left ventricular hypertrophy or dilation. The harvesting team communicates the decision to the recipient hospital's transplant team, so that the recipient may be prepared for surgery.

One of the main reasons thought to be responsible for early graft failure after transplant is inadequate myocardial protection during prolonged ischemic transport.[1,44,45] Current myocardial preservation techniques allow interventions to be made during five different phases of the transplant procedure: donor cardiovascular management; protection during explantation; protection during transportation to the recipient center; protection during implantation; and protection during the immediate reperfusion period.[46,47] Ideally, optimal protection of donor hearts will ultimately expand the potential donor pool and enhance early graft function. Moreover, endothelial injury that occurs during organ procurement, preservation, and reperfusion, as well as ongoing injury during the lifespan of the cardiac allograft, results in endothelial activation.[48] If protection strategies can successfully reduce ischemia-reperfusion damage, there may also be a beneficial effect on long-term heart transplant outcomes by the protective effects on endothelial cells, reducing the subsequent development of cardiac allograft vasculopathy. This goal has spurred the development of new devices that are designed to further protect the harvested heart during transport by continuous bloodless circulation or autologous blood–perfused systems.[44]

Surgical Considerations

The two most common surgical approaches for the implantation of the donor heart are the biatrial and the bicaval anastomoses (**Figure 40-3**). The biatrial anastomosis technique has long enjoyed the reputation of being simple, safe, and reproducible. It consists of four suture lines: left atrium, pulmonary artery, aorta, and right atrium. The bicaval

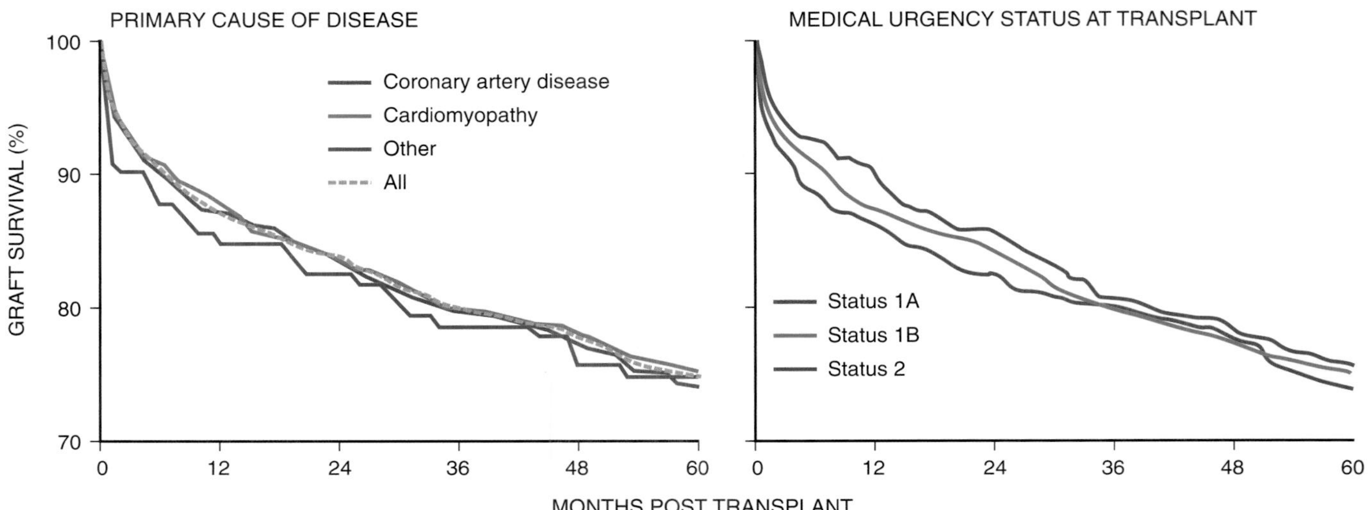

FIGURE 40-2 Survival of heart transplant patients in the United States based on primary cause of disease and UNOS medical urgency status at time of transplant. *From the Scientific Registry of Transplant Recipients website 2011 Annual Data Report, accessed March 25, 2013.*

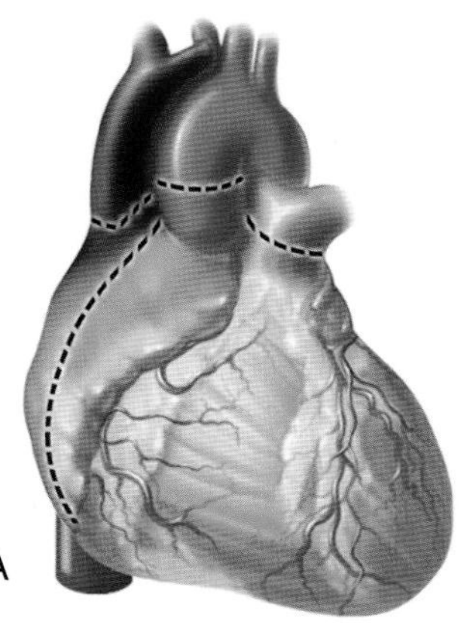

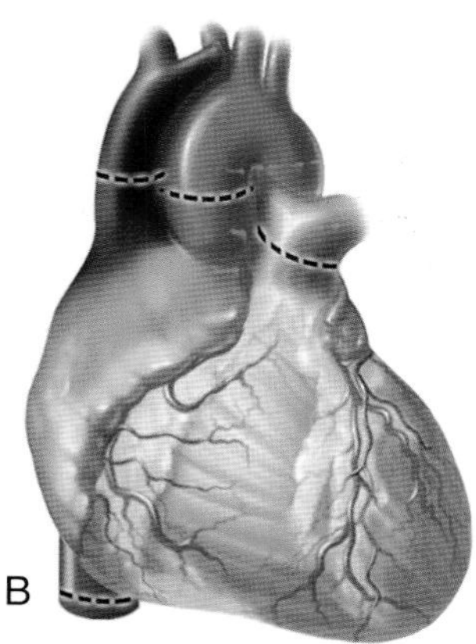

FIGURE 40-3 Surgical techniques for cardiac transplantation. **A,** Traditional Shumway (biatrial) technique of orthotopic heart transplantation. **B,** Bicaval technique of orthotopic heart transplantation. *Modified from Al Khaldi A, Robbins RC: New directions in cardiac transplantation. Ann Rev Med 57:455, 2006.*

anastomosis technique was introduced in the early 1990s with the intention to reduce right atrial size to minimize distortion of the recipient heart, to preserve atrial conduction pathways, and to decrease tricuspid regurgitation. In this alternative procedure, there are five anastomoses: left atrium, pulmonary artery, aorta, inferior vena cava, and the superior vena cava. Although there has been no prospective trial to establish the superiority of either technique, the bicaval technique is now being done most often in the United States, primarily because it appears to decrease the need for permanent pacemakers in transplanted recipients.[49-51] Some surgeons have become increasingly interested in techniques to minimize subsequent tricuspid regurgitation and have described tricuspid annuloplasty done simultaneously with the transplant surgery.[52]

Transplant candidates will often have had pacemaker or cardiac defibrillator devices implanted during the years leading up to their need for a transplant. These devices are typically surgically removed at the end of the operation after the chest has been closed. Similarly, previous heart surgery, most commonly coronary artery bypass graft procedures, will lengthen the time it takes to prepare the recipient to receive the donor heart and increase the risk of bleeding during and after surgery. Just as the age at the time of transplant has increased in the past decade, so too has the number of patients with previous heart surgery. Most importantly, the number of patients coming to transplant with VADs in place has steadily increased, so that transplant procedures are riskier and result in more bleeding.[53-58] But the long-term outcomes for heart transplant following VAD insertion have demonstrated excellent results,[59] with 87% 1-year and 82% 3-year survival for patients bridged to transplant with a VAD.

The most common reason for failure to wean a heart transplant patient from cardiopulmonary bypass is right-heart failure, evidenced by a low cardiac output despite a rising central venous pressure. The right heart can be seen in the surgical field to dilate and contract poorly. Intraoperative transesophageal echocardiography (TEE) shows a dilated, poorly contracting right ventricle and an underfilled, vigorously contracting left ventricle. Right ventricular function may be enhanced with inotropes and pulmonary vasodilators, but the prognostic importance of preoperative pulmonary vascular resistance becomes obvious in these first few hours after surgery.[60,61]

EARLY POSTOPERATIVE MANAGEMENT

Cardiovascular Issues

In general, the management of the heart transplant patient early after surgery does not differ substantially from other open-heart procedures, although the recipient is generally debilitated after suffering severe heart failure for weeks or months before surgery. Cardiac transplant recipients often go into surgery with profoundly disturbed hemodynamics and significant renal insufficiency. Postoperative management has to be undertaken with close scrutiny of the urine output and renal function, as a rising creatinine may require a change in the immunosuppressive regimen. The resultant fluid overload may serve to further overdistend a struggling right ventricle. Many patients will manifest generalized edema within the first week after surgery that generally responds to intravenous diuretics. This is in part related to vasomotor alterations of the peripheral vasculature that result in tissue edema.

Because the donor heart will be denervated after surgical implantation, bradycardia is a frequent problem, and a direct acting β-agonist drug should be available. Temporary pacing leads are necessary for all patients, as most will be dependent on external pacemakers for a number of days after the operation. As many as 10% to 15% of patients require a permanent pacemaker after transplant surgery.[58] Cardiac transplant patients typically need chronotropic and inotropic support for a few days in the intensive care unit after which time the infusions are weaned as tolerated. Many centers use isoproterenol for this purpose because of its lack of alpha and vasoconstrictive effects on the pulmonary vasculature. Inhaled agents have been used to achieve selective pulmonary vasodilation in cardiac transplant patients, especially those with preoperative pulmonary hypertension. Inhaled nitric oxide (NO) is a potent vasodilator that has a selective effect on the pulmonary vasculature because of its rapid breakdown in the lung.[60] Administration of NO in heart transplant recipients with pulmonary hypertension has been shown to reduce pulmonary vascular resistance and improve right ventricular function. Iloprost, a carbacyclin analog of prostaglandin I2, can be aerosolized and has been given in an inhaled form to treat severe pulmonary hypertension. Frequently, the inhaled agents, delivered via the ventilator, are initiated in the operating room and continued until right ventricular function has stabilized.

Immunosuppression

Cardiac transplant centers throughout the world have individual approaches to the management of immune modulation for transplant recipients so that the donor heart is accepted immunologically. All adhere to the principle that there is no patient undergoing heart transplant at low risk for rejection. Instead, it is more appropriate to stratify patients into those with average risk and those at high risk for subsequent rejection. Before transplant surgery, patients at high risk for rejection include those with preformed antibodies (e.g., the sensitized patient), usually secondary to previous surgery requiring transfusions, pregnancy, patients waiting on mechanical circulatory assist devices, and possibly the African American patient.[55] In addition, it is useful to characterize patients as higher risk to develop important comorbidities after transplant, including infection, acute renal failure, or worsening diabetes, because this may dictate modification of an immunosuppressive regimen. Postoperatively, a risk profile may be additionally tailored by the retrospective crossmatch information and donor/recipient cytomegalovirus (CMV) status. Accordingly, an immunosuppression strategy is developed for each patient based on his or her risk for rejection and for developing important complications of the immunosuppressive drug therapy.[1,62-65] Nevertheless, most immunosuppressive regimens begin with the simultaneous use of three classes of drugs: glucocorticoids, calcineurin inhibitors, and antiproliferative agents. In a subset of patients, transplant teams use a variety of drugs for induction therapy, with the idea to rapidly enhance immune tolerance.

Induction Therapy in the Perioperative Period

Induction therapy is a heterogeneous application of perioperative antibody drugs used in combination with a foundation immunosuppressive regimen in solid-organ transplantation. The ultimate aim of induction is to inhibit only those T cells that respond to donor antigen. Ideally, induction treatment achieves immunologic unresponsiveness in the recipient to the transplant in the face of a fully functioning immune system, called *donor-specific tolerance*. Both polyclonal and monoclonal antibodies have been used for this form of therapy; the practice is institutional as well as country dependent. Induction therapy is currently used in approximately 40% of heart transplant recipients.[66-68] Induction agents have included high-dose steroids or specialized induction agents (immunoglobulins or antibodies). Theoretically, induction agents should reduce acute rejection and hence overall rejection. Their primary benefit seems to be to delay cellular rejection in the first 4-8 weeks of the early postoperative period when renal dysfunction is most worrisome. Induction therapy may allow the less aggressive use of calcineurin inhibitors, thereby sparing renal function initially during the most vulnerable period. The benefit of induction therapy versus a standard immunosuppressive protocol without induction remains unclear.

Drugs used for induction include the polyclonal antibodies, antithymocyte globulins, and the monoclonal agents: the anti-CD3 antibody OKT3 and the IL-2 receptor antagonists daclizumab and basiliximab. OKT3 was widely used in induction in years past, but has virtually vanished as an option because of the subsequent occurrence of increased rejection and lymphomas.[69] In fact, manufacturing has been discontinued for OKT3 and daclizumab. The polyclonal antibodies, antithymocyte globulins, are more commonly used currently, for the first 3 to 7 or even 14 days after transplant, despite a paucity of efficacy data in the heart transplant population. The use of basiliximab has been explored in three trials: one where the drug was compared with OKT3 induction[70] and two studies where basiliximab was randomized against a placebo.[71,72] Although basiliximab was less toxic than OKT3, it did not alter outcome with respect to rejection, infection, or survival. In comparison to a placebo, a significant delay in rejection occurred with basiliximab, but at a possible expense of increased late rejection. Moreover, basiliximab was found to be noninferior to rabbit antithymocyte globulin for the prevention of acute rejection in a trial of 35 patients.[73] Daclizumab was shown, as compared with no induction, to reduce rejection without an attendant increase in mortality.[74] Thus there may be some rationale to use the induction agents for select, high-risk patients (e.g., with preformed antibodies, renal dysfunction, or a worrisome retrospective crossmatch), but there is no compelling data as of yet in the heart transplant population and they are the source of considerable controversy.[66,75,76]

Maintenance Immunosuppression

Immunosuppressive regimens begin with the simultaneous use of three classes of drugs: glucocorticoids, calcineurin inhibitors, and antiproliferative agents. In the immediate postoperative period, they are given parenterally with a quick transition to oral formulations. *Corticosteroids* are nonspecific anti-inflammatory agents that work primarily by lymphocyte depletion. Patients initially receive high doses of intravenous and then oral steroids that are gradually tapered over the next 6 months; often the goal is to completely withdraw steroid therapy. At many centers, steroids are given several hours before the transplant surgery. Side effects include cushingoid appearance, hypertension, dyslipidemia, weight gain with central obesity, peptic ulcer formation and gastrointestinal bleeding, pancreatitis, personality changes, cataract formation, hyperglycemia progressing to steroid diabetes, and osteoporosis with avascular necrosis of bone. The well-appreciated adverse profile of the corticosteroids has led to a number of innovative strategies to eliminate them as early as possible after the transplant surgery. Corticosteroids are usually the drug of first choice to treat acute rejection as well.[77,78]

There are two *calcineurin inhibitors*, cyclosporine and tacrolimus. Their main mechanism of action involves binding to specific proteins to form complexes that block the action of calcineurin, a key participant in T-cell activation. The calcineurin inhibitors serve to block the signal transduction pathways responsible for T-cell and B-cell activation and therefore act specifically on the immune system and do not affect other rapidly proliferating cells. Critical and often limiting adverse effects include nephrotoxicity in as many as 40% to 70% of patients, and hypertension with the development of left ventricular hypertrophy; both drugs cause a roughly equivalent incidence of these untoward events.[77,79] Hirsutism, gingival hyperplasia, and hyperlipidemia are more frequent with cyclosporine, and diabetes and neuropathy are more frequent with tacrolimus.[73] There is also an increased incidence of deep vein thrombosis, tremor, headache, convulsions, and paresthesia of the limbs with both drugs.[77,78] There are target therapeutic levels for both drugs; these goals are also adjusted over the subsequent months and years following transplant. Therapeutic levels have been typically performed on trough blood draws, but it has been shown that cyclosporine concentration 2 hours postdose (C2) is a more accurate predictor of total cyclosporine exposure.[80] It remains to be demonstrated whether the short- or long-term efficacy of cyclosporine in heart transplant will be further improved by using C2 monitoring. In the United States, tacrolimus is now available in generic formulations, so the drug tends to be the calcineurin inhibitor of choice in most centers.[81,82] As discussed below, progressive renal insufficiency is a major limitation of the calcineurin inhibitors, and investigators continue to explore successful methods to minimize their use or withdraw it all together.[75,79]

Antiproliferative agents work to either directly or indirectly inhibit the expansion of alloactivated T-cell and

B-cell clones. Azathioprine was the earlier agent used in this class and served as the mainstay of immunosuppression even before the routine use of cyclosporine. In the past decade, mycophenolate mofetil (MMF) has replaced azathioprine as the first-line antiproliferative drug, with several randomized trials demonstrating superiority compared to azathioprine.[83-86] MMF is hydrolyzed to mycophenolic acid (MPA) that inhibits de novo purine synthesis. Both azathioprine and MMF cause leukopenia as their major adverse effect; the use of MMF can be limited by debilitating diarrhea or nausea. It is likely that the combination of MMF and tacrolimus potentiates their individual adverse effects.

Sirolimus (often called rapamycin) and everolimus are two newer agents that block activation of T cells following autocrine stimulation by interleukin-2. They also are known to inhibit proliferation of endothelial cells and fibroblasts. Their action is complementary to calcineurin inhibitors, and both sirolimus and everolimus have been used as maintenance immunosuppression, as alternatives to standard immunosuppression, and as rescue drugs for rejection. Sirolimus, an m-TOR inhibitor, has been shown to slow progression of cardiac allograft vasculopathy (CAV) with established disease,[87-89] and everolimus has been demonstrated to reduce both acute rejection and CAV.[90] In one randomized trial, sirolimus, compared to azathioprine, with cyclosporine and steroids, decreased by half the number of patients with acute rejection, which resulted in less subsequent development of CAV.[85,86] Because the drugs inhibit the proliferation of fibroblasts, they may cause significant difficulties with wound healing. Most centers do not use them as initial therapy immediately after the transplant surgery. The drugs have also been associated with the development of significant pericardial effusions. Sirolimus has been increasingly used to replace the calcineurin inhibitors as a strategy to improve renal dysfunction or reverse left ventricular hypertrophy.[79,91,92]

The long-standing use of the maintenance combination of cyclosporine, azathioprine, and steroids has been challenged in a number of trials. Tacrolimus plus MMF, or tacrolimus plus sirolimus, was evaluated against cyclosporine plus MMF in a multicenter trial.[84] Overall, 1-year survival did not differ among the three regimens, but there was statistically less significant rejection with or without hemodynamic compromise in the tacrolimus plus MMF arm compared with the cyclosporine plus MMF arm. Moreover, the tacrolimus plus MMF group had better renal function and triglyceride levels at 1 year. This trial has been pivotal in moving tacrolimus as the primary calcineurin inhibitor used worldwide. Later studies have explored the use of converting a calcineurin inhibitor to sirolimus or everolimus for a renal-sparing effect, or even limiting the use of calcineurin inhibitors and only using MMF or sirolimus/everolimus.[93-96] Unfortunately, many of these newer approaches are being implemented without the benefit of rigorous, controlled trials.

Other Potential Perioperative Management Issues

In addition to the common postoperative problems encountered after heart surgery, the transplant recipient is frequently debilitated and may be malnourished, particularly in the patient who has not been supported by a VAD. Issues surrounding exercise rehabilitation and nutrition can be time-consuming for the transplant team and challenging for the patient and family. Depression in patients with chronic heart failure is a regular occurrence, and is not immediately alleviated by the transplant procedure.[97-99] In addition, there is commonly a marked emotional lability in the recipient that is aggravated by the high-dose steroids used. As a result, successful heart transplant teams must focus on more than the physical needs of the recently transplanted patient. In an occasional patient, the stress of the wait for transplant often depletes the family of financial resources and emotional resiliency. On the other hand, patients are often rehabilitated much faster if they were allowed time to recover from the heart failure syndrome by the use of VAD support pretransplant. It is critical that a transplant center have dedicated physical therapists, nutritionists, and social workers or psychologists who can act in concert to address these noncardiovascular demands.

CHRONIC MANAGEMENT OF THE CARDIAC TRANSPLANT PATIENT

Rejection

Rejection involves cell- and/or antibody-mediated cardiac injury occurring as the result of recognition of the cardiac allograft as non-self. This process is categorized into three major types of rejection, using histologic and immunologic criteria: hyperacute, acute, and chronic.[62,100-103] *Hyperacute rejection* results when an abrupt loss of allograft function occurs within minutes to hours after circulation is reestablished in the donor heart, and is rare in modern day transplant. The phenomenon is mediated by preexisting antibodies to allogeneic antigens on the vascular endothelial cells of the donor organ, which is mostly avoided with current HLA typing techniques. These antibodies fix complement that promotes intravascular thrombosis. Subsequently there is rapid occlusion of graft vasculature and swift and overwhelming failure of the cardiac graft. Within minutes after reperfusion, the heart will stop contracting, resulting in what many surgeons have described as a "stone heart." In this scenario, the only option is to maintain biventricular mechanical circulatory support with either ECMO (extracorporeal membrane oxygenation) or BIVADs.

Acute cellular rejection or *cell-mediated rejection* (CMR) is a mononuclear inflammatory response, predominantly lymphocytic, directed against the donor heart that most commonly occurs from the first week to several years after transplantation and occurs in up to 40% of patients during the first year following surgery. The key event in both the initiation and the coordination of the rejection response is T-cell activation, moderated by interleukin-2, a cytokine. Interleukin-2 is produced by CD4 cells and to a lesser extent by CD8 cells and exerts both an autocrine and a paracrine response. Unlike renal and liver transplants, there are no reliable serologic markers for rejection in cardiac transplant. Therefore, the endomyocardial biopsy remains the gold standard for the diagnosis of acute rejection. Biopsies are performed via a transjugular approach weekly, then every other week for several months; monthly biopsies continue for 6 to 12 months in many programs, and for years thereafter in some. CMR is graded according to a universally agreed on system that is periodically reviewed, as shown in **Table 40-1**.[104]

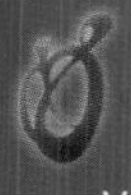

TABLE 40-1 Current and Previous Grading Systems for Cell-Mediated Rejection in Heart Transplantation

2004		1990	
Grade 0 R	No rejection	Grade 0	No rejection
Grade 1 R, mild	Interstitial and/or perivascular infiltrate with up to one focus of myocyte damage	Grade 1, mild	
		A: Focal	Focal perivascular and/or interstitial infiltrate without myocyte damage
		B: Diffuse	Diffuse infiltrate without myocyte damage
Grade 2 R, moderate	Two or more foci of infiltrate with associated myocyte damage	Grade 2, moderate (focal)	One focus of infiltrate with associated myocyte damage
Grade 3 R, severe	Diffuse infiltrate with multifocal myocyte damage ± edema ± hemorrhage ± vasculitis	Grade 3, moderate	
		A: Focal	Multifocal infiltrate with myocyte damage
		B: Diffuse	Diffuse infiltrate with myocyte damage
		Grade 4, severe	Diffuse, polymorphous infiltrate with extensive myocyte damage ± hemorrhage + vasculitis

From Stewart S, Winters GL, Fishbein MC, et al: Revision of the 1990 working formulation for the standardization of nomenclature in the diagnosis of heart rejection. J Heart Lung Transplant 24:1710–1720, 2005.

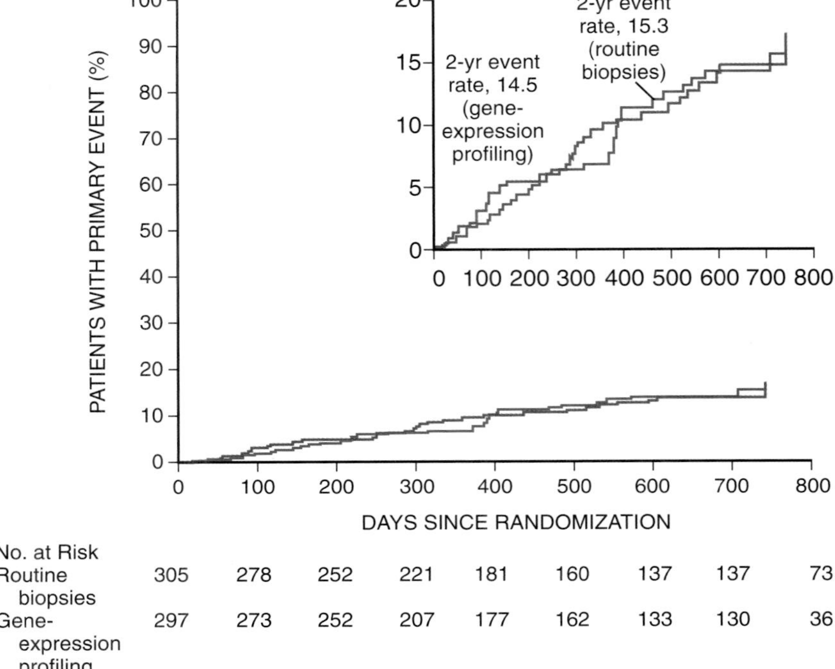

FIGURE 40-4 Time to first occurrence of rejection with hemodynamic compromise, graft dysfunction due to other causes, death, or retransplantation. Comparison is made between AlloMap genetic surveillance and routine endomyocardial biopsies (IMAGE trial). *Modified from Pham MX, Teuteberg JJ, Kfoury AG, et al: Gene-expression profiling for rejection surveillance after cardiac transplantation. N Eng J Med 362:1890–1900, 2010.*

More recent studies have attempted to use additional markers as well as serologic and immunologic methods to more accurately determine CMR.[105] Noninvasive analysis of gene expression has demonstrated reasonable efficacy as a surveillance tool to screen for CMR among patients who are more than 6 months past transplant with a low likelihood of rejection.[106-110] A randomized prospective study (602 patients) evaluating AlloMap (XDx) versus routine endomyocardial biopsy found no difference in serious adverse events, including hemodynamic compromise, graft dysfunction, retransplant, or death[111] (**Figure 40-4**). AlloMap is a panel of 20 gene expression assays used in the calculation of an overall score from 1 to 40; the lower the score the lower the risk of rejection, permitting the stratification of patients into low- (≤20), intermediate- (21-30), and high-risk (>30) categories for rejection. The clinician uses this score in conjunction with the patient's clinical picture in deciding on the need for subsequent invasive testing/biopsy and management of rejection. The AlloMap assay was approved by the FDA in 2008. Posttransplant ischemic injury, including coronary allograft vasculopathy, has been associated with a false-positive AlloMap score.[107,112]

Risk factors for early rejection include younger recipient age, female gender, female donor, positive CMV serology, prior infection, black recipient race, and number of HLA mismatches.[55,113] Most importantly, patients who fail to take or tolerate their immunosuppressant drugs, especially early in their postoperative course, are at very high risk for severe or recurrent cellular rejection. The occurrence of one or more episodes of treated rejections during the first year is a risk factor for both a 5-year survival and development of transplant coronary disease.[114] Similarly, treatment for acute rejection in the first 6 months following transplant contributes to a slower overall rehabilitation of the patient.

The aggressiveness of treatment for CMR depends on the biopsy grade, clinical correlation, patient risk factors, rejection history, length of time after transplant, and whether or not target levels are achieved for the immunosuppressant drugs. For example, an asymptomatic, moderate rejection in a patient soon after transplant who is at or above target levels of immunosuppressants or who has one or more risk

TABLE 40-2 Diagnostic Criteria for Antibody-Mediated Rejection

CRITERIA	FINDING	COMMENT
Clinical	Graft dysfunction	Required
Histologic	Capillary endothelial changes: swelling, denudation, congestion	Required
	Macrophages in capillaries	More severe cases
	Neutrophils in capillaries	More severe cases
	Interstitial changes: edema and/or hemorrhage	
Immunopathologic	Immunoglobulin (G, M, and/or A) plus C3d and/or C4d or C1q staining (2 to 2+) in capillaries by immunofluorescence	One of the first two immunopathologic criteria is required
	CD68 positivity for macrophages in capillaries and/or C4D staining of capillaries with 2 to 3+ intensity by paraffin immunohistochemistry	
	Fibrin in vessels	More severe cases
Serologic	Evidence of anti–human leukocyte antigen class I and/or class II antibodies or other anti–donor antibody at time of biopsy	Supports other findings

Adapted from Stewart S, Winters GL, Fishbein MC, et al: Revision of the 1990 working formulation for the standardization of nomenclature in the diagnosis of heart rejection. J Heart Lung Transplant 24:1710–1720, 2005.

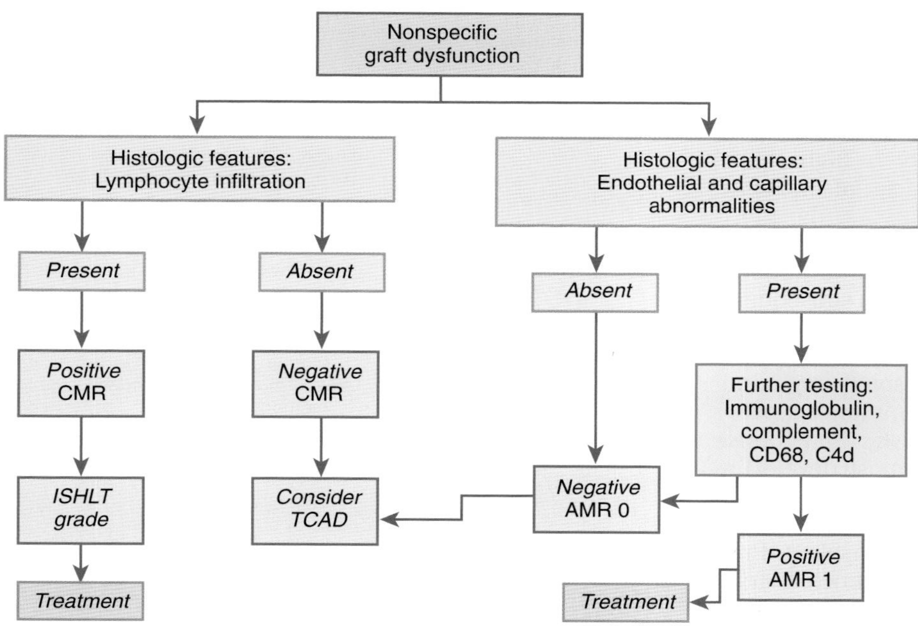

FIGURE 40-5 Diagnostic algorithm for the heart transplant patient with nonspecific graft dysfunction. *AMR,* Antibody-mediated rejection; *CMR,* cell-mediated rejection; *ISHLT,* International Society for Heart and Lung Transplant; *TCAD,* transplant coronary artery disease. *From Jessup M, Brozena S: State-of-the-art strategies for immunosuppression. Curr Opin Organ Transplant 12:536–542, 2007.*

factors for early rejection would be treated more aggressively than a low-risk patient with no prior history of CMR.

Another form of acute rejection is *acute humoral rejection,* or antibody-mediated rejection (AMR), which occurs days to weeks after transplant and is initiated by antibodies rather than T cells. The alloantibodies are directed against donor HLA or endothelial cell antigens. AMR is a serious complication after heart transplantation and presents as "graft dysfunction" or hemodynamic abnormalities in the absence of cellular rejection on biopsy. AMR is now recognized as a distinct clinical entity, and strict histopathologic and immunologic criteria for its diagnosis have been established, as shown in **Table 40-2**.[104,115] Further testing, including immunofluorescent staining of specially prepared myocardial tissue, is often necessary to elucidate the presence of AMR and is an important consideration in the evaluation of the post-transplant patient with left ventricular dysfunction. The pathologic markers of AMR identifiable in endomyocardial biopsy tissue include deposits of IgM, IgG, or complement in the microvasculature or myocytes. Evidence for antibodies in the circulation with specificity for non-HLA antigens on the graft is also a possibility and should support the diagnosis of AMR. Patients at greatest risk for AMR are women, patients with a high PRA screen, and/or patients with a positive crossmatch. It is estimated that significant AMR occurs in about 7% of patients, but may be as high as 20%. Because antibody assays are becoming more precise, it is probable that more AMR will be recognized, with a correlating need for newer treatment algorithms.[100,116,117]

Chronic rejection, or late graft failure, is an irreversible gradual deterioration of graft function that occurs in many allografts months to years after transplant. Current concepts suggest that donor heart dysfunction in the chronic stages of maintenance immunosuppression is either related to chronic rejection, mediated by antibodies, or as a result of progressive graft loss from ischemia. The latter process is characterized by intimal thickening and fibrosis leading to luminal occlusion of the graft vasculature, and is often referred to as *cardiac allograft vasculopathy* (CAV), or transplant coronary artery disease. An approach to the patient with nonspecific graft dysfunction is outlined in **Figure 40-5**, and is primarily focused on the diagnosis of AMR versus the presence of CAV.[118] Interestingly, it has been recently demonstrated that a large number of patients with graft dysfunction will actually manifest non-descript unexplained pathology. These patients have been found to have a significantly worse prognosis and limited therapy.[119]

More recently, attention has focused on noninvasive methods to detect rejection. Gene expression assays have been developed by identifying a number of candidate gene markers from a pool of over 25,000 genes of interest using gene-chip array technology. Subsequently, real-time PCR technologies are used in the peripheral blood to identify a pattern of gene activation that may correlate with allograft rejection. One such assay is available for clinical use, but it is not yet clear how the information obtained can be best used in a wide range of post-transplant patients.[108]

Infection

Despite the advances in immunosuppressive management, a major untoward consequence remains the occurrence of life-threatening infections. Infections cause approximately 20% of deaths within the first year of transplant, and continue to be a common cause of morbidity and mortality throughout the recipient's life. The most common infections seen in the first month after surgery are nosocomial: bacterial and fungal infections related to mechanical ventilation, catheters, and the surgical site. Mortality is highest for fungal infections, followed by protozoal, bacterial, and viral infections. *Aspergillus* and *Candida* species are the most common fungal infections after heart transplant. In addition, a higher number of infections of any type during the first month after transplant increase the risk of a subsequent fatal cytomegalovirus (CMV) infection, a rejection, because immunosuppression frequently has to be decreased for the infection to be treated, or a prolonged hospital stay. Viral infections, especially CMV, can enhance immunosuppression, resulting in additional opportunistic infections. Accordingly, each heart transplant team must develop a prophylactic regimen against CMV, *Pneumocystis carinii* (PCP), herpes simplex virus, and oral candidiasis to be used during the first 6 to 12 months after transplant. Prophylactic intravenous ganciclovir or oral valganciclovir is generally given for variable amounts of time in the CMV-seronegative recipient of a CMV-positive donor. Optimal prophylaxis regimens and timing have not been completely standardized, and some of the decisions to be made about prophylaxis are outlined in **Table 40-3**.[120] The necessity of routine prophylaxis, however, has withstood the test of time. The regimen increases substantially the number of medications and potential drug interactions the recipient may experience. Some of the important drug interactions are listed in **Table 40-4**.[77,78,121]

TABLE 40-3 Usual Care and Individual Decisions in the Management of Patients after Heart Transplantation

USUAL CARE	INDIVIDUAL DECISIONS
Maintenance immunosuppression • Corticosteroids • Calcineurin inhibitors • Antiproliferative agents	Wean from prednisone completely? Cyclosporine or tacrolimus? Azathioprine or mycophenolate mofetil? Induction of immunosuppression? • Polyclonal antibodies: antithymocyte globulins • Monoclonal antibodies: OKT3, basiliximab, daclizumab
Viral prophylaxis • Ganciclovir, acyclovir, valacyclovir	Duration of prophylaxis? Drug choice for risk profile?
Fungal prophylaxis • Fluconazole • Trimethoprim/sulfamethoxazole, dapsone, pentamidine	Duration of prophylaxis? Reinstitution during intensified immunosuppression?
Vascular protection • Pravastatin, simvastatin	Efficacy of other statins? Role of aspirin? Role of rapamycin and everolimus? Target lipid levels?
Antihypertension therapy • Goal: optimal blood pressure control	First-line drug or drugs of choice?
Surveillance for rejection • Endomyocardial biopsy	Role of echocardiography or other noninvasive tools? Role of biomarkers or gene expression assays? How long and how often to perform biopsy? Role of humoral rejection and methods to detect it?
Surveillance for vasculopathy of transplanted heart • Coronary arteriography	Role of noninvasive testing? Role of intravascular ultrasonography? Role of computed tomographic angiography?
Surveillance for malignancy • Annual examination • Chest radiography • Colonoscopy, mammography, other imaging tests* • Dermatologic examinations	Role of primary care team versus transplantation team?

**Recommended adult immunization schedule: United States. Ann Intern Med 152:36–39, 2010. Screening for breast cancer: U.S. Preventive Services task force recommendation statement. Ann Intern Med 151:716–726, 2009. Clinical guideline: screening for ovarian cancer: recommendations and rationale. Ann Intern Med 121:141–142, 1994. Clinical guideline: Part I: Suggested technique for fecal occult blood testing and interpretation in colorectal cancer screening. Ann Intern Med 126:808–810, 1997. Clinical guideline: Part III: screening for prostate cancer. Ann Intern Med 126:480–484, 1997.*

Medical Complications and Comorbidities

The complications following heart transplant reflect in part the premorbid status of most transplant recipients who have vascular disease and other significant medical conditions. After 5 years, over 90% of recipients have hypertension, at least 80% have hyperlipidemia, and more than 30% of patients have diabetes, as shown in **Table 40-5**.[122] Each year following transplant, a larger number of patients will develop clinically significant CAV, which is the major limitation to long life following transplant. By 5 years, almost 30% of recipients will have CAV, and at least half will be so afflicted at 10 years. Similarly, progressive renal insufficiency is an insidious problem that is only recently being addressed by substitution protocols to limit the administration of calcineurin inhibitors.[91,123]

Malignancy

The magnitude of overimmunosuppression in many transplant recipients is illustrated by the prediction of a 30% to 40% incidence of neoplasia in transplant patients over the period of the past 30 years. The risk of fatal malignancy progressively increases in the years following transplantation, and there is a substantially higher risk in immunosuppressed patients compared with the normal population. Post-transplant lymphoproliferative disease and lung cancer are the most common fatal malignancies, as shown in **Table 40-6**.[122]

Risk factors for malignancy are multifactorial and include impaired immunoregulation, a synergistic effect with other carcinogens such as nicotine or ultraviolet light exposure, and oncogenic causes such as the Epstein-Barr

TABLE 40-4 Commonly Used Drugs and Potential Drug Interactions with Immunosuppressants

DRUG	POTENTIAL INTERACTION
Acyclovir	Increased nephrotoxicity with calcineurin inhibitors
Allopurinol	Increased bone marrow suppression with azathioprine
Amlodipine or felodipine	Increased levels of calcineurin inhibitor
Antacids	Decreased levels of mycophenolate mofetil
Antidepressants	Increased levels of calcineurin inhibitor
Cimetidine	Increased levels of calcineurin inhibitor
Calcineurin inhibitors	Increased levels of mycophenolate mofetil
Clotrimazole	Increased levels of calcineurin inhibitor
Colchicine	Increased toxicity of colchicine
Diltiazem	Increased level of calcineurin inhibitor; increased neurotoxicity
Erythromycin or clarithromycin	Increased level of calcineurin inhibitor; prolonged QT intervals
Ganciclovir or valganciclovir	Increased nephrotoxicity with calcineurin inhibitors; leukopenia
Iron	Decreased levels of mycophenolate mofetil
Ketoconazole	Increased levels of calcineurin inhibitor
Phenobarbital	Decreased levels of calcineurin inhibitor
Phenytoin	Decreased levels of calcineurin inhibitor, increased levels of phenytoin
Primidone	Decreased levels of calcineurin inhibitor
Rifampin	Decreased levels of calcineurin inhibitor
Statin drugs	Increased risk for myopathy/rhabdomyolysis
St. John's wort	Decreased levels of calcineurin inhibitor levels
Target of rapamycin inhibitors	Increased nephrotoxicity with calcineurin inhibitors
Trimethoprim-sulfamethoxazole	Increased nephrotoxicity with calcineurin inhibitors
Verapamil	Increased levels of calcineurin inhibitor

and papilloma viruses. The cumulative amount of immunosuppression is positively correlated with risk of malignancy. Lymphoproliferative disease, skin, and lip cancers and Kaposi's sarcoma have a particularly high incidence. Malignancies account for 24% of deaths after 5 years. Accordingly, as illustrated in Table 40-6, transplant teams must ensure that the transplant recipient is adequately screened on a regular basis for the development of cancer.[124,125]

Diabetes

Patients who develop new-onset diabetes mellitus after transplant are at increased risk for morbidity and mortality. Accumulating evidence suggests that their long-term outcomes, including patient survival and/or graft survival, may be adversely affected. Decreased B-cell insulin secretion and increased insulin resistance secondary to the effects of immunosuppression characterize new-onset diabetes. Much of the diabetes that occurs is attributed to the high-dose steroids used early after transplant surgery, but it is now appreciated that the calcineurin inhibitors play an important role as well. Impaired B-cell function appears to be the primary mechanism of calcineurin inhibitor–induced new-onset diabetes.[126,127] Unfortunately there are very few data on specific drugs to be used in the management of patients with new-onset diabetes following cardiac transplantation.

Hypertension

The excess risk of hypertension is primarily related to the use of calcineurin inhibitors, because of both direct effects of the drugs on the kidney and the associated renal insufficiency that is also highly prevalent. The incidence of hypertension may be lower with tacrolimus as compared to

TABLE 40-5 Morbidity after Heart Transplantation for Adults

	Within 5 Years		*Within 10 Years*	
OUTCOME	PERCENTAGE WITH KNOWN RESPONSE	TOTAL *N* WITH KNOWN RESPONSE	PERCENTAGE WITH KNOWN RESPONSE	TOTAL *N* WITH KNOWN RESPONSE
Hypertension	93.8%	8266	98.5%	1586
Renal dysfunction	32.6%	8859	38.7%	1829
Abnormal creatinine level (<2.5 mg/dL)	21.2%		24.4%	
Creatinine level >2.5 mg/dL	8.4%		8.2%	
Chronic dialysis	2.5%		4.9%	
Renal transplantation	0.5%		1.2%	
Hyperlipidemia	87.1%	9237	93.3%	1890
Diabetes	34.8%	8219	36.7%	1601
Cardiac allograft vasculopathy	31.5%	5944	52.7%	896

Cumulative prevalence in survivors 5 and 10 years after transplantation (follow-up assessments: April 1994 to June 2006).
Modified from Hertz MI, Aurora P, Christie JD, et al: Registry of the International Society for Heart and Lung Transplantation: a quarter century of thoracic transplantation. J Heart Lung Transplant 27:937–942, 2008.

TABLE 40-6 Malignancy after Heart Transplantation in Adults

MALIGNANCY/TYPE	1-YEAR SURVIVORS	5-YEAR SURVIVORS	10-YEAR SURVIVORS
No malignancy	20,442 (97.1%)	7780 (84.9%)	1264 (68.1%)
Malignancy (all types combined)	612 (2.9%)	1389 (15.1%)	592 (31.9%)
Skin	282	937	360
Lymph	142	127	38
Other	132	359	108
Type not reported	56	40	126

Cumulative prevalence in survivors (follow-up assessments: April 1994 to June 2006).
From Hertz MI, Aurora P, Christie JD, et al: Registry of the International Society for Heart and Lung Transplantation: a quarter century of thoracic transplantation. J Heart Lung Transplant 27:937–942, 2008.

cyclosporine.[128] Blood pressure elevation in this population is characterized by a disturbed circadian rhythm without the normal nocturnal blood pressure fall and with a greater 24-hour hypertensive burden. Post-transplant hypertension is difficult to control and often requires a combination of several antihypertensive agents.

Renal Insufficiency

In a large registry of almost 70,000 nonrenal solid organ transplant recipients, the risk of developing chronic renal failure was 16% at 10 years.[129] There are a variety of postulated causes for calcineurin inhibitor-associated early renal insufficiency, including direct calcineurin inhibitor-mediated renal arteriolar vasoconstriction; increased levels of endothelin-1, a potent vasoconstrictor; as well as decreased NO production and alterations in the kidney's ability to adjust to changes in serum tonicity. Once early renal insufficiency occurs, progressive renal failure has appeared to be inexorable until recently. A number of new trials are in progress to evaluate the effects of substituting a TOR inhibitor, sirolimus, or everolimus for a calcineurin inhibitor on renal function, as well as rejection episodes.[91,123]

Hyperlipidemia

Hyperlipidemia is a common occurrence in post-transplant recipients, as it is in the general population. The concern has been that many studies have associated hyperlipidemia with the development of CAV, cerebrovascular, and peripheral vascular disease, with the attendant morbidity and mortality of these vascular disorders. Typically, total cholesterol, LDL cholesterol, and triglycerides increase by 3 months post-transplant and then generally fall somewhat after the first year. A number of drugs commonly used after transplant contribute to the hyperlipidemia observed.[77,121]

Lipid lowering therapy with any statin, or HMG-CoA reductase inhibitor, was strongly associated with a marked improvement in 1-year survival in the Heart Transplant Lipid registry.[130] In heart transplant recipients, pravastatin and simvastatin have been associated with outcome benefits in survival, severity of rejection, and cardiac allograft vasculopathy.[55,131] However, there are no long-term trials or data in this population demonstrating that lowering LDL-C levels to a specific target with more potent or higher dose statin therapy results in improved outcomes. Statins are metabolized differently, some by the cytochrome cyproheptadine (CYP) 3A4 and some by CYP2C9, and others are metabolized by a non-CYP mechanism in the liver. Thus caution must be used in the indiscriminate use of statin drugs beyond the doses used in the randomized trials of simvastatin and pravastatin.[121]

Cardiac Allograft Vasculopathy

The development of transplant vasculopathy remains the most disheartening long-term complication of heart transplant, with an annual incidence rate of 5% to 10%. The prognosis of heart transplant recipients is largely determined by the occurrence of CAV; after the first postoperative year, CAV becomes increasingly important as a cause of death. CAV can develop as early as 3 months after transplant and is detected angiographically in 20% of grafts at 1 year and 40% to 50% at 5 years.[132,133] In contrast to eccentric lesions seen in atheromatous disease, CAV results from neointimal proliferation of vascular smooth muscle cells so that it is a generalized process. Typically, the condition is characterized by concentric narrowing that affects the entire length of the coronary tree, from the epicardial to intramyocardial segments, leading to rapid tapering, pruning, and obliteration of third order branch vessels. Most patients will not experience anginal symptoms because of denervation of coronary arteries. The first clinical manifestation of CAV may include myocardial ischemia and infarction, heart failure, ventricular arrhythmia, or sudden death.

The causes of transplant vasculopathy are multifactorial. The risk of CAV increases as the number of HLA mismatches and the number and duration of rejection episodes increase. Various nonimmunologic factors have been associated with the development of CAV, including CMV infection, donor or recipient factors (e.g., age, gender), and surgical factors (e.g., ischemia-reperfusion injury). Classic risk factors for vascular disease, such as smoking, obesity, diabetes, dyslipidemia, and hypertension, increase CAV as well.

In an effort to detect the development of CAV, transplant teams must devise an approach to screen for the disease and, when found, control its progression. Coronary angiography is limited by the fact that CAV produces concentric lesions that affect the distal and small vessels, often before becoming apparent in the main epicardial vessels. Intravascular ultrasound, IVUS, is currently the most sensitive imaging technique to study early transplant vasculopathy. IVUS provides quantitative information on vessel wall morphology and lumen dimensions. An increase in intimal thickness of at least 0.5 mm in the first year after transplant is a reliable indicator of both CAV development and 5-year mortality.[134,135] However, increased invasiveness and cost of IVUS preclude its widespread application. Dobutamine stress echocardiography has a high sensitivity (83%-95%) and specificity (between 53% and 91%) when compared with angiographic CAV or even greater specificity when compared with IVUS-detected disease.[136] Most transplant centers do one of the above screening tests on an annual basis to assess the risk of new CAV.

The only definitive treatment of transplant vasculopathy is a second heart transplant procedure. Other approaches, such as PCI and CABG, may have a high restenosis rate, and are unlikely to be effective because of the diffuse nature of the process.[137,138] Another approach to the prevention of transplant vasculopathy is the use of the statins pravastatin and simvastatin. The drugs effectively repress the induction of MHC-II expression by interferon-γ and thereby inhibit T-cell proliferation. In addition, statins have a direct influence on the expression of genes for growth factors that are essential for the proliferation of smooth muscle cells. Randomized controlled trials have shown that both drugs result in significantly lower cholesterol levels, as well as significantly improved survival rates, significantly fewer severe rejections, and a significantly lower incidence of transplant vasculopathy.[135,139] It is not clear whether all statin drugs have the same benefit in this population.

Recently, there have been an increased number of trials examining the efficacy of sirolimus or everolimus to prevent the development or progression of CAV in heart transplant recipients. The precise role of the two drugs in maintenance immunosuppression has not yet been determined, but they are frequently used and are promising in their reduction of coronary intimal thickening once CAV has been detected.[132]

New Health Problems

Patients waiting for heart transplant should have an updated review of immunizations, and yearly influenza vaccines should be encouraged thereafter, along with the periodic pneumococcal vaccine.[140] Newer vaccines must be considered carefully before the routine administration to the immune-compromised transplant patient to avoid those with live viral particles. Generally, a comprehensive visit is scheduled at the anniversary of the transplant procedure so that annual issues may be reviewed beyond the typical cardiovascular problems addressed so frequently in the first year. These include a thorough skin and eye examination and recommended screening examinations, such as mammography, colonoscopy, and rectal and pelvic examinations, according to guidelines. This is the opportune time to reinforce the necessity of regular physical exercise, maintenance of ideal body weight, abstinence from tobacco, and moderation with alcohol. The annual examination is also when many transplant teams look more carefully for the presence of CAV.

In many centers, recipients are given daily aspirin to prevent further vascular disease, but there are no randomized trials evaluating the benefits of antiplatelet therapy in heart transplant patients. Similarly, most recipients are given vitamins, stool softeners, iron supplements, and proton pump inhibitors early after surgery, primarily from an empiric basis. These are parts of the decisions that must be made on a programmatic basis for the transplant recipient.

The development of osteoporosis is a major problem in the transplant population, and prophylaxis with calcium and vitamin D is usually initiated; vertebral fractures are common and result in marked debilitation. At least 50% of patients pretransplant have evidence of osteopenia, and osteoporosis is frequent in patients with advanced heart failure.[141] Glucocorticoids given post-transplant surgery are a major factor of additional bone loss; most bone loss occurs in the first 6 to 12 months.

Depression, a common finding in heart failure, occurs in up to 25% of transplant recipients, and can remarkably interfere with a satisfactory recovery. A number of antidepressants may be used, but the potential for adverse drug interactions must be considered (see Table 40-4). The management of gout may similarly be difficult because of drug-drug interactions. Colchicine may have increased risk of myoneuropathy, and nonsteroidal anti-inflammatory drugs often result in worsening renal insufficiency and hyperkalemia. Allopurinol and azathioprine administered together can cause life-threatening neutropenia. Thus transplant recipients must be instructed to discuss any new medicines prescribed to them with the transplant team before ingestion.[77,121,142]

Physicians outside the transplant hospital may be reluctant to care for the heart transplant recipient, complicating the comprehensive management of these patients. Ideally, primary care doctors could provide a very important and early intervention that might be lifesaving. The most common errors referring physicians make, unaware of normal transplant procedures, are the addition of new drugs that result in adverse drug interactions, as shown in Table 40-4. Both calcineurin inhibitors are metabolized in the liver by the cytochrome P-450 enzyme system. The activity of this cytochrome system is influenced by hepatic dysfunction. Inducers of CYP 3A4 include amiodarone, rifampin, and phenytoin; the use of these drugs has the potential to lower the levels of calcineurin inhibitors. Agents that inhibit the CYP 3A4, and raise levels of the immunosuppression regimen, include antifungals, macrolide antibacterials, calcium channel antagonists, and grapefruit juice.[142]

A higher index of suspicion must be used when evaluating the possibility of infection in a transplant recipient who must always be considered an immune-compromised host. Physicians unaccustomed to caring for the infection-prone transplant patient may inadvertently miss an important manifestation of an infectious disease, especially early in the post-transplant course. Again, communication with the transplant team should be fostered as a strategy to prevent these and countless other mishaps.

OUTCOMES FOLLOWING HEART TRANSPLANTATION

Survival

Figure 40-6 depicts the data from the International Society for Heart and Lung Transplantation on overall transplant survival.[59] During the first year after transplant, early causes of death are graft failure, infection, and rejection. Overall survival depends largely on the indication for transplant with patients with valvular cardiomyopathy (79% 1-year survival), congenital heart disease (79% 1-year survival), retransplantation (81% 1-year survival), ischemic cardiomyopathy (84% 1-year survival), and nonischemic cardiomyopathy (86% 1-year survival). Beyond 3 years, allograft vasculopathy and malignancy are the leading causes of mortality. Interestingly, although approaches to the management of the cardiac transplant recipient worldwide are substantially different from center to center, the outcomes are surprisingly similar. Nonspecific graft failure accounted for 41% of deaths during the first 30 days post-transplant, whereas non-cytomegalovirus infection was the primary cause of death during the first year. After 5 years, CAV and late graft failure (31% together), malignancy (24%), and non-cytomegalovirus infection (10%) are the most prominent causes of death.[21,56,143]

Functional Outcomes

By the first year following transplant surgery, 90% of surviving patients report no functional limitations and approximately 35% return to work.[144] These figures may change as the demographics of cardiac transplant recipients evolve. There are numerous challenges to ensure optimal functional outcomes, not the least of which is nonreimbursement for cardiac rehabilitation programs by many third-party payers in the United States and reluctance of employers in the United States to hire the transplant survivor. Adapting to life after transplant involves a variety of pretransplant factors, including the patient's duration of illness, personality, intelligence, social support, and financial well-being.

The heart transplant procedure markedly reduces cardiac filling pressures observed in the recipient before transplant and augments cardiac output. There may be an abnormal maximal cardiac output during exercise secondary to denervation, limited atrial function, decreased myocardial compliance from rejection or ischemic injury, and donor-recipient size mismatch.[145] Much of this hemodynamic abnormality may be normalized with regular exercise.[146,147]

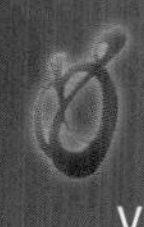

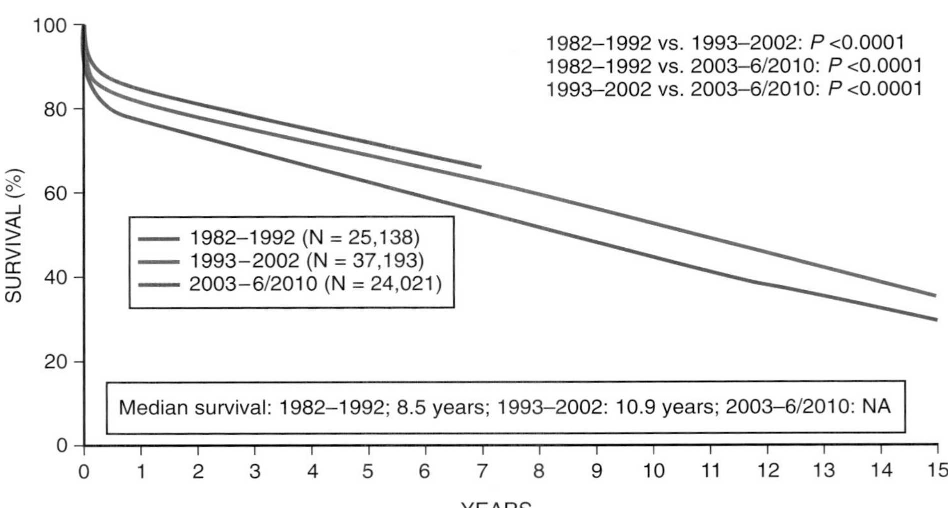

FIGURE 40-6 Survival of heart transplants by year of implant. Note: This figure includes only the heart transplants that are reported to the heart transplant registry of the ISHLT. *From Stehlik J, Edwards LB, Kucheryavaya AY, et al: The registry of the International Society for Heart and Lung Transplantation: 29th official adult heart transplant report—2012. J Heart Lung Transplant 31:1052–1064, 2012.*

Immediately after surgery, a restrictive hemodynamic pattern is frequently observed that gradually improves over a few days to weeks. Some 10% to 15% of recipients develop a chronic restrictive-type response during exercise that may produce fatigue and breathlessness. In the absence of parasympathetic innervation that normally lowers the heart rate, the resting heart rate of a recipient is typically 90 to 115 bpm. Similarly, β-blockers may further impair exercise response in the transplant patient, and should not be first-line therapy for hypertension in this group.

FUTURE DIRECTIONS

Heart transplant as a therapy has multiple, competing therapeutic options for advanced heart failure, including "destination" or permanent mechanical circulatory support. As newer therapies such as cell transplantation and better permanent mechanical devices become available, heart transplant's role will need to be redefined as the therapy of choice. Moreover, the cost-effectiveness of the transplant procedure will move in the wrong direction if 40% to 50% of patients require a VAD preoperatively. Organ allocation may need to be reconsidered in this era of rapid HLA typing and virtual crossmatches.

An ideal cardiac transplant immunosuppressive regimen will prevent cellular rejection, retard the development of CAV, have no nephrotoxicity, and negligible morbidity with respect to lymphoproliferative disease and opportunistic infections. The development of renal sparing strategies in transplant recipients is one of the most significant therapeutic challenges. This and other modifications of the standard regimen must be explored in future trials. Trial networks to investigate some of these newer ideas or therapies must be established to facilitate research in this fragile population.

In the United States, there is now an acknowledged and accredited secondary subspecialty in medicine specifically for cardiologists who want to acquire expertise in the care of the heart transplant recipient.[148] Surgical training has allowed for the increased skill required to manage the wide array of mechanical circulatory support devices used to sustain the patient with advanced heart failure. Mechanisms to fund the prolonged training of these transplant specialists, and other transplant personnel, must be found in an increasingly impoverished health care system.

References

1. Hunt SA, Haddad F, Hunt SA, et al: The changing face of heart transplantation. *J Am Coll Cardiol* 52:587–598, 2008.
2. Hunt SA, Hunt SA: Taking heart–cardiac transplantation past, present, and future [erratum appears in N Engl J Med. 2006 Aug 31;355(9):967]. *NEJM* 355:231–235, 2006.
3. Butler J, Khadim G, Paul KM, et al: Selection of patients for heart transplantation in the current era of heart failure therapy [see comment]. *J Am Coll Cardiol* 43:787–793, 2004.
4. Mehra MR, Kobashigawa J, Starling R, et al: Listing criteria for heart transplantation: International Society for Heart and Lung Transplantation guidelines for the care of cardiac transplant candidates-2006. *J Heart Lung Transplant* 25:1024–1042, 2006.
5. Slaughter MS, Rogers JG, Milano CA, et al: Advanced heart failure treated with continuous-flow left ventricular assist device. *N Engl J Med* 361:2241–2251, 2009.
6. Hansky B, Vogt J, Zittermann A, et al: Cardiac resynchronization therapy: long-term alternative to cardiac transplantation? [see comment]. *Ann Thorac Surg* 87:432–438, 2009.
7. John R: Donor management and selection for heart transplantation. *Semin Thorac Cardiovasc Surg* 16:364–369, 2004.
8. Goldberg LR, Jessup M: A time to be born and a time to die. *Circulation* 116:360–362, 2007.
9. Levy WC, Mozaffarian D, Linker DT, et al: Can the Seattle heart failure model be used to risk-stratify heart failure patients for potential left ventricular assist device therapy? *J Heart Lung Transplant* 28:231–236, 2009.
10. Schulze PC, Jiang J, Yang J, et al: Preoperative assessment of high-risk candidates to predict survival after heart transplantation. *Circ Heart Fail* 6:527–534, 2013.
11. Kilic A, Allen JG, Weiss ES: Validation of the United States-derived Index for Mortality Prediction After Cardiac Transplantation (IMPACT) using international registry data. *J Heart Lung Transplant* 32:492–498, 2013.
12. Stevenson LW, Pagani FD, Young JB, et al: INTERMACS profiles of advanced heart failure: the current picture. *J Heart Lung Transplant* 28:535–541, 2009.
13. Simmonds J, Burch M, Dawkins H, et al: Heart transplantation after congenital heart surgery: improving results and future goals. *Eur J Cardiothorac Surg* 34:313–317, 2008.
14. Bhama JK, Shulman J, Bermudez CA, et al: Heart transplantation for adults with congenital heart disease: results in the modern era. *J Heart Lung Transplant* 32:499–504, 2013.
15. Mancini DM, Eisen H, Kussmaul W, et al: Value of peak exercise oxygen consumption for optimal timing of cardiac transplantation in ambulatory patients with heart failure. *Circulation* 83:778–786, 1991.
16. Lund LH, Aaronson KD, Mancini DM, et al: Validation of peak exercise oxygen consumption and the Heart Failure Survival Score for serial risk stratification in advanced heart failure. *Am J Cardiol* 95:734–741, 2005.
17. Allen LA, Rogers JG, Warnica JW, et al: High mortality without ESCAPE: the registry of heart failure patients receiving pulmonary artery catheters without randomization. *J Card Fail* 14:661–669, 2008.
18. Nohria A, Hasselblad V, Stebbins A, et al: Cardiorenal interactions: insights from the ESCAPE trial.[see comment]. *J Am Coll Cardiol* 51:1268–1274, 2008.
19. Chen JM, Russo MJ, Hammond KM, et al: Alternate waiting list strategies for heart transplantation maximize donor organ utilization. *Ann Thorac Surg* 80:224–228, 2005.
20. Tjang YS, van der Heijden GJ, Tenderich G, et al: Impact of recipient's age on heart transplantation outcome.[see comment]. *Ann Thorac Surg* 85:2051–2055, 2008.
21. Weiss ES, Nwakanma LU, Patel ND, et al: Outcomes in patients older than 60 years of age undergoing orthotopic heart transplantation: an analysis of the UNOS database. *J Heart Lung Transplant* 27:184–191, 2008.
22. Russo MJ, Rana A, Chen JM, et al: Pretransplantation patient characteristics and survival following combined heart and kidney transplantation: an analysis of the United Network for Organ Sharing Database. *Arch Surg* 144:241–246, 2009.
23. Gill J, Shah T, Hristea I, et al: Outcomes of simultaneous heart-kidney transplant in the US: a retrospective analysis using OPTN/UNOS data. *Am J Transplant* 9:844–852, 2009.
24. Cannon RM, Hughes MG, Jones CM, et al: A review of the United States experience with combined heart-liver transplantation. *Transpl Int* 25:1223–1228, 2012.
25. Topilsky Y, Raichlin E, Hasin T, et al: Combined heart and liver transplant attenuates cardiac allograft vasculopathy compared with isolated heart transplantation. *Transplantation* 95:859–865, 2013.

26. Klotz S, Wenzelburger F, Stypmann J, et al: Reversible pulmonary hypertension in heart transplant candidates: to transplant or not to transplant. *Ann Thorac Surg* 82:1770–1773, 2006.
27. Kutty RS, Parameshwar J, Lewis C, et al: Use of centrifugal left ventricular assist device as a bridge to candidacy in severe heart failure with secondary pulmonary hypertension. *Eur J Cardiothorac Surg* 43:1237–1242, 2013.
28. Zimpfer D, Zrunek P, Roethy W, et al: Left ventricular assist devices decrease fixed pulmonary hypertension in cardiac transplant candidates. *J Thorac Cardiovasc Surg* 133:689–695, 2007.
29. Zimpfer D, Zrunek P, Sandner S, et al: Post-transplant survival after lowering fixed pulmonary hypertension using left ventricular assist devices. *Eur J Cardiothorac Surg* 31:698–702, 2007.
30. Lorenz KA, Lynn J, Dy SM, et al: Evidence for improving palliative care at the end of life: a systematic review [see comment]. *Ann Intern Med* 148:147–159, 2008.
31. Kobashigawa J, Mehra M, West L, et al: Report from a Consensus Conference on the Sensitized Patient Awaiting Heart Transplantation. *J Heart Lung Transplant* 28:213–225, 2009.
32. Tait BD, Hudson F, Cantwell L, et al: Review article: Luminex technology for HLA antibody detection in organ transplantation. *Nephrology* 14:247–254, 2009.
33. Fuggle SV, Martin S: Tools for human leukocyte antigen antibody detection and their application to transplanting sensitized patients. *Transplantation* 86:384–390, 2008.
34. Zachary AA, Eng HS: Desensitization: achieving immune detente. *Tissue Antigens* 77:3–8, 2011.
35. Reinsmoen NL: New approaches for optimizing transplant of sensitized patients. *Curr Opin Organ Transplant* 17:406–408, 2012.
36. Reinsmoen NL, Lai CH, Vo A, et al: Evolving paradigms for desensitization in managing broadly HLA sensitized transplant candidates. *Discov Med* 13:267–273, 2012.
37. Patel J, Everly M, Chang D, et al: Reduction of alloantibodies via proteasome inhibition in cardiac transplantation. *J Heart Lung Transplant* 30:1320–1326, 2011.
38. Vega J, Moore J, Murray S, et al: Heart transplantation in the United States, 1998-2007. *Am J Transplant* 9(Pt 2):932–941, 2009.
39. Cleveland JC, Jr, Grover FL, Fullerton DA, et al: Left ventricular assist device as bridge to transplantation does not adversely affect one-year heart transplantation survival. *J Thorac Cardiovasc Surg* 136:774–777, 2008.
40. Hoercher KJ, Nowicki ER, Blackstone EH, et al: Prognosis of patients removed from a transplant waiting list for medical improvement: implications for organ allocation and transplantation for status 2 patients. *J Thorac Cardiovasc Surg* 135:1159–1166, 2008.
41. Halpern SD, Shaked A, Hasz RD, et al: Informing candidates for solid-organ transplantation about donor risk factors [see comment]. *N Eng J Med* 358:2832–2837, 2008.
42. Khasati NH, Machaal A, Barnard J, et al: Donor heart selection: the outcome of "unacceptable" donors. *J Cardiothorac Surg* 2:13, 2007.
43. Gupta D, Piacentino V, 3rd, Macha M, et al: Effect of older donor age on risk for mortality after heart transplantation. *Annals of Thoracic Surgery* 78:890–899, 2004.
44. Collins MJ, Moainie SL, Griffith BP, et al: Preserving and evaluating hearts with ex vivo machine perfusion: an avenue to improve early graft performance and expand the donor pool. *Eur J Cardiothorac Surg* 34:318–325, 2008.
45. Mehra MR: The cardiac allograft is going up in smoke: a call to action. *Am J Transplant* 8:737–738, 2008.
46. Rosendale JD, Kauffman HM, McBride MA, et al: Aggressive pharmacologic donor management results in more transplanted organs. *Transplantation* 75:482–487, 2003.
47. Zaroff JG, Rosengard BR, Armstrong WF, et al: Consensus conference report: maximizing use of organs recovered from the cadaver donor: cardiac recommendations, March 28-29, 2001, Crystal City, VA. *Circulation* 106:836–841, 2002.
48. Kubrich M, Petrakopoulou P, Kofler S, et al: Impact of coronary endothelial dysfunction on adverse long-term outcome after heart transplantation. *Transplantation* 85:1580–1587, 2008.
49. Grande AM, Gaeta R, Campana C, et al: Comparison of standard and bicaval approach in orthotopic heart transplantation: 10-year follow-up. *J Cardiovasc Med* 9:493–497, 2008.
50. Morgan JA, Edwards NM: Orthotopic cardiac transplantation: comparison of outcome using biatrial, bicaval, and total techniques. *J Card Surg* 20:102–106, 2005.
51. Schnoor M, Schafer T, Luhmann D, et al: Bicaval versus standard technique in orthotopic heart transplantation: a systematic review and meta-analysis. *J Thorac Cardiovasc Surg* 134:1322–1331, 2007.
52. Fiorelli AI, Stolf NA, Abreu Filho CA, et al: Prophylactic donor tricuspid annuloplasty in orthotopic bicaval heart transplantation. *Transplant Proc* 39:2527–2530, 2007.
53. Christiansen S, Klocke A, Autschbach R, et al: Past, present, and future of long-term mechanical cardiac support in adults. *J Card Surg* 23:664–676, 2008.
54. Miller LW, Pagani FD, Russell SD, et al: Use of a continuous-flow device in patients awaiting heart transplantation [see comment] [reprint in *Nat Clin Pract Cardiovasc Med* 5(2): 80–81, 2008]. *N Eng J Med* 357:885–896, 2007.
55. Kobashigawa JA, Starling RC, Mehra MR, et al: Multicenter retrospective analysis of cardiovascular risk factors affecting long-term outcome of de novo cardiac transplant recipients. *J Heart Lung Transplant* 25:1063–1069, 2006.
56. Marelli D, Kobashigawa J, Hamilton MA, et al: Long-term outcomes of heart transplantation in older recipients. *J Heart Lung Transplant* 27:830–834, 2008.
57. Russo MJ, Chen JM, Sorabella RA, et al: The effect of ischemic time on survival after heart transplantation varies by donor age: an analysis of the United Network for Organ Sharing database. *J Thorac Cardiovasc Surg* 133:554–559, 2007.
58. Sezgin A, Akay TH, Ozcobanoglu S, et al: Surgery-related complications in cardiac transplantation patients. *Transplant Proc* 40:255–258, 2008.
59. Stehlik J, Edwards LB, Kucheryavaya AY, et al: The registry of the International Society for Heart and Lung Transplantation: 29th official adult heart transplant report–2012. *J Heart Lung Transplant* 31:1052–1064, 2012.
60. Novick RJ: Immediate postoperative care of the heart transplant recipient: perils and triumphs. *Semin Cardiothorac Vasc Anesth* 13:95–98, 2009.
61. Ramakrishna H, Jaroszewski DE, Arabia FA, et al: Adult cardiac transplantation: a review of perioperative management Part-I. *Ann Card Anaesth* 12:71–78, 2009.
62. Khush KK, Valantine HA, Khush KK, et al: New developments in immunosuppressive therapy for heart transplantation. *Expert Opin Emerg Drugs* 14:1–21, 2009.
63. Mehra MR, Uber PA, Kaplan B: Immunosuppression in cardiac transplantation: science, common sense and the heart of the matter. *Am J Transplant* 6:1243–1245, 2006.
64. Mueller XM: Drug immunosuppression therapy for adult heart transplantation. Part 2: clinical applications and results. *Ann Thorac Surg* 77:363–371, 2004.
65. Mueller XM: Drug immunosuppression therapy for adult heart transplantation. Part 1: immune response to allograft and mechanism of action of immunosuppressants. *Ann Thorac Surg* 77:354–362, 2004.
66. Goland S, Czer LS, Coleman B, et al: Induction therapy with thymoglobulin after heart transplantation: impact of therapy duration on lymphocyte depletion and recovery, rejection, and cytomegalovirus infection rates. *J Heart Lung Transplant* 27:1115–1121, 2008.
67. Issa NC, Fishman JA, Issa NC, et al: Infectious complications of antilymphocyte therapies in solid organ transplantation. *Clin Infect Dis* 48:772–786, 2009.
68. Uber PA, Mehra MR: Induction therapy in heart transplantation: is there a role? *J Heart Lung Transplant* 26:205–209, 2007.
69. Opelz G, Henderson R: Incidence of non-Hodgkin lymphoma in kidney and heart transplant recipients. *Lancet* 342:1514–1516, 1993.
70. Segovia J, Rodriguez-Lambert JL, Crespo-Leiro MG, et al: A randomized multicenter comparison of basiliximab and muromonab (OKT3) in heart transplantation: SIMCOR study. *Transplantation* 81:1542–1548, 2006.
71. Hershberger RE, Starling RC, Eisen HJ, et al: Daclizumab to prevent rejection after cardiac transplantation [see comment]. *N Eng J Med* 352:2705–2713, 2005.
72. Mehra MR, Zucker MJ, Wagoner L, et al: A multicenter, prospective, randomized, double-blind trial of basiliximab in heart transplantation. *J Heart Lung Transplant* 24:1297–1304, 2005.
73. Carrier M, Leblanc MH, Perrault LP, et al: Basiliximab and rabbit anti-thymocyte globulin for prophylaxis of acute rejection after heart transplantation: a non-inferiority trial. *J Heart Lung Transplant* 26:258–263, 2007.
74. Kobashigawa J, David K, Morris J, et al: Daclizumab is associated with decreased rejection and no increased mortality in cardiac transplant patients receiving MMF, cyclosporine, and corticosteroids. *Transplant Proc* 37:1333–1339, 2005.
75. Patel J, Kobashigawa JA, Patel J, et al: Minimization of immunosuppression: transplant immunology. *Transpl Immunol* 20:48–54, 2008.
76. Moller CH, Gustafsson F, Gluud C, et al: Interleukin-2 receptor antagonists as induction therapy after heart transplantation: systematic review with meta-analysis of randomized trials. *J Heart Lung Transplant* 27:835–842, 2008.
77. Lindenfeld J, Miller GG, Shakar SF, et al: Drug therapy in the heart transplant recipient: part II: immunosuppressive drugs. *Circulation* 110:3858–3865, 2004.
78. Lindenfeld J, Miller GG, Shakar SF, et al: Drug therapy in the heart transplant recipient: part I: cardiac rejection and immunosuppressive drugs. *Circulation* 110:3734–3740, 2004.
79. Flechner SM, Kobashigawa J, Klintmalm G, et al: Calcineurin inhibitor-sparing regimens in solid organ transplantation: focus on improving renal function and nephrotoxicity. *Clin Transplant* 22:1–15, 2008.
80. Solari SG, Goldberg LR, DeNofrio D, et al: Cyclosporine monitoring with 2-hour postdose levels in heart transplant recipients. *Ther Drug Monit* 27:417–421, 2005.
81. Grimm M, Rinaldi M, Yonan NA, et al: Superior prevention of acute rejection by tacrolimus vs. cyclosporine in heart transplant recipients–a large European trial. *Am J Transplant* 6:1387–1397, 2006.
82. Kobashigawa JA, Patel J, Furukawa H, et al: Five-year results of a randomized, single-center study of tacrolimus vs microemulsion cyclosporine in heart transplant patients. *J Heart Lung Transplant* 25:434–439, 2006.
83. Lehmkuhl H, Hummel M, Kobashigawa J, et al: Enteric-coated mycophenolate-sodium in heart transplantation: efficacy, safety, and pharmacokinetic compared with mycophenolate mofetil. *Transplant Proc* 40:953–955, 2008.
84. Kobashigawa JA, Miller LW, Russell SD, et al: Tacrolimus with mycophenolate mofetil (MMF) or sirolimus vs. cyclosporine with MMF in cardiac transplant patients: 1-year report. [see comment]. *Am J Transplant* 6:1377–1386, 2006.
85. Kobashigawa JA, Tobis JM, Mentzer RM, et al: Mycophenolate mofetil reduces intimal thickness by intravascular ultrasound after heart transplant: reanalysis of the multicenter trial. *Am J Transplant* 6:993–997, 2006.
86. Eisen HJ, Kobashigawa J, Keogh A, et al: Three-year results of a randomized, double-blind, controlled trial of mycophenolate mofetil versus azathioprine in cardiac transplant recipients. *J Heart Lung Transplant* 24:517–525, 2005.
87. Raichlin E, Chandrasekaran K, Kremers WK, et al: Sirolimus as primary immunosuppressant reduces left ventricular mass and improves diastolic function of the cardiac allograft. *Transplantation* 86:1395–1400, 2008.
88. Mudge GH, Jr, Mudge GH, Jr: Sirolimus and cardiac transplantation: is it the "magic bullet"? [comment]. *Circulation* 116:2666–2668, 2007.
89. Raichlin E, Bae JH, Khalpey Z, et al: Conversion to sirolimus as primary immunosuppression attenuates the progression of allograft vasculopathy after cardiac transplantation [see comment]. *Circulation* 116:2726–2733, 2007.
90. Sanchez-Fructuoso AI, Sanchez-Fructuoso AI: Everolimus: an update on the mechanism of action, pharmacokinetics and recent clinical trials. *Expert Opin Drug Metab Toxicol* 4:807–819, 2008.
91. Groetzner J, Kaczmarek I, Schulz U, et al: Mycophenolate and sirolimus as calcineurin inhibitor-free immunosuppression improves renal function better than calcineurin inhibitor-reduction in late cardiac transplant recipients with chronic renal failure. *Transplantation* 87:726–733, 2009.
92. Kushwaha SS, Raichlin E, Sheinin Y, et al: Sirolimus affects cardiomyocytes to reduce left ventricular mass in heart transplant recipients [see comment]. *Eur Heart J* 29:2742–2750, 2008.
93. Stypmann J, Engelen MA, Eckernkemper S, et al: Calcineurin inhibitor-free immunosuppression using everolimus (Certican) after heart transplantation: 2 years' follow-up from the University Hospital Munster. *Transplant Proc* 43:1847–1852, 2011.
94. Rothenburger M, Zuckermann A, Bara C, et al: Recommendations for the use of everolimus (Certican) in heart transplantation: results from the second German-Austrian Certican Consensus Conference. *J Heart Lung Transplant* 26:305–311, 2007.
95. Kaczmarek I, Zaruba MM, Beiras-Fernandez A, et al: Tacrolimus with mycophenolate mofetil or sirolimus compared with calcineurin inhibitor-free immunosuppression (sirolimus/mycophenolate mofetil) after heart transplantation: 5-year results. *J Heart Lung Transplant* 32:277–284, 2013.
96. Gullestad L, Mortensen SA, Eiskjaer H, et al: Two-year outcomes in thoracic transplant recipients after conversion to everolimus with reduced calcineurin inhibitor within a multicenter, open-label, randomized trial. *Transplantation* 90:1581–1589, 2010.
97. Dobbels F, Vanhaecke J, Dupont L, et al: Pretransplant predictors of posttransplant adherence and clinical outcome: an evidence base for pretransplant psychosocial screening. *Transplantation* 87:1497–1504, 2009.
98. Saeed I, Rogers C, Murday A, et al: Health-related quality of life after cardiac transplantation: results of a UK National Survey with Norm-based Comparisons. *J Heart Lung Transplant* 27:675–681, 2008.
99. Fusar-Poli P, Picchioni M, Martinelli V, et al: Anti-depressive therapies after heart transplantation. *J Heart Lung Transplant* 25:785–793, 2006.
100. Singh N, Pirsch J, Samaniego M, et al: Antibody-mediated rejection: treatment alternatives and outcomes. *Transplant Rev* 23:34–46, 2009.
101. Fedson SE, Daniel SS, Husain AN, et al: Immunohistochemistry staining of C4d to diagnose antibody-mediated rejection in cardiac transplantation. *J Heart Lung Transplant* 27:372–379, 2008.
102. Tan CD, Baldwin WM, 3rd, Rodriguez ER, et al: Update on cardiac transplantation pathology. *Arch Pathol Lab Med* 131:1169–1191, 2007.
103. Patel JK, Kobashigawa JA, Patel JK, et al: Should we be doing routine biopsy after heart transplantation in a new era of anti-rejection? *Curr Opin Cardiol* 21:127–131, 2006.
104. Stewart S, Winters GL, Fishbein MC, et al: Revision of the 1990 working formulation for the standardization of nomenclature in the diagnosis of heart rejection [see comment]. *J Heart Lung Transplant* 24:1710–1720, 2005.
105. Mirabet S, Gelpi C, Roldan C, et al: Assessment of immunological markers as mediators of graft vasculopathy development in heart transplantation. *Transplant Proc* 43:2253–2256, 2011.

106. Pham MX, Deng MC, Kfoury AG, et al: Molecular testing for long-term rejection surveillance in heart transplant recipients: design of the Invasive Monitoring Attenuation Through Gene Expression (IMAGE) trial. *J Heart Lung Transplant* 26:808–814, 2007.
107. Yamani MH, Taylor DO, Rodriguez ER, et al: Transplant vasculopathy is associated with increased AlloMap gene expression score. *J Heart Lung Transplant* 26:403–406, 2007.
108. Deng MC, Eisen HJ, Mehra MR, et al: Noninvasive discrimination of rejection in cardiac allograft recipients using gene expression profiling. *Am J Transplant* 6:150–160, 2006.
109. Mehra MR, Kobashigawa JA, Deng MC, et al: Transcriptional signals of T-cell and corticosteroid-sensitive genes are associated with future acute cellular rejection in cardiac allografts. *J Heart Lung Transplant* 26:1255–1263, 2007.
110. Mehra MR, Kobashigawa JA, Deng MC, et al: Clinical implications and longitudinal alteration of peripheral blood transcriptional signals indicative of future cardiac allograft rejection. *J Heart Lung Transplant* 27:297–301, 2008.
111. Pham MX, Teuteberg JJ, Kfoury AG, et al: Gene-expression profiling for rejection surveillance after cardiac transplantation. *N Engl J Med* 362:1890–1900, 2010.
112. Yamani MH, Taylor DO, Haire C, et al: Post-transplant ischemic injury is associated with up-regulated AlloMap gene expression. *Clin Transplant* 21:523–525, 2007.
113. Jarcho J, Naftel DC, Shroyer TW, et al: Influence of HLA mismatch on rejection after heart transplantation: a multiinstitutional study. The Cardiac Transplant Research Database Group. *J Heart Lung Transplant* 13:583–595, discussion 95–96, 1994.
114. Taylor DO, Edwards LB, Boucek MM, et al: Registry of the International Society for Heart and Lung Transplantation: twenty-second official adult heart transplant report—2005. *J Heart Lung Transplant* 24:945–955, 2005.
115. Reed EF, Demetris AJ, Hammond E, et al: Acute antibody-mediated rejection of cardiac transplants. *J Heart Lung Transplant* 25:153–159, 2006.
116. Kfoury AG, Hammond ME, Snow GL, et al: Cardiovascular mortality among heart transplant recipients with asymptomatic antibody-mediated or stable mixed cellular and antibody-mediated rejection. *J Heart Lung Transplant* 28:781–784, 2009.
117. Turgeon NA, Kirk AD, Iwakoshi NN, et al: Differential effects of donor-specific alloantibody. *Transplant Rev* 23:25–33, 2009.
118. Jessup M, Brozena S: State-of-the-art strategies for immunosuppression. *Curr Opin Organ Transplant* 12:536–542, 2007.
119. Shahzad K, Aziz QA, Leva JP, et al: New-onset graft dysfunction after heart transplantation–incidence and mechanism-related outcomes. *J Heart Lung Transplant* 30:194–203, 2011.
120. Potena L, Grigioni F, Magnani G, et al: Prophylaxis versus preemptive anti-cytomegalovirus approach for prevention of allograft vasculopathy in heart transplant recipients. *J Heart Lung Transplant* 28:461–467, 2009.
121. Lindenfeld J, Page RL, 2nd, Zolty R, et al: Drug therapy in the heart transplant recipient: Part III: common medical problems. *Circulation* 111:113–117, 2005.
122. Hertz MI, Aurora P, Christie JD, et al: Registry of the International Society for Heart and Lung Transplantation: a quarter century of thoracic transplantation. *J Heart Lung Transplant* 27:937–942, 2008.
123. Gonzalez-Vilchez F, de Prada JA, Exposito V, et al: Avoidance of calcineurin inhibitors with use of proliferation signal inhibitors in de novo heart transplantation with renal failure. *J Heart Lung Transplant* 27:1135–1141, 2008.
124. Crespo-Leiro MG, Alonso-Pulpon L, Vazquez de Prada JA, et al: Malignancy after heart transplantation: incidence, prognosis and risk factors. *Am J Transplant* 8:1031–1039, 2008.
125. Roussel JC, Baron O, Perigaud C, et al: Outcome of heart transplants 15 to 20 years ago: graft survival, post-transplant morbidity, and risk factors for mortality. *J Heart Lung Transplant* 27:486–493, 2008.
126. Russo MJ, Chen JM, Hong KN, et al: Survival after heart transplantation is not diminished among recipients with uncomplicated diabetes mellitus: an analysis of the United Network of Organ Sharing database. *Circulation* 114:2280–2287, 2006.
127. Wilkinson A, Davidson J, Dotta F, et al: Guidelines for the treatment and management of new-onset diabetes after transplantation. *Clin Transplant* 19:291–298, 2005.
128. Ye F, Ying-Bin X, Yu-Guo W, et al: Tacrolimus versus cyclosporine microemulsion for heart transplant recipients: a meta-analysis. *J Heart Lung Transplant* 28:58–66, 2009.
129. Lonze BE, Warren DS, Stewart ZA, et al: Kidney transplantation in previous heart or lung recipients. *Am J Transplant* 9:578–585, 2009.
130. Wu AH, Ballantyne CM, Short BC, et al: Statin use and risks of death or fatal rejection in the Heart Transplant Lipid Registry. *Am J Cardiol* 95:367–372, 2005.
131. Bilchick KC, Henrikson CA, Skojec D, et al: Treatment of hyperlipidemia in cardiac transplant recipients. *Am Heart J* 148:200–210, 2004.
132. Delgado JF, Manito N, Segovia J, et al: The use of proliferation signal inhibitors in the prevention and treatment of allograft vasculopathy in heart transplantation. *Transplant Rev* 23:69–79, 2009.
133. Schmauss D, Weis M, Schmauss D, et al: Cardiac allograft vasculopathy: recent developments. *Circulation* 117:2131–2141, 2008.
134. Tuzcu EM, Kapadia SR, Sachar R, et al: Intravascular ultrasound evidence of angiographically silent progression in coronary atherosclerosis predicts long-term morbidity and mortality after cardiac transplantation. *J Am Coll Cardiol* 45:1538–1542, 2005.
135. Kobashigawa JA, Tobis JM, Starling RC, et al: Multicenter intravascular ultrasound validation study among heart transplant recipients: outcomes after five years. *J Am Coll Cardiol* 45:1532–1537, 2005.
136. Bacal F, Moreira L, Souza G, et al: Dobutamine stress echocardiography predicts cardiac events or death in asymptomatic patients long-term after heart transplantation: 4-year prospective evaluation. *J Heart Lung Transplant* 23:1238–1244, 2004.
137. Bhama JK, Nguyen DQ, Scolieri S, et al: Surgical revascularization for cardiac allograft vasculopathy: Is it still an option? *J Thorac Cardiovasc Surg* 137:1488–1492, 2009.
138. Gupta A, Mancini D, Kirtane AJ, et al: Value of drug-eluting stents in cardiac transplant recipients [see comment]. *Am J Cardiol* 103:659–662, 2009.
139. Kobashigawa JA, Kobashigawa JA: Cardiac allograft vasculopathy in heart transplant patients: pathologic and clinical aspects for angioplasty/stenting [comment]. *J Am Coll Cardiol* 48:462–463, 2006.
140. Magnani G, Falchetti E, Pollini G, et al: Safety and efficacy of two types of influenza vaccination in heart transplant recipients: a prospective randomised controlled study. *J Heart Lung Transplant* 24:588–592, 2005.
141. Ebeling PR, Ebeling PR: Approach to the patient with transplantation-related bone loss. *J Clin Endocrinol Metab* 94:1483–1490, 2009.
142. Page RL, 2nd, Miller GG, Lindenfeld J: Drug therapy in the heart transplant recipient: part IV: drug-drug interactions. *Circulation* 111:230–239, 2005.
143. Vaseghi M, Lellouche N, Ritter H, et al: Mode and mechanisms of death after orthotopic heart transplantation [see comment]. *Heart Rhythm* 6:503–509, 2009.
144. Grady KL, Naftel DC, Young JB, et al: Patterns and predictors of physical functional disability at 5 to 10 years after heart transplantation. *J Heart Lung Transplant* 26:1182–1191, 2007.
145. Scott JM, Esch BT, Haykowsky MJ, et al: Cardiovascular responses to incremental and sustained submaximal exercise in heart transplant recipients. *Am J Physiol Heart Circ Physiol* 296:H350–H358, 2009.
146. Roten L, Schmid JP, Merz F, et al: Diastolic dysfunction of the cardiac allograft and maximal exercise capacity. *J Heart Lung Transplant* 28:434–439, 2009.
147. Haykowsky M, Taylor D, Kim D, et al: Exercise training improves aerobic capacity and skeletal muscle function in heart transplant recipients. *Am J Transplant* 9:734–739, 2009.
148. Konstam MA, Jessup M, Francis GS, et al: Advanced heart failure and transplant cardiology: a subspecialty is born. *J Am Coll Cardiol* 53:834–836, 2009.

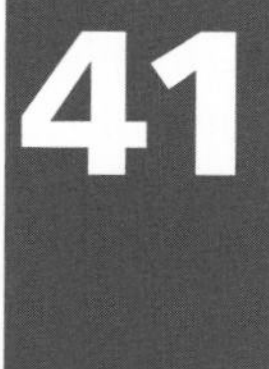

Surgical Treatment of Chronic Congestive Heart Failure

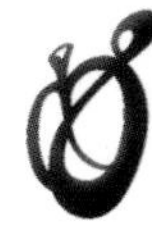

Wilfried Mullens, Frederik H. Verbrugge, and Randall C. Starling

Cardiac surgical interventions have been performed for decades on patients with congestive heart failure, albeit with a high perioperative morbidity and mortality as observed in the 1970s and 1980s. For that reason, the role of surgery was initially limited to cases of failed medical management. Fortunately, a real resurgence of interest into surgical options for heart failure has emerged as a result of evolving surgical techniques and devices that treat both ischemic and nonischemic heart failure.

Because of the aging of the population, the significant increase in the prevalence, morbidity, and mortality from heart failure is a compelling problem (see also Chapter 17). Advances in the treatment of acute myocardial infarction and nonischemic cardiomyopathy have led to an increased survival of patients. However, this has resulted in a continuous increase in the number of patients ultimately presenting with heart failure. Although cardiac transplantation remains a valuable therapeutic option for advanced end-stage heart failure (see also Chapter 40), the field of transplantation will continue to be plagued by a finite number of organ donors. The advent of axial flow implantable left ventricular assist devices (LVADs) as a bridge to transplantation or destination therapy has markedly improved outcomes for recipients and already resulted in more widespread use (see also Chapter 42). However, LVADs remain expensive, and still have a high incidence of adverse events, and therefore have not yet achieved their goal as a readily available alternative to most patients with advanced heart failure. As the number of patients suffering from advanced heart failure continues to expand and the availability and feasibility of cardiac transplantation and assist devices does not meet that growing demand, it is imperative that a substantial number of heart failure patients will become candidates for and derive benefit from heart failure surgery.

Because heart failure as a continuous disease process with ongoing detrimental reverse remodeling of the ventricles, insights into its pathophysiologic features have led to major advances in surgical therapies. Contemporary surgical heart failure techniques and devices try to restore the geometry of the failing ventricle, and thereby arrest or reverse the negative remodeling processes. As a result, cardiac function and subsequent clinical outcome have improved. Major advances in pharmacotherapy and imaging modalities have helped the surgical team to select those patients who will benefit most from surgical treatment of advanced heart failure. Finally, the management of chronic heart failure yields the best results through a combined medical and surgical approach, both of which are possible with a multidisciplinary team.

In this chapter, current and evolving surgical strategies for treating congestive heart failure will be reviewed, with a focus on three major areas: revascularization for ischemic cardiomyopathy, valve surgery in the presence of LV dysfunction, and ventricular remodeling surgery. Of course these three areas often overlap in patients; for example, an ischemic cardiomyopathy patient may undergo coronary artery bypass grafting (CABG), mitral valve repair, and reconstruction of scarred dyskinetic infarcted segments.

CORONARY REVASCULARIZATION FOR ISCHEMIC CARDIOMYOPATHY (see also Chapter 18)

Definition and Epidemiology

The definition of ischemic cardiomyopathy is currently applied to patients with significantly impaired LV dysfunction (LV ejection fraction ≤ 35%-40%) that results from coronary artery disease.[1] Importantly, in a review of 2000 patients with symptomatic heart failure, those with ischemic cardiomyopathy had a significantly worse outcome than those with nonischemic cardiomyopathy. In contrast, patients with single-vessel disease who had no history of myocardial infarction or revascularization had a similar prognosis compared with those with nonischemic cardiomyopathy.[1] Recent data show that the prevalence of heart failure after myocardial infarction ranges from 10% after 2 years to more than 40% after 6.5 years.[2,3] Improved early revascularization, intensive care strategies, and heart failure therapies (medications and device therapies, such as cardiac resynchronization therapy and implantable cardioverter-defibrillators) have led to an increased survival of patients admitted with extensive myocardial infarcts, leading to a higher incidence of subsequent systolic heart failure. Importantly, the development of heart failure late after myocardial infarction is related to a variety of factors, including the size and location of the infarct, the presence of ischemic mitral valve regurgitation (IMR), and perhaps inflammatory status as assessed by serum C-reactive protein.[2-4] In addition, the risk of developing heart failure is also increased two to three times in patients with persistent angina, suggesting potentially a contributing role of myocardial ischemia to progressive LV dysfunction.[5] Therefore, strategies must be in place to detect and treat heart failure and ongoing, potentially reversible ischemia in patients who might benefit from coronary revascularization.

Pathophysiology of Ischemic Cardiomyopathy

The most commonly involved mechanism in myocardial dysfunction secondary to ischemic cardiomyopathy is loss of cardiac myocytes, which eventually leads to progressive remodeling of the heart.[6] The LV remodeling process following myocardial infarction is complex, involving myocyte stretch and slippage, a phenomenon that also occurs in the adjacent remote viable myocardium.[7] Ischemia-induced cellular changes include loss of myofibrils and disorganization of the structural proteins within the myocytes. In addition, extracellular changes including fibrosis and alterations in the fiber orientation cause changes in the geometric shape of the heart.[8] Eventually, these processes lead to a progressive dilation of the ventricles with subsequent increased wall tension and impaired systolic function. Thus the progressive loss of viable myocardium over time following a myocardial infarction is a continuous process, which ultimately might be accompanied by the clinical heart failure syndrome.[9] However, it is well known that restoration of myocardial blood flow might reverse the detrimental process of progressive cardiac remodeling.

Insights into myocardial ischemia-induced changes on a cellular level help physicians to better select patients who will benefit most from revascularization strategies. Although transient ischemia can lead to a period of prolonged contractile dysfunction of cardiac myocytes, even after the restoration of flow ("stunning"), persistent but asymptomatic ischemia might induce LV dysfunction ("hibernation") that can mimic nonischemic causes of heart failure. Stunned myocardium is used to describe a condition in which a *short-term*, total or near total reduction of coronary blood flow produces an abnormality in regional LV wall motion of limited duration (hours to days) following reperfusion.[10-12] In contrast, hibernating myocardium is a state of persistently impaired myocardial and LV function at rest due to *chronically* reduced coronary blood flow that can be partially or completely restored to normal either by improving blood flow or reducing oxygen demand.[10-13] On the other hand, if hibernating myocardium is not treated in a timely manner, it may be associated with progressive cellular damage, recurrent myocardial ischemia, myocardial infarction, heart failure, and death.[14] Positron emission tomography (PET) has been demonstrated to be able to guide patient selection for revascularization strategies, because it has shown that regions with abnormal wall motion may still be metabolically active and might therefore improve after revascularization.[15] Such regions are likely to be hypokinetic rather than akinetic or dyskinetic during routine echocardiographic examination. In addition, the reduction in resting coronary blood flow in hibernating segments and the improvement following coronary intervention can also be visualized by cardiovascular magnetic resonance imaging (CMR).[16] Although in the clinical setting, stunned myocardium is often superimposed on hibernation, or irreversible contractile dysfunction, earlier identification of hibernating myocardial regions with prompt myocardial revascularization is crucial in preventing and reversing the ongoing remodeling process of the heart.

Natural History of Ischemic Cardiomyopathy

The prognosis of patients after myocardial infarction depends upon the extent of LV damage.[17] In the Coronary Artery Surgery Study (CASS) registry, long-term survival of medically treated patients with an LV ejection fraction less than 35% was 21% after 12 years, compared with 54% survival in patients with an ejection fraction that remained between 35% and 50%.[18] With current interventional techniques, survival has improved, especially with the addition of angiotensin-converting enzyme inhibitors, β-blockers, spironolactone, statins, ICDs, and CRTs to the armamentarium of heart failure therapy. However, in a more recent study all-cause mortality was still 34% after a mean follow-up of 4.4 years in patients who had developed an ischemic cardiomyopathy, whereas 4.6% had undergone cardiac transplantation.[19] Outcomes were worse compared with those patients with an idiopathic or peripartum cardiomyopathy, but considerably better than those with infiltrative, chemotherapy or HIV-induced cardiomyopathies (**Figure 41-1**).

Selection of Appropriate Candidates for Revascularization

Clinical Trials

Currently, only one randomized, multicenter, international, prospective clinical trial has compared the outcome of contemporary medical therapy plus CABG, medical therapy alone, and CABG with or without surgical ventricular restoration for patients with congestive heart failure and coronary heart disease. The hypothesis 1 group consisted of 1212 patients with ischemic cardiomyopathy (LV ejection fraction <35% and coronary artery disease amenable to CABG), recruited in 99 centers (22 countries), of whom 602 were randomly assigned to receive medical therapy alone and 610 were randomly assigned to receive medical therapies plus CABG.[20] The STICH trial did not demonstrate a statistically significant difference in the occurrence of the

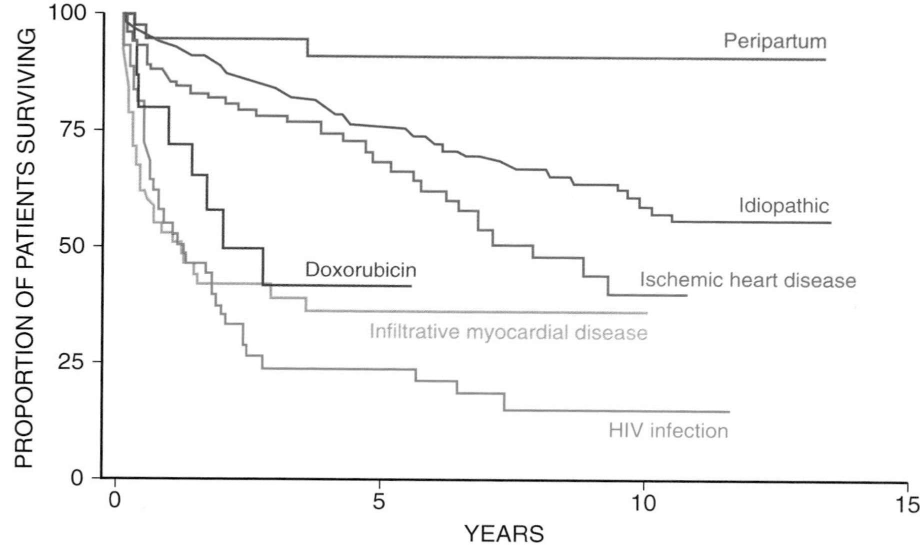

FIGURE 41-1 Survival of patients with cardiomyopathies stratified by cause. *Modified from Felker GM, Thompson RE, Hare JM, et al: Underlying causes and long-term survival in patients with initially unexplained cardiomyopathy. N Engl J Med 342:1077–1084, 2000.*

primary endpoint of all-cause mortality among groups after a median follow-up of 56 months, although the incidence was numerically lower in patients of the CABG group (36% versus 41%). In addition, CABG was associated with an increased early mortality risk after 30 days, but a significant 16% risk reduction of death or heart failure admission at follow-up, which was a prespecified secondary outcome. The trial was well conducted, with all participating surgeons demonstrating surgical expertise (operative mortality <5% in patients with ischemic cardiomyopathy) and more than 90% of patients randomized to CABG undergoing the procedure within a window of 10 days after randomization. However, some important limitations should be noted when interpreting the results of the STICH trial. The crossover rate of 17% from the medical therapy to the CABG group was substantial and might have diluted the benefits of the procedure. Therefore, the positive findings with CABG on several secondary outcomes (death or heart failure admission, death or hospital admission for cardiovascular cause, death or any rehospitalization, death or revascularization) remain to be confirmed in a new trial. In addition, it should be noted that the patients studied in the STICH trial were at relatively low surgical risk, as demonstrated by a mean age of 60 years and a New York Heart Association (NYHA) functional class I or II in more than 60% of patients. More importantly, an important selection bias might have confounded the data as the number of patients enrolled per participating center was very low, which illustrates the difficulties in conducting a trial for which many clinicians believe there is no real clinical equipoise.

Three major randomized clinical trials of CABG versus medical management, the Veterans Administration Cooperative Study, the CASS registry, and the European Coronary Surgery Study have all excluded patients with severe LV dysfunction.[21-23] Such patients have traditionally been considered too "high risk" and were deemed inoperable. This category of patients with end-stage ischemic cardiomyopathy accounts for 40% to 50% of heart transplants performed.[24] However, as many as 20% to 30% of these patients die while awaiting heart transplantation; because of existing comorbid conditions, organ shortage, or both, most will never undergo transplantation.[25] However, even in patients with advanced ischemic cardiomyopathy, it has been demonstrated that survival is reduced if revascularization of viable myocardium is not undertaken.[26] Therefore, each patient with ischemic cardiomyopathy must be carefully evaluated to determine the suitability for revascularization.

Clinical Factors

In the selection of candidates for revascularization, several clinical factors might play a role, including the presence of angina, suitability of target vessels for bypass grafting, heart failure symptoms, LV dimension, and the severity of hemodynamic compromise.[27] The absence of angina should not preclude consideration for surgical revascularization; however, there is little information about the percentage of patients with heart failure who have silent ischemia that might be ameliorated by revascularization.

Myocardial Viability

Patients with ischemic cardiomyopathy are heterogeneous with regard to adequacy of target vessels for revascularization, ischemic jeopardy, and myocardial viability. It is therefore of utmost importance to preoperatively select those patients who will benefit most from revascularization. Some retrospective, nonrandomized studies provide evidence that revascularization of hibernating myocardium in patients with ischemic cardiomyopathy improves both survival and LV function compared with medical therapy alone, irrespective of the preoperative degree of LV dysfunction.[15,28-33] However, in many of these studies, the presence of angina was a prerequisite, which might have served as a clinical indicator of extensive myocardial viability. Moreover, these type of studies have important limitations, including selection bias in patients who undergo CABG, publication bias, and uncertain applicability to current practice because of the lack of use of contemporary standard medical therapies (e.g., statins) and underuse of internal mammary artery grafts. Importantly, the STICH trial investigators have reported a subgroup analysis of 601 patients (from the original 1212) who underwent myocardial viability testing by single-photon-emission computed

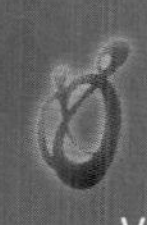

tomography (SPECT), dobutamine stress echocardiography (DSE), or both.[34] Myocardial viability on a per-patient basis was prospectively defined as the presence of 11/17 or more viable segments on SPECT or 5/16 or more viable segments on DSE. As expected, patients with myocardial viability had lower all-cause mortality with a highly significant relative risk reduction of 36%. However, after correction for baseline variables in a multivariate model, this result was no longer significant. Surprisingly, the authors found no differential survival benefit in patients undergoing CABG with versus without myocardial viability. A major limitation of the trial was that viability testing was performed at the discretion of the investigators, which might have created substantial bias. Indeed baseline characteristics between patients who were tested and those who were not differed significantly. Yet the study findings do raise reasonable questions about the most appropriate method to assess myocardial viability. Because most of the patients had angina, one could speculate whether this simple question is enough. However, because of the paucity of literature identifying the percentage of patients with heart failure who have silent ischemia, the absence of angina should not preclude at least a consideration for surgical revascularization, because augmentation of coronary flow to viable ischemic or hibernating myocardium will improve LV function and survival. Hence, a clinician should not require the presence of "viability" as a criterion to determine eligibility for revascularization.

Several noninvasive imaging modalities have emerged that might identify patients who have ischemic or hibernating myocardium amenable to revascularization surgery if adequate target vessels exist (see also Chapter 29). The information they can provide concerning myocardial viability differs because different modalities depend on inotropic reserve (DSE), demonstration of cell membrane integrity (SPECT), preserved myocardial metabolism (PET), or absence of scar tissue (gadolinium-enhanced CMR) in areas of dysfunctional myocardium.

Dobutamine stress echocardiography has a sensitivity of 69% and a specificity of 78% (overall accuracy 75%) for the prediction of segmental recovery after surgery.[35] DSE examines the "inotropic reserve" of dysfunctional but viable myocardium. Viable myocardium shows improved regional contractile function (inotropic reserve), assessed by simultaneous transthoracic echocardiography, in response to dobutamine. Segmental wall motion is monitored during dobutamine infusion at increasing dosages. Augmentation of segmental wall motion beginning at low dose and continuing during higher doses of dobutamine (uniphasic response) is suggestive of myocardial stunning. However, augmentation at lower doses, followed by a reduction in contractile function at higher doses (biphasic response), is indicative of ischemia and hibernation. Importantly, the prevalence of contractile reserve in patients with ischemic cardiomyopathy is independent of the angiographic extent and severity of coronary disease.[36] A contractile response to dobutamine appears to require at least 50% viable myocytes in a given segment and correlates inversely with the extent of interstitial fibrosis on myocardial biopsy.[37]

SPECT uses thallium-201 as a perfusion tracer because of its high (80%) first-pass myocardial extraction fraction across physiologic ranges of myocardial blood flow. The myocardial uptake is a process requiring cell membrane integrity, and is therefore indicative of regional perfusion, as well as myocardial viability. Several approaches have been used to optimize the information obtained from thallium-201 scintigraphy, mostly involving a baseline stress image and one or two delayed images (4-hour redistribution and 24-hour late-delayed imaging). Regional thallium redistribution activity represents the extent of regional myocardial viability. As a result, stress-redistribution thallium imaging following a single stress injection has become the standard imaging. The demonstration of reversible ischemia by the conventional stress 4-hour redistribution protocol implies the presence of viable myocardium. However, up to 50% of segments that have fixed defects at 4 hours might still recover either perfusion or function following revascularization.[38,39] Therefore, several modifications of the stress 4-hour redistribution protocol were developed to improve the accuracy of viability detection. Late redistribution (24 hours) or reinjection of a second, smaller dose of thallium-201 immediately following the redistribution images, often leads to visualization of segments in a significant number of perfusion defects deemed fixed by imaging at 4 hours only. In comparison with DSE, SPECT can identify segments with fewer viable myocytes. In one series, for example, DSE and SPECT showed equivalent sensitivity among segments with more than 75% viable myocytes (78% versus 87%), but DSE was much less sensitive among segments with 25-50% viable myocytes (15% versus 82%).[40] However, compared with SPECT, DSE was found to have greater specificity and positive predictive value in forecasting functional recovery after revascularization.[41]

PET is often considered the "gold standard" to evaluate myocardial perfusion and viability.[42] It has the advantage of being able to assess perfusion and metabolism simultaneously. PET requires the use of positron-emitting elements, which are incorporated into physiologically active molecules. Ischemia shifts myocyte metabolism away from fatty acids to glucose. Thus uptake of the glucose analog, fluorine-18 labeled deoxyglucose (FDG) by cardiac myocytes in an area of dysfunctional myocardium indicates metabolic activity and thus viability. Regional perfusion can be simultaneously assessed with an agent that remains in the vascular space, demonstrating blood flow (such as N-13 ammonia or Rb-82). As a result, PET imaging has the potential to differentiate among normal, stunned, hibernating, and necrotic myocardium. The presence of enhanced FDG uptake in regions of decreased blood flow ("PET mismatch") defines hibernating myocardium, whereas a concordant reduction in both metabolism and flow ("PET match") is thought to represent predominantly necrotic myocardium. Regional dysfunction in the presence of normal perfusion is indicative of stunning. Importantly, myocardial segments with significant reductions in both blood flow and FDG uptake only have a 20% chance of functional improvement after revascularization, whereas dysfunctional hibernating territories have an approximately 85% chance.[15,43-45] The greater the number of viable myocardial segments, the greater the likelihood that revascularization will improve global LV function and consequently improve heart failure symptoms and survival. The ability to improve survival based upon the demonstration of viability, however, has recently been challenged by the STICH data already described.

Gadolinium-enhanced cardiac magnetic resonance imaging can also be used to establish the presence of hibernating myocardium. Regions of myocardium exhibiting late (or delayed) enhancement 10 minutes after injection of Gd-DTPA coincide with regions of myocardial necrosis and irreversible injury; regions that fail to hyperenhance are viable. In addition, quantitative perfusion assessment can document the reduction in resting coronary blood flow in hibernating segments. The degree and transmural extent of enhancement with gadolinium-enhanced CMR are inversely related to the potential of LV functional recovery after revascularization.[46,47] In addition, myocardial tagging is another CMR method that quantifies local myocardial segment shortening throughout the LV myocardium and across the LV wall thickness. This technique can be combined with low-dose dobutamine to quantify the amount of myocardial viability, based upon myocardial shortening and thickening, which provides prognostic information as well. For example, a preoperative end-diastolic wall thickness greater than 15 mm correlates well with postoperative functional improvement, whereas only 4% of the segments with an end-diastolic wall thickness less than 6 mm will improve.[48] Compared with DSE, dobutamine CMR has a higher sensitivity (86% versus 74%) and specificity (86% versus 70%), although it is more labor intensive and technically challenging.[49] Unlike SPECT and DSE, which appear to have limited predictive accuracy if more severe systolic dysfunction is present, gadolinium-enhanced CMR has greater accuracy in segments with the most severe dysfunction, which represents another advantage of this technique.[50] In most centers, CMR has therefore an established role to detect the extent of viable myocardium and areas of scar that might be amenable to reperfusion and/or ventricular reconstruction strategies.

Risk of Revascularization

The most effective way of stratifying operative risk for cardiac surgical patients is to use a risk prediction algorithm that incorporates multiple variables to derive a risk score. The most widely used algorithms for this purpose in the United States and Europe are the Society of Thoracic Surgeons (STS) risk score and the additive or logistic EuroSCORE, which has been updated to increase its predictive accuracy.[51-55] Both algorithms incorporate patient age, sex, and comorbidities, as well as the severity and acuity of cardiac disease and can fairly accurately predict 30-day operative mortality. One important limitation of such risk prediction algorithms is their dependence upon the patient data from which they were derived. As the population and surgical techniques are changing over time, risk calculators might soon become outdated.[56]

The presence of LV dysfunction and heart failure remains one of the most important independent predictors of operative mortality and other major adverse events after CABG (**Figure 41-2**).[57] In a prospective observational study of over 8600 patients undergoing CABG between 1992 and 1997, the rate of operative mortality varied: less than 2% of patients with LVEF higher than 40%, 4% of those with LVEF of 20% to 40%, and 8% of those with LVEF lower than 20%.[58] However, the Cleveland Clinic has reported lower in-hospital mortality rates for patients with normal (1.5%), moderately (2.5%), or severely (3.2%) impaired LV function when they reviewed more than 14,000 patients who underwent isolated CABG between 1990 and 1999. In addition, they have also reported that the prevalence of high-risk patients increased, yet surgical morbidity rates adjusted for preoperative risk score had fallen significantly from 1986 to 1994 (14.5% to 8.8%).[59] Additional determinants of mortality and morbidity risk include advanced age, female sex, comorbid conditions (e.g., diabetes mellitus, cerebrovascular disease, renal dysfunction, chronic lung disease) and need for emergent CABG or concomitant valve surgery.[60,61] However, improved surgical techniques with better myocardial protection and routine use of retrograde coronary sinus cardioplegia, together with a high level of experience, and optimization of preoperative conditions, have led to improved outcomes, especially when combined through a multidisciplinary approach.

Benefits of Revascularization

Considering the advances in the pharmacologic treatment of ischemic cardiomyopathy and the current widespread use of implantable defibrillators and cardiac resynchronization therapy devices, it has been suggested that that surgical revascularization may not provide additional benefit for some patients with ischemic cardiomyopathy. However, unless the nonsurgical approaches can prevent further ischemic events from occurring and reverse the detrimental remodeling process, the presence of uncorrected coronary stenoses still threatens the survival of patients with ischemic cardiomyopathy. In addition, angina control seems to be best achieved by surgical revascularization in eligible patients. Surgically improving blood flow to hypoperfused but viable myocardium leads to functional

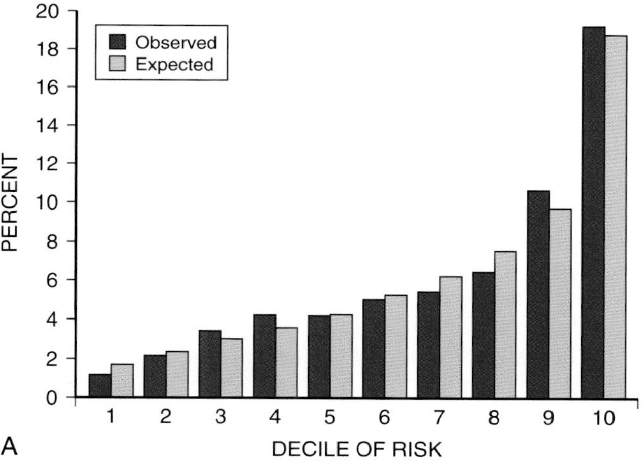

CORRELATE	POINTS
Pre-CABG creatinine ≥ 3.0 mg/dL (265 μmol/L)	12
Age ≥ 80 yrs	11
Cardiogenic shock	10
Emergent operation	9
Age 70 to 79 yrs	8
Prior CABG	7
Left ventricular section fraction <30%	6
Liver disease (history)	6
Age 60 to 69 yrs	5
Pre-CABG creatinine 1.5 to 3.0 mg/dL (133 to 265 μmol/L)	5
Stroke or transient ischemic attack (history)	4
Left ventricular ejection fraction 30% to 49%	3
Chronic obstructive pulmonary disease (history)	3
Female gender	3
Hypertension (history)	2
Urgent operation	2

B

FIGURE 41-2 Predictive model for outcomes after coronary artery bypass grafting (CABG). *Modified from Kolh P: Importance of risk stratification models in cardiac surgery. Eur Heart J 27:768–769, 2006.*

improvement of the myocardium, with secondary effects of retarding or reversing ventricular remodeling, reducing the substrate for malignant ventricular arrhythmias, and ameliorating symptoms. For example, the placement of an internal mammary graft to the left anterior descending artery provides a durable long-term, effective treatment for anterior wall ischemia.

Improvement of Congestive Heart Failure Symptoms and Functional Capacity

Several small-scale studies in ischemic cardiomyopathy patients revealed significant improvements in heart failure symptoms following revascularization.[62-65] Apart from a reduction in angina, the improvement in NYHA functional class or heart failure symptoms is related to the amount of "viable" myocardium, which serves as a surrogate to predict reverse remodeling after CABG. For example, a blood flow–metabolism mismatch greater than 18% on PET was associated with a sensitivity of 76% and a specificity of 78% to predict a change in functional status after revascularization.[62] Another study showed similar significant improvements in functional capacity after revascularization, as reflected by an increase in metabolic equivalents (METs) from 5.6 to 7.5 in patients with significant PET mismatch before surgery.[64] Other investigators have demonstrated a significant increase in peak oxygen consumption (15 mL/kg/min to 22 mL/kg/min) in a group of 34 patients with ischemic cardiomyopathy undergoing CABG.[65]

Improvement of Left Ventricular Function

The improvement in LV ejection fraction after revascularization in patients with ischemic cardiomyopathy is typically related to the presence of myocardial viability. A recent review of 29 studies assessing 758 patients nicely showed that there was an increase in LV ejection fraction of 8% after revascularization when myocardial viability was present, whereas no improvement in LV ejection fraction was noticed in the absence of viability.[66] Importantly, recovery of contractile function after restoration of normal blood flow to areas of hibernating myocardium might take several days, weeks, or even months.[28] In addition, improvements in LV ejection fraction are often associated with reverse LV remodeling, characterized by reductions in LV end-systolic and end-diastolic dimensions, with a less spherical shape of the LV.[67,68] The degree of improvement is significantly correlated with the number of segments that recover function after revascularization.[67] However, despite evidence of viability through noninvasive imaging techniques, late revascularization may not always result in measurable improvements in contractility.

LV end-diastolic dimension is another potential predictor of improvement in LV ejection fraction and reverse remodeling after CABG in patients with ischemic cardiomyopathy. If LV end-diastolic dimension is greater than 7.0 cm (>4.0 cm/m^2), patients do not only experience higher operative mortality rates but also have a lower chance of reverse ventricular remodeling. The impact of LV enlargement on improvement of LV function after surgery was illustrated in a review of 61 patients with ischemic cardiomyopathy (mean LV ejection fraction 28%), all of whom had evidence of substantial myocardial viability.[69] In this study, one third of patients did not exhibit any improvement in LV ejection fraction or reduction in LV dimensions. In contrast, the other two thirds of the patients, who did experience significant improvement in LVEF, all had smaller LV end-systolic volumes.[69]

There is some evidence that concomitant medical therapy with β-blockers might increase the likelihood that surgical revascularization will cause reverse ventricular remodeling and improve clinical outcome. In the Carvedilol Hibernation Reversible Ischaemia (CHRISTMAS) trial, 387 patients with ischemic cardiomyopathy were included and randomized to treatment with carvedilol versus a placebo. A significant linear correlation between the number of cardiac segments with hibernating myocardium at baseline and improvement in LV ejection fraction after 6 months was seen in the carvedilol group, whereas placebo-treated patients did not demonstrate any significant improvement in LV ejection fraction.[70] It was hypothesized that β-blockade might improve the function of hibernating myocardium by reducing myocardial oxygen consumption and increasing diastolic perfusion, ultimately leading to improved reverse ventricular remodeling.[70] Finally, although it has been suggested that improved survival after CABG may not require an improvement in LV ejection fraction, it is well established that any therapy capable of inducing reverse remodeling will ultimately lead to improved survival.[30] All heart failure guidelines (American College of Cardiology/American Heart Association [ACC/AHA], European Society of Cardiology [ESC], Heart Failure Society of America [HFSA]) advocate the concomitant use of evidence-based medical therapy in addition to revascularization (when applicable) with an assessment of the need for ICD and or CRT postrevascularization.

Improved Survival

Initial large observational studies, such as the CASS registry and a post hoc analysis from the Studies of Left Ventricular Dysfunction (SOLVD) trial, have suggested that CABG improves clinical outcome compared with optimal medical therapy alone in patients with coronary artery disease and LV dysfunction.[22,71,72] However, those studies did not evaluate myocardial viability and, in the case of the CASS registry, largely excluded patients with heart failure. Subsequent small, retrospective, observational studies have shown that survival benefits with revascularization in patients with ischemic cardiomyopathy are mainly limited to those patients with viable myocardium[31,33,73-75] as illustrated in **Figure 41-3**. The potential survival benefit with CABG was best demonstrated in a 2002 meta-analysis of 24 nonrandomized viability studies involving 3088 patients with coronary artery disease and LV dysfunction (mean LV ejection fraction 32%).[31] Patients with myocardial viability had a significant 80% reduction in annual mortality with revascularization (3.2% versus 16% with optimal medical therapy). In addition, a direct relationship between the severity of LV dysfunction and the magnitude of this benefit was noted. However, no difference in annual mortality with revascularization was noticed in patients without myocardial viability (annual mortality 7.7% versus 6.2% with optimal medical therapy).

In contrast, as explained, the only randomized clinical trial currently available is STICH, and it did not demonstrate a benefit for CABG over optimal medical therapy in patients with ischemic cardiomyopathy. Moreover, no correlation was found between the treatment effect of CABG and myocardial viability assessed by SPECT or DSE.[20,34] However, in the STICH trial, patients with left main disease or severe

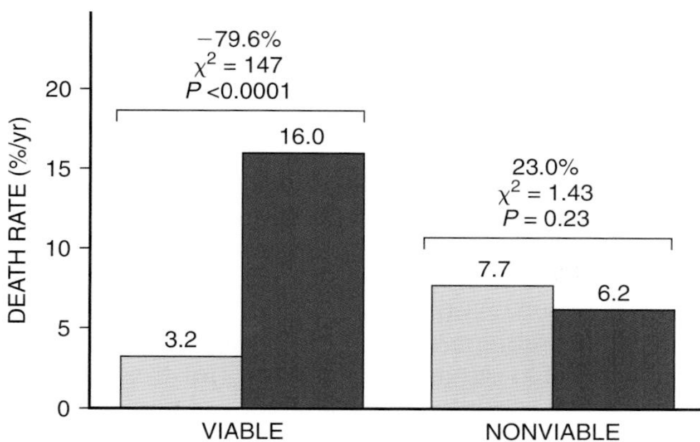

FIGURE 41-3 All-cause mortality, stratified according to the presence of viable myocardium in medically treated *(red bars)* versus surgically revascularized *(blue bars)* patients. *Modified from Chareonthaitawee P, Gersh BJ, Araoz PA, et al: Revascularization in severe left ventricular dysfunction: the role of viability testing. J Am Coll Cardiol 46:567–574, 2005.*

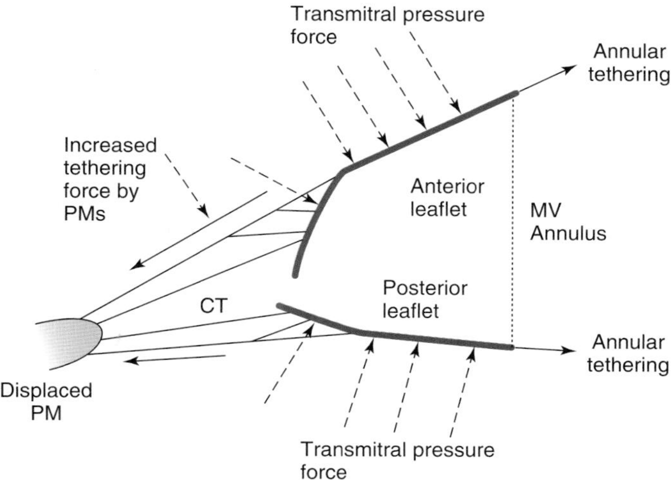

FIGURE 41-4 Pathophysiology of functional mitral valve regurgitation. *CT,* Chordae tendineae; *MV,* mitral valve; *PM,* papillary muscle. *Modified from Bursi F, Enriquez-Sarano M, Nkomo VT, et al: Heart failure and death after myocardial infarction in the community: the emerging role of mitral regurgitation. Circulation 111:295–301, 2005.*

angina were not eligible for randomization, and therefore such patients should continue to be revascularized. However, in the absence of these conditions, aggressive medical therapy should be initiated and optimized first, according to evidence-based guidelines. The decision to perform CABG in this group remains an individual one, balancing potential benefits in case of symptoms or myocardial viability versus the risk of cardiac surgery. A multidisciplinary cooperation between cardiologists, imaging specialists, and surgeons is therefore highly recommended and supported by the most recent guidelines.[76]

Conclusion

In the current era, CABG remains an important treatment option for ischemic cardiomyopathy. The use of evidence-based medical therapy may provide equivalent outcomes in some patient groups. However, CABG in the presence of angina, viability, and suitable vessels as targets may yield improved patient outcomes and reduce the need for subsequent revascularization. The absence of viability should not exclude a patient for consideration of CABG.

VALVE SURGERY IN THE PRESENCE OF LEFT VENTRICULAR DYSFUNCTION (see also Chapter 24)

Many patients with heart failure or LV dysfunction have clinically significant valvular lesions. It is estimated that almost 50% of patients with an LV ejection fraction less than 35% have grades 3 to 4+ mitral valve regurgitation (MR), and 35% have grades 3 to 4+ tricuspid valve regurgitation (TR).[77] Importantly, severe MR and/or TR have been linked to adverse outcome and increased mortality.[77,78] Valvular disease also frequently causes heart failure, and surgical treatment of many valvular lesions is a well-accepted therapy, especially for the aortic valve. However, other combinations of valve disorders with LV dysfunction are more controversial, and many patients have been thought too sick to withstand surgery. Historically, clinicians were taught that mitral valve replacement in patients with an LV ejection fraction less than 40% should not be performed because of the high perioperative mortality.[79] However, at that time the attitude was to replace the mitral valve with a ball-in-cage prosthesis, together with removal of both papillary muscles and the entire subvalvular apparatus. Nowadays, the importance of an intact "valvulo-ventricular" interaction is recognized. Together with changing surgical opinion more in favor of mitral repairs instead of replacements, interest has resurged in the field of valvular surgery as part of the treatment strategy for LV dysfunction. Moreover, rapid advances in percutaneous valvular treatment strategies will probably continue to evolve the field, making interventions possible in even advanced heart failure patients.

Functional Mitral Valve Regurgitation in Patients with Severe Left Ventricular Dysfunction

Pathophysiology

The integrity of the saddle-shaped mitral valve is sustained by coaptation of the anterior and posterior leaflets in the annular plane during ventricular systole, in a design that decreases leaflet, annular, and chordal strain.[80] There are six components responsible for an optimal valve function: the valve annulus, leaflets, chordae tendineae, papillary muscles, LV muscle, and the left atrium, and any one of these might exhibit defects leading to mitral valve pathology. In both ischemic and nonischemic cardiomyopathy, functional MR usually results from geometric abnormalities of the LV, leading to dysfunction of a structurally normal mitral valve. Enlargement of the LV causes functional MR through annular dilation, an increase in interpapillary muscle distance, increased leaflet tethering (elongation and stretch on the chordae tendineae because of cardiac enlargement), and decreased closing forces from muscle weakness, in addition to dyssynchrony of papillary muscle contractile timing.[80-82] This ultimately results in coaptation failure of the structurally normal leaflets and central MR jet (**Figure 41-4**). There is clear overlap between functional MR and ischemic MR, and reports of functional MR often include patients with ischemic cardiomyopathy. Nevertheless, the clinical features and management of IMR,

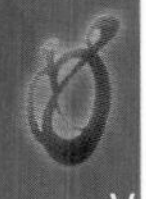

including MR in association with myocardial infarction, are different and will be discussed separately.

Nonsurgical Treatment Options

As with mitral regurgitation resulting from primary valve disease, functional mitral regurgitation imposes an important hemodynamic load on the left ventricle, which contributes to further eccentric hypertrophy and dilation, which increases the degree of mitral regurgitation and heart failure; thus a vicious cycle exists.[83,84] Fortunately, the treatment of heart failure has evolved from symptom-directed therapy to treatments capable of altering the natural history of the disease. Optimized pharmacologic therapy and cardiac resynchronization therapy, in patients with interventricular and intraventricular conduction delay, are nowadays the first-line treatment strategies in patients with functional MR. Neurohumoral blockers such as angiotensin-converting enzyme inhibitors, angiotensin II receptor blockers, mineralocorticoid receptor blockers, and β-blockers have all proven to induce reverse ventricular remodeling in heart failure with favorable effects on all-cause mortality and heart failure morbidity.[85] Especially β-blockers have demonstrated that they might prolong preservation of LV function in the presence of chronic MR and therefore potentially delay or defer the necessity for surgery.[86] In addition, in selected patients with electromechanical dyssynchrony, cardiac resynchronization therapy has led to impressive reverse ventricular remodeling with ultrastructural changes in cardiac myocytes and a favorable impact on clinical outcome.[87,88] Therefore, by judiciously applying those therapies, the degree of MR can often be reduced. However, patients with advanced heart failure commonly present with significant mitral regurgitation despite use of these therapies and are therefore often referred for cardiovascular surgical treatment.

Mitral Valve Repair

Until recently, the risk associated with surgical correction of MR in the setting of severe LV dysfunction was considered prohibitive. However, Bolling and colleagues were the first to demonstrate that this approach was feasible and could be conducted with reasonably low morbidity.[89] They used an undersized annuloplasty repair, which effectively corrects functional MR in heart failure patients. In more than 200 patients with an LV ejection fraction less than 20% and severe functional MR, mitral valve repair was associated with 1-, 2-, and 5-year actuarial survival rates of 82%, 71%, and 52%, respectively.[90] In addition, NYHA functional class improved for all patients, and most patients also demonstrated an improvement in LV ejection fraction, end-diastolic volume, and cardiac index together with a reduction in sphericity index after 24 months of follow-up.[90] These results were confirmed by a case series at the Cleveland Clinic, which also reported improved survival and positive effects on reverse ventricular remodeling with mitral valve repair, in addition to a reduced need for heart failure hospitalizations during follow-up.[91] However, the most convincing data for the safety and efficacy of mitral valve repair for functional MR come from the mitral valve surgery arm of the prospective CorCap study.[92] In this study, 193 medically optimized patients with significant functional MR, mean LV ejection fraction of 24%, mean LV end-diastolic diameter of 7 cm, and NYHA functional class III or IV heart failure underwent mitral valve repair with an undersized annuloplasty ring (84%) or valve replacement surgery (16%). Most patients (94%) had an idiopathic cardiomyopathy. Survival at 30 days was 98.4% and 85.2% after 24 months. Moreover, there was evidence of progressive and sustained reverse ventricular remodeling after surgery. The important outcomes were that mitral regurgitation was successfully abolished and the mitral valve repair was durable; 88.4% of patients had grade 0 or 1 mitral regurgitation after 2 years, and reoperation was required by only 2% of patients.

A weakness of all the aforementioned studies was that they lacked a comparable control group of subjects who did not undergo surgery. The findings of these observational surgical series were subsequently challenged by Wu and associates.[93] In a propensity-matched, nonrandomized analysis, 126 patients who underwent mitral valve annuloplasty were compared with 293 who did not. Although both groups had similar degrees of severe functional mitral regurgitation, no net improvement in long-term survival (or in the combined endpoint of mortality or urgent transplantation) was evident in the patients who underwent surgery, regardless of the cause of heart failure (either ischemic or nonischemic) surgery. These results are provocative, but reliance on propensity-matching in a retrospective study does not substitute the need for a proper prospectively conducted randomized clinical trial. Moreover, the study lacked information on indices of reverse ventricular remodeling and symptom improvement, included patients who were not on optimal medical therapy, and provided little information on durability of the repair.

Together, these experiences demonstrate that mitral valve repair, with an undersized complete rigid annuloplasty ring, and without altering the subvalvular apparatus, can be performed safely with low operative mortality (<2%) in patients with congestive heart failure and functional MR. This probably also has positive effects on reverse remodeling, if performed by surgeons experienced in mitral valve repair. However, only a randomized clinical trial can definitively determine whether or not surgery is associated with a mortality benefit. The lack of such a trial is reflected in published guidelines from major societies. The 2009 focused update of the ACC/AHA heart failure guidelines states that the effectiveness of mitral valve repair or replacement for severe secondary MR in refractory end-stage HF is *not established* (class IIb, level of evidence C), while it is *not generally recommended* by the 2010 Heart Failure Society of America (HFSA) practice guidelines (level of evidence C).[94,95] Therefore, if mitral valve repair is considered as an alternative to transplantation, the patient should be informed that, although symptoms are often improved, there is no clear evidence of a long-term mortality benefit. Also, factors that generally preclude mitral valve repair in patients with heart failure include structural mitral valve dysfunction, significant aortic valve regurgitation (AR), and long-standing MR antedating the onset of LV dysfunction with marked LV enlargement or dependence on inotropic therapy.

Percutaneous Alternatives to Mitral Valve Repair

Percutaneous valvular repair or replacement is a rapidly evolving field. The Endovascular Valve Edge-to-Edge Repair Study (EVEREST) demonstrated feasibility of the MitraClip system (Abbott Vascular), which replicates the Alfieri stitch (approximation of the mitral leaflets with a suture to create a double orifice) by percutaneous application of a clip.[96,97] Subsequently EVEREST II was conducted, and demonstrated that delivery of the MitraClip system has a low periprocedural risk, leads to significant reverse remodeling, and improves quality of life and functional capacity of patients with significant MR at baseline.[98] However, EVEREST II included mostly patients with structural MR and normal LV ejection fraction, and percutaneous mitral valve repair was less effective than conventional surgery. Nevertheless, one might speculate that advanced heart failure patients with functional MR constitute a higher-risk group that could benefit from a low-risk procedure such as the MitraClip. Therefore, the Clinical Outcomes Assessment of the MitraClip Therapy Percutaneous Therapy for High Surgical Risk Patients (COAPT) study (NCT01626079) is currently enrolling patients who are deemed inoperable because of a high anticipated procedural risk, and it is believed that a significant number of those patients probably suffer from advanced heart failure.

Ischemic Mitral Regurgitation in Patients with Severe Left Ventricular Dysfunction

Pathophysiology

IMR is a complication most often occurring after prior myocardial infarction with permanent damage to the papillary muscle or the adjacent myocardium. In addition, it might also be seen with acute ischemia, but it typically disappears after the ischemia resolves. However, preexisting MR may become more severe in the presence of superimposed ischemia. Although IMR is, in rare cases, caused by a papillary muscle rupture, which always mandates urgent surgery, most affected patients have "functional" IMR, similar to the functional mitral regurgitation in dilated cardiomyopathy in which the papillary muscles, chordae, and valve leaflets are normal but there is poor coaptation of the leaflets, and restricted leaflet motion is frequently noted on echocardiography. However, there are two important differences between the conditions. First, in comparison with patients who have dilated cardiomyopathy, many patients with IMR are in need of CABG, and so clinicians often must decide whether the mitral valve should be treated. Second, whereas the LV dilation in dilated cardiomyopathy is more spherical, patients with ischemic cardiomyopathy have one or more segments of hypokinesia, akinesia, or dyskinesia that lead to local LV remodeling, thereby altering the geometric shape of the left ventricle in a different way. Many clinicians still use the term *papillary muscle dysfunction* to describe patients with IMR, but this is a misnomer because papillary muscle dysfunction alone does not explain the mechanism of this disorder. The papillary muscle is dysfunctional because the LV wall—especially the posterolateral segment on which it is implanted—is dysfunctional and the geometry of the ventricle is disturbed. Therefore, IMR is a more complex pathology that is consequently more challenging to repair successfully.

Mitral Valve Repair

Patients with an ischemic cardiomyopathy should be treated with the usual therapies for heart failure, including medical and pacing therapies. However, medical therapy does not play a major role in the management of IMR itself. Among patients who have IMR associated with an acute myocardial infarction, reperfusion can sometimes reduce localized LV remodeling and prevent/treat concomitant IMR, especially in acute situations. However, the optimal surgical treatment of IMR long after myocardial infarction is a matter of controversy and there is wide variation in practice among cardiovascular surgeons. Much of this controversy stems from the lack of good data addressing this issue. Although there is a consensus that mitral valve repair is preferred over mitral valve prosthesis, there have been few randomized clinical trials comparing CABG with CABG plus mitral valve repair. The Randomized Ischemic Mitral Evaluation (RIME) trial randomized 73 patients with moderate MR and a mean LV ejection fraction of 40% to CABG versus CABG plus mitral valve repair.[99] After 1 year, improvements in peak oxygen consumption during exercise were significantly higher in the group with mitral valve repair (3.3 mL/kg/min versus 0.8 mL/kg/min in the CABG-only group). In a similar study design involving 102 patients with moderate MR and a mean LV ejection fraction of 42%, Fattouch and colleagues have demonstrated improved functional capacity and beneficial effects on reverse remodeling with mitral valve repair.[100] However, both studies were not powered to evaluate clinical outcome including all-cause mortality.

Observational studies suffer from selection bias and the lack of an adequate control group despite the use of propensity matching to account for differences in baseline characteristics. They have generated conflicting results about the effect of late revascularization with or without mitral valve surgery for the reduction of IMR. Reviewing 136 CABG patients with moderate to severe IMR, 40% continued to have moderate to severe MR, whereas 51% had some improvement to mild MR, and 9% even had a total disappearance of MR.[101] In contrast, another group has reported that among patients with moderate to severe IMR, mitral valve surgery at the time of CABG did not improve symptoms nor survival compared with CABG alone.[102] The Cleveland Clinic recently reported the largest series so far comparing CABG plus mitral valve annuloplasty (n = 290) with CABG alone (n = 100) in patients with ischemic cardiomyopathy and moderate/severe IMR.[103] Groups were propensity-matched using demographics, extent of coronary disease, regional wall motion, and quantitative electrocardiography. The 1-, 5-, and 10-year survival rates were 88%, 75%, and 47% after CABG alone and 92%, 74%, and 39% after CABG plus mitral valve annuloplasty (P = 0.6) (**Figure 41-5**). However, patients undergoing CABG alone were more likely to have grade 3+ or 4+ postoperative mitral regurgitation than were those undergoing CABG with mitral valve annuloplasty (48% vs. 12% at 1 year; P <0.0001) (**Figure 41-6**). Nevertheless, NYHA functional class improved substantially in both groups, which remained so after 5 years without differences between groups. The authors therefore concluded that although CABG with mitral valve annuloplasty reduces postoperative IMR and improves early symptoms in comparison with CABG alone, it does not improve long-term functional status or survival in patients with severe functional IMR. They hypothesized that mitral valve annuloplasty alone, without addressing the underlying ventricular disease, was probably insufficient to improve long-term clinical outcomes. Therefore, although revascularization with mitral valve repair probably does improve symptoms and reduces IMR more than does CABG alone in patients with ischemic cardiomyopathy, no data confirm that long-term outcomes are better. Acker recently reported equivalent outcomes (LVESVI and survival) in a randomized controlled trial of replacement versus repair in a patient

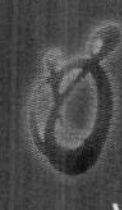

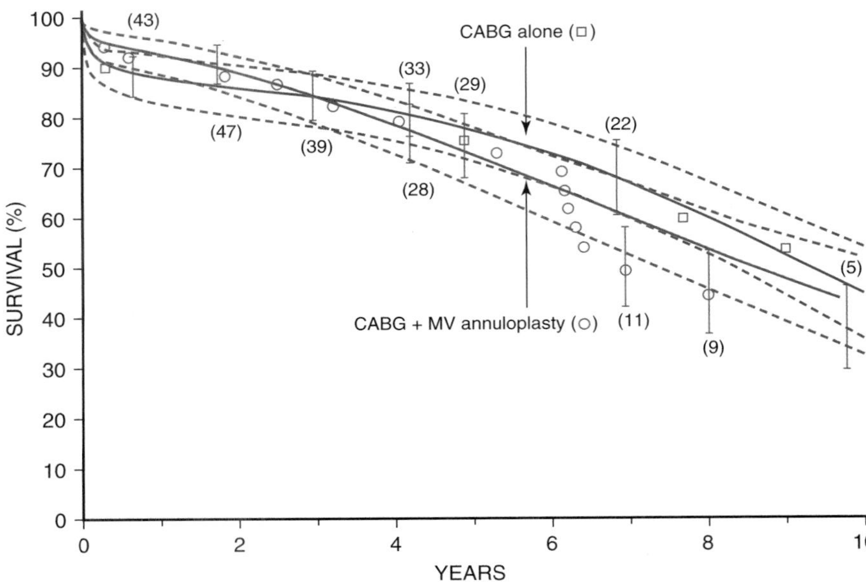

FIGURE 41-5 Outcomes after coronary artery bypass grafting (CABG) or CABG plus mitral valve annuloplasty in patients with ischemic cardiomyopathy and ischemic mitral valve regurgitation. *MV,* Mitral valve. *Modified from Aklog L, Filsoufi F, Flores KQ, et al: Does coronary artery bypass grafting alone correct moderate ischemic mitral regurgitation? Circulation 104:168–75, 2001.*

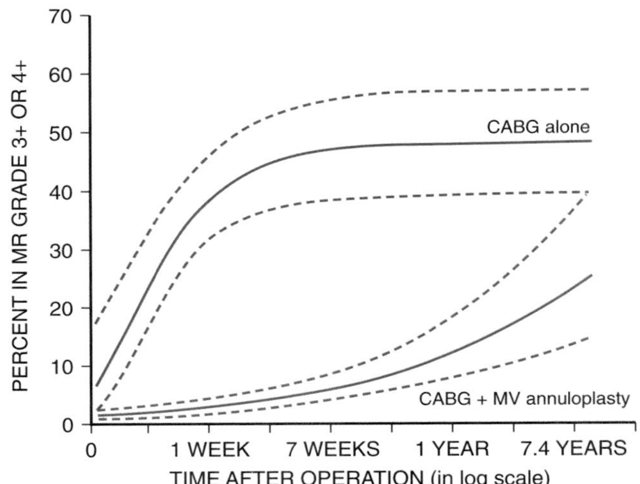

FIGURE 41-6 Moderate/severe mitral valve regurgitation after coronary artery bypass grafting (CABG) or CABG plus mitral valve annuloplasty in patients with ischemic cardiomyopathy and ischemic mitral valve regurgitation. *MV,* Mitral valve. *Modified from Aklog L, Filsoufi F, Flores KQ, et al: Does coronary artery bypass grafting alone correct moderate ischemic mitral regurgitation? Circulation 104:168–75, 2001.*

population with ischemic mitral regurgitation (effective regurgitant orifice area ≈0.4).[104]

Given the limited life expectancy of patients with IMR and ischemic cardiomyopathy, even after valve surgery, it is reasonable to use a tissue valve rather than mechanical prosthesis for patients undergoing valve replacement because few patients will live long enough to have significant structural deterioration of the bioprosthesis. In addition, saving the subvalvular apparatus is technically less demanding and associated with fewer valve-related complications when a bioprosthesis is used.

Tricuspid Valve Surgery in Patients with Severe Left Ventricular Dysfunction

TR is very common in heart failure patients and frequently not addressed during cardiac surgery. Importantly, regardless of the cause, TR is associated with decreased survival.[77,105] In a patient with heart failure, the type of tricuspid regurgitation is almost always functional, being caused by dilation of the right ventricle and the tricuspid annulus as a result of high pulmonary artery pressures induced by left-sided heart failure. It leads to backward flow of blood into the right atrium during systole. When the tricuspid regurgitation is only mild or moderate, this has no major hemodynamic consequences because the right atrium is very compliant. However, when tricuspid regurgitation is severe, right atrial and central venous pressure rise, which results in signs and symptoms of right-sided heart failure and eventually a reduced forward cardiac output.

There is a preconceived notion that correction of high pulmonary artery pressures can result in TR improvement, even if severe, if TR is functional and valvular disease is not present. Importantly, data from the Cleveland Clinic have shown that in 845 patients with moderate to severe TR undergoing isolated mitral valve surgery, more than half of patients still had moderate to severe TR postoperatively, with a tendency to increase even more over time, suggesting that tricuspid valve surgery should have been performed as well. In addition, observational studies suggest that following successful TR surgery, the right ventricle will remodel with subsequent improvement in its function in most patients, but 10% to 20% of such patients will continue to have persistent moderate to severe TR soon after surgery.[106,107] Nevertheless, the risk of early death or subsequent heart failure hospitalizations remains high after tricuspid valve annuloplasty performed concomitantly with mitral valve surgery, and patients should be followed rigorously through a multidisciplinary approach with strong emphasis on optimal heart failure management.[108]

Aortic Valve Surgery in Patients with Severe Left Ventricular Dysfunction

Aortic Valve Stenosis

The results of valve replacement in patients with normal ventricular function are similar to those in patients with mild or moderately reduced LV function. Moreover, the reduced LVEF, which is secondary to the excessive afterload, is often immediately corrected by valve replacement.[109,110] In comparison, patients with severely reduced LV ejection fraction in the range of 25% to 35% often experience incomplete resolution of symptoms after valve replacement. However, survival is still improved in this setting although surgery is associated with a higher operative mortality.[111]

When the ventricular function is extremely reduced (<25%), the cardiologist is challenged to carefully select patients who might still benefit from surgery. This group of patients might not be able to generate a high gradient across the aortic valve despite significant valve narrowing and need further diagnostic testing. Some patients with such low gradient aortic valve stenosis (AS) have true severe AS, whereas others have pseudo-AS with a low transvalvular pressure gradient because of the combination of moderate AS and low cardiac output. True stenosis is distinguished from pseudo–aortic valve stenosis through evaluation of echocardiographic changes in hemodynamic and structural measurements in response to dobutamine, which normally augments cardiac output. In pseudo–aortic valve stenosis, the aortic valve area usually increases as ventricular function improves, whereas in true aortic valve stenosis, this area does not increase. In addition, patients with contractile reserve in response to dobutamine have a much better outcome after surgery. Although patients with low-gradient, true aortic valve stenosis have high perioperative and postoperative mortality rates, surgery is still recommended because valve replacement is associated with better outcomes than is continued medical therapy.[112] Indeed, the 1- and 4-year survival rates were markedly improved among patients who underwent surgery (82% and 78%), in comparison with those among patients who received medical therapy (41% and 15%; $P < 0.0001$).

Some critically ill patients with true AS are hemodynamically too unstable before surgery and have a perioperative mortality risk that is deemed too high to warrant surgery. Stabilizing such patients before surgery through judicious medical intervention or interventional procedures might be considered. The use of nitroprusside during continuous hemodynamic monitoring with a pulmonary artery catheter has been reported to significantly increase cardiac index and reduce mean pulmonary arterial pressure and systemic vascular resistance, allowing hemodynamic stabilization with subsequent safer aortic valve replacement.[113] Percutaneous balloon valvotomy with or without placement of a valve prosthesis may reduce the aortic valve gradient and can potentially improve symptoms as well. Experience with transcatheter aortic valve replacement is increasing and promising results have been reported in patients at very high (mostly noncardiac related) surgical risk, which makes this technique an attractive modality to treat patients with advanced heart failure.[114,115] However, the optimal selection of patients and cost-efficient use of transcatheter aortic valve replacement is yet to be defined. Occasionally, our practice is to prepare the patient to receive an LVAD (if needed) at the time of surgery when profound low cardiac output prevents separation from cardiopulmonary bypass.

Aortic Valve Regurgitation

The volume load and subsequent LV dilation in patients with chronic AR is similar to the volume load of MR and can be affected by pharmacologic therapy (i.e., vasodilators such as nifedipine and angiotensin-converting enzyme inhibitors) and reversed by valve replacement. Importantly, evaluation of LV size and function is important because there is not always a correlation between these parameters and symptoms.[116,117] However, the prognosis of patients with aortic regurgitation is determined largely by symptom status and by LV size and function.[116,117] An LV end-systolic volume greater than 60 mL/m^2, an LV end-systolic dimension greater than 50 mm, or an LV ejection fraction less than 50% usually indicates serious depression of LV systolic function with adverse outcome if not surgically corrected. Surgical correction of the regurgitant lesion usually produces at least some improvements in symptoms, regardless of the functional state of the ventricle.[118,119] In addition, whereas earlier studies indicated a high mortality risk for patients with severely depressed LV ejection fraction, the projected survival for patients operated in the current era indicates that early and 5-year survival are similar to those with better LV function.[120] Moreover, many of the reported poor results with aortic valve replacement for AR and severe LV impairment come from an era in which myocardial protection was less sophisticated, and valve prostheses (such as the Starr-Edwards mechanical valve) had high gradients, which substantially decreased the possibility of late LV recovery.

Because of the improved outcomes, aortic valve surgery for AS or AR should be considered for many patients with severe LV dysfunction, often with excellent clinical outcome, obviating the need for cardiac transplantation. Although some centers experiment with aortic valve repair, most still replace the aortic valve with either a mechanical or bioprosthetic valve. The choice between these valves is discussed in detail by the 2008 focused update of the 2006 ACC/AHA guidelines for the management of patients with valvular heart disease, which recommended that the patient's age, ability to tolerate warfarin, and personal preference should all be taken into account.[121] The guidelines advocate that patients with a projected long lifespan generally receive a mechanical valve because of the greater durability and improved patient survival after 15 years. To the contrary, patients who cannot tolerate warfarin have potential compliance problems, or patients $\geq$ 65 years of age have a stronger indication for a bioprosthesis because valve durability is less of an issue in these cases. The prospect of a percutaneous valve later on in a previously surgically degenerated valve might also favor the use of a bioprosthesis.

LEFT VENTRICULAR RECONSTRUCTION SURGERY

Surgical ventricular restoration (SVR), or volume reduction, is the active surgical attempt to restore the shape of the pathologically remodeled ventricle to one that is physiologically superior. It has long been recognized that ventricular reconstruction alone can improve cardiac function and a patient's functional status.[122] In the setting of heart failure with reduced ejection fraction, the heart enlarges to maintain stroke volume, at the expense of several physiologic and mechanical disadvantages. These include increased myocardial wall stress, subendocardial hypoperfusion, increased myocardial oxygen consumption, afterload mismatch, and activation of compensatory neurohumoral mechanisms. Changes in LV size and geometry will lead to progressive LV dysfunction and worsening heart failure.

Sometimes it is possible to surgically remove or exclude portions of the dysfunctional myocardium, infarcted territories, or both to return the LV cavity to a smaller chamber with more normal geometry and physiologic properties. Reduction of internal cavity dimensions on the basis of Laplace's law help reduce end-systolic and end-diastolic wall stress, which results in reduced myocardial oxygen consumption and helps improve myocardial efficiency, which has been shown to ameliorate heart failure symptoms and improve outcomes.[123-125] Importantly, the surgical remodeling has beneficial effects on areas of the left ventricle remote from the scar, which results in improved performance of the lateral wall in the case of surgical anterior LV reconstruction.[123]

Four developments, however, have affected the current surgical LV reconstruction techniques for ischemic cardiomyopathy. First, classic ventricular aneurysms are much less common than decades ago because of aggressive interventions following myocardial infarction, and the widespread use of neurohumoral blockers after myocardial infarction.[126-131] Second, the technique of ventricular reconstruction has evolved from linear repair involving the free wall, to a more complete infarct exclusion technique that includes repair of the scarred septum.[132-135] Third, the concept of reconstruction for dyskinesia (aneurysms) has been extended to include akinetic, scarred but nonaneurysmal, areas of the LV.[136-140] Finally, ablation can now be used to eliminate foci of tachyarrhythmias and often reconstruction procedures are combined with valvular surgery. The surgeon must exhibit extreme care to ensure that the LV cavity is not too small after SVR and that the mitral valve remains competent. On occasion the patient must go back on cardiopulmonary bypass to increase the LV volume or to undergo repair on the mitral valve after SVR. Hence, perioperative transesophageal echocardiography plays a very important role in the surgical management of patients undergoing SVR.

Indications for Ventricular Reconstruction Surgery in Ischemic Cardiomyopathy

The classic indications included congestive heart failure, embolism originating from a thrombus contained in the aneurysm, and persistent malignant ventricular arrhythmias, despite optimal medical therapy. However, many patients undergo remodeling surgery only because the surgeon is committed and experienced in this type of difficult surgery. In the Cleveland Clinic experience, a thin-walled aneurysm that collapses with venting of the aorta or left atrium must be present, most often in the vicinity of the left anterior descending coronary artery. If diffuse scar is mixed with muscle in all three coronary arteries' territories, often no reconstruction is undertaken because there is no discrete area to resect. As explained previously, viability studies are only 80% to 90% accurate; therefore, areas that are found to be thick-walled muscle intraoperatively are not resected, even though the "scar" was indicated on the viability study. All efforts are undertaken to optimally revascularize areas with preserved wall thickness. Most often, reconstruction is performed for a true dyskinetic aneurysm, although transmural scar in a thin-walled akinetic segment might be resected as well. In 2002, Dor proposed similar indications in asymptomatic patients for ventricular reconstructive surgery after anteroseptal myocardial infarction: a dilated LV (end-diastolic volume index >100 mL/m^2), LV ejection fraction less than 20%, LV regional dyskinesis or akinesis greater than 30% of the ventricular perimeter, and symptoms of angina, heart failure, arrhythmias, or inducible ischemia on provocative tests.[124] Relative contraindications were systolic pulmonary artery pressure less than 60 mm Hg, severe right ventricular dysfunction and regional dyskinesis or akinesis without dilation of the ventricle.[124] At the Cleveland Clinic, ventricular reconstruction surgery is also not performed in patients with stage D inotrope-dependent heart failure, because these patients usually do not benefit any more from the procedure. In addition, it is prudent that patients who are candidates for LV reconstruction surgery are screened for cardiac transplantation or implantation of a ventricular assist device before remodeling surgery. After the completion of the STICH trial, which demonstrated lack of benefit with reconstruction, the frequency of LV resection has decreased markedly.

Techniques for Remodeling Surgery in Ischemic Cardiomyopathy

The Dor Procedure

The Dor procedure, also called *endoventricular circular patch plasty*, is only indicated when an aneurysm has formed after a myocardial infarction.[141] A pursestring stitch is created around a nonviable scarred aneurysm. Afterward, the aneurysm is excluded and the residual defect is covered by a patch made from Dacron, pericardium, or an autologous tissue flap. The remaining aneurysmal scar is subsequently closed over the outside of the patch to give additional stability to the repair. The result is a restored "normal" LV chamber geometry and improved LV function. The operation shortens the long axis, but leaves the short axis length unchanged, producing an increase in ventricular diastolic sphericity while the systolic shape becomes more elliptical.[142] The first 661 patients who underwent the Dor procedure had an overall operative mortality of 8% (16.3% versus 6.2% when performed urgently versus planned). A dramatic improvement in LV ejection fraction (33% versus 50%) with subsequent improvements in NYHA functional class in 92% of patients (58% in NYHA functional class I and 33% in NYHA functional class II) and disappearance of ventricular arrhythmias in more than 90% of patients was seen at 1 week and maintained after 1 year.[142] At 3 years, the survival rate was 89.4% ± 1.3% and 88.7% avoided readmission to the hospital for heart failure.

Cleveland Clinic Approach

At the Cleveland Clinic, most of the patients scheduled for LV reconstruction surgery for ischemic cardiomyopathy also undergo CABG (89%), and almost 50% undergo concomitant mitral valve surgery, especially if MR is ≥ 2/4.[143] The operation is performed through a full sternotomy on cardiopulmonary bypass. After the coronary grafts are established, the mitral valve is repaired, and a modified Maze procedure is performed if the patient has a history of atrial fibrillation. The left atrial appendage is closed or resected to prevent future embolism. The LV scar is opened 2 cm lateral to the left anterior descending artery, any underlying LV thrombus is removed, and sutures are placed to retract the thin LV walls and thereby facilitate exposure of the septum, the papillary muscles, and the border zone of the infarcted and normal appearing myocardium.

Subsequently, the aneurysm or scarred area is resected subendocardially, and cryolesions are applied along the entire border zone in patients with a history of ventricular arrhythmias. With the heart beating, a first pursestring suture is placed in the border zone, and each bite is placed deep in the scarred tissue. This suture is then tightened to create a "neck." In contrast to the DOR procedure, a patch is not routinely sewed over this opening because the dyskinetic or akinetic area will simply be replaced with another akinetic area; a patch is used only when the LV cavity would be too small. Therefore, an intraventricular balloon filled to a known volume of 60 mL/m^2 is inserted to ensure that the residual chamber size is adequate. Thus in 95% of patients, simply a second pursestring suture a few millimeters above the first suture closes this opening. The resulting "neck" is less than 1 cm in length but is often completely obliterated once the sutures are tightened. Finally, two strips of felt are then placed on the epicardial surface, and horizontal mattress sutures passing through the free wall of the left ventricle are applied to approximate the border zone between normal and infarcted myocardium. The ventricular cavity beneath the pursestring sutures is almost completely surrounded by normal myocardium. This technique can be viewed at http://cvbook.nmh.org.

Thirty-day and 1-, 2-, and 3-year survival in 84 patients with NYHA functional class III-IV heart failure undergoing this procedure at the Cleveland Clinic was 100%, 90%, 85%, and 83%, respectively. Mean NYHA functional class decreased from 3.4 to 1.4, with significant improvements in levels of neurohumoral markers as well. Although mitral valve surgery was clearly associated with more pronounced symptomatic improvement, no differences in mortality were seen between patients who did and did not undergo mitral valve surgery in addition to remodeling surgery.

The aforementioned STICH trial was the first prospective, randomized clinical trial in which medical therapy only, medical therapy with CABG, and medical therapy with CABG and remodeling surgery were compared. The Hypothesis 2 group consisted of 1000 patients with ischemic cardiomyopathy, an LV ejection fraction of ≤ 35%, coronary artery disease that was amenable to CABG, and dominant anterior left ventricular dysfunction that was amenable to surgical LV reconstruction. Patients were randomized to either CABG alone or CABG plus LV reconstruction surgery.[144] LV reconstruction reduced the end-systolic volume index by 19%, as compared with a reduction of 6% with CABG alone. In both groups, there were significant improvements in symptoms and exercise tolerance. However, the incidence of the primary endpoint of all-cause mortality or any cardiovascular hospitalization was similar among groups after 48 months of follow-up (59% in the CABG alone group versus 58% in the LV reconstruction group). In conclusion, the addition of SVR to CABG reduced the LV volume, in comparison with CABG alone, but the seemingly beneficial ventricular remodeling was not associated with a greater improvement in symptoms or exercise tolerance or with a reduction in the rate of death or hospitalization for cardiac causes. On the basis of this trial, routine use of LV reconstruction surgery in addition to CABG cannot be justified in such patients. Potential explanations for the lack of added efficacy of the combined procedure include the fact that current heart failure therapies are very effective at limiting adverse LV remodeling. Moreover, the addition of CABG may further enhance this process, leaving little room for additional benefits from ventricular reconstruction surgery. Most probably, there are patients who might benefit from the combined procedure, but the STICH trial lacked the necessary information to define this important subgroup. Given the diversity of the study population and complexity of the surgical technique, one might wonder if a randomized clinical trial will ever be able to definitely determine the population that benefits from LV reconstruction surgery over CABG alone. Therefore, individual cardiac surgeons and cardiothoracic centers that have extensive experience and good outcomes with SVR will probably continue to apply this procedure in patients with dyskinetic segments, who undergo CABG (+/– MVR) and meet their proven selection criteria.

Indications for Left Ventricular Reconstruction Surgery in Nonischemic Cardiomyopathy

Patients with idiopathic dilated cardiomyopathy and extreme ventricular dilation have always been deemed inoperable, and are usually referred for cardiac transplantation. However, Randas Batista, a Brazilian cardiac surgeon, popularized a radical technique of "partial left ventriculectomy" to remove part of the ventricular wall and restore the dilated ventricle to an almost normal size and shape.[145] The Batista procedure involves the removal of a section of the LV free wall, between both papillary muscles extending from the apex to the mitral annulus. The remaining free edges are reapproximated and stitched together. The mitral valve and subvalvular apparatus are preserved, repaired, or replaced, depending upon the amount of tissue that needs to be removed. Several centers, including in the United States, have published their experience with the Batista procedure. All have demonstrated an initial increase in LV ejection fraction, a reduction in LV dimensions, and improvements in functional status in survivors over the short- and mid-term.[146-148] However, despite this apparent clinical success, there was an unacceptably high recurrence rate of symptomatic heart failure in patients undergoing the Batista procedure.[149,150] Even more important, one third of patients did not have any benefit and up to another one third were even worse after surgery. In addition, the Batista procedure was associated with a high incidence of late fatal arrhythmias.[147,149] As a consequence, the Batista procedure is no longer considered to be an appropriate option for patients with advanced heart failure, and both the 2009 focused update of the ACC/AHA heart failure guidelines and the 2010 Heart Failure Society of America (HFSA) practice guidelines state that partial left ventriculectomy is *not recommended* in nonischemic cardiomyopathy.[94,95]

Another historical surgical therapy for nonischemic cardiomyopathy—referred to as *dynamic cardiomyoplasty*, in which the latissimus dorsi muscle is wrapped around the heart and paced during ventricular systole—initially gained a lot of interest.[151] The physiologic reasoning behind this technique was to provide an auxiliary pump for the failing LV, aiming to improve cardiac output and functional status. Symptomatic improvement occurred after dynamic cardiomyoplasty, although the mechanism of benefit was not clear. A large randomized clinical trial of dynamic cardiomyoplasty was started. However, only patients with NYHA functional class III heart failure were considered suitable for recruitment, because surgical mortality was deemed too high for patients with more advanced heart failure (30% for patients residing in NYHA functional class IV). Low enrollment and marginal overall clinical improvements resulted in the premature termination of the study. In addition, it appeared that those who can survive the operation do not need it and those who need it cannot survive it.[151-153] For these reasons, cardiomyoplasty is not a viable surgical strategy for the management of heart failure.

Device Therapies for Nonischemic Cardiomyopathy

The cardiomyoplasty and volume reduction (Batista) experience has led to other novel approaches to treat heart failure because postoperative observations suggested that some patients benefited from the diastolic "girdling" effect of the muscle wrap and consequently progressive LV dilation could be slowed.[152] Several devices to prevent further LV dilation have been developed.

The Acorn Device

The Acorn CorCap is a compliant polyester mesh jacket placed around the ventricles of the heart. It does not interfere with diastolic function but acts as an external constraint device, thereby preventing further dilation of the heart (**Figure 41-7**). Based on results of animal studies and small human case series demonstrating positive effects on reverse ventricular remodeling and clinical symptoms, a multicenter randomized clinical trial was performed comparing the CorCap to medical therapy, and the CorCap with concomitant mitral valve repair versus mitral valve repair alone.[154] Results were in favor of the CorCap cardiac support device, with 38% versus 27% of patients improving their heart failure status.[92] Moreover, mitral valve repair was associated with progressive reductions in LV volumes and mass, and increases in LV ejection fraction and sphericity index, all consistent with reverse ventricular remodeling. Recurrence of clinically significant MR was uncommon. Quality of life, exercise performance, and NYHA functional class were all improved. The addition of the CorCap cardiac support device led to greater decreases in LV volumes, a more elliptical shape, a trend for a reduction in subsequent major cardiac procedures, and improvements in quality of life, compared with mitral valve repair alone. Importantly, beneficial effects on LV remodeling were sustained at long-term follow-up.[155] These findings indicate that there might be additional benefit with the CorCap cardiac support device compared with mitral valve surgery alone in patients with nonischemic cardiomyopathy. Given the improvement in LV structure and function, along with a low mortality rate, offering mitral valve surgery in combination with the CorCap cardiac support device to patients with heart failure who are on an optimal medical regimen is an appealing treatment strategy. In the United States, the device was not approved despite the positive findings in the clinical trial. Regrettably, the company that developed the CorCap cardiac support device has opted to withdraw the device, not seeking market approval.

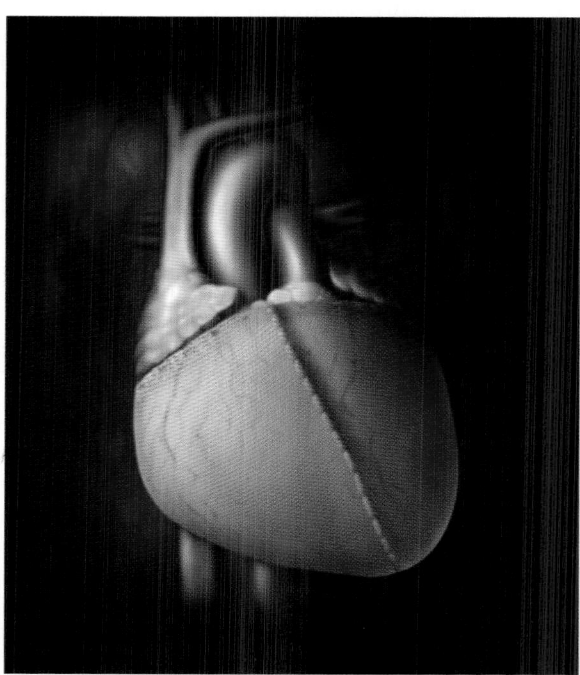

FIGURE 41-7 CorCap device.

The Myocor Myosplint device is also aimed at inhibiting negative LV remodeling. The device consists of a transventricular splint with epicardial pads that are adjusted to decrease the LV radius, creating a smaller, more energetically efficient LV with decreased wall tension (by the law of Laplace). The transventricular splints are placed on the beating heart without cardiopulmonary bypass, typically from the lateral LV through the posterior interventricular septum. After the splints are tightened, the final ventricle has a bilobular shape. Animal and small human case series have also shown positive effects on ventricular remodeling and clinical symptoms. The company recently developed a new product (Coapsys) that is designed to achieve off-pump mitral valve repair along with ventricular volume reduction (**Figure 41-8**). The device includes a single transventricular splint and pads on the outer surface of the LV. Under continuous echocardiography monitoring, the pads are tightened until mitral regurgitation is reduced and eventually eliminated. One pad on the LV is positioned at the level of the mitral valve apparatus and pulls the posterior annulus toward the anterior leaflet during tightening. The other pad on the LV free wall changes the ventricular shape during tightening. In humans who had Myosplint placement (immediately before heart transplant), an acute reduction in LV end-diastolic and end-systolic volumes was similar to that seen in animal experiments. A safety/feasibility study has been carried out with encouraging results, but again the company opted to not pursue market approval.[156]

CONCLUSIONS

Surgical treatments for heart failure are used in a small percentage of the heart failure population. Surgery when indicated may alter the natural history of ventricular dysfunction and prevent or ameliorate heart failure. High-risk surgery should be pursued at experienced referral centers in lieu of transplantation or ventricular assist devices. A large series at the Cleveland Clinic has shown that risk stratification models will identify when conventional surgical approaches (CABG, MVR) will yield superior survival versus transplantation.[157] Modern techniques yield a low perioperative morbidity and mortality and have led to improved long-term ventricular function and outcomes. Many patients referred for transplantation can now be

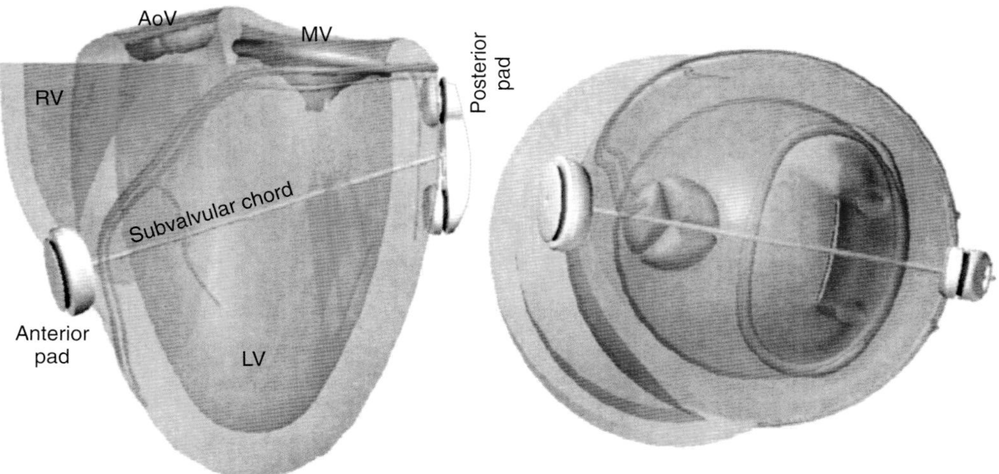

FIGURE 41-8 Myosplint device. *AoV,* Aortic valve; *LV,* left ventricle; *MV,* mitral valve; *RV,* right ventricle.

treated surgically that may delay or even preclude the need for cardiac transplantation. For patients who have severe LV dysfunction but a considerable amount of viable myocardial tissue, coronary bypass surgery should be the first option. Mitral valve repair in the presence of severe LV dysfunction appears to be effective for symptomatic relief and might carry improved survival, especially if combined with therapies that also directly address LV remodeling. Direct ventricular reconstruction for ischemic cardiomyopathy with resection of delineated areas of dyskinetic or akinetic scar can be performed with acceptable perioperative mortality, and will lead to improved ventricular function, but effects on long-term clinical outcome remain undetermined. Patients with nonischemic cardiomyopathy might benefit from alternative device strategies aiming to halt or reverse the detrimental ventricular remodeling process. Several ongoing prospective randomized clinical trials should make the role of surgery in both ischemic and nonischemic cardiomyopathy clearer. The cardiologist must be diligent to consider appropriate surgical procedures and refer for transplantation or LVAD only when no other option exists.

References

1. Felker GM, Shaw LK, O'Connor CM: A standardized definition of ischemic cardiomyopathy for use in clinical research. *J Am Coll Cardiol* 39:210–218, 2002.
2. Hellermann JP, Jacobsen SJ, Redfield MM, et al: Heart failure after myocardial infarction: clinical presentation and survival. *Eur J Heart Fail* 7:119–125, 2005.
3. Suleiman M, Khatib R, Agmon Y, et al: Early inflammation and risk of long-term development of heart failure and mortality in survivors of acute myocardial infarction predictive role of C-reactive protein. *J Am Coll Cardiol* 47:962–968, 2006.
4. Bursi F, Enriquez-Sarano M, Nkomo VT, et al: Heart failure and death after myocardial infarction in the community: the emerging role of mitral regurgitation. *Circulation* 111:295–301, 2005.
5. Kannel WB, Cupples A: Epidemiology and risk profile of cardiac failure. *Cardiovasc Drugs Ther* 2(Suppl 1):387–395, 1988.
6. Poole-Wilson PA: Relation of pathophysiologic mechanisms to outcome in heart failure. *J Am Coll Cardiol* 22:22A–29A, 1993.
7. Weisman HF, Bush DE, Mannisi JA, et al: Cellular mechanisms of myocardial infarct expansion. *Circulation* 78:186–201, 1988.
8. Gerdes AM, Capasso JM: Structural remodeling and mechanical dysfunction of cardiac myocytes in heart failure. *J Mol Cell Cardiol* 27:849–856, 1995.
9. Fragasso G, Margonato A, Chierchia SL: Assessment of viability after myocardial infarction. Clinical relevance and methodological problems. *Int J Card Imaging* 9(Suppl 1):3–10, 1993.
10. Heyndrickx GR, Baig H, Nellens P, et al: Depression of regional blood flow and wall thickening after brief coronary occlusions. *Am J Physiol* 234:H653–H659, 1978.
11. Braunwald E, Kloner RA: The stunned myocardium: prolonged, postischemic ventricular dysfunction. *Circulation* 66:1146–1149, 1982.
12. Marban E: Myocardial stunning and hibernation. The physiology behind the colloquialisms. *Circulation* 83:681–688, 1991.
13. Bristow JD, Arai AE, Anselone CG, et al: Response to myocardial ischemia as a regulated process. *Circulation* 84:2580–2587, 1991.
14. Knight C, Fox K: The vicious circle of ischemic left ventricular dysfunction. *Am J Cardiol* 75:10E–15E, 1995.
15. Tillisch J, Brunken R, Marshall R, et al: Reversibility of cardiac wall-motion abnormalities predicted by positron tomography. *N Engl J Med* 314:884–888, 1986.
16. Selvanayagam JB, Jerosch-Herold M, Porto I, et al: Resting myocardial blood flow is impaired in hibernating myocardium: a magnetic resonance study of quantitative perfusion assessment. *Circulation* 112:3289–3296, 2005.
17. Risk stratification and survival after myocardial infarction. *N Engl J Med* 309:331–336, 1983.
18. Emond M, Mock MB, Davis KB, et al: Long-term survival of medically treated patients in the Coronary Artery Surgery Study (CASS) Registry. *Circulation* 90:2645–2657, 1994.
19. Felker GM, Thompson RE, Hare JM, et al: Underlying causes and long-term survival in patients with initially unexplained cardiomyopathy. *N Engl J Med* 342:1077–1084, 2000.
20. Velazquez EJ, Lee KL, Deja MA, et al: Coronary-artery bypass surgery in patients with left ventricular dysfunction. *N Engl J Med* 364:1607–1616, 2011.
21. Murphy ML, Hultgren HN, Detre K, et al: Treatment of chronic stable angina. A preliminary report of survival data of the randomized Veterans Administration cooperative study. *N Engl J Med* 297:621–627, 1977.
22. Alderman EL, Fisher LD, Litwin P, et al: Results of coronary artery surgery in patients with poor left ventricular function (CASS). *Circulation* 68:785–795, 1983.
23. Varnauskas E: Twelve-year follow-up of survival in the randomized European Coronary Surgery Study. *N Engl J Med* 319:332–337, 1988.
24. Primo G, Le Clerc JL, Goldstein JP, et al: Cardiac transplantation for the treatment of end-stage ischemic cardiomyopathy. *Adv Cardiol* 36:293–297, 1988.
25. McManus RP, O'Hair DP, Beitzinger JM, et al: Patients who die awaiting heart transplantation. *J Heart Lung Transplant* 12:159–171, discussion 172, 1993.
26. Elefteriades JA, Kron IL: CABG in advanced left ventricular dysfunction. *Cardiol Clin* 13:35–42, 1995.
27. Wechsler AS, Junod FL: Coronary bypass grafting in patients with chronic congestive heart failure. *Circulation* 79:192–196, 1989.
28. Ragosta M, Beller GA, Watson DD, et al: Quantitative planar rest-redistribution 201Tl imaging in detection of myocardial viability and prediction of improvement in left ventricular function after coronary bypass surgery in patients with severely depressed left ventricular function. *Circulation* 87:1630–1641, 1993.
29. Pagley PR, Beller GA, Watson DD, et al: Improved outcome after coronary bypass surgery in patients with ischemic cardiomyopathy and residual myocardial viability. *Circulation* 96:793–800, 1997.
30. Samady H, Elefteriades JA, Abbott BG, et al: Failure to improve left ventricular function after coronary revascularization for ischemic cardiomyopathy is not associated with worse outcome. *Circulation* 100:1298–1304, 1999.
31. Allman KC, Shaw LJ, Hachamovitch R, et al: Myocardial viability testing and impact of revascularization on prognosis in patients with coronary artery disease and left ventricular dysfunction: a meta-analysis. *J Am Coll Cardiol* 39:1151–1158, 2002.
32. Wellnhofer E, Olariu A, Klein C, et al: Magnetic resonance low-dose dobutamine test is superior to SCAR quantification for the prediction of functional recovery. *Circulation* 109:2172–2174, 2004.
33. Chareonthaitawee P, Gersh BJ, Araoz PA, et al: Revascularization in severe left ventricular dysfunction: the role of viability testing. *J Am Coll Cardiol* 46:567–574, 2005.
34. Bonow RO, Maurer G, Lee KL, et al: Myocardial viability and survival in ischemic left ventricular dysfunction. *N Engl J Med* 364:1617–1625, 2011.
35. Pasquet A, Williams MJ, Secknus MA, et al: Correlation of preoperative myocardial function, perfusion, and metabolism with postoperative function at rest and stress after bypass surgery in severe left ventricular dysfunction. *Am J Cardiol* 84:58–64, 1999.
36. Main ML, Grayburn PA, Landau C, et al: Relation of contractile reserve during low-dose dobutamine echocardiography and angiographic extent and severity of coronary artery disease in the presence of left ventricular dysfunction. *Am J Cardiol* 79:1309–1313, 1997.
37. Nagueh SF, Mikati I, Weilbaecher D, et al: Relation of the contractile reserve of hibernating myocardium to myocardial structure in humans. *Circulation* 100:490–496, 1999.
38. Gibson RS, Watson DD, Taylor GJ, et al: Prospective assessment of regional myocardial perfusion before and after coronary revascularization surgery by quantitative thallium-201 scintigraphy. *J Am Coll Cardiol* 1:804–815, 1983.
39. Liu P, Kiess MC, Okada RD, et al: The persistent defect on exercise thallium imaging and its fate after myocardial revascularization: does it represent scar or ischemia? *Am Heart J* 110:996–1001, 1985.
40. Baumgartner H, Porenta G, Lau YK, et al: Assessment of myocardial viability by dobutamine echocardiography, positron emission tomography and thallium-201 SPECT: correlation with histopathology in explanted hearts. *J Am Coll Cardiol* 32:1701–1708, 1998.
41. Grayburn PA: How good is echocardiography at assessing myocardial viability? *Am J Cardiol* 76:1183–1184, 1995.
42. Schelbert HR: Metabolic imaging to assess myocardial viability. *J Nucl Med* 35:8S–14S, 1994.
43. Lucignani G, Paolini G, Landoni C, et al: Presurgical identification of hibernating myocardium by combined use of technetium-99m hexakis 2-methoxyisobutylisonitrile single photon emission tomography and fluorine-18 fluoro-2-deoxy-D-glucose positron emission tomography in patients with coronary artery disease. *Eur J Nucl Med* 19:874–881, 1992.

44. Marwick TH, MacIntyre WJ, Lafont A, et al: Metabolic responses of hibernating and infarcted myocardium to revascularization. A follow-up study of regional perfusion, function, and metabolism. *Circulation* 85:1347–1353, 1992.
45. Tamaki N, Kawamoto M, Tadamura E, et al: Prediction of reversible ischemia after revascularization. Perfusion and metabolic studies with positron emission tomography. *Circulation* 91:1697–1705, 1995.
46. Kim RJ, Wu E, Rafael A, et al: The use of contrast-enhanced magnetic resonance imaging to identify reversible myocardial dysfunction. *N Engl J Med* 343:1445–1453, 2000.
47. Selvanayagam JB, Kardos A, Francis JM, et al: Value of delayed-enhancement cardiovascular magnetic resonance imaging in predicting myocardial viability after surgical revascularization. *Circulation* 110:1535–1541, 2004.
48. Baer FM, Theissen P, Schneider CA, et al: Dobutamine magnetic resonance imaging predicts contractile recovery of chronically dysfunctional myocardium after successful revascularization. *J Am Coll Cardiol* 31:1040–1048, 1998.
49. Gunning MG, Anagnostopoulos C, Knight CJ, et al: Comparison of 201Tl, 99mTc-tetrofosmin, and dobutamine magnetic resonance imaging for identifying hibernating myocardium. *Circulation* 98:1869–1874, 1998.
50. Beller GA: Noninvasive assessment of myocardial viability. *N Engl J Med* 343:1488–1490, 2000.
51. Edwards FH, Clark RE, Schwartz M: Coronary artery bypass grafting: the Society of Thoracic Surgeons National Database experience. *Ann Thorac Surg* 57:12–19, 1994.
52. Hattler BG, Madia C, Johnson C, et al: Risk stratification using the Society of Thoracic Surgeons Program. *Ann Thorac Surg* 58:1348–1352, 1994.
53. Roques F, Nashef SA, Michel P, et al: Risk factors and outcome in European cardiac surgery: analysis of the EuroSCORE multinational database of 19030 patients. *Eur J Cardiothorac Surg* 15:816–822, discussion 822–823, 1999.
54. Nashef SA, Roques F, Hammill BG, et al: Validation of European System for Cardiac Operative Risk Evaluation (EuroSCORE) in North American cardiac surgery. *Eur J Cardiothorac Surg* 22:101–105, 2002.
55. Roques F, Michel P, Goldstone AR, et al: The logistic EuroSCORE. *Eur Heart J* 24:881–882, 2003.
56. Kolh P: Importance of risk stratification models in cardiac surgery. *Eur Heart J* 27:768–769, 2006.
57. Fortescue EB, Kahn K, Bates DW: Development and validation of a clinical prediction rule for major adverse outcomes in coronary bypass grafting. *Am J Cardiol* 88:1251–1258, 2001.
58. Yau TM, Fedak PW, Weisel RD, et al: Predictors of operative risk for coronary bypass operations in patients with left ventricular dysfunction. *J Thorac Cardiovasc Surg* 118:1006–1013, 1999.
59. Estafanous FG, Loop FD, Higgins TL, et al: Increased risk and decreased morbidity of coronary artery bypass grafting between 1986 and 1994. *Ann Thorac Surg* 65:383–389, 1998.
60. Fisher LD, Kennedy JW, Davis KB, et al: Association of sex, physical size, and operative mortality after coronary artery bypass in the Coronary Artery Surgery Study (CASS). *J Thorac Cardiovasc Surg* 84:334–341, 1982.
61. O'Connor GT, Plume SK, Olmstead EM, et al: Multivariate prediction of in-hospital mortality associated with coronary artery bypass graft surgery. Northern New England Cardiovascular Disease Study Group. *Circulation* 85:2110–2118, 1992.
62. Di Carli MF, Asgarzadie F, Schelbert HR, et al: Quantitative relation between myocardial viability and improvement in heart failure symptoms after revascularization in patients with ischemic cardiomyopathy. *Circulation* 92:3436–3444, 1995.
63. Yamaguchi A, Ino T, Adachi H, et al: Left ventricular volume predicts postoperative course in patients with ischemic cardiomyopathy. *Ann Thorac Surg* 65:434–438, 1998.
64. Eitzman D, al-Aouar Z, Kanter HL, et al: Clinical outcome of patients with advanced coronary artery disease after viability studies with positron emission tomography. *J Am Coll Cardiol* 20:559–565, 1992.
65. Marwick TH, Nemec JJ, Lafont A, et al: Prediction by postexercise fluoro-18 deoxyglucose positron emission tomography of improvement in exercise capacity after revascularization. *Am J Cardiol* 69:854–859, 1992.
66. Bax JJ, van der Wall EE, Harbinson M: Radionuclide techniques for the assessment of myocardial viability and hibernation. *Heart* 90(Suppl 5):v26–v33, 2004.
67. Carluccio E, Biagioli P, Alunni G, et al: Patients with hibernating myocardium show altered left ventricular volumes and shape, which revert after revascularization: evidence that dyssynergy might directly induce cardiac remodeling. *J Am Coll Cardiol* 47:969–977, 2006.
68. Rahimtoola SH, La Canna G, Ferrari R: Hibernating myocardium: another piece of the puzzle falls into place. *J Am Coll Cardiol* 47:978–980, 2006.
69. Schinkel AF, Poldermans D, Rizzello V, et al: Why do patients with ischemic cardiomyopathy and a substantial amount of viable myocardium not always recover in function after revascularization? *J Thorac Cardiovasc Surg* 127:385–390, 2004.
70. Cleland JG, Pennell DJ, Ray SG, et al: Myocardial viability as a determinant of the ejection fraction response to carvedilol in patients with heart failure (CHRISTMAS trial): randomised controlled trial. *Lancet* 362:14–21, 2003.
71. Bounous EP, Mark DB, Pollock BG, et al: Surgical survival benefits for coronary disease patients with left ventricular dysfunction. *Circulation* 78:I151–I157, 1988.
72. Veenhuyzen GD, Singh SN, McAreavey D, et al: Prior coronary artery bypass surgery and risk of death among patients with ischemic left ventricular dysfunction. *Circulation* 104:1489–1493, 2001.
73. Underwood SR, Bax JJ, vom Dahl J, et al: Imaging techniques for the assessment of myocardial hibernation. Report of a Study Group of the European Society of Cardiology. *Eur Heart J* 25:815–836, 2004.
74. Desideri A, Cortigiani L, Christen AI, et al: The extent of perfusion-F18-fluorodeoxyglucose positron emission tomography mismatch determines mortality in medically treated patients with chronic ischemic left ventricular dysfunction. *J Am Coll Cardiol* 46:1264–1269, 2005.
75. Tarakji KG, Brunken R, McCarthy PM, et al: Myocardial viability testing and the effect of early intervention in patients with advanced left ventricular systolic dysfunction. *Circulation* 113:230–237, 2006.
76. Hillis LD, Smith PK, Anderson JL, et al: 2011 ACCF/AHA guideline for coronary artery bypass graft surgery: executive summary: a report of the American College of Cardiology Foundation/American Heart Association Task Force on Practice Guidelines. *J Thorac Cardiovasc Surg* 143:4–34, 2012.
77. Koelling TM, Aaronson KD, Cody RJ, et al: Prognostic significance of mitral regurgitation and tricuspid regurgitation in patients with left ventricular systolic dysfunction. *Am Heart J* 144:524–529, 2002.
78. Mullens W, Abrahams Z, Skouri HN, et al: Prognostic evaluation of ambulatory patients with advanced heart failure. *Am J Cardiol* 101:1297–1302, 2008.
79. Braunwald E: *Heart disease: a textbook of cardiovascular medicine*, Philadelphia, 1980, Saunders, pp 1095–1165.
80. Jimenez JH, Soerensen DD, He Z, et al: Effects of a saddle shaped annulus on mitral valve function and chordal force distribution: an in vitro study. *Ann Biomed Eng* 31:1171–1181, 2003.
81. Nielsen SL, Nygaard H, Mandrup L, et al: Mechanism of incomplete mitral leaflet coaptation–interaction of chordal restraint and changes in mitral leaflet coaptation geometry. Insight from in vitro validation of the premise of force equilibrium. *J Biomech Eng* 124:596–608, 2002.
82. Karagiannis SE, Karatasakis GT, Koutsogiannis N, et al: Increased distance between mitral valve coaptation point and mitral annular plane: significance and correlations in patients with heart failure. *Heart* 89:1174–1178, 2003.
83. He S, Fontaine AA, Schwammenthal E, et al: Integrated mechanism for functional mitral regurgitation: leaflet restriction versus coapting force: in vitro studies. *Circulation* 96:1826–1834, 1997.
84. Trichon BH, O'Connor CM: Secondary mitral and tricuspid regurgitation accompanying left ventricular systolic dysfunction: is it important, and how is it treated? *Am Heart J* 144:373–376, 2002.
85. Mehra MR, Uber PA, Francis GS: Heart failure therapy at a crossroad: are there limits to the neurohormonal model? *J Am Coll Cardiol* 41:1606–1610, 2003.
86. Ahmed MI, Aban I, Lloyd SG, et al: A randomized controlled phase IIb trial of beta(1)-receptor blockade for chronic degenerative mitral regurgitation. *J Am Coll Cardiol* 60:833–838, 2012.
87. Cleland JG, Daubert JC, Erdmann E, et al: The effect of cardiac resynchronization on morbidity and mortality in heart failure. *N Engl J Med* 352:1539–1549, 2005.
88. Vanderheyden M, Mullens W, Delrue L, et al: Myocardial gene expression in heart failure patients treated with cardiac resynchronization therapy responders versus nonresponders. *J Am Coll Cardiol* 51:129–136, 2008.
89. Bolling SF, Deeb GM, Brunsting LA, et al: Early outcome of mitral valve reconstruction in patients with end-stage cardiomyopathy. *J Thorac Cardiovasc Surg* 109:676–682, discussion 682–683, 1995.
90. Romano MA, Bolling SF: Update on mitral repair in dilated cardiomyopathy. *J Card Surg* 19:396–400, 2004.
91. Bishay ES, McCarthy PM, Cosgrove DM, et al: Mitral valve surgery in patients with severe left ventricular dysfunction. *Eur J Cardiothorac Surg* 17:213–221, 2000.
92. Acker MA, Bolling S, Shemin R, et al: Mitral valve surgery in heart failure: insights from the Acorn Clinical Trial. *J Thorac Cardiovasc Surg* 132:568–577, 577.e1–577.e4, 2006.
93. Wu AH, Aaronson KD, Bolling SF, et al: Impact of mitral valve annuloplasty on mortality risk in patients with mitral regurgitation and left ventricular systolic dysfunction. *J Am Coll Cardiol* 45:381–387, 2005.
94. Jessup M, Abraham WT, Casey DE, et al: 2009 focused update: ACCF/AHA Guidelines for the Diagnosis and Management of Heart Failure in Adults: a report of the American College of Cardiology Foundation/American Heart Association Task Force on Practice Guidelines: developed in collaboration with the International Society for Heart and Lung Transplantation. *Circulation* 119:1977–2016, 2009.
95. Lindenfeld J, Albert NM, Boehmer JP, et al: HFSA 2010 comprehensive heart failure practice guideline. *J Card Fail* 16:e1–e194, 2010.
96. Alfieri O, Maisano F, De Bonis M, et al: The double-orifice technique in mitral valve repair: a simple solution for complex problems. *J Thorac Cardiovasc Surg* 122:674–681, 2001.
97. Feldman T, Wasserman HS, Herrmann HC, et al: Percutaneous mitral valve repair using the edge-to-edge technique: six-month results of the EVEREST Phase I Clinical Trial. *J Am Coll Cardiol* 46:2134–2140, 2005.
98. Feldman T, Foster E, Glower DD, et al: Percutaneous repair or surgery for mitral regurgitation. *N Engl J Med* 364:1395–1406, 2011.
99. Chan KM, Punjabi PP, Flather M, et al: Coronary artery bypass surgery with or without mitral valve annuloplasty in moderate functional ischemic mitral regurgitation: final results of the Randomized Ischemic Mitral Evaluation (RIME) trial. *Circulation* 126:2502–2510, 2012.
100. Fattouch K, Guccione F, Sampognaro R, et al: POINT: Efficacy of adding mitral valve restrictive annuloplasty to coronary artery bypass grafting in patients with moderate ischemic mitral valve regurgitation: a randomized trial. *J Thorac Cardiovasc Surg* 138:278–285, 2009.
101. Aklog L, Filsoufi F, Flores KQ, et al: Does coronary artery bypass grafting alone correct moderate ischemic mitral regurgitation? *Circulation* 104:I68–I75, 2001.
102. Diodato MD, Moon MR, Pasque MK, et al: Repair of ischemic mitral regurgitation does not increase mortality or improve long-term survival in patients undergoing coronary artery revascularization: a propensity analysis. *Ann Thorac Surg* 78:794–799, discussion 794–799, 2004.
103. Mihaljevic T, Lam BK, Rajeswaran J, et al: Impact of mitral valve annuloplasty combined with revascularization in patients with functional ischemic mitral regurgitation. *J Am Coll Cardiol* 49:2191–2201, 2007.
104. Acker MA, Parides MK, Perrault LP, et al: Mitral-valve repair versus replacement for severe ischemic mitral regurgitation. *N Engl J Med* 370:23–32, 2014.
105. Nath J, Foster E, Heidenreich PA: Impact of tricuspid regurgitation on long-term survival. *J Am Coll Cardiol* 43:405–409, 2004.
106. McCarthy PM, Bhudia SK, Rajeswaran J, et al: Tricuspid valve repair: durability and risk factors for failure. *J Thorac Cardiovasc Surg* 127:674–685, 2004.
107. Fukuda S, Song JM, Gillinov AM, et al: Tricuspid valve tethering predicts residual tricuspid regurgitation after tricuspid annuloplasty. *Circulation* 111:975–979, 2005.
108. Koppers G, Verhaert D, Verbrugge FH, et al: Clinical outcomes after tricuspid valve annuloplasty in addition to mitral valve surgery. *Congest Heart Fail* 19:70–76, 2013.
109. Villari B, Vassalli G, Betocchi S, et al: Normalization of left ventricular nonuniformity late after valve replacement for aortic stenosis. *Am J Cardiol* 78:66–71, 1996.
110. Lund O, Flo C, Jensen FT, et al: Left ventricular systolic and diastolic function in aortic stenosis. Prognostic value after valve replacement and underlying mechanisms. *Eur Heart J* 18:1977–1987, 1997.
111. Connolly HM, Oh JK, Orszulak TA, et al: Aortic valve replacement for aortic stenosis with severe left ventricular dysfunction. Prognostic indicators. *Circulation* 95:2395–2400, 1997.
112. Pereira JJ, Lauer MS, Bashir M, et al: Survival after aortic valve replacement for severe aortic stenosis with low transvalvular gradients and severe left ventricular dysfunction. *J Am Coll Cardiol* 39:1356–1363, 2002.
113. Khot UN, Novaro GM, Popovic ZB, et al: Nitroprusside in critically ill patients with left ventricular dysfunction and aortic stenosis. *N Engl J Med* 348:1756–1763, 2003.
114. Makkar RR, Fontana GP, Jilaihawi H, et al: Transcatheter aortic-valve replacement for inoperable severe aortic stenosis. *N Engl J Med* 366:1696–1704, 2012.
115. Kodali SK, Williams MR, Smith CR, et al: Two-year outcomes after transcatheter or surgical aortic-valve replacement. *N Engl J Med* 366:1686–1695, 2012.
116. Bonow RO, Lakatos E, Maron BJ, et al: Serial long-term assessment of the natural history of asymptomatic patients with chronic aortic regurgitation and normal left ventricular systolic function. *Circulation* 84:1625–1635, 1991.
117. Chaliki HP, Mohty D, Avierinos JF, et al: Outcomes after aortic valve replacement in patients with severe aortic regurgitation and markedly reduced left ventricular function. *Circulation* 106:2687–2693, 2002.
118. Daniel WG, Hood WP, Jr, Siart A, et al: Chronic aortic regurgitation: reassessment of the prognostic value of preoperative left ventricular end-systolic dimension and fractional shortening. *Circulation* 71:669–680, 1985.
119. Carabello BA, Usher BW, Hendrix GH, et al: Predictors of outcome for aortic valve replacement in patients with aortic regurgitation and left ventricular dysfunction: a change in the measuring stick. *J Am Coll Cardiol* 10:991–997, 1987.

120. Carabello BA: Is it ever too late to operate on the patient with valvular heart disease? *J Am Coll Cardiol* 44:376–383, 2004.
121. Bonow RO, Carabello BA, Chatterjee K, et al: 2008 Focused update incorporated into the ACC/AHA 2006 guidelines for the management of patients with valvular heart disease: a report of the American College of Cardiology/American Heart Association Task Force on Practice Guidelines (Writing Committee to Revise the 1998 Guidelines for the Management of Patients with Valvular Heart Disease): Endorsed by the Society of Cardiovascular Anesthesiologists, Society for Cardiovascular Angiography and Interventions, and Society of Thoracic Surgeons. *Circulation* 118:e523–e661, 2008.
122. Cooley DA, Henly WS, Amad KH, et al: Ventricular aneurysm following myocardial infarction: results of surgical treatment. *Ann Surg* 150:595–612, 1959.
123. Di Donato M, Sabatier M, Toso A, et al: Regional myocardial performance of non-ischaemic zones remote from anterior wall left ventricular aneurysm. Effects of aneurysmectomy. *Eur Heart J* 16:1285–1292, 1995.
124. Dor V: Left ventricular reconstruction: the aim and the reality after twenty years. *J Thorac Cardiovasc Surg* 128:17–20, 2004.
125. Dang AB, Guccione JM, Zhang P, et al: Effect of ventricular size and patch stiffness in surgical anterior ventricular restoration: a finite element model study. *Ann Thorac Surg* 79:185–193, 2005.
126. Favaloro RG, Effler DB, Groves LK, et al: Ventricular aneurysm–clinical experience. *Ann Thorac Surg* 6:227–245, 1968.
127. Effects of enalapril on mortality in severe congestive heart failure. Results of the Cooperative North Scandinavian Enalapril Survival Study (CONSENSUS). The CONSENSUS Trial Study Group. *N Engl J Med* 316:1429–1435, 1987.
128. Konstam MA, Rousseau MF, Kronenberg MW, et al: Effects of the angiotensin converting enzyme inhibitor enalapril on the long-term progression of left ventricular dysfunction in patients with heart failure. SOLVD Investigators. *Circulation* 86:431–438, 1992.
129. Gaudron P, Eilles C, Kugler I, et al: Progressive left ventricular dysfunction and remodeling after myocardial infarction. Potential mechanisms and early predictors. *Circulation* 87:755–763, 1993.
130. Cohn JN: Structural basis for heart failure. Ventricular remodeling and its pharmacological inhibition. *Circulation* 91:2504–2507, 1995.
131. St John Sutton M, Pfeffer MA, Moye L, et al: Cardiovascular death and left ventricular remodeling two years after myocardial infarction: baseline predictors and impact of long-term use of captopril: information from the Survival and Ventricular Enlargement (SAVE) trial. *Circulation* 96:3294–3299, 1997.
132. Mills NL, Everson CT, Hockmuth DR: Technical advances in the treatment of left ventricular aneurysm. *Ann Thorac Surg* 55:792–800, 1993.
133. Cox JL: Left ventricular aneurysms: pathophysiologic observations and standard resection. *Semin Thorac Cardiovasc Surg* 9:113–122, 1997.
134. Cox JL: Surgical management of left ventricular aneurysms: a clarification of the similarities and differences between the Jatene and Dor techniques. *Semin Thorac Cardiovasc Surg* 9:131–138, 1997.
135. Shapira OM, Davidoff R, Hilkert RJ, et al: Repair of left ventricular aneurysm: long-term results of linear repair versus endoaneurysmorrhaphy. *Ann Thorac Surg* 63:701–705, 1997.
136. Mangschau A: Akinetic versus dyskinetic left ventricular aneurysms diagnosed by gated scintigraphy: difference in surgical outcome. *Ann Thorac Surg* 47:746–751, 1989.
137. Dor V, Sabatier M, Di Donato M, et al: Late hemodynamic results after left ventricular patch repair associated with coronary grafting in patients with postinfarction akinetic or dyskinetic aneurysm of the left ventricle. *J Thorac Cardiovasc Surg* 110:1291–1299, discussion 1300–1301, 1995.
138. Di Donato M, Sabatier M, Dor V, et al: Akinetic versus dyskinetic postinfarction scar: relation to surgical outcome in patients undergoing endoventricular circular patch plasty repair. *J Am Coll Cardiol* 29:1569–1575, 1997.
139. Dor V: Left ventricular aneurysms: the endoventricular circular patch plasty. *Semin Thorac Cardiovasc Surg* 9:123–130, 1997.
140. Dor V, Sabatier M, Di Donato M, et al: Efficacy of endoventricular patch plasty in large postinfarction akinetic scar and severe left ventricular dysfunction: comparison with a series of large dyskinetic scars. *J Thorac Cardiovasc Surg* 116:50–59, 1998.
141. Di Donato M, Sabatier M, Dor V, et al: Effects of the Dor procedure on left ventricular dimension and shape and geometric correlates of mitral regurgitation one year after surgery. *J Thorac Cardiovasc Surg* 121:91–96, 2001.
142. Dor V, Sabatier M, Montiglio F, et al: Endoventricular patch reconstruction of ischemic failing ventricle. A single center with 20 years experience. Advantages of magnetic resonance imaging assessment. *Heart Fail Rev* 9:269–286, 2004.
143. Batista RJ, Santos JL, Takeshita N, et al: Partial left ventriculectomy to improve left ventricular function in end-stage heart disease. *J Card Surg* 11:96–97, discussion 98, 1996.
144. Jones RH, Velazquez EJ, Michler RE, et al: Coronary bypass surgery with or without surgical ventricular reconstruction. *N Engl J Med* 360:1705–1717, 2009.
145. Batista RJ, Verde J, Nery P, et al: Partial left ventriculectomy to treat end-stage heart disease. *Ann Thorac Surg* 64:634–638, 1997.
146. Angelini GD, Pryn S, Mehta D, et al: Left-ventricular-volume reduction for end-stage heart failure. *Lancet* 350:489, 1997.
147. Etoch SW, Koenig SC, Laureano MA, et al: Results after partial left ventriculectomy versus heart transplantation for idiopathic cardiomyopathy. *J Thorac Cardiovasc Surg* 117:952–959, 1999.
148. Franco-Cereceda A, McCarthy PM, Blackstone EH, et al: Partial left ventriculectomy for dilated cardiomyopathy: is this an alternative to transplantation? *J Thorac Cardiovasc Surg* 121:879–893, 2001.
149. Gradinac S, Miric M, Popovic Z, et al: Partial left ventriculectomy for idiopathic dilated cardiomyopathy: early results and six-month follow-up. *Ann Thorac Surg* 66:1963–1968, 1998.
150. Starling RC, McCarthy PM, Buda T, et al: Results of partial left ventriculectomy for dilated cardiomyopathy: hemodynamic, clinical and echocardiographic observations. *J Am Coll Cardiol* 36:2098–2103, 2000.
151. Acker MA: Dynamic cardiomyoplasty: at the crossroads. *Ann Thorac Surg* 68:750–755, 1999.
152. Kass DA, Baughman KL, Pak PH, et al: Reverse remodeling from cardiomyoplasty in human heart failure. External constraint versus active assist. *Circulation* 91:2314–2318, 1995.
153. Leier CV: Cardiomyoplasty: is it time to wrap it up? *J Am Coll Cardiol* 28:1181–1182, 1996.
154. Mann DL, Acker MA, Jessup M, et al: Rationale, design, and methods for a pivotal randomized clinical trial for the assessment of a cardiac support device in patients with New York health association class III-IV heart failure. *J Card Fail* 10:185–192, 2004.
155. Starling RC, Jessup M, Oh JK, et al: Sustained benefits of the CorCap Cardiac Support Device on left ventricular remodeling: three year follow-up results from the Acorn clinical trial. *Ann Thorac Surg* 84:1236–1242, 2007.
156. Grossi EA, Saunders PC, Woo YJ, et al: Intraoperative effects of the Coapsys annuloplasty system in a randomized evaluation (RESTOR-MV) of functional ischemic mitral regurgitation. *Ann Thorac Surg* 80:1706–1711, 2005.
157. Yoon DY, Smedira NG, Nowicki ER, et al: Decision support in surgical management of ischemic cardiomyopathy. *J Thorac Cardiovasc Surg* 139(2):283–293, 2010.

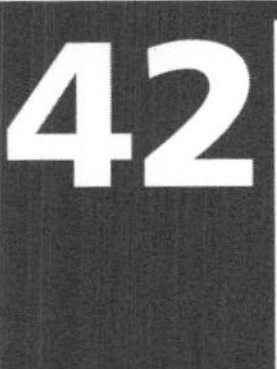

Circulatory Assist Devices in Heart Failure

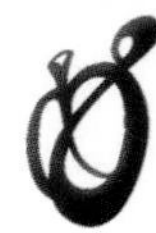

Gregory A. Ewald, Carmelo A. Milano, and Joseph G. Rogers

Management of advanced heart failure is often less evidence-based than management of earlier stages of disease. Few clinical trials have targeted this population; and by definition, these patients are failing contemporary medical and electrical heart failure therapies. Knowledge accumulation has been hampered by lack of a standardized definition of "advanced" heart failure. The European Society of Cardiology developed a framework to identify patients with advanced heart failure that integrates key domains including (1) New York Heart Association (NYHA) class III-IV symptoms; (2) episodic evidence of volume overload or hypoperfusion; (3) evidence of severe left ventricular (LV) dysfunction, including an ejection fraction less than 30%, invasive or noninvasive evidence of abnormal ventricular filling, elevated intracardiac filling pressures, or elevated B-type natriuretic peptide; (4) impaired functional capacity based on a 6-minute walk distance less than 300 m or a maximal oxygen consumption less than 12 to 14 mL/kg/min; (5) at least one hospitalization in the past 6 months; and (6) the above occurring in the setting of optimal therapies.[1] The size of the population that fulfills the definition of "advanced" heart failure is unknown but may exceed 250,000 in the United States (**see also Chapter 17**).[2] However, the morbidity and mortality associated with advanced heart failure are clear: 4-month readmission rates approximate 50% and the annualized mortality is 80% to 90%.[3-6]

Patients with advanced heart failure have limited therapeutic options. Positive inotropic agents may be used to stabilize patients with hemodynamic compromise or cardiogenic shock (**see also Chapter 33**), but longer-term use of these drugs is associated with 6-month mortality rates that exceed 50%.[3,7] Cardiac transplantation (**see also Chapter 40**) is offered to a highly selected cohort that distinguishes itself as younger with less comorbidity than the larger advanced heart failure population. Further, transplantation is limited to approximately 2200 patients annually in the United States and less than 4000 worldwide.[8] The limitations of transplantation in terms of the clinician's ability to provide acute therapy coupled with the limited supply of donor organs provides the rationale for alternatives such as mechanically assisted circulation.

In this chapter, we will discuss the role of mechanical therapies designed to improve cardiac output and lower cardiac filling pressures in patients with acute and chronic advanced systolic heart failure. In the past decade, this strategy has gained wide acceptance as an important approach to the care of advanced heart failure patients.

ACUTE CARDIOGENIC SHOCK

Acute cardiogenic shock remains an important cause of cardiovascular morbidity and mortality. Most commonly, cardiogenic shock results from LV failure following acute myocardial infarction (MI) or from a mechanical complication following MI such as ventricular septal defect or mitral insufficiency as a result of papillary muscle rupture (**see also Chapter 18**).[9] However, other conditions may present with similarly deranged hemodynamics, such as acute myocarditis (**see also Chapter 26**), giant cell myocarditis, or acute aortic insufficiency (**see also Chapter 24**). Postcardiotomy shock has been reported as a complication of cardiac surgery in 0.2% to 6% of cases (**see also Chapter 41**) and is associated with high short-term mortality risk without mechanically assisted circulation.[10]

Despite important advances in coronary reperfusion, including a focus on early intervention, acute cardiogenic shock following myocardial infarction remains associated with high short-term mortality. The SHOCK II-IABP trial examined the impact of the intra-aortic balloon pump (IABP) in patients with clinically diagnosed cardiogenic shock following acute MI. The 30-day mortality rate was 40% in both the IABP and medical therapy arms of the trial despite revascularization and contemporary adjuvant medical therapy.[11]

The general approach to acute cardiogenic shock includes rapid integration of clinical information targeted at determining the cause of the condition and the severity of hemodynamic compromise that is subsequently linked

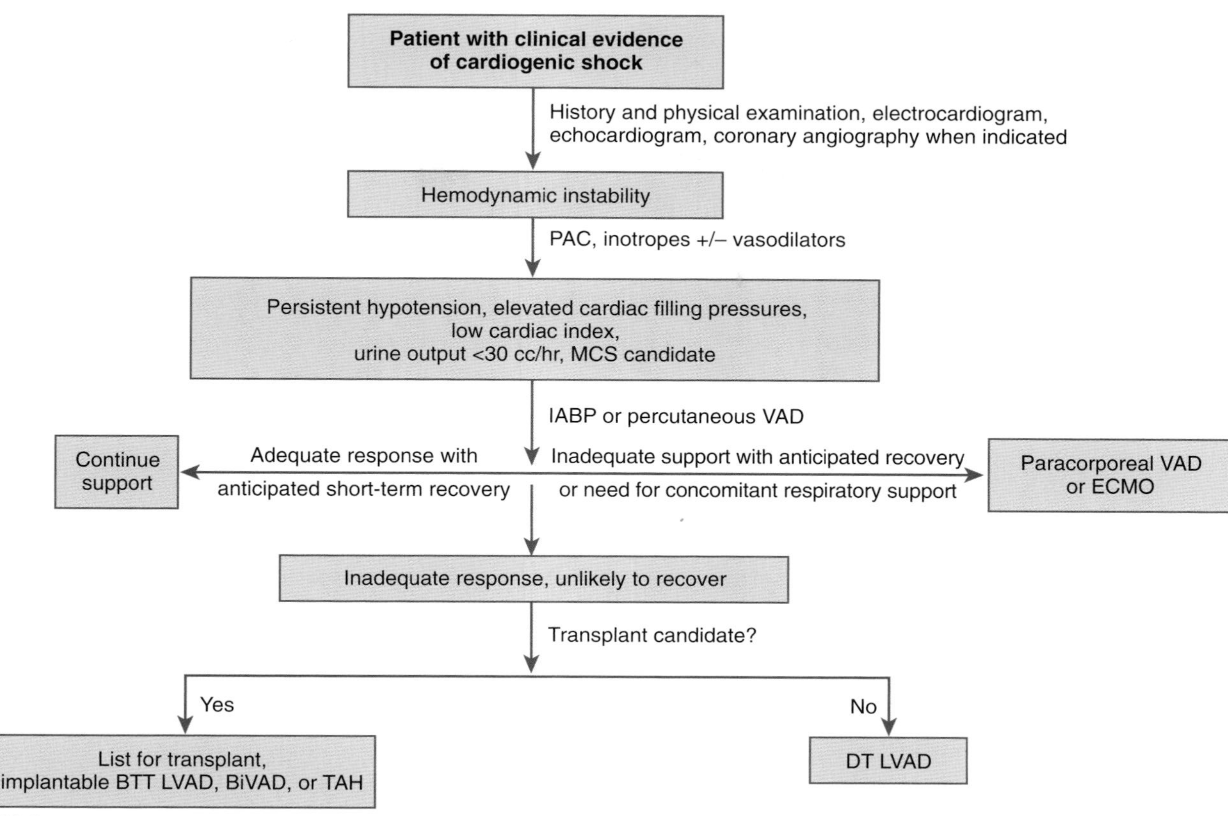

FIGURE 42-1 Approach to the patient with cardiogenic shock using multimodality diagnostics and therapeutics. *BiVAD,* Biventricular assist device; *BTT,* bridge to transplant; *DT,* destination therapy; *ECMO,* extracorporeal membrane oxygenator; *IABP,* intra-aortic balloon pump; *MCS,* mechanically assisted circulation; *PAC,* pulmonary artery catheter; *TAH,* total artificial heart; *VAD,* ventricular assist device.

to a therapy that addresses the physiologic needs of the individual patient (**Figure 42-1**). A directed history and physical examination and electrocardiogram are critical elements of the evaluation and should be rapidly obtained. If the cause or severity of the heart failure is not evident following the above, echocardiography and/or coronary angiography should be performed to evaluate ventricular and valvular function. Endomyocardial biopsy should also be considered in new-onset, nonischemic cardiomyopathy but should probably be limited to centers with expertise in the performance of the procedure and interpretation of the histology.[12]

Initial interventions should include appropriate volume resuscitation, vasodilators in selected patients, and inotropic agents if the patient remains in shock. Placement of a pulmonary artery catheter (see also Chapters 31 and 33) has been advocated to guide volume administration and vasoactive drug therapy.[13] Mechanical circulatory support should be considered in patients with persistent evidence of shock despite the above interventions. Device selection should be tailored to each patient's unique hemodynamic abnormalities, as well as the need for univentricular or biventricular and respiratory support.

Devices

IABP

Over the past 50 years, the IABP has been the most commonly used mechanical circulatory support device. The IABP is generally inserted retrograde in the aorta via the femoral artery and positioned with the distal tip just beyond the left subclavian artery (**Figure 42-2**). Balloon filling is triggered from the electrocardiogram (ECG) and inflates during diastole and deflates during systole. The favorable physiologic effects of diastolic augmentation include enhanced coronary blood flow and reduced left ventricular afterload.[14]

The effectiveness of the IABP is highly dependent on proper timing of the balloon inflation and deflation (**Figure 42-3**).[15] Optimal timing results in IABP inflation just after the dicrotic notch in the aortic pressure tracing and deflation before the pressure upstroke of ventricular systole. The hemodynamic and physiologic benefits of IABP support include elevation of systemic blood pressure relative to unassisted beats, and reduction of LV afterload, LV wall stress, and myocardial oxygen demand.[14,16] Inappropriate timing with early inflation or late deflation results in the balloon expansion during ventricular systole increasing the afterload against which the ventricle is ejecting. Late balloon inflation or early deflation limits the hemodynamic benefits of the therapy.[15] The hemodynamic effectiveness of the IABP may be limited by tachycardia, such as atrial fibrillation with rapid ventricular response. More than mild aortic valve insufficiency is likely to limit the hemodynamic benefits of IABP therapy by increasing LV loading and is a contraindication to therapy. Significant aortic or iliofemoral atherosclerotic disease is also a relative contraindication to IABP support and has led some to propose

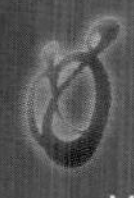

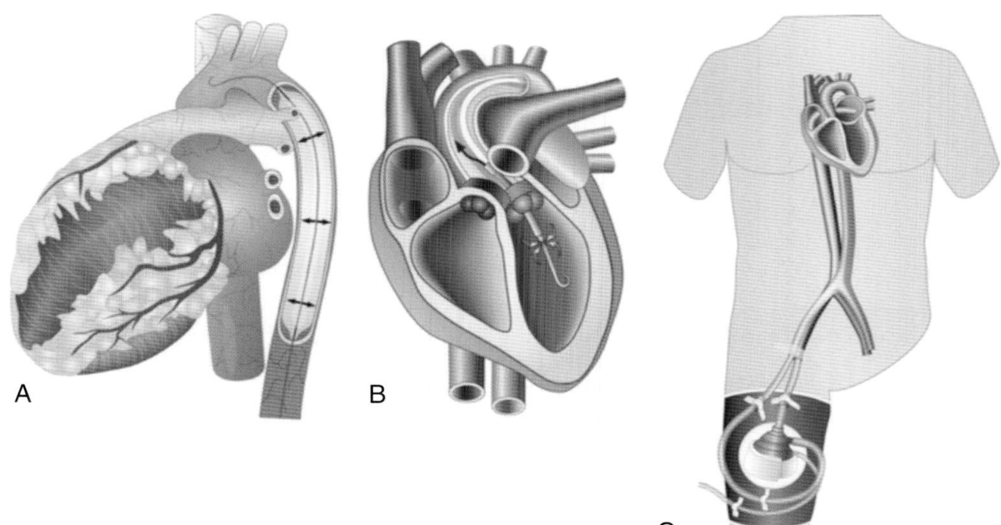

FIGURE 42-2 Percutaneous devices for mechanically assisted circulation. The intra-aortic balloon pump **(A)** is inserted retrograde in the aorta and functions as a counterpulsation device with balloon inflation during diastole and deflation during systole. The Impella **(B)** is a microaxial flow device that is inserted across the aortic valve and withdraws blood from the left ventricle and delivers it in to the aortic root. The TandemHeart **(C)** is a paracorporeal centrifugal flow pump that withdraws blood from the left atrium via a transseptal catheter and returns blood to the iliofemoral system. *From Desai NR, Bhatt DL: Evaluating percutaneous support for cardiogenic shock: data shock and sticker shock. Eur Heart J 30:2073–2075, 2009.*

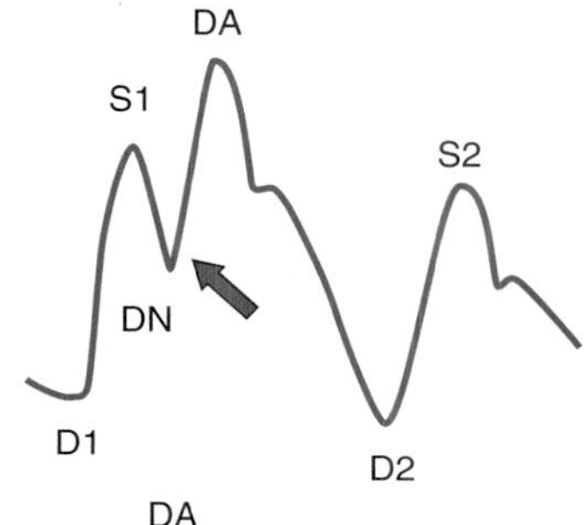

Normal timing of the IABP (arrow) with inflation at the dicrotic notch (DN) and good diastolic augmentation (DA). Unassisted end-diastolic pressure (D1) is higher than assisted end-diastolic pressure (D2). Assisted peak systolic pressure (S2) is lower than unassisted peak systolic pressure (S1).

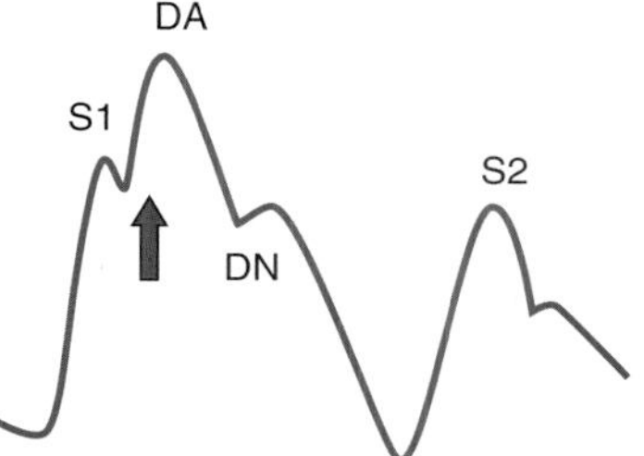

Early inflation—rapid rise in diastolic pressure with dicrotic notch after IABP deflation; causes increased afterload.

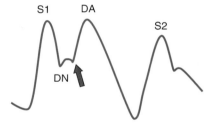

Late inflation—prolonged dip before a decreased diastolic augmentation reduces effectiveness.

FIGURE 42-3 Appropriate and inappropriate timing of intra-aortic balloon pump (IABP). *From Santa-Cruz RA, Cohen MG, Ohman EM: Aortic counterpulsation: A review of the hemodynamic effects and indications for use. Cathet Cardiovasc Interv 67:68–77, 2006.*

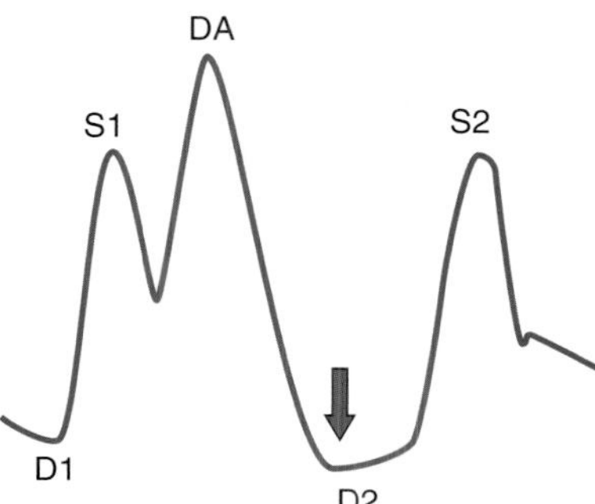

Early deflation—prolonged dip of assisted end-diastolic pressure and no decrease in assisted systolic pressure; no afterload reduction.

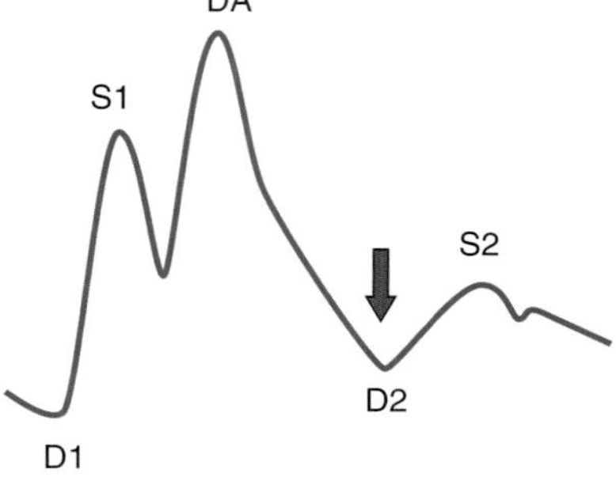

Late deflation—the assisted end-diastolic pressure is higher than the unassisted end-diastolic pressure; causes increased afterload.

alternative insertion strategies, including subclavian artery or direct aortic access used in the context of cardiac surgery.[17]

The IABP has been used as an adjunctive therapy for many cardiac conditions, including acute myocardial infarction, ruptured VSD, acute mitral insufficiency with compromised hemodynamics, and cardiogenic shock.[18] However, improved outcomes with IABP therapy in clinical trials have been difficult to demonstrate. Perhaps the most validated use of the IABP is as adjunctive therapy for the treatment of acute myocardial infarction treated with thrombolytic therapy. In this setting, the use of prophylactic IABP was shown to be associated with an 18% reduction in all-cause mortality.[19] As noted above, the SHOCK II-IABP trial failed to demonstrate improved survival in a cohort of patients with acute MI and cardiogenic shock treated with IABP compared with those supported medically.[11]

The limitations of the IABP coupled with a lack of positive outcome studies has resulted in the proliferation of other percutaneous approaches for the treatment of cardiogenic shock and support of complex cardiac procedures, such as high-risk percutaneous coronary interventions and ventricular tachycardia ablations. These devices, which are designed to increase cardiac output and lower intracardiac filling pressures, can be rapidly inserted and are approved for short-term (hours) support.

TandemHeart

The TandemHeart (CardiacAssist, Pittsburgh, Pa.) is an extracorporeal centrifugal continuous flow pump that receives blood from a 21F cannula inserted in the femoral vein and passed into the left atrium via a transseptal puncture (see Figure 42-2). The TandemHeart returns the blood to the arterial circulation via a 17F catheter inserted in the iliofemoral system. In this configuration, the device can provide up to 5 L/min of flow and is approved for short-term support. The hemodynamic effects of the TandemHeart were compared with IABP in two small, randomized clinical trials that demonstrated superior improvements in cardiac index and the lowering of intracardiac filling pressures with the TandemHeart pump.[20,21] A nonrandomized, experiential series described the potential benefits of the TandemHeart in patients with cardiogenic shock. In this series, 117 patients with clinical evidence of shock (including almost 50% who were receiving or had just received cardiopulmonary resuscitation) were treated with the device. The median cardiac index increase from 0.5 to 3.0 L/min/m^2 was associated with improvement in serum lactate and creatinine. The 30-day survival in this cohort was 60% and largely dependent on candidacy for another treatment such as implantable left ventricular assist device.[22] Limitations of the TandemHeart device include the transseptal puncture, which adds technical complexity and may require surgical closure if the patient is transitioned to surgical left ventricular assist device (LVAD). In addition, the 17F arterial cannula in the femoral artery can result in limb ischemia and often requires surgical closure.

Impella

This miniaturized, microaxial flow pump is incorporated into a catheter-based technology and is available in several sizes capable of producing flows from 2.5 to 5.0 L/min (see Figure 42-2). The smaller Impella (ABIOMED, Danvers, Mass.) pumps (9F) can be inserted percutaneously via the femoral artery, whereas the larger device capable of greater blood flow requires surgical implantation techniques. Impella withdraws blood from the distal port in the LV and delivers it to the ascending aorta. This device has been demonstrated to improve cardiac output and reduce left ventricular filling pressures to a greater degree than IABP.[23] Impella 2.5 was compared to IABP in 452 patients with LV dysfunction undergoing percutaneous intervention for complex three-vessel disease or left main coronary artery disease.[24] The primary endpoint of the trial was intraprocedural and postprocedural major adverse events, including death, MI, stroke/transient ischemic attack, repeat coronary revascularization, lower extremity vascular injury, acute renal failure, intraprocedural hypotension, cardiopulmonary resuscitation, or ventricular tachycardia requiring cardioversion, aortic insufficiency, and angiographic failure of the PCI. Enrollment in this trial was halted prematurely because the primary endpoint was no different between study groups. The Impella-treated cohort had a significant improvement in cardiac power output. Impella 5.0 was also recently studied in a prospective registry that included 16 patients with postcardiotomy shock.[25] Following implantation, the mean arterial pressure increased by 12 mm Hg and the mean cardiac index increased from 1.65 to 2.7 L/min/m^2. There were two primary safety events in this study, one stroke and one death, and the 30- and 180-day survival rates were 94% and 81%, respectively. Finally, the Impella EUROSHOCK Registry retrospectively examined 120 patients with cardiogenic shock following a myocardial infarction treated with Impella 2.5.[26] Less than half of the patients were able to be weaned from support with an associated 30-day mortality rate of 64%. Further, 15% of the patients experienced a major cardiac or cerebrovascular adverse event.

The design of Impella has been reconfigured to allow percutaneous right-sided support. The Impella RP features a 22F pump mounted on an 11F catheter that withdraws blood from the right atrial/inferior vena caval junction and delivers the blood to the pulmonary artery. It is currently undergoing clinical trial as a strategy to treat acute right heart failure resulting from acute MI, postcardiotomy syndrome, or following cardiac transplant or left-sided mechanical circulatory support.

PHP

The PHP (Thoratec, Pleasanton, Calif.) device is a small catheter-based microaxial flow pump that is conceptually similar to Impella. It is a 12F catheter capable of providing 4 to 4.5 L/min of flow. There is limited clinical experience with this device but it is being tested in a randomized, controlled clinical trial versus the IABP in patients with cardiogenic shock.

Extracorporeal Membrane Oxygenation

Extracorporeal membrane oxygenation (ECMO) is a temporary strategy to provide circulatory and/or respiratory support to critically ill patients. The ECMO circuit consists of a cannula inserted either percutaneously or centrally in the venous system for device inflow. A centrifugal flow pump moves the blood through an oxygenator and returns it to the body via a cannula placed in the arterial system (venoarterial ECMO for cardiorespiratory failure) or to the venous system (venovenous ECMO for respiratory failure). Flow rates of 4 to 6 L/minute are typical for most adult patients. ECMO can be initiated rapidly, and peripheral cannulation allows its use in many settings, including the cardiac catheterization laboratory, the intensive care unit, and the operating room. In the setting of cardiogenic shock, establishing hemodynamic stability with ECMO allows time to assess cardiopulmonary recovery and improvement in end-organ function. ECMO is generally considered useful for short periods of time (days to weeks). An important complication of peripheral ECMO that limits longer term benefit is a lack of direct LV unloading, with resultant ventricular distention and pulmonary venous hypertension. Further, extended support is undesirable as the patient is typically confined to bed and the incidence of adverse events including bleeding, hemolysis, thrombocytopenia, limb ischemia, vascular injury, and stroke are related to the duration of support. Thus, after stabilization of the patient for a brief period of time, the clinical team must decide on the next step in the patient's care. In some cases, ECMO can be weaned and the patient separated from the system. In other cases, it is a bridge to another procedure, including permanent mechanical circulatory support or transplantation. There are limited outcomes data examining the role of ECMO for the treatment of heart failure, and much of the reported literature is from single centers and small experiences.[27] Survival following ECMO support appears to be strongly related to the underlying cause of the ventricular dysfunction, with myocarditis patients having better outcomes than patients with postcardiotomy syndrome or those who experienced a cardiac arrest.

INDICATIONS FOR IMPLANTABLE MECHANICAL CIRCULATORY SUPPORT DEVICES

Decision making regarding implantation of durable mechanical circulatory support devices is dependent on the clinical status of the patient and the recognized indications for the therapy defined by clinical trials. Although seemingly congruous, unique aspects of the individual patient often are misaligned with a two-tiered system that artificially defines candidacy based upon candidacy for transplantation.[28] Commonly used clinical nomenclature for mechanically assisted circulation indications will be presented. However, there are only two recognized indications for implantable left ventricular assist devices: as a means to support critically ill patients until they can receive cardiac transplantation (bridge to transplant) or as permanent therapy in nontransplant candidates (destination therapy).

Bridge to bridge is a strategy in which a short-term circulatory support device is used until a more definitive procedure can be performed. This strategy is typically used for patients in cardiogenic shock who require rapid hemodynamic restoration to reverse the shock state and/or improve end-organ function. Device selection depends on the severity of hemodynamic compromise, the presence or absence of biventricular heart failure, and the anticipated duration of this approach. In many cases, the percutaneous devices or ECMO may be used.

Bridge-to-recovery mechanical circulatory support may be used in patients with a disease process anticipated to recover with a period of hemodynamic support, such as acute myocarditis (see also Chapter 26), peripartum cardiomyopathy (see also Chapter 19), cardiac transplant rejection with hemodynamic compromise (see also Chapter 40), or following cardiac surgery (see also Chapter 41). Selection of the most appropriate device typically involves determination of the need to provide partial or full support of the hemodynamics and the projected duration of therapy.

Bridge to decision is the most commonly cited indication by clinicians at the time of device implantation despite its lack of formal recognition by regulators and payers.[29] Transplant candidacy is frequently confounded by potentially reversible comorbidities when the decision for mechanical circulatory support (MCS) is made. The favorable hemodynamic impact of LVAD support, including increased cardiac output and reduction of left-sided filling pressures, improves end-organ function, lowers pulmonary artery pressures, and allows the patient to become physically and nutritionally rehabilitated before consideration of transplantation. However, if the patient does not achieve these milestones he or she may remain on mechanically assisted circulation for prolonged periods of time or indefinitely.

Bridge to transplant (BTT) is reserved for device implantation in patients listed for transplant at high priority (status 1A or 1B) who are failing optimal therapies. Qualification for this priority on the transplant waiting list requires the use of continuous infusion inotropic therapy, mechanical ventilation, or an intra-aortic balloon pump, so by definition this is a high-risk population with deranged hemodynamics and evidence of cardiogenic shock.

Destination therapy (DT) designates LVAD implantation in a patient with advanced heart failure who is ineligible for transplantation. The regulatory and payer DT criteria are aligned with the inclusion criteria from clinical trials and include an ejection fraction less than 25%, NYHA class IIIb-IV symptoms, objective functional impairment with a maximal oxygen consumption of less than 14 mL/kg/min (or <50% predicted), and treatment with either optimal medical therapy for 45 of the past 60 days, IV inotropic support for 14 days, or an intra-aortic balloon pump for 7 days. During deliberations for LVAD financial coverage in the United States, the Center for Medicare and Medicaid Services was unable to agree on the definition of NYHA class IIIb symptoms and subsequently only supports payment for patients with NYHA class IV functional limitations.

PATIENT SELECTION FOR MECHANICAL CIRCULATORY SUPPORT

In general, patients considered for mechanically assisted circulation have severely depressed ventricular function, marked limitation in functional capacity, are treated with evidence-based medical and electrical therapies, and have a high residual mortality risk within the ensuing 1 to 2 years. Patient selection is critically important to achieving optimal postoperative outcomes. Selection criteria should identify patients with sufficient severity of illness to derive benefit from mechanical circulatory support while simultaneously avoiding those with a severity of illness or comorbidities that would compromise survival following implantation. Baseline characteristics of patients enrolled in the HeartMate II BTT and DT trials demonstrated end-organ dysfunction with hyponatremia and elevated serum blood urea nitrogen and creatinine levels.[30,31] In addition, the mean ejection fraction was less than 0.20 with elevated right- and left-sided cardiac filling pressures and mean cardiac index of 2.0 L/min/m^2 despite treatment with continuous infusion intravenous inotropes in 80% to 90% of patients and intra-aortic balloon pump support in 20% to 40%.

Destination therapy was originally conceived as a treatment for patients with end-stage heart failure ineligible for cardiac transplantation. As a result, many of those being referred for DT LVAD are older than 65 years. Older age has been identified as an important predictor of adverse outcomes in the VAD population. The HeartMate II risk score demonstrated an increased postimplant mortality risk of 32% per decade.[32] Data from the Interagency Registry for Mechanically Assisted Circulation (INTERMACS) also described older age as a risk factor for early mortality following LVAD placement and highlighted the important interaction between age and other and risk factors for mortality such as severity of illness.[33] However, carefully selected patients over 70 years appear to derive similar benefits with VAD as a younger cohort,[34] raising the important concept of chronologic versus physiologic age in patient selection. Chronologic age is likely an imperfect surrogate for the true predictors of adverse outcomes in this population, which are more likely measures of frailty and debilitation.[35]

Beyond age, other contraindications to implantable VAD therapy appear to influence short- and long-term outcomes and must be considered in the overall risk assessment of the candidate. INTERMACS developed a new nomenclature for classification of advanced heart failure that has been used to understand the impact of severity of illness on outcomes (**Table 42-1**).[36] Patients with INTERMACS profile 1 and 2 have a high early mortality hazard relative to MCS patients with lesser degrees of hemodynamic compromise, leading many centers to be highly selective in the use of durable implantable LVADs in these patient cohorts.[33]

Right ventricular (RV) failure, defined as the need for prolonged inotropic therapy to support the right heart or a right ventricular assist device, remains an Achilles heel of LVAD therapy and is associated with multisystem organ failure, prolonged hospitalization, and increased morbidity and mortality following LVAD implantation.[37,38] Unfortunately, prediction of post-LVAD RV failure is challenging despite identification of individual parameters and multivariable models that provide insights into the likelihood of RV failure in larger patient populations. Predictors of RV failure following LVAD fall into three general categories: (1) echocardiographic measurements; (2) hemodynamic parameters; and (3) clinical features before LVAD insertion. Increased right ventricular size and severe RV systolic function are associated with post-LVAD RV failure.[39,40] Quantitative measures of RV performance such as a tricuspid annular motion (TAPSE) of less than 7.5 mm, reduced right ventricular peak longitudinal strain, and the severity of tricuspid insufficiency have been shown to be useful markers in the prediction of RV failure after LVAD.[41-43] Hemodynamic variables such as a CVP: PCWP of greater than 0.63 or a right ventricular stroke work index of less than 250 to 300 mm Hg × mL/m^2 are linked to worse outcomes following LVAD placement.[38,44,45] Finally, general clinical features such as preoperative mechanical ventilation and abnormal renal and hepatic function have been identified as risk factors for RV failure.[38,45] Matthews and colleagues derived a multivariable model for predicting RV failure that included abnormal serum creatinine, aspartate aminotransferase, and bilirubin in conjunction with the use of vasopressors. The incremental presence of these was associated with a higher risk for RV failure and death following LVAD.[46]

Renal failure requiring dialysis is considered a strong relative contraindication to durable MCS. Significant renal dysfunction was an exclusion criterion in the clinical trials, so the benefit and potential incremental complications of implanting an LVAD in dialysis patients is unknown. Further, support with newer generation LVADs that provide continuous flow results in a minimal (and often imperceptible) pulse pressure, making measurement of blood pressure difficult during hemodialysis.

Active systemic infection is a strong relative contraindication to LVAD implantation. Patients with fever or unexplained leukocytosis should undergo thorough evaluation, including blood and urine cultures, chest x-ray, and other diagnostic testing directed at potential sites of infection. Hospitalized patients and those with chronic indwelling catheters should have intravenous cannulae removed. Patients with pacing systems and unexplained bacteremia may require chest wall or transesophageal echocardiography to rule out pacemaker-associated endocarditis.

TABLE 42-1 INTERMACS Patient Profiles

ADULT PROFILES	CURRENT CMS DT INDICATION?	IV INOTROPES	OFFICIAL PARLANCE	NYHA CLASS	MODIFIER OPTION
INTERMACS Level 1	Yes	Yes	"Crash and burn"	IV	A, TCS
INTERMACS Level 2	Yes	Yes	"Sliding fast" on inotropes	IV	A, TCS
INTERMACS Level 3	Yes	Yes	"Stable" on inotropes	IV	A, FF, TCS
INTERMACS Level 4	+peak $V_{O_2} \leq 14$	No	Resting symptoms on oral therapy at home	Ambulatory IV	A, FF
INTERMACS Level 5	+peak $V_{O_2} \leq 14$	No	"Housebound," comfortable at rest, symptoms with minimal activity or ADLs	Ambulatory IV	A, FF
INTERMACS Level 6	No	No	"Walking wounded," ADLs possible but meaningful activity limited	IIIb	A, FF
INTERMACS Level 7	No	No	Advanced class III	III	A, FF

A, Arrhythmia; *ADL,* activities of daily living; *CMS,* Centers for Medicare and Medicaid Services; *DT,* destination therapy; *FF,* frequent flier; *IV,* intravenous; *NYHA,* New York Heart Association; *TCS,* temporary circulatory support; V_{O_2}, maximal oxygen consumption.

From Stewart GC, Stevenson LW: Keeping left ventricular assist device acceleration on track. Circulation 123:1559–1568, 2011.

An evaluation for cerebrovascular disease should be performed in at-risk patients using noninvasive imaging.[47] The presence of a prior stroke does not preclude implantation of an LVAD, but consideration must be given to the potential for meaningful rehabilitation and the patient's ability to interact with the device. For example, an individual with hemiparesis of a dominant arm may have difficulty making the electrical connections required to operate the VAD.

Other end-organ dysfunction may also limit favorable outcomes with VAD therapy and should be considered during the evaluation. Individuals with clinically significant chronic obstructive pulmonary disease whose FEV1 is less than 1 L are likely to have residual dyspnea despite hemodynamic improvement and may have difficulty weaning from the ventilator post-operatively. A VE/MVV ratio of more than 80% on a pre-operative cardiopulmonary exercise test suggests a pulmonary component to dyspnea.[48] Patients with long-standing right heart failure or other conditions associated with liver injury should undergo an evaluation for hepatic insufficiency.[49] Serum transaminases, albumin, and imaging studies to examine the texture and contour of the liver may provide insights about the necessity for liver biopsy. The presence of an elevated model for end-stage liver disease (MELD) score has been linked to higher post-LVAD mortality.[50] Careful evaluation of the coagulation system is warranted in individuals with a history of a bleeding diathesis or in those with unexplained thrombotic or thromboembolic events. Patients with a low platelet count and exposure to heparin should be screened for heparin-induced thrombocytopenia with a PF4 antibody and a serotonin release assay.[51] To the extent possible, patients should have a normal coagulation profile before MCS surgery as an elevated international normalized ratio (INR) at the time of LVAD implantation was identified as a risk factor for mortality.[32] Correction of coagulopathy will reduce the likelihood of bleeding complications and associated perioperative morbidity. Malnutrition is considered an important risk factor for adverse outcomes, including infection, prolonged debilitation, and mortality. However, the ability to favorably impact nutrition in a critically ill heart failure patient is unclear. Instead, nutrition management should be a primary focus of the entire VAD team following device implantation.[52] Supplemental enteral feedings may be required perioperatively, with additional support in the outpatient setting until nutritional deficits are corrected.

Disease processes with an anticipated survival of less than 3 years were an exclusion criterion in the DT clinical trials, so there are no data supporting the role for mechanically assisted circulation in the management of these patients.

Psychosocial factors also play a pivotal role in VAD outcomes. As part of the evaluation, patients should be seen by multiple health care providers, including those who focus primarily on prior history of compliance, substance use, health literacy, and the availability and abilities of family and friends who will participate in the ongoing outpatient management of the patient and the device. There is a relatively high caregiver burden with MCS, including the need for device training, care of the percutaneous driveline, and companionship. These issues and expectations need to be clearly articulated by the team and agreed on by the patient and his or her caregivers.

Two multivariable models have been developed to assist the clinician in risk stratification. The Leitz-Miller model was developed in the era of pulsatile LVADs and consisted of nine variables that stratified 1-year survival rates between 10% and 80%.[53] However, in a contemporary cohort of patients managed with a continuous flow LVAD, the Leitz-Miller model did not retain predictive accuracy.[54] The HeartMate II Risk Model was recently published and demonstrated that age, elevated INR, increased serum creatinine, and lower serum albumin were predictive of postimplant mortality.[32]

MECHANICAL CIRCULATORY ASSIST DEVICES

Recent successes in mechanically assisted circulation have resulted in acceptance of this approach as a useful therapy for the treatment of selected patients with advanced heart failure. The INTERMACS registry has captured almost all implants using FDA-approved MCS devices in the United States since 2006, and has carefully documented the growth of this field following the introduction of the new-generation continuous flow devices (**Figure 42-4**).[33] The number of centers implanting long-term devices is increasing and has expanded from the traditional transplant centers to programs that do not perform transplantation. Preliminary evidence suggests that this proliferation has been associated with outcomes similar to more established centers, although low center volume appears to be associated with higher mortality risk.[55]

Mechanical circulatory support devices can be characterized in several ways: temporary versus permanent, intracorporeal versus extracorporeal, and pulsatile versus continuous flow.

Temporary Pulsatile Flow Devices

ABIOMED AB5000

ABIOMED has developed an extracorporeal pulsatile pump for temporary support of the LV, RV, or both ventricles (**Figure 42-5**). The AB5000 pump is designed to lie on the anterior abdominal wall and attach directly to tunneled cannulae that exit the body just inferior to the sternotomy incision. The drainage cannula is placed through pursestring sutures into either the right atrium for right heart drainage or the left atrium or left ventricle for left-sided drainage. The outflow cannula is a 14-mm Hemashield graft that is sutured to either the aorta or the main pulmonary artery for left and right heart support, respectively. The AB5000 is pneumatically actuated to provide compressed air to eject blood from a polyurethane blood chamber. The pump contains prosthetic valves to ensure unidirectional flow. The ABIOMED has been FDA approved for bridge to transplant.

Thoratec PVAD

The Thoratec PVAD can also be configured as a univentricular or biventricular support device (**Figure 42-6**). It is a pulsatile device intended for inpatient use, although it has been less commonly used in the outpatient setting. The device is composed of inflow and outflow cannulae attached to a pump that houses a polyurethane blood sac

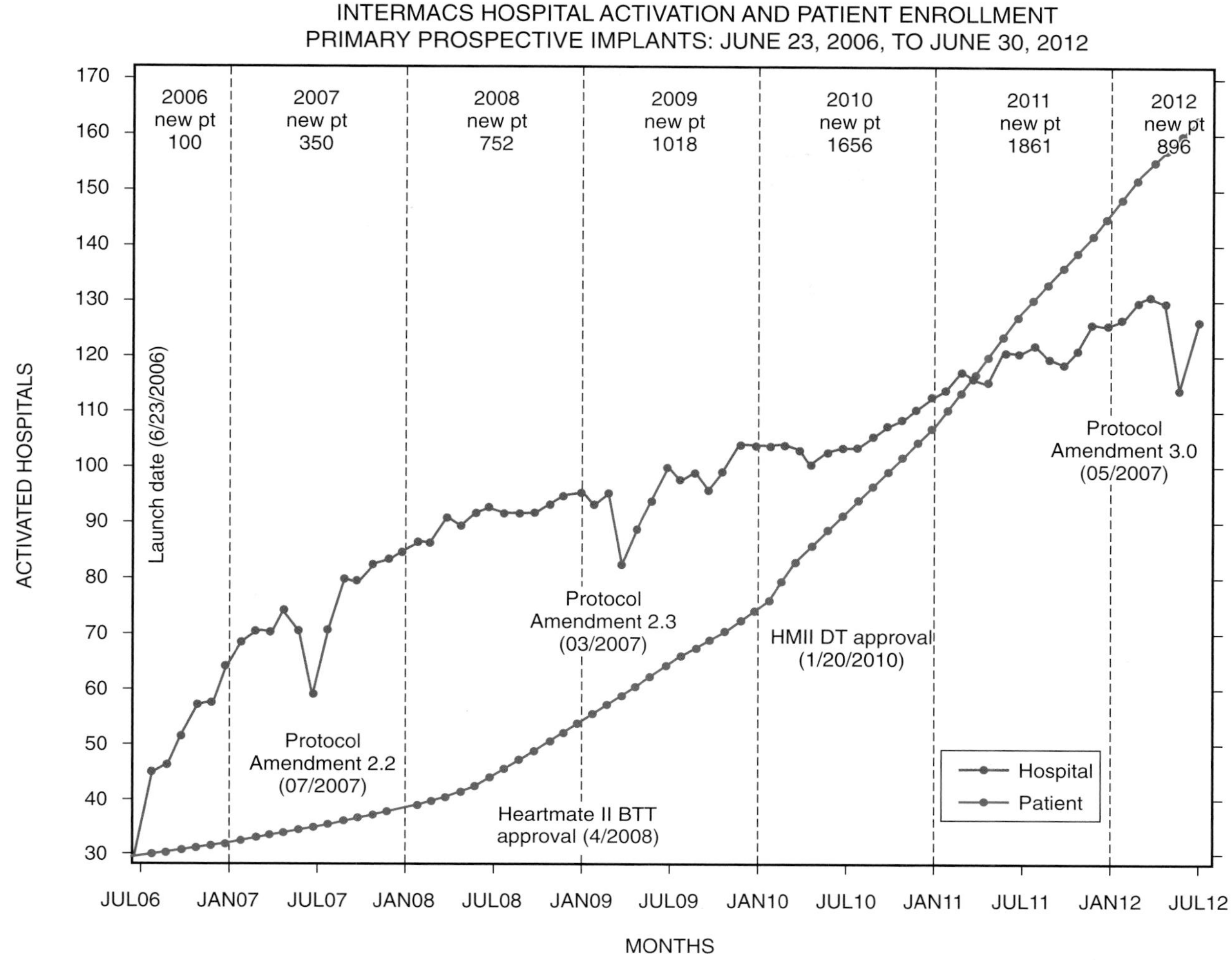

INTERMACS HOSPITAL ACTIVATION AND PATIENT ENROLLMENT
PRIMARY PROSPECTIVE IMPLANTS: JUNE 23, 2006, TO JUNE 30, 2012

2006 new pt 100
2007 new pt 350
2008 new pt 752
2009 new pt 1018
2010 new pt 1656
2011 new pt 1861
2012 new pt 896

ACTIVATED HOSPITALS
170
160
150
140
130
120
110
100
90
80
70
60
50
40
30

PATIENT ACCRUAL
7000
6500
6000
5500
5000
4500
4000
3500
3000
2500
2000
1500
1000
500
0

Launch date (6/23/2006)
Protocol Amendment 2.2 (07/2007)
Protocol Amendment 2.3 (03/2007)
Heartmate II BTT approval (4/2008)
HMII DT approval (1/20/2010)
Protocol Amendment 3.0 (05/2007)

Hospital
Patient

JUL06 JAN07 JUL07 JAN08 JUL08 JAN09 JUL09 JAN10 JUL10 JAN11 JUL11 JAN12 JUL12

MONTHS

FIGURE 42-4 Total patient enrollment and implanting centers in the INTERMACS registry. The INTERMACS registry began collecting data on implantable ventricular assist devices in July 2006. During the ensuing 6 years, the outcomes of more than 6500 patients from 131 centers have been catalogued. *From Kirklin JK, Naftel DC, Kormos RL, et al: Fifth INTERMACS annual report: risk factor analysis from more than 6,000 mechanical circulatory support patients. J Heart Lung Transplant 32:141–156, 2013.*

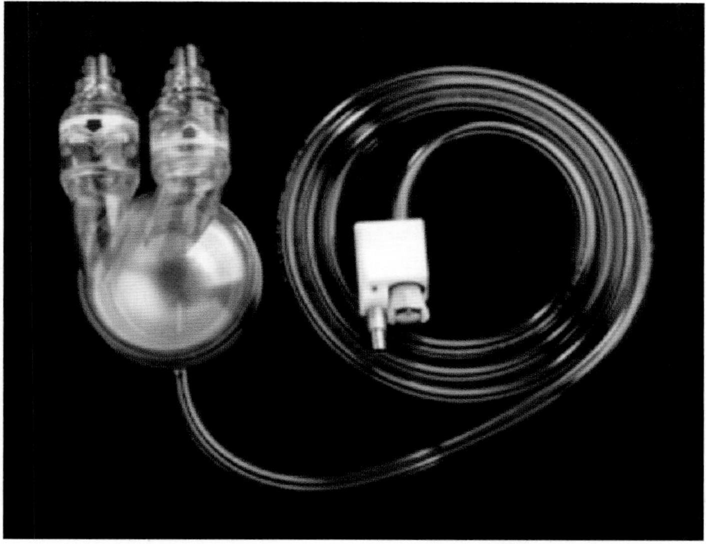

FIGURE 42-5 The ABIOMED AB5000 is a pulsatile flow VAD intended for short- to intermediate-term use. It can be implanted as an LVAD, RVAD, or in the biventricular configuration. *ABIOMED, Danvers, MA.*

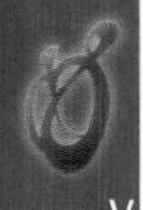

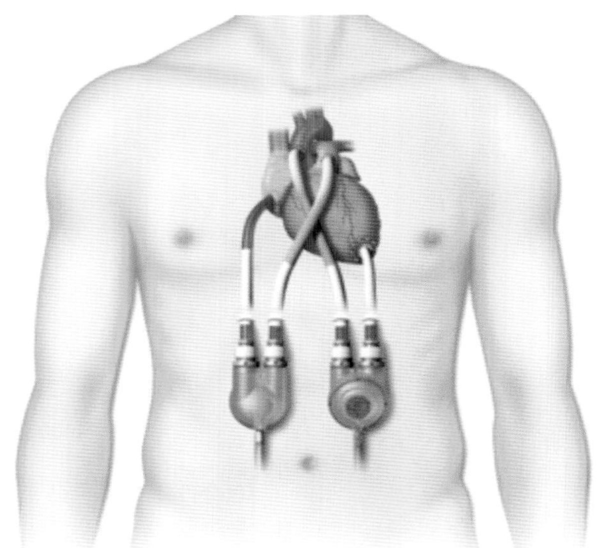

FIGURE 42-6 Thoratec paracorporeal ventricular assist device (PVAD). The Thoratec PVAD is a paracorporeal, pneumatically driven pulsatile flow device capable of providing univentricular or biventricular support. *Omnimedics CZ.*

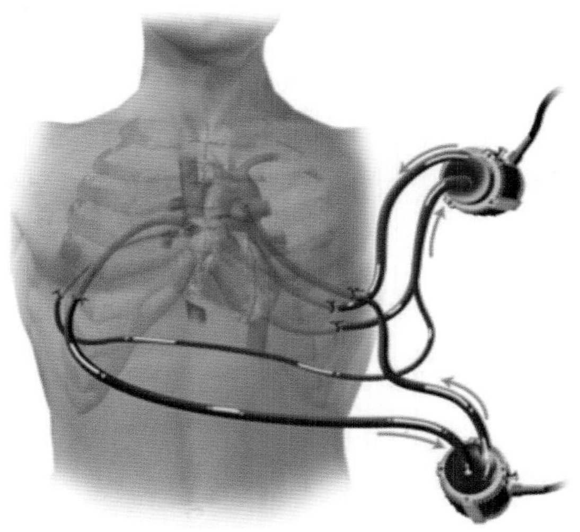

FIGURE 42-7 CentriMag continuous flow ventricular assist devices (VADs). The CentriMag VAD is shown in a biventricular support strategy. In this figure, please note the cannulation of both the right superior pulmonary vein and the left ventricular apex in an attempt to more completely unload the left ventricle. *From cardiothoracicsurgery.org.*

within a hard plastic chamber. The blood pump is attached to a pneumatic driver that detects filling of the blood sac and provides compressed air into the sealed housing to compress the sac and propel the blood forward. This device also has an active filling phase in which negative pressure is applied to the system to promote filling. Two tilting disk mechanical valves ensure unidirectional blood flow. The Thoratec PVAD can provide 4 to 6 L of flow and has been used in postcardiotomy shock and other conditions in which short- to intermediate-term support is required.

Temporary Continuous Flow Devices

CentriMag

The CentriMag (Thoratec) pump is an extracorporeal device approved for short-term support in the United States and can be configured to provide univentricular (either right or left) or biventricular support (**Figure 42-7**). It is a magnetically levitated centrifugal flow device capable of delivering 10 L/min, although the standard clinical flows are 4 to 6 L/min. PediaMag is a smaller version of the same device capable of flows to 1.5 L/min.

Implantable Pulsatile Flow Pumps

Three implantable pulsatile VADs were developed and tested in patients as a means to bridge critically ill patients to transplant or as destination therapy. The principle underlying these devices was that each pump "contraction" should provide a normal stroke volume. As a result, the devices were large enough to contain an adult stroke volume, mechanically complex and prone to failure. Of these pumps, only the Thoratec IVAD is still available but is rarely used.

Thoratec IVAD

The Thoratec IVAD is conceptually the same as the PVAD, except that it is designed such that the blood pump is implanted in the anterior abdominal wall posterior to the rectus muscle. Its clinical usefulness has been limited, largely because of its relatively large transcutaneous drive cord and the size of the pneumatic driver required to actuate this pulsatile device.

HeartMate XVE

Several innovations in VAD design were hallmarks of the HeartMate XVE (Thoratec). The initial iteration of this pump was pneumatic (HeartMate IP), requiring the patient to be tethered to a relatively large driver and confining its use as a bridge to transplant in hospitalized patients. Subsequent conversion to an electric motor and development of externally worn batteries permitted patients to become more ambulatory and allowed for out-of-hospital management. Further, the blood-contacting surface of HeartMate VE was made of sintered titanium that promoted deposition of a pseudointima that eliminated the requirement for chronic anticoagulation. This device was tested as a bridge to transplant in a multicenter trial of 280 patients with advanced heart failure failing optimal medical therapy and compared with a control cohort managed medically with or without IABP support.[56] HeartMate VE–treated patients had superior survival to transplant relative to the control population with post-transplant survival that was similar to patients who did not require LVAD support. Based on this study, the device was approved for bridge to transplantation. Following device modifications designed to reduce the risk of inflow valve failure, the HeartMate XVE was tested in the Randomized Evaluation of Mechanical Assistance in Congestive Heart Failure (REMATCH) trial.[6] This trial screened almost 1000 patients to achieve a final enrollment of 129 patients with severe heart failure who were failing optimal medical therapy, ineligible for transplant, and who were willing to accept randomization to either a permanent LVAD or remain on medical therapy. The LVAD-treated patients had 1- and 2-year survival rates of 50% and 23%, respectively, compared with 25% and 8% at the same time points in the medically treated arm. In addition,

LVAD-treated patients experienced superior improvements in functional capacity and quality of life. The benefits of mechanically assisted circulation demonstrated in REMATCH resulted in approval of the HeartMate XVE as the first device for chronic use in patients ineligible for transplant. There are no longer any patients supported on the HeartMate XVE, and this device is no longer being produced.

Novacor LVAD

The Novacor LVAD was an electrically driven, implantable, pulsatile device intended for long-term use as either bridge to transplant or DT. The device was FDA approved as a bridge to transplant based on a clinical trial supporting this indication that was never published. The Investigation of Nontransplant-Eligible Patients who are Inotrope Dependent (INTrEPID) trial was a nonrandomized, controlled clinical trial to assess the safety and efficacy of the Novacor device as DT.[5] Thirty-seven patients received an LVAD and 18 patients were treated with optimal medical therapy. The LVAD patients had a superior survival, although the 1-year survival was only 27% in the VAD cohort. Despite the need for chronic anticoagulation and antiplatelet therapy, the stroke rate was higher with the Novacor LVAD than that reported with the HeartMate XVE. The smooth interior of the device coupled with a relatively long inflow cannula resulted in more thromboembolic and particuloembolic events in patients supported with this device. In 2007, production and clinical application of the Novacor LVAD were halted.

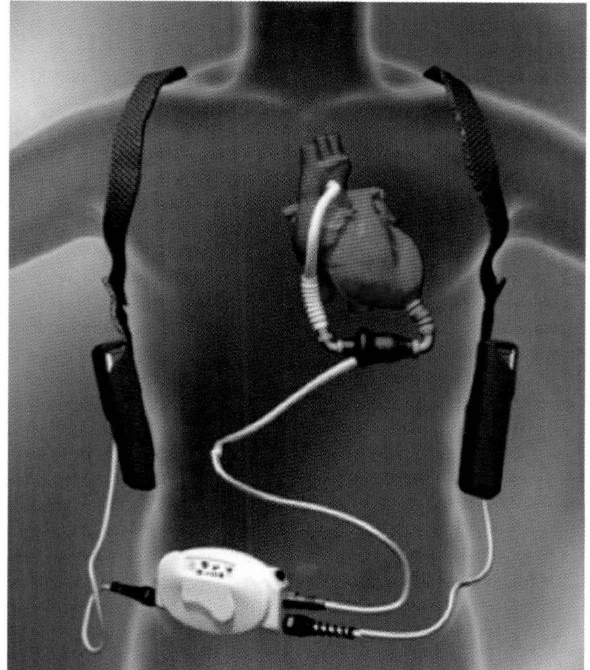

FIGURE 42-8 Implant configuration of the HeartMate II LVAD. The HeartMate II LVAD is implanted in a preperitoneal pocket with the inflow cannula attached to the LV apex and the outflow graft connected to the ascending aorta. A subcutaneous drive line connects the LVAD to the controller. Two batteries supply power to the controller. *Thoratec Corp. Pleasanton, Calif.*

Continuous Flow Pumps

A pivotal innovation in mechanically assisted circulation came with the observation that the human body did not require a "normal" pulse pressure. This led to the development of LVAD pumps with rotary mechanisms that produced continuous rather than pulsatile blood flow. These devices are nonvalved systems that draw blood from the LV apex and return the blood to the circulation via an outflow graft generally attached to the ascending aorta. The devices are electrically driven by external battery or AC power delivered to the pump via a subcutaneous driveline that exits the skin and is attached to a wearable controller that regulates and monitors pump function (**Figure 42-8**). The blood-propelling mechanism in these devices rotates at a constant set speed and operates to maximally reduce LV size with minimal or no aortic valve opening. As a result, there may not be a detectable pulse in patients supported with a continuous flow device (**Figure 42-9**), and most of the observed pulsatility is derived from the contribution of native ventricular systole to LVAD filling.

Cardiopulmonary bypass provided an extensive experience with short-duration nonpulsatile blood flow. The clinical trials of continuous flow LVADs provided the opportunity to explore the impact of chronic minimally pulsatile flow on end-organ function. Russell and colleagues were unable to demonstrate deterioration of renal and hepatic function over a 6-month observation period.[57] Similarly, neurocognitive function was examined over 24 months of continuous flow support with no evidence of decline in executive cognitive function.[58] Finally, submaximal exercise performance was serially evaluated and shown to statistically improve during the first 3 months following LVAD implantation and remain stable throughout a 24-month follow-up period, suggesting no detrimental impact on peripheral muscle function.[59] Thus there is no evidence from clinical trials to suggest a decline in end-organ function resulting from chronic circulatory support with minimal (or no) pulsatility.

HeartMate II

HeartMate II (HMII, Thoratec) is an axial flow LVAD that is implanted in a subcutaneous pocket beneath the left costal margin. It is small, operates in a quiet mode, and is capable of flows up to 10 L/min, although clinical flows are primarily 4 to 6 L/min. The HeartMate II is approved in the United States for bridge to transplant and DT. The pivotal HeartMate II BTT trial used a unique trial design that compared the outcomes of 133 patients supported on the device to objective performance criteria.[30] The primary composite endpoint of the study was survival on support to 180 days, transplant, or ventricular recovery that permitted device removal. Seventy-five percent of patients successfully achieved this endpoint with a 12-month actuarial survival of 68%. Following enrollment of the primary patient cohort, additional patients (n = 336) were enrolled in a continued access protocol. Evaluation of this extended population demonstrated improvement in the primary composite endpoint to 79% and a 12-month actuarial survival of 73%.[60]

The HeartMate II destination therapy trial compared the rates of survival free from disabling stroke and reoperation to repair or replace the device in 200 patients randomized to either HeartMate II or HeartMate XVE.[31] There was a fourfold increase in successful achievement of the primary endpoint at 24 months in the HMII cohort. Actuarial survival at 24 months was 58% and 24% in the

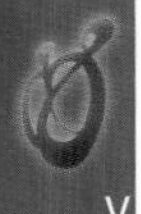

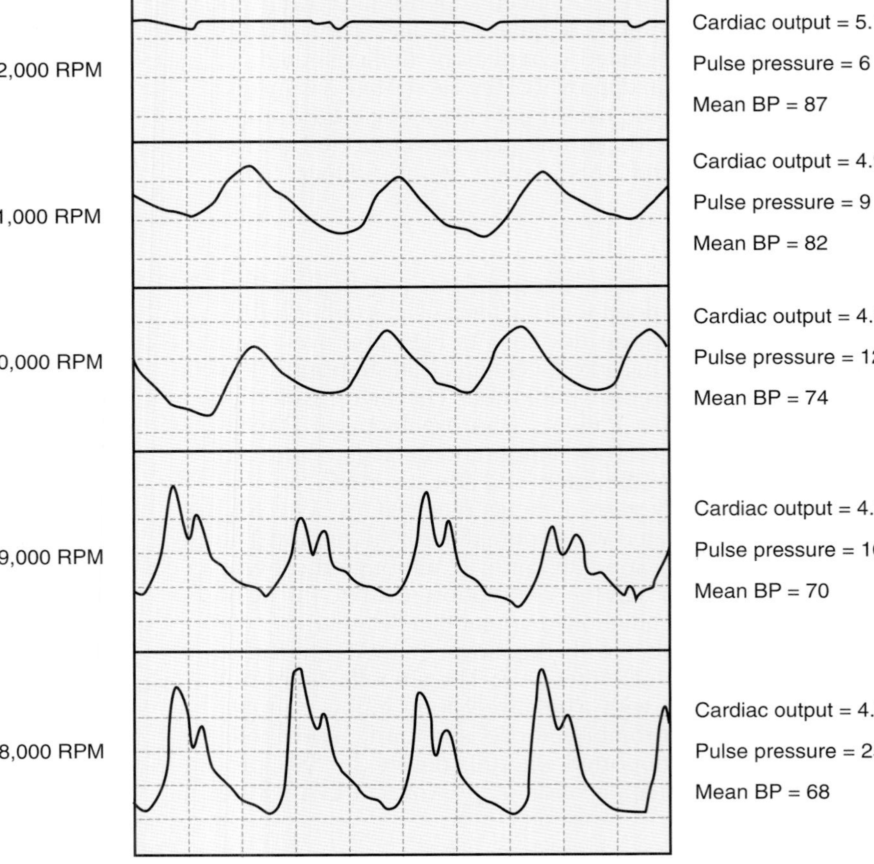

FIGURE 42-9 Pulse pressure in continuous flow left ventricular assist device (LVAD). The pulse pressure in a continuous flow LVAD is dependent on the speed. At slower speeds (8000-9000) a dicrotic notch can be seen in the arterial pressure tracing. As the VAD speed is increased further, the pulse pressure narrows as the cardiac output increases. These very low pulse pressures are often clinically imperceptible. *From Frazier OH, Jacob LP: Small pumps for ventricular assistance: progress in mechanical circulatory support. Cardiology Clinics 25: 553–564, 2007.*

continuous flow and pulsatile flow cohorts, respectively. When the components of the primary endpoint were examined, device replacement and death were statistically less common in the HMII cohort and there was a trend toward fewer strokes. Quality of life and functional capacity were not different between study groups, suggesting that the hemodynamic benefits of mechanical circulatory support were more important determinants of these outcomes than the mode of circulatory support (pulsatile vs. continuous flow). Like the BTT trial, a continued access protocol allowed enrollment in the study, while the primary cohort completed follow-up. This resulted in an expanded patient population of 281 patients. Analysis of the HeartMate II–treated patients in this cohort demonstrated a 2-year survival of 63%.[61]

HeartWare HVAD

HeartWare HVAD (HeartWare Corp., Framingham, Mass.) is a bearingless centrifugal flow pump capable of providing up to 10 L of blood flow. Its small size and design allow placement in the pericardium (**Figure 42-10**). The HVAD was studied as a bridge to transplant in a noninferiority trial that used concomitantly enrolled patients in the INTERMACS registry implanted with a commercially available device as a control group.[62] The primary endpoint was survival to 180 days on the originally implanted device, transplant, or device removal for recovery. Ninety-two percent of the HVAD population successfully achieved the primary endpoint compared with 90.7% of the control group

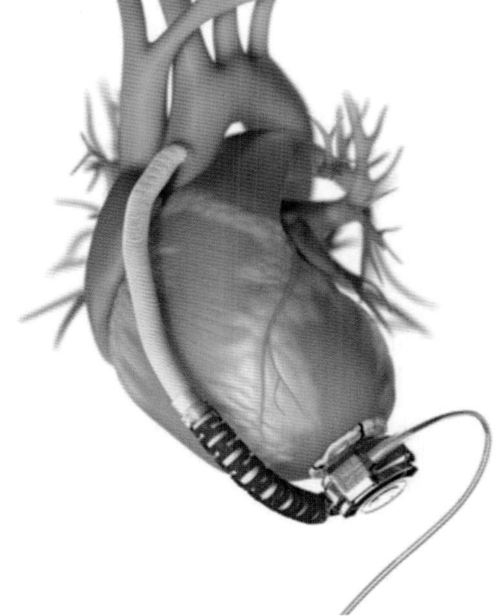

FIGURE 42-10 HeartWare HVAD. The HeartWare HVAD (HeartWare Corp. Framingham, MA) is a centrifugal flow pump with a size sufficiently small to be implanted in the pericardial space. The remainder of the implant configuration is similar to that shown in Figure 42-8. *HeartWare Corp.*

(noninferiority, $P < 0.001$). On the basis of this trial, HVAD was approved as a bridge to transplant by the FDA.

The HVAD is currently undergoing evaluation in the DT application in 433 patients randomized in a 2:1 fashion to receive the HVAD or the HMII. The primary endpoint is survival to 2 years on the originally implanted device without a disabling stroke.

Several other devices are in various stages of development and testing. The Jarvik 2000 is a small axial flow device with several interesting innovations, including implantation of the pump directly into the left ventricle, variable speed control that can be manipulated by the patient, and novel power cord implantation. The bridge-to-transplant trial with this device has completed enrollment and is in the follow-up phase.

Management Issues of a Continuous Flow Pump

Beyond the unique physiology associated with continuous flow VADs, management of patients on these devices is nuanced. The minimally pulsatile blood flow can make standard blood pressure monitoring difficult. Doppler appears to be superior to auscultation or the use of automated blood pressure cuffs to assess blood pressure.[63] Hypertension is common following a period of support on a continuous flow VAD. Careful assessment and management of hypertension may have a favorable impact on the risk of stroke in this patient population, particularly with the HVAD.

Systemic anticoagulation with warfarin and an antiplatelet agent are recommended with all commercially available devices. However, the target INR varies from device to device. The newer anticoagulants have not been tested with the LVADs and their efficacy is unknown at present.

Thoughtful management of LVAD settings is also an important component of ongoing device care. The LVAD creates negative pressure at the LV apex. Excessive speed or intravascular volume depletion may result in the device pulling the ventricular septum toward the inflow cannula (**Figure 42-11**). When this is severe, the myocardium may partially occlude flow into the VAD, causing a "suction" event. Contemporary devices will recognize this phenomenon and sound an alarm or reduce the speed of the pump temporarily to allow greater LV filling that moves the inflow cannula away from the myocardium. Excessive pump speeds should be considered as a cause when a patient presents with ventricular tachycardia.

Multimodality imaging is a critical component of the ongoing care of VAD patients (**Figure 42-12**). Chest x-ray and echocardiography are useful tools to evaluate inflow cannula positioning, which should optimally be centered in the LV cavity, directed toward the mitral valve, and not in opposition to the ventricular myocardium. Chest wall echocardiography is also used to determine the most appropriate speed for the device.[47,64] The ramp study has been proposed as an objective test to determine optimal pump speed and to detect evidence of VAD thrombosis.[64] In a ramp study, the VAD speed is decreased to a minimal level such that the LV dilates and the aortic valve opens, signifying inadequate left ventricular unloading. The speed of the VAD is then incrementally increased with simultaneous monitoring of symptoms, vital signs, left ventricular size, and aortic valve movement using transthoracic echocardiography. The optimal speed results in maximal pump output and reduction of left ventricular diastolic diameter, maintenance of the ventricular septum in the "midline," and either intermittent or no aortic valve opening. Many programs perform the ramp study early after device implant and again with changes in the clinical status including worsening dyspnea, ventricular tachycardia, or evidence that the device is unloading the LV excessively. Cine CT can be useful to identify inflow cannula malposition when other imaging studies result in diagnostic uncertainty. CT is also useful to evaluate the outflow graft. Finally, cardiac catheterization may be particularly useful in patients presenting with dyspnea. An appropriately functioning LVAD will lower the LVEDP/PCWP into a normal or near normal range. Elevated left ventricular filling pressures should raise the possibility of inadequate device speed, aortic insufficiency, or device malfunction.

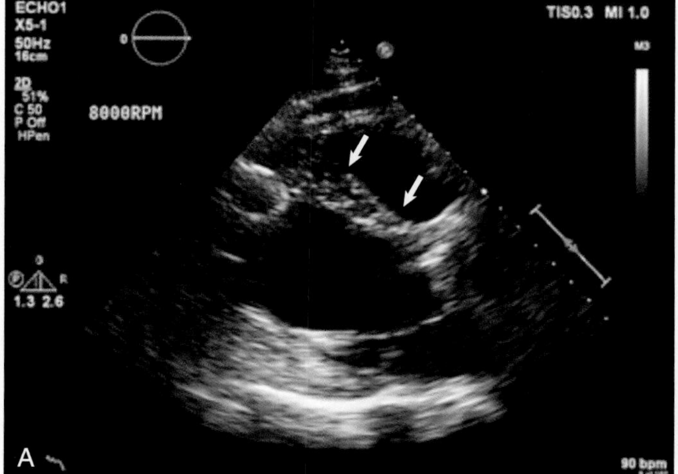

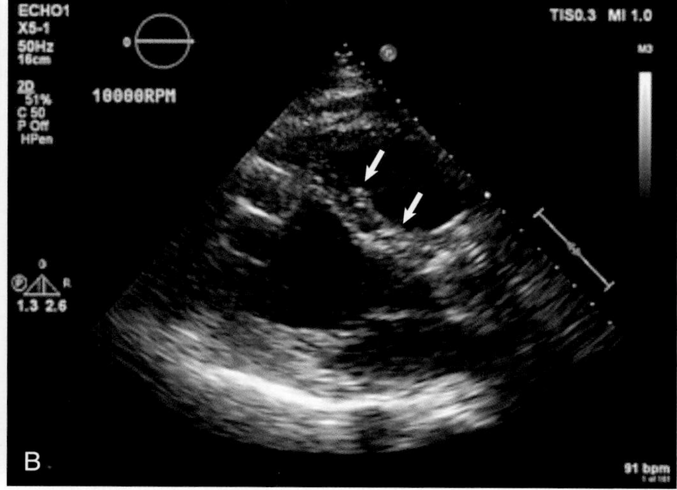

FIGURE 42-11 The impact of excessive ventricular assist device (VAD) speed on ventricular septal position. The impact of varying LVAD speed is demonstrated. At a pump speed of 8000 RPM **(A)** the ventricular septum *(arrows)* is positioned in the midline. When the speed is increased to 10,000 RPM **(B)** the ventricular septum is shifted toward the posterior wall.

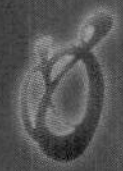

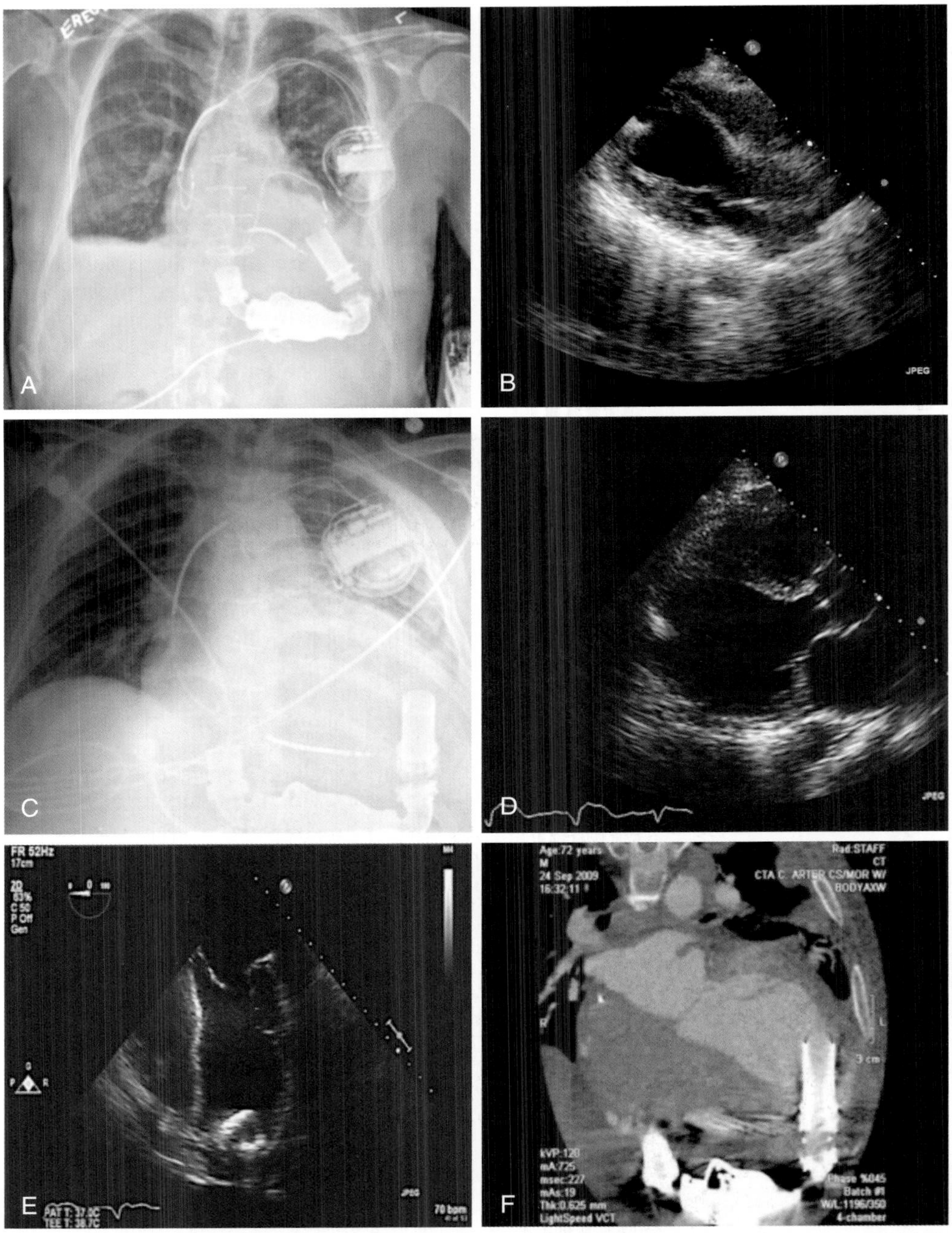

FIGURE 42-12 The role of chest radiography, echocardiography, and chest computed tomography to evaluate proper left ventricular assist device positioning. A normally positioned inflow cannula is directed in the long axis of the ventricle at the mitral valve **(A** and **B)**. Misdirected inflow cannulae are seen by chest x-ray **(C)**, transthoracic echo **(D)**, transesophageal echo **(E)**, and cardiac computed tomography **(F)**.

Adverse Events

Adverse events following left ventricular assist device placement are common. A recent analysis demonstrated that 70% of patients have a major adverse event within 12 months of device implantation.[33] Most adverse events occur early after device implantation. However, some complications such as infections are time-dependent with progressive risk the longer the patient has an LVAD in place. One of the important challenges in understanding the rate of device-related complications was the lack of standardized definitions. The INTERMACS registry has developed standardized definitions for common adverse events that are now being used in the registry and in clinical trials.

Right Heart Failure

Right heart failure following LVAD implantation is associated with incremental morbidity and mortality. The need for continuous infusion inotropes to support right ventricular (RV) performance for more than 2 weeks or a right ventricular assist device following LVAD reduced 180-day survival from 87% to 66% in the HeartMate II BTT trial.[38] Further, many of the events categorized as multisystem organ failure in the clinical LVAD trials can be traced back to right ventricular failure. The clinical presentation is typically in the first hours following LVAD implantation and is characterized by systemic hypotension, elevated right atrial pressure, and poor VAD filling. Echo may demonstrate a

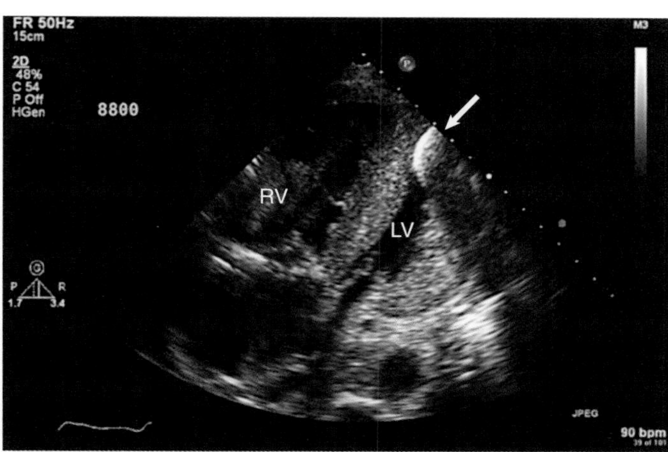

FIGURE 42-13 Echocardiographic diagnosis of right ventricular failure. Apical four-chamber view from transthoracic echocardiography showing the left ventricular assist device (LVAD) cannula in the left ventricular apex *(arrow)*. The left ventricle (LV) is small and underfilled, whereas the right ventricle (RV) is markedly dilated.

dilated and dysfunctional right ventricle with or without tricuspid insufficiency, and a small and underfilled left ventricle (**Figure 42-13**). Prevention of RV failure by careful patient selection is desirable, but the available tools lack high predictive accuracy. Integration of clinical parameters, imaging measures of right ventricular performance, and hemodynamic variables may assist the clinician in prognostication. Treatment of post-LVAD RV failure includes the use of pharmacologic agents that increase cardiac contractility such as dobutamine or milrinone, drugs that lower pulmonary artery pressures such as inhaled nitric oxide, prostacycline, or oral phosphodiesterase-5 inhibitors such as sildenafil. If these agents are ineffective, a right ventricular assist device such as CentriMag or PVAD may be required. Determination of significant right heart failure after LVAD should prompt the clinician to consider early transplant in eligible patients.

Neurologic Events

In the clinical trials of mechanical circulatory support devices, neurologic event reporting has ranged in severity from metabolic encephalopathy to ischemic and hemorrhagic stroke. Hemorrhagic strokes have the highest associated mortality and result from the requisite use of anticoagulants and antiplatelet agents, the presence of acquired von Willebrand factor deficiency, and systemic hypertension (see later discussion). The stroke rate appears to be device specific and ranges from 8% to 17%/year.[60,65] The role for enhanced blood pressure management to decrease the incidence of stroke is being tested in a clinical trial.

Infection

The diagnosis and management of infections in patients supported on a mechanically circulatory support device can be challenging, relating to the complexity of intracorporeal foreign materials and their anatomic position, the presence of a percutaneous driveline, the surgical implant procedure, and the poor general health of many of the heart failure patients undergoing the procedure. Standardized definitions for device-specific, device-related, and non-VAD infections in device-supported patients have been described.[66] During the early perioperative period, infectious complications are typically related to the surgical procedure and nosocomial infections, such as pneumonia, urinary tract infections, and wound infections.[67] Development of a sternal infection following VAD implantation can be a devastating complication because of the proximity of the VAD components. Infection of device components is almost impossible to correct without replacement of the pump. In many cases, long-term suppressive antibiotic therapy is used and transplant should be considered if the infection is controlled and the patient is otherwise an acceptable candidate. Later infectious complications are more likely related to the percutaneous driveline. Trauma to the exit site can result in disruption of the driveline-tissue barrier, leading to an ascending infection that tracks proximally toward the device. The diagnosis is often made clinically by the identification of purulent drainage from the exit site coupled with erythema and tenderness along the driveline (which is commonly palpable). In some cases, CT imaging can identify areas along the driveline surrounded by fluid or stranding in the subcutaneous tissues. Antimicrobial therapy should be directed against the cultured organism. However, surgical débridement is often required with fashioning of a new exit site.

Bleeding

Bleeding is the most common adverse event early following LVAD implantation.[68,69] Early bleeding complications are primarily surgical and are treated with correction of operative coagulopathies, as well as identification and management of anastomotic bleeding sources. Late bleeding rates are estimated to be 13% to 30%, are more common with continuous flow VADs than pulsatile pumps, and are typically mucosal.[70-72] There appear to be at least three critical components to late bleeding following LVAD. First, all patients on contemporary continuous flow devices develop acquired von Willebrand disease caused by the sheer stress applied to the von Willebrand molecules by the device, resulting in exposure of a cleavage site for the ADAMTS13 enzyme.[71,73,74] Subsequent degradation of the large molecular weight von Willebrand multimers into smaller fragments that are less efficient at crosslinking platelets and clot stabilization increase bleeding risk. Second, small arteriovenous malformations (AVM) occur primarily in the small intestine but may also be present in the large bowel or nasal mucosa. Although the cause of this observation is not clearly understood, the pathophysiology is thought to be similar to the mucosal AVM development in Heyde syndrome associated with AVM formation in patients with hemodynamically significant aortic stenosis. The commonality between AS and a continuous flow LVAD is a reduced pulse pressure and increased sheer force applied to blood elements, but the mechanism by which this physiologic alteration is associated with the development of AVMs is not clear. Finally, the requisite use of antiplatelet agents and anticoagulation associated with MCS use contributes to bleeding complications.

Valvular Heart Disease

Several valvular lesions can impact the performance of an LVAD. The presence of hemodynamically significant mitral stenosis will limit LVAD filling and should be addressed at the time of LVAD implantation. A previously implanted, undersized mitral annuloplasty ring may need

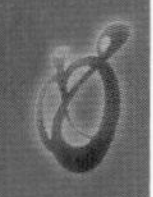

to be removed at the time of VAD implantation if it is causing significant limitation of flow across the mitral annulus. Mitral regurgitation is not thought to be an important valvular lesion in LVAD patients. In most cases, a normally functioning LVAD will reduce the residual blood volume in the LV to such an extent that secondary MR will be significantly reduced. Despite the observation that persistent moderate to severe mitral insufficiency following LVAD does not appear to impact survival, some have advocated the repair of mitral insufficiency to incrementally reduce pulmonary vascular resistance.[75,76] Aortic stenosis without insufficiency tends not to be a lesion that requires intervention as the LVAD circumvents this valve. De novo aortic stenosis has been reported in LVAD-supported patients and is thought to result from limited opening of the aortic valve with subsequent scarring and fusion of the aortic valve cusps.[77] As a result, some advocate setting the pump speed to allow intermittent opening of the aortic valve. The presence of greater than mild aortic insufficiency at the time of LVAD implantation should be corrected.[78] The optimal surgical technique has not been defined, but many surgeons favor the Park stitch that consists of a central oversewing of the three valve leaflets with sutures placed in the nodules of Arantius.[79] An alternative is replacement of the valve with a bioprosthesis. Development of clinically significant de novo aortic insufficiency (AI) following LVAD appears to be time-dependent and may result in symptomatic heart failure if the regurgitant volume becomes sufficient.[80-82] To date, correction of AI in the VAD population has typically required redo sternotomy with placement of an aortic bioprosthesis, but eventually catheter-based approaches may prove beneficial with less comorbidity.[83] Presence of a mechanical aortic prosthesis must be addressed at the time of LVAD implantation because of the risk of thrombus development with reduced leaflet movement. The surgical approach to these patients has been to either replace the valve with a bioprosthesis or alternatively occlude the valve with a circular felt patch.[84]

Hemolysis/Pump Thrombosis

Subtle alterations in the flow characteristics in the LVAD or its inflow or outflow cannulae may result in hemolysis. This can be caused by the development of thrombus on the blood-contacting components of the pump, twisting of the pliable outflow graft, or any other change in the VAD anatomy that alters the normal rheology. The clinical presentation is often asymptomatic and detected with serologic measures of red blood cell trauma including elevated levels of serum lactate dehydrogenase (LDH) or plasma free hemoglobin or a low serum haptoglobin. Recently, LDH level has been validated as a predictor of hemolysis, and elevated levels predate other manifestations of device thrombosis.[85,86] Patients are frequently asymptomatic, although they may complain of nausea and vomiting or abdominal pain.[87] In addition, hemoglobinuria may be seen in cases of more significant hemolysis. Paradoxically, the VAD flow may appear elevated on the system monitor associated with high power consumption. Imaging of the device is a critical component of the evaluation. Transthoracic echocardiography should be performed to assess LV size and valvular function. Left ventricular enlargement, frequent opening of a previously closed aortic valve, and worsening mitral insufficiency all suggest increased left ventricular volume and pressure and abnormal LVAD function. A ramp study (previously described) may also be useful in patients with a HeartMate II. Failure of the LV end-diastolic dimension to decrease with increasing pump speed is highly correlated with VAD thrombosis.[64] Cine CT of the chest allows careful determination of the LV inflow cannula position, as well as examination of the LV outflow graft. Finally, determination of invasive hemodynamics may provide useful information in unclear cases. Demonstration of elevated pulmonary capillary wedge pressure and a low cardiac output (that may be discrepant from the system monitor) are also suggestive of device malfunction. Treatment of hemolysis and VAD thrombosis should be directed at the cause. If the inflow cannula is in continuity with the left ventricular myocardium, surgical repositioning may be required. If the outflow graft is twisted, surgical manipulation will be required to either untwist or replace the graft. Medical management of device thrombosis is more controversial. Some have advocated a stepped approach that includes the administration of unfractionated heparin, direct thrombin inhibitors, glycoprotein 2B/3A antagonists, or tissue plasminogen activator inhibitor.[88] If ineffective, LVAD replacement should be rapidly considered if the patient is a suitable candidate. Two-year survival following device exchange for thrombosis is reduced relative to primary LVAD implant (56% vs. 69%, P <0.0001).[89]

Support for Biventricular Heart Failure

Managing biventricular heart failure with mechanical circulatory support requires use of devices that were not intended for long-term, out-of-hospital use in the biventricular configuration, the use of continuous flow VADs implanted in both ventricles, or the total artificial heart. INTERMACS has provided important insights about the outcome of patients requiring biventricular support.[33] One-year survival in LVAD-treated patients was 80% versus 64% and 48% in patients treated with a continuous flow or pulsatile BiVADs, respectively (P<0.0001). The Thoratec PVAD system can be used outside the hospital with a portable driver; however, experience with this approach is limited.[90] A small series of patients treated with centrifugal flow devices in both ventricles demonstrated a 30-day survival rate of 82%.[91]

The total artificial heart (TAH) can be used to support patients with severe biventricular failure and is approved as a bridge to transplant. The surgical approach requires a cardiectomy and attachment of the TAH to atrial cuffs and the great vessels. The SynCardia TAH (SynCardia Systems, Tucson, Ariz.) is available as both a 50-mL and 70-mL ventricle to accommodate a variety of patient body sizes (**Figure 42-14**). In a prospective clinical trial comparing TAH to optimal medical therapy and IABP, patients supported with TAH had a significantly better survival to transplantation (79% vs. 46%, P <0.001) than the control group.[92] Previously the SynCardia TAH was limited to use in the hospital because of the size of the pneumatic driver used to actuate the device. Recently, a smaller version of the driver has been developed that allows enhanced patient mobility and the ability to be managed outside the hospital.

Mechanical Circulatory Support in Children

The use of mechanical blood pumps in children poses several challenges beyond those encountered with adults.

An array of devices must be available to accommodate body sizes from infant to adolescent. In addition, as body size increases, the need for higher device output may exceed the capabilities of an implanted pump. Many children with failing ventricles have structurally abnormal hearts or prior cardiac procedures that add technical limitations to MCS (see also Chapter 25). Further, the daily interaction of a child with a VAD and the impact on physical and psychosocial growth is understudied. Finally the paucity of small donor hearts for transplantation predictably results in relatively long support times.

The most commonly used mechanical device to support the circulation of children remains ECMO.[93] The versatility of ECMO, including its ability to support both cardiac and pulmonary systems, the ease and rapidity of implantation, and limited alternatives for mechanically assisted circulation in children, has resulted in the widespread adoption of this technology. The majority of pediatric patients are supported on ECMO for short durations, although a series of patients supported for more than 30 days has been reported.[94,95] Neurologic complications remain an important adverse event in ECMO-supported children. Twenty-four percent of children in the Extracorporeal Life Support Organization (ELSO) registry had a neurologic event.[96] Low birth weight, gestational age less than 34 weeks, the need for pre-ECMO cardiopulmonary resuscitation, systemic acidosis or the use of bicarbonate, and recurrent need for ECMO were important predictors of mortality.

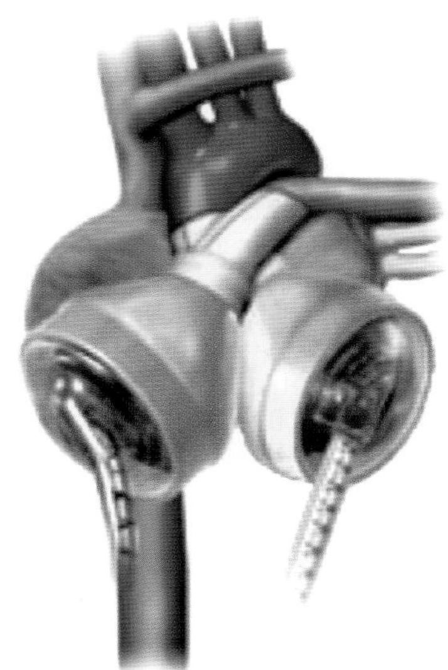

FIGURE 42-14 SynCardia total artificial heart. The SynCardia total artificial heart replaces the function of both the right and left ventricles and requires a cardiectomy for implantation. The device is approved in the United States as a bridge to transplantation. *Reprinted with permission, syncardia.com.*

Recently, a novel, extracorporeal, pulsatile pump has been introduced for use in children. The Excor Pediatric VAD (Berlin Heart, Woodlands, Tex.) is manufactured in multiple sizes to accommodate children across a broad spectrum of body sizes (**Figure 42-15**). This device was recently tested in a single-arm trial of children less than 17 years of age who weighed 3 to 60 kg and had two-ventricle circulation and severe heart failure.[97] Study participants were enrolled in to one of two cohorts based on body surface area (cohort 1 <0.7 m^2; cohort 2 = 0.7-1.5 m^2) and compared with a historical control group supported with ECMO. The primary endpoint of the VAD-treated patients was death, withdrawal of support with an unacceptable neurologic outcome, or unsuccessful weaning from the device. The primary endpoint for the ECMO-treated control cohort was all-cause mortality. Both VAD-treated study cohorts had superior freedom from the primary endpoint compared with controls. Adverse events with the Excor device included bleeding, infection, stroke, and hypertension. In addition, pump exchange was common and most often resulted from device thrombosis. Based on the results of this clinical trial, the Excor was approved by the FDA as a bridge to transplantation in children.

The DeBakey Child VAD is the other FDA-approved device for supporting children to transplant. Clinical application of this device has been limited by a relatively high risk of thrombosis.[98]

FUTURE DIRECTIONS

Partial Support Devices

An evolving innovation in the field of mechanically assisted circulation is the development and clinical assessment of partial support devices. Currently used VADs are designed to replace the entirety of the cardiac output. However, a larger population exists that would benefit from cardiac output augmentation and reduction in the left-sided filling pressures. The CircuLite Synergy (HeartWare) axial flow device is designed to be implanted in a pacemaker-like

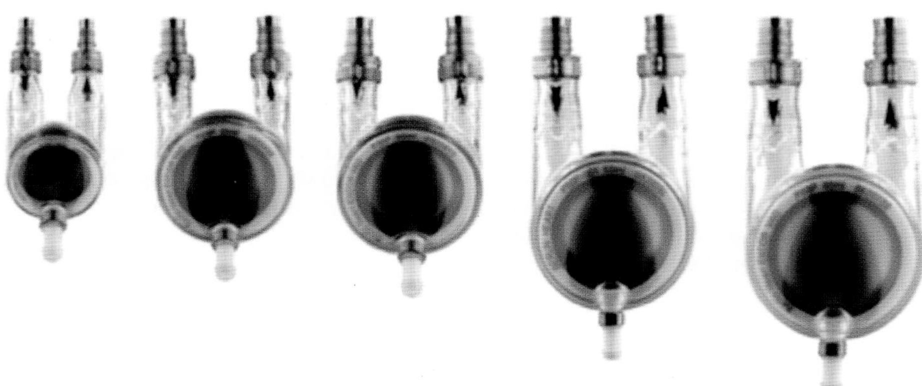

FIGURE 42-15 The Berlin heart pediatric ventricular assist device (VAD). The Berlin heart VAD is an extracorporeal device that is manufactured with various chamber sizes (10, 25, 30, 50, and 60 mL) to accommodate a range of pediatric patients.

pocket fashioned in the infraclavicular subcutaneous tissues with pump inflow obtained through a minithoracotomy to access the right superior pulmonary vein and cannulation of the subclavian artery for device outflow. Eventually, inflow may be obtained by placing the cannula retrograde through the subclavian vein into the left atrium via a transseptal puncture. This device has been shown to augment cardiac index by 0.5 to 1.0 L/min/m^2 and reduce the left atrial pressure by 8 to 10 mm Hg.[99]

The C-Pulse (Sunshine Heart, Eden Prairie, Minn.) is a pneumatically driven inflatable cuff that is surgically implanted on the ascending aorta and synchronized with the ECG to fill during diastole and empty during systole. In this manner it functions like an intra-aortic balloon pump. Since there is no blood-contacting surface, the device can be used intermittently and could be turned off for prolonged periods of time. The C-Pulse has entered a U.S. pivotal trial in patients with NYHA class III symptoms.

Totally Implantable Systems

Development of reliable totally implantable systems is anticipated to have an important impact on patient acceptance of the therapy, as well as to reduce the infection rates associated with these devices. As currently envisioned, patients would have a capacitor implanted in the soft tissue of the abdominal wall that would allow several hours of untethered use. Tethering would involve wearing a vest containing an energy transmission coil that would transfer energy from batteries to the subcutaneous capacitor. Other novel methods of battery charging are being explored, including the use of electrically charged rooms capable of charging battery-operated devices.

Novel Patient Populations

Approximately 80% of patients currently implanted with an LVAD have a severity of illness that requires treatment with intravenous inotropic therapy.[33] In this cohort, LVAD has been shown to provide important improvements in both quality of life and survival. The use of these devices in patients with less advanced heart failure remains speculative. Two trials are under way to address the role of LVADs in patients with advanced heart failure who have NYHA class III or ambulatory class IV symptoms and are not treated with inotropic support. The Risk Assessment and Comparative Effectiveness of Left Ventricular Assist Device and Medical Management (ROADMAP) study is a nonrandomized evaluation of the HeartMate II device compared with optimal medical therapy in patients who are ineligible for transplantation, meet current indications for DT, and are not yet treated with inotropic therapy. The primary endpoint of ROADMAP is a composite of survival and functional improvement at 12 months. The Randomized Evaluation of VAD Intervention before Inotropic Therapy (REVIVE IT) is an NIH-sponsored evaluation of HeartMate II versus optimal medical therapy in patients selected to have a predicted annualized mortality of approximately 25% using the Seattle Heart Failure Model.

Myocardial Recovery

An important promise of MCS is the opportunity to support the circulation sufficiently to allow recovery of native heart function, either by reversal of the process causing ventricular dysfunction, such as acute myocarditis, or allowing the use of adjuvant therapies that promote myocardial functional recovery. Clinical trial and contemporary registry data demonstrate a recovery rate with successful LVAD removal in approximately 1% to 2% of the implanted population.[30,100] Predictors of recovery include younger age, nonischemic cause, and shorter duration of heart failure before device implantation.[100] Generally, the management strategy to promote myocardial recovery has included maintaining the device speed such that the heart size is maximally reduced and the use of standard heart failure therapies. Serial assessment of intrinsic myocardial function typically includes measurement of cardiac structure and function using echocardiography, submaximal and maximal exercise testing, and evaluation of hemodynamics. The above studies are performed with the pump speed turned down to achieve a net neutral flow such that there is no backflow through the outflow graft into the pump and left ventricle.

Standard heart failure pharmacotherapy consisting of angiotensin antagonists, mineralocorticoid antagonists, and β-adrenergic blockers is typically used.[101] Clenbuterol, a β_2-adrenergic agonist with anabolic steroid properties, has been systematically tested as adjuvant therapy in both pulsatile and continuous flow devices. Addition of clenbuterol was shown to result in sustained improvements of LV structure and normalization of LV function in a greater proportion than previously reported in clinical trial databases and registries.[102,103]

Stem cell therapy may also prove to be an important adjuvant to mechanically assisted circulation (see also Chapter 38). An NIH-sponsored clinical trial using allogeneic mesenchymal precursor cells was recently reported.[104] This safety trial included 30 patients randomized to administration of either 25 million allogeneic stem cells or control medium directly injected into the left ventricular myocardium during LVAD implantation. There were no safety events associated with direct myocardial injection of stem cells nor was there evidence of immunologic sensitization. Injection of mesenchymal precursor cells did not increase the likelihood of temporary VAD weaning at 90 days or 1 year, nor did it improve the ejection fraction in this small trial.

The field of mechanically assisted circulation is growing and evolving rapidly with proliferation of new devices designed for short- and long-term circulatory support. Clinical trials in the past several years have clearly demonstrated reduced mortality and quality of life improvements in patients with advanced heart failure. However, the persistently high mortality rates associated with cardiogenic shock following acute myocardial infarction demands careful evaluation and innovative solutions that may require multiple devices to improve survival. The role of mechanically assisted circulation in expanded patient populations such as children, NYHA class III, and right heart failure will require new device design and thoughtful clinical trials. Moving forward, centers invested in mechanically assisted circulation will have clinical expertise with a broad array of VADs that can be tailored to the specific needs of the individual patient. Newer generation continuous flow pumps with smaller size, more durable design, and novel blood-contacting surfaces are likely to have favorable and incremental impact on the long-term outcomes for MCS patients. Concerns that prolonged exposure to reduced pulsatility plays a role in some of the adverse events associated with these devices are likely to result in innovative device design and management strategies to restore a higher degree of pulsatility. Finally, there will be an even greater focus on the patient and caregiver experience as more patients live for prolonged periods of time on mechanical circulatory support devices.

References

1. Metra M, Ponikowski P, Dickstein K, et al: Advanced chronic heart failure: A position statement from the study group on advanced heart failure of the Heart Failure Association of the European Society of Cardiology. *Eur J Heart Fail* 9:684–694, 2007.
2. Miller LW, Guglin M, Rogers JG: Cost of ventricular assist devices: Can we afford the progress? *Circulation* 127:743–748, 2013.
3. Gorodeski EZ, Chu EC, Reese JR, et al: Prognosis on chronic dobutamine or milrinone infusions for stage D heart failure. *Circ Heart Fail* 2:320–324, 2009.
4. Hershberger RE, Nauman D, Walker T, et al: Care processes and clinical outcomes of continuous outpatient support with inotropes (COSI) in patients with refractory end-stage heart failure. *J Card Fail* 9:180–187, 2003.
5. Rogers JG, Butler J, Lansman S, et al, for the INTrEPID Investigators: Chronic mechanical circulatory support for inotrope-dependent heart failure patients who are not transplant candidates. *J Am Coll Cardiol* 50:741–747, 2007.
6. Rose EA, Gelijns AC, Moskowitz AJ, et al, for the Randomized Evaluation of Mechanical Assistance for the Treatment of Congestive Heart Failure (REMATCH) Study Group: Long-term use of a left ventricular assist device for end-stage heart failure. *N Engl J Med* 345:1435–1443, 2001.
7. Stevenson LW: Clinical use of inotropic therapy for heart failure: Looking backward or forward?: Chronic inotropic therapy. *Circulation* 108:492–497, 2003.
8. Stehlik J, Edwards LB, Kucheryavaya AY, et al, for the International Society of Heart and Lung Transplantation: The Registry of the International Society for Heart and Lung Transplantation: 29th official adult heart transplant report – 2012. *J Heart Lung Transplant* 31:1052–1064, 2012.
9. Hochman JS, Buller CE, Sleeper LA, et al, for the SHOCK Investigators: Cardiogenic shock complicating acute myocardial infarction—Etiologies, management and outcomes: A report from the SHOCK Trial Registry. *J Am Coll Cardiol* 36:1063–1070, 2000.
10. Sylvin EA, Stern DR, Goldstein D: Mechanical support for postcardiotomy cardiogenic shock: Has progress been made? *J Card Surg* 25:442–454, 2010.
11. Thiele H, Zeymer U, Neumann FJ, et al: Intraaortic balloon support for myocardial infarction with cardiogenic shock. *N Engl J Med* 367:1287–1296, 2012.
12. Cooper LT, Baughman KL, Feldman A, et al: The role of endomyocardial biopsy in the management of cardiovascular disease. A scientific statement from the American Heart Association, the American College of Cardiology and the European Society of Cardiology. *Circulation* 116:2216–2233, 2007.
13. Rogers JG, Milano CA: The role for mechanical circulatory support for cardiogenic shock. In Hochman JS, Ohman EM, editors: *Cardiogenic Shock*. Oxford, UK, 2009, Wiley-Blackwell.
14. Williams DO, Korr KS, Gewirtz H, et al: The effect of intraaortic balloon counterpulsation on regional myocardial blood flow and oxygen consumption in the presence of coronary artery stenosis in patients with unstable angina. *Circulation* 66:593–597, 1982.
15. Santa-Cruz RA, Cohen MG, Ohman EM: Aortic counterpulsation: A review of the hemodynamic effects and indications for use. *Catheter Cardiovasc Interv* 67:68–77, 2006.
16. Trost JC, Hillis LD: Intra-aortic balloon counterpulsation. *Am J Cardiol* 97:1391–1398, 2006.
17. Estep JD, Cordero-Reyes AM, Bhimaraj A, et al: Percutaneous placement of an intra-aortic balloon pump in the left axillary/subclavian position provides safe, ambulatory long-term support as bridge to heart transplantation. *JACC Heart Fail* 1:382–388, 2013.
18. Roger J, Baskett F, Ghali WA, et al: The intraaortic balloon pump in cardiac surgery. *Ann Thorac Surg* 74:1276–1287, 2002.
19. Barron HV, Every NR, Parsons LS, et al: The use of intra-aortic balloon counterpulsation in patients with cardiogenic shock complication acute myocardial infarction: Data from the National Registry of Myocardial Infarction 2. *Am Heart J* 141:933–939, 2001.
20. Burkhoff D, Cohen H, Brunckhorst C, et al: A randomized multicenter clinical study to evaluate the safety and efficacy of the TandemHeart percutaneous ventricular assist device versus conventional therapy with intraaortic balloon pumping for treatment of cardiogenic shock. *Am Heart J* 152:469.e1–469.e1-8, 2006.
21. Thiele H, Sick P, Boudriot E, et al: Randomized comparison of intra-aortic balloon support with a percutaneous left ventricular assist device in patients with revascularized acute myocardial infarction complicated by cardiogenic shock. *Eur Heart J* 26:1276–1283, 2005.
22. Kar B, Gregoric ID, Basra SS, et al: The percutaneous ventricular assist device in severe refractory cardiogenic shock. *J Am Coll Cardiol* 57:688–696, 2011.
23. Reesink KD, Dekker AL, Ommen VV, et al: Miniature intracardiac assist device provides more effective cardiac unloading and circulatory support during severe left heart failure than intraaortic balloon pumping. *Chest* 126:896–902, 2004.
24. O'Neill WW, Kleiman NS, Moses J, et al: A prospective, randomized clinical trial of hemodynamic support with Impella 2.5 versus intra-aortic balloon pump in patients undergoing high-risk percutaneous coronary intervention The PROTECT II Study. *Circulation* 126:1717–1727, 2012.
25. Griffith BP, Anderson MB, Samuels LE, et al: The RECOVER I: A multicenter prospective study of Impella 5.0/LD for postcardiotomy circulation support. *J Thorac Cardiovasc Surg* 145:548–554, 2013.
26. Lauten A, Engstrom E, Jung C, et al: Percutaneous left-ventricular support with the Impella 2.5-assist device in acute cardiogenic shock: Results of the Impella–EUROSHOCK Registry. *Circ Heart Fail* 6:23–30, 2013.
27. Allen S, Holena D, McCunn M, et al: A review of the fundamental principles and evidence base in the use of extracorporeal membrane oxygenation (ECMO) in critically ill adult patients. *J Intensive Care Med* 26:13–26, 2011.
28. Felker MG, Rogers JG: Same bridge, new destinations. Rethinking paradigms for mechanical cardiac support in heart failure. *J Am Coll Cardiol* 47:930–932, 2006.
29. Kirklin JK, Naftel DC, Kormos RL, et al: The fourth INTERMACS annual report: 4,000 implants and counting. *J Heart Lung Transplant* 31:117–126, 2012.
30. Miller LW, Pagani FD, Russell SD: Use of a continuous-flow device in patients awaiting heart transplantation. *N Engl J Med* 357:885–896, 2007.
31. Slaughter MS, Rogers JG, Milano CA, et al: Advanced heart failure treated with continuous-flow ventricular assist device. *N Engl J Med* 361:2241–2251, 2009.
32. Cowger J, Sundareswaran K, Rogers JG, et al: Predicting survival in patients receiving continuous flow left ventricular assist devices. *J Am Coll Cardiol* 61:313–321, 2013.
33. Kirklin JK, Naftel DC, Kormos RL, et al: Fifth INTERMACS annual report: Risk factor analysis from more than 6,000 mechanical circulatory support patients. *J Heart Lung Transplant* 32:141–156, 2013.
34. Adamson RM, Stahovich M, Chillcott S, et al: Clinical strategies and outcomes in advanced heart failure patients older than 70 years of age receiving the HeartMate II left ventricular assist device. *J Am Coll Cardiol* 57:2487–2495, 2011.
35. Flint KM, Matlock DD, Lindenfeld J, et al: Frailty and the selection of patients for destination therapy left ventricular assist device. *Circ Heart Fail* 5:286–293, 2012.
36. Stewart GC, Stevenson LW: Keeping left ventricular assist device acceleration on track. *Circulation* 123:1559–1568, 2011.
37. Schenk S, McCarthy PM, Blackstone EH, et al: Duration of inotropic support after left ventricular assist device implantation: Risk factors and impact on outcome. *J Thorac Cardiovasc Surg* 131:447–454, 2006.
38. Kormos RL, Teuteberg JL, Pagani FD, et al: Right ventricular failure in patients with the HeartMate II continuous-flow left ventricular assist device: Incidence, risk factors, and effect on outcomes. *J Thorac Cardiovasc Surg* 139:1316–1324, 2010.
39. Vivo RP, Cordero-Reyes AM, Qamar U, et al: Increased right-to-left ventricular diameter ratio is a strong predictor of right ventricular failure after left ventricular assist device. *J Heart Lung Transplant* 32:792–799, 2013.
40. Atluri P, Goldston AB, Fairman A, et al: Predicting right ventricular failure in the modern continuous flow left ventricular assist device era. *Ann Thorac Surg* 96:857–864, 2013.
41. Puwanant S, Hamilton K, Klodell CT, et al: Tricuspid annular motion as a predictor of severe right ventricular failure after left ventricular assist device implantation. *J Heart Lung Transplant* 27:1102–1107, 2008.
42. Grant AD, Smedira NG, Starling RC, et al: Independent and incremental role of quantitative right ventricular evaluation for the prediction of right ventricular failure after left ventricular assist device implantation. *J Am Coll Cardiol* 60:521–528, 2012.
43. Piacentino V, Williams ML, Depp T, et al: Impact of tricuspid valve regurgitation in patients treated with implantable left ventricular assist devices. *Ann Thorac Surg* 91:1342–1347, 2011.
44. Ochiai Y, McCarthy PM, Smedira NG, et al: Predictors of severe right ventricular failure after implantable left ventricular assist device insertion: Analysis of 245 patients. *Circulation* 106:I-198–I-202, 2002.
45. Fitzpatrick JR, Frederick JR, Hsu VM, et al: Risk score derived from pre-operative data analysis predicts the need for biventricular mechanical circulatory support. *J Heart Lung Transplant* 27:1286–1292, 2008.
46. Matthews JC, Koelling TM, Pagani FD, et al: The right ventricular failure risk score. A pre-operative tool for assessing the risk of right ventricular failure in left ventricular assist device candidates. *J Am Coll Cardiol* 51:2163, 2008.
47. Slaughter MS, Pagani FD, Rogers JG, et al: Clinical management of continuous-flow left ventricular assist devices in advanced heart failure. *J Heart Lung Transplant* 29:S1–S39, 2010.
48. Balady GJ, Arena R, Sietsema K, et al: Clinician's guide to cardiopulmonary exercise testing in adults: A scientific statement from the American Heart Association. *Circulation* 122:191–225, 2010.
49. Samsky MD, Patel CP, DeWald TA, et al: Cardiohepatic interactions in heart failure. *J Am Coll Cardiol* 61:2397–2405, 2013.
50. Yang JA, Kato TS, Shulman BP, et al: Liver dysfunction as a predictor of outcomes in patients with advanced heart failure requiring ventricular assist device support: Use of the model of end-stage liver disease (MELD) and MELD excluding INR (MELD-XI) scoring system. *J Heart Lung Transplant* 31:601–610, 2012.
51. Schenk S, El-Banayosy A, Prohaska W, et al: Heparin-induced thrombocytopenia in patients receiving mechanical circulatory support. *J Thorac Cardiovasc Surg* 131:1373–1381, 2006.
52. Holdy K, Dembitsky W, Eaton LL, et al: Nutrition assessment and management of left ventricular assist device patients. *J Heart Lung Transplant* 24:1690–1696, 2005.
53. Lietz K, Long JW, Kfoury AG, et al: Outcomes of left ventricular assist device implantation as destination therapy in the post-REMATCH era: Implications for patient selection. *Circulation* 116:497–505, 2007.
54. Teuteberg J, Ewald GA, Adamson RM, et al: Risk assessment for continuous flow left ventricular assist devices: Does the destination therapy risk score work? *J Am Coll Cardiol* 60:44–51, 2012.
55. Lietz K, Long JW, Kfoury AG, et al: Impact of center volume on outcomes of left ventricular assist device implantation as destination therapy: Analysis of the Thoratec HeartMate registry, 1998–2005. *Circ Heart Fail* 2:3–10, 2009.
56. Frazier OH, Rose EA, Oz MC, et al: Multicenter clinical evaluation of the HeartMate vented electric left ventricular assist system in patients awaiting heart transplantation. *J Thorac Cardiovasc Surg* 122:1186–1195, 2001.
57. Russell SD, Rogers JG, Milano CA, et al: Renal and hepatic function improve in advanced heart failure patients during continuous-flow support with the HeartMate II left ventricular assist device. *Circulation* 120:2352–2357, 2009.
58. Petrucci RJ, Rogers JG, Blue L, et al: Neurocognitive function in destination therapy patients receiving continuous-flow vs pulsatile-flow left ventricular assist device support. *J Heart Lung Transplant* 31:27–36, 2012.
59. Rogers JG, Aaronson KD, Boyle AJ, et al: Continuous flow ventricular assist device improves functional capacity and quality of life of advanced heart failure patients. *J Am Coll Cardiol* 55:1826–1834, 2010.
60. Pagani FD, Miller LW, Russell SD, et al: Extended mechanical circulatory support with a continuous-flow rotary left ventricular assist device. *J Am Coll Cardiol* 54:312–321, 2009.
61. Park S, Milano C, Tatooles AJ, et al: Outcomes in advanced heart failure patients with left ventricular assist devices for destination therapy. *Circ Heart Fail* 5:241–248, 2012.
62. Aaronson KD, Slaughter MS, Miller LW, et al: Use of an intrapericardial, continuous-flow, centrifugal pump in patients awaiting heart transplantation. *Circulation* 125:3191–3200, 2012.
63. Bennett MK, Roberts CA, Dordunoo D, et al: Ideal methodology to assess systemic blood pressure in patients with continuous-flow left ventricular assist devices. *J Heart Lung Transplant* 29:593–594, 2012.
64. Uriel N, Morrison KA, Garan AR, et al: Development of a novel echocardiography ramp test for speed optimization and diagnosis of device thrombosis in continuous-flow left ventricular assist devices. *J Am Coll Cardiol* 60:1764–1775, 2012.
65. HeartWare Ventricular Assist System: Instructions for Use. HeartWare. www.heartware.com/clinicians/instructions-use.
66. Hannan MM, Husain S, Mattner F, et al: Working formulation for the standardization of definitions of infections in patients using ventricular assist devices. *J Heart Lung Transplant* 30:375–384, 2011.
67. Gordon RJ, Weinberg A, Pagani F, et al: Prospective multicenter study of ventricular assist device infections. *Circulation* 127:691–702, 2013.
68. Genovese EA, Dew MA, Teuteberg JJ, et al: Incidence and patterns of adverse event onset during the first 60 days after ventricular assist device implantation. *Ann Thorac Surg* 88:1162–1170, 2009.
69. Holman WL, Pae WE, Teutenberg JJ, et al: INTERMACS: Interval Analysis of Registry Data. *J Am Coll Surg* 208:755–762, 2009.
70. Crow S, John R, Boyle A, et al: Gastrointestinal bleeding rates in recipients of nonpulsatile and pulsatile left ventricular assist devices. *J Thorac Cardiovasc Surg* 137:208–215, 2009.

71. Suarez J, Patel CB, Felker M, et al: Mechanisms of bleeding and approach to patients with axial-flow left ventricular assist devices. *Circ Heart Fail* 4:779–784, 2011.
72. Demirozu ZT, Radovancevic R, Hochman LF, et al: Arteriovenous malformation and gastrointestinal bleeding in patients with the HeartMate II left ventricular assist device. *J Heart Lung Transplant* 30:849–853, 2011.
73. Uriel N, Pak SW, Jorde UP, et al: Acquired von Willebrand syndrome after continuous-flow mechanical device support contributes to a high prevalence of bleeding during long-term support and at the time of transplantation. *J Am Coll Cardiol* 56:1207–1213, 2010.
74. Crow S, Chen D, Milano C, et al: Acquired von Willebrand syndrome in continuous-flow ventricular assist device recipients. *Ann Thorac Surg* 90:1263–1269, 2010.
75. Kitada S, Kato TS, Thomas SS, et al: Pre-operative echocardiographic features associated with persistent mitral regurgitation after left ventricular assist device implantation. *J Heart Lung Transplant* 32:897–904, 2013.
76. Taghavi S, Hamad E, Wilson L, et al: Mitral valve repair at the time of continuous-flow ventricular assist device implantation confers meaningful decrement in pulmonary vascular resistance. *ASAIO J* 59(5):469–473, 2013.
77. Mudd JO, Cuda JD, Halushka M, et al: Fusion of aortic valve commissures in patients supported by a continuous axial flow left ventricular assist device. *J Heart Lung Transplant* 27:1269–1274, 2008.
78. Arabia F, Bauman ME, Buchholz HW, et al: The 2013 International Society for Heart and Lung Transplantation guidelines for mechanical circulatory support: Executive summary. *J Heart Lung Transplant* 32:157–187, 2013.
79. Park SJ, Liao KK, Segurola R, et al: Management of aortic insufficiency in patients with left ventricular assist devices: A simple coaptation stitch method (Park's stitch). *J Thorac Cardiovasc Surg* 127:264–266, 2004.
80. Pak SW, Uriel N, Takayama H, et al: Prevalence of de novo aortic insufficiency during long-term support with left ventricular assist devices. *J Heart Lung Transplant* 29:1172–1176, 2010.
81. Cowger J, Pagani FD, Haft JW, et al: The development of aortic insufficiency in left ventricular assist device-supported patients. *Circ Heart Fail* 3:668–674, 2010.
82. Rajagopal K, Daneshmand MA, Patel CB, et al: Natural history and clinical effect of aortic valve regurgitation after left ventricular assist device implantation. *J Thorac Cardiovasc Surg* 145:1373–1379, 2013.
83. Atkins BZ, Hashmi ZA, Ganapathi AM, et al: Surgical correction of aortic valve insufficiency after left ventricular assist device implantation. *Cardiovasc Surg* 146:1247–1252, 2013.
84. Cohn WE, Frazier OH: The sandwich plug technique: Simple, effective, and rapid closure of a mechanical aortic valve prosthesis at left ventricular assist device implantation. *J Thorac Cardiovasc Surg* 142:455–457, 2011.
85. Shah P, Mehta VM, Cowger JA, et al: Diagnosis of hemolysis and device thrombosis with lactate dehydrogenase during left ventricular assist device support. *J Heart Lung Transplant* 33:102–104, 2014.
86. Starling RC, Moazami N, Silvestry SC, et al: Unexpected abrupt increase in left ventricular assist device thrombosis. *N Engl J Med* 370:33–40, 2014.
87. Mentz RJ, Schlendorf K, Hernandez AF, et al: Dysphagia in the setting of left ventricular assist device hemolysis. *ASAIO J* 59(3):322–323, 2013.
88. Goldstein DJ, John R, Salerno C, et al: Algorithm for the diagnosis and management of suspected pump thrombus. *J Heart Lung Transplant* 32:667–670, 2013.
89. Kirklin JK, Naftel DC, Kormos RL, et al: INTERMACS analysis of pump thrombosis in the HeartMate II left ventricular assist device. *J Heart Lung Transplant* 33:12–22, 2014.
90. Slaughter MS, Sobieski MA, Martin M, et al: Home discharge experience with the Thoratec TLC-II portable driver. *ASAIO J* 53(2):132–135, 2007.
91. Krabatsch T, Potapov E, Stepanenko A, et al: Biventricular circulatory support with two miniaturized implantable assist devices. *Circulation* 124:S179–S186, 2011.
92. Copeland JG, Smith RG, Arabia FA, et al: Cardiac replacement with a total artificial heart as a bridge to transplantation. *N Engl J Med* 351:859–867, 2004.
93. Chrysostomou C, Morell VO, Kuch BA, et al: Short and intermediate-term survival after extracorporeal membrane oxygenation in children with cardiac disease. *J Thorac Cardiovasc Surg* 146:317–325, 2013.
94. Gupta P, McDonald R, Chipman CW, et al: 20-year experience of prolonged extracorporeal membrane oxygenation in critically ill children with cardiac or pulmonary failure. *Ann Thorac Surg* 93:1584–1591, 2012.
95. Merrill ED, Schoeneberg L, Sandesara P, et al: Outcomes after prolonged extracorporeal membrane oxygenation support in children with cardiac disease—Extracorporeal Life Support Organization registry study. *J Thorac Cardiovasc Surg* 1–7, 2013.
96. Polito A, Barrett CS, Wypij D, et al: Neurologic complications in neonates supported with extracorporeal membrane oxygenation. An analysis of ELSO registry data. *Intensive Care Med* 39:1594–1601, 2013.
97. Fraser CD, Jaquiss R, Rosenthal DN, et al: Prospective trial of a pediatric ventricular assist device. *N Engl J Med* 367:532–541, 2012.
98. Fraser CD, Carberry KE, Owens WR, et al: Preliminary experience with the MicroMed DeBakey pediatric ventricular assist device. *Semin Thorac Cardiovasc Surg Pediatr Card Surg Annu* 9:109–114, 2006.
99. Klotz S, Meyns B, Simon A, et al: Partial mechanical long-term support with the CircuLite synergy pump as bridge-to-transplant in congestive heart failure. *Thorac Cardiovasc Surg* 58(Suppl 2):S173–S178, 2010.
100. Goldstein DJ, Maybaum S, Macgillivray TE, et al: Young patients with nonischemic cardiomyopathy have higher likelihood of left ventricular recovery during left ventricular assist device support. *J Card Fail* 18:392–395, 2012.
101. Patel SR, Saeed O, Murthy S, et al: Combining neurohormonal blockade with continuous-flow left ventricular assist device support for myocardial recovery: A single-arm prospective study. *J Heart Lung Transplant* 32:305–312, 2013.
102. Birks E, Tansley PD, Hardy J, et al: Left ventricular assist device and drug therapy for the reversal of heart failure. *N Engl J Med* 355:1873–1884, 2006.
103. Birks EJ, George RS, Hedger M, et al: Reversal of severe heart failure with a continuous-flow left ventricular assist device and pharmacological therapy: A prospective study. *Circulation* 123:381–390, 2011.
104. Ascheim D, Gelijns AC, Goldstein D, et al: Mesenchymal precursor cells as adjunctive therapy in recipients of contemporary LVADs. *Circulation* 129:2287–2296, 2014.

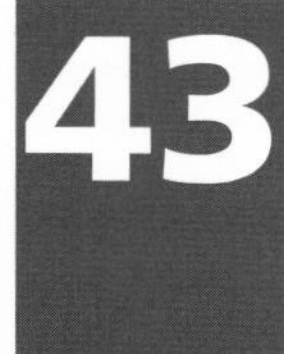

Managing Heart Failure in Cancer Patients

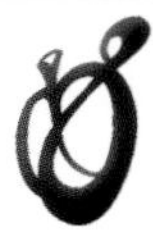

Douglas B. Sawyer and Daniel Lenihan

Heart failure as a consequence of cancer treatment is a well-known clinical challenge, with a history as old as the earliest days of cytotoxic chemotherapies and radiation-based treatment. During the past several decades of advancement in cancer treatment and overall improvements in the detection of cancer, cardiovascular toxicities, specifically heart failure (HF), have become more commonly recognized. One long-term vexing issue is the relatively unpredictable lag time from the exposure of a patient with cancer to potentially cardiotoxic treatments and the clinical manifestations of cardiovascular disease. Recent evidence suggests that many of these effects may be preventable with careful control of known cardiovascular risk factors at the time of cancer treatment. A more recent issue is the recognition that newer "targeted" cancer therapies may have effects on the cardiovascular system in general, and the cardiomyocyte in particular, that can manifest as HF and myocardial dysfunction. A more detailed understanding of the interaction between HF and cancer is rapidly evolving and gaining increased attention by basic and clinical scientists. In this chapter, we will cover the most critical issues that should be understood by the practicing cardiologist. For more in-depth coverage of this topic, see recent consensus statements and expert recommendations.[1-4]

EPIDEMIOLOGY OF CANCER AND HEART FAILURE

The population of patients experiencing both cardiovascular disease, including HF, and cancer grows each year (see also Chapter 17). This increase is driven by several factors, including the success of both cardiac treatment and cancer therapies leading to greater survivorship, the age-associated risk of heart disease and malignancy in an aging population, the overlap in risk factors between heart disease and malignancy, and the cardiovascular effects of cancer therapy. Cancer survivors are at increased risk compared with persons without malignancy for developing ischemic heart disease and HF throughout their lives.[5] Health behavior, such as tobacco use and alcohol abuse, as well as obesity and associated metabolic disorder, increases the risk of both HF and certain cancers. In addition, cardiovascular disease and HF are known consequences of certain cancer therapies. The improvements in outcome for pediatric cancer patients have been tremendous, and result in a growing population of adults at risk for HF who will benefit from attention throughout their lives.[2] A striking example of this is the apparent rise in incidence of heart transplant patients with a history of anthracycline cardiomyopathy.[6] Additionally, although radiation therapy has improved over the decades, chest radiation remains an important cause of significant heart disease, including complex vascular and valvular disease that may result in HF.[7,8] Newer emerging cancer therapies, although offering hope to previously untreatable malignancies such as metastatic breast cancer and multiple myeloma, do have direct deleterious effects on cardiovascular tissues in susceptible patients, and this concept needs to be understood by both oncologists and cardiologists.

HEART FAILURE SECONDARY TO CANCER THERAPY

A growing number of cancer therapies are known to cause cardiac dysfunction and HF (**Table 43-1**). Thus a patient being treated with these should considered a stage A HF patient per American College of Cardiology/American Heart Association (ACC/AHA) guidelines.[9] The risk of HF varies by chemotherapeutic agent and individual risk factors, and there can be a considerable time delay between exposure and clinical presentation. For some older chemotherapeutics, a great deal is known about cardiovascular safety and toxicity, whereas for newer therapies the risks may be largely unidentified. Moreover, many lifesaving cancer therapies gain approval with relatively limited supporting data. When HF or other cardiovascular disease is detected in a cancer patient during or after treatment with a novel therapy, some degree of suspicion that the cancer treatment is promoting the cardiovascular disease is warranted.

TABLE 43-1 Common Cancer Treatments Known to Be Associated with Development of Heart Failure

CLASS OF THERAPY	GENERIC NAMES	TIMING	RISK FACTORS FOR HEART FAILURE
Anthracyclines	doxorubicin daunorubicin epirubicin idarubicin mitoxantrone	Concurrent and delayed	Cumulative dose Concurrent radiation therapy, cyclophosphamide, or ErbB2 targeted therapies Age (young and old) Hypertension Known heart disease
Alkylating agent	cyclophosphamide	Early	Dose, age, concurrent anthracyclines
HER2 (ErbB2)-targeted therapies	trastuzumab pertuzumab lapatinib	Concurrent	Hypertension, age, low pretreatment LVEF
VEGF/angiogenesis-targeted therapies	sunitinib sorafenib pazopamib bevacizumab	Concurrent	Hypertension
BCR-ABL inhibitors	imatinib ponatinib	Concurrent	
Proteasome inhibitors	bortezomib carfilzomib	Concurrent	Prior anthracyclines
Mediastinal/chest radiation		Delayed	Cumulative dose Concurrent anthracyclines Age (young) Hypertension

LVEF, Left ventricular ejection fraction; *VEGF,* vascular endothelial growth factor.

Guidelines developed by both oncologists and cardiologists recommend echocardiography or multiple-gated acquisition (MUGA) radionuclide ventriculography to screen for left ventricular (LV) dysfunction in patients being treated with potentially cardiotoxic chemotherapy.[1,2] These recommendations have largely been developed from oncology clinical trial data and expert opinion. There remain significant gaps in our knowledge over best practices to optimize outcome for these patients. No definitive guideline exists as to how often assessments of ventricular function should be performed, particularly after completion of therapy. Measurement of cardiac function and decisions over continuation of potentially cardiotoxic cancer therapy have primarily focused on left ventricular ejection fraction (LVEF) as a marker of cardiac damage in detecting cancer effects on the myocardium.[1] However, changes in diastolic dysfunction are widely acknowledged to contribute to HF in cancer patients, and in some cancer populations occur more commonly than reduced systolic function.[10] Moreover, a significant reduction in LVEF is not a sensitive screen for HF given that the heart can adapt to substantial injury without a major change in LVEF. With this in mind, improved methods to screen for cardiac effects of cancer therapy are clearly needed.[11] In patients with significant chest radiation exposure, periodic assessment of cardiac valve function may also be warranted. In addition to baseline screening, all patients receiving potentially cardiotoxic cancer therapy should undergo careful clinical assessment and repeat assessment of LVEF at some interval during and at the conclusion of cardiotoxic therapy. Furthermore, in patients who have received cancer treatments associated with delayed cardiac effects (e.g., anthracyclines, radiation) periodic assessment throughout their life has been recommended.[1,2]

Due to variability in techniques of the measurement of LVEF, it is generally recommended that the same technique be used serially for an individual patient to optimize comparison with previous measurements. It is also recognized that echocardiography provides substantial additional information on cardiac structure, hemodynamics, and physiology not typically found with MUGA. The use of magnetic resonance imaging (MRI) is increasing and is able to detect early changes that predict late outcomes,[12] but limitations in availability, expertise, and contrast usage to look for delayed enhancement of the lateral wall may impede a wide adoption of this technique.[13]

Treatment of HF secondary to cancer therapy in general should follow the guidelines established for other forms of HF. Consistent with other categories of stage A HF, there is some evidence to suggest that antihypertensive agents with known benefits, such as angiotensin-converting enzyme inhibitors (ACEI) or selected β-adrenergic receptor blockers (BB), may prevent or reduce the risk of progression to more advanced stages of HF.[14,15] In later stage HF, guideline-directed medical therapy is associated with improvements in outcome, including improved cardiac function.[16] In advanced chemotherapy-induced HF, cardiac transplant and mechanical circulatory support have been used in cancer survivors achieving complete remission with comparable outcomes to other forms of HF.[17,18]

SPECIFIC CANCER THERAPIES, THEIR MECHANISMS OF CARDIOTOXICITY, AND IMPLICATIONS FOR CLINICAL PRACTICE

Anthracyclines

Anthracyclines are a mainstay of cancer treatment, and a well-recognized cause of cardiomyopathy and HF. Anthracyclines intercalate into nucleic acids and cause oxidative damage to lipids, proteins, and nucleic acids, along with inhibition of DNA and RNA synthesis and repair in all cells including cardiac myocytes (**Figure 43-1**). Myocyte death can be detected after anthracycline exposure in the form of elevated cardiac troponins (**see also Chapter 30**). It is well established that an individual's risk of HF secondary to anthracyclines is directly related to the cumulative drug exposure,[19] which is consistent with the concept that every anthracycline dose causes some degree of irreversible cardiac damage. General guidance for anthracycline

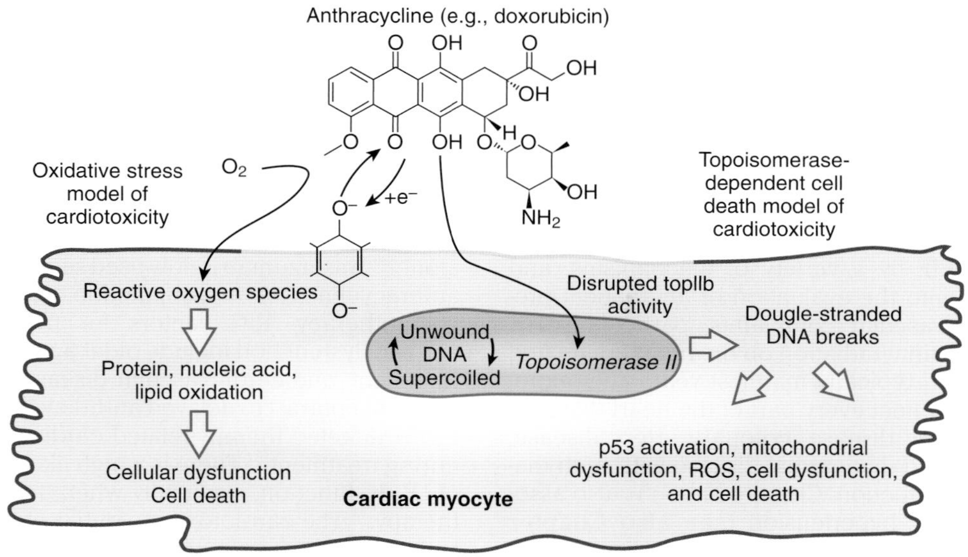

FIGURE 43-1 Proposed mechanisms of anthracycline cardiotoxicity. Anthracyclines are directly toxic to cardiac myocytes. The quinone moiety can redox cycle and reduce molecular oxygen to superoxide anion, leading to an increase in reactive oxygen species, and resulting oxidant stress can lead to direct damage to cellular elements. Recent experimental studies in mice supports a mechanism where alteration in topoisomerase IIb (TopIIb) function leads to DNA damage upstream of mitochondrial function and oxidant stress.

cumulative dosing is to avoid cumulative doses of greater than 500 mg/m^2. Other known risk factors for anthracycline HF include age (both young and elderly), hypertension, preexisting cardiac conditions, concurrent mediastinal radiation, and/or other therapies with cardiac effects, including cyclophosphamide, paclitaxel, and trastuzumab (see later discussion).

Despite the probable immediate loss of myocardium during anthracycline treatment, cancer patients frequently remain asymptomatic or only minimally symptomatic for months to years. Contractile reserve and compensatory mechanisms on the cellular and subcellular levels presumably maintain cardiac function. One of the survival factors implicated in the modulation of anthracycline cardiotoxicity is the neuregulin/ErbB signaling system, explaining the increased toxicity when anthracyclines are used concomitantly with ErbB2-targeted therapeutics.[20]

The oxidative stress induced by the quinone moiety of anthracyclines has long been the target of strategies to prevent cardiotoxicity. Numerous antioxidant strategies have been explored, with limited success. Dexrazoxane is the only approved agent for prevention of anthracycline treatment–related HF, which was developed with the concept that its iron-chelating properties will limit Fenton chemistry and generation of cytotoxic reactive oxygen species. Recently, an alternative mechanism for the cardiotoxicity of anthracyclines and the cardioprotective properties of dexrazoxane has emerged. Both drugs interact with topoisomerase II (topII), enzymes that wind and unwind DNA to allow for the packing and unpacking critical for normal cellular function. Mice lacking topIIb, the form of topII expressed in myocardium, are resistant to the cardiotoxicity of anthracyclines.[20a] Dexrazoxane interacts with topII and prevents topII-dependent anthracycline myocytotoxicity. This finding raises the question of whether dexrazoxane is protecting the heart through inhibition of oxidative stress as has been previously proposed. This may also lead to new strategies to predict and prevent the deleterious effects of anthracyclines on the heart.

Genetic analysis of cohorts by genomewide association studies have identified a number of genetic loci that speak to the importance of cellular uptake mechanisms and carbonyl redox cycling in the cardiotoxicity of anthracyclines. Loci associated with genes encoding protein components of cellular transport systems, including the ATP-cassette transporters in the multi-drug resistance family, are associated with risk of cardiotoxicity.[21-23] Animal work supports the notion that these transporters regulate the uptake of anthracyclines. This has important implications for patients undergoing treatment with anthracyclines that are typically underappreciated by most practitioners. Commonly prescribed medications, including antihypertensives diltiazem and verapamil, are competitively transported by these same proteins, and concomitant treatment with these or other similarly transported pharmaceuticals will raise the cytoplasmic anthracycline concentration.[24] Other antihypertensives, such as BB and ACEI, are not handled by this transporter and therefore will not alter intracellular anthracycline concentrations. Recent evidence supports the concept that BB and ACEI may be cardioprotective against anthracyclines, particularly in higher risk patients.[25,26] With this knowledge, a change in the antihypertensive regimen of some patients may have an important impact on their risk for cardiomyopathy. Other less commonly prescribed medications, such as cyclosporine and digoxin, are similarly transported and may raise the cytoplasmic anthracycline concentration. Thus all patients should have a careful review of their medication list with a focus on identifying substrates for the p-glycoprotein/MDR/ATP-cassette transporters, and consider a change in medication class if appropriate.

Recent evidence supports the concept that careful monitoring of patients during anthracycline-based chemotherapy will reduce the likelihood of development of chronic HF. Early detection and initiation of neurohormonal antagonist therapy is associated with a greater likelihood of improving cardiac function after anthracycline exposure. Cardiac biomarker-based strategies to screen for cardiac injury at the time of chemotherapy are also likely to lead to earlier intervention and improved outcome (see Chapter 30).[27] There is also emerging evidence that statins, one of the most commonly prescribed class of cardiovascular medications, may limit anthracycline cardiotoxicity.[28]

Radiation Therapy

Radiation therapy remains an important component of therapy for specific cancers. A history of mediastinal radiation may result in HF by a variety of mechanisms, and should be factored into the evaluation of any patient presenting with cardiovascular complaints, particularly HF. The effects of mediastinal radiation on the heart are related to radiation dose, and typically manifest years after exposure.[29] Radiation can affect every part of the heart that is in the path, causing valve disease, coronary artery disease, pericardial disease, and myocardial disease with both diastolic and systolic dysfunction. Chest radiation is also associated with pulmonary hypertension (see also Chapter 39).[30] The only known strategies to prevent cardiac disease during radiation treatment are to limit cardiovascular exposure and to control cardiovascular risk factors optimally and hopefully reduce the risk of subsequent cardiovascular injury.

Other Chemotherapeutics

Acute cardiac injury in the form of myocarditis and pericarditis is a known complication of cyclophosphamide, particularly when used at high doses during induction therapy for some bone marrow transplant regimens. HF occurs in some 7% to 28% of patients receiving high-dose cyclophosphamide. Pathologic examination shows disruption of endothelial cells, hemorrhagic myocarditis, and disrupted myocyte ultrastructure. Risk factors identified include age, dose, and concurrent treatment with anthracyclines. Fulminant HF refractory to treatment has been reported in this setting. There are no current practice guidelines for monitoring of cardiac function after cyclophosphamide induction therapy and no accepted practices for prevention. Careful monitoring by physical examination for signs of fluid retention, with maintenance of high suspicion for cardiac contribution to nonspecific symptoms of fatigue and malaise in the early weeks/months after induction therapy with cyclophosphamide, is clinically prudent.

Targeted Therapies

Recent advances in cancer therapy have occurred through the discovery of specific signaling cascades contributing to cancer progression and the development of novel agents that target these processes. Several of these therapies have been associated with development of HF and are highlighted below.

ErbB2-Targeted Therapies: Trastuzumab, Lapatinib, Pertuzumab

Trastuzumab (Herceptin, Genentech/Roche) and pertuzumab (Perjeta, Roche), are recombinant humanized monoclonal antibodies against the human epidermal growth factor receptor 2 (HER2, a.k.a. ErbB2) protein, an oncogene that when overexpressed in tumor cells promotes cell proliferation through constitutive activation of growth signaling pathways. Lapatinib (Tykerb/ Tyverb, GlaxoSmithKline) is a small molecule dual tyrosine kinase inhibitor (TKI) of the epidermal growth factor (EGF) and ErbB2 receptors that blocks receptor activation of intracellular signaling. These therapies are used for the treatment of ErbB2-overexpressing tumors, including breast and gastric cancers. Cardiac side effects of ErbB2-targeted therapeutics were first detected in the pivotal trastuzumab breast cancer trials, where trastuzumab combined with anthracyclines showed greater cardiotoxicity compared with anthracycline alone.[20] Trastuzumab is now used sequentially after or before anthracyclines or in conjunction with anthracycline-free chemotherapy. Risk factors for trastuzumab-associated cardiac dysfunction include older age, lower LVEF at time of treatment, and cardiovascular disease including hypertension.[31] In contrast to delayed anthracycline cardiomyopathy, ErbB2-targeted therapy-related cardiac dysfunction occurs during treatment.[32] There is a high likelihood of reversibility of LV dysfunction, especially when treated with typical HF therapy.[33] The cardiotoxic potential of lapatinib appears to be less than trastuzumab, perhaps due to the shorter half-life of this small molecule.[34] Pertuzumab also appears to be associated with less LV dysfunction and HF.[35] Although this may be due to differences in the biologic properties of these ErbB2-targeted therapies, there has also been much greater scrutiny of cardiac function in patients being considered for treatment with ErbB2-targeted therapies since the initial trials.

The cardiac side effects of anti-ErbB2 therapeutics might be explained by studies examining the biology of neuregulin, an EGF-family ligand and ErbB receptor in the cardiovascular system (**Figure 43-2**). Neuregulin, ErbB2, and ErbB4 receptor tyrosine kinases play an important role in cell-cell crosstalk and mediate cellular responses to stress in the heart (for review see Odiete et al[36]). ErbB2 is expressed in the adult cardiomyocytes, and disruption of its expression through genetic engineering in mice leads to progressive dilated cardiomyopathy.[37] Myocardial stress induced by ischemia activates neuregulin/ErbB signaling in the heart,[38] and suppressing signaling prevents recovery from ischemic injury.[39]

Like anthracycline-treated cancer patients, those anticipating treatment with ErbB2-targeted therapies should be considered stage A HF patients. Pretreatment screening, including measurement of LV function, is recommended to detect more advanced HF, and current practice is to not use ErbB2-targeted therapies in patients with stage B or greater HF. Current practice also includes monitoring of cardiac function with periodic reassessment of LV function during treatment with ErbB2-targeted therapy, particularly in patients at higher risk for cardiac dysfunction. Patients developing advanced HF appear to respond to established HF therapy, and in some patients continued treatment with ErbB2-targeted therapy appears to be tolerated.[33] Whether neurohormonal blockade has any role in preventing LV dysfunction in this setting is not yet known.

Angiogenesis Inhibitors

Cancer treatments targeting vascular endothelial growth factor (VEGF) and angiogenesis are an important class of compounds that have been associated with development of HF. VEGF regulates angiogenesis, endothelial cell survival, vasodilation, and cardiac contractile function.[40] The VEGF-targeted angiogenesis inhibitors, such as ErbB2-targeted therapy, are either antibody-based, which bind

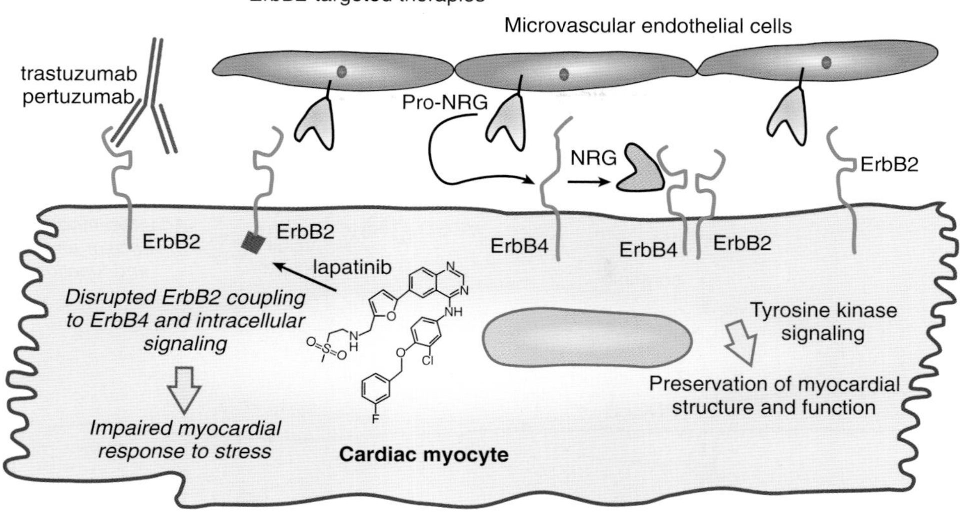

FIGURE 43-2 Potential mechanisms of ErbB2-targeted therapy associated cardiac dysfunction. The ErbB2 receptor tyrosine kinase is expressed in cardiac myocytes where it is activated by the ligand neuregulin (NRG) through heterodimerization with ErbB4 receptors. ErbB activation in cardiac myocytes is associated with a number of effects on cardiac myocytes, including regulating cell structure, adaptations in Ca^{++} handling, and metabolism. ErbB2-targeted therapies interrupt NRG/ErbB signaling and prevent this pathway from regulating cardiac response to stress.

and neutralize VEGF (e.g., bevacizumab), or small molecular inhibitors of VEGF tyrosine kinase receptors (e.g., sunitinib, sorafenib). These are now used in the treatment of a variety of cancers.

A general cardiovascular class effect of these compounds is the augmentation of blood pressure.[41,42] VEGF-targeted therapy–associated hypertension appears to occur through several mechanisms, including increased vascular stiffness that may be mediated by increased activity of the renin-angiotensin system.[43] A preeclampsia-like syndrome with proteinuria and thrombotic microangiopathy has been reported in a subset of patients.[44,45] VEGF activates vascular eNOS via the PI3-kinase/PKB/Akt pathway, and this is one mechanism for VEGF-mediated vasorelaxation. Mice lacking VEGF demonstrate glomerular pathology, with loss of podocytes and disruption of the basement membrane.[46] VEGF-targeted therapies are also associated with a threefold increase in risk for arterial thromboembolic events (stroke, transient ischemic attacks, myocardial infarction, angina, and other arterial events),[47,48] which appears to be an additional consequence of disrupting endothelial homeostasis.[49]

LV dysfunction and HF occur in bevacizumab-treated patients, although they appear to be more common in those treated with VEGF-targeted TKIs. VEGF signaling mediates the adaptation of the heart to pressure overload. Suppressing VEGF signaling in the setting of pressure overload leads to more rapid deleterious cardiac remodeling and HF in mice.[50] This may involve VEGF's angiogenic activity that regulates growth of microvasculature in proportion to that of cardiac myocytes during adaptation of the heart to increased load.

Retrospective analyses of sunitinib-associated cardiac dysfunction report that up to 10% of patients receiving sunitinib experience some degree of HF,[51,52] although larger meta-analyses have reported an incidence of 4%.[53] Sunitinib induces mitochondrial injury and cardiomyocyte apoptosis in both mice and cultured rat cardiomyocytes.[54] Sunitinib inhibits several tyrosine kinases, including AMPK and PDGFR, which may explain the higher rate of clinical cardiac toxicity (**Figure 43-3**). Mice lacking PDGF receptor expression respond to pressure overload induced by surgical aortic constriction with accelerated cardiac remodeling associated with impaired vascular growth and function.[55] Mice lacking AMPKa2 similarly are normal in the unstressed condition, but experience accelerated remodeling and HF after pressure overload.[56] It is interesting that in each of these animals the phenotype of cardiac dysfunction is not manifested unless the animals are subjected to pressure overload. This would suggest that the hypertensive effect of VEGF-targeted TKIs may be requisite for induction of contractile dysfunction.

It is yet unclear whether cardiac dysfunction induced by angiogenesis inhibitors is reversible. In early reports, patients with HF and LV dysfunction generally responded to temporary suspension of sunitinib and medical management.[54] However, the preclinical data in animals and cells support a pro-apoptotic effect of sunitinib that would be associated with some degree of irreversible cardiac damage. Persistent cardiac dysfunction has been noted in some persons treated with sunitinib.[52] Predicting and preventing HF in these patients remains a challenge for the future.

BCR-ABL Inhibitors

Inhibitors of "Philadelphia chromosome" BCR-ABL have become the first-line therapy for the approximately 90% of patients with chronic myelogenous leukemia, as well as other tumors with this oncogene. Imatinib (Gleevec) was the first BCR-ABL inhibitor developed. Imatinib-associated systolic HF has been reported[57] and may occur because of inhibition of Abl in cardiac myocytes where it regulates endoplasmic reticulum stress responses. Second- and third-generation BCR-ABL inhibitors have been developed that have distinct properties, most important the ability to overcome imatinib resistance via a number of strategies. These newer BCR-ABL inhibitors have been linked to higher rates of peripheral arterial occlusive disease (nilotinib).[58] Most recently, a unique BCR-ABL inhibitor that is able to block a specific mutant form of BCR-ABL, ponatinib, has

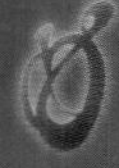

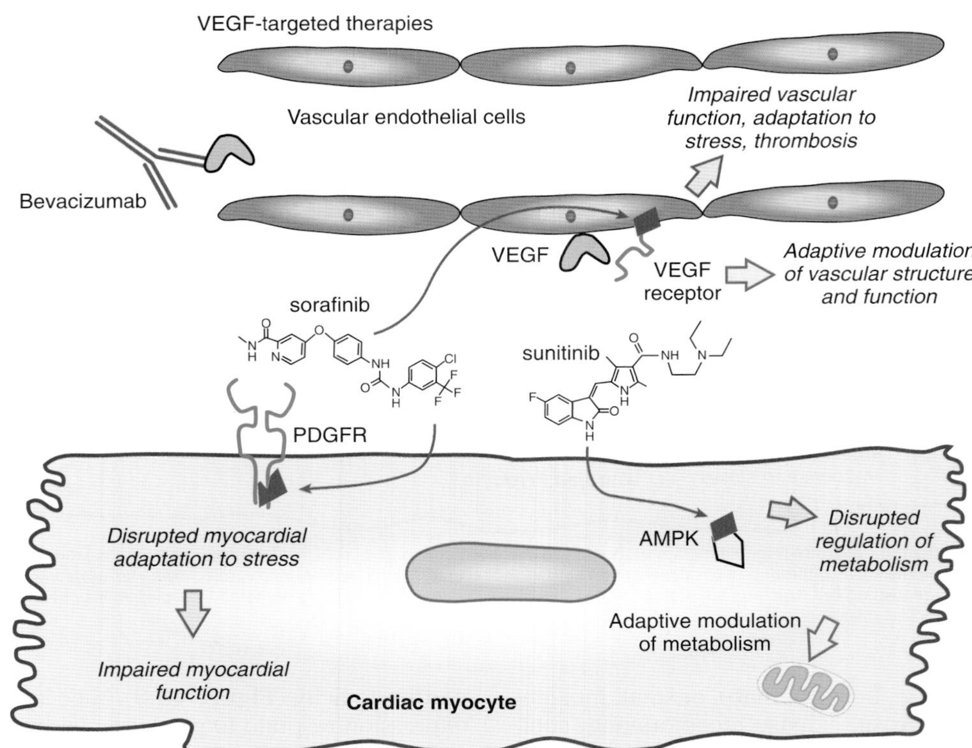

FIGURE 43-3 Potential mechanisms of angiogenesis inhibitor–associated heart failure. Bevacizumab, and other drugs that bind and inhibit VEGF (VEGF trap), block VEGF activity. Inhibition of VEGF receptor activation will reduce vascular reactivity, as well as promote platelet activation. Sunitinib and sorafenib are small molecule inhibitors of tyrosine kinases that block the activity of not only VEGF receptor, but also kinases such as platelet-derived growth factor receptors (PDGFR) and AMP-activated kinase (AMPK). These other effects may explain why heart failure is more common in patients treated with these multityrosine kinase inhibitors.

been linked to high rates of thromboemboli, arterial occlusion, and HF.[59]

Proteasome Inhibitors

The ubiquitin–proteasome system (UP-S) is a cellular protein degradation system that is vital to normal cellular function, and in some tumors critical for proliferation. Preclinical studies have shown that proteasome disruption inhibits proliferation, induces apoptosis, reverses chemoresistance, and enhances chemotherapy and radiation efficacy in some tumors. The proteasome pathway is also critical for maintenance of cardiac structure and function, and altered proteasome function is associated with cardiac pathophysiology.[60]

Bortezomib (Velcade) was the first proteasome inhibitor to be developed successfully as a cancer therapeutic. Bortezomib blocks proliferation and induces apoptosis of plasma cells.[61] It also inhibits the proteasomal degradation of signaling molecules that regulate cell survival, leading to enhancement of chemotherapy sensitivity. Bortezomib is used for initial treatment of patients with multiple myeloma based on its effects on plasma cell proliferation. The side effects reported include asthenia, peripheral neuropathy, gastrointestinal symptoms, and anorexia. There are a few reports of cardiac failure occurring in patients during treatment with bortezomib,[62] suggesting that under some circumstances inactivation of the cardiac proteasome can result in adverse effects on the heart.

Because of the success of generally well-tolerated bortezomib, newer proteasome inhibitors are being developed. Carfilzomib, an irreversible proteasome inhibitor, is now approved as second-line therapy for relapsed multiple myeloma. Although this therapy appears to be more active in resistant myeloma cases than previous treatments, there may be a greater likelihood of cardiac events including HF, sudden cardiac death, and acute coronary syndrome.[63] The cardiac safety of carfilzomib and other proteasome inhibitors will become clearer as greater experience accumulates with these therapies.

Emerging Cancer Therapies

There are many oncogenic proteins that regulate tumor growth and are targets of ongoing efforts to develop new therapies for cancer. To the extent that these targets serve functions in cardiovascular homeostasis, one might anticipate adverse cardiovascular effects including HF.[64] An obvious challenge for development of drugs targeting these pathways will be selection of timing and delivery strategies that will limit this potential. It appears that the normal myocardium can escape brief interruptions in pathways regulating metabolism as long as fatty acid, oxygen, and glucose are in ready supply, allowing for adaptive changes in substrate use. However, longer interruptions of these cascades, and/or alterations during times of metabolic stress (e.g., ischemia, hemodynamic stress, or chronic increases in rate-pressure product) may increase the likelihood that suppressing the activity of kinases required for metabolic adaptation, such as AMPK and PI3-kinase, will result in cardiovascular dysfunction including HF. Similarly, cancer therapies targeting proteins involved in regulating cell survival may have no deleterious effects in the absence of stressors promoting cell death.

HEART FAILURE AS A CONSEQUENCE OF CANCER

There are several situations where HF is a direct consequence of malignancy, rather than therapy. Infiltrative cardiomyopathy secondary to primary amyloid light-chain (AL) amyloidosis occurs in the setting of multiple myeloma and plasma cell dyscrasia. The unique challenges this condition presents to the HF clinician are covered in detail elsewhere (see Chapter 20).

MANAGING HEART FAILURE DURING CANCER TREATMENT

Increasing numbers of patients with HF are surviving cardiac disease, such as myocardial infarction (MI), only to develop malignancies, and these patients pose a special challenge to their cardiology and oncology providers. Preexisting HF in a patient newly diagnosed with cancer is likely to change the treatment options offered by some medical and surgical oncologists. A careful cardiac assessment should be done at that time and considerable discussion between the cardiology and oncology provider is ideal to help the oncologist understand the HF history, prognosis, and how this might influence oncologic treatment plans.

As cancer treatment ensues, challenges for the cardiologist to consider are managing fluid status, neurohormonal blockade, and thromboembolic risk during cycles of cancer therapy that may promote fluid retention, change hemodynamics, and increase thrombosis or bleeding risk (**Table 43-2**). Some familiarity with the medications used in oncology may improve the likelihood that a patient with HF can be managed effectively during cancer treatment without a HF exacerbation. Typically, this requires more intensive attention to volume status and hemodynamics, with frequent HF clinic visits during active cancer treatment.

Anticipating changes in fluid status induced during steroid-containing regimens in patients prone to fluid retention may help reduce the likelihood that acute HF becomes a complication of cancer treatment. Anticipating fluid shifts that occur with some therapies such as granulocyte colony-stimulating factor (GCSF) may similarly reduce the likelihood of acute HF exacerbation. Changes in blood pressure frequently occur during cancer treatment, and this may lead to changes in the HF medical therapy, which will obviously require close monitoring and readjustment when patients regain hemodynamic stability.

Standard therapy for cardiovascular disease and HF may interact with cancer outcomes based on a number of observations, mostly retrospective analysis of large cancer registry data sets (**Table 43-3**). Although further work is clearly needed before any firm conclusions should be drawn or recommendations made, many patients are aware of these data. The use of ACEI or angiotensin receptor blockers (ARBs) has been associated with higher rates of relapse of breast cancer, whereas use of β-blockers appears to improve cancer outcomes.[65-67] Aspirin and cholesterol-lowering statins have also been associated with the reduced likelihood of relapse for some malignancies,[68,69] and for statins a reduced likelihood of development of HF.[28] Digoxin is a phytoestrogen, and its use has been associated with increased risk of estrogen-sensitive malignancies.[70,71]

TABLE 43-2 Common Cancer Treatments and Treatment Effects That May Exacerbate Heart Failure

CLASS OF THERAPY	EFFECT	STRATEGY
Steroids	Subacute fluid retention	Careful monitoring of fluid status Adjustable diuretic dosing
GCSF	Acute capillary leak	Optimize volume status pre-GCSF
Antiangiogenics	Hypertension	Adjust vasodilators/antihypertensives
Vomiting, diarrhea	Dehydration, sensitivity to HF medications	Sliding scale diuretic plan, close monitoring by HF provider
Anemia, thrombocytopenia requiring transfusion	Volume load	Careful monitoring of fluid status Adjustable diuretic dosing
Sepsis syndrome	Sensitivity to HF medications	Careful hemodynamic monitoring and medication adjustment

GCSF, Granulocyte colony-stimulating factor; *HF,* heart failure.

ADVANCED THERAPIES IN THE CANCER PATIENT WITH HEART FAILURE

Advanced therapies including electrophysiologic devices (see Chapter 35), mechanical circulatory support (see Chapter 42), and heart transplant (see Chapter 40) have all been used with success in cancer survivors with HF refractory to medical therapy. The most experience is with cardiomyopathy secondary to anthracycline. Over 20 years of outcome data collected by the United Network of Organ Sharing (UNOS) reveal that heart transplant outcomes are as similar for anthracycline cardiomyopathy patients as they are for other causes of HF.[6,18] Rates of infection and malignancy, as well as the likelihood of needing a right ventricular assist device, were higher in chemotherapy-associated HF compared with nonischemic HF patients.[18] Although this supports the use of heart transplant as a treatment in this group of patients, a disturbing trend was noted for increased numbers of heart transplants being done in cancer survivors,[6] suggesting that HF resulting from cancer treatment is potentially an emerging cause of refractory HF.

The efficacy of biventricular pacemakers in appropriate patients with anthracycline cardiomyopathy and HF has similarly been demonstrated in a very selected group.[72] It

TABLE 43-3 Potential Effects of Therapies Used in Heart Failure on Cancer Outcomes

CLASS OF THERAPY	EFFECT	EVIDENCE
ACEI, ARB	May raise rate of relapse	Retrospective databases[65]
β-blocker	May lower rate of relapse	Retrospective databases[65,66, 73]
Aldosterone blocker	No effect	Retrospective database[74]
Aspirin	May lower rate of relapse	Prospective cohort[68]
HMG-CoA reductase I	May lower rate of relapse	Retrospective[69]
Digoxin	Increased risk of breast/ovarian cancer	Retrospective[70, 71]

ACEI, Angiotensin-converting enzyme inhibitors; *ARB,* angiotensin receptor blocker.

certainly appears that the expected benefit of cardiac resynchronization in all HF patients who qualify is applicable to those cancer survivors who have typical clinical characteristics that warrant device implantation.

References

1. Curigliano G, Cardinale D, Suter T, et al: Cardiovascular toxicity induced by chemotherapy, targeted agents and radiotherapy: ESMO Clinical Practice Guidelines. *Ann Oncol* 23(Suppl 7):vii155–vii166, 2012.
2. Lipshultz SE, Adams MJ, Colan SD, et al: Long-term cardiovascular toxicity in children, adolescents, and young adults who receive cancer therapy: pathophysiology, course, monitoring, management, prevention, and research directions: a scientific statement from the American Heart Association. *Circulation* 128(17):1927–1995, 2013.
3. Steingart RM, Yadav N, Manrique C, et al: Cancer survivorship: cardiotoxic therapy in the adult cancer patient; cardiac outcomes with recommendations for patient management. *Semin Oncol* 40(6):690–708, 2013.
4. Lenihan DJ, Cardinale DM: Late cardiac effects of cancer treatment. *J Clin Oncol* 30(30):3657–3664, 2012.
5. Tashakkor AY, Moghaddamjou A, Chen L, et al: Predicting the risk of cardiovascular comorbidities in adult cancer survivors. *Curr Oncol* 20(5):e360–e370, 2013.
6. Lenneman AJ, Wang L, Wigger M, et al: Heart transplant survival outcomes for Adriamycin-dilated cardiomyopathy. *Am J Cardiol* 111(4):609–612, 2013.
7. Adams MJ, Lipshultz SE, Schwartz C, et al: Radiation-associated cardiovascular disease: manifestations and management. *Semin Radiat Oncol* 13(3):346–356, 2003.
8. Darby SC, Ewertz M, McGale P, et al: Risk of ischemic heart disease in women after radiotherapy for breast cancer. *N Engl J Med* 368(11):987–998, 2013.
9. Yancy CW, Jessup M, Bozkurt B, et al: 2013 ACCF/AHA guideline for the management of heart failure: a report of the American College of Cardiology Foundation/American Heart Association Task Force on Practice Guidelines. *J Am Coll Cardiol* 62(16):e147–e239, 2013.
10. Brouwer CA, Gietema JA, van den Berg MP, et al: Long-term cardiac follow-up in survivors of a malignant bone tumour. *Ann Oncol* 17(10):1586–1591, 2006.
11. Ewer MS, Lenihan DJ: Left ventricular ejection fraction and cardiotoxicity: is our ear really to the ground? *J Clin Oncol* 26(8):1201–1203, 2008.
12. Wassmuth R, Lentzsch S, Erdbruegger U, et al: Subclinical cardiotoxic effects of anthracyclines as assessed by magnetic resonance imaging—a pilot study. *Am Heart J* 141(6):1007–1013, 2001.
13. Vasu S, Hundley WG: Understanding cardiovascular injury after treatment for cancer: an overview of current uses and future directions of cardiovascular magnetic resonance. *J Cardiovasc Magn Reson* 15(1):66, 2013.
14. Cardinale D, Colombo A, Sandri MT, et al: Prevention of high-dose chemotherapy-induced cardiotoxicity in high-risk patients by angiotensin-converting enzyme inhibition. *Circulation* 114(23):2474–2481, 2006.
15. Kalay N, Basar E, Ozdogru I, et al: Protective effects of carvedilol against anthracycline-induced cardiomyopathy. *J Am Coll Cardiol* 48(11):2258–2262, 2006.
16. Cardinale D, Bacchiani G, Beggiato M, et al: Strategies to prevent and treat cardiovascular risk in cancer patients. *Semin Oncol* 40(2):186–198, 2013.
17. Geisberg CA, Abdallah WM, da Silva M, et al: Circulating neuregulin during the transition from stage A to stage B/C heart failure in a breast cancer cohort. *J Card Fail* 19(1):10–15, 2013.
18. Oliveira GH, Hardaway BW, Kucheryavaya AY, et al: Characteristics and survival of patients with chemotherapy-induced cardiomyopathy undergoing heart transplantation. *J Heart Lung Transplant* 31(8):805–810, 2012.
19. Swain SM, Whaley FS, Ewer MS: Congestive heart failure in patients treated with doxorubicin: a retrospective analysis of three trials. *Cancer* 97(11):2869–2879, 2003.
20. Slamon DJ, Leyland-Jones B, Shak S, et al: Use of chemotherapy plus a monoclonal antibody against HER2 for metastatic breast cancer that overexpresses HER2. *N Engl J Med* 344(11):783–792, 2001.
20a. Zhang S, Liu X, Bawa-Khalfe T, et al: Identification of the molecular basis of doxorubicin-induced cardiotoxicity. *Nat Med* 18(11):1639–1642, 2012.
21. Blanco JG, Sun CL, Landier W, et al: Anthracycline-related cardiomyopathy after childhood cancer: role of polymorphisms in carbonyl reductase genes–a report from the Children's Oncology Group. *J Clin Oncol* 30(13):1415–1421, 2012.
22. Visscher H, Ross CJ, Rassekh SR, et al: Pharmacogenomic prediction of anthracycline-induced cardiotoxicity in children. *J Clin Oncol* 30(13):1422–1428, 2012.
23. van der Pal HJ, van Dalen EC, van Delden E, et al: High risk of symptomatic cardiac events in childhood cancer survivors. *J Clin Oncol* 30(13):1429–1437, 2012.
24. Couture L, Nash JA, Turgeon J: The ATP-binding cassette transporters and their implication in drug disposition: a special look at the heart. *Pharmacol Rev* 58(2):244–258, 2006.
25. Cardinale D, Colombo A, Cipolla CM: Prevention and treatment of cardiomyopathy and heart failure in patients receiving cancer chemotherapy. *Curr Treat Options Cardiovasc Med* 10(6):486–495, 2008.
26. Bosch X, Rovira M, Sitges M, et al: Enalapril and carvedilol for preventing chemotherapy-induced left ventricular systolic dysfunction in patients with malignant hemopathies: the OVERCOME trial (preventiOn of left Ventricular dysfunction with Enalapril and caRvedilol in patients submitted to intensive ChemOtherapy for the treatment of Malignant hEmopathies). *J Am Coll Cardiol* 61(23):2355–2362, 2013.
27. Ky B, Putt M, Sawaya H, et al: Early increases in multiple biomarkers predict subsequent cardiotoxicity in patients with breast cancer treated with doxorubicin, taxanes, and trastuzumab. *J Am Coll Cardiol* 63:809–816, 2014.
28. Seicean S, Seicean A, Plana JC, et al: Effect of statin therapy on the risk for incident heart failure in patients with breast cancer receiving anthracycline chemotherapy: an observational clinical cohort study. *J Am Coll Cardiol* 60(23):2384–2390, 2012.
29. Galper SL, Yu JB, Mauch PM, et al: Clinically significant cardiac disease in patients with Hodgkin lymphoma treated with mediastinal irradiation. *Blood* 117(2):412–418, 2011.
30. Armstrong GT, Joshi VM, Zhu L, et al: Increased tricuspid regurgitant jet velocity by Doppler echocardiography in adult survivors of childhood cancer: a report from the St Jude Lifetime Cohort Study. *J Clin Oncol* 31(6):774–781, 2013.
31. Perez EA, Suman VJ, Davidson NE, et al: Cardiac safety analysis of doxorubicin and cyclophosphamide followed by paclitaxel with or without trastuzumab in the North Central Cancer Treatment Group N9831 adjuvant breast cancer trial. *J Clin Oncol* 26(8):1231–1238, 2008.
32. Procter M, Suter TM, de Azambuja E, et al: Longer-term assessment of trastuzumab-related cardiac adverse events in the Herceptin Adjuvant (HERA) trial. *J Clin Oncol* 28(21):3422–3428, 2010.
33. Ewer MS, Vooletich MT, Durand JB, et al: Reversibility of trastuzumab-related cardiotoxicity: new insights based on clinical course and response to medical treatment. *J Clin Oncol* 23(31):7820–7826, 2005.
34. Perez EA, Koehler M, Byrne J, et al: Cardiac safety of lapatinib: pooled analysis of 3689 patients enrolled in clinical trials. *Mayo Clin Proc* 83(6):679–686, 2008.
35. Lenihan D, Suter T, Brammer M, et al: Pooled analysis of cardiac safety in patients with cancer treated with pertuzumab. *Ann Oncol* 23(3):791–800, 2012.
36. Odiete O, Hill MF, Sawyer DB: Neuregulin in cardiovascular development and disease. *Circ Res* 111(10):1376–1385, 2012.
37. Crone SA, Zhao YY, Fan L, et al: ErbB2 is essential in the prevention of dilated cardiomyopathy. *Nat Med* 8(5):459–465, 2002.
38. Kuramochi Y, Cote GM, Guo X, et al: Cardiac endothelial cells regulate reactive oxygen species-induced cardiomyocyte apoptosis through neuregulin-1beta/ErbB4 signaling. *J Biol Chem* 279(49):51141–51147, 2004.
39. Hedhli N, Huang Q, Kalinowski A, et al: Endothelium-derived neuregulin protects the heart against ischemic injury. *Circulation* 123(20):2254–2262, 2011.
40. Yla-Herttuala S, Rissanen TT, Vajanto I, et al: Vascular endothelial growth factors: biology and current status of clinical applications in cardiovascular medicine. *J Am Coll Cardiol* 49(10):1015–1026, 2007.
41. Launay-Vacher V, Deray G: Hypertension and proteinuria: a class-effect of antiangiogenic therapies. *Anticancer Drugs* 20(1):81–82, 2009.
42. Kruzliak P, Novak J, Novak M: Vascular endothelial growth factor inhibitor-induced hypertension: from pathophysiology to prevention and treatment based on long-acting nitric oxide donors. *Am J Hypertens* 27(1):3–13, 2014.
43. Belcik JT, Qi Y, Kaufmann BA, et al: Cardiovascular and systemic microvascular effects of anti-vascular endothelial growth factor therapy for cancer. *J Am Coll Cardiol* 60(7):618–625, 2012.
44. Eremina V, Jefferson JA, Kowalewska J, et al: VEGF inhibition and renal thrombotic microangiopathy. *N Engl J Med* 358(11):1129–1136, 2008.
45. Vigneau C, Lorcy N, Dolley-Hitze T, et al: All anti-vascular endothelial growth factor drugs can induce "pre-eclampsia-like syndrome": a RARe study. *Nephrol Dial Transplant* 29:325–332, 2014.
46. Eremina V, Sood M, Haigh J, et al: Glomerular-specific alterations of VEGF-A expression lead to distinct congenital and acquired renal diseases. *J Clin Invest* 111(5):707–716, 2003.
47. Scappaticci FA, Skillings JR, Holden SN, et al: Arterial thromboembolic events in patients with metastatic carcinoma treated with chemotherapy and bevacizumab. *J Natl Cancer Inst* 99(16):1232–1239, 2007.
48. Choueiri TK, Schutz FA, Je Y, et al: Risk of arterial thromboembolic events with sunitinib and sorafenib: a systematic review and meta-analysis of clinical trials. *J Clin Oncol* 28(13):2280–2285, 2010.
49. Ferroni P, Formica V, Roselli M, et al: Thromboembolic events in patients treated with anti-angiogenic drugs. *Curr Vasc Pharmacol* 8(1):102–113, 2010.
50. Izumiya Y, Shiojima I, Sato K, et al: Vascular endothelial growth factor blockade promotes the transition from compensatory cardiac hypertrophy to failure in response to pressure overload. *Hypertension* 47(5):887–893, 2006.
51. Schmidinger M, Zielinski CC, Vogl UM, et al: Cardiac toxicity of sunitinib and sorafenib in patients with metastatic renal cell carcinoma. *J Clin Oncol* 26(32):5204–5212, 2008.
52. Khakoo AY, Kassiotis CM, Tannir N, et al: Heart failure associated with sunitinib malate: a multitargeted receptor tyrosine kinase inhibitor. *Cancer* 112(11):2500–2508, 2008.
53. Richards CJ, Je Y, Schutz FA, et al: Incidence and risk of congestive heart failure in patients with renal and nonrenal cell carcinoma treated with sunitinib. *J Clin Oncol* 29(25):3450–3456, 2011.
54. Chu TF, Rupnick MA, Kerkela R, et al: Cardiotoxicity associated with tyrosine kinase inhibitor sunitinib. *Lancet* 370(9604):2011–2019, 2007.
55. Chintalgattu V, Ai D, Langley RR, et al: Cardiomyocyte PDGFR-beta signaling is an essential component of the mouse cardiac response to load-induced stress. *J Clin Invest* 120(2):472–484, 2010.
56. Zhang P, Hu X, Xu X, et al: AMP activated protein kinase-alpha2 deficiency exacerbates pressure-overload-induced left ventricular hypertrophy and dysfunction in mice. *Hypertension* 52(5):918–924, 2008.
57. Kerkela R, Grazette L, Yacobi R, et al: Cardiotoxicity of the cancer therapeutic agent imatinib mesylate. *Nat Med* 12(8):908–916, 2006.
58. Kim TD, Rea D, Schwarz M, et al: Peripheral artery occlusive disease in chronic phase chronic myeloid leukemia patients treated with nilotinib or imatinib. *Leukemia* 27(6):1316–1321, 2013.
59. Ponatinib prescribing information. www.fda.gov/safety/medwatch/safetyinformation/safetyalertsforhumanmedicalproducts/ucm370971.htm.
60. Mearini G, Schlossarek S, Willis MS, et al: The ubiquitin-proteasome system in cardiac dysfunction. *Biochim Biophys Acta* 1782(12):749–763, 2008.
61. Esparis-Ogando A, Alegre A, Aguado B, et al: Bortezomib is an efficient agent in plasma cell leukemias. *Int J Cancer* 114(4):665–667, 2005.
62. Enrico O, Gabriele B, Nadia C, et al: Unexpected cardiotoxicity in haematological bortezomib treated patients. *Br J Haematol* 138(3):396–397, 2007.
63. Herndon TM, Deisseroth A, Kaminskas E, et al: U.S. Food and Drug Administration approval: carfilzomib for the treatment of multiple myeloma. *Clin Cancer Res* 19(17):4559–4563, 2013.
64. Peng X, Pentassuglia L, Sawyer DB: Emerging anticancer therapeutic targets and the cardiovascular system: is there cause for concern? *Circ Res* 106(6):1022–1034, 2010.
65. Ganz PA, Habel LA, Weltzien EK, et al: Examining the influence of beta blockers and ACE inhibitors on the risk for breast cancer recurrence: results from the LACE cohort. *Breast Cancer Res Treat* 129(2):549–556, 2011.
66. Melhem-Bertrandt A, Chavez-Macgregor M, Lei X, et al: Beta-blocker use is associated with improved relapse-free survival in patients with triple-negative breast cancer. *J Clin Oncol* 29(19):2645–2652, 2011.
67. Grytli HH, Fagerland MW, Fossa SD, et al: Use of beta-blockers is associated with prostate cancer-specific survival in prostate cancer patients on androgen deprivation therapy. *Prostate* 73(3):250–260, 2013.
68. Holmes MD, Chen WY, Li L, et al: Aspirin intake and survival after breast cancer. *J Clin Oncol* 28(9):1467–1472, 2010.
69. Brewer TM, Masuda H, Liu DD, et al: Statin use in primary inflammatory breast cancer: a cohort study. *Br J Cancer* 109(2):318–324, 2013.
70. Ahern TP, Lash TL, Sorensen HT, et al: Digoxin treatment is associated with an increased incidence of breast cancer: a population-based case-control study. *Breast Cancer Res* 10(6):R102, 2008.
71. Biggar RJ, Wohlfahrt J, Oudin A, et al: Digoxin use and the risk of breast cancer in women. *J Clin Oncol* 29(16):2165–2170, 2011.
72. Rickard J, Kumbhani DJ, Baranowski B, et al: Usefulness of cardiac resynchronization therapy in patients with Adriamycin-induced cardiomyopathy. *Am J Cardiol* 105(4):522–526, 2010.
73. Grytli HH, Fagerland MW, Fossa SD, et al: Association between use of beta-blockers and prostate cancer-specific survival: a cohort study of 3561 prostate cancer patients with high-risk or metastatic disease. *Eur Urol* 65:635–641, 2014.
74. Mackenzie IS, Macdonald TM, Thompson A, et al: Spironolactone and risk of incident breast cancer in women older than 55 years: retrospective, matched cohort study. *BMJ* 345:e4447, 2012.

Disease Management in Heart Failure

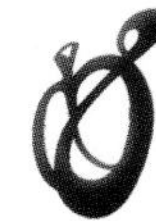

David Whellan, Kariann Abbate, and Efstathia Andrikopoulou

Heart failure currently affects more than 5 million Americans, and because of the aging population and the expected growth of the U.S. population, the prevalence of heart failure (HF) is expected to increase to more than 8 million Americans by 2030 (see also Chapter 17). Between 2012 and 2030, real (2010 dollars) total direct medical costs of heart failure are projected to increase from $23 billion to $53 billion per year.[1] Heart failure is the leading cause of hospitalization in patients older than 65 years of age.[2] Due to the high cost and increasing prevalence of heart failure hospitalizations, starting in 2012 the Centers for Medicare and Medicaid Services have implemented the Hospital Readmission Reduction Program, which reduces hospitals' Medicare payments up to 1% for higher than expected 30-day readmission rates for heart failure patients. Many hospitals have responded to this potential financial penalty by initiating heart failure disease management and care coordination programs or processes that target high-risk HF patients.

Early studies demonstrate that heart failure disease management, defined as an integrative approach that aims to enhance quality of health care and its cost-effectiveness for patients with chronic conditions, decreases hospital readmission rates, improves quality of life, and decreases costs.[3-9] Rich and colleagues published a landmark multicenter randomized controlled trial examining heart failure disease management in 1995. The intervention consisted of intense education about heart failure (HF) and its treatment by an experienced cardiovascular team, including a geriatric cardiologist, clinic nurse, dietitian, case manager, and home care provider. The study demonstrated that survival for 90 days without readmission (the primary endpoint) occurred in 54% of the control group versus 64% in the treatment group ($P = 0.09$). The difference was not statistically significant. However, when the analysis was restricted to survivors of the initial hospitalization, a significant difference in survival for 90 days without readmission was noted (risk ratio = 0.56, $P = 0.02$). The study also showed a significant improvement in the quality of life and a decrease in the total cost of care in the treatment group versus the control group.[3] A limitation of the Rich study is that current guidelines for evidence-based heart failure background therapy were not the standard of care at that time. Although the average ejection fractions in the control and treatment groups were 40% and 44%, respectively, only 11% of controls and 13% of patients in the treatment group were receiving β-blocker therapy.

Common features of early studies on heart failure disease management are that they were based at health care systems, traditionally enrolled inpatients, and had small, single-center trial designs. Because most heart failure patients receive their care in a community setting, it is unclear if trials performed at large health care centers can be replicated in a more "real world" setting. There are many limitations to single-center trial designs, namely limited external validity (interventions tested in a single clinical environment are not necessarily generalizable to a broader population), implausible effect size, and unequal allocation of resources (often single-center trials are performed by an investigator with highly atypical expertise and commitment).[10] Along those lines, several meta-analyses were performed on disease management programs for heart failure.[11-18] Although these studies show favorable results for heart failure disease management programs, because these meta-analyses are based on small, single-center trials, we must use caution when interpreting these results.

More recently, several large, multicenter, randomized controlled trials have been published related to heart failure disease management programs.[19-30] The results of these trials have been mixed, with many being neutral. The reason for the lack of benefit in many of these heart failure disease management trials is unclear. There was significant heterogeneity among these trials; each targeted a different patient population, provided varying quality of usual care, and used different program designs and interventions. In this chapter, we will explore types of heart failure disease management and target patient populations and discuss how the approach to heart failure disease management may change in the future.

DEFINING DISEASE MANAGEMENT

Disease management is an approach to patient care that coordinates medical resources for patients across the entire health care delivery system.[31] A critical distinction between disease management and other approaches to traditional medical care is a shift in focus from treating patients during discrete episodes of care (i.e., hospital or clinic) to provisions of high-quality care across the continuum of care.[32] Disease management involves practice redesign with increased availability to experts, use of evidence-based guidelines, improved education and counseling, and use of monitored outcomes to improve care processes. The goals of disease management are to (1) improve patients' knowledge about their disease state; (2) facilitate health behavior change that improves self-care, including adherence to treatment and management of symptoms; and (3) improve clinical outcomes, such as lower hospitalization costs and lower rates of mortality.[33]

Heart failure is a prime target for implementation of disease management programs because of its increasing prevalence, high costs to patients and society, high mortality and hospitalization rates, availability of evidence-based therapies, and need for timely identification of symptom progression and clinical deterioration. Heart failure is often accompanied by a multitude of comorbidities and barriers to care, including advanced age, cognitive deficits, depression, low socioeconomic class, and low health literacy. Heart failure patients also have multiple baseline risk factors such as medication or dietary nonadherence and propensity to ischemia, infection, and arrhythmias that may cause a perturbation of their already tenuous state and trigger deterioration that requires a hospitalization. These factors must be taken into account when conceptualizing a heart failure disease management program. Heart failure disease management aims at detecting instability before the point of clinical deterioration severe enough to warrant admission to the hospital by (1) implementing strategies that modify patients' baseline risk; (2) monitoring for worsening signs and symptoms of decompensation; and (3) encouraging patient participation in their own care (**Figure 44-1**).

THE SELF-CARE PARADIGM

Self-care is the foundation upon which successful management of heart failure is built.[33] The self-care process includes both maintenance and management components.[34] Examples of self-care maintenance are adhering to prescribed medications, diets, exercise regimens, and doctor's appointments. Self-care management involves more complex skills, including monitoring symptoms and making decisions regarding their severity, identifying possible treatment options, and assessing whether the treatment implemented was effective. Since the initial symptoms of a heart failure exacerbation are often subtle, health care management is often difficult for patients to perform successfully, especially in situations involving cognitive deficits and depression. A major factor that influences patients' skills at self-care management activities is self-efficacy, or confidence in one's ability to perform self-care.[34] Most heart failure disease management programs involve an education component (provided in either the inpatient or outpatient settings) designed to provide knowledge so that patients can successfully perform self-care maintenance. Additionally, heart failure disease management programs typically include a monitoring component in the outpatient setting, such as specialized heart failure clinics, home visits by nurses, structured telephone support, or telemonitoring to help patients with self-care management.

HEART FAILURE DISEASE MANAGEMENT CLASSIFICATION SCHEMES

Considerable variability exists among disease management programs in the literature. Significantly different populations have been targeted, and the spectrum of interventions studied has been wide. This heterogeneity has made comparison of heart failure disease management programs difficult. Grady and colleagues developed a classification scheme in an attempt to better categorize heart failure management programs. They identified the following settings for disease management: inpatient, specialty heart failure care outside the clinic setting (home visits, telephone calls, or telemonitoring), and primary care clinic.[35,36] In 2006, the American Heart Association's Disease Management Taxonomy Writing Group developed a system of classification that can be used both to categorize and compare disease

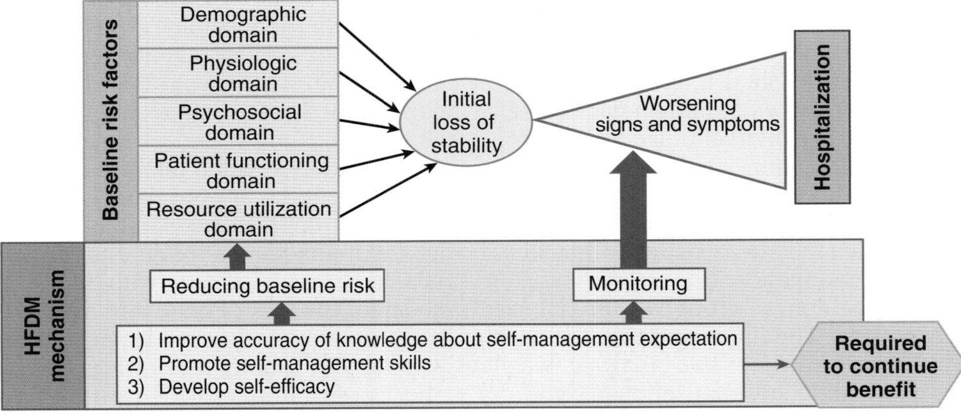

FIGURE 44-1 Conceptual model for heart failure disease management (HFDM) and mechanisms by which HFDM interventions reduce hospitalizations. *From Andrikopoulou E, Abbate K, Whellan DJ: Conceptual model for heart failure disease management. Can J Cardiol 30:304, 2014.*

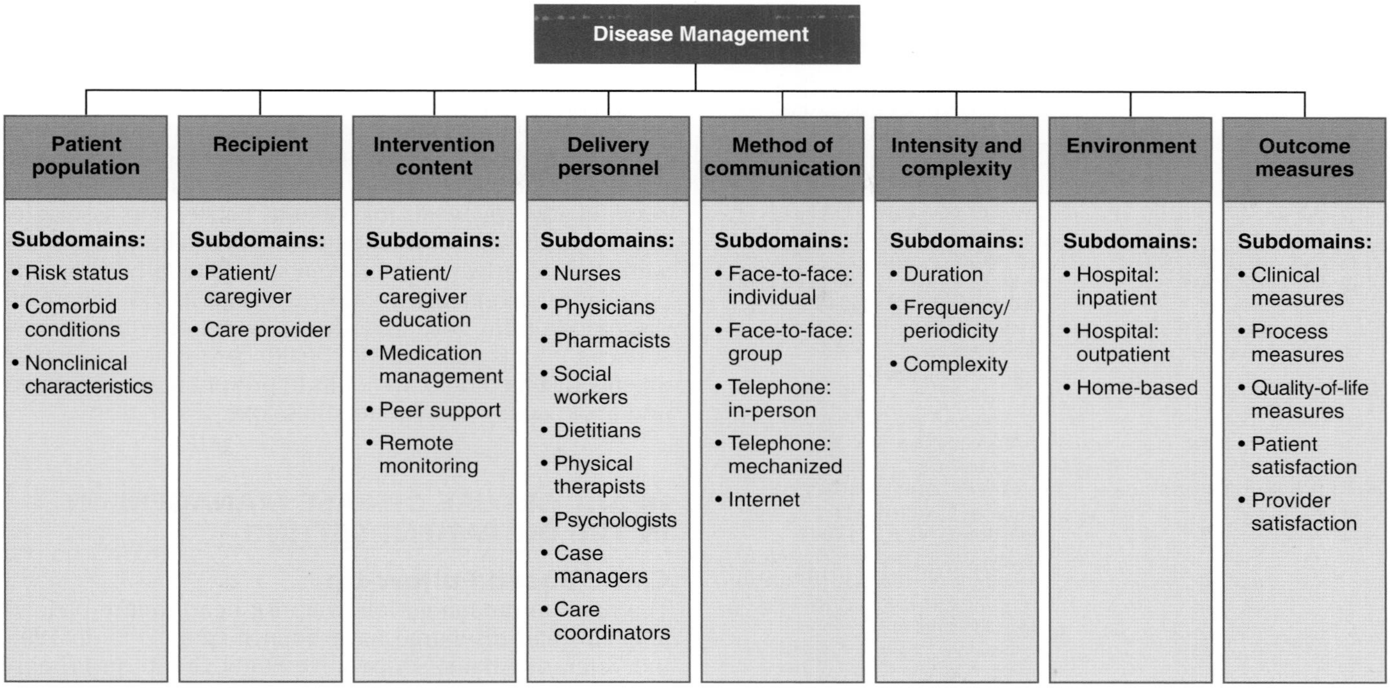

Disease Management

Patient population	Recipient	Intervention content	Delivery personnel	Method of communication	Intensity and complexity	Environment	Outcome measures
Subdomains: • Risk status • Comorbid conditions • Nonclinical characteristics	**Subdomains:** • Patient/ caregiver • Care provider	**Subdomains:** • Patient/ caregiver education • Medication management • Peer support • Remote monitoring	**Subdomains:** • Nurses • Physicians • Pharmacists • Social workers • Dietitians • Physical therapists • Psychologists • Case managers • Care coordinators	**Subdomains:** • Face-to-face: individual • Face-to-face: group • Telephone: in-person • Telephone: mechanized • Internet	**Subdomains:** • Duration • Frequency/ periodicity • Complexity	**Subdomains:** • Hospital: inpatient • Hospital: outpatient • Home-based	**Subdomains:** • Clinical measures • Process measures • Quality-of-life measures • Patient satisfaction • Provider satisfaction

FIGURE 44-2 Disease management. *From Krumholz HM, Currie PM, Riegel B, et al. A taxonomy for disease management: a scientific statement from the American Heart Association Disease Management Taxonomy Writing Group. Circulation 114:1432–1445, 2006.*

management programs and to inform efforts to identify specific factors associated with effectiveness (**Figure 44-2**).[37] The goal of this taxonomy is to establish a common language for evaluation of disease management. The authors hope that it will ultimately facilitate more rapid identification of effective program components.

HEART FAILURE DISEASE MANAGEMENT IN THE INPATIENT SETTING

Despite the opportunity to closely assess patients, modify therapy under observation, and provide intensive education during hospitalization for an acute exacerbation, the preponderance of evidence suggests that heart failure management during hospitalization is inadequate.[38] Approximately 20% of unplanned hospital readmissions for heart failure have been attributed to substandard inpatient care.[38]

In 1996, the Centers for Medicare & Medicaid Services (CMS) first implemented a program to track and improve the quality of heart failure care in hospitals (**see also Chapter 46**). The CMS subsequently aligned with The Joint Commission to create a national standardized "core" set of four heart failure performance metrics: measuring left ventricular function; using angiotensin-converting enzyme (ACE) inhibitors in patients with left ventricular systolic dysfunction; providing complete heart failure discharge instructions; and providing smoking cessation counseling in current or recent smokers. The original heart failure process measures have been modified only once since then by adding use of angiotensin II receptor blockers as an alternative to ACE inhibitors.[39] From 2002 to 2007, provision of discharge instructions improved from 31% to 78%, left ventricular function measures improved from 82% to 95%, use of ACE inhibitors or angiotensin II receptor blockers for left ventricular systolic dysfunction improved from 74% to 90%, and provision of smoking cessation advice improved from 42% to 96%.[39] Unfortunately, these improvements in performance measures did not correlate with improvements in 30-day or 1-year mortality or rehospitalization.[39,40]

It is unclear why an improvement in compliance with performance metrics did not correlate with improvement in clinical outcomes, but one hypothesis is that the perceived improvement in core metrics may simply have been better documentation of care that hospitals have been providing all along. Conversely, it may appear that hospitals have improved adherence with core metrics by "checking the appropriate boxes."[39] The reason for lack of clinically meaningful improvement could also be due to poorly chosen metrics. Of the four CMS-mandated heart failure performance measures, only prescription of an ACE inhibitor or ARB is supported by direct clinical trial evidence (**Table 44-1**).[41] Data from the Organized Program to Initiate Lifesaving Treatment in Hospitalized Patients With Heart Failure (OPTIMIZE-HF), a registry and performance improvement program for patients hospitalized with heart failure, β-blockade at the time of hospital discharge, currently not a heart failure performance measure, was strongly associated with reduced risk of mortality (hazard ratio [HR] 0.48; 95% confidence interval [CI] 0.30-0.79; $P = 0.004$) and mortality/rehospitalization during follow-up.[41]

Although most evidence-based heart failure therapies are not represented by the CMS outcome metrics, a heart failure hospitalization is an opportune time to ensure patients are prescribed these life-saving therapies (**see also Chapter 33**). It is also an excellent time to initiate and/or reinforce patient education on topics such as dietary recommendations, medications, activity and exercise, risk factor modification, and symptom monitoring and recognition.[33] In 2005, the American Heart Association launched the Get With The Guidelines-HF (GWTG-HF) program. This is an in-hospital quality improvement program to ensure that every patient with heart failure receives the best care.

TABLE 44-1 ACC/AHA Heart Failure Performance Measures: Inpatient Measure Descriptions

PERFORMANCE MEASURE NAME	MEASURE DESCRIPTION
1. Evaluation of left ventricular systolic (LVS) function	Heart failure patients with documentation in the hospital record that LVS function was assessed before arrival, during hospitalization, or is planned after discharge.
2. ACE inhibitor (ACEI), or angiotensin receptor blocker (ARB) for LVS dysfunction (LVSD)	Heart failure patients with LVSD and without both ACEI and ARB contraindications, who are prescribed an ACEI or ARB at hospital discharge.
3. Anticoagulant at discharge for HF patients with atrial fibrillation (AF)	Heart failure patients with chronic/recurrent AF and without warfarin contraindications who are prescribed warfarin at discharge.
4. Discharge instructions	Heart failure patients discharged home with written instructions or educational material given to patient or caregiver at discharge or during the hospital stay addressing all of the following: activity level, diet, discharge medications, follow-up appointment, weight monitoring, and what to do if symptoms worsen.
5. Adult smoking cessation advice/counseling	Heart failure patients with a history of smoking cigarettes, who are given smoking cessation advice or counseling during hospital stay.

From Bonow RO, Bennett S, Casey DE, Jr, et al: ACC/AHA clinical performance measures for adults with chronic heart failure: a report of the American College of Cardiology/American Heart Association task force on performance measures (Writing Committee to Develop Heart Failure Clinical Performance Measures) endorsed by the Heart Failure Society of America. J Am Coll Cardiol 46:1144–1178, 2005.

The GWTG-HF module has a patient management tool that provides patient-specific guideline recommendations, allows for real-time data validation, and enables each institution to track its adherence to the guidelines individually and against national benchmarks.[42] The GWTG-HF program facilitates data collection and provides quality improvement tools to hospitals, including clinical decision support and dissemination of best practices, and regularly reports performance back to the participating hospitals.[42] Heidenreich and associates demonstrated that process of care, as defined by CMS performance measures, is higher in the GWTG-HF–participating hospitals than in other U.S. hospitals. In addition, readmission rates, but not mortality, were lower in GWTG-HF hospitals.[42]

Hospital discharge planning is an important component of heart failure disease management. Naylor and colleagues conducted a prospective randomized clinical trial evaluating hospital readmission in elderly patients after initiation of a comprehensive, multidisciplinary discharge program.[43] During the initial 2-week period after discharge, 3 patients (4%) in the intervention group were readmitted, compared with 11 patients (16%) in the control group ($P = 0.02$). For the intervals from 2 to 6 weeks and from 6 to 12 weeks after discharge, the percentages of patients readmitted were similar for the intervention and control groups.[43] Based on this trial, it appears that a comprehensive discharge plan for elderly heart failure patients is helpful in preventing readmission immediately after discharge, but to prevent readmission beyond 2 weeks postdischarge, further outpatient intervention is needed.

Transition of care from one health care venue (inpatient) to the next (outpatient: home, nursing home, etc.) can be difficult in heart failure patients. Poor communication between inpatient teams and outpatient caregivers can result in medication errors and other mistakes that can result in adverse events for patients. Forster and associates found that 66% of untoward outcomes in discharged patients were due to adverse drug events.[44,45] Similarly, Gray and colleagues identified adverse drug events in 20% of patients discharged from hospital to home with home health care services.[45,46] It is important for health care systems to devise an effective method of handoffs to prevent harm to patients and avoid costly hospital readmissions.

HEART FAILURE DISEASE MANAGEMENT IN THE OUTPATIENT SETTING

Clinic-Based Follow-Up

The data on outpatient follow-up for heart failure patients after hospital discharge have been mixed.[17,18,47-51] In 1996, the Veterans Affairs Cooperative Study Group on Primary Care and Hospital Readmission conducted a multicenter randomized, controlled trial at nine Veterans Affairs Medical Centers.[47] The investigators randomized 1396 veterans hospitalized with diabetes, chronic obstructive pulmonary disease, or congestive heart failure to receive either usual care or an intensive primary care intervention. The intervention involved close follow-up by a nurse and a primary care physician, beginning before discharge and continuing for the next 6 months. The outpatient component of the intervention included telephone calls by nurses and regular visits with a primary care physician. The population studied consisted of a disadvantaged class of men who were quite ill, as demonstrated by the patients' multiple comorbidities. Half of the patients with congestive heart failure (504 patients) had disease in New York Heart Association (NYHA) class III or IV; 30% of those with diabetes (751 patients) had end-organ damage; and a quarter of those with chronic obstructive pulmonary disease (583 patients) required home oxygen treatment or oral corticosteroids. Although they received more intensive primary care than the controls, the patients in the intervention group had significantly higher rates of readmission (0.19 vs. 0.14 per month, $P = 0.005$) and more days of rehospitalization (10.2 vs. 8.8, $P = 0.041$). The patients in the intervention group were more satisfied with their care ($P<0.001$), but there was no difference between the study groups in quality-of-life scores, which remained very low ($P = 0.53$). The reason for increased hospital readmission in the intervention group could be that additional primary care offered to seriously ill patients may have led to the detection and treatment of previously undetected medical problems. It is also possible that patients with such advanced disease (i.e., patients with NYHA class III and IV heart failure symptoms with multiple co-morbidities) may not be the most ideal patients to target for outpatient heart failure disease management. Despite intensive outpatient management, it may not be possible to prevent rehospitalization of these severely ill patients.

McAlister and associates published a meta-analysis of heart failure disease management programs through 1999. Eleven trials involving a total of 2067 patients were identified. Hospitalizations (risk ratio [RR] 0.87, 95% CI 0.79-0.96), but not all-cause mortality (RR 0.94, 95% CI 0.75-1.19), were reduced by heart failure disease management programs. However, there were considerable differences in the effects of various interventions on hospitalization rates; specialized follow-up by a multidisciplinary team led to a substantial reduction in the risk of hospitalization (RR 0.77, 95% CI 0.68-0.86, $n = 1366$), whereas trials employing telephone contact with improved coordination of primary care services failed to find any benefit (RR 1.15, 95% CI 0.96-1.37, $n = 646$). In an updated meta-analysis by McAlister and colleagues, the investigators determined that strategies incorporating follow-up by a specialized multidisciplinary team reduced mortality (RR 0.75, 95% CI 0.59-0.96), HF hospitalizations (RR 0.74, 95% CI 0.63-0.87), and all-cause hospitalizations (RR 0.81, 95% CI 0.71-0.92). Programs that focused on enhancing patient self-care activities reduced HF hospitalizations (RR 0.66, 95% CI 0.52-0.83) and all-cause hospitalizations (RR 0.73, 95% CI 0.57-0.93) but had no effect on mortality (RR 1.14, 95% CI 0.67-1.94). Strategies that employed telephone contact and advised patients to contact their primary care physician in the event of deterioration reduced HF hospitalizations (RR 0.75, 95% CI 0.57-0.99) but not mortality (RR 0.91, 95% CI 0.67-1.29) or all-cause hospitalizations (RR 0.98, 95% CI 0.80-1.20). In 15 of 18 trials that evaluated cost, multidisciplinary strategies were cost saving (**Table 44-2**).[17]

Phillips and associates conducted a meta-analysis to determine the efficacy of interventions consisting of comprehensive discharge planning plus postdischarge support for older inpatients with HF. Eighteen studies with a total of 3304 patients were evaluated. During a pooled mean observation period of 8 months (range, 3-12 months), fewer intervention patients were readmitted compared with controls (555/1590 vs. 741/1714, number needed to treat = 12; RR 0.75; 95% CI 0.64-0.88). There was no statically significant difference in mortality between the control versus the intervention groups.[18]

Based on these data, a multidisciplinary approach to outpatient heart failure disease management may help to reduce hospital readmission. Unfortunately, the need for intense face-to-face follow-up strategies limits the number of patients who can participate in these programs.[52] Heart failure patients with decreased mobility may find it difficult to frequently commute to the doctor's office, especially if they live in rural areas. Given these limitations, alternative heart failure disease management approaches have been studied, including visiting home nurses, telephone monitoring, and telemonitoring.

Home Nursing Visits

In specialty heart failure care outside the clinic setting that involves community outreach, care is delivered primarily in patients' homes. Patients do not routinely go to a clinic or other outpatient setting to receive care; rather, the health care provider calls on the telephone or comes to the home.[35] There are many advantages to implementing a home-based heart failure disease management program. The home is the most important context of care for individuals with chronic heart failure. Patients often struggle to manage a complex regimen of medications, follow an unfamiliar diet, monitor weight and vital signs, and work to coordinate care among various providers who, in some cases, fail to communicate effectively.[53] Intuitively, it would seem that a home-based heart failure disease management approach would improve outcomes and reduce costs. Based on current available data,[45,54,55] however, it is unclear if a home-based approach is superior to other types of heart failure disease management programs.

In 2012, Stewart and associates published the Which Heart Failure Intervention is Most Cost-Effective & Consumer-Friendly in Reducing Hospital Care (WHICH) trial comparing a home-based intervention (HBI) with a clinic-based intervention (CBI). This was a prospective, multicenter, randomized controlled trial that enrolled 280 patients with HF being discharged from the hospital. The primary endpoint was all-cause, unplanned hospitalization or death during a 12- to 18-month follow-up. The primary endpoint occurred in 102 of 143 (71%) HBI versus 104 of 137 (76%) CBI patients (adjusted HR 0.97; 95% CI 0.73-1.30; $P = 0.861$). Ninety-six (67.1%) HBI versus 95 (69.3%) CBI patients had an unplanned hospitalization ($P = 0.887$), and 31 (21.7%) versus 38 (27.7%) died ($P = 0.252$).[45,54] Based on this trial, it appears that an HBI is not superior to a CBI in reducing all-cause mortality and hospitalization.

In a smaller, single-center study published by Stewart and associates in 1998, 97 patients were randomized to either usual care or an HBI 1 week after hospital discharge. The primary endpoint was frequency of unplanned readmissions, plus out-of-hospital deaths within 6 months of discharge. Secondary endpoints included duration of hospital stay and overall mortality. During follow-up, patients in the HBI group had fewer unplanned readmissions (36 vs. 63; $P = 0.03$) and fewer out-of-hospital deaths (1 vs. 5; $P = 0.11$): 0.8 ± 0.9 vs. 1.4 ± 1.8 (mean ± SD) events per patient assigned to HBI and usual care, respectively ($P = 0.03$). Patients in the HBI group also had fewer days of hospitalization (261 vs. 452; $P = 0.05$) and fewer total deaths (6 vs. 12; $P = 0.11$).[55]

Despite the merits of a home-based heart failure disease management program, it may not be feasible to conduct on a large scale due to limited nursing personnel and costs. Therefore, alternative methods of heart failure disease management have been explored, such as telephone-based interventions and telemonitoring.

Telephone Interventions and Telemonitoring

Structured telephone support (STS) consists of a health care provider, most often a nurse, calling patients after hospital discharge to confirm adherence to treatment, enhance patient education, and manage symptoms. Telemonitoring (TM) is a digital, broadband, satellite, wireless, or Bluetooth transmission of physiologic data (e.g., electrocardiogram, blood pressure, weight, pulse oximetry, and respiratory rate). Both models of care have the potential to provide access to specialist care for a much larger number of patients across a much greater geography and might reduce the cost of care.[53] However, as in heart failure disease management trials of multidisciplinary clinics and home nursing visits, the results of trials in STS and TM are mixed.[20,52,56-71]

The WHARF trial, published in 2003, randomized 280 patients in a multicenter randomized controlled trial to receive either heart failure standard of care or heart failure standard of care plus the AlereNet system. NYHA stage III or IV patients were enrolled in the study. Patients

TABLE 44-2 Impact of Interventions on All-Cause Mortality, All-Cause Hospitalization Rates, and Heart Failure Hospitalization Rates

		All-Cause Mortality (No. Events/Total No. Patients)			*All-Cause Hospitalization Rates (No. Re-Admitted at Least Once/Total No. Patients)*			*Heart Failure Hospitalization Rates (No. Readmitted at Least Once/Total No. Patients)*		
STUDY (YEAR)	**LENGTH OF FOLLOW-UP (MOS)**	**INTERVENTION ARM**	**CONTROL ARM**	**RISK RATIO (95% CI)**	**INTERVENTION ARM**	**CONTROL ARM**	**RISK RATIO (95% CI)**	**INTERVENTION ARM**	**CONTROL ARM**	**RISK RATIO (95% CI)**
Multidisciplinary Heart Failure Clinic										
Cline et al (1998)*	12	24/80	31/110	1.06 (0.68, 1.67)	22/56	43/79	0.72 (0.49, 1.06)	NR	NR	NR
Ekman et al (1998)	6	21/79	17/79	1.24 (0.71, 2.16)	48/79	45/79	1.07 (0.82, 1.38)	36/79	38/79	0.95 (0.68, 1.32)
Doughty et al (2002)	12	19/100	24/97	0.77 (0.45, 1.31)	64/100	59/97	1.05 (0.85, 1.31)	21/100	23/97	0.89 (0.53, 1.49)
Kasper et al (2002)	6	7/102	13/98	0.52 (0.22, 1.24)	40/102	42/98	0.92 (0.66, 1.28)	26/102	35/98	0.71 (0.47, 1.09)
Capomolla et al (2002)	12	3/112	21/122	0.16 (0.05, 0.51)	9/112	37/122	0.26 (0.13, 0.52)	NR	NR	NR
Stromberg et al (2003)	12	7/52	20/54	0.36 (0.17, 0.79)	28/52	37/54	0.79 (0.58, 1.07)	17/52	27/54	0.65 (0.41, 1.05)
Ledwidge et al (2003)	3	3/51	3/47	0.92 (0.20, 4.34)	2/51	12/47	0.15 (0.04, 0.65)	2/51	10/47	0.18 (0.04, 0.80)
Subtotal		0.66 (0.42, 1.05)			0.76 (0.58, 1.01)			0.76 (0.58, 0.99)		
Multidisciplinary Team Providing Specialized Follow-up in Nonclinic Setting										
Hanchett and Torrens (1967)[†]	30	NR	NR	NR	NR	NR	NR	NR	NR	NR
Rich et al (1993)	3	NR	NR	NR	21/63	16/35	0.73 (0.44, 1.20)	NR	NR	NR
Rich et al (1995)	3	13/142	17/140	0.75 (0.38, 1.49)	41/142	59/140	0.69 (0.50, 0.95)	NR	NR	NR
Stewart et al (1998)	6	6/49	12/48	0.49 (0.20, 1.20)	24/49	31/48	0.76 (0.53, 1.08)	12/49	18/48	0.65 (0.35, 1.20)
Stewart et al (1999)	6	18/100	28/100	0.64 (0.38, 1.08)	40/100	51/100	0.78 (0.58, 1.07)	21/100	27/100	0.78 (0.47, 1.28)
Naylor et al (1999)	6	NR	NR	NR	18/52	26/56	0.75 (0.47, 1.19)	NR	NR	NR
Blue et al (2001)	12	25/84	25/81	0.96 (0.61, 1.53)	47/84	49/81	0.92 (0.71, 1.20)	12/84	26/81	0.45 (0.24, 0.82)
Trochu et al (2004)	12	38/102	42/100	0.89 (0.63, 1.25)	58/95	71/100	0.86 (0.70, 1.05)	47/95	64/100	0.77 (0.60, 0.99)
Subtotal		0.81 (0.65, 1.01)			0.81 (0.72, 0.91)			0.72 (0.59, 0.87)		
Summary for Specialized Multidisciplinary Team Follow-up (Clinic or Nonclinic Settings)										
Subtotal		0.75 (0.59, 0.96)			0.81 (0.71, 0.92)			0.74 (0.63, 0.87)		

Telephone Follow-up and Attendance with Primary Care Physician if Deteriorates										
Naylor et al (1994)	3	NR	NR	NR	16/72	23/70	0.68 (0.39, 1.17)	NR	NR	NR
Weinberger et al (1996)	6	NR	NR	NR	130/249	106/255	1.26 (1.04, 1.52)	NR	NR	NR
PHARM (1999)	6	3/90	5/91	0.61 (0.15, 2.46)	NR	NR	NR	NR	NR	NR
Rainville et al (1999)	12	1/17	4/17	0.25 (0.03, 2.01)	NR	NR	NR	4/17	10/17	0.40 (0.16, 1.03)
Pugh et al (2001)	6	NR	NR	NR	NR	NR	NR	9/25	11/30	0.98 (0.49, 1.98)
Jerant et al (2001)	6	2/25	0/12	2.50 (0.13, 48.36)	8/25	7/12	0.55 (0.26, 1.16)	2/25	4/12	0.24 (0.05, 1.13)
de Lusignan et al (2001)	12	2/10	3/10	0.67 (0.14, 3.17)	NR	NR	NR	NR	NR	NR
Riegel et al (2002)	6	16/130	32/228	0.88 (0.50, 1.54)	56/130	114/228	0.86 (0.68, 1.09)	23/130	63/228	0.64 (0.42, 0.98)
Laramee et al (2003)	3	13/141	15/146	0.90 (0.44, 1.82)	49/134	46/130	1.03 (0.75, 1.43)	18/134	21/130	0.83 (0.46, 1.49)
Tsuyuki et al (2004)	6	16/140	12/136	1.30 (0.64, 2.64)	59/140	51/136	1.12 (0.84, 1.50)	37/140	38/136	0.95 (0.64, 1.39)
Subtotal		0.91 (0.67, 1.29)			0.98 (0.80, 1.20)			0.75 (0.57, 0.99)		
Enhanced Patient Self-Care Activities										
Serxner et al (1998)	6	NR	NR	NR	NR	NR	NR	15/55	27/54	0.55 (0.33, 0.91)
Jaarsma et al (1999)	9	22/84	16/95	1.56 (0.88, 2.76)	31/84	47/95	0.75 (0.53, 1.05)	24/84	37/95	0.73 (0.48, 1.12)
Harrison et al (2002)	5	6/92	5/100	1.30 (0.41, 4.13)	21/92	31/100	0.74 (0.46, 1.19)	18/92	24/100	0.82 (0.47, 1.40)
Krumholz et al (2002)	12	9/44	13/44	0.69 (0.33, 1.45)	16/44	23/44	0.70 (0.43, 1.13)	18/44	30/44	0.60 (0.40, 0.90)
Subtotal		1.14 (0.67, 1.94)			0.73 (0.57, 0.93)			0.66 (0.52, 0.83)		
Total		0.83 (0.70, 0.99)			0.84 (0.75, 0.93)			0.73 (0.66, 0.82)		

*The hospitalization data in this study were reported only for those patients who did not die during follow-up.

†This study reported total number of hospitalizations (all-cause and heart failure) and was included in those analyses.

CI, Confidence interval; *NR,* not reported; *PHARM,* Pharmacist in Heart failure Assessment Recommendation and Monitoring study.

From McAlister FA, Stewart S, Ferrua S, et al: Multidisciplinary strategies for the management of heart failure patients at high risk for admission: a systematic review of randomized trials. J Am Coll Cardiol 44:810–819, 2004.

randomized to standard of care were instructed to weigh themselves daily and bring a copy of their weight log to their physician visits. Patients randomized to use the Alere DayLink monitor were asked to respond to daily questions regarding their HF symptoms via the monitoring system and received a scale that transmitted daily weights to trained cardiac nurses. Patients were followed for 6 months. Although no difference in rehospitalization rates was found, the AlereNet group had a 56.2% reduction in mortality rate ($P < 0.003$) without increased use.[72]

In 2004, Galbreath and colleagues[73] reported on a single-center randomized controlled trial of a telephonically administered intervention. A total of 1069 patients with symptoms of heart failure and documented systolic or diastolic dysfunction were enrolled. The disease management program was administered via a commercial vendor that was distinct from each patient's usual source of medical care. The intervention patients were shown to have a reduced mortality rate ($P = 0.037$), and the beneficial outcomes were most apparent in patients with systolic heart failure. Total health care consumption was not decreased by disease management.[73]

In 2005, the GESICA Investigators published the Randomized Trial of Telephone Interventions in Chronic Heart Failure: DIAL Trial. This was a multicenter, randomized controlled trial conducted in Argentina that enrolled 1518 patients. Outpatients with stable, chronic heart failure were randomized to receive usual care versus education, counseling, and monitoring by nurses through frequent telephone follow-up. It is unclear how much telephone contact per patient occurred. Heart failure hospitalizations and mortality were higher in the usual care group compared with the intervention group (relative risk reduction = 20%; 95% CI 3-34; $P = 0.026$). The difference was mostly due to a reduction in heart failure hospitalizations (relative risk reduction = 29%; $P = 0.005$). Mortality was similar in both groups. The intervention group reported an improved quality of life.[20] A report of long-term follow-up from the DIAL trial observed a reduction in the rate of death or hospitalization for heart failure in the intervention group at both 1 and 3 years, driven by a reduction in hospitalizations.[74]

In 2005, the Trans-European Network-Home-Care Management System (TEN-HMS) Study[19] was published, evaluating whether home telemonitoring (HTM) improves outcomes compared with nurse telephone support (NTS) and usual care (UC). Four hundred twenty-six patients from hospitals in Germany, the Netherlands, and the United Kingdom were randomly assigned to HTM (consisting of twice daily patient self-measurement of weight, blood pressure, heart rate and rhythm), NTS, or UC. The primary endpoint was days dead or hospitalized. During the 240-day follow-up, there was no significant difference between death or hospitalization for the UC, NTS, and HTM groups. Patients randomly assigned to receive UC had higher 1-year mortality than patients assigned to receive NTS or HTM ($P = 0.032$).[19]

The Alere Trial (Heart Failure Home Care Trial), published in 2008, was a multicenter randomized controlled trial examining a computer-based home disease management program among older minority and female Medicare beneficiaries with HF receiving care in a community-based primary care setting. The study randomized 315 patients to examine the effect of the Alere DayLink Monitoring System in a resource-limited, diverse population. The HFMS system was compared with standard HF care, including enhanced patient education, education to clinicians, and follow-up. The primary endpoint of treatment failure, defined as the composite of cardiovascular death or rehospitalization within 6 months of enrollment, was compared between groups. No statistically significant difference was found between groups.[22]

The Home or Hospital in Heart Failure (HHH) study was a multinational, randomized controlled clinical trial, conducted in the United Kingdom, Poland, and Italy. Across these 11 centers, 461 heart failure patients were enrolled and randomized to either the usual outpatient care or HTM administered as three randomized strategies: (1) monthly telephone contact; (2) strategy 1 plus weekly transmission of vital signs; and (3) strategy 2 plus monthly 24-hour recording of cardiorespiratory activity.[52] Over a 12-month follow-up, there was no significant effect of HTM in reducing bed-days occupancy for heart failure or cardiac death plus heart failure hospitalization.[52] In 2012, the Interdisciplinary Network for Heart Failure (INH) study developed and evaluated in a randomized, controlled trial a nurse-coordinated disease management program (HeartNetCare-HF, HNC)[75]; 715 patients hospitalized for systolic heart failure were randomly assigned to HNC or UC. Besides telephone-based monitoring and education, HNC addressed individual problems raised by patients, pursued networking of health care providers, and provided training for caregivers. Endpoints were time to death or rehospitalization. Within 180 days, 130 HNC and 137 UC patients reached the primary endpoint (HR 1.02; 95% CI 0.81-1.30; $P = 0.89$), because more HNC patients were readmitted. Overall, 32 HNC and 52 UC patients died. Uncensored HR was 0.62 (0.40-0.96; $P = 0.03$). HNC patients improved more regarding NYHA class ($P = 0.05$), physical functioning ($P = 0.03$), and physical health component ($P = 0.03$).[75]

In 2010, Chaudhry and colleagues published the Tele-HF study,[27] a multicenter, randomized controlled trial to determine whether telemonitoring would reduce the combined endpoint of readmission or death from any cause among patients recently hospitalized for heart failure; 1653 patients were randomized to telemonitoring versus usual care. The intervention consisted of an interactive voice response system that collected data but did not provide education. Adherence with the system was poor, suggesting that patients did not engage with the service, perhaps because of the nature of the technology.[53] There was no significant difference between the two groups with respect to readmission for any cause or death.[27,53]

In 2011, Koehler and associates published Impact of Remote Telemedical Management on Mortality and Hospitalization in Ambulatory Patients with Chronic Heart Failure: the Telemedical Interventional Monitoring In Heart Failure Study (TIM-HF).[28] This was a multicenter, randomized controlled trial designed to determine whether physician-led remote telemedical management (RTM) compared with UC would result in reduced mortality in ambulatory patients with chronic heart failure (HF); 710 stable heart failure patients (NYHA class II and III) were randomly assigned to RTM or UC. RTM used portable devices for electrocardiogram, blood pressure, and body weight measurements connected to a personal digital assistant that sent automated encrypted transmission via cell phones to the telemedical centers. The primary endpoint was death from any cause. The first secondary endpoint was a composite of cardiovascular death and hospitalization for HF. Compared with UC, RTM had no significant effect on all-cause mortality (HR 0.97; 95% CI 0.67-1.41; $P = 0.87$) or on cardiovascular death or HF hospitalization (HR 0.89; 95% CI 0.67-1.19; $P = 0.44$).[28] The lack of significant clinical improvement in TIM-HF may be related to the target population. Stable patients who are exceptionally well managed may not obtain as much benefit from TM as a group of patients who may not have exposure to such high-quality care at baseline. The Weight Monitoring In Patients with Severe Heart Failure (WISH) Trial was published in 2012.[76] This was a multicenter, randomized controlled trial designed to determine if daily electronic transmission of body weight to a heart failure clinic would reduce cardiac hospitalization in patients recently hospitalized with heart failure. A total of 344 patients were randomized to the intervention group versus the control group. No significant differences were found for the primary endpoint, cardiac rehospitalization (HR 0.90; 95% CI 0.65-1.26; $P = 0.54$), or for the secondary endpoints, which included all-cause hospitalization (HR 0.83; 95% CI 0.61-1.13; $P = 0.24$), death from any cause (HR 0.57; 95% CI 0.19-1.73; $P = 0.32$), or the composite endpoint of cardiac hospitalization and death from any cause (HR 0.90; 95% CI 0.65-1.26; $P = 0.54$).[76]

A Cochrane Review evaluating the effectiveness of STS and TM as a primary component of a chronic heart failure disease management program was published in 2011.[53,56] They included randomized controlled trials comparing TM or STS to UC in patients with HF. The primary outcomes analyzed were mortality and hospitalizations. Twenty-five peer-reviewed studies were included (11 evaluated TM and 16 evaluated STS with 2 studies testing both TM and STM). Tele-HF, TIM-HF, and WISH were not included, because they were reported after the meta-analysis was completed. Telemonitoring reduced all-cause mortality (RR 0.66; 95% CI 0.54-0.81; $P<0.0001$). STS showed a similar but nonsignificant trend (RR 0.77; 95% CI 0.76-1.01; $P = 0.08$) (**Figure 44-3**). Both TM (RR 0.79; 95% CI 0.76-0.940; $P = 0.008$) and STM (RR 0.77; 95% CI 0.68-0.87; $P <0.0001$) reduced HF-related hospitalizations.[53,56] Although this meta-analysis is positive, we must use caution when interpreting the results. The quality of the methods used in the studies was variable, and many of the studies were small.[27]

Invasive Telemonitoring

Invasive telemonitoring measurements include intrathoracic impedance, right-sided cardiac pressure, left atrial pressure, and pulmonary artery pressure. Bourge and colleagues conducted the COMPASS-HF (Chronicle Offers Management to Patients with Advanced Signs and Symptoms of Heart Failure) Trial[29] to determine whether a heart failure management strategy using continuous right-sided intracardiac pressure monitoring could decrease heart failure morbidity. The study was a prospective, multicenter, randomized, single-blinded, parallel-controlled trial of 274 New York Heart Association functional class III or IV heart failure patients who received an implantable continuous hemodynamic monitor. Patients were randomized to a Chronicle (Medtronic Inc., Minneapolis, Minn.) or control group. All patients received optimal medical therapy, but the hemodynamic information from the monitor was used to guide patient management only in the Chronicle group. Primary endpoints included freedom from system-related complications (DSRC), freedom from pressure-sensor failure, and reduction in the rate of HF-related events (hospitalizations and emergency or urgent care visits requiring intravenous therapy). The two safety endpoints were achieved, but the primary efficacy endpoint was not met because the Chronicle group had a nonsignificant 21% lower rate of all HF-related events compared with the control group ($P = 0.33$).[29]

A number of potential factors contributed to there being no difference between monitoring or usual care. The study demonstrated chronically elevated filling pressures in many patients that increased the risk of HF events. Additionally, patients enrolled had a progressive increase in risk for heart failure events with higher chronic 24-hour estimated pulmonary artery pressure (event risk 20% at 18 mm Hg, 34% at 25 mm Hg, and 56% at 30 mm Hg).[29,74] In addition to these difficulties in reducing pressures, HF patients in UC received a similar number of calls allowing for changes in therapy.

Reducing Events in Patients with Chronic Heart Failure (REDUCEhf)[77] also evaluated the use of the Chronicle device that was attached to an ICD to monitor right-sided intracardiac pressures. Endpoints were the same as for COMPASS-HF. REDUCEhf was prematurely stopped due to issues with the device, but analysis of available data did not show significant benefit in using intracardiac monitoring.[77] In March 2007, FDA's Circulatory System Devices Panel voted against the approval of Medtronic's implantable hemodynamic monitor because its use did not significantly improve clinical outcomes for HF patients.

In Sensitivity and Positive Predictive Value of Implantable Intrathoracic Impedance Monitoring as a Predictor of Heart Failure Hospitalizations: the SENSE-HF Trial,[78] Conraads and colleagues investigated the performance of OptiVol intrathoracic fluid monitoring for the prediction of HF events in chronic HF patients newly implanted with an implantable cardiac defibrillator (ICD). This was a prospective, multicenter study that enrolled 501 patients. The authors concluded that an intrathoracic impedance-derived fluid index had low sensitivity and PPV in the early period after implantation of a device in chronic HF patients. Sensitivity improved within the first 6 months after implant.[78]

In the PARTNERS HF (Program to Access and Review Trending Information and Evaluate Correlation to Symptoms in Patients With Heart Failure) Study,[26] Whellan and associates sought to determine the utility of combined heart failure device diagnostic information to predict clinical deterioration of HF in patients with systolic left ventricular dysfunction. This was a prospective, multicenter observational study in patients receiving cardiac resynchronization therapy (CRT) implantable cardioverter-defibrillators. A combined HF device diagnostic algorithm was developed on an independent dataset. The algorithm was considered positive if a patient had two of the following abnormal criteria during a 1-month period: long atrial fibrillation duration, rapid ventricular rate during atrial fibrillation, high (≥60) fluid index, low patient activity, abnormal autonomics (high night heart rate or low heart rate variability), or notable device therapy (low CRT pacing or implantable cardioverter-defibrillator shocks), or if they only had a very high (≥100) fluid index. The authors found that patients with a positive combined heart failure device diagnostics had a 5.5-fold increased risk of HF hospitalization with pulmonary signs or symptoms within the next month (HR 5.5; 95% CI 3.4-8.8;

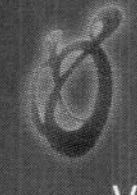

STRUCTURED TELEPHONE SUPPORT

Study or subgroup	Intervention Events	Intervention Total	Usual care Events	Usual care Total	Weight	Risk ratio M-H, fixed, 95% CI
Barth 2001	0	17	0	17		Not estimable
Cleland 2005 (Struct Tele)	27	173	20	85	7.8%	0.66 (0.40, 1.11)
DeBusk 2004	21	228	29	234	8.3%	0.74 (0.44, 1.26)
DeWalt 2006	3	62	4	65	1.1%	0.79 (0.18, 3.37)
Galbreath 2004	54	710	39	359	15.0%	0.70 (0.47, 1.04)
Gattis 1999 (PHARM)	3	90	5	91	1.4%	0.61 (0.15, 2.46)
GESICA 2005 (DIAL)	116	760	122	758	35.4%	0.95 (0.75, 1.20)
Laramee 2003	13	141	15	146	4.3%	0.90 (0.44, 1.82)
Mortara 2009 (Struct Tele)	9	106	9	160	2.1%	1.51(0.62, 3.68)
Rainville 1999	1	19	4	19	1.2%	0.25 (0.03, 2.04)
Riegel 2002	16	130	32	228	6.7%	0.88 (0.50, 1.54)
Riegel 2006	6	70	8	65	2.4%	0.70 (0.26, 1.90)
Sisk 2006	22	203	22	203	6.4%	1.00 (0.57, 1.75)
Tsuyuki 2004	16	140	12	136	3.5%	1.30 (0.64, 2.64)
Wakefield 2008	25	99	11	49	4.3%	1.12 (0.60, 2.09)
Total (95% CI)		**2948**		**2615**	**100.0%**	**0.88 (0.76, 1.01**
Total events	332		332			

Heterogeneity: $Chi^2 = 8.48$, df = 13 ($P = 0.81$), $I^2 = 0\%$
Test for overall effect Z = 1.78 ($P = 0.08$)

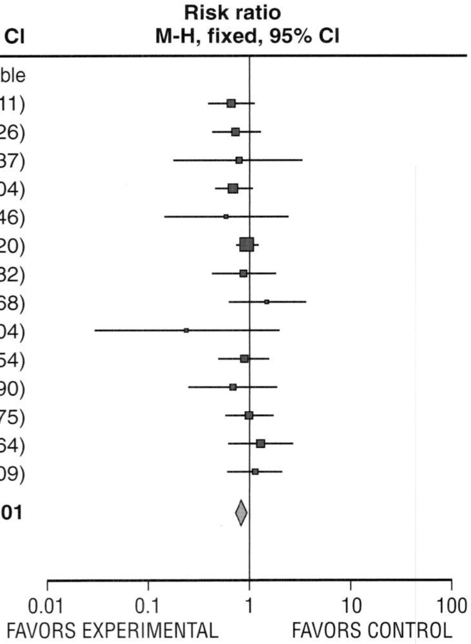

TELEMONITORING

Study or subgroup	Intervention Events	Intervention Total	Usual care Events	Usual care Total	Weight	Risk ratio M-H, fixed, 95% CI
Antonicelli 2008	3	28	5	29	2.4%	0.62 (0.16, 2.36)
Balk 2008	9	101	8	113	3.6%	1.26 (0.50, 3.14)
Capomolla 2004	5	67	7	66	3.4%	0.70 (0.24, 2.11)
Cleland 2005 (Telemon)	28	168	20	85	12.8%	0.71 (0.42, 1.18)
de Lusignan 2001	2	10	3	10	1.4%	0.67 (0.14, 3.17)
Giordano 2009	21	230	32	230	15.5%	0.66 (0.39, 1.10)
Goldberg 2003 (WHARF)	11	138	26	142	12.4%	0.44 (0.22, 0.85)
Kielblock 2007	37	251	69	251	33.3%	0.54 (0.37, 0.77)
Mortara 2009 (Telemon)	15	195	9	160	4.8%	1.37 (0.61, 3.04)
Soran 2008	11	160	17	155	8.3%	0.63 (0.30, 1.29)
Woodend 2008	5	62	4	59	2.0%	1.19 (0.34, 4.22)
Total (95% CI)		**1410**		**1300**	**100.0%**	**0.66 (0.54, 0.81**
Total events	147		200			

Heterogeneity: $Chi^2 = 8.84$, df=10 ($P = 0.55$), $I^2 = 0\%$
Test for overall effect Z = 4.07 ($P < 0.00001$)

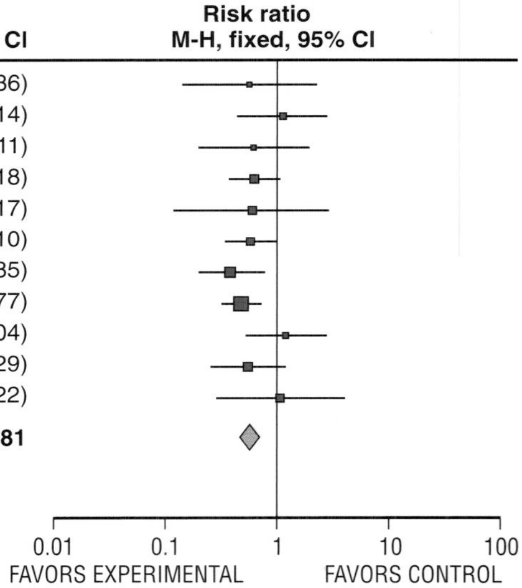

FIGURE 44-3 Effect of structured telephone support and telemonitoring on all-cause mortality. *From Inglis SC, Clark RA, McAlister FA, et al: Which components of heart failure programmes are effective? A systematic review and meta-analysis of the outcomes of structured telephone support or telemonitoring as the primary component of chronic heart failure management in 8323 patients: Abridged Cochrane Review. Eur J Heart Fail 13:1028–1040, 2011.*

P <0.0001), and the risk remained high after adjusting for clinical variables (HR 4.8; 95% CI 2.9-8.1; *P* <0.0001). The authors concluded that monthly review of HF device diagnostic data identifies patients at a higher risk of HF hospitalizations within the subsequent month.[26]

The CHAMPION (CardioMEMS Heart Sensor Allows Monitoring of Pressure to Improve Outcomes in NYHA class III heart failure patients)[30] trial was a prospective, multicenter, randomized, single-blinded study designed to evaluate whether pulmonary artery pressure–guided treatment of heart failure was better than usual care. All patients underwent implantation of the device, but no pulmonary artery pressure measurements were performed in the control group. In the treatment group, clinicians used daily measurement of pulmonary artery pressures in addition to standard of care versus standard of care alone in the control group. The primary efficacy endpoint was the rate of heart failure–related hospitalizations at 6 months. The safety endpoints assessed at 6 months were freedom from device-related or DSRC and freedom from pressure-sensor failures. At 6 months, 84 heart failure–related hospitalizations were reported in the treatment group (*n* = 270) compared with 120 in the control group (*n* = 280; rate 0.32 vs. 0.44; HR 0.72; 95% CI 0.60-0.85; *P* = 0.0002) (**Figure 44-4**). During the entire follow-up (mean 15 months [SD 7]), the treatment group had a 37% reduction in heart failure–related hospitalization compared with the control group (158 vs. 254; HR 0.63; 95% CI 0.52-0.77; *P* <0.0001). Eight patients had DSRC

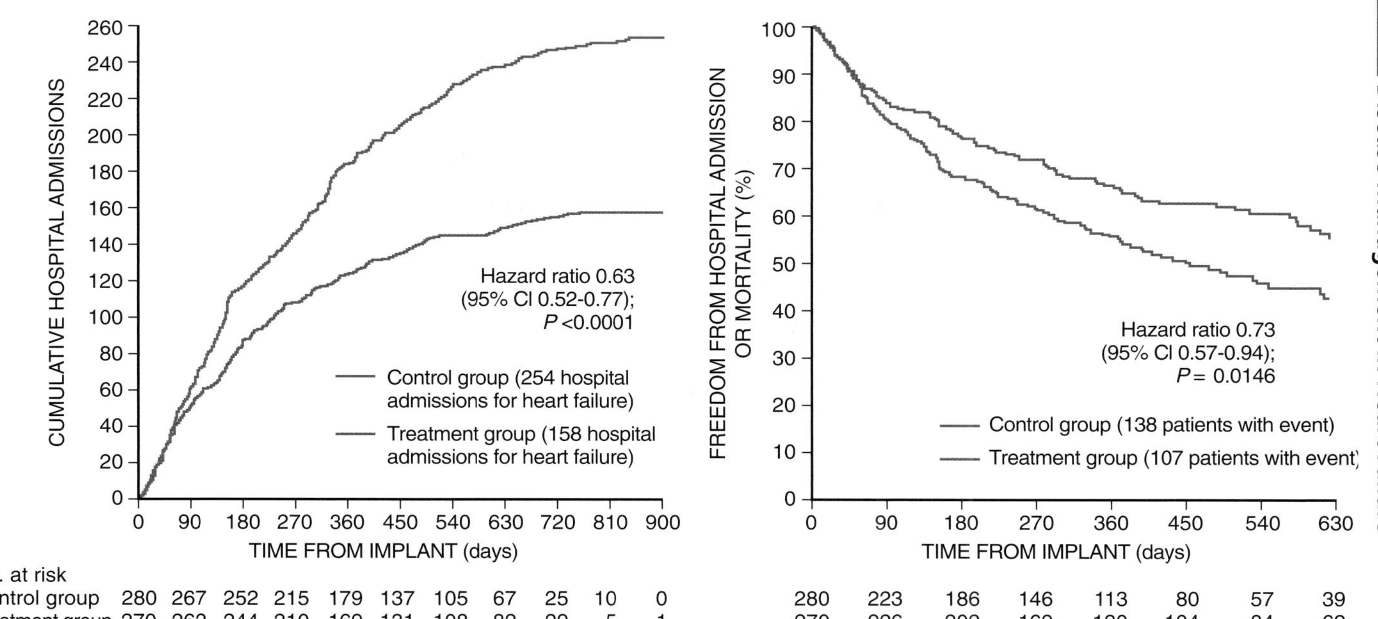

No. at risk

Control group	280	267	252	215	179	137	105	67	25	10	0
Treatment group	270	262	244	210	169	131	108	82	29	5	1

Control group	280	223	186	146	113	80	57	39
Treatment group	270	226	202	169	130	104	84	62

FIGURE 44-4 Cumulative heart failure–related hospitalizations during entire period of randomized single-blind follow-up **(A)**, and freedom from first heart failure–related hospitalization or mortality during the entire period of randomized follow-up **(B)**. *From Abraham WT, Adamson PB, Bourge RC, et al: Wireless pulmonary artery haemodynamic monitoring in chronic heart failure: a randomised controlled trial. Lancet 377:658–666, 2011.*

and overall freedom from DSRC was 98.6% (97.3-99.4) compared with a prespecified performance criterion of 80% (P <0.0001), and overall freedom from pressure-sensor failures was 100% (99.3-100.0). The authors concluded that wireless, implantable hemodynamic monitors in patients with NYHA class III heart failure significantly improved heart failure management.[30]

Despite the apparent benefit of the CardioMEMS device based on results of the CHAMPION trial, in December 2011 the FDA decided that there was not reasonable assurance that the CardioMEMS monitoring system was effective and decided not to approve the device.[79] The FDA committee members based their decision not to approve the device on concerns regarding analysis of the primary endpoint, differential interaction between the sponsor and principal investigator (PI) with centers regarding management of enrolled patients, and concerns regarding efficacy in subpopulations. The device has undergone further evaluation in response to the FDA review. Following a review to determine the effect of the differential interaction and an independent statistical analysis plan, the device was approved after a second review. Revised analyses confirmed a 28% lower rate of heart failure hospitalizations between the treatment and control groups during the first 6 months of the trial (84 vs. 120; P = 0.0002) and a 33% lower rate of heart failure hospitalizations during the entire randomized access part of the trial (182 vs. 279; P = 0.0002).[80]

WHY HAVE WE NOT SEEN CLEAR BENEFIT WITH HEART FAILURE DISEASE MANAGEMENT PROGRAMS?

Are We Targeting the Correct Patient Population?

Many of the recent multicenter, randomized, controlled trials on heart failure disease management programs have been neutral. There are several theories as to why these high-quality studies failed to demonstrate benefit. It is possible that some trials have targeted patient populations that may not necessarily benefit from a structured disease management program. For example, DeBusk and associates published a randomized controlled trial of a nurse case management system for heart failure patients immediately following a heart failure hospitalization in the Kaiser Permanente System.[58] In addition to usual care, patients in the intervention group received a physician-directed, nurse-managed, home-based program. The intervention included an initial educational session; baseline telephone counseling session; nurse-initiated follow-up telephone contacts; pharmacologic management; and nurse-initiated communication with physicians.[58] The authors found no statistically significant differences between usual care alone and usual care supplemented with nurse care management in the rate of rehospitalizations or in the combined outcome of rehospitalization, emergency department visits, or death. The investigators believed that the inclusion of patients newly diagnosed with heart failure lowered the overall risk for heart failure readmission. In addition, the study was performed in a health system that provided a high level of follow-up and excellent communication during care transition.

In contrast, Sisk and associates conducted a randomized controlled trial evaluating the benefits of a nurse case management system for a group of non-Hispanic black and Hispanic patients of a low socioeconomic class from four hospitals in Harlem.[68] The design of the intervention was based on the nurse case management model designed for the Kaiser Permanente trial conducted by DeBusk and colleagues.[58] Sisk and associates found that compared with usual care patients, nurse management patients had significantly fewer hospitalizations and better functioning.[68] Based on these trials, it appears that heart failure disease management programs may be more efficacious in settings

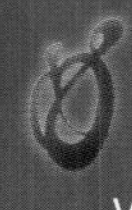

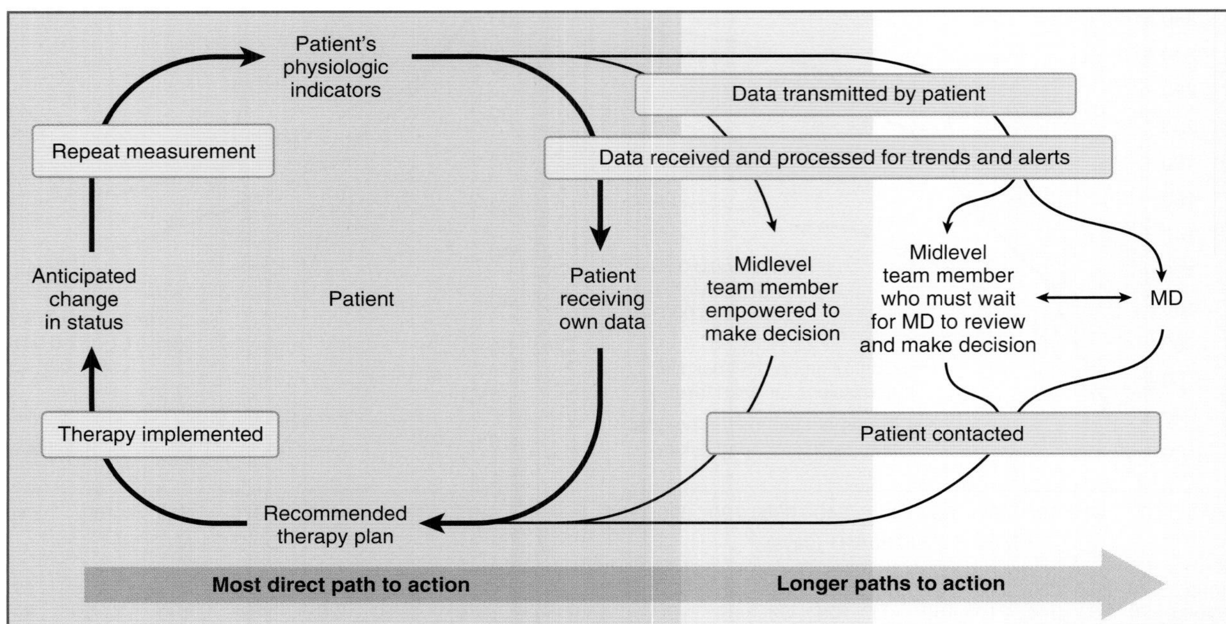

FIGURE 44-5 The circle of home management of heart failure. *From Desai AS, Stevenson LW: Connecting the circle from home to heart failure disease management. N Engl J Med 363:2364–2367, 2010.*

where background therapy has yet to be optimized in vulnerable populations.

There may be a tipping point when patients may be too sick to benefit from a heart failure disease management program. As demonstrated in the VA study conducted by Weinberger and associates,[47] patients with NYHA class III and IV heart failure with multiple comorbidities may require frequent hospitalizations despite our best efforts. The optimum acuity of illness to target may be NYHA class II and III, though further research is needed in this area. In the era of limited health care dollars, it is imperative that we focus our resources in areas where we will derive the most benefit.

Do We Have the Correct Health Care Providers on the Team?

Generalists rather than cardiologists manage most patients with HF.[81] However, HF is a complex problem, with a high rate of treatment failures and rehospitalizations and therefore may be more optimally managed with the guidance of specialists or subspecialists.[82] Edep and associates conducted a study designed to characterize physician practices in the management of HF and to determine whether these practices vary by specialty and how they relate to guideline recommendations. They found that cardiologists report practices more in conformity with published guidelines for HF than do internists and family practitioners. Because of the large numbers of patients with HF and their substantial mortality, morbidity, and cost of care, these differences may have a major impact on outcomes and health care costs.[82]

In many of the heart failure disease management programs discussed in this chapter, heart failure nurse specialists, nurse practitioners, and/or other midlevel providers played integral roles in implementation and day-to-day management of these programs. To manage the growing number of heart failure patients in the United States, the number of trained midlevel providers will need to increase dramatically. According to Desai and Stevenson,[83] one of the most urgent needs in cardiology is to design training, reimbursement, and a hub-and-spoke regional system incorporating a personnel force on the order of 10,000 nurses, nurse practitioners, and physicians' assistants to offer heart failure management to the 2 million patients with advanced heart failure. This goal might be achievable for less than a third of the cost associated with the number of cardioverter-defibrillators implanted annually.[83,84]

A barrier to effective care in heart failure disease management is the time delay between identification of a problem and initiation of a treatment. The requirement that heart failure coordinators review data with physicians can introduce delays in care. Small studies have suggested that the team member receiving the data should be empowered to contact the patient directly with a treatment plan, without having to "triangulate" the discussion with a physician before recommending a plan to the patient[83] (**Figure 44-5**).

Are We Measuring the Right Parameters?

Remote-monitoring approaches rely on the premise that routine surveillance of selected physiologic indicators will facilitate early detection of clinical deterioration and direct timely intervention to prevent adverse outcomes.[83] In regard to the Tele-HF trial, Desai and Stevenson hypothesize that an increase in weight and symptoms (the parameters monitored in the study) may not provide adequate warning. Results from trials of ambulatory hemodynamic monitoring in patients with heart failure suggest that weight is a poor surrogate for filling pressures and may be inadequate to anticipate the onset of decompensation.[85] The association between body weight and volume status lessens as the time since hospital discharge increases, because the target dry weight changes on the basis of caloric intake.[83] Although thoracic impedance alone was shown to be insensitive at predicting heart failure decompensation in patients with newly implanted ICDs, this parameter has been demonstrated to predict hospital readmission in PARTNERS-HF when viewed in combination with other parameters or when the threshold was set at a very high fluid index.[26] Although as clinicians we have been trained to treat the patients' symptoms and not a set of numbers or laboratory values, if markers are identified that predict decompensation before symptoms occur, early initiation of treatment may ward off deterioration and need for hospitalization.

FUTURE DIRECTION OF HEART FAILURE DISEASE MANAGEMENT PROGRAMS

The most expensive aspect of health care in high-income countries is staff to run services and deliver care. Delivering care by increasing direct one-to-one interactions is likely to be an expensive long-term strategy.[53] Therefore, telemonitoring is likely to become a more prevalent component of heart failure disease management programs. An advantage of telemonitoring is that it is a direct investment in the patient rather than in health care services. The patient is less likely to be a passive recipient of services and more likely to become an active participant in his or her own health care.[53] Diabetes is a good example of a chronic disease that is successfully managed by empowering patients to use technology to monitor and treat their conditions. In the future, patients may be able to adjust their own diuretic regimen on the basis of daily readings from internal monitors. Similar to the insulin pump, "smart" drug-delivery systems can perhaps be developed to trigger the automated release of medications in response to cardiorenal indicators.[83] Further research is needed to develop accurate, user-friendly technology to provide patients with real-time feedback regarding their clinical status. We also need to develop mechanisms to allow relevant data to be transmitted to health care providers in a timely manner so that appropriate treatments can be initiated quickly. A downside to telemonitoring is the daily generation of reams of data, most of which is irrelevant to patient care. Managing this volume of information will likely increase the need for mid-level personnel specialized in heart failure management and may also create new concerns about liability for unread transmissions.[83] Data management will be an important component of heart failure disease management in the future. Until we determine the most efficacious way of delivering heart failure disease management to all patients, we must be judicious and use it in patients who will likely derive the most benefit, such as elderly, vulnerable, and underserved populations.

References

1. Heidenreich PA, Albert NM, Allen LA, et al: Forecasting the impact of heart failure in the United States: a policy statement from the American Heart Association. *Circ Heart Fail* 6(3):606–619, 2013.
2. Adams KF, Jr, Fonarow GC, Emerman CL, et al: Characteristics and outcomes of patients hospitalized for heart failure in the United States: rationale, design, and preliminary observations from the first 100,000 cases in the Acute Decompensated Heart Failure National Registry (ADHERE). *Am Heart J* 149(2):209–216, 2005.
3. Rich MW, Beckham V, Wittenberg C, et al: A multidisciplinary intervention to prevent the readmission of elderly patients with congestive heart failure. *N Engl J Med* 333(18):1190–1195, 1995.
4. Fonarow GC, Stevenson LW, Walden JA, et al: Impact of a comprehensive heart failure management program on hospital readmission and functional status of patients with advanced heart failure. *J Am Coll Cardiol* 30(3):725–732, 1997.
5. Hanumanthu S, Butler J, Chomsky D, et al: Effect of a heart failure program on hospitalization frequency and exercise tolerance. *Circulation* 96(9):2842–2848, 1997.
6. Stewart S, Marley JE, Horowitz JD: Effects of a multidisciplinary, home-based intervention on unplanned readmissions and survival among patients with chronic congestive heart failure: a randomised controlled study. *Lancet* 354(9184):1077–1083, 1999.
7. Gattis WA, Hasselblad V, Whellan DJ, et al: Reduction in heart failure events by the addition of a clinical pharmacist to the heart failure management team: results of the Pharmacist in Heart Failure Assessment Recommendation and Monitoring (PHARM) Study. *Arch Intern Med* 159(16):1939–1945, 1999.
8. West JA, Miller NH, Parker KM, et al: A comprehensive management system for heart failure improves clinical outcomes and reduces medical resource utilization. *Am J Cardiol* 79(1):58–63, 1997.
9. Shah NB, Der E, Ruggerio C, et al: Prevention of hospitalizations for heart failure with an interactive home monitoring program. *Am Heart J* 135(3):373–378, 1998.
10. Bellomo R, Warrillow SJ, Reade MC: Why we should be wary of single-center trials. *Crit Care Med* 37(12):3114–3119, 2009.
11. Clark RA, Inglis SC, McAlister FA, et al: Telemonitoring or structured telephone support programmes for patients with chronic heart failure: systematic review and meta-analysis. *BMJ* 334(7600):942, 2007.
12. Gohler A, Januzzi JL, Worrell SS, et al: A systematic meta-analysis of the efficacy and heterogeneity of disease management programs in congestive heart failure. *J Card Fail* 12(7):554–567, 2006.
13. Holland R, Battersby J, Harvey I, et al: Systematic review of multidisciplinary interventions in heart failure. *Heart* 91(7):899–906, 2005.
14. Yu DS, Thompson DR, Lee DT: Disease management programmes for older people with heart failure: crucial characteristics which improve post-discharge outcomes. *Eur Heart J* 27(5):596–612, 2006.
15. Whellan DJ, Hasselblad V, Peterson E, et al: Metaanalysis and review of heart failure disease management randomized controlled clinical trials. *Am Heart J* 149(4):722–729, 2005.
16. Gwadry-Sridhar FH, Flintoft V, Lee DS, et al: A systematic review and meta-analysis of studies comparing readmission rates and mortality rates in patients with heart failure. *Arch Intern Med* 164(21):2315–2320, 2004.
17. McAlister FA, Stewart S, Ferrua S, et al: Multidisciplinary strategies for the management of heart failure patients at high risk for admission: a systematic review of randomized trials. *J Am Coll Cardiol* 44(4):810–819, 2004.
18. Phillips CO, Wright SM, Kern DE, et al: Comprehensive discharge planning with postdischarge support for older patients with congestive heart failure: a meta-analysis. *JAMA* 291(11):1358–1367, 2004.
19. Cleland JG, Louis AA, Rigby AS, et al: Noninvasive home telemonitoring for patients with heart failure at high risk of recurrent admission and death: the Trans-European Network-Home-Care Management System (TEN-HMS) study. *J Am Coll Cardiol* 45(10):1654–1664, 2005.
20. GESICA Investigators: Randomised trial of telephone intervention in chronic heart failure: DIAL trial. *BMJ* 331(7514):425, 2005.
21. Ferrante D, Varini S, Macchia A, et al: Long-term results after a telephone intervention in chronic heart failure: DIAL (Randomized Trial of Phone Intervention in Chronic Heart Failure) follow-up. *J Am Coll Cardiol* 56(5):372–378, 2010.
22. Soran OZ, Pina IL, Lamas GA, et al: A randomized clinical trial of the clinical effects of enhanced heart failure monitoring using a computer-based telephonic monitoring system in older minorities and women. *J Card Fail* 14(9):711–717, 2008.
23. Soran OZ, Feldman AM, Pina IL, et al: Cost of medical services in older patients with heart failure: those receiving enhanced monitoring using a computer-based telephonic monitoring system compared with those in usual care: the Heart Failure Home Care trial. *J Card Fail* 16(11):859–866, 2010.
24. Jaarsma T, van der Wal MH, Lesman-Leegte I, et al: Effect of moderate or intensive disease management program on outcome in patients with heart failure: Coordinating Study Evaluating Outcomes of Advising and Counseling in Heart Failure (COACH). *Arch Intern Med* 168(3):316–324, 2008.
25. Jaarsma T, Lesman-Leegte I, Hillege HL, et al: Depression and the usefulness of a disease management program in heart failure: insights from the COACH (Coordinating study evaluating Outcomes of Advising and Counseling in Heart failure) study. *J Am Coll Cardiol* 55(17):1837–1843, 2010.
26. Whellan DJ, Ousdigian KT, Al-Khatib SM, et al: Combined heart failure device diagnostics identify patients at higher risk of subsequent heart failure hospitalizations: results from PARTNERS HF (Program to Access and Review Trending Information and Evaluate Correlation to Symptoms in Patients With Heart Failure) study. *J Am Coll Cardiol* 55(17):1803–1810, 2010.
27. Chaudhry SI, Mattera JA, Curtis JP, et al: Telemonitoring in patients with heart failure. *N Engl J Med* 363(24):2301–2309, 2010.
28. Koehler F, Winkler S, Schieber M, et al: Impact of remote telemedical management on mortality and hospitalizations in ambulatory patients with chronic heart failure: the telemedical interventional monitoring in heart failure study. *Circulation* 123(17):1873–1880, 2011.
29. Bourge RC, Abraham WT, Adamson PB, et al: Randomized controlled trial of an implantable continuous hemodynamic monitor in patients with advanced heart failure: the COMPASS-HF study. *J Am Coll Cardiol* 51(11):1073–1079, 2008.
30. Abraham WT, Adamson PB, Bourge RC, et al: Wireless pulmonary artery haemodynamic monitoring in chronic heart failure: a randomised controlled trial. *Lancet* 377(9766):658–666, 2011.
31. The Boston Consulting Group: *The Promise of Disease Management*, Boston, Mass., 1995, The Boston Consulting Group Inc.
32. Ellrodt G, Cook DJ, Lee J, et al: Evidence-based disease management. *JAMA* 278(20):1687–1692, 1997.
33. Moser DK, Riegel B: Disease management in heart failure. In Mann DL, editor: *Heart failure: a companion to Braunwald's heart disease*, ed 2, St. Louis, 2011, Saunders, pp 854–864.
34. Riegel B, Carlson B, Glaser D: Development and testing of a clinical tool measuring self-management of heart failure. *Heart Lung* 29(1):4–15, 2000.
35. Grady KL, Dracup K, Kennedy G, et al: Team management of patients with heart failure: a statement for healthcare professionals from the Cardiovascular Nursing Council of the American Heart Association. *Circulation* 102(19):2443–2456, 2000.
36. Whellan D: Disease management in the advanced heart failure patient. In O'Connor CSW, Gheorghiade M, Kirkwood FA, Jr, editors: *Managing acute decompensated heart failure*, Oxford, 2005, Taylor & Francis Publishers, pp 555–568.
37. Krumholz HM, Currie PM, Riegel B, et al: A taxonomy for disease management: a scientific statement from the American Heart Association Disease Management Taxonomy Writing Group. *Circulation* 114(13):1432–1445, 2006.
38. Ashton CM, Kuykendall DH, Johnson ML, et al: The association between the quality of inpatient care and early readmission. *Ann Intern Med* 122(6):415–421, 1995.
39. Fonarow GC, Peterson ED: Heart failure performance measures and outcomes: real or illusory gains. *JAMA* 302(7):792–794, 2009.
40. Curtis LH, Greiner MA, Hammill BG, et al: Early and long-term outcomes of heart failure in elderly persons, 2001-2005. *Arch Intern Med* 168(22):2481–2488, 2008.
41. Fonarow GC, Abraham WT, Albert NM, et al: Association between performance measures and clinical outcomes for patients hospitalized with heart failure. *JAMA* 297(1):61–70, 2007.
42. Heidenreich PA, Hernandez AF, Yancy CW, et al: Get With The Guidelines program participation, process of care, and outcome for Medicare patients hospitalized with heart failure. *Circ Cardiovasc Qual Outcomes* 5(1):37–43, 2012.

43. Naylor M, Brooten D, Jones R, et al: Comprehensive discharge planning for the hospitalized elderly. A randomized clinical trial. *Ann Intern Med* 120(12):999–1006, 1994.
44. Forster AJ, Murff HJ, Peterson JF, et al: The incidence and severity of adverse events affecting patients after discharge from the hospital. *Ann Intern Med* 138(3):161–167, 2003.
45. Gorodeski EZ, Chlad S, Vilensky S: Home-based care for heart failure: Cleveland Clinic's "Heart Care at Home" transitional care program. *Cleve Clin J Med* 80(Electronic Suppl 1):eS20–eS26, 2013.
46. Gray SL, Mahoney JE, Blough DK: Adverse drug events in elderly patients receiving home health services following hospital discharge. *Ann Pharmacother* 33(11):1147–1153, 1999.
47. Weinberger M, Oddone EZ, Henderson WG: Does increased access to primary care reduce hospital readmissions? Veterans Affairs Cooperative Study Group on Primary Care and Hospital Readmission. *N Engl J Med* 334(22):1441–1447, 1996.
48. Abraham WT, Bristow MR: Specialized centers for heart failure management. *Circulation* 96(9):2755–2757, 1997.
49. Doughty RN, Wright SP, Pearl A, et al: Randomized, controlled trial of integrated heart failure management: the Auckland Heart Failure Management Study. *Eur Heart J* 23(2):139–146, 2002.
50. Cline CM, Israelsson BY, Willenheimer RB, et al: Cost effective management programme for heart failure reduces hospitalisation. *Heart* 80(5):442–446, 1998.
51. McAlister FA, Lawson FM, Teo KK, et al: A systematic review of randomized trials of disease management programs in heart failure. *Am J Med* 110(5):378–384, 2001.
52. Mortara A, Pinna GD, Johnson P, et al: Home telemonitoring in heart failure patients: the HHH study (Home or Hospital in Heart Failure). *Eur J Heart Fail* 11(3):312–318, 2009.
53. Inglis SC, Clark RA, McAlister FA, et al: Which components of heart failure programmes are effective? A systematic review and meta-analysis of the outcomes of structured telephone support or telemonitoring as the primary component of chronic heart failure management in 8323 patients: Abridged Cochrane Review. *Eur J Heart Fail* 13(9):1028–1040, 2011.
54. Stewart S, Carrington MJ, Marwick TH, et al: Impact of home versus clinic-based management of chronic heart failure: the WHICH? (Which Heart Failure Intervention Is Most Cost-Effective & Consumer Friendly in Reducing Hospital Care) multicenter, randomized trial. *J Am Coll Cardiol* 60(14):1239–1248, 2012.
55. Stewart S, Pearson S, Horowitz JD: Effects of a home-based intervention among patients with congestive heart failure discharged from acute hospital care. *Arch Intern Med* 158(10):1067–1072, 1998.
56. Inglis SC, Clark RA, McAlister FA, et al: Structured telephone support or telemonitoring programmes for patients with chronic heart failure. *Cochrane Database Syst Rev* (8):CD007228, 2010.
57. Barth V: A nurse-managed discharge program for congestive heart failure patients: outcomes and costs. *Home Health Care Manage Pract* 13(6):436–443, 2001.
58. DeBusk RF, Miller NH, Parker KM, et al: Care management for low-risk patients with heart failure: a randomized, controlled trial. *Ann Intern Med* 141(8):606–613, 2004.
59. Laramee AS, Levinsky SK, Sargent J, et al: Case management in a heterogeneous congestive heart failure population: a randomized controlled trial. *Arch Intern Med* 163(7):809–817, 2003.
60. Rainville EC: Impact of pharmacist interventions on hospital readmissions for heart failure. *Am J Health Syst Pharm* 56(13):1339–1342, 1999.
61. Ramachandran K, Husain N, Maikhuri R, et al: Impact of a comprehensive telephone-based disease management programme on quality-of-life in patients with heart failure. *Natl Med J India* 20(2):67–73, 2007.
62. Riegel B, Carlson B, Kopp Z, et al: Effect of a standardized nurse case-management telephone intervention on resource use in patients with chronic heart failure. *Arch Intern Med* 162(6):705–712, 2002.
63. Riegel B, Carlson B, Glaser D, et al: Standardized telephonic case management in a Hispanic heart failure population. *Dis Manage Health Outcomes* 10(4):241–249, 2002.
64. Riegel B, Carlson B, Glaser D, et al: Randomized controlled trial of telephone case management in Hispanics of Mexican origin with heart failure. *J Card Fail* 12(3):211–219, 2006.
65. Hebert PL, Sisk JE, Wang JJ, et al: Cost-effectiveness of nurse-led disease management for heart failure in an ethnically diverse urban community. *Ann Intern Med* 149(8):540–548, 2008.
66. Sisk JE, Horowitz CR, McLaughlin MA, et al: Effectiveness and cost-effectiveness of nurse-management to improve heart-failure care in minority communities. Proceedings of the First Annual Meeting of the Health Technology Assessment International (HTAi) 1(111), 2004.
67. Tsuyuki RT, Fradette M, Johnson JA, et al: A multicenter disease management program for hospitalized patients with heart failure. *J Card Fail* 10(6):473–480, 2004.
68. Sisk JE, Hebert PL, Horowitz CR, et al: Effects of nurse management on the quality of heart failure care in minority communities: a randomized trial. *Ann Intern Med* 145(4):273–283, 2006.
69. Giordano A, Scalvini S, Zanelli E, et al: Multicenter randomised trial on home-based telemanagement to prevent hospital readmission of patients with chronic heart failure. *Int J Cardiol* 131(2):192–199, 2009.
70. Blasius M, editor: *Impact of telemetric management on overall treatment costs and mortality rate among patients with chronic heart failure*, European Heart Journal, Oxford, 2008, Oxford Univ Press.
71. Pare G, Jaana M, Sicotte C: Systematic review of home telemonitoring for chronic diseases: the evidence base. *J Am Med Inform Assoc* 14(3):269–277, 2007.
72. Goldberg LR, Piette JD, Walsh MN, et al: Randomized trial of a daily electronic home monitoring system in patients with advanced heart failure: the Weight Monitoring in Heart Failure (WHARF) trial. *Am Heart J* 146(4):705–712, 2003.
73. Galbreath AD, Krasuski RA, Smith B, et al: Long-term healthcare and cost outcomes of disease management in a large, randomized, community-based population with heart failure. *Circulation* 110(23):3518–3526, 2004.
74. Owens AT, Jessup M: The year in heart failure. *J Am Coll Cardiol* 60(5):359–368, 2012.
75. Angermann CE, Stork S, Gelbrich G, et al: Mode of action and effects of standardized collaborative disease management on mortality and morbidity in patients with systolic heart failure: the Interdisciplinary Network for Heart Failure (INH) study. *Circ Heart Fail* 5(1):25–35, 2012.
76. Lynga P, Persson H, Hagg-Martinell A, et al: Weight monitoring in patients with severe heart failure (WISH). A randomized controlled trial. *Eur J Heart Fail* 14(4):438–444, 2012.
77. Adamson PB, Conti JB, Smith AL, et al: Reducing events in patients with chronic heart failure (REDUCEhf) study design: continuous hemodynamic monitoring with an implantable defibrillator. *Clin Cardiol* 30(11):567–575, 2007.
78. Conraads VM, Tavazzi L, Santini M, et al: Sensitivity and positive predictive value of implantable intrathoracic impedance monitoring as a predictor of heart failure hospitalizations: the SENSE-HF trial. *Eur Heart J* 32(18):2266–2273, 2011.
79. Loh JP, Barbash IM, Waksman R: Overview of the 2011 Food and Drug Administration Circulatory System Devices Panel of the Medical Devices Advisory Committee Meeting on the CardioMEMS Champion Heart Failure Monitoring System. *J Am Coll Cardiol* 61(15):1571–1576, 2013.
80. The CardioMEMS Champion HF Monitoring System for Patients with NYHA Class III Heart Failure Briefing Document for the Circulatory System Devices Panel FDA Advisory Committee. In Administration UFaD, editor: *CardioMEMS Champion HF Monitoring System PMA Amendment P100045*, 2013.
81. Borowsky SJ, Kravitz RL, Laouri M, et al: Effect of physician specialty on use of necessary coronary angiography. *J Am Coll Cardiol* 26(6):1484–1491, 1995.
82. Edep ME, Shah NB, Tateo IM, et al: Differences between primary care physicians and cardiologists in management of congestive heart failure: relation to practice guidelines. *J Am Coll Cardiol* 30(2):518–526, 1997.
83. Desai AS, Stevenson LW: Connecting the circle from home to heart-failure disease management. *N Engl J Med* 363(24):2364–2367, 2010.
84. Hammill SC, Kremers MS, Stevenson LW, et al: Review of the Registry's second year, data collected, and plans to add lead and pediatric ICD procedures. *Heart Rhythm* 5(9):1359–1363, 2008.
85. Zile MR, Bennett TD, St John Sutton M, et al: Transition from chronic compensated to acute decompensated heart failure: pathophysiological insights obtained from continuous monitoring of intracardiac pressures. *Circulation* 118(14):1433–1441, 2008.

Management of Comorbidities in Heart Failure

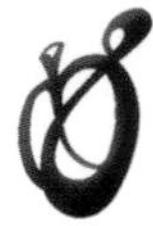

Justin A. Ezekowitz

Heart failure patients often have multiple comorbid conditions that may interact with heart failure syndrome and/or the choice of therapies. Research into the common comorbid conditions has furthered the understanding of the pathophysiologic basis for symptoms or structural abnormalities of heart failure (HF), aided in the refinement of the often complicated management because of the competing therapies, and provided clarity regarding the diagnostic certainty (or uncertainty) as a result of competing causes for signs and symptoms of disease. In clinical practice, this is seen on a day-to-day basis, and thus understanding the management of HF requires consideration of all aspects of human health.

In most chronic HF registry, administrative, or trial data, the number of comorbid conditions exceeds five (including other related components of cardiovascular disease [e.g., atrial fibrillation]) for many patients.[1] From the major registry data, the most common comorbid conditions and their approximate prevalence are depression (22%),[2] chronic obstructive pulmonary disease (COPD; 20%-30%),[3,4] diabetes (30%),[5] and sleep-disordered breathing (40%).[6] Other important cardiovascular conditions that interact with heart failure, such as atrial fibrillation (see Chapter 35) or coronary artery disease (see Chapter 18), are discussed elsewhere.

Importantly, although all of these comorbid conditions have a significant impact on prognosis, the specific treatment of the comorbid condition has generally not been shown to improve major clinical outcomes. For example, treating depression with sertraline did not lead to a reduction in cardiovascular events.[7] This creates a unique situation for clinicians caring for patients with HF because they require expert management beyond the disease-disease and drug-drug interactions. Each disease (HF and a comorbid condition) can exacerbate or be a trigger for the other, or complicate the treatment course because therapies typically used for the comorbid condition of interest may indeed exacerbate HF (e.g., etanercept for rheumatoid arthritis). Likewise, some therapies can be used for both, allowing for rational selection of therapy (e.g., ACE inhibitors for HF and diabetes) or potentially synergistic effects (CPAP for sleep apnea may induce better control of atrial fibrillation and HF symptoms). Thus the interaction is often far more complex than first anticipated and clinicians should be aware and ask five simple questions when faced with this situation (**Table 45-1**). Each situation will be unique, however, and where possible, an informed choice can be made by integrating information from the published literature, patient preferences, and in consultation with other health professionals.

ANEMIA

Definitions, Prevalence, and Outcomes

Anemia is defined by the World Health Organization as a hemoglobin <13.0 g/dL in men and <12.0 g/dL in women. Additional other definitions are available, including those of the Centers for Disease Control (<13.0 g/dL in men and <12.5 g/dL in women)[8] and National Kidney Foundation (<13.5 g/dL in males and <12.0 g/dL in females).[9] Others have defined anemia by chart abstract coding of anemia[10] or have devised their own cut-point based on the lowest quartile. Using these definitions, the prevalence of anemia in patients with chronic heart failure has been found to be very substantially based on the location or context surveyed, severity of illness, age, gender, race, and whether or not they were acute or chronic heart failure patients. Given the limitations listed previously, the prevalence in larger population studies is approximately 15% to 20%[10,11] and approximately 30% to 50% in either acute HF populations or specialized clinics,[12,13] summarized elsewhere.[14]

Anemia has been associated with poor clinical outcomes. Regardless of the definitions used to define the

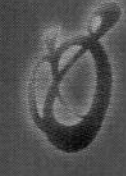

TABLE 45-1 Five Questions to Ask When Reviewing the Comorbid Condition in a Patient with Heart Failure

	QUESTION	CONSIDERATIONS	EXAMPLE
1.	Does the comorbid condition affect the characteristics of a test used to diagnosis or manage HF?	Test sensitivity or specificity modified due to known or unknown confounders because of the comorbid condition	BNP levels in patients who are obese are lower than nonobese patients.
2.	Does HF affect the characteristics of a test used to diagnosis or manage a comorbid condition?	HF may modify the underlying pathophysiology upon which the test is based.	Pulmonary function tests can be abnormal for patients with HF even in the absence of COPD.
3.	Did this comorbid condition or its related therapies "cause" or exacerbate HF in this patient?	Some disease-disease links are strong, whereas others are putative.	Diabetic cardiomyopathy; anthracyclines for cancer
4.	Does the comorbid condition modify the options for treatment of HF?	Some therapies used in HF need to be carefully selected so as not to worsen a comorbid condition.	The risk/benefit of ACE inhibitors in end-stage renal disease; volume management with diuretics in COPD; appropriateness of cardiac resynchronization therapy in advanced COPD
5.	Should we modify the management of the comorbid condition due to the presence of HF?	Known risks for some therapies may include exacerbating HF.	Etanercept for rheumatoid arthritis; Herceptin for breast cancer

ACE, Angiotensin-converting enzyme; *BNP,* B-type natriuretic peptide; *COPD,* chronic obstructive pulmonary disease; *HF,* heart failure.

TABLE 45-2 Diagnostic Assays of Clinical Use for the Cause of Anemia

CATEGORY	ETIOLOGY	TEST	POSSIBLE RESULTS	OTHER NOTES
General		Peripheral smear	Microcytic, normocytic, or macrocytic	Nondiagnostic but helpful for further testing
		Reticulocyte count/index	RI 1%-2% = normal; RI <2% with anemia = blood loss or inadequate bone marrow response; RI >3% bone marrow compensation	Helpful for determining bone marrow response to therapy
		Bone marrow biopsy	Variable	Invasive; often used for diagnosis in selected diseases
Blood loss	Gastrointestinal	Endoscopy	Ulcers, erosions, masses, polyps	Consider all anti-platelet, anti-coagulant, and NSAID use
		Fecal occult blood	Positive compatible with IDA or blood loss	Consider further testing to identify source
Nutritional deficiency	Folate	Serum folate	<4 ng/mL	Can drop in acute illness
		RBC folate	Variable based on assay	Indicative of folate deficiency
		Serum B_{12}	<200 pg/mL	May need additional testing for pernicious anemia
	Iron	Serum transferrin saturation	<20% compatible with IDA	
		Ferritin	<50 ng/mL compatible with IDA	Can be elevated due to inflammation in HF
Sickle-cell		Hemoglobin electrophoresis	HbSS, HbSC	
Thalassemia		Hemoglobin electrophoresis	% $\alpha\beta\delta$ Hb	
Other		Ultrasound of kidneys, liver, spleen	Medicorenal disease; cirrhosis; splenomegaly	

Hb, Hemoglobin; *HF,* heart failure; *IDA,* iron-deficiency anemia; *RBC,* red blood cell; *RI,* reticulocyte index.

prevalence, the clinical importance may matter more on the interaction of multiple factors for individual patients. The within-person changes to hemoglobin over time may be more important than the overall hemoglobin level. In the Val-HEFT trial, 16.9% of patients developed new-onset anemia, and a decline in hemoglobin over 12 months was strongly related to subsequent clinical outcomes even after adjusting for powerful prognostic markers such as B-type natriuretic peptide (BNP) and estimated glomerular filtration rate (eGFR).[15] Most of the studies of patients with anemia and heart failure highlight a 1.5- to 2-fold increase in short- and long-term mortality even after adjustment for other clinical variables.

Diagnosis of Anemia

The diagnosis of anemia is a combination of symptoms, signs, and biomarkers related to the hematopoietic system. Given the substantial overlap of symptoms of heart failure and anemia (e.g., fatigue, shortness of breath), there are no specific symptoms that appear to aid diagnosis. Similarly, given the lack of specificity of physical signs of anemia, there are no additional signs to aid in the diagnosis of anemia in a patient with heart failure.

The biomarkers for diagnosing and exploring the cause or subtype of anemia are multiple and well developed (**Table 45-2**). They are aimed at diagnosing the most common conditions (nutritional deficiency or blood loss), ruling out other related diseases (bone-related malignancy, thyroid disease, sickle-cell anemia, thalassemia) or establishing a diagnosis of anemia of chronic disease related to heart failure. Most patients will require some combination of the testing and repeat testing if an intervention is done (e.g., iron therapy should be followed by a repeat hemoglobin, iron saturation, and possibly a ferritin).

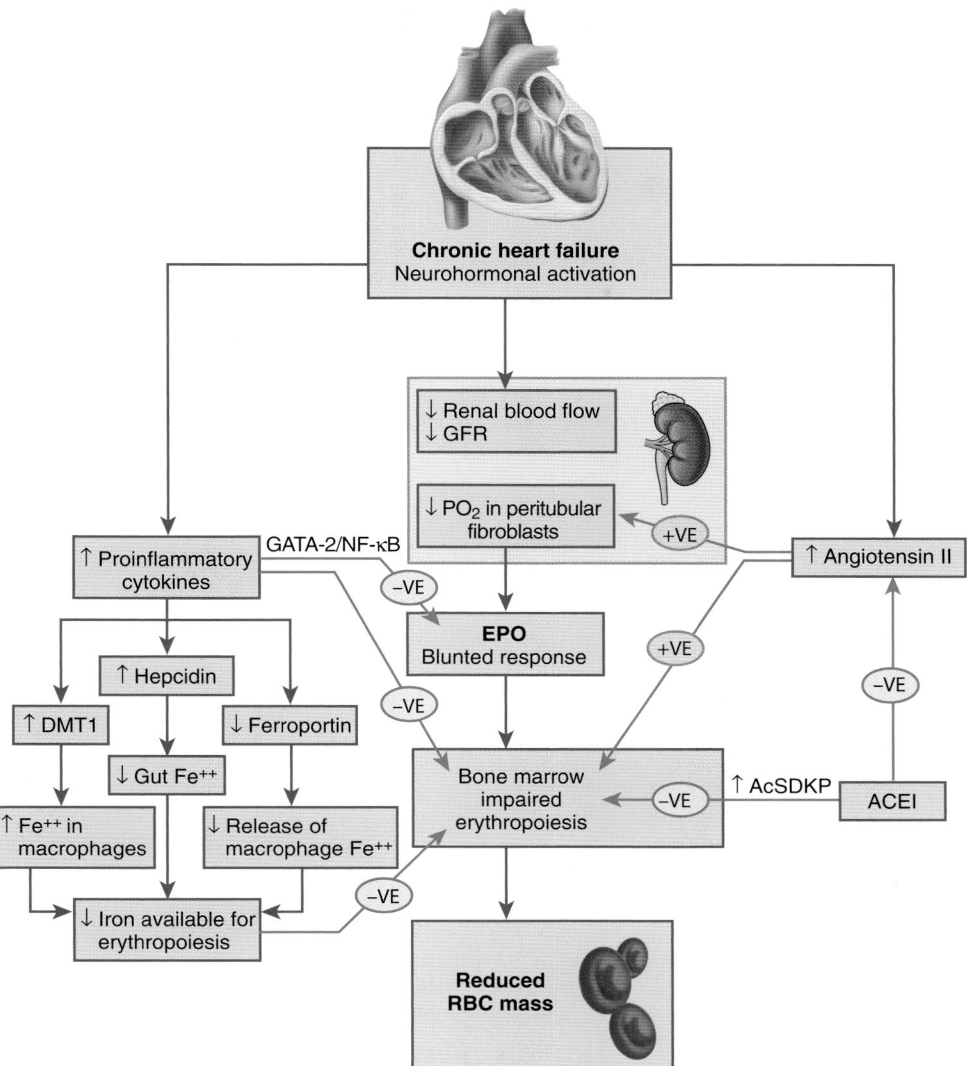

FIGURE 45-1 Possible mechanisms involved in the genesis of anemia in heart failure. Shown is a diagram of the possible mechanisms of anemia in patients with heart failure. *ACEI,* Angiotensin-converting enzyme inhibitor; *AcSDKP, N*-acetyl-seryl-aspartyl-lysyl-proline; *DMT1,* divalent metal transporter 1; *EPO,* epoetin; *GFR,* glomerular filtration rate; *NF-κB,* nuclear factor-kappa B; *RBC,* red blood cell mass. *From Anand IS: Anemia and chronic heart failure. J Am Coll Cardiol 52:501–511, 2008. Illustration by Rob Flewell.*

Given the variety of causes for anemia, targeted diagnosis and therapy are important (**Figure 45-1**). However, many patients (up to 46% in one series[16]) may have hemodilution as a cause of their anemia, so judicious measurement of hemoglobin after euvolemia is attained is essential when evaluating patients with anemia.

Treatment

Once a clear or working diagnosis is obtained, therapy will be targeted to the potential cause. The general approach to the treatment of anemia is beyond the scope of this chapter; thus the remainder of this section will focus on the results of randomized controlled trials that specifically enrolled patients with HF.

Iron therapy has remained the mainstay of therapy for iron deficiency anemia. Many guidelines recommend a trial of oral iron therapy, although this has never been subjected to rigorous study in patients with cardiovascular disease. However, intravenous iron injections have recently been the subject of randomized controlled trials (RCTs). The Ferinject Assessment in Patients with Iron Deficiency and Chronic Heart Failure (FAIR-HF) trial assessed patients with New York Heart Association (NYHA) class II or III, left ventricular ejection fraction (LVEF) of 45% or less, a hemoglobin between 95 and 135 g/dL, with iron deficiency anemia (ferritin <100 μg/L or was between 100 and 299 μg/L and transferrin saturation <20%).[17] For the primary endpoint at 24 weeks of Patient Global Assessment (PGA) and compared with a placebo, patients randomized to intravenous iron (and titrated to iron indices) had an odds ratio of 2.51 (95% confidence interval [CI] 1.75-3.61) of being improved by PGA and an odds ratio of 2.4 (95% CI 1.55-3.71) of improving one NYHA class. Similar positive outcomes were seen for the EQ-5D, KCCQ, and 6-minute walk test without any significant safety signal (or efficacy for clinical events) (**Figure 45-2**). Three other small trials have had similar results, summarized elsewhere,[18] and there are ongoing small studies (clinicaltrials.gov: NCT00386126, NCT00384657, NCT01453608). Adequately powered RCTs will be required to assess if the effect size and clinical outcomes are seen in truly blinded trials, with important clinical outcomes as

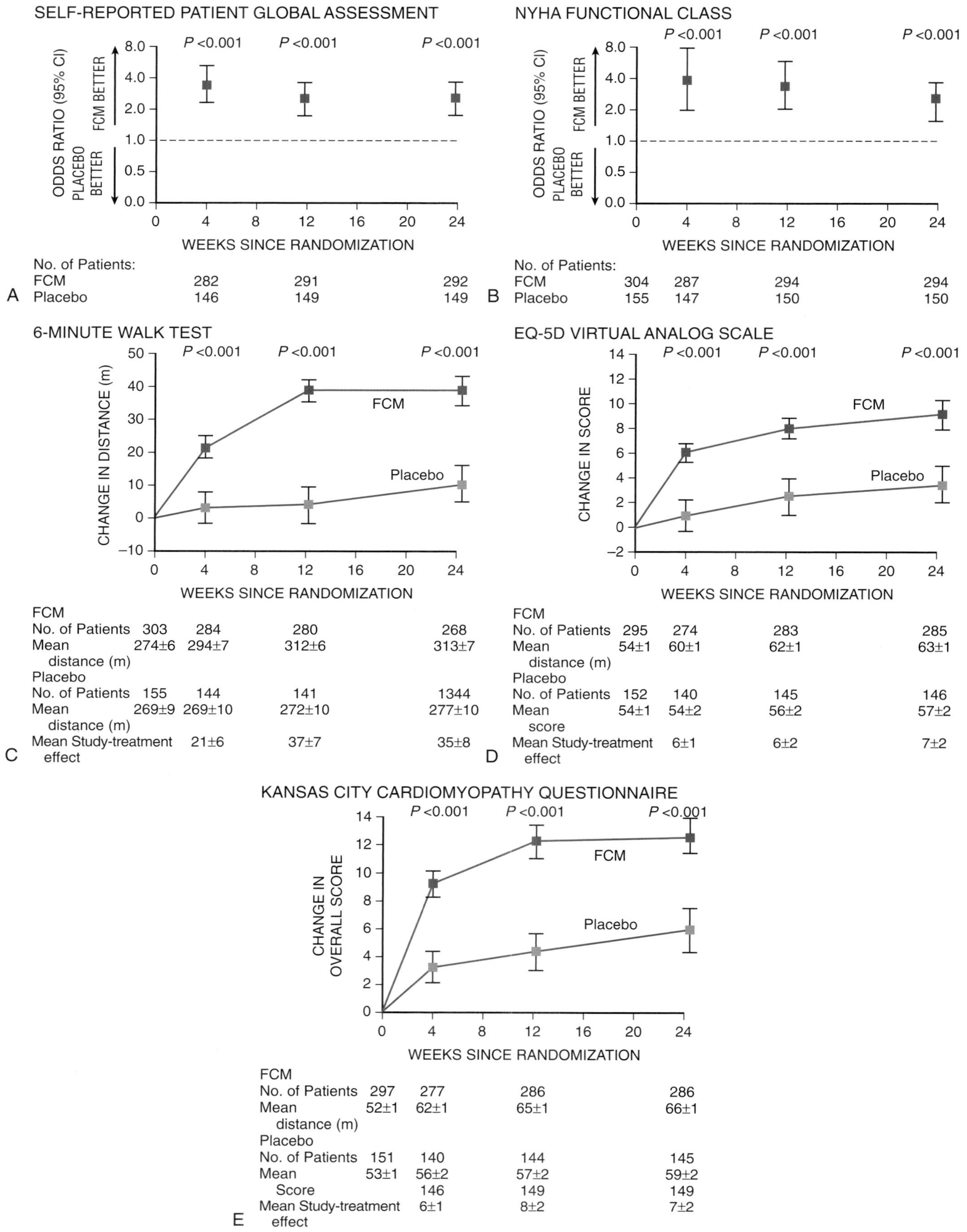

SELF-REPORTED PATIENT GLOBAL ASSESSMENT

ODDS RATIO (95% CI) — FCM BETTER / PLACEBO BETTER

8.0, 4.0, 2.0, 1.0, 0.5, 0.0

P <0.001 P <0.001 P <0.001

0 4 8 12 16 20 24

WEEKS SINCE RANDOMIZATION

No. of Patients:	4	12	24
FCM	282	291	292
Placebo	146	149	149

A

NYHA FUNCTIONAL CLASS

ODDS RATIO (95% CI) — FCM BETTER / PLACEBO BETTER

8.0, 4.0, 2.0, 1.0, 0.5, 0.0

P <0.001 P <0.001 P <0.001

0 4 8 12 16 20 24

WEEKS SINCE RANDOMIZATION

No. of Patients:	0	4	12	24
FCM	304	287	294	294
Placebo	155	147	150	150

B

6-MINUTE WALK TEST

CHANGE IN DISTANCE (m)

50, 40, 30, 20, 10, 0, −10

P <0.001 P <0.001 P <0.001

FCM

Placebo

0 4 8 12 16 20 24

WEEKS SINCE RANDOMIZATION

	0	4	12	24
FCM				
No. of Patients	303	284	280	268
Mean distance (m)	274±6	294±7	312±6	313±7
Placebo				
No. of Patients	155	144	141	1344
Mean distance (m)	269±9	269±10	272±10	277±10
Mean Study-treatment effect		21±6	37±7	35±8

C

EQ-5D VIRTUAL ANALOG SCALE

CHANGE IN SCORE

14, 12, 10, 8, 6, 4, 2, 0, −2

P <0.001 P <0.001 P <0.001

FCM

Placebo

0 4 8 12 16 20 24

WEEKS SINCE RANDOMIZATION

	0	4	12	24
FCM				
No. of Patients	295	274	283	285
Mean distance (m)	54±1	60±1	62±1	63±1
Placebo				
No. of Patients	152	140	145	146
Mean score	54±1	54±2	56±2	57±2
Mean Study-treatment effect		6±1	6±2	7±2

D

KANSAS CITY CARDIOMYOPATHY QUESTIONNAIRE

CHANGE IN OVERALL SCORE

14, 12, 10, 8, 6, 4, 2, 0

P <0.001 P <0.001 P <0.001

FCM

Placebo

0 4 8 12 16 20 24

WEEKS SINCE RANDOMIZATION

	0	4	12	24
FCM				
No. of Patients	297	277	286	286
Mean distance (m)	52±1	62±1	65±1	66±1
Placebo				
No. of Patients	151	140	144	145
Mean	53±1	56±2	57±2	59±2
Score		146	149	149
Mean Study-treatment effect		6±1	8±2	7±2

E

FIGURE 45-2 The Ferinject Assessment in Patients with Iron Deficiency and Chronic Heart Failure trial results. *FCM,* Ferric carboxymaltose; *NYHA,* New York Heart Association. *From Anker SD, Comin Colet J, Filippatos G, et al: Ferric carboxymaltose in patients with heart failure and iron deficiency. N Engl J Med 361:2436–2448, 2009.*

the endpoint. In the interim, it appears that intravenous iron is a reasonable therapeutic choice for carefully selected patients with the goal of improving symptoms.

Erythropoiesis-stimulating agents (ESA) including erythropoietin and darbepoetin are used in patients with chronic kidney disease to increase the hemoglobin level. Although RCT evidence has not been overwhelmingly supportive of this strategy, and most guidelines recommend only cautious use for much lower hemoglobin targets, ESA have been subjected to multiple small and one large RCT including patients with HF. In the RED-HF trial, 2278 patients with a low ejection fraction (LVEF ≤ 40%), NYHA II-IV, and a hemoglobin between 9.0 and 12.0 g/dL were randomized to darbepoetin or a placebo and a target hemoglobin of 13.0 g/dL and followed for a median of 28 months.[19] Overall, there was no meaningful difference between the groups for important clinical outcomes, including quality of life, symptoms, death, or rehospitalization; thus there was no additional benefit in a strategy of increasing hemoglobin via an ESA for clinical outcomes.

Summary/Conclusions

Ongoing trials of intravenous iron replacement for anemic patients or as an agent to improve clinical outcomes even in nonanemic patients are key steps in understanding if the correction of anemia can alter clinical outcomes. Key interactions between the bone marrow, the hematologic system, and the vasculature have both shed light on the mechanisms of anemia and helped in the understanding of other pathophysiologic roles of new molecules (e.g., hepcidin),[20] "old" systems (e.g., renin-angiotensin-aldosterone), or new targets (iron receptors).[21]

CHRONIC OBSTRUCTIVE PULMONARY DISEASE

Definitions, Prevalence, and Outcomes

The diagnosis of COPD is done by a combination of clinical history and physical examination findings, and is confirmed by spirometry. The most commonly used criteria are the Global Initiative for Chronic Obstructive Lung Disease (GOLD) criteria that define COPD as a postbronchodilator fixed ratio of FEV_1/FVC of 0.70 or less (**Table 45-3**).[22] Both obstructive and restrictive components of COPD are recognized as important, and can coexist.

Given the significant overlap in symptoms, such as shortness of breath, fatigue, and other descriptors, studies have not shown that the two diseases can be distinguished based on symptoms.[23] Studies using the Framingham or other diagnostic symptom-based criteria are less useful given this overlap and can provide erroneous estimates of incidence, prevalence, or outcome relationships.[24] Similarly, the physical signs of HF may overlap, and specifically right ventricular failure signs may be evident in both diseases related to secondary pulmonary hypertension and direct myocardial effects. The overlap is summarized elsewhere.[25]

TABLE 45-3 Classification of Chronic Obstructive Lung Disease

STAGE	FEV_1/FVC	PREDICTED FEV_1
Stage I: mild	<0.70	>80%
Stage II: moderate	<0.70	50% to 79%
Stage III: severe	<0.70	30% to 49%
Stage IV: very severe	<0.70	<30% or <50% plus chronic respiratory failure*

*Respiratory failure: arterial partial pressure of oxygen (Pa_{O_2}), 8.0 kPa (60 mm Hg) with or without arterial partial pressure of CO_2 (Pa_{CO_2}). 6.7 kPa (50 mm Hg) while breathing air at sea level.

FEV_1, Forced expiratory volume in one second; *FVC,* forced vital capacity.
Adapted from Rabe KF, Hurd S, Anzueto A, et al: Global strategy for the diagnosis, management, and prevention of chronic obstructive pulmonary disease: GOLD executive summary. Am J Respir Crit Care Med 176:532–555, 2007.

As a comorbidity in community-based surveys, the COPD is present in up to one third of outpatients,[3,4] distributed relatively between those with a reduced or preserved ejection fraction.[26] Importantly, many clinical trials of current evidence-based therapy excluded COPD or other respiratory disorders, so estimates of prevalence from RCT should be evaluated cautiously. Hence, establishing the diagnosis of COPD in a patient with HF, or HF in a patient with COPD, requires clinical vigilance, understanding the overlapping risk factors (e.g., smoking) and testing for both diseases.

Pulmonary Function Tests and Heart Failure

Pulmonary function tests (PFTs) and spirometry involve establishing the key parameters of FEV_1, FVC, DLCO, and peak expiratory flow rate. As discussed previously, the diagnosis of COPD may be evident as per the GOLD criteria, but there are limitations to consider. For example, interstitial edema may cause partial obstruction and increased bronchial sensitivity leading to an obstructive pattern on PFTs.[27] This may partially or fully resolve after a patient diuresis if they were acutely ill.[28] Interestingly, peak expiratory flow has recently been assessed for its use as a clinical endpoint for trials of acute heart failure therapy given the relatively dynamic change seen over the first 24 hours of therapy.[29] Restrictive defects are also commonly evident[30] and may be caused by underlying lung disease, respiratory muscle weakness, secondary drug effects (e.g., amiodarone), or concomitant diseases (e.g., sarcoidosis).

The diffusion capacity is measured by the DLCO (lung diffusion of carbon monoxide) and reflects both the ability of gases to go across the membrane and the volume of blood in the capillary bed. It can change acutely and is linked to abnormal lung mechanics and severity of HF and should be interpreted with caution.[31] Nevertheless, PFTs should be done once the patient is clinically stable and preferably once adequately diuresed if the comorbid condition of COPD is being considered.

Treatment

HF-Related Treatment in Patients with COPD

The mainstay of therapy, including renin-angiotensin-aldosterone axis agents (e.g., ACE inhibitors, ARBs, MRAs), have all been shown to be effective in patients with lung disease in the large RCTs and should be initiated and titrated accordingly. Other therapies, including defibrillators, cardiac resynchronization therapy, digoxin, nitrates, and diuretics, have limited data because of the limited enrollment in trials, and thus the results of RCTs should be applied with caution.

β-blockers and COPD have been controversial in terms of their use, effect on respiratory function, and clinical outcomes. Most of the earlier β-blocker RCTs excluded patients with known COPD given the concern of β-receptor stimulation versus blockade in patients with reactive airways

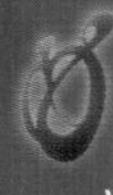

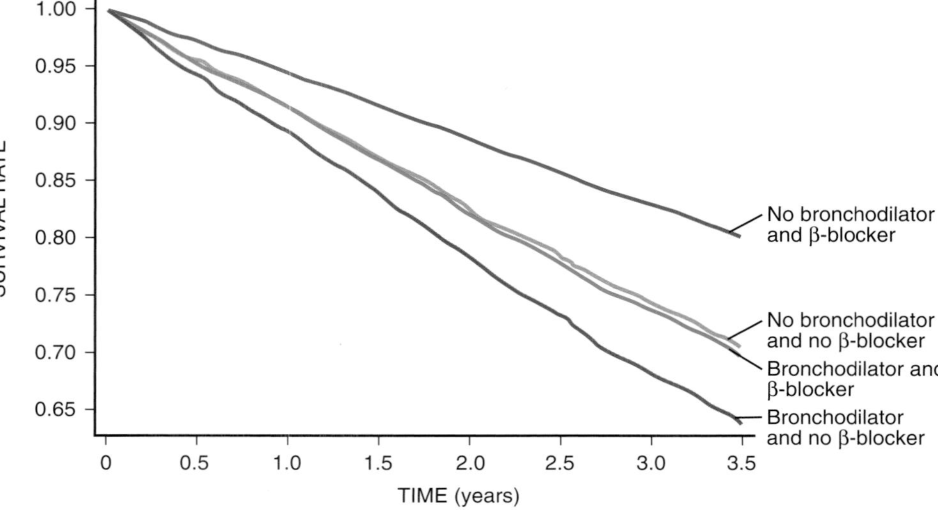

FIGURE 45-3 Characteristics and outcomes of patients with heart failure receiving bronchodilators. *Adapted from Hawkins NM, Wang D, Petrie MC, et al: Baseline characteristics and outcomes of patients with heart failure receiving bronchodilators in the CHARM programme. Eur J Heart Fail 12:557–565, 2010.*

disease. As such, the RCT experience is limited but no overt "risk" has been seen[32] and the small subgroups have shown a preserved (although vastly underpowered) treatment effect in the larger RCTs. Large population-based analyses have shown that, after propensity matching,[33] β-blockers were associated with a reduced risk of mortality when used in patients with COPD and concomitant HF.

A small mechanistic trial of patients with severe COPD (baseline FEV_1 = 1.3 L) tested the β_1-selective β-blocker bisoprolol versus a placebo on the FEV_1 and noted a significant, small reduction in FEV_1 but no alteration of the reversibility following β-agonists and overall lung volumes and no negative symptoms, impairment of quality of life, or clinical events.[34] One conclusion, given the limited sample size and large treatment effect in other populations, is that this reduction in FEV_1 is of minimal clinical importance and overweighed by the potential reduction in clinical events related to HF. Thus, selection of a β_1-selective β-blocker with clinical trial evidence is limited to that of bisoprolol[34,35] and metoprolol succinate[36] and could be considered in preference to carvedilol in this select population.

New agents such as ivabradine may be an option for patients with concomitant COPD who are unable to tolerate a β-blocker. In the SHIFT trial, 10% of patients with a clear indication for a β-blocker and were not on any β-blocker, and of these, one third identified COPD as the principal reason.[37] Additionally, in multivariable analysis, COPD was associated with being on a β-blocker at less than 50% of target dose (odds ratio 0.67 [95% CI 0.55-0.80]),[38] whereas the effects of ivabradine versus the placebo were still preserved. This indicates that for many patients with concomitant COPD and HF, ivabradine may be an option for reducing morbidity or mortality.

COPD Treatment in Patients with HF

Concomitant inhaled bronchodilators, anticholinergic agents, and steroids form the therapeutic strategy for most patients with COPD. The controversy and an updated systematic review have summarized this elsewhere.[39] Bronchodilators, specifically the β_2-agonists (e.g., formoterol, salbutamol, salmeterol, terbutaline) have efficacy in patients with COPD, but the trials have systematically excluded patients with HF.[40] Whether or not the association of harm for the use of these agents in patients with HF seen in observational studies is replicated in prospective randomized trials is uncertain (**Figure 45-3**).[41] Given the overlap in symptoms and difficulty in separating out the shared risk factors and similarity in patterns for hospitalization along with the confounding by indication of the use of β-agonists, caution should be exercised before restricting the use of β-agonists for patients with concomitant COPD and HF. Nevertheless, it would appear given there are choices for initial therapy that an anticholinergic may be a better first-line choice. The anticholinergic agents (ipratropium, tiotropium) principally act via the cholinergic system. Tiotropium has been tested versus salmeterol and appears to have better efficacy in patients with at least moderate COPD to prevent exacerbations of COPD and has demonstrated relatively neutral safety outcomes.[42] Thus the strategy of a long-acting anticholinergic agent would appear to be the appropriate strategy for patients with HF until further clinical trial information is available.

Inhaled steroids appear to have a relatively neutral safety profile and positive effect for clinical outcomes; however, oral steroids should be considered carefully. Oral steroids can produce intense sodium (and fluid) retention, and thus should be used with caution.

Summary/Conclusions

The diagnosis of COPD in a patient with HF and vice versa is challenging despite clinical acumen, chest x-rays, and standard biomarkers. When COPD is present in a patient with heart failure, it conveys a negative prognosis and treatment should be targeted toward maximizing evidence-based therapies for HF and encouraging appropriate use of COPD therapies where applicable.

SLEEP-DISORDERED BREATHING

Definitions, Prevalence, and Outcomes

Sleep-disordered breathing is a complex interaction of neurologic, respiratory, cardiac, and mechanical events that create "apneic episodes." Apnea is typically defined as cessation of air flow for more than 10 seconds, whereas hypopnea is a 50% reduction in air flow.[43] The diagnosis of either obstructive sleep apnea (OSA) or central sleep apnea (CSA) involves quantifying the apnea-hypopnea index (AHI), typically expressed as a ratio of events per hour: mild (5 to 15 events), moderate (15 to 30 events), or severe (>30 events). Typically, to diagnose OSA or CSA, a full laboratory-based polysomnography study is needed and ambulatory methods considered best for areas where access is limited or for screening in patients at risk.

OSA is often a combination of reduced muscle tone, complemented by fluid shifts and increased tissue in the oropharynx (**Figure 45-4A**).[44] CSA is complex interaction of a reduction in $PaCO_2$, leading to loss of the central drive for breathing, and involves the chemoreceptors, changes in venous blood flow, and vagal nerve activity in addition to other elements (see Figure 45-4B).[45]

Up to 50% of patients with systolic HF have either CSA or OSA when formally assessed by laboratory-based polysomnography.[6] Importantly, most of these patients have moderate to severe OSA or CSA, and the diagnosis tracks with the severity of illness. Patients with HF who are over 60 years of age, male, and have atrial fibrillation have been consistently shown to be at risk for CSA.[6,46] In patients with HF and preserved systolic function, 69% were found to have OSA (40%) or CSA (29%), and this was related to the diastolic function by echocardiogram, performance on a 6-minute walk test, or cardiopulmonary exercise test and higher NT-proBNP levels.[47] When present, OSA or CSA was found to be a risk factor for ventricular arrhythmias in 472 patients with a cardiac resynchronization therapy–defibrillator (CRT-D) device, and as the AHI increased the risk also increased, thus postulating the cause behind the relationship between OSA or CSA and mortality.[48]

Treatment

The treatment of OSA and CSA remain controversial. OSA is typically treated with nasal continuous positive airway pressure (CPAP), and surrogate outcomes show general improvement in smaller RCTs testing this hypothesis for patients with HF.[49-51] No longer term studies have shown a reduction in the morbidity or mortality.

Early trials showed promise for nasal CPAP to effectively improve LVEF in patients with HF and Cheyne-Stokes respiration,[52] but a larger and longer duration trial did not demonstrate a significant reduction in clinical events.[53] However, patients randomized to CPAP had a lower resultant AHI and a higher nocturnal oxygen level, LVEF, and 6-minute walk test. Those who had suppression of the AHI by CPAP had improved outcomes.[54] This would suggest that if CPAP is to be used for patients with CSA, a repeat sleep study 3 months after therapy initiation may help identify those patients who will get a sustained benefit.

Other therapies such as nocturnal or 24-hour oxygen, dental or mandibular devices or manipulation, atrial pacing, or even CRT have not shown to be beneficial. Ongoing trials (NCT01128816, NCT00733343) testing adaptive seroventilation may help guide future therapy for this population; however, adequately powered clinical trials and cost-effectiveness will be required before widespread adoption could be considered.

Summary/Conclusions

OSA or CSA may be present in patients with HF, and patients should be screened and tested appropriately. Specific subgroups to pay particular attention to include those unresponsive to therapy, with pulmonary hypertension, increased body mass index, hypertension, and those at risk on sleepiness scales. Treatment of patients with a formal diagnosis from a laboratory-based polysomnography test is best introduced and titrated by those with formal training and expertise in sleep medicine and caring for patients with HF.

DIABETES

Definitions, Prevalence, and Outcomes

Diabetes and heart failure share a number of features: they are both common, chronic, and increasing in prevalence. Worldwide, an estimated 10% of the adult population has diabetes[55] and is a well-established risk factor for coronary artery disease, a major cause of heart failure. Additionally, diabetes alone can produce a "diabetic cardiomyopathy," and 6% of patients with new-onset diabetes will develop HF within 5 years (**Figure 45-5**).[5] Accordingly, up to 30% of patients with HF have diabetes, making it one of the most common chronic comorbid conditions that a cardiovascular practitioner will deal with over the lifespan of a patient. Diabetes can be defined using a hemoglobin A_{1c} of 6.5% or more, fasting plasma glucose of 7.0 mmol/L or more, random plasma glucose of 11.1 mmol/L or more, or with a 2-hour plasma glucose with oral glucose tolerance test of 11.1 mmol/L or more.[56] Regardless of the definitions used by various guidelines across the world, the presence or absence of diabetes or the risk factors for diabetes is important for those with or at risk for heart failure.

Treatment

Treatment of Heart Failure for Patients with Diabetes

Patients with diabetes should be afforded the same options for treatment as those without diabetes given the similarities in efficacy and safety of commonly used HF therapies between those with and without diabetes. Patients should be treated with HF guideline-endorsed therapies, including blockade of the renin-angiotensin-aldosterone axis, β-blockers, implantable devices, and other therapies where appropriate.

Treatment of Diabetes for Patients with Heart Failure

There are many established and novel medications available to treat diabetes. It is unclear that treatment of diabetes itself modifies the natural history of heart failure or what targets (e.g., hemoglobin A_{1c} <7%) are both realistic and will modify clinical outcomes. Nevertheless, the medications listed below have been tested typically in a non-HF population and it is reasonable (although not ideal) to consider each of the following for a patient with diabetes.

Biguanides (Metformin)

Biguanides are the first-line therapy for many patients with diabetes given their established efficacy and safety. They act by increasing insulin sensitivity in tissues and reduce gluconeogenesis. For patients with HF, most guidelines support this strategy despite the lack of RCT evidence.[57] Earlier concerns regarding the risk of lactic acidosis have not been borne out by thorough population-based analysis and systematic review.[58,59]

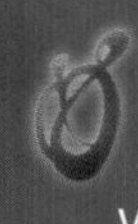

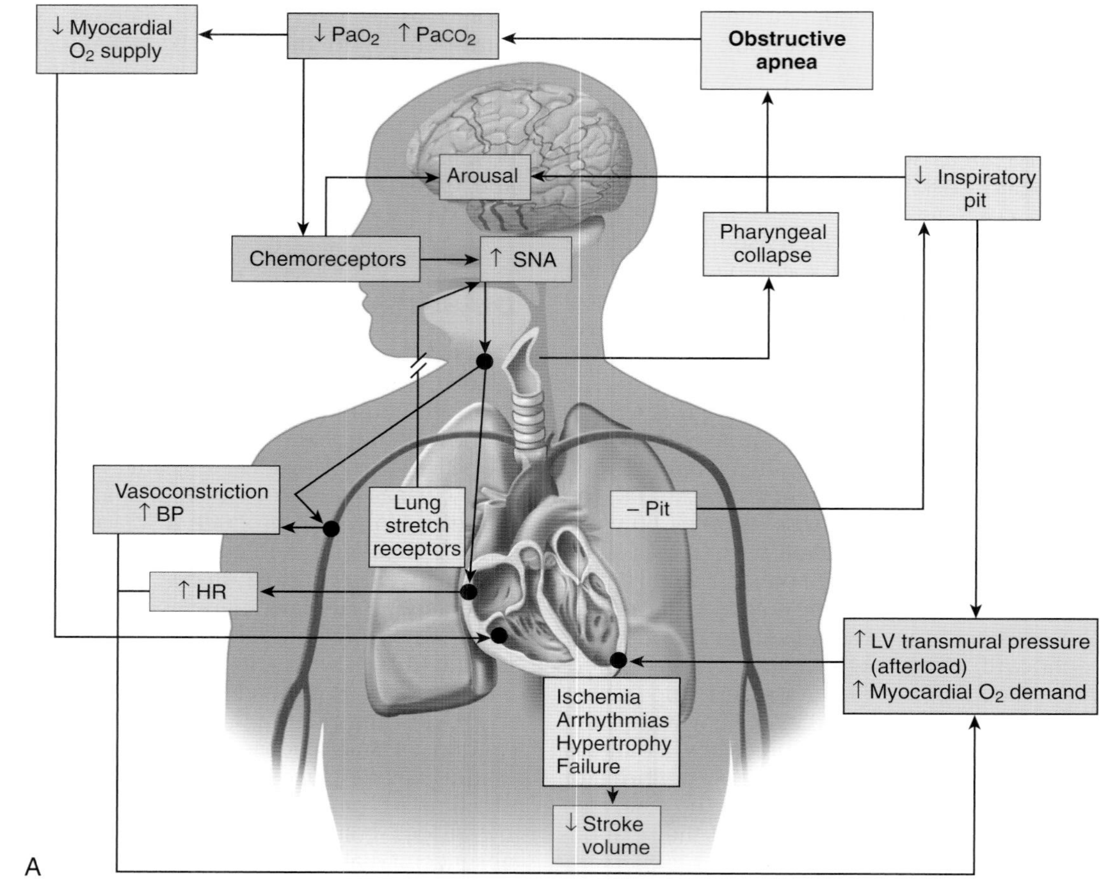

↓ Myocardial O_2 supply

↓ PaO_2 ↑ $PaCO_2$

Obstructive apnea

Arousal

↓ Inspiratory pit

Pharyngeal collapse

Chemoreceptors

↑ SNA

Vasoconstriction ↑ BP

Lung stretch receptors

– Pit

↑ HR

↑ LV transmural pressure (afterload)
↑ Myocardial O_2 demand

Ischemia
Arrhythmias
Hypertrophy
Failure

↓ Stroke volume

A

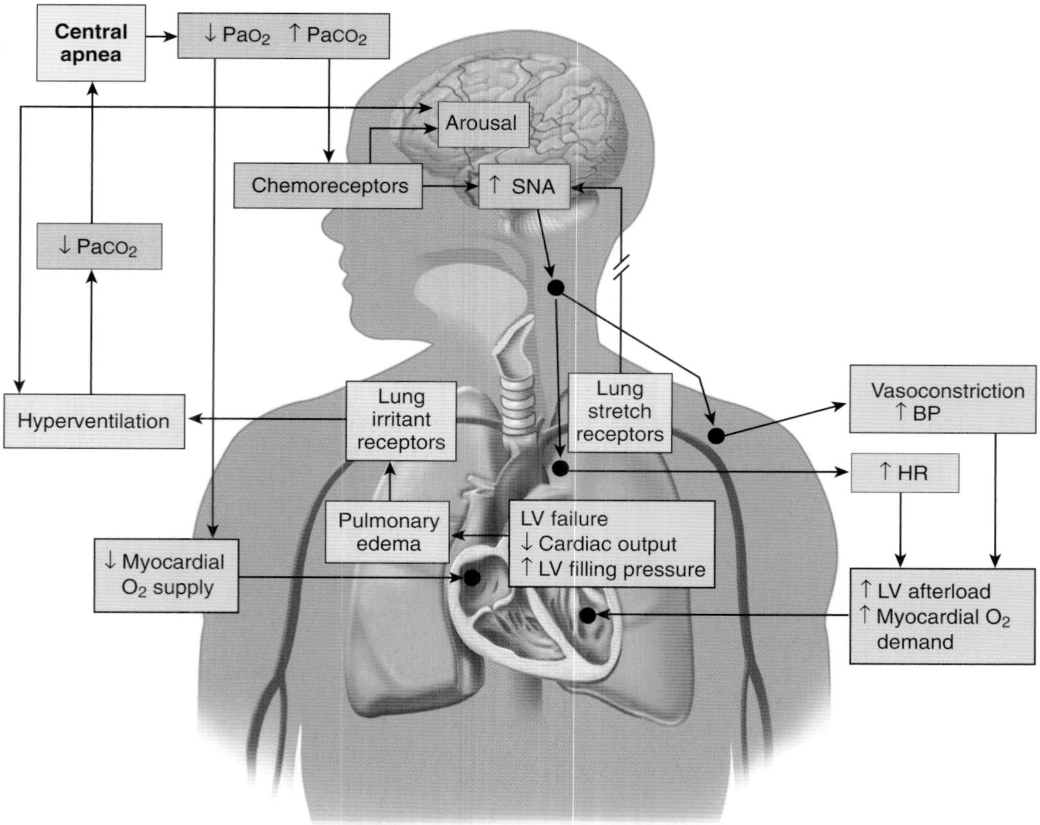

Central apnea

↓ PaO_2 ↑ $PaCO_2$

Arousal

Chemoreceptors

↑ SNA

↓ $PaCO_2$

Hyperventilation

Lung irritant receptors

Lung stretch receptors

Vasoconstriction ↑ BP

↑ HR

Pulmonary edema

LV failure
↓ Cardiac output
↑ LV filling pressure

↓ Myocardial O_2 supply

↑ LV afterload
↑ Myocardial O_2 demand

B

FIGURE 45-4 A, Pathophysiologic effects of obstructive sleep apnea on the cardiovascular system. Obstructive apneas increase left ventricular (LV) transmural pressure (i.e., afterload) through the generation of negative intrathoracic pressure (Pit) and elevations in systemic blood pressure (BP) secondary to hypoxia, arousals from sleep, and increased sympathetic nervous system activity (SNA). Apnea also suppresses the sympathetic inhibitory effects of lung stretch receptors, further enhancing SNA. The combination of increased LV afterload and increased heart rate (HR) secondary to increased SNA increases myocardial O_2 demand in the face of a reduced myocardial O_2 supply. These conditions predispose a patient acutely to cardiac ischemia and arrhythmias, and chronically could contribute to LV hypertrophy and, ultimately, failure. The resultant fall in stroke volume will further augment SNA. **B,** Pathophysiology of central sleep apnea in heart failure (HF). HF leads to increased LV filling pressure. The resulting pulmonary congestion activates lung vagal irritant receptors, which stimulate hyperventilation and hypocapnia. Superimposed arousals cause further abrupt increases in ventilation and drive Pa_{CO_2} below the threshold for ventilation, triggering a central apnea. Central sleep apneas are sustained by recurrent arousals resulting from apnea-induced hypoxia and the increased effort to breathe during the ventilatory phase because of pulmonary congestion and reduced lung compliance. Although central apneas have a different pathophysiology than obstructive apneas and are not associated with the generation of exaggerated negative intrathoracic pressure, they both increase sympathetic SNA. The consequent increases in BP and HR increase myocardial O_2 demand in the face of reduced supply. This chain of events contributes to a pathophysiologic vicious cycle. *From Bradley TD, Floras JS: Sleep apnea and heart failure: Part I: obstructive sleep apnea. Circulation 107:1671–1678, 2003; and Bradley TD, Floras JS: Sleep apnea and heart failure: Part II: central sleep apnea. Circulation 107:1822–1826, 2003.*

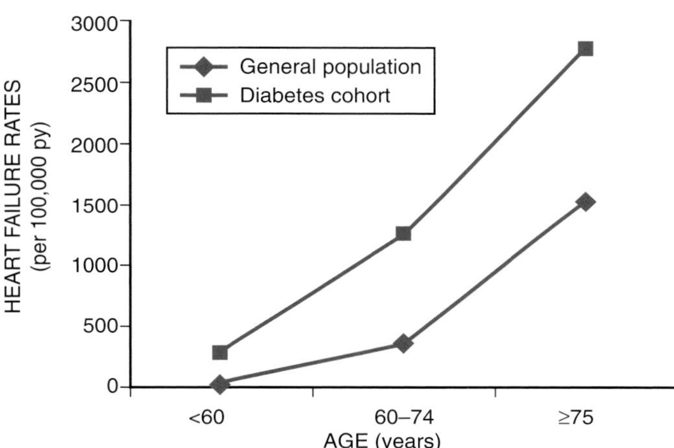

FIGURE 45-5 Age and sex standardized rates of incident heart failure in patients with recent-onset type 2 diabetes compared with a general population. *py,* Person-years. *Adapted from Leung AA, Eurich DT, Lamb DA, et al: Risk of heart failure in patients with recent-onset type 2 diabetes: population-based cohort study. J Card Fail 15:152–157, 2009.*

Sulfonylureas and Meglitinides (e.g., Gliclazide, Glimepiride, Glyburide, Repaglinide)

These agents stimulate the release of preformed insulin by binding to the potassium ATP channel on the β-cell and therefore may induce hypoglycemia, a significant limitation in clinical practice considering the older population with HF. These also can induce weight gain from uncertain mechanisms that may provide additional challenges to assessing a HF patient in terms of the cause of weight gain.

Thiazolidinediones (e.g., Rosiglitazone)

These agents act by increasing insulin sensitivity especially in skeletal muscle and adipose tissue. These agents are also responsible for significant fluid retention and thus have been associated with an increase in HF incidence.[60,61] Most guidelines are now recommending against using these agents in patients with known HF or at risk for HF.

DPP-IV Inhibitors (e.g., Sitagliptin, Saxagliptin)

These agents block the breakdown of GLP-1 via blocking the breakdown via DPPIV, which in turn increases insulin secretion while suppressing glucagon secretion, all in response to the presence of glucose. These agents have not been extensively studied in HF (an ongoing study has yet to be published, NCT00894868), but three large-scale trials are ongoing to test if new-onset HF and/or cardiovascular outcomes can be improved by these agents.

Incretin Mimetics (GLP-1 "Agonists" [e.g., Exanatide, Liraglutide])

These agents act as GLP agonists by mimicking the effect of naturally occurring GLP-1. Also the subject of large ongoing clinical trials, the HF experience is limited. Liraglutide and exanatide are both the subject of one HF-focused clinical trial (NCT01800968, NCT00766857, NCT01472640, NCT00799435, NCT01425580) to see if it can improve clinical HF outcomes in patients with or without concomitant diabetes and acute or chronic HF.

Insulin

Insulin is the mainstay of therapy for patients with poorly controlled diabetes. There are no large-scale trials supporting the use (or calling into question safety). Some observational analyses have highlighted the use of insulin as an independent predictor of poor outcomes, but this may indeed be a risk marker instead of a causal factor.

Summary/Conclusions

Diabetes and heart failure are two highly prevalent diseases and their intersection complicates both diseases. Further work on the best strategies for treatment and targets for both day-to-day glucose management and long-term vascular prevention are clearly needed.

LIPIDS

Definitions, Prevalence, and Outcomes

Patients with HF often have risk factors for or concomitant coronary artery or other vascular disease. Given the high prevalence of these vascular risk factors, patients often have screening fasting lipids and are placed on a lipid-lowering agent.

The prevalence of hyperlipidemia varies substantially depending on the era of the study, the definitions used (e.g., LDL vs. total cholesterol) and HF population surveyed (e.g., chronic vs. acute, NYHA class, duration of disease). Much of the earlier work focused on the presence or absence of hyperlipidemia and the interaction with vascular disease. It has been noted that the overall prevalence of coronary artery disease in patients with HF exceeds 50% for most populations, and in Western Europe and North America this generally exceeds 60%.[62,63]

Treatment

Of significant interest is the following clinical question: Could patients with the combination of coronary artery disease (CAD) and HF have fewer future CAD-related events with treatment of lipid abnormalities? Within most HF trials, HF admissions and mortality far exceed the risk for a new myocardial infarction and despite events being adjudicated, many myocardial infarctions may be mislabeled as a sudden death or a HF-related admission. Many large RCTs

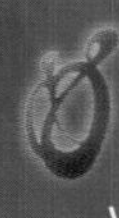

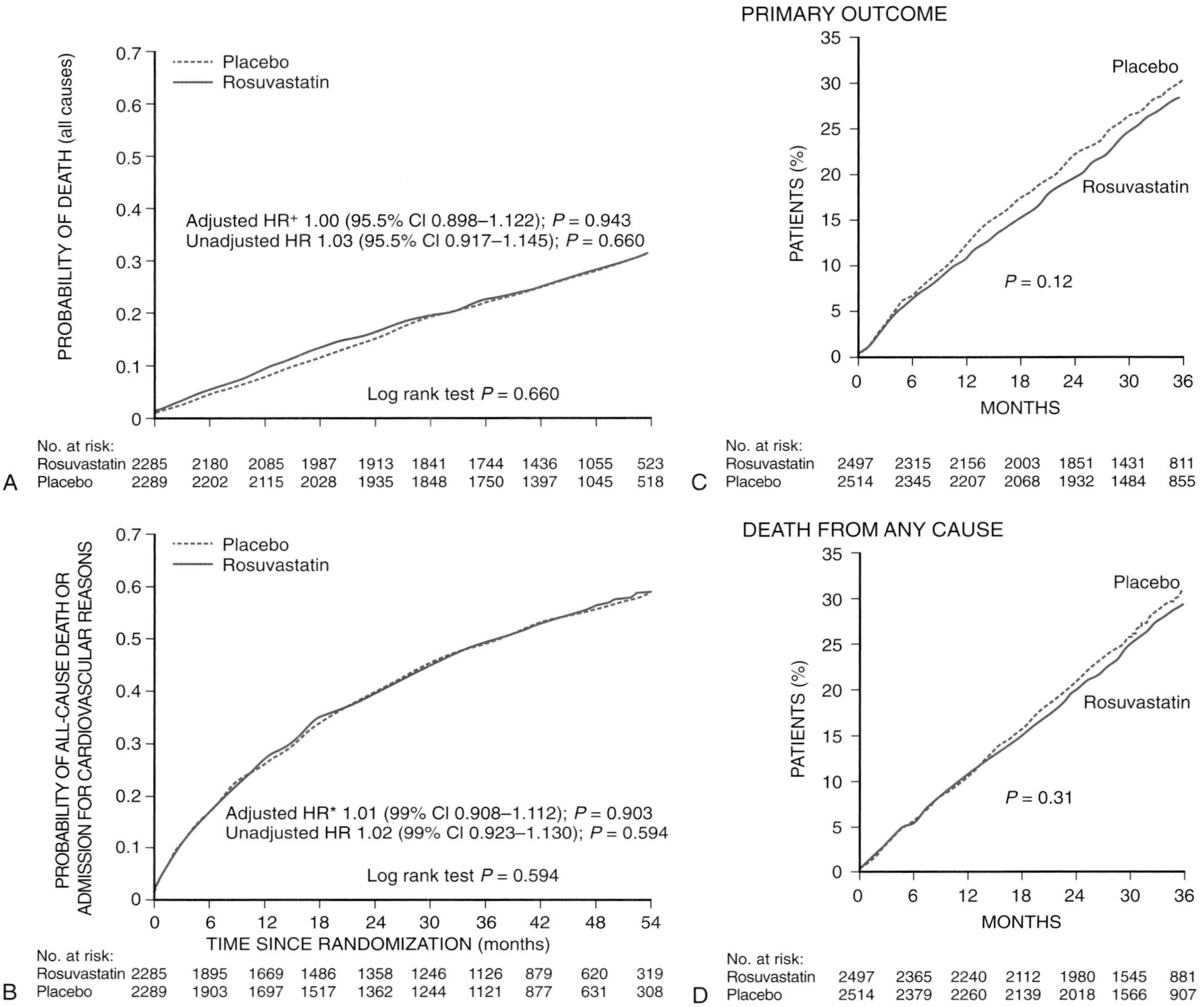

A

No. at risk:										
Rosuvastatin	2285	2180	2085	1987	1913	1841	1744	1436	1055	523
Placebo	2289	2202	2115	2028	1935	1848	1750	1397	1045	518

B

No. at risk:										
Rosuvastatin	2285	1895	1669	1486	1358	1246	1126	879	620	319
Placebo	2289	1903	1697	1517	1362	1244	1121	877	631	308

C — PRIMARY OUTCOME

No. at risk:							
Rosuvastatin	2497	2315	2156	2003	1851	1431	811
Placebo	2514	2345	2207	2068	1932	1484	855

D — DEATH FROM ANY CAUSE

No. at risk:							
Rosuvastatin	2497	2365	2240	2112	1980	1545	881
Placebo	2514	2379	2260	2139	2018	1566	907

FIGURE 45-6 The results of the CORONA67 **(A, B)** and GISSI-HF68 **(C, D)** trials. Neither trial shows a significant difference in all-cause mortality **(A** and **D)** or in the principal secondary outcomes **(B** and **C).** *Parts A and B adapted from Gissi-HF Investigators, Tavazzi L, Maggioni AP, et al: Effect of rosuvastatin in patients with chronic heart failure (the GISSI-HF trial): a randomised, double-blind, placebo-controlled trial. Lancet 372:1231–1239, 2008; Parts C and D adapted from Kjekshus J, Apetrei E, Barrios V, et al: Rosuvastatin in older patients with systolic heart failure. N Engl J Med 357:2248–2261, 2007.*

have shown benefit for chronic therapy in patients with CAD or post–acute coronary syndrome (ACS); however, patients with systolic dysfunction or heart failure symptoms were excluded from statin trials or recruited in low numbers. Observational data using propensity-matched cohorts drew an association between treatment with a statin and a 21% relative risk "reduction" in clinical events.[64] Initial subgroup analyses of larger RCTs have been underpowered[65] to sufficiently answer the important clinical (and controversial[66]) question of whether or not patients with systolic dysfunction and HF would benefit from statin therapy. Additional pathophysiologic rationale for and against the use of statins is summarized elsewhere[66] and lead to the testing of this in large RCTs.

Two large RCTs tested this hypothesis: CORONA and GISSI-HF.[67,68] In the CORONA trial, 5011 patients older than 60 years of age, with NYHA II-IV symptoms and an EF less than 40% were enrolled.[67] Patients were randomized to rosuvastatin 10 mg daily or a placebo and followed for a median of 32.8 months for the primary outcome of death from cardiovascular causes, nonfatal myocardial infarction, or stroke. The mean LDL declined from 3.5 mmol/L to 1.96 mmol/L (44% decline), and C-reactive protein also declined by 32%. Despite the aggressive LDL and CRP lowering, good tolerability, and generally good safety profile, there was no clinical or statistical difference in clinical outcomes between the placebo and rosuvastatin groups. There was no significant difference in myocardial infarction (the principal event thought to be prevented by statins) and no reduction in all-cause mortality. Notably, patients were on good evidence-based medical therapy for heart failure, and patients were not on a statin at baseline.

The second trial, GISSI-HF,[68] enrolled 4574 patients with NYHA II-IV symptoms and any EF were enrolled. Patients were randomized to rosuvastatin 10 mg daily or a placebo and followed for a median of 3.9 years for the primary outcome of death or hospitalization for cardiovascular causes. As with CORONA, there was no difference in the primary outcome or any of the principal secondary outcomes of clinical importance (**Figure 45-6**).

Summary/Conclusions

Reconciling these results with those of patients with acute coronary syndromes has been the subject of intense debate. Nevertheless, as tested in an RCT enrolling approximately 10,000 patients with chronic HF, none of the major international guidelines strongly recommends initiating a statin if a patient has HF.[69-71]

OVERALL SUMMARY

Patients with heart failure carry with them significant comorbid conditions and the risk for developing new medical problems that will require diagnosis and management. Given the high prevalence of anemia, diabetes, COPD, sleep-disordered breathing, and dyslipidemia, the clinician caring for this population requires expertise in many fields. Concomitant medications such as bronchodilators or diabetes therapies may improve or worsen heart failure, and much remains to be learned. Newer therapies hold promise for improving the outcomes of these patients with complex heart disease.

References

1. Braunstein JB, Anderson GF, Gerstenblith G, et al: Noncardiac comorbidity increases preventable hospitalizations and mortality among Medicare beneficiaries with chronic heart failure. *J Am Coll Cardiol* 42(7):1226–1233, 2003.
2. Rutledge T, Reis VA, Linke SE, et al: Depression in heart failure: a meta-analytic review of prevalence, intervention effects, and associations with clinical outcomes. *J Am Coll Cardiol* 48(8):1527–1537, 2006.
3. Fonarow GC, Stough WG, Abraham WT, et al: Characteristics, treatments, and outcomes of patients with preserved systolic function hospitalized for heart failure: a report from the OPTIMIZE-HF Registry. *J Am Coll Cardiol* 50(8):768–777, 2007.
4. Ather S, Chan W, Bozkurt B, et al: Impact of noncardiac comorbidities on morbidity and mortality in a predominantly male population with heart failure and preserved versus reduced ejection fraction. *J Am Coll Cardiol* 59(11):998–1005, 2012.
5. Leung AA, Eurich DT, Lamb DA, et al: Risk of heart failure in patients with recent-onset type 2 diabetes: population-based cohort study. *J Card Fail* 15(2):152–157, 2009.
6. Yumino D, Wang H, Floras JS, et al: Prevalence and Physiological Predictors of Sleep Apnea in Patients With Heart Failure and Systolic Dysfunction. *J Card Fail* 15(4):279–285, 2009.
7. O'Connor CM, Jiang W, Kuchibhatla M, et al: Safety and efficacy of sertraline for depression in patients with heart failure: results of the SADHART-CHF (Sertraline Against Depression and Heart Disease in Chronic Heart Failure) trial. *J Am Coll Cardiol* 56(9):692–699, 2010.
8. Recommendations to prevent and control iron deficiency in the United States. Centers for Disease Control and Prevention. *MMWR Recomm Rep* 47(RR-3):1–29, 1998.
9. National Kidney Foundation: II. Clinical practice guidelines and clinical practice recommendations for anemia in chronic kidney disease in adults. *Am J Kidney Dis* 47(5 Suppl 3):S16–S85, 2006.
10. Ezekowitz JA, McAlister FA, Armstrong PW: Anemia is common in heart failure and is associated with poor outcomes: insights from a cohort of 12065 patients with new-onset heart failure. *Circulation* 107(2):223–225, 2003.
11. Maggioni AP, Opasich C, Anand I, et al: Anemia in patients with heart failure: prevalence and prognostic role in a controlled trial and in clinical practice. *J Card Fail* 11(2):91–98, 2005.
12. Ezekowitz JA, McAlister FA, Armstrong PW: The interaction among sex, hemoglobin and outcomes in a specialty heart failure clinic. *Can J Cardiol* 21(2):165–171, 2005.
13. Horwich TB, Fonarow GC, Hamilton MA, et al: Anemia is associated with worse symptoms, greater impairment in functional capacity and a significant increase in mortality in patients with advanced heart failure. *J Am Coll Cardiol* 39(11):1780, 2002.
14. Tang YD: Anemia in chronic heart failure: prevalence, etiology, clinical correlates, and treatment options. *Circulation* 113(20):2454–2461, 2006.
15. Anand ISI, Kuskowski MA, Rector TS, et al: Anemia and change in hemoglobin over time related to mortality and morbidity in patients with chronic heart failure: results from Val-HeFT. *Circulation* 112(8):1121–1127, 2005.
16. Androne ASI, Katz SD, Lund L, et al: Hemodilution is common in patients with advanced heart failure. *Circulation* 107(2):226–229, 2003.
17. Anker SD, Comin Colet J, Filippatos G, et al: Ferric carboxymaltose in patients with heart failure and iron deficiency. *N Engl J Med* 361(25):2436–2448, 2009.
18. Avni T, Leibovici L, Gafter-Gvili A: Iron supplementation for the treatment of chronic heart failure and iron deficiency: systematic review and meta-analysis. *Eur J Heart Fail* 14(4):423–429, 2012.
19. Swedberg K1, Young JB, Anand IS, et al: Treatment of anemia with darbepoetin alfa in systolic heart failure. *N Engl J Med* 368(13):1210–1219, 2013.
20. Ganz T: Hepcidin, a key regulator of iron metabolism and mediator of anemia of inflammation. *Blood* 102(3):783–788, 2003.
21. Oudit GY, Sun H, Trivieri MG, et al: L-type Ca2+ channels provide a major pathway for iron entry into cardiomyocytes in iron-overload cardiomyopathy. *Nat Blood* 9(9):1187–1194, 2003.
22. Rabe KF, Hurd S, Anzueto A, et al: Global strategy for the diagnosis, management, and prevention of chronic obstructive pulmonary disease: GOLD executive summary. *Am J Respir Crit Care Med* 176(6):532–555, 2007.
23. Caroci Ade S, Lareau SC: Descriptors of dyspnea by patients with chronic obstructive pulmonary disease versus congestive heart failure. *Heart Lung* 33(2):102–110, 2004.
24. Schellenbaum GD1, Rea TD, Heckbert SR, et al: Survival associated with two sets of diagnostic criteria for congestive heart failure. *Am J Epidemiol* 160(7):628–635, 2004.
25. Howlett JG, McKelvie RS, Arnold JMO, et al: Canadian Cardiovascular Society Consensus Conference guidelines on heart failure, update 2009: diagnosis and management of right-sided heart failure, myocarditis, device therapy and recent important clinical trials. *Can J Cardiol* 25(2):85–105, 2009.
26. Hawkins NM, Petrie MC, Jhund PS, et al: Heart failure and chronic obstructive pulmonary disease: diagnostic pitfalls and epidemiology. *Eur J Heart Fail* 11(2):130–139, 2009.
27. Petermann W, Barth J, Entzian P: Heart failure and airway obstruction. *Int J Cardiol* 17(2):207–209, 1987.
28. Pison C, Malo JL, Rouleau JL, et al: Bronchial hyperresponsiveness to inhaled methacholine in subjects with chronic left heart failure at a time of exacerbation and after increasing diuretic therapy. *Chest* 96(2):230–235, 1989.
29. Ezekowitz JA, Hernandez AF, O'Connor CM, et al: Assessment of dyspnea in acute decompensated heart failure. *JAC* 59(16):1441–1448, 2012.
30. Wasserman K, Zhang YY, Gitt A, et al: Lung function and exercise gas exchange in chronic heart failure. *Circulation* 96(7):2221–2227, 1997.
31. Agostoni P, Bussotti M, Cattadori G, et al: Gas diffusion and alveolar-capillary unit in chronic heart failure. *Eur Heart J* 27(21):2538–2543, 2006.
32. Ni Y, Shi G, Wan H: Use of cardioselective beta-blockers in patients with chronic obstructive pulmonary disease: a meta-analysis of randomized, placebo-controlled, blinded trials. *J Int Med Res* 40(6):2051–2065, 2012.
33. Sin DD, McAlister FA: The effects of beta-blockers on morbidity and mortality in a population-based cohort of 11,942 elderly patients with heart failure. *Am J Med* 113(8):650–656, 2002.
34. Hawkins NM, MacDonald MR, Petrie MC, et al: Bisoprolol in patients with heart failure and moderate to severe chronic obstructive pulmonary disease: a randomized controlled trial. *Eur J Heart Fail* 11(7):684–690, 2009.
35. CIBIS-II Investigators and Committees: The Cardiac Insufficiency Bisoprolol Study II (CIBIS-II): a randomised trial. *Lancet* 353(9146):9–13, 1999.
36. Hjalmarson A, Goldstein S, Fagerberg B, et al: Effects of controlled-release metoprolol on total mortality, hospitalizations, and well-being in patients with heart failure: the Metoprolol CR/XL Randomized Intervention Trial in congestive heart failure (MERIT-HF). MERIT-HF Study Group. *JAMA* 283(10):1295–1302, 2000.
37. Swedberg K, Komajda M, Böhm M, et al: Ivabradine and outcomes in chronic heart failure (SHIFT): a randomised placebo-controlled study. *Lancet* 376(9744):875–885, 2010.
38. Swedberg K, Komajda M, Böhm M, et al: Effects on outcomes of heart rate reduction by ivabradine in patients with congestive heart failure: is there an influence of beta-blocker dose?: findings from the SHIFT (Systolic Heart failure treatment with the I(f) inhibitor ivabradine Trial) study. *J Am Coll Cardiol* 59(22):1938–1945, 2012.
39. Hawkins NM, Petrie MC, Macdonald MR, et al: Heart failure and chronic obstructive pulmonary disease: the quandary of beta-blockers and beta-agonists. *J Am Coll Cardiol* 57(21):2127–2138, 2011.
40. Mentz RJ, Fiuzat M, Kraft M, et al: Bronchodilators in heart failure patients with COPD: is it time for a clinical trial? *J Card Fail* 18(5):413–422, 2012.
41. Hawkins NM, Wang D, Petrie MC, et al: Baseline characteristics and outcomes of patients with heart failure receiving bronchodilators in the CHARM programme. *Eur J Heart Fail* 12(6):557–565, 2010.
42. Vogelmeier C, Hederer B, Glaab T, et al: Tiotropium versus salmeterol for the prevention of exacerbations of COPD. *N Engl J Med* 364(12):1093–1103, 2011.
43. Fleetham J, Ayas N, Bradley D, et al: Canadian Thoracic Society guidelines: diagnosis and treatment of sleep disordered breathing in adults. *Can Respir J* 13(7):387–392, 2006.
44. Bradley TD, Floras JS: Sleep apnea and heart failure: Part I: obstructive sleep apnea. *Circulation* 107(12):1671–1678, 2003.
45. Bradley TD, Floras JS: Sleep apnea and heart failure: Part II: central sleep apnea. *Circulation* 107(13):1822–1826, 2003.
46. Sin DD, Fitzgerald F, Parker JD, et al: Risk factors for central and obstructive sleep apnea in 450 men and women with congestive heart failure. *Am J Respir Crit Care Med* 160(4):1101–1106, 1999.
47. Bitter T, Faber L, Hering D, et al: Sleep-disordered breathing in heart failure with normal left ventricular ejection fraction. *Eur Heart J Fail* 11(6):602–608, 2009.
48. Bitter T, Westerheide N, Prinz C, et al: Cheyne-Stokes respiration and obstructive sleep apnoea are independent risk factors for malignant ventricular arrhythmias requiring appropriate cardioverter-defibrillator therapies in patients with congestive heart failure. *Eur Heart J* 32(1):61, 2011.
49. Kaneko Y, Floras JS, Usui K, et al: Cardiovascular effects of continuous positive airway pressure in patients with heart failure and obstructive sleep apnea. *N Engl J Med* 348(13):1233–1241, 2003.
50. Usui K, Bradley TD, Spaak J, et al: Inhibition of awake sympathetic nerve activity of heart failure patients with obstructive sleep apnea by nocturnal continuous positive airway pressure. *J Am Coll Cardiol* 45(12):2008–2011, 2005.
51. Smith LA, Vennelle M, Gardner RS, et al: Auto-titrating continuous positive airway pressure therapy in patients with chronic heart failure and obstructive sleep apnoea: a randomized placebo-controlled trial. *Eur Heart J* 28(10):1221–1227, 2007.
52. Naughton MT, Liu PP, Bernard DC, et al: Treatment of congestive heart failure and Cheyne-Stokes respiration during sleep by continuous positive airway pressure. *Am J Respir Crit Care Med* 151(1):92–97, 1995.
53. Bradley TD, Logan AG, Kimoff RJ, et al: Continuous positive airway pressure for central sleep apnea and heart failure. *N Engl J Med* 353(19):2025–2033, 2005.
54. Artz M, Floras JS, Logan AG, et al: Suppression of central sleep apnea by continuous positive airway pressure and transplant-free survival in heart failure. *Circulation* 115:3173–3180, 2007.
55. Mathers CD, Loncar D: Projections of global mortality and burden of disease from 2002 to 2030. *PLoS Med* 3(11):e442, 2006.
56. Ronald G, Zubin P: Definition, classification and diagnosis of diabetes, prediabetes and metabolic syndrome. *Can J Diabetes* 37:S8–S11, 2013.
57. Eurich DT, Tsuyuki RT, Majumdar SR, et al: Metformin treatment in diabetes and heart failure: when academic equipoise meets clinical reality. *Trials* 10:12, 2009.
58. Eurich DT, McAlister FA, Blackburn DF, et al: Benefits and harms of antidiabetic agents in patients with diabetes and heart failure: systematic review. *BMJ* 335(7618):497, 2007.
59. Eurich DT, Weir DL, Majumdar SR, et al: Comparative safety and effectiveness of metformin in patients with diabetes mellitus and heart failure: systematic review of observational studies involving 34,000 patients. *Circ Heart Fail* 6:395–402, 2013.
60. Kahn SE, Haffner SM, Heise MA, et al: Glycemic durability of rosiglitazone, metformin, or glyburide monotherapy. *N Engl J Med* 355(23):2427–2443, 2006.
61. Dormandy JA, Charbonnel B, Eckland DJ: Secondary prevention of macrovascular events in patients with type 2 diabetes in the PROactive Study (PROspective pioglitAzone Clinical Trial In macroVascular Events): a randomised controlled trial. *Lancet* 366(9493):1279–1289, 2005.
62. Nieminen MS, Brutsaert D, Dickstein K, et al: EuroHeart Failure Survey II (EHFS II): a survey on hospitalized acute heart failure patients: description of population. *Eur Heart J* 27(22):2725–2736, 2006.

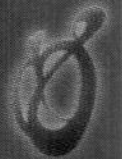

63. Fonarow GC, Albert NM, Curtis AB, et al: Improving evidence-based care for heart failure in outpatient cardiology practices: primary results of the Registry to Improve the Use of Evidence-Based Heart Failure Therapies in the Outpatient Setting (IMPROVE HF). *Circulation* 122(6):585–596, 2010.
64. Go AS, Lee WY, Yang J, et al: Statin therapy and risks for death and hospitalization in chronic heart failure. *JAMA* 296(17):2105–2111, 2006.
65. Scandinavian Simvastatin Survival Study Group: Randomised trial of cholesterol lowering in 4444 patients with coronary heart disease: the Scandinavian Simvastatin Survival Study (4S). *Lancet* 344(8934):1383–1389, 1994.
66. Krum H, McMurray JJ: Statins and chronic heart failure: do we need a large-scale outcome trial? *J Am Coll Cardiol* 39(10):1567–1573, 2002.
67. Kjekshus J, Apetrei E, Barrios V, et al: Rosuvastatin in older patients with systolic heart failure. *N Engl J Med* 357(22):2248–2261, 2007.
68. Gissi-HF Investigators, Tavazzi L, Maggioni AP, et al: Effect of rosuvastatin in patients with chronic heart failure (the GISSI-HF trial): a randomised, double-blind, placebo-controlled trial. *Lancet* 372(9645):1231–1239, 2008.
69. Authors/Task Force Members, McMurray JJV, Adamopoulos S, et al: ESC Guidelines for the diagnosis and treatment of acute and chronic heart failure 2012: The Task Force for the Diagnosis and Treatment of Acute and Chronic Heart Failure 2012 of the European Society of Cardiology. Developed in collaboration with the Heart Failure Association (HFA) of the ESC. *Eur Heart J* 33(14):1787–1847, 2012.
70. McKelvie RS, Moe GW, Ezekowitz JA, et al: The 2012 Canadian Cardiovascular Society Heart Failure Management Guidelines Update: Focus on Acute and Chronic Heart Failure. *Can J Cardiol* 29:168–181, 2013.
71. Heart Failure Society of America, Lindenfeld J, Albert NM, et al: HFSA 2010 Comprehensive Heart Failure Practice Guideline. *J Card Fail* 16(6):e1–e194, 2010.

46 Quality and Outcomes in Heart Failure

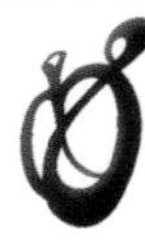

Adam D. DeVore and Adrian F. Hernandez

Because of the prevalence and major morbidity of heart failure (HF), as well as its associated public health burden with regard to total health care expenditures, HF serves as one of the top conditions targeted for quality of care improvement.[1,2] Randomized clinical trials have established the efficacy of several therapies to reduce all-cause mortality and reduce the risk of other adverse outcomes for patients with HF and reduced left ventricular ejection fraction (LVEF) (**see Chapter 34**).[3] This evidence has been translated into professional society guideline recommendations including many class I recommendations for HF treatments, such as use of angiotensin-converting enzyme inhibitors (ACEIs)/angiotensin receptor blockers (ARBs), β-blockers, hydralazine/isosorbide dinitrate, aldosterone antagonists, implantable cardioverter-defibrillators (ICDs), and resynchronization therapy. However, there has been wide variation in the implementation of evidence into practice; often years go by before guideline-recommended therapies are routinely applied to clinical practice.[4] This 15- to 20-year gap between evidence and routine practice is often referred to as the *quality chasm,* which received national attention in a landmark report published by the Institute of Medicine (IOM).[5] Beyond the gap between evidence and care, there are also substantial disparities in care based on age, sex, race, ethnicity, and socioeconomic backgrounds.[6,7] While there are multiple reasons for this quality gap, clinical inertia has most often been noted as a major barrier.[8] In order to overcome inertia and other barriers, attention has increasingly turned toward aligning incentives in the delivery of health care by measuring and improving quality of care.

Historically, the pursuit of high quality of care has been challenging. Until receiving scrutiny from the IOM, payers, and government agencies, the need to translate life-prolonging therapies into practice did not receive due attention. Systems and strategies for improving quality of care were not routinely in place until early to mid-2000. Unfortunately, the lack of systematic efforts for improving quality of care leaves a substantial proportion of patients at risk for hospitalizations and deaths that could be prevented by better implementation of evidence-based therapies.[9] This chapter will review the existing framework for quality of care and how to integrate quality of care into everyday practice through performance improvement systems that are designed to facilitate the use of evidence-based therapy and improve outcomes for patients with HF in the inpatient and outpatient setting.

GENERAL PRINCIPLES OF QUALITY MEASUREMENT

Defining Quality

Defining quality of care is often controversial. While stakeholders such as patients, providers, and payers agree that quality is an important value for health care, it is often difficult to precisely define how quality is measured and what its limits may be. Recognizing that quality is a difficult value to conceptualize, the IOM proposed a definition of quality health care based on six dimensions. This definition is now widely accepted as the means by which health care quality can be characterized.[5]

Institute of Medicine Principles

The IOM defines health care quality as the degree to which health care services increase the likelihood of desired health outcomes and are consistent with current professional knowledge. Put simply, high-quality health care involves the delivery of appropriate care, from which patients benefit.

In the influential IOM report *Crossing the Quality Chasm: A New Health System for the 21st Century,* six aims are outlined for health care improvement.[5] Health care should be safe, effective, patient-centered, timely, efficient, and equitable. As a result, efforts for improving quality of care generally target these six aims (**Table 46-1**).[5]

Framework

Although the goal of quality care is directed toward having optimal outcomes, there needs to be a supportive framework capable of evaluating the steps toward these ideal outcomes. Most often referenced is the Donabedian Model

(**Table 46-2**), which is a conceptual model that provides a framework for examining health services and evaluating quality of care.[10] This model highlights three specific areas that may be targeted for quality measurement and improvement: structure, process, and outcomes.

Structure

Structure generally includes the context in which the care is delivered, such as the physical facility and organizational characteristics (i.e., staff, equipment, and human resources). While these structural factors of a health system such as number of critical care beds or access to invasive procedures are easy to measure and observe, they are often more difficult to change. Structure may represent the overall ability to provide quality of care and sometimes can be identified as a potential problem upstream for a problematic process of care. An example of a potential structural problem is the financial ability of a health system to leverage health information technology or other resource intensive services. This can be particularly troublesome for health systems that serve socioeconomically disadvantageous populations where health policy may penalize organizations that have high readmission rates.[11,12] In health systems that serve vulnerable populations, there are many different factors that need to be overcome for high-quality care, one of which being access to financial resources, staff, clinical access, and other structural improvements that will prevent readmission for worsening HF. Procedural volume is a classic example of a structural relationship with outcome. Implantation and care for patients with ventricular assist devices is quite complex for health systems. In general, hospitals with higher procedural volume have better survival outcomes, which may represent the overall ability of the health system to deliver the service, as well as having the infrastructure to support care demands.[13] Despite their intimate relationship, the connection between structure and optimal outcomes is often difficult to demonstrate, given that the observed relationship is often modest, if observed at all. In the case of ventricular assist devices, there appears to be a modest volume-outcome relationship for mortality but not readmission, making it difficult to determine what volume may be most appropriate for optimal outcomes. This is particularly difficult for structural relationships such as procedural volume with readmission—an outcome putatively expected to be influenced by infrastructural support.

TABLE 46-1 Institute of Medicine Aims for Health Care Improvement

AIM	DEFINITION
Safe	Avoiding injuries to patients from the care that is intended to help them
Effective	Providing services based on scientific knowledge to all who could benefit and refraining from providing services to those not likely to benefit (avoiding underuse and overuse, respectively)
Patient-centered	Providing care that is respectful of and responsive to individual patient preferences, needs, and values and ensuring that patient values guide all clinical decisions
Timely	Reducing waits and sometimes harmful delays for both those who receive and those who give care
Efficient	Avoiding waste, including waste of equipment, supplies, ideas, and energy
Equitable	Providing care that does not vary in quality because of personal characteristics such as gender, ethnicity, geographical location, and socioeconomic status

Institute of Medicine: Crossing the quality chasm: a new health system for the 21st century. The National Academies Press, 2001, Washington DC.

Process

Process is the second area highlighted by the Donabedian Model as a target for quality measurement and improvement, and is most often the focus of development. In general, process represents the transactions or services that sum up health care, like diagnosis, treatment, or other actions of care delivery. Measuring process is common, due to the difficulty of using outcome measures for quantifying quality of care. For most processes of care to be considered a measure of quality care, they typically must have a strong link to an important health outcome. Nevertheless, there are some process measures that are so fundamental to care (such as defining a HF patient's ejection fraction), that they serve as a means to systematical, define potential patient populations in which evidence-based therapies are targeted. Perhaps most important, a process measure must be actionable by a health care provider or a health system.

Process measures are defined by the percentage of eligible patients receiving a given treatment or service, with the numerator indicating which patients received the treatment or service and the denominator defining the eligible population. Typically, for a process measure to be considered important for defining quality of care as a performance measure, the measure usually needs to undergo a thorough review and endorsement by national bodies. The criteria for selecting quality evaluation process measures include

TABLE 46-2 Donabedian Model of Quality

MEASURE	DEFINITION	ADVANTAGES	DISADVANTAGES
Structure	Components or characteristics of the care delivery system thought to have an influence on health care delivery or health-related outcomes (i.e., physical facilities, staff qualifications, case volume, or use of electronic health records)	Easily defined	Weakest link to outcomes; some structural components difficult to rapidly alter
Process	What is actually done for a patient in terms of diagnosis, treatment, and other services	Discrete and actionable; Innumerable potential measures	Outcome-link may vary, especially across duration of exposure; requires precise medical record collection
Outcomes	Clinical events such as mortality, morbidity, and quality of life	Self-evident validity and easily defined	Sample size may be limiting for rare events; risk adjustment is key and may still be incomplete; not directly actionable

TABLE 46-3 Criteria for Process Measures in Quality

CRITERION	DEFINITION
Interpretable	The degree to which a health care provider is likely to understand what the results mean and address if necessary
Actionable	The degree to which the process measure is under the control of the health care provider
Feasible	The ease with which the data can be collected and reproducible across health systems

whether the measure is easily interpretable, actionable, and feasible (**Table 46-3**). Professional societies (i.e., American Heart Association [AHA], American College of Cardiology [ACC], etc.) will typically form a task force dedicated to defining process measures that may be considered quality performance measures. Programs such as the AHA's Get With The Guidelines (GWTG) will define process measures from class I recommendations of care guidelines.[3] For process measures to be tied to either payment or public reporting, they normally must meet approval by national organizations that are dedicated to quality, such as the National Quality Forum or The Joint Commission. These quality-focused organizations review a proposed measure based on its importance, feasibility, and evidence as a best care allotment. Payers such as the Centers for Medicare & Medicaid Services (CMS) ultimately impact health care once a process measure is implemented for performance of a health care system.

Challenges for defining process measures as a measure of quality of care include the link to outcome, the trade-off between specificity and sensitivity, and how to combine measures for an overall quality measure. Ideally, the definition yields a strong link to outcome, but as noted earlier, there are some fundamental process measures that may be important for quality of care that have high variability in delivery (such as measurement of ejection fraction). These basic measures may be difficult to link to outcome because of confounding factors or ceiling effects. For example, the basic measures of HF quality (LVEF, smoking cessation counseling, ACEI/ARB use in left ventricular systolic dysfunction [LVSD], and discharge summaries) do not have a strong link to short- or long-term outcomes.[14] In contrast, other emerging measures, such as prescribing a β-blocker for patients with LVSD, have a strong link to outcomes.[15]

For any process measure, there will be a trade-off between sensitivity and specificity. For example, the evidence and guidelines strongly support the use of ACEIs or ARBs, because of the risk reduction for mortality and other important outcomes among patients with HF and reduced ejection fraction. One could apply this evidence across all patients with HF and reduced ejection fraction, thereby creating a very sensitive process measure. To be more specific and undeniable, the measure with widespread endorsement and used by payers should include absolute contraindications for ACEIs or ARBs. To be even more specific, then further restriction of the eligible population to precisely those patients studied in clinical trials could be considered; however, applying such stringent standards would limit the general applicability of a process measure, as well as its potential impact on quality of care.

Another area of debate is how to measure the overall quality of health systems, particularly when multiple process measures may be available for evaluation. Although outcome measures can provide an overall assessment of quality, they are often difficult to use because of their inability to fully address potential confounding factors, such as patient case mix or severity of illness. Furthermore, there is a need to summarize process measures that are considered more actionable. To address this need, an alternative approach to quantifying overall quality is to use composite measures that combine two or more measures, most often process measures.[16] These composite performance measures allow data reduction when there is a large array of individual indicators. They also allow for combining measures into a summary measure to better profile or inform decisions on provider performance, such as pay-for-performance programs.

The most commonly used composite measures are "opportunity" scoring and "any-or-none" scoring. Opportunity scoring counts the number of times a given care process was actually performed (numerator), divided by the number of chances a provider had to give this care correctly (denominator). Unlike simple averaging, each item is based on the percentage of eligible patients, which may vary from provider to provider. Any-or-none scoring is similar to composite outcomes for a clinical trial where a patient counts once toward the primary endpoint as an event regardless of how many events the patient may have had during the observation period. In this method, a patient is counted as failing if he or she experiences at least one missed process from a list of two or more processes. Use of any-or-none composites may be misleading, because this method is driven by the processes most commonly failed and, therefore, may not be representative of the overall number and range of processes that can occur during the health care process.[17]

Outcomes

Outcomes are the third area highlighted by the Donabedian Model as a target for quality measurement and improvement. Outcomes are easily understood as the all-encompassing measure of quality and represent the end-effects of health care on patients or populations. Outcome measures may include mortality, morbidity, readmission, and quality of life. The rationale behind outcome measures such as 30-day mortality or 30-day readmission after a hospital stay for HF is three-fold. First, process measures typically focus on narrow aspects of care; the number of process measures that can be feasibly measured is finite. Second, due to eligibility criteria, process measures may only apply to a small segment of the population, yet there remains the need to fully assess the overall quality of the health system. Finally, the existing or typical process measures may have a limited relationship to the most meaningful outcomes that matter most to patients.[17] Therefore, outcome measures can provide a broad perspective on health system performance and spur local innovation to improve the end results desired for quality of care.

Accurately measuring outcomes in a manner that is fair across health systems for performance profiling is challenging due to measured and unmeasured confounding factors such as patient case mix. Making conclusions on quality due to outcome measurements requires large sample sizes, as well as rigorous adjustment methods for case mix and other factors. The challenge of using outcome as a quality measure may be best illustrated by considering HF mortality. At face value, mortality is an important outcome; however, for a group of patients under

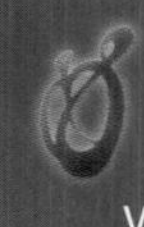

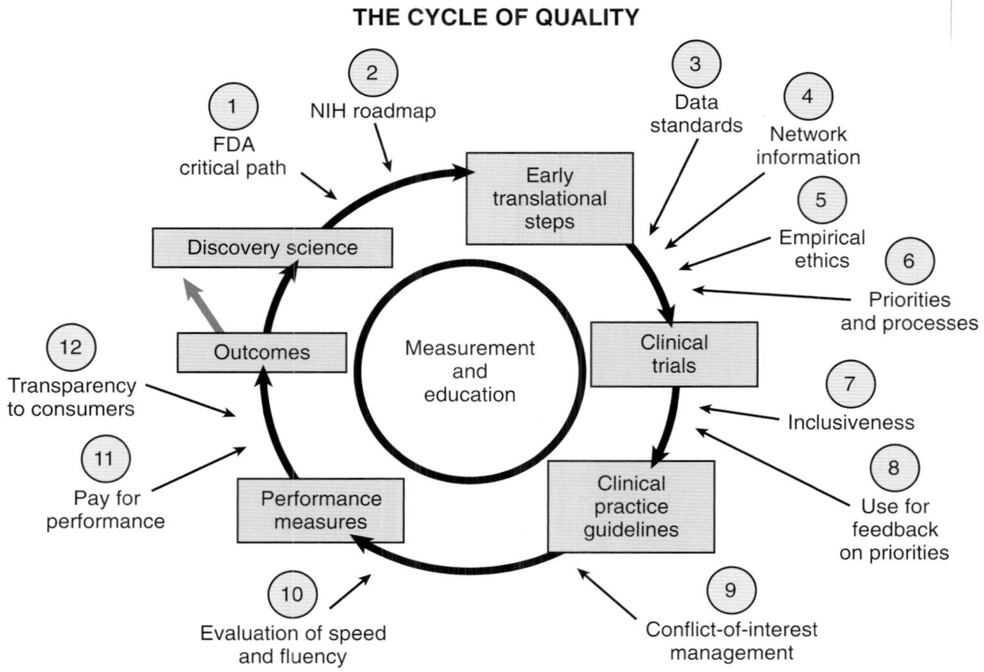

THE CYCLE OF QUALITY

1 FDA critical path
2 NIH roadmap
3 Data standards
4 Network information
5 Empirical ethics
6 Priorities and processes
7 Inclusiveness
8 Use for feedback on priorities
9 Conflict-of-interest management
10 Evaluation of speed and fluency
11 Pay for performance
12 Transparency to consumers
Discovery science
Early translational steps
Clinical trials
Clinical practice guidelines
Performance measures
Outcomes
Measurement and education

FIGURE 46-1 The cycle of quality. This figure displays the cycle of quality and the consequent relationship between early translational steps, clinical trials, clinical practice guidelines, performance measures, outcomes, and discovery science. *FDA,* U.S. Food & Drug Administration; *NIH,* National Institutes of Health. *From Califf RM, Harrington RA, Madre LK, et al: Curbing the cardiovascular disease epidemic: aligning industry, government, payers, and academics. Health Aff (Millwood) 26:62–74, 2007.*

a single health care provider that has different referral patterns (e.g., a cardiac transplant physician), mortality comparisons would be generally unfair. At the health system level, case mix may still be a factor, but it is more easily addressable due to a larger sample size and analytic methods that provide greater ability to conservatively draw comparisons between health systems, particularly when considering outliers.

Selecting the duration of exposure for an outcome can also be difficult and depends on the overall goal. For example, how far out from an admission should a hospital be accountable for a patient's outcome? Although 30 days may seem a reasonable amount of time to hold a hospital accountable, there is increasing pressure for health systems to be held accountable for outcomes up to 1 year. The more time that passes after a hospital admission, the more actionable factors become difficult to define. Long-term outcomes more than 1 year post hospital admission are likely affected by care during the index hospitalization, outpatient care, and potentially care outside of the index hospital at other institutions, including other hospitals and skilled nursing facilities. On the other hand, shorter observation periods may not allow enough time to accurately assess the potential benefit of a given process, such as ICD implantation or β-blocker therapy.

Notably, measuring outcomes is generally an insufficient means of improving quality, as efforts often have to be isolated into discrete processes or segments of care such as admission, discharge, and transitional care. Another challenge with measuring outcomes is that organizations using continuous quality improvement techniques need to assess performance measures at relatively frequent intervals because some outcome measures may be too small, occurring over short periods of time or varying considerably (similar to day-to-day changes in the stock market). Receiving reliable outcome data in a timely fashion may also be a challenge, especially for health systems that are not integrated or have patient care spread across disparate organizations.

In the end, quality is measured in a variety of ways. For many, quality needs to be summarized across different domains into a composite measure. The most publicized example of a composite measure that includes structural, process, and outcome measures is the annual U.S. News & World Report Annual Index of Hospital Quality, yet whether this report reflects "true" quality is of considerable debate.[18] Looking toward the future, value of care will also become increasingly emphasized, and for some measures, value of care will be directly incorporated depending on the cost-effectiveness of a given therapy.[19]

KEY COMPONENTS FOR QUALITY: INTEGRATIVE MODEL FOR QUALITY

The "cycle of quality" has been proposed, as attention to quality of care has evolved, along with the recognition of the need for a continuous cycle of quality improvement that takes into account the roles of different stakeholders including public, private, and governmental organizations. The cycle of quality model connects the innovation of initial scientific discovery with validated methods of translating research into effective care delivery (**Figure 46-1**).[20] This model serves as a basis for accelerating development, encouraging appropriate adoption of new treatments, and achieving greater penetration of effective behavioral therapies and established technologies, with the ultimate goal being major improvements in patient health. The cycle of quality is a model that has been built on the traditional quality framework that was first proposed by Donabedian. Key components for a cycle of quality include the roles of the health care system and health information technology accompanied by a learning environment.[21]

Health Care System

Health care systems are often characterized by how well the different service components are integrated. The fragmented nature of the U.S. health care system serves as a prime example of the difficulties in enacting high-quality affordable care. Our health system is comprised of a variety of different systems responsible for care with and without direct links to payment. Furthermore, in most settings, no single group (whether it be physicians, hospitals, public payers, or private payers) has the full responsibility of a population's health. Patients often encounter many groups inside and outside of a health care system. Even within a single health care system, integration is challenging, as there are barriers with regard to information exchange for the most basic functions between inpatient and outpatient care, which leads to waste, duplication, and inevitable, higher costs. This fragmentation of information has highlighted the need for more accountable care organizations.[22]

Although there are examples of integrated health care delivery systems, the pressure for all health care systems to be more integrated has generated consolidation, with hospitals purchasing provider practices and strategic alliances across different components of health care delivery. For example, primary care physicians and cardiologists frequently deliver HF care, but they may not have access to common medical records or other functions. Often, the care of patients hospitalized with HF covers the full spectrum of providers, from hospitalists to consulting cardiologists to outpatient providers.[23] These providers and their affiliated hospitals may not be associated with each other, so follow-up after a hospital admission is often quite different from the care provided during a hospital episode.[24] Other components of the health system add to the complexity of care, including pharmacies, home health agencies, rehabilitation services, and skilled nursing facilities. Patients navigating these systems—particularly those who have frequent comorbidities—present enormous difficulties in ensuring that the right care is delivered at the right time. With such a diffuse system, consisting of so many different components in action, it is difficult to discern who is actually responsible for quality. Heart failure care uses a variety of health care system components, thereby serving as a prime example of policy development to align incentives under an accountable care organization. For example, a bundled payment across the inpatient to outpatient care environment is an incentive intended to force individual components to become more integrated and efficient. Whether or not this emphasis on improved health system accountability actually leads to higher quality of care remains to be seen, especially if cost reduction is a key component.[25]

Health Information Technology

Data drive the decisions and actions for improving quality of care. In order to be as close to real time as possible, health information technology and its associated analytics become central to driving quality improvement. As described previously, process measures require data collection to define an eligible population, as well as those who receive a given care process. Collection of such data is necessary, but can be labor intensive if it is not integrated into the normal workflow or through the health record. With the requirement that health systems use electronic health records, health information technology becomes a platform to measure, evaluate, and act on key processes of care. More important, health information technology may allow for the development of real-time tools, such as integrated risk assessment models for outcome measures.[26]

Despite the promise of health information technology, the impact on outcomes remains to be seen.[27,28] Electronic health records are often complex and the number of potential automated reporting functions can be overwhelming for providers. Users may "click" through reminders because of time constraints or simply the sheer number of reminders that are generated. In the early development of electronic health records, the Veterans Administration demonstrated improved quality through a variety of tools such as computerized order entry.[29] Many hospitals still only have the most basic electronic health record systems. Furthermore, many hospitals with higher functioning systems do not use them to their fullest capability.[30] Health information technology cannot sit in isolation; for any data generated or tools used, providers must act on the information in a timely and consistent manner.

STATUS OF HEART FAILURE QUALITY MEASURES

Public Reporting

Public reporting of health care quality began as an attempt to not only incentivize health care systems to improve performance on quality metrics, but to increase transparency for patients and empower them as consumers in the health care marketplace. Public reporting in HF care began shortly after individual states started reporting outcomes for patients undergoing coronary artery bypass surgery and percutaneous coronary intervention.

The first large-scale HF reporting effort began with the launch of Hospital Compare, a public reporting database founded by CMS. In 2005, Hospital Compare began reporting information on quality process measures related to the care of patients with HF, as well as acute myocardial infarction and pneumonia. In June 2007, the database began reporting risk-adjusted mortality.[31]

Given that almost all hospitals in the United States participated in the Hospital Compare program, there is a limited number of available control groups for comparison purposes, thereby making the impact assessment of public reporting on HF mortality somewhat challenging. An analysis that adjusted for previous secular trends in HF care and changes in other related chronic conditions found a very modestly adjusted relative risk reduction of 0.97 (95% confidence interval [CI] 0.95-0.99) in 30-day mortality for Medicare patients with HF, but there was no improvement over time of the adjusted risk ratio for acute myocardial infarction or pneumonia.[32]

In July 2009, CMS began publicly reporting risk-standardized readmission rates for HF along with two other common conditions: acute myocardial infarction and pneumonia. In October 2012, CMS extended this policy through the Hospitals Readmissions Reduction Program by imposing cuts in total Medicare reimbursements for higher than predicted readmission rates. The impact of these two policy changes has yet to be determined.

TABLE 46-4 Heart Failure Performance Measures over Time

2001 The Joint Commission[33]	*2005 ACCF/AHA*[2]		*2011 ACCF/AHA*[34]	
INPATIENT	**INPATIENT**	**OUTPATIENT**	**INPATIENT**	**OUTPATIENT**
1. LVEF assessment 2. ACEI use for LVSD* 3. Discharge instructions 4. Smoking cessation counseling	1. LVEF assessment 2. ACEI/ARB use for LVSD 3. Discharge instructions 4. Smoking cessation counseling 5. Anticoagulant for patients with a-fib	1. LVEF assessment 2. ACEI/ARB use for LVSD 3. β-blocker use for LVSD 4. Symptom assessment 5. Activity assessment 6. Patient education 7. Anticoagulant for patients with a-fib 8. Physical examination for volume status 9. Laboratory testing with new diagnosis 10. BP measurement 11. Weight measurement	1. LVEF assessment 2. ACEI/ARB use for LVSD 3. β-blocker use for LVSD 4. Follow-up after discharge	1. LVEF assessment 2. ACEI/ARB use for LVSD 3. β-blocker use for LVSD 4. Symptom and activity assessment 5. Symptom management 6. Patient education 7. ICD counseling for LVSD

*ARB later added as an acceptable alternative.

ACCF, American College of Cardiology Foundation; *ACEI,* angiotensin-converting enzyme inhibitor; *a-fib,* atrial fibrillation; *AHA,* American Heart Association; *ARB,* angiotensin receptor blocker; *BP,* blood pressure; *ICD,* implantable cardioverter-defibrillator; *LVEF,* left ventricular ejection fraction; *LVSD,* left ventricular systolic dysfunction.

Process Measures

In an attempt to improve outcomes for patients with HF, stakeholders developed specific processes measures that could be quantified and modified. These process measures cover both the inpatient and outpatient domains of HF care and have been modified over time (**Table 46-4**). In 2002, The Joint Commission began providing quarterly feedback to sites on specific quality metrics and allowed sites to compare individual performance to national rates.[35] This process has also been utilized in HF-specific registries, including the Organized Program to Initiate Lifesaving Treatment in Hospitalized Patients with HF (OPTIMIZE-HF)[36] and most recently, the GWTG-HF program.[37] Improvement in these process measures has been a remarkable achievement in HF care, but the association between improvement in process measures and improved outcomes for patients with HF is modest.

The first large analysis of the process-outcome link examined the association between hospital-level performance in CMS's Hospital Compare program and risk-adjusted mortality.[38] The authors looked at differences in risk-adjusted mortality rates (inpatient, 30 day, and 1 year) for hospitals performing in the 25th and 75th percentile for assessment of LVSD and ACEI use for LVSD and found few to no differences between the hospital mortality rates.

An analysis of data from OPTIMIZE-HF, which was a national quality improvement initiative designed to enhance guideline adherence in patients hospitalized with HF,[36] looked at outcomes associated with specific HF performance measures. This analysis specifically examined conformity to the 2005 ACC/AHA HF inpatient performance measures[2] (see Table 46-4), β-blocker use for LVSD, and associated mortality or all-cause rehospitalization 60 to 90 days post discharge.[39] β-blocker use was associated with a reduced risk of mortality and mortality/rehospitalization, whereas ACEI/ARB use in eligible patients was only associated with reduced mortality/rehospitalization. There was no association with improved outcomes for the other individual measures.

A more contemporary analysis compared hospitals participating in the GWTG-HF program, which was a voluntary in-hospital quality improvement initiative for patients hospitalized with HF[37] to those who were not. Hospitals participating in the program had improved process of care performance on four measures (discharge instructions, assessment of LVSD, smoking cessation, and ACEI/ARB use in eligible patients); for every 10% increase in a composite of these four measures, there was an associated 0.1% decrease in all-cause 30-day readmission with no associated change in 30-day mortality.

Similar findings were seen in outpatients. An analysis of data from the registry to Improve the Use of Evidence-Based HF Therapies in the Outpatient Setting (IMPROVE HF) found an association among various performance measures (ACEI/ARB use, β-blocker use, aldosterone antagonist use, anticoagulant for atrial fibrillation, cardiac resynchronization therapy [CRT], ICD, and HF education) and reduced adjusted mortality.[40] The authors specifically noted that for every 10% increase in a composite score of the eligible measures, there was an associated 13% lower adjusted odds of 24-month mortality (adjusted odds ratio [OR] 0.87, 95% CI 0.84-0.90).

Perhaps the best evidence of modest gains from improvements in processes of care comes from the very small improvements in HF-related mortality and readmissions seen over the past two decades. As previously noted,[41] process measures in HF made remarkable improvements from 2000 to 2010; in contrast, readmission and mortality rates were disappointingly stagnant.[42,43]

Most quality improvement efforts in the United States are targeted at patients hospitalized with a primary diagnosis of HF, though as discussed previously, outpatient quality improvement initiatives do exist. Most hospitalizations for patients with HF are for reasons other than HF,[44] and care during these other hospitalizations is measurably worse.[45]

Outcome Measures

Mortality is the most commonly analyzed outcome in the attempt to understand the impact of a quality intervention on HF patients. Mortality analysis is appropriate given the high associated mortality[1] of HF, as well as the fact that mortality is an outcome that most clinical trial and observational databases can accurately quantify. There is also a growing interest in reporting the impact of quality interventions on hospitalization rates. Nonetheless, mortality and readmission rates may not be the best measures to evaluate quality of care, as outcome measurements do not provide information on the modifiable steps in the process of care. A sports analogy would be a baseball team that is trying to improve performance, but only focuses on wins and losses without considering the individual components of the game, such as team batting average, pitching performance, and errors on the field. Analyzing these individual components allows for quantifiable and actionable changes; hence the interest in process measures when considering improving HF quality-of-care performance. Additionally, focusing only on mortality and hospitalization rates may under-recognize patient-centered outcomes[47] and values in health care.[48]

Pay-for-Performance

Initial programs for pay-for-performance incentives began at the state level.[49,50] The first nationwide program, the CMS Premier Hospital Quality Incentives Demonstration, began in 2003.[51] The program incentivizes participating hospitals through bonus payments for process measure performance for a number of conditions including HF. The highest performing hospitals for these measures (LVEF assessment, ACEI/ARB use for LVSD, discharge instructions, and smoking cessation counseling) receive a financial bonus while the lowest performing hospital receives a financial penalty. The impact on outcomes has not been assessed, and efforts to expand this program are not yet clear, though as noted above, CMS recently began imposing cuts on total Medicare reimbursements for higher-than-predicted readmission rates for HF and other chronic conditions.

Effectiveness

One measure of the evidence base supporting HF treatment comes from clinical practice guidelines. The most recent ACC/AHA guidelines recognize 22.1% of recommendations at level of evidence A,[3] whereas in 2005, it was 26.4%[52]; this lack of improvement highlights the need for an evidence base for this common and expensive medical condition.

In addition to high-quality evidence from clinical trials, disease-specific registries have afforded the opportunity to examine the real-world effectiveness of therapies outside of trial settings. For patients not included in trials, this is an important step in integrating quality in the development cycle.[53] A recent analysis of the National Cardiovascular Data Registry's ICD Registry demonstrated that survival after primary prevention ICD was similar in a real-world setting compared with the findings from the Multicenter Automatic Defibrillator Implantation Trial (MADIT-II) and the Sudden Cardiac Death in Heart Failure Trial (SCD-HeFT).[54] An analysis of the OPTIMIZE-HF registry linked with Medicare claims data also showed that β-blockers improved outcomes in elderly patients with LVSD.[55]

Patient-Centeredness

Clinical trials in cardiology have largely focused on mortality as a primary outcome. While using mortality as a primary outcome is both necessary and scientifically appropriate, it often compromises our understanding of the impact of cardiovascular care on patient-reported outcomes. In the field of HF, the Kansas City Cardiomyopathy Questionnaire is one of many disease-specific tools validated for purposes of understanding cardiovascular care impact on patient-reported outcomes,[56] yet this tool is rarely used in clinical practice. Since our application of HF therapies to treat patient symptoms is poorly understood, we are hopeful that current initiatives, such as the Patient-Centered Outcomes Research Institute (PCORI), may help address some of these gaps for patients with HF.[47]

Equity

Equitable care for patients with HF implies that care is at least offered to all eligible patients regardless of gender, ethnicity, geographical location, or socioeconomic status.[5] Previous variations in HF practice and outcomes have been well documented[43,57-64] (see Chapter 37), and while these differences are striking, not all variations in care are due to health care disparities. Unfortunately, the United States is currently lacking the research platform that would enable us to better understand these differences and address treatment disparities. Disease-based registries are typically voluntary, so limited information is available on patients treated at hospitals not participating in these registries, as well as patients without Medicare insurance. Nevertheless, there is hope that national efforts to address disparities in HF treatment may be effective. A previous analysis of the OPTIMZE-HF program suggested that African-Americans received evidence-based HF care in the setting of a quality improvement intervention.[65]

IMPROVING QUALITY OF CARE (IMPLEMENTATION)

Measuring quality of care is not, in and of itself, an end result; rather, it is necessary to improve care via evidence implementation through a variety of methods. **Table 46-5** describes different care goals and the quality improvement tools that are often available.[66] A variety of reports and tools can be used. In programs focusing on quality of care, there has been remarkable success in improving quality of care over time.[67]

Quality Improvement Registries

Heart failure has been a leading example of registry-based systems delivering provider feedback guideline-recommended therapies, educational materials oriented to patients and providers, and abilities to benchmark against local, regional, and national norms. Through clinical decision support tools, patients receive more consistent delivery of care and also identify opportunities for standardizing care. Examples of registries include the Acute Decompensated HF National Registry (ADHERE), OPTIMIZE-HF, and the AHA's GWTG-HF Registry. Data from GWTG-HF have helped define disparities in care,[7] gaps in transitional care,[24] and potential methods for systematically improving readmission rates.[31]

TABLE 46-5 Potential Methods for Quality Improvement

MAJOR QUALITY GOAL	QI TOOL	DESCRIPTION
Care delivery and coordination	Patient lists	Lists of patients with a particular condition who may be due for an examination, procedure, etc.
	Patient-level reports	Summarize data on an individual patient (e.g., longitudinal data on blood pressure readings)
	Automated notifications	Prompts provider or patient when an examination or other action is needed
	Automated communications	Summarizes patient information in a format that can be shared with the patient or other providers
	Decision support tools	Provide recommendations for care for an individual patient using evidence-based guidelines
Population measurement	Population-level standardized reports	Provides an analysis of population-level compliance with QI measures or other summaries (e.g., patient outcomes across the population)
	Benchmarking reports	Compares population-level data for various types of providers
	Ad-hoc reports	Enables participants to analyze registry data to explore their own questions
	Population-level dashboards	Provides snapshot look at QI progress and areas for continued improvement
	Third-party quality reporting	Enables registry data to be leveraged for reporting to third-party quality reporting initiatives

QI, Quality improvement.
From Gliklich RE, Dreyer NA, Matchar D, et al: Registries for evaluating patient outcomes: a user's guide, ed 3, prepared by Outcome DEcIDE Center (Outcomes Sciences, Inc. dba Outcome) under Contract No. HHSA29020050035I TO1. AHRQ Publication No. 07-EHC001-1. Agency for Healthcare Research and Quality, 2014, Rockville, Md.

Health Care Delivery Models

Due to the attention toward more integrated or accountable care, health systems are developing new care models. The hallmarks of these new delivery systems can be traced to disease management programs, which are multidisciplinary systems of coordinated care (**see also Chapter 44**).[68] Disease management programs traditionally focus on discharge planning, formal patient education, frequent patient assessment, and easy access to care providers through telephone monitoring, nurse visits, or drop-in clinics. The programs are effective in promoting self-care and recognition of early signs or systems. As health systems develop strategies for preventing readmission, features of disease management programs are being harnessed in different models of care. Specifically, creating same-day access clinics to allow patients access to therapy without having to go to the emergency department is being done more often in the United States. These new models also leverage multidisciplinary systems to provide coordinated care through dietitians, nurse educators, pharmacists, and other health care providers. These new models will need to be formally evaluated as prior studies have found that depending on the size, design, and intensity of the program, outcomes improvement may vary significantly.[69]

Future Directions for Quality of Care

Patients, providers, and payers all agree that evaluating and improving quality of care is an essential goal for health care, yet key questions for the future include (1) which measures should be used?; (2) how should these measures be enforced or how should incentives be tied to improvement?; and (3) what are the most effective strategies for improving quality of care? In some cases, randomized trials should be considered to evaluate the positive or negative implications for policies designed to improve quality, particularly when there are potential financial rewards or penalties.

Understanding the best method for improving quality via public reporting or pay-for-performance remains an unknown. For example, initial reports of outcomes public reporting after coronary artery bypass graft surgery in New York state were encouraging,[70] but these outcomes were later attributed to secular trends unrelated to the intervention of public reporting.[71] This cautionary tale highlights the need for rigorous scientific investigations of quality metrics and improvement initiatives.

The stakes are large for translating evidence into practice. As many as 68,000 deaths could be delayed or prevented annually if all six guideline class I evidence-based therapies were used optimally.[9] Achieving optimal implementation of these therapies will require substantial commitment toward improving quality in HF treatment, including the application and evaluation of collaborative performance improvement systems that report on quality of care, providing clinical decision support, and supplying data feedback. Developing and expanding technologies to better implement practice standards, providing better patient interfaces, and supplying a learning environment focused on improving quality in HF care will especially be needed as patients turn to easily accessible resources using mobile technology.

References

1. Go AS, Mozaffarian D, Roger VL, et al: Heart disease and stroke statistics–2014 update: a report from the American Heart Association. *Circulation* 129:e28–e292, 2014.
2. Bonow RO, Bennett S, Casey DE, Jr, et al: ACC/AHA clinical performance measures for adults with chronic heart failure: a report of the American College of Cardiology/American Heart Association Task Force on Performance Measures (Writing Committee to Develop Heart Failure Clinical Performance Measures) endorsed by the Heart Failure Society of America. *J Am Coll Cardiol* 46:1144–1178, 2005.
3. Yancy CW, Jessup M, Boskurt B, et al: 2013 ACCF/AHA guideline for the management of heart failure: a report of the American College of Cardiology Foundation/American Heart Association Task Force on Practice Guidelines. *J Am Coll Cardiol* 62:e147–e239, 2013.
4. Fonarow GC, Yancy CW, Heywood JT: Adherence to heart failure quality-of-care indicators in US hospitals: analysis of the ADHERE Registry. *Arch Intern Med* 165:1469–1477, 2005.
5. Institute of Medicine: *Crossing the quality chasm: a new health system for the 21st century*, Washington, DC, 2001, The National Academies Press.
6. Rathore SS, Foody JM, Wang Y, et al: Race, quality of care, and outcomes of elderly patients hospitalized with heart failure. *JAMA* 289:2517–2524, 2003.
7. Hernandez AF, Fonarow GC, Liang L, et al: Sex and racial differences in the use of implantable cardioverter-defibrillators among patients hospitalized with heart failure. *JAMA* 298:1525–1532, 2007.
8. Phillips LS, Branch WT, Cook CB, et al: Clinical inertia. *Ann Intern Med* 135:825–834, 2001.
9. Fonarow GC, Yancy CW, Hernandez AF, et al: Potential impact of optimal implementation of evidence-based heart failure therapies on mortality. *Am Heart J* 161:1024–1030.e3, 2011.
10. Donabedian A: The quality of medical care. *Science* 200:856–864, 1978.
11. Joynt KE, Orav EJ, Jha AK: Thirty-day readmission rates for Medicare beneficiaries by race and site of care. *JAMA* 305:675–681, 2011.
12. Hernandez AF, Curtis LH: Minding the gap between efforts to reduce readmissions and disparities. *JAMA* 305:715–716, 2011.
13. Khazanie P, Hammill BG, Patel CB, et al: Trends in the use and outcomes of ventricular assist devices among Medicare beneficiaries, 2006 through 2011. *J Am Coll Cardiol* 63:1395–1404, 2014.
14. Patterson ME, Hernandez AF, Hammill BG, et al: Process of care performance measures and long-term outcomes in patients hospitalized with heart failure. *Med Care* 48:210–216, 2010.
15. Hernandez AF, Hammill BG, Peterson ED, et al: Relationships between emerging measures of heart failure processes of care and clinical outcomes. *Am Heart J* 159:406–413, 2010.

16. Peterson ED, DeLong ER, Masoudi FA, et al: ACCF/AHA 2010 Position Statement on Composite Measures for Healthcare Performance Assessment: a report of American College of Cardiology Foundation/American Heart Association Task Force on Performance Measures (Writing Committee to Develop a Position Statement on Composite Measures). *J Am Coll Cardiol* 55:1755–1766, 2010.
17. Hernandez AF, Fonarow GC, Liang L, et al: The need for multiple measures of hospital quality: results from the Get with the Guidelines-Heart Failure Registry of the American Heart Association. *Circulation* 124:712–719, 2011.
18. Mulvey GK, Wang Y, Lin Z, et al: Mortality and readmission for patients with heart failure among U.S. News & World Report's top heart hospitals. *Circ Cardiovasc Qual Outcomes* 2:558–565, 2009.
19. Anderson JL, Heidenreich PA, Barnett PG, et al: ACC/AHA Statement on Cost/Value Methodology in Clinical Practice Guidelines and Performance Measures: a report of the American College of Cardiology/American Heart Association Task Force on Performance Measures and Task Force on Practice Guidelines. *J Am Coll Cardiol* 63:2304–2322, 2014.
20. Califf RM, Harrington RA, Madre LK, et al: Curbing the cardiovascular disease epidemic: aligning industry, government, payers, and academics. *Health Aff (Millwood)* 26:62–74, 2007.
21. Dzau VJ, Ackerly DC, Sutton-Wallace P, et al: The role of academic health science systems in the transformation of medicine. *Lancet* 375:949–953, 2010.
22. Berwick DM: Launching accountable care organizations–the proposed rule for the Medicare Shared Savings Program. *N Engl J Med* 364:e32, 2011.
23. Kociol RD, Hammill BG, Fonarow GC, et al: Associations between use of the hospitalist model and quality of care and outcomes of older patients hospitalized for heart failure. *JACC Heart Fail* 1:445–453, 2013.
24. Hernandez AF, Greiner MA, Fonarow GC, et al: Relationship between early physician follow-up and 30-day readmission among Medicare beneficiaries hospitalized for heart failure. *JAMA* 303:1716–1722, 2010.
25. Eapen ZJ, Reed SD, Curtis LH, et al: Do heart failure disease management programs make financial sense under a bundled payment system? *Am Heart J* 161:916–922, 2011.
26. Eapen ZJ, Liang L, Fonarow GC, et al: Validated, electronic health record deployable prediction models for assessing patient risk of 30-day rehospitalization and mortality in older heart failure patients. *JACC Heart Fail* 1:245–251, 2013.
27. Chaudhry B, Wang J, Wu S, et al: Systematic review: impact of health information technology on quality, efficiency, and costs of medical care. *Ann Intern Med* 144:742–752, 2006.
28. Walsh MN, Albert NM, Curtis AB, et al: Lack of association between electronic health record systems and improvement in use of evidence-based heart failure therapies in outpatient cardiology practices. *Clin Cardiol* 35:187–196, 2012.
29. Jha Ak, Perlin JB, Kizer KW, et al: Effect of the transformation of the Veterans Affairs Health Care System on the quality of care. *N Engl J Med* 348:2218–2227, 2003.
30. DesRoches CM, Charles D, Furukawa MF, et al: Adoption of electronic health records grows rapidly, but fewer than half of US hospitals had at least a basic system in 2012. *Health Aff (Millwood)* 32:1478–1485, 2013.
31. Kociol RD, Peterson ED, Hammill BG, et al: National survey of hospital strategies to reduce heart failure readmissions: findings from the Get With the Guidelines-Heart Failure registry. *Circ Heart Fail* 5:680–687, 2012.
32. Ryan AM, Nallamothu BK, Dimick JB: Medicare's public reporting initiative on hospital quality had modest or no impact on mortality from three key conditions. *Health Aff (Millwood)* 31:585–592, 2012.
33. Hernandez AF, Mi X, Hammill BG, et al: Associations between aldosterone antagonist therapy and risks of mortality and readmission among patients with heart failure and reduced ejection fraction. *JAMA* 308:2097–2107, 2012.
34. Bonow RO, Ganiats TG, Beam CT, et al: ACCF/AHA/AMA-PCPI 2011 performance measures for adults with heart failure: a report of the American College of Cardiology Foundation/American Heart Association Task Force on Performance Measures and the American Medical Association–Physician Consortium for Performance Improvement. *J Am Coll Cardiol* 59:1812–1832, 2012.
35. Williams SC, Schmaltz SP, Morton DJ, et al: Quality of care in U.S. hospitals as reflected by standardized measures, 2002–2004. *N Engl J Med* 353:255–264, 2005.
36. Fonarow GC, Abraham WT, Albert NM, et al: Organized Program to Initiate Lifesaving Treatment in Hospitalized Patients with Heart Failure (OPTIMIZE-HF): rationale and design. *Am Heart J* 148:43–51, 2004.
37. Ellrodt AG, Fonarow GC, Schwamm LH, et al: Synthesizing lessons learned from Get With The Guidelines: the value of disease-based registries in improving quality and outcomes. *Circulation* 128:2447–2460, 2013.
38. Werner RM, Bradlow ET: Relationship between Medicare's Hospital Compare performance measures and mortality rates. *JAMA* 296:2694–2702, 2006.
39. Fonarow GC, Abraham WT, Albert NM, et al: Association between performance measures and clinical outcomes for patients hospitalized with heart failure. *JAMA* 297:61–70, 2007.
40. Fonarow GC, Albert NM, Curtis AB, et al: Associations between outpatient heart failure process-of-care measures and mortality. *Circulation* 123:1601–1610, 2011.
41. Fonarow GC, Peterson ED: Heart failure performance measures and outcomes: real or illusory gains. *JAMA* 302:792–794, 2009.
42. Ross JS, Chen J, Lin Z, et al: Recent national trends in readmission rates after heart failure hospitalization. *Circ Heart Fail* 3:97–103, 2010.
43. Chen J, Normand SL, Wang Y, et al: National and regional trends in heart failure hospitalization and mortality rates for Medicare beneficiaries, 1998-2008. *JAMA* 306:1669–1678, 2011.
44. Blecker S, Paul M, Taksler G, et al: Heart failure-associated hospitalizations in the United States. *J Am Coll Cardiol* 61:1259–1267, 2013.
45. Blecker S, Agarwal SK, Chang PP, et al: Quality of care for heart failure patients hospitalized for any cause. *J Am Coll Cardiol* 63:123–130, 2014.
46. Deleted in page proofs.
47. Selby JV, Beal AC, Frank L: The Patient-Centered Outcomes Research Institute (PCORI) national priorities for research and initial research agenda. *JAMA* 307:1583–1584, 2012.
48. Anderson JL, Heidenreich PA, Barnett PG, et al: ACC/AHA statement on cost/value methodology in clinical practice guidelines and performance measures: a report of the American College of Cardiology/American Heart Association Task Force on Performance Measures and Task Force on Practice Guidelines. *J Am Coll Cardiol* 63:2304–2322, 2014.
49. Berthiaume JT, Chung RS, Ryskina KL, et al: Aligning financial incentives with quality of care in the hospital setting. *J Healthc Qual* 28:36–44, 51, 2006.
50. Nahra TA, Reiter KL, Hirth RA, et al: Cost-effectiveness of hospital pay-for-performance incentives. *Med Care Res Rev* 63:49S–72S, 2006.
51. Shahian DM, Edwards FH, Ferraris VA, et al: Quality measurement in adult cardiac surgery: part 1—Conceptual framework and measure selection. *Ann Thorac Surg* 83:S3–S12, 2007.
52. Tricoci P, Allen JM, Kramer JM, et al: Scientific evidence underlying the ACC/AHA clinical practice guidelines. *JAMA* 301:831–841, 2009.
53. Califf RM, Peterson ED, Gibbons RJ, et al: Integrating quality into the cycle of therapeutic development. *J Am Coll Cardiol* 40:1895–1901, 2002.
54. Al-Khatib SM, Hellkamp A, Bardy GH, et al: Survival of patients receiving a primary prevention implantable cardioverter-defibrillator in clinical practice vs clinical trials. *JAMA* 309:55–62, 2013.
55. Hernandez AF, Hammill BG, O'Connor CM, et al: Clinical effectiveness of beta-blockers in heart failure: findings from the OPTIMIZE-HF (Organized Program to Initiate Lifesaving Treatment in Hospitalized Patients with Heart Failure) Registry. *J Am Coll Cardiol* 53:184–192, 2009.
56. Green CP, Porter CB, Bresnahan DR, et al: Development and evaluation of the Kansas City Cardiomyopathy Questionnaire: a new health status Measure for heart failure. *J Am Coll Cardiol* 35:1245–1255, 2000.
57. Hernandez AF, Fonarow GC, Liang L, et al: Sex and racial differences in the use of implantable cardioverter-defibrillators among patients hospitalized with heart failure. *JAMA* 298:1525–1532, 2007.
58. Yancy CW, Fonarow GC, Albert NM, et al: Influence of patient age and sex on delivery of guideline-recommended heart failure care in the outpatient cardiology practice setting: findings from IMPROVE HF. *Am Heart J* 157:754–762.e2, 2009.
59. Fonarow GC, Abraham WT, Albert NM, et al: Age- and gender-related differences in quality of care and outcomes of patients hospitalized with heart failure (from OPTIMIZE-HF). *Am J Cardiol* 104:107–115, 2009.
60. Forman DE, Cannon CP, Hernandez AF, et al: Influence of age on the management of heart failure: findings from Get With the Guidelines-Heart Failure (GWTG-HF). *Am Heart J* 157:1010–1017, 2009.
61. Hernandez AF, Greiner MA, Fonarow GC, et al: Relationship between early physician follow-up and 30-day readmission among Medicare beneficiaries hospitalized for heart failure. *JAMA* 303:1716–1722, 2010.
62. Kapoor JR, Kapoor R, Hellkamp AS, et al: Payment source, quality of care, and outcomes in patients hospitalized with heart failure. *J Am Coll Cardiol* 58:1465–1471, 2011.
63. Al-Khatib SM, Hellkamp AS, Hernandez AF, et al: Trends in use of implantable cardioverter-defibrillator therapy among patients hospitalized for heart failure: have the previously observed sex and racial disparities changed over time? *Circulation* 125:1094–1101, 2012.
64. Allen LA, Fonarow GC, Grau-Sepulveda MV, et al: Hospital variation in intravenous inotrope use for patients hospitalized with heart failure: insights from Get With The Guidelines. *Circ Heart Fail* 7:251–260, 2014.
65. Yancy CW, Abraham WT, Albert NM, et al: Quality of care of and outcomes for African Americans hospitalized with heart failure: findings from the OPTIMIZE-HF (Organized Program to Initiate Lifesaving Treatment in Hospitalized Patients With Heart Failure) registry. *J Am Coll Cardiol* 51:1675–1684, 2008.
66. Gliklich RE, Dreyer NA, Matchar D, et al: *Registries for evaluating patient outcomes: a user's guide*, ed 3, Prepared by Outcome DEcIDE Center (Outcomes Sciences, Inc. dba Outcome) under Contract No. HHSA29020050035I TO1. AHRQ Publication No. 07-EHC001-1, Rockville, MD, 2014, Agency for Healthcare Research and Quality.
67. Ellrodt AG, Fonarow GC, Schwamm LH, et al: Synthesizing lessons learned from Get With The Guidelines: the value of disease-based registries in improving quality and outcomes. *Circulation* 128:2447–2460, 2013.
68. Krumholz HM, Currie PM, Riegel B, et al: A taxonomy for disease management: a scientific statement from the American Heart Association Disease Management Taxonomy Writing Group. *Circulation* 114:1432–1445, 2006.
69. Whellan DJ, Hasselblad V, Peterson E, et al: Metaanalysis and review of heart failure disease management randomized controlled clinical trials. *Am Heart J* 149:722–729, 2005.
70. Hannan EL, Kilburn H, Jr, Racz M, et al: Improving the outcomes of coronary artery bypass surgery in New York State. *JAMA* 271:761–766, 1994.
71. Ghali WA, Ash AS, Hall RE, et al: Statewide quality improvement initiatives and mortality after cardiac surgery. *JAMA* 277:379–382, 1997.

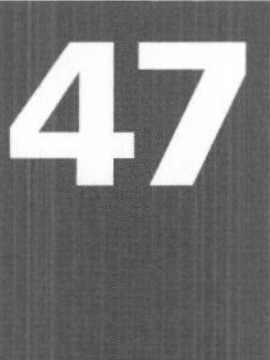

Decision Making and Palliative Care in Advanced Heart Failure

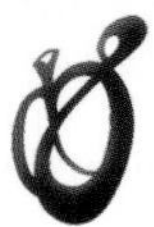

Larry A. Allen and Daniel D. Matlock

Heart failure affects more than 5 million Americans, half of whom are older than 74 years of age.[1] Existing therapies slow, but infrequently reverse, disease progression. As a result, the prevalence of symptomatic heart failure has increased, as has the length of time that people spend in an advanced phase of the disease.[2] At the far end of the heart failure spectrum are a group of patients with advanced (stage D) heart failure for whom symptoms limit daily life despite the usual recommended therapies, and for whom lasting remission into less symptomatic disease is unlikely.[3,4] The increasing prevalence and high symptom burden of advanced heart failure have broadened the need for palliative care services. Simultaneously, the possibility of high-intensity therapies with complex trade-offs mandate a systematic and thoughtful approach to medical decision making.

This chapter highlights how decision making and palliative care play a central role in the care of patients with advanced heart failure. Specifically, the chapter aims to describe theoretical foundations of medical decision making, summarize issues around risk assessment, outline a framework for major medical decisions faced by advanced heart failure patients and their clinicians, and detail how palliative measures and communication can be better integrated into the care of these complex patients. The goals are to both emphasize the inclusion of formal palliative care services into the management of patients with advanced heart failure, and to help health care providers of all types incorporate these concepts into routine practice. The chapter draws from the prior work of researchers, clinicians, and policy experts in the fields of heart failure, palliative care, and medical decision making,[5-11] with particular benefit from the writing group that crafted the American Heart Association's Scientific Statement on "Decision Making in Advanced Heart Failure."[12]

MEDICAL DECISION MAKING

Health care decisions almost always involve uncertainty and are made within the context of incomplete knowledge of the future. How potential risks and benefits of various options are weighed against each other depends on the perspective of the decision maker. With growing emphasis on evidence-based medicine, shared decision making, and patient-centered care, improving processes for making complex decisions with difficult trade-offs has garnered increasing attention, particularly in disease states such as advanced heart failure.[12]

Health care providers have an ethical and legal mandate to involve patients in medical decisions. Judicial decisions (e.g., *Cruzan v. Missouri Department of Health*[13]) and legislative actions (e.g., the Patient Self-Determination Act[14]) have repeatedly affirmed the rights of patients, or duly appointed surrogates, to choose their medical therapy from among reasonable options. The process of informed consent before procedural interventions is an embodiment of the ethical principle of autonomy in that it underscores the clinician's obligation to ensure that the patient is aware of the diagnosis and prognosis, the nature of the proposed intervention, the risks and benefits of that intervention, and all reasonable alternatives and their associated risks and benefits.[15] A gold standard for informed consent would entail a high-functioning health care system that is able to provide the resources with which an activated, informed patient can engage in productive discussions with a proactive, prepared health care team.

Shared decision making builds on the principles that guide informed consent. It asks that clinicians and patients *share information with each other* and *work toward patient-centered decisions* about treatment.[16] Shared decision making incorporates the perspective of the patient, who is responsible for articulating goals, values, and preferences as they relate to his or her health care. Shared decision making also incorporates the perspective of the clinician, who is responsible for narrowing the diagnostic and treatment options to those that are medically reasonable. Shared decision making is most naturally applied to preference-sensitive decisions, where both clinicians and patients generally agree that equipoise exists, and decision support helps patients think through, forecast, and deliberate their options. Shared decision making aims to uphold the ideal that patients' values, goals, and preferences should guide the medical decision-making process. It should be assumed that discussions and decision making with patients also include, when appropriate, the family and other individuals involved, such as caregivers and companions. Thus shared decision making puts into practice the principle of "patient-centered care," which the U.S. Institute of Medicine has identified as one of the six pillars of quality.[17]

Not all medical decisions are considered to be sensitive to patient preferences or appropriate for shared decision making. In situations where clinicians hold the view that scientific evidence for benefit strongly outweighs harm (e.g., smoking cessation counseling), behavioral support designed to describe, justify, and recommend may also be appropriate.[18] Separately, certain therapeutic options may be considered unreasonable (transplantation or permanent mechanical circulatory support above a certain age or comorbidity burden) and therefore independent of patient demands. Situations of medical futility can be difficult to define but have legal precedent.[19]

Finally, it should also be noted that health policy makers and societal considerations also play a role in medical decision making. Rules and regulations often help promote distributive justice and optimal resource allocation. Patient-clinician discussions regarding treatment options occur within the context of these societal rules and regulations. With the costs of care rising, these policy discussions will almost certainly become more common.[20] Although clinicians should play a crucial role in these broader policy decisions, clinicians should simultaneously avoid allowing their own interpretation of societal considerations about cost in the absence of policy to dictate individual decisions at the bedside.

RISK ASSESSMENT AND EXPECTATIONS FOR THE FUTURE

Medical therapies tend to derive their indications and risk-benefit ratios from the nature and severity of the disease for which they are being considered. Therefore, assessment of prognosis provides the context for selecting among therapies for life-threatening disease. Frequent reappraisal of a patient's clinical trajectory helps calibrate future expectations, guide communication, and inform rational decisions. Recognizing when patients have entered into a state of advanced heart failure—American Heart Association Stage D "refractory end-stage heart failure"[3,4] (**Table 47-1**)—is important for considering and applying advanced therapies in an appropriate and timely manner.

Unfortunately, estimating prognosis is particularly challenging for heart failure (see also Chapter 28). The clinical course varies dramatically across the spectrum of disease severity and is relatively unpredictable for individual patients (**Figure 47-1**).[7] This contrasts with the more linear decline of patients with advanced cancer, which has traditionally been the model for decision making and palliative care in end-stage disease. Even late in heart failure, patients often enjoy "good days" and brief interludes of apparent stability, which can lull them and their care providers into postponing vital decisions. Prognosis is further clouded by the unique contrast between unexpected sudden death (i.e., lethal arrhythmia) and lingering death with congestive symptoms (i.e., progressive pump failure).

TABLE 47-1 Criteria for Advanced Chronic Heart Failure, as Defined by the European Society of Cardiology[3]

1. Moderate to severe symptoms of dyspnea and/or fatigue at rest or with minimal exertion (NYHA functional class III or IV)
2. Episodes of fluid retention and/or reduced cardiac output
3. Objective evidence of severe cardiac dysfunction demonstrated by at least one of the following:
   - Left ventricular ejection fraction <30%;
   - Pseudo-normal or restrictive mitral inflow pattern by Doppler;
   - High left and/or right ventricular filling pressures; or
   - Elevated B-type natriuretic peptide
4. Severe impairment of functional capacity as demonstrated by either inability to exercise, 6-minute walk distance <300 meters, or peak oxygen uptake <12-14 mL/g/min
5. History of at least 1 hospitalization in the past 6 months
6. Characteristics should be present despite optimal medical therapy

NYHA, New York Heart Association.

Hundreds of factors have been shown to predict mortality and hospitalization in heart failure. These include demographics, comorbidities (see Chapter 45), exercise capacity, functional status, health-related quality of life, cardiac structure and function (see Chapters 28 and 29), ventricular filling pressures, natriuretic and inflammatory biomarkers (see Chapter 30), end-organ function (renal, liver, bone marrow), arrhythmias (see Chapter 35), depression, behavior, and social-environmental factors. A variety of multivariable risk models have been published, for both ambulatory[21-23] and hospitalized settings[24-27] (**Table 47-2**). Elevated natriuretic peptides, renal dysfunction, and low blood pressure have particularly strong association with survival in patients hospitalized for heart failure.[28] Most prognostic factors tend to function similarly independent of LVEF.[29] The Seattle Heart Failure Model (SHFM) has gained popularity for risk prediction in the ambulatory setting, although in the advanced heart failure population it can result in miscalibrated estimates of life expectancy (with significant underestimation of risk).[30] The increasing use of health information technology in the delivery of care offers the potential to automatically generate risk profiles from the electronic health record. In the meantime, a number of clinical events are known to herald worsening disease (**Table 47-3**), which should prompt reassessment of patient goals of care as well as consideration of therapy options for advanced heart failure.

Most prognostic models in heart failure focus on the singular outcome of mortality. Hospitalization and readmission have gained increasing favor in recent years as another outcome measure. However, other clinical outcomes also rank high in importance to individual patients (**Figure 47-2**). Multiple studies have documented patients' willingness to sacrifice survival in exchange for symptom relief, a trade-off that varies among patients[31] and within the same patient over time.[32] This is correlated loosely with disease severity but strongly with do not resuscitate (DNR) status.[33]

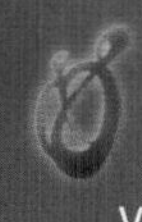

A full discussion of prognosis therefore includes not only the risks of death but also the patient's goals and values, including potential burdens of worsening symptoms, limited functional capacity, loss of independence, reduced social functioning, decreased quality of life, and increased caregiver commitment. Unfortunately, much less is known about risk prediction for these latter outcomes. The only existing heart failure risk model that estimates the risk of unfavorable future quality of life shows important differences from risk models for death or hospitalization.[27] Even less is known about the relative impact of disease and therapies on caregiver burden and quality of life for family members.[34]

Further complicating practical use, risk prediction models represent averages for populations of patients, which are much more helpful for population management than for individual patient decisions. For example, an 80% chance of 1-year survival does not directly translate to an individual who will instead be 100% either alive or dead at 1 year. Patients themselves tend not to think in terms of average survival rates at fixed points in time, but rather ask the question, "How long do I have?" Statistically, point predictions of median survival time are difficult to estimate from most existing models.[35] Such estimates also are prone to significant error because of wide confidence intervals,[36,37]

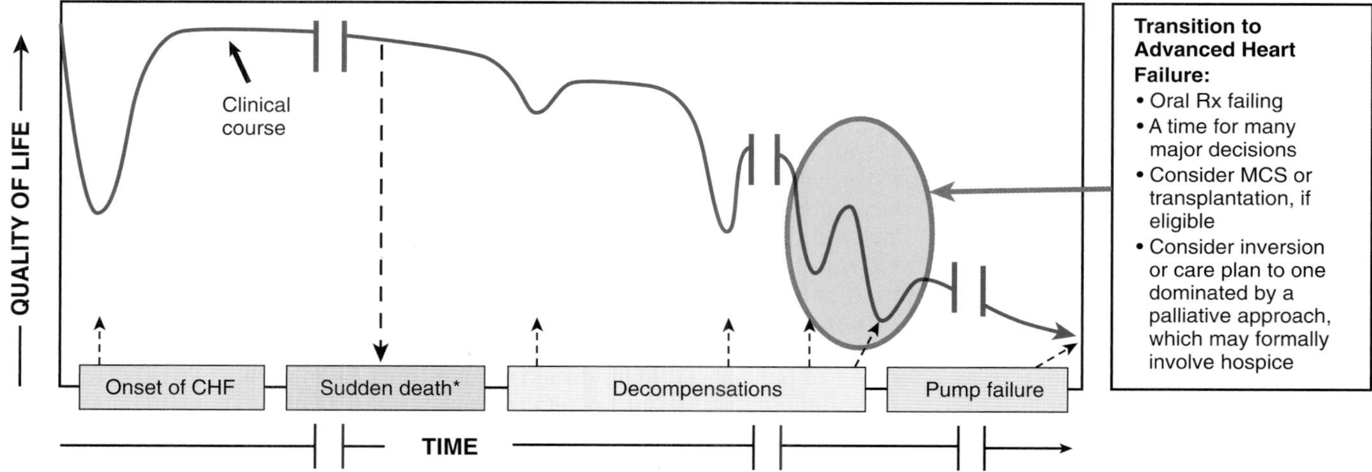

FIGURE 47-1 A depiction of the varied and undulating clinical course of heart failure. Most patients experience a progressive, albeit nonlinear, increase in symptoms and decrease in functional capacity, resulting in a general decline in health-related quality of life over time. This course can be interrupted by sudden cardiac death from arrhythmia (or other cause) or can end in a more delayed death from progressive pump failure. Clinicians should be attentive to the transition from stable symptomatic heart failure to advanced heart failure, when standard therapies begin to fail and multiple major decisions arise.[7,12] *CHF,* Congestive heart failure; *MCS,* mechanical circulatory support.

TABLE 47-2 Selected Prognostic Models in Heart Failure

	KEY COVARIATES	OUTCOME
Ambulatory		
Heart Failure Survival Score[21]	Peak Vo_2, LVEF, serum sodium, mean BP, HR, ischemic etiology, QRS duration/morphology	All-cause mortality
Seattle Heart Failure Model[22] (depts.washington.edu/shfm)	Diuretic dose, SBP, percent lymphocytes, hemoglobin, ischemic etiology, LVEF, serum cholesterol, serum uric acid, allopurinol, serum sodium, statin, NYHA class, age, gender	All-cause mortality, urgent transplantation, or LVAD implantation
Meta-Analysis Global Group in Chronic Heart Failure (MAGGIC)[23] (www.heartfailurerisk.org)	Age, LVEF, NYHA class, serum creatinine, diabetes, not prescribed β-blocker, lower SBP, lower body mass, time since diagnosis, current smoker, COPD, gender, not prescribed ACE inhibitor or angiotensin receptor blocker	All-cause mortality
Hospitalized		
EFFECT Risk Model[24] (www.ccort.ca/Research/CHFRiskModel.aspx)	Age, SBP, respiratory rate, sodium, hemoglobin, BUN, h/o CVA, h/o dementia, h/o COPD, h/o cirrhosis, h/o cancer	30-day and 1-year mortality
ADHERE Risk Model[25]	BUN, SBP, serum creatinine	In-hospital mortality
ESCAPE Discharge Score[26]	BNP, cardiopulmonary resuscitation or mechanical ventilation during hospitalization, BUN, sodium, age >70 years, daily loop diuretic dose, lack of β-blocker, 6-minute walk distance	6-month mortality
EVEREST Risk Model[27]	Age, diabetes, h/o stroke, h/o arrhythmia, β-blocker use, BUN, serum sodium, BNP, KCCQ score	Mortality or persistently poor quality of life (KCCQ <45) over the 6 months after discharge

ACE, Angiotensin-converting enzyme; *ADHERE,* Registry for Acute Decompensated Heart Failure Patients; *BNP,* B-type natriuretic peptide; *BP,* blood pressure; *BUN,* blood urea nitrogen; *COPD,* chronic obstructive pulmonary disease; *CVA,* cerebrovascular accident; *EFFECT,* Enhanced Feedback for Effective Cardiac Treatment; *ESCAPE,* Evaluation Study of Congestive Heart Failure and Pulmonary Artery Catheterization Effectiveness; *EVEREST,* Efficacy of Vasopressin Antagonism in Heart Failure Outcome Study with Tolvaptan; *h/o,* medical history of; *HR,* heart rate; *KCCQ,* Kansas City Cardiomyopathy Questionnaire; *LVAD,* left ventricular assist device; *LVEF,* left ventricular ejection fraction; *NYHA,* New York Heart Association; *SBP,* systolic BP; *Vo_2,* oxygen consumption.

TABLE 47-3 Factors That Herald Worsening Disease, Which Should Prompt Reassessment of Patient Goals of Care as Well as Consideration of Therapy Options for Advanced Heart Failure[12]

Progressive increases in symptom burden and/or decreased quality of life
Significant decrease in functional capacity
Loss of ADLs
Falls
Transition in living situation (independent to assisted living or long-term care)
Worsening heart failure prompting hospitalization, particularly if recurrent
Increasing natriuretic peptide levels or worsening measures of left ventricular remodeling (LVEF, LV volumes, restrictive physiology, etc.)
Serial increases of maintenance diuretic dose
Symptomatic hypotension, azotemia, or refractory fluid retention necessitating neurohormonal medication (ACEI/ARB, β-blocker) underdosing or withdrawal
First or recurrent ICD shock for VT/VF
Initiation of intravenous inotropic support
Consideration of renal replacement therapy (i.e., dialysis)
Other important comorbidities (e.g., new cancer, etc.)
Major life events (e.g., death of a spouse)

ACEI, Angiotensin-converting enzyme inhibitor; *ADL,* activities of daily living; *ARB,* angiotensin receptor blocker; *ICD,* implantable cardioverter-defibrillator; *LVEF,* left ventricular ejection fraction; *VF,* ventricular fibrillation; *VT,* ventricular tachycardia.

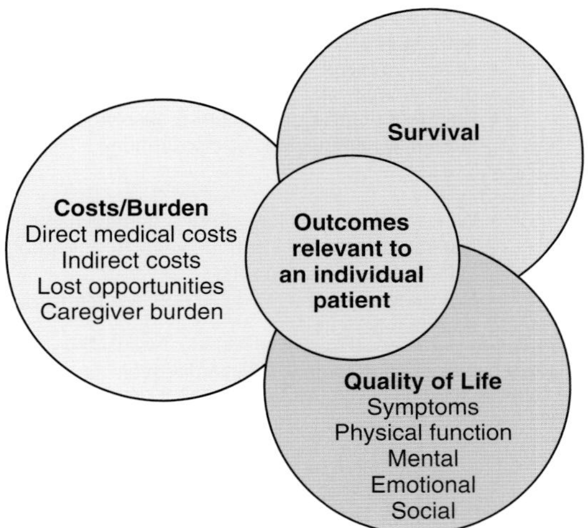

FIGURE 47-2 Multiple outcomes that are of varying importance to individual patients. Discussions about the potential risks and benefits of therapy options should extend beyond survival to consider the full range of patient-centered outcomes.[12]

which is exacerbated in the case of heart failure risk models that have only modest accuracy. For example, if a patient died 12 months from the time a model was used to estimate survival time, the probability that the model prediction would have a greater than twofold error (a model-predicted median survival of >24 months or <6 months) remains almost 50% for most survival models. Ultimately the stochastic nature of heart failure conveys a high level of prognostic uncertainty for most individual patients. It is therefore vital to acknowledge and incorporate uncertainty in discussions about future care.

Despite limitations of prognostic models, they are generally more accurate than biased clinical intuition. Among terminally ill cancer patients, physicians consistently overestimated survival.[38] For patients discharged from the hospital with advanced heart failure, both physicians' and nurses' survival estimates had modest ability to discriminate those who subsequently died from those who lived (with nurses outperforming physicians), and absolute estimates significantly overestimating survival.[39] In patients with chronic heart failure, patient self-predictions also tended to overestimate survival versus model-based predictions and actual survival, particularly for younger patients.[40] Clinicians can leverage objective risk models to minimize their own human biases, while recognizing risk model limitations and uncertainties.

CATEGORIES OF MAJOR TREATMENT DECISIONS

In the face of the increasing complexity of diagnostic and treatment options for heart failure, a framework for classifying various medical decisions can help clinicians and their patients better anticipate and manage those decisions most likely to occur as the disease progresses to an advanced stage (**Table 47-4**). Clinicians should take an active role in defining the set of interventions that are medically reasonable, and from these clinicians and patients can work together to determine which option is most consistent with patient values, goals, and preferences. The more that clinicians can anticipate medical decisions in advance (see Risk Assessment section), the more they can help patients have adequate time to consider their likely options.

Low-Intensity Interventions That May Improve Quantity and Quality of Life

In addition to anticipating and addressing new management options that accompany the transition to advanced heart failure, clinicians should work to optimize background medical therapy for heart failure and other comorbidities.[4,41,42] In order for patients to be defined as advanced stage D heart failure, patients must have failed optimal medical therapy (see Table 47-1). The need to decrease or discontinue neurohormonal antagonists (e.g., β-blockers—see Table 47-3) may be necessary in advanced heart failure, and generally signals worsening disease.

High-Intensity Interventions That May Improve Quantity and Quality of Life

A variety of invasive procedures exist that have the potential to improve cardiac function, thereby increasing both survival and quality of life. However, they also have the potential to cause harm and patient burden, particularly among patients with advanced heart failure who are older and have greater multimorbidity than patients studied in randomized trials. Therefore, decisions about such therapies should include detailed informed consent and shared decision making, even if the therapies are generally supported by a strong evidence base. Additionally, careful consideration of a range of potential complications should be addressed with patients preprocedurally ("What if?") so that contingency plans are in place in case rare but serious events do occur.

Patients with heart failure may be considered for cardiac surgery for coronary, valvular, and pericardial disease (see also Chapter 41). Cardiac surgeries involving general anesthesia, thoracic access, and cardiopulmonary bypass are higher risk as a consequence of underlying severe cardiac dysfunction. To consider cardiac surgery as an option, the surgery should be expected to convey

TABLE 47-4 Framework of Major Medical Decisions in Advanced Heart Failure Faced by Patients and Their Clinicians

TYPES OF OPTIONS	EXAMPLES OF INTERVENTIONS	EXAMPLES OF ADVERSE OUTCOMES THAT SHOULD BE ANTICIPATED IN HIGH-RISK PATIENTS
Low-Intensity Interventions that Might Improve Quantity and Quality of Life		
Medical therapy	β-blocker, ACEI/ARB, MRA, diuretics, control of hypertension and other comorbidities	• Hypotension, azotemia: threshold for accepting intolerance and considering advanced therapies?
High-Intensity Interventions that Might Improve Quantity and Quality of Life		
Procedures with the potential to improve cardiac function	CABG Valve surgery Pericardial stripping Percutaneous valve intervention PCI CRT	• Inability to come off bypass: place mechanical circulatory support? • Ventilator dependence: tracheostomy versus extubate? • Stroke: feeding tube? Institutional care? • Coronary occlusion: revert to CABG? • Unable to place coronary sinus lead: convert to thoracotomy?
Replacement of cardiac function	Transplantation	• Early graft failure or other serious postoperative complications: mechanical circulatory support or withdraw support? • Later graft failure: list for retransplantation?
	Permanent MCS/LVAD	• Stroke, infection, or recurrent bleeding: turn off device?
High-Intensity Interventions that Might Improve Quantity but *Not* Quality of Life		
Procedures to reduce the risk of sudden cardiac death	ICD	• Worsening pump failure disease: ICD deactivation?
Temporary Therapies to Stabilize Patients That Can Lead to Dependence		
Adjunctive therapies instituted during acute decompensation with potential chronic dependence	Temporary mechanical circulatory support devices (IABP, percutaneous VAD, ECMO)	• Unable to wean: convert to permanent LVAD or withdraw?
	IV inotropes	• Unable to wean: transition to home inotropes or discontinue?
	Renal replacement therapy (dialysis or ultrafiltration)	• Failure of acute kidney injury to resolve: initiate indefinite hemodialysis or discontinue?
Noncardiac Procedures with Increased Risk and Potentially Decreased Benefit		
	Joint replacement Hernia repair	• Worsening heart failure causing hemodynamic and/or respiratory collapse: continue ventilatory support and/or initiate circulatory support?
	Resection of pulmonary nodule, routine screening colonoscopy	• Not generally to be done, as risks are felt to outweigh potential benefit

ACE, Angiotensin-converting enzyme inhibitor; *ARB,* angiotensin receptor blocker; *CABG,* coronary artery bypass grafting surgery; *CRT,* cardiac resynchronization therapy; *ECMO,* extracorporeal membranous oxygenation; *IABP,* intra-aortic balloon pump; *ICD,* implantable cardioverter-defibrillator; *MCS,* mechanical circulatory support; *MRA,* mineralocorticoid receptor antagonist; *PCI,* percutaneous coronary intervention; *VAD,* ventricular assist device.

significant long-term benefit. However, the benefit of many cardiac procedures in advanced chronic heart failure is not well established.[43] The potential for residual cardiac dysfunction, perioperative death, protracted postoperative rehabilitation, and loss of independence must be considered and included thoughtfully in the shared decision, because surgery inherently increases short-term risk for the prospect of longer term benefit. Unfortunately, there is limited information about the frequency of these outcomes beyond general estimates of perioperative death and prolonged hospitalization.[44]

Less invasive percutaneous approaches for the treatment of coronary and valvular disease may be appealing in advanced heart failure. Catheter approaches to both aortic[45] and mitral[46] disease have now been shown to be reasonable alternatives to surgery in certain populations (see also Chapter 24). However, the benefits of valve repair or replacement are less well established in patients with significant heart failure, especially when treating functional (secondary) mitral regurgitation for patients with a dilated left ventricle.[47] Additionally, potential benefits depend on a variety of factors, and risks of contrast-induced nephropathy, stroke, and 30-day mortality are increased in the advanced heart failure population. Patient-clinician discussions regarding percutaneous interventions should also include preprocedural consideration of whether emergency surgery would be appropriate and feasible.

Device-based therapy for bradycardia and cardiac resynchronization (CRT) can improve cardiac function but require minor surgery, include risk of infection, and require long-term follow up (see also Chapter 35). Additionally, patients with advanced heart failure (New York Heart Association [NYHA] functional class IV) have represented a small fraction of patients included in randomized trials of CRT.[48] Although there are some reports suggesting that CRT can improve outcomes for patients on intravenous inotropes, these findings have not been consistent and have methodological limitations.[49,50] Additionally, the care team should plan for contingencies, such as consideration of an open thoracotomy for perforation or unsuccessful coronary sinus lead placement. Factors likely to modify the risk-benefit ratio of device implantation, such as noncardiovascular morbidity and acute decompensation, should also be recognized and incorporated into these discussions.[51] Although CRT and implantable cardioverter-defibrillators (ICD) are often packaged together, their purposes are quite different; CRT, like neurohormonal antagonist therapy, is designed to improve cardiac performance and can improve quality of life; ICDs do not. Therefore, a recommendation for combined CRT-D should prompt separate discussions about the indications for defibrillation versus CRT, as well as differences in need for monitoring, chances for inappropriate shocks and worsening heart failure, risks for infection and lead malfunction, and options for deactivation.

Cardiac transplantation and mechanical circulatory support offer the potential to fundamentally change the clinical course of heart failure by exchanging it for surgical therapy and a different set of benefits, risks, and burdens (see also Chapters 40 and 42). In the case of transplantation, patients are asked to weigh their current clinical course against a post-transplant estimated mean survival of approximately 12 years, as well as the risks of surgery, graft rejection, infection, and other side effects of immunosuppression. For permanently implanted mechanical circulatory support, 2-year survival is increased from 10% to approximately 70% with a near doubling in quality of life measures among survivors, but at the risk of reoperation to replace a malfunctioning pump (10%), disabling stroke (11%), device infection, bleeding, and recurrent hospitalizations. Even in the setting of successful destination therapy left ventricular assist device (DT LVAD), patients must maintain a constant power source, perform vigilant driveline care, and manage other chronic diseases; and these issues spill over to caregivers. Thus, for eligible patients, whether to pursue transplantation and/or mechanical circulatory support involves complex trade-offs and major uncertainties. For most patients with heart failure, these advanced therapies are not an option, because of the predominance of heart failure with normal ejection fraction, multiple comorbidities, or very advanced age.[1] Detailed clinical practice guidelines are available that address the use of these advanced therapies,[52,53] and are covered in detail in other chapters.

High-Intensity Interventions That May Improve Quantity but Not Quality of Life

ICDs are fundamentally different from many lifesaving therapies for patients with chronic heart failure with reduced ejection fraction. ICDs improve survival by aborting lethal arrhythmias, but do not improve cardiac function or heart failure symptoms. Additionally, ICDs can create an additional burden for patients, particularly from inappropriate discharges and prevention of a rapid death. Because ICDs involve this trade-off between reduced risk of sudden cardiac death for an increased risk of hospitalization,[54] potential decrease in quality of life,[55] and higher likelihood of death from progressive pump failure, meticulous discussion of absolute risks with and without ICDs are particularly important for informed consent and shared decision making.[56]

Temporary Therapies with Potential Dependence

Some therapies are intended for short-term use to stabilize patients, thereby allowing for recovery from potentially reversible insults or transition to more definitive therapy. Although initially intended as a temporary intervention, such stabilizing therapies can create indefinite dependence if the patient does not improve as hoped or develops an adverse event (e.g., stroke, progressive renal failure) that compromises previously anticipated options.

Short-term circulatory support with intra-aortic balloon pumps or percutaneous ventricular assist devices may be initiated when acute hemodynamic instability requires urgent intervention to avoid permanent end-organ dysfunction and/or death. It may be instituted with the hope of supporting a reversible underlying condition, such as fulminate myocarditis or right heart failure after acute myocardial infarction. It may also be initiated in patients who might be potential candidates for transplantation or permanent circulatory support in whom (1) there has not been opportunity to appropriately evaluate a patient's candidacy or preferences for more definitive high-dependence therapies, (2) reversibility of end-organ dysfunction is uncertain, or (3) socioeconomic contraindications to more definitive therapies may resolve in the near future. If device dependency persists and contraindications to definitive therapies do not resolve, a decision will need to be made about discontinuation. To whatever degree possible, these issues should be addressed before the initiation of short-term support.

Intravenous inotropic agents are commonly initiated in the acute setting for hemodynamic stabilization and to improve end-organ perfusion. Use is most often anticipated to be temporary, with the hope of either clinical improvement or eligibility for more definitive therapies as above. Regardless of intent, initiation of inotropic support for exacerbation of chronic heart failure should be considered a harbinger of severe heart failure (see Table 47-3). When patients fail to wean from intravenous inotropic support, decisions arise regarding continued chronic use. Therefore, the goals of temporary inotrope use should be clearly established before initiation, and unexpected dependence on this therapy should prompt direct discussions about overall goals of care. The decision to arrange for chronic continuous infusions after hospital discharge should be guided by the patient's goals and preferences, including the need for symptom relief. Nonrandomized data suggest that the number of hospital days may decrease following initiation of chronic inotrope infusion,[57] with an increased risk of sudden cardiac death.[58] However, most patients require hospital readmission after initiation of chronic intravenous inotropic therapy, even if begun with the hope of helping patients to stay at home until death. The use of intermittent infusions to control symptoms is currently not recommended by practice guidelines (class III recommendation).[4] Most patients on home inotropic infusions die by 6 months, most often from terminal hemodynamic decompensation.[59]

The prevalence of advanced kidney disease increases dramatically with worsening heart failure, and measures of renal dysfunction are strong predictors of adverse outcomes in patients with heart failure (see Table 47-2). Dialysis in the setting of advanced heart failure, especially in older patients with other comorbidities or frailty, has been shown to add to patient burden, and in high-risk patients may not extend life.[60] Therefore, the decision to initiate renal replacement therapies (e.g., hemodialysis, ultrafiltration) in patients with advanced heart failure should only be made after a clear discussion with the patient about the risks and benefits of dialysis on the patient's quality of life and prognosis.[61]

Feeding tubes, placement of permanent peritoneal and pleural catheters for the control of volume status, and intensive care provide additional examples of therapies with questionable long-term value in patients with irreversible

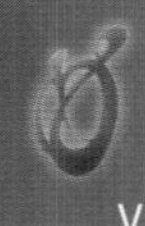

underlying disease. When such situations are anticipated, these types of near end-of-life interventions can be considered as part of a healthy discussion about end-of-life care, ideally before the occurrence of a near-terminal event.

Noncardiac Procedures in Patients with Advanced Heart Failure

The risks and benefits of interventions for noncardiac conditions may be significantly altered in patients with advanced heart failure. When the likelihood of meaningful recovery without the procedure is small, the increase in procedural risk in patients with advanced heart failure may be considered acceptable. Examples include both emergent (e.g., laparotomy for perforated viscous) and urgent (e.g., hip arthroplasty for fracture) surgical procedures. However, most noncardiac procedures, such as knee replacement for degenerative joint disease, must be carefully considered in the context of patient preferences, because complications of the procedure may or may not outweigh the potential benefit. Major procedures should generally be discouraged when they do not offer a tangible improvement in quality of life (e.g., repair of asymptomatic abdominal aortic aneurysm). Routine screening tests (e.g., mammography, colonoscopy) are generally not appropriate in the context of a significant competing risk of mortality from advanced heart failure, yet such tests are frequently ordered at the end of life.[62]

PALLIATIVE CARE

Palliative care is interdisciplinary care aimed at preventing and relieving suffering, while also supporting families and caregivers. The Centers for Medicare and Medicaid Services (CMS) defines palliative care as treatment for the relief of pain and other uncomfortable symptoms through the appropriate coordination of all aspects of care needed to maximize personal comfort and relieve distress.[63] The World Health Organization (WHO) provides an expanded definition that includes a supportive role, as well as a role in communicating and anticipating end-of-life needs.[64] Thus palliative care interventions are those in which the principal aim is to improve symptomatology and quality of life, in contrast to interventions that are primarily meant to be curative or prolong life (**Figure 47-3**). Palliative care can be offered simultaneously with other appropriate medical therapies and can be integrated at any point in the care of those afflicted with serious illness (**Figure 47-4**). In the treatment of heart failure, many traditional therapies are aimed at treating the physiologic causes of symptoms (e.g., diuretics), and by definition, are palliative. Palliative care is *not* synonymous with end-of-life care or hospice, but often includes these more specific interventions as disease advances. Palliative care allows for continued disease-modifying therapies while ensuring symptom relief and interventions that address psychosocial, physical, and spiritual needs. This is done in two primary ways: by treating symptoms and by ensuring that patients' treatment plans match their values and goals.[65] The process of shared decision making is a central tenet of palliative care: that the patient and clinician reach an understanding about preferences for life-prolonging therapy, symptom relief, pain control, and end-of-life care. Unlike hospice care (see later discussion), the application

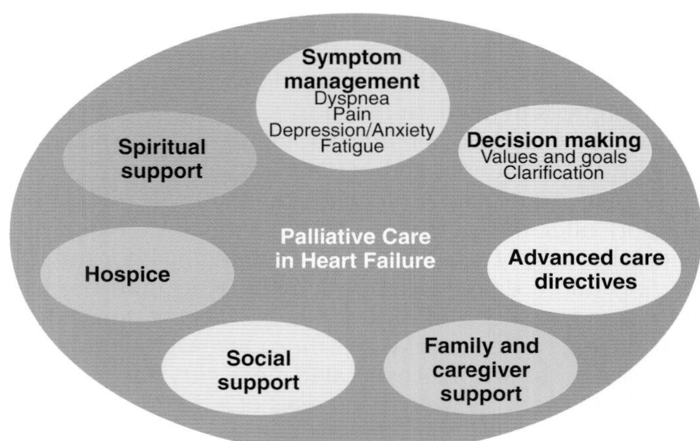

FIGURE 47-3 Palliative care includes many domains.

of palliative care is based on patient need rather than prognosis or life expectancy.

Although data on palliative care in patients with heart failure are limited, several guidelines and reviews recommend integration of palliative care for all patients with advanced heart failure.[5-11] Primary palliative care can and should be done by all clinicians involved in the care of these patients.[66] However, referral to a tertiary palliative care team should be considered for assistance with difficult decision making and refractory symptom management in advanced disease, even as patients continue to receive disease-modifying therapies. Palliative care teams can consist of physicians, nurses, social workers, chaplains, and other professionals who work to ensure that patient and caregiver needs are assessed and met. Because of the complex and changing nature of heart failure, as well as the complexity of conversations, it is important to integrate palliative care into the care of patients with heart failure before they are frankly advanced stage D. Even as patients are being considered for transplantation and/or mechanical circulatory support, palliative consultation could be considered to ensure that patients' symptoms are appropriately controlled and that patients understand the nature of these interventions, as well as the full complement of alternative therapies.[11,67]

Symptom Palliation

The most prevalent complaints for patients with heart failure are dyspnea, pain, edema, depression, and fatigue. Other sources of suffering that have been identified include isolation, difficulty navigating the health care system, and the feeling of uncertainty surrounding prognosis and longevity.[68] Because many of the symptomatic complaints expressed by patients with advanced heart failure are the result of the underlying cardiac dysfunction, most evidence-based traditional therapies actually form the foundation of symptom palliation for patients with heart failure. For example, if patients had diuretics or vasodilators stopped at the time of transition to hospice care, they may experience an increase in congestive symptoms. In addition, patients with advanced heart failure often have other medical comorbidities that contribute to their symptoms and suffering (e.g., osteoarthritis). It is important to consider all sources of suffering, and address any treatable issues that may be contributing to the spectrum of suffering. Therefore, beyond

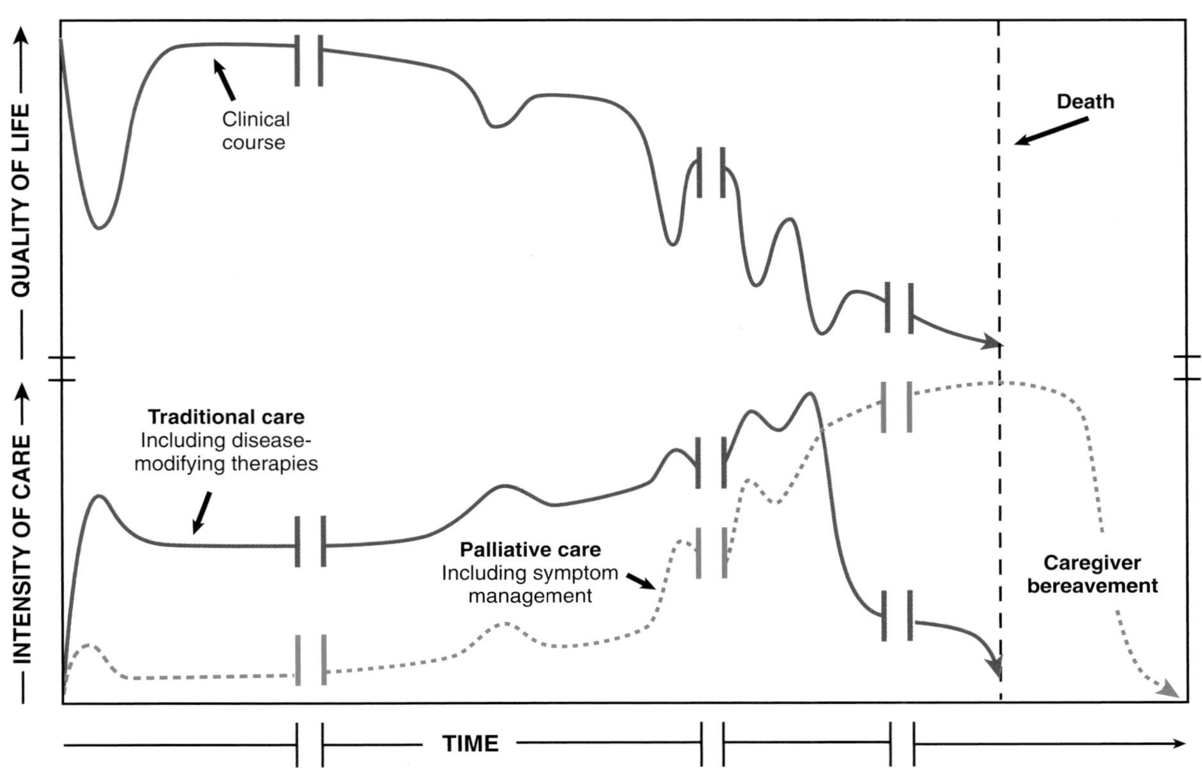

FIGURE 47-4 A depiction of the types and intensities of therapies throughout the clinical course of heart failure. *Top, blue line:* Many patients tend to follow an undulating but eventually progressive decline, ultimately ending in refractory pump failure. *Middle, red line:* At disease onset multiple oral therapies are prescribed for cardiac dysfunction and/or treatment of comorbidities (e.g., diuretics, vasodilators, β-blockers). As disease severity increases the intensity of care will increase in parallel, with intensification of diuretics, addition of ICD/CRT for those eligible, and increased interaction with the medical system through ambulatory visits and hospitalizations. *Bottom, dotted line:* Palliative therapies to control symptoms, address quality of life, and enhance communication are relevant throughout the course of heart failure, not just in advanced disease; palliative therapies work hand in hand with traditional therapies designed to prolong survival. Once patients reach a terminal phase of the illness, there is often a transition in goals of care from life sustaining to symptom relief, seen as an inflection in the relative use of palliative compared with traditional therapies. After the patient is deceased, palliative interventions often continue to aid with family/caregiver bereavement.[12,109]

continuing a medical regimen appropriate for advanced heart failure, adjuvant therapies for symptom management should be considered on an individual basis. Medications and nonpharmacologic therapies are generally added in a stepwise and complementary fashion, which generally involves first optimizing therapies for underlying disease, removing exacerbating factors, and then adding palliative treatments for specific symptomatology (**Figure 47-5**).

Dyspnea

Dyspnea is the most common symptom experienced in advanced heart failure. The mainstay of therapy is diuresis and vasodilation to decrease pulmonary congestion.[4,41,42] However, patients with advanced heart failure may have hypotension, renal dysfunction, or other factors that may limit the effective use of these therapies to diminish dyspnea. In the circumstance of refractory dyspnea, low-dose opiates are the mainstay of therapy, although existing data come largely from the treatment of primary pulmonary disease.[69] An additional benefit of opiates is that they may aid in the control of pain symptoms, which often overlap with symptoms of dyspnea. Benzodiazepines have also been tested for control of breathlessness, but have been found to be inferior to opiates.[70,71] Oxygen is only beneficial in reducing dyspnea in hypoxic patients and has no role in the nonhypoxic patient.[72]

Pain

The general sensation of pain is a shared complaint of many patients with advanced heart failure.[73] Most patients with symptomatic heart failure report some form of pain, which increases with NYHA functional class; 69% of class III patients and 89% of class IV patients report pain.[74] Though pain syndromes in heart failure are not well described, it is thought that both heart failure itself and underlying medical comorbidities and psychosocial stressors contribute to the experience of pain. Unfortunately, there are few high-quality data to guide the management of pain in advanced heart failure. As a first step, providers should do all they can to treat heart failure and comorbidities, as well as screen for and treat coexistent depression and anxiety, because these can exacerbate pain. If pain persists, opiates should be

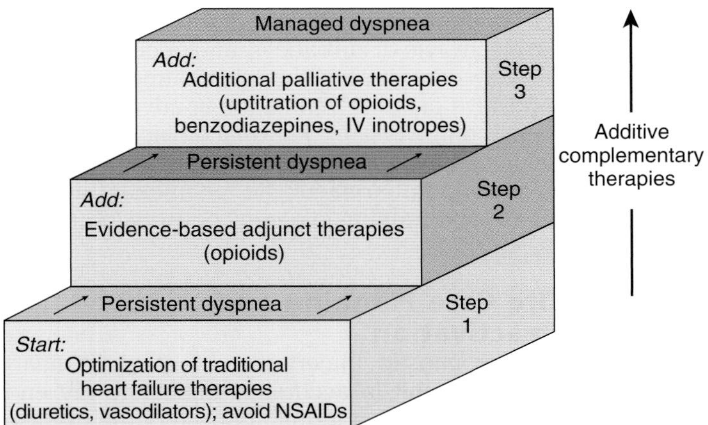

FIGURE 47-5 A stepwise approach to the palliation of dyspnea in patients with heart failure.

considered and up-titrated.[75] In choosing opiates, special caution should be given to methadone, which can prolong the QT interval.[76] Nonsteroidal anti-inflammatory drugs should be avoided in patients with heart failure because of their propensity to cause sodium and fluid retention.[77] Though there is a high prevalence of pain among the advanced heart failure population, usage of opiates appears to be disproportionately low among these patients. One study demonstrated that the usage of opiates was only 22% among patients with advanced heart failure compared with almost 50% among patients with cancer.[78]

Depression

Depression is highly prevalent among patients with advanced heart failure. Approximately 20% of patients meet the criteria for a major depressive disorder, and a greater percentage report depressive symptoms.[79] Even when adjusting for covariates, it has been found that patients with worsening depression have worsened clinical outcomes. Additionally, depressive symptoms are highly correlated with decreased quality of life and increased pain. Despite the obvious need to treat depression in patients with advanced heart failure, there is limited high-quality evidence to guide therapy. To date, the only large randomized controlled trial with specific pharmacologic intervention for the treatment of depression in heart failure was negative for its primary endpoint.[80] Tricyclic antidepressants should be used even more cautiously in heart failure because they can cause QTc prolongation and promote anticholinergic effects, such as dry mouth and orthostatic hypotension.

Fatigue

As with other symptoms, the primary approach to fatigue is the identification and treatment of all potential secondary causes, such as depression, thyroid dysfunction, anemia, overdiuresis, electrolyte disturbances, and occult infection. Sleep apnea may contribute, although treatment of sleep apnea with positive pressure ventilation in advanced heart failure remains controversial.[81] Pharmacologic options for primary fatigue can include stimulants, such as methylphenidate, as well as nonpharmacologic techniques, such as aerobic exercise and training in energy conservation.

End-of-Life Care Planning and Device Deactivation

Although the prognostic uncertainty inherent in heart failure makes it difficult to accurately anticipate the end of life, some patients enter a terminal phase of the disease that may be relatively apparent to the patients, caregivers, and/or clinicians. In such situations, where the goals of care often transition from a focus on survival to quality of life and ensuring a good death, clinicians should take responsibility for initiating and coordinating a comprehensive plan of care consistent with patient values, preferences, and goals.

The option and ease of ICD deactivation should be discussed before implantation and again for major changes in clinical status or transitions in goals of care.[82] At present, this is done only rarely, thus leaving many patients vulnerable to inappropriate device discharge and unnecessary suffering. A recent survey found that only 1 in 4 next of kin reported that a physician had discussed device deactivation with their deceased family member before death.[83] Concordant with those findings, a national survey of hospices found that less than 10% of hospices have a policy regarding deactivation of ICDs, and more than 50% of hospices had at least one patient who had been shocked within the past year.[84] For a device near end of battery life, the generator should not be changed without careful review of whether or not active defibrillation is consistent with overall goals of care and anticipated duration of good quality survival.

Although the legal construct of patient autonomy does not recognize different degrees of dependence on therapies to be withdrawn, clinicians, patients, and caregivers/families may view scenarios in which proactive withdrawal leads to direct patient demise as unique and emotionally difficult. Examples include withdrawal of renal replacement therapy, feeding tubes, or pacemaker support for patients dependent on cardiac pacing. An increasingly common scenario is the withdrawal of mechanical circulatory support devices, either temporary or durable, in patients who are not expected to recover to return to an acceptable quality of life.[11] With improvements in medical technology and associated outcomes, patients maintained with mechanical circulatory support may not only be susceptible to death from cardiovascular causes and pump complications but from other life-limiting disease as well. The discussion about discontinuing device therapy should be part of the consent process before implantation. The most common triggers for LVAD discontinuation include sepsis, stroke, cancer, renal failure, and impending pump failure.[85] Device deactivation can be done in the hospital or at home, attended by a device-trained individual and others as requested (hospice nurse, chaplain, etc.). Discontinuation of power to valveless continuous flow devices typically results in an immediate and marked reduction in systemic blood flow, with most deaths occurring in less than 20 minutes. This clinical scenario has been likened to withdrawal of endotracheal intubation and ventilatory support, although patients with LVAD support are more likely to be awake and alert at the time of decision to discontinue support. Patients on multiple forms of support (e.g., LVAD support, mechanical ventilatory support, and ICD) should have all of their therapies discontinued in a thoughtful and orderly manner.

Hospice Services

Hospice describes a subset of palliative care services that have specific legal, administrative, and financial definitions. For patients approaching the end of life, hospice may be a viable option to provide symptom relief and supportive services, while also ensuring that patients are able to die in their preferred environment. In the United States, the Medicare hospice benefit requires that two physicians or a physician and a nurse practitioner (one of whom is often the hospice medical director) certify that the patient is expected to have 6 months or less to live, and the patient must be willing to forego usual medical services aimed at curing the underlying terminal diagnosis.[63] Although hospice is provided in a variety of environments, it is most commonly provided for patients at home with the goal of keeping them in their home until death.[86] Hospice can offer a number of benefits to enrollees and their families, including interdisciplinary team management, home visits, respite care, and provision of medications and durable medical equipment.

Hospice also includes a nurse who can always be contacted to advise on urgent symptom needs and provide reassurance that such interventions are appropriate.

Customized care plans may provide comfort and relief for some patients unwilling to accept formal hospice support. In many cases patients feel they are "not ready for hospice." Where available, patients can be referred to outpatient palliative care to ensure expert control of their symptoms and provide additional support for the family. Likewise, continued education about the benefits of hospice and the fact that families are often more satisfied with hospice care than care provided in the hospital may also help elucidate its benefits.[87] One study of Medicare beneficiaries who received hospice demonstrated a longer survival (by 81 days) as compared with those heart failure patients who did not receive hospice, such that enrollment in hospice should not be equated with accelerated death or "giving up."[88]

Hospice services have been shown to improve patient and family satisfaction with care. Families of those dying with hospice services were more likely to rate their dying experience as "favorable or excellent" as compared with those who died in an institution or at home with only home health services.[87] Less than half of all patients with heart failure receive hospice.[86] This is, however, a marked increase from less than 20% of heart failure patients being enrolled in hospice a decade ago. Appropriate timing of referral to hospice is important, as the family's perception of being referred "too late" is associated with greater dissatisfaction and unmet needs.[89]

DECISION-MAKING APPROACHES AND COMMUNICATION SKILLS

Advanced heart failure—with its high degree of prognostic uncertainty and complex trade-offs in the choice of medical care—demands a thoughtful approach to communication and decision making. Most patients and families want accurate and honest conversations with their clinicians.[90,91] One study found that 93% of surrogate decision makers felt that avoiding discussions about prognosis was unacceptable.[92] Ideally, these interactions are not one-time events but occur as an evolving series of discussions over time, particularly as a patient's condition changes.[12] Such interactions may be difficult and time-consuming, and they often require planning to create a supportive environment for effective communication. These discussions require careful attention to both cognitive and emotional needs. Clinicians must determine how much quantitative information patients desire. At the same time, clinicians must attend to the emotional nature of conversations with patients to build trust and clarify core values.

Timing of Discussions

Finding appropriate time to discuss preferences, prognosis, and medical options is a formidable challenge in routine clinical practice. Such discussions require a major commitment of time, focus, and emotional energy. Current organizational and reimbursement structures tend to disincentivize such encounters. As a result, formal discussions about prognosis and decision making are often deferred until more emergent occasions, when thoughtful decision making may be impaired.

It has been shown that patients deciding resuscitation preferences during an acute hospitalization frequently reverse their decisions over the next few months.[93] Therefore, the day of hospital admission is a time to review and possibly update—rather than introduce—advanced care planning. On the other hand, once the clinical course has become apparent during hospitalization, clinicians can take advantage of the substantial time they have with the patient and family to further address complex medical decisions before discharge. When the expected survival or quality of life is very limited, hospitalization may also afford better access to multidisciplinary teams, palliative care, and other resources than can be marshaled in the outpatient setting.

All of these considerations underscore the importance of a proactive, anticipatory, and iterative approach to soliciting patients' preferences. This should occur both routinely and at the occurrence of major clinical events that herald a worsening prognosis (see Table 47-3). Some have argued for an "Annual Heart Failure Review," modeled after primary care annual wellness visits, to routinize decision making and ensure anticipatory guidance.[12] In addition to "voluntary advance care planning," including formal designation of a health care proxy and DNR status, such reviews could also include values clarification, formal assessment of prognosis, review of existing therapies, and discussions about possible future events. Understandably, such a review would require considerable face-to-face time between the patient, family, and physician, and thus requires a commitment by individual clinicians, as well as the health care delivery system.

Optimal Communication Techniques

Open, clear, and accurate communication with patients with heart failure is important for several reasons. First, most patients with serious illness want information about their illness and to be included in the decision-making process.[91] Second, when clinicians have conversations with patients about their prognosis and desires, patients are more likely to receive care that is aligned with their goals and preferences.[94,95] These conversations also improve the patient-clinician relationship. Finally, when conversations occur, families of deceased patients have better outcomes in terms of the manner in which they cope with the loss of their loved one, as well as their own psychological outcome.[96] How to communicate with patients with advanced illness is a field unto its own.[97] There is no single best way to have these conversations, and they must be tailored to individual patients under existing circumstances. However, there are practices that can help optimize communication. **Table 47-5** outlines specific tasks, steps, and phrases that can be used to facilitate better communication. Although much of the data regarding communication strategies in advanced illness are from the field of oncology, the evidence base demonstrating similar results in cardiology is increasing.[8,12]

Before one can embark on conversations with patients and their families, it is important to establish the right context for the conversation. This includes asking if patients want to have the conversation by themselves or would like other individuals present, remembering that patients often define family in a myriad of ways. Creating the right setting also involves ensuring that the right clinicians are present,

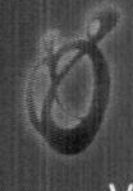

TABLE 47-5 Core Tasks, Skills, and Sample Phrases to Improve Clinician-Patient Communication in Advanced Heart Failure[12]

STEPS IN THE ROADMAP	ELEMENTS OF THE STEP	SAMPLE PHRASES
Establish the setting and participants	Determine who should be present and ensure that all appropriate clinicians are present as well.	"In preparation for our meeting tomorrow, I'm going to have the cardiothoracic surgeon there to be a part of our conversation. In terms of your family or support network, who is it important that we make sure is there?"
Determine what patients know and want to know	ASK what patients/families know.	"Tell me about your heart disease; how have you been doing lately?" "What is your understanding of what is occurring now and why we are considering the treatment that we have been discussing?"
	ASK what patients/families want to know.	"Sometime patients want to know all the details, whereas other times they just want to know a general outline. What kind of person are you?" "How much information would you like to know about what is happening with your heart disease?"
	TELL the patient/family the information in a sympathetic and thoughtful manner while also clearing up any misconceptions or unanswered questions.	"I think you have a pretty good understanding of what is happening with your heart, but there are a few points I'd like to review and clarify."
	ASK the patient or family to repeat back the information that has been delivered.	"Now that I've clarified a few things about your illness, I want to make sure you understand what I've said. Tell me in your own words what we've been talking about."
Establish goals and preferences	Use open-ended questions to gain understanding of the patient's values to determine what is most important to them.	"Help me to understand what is important to you. Some patients say they want to live as long as possible, regardless of quality of life. Sometimes patients tell me they are worried that they will be in a great deal of pain or have other uncontrolled symptoms. What is important to you at this point in terms of your health care?" "What are you hoping for?" "What is important to you now?" "What is your biggest concern right now?" "When you think about the future, what are the things you want to avoid?" In cases where the patient is not involved in the conversation, a useful phrase might be, "What would your loved one say right now if he or she was hearing what we are discussing?"
Work with patient and family to tailor treatments and decisions to goals	Tailor explanation of benefits/burdens of a particular therapy based on goals established.	"I think I understand what is important to you now, and it helps me better explain to you the decisions and treatments at hand now. I'd like to take a moment to review the benefits and burdens of each of the treatments based on what you've said is important to you at this point. ..."
	Be willing to make a recommendation based on the patient's goals.	"Would it be helpful if I made a recommendation based on what you've said the overall focus of care should be now?" "Based on what you have told me, if you get sicker and need to go back on a breathing machines again to stay alive, that is very unlikely to provide the kind of life you want to lead. Therefore, I think you should not go back on those machines."
	Acknowledge that there is uncertainty in the course of heart failure.	"One of the most difficult things about heart disease is that we can never know for sure exactly what will happen in the next (hours, days, weeks, etc.). We must make our best guess and decide what to do based on that information. If things change, we can always readdress this discussion at any time in the future."

or at least have been consulted, before the conversation begins. The individual leading the meeting ideally will have spoken to all the clinicians involved in the care of the patient so all points of view are represented and everyone is "on the same page."

A helpful beginning is often created by asking the patient and family what they know and want to know. In this system, often called Ask-Tell-Ask,[98] the clinician begins by asking patients and their families both what they know about their disease or the treatment being considered as well as how much information they want. This provides the patient this locus of control, which generates trust that is essential for collaborative decision making. An explicit way to ask is "Would you want to know everything about your illness or the treatments we are considering, even if it wasn't good news?" Denial and other defense mechanisms should not be ignored but instead carefully addressed and managed (see Overcoming Barriers to Optimal Communication, later). Once basic expectations for information exchange have been established, clinicians give information to the patient and family in a clear and thoughtful manner, while also clearing up any misconceptions or unanswered questions they might have. It is important to initially focus on the larger picture of the patient's health, as the ability to cognitively hear information, particularly in stressful situations, is limited.[99] Information should be delivered in simple language. Finally, clinicians should ask the patient or family to repeat back the information that has been delivered in order to assess their understanding. This allows the clinician to determine the level of understanding the patient and/or family have, as well as clarify any elements that may remain unclear in their minds.

One of the core elements of good communication is that it assesses patients' values, goals, and desired outcomes.

Optimal communication with patients with advanced heart failure should not begin with questions about treatments. Open-ended questions to gain insight into the patient's life are a useful "What are you hoping for?" or "What is important outside of the hospital?" or "What is your biggest concern right now?" After clarifying the patient's goals, it is often useful for the clinician to summarize what has been expressed. In addition to ensuring that the clinician has heard and understood these hopes correctly, doing this also demonstrates empathy and attending to patient needs. This may start with phrases such as "Let me see if I understand what you are saying."

After goals are clarified, the conversation can then move to discussing the role of specific treatments within the context of the desired outcomes. This involves working with the patient and family to (1) summarize the range of medically reasonable treatments for this particular patient at this particular time and then (2) explain the risks and benefits of each treatment option within the context of the personalized goals and desires set forth by the patient and family. Working within this context, the clinician helps the patient understand which treatments are most appropriate or inappropriate, based on their likelihood of getting the patient to the desired outcome. Uncertainty about outcomes of specific treatments should be communicated honestly and openly with patients and their families.

Overcoming Barriers to Optimal Communication

Complex conversations about prognosis and medical decision making with patients and families include serious challenges. Difficult decision making in the setting of severe illness can stimulate complex emotions. Engaging patients in selecting treatments aligned with their informed goals and values requires that clinicians not only present the options clearly, but that they are also attentive to patients' emotional needs and impaired decision-making capacities. In such settings cognitive information is often not accurately processed.[99] Attending to patients' emotions may improve their ability to process cognitive data and make better decisions. In addition, responding empathetically has been show to strengthen the patient-clinician relationship, increase patient satisfaction, and make patients more likely to disclose future worries. One useful mnemonic device that can help clinicians respond empathetically in conversations is the mnemonic N-U-R-S-E: Naming the emotion expressed in the conversation, demonstrating Understanding of the emotion, Respecting the emotion displayed by the patient or family, Supporting the patient/family, and Exploring the emotion in the context of the discussion.[100] This assists clinicians in demonstrating verbal empathy and ensures that the complex emotional components of the conversation are addressed.

Cognitive impairments compound difficulties with communication, comprehension, and decision making. Mild cognitive decline is seen in 25% to 50% of adults with heart failure.[101] Heart failure patients tend to have poorer memory, psychomotor speed, and executive function; patients most likely to experience cognitive decline are those with the worst heart failure severity. Limitations in health literacy and numeracy further interfere with understanding and integration of the information discussed as it relates to decision making. Almost 10% of the U.S. population is functioning at below basic literacy levels.[102]

Sensitivity to cultural, religious, and language differences can facilitate understanding of patient choices when discussing treatment options.[103] Although clinicians are not expected to be experts in cultural or religious issues relating to decision making, it is important that they are aware of the influence of these elements on decision making.

Decision Support to Assist with Particularly Difficult Conversations

In many cases, the decision at hand may be particularly complex or may require assistive methods to help patients and caregivers understand the potential risks and benefits. In these cases, a decision support intervention, such as a decision aid or a decision coach, can help enhance conversations between patients and clinicians.

Decision aids are tools that help patients and caregivers become involved in decision making by providing information about the options and outcomes and by assisting patients in clarifying their personal values. Decision aids come in various forms including booklets, pamphlets, videos, and web-based systems (see http://decisionaid.ohri.ca/) and are designed to complement, not replace, a clinical encounter. They can be conceptualized broadly as either aids to assist the patient during or independently from the face-to-face encounter.[18] Decision aids attempt to present probabilities of the risks and benefits in ways that patients can understand. Recent innovations have included the calculation and presentation of patient-specific outcomes generated from multivariable models.[104] A key difference between decision aids and a simple information pamphlet is that decision aids do not just provide data about the anticipated risks and benefits but also provide guidance to help patients clarify their personal values and make a decision. Decision aids can help patients clarify their values explicitly through a simple pro/con list or implicitly through an "imagined future" exercise. A Cochrane review of 55 randomized trials of patient decision aids demonstrated that decision aids improved patient knowledge, reduced decisional conflict, increased patients' participation in decision making, and reduced the number of people remaining undecided with no associated adverse health outcomes.[105] However, only one trial in this Cochrane review was related to ischemic heart disease, and none was related to heart failure.

An alternative or adjunctive model to decision aids is the "decision coach," a trained professional, often a nurse, who assists patients in making medical decisions by helping them prepare for a consultation and by empowering them to ask questions of their provider. Early research suggests that coaching interventions may have modest effects on knowledge and participation in decision making.[106] Although coaches have not been studied in patients with advanced heart failure, nurses and other providers working with heart failure patients could be trained in decision coaching techniques.

UNMET NEEDS AND DIRECTIONS FOR THE FUTURE

The unique role of clinicians asks that they assume the primary responsibility for medical decision making and end-of-life care. Yet, the diverse tasks and clinical demands of health care providers involved in primary care, general cardiology, and advanced heart failure limit the capacity to conduct thorough prognostication and shared decision making. As such, the routine conduct of these activities must be efficiently integrated into routine care. The more clinicians perform shared decision making, the better they will be at making it a natural part of their routine practice of care. Ultimately, this approach to care can only occur within health systems that support clinicians not just for doing things but also for deciding which things should and should not be done.

Multiple studies have shown variation and deficiencies in the ability of clinicians to communicate with patients and address end-of-life issues. Given the important yet difficult task of communication in clinical practice, improving communication should be a core element of the performance-based training and certification processes. Several interventions have successfully improved communication skills for clinicians, particularly around end-of-life care.[107]

Useful decision aids for commonly encountered medical decisions in heart failure are largely underdeveloped and/or unavailable. One company has developed decision aids for patients considering ICD and CRT therapy (www.healthwise.org) and another has developed a general decision aid for patients with heart failure (www.healthdialog.com), but these have not been formally studied in real-world settings. The Patient Centered Outcomes Research Institute has funded the development and evaluation of a variety of decision aids for patients with heart failure, but the results of this work are several years away.

At a more basic level, our understanding of how patients with advanced heart failure make choices is limited. There is also no consensus in the literature on the best way to measure whether a medical decision was a "good" one. Decisional quality, defined as "the extent to which the implemented decision reflects the considered preferences of a well-informed patient," is emerging as another possible measure to assess the quality of decision making, but validated measures to quantify decisional quality tend to be decision specific.[108]

Finally, our understanding of health-related quality of life for patients with advanced heart disease is limited. Although health-related quality of life measurements have been developed for patients with symptomatic heart failure, questions remain about their sensitivity in very advanced stages of disease and their relevance after major interventions such as LVAD. Our understanding of the burden and quality of life of caregivers of heart failure patients is even more limited, as is knowledge about how best to improve caregiver quality of life.

CONCLUSIONS

The importance of decision making and palliative care in advanced heart failure cannot be overstated given the complex myriad of treatment options that confront patients, families, and caregivers. Although the promotion of shared decision making and incorporation of palliative care into the management of patients with advanced heart failure may seem daunting to busy practicing clinicians, guiding principles and simple tools can help set future expectations, anticipate major decisions, and promote productive conversations.

Acknowledgment

The authors of this chapter would like to specifically acknowledge the collective efforts of all of the authors who participated in the AHA scientific statement "Decision Making in Advanced Heart Failure," which greatly informed the writing of this chapter.[12]

References

1. Go AS, Mozaffarian D, Roger VL, et al: Heart disease and stroke statistics–2013 update: a report from the American Heart Association. *Circulation* 127:e6–e245, 2013.
2. Cubbon RM, Gale CP, Kearney LC, et al: Changing characteristics and mode of death associated with chronic heart failure caused by left ventricular systolic dysfunction: a study across therapeutic eras. *Circ Heart Fail* 4:396–403, 2011.
3. Metra M, Ponikowski P, Dickstein K, et al: Advanced chronic heart failure: a position statement from the study group on advanced heart failure of the Heart Failure Association of the European Society of Cardiology. *Eur J Heart Fail* 9:684–694, 2007.
4. Yancy CW, Jessup M, Bozkurt B, et al: 2013 ACCF/AHA Guideline for the Management of Heart Failure: a report of the American College of Cardiology Foundation/American Heart Association Task Force on Practice Guidelines. *Circulation* 128:e240–e319, 2013.
5. Jaarsma T, Beattie JM, Ryder M, et al: Palliative care in heart failure: a position statement from the Palliative Care Workshop of the Heart Failure Association of the European Society of Cardiology. *Eur J Heart Fail* 11:433–443, 2009.
6. Adler ED, Goldfinger JZ, Kalman J, et al: Palliative care in the treatment of advanced heart failure. *Circulation* 120:2597–2606, 2009.
7. Goodlin SJ, Hauptman PJ, Arnold R, et al: Consensus statement: palliative and supportive care in advanced heart failure. *J Cardiac Fail* 10:200–209, 2004.
8. Goodlin SJ, Quill TE, Arnold RM: Communication and decision-making about prognosis in heart failure care. *J Cardiac Fail* 14:106–113, 2008.
9. Goodlin SJ: Palliative care in congestive heart failure. *J Am Coll Cardiol* 54:386–396, 2009.
10. Pantilat SZ, Steimle AE: Palliative care for patients with heart failure. *JAMA* 291:2476–2482, 2004.
11. Goldstein NE, May CW, Meier DE: Comprehensive care for mechanical circulatory support: a new frontier for synergy with palliative care. *Circ Heart Fail* 4:519–527, 2011.
12. Allen LA, Stevenson LW, Grady KL, et al: Decision making in advanced heart failure: a scientific statement from the American Heart Association. *Circulation* 125:1928–1952, 2012.
13. Cruzan V: Director, Missouri Department of Health. 497 US 261, 1990.
14. The Patient Self-Determination Act of 1990. 42 USC 1395 cc (a), 1990.
15. Krumholz HM: Informed consent to promote patient-centered care. *JAMA* 303:1190–1191, 2010.
16. Charles C, Gafni A, Whelan T: Shared decision-making in the medical encounter: what does it mean? (or it takes at least two to tango). *Soc Sci Med* 44:681–692, 1997.
17. Institute of Medicine Committee on Quality of Health Care in America: *Crossing the quality chasm: a new health system for the 21st century*, Washington, DC, 2001, National Academy Press.
18. Elwyn G, Frosch D, Volandes AE, et al: Investing in deliberation: a definition and classification of decision support interventions for people facing difficult health decisions. *Med Dec Making* 30:701–711, 2010.
19. Schneiderman LJ: Defining medical futility and improving medical care. *J Bioeth Inq* 8:123–131, 2011.
20. Oshima Lee E, Emanuel EJ: Shared decision making to improve care and reduce costs. *New Engl J Med* 368:6–8, 2013.
21. Aaronson KD, Schwartz JS, Chen TM, et al: Development and prospective validation of a clinical index to predict survival in ambulatory patients referred for cardiac transplant evaluation. *Circulation* 95:2660–2667, 1997.
22. Levy WC, Mozaffarian D, Linker DT, et al: The Seattle Heart Failure Model: prediction of survival in heart failure. *Circulation* 113:1424–1433, 2006.
23. Pocock SJ, Ariti CA, McMurray JJ, Meta-Analysis Global Group in Chronic Heart Failure, et al: Predicting survival in heart failure: a risk score based on 39372 patients from 30 studies. *Eur Heart J* 34:1404–1413, 2013.
24. Lee DS, Austin PC, Rouleau JL, et al: Predicting mortality among patients hospitalized for heart failure: derivation and validation of a clinical model. *JAMA* 290:2581–2587, 2003.
25. Fonarow GC, Adams KF, Jr, Abraham WT, et al: Risk stratification for in-hospital mortality in acutely decompensated heart failure: classification and regression tree analysis. *JAMA* 293:572–580, 2005.
26. O'Connor CM, Hasselblad V, Mehta RH, et al: Triage after hospitalization with advanced heart failure: the escape (evaluation study of congestive heart failure and pulmonary artery catheterization effectiveness) risk model and discharge score. *J Am Coll Cardiol* 55:872–878, 2010.
27. Allen LA, Gheorghiade M, Reid KJ, et al: Identifying patients hospitalized with heart failure at risk for unfavorable future quality of life. *Circ Cardiovasc Qual Outcomes* 4:389–398, 2011.
28. Fonarow GC: Epidemiology and risk stratification in acute heart failure. *Am Heart J* 155:200–207, 2008.
29. Allen LA, Magid DJ, Gurwitz JH, et al: Risk factors for adverse outcomes by left ventricular ejection fraction in a contemporary heart failure population. *Circ Heart Fail* 6:635–646, 2013.
30. Gorodeski EZ, Chu EC, Chow CH, et al: Application of the Seattle Heart Failure Model in ambulatory patients presented to an advanced heart failure therapeutics committee. *Circ Heart Fail* 3:706–714, 2010.
31. Stevenson LW, Hellkamp AS, Leier CV, et al: Changing preferences for survival after hospitalization with advanced heart failure. *J Am Coll Cardiol* 52:1702–1708, 2008.
32. Lewis EF, Johnson PA, Johnson W, et al: Preferences for quality of life or survival expressed by patients with heart failure. *J Heart Lung Transplant* 20:1016–1024, 2001.
33. Dev S, Clare RM, Felker GM, et al: Link between decisions regarding resuscitation and preferences for quality over length of life with heart failure. *Eur J Heart Fail* 14:45–53, 2012.
34. Pressler SJ, Gradus-Pizlo I, Chubinski SD, et al: Family caregiver outcomes in heart failure. *Am J Crit Care* 18:149–159, 2009.
35. Henderson R, Jones M, Stare J: Accuracy of polntern predictions in survival analysis. *Stats Med* 20:3083–3096, 2001.
36. Glare P, Sinclair C, Downing M, et al: Predicting survival in patients with advanced disease. *Eur J Cancer* 44:1146–1156, 2008.
37. Siontis GC, Tzoulaki I, Ioannidis JP: Predicting death: an empirical evaluation of predictive tools for mortality. *Arch Intern Med* 171:1721–1726, 2011.
38. Glare P, Virik K, Jones M, et al: A systematic review of physicians' survival predictions in terminally ill cancer patients. *BMJ* 327:195–198, 2003.
39. Yamokoski LM, Hasselblad V, Moser DK, et al: Prediction of rehospitalization and death in severe heart failure by physicians and nurses of the ESCAPE trial. *J Card Fail* 13:8–13, 2007.

40. Allen LA, Yager JE, Funk MJ, et al: Discordance between patient-predicted and model-predicted life expectancy among ambulatory patients with heart failure. *JAMA* 299:2533–2542, 2008.
41. Lindenfeld J, Albert NM, Boehmer JP, et al: HFSA 2010 comprehensive heart failure practice guideline. *J Card Fail* 16:e1–e194, 2010.
42. McMurray JJ, Adamopoulos S, Anker SD, et al: ESC Guidelines for the diagnosis and treatment of acute and chronic heart failure 2012: the task force for the diagnosis and treatment of acute and chronic heart failure 2012 of the European Society of Cardiology. Developed in collaboration with the Heart Failure Association of the ESC. *Eur Heart J* 33:1787–1847, 2012.
43. Velazquez EJ, Lee KL, Deja MA, et al: Coronary-artery bypass surgery in patients with left ventricular dysfunction. *N Engl J Med* 364:1607–1616, 2011.
44. The Society of Thoracic Surgeons national database. http://www.STS.org/national-database. Accessed June 1, 2013.
45. Makkar RR, Fontana GP, Jilaihawi H, et al: Transcatheter aortic-valve replacement for inoperable severe aortic stenosis. *N Engl J Med* 366:1696–1704, 2012.
46. Mauri L, Foster E, Glower DD, et al: Four-year results of a randomized controlled trial of percutaneous repair versus surgery for mitral regurgitation. *J Am Coll Cardiol* 62:317–328, 2013.
47. Franzen O, van der Heyden J, Baldus S, et al: Mitraclip(r) therapy in patients with end-stage systolic heart failure. *Eur J Heart Fail* 13:569–576, 2011.
48. Lindenfeld J, Feldman AM, Saxon L, et al: Effects of cardiac resynchronization therapy with or without a defibrillator on survival and hospitalizations in patients with New York Heart Association class IV heart failure. *Circulation* 115:204–212, 2007.
49. Bhattacharya S, Abebe K, Simon M, et al: Role of cardiac resynchronization in end-stage heart failure patients requiring inotrope therapy. *J Card Fail* 16:931–937, 2010.
50. Begg GA, Witte KK: Closing the door after the horse has bolted: device therapy in patients with end-stage heart failure. *J Card Fail* 16:938–939, 2010.
51. Swindle JP, Rich MW, McCann P, et al: Implantable cardiac device procedures in older patients: use and in-hospital outcomes. *Arch Intern Med* 170:631–637, 2010.
52. Costanzo MR, Dipchand A, Starling R, et al: The International Society of Heart and Lung Transplantation guidelines for the care of heart transplant recipients. *J Heart Lung Tranplant* 29:914–956, 2010.
53. Feldman D, Pamboukian SV, Teuteberg JJ, et al: The 2013 International Society for Heart and Lung Transplantation guidelines for mechanical circulatory support: executive summary. *J Heart Lung Transplant* 32:157–187, 2013.
54. Nazarian S, Maisel WH, Miles JS, et al: Impact of implantable cardioverter defibrillators on survival and recurrent hospitalization in advanced heart failure. *Am Heart J* 150:955–960, 2005.
55. Passman R, Subacius H, Ruo B, et al: Implantable cardioverter defibrillators and quality of life: results from the defibrillators in nonischemic cardiomyopathy treatment evaluation study. *Arch Intern Med* 167:2226–2232, 2007.
56. Matlock DD, Stevenson LW: Life-saving devices reach the end of life with heart failure. *Prog Cardiovasc Dis* 55:274–281, 2012.
57. Hauptman PJ, Mikolajczak P, George A, et al: Chronic inotropic therapy in end-stage heart failure. *Am Heart J* 152:1096, e1091–1098, 2006.
58. Thackray S, Easthaugh J, Freemantle N, et al: The effectiveness and relative effectiveness of intravenous inotropic drugs acting through the adrenergic pathway in patients with heart failure—a meta-regression analysis. *Eur J Heart Fail* 4:515–529, 2002.
59. Hershberger RE, Nauman D, Walker TL, et al: Care processes and clinical outcomes of continuous outpatient support with inotropes (COSI) in patients with refractory endstage heart failure. *J Card Fail* 9:180–187, 2003.
60. Murtagh FE, Marsh JE, Donohoe P, et al: Dialysis or not? A comparative survival study of patients over 75 years with chronic kidney disease stage 5. *Nephrol Dial Transplant* 22:1955–1962, 2007.
61. Moss AH: Ethical principles and processes guiding dialysis decision-making. *Clin J Am Soc Nephrol* 6:2313–2317, 2011.
62. Sima CS, Panageas KS, Schrag D: Cancer screening among patients with advanced cancer. *JAMA* 304:1584–1591, 2010.
63. Department of Health and Human Services, Centers for Medicare and Medicaid Services: 42 CFR part 418: Medicare and Medicaid programs: hospice conditions of participation; final rule. *Fed Reg* 73(109):32088–32220, 2008.
64. World Health Organization: WHO definition of palliative care. http://www.who.int/cancer/palliative/definition/en/. Accessed September 19, 2014.
65. Morrison RS, Meier DE: Clinical practice. Palliative care. *N Engl J Med* 350:2582–2590, 2004.
66. Quill TE, Abernethy AP: Generalist plus specialist palliative care–creating a more sustainable model. *N Engl J Med* 368:1173–1175, 2013.
67. Swetz KM, Freeman MR, AbouEzzeddine OF, et al: Palliative medicine consultation for preparedness planning in patients receiving left ventricular assist devices as destination therapy. *Mayo Clin Proc* 86:493–500, 2011.
68. Blinderman CD, Homel P, Billings JA, et al: Symptom distress and quality of life in patients with advanced congestive heart failure. *J Pain Symptom Manage* 35:594–603, 2008.
69. Abernethy AP, Currow DC, Frith P, et al: Randomised, double blind, placebo controlled crossover trial of sustained release morphine for the management of refractory dyspnoea. *BMJ* 327:523–528, 2003.
70. Rocker G, Horton R, Currow D, et al: Palliation of dyspnoea in advanced COPD: revisiting a role for opioids. *Thorax* 64:910–915, 2009.
71. Simon ST, Higginson IJ, Booth S, et al: Benzodiazepines for the relief of breathlessness in advanced malignant and non-malignant diseases in adults. *Cochrane Database Syst Rev* CD007354, 2010.
72. Clemens KE, Quednau I, Klaschik E: Use of oxygen and opioids in the palliation of dyspnoea in hypoxic and non-hypoxic palliative care patients: a prospective study. *Support Care Cancer* 17:367–377, 2009.
73. Light-McGroary K, Goodlin SJ: The challenges of understanding and managing pain in the heart failure patient. Current opinion in supportive and palliative care. *Curr Opin Support Palliat Care* 7:14–20, 2013.
74. Evangelista LS, Sackett E, Dracup K: Pain and heart failure: unrecognized and untreated. *Eur J Cardiovasc Nurs* 8:169–173, 2009.
75. Goodlin SJ, Wingate S, Albert NM, et al: Investigating pain in heart failure patients: the pain assessment, incidence, and nature in heart failure (PAIN-HF) study. *J Card Fail* 18:776–783, 2012.
76. Krantz MJ, Martin J, Stimmel B, et al: QTc interval screening in methadone treatment. *Ann Intern Med* 150:387–395, 2009.
77. Page J, Henry D: Consumption of NSAIDs and the development of congestive heart failure in elderly patients: an underrecognized public health problem. *Arch Intern Med* 160:777–784, 2000.
78. Setoguchi S, Glynn RJ, Stedman M, et al: Hospice, opiates, and acute care service use among the elderly before death from heart failure or cancer. *Am Heart J* 160:139–144, 2010.
79. Rutledge T, Reis VA, Linke SE, et al: Depression in heart failure a meta-analytic review of prevalence, intervention effects, and associations with clinical outcomes. *J Am Coll Cardiol* 48:1527–1537, 2006.
80. O'Connor CM, Jiang W, Kuchibhatla M, et al: Safety and efficacy of sertraline for depression in patients with heart failure: results of the SADHART-CHF (sertraline against depression and heart disease in chronic heart failure) trial. *J Am Coll Cardiol* 56:692–699, 2010.
81. Sun H, Shi J, Li M, et al: Impact of continuous positive airway pressure treatment on left ventricular ejection fraction in patients with obstructive sleep apnea: a meta-analysis of randomized controlled trials. *PLoS ONE* 8:e62298, 2013.
82. Padeletti L, Arnar DO, Boncinelli L, et al: EHRA expert consensus statement on the management of cardiovascular implantable electronic devices in patients nearing end of life or requesting withdrawal of therapy. *Europace* 12:1480–1489, 2010.
83. Kelley AS, Reid MC, Miller DH, et al: Implantable cardioverter-defibrillator deactivation at the end of life: a physician survey. *Am Heart J* 157:702–708, 2009.
84. Goldstein N, Carlson M, Livote E, et al: Brief communication: management of implantable cardioverter-defibrillators in hospice: a nationwide survey. *Ann Intern Med* 152:296–299, 2010.
85. Brush S, Budge D, Alharethi R, et al: End-of-life decision making and implementation in recipients of a destination left ventricular assist device. *J Heart Lung Transplant* 29:1337–1341, 2010.
86. *NHPCO facts and figures: Hospice care in America*, Alexandria, VA, 2012, National Hospice and Palliative Care Organization.
87. Teno JM, Clarridge BR, Casey V, et al: Family perspectives on end-of-life care at the last place of care. *JAMA* 291:88–93, 2004.
88. Connor SR, Pyenson B, Fitch K, et al: Comparing hospice and nonhospice patient survival among patients who die within a three-year window. *J Pain Symptom Manage* 33:238–246, 2007.
89. Teno JM, Shu JE, Casarett D, et al: Timing of referral to hospice and quality of care: length of stay and bereaved family members' perceptions of the timing of hospice referral. *J Pain Symptom Manage* 34:120–125, 2007.
90. Golin CE, Wenger NS, Liu H, et al: A prospective study of patient-physician communication about resuscitation. *J Am Geriatr Soc* 48:S52–S60, 2000.
91. Singer PA, Martin DK, Kelner M: Quality end-of-life care: patients' perspectives. *JAMA* 281:163–168, 1999.
92. Apatira L, Boyd EA, Malvar G, et al: Hope, truth, and preparing for death: perspectives of surrogate decision makers. *Ann Intern Med* 149:861–868, 2008.
93. Krumholz HM, Phillips RS, Hamel MB, et al: Resuscitation preferences among patients with severe congestive heart failure: results from the support project. Study to understand prognoses and preferences for outcomes and risks of treatments. *Circulation* 98:648–655, 1998.
94. Silveira MJ, Kim SY, Langa KM: Advance directives and outcomes of surrogate decision making before death. *N Engl J Med* 362:1211–1218, 2010.
95. Detering KM, Hancock AD, Reade MC, et al: The impact of advance care planning on end of life care in elderly patients: randomised controlled trial. *BMJ* 340:c1345, 2010.
96. Wright AA, Zhang B, Ray A, et al: Associations between end-of-life discussions, patient mental health, medical care near death, and caregiver bereavement adjustment. *JAMA* 300:1665–1673, 2008.
97. Back AL, Arnold R, Tulsky JA: *Mastering communication with seriouly ill patients*, Cambridge, 2009, Cambridge University Press.
98. Back AL, Arnold RM, Baile WF, et al: Approaching difficult communication tasks in oncology. *CA Cancer J Clin* 55:164–177, 2005.
99. Knight SJ, Emanuel L: Processes of adjustment to end-of-life losses: a reintegration model. *J Palliat Med* 10:1190–1198, 2007.
100. Back AL, Anderson WG, Bunch L, et al: Communication about cancer near the end of life. *Cancer* 113:1897–1910, 2008.
101. Pressler SJ, Subramanian U, Kareken D, et al: Cognitive deficits in chronic heart failure. *Nurs Res* 59:127–139, 2010.
102. Kutner M, Greenberg E, Yin T, et al, editors: *Results from the 2003 national assessment of adult literacy*, Washington, DC, 2006, U.S. Department of Education.
103. Blackhall LJ, Frank G, Murphy ST, et al: Ethnicity and attitudes towards life sustaining technology. *Soc Sci Med* 48:1779–1789, 1999.
104. Decker C, Arnold SV, Olabiyi O, et al: Implementing an innovative consent form: the predict experience. *Implement Sci* 3:58, 2008.
105. O'Connor AM, Bennett CL, Stacey D, et al: Decision aids for people facing health treatment or screening decisions. *Cochrane Database Syst Rev* CD001431, 2009.
106. O'Connor AM, Stacey D, Legare F: Coaching to support patients in making decisions. *BMJ* 336:228–229, 2008.
107. Robinson K, Sutton S, von Gunten CF, et al: Assessment of the education for physicians on end-of-life care (EPEC) project. *J Palliat Med* 7:637–645, 2004.
108. Sepucha KR, Fowler FJ, Jr, Mulley AG, Jr: Policy support for patient-centered care: The need for measurable improvements in decision quality. *Health Aff (Millwood)* Suppl Variation:VAR54-62, 2004.
109. Lanken PN, Terry PB, Delisser HM, et al: An official American Thoracic Society Clinical Policy statement: palliative care for patients with respiratory diseases and critical illnesses. *Am J Respir Crit Care Med* 177:912–927, 2008.

Index

Page numbers followed by f indicate figures; t, tables; b, boxes.

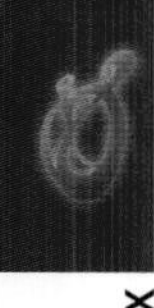

D

E

F

G

H

I

J

K

L

N

Q

R

T

U

V

W

X

Z

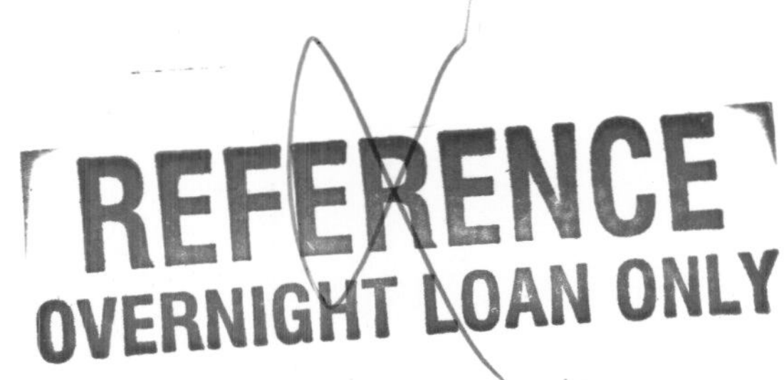